Comprehensive
Medical
Assisting

Administrative and
Clinical Competencies

Comprehensive
Medical
Assisting

Administrative and Clinical Competencies

WILBURTA Q. LINDH, CMA (AAMA)

CAROL D. TAMPARO, CMA (AAMA), PHD

BARBARA M. DAHL

JULIE A. MORRIS, RN, BSN, CBCS, CCMA, CMAA

CINDY CORREA, AHI (AMT)

Sixth Edition

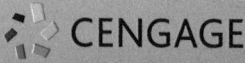

Australia • Brazil • Mexico • Singapore • United Kingdom • United States

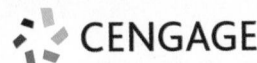

Comprehensive Medical Assisting: Administrative and Clinical Competencies, Sixth Edition

Wilburta Q. Lindh, Carol D. Tamparo, Barbara M. Dahl, Julie A. Morris, Cindy Correa

SVP, GM Skills & Global Product Management: Jonathan Lau

Product Director: Matthew Seeley

Product Team Manager: Stephen Smith

Senior Director, Development: Marah Bellegarde

Product Development Manager: Juliet Steiner

Senior Content Developer: Lauren Whalen

Product Assistant: Mark Turner

Vice President, Marketing Services: Jennifer Ann Baker

Marketing Manager: Jonathan Sheehan

Senior Production Director: Wendy Troeger

Production Director: Andrew Crouth

Senior Content Project Manager: Thomas Heffernan

Senior Art Director: Jack Pendleton

Media Producer: Jim Gilbert

Cover image(s): My Portfolio/Shutterstock.com
Vikpit/Shutterstock.com
Svetlana_Okeana/Shutterstock.com

© 2018, 2014, 2010, 2006, 2002, 1997 Cengage Learning, Inc.

WCN: 01-100-101

For product information and technology assistance, contact us at
Cengage Customer & Sales Support, 1-800-354-9706

For permission to use material from this text or product, submit all requests online at **www.cengage.com/permissions.**
Further permissions questions can be e-mailed to
permissionrequest@cengage.com

Library of Congress Control Number: 2016953587

ISBN: 978-1-305-96479-2

Cengage
200 Pier 4 Boulevard
Boston, MA 02210
USA

Cengage is a leading provider of customized learning solutions with employees residing in nearly 40 different countries and sales in more than 125 countries around the world. Find your local representative at **www.cengage.com.**

Cengage products are represented in Canada by Nelson Education, Ltd.

To learn more about Cengage platforms and services, register or access your online learning solution, or purchase materials for your course, visit **www.cengage.com.**

Notice to the Reader

Publisher does not warrant or guarantee any of the products described herein or perform any independent analysis in connection with any of the product information contained herein. Publisher does not assume, and expressly disclaims, any obligation to obtain and include information other than that provided to it by the manufacturer. The reader is expressly warned to consider and adopt all safety precautions that might be indicated by the activities described herein and to avoid all potential hazards. By following the instructions contained herein, the reader willingly assumes all risks in connection with such instructions. The publisher makes no representations or warranties of any kind, including but not limited to, the warranties of fitness for particular purpose or merchantability, nor are any such representations implied with respect to the material set forth herein, and the publisher takes no responsibility with respect to such material. The publisher shall not be liable for any special, consequential, or exemplary damages resulting, in whole or part, from the readers' use of, or reliance upon, this material.

Printed in the United States of America
Print Number: 07   Print Year: 2021

TABLE OF CONTENTS

SECTION I
General Procedures   1

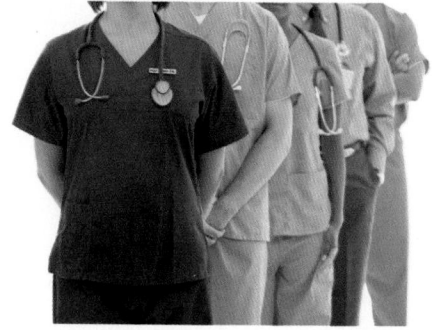

UNIT I: INTRODUCTION TO MEDICAL ASSISTING AND HEALTH PROFESSIONS   2

CHAPTER 1: The Medical Assisting Profession   4

CHAPTER 2: Health Care Settings and the Health Care Team   20

SECTION II
Administrative Procedures   179

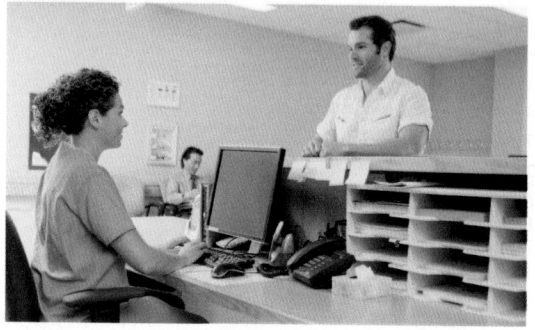

UNIT IV: INTEGRATED ADMINISTRATIVE PROCEDURES   180

SECTION III
Clinical Procedures 469

UNIT VI: INTEGRATED CLINICAL PROCEDURES 470

CHAPTER 21: Infection Control and Medical Asepsis 472

CHAPTER 22: The Patient History and Documentation 536

UNIT IX: **LABORATORY PROCEDURES** 1192

CHAPTER 37: Regulatory Guidelines for Safety and Quality in the Medical Laboratory 1194

CHAPTER 38: Introduction to the Medical Laboratory 1210

CHAPTER 39: Phlebotomy: Venipuncture and Capillary Puncture 1234

CHAPTER 40: Hematology 1280

SECTION IV
Professional Procedures   1397

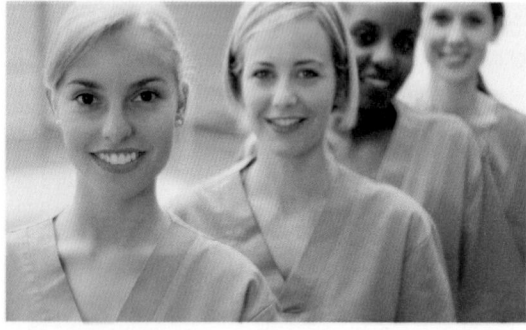

UNIT X: CLINIC AND HUMAN RESOURCES MANAGEMENT   1398

CHAPTER 44: The Medical Assistant as Clinic Manager   1400

CHAPTER 45: The Medical Assistant as Human Resources Manager   1438

LIST OF PROCEDURES

PREFACE

The world of health care continues to change rapidly, and, as medical assistants, you will be called on to do more and respond to an increasing number of clinical and administrative responsibilities. Now is the time to equip yourself with the skills you will need to excel in the field to maximize your potential, expand your base of knowledge, and dedicate yourself to becoming the best multifaceted, multiskilled medical assistant that you can be.

The new edition of *Comprehensive Medical Assisting: Administrative and Clinical Competencies* will guide you on this journey. The word *comprehensive* is not used lightly here, for this text is part of a dynamic learning system that includes software, a study guide, and online materials. Together, this learning package includes coverage of the most current entry-level competencies identified by the Accrediting Bureau of Health Education Schools (ABHES) and the Commission on Accreditation of Allied Health Education Programs (CAAHEP). It will also help you prepare for certification examinations from the American Association of Medical Assistants (AAMA), the American Medical Technologists (AMT), and the National Healthcareer Association (NHA).

You will find this edition continues to provide you with opportunities to use your critical thinking skills through case studies, critical thinking boxes, patient education boxes, and scenarios. You will also see that the text addresses topics that will make you workplace-ready, including electronic health records (EHR), Practice Management (PM) software, ICD-10, professionalism, and confidentiality and privacy issues.

Some of the special new features and updates to this edition include:

- Increased emphasis on EHR and PM software, including many visual examples of EHR and PM systems, and sample electronic documentation
- Expanded coverage of ICD-10-CM and ICD-10-PCS, and their implementation
- Refreshed learning outcomes that map to the most current ABHES and CAAHEP competencies

- A refreshed *Attributes of Professionalism* feature in each unit opener that emphasizes behavioral skills
- A new *Quick Reference Guide* feature that highlights critical information in each chapter through a combination of photos, graphics, illustrations, and narrative text
- Dozens of new photos and illustrations portraying a greater number of procedures and showing the latest equipment
- Updated procedures that include language emphasizing professionalism skills
- Updated end of chapter content, including an expanded *Certification Review* section with multiple-choice questions that mimic the medical assisting certification examinations
- Updated certification and examination information for AAMA, AMT, and NHA
- Additional *Critical Thinking* boxes throughout the text

HOW THE TEXT IS ORGANIZED

Section I, "General Procedures" (Chapters 1 through 8), provides the groundwork for understanding the role and responsibilities of the medical assistant. Topics include the medical assisting profession, the health care team, communication skills, legal and ethical issues, and emergency and first aid procedures.

New material in this section includes:

- Quick Reference Guides
- Updated Attributes of Professionalism feature
- Expansion of factors causing stress in the work environment
- Patient coaching and navigation
- Americans with Disabilities Act
- Definition of expressed consent
- New Chapter 4 procedure that covers patient coaching
- New Chapter 6 procedures covering locating a state's legal scope of practice for medical assistants, and performing compliance-based reporting on public health statutes

- New Chapter 7 procedure that covers developing a plan for separating personal and professional ethics
- New Chapter 8 procedures covering performing first aid procedures for insulin shock, seizures, shock, and syncope
- New topics in Section I: patient-centered medical homes; accountable care organizations (ACO); influence of technology on communication; communication in end-of-life care; Affordable Care Act and Patients' Bill of Rights and Responsibilities

Section II, "Administrative Procedures" (Chapters 9 through 20), provides up-to-date information on all administrative competencies required of medical assistants. Topics include the facility environment, using computers and technology, clinic communications, scheduling, creating and managing medical records, insurance and coding, and financial practices.

New material in this section includes:

- Quick Reference Guides
- Expanded coverage of electronic health records (EHR) and related figures
- Expanded coverage of ICD-10-CM and ICD-10-PCS
- Expanded information on community resources
- New Chapter 11 procedures covering developing a list of community resources, and facilitating referrals to community resources
- New topics in Section II: patient portal systems; telemedicine; online scheduling; do-it-yourself appointments; traditional indemnity insurance

Section III, "Clinical Procedures" (Chapters 21 through 43), provides a thorough understanding of the clinical, diagnostic, and laboratory procedures you will be performing and assisting with in the medical clinic. Topics include asepsis, patient history, vital signs, body system examinations, specialty examinations, minor surgery, diagnostic imaging, nutrition, ECG, pharmacology, dosage calculation, venipuncture, urinalysis, and laboratory tests.

New material in this section includes:

- Quick Reference Guides
- A greater emphasis on the use of electronic health records (EHR) when taking a patient history

- Chapters 25 and 42 have been internally reorganized to improve the flow of content
- Additional coverage of common childhood illnesses
- Expanded coverage of laboratory sample collection procedures
- Updated laboratory procedures to reflect the latest equipment technology and processes
- New Chapter 42 procedure that covers wound cultures
- Updated immunization guidelines
- New topics in Section III: SOAPIE and SOAPIER methods of charting

Section IV, "Professional Procedures" (Chapters 44 through 47), examines the role of the medical assistant as clinic manager and human resources manager and provides tools and techniques to use when preparing for student practicums, medical assistant credentialing, and finding employment opportunities.

New material in this section includes:

- Quick Reference Guides
- Updated certification and examination information
- Revised section on using social media in the job search
- New Chapter 47 procedures covering how to write a résumé, and how to follow up on a job interview effectively
- New topics in Section IV: generational expectations of employment; evaluating employees; online profiles

THE COMPLETE LEARNING PACKAGE: STUDENT SUPPLEMENTS

Study Guide (ISBN 978-1-3059-6485-3)

Explore the text content through Vocabulary Builder, Learning Review, Certification Review, and Application Activities for each chapter. The Study Guide has been fully revised to align with the content in the sixth edition.

Student Companion Website
(www.cengagebrain.com)

This student website is designed to provide students with the resources they will need to complete the text procedures. Editable Competency Checklists and Procedure Forms can be downloaded from the Student Companion Website.

Competency Checklists have been streamlined for ease of use and evaluation, and provide instructions on the specific scenario information needed to complete the procedure, as well as any forms to be used.

Procedure Forms are provided for the relevant checklists. The forms can be completed electronically and saved, or printed and completed manually.

Detailed instructions for accessing the Student Companion Website can be found on the Instructor Companion Website.

Critical Thinking Challenge 3.0
(ISBN 978-1-1339-3330-4 or 978-1-1339-3324-3)

The Critical Thinking Challenge 3.0 software simulates a 3-month practicum in a medical clinic. You will be confronted with a series of situations in which you must use your critical thinking skills to choose the most appropriate action in response to the situation. Your decisions will be evaluated in three categories: how your decisions affect the practice, the patient, and your career. The 3.0 version includes 12 all-new video-based scenarios with more branching options. After successfully completing the program, a Certification of Completion may be printed.

Learning Lab
(ISBN 978-1-1336-0956-8 or 978-1-1336-0953-7)

Learning Lab maps to learning objectives and includes interactive activities and case scenarios to build students' critical thinking skills and help retain the more difficult concepts. This simulated, immersive environment engages users with its real-life approach. Each Learning Lab has a pre-assessment quiz, three to five learning activities, and post-assessment quiz. The post-assessment scores can be posted to the instructor grade book in any learning management system.

MindTap to Comprehensive Medical Assisting: Administrative and Clinical Competencies, Sixth Edition

MindTap is a fully online, interactive learning experience built upon authoritative Cengage Learning content. By combining readings, multimedia, activities, and assessments into a singular learning path, MindTap elevates learning by providing real-world application to better engage students. Instructors customize the learning path by selecting Cengage Learning resources and adding their own content via apps that integrate into the MindTap framework seamlessly with many learning management systems.

The guided learning path demonstrates the importance of the medical assistant through engagement activities and interactive exercises. Learners can apply their understanding of the material through interactive activities taken from Critical Thinking Challenge 3.0 and the Medical Assisting Learning Lab, in addition to certification style quizzing and case studies. These simulations elevate the study of medical assisting by challenging students to apply concepts to practice.

To learn more, visit www.cengage.com/mintdtap

THE COMPLETE LEARNING PACKAGE: INSTRUCTOR SUPPLEMENTS

Instructor Companion Site
(ISBN 978-1-3059-6482-2)

(Access at www.cengage.com/login)

Spend less time planning and more time teaching with Cengage Learning's Instructor Resources. Log on to the Instructor Companion Site to gain access to the Instructor's Manual, Cognero Test Bank, and PowerPoint slides. Access at www.cengage.com/login with your Cengage instructor account. If you are a first-time user, click Create a New Faculty Account and follow the prompts.

Instructor's Manual The Instructor's Manual provides mapping to the most current ABHES and CAAHEP curriculum, lesson outlines, suggestions for classroom activities, and answer keys for the text and Study Guide.

Online Cognero Test Bank An electronic test bank makes and generates tests and quizzes in an instant. With a variety of question types, including multiple choice and matching exercises, creating challenging exams will be no barrier in your classroom. This test bank includes a rich bank of over 2,000 questions that test students on retention and application of what they have learned in the course. Answers are provided for all questions so instructors can focus on teaching, not grading. Each question also contains a reference to the text page number and ABHES and CAAHEP curriculum standard.

Instructor PowerPoint Slides A comprehensive offering of more than 1,800 instructor support slides created in Microsoft PowerPoint outlines concepts and objectives to assist instructors with lectures.

ABOUT THE AUTHORS

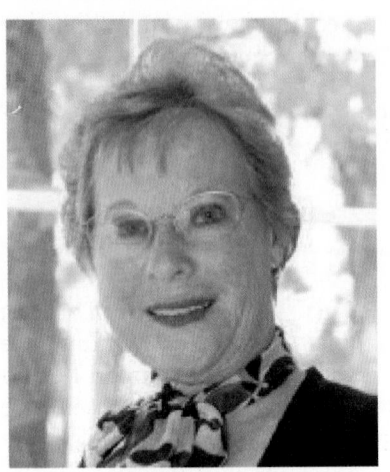

Wilburta (Billie) Q. Lindh, CMA, (AAMA), is Professor Emerita at Highline College in Des Moines, Washington, where she served as Program Director and consultant to the Medical Assistant Program. She received the Outstanding Faculty Member of the Year award for her efforts in revamping the program. An active member of SeaTac Chapter of the American Association of Medical Assistants (AAMA), and the National American Association of Medical Assistants, Ms. Lindh conducted workshops and lectured across the country. She is the co-author of several textbooks on medical assisting.

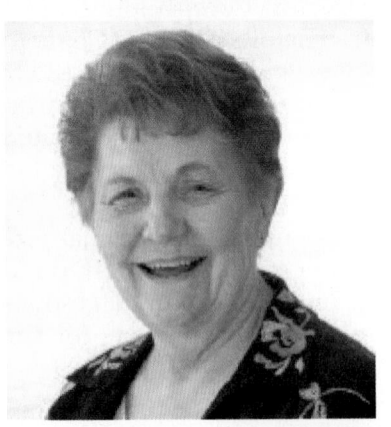

Carol D. Tamparo, CMA (AAMA), PhD, is the former Dean of Business and Allied Health at the Lake Washington Institute of Technology in Kirkland, Washington, and founder of the Medical Assistant program at Highline Community College. Author and Co-author of four texts for allied health professionals, she is also a member of the SeaTac American Association of Medical Assistants and the National American Association of Medical Assistants.

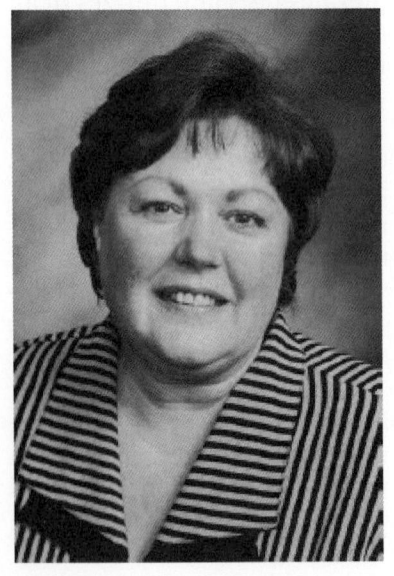

Barbara M. Dahl, served as a tenured faculty member and coordinator of the Medical Assisting Program at Whatcom Community College in Bellingham, Washington, for over 20 years. She was a very active member of several professional organizations, including the Whatcom County Chapter of Medical Assistants, the Washington State Society of Medical Assistants, the American Association of Medical Assistants (AAMA), and the Washington State Medical Assisting Educators and the American Academy of Professional Coders (AAPC). Ms. Dahl is currently involved in medical management and personnel consulting, curriculum development, and program accreditation advising, as well as advocating for medical assistants to enjoy the right to practice in Washington.

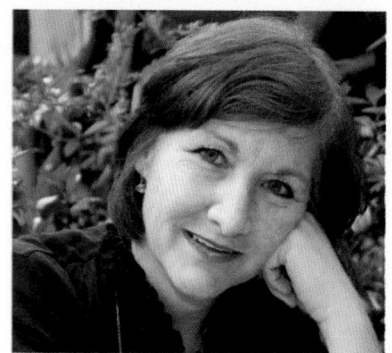

Julie A. Morris, RN, BSN, CBCS, CCMA, CMAA, decided to become a nurse at the age of 16. Ms. Morris has been involved in health care for more than four decades. She graduated from the Lurleen B. Wallace School of Nursing at Jacksonville State University with a Bachelor of Science degree in nursing. Her career has included directorship positions in case management, home infusion care, clinical education and clinic management. She has spent the last ten years pursuing her dream of educating adults in the allied healthcare field; holding positions as Instructor, Program Director, Externship Coordinator, and Director of Career Services. Currently, Ms. Morris is involved in integrating active learning in the classroom, curriculum development, and strategies to engage students and assist them in successful completion of educational programs. She is an active member of the Cobb Chapter of the American Association of Medical Assistants in Georgia.

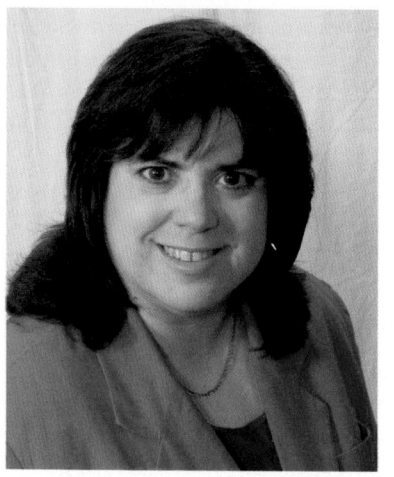

Cindy Correa, AHI (AMT), is the former Allied Health Educational Coordinator at City University of New York at Queens College. Cindy was responsible for the initial creation and curricula development of at least seven certificate programs of the Allied Health Program, including the Medical Assistant program at Queens College. She has extended her expertise to satellite courses in adult education programs. Her experience working in the private practice and administrative hospital environments includes oncology, cardiovascular surgery, pulmonology, and thoracic surgery. Cindy is actively involved in technical writing, software development projects, and serves on advisory boards of technical colleges in her home state of Colorado.

ACKNOWLEDGMENTS

A special thank you to my husband, DeVere, who continually supports, encourages, and assists me in so many ways. Thank you to my family and friends, who understood when I was not available for activities, but continually accepted and encouraged my commitment to excellence. Collaborating with the author team and those at Cengage Learning encouraged forward thinking and a 6th edition that is progressive and current with technology to ensure that medical assisting students are well prepared for tomorrow's challenges.

—Billie Q. Lindh

Many thanks are expressed to my husband, Tom, who assumed many household chores and took us out to dinner at just the right times. Writing a textbook, even the revision of a textbook, requires the input and dedication of many individuals, especially in the field of health care where changes occur almost daily. Collaborating with the other authors on this edition has ensured that the most recent information is included in this text. Thank you Stephen Smith and Lauren Whalen for your vision and guidance.

—Carol D. Tamparo

First I would like to thank my husband, Ed, for his continued support and encouragement during this 6th edition revision. It has been an exciting experience—making sure our textbook is the best and most current representation of what today's medical assistant student needs to know to enter the profession; covering the cognitive, psychomotor, and affective domains; as well as using the most current technology and new clinical diagnostics and equipment. I appreciate the opportunity to continue working with my diversely talented team members, Billie and Carol, and I welcome the fresh perspective of our new team members, Julie and Cindy. I also have a great deal of appreciation for the expertise and patience of Lauren Whalen, Stephen Smith, as well as the rest of our Cengage Learning team and Aravinda Doss with Lumina Datamatics in updating this nationally respected resource.

—Barbara M. Dahl

Of the things that I revere and find valuable in the profession of medical assisting, expanding knowledge and the delivery of quality patient care rank at the top. It is my hope that this text provides a guide to attain essential knowledge and the tools to apply that knowledge to the care of every patient. Each minute that was spent on the revision of this text will result in hours, days, months, and years of teaching and learning. That thought makes it all worth it! Dear future medical assistant, I wish you success and satisfaction in this career that you have chosen.

Thank you, co-authors and the team at Cengage. The sixth edition is a result of amazing collaboration. Specifically, Lauren Whalen and Stephen Smith, thank you for the kindness and support you have shown me during this and other Cengage projects.

Special thanks and appreciation to my family. Phillip Rutledge; Bryan, Casey, and Arleigh Mountjoy; and Sam Huckaby, you fill my heart with gratitude and love. Thank you for caring for me, supporting me, and always being around for a diversion when one is desperately needed.

—Julie A. Morris

Many thanks to Lauren Whalen for her guidance and support, and always having a sharp eye, valuable suggestions, and a helping hand. I appreciate the patience from the entire team during some challenging personal experiences during this project. I especially owe a tremendous debt to Audrey Theisen for her generous assistance and expertise— thank you! Billie, Carol, Barbara, and Julie, it was a pleasure working with such a professional team of authors. I am grateful to Stephen Smith and everyone at Cengage Learning for the opportunities extended and allowing me to be part of your ongoing projects. To my family and friends, who have propped me up and have made it possible for me to focus on my work by taking care of all the other details when needed, it would never have gotten done without you.

—Cindy Correa

CONTRIBUTOR

The authors and publisher would like to acknowledge the following professional for contributing to the content of this book:

Audrey Theisen, BS, RHIA, MSCIS, PhD
HIM Professor
Contributing author for Chapter 17

REVIEWERS

Deneen Dotson, CCMA (NHA)
Clinical Medical Assistant Program Director
Brookline College
Tucson, AZ

Alicia C. Dumas-Pace, MA, PA, AHI
College Administrator & Consultant/Instructor
Masters Vocational College
Riverside, CA

Amy Eady, MT(ASCP), MS, RMA (AMT)
Dean of Health Occupation
Montcalm Community College
Sidney, MI

Lisa Graese, CHDS
Intructor, Medical Office Careers
Spokane Community College
Spokane, WA

Karon Green-Walton, CMA (AAMA), BS
Program Director
Augusta Technical College
Augusta, GA

Kim Hashem-Dugal, MBA, NCMA (NCCT)
Medical Assisting Training Program Developer,
    Consultant
Great Bay Community College
Portsmouth, NH

Susan Holler, MSEd, CPC, CMRS
Medical Administrative Assistant, Medical
    Reimbursement & Coding
Bryant & Stratton College
Orchard Park, NY

Judith Hurtt, M.Ed.
Instructor
East Central Community College
Decatur, MS

Madeline Y. Jones, BSN, MBA, RN
Regional Director, Health Science Programs for
    VA, WV, and TN
American National University
Roanoke, VA

Michelle McCranie, A.A.S., CPhT, CMA (AAMA)
Medical Assisting Instructor
Ogeechee Technical College
Statesboro, GA

Nancy Measell, BS, AAS, CMA (AAMA)
Assistant Professor
Ivy Tech Community College
South Bend, IN

Janet Melton, MBA
VP of Education
Brookline College
Phoenix, AZ

Sandra Metcalf, M.Ed.
Professor and Program Director of Office &
    Computer Technology
Grayson College
Denison, TX

Karen Minchella, Ph.D., CMA (AAMA)
Educational Consultant
Consulting Management Associates, LCC
Warren, MI

Pamela Neu, CMA (AAMA), MBA
Medical Assisting Program Chair
Ivy Tech Community College
Fort Wayne, IN

Margaret Noirjean, BSN, RN
Medical Assistant Program Instructor
Dakota County Technical College
Rosemount, MN

Linda Pace, BS, CMA (AAMA)
Director of Medical Assisting and Phlebotomy
Red Rocks Community College
Arvada, CO

Cathy Salazar, MS, MA, EdS
Director
ITT Technical Institute
Pensacola, FL

Patricia Seydlitz, RHIT
Professor
Clark College
Vancouver, WA

Loreane Sheets, CMA (AAMA), BSH, BLS-I
Assistant Professor, Program Chair Medical
    Assisting
Belmont College
St. Clairsville, OH 43950

Deanna Stephens, AABA, RMA (AMT), CMOA
Instructor
Virginia College
Baton Rouge, LA

Gayla Taylor, MSM
Director of Education
PCI Health Training Center
Dallas, TX

Kathleen Tettam, CMA (AAMA), PBT (ASCP)
Medical Assistant Instructor
Dakota County Technical College
Rosemount, MN

Holly Tumbarello, RN, BSN
Certified Allied Health Instructor, MA
    Coordinator
Clatsop Community College
Astoria, OR

Marilyn Turner, RN, CMA (AAMA)
Medical Assisting Program Director
Ogeechee Technical College
Statesboro, GA

Jeanne Von Ohlsen, CMA (AAMA)
Program Chair, Medical Assisting
Hodges University
Naples, FL

Barb Westrick, AAS, CMA (AAMA), CPC
Program Chair, Medical Assisting and Medical
    Billing
Ross Education, LLC
Brighton, MI

Micheline B. Wheeler, ADN, RN, RMA (AMT)
Medical Assisting Program Manager
Central Carolina Technical College
Sumter, SC

Aprilan F. Woolworth, RHIT, CPC, CRC
Education Manager
Os2 Healthcare Solutions
Killeen, TX

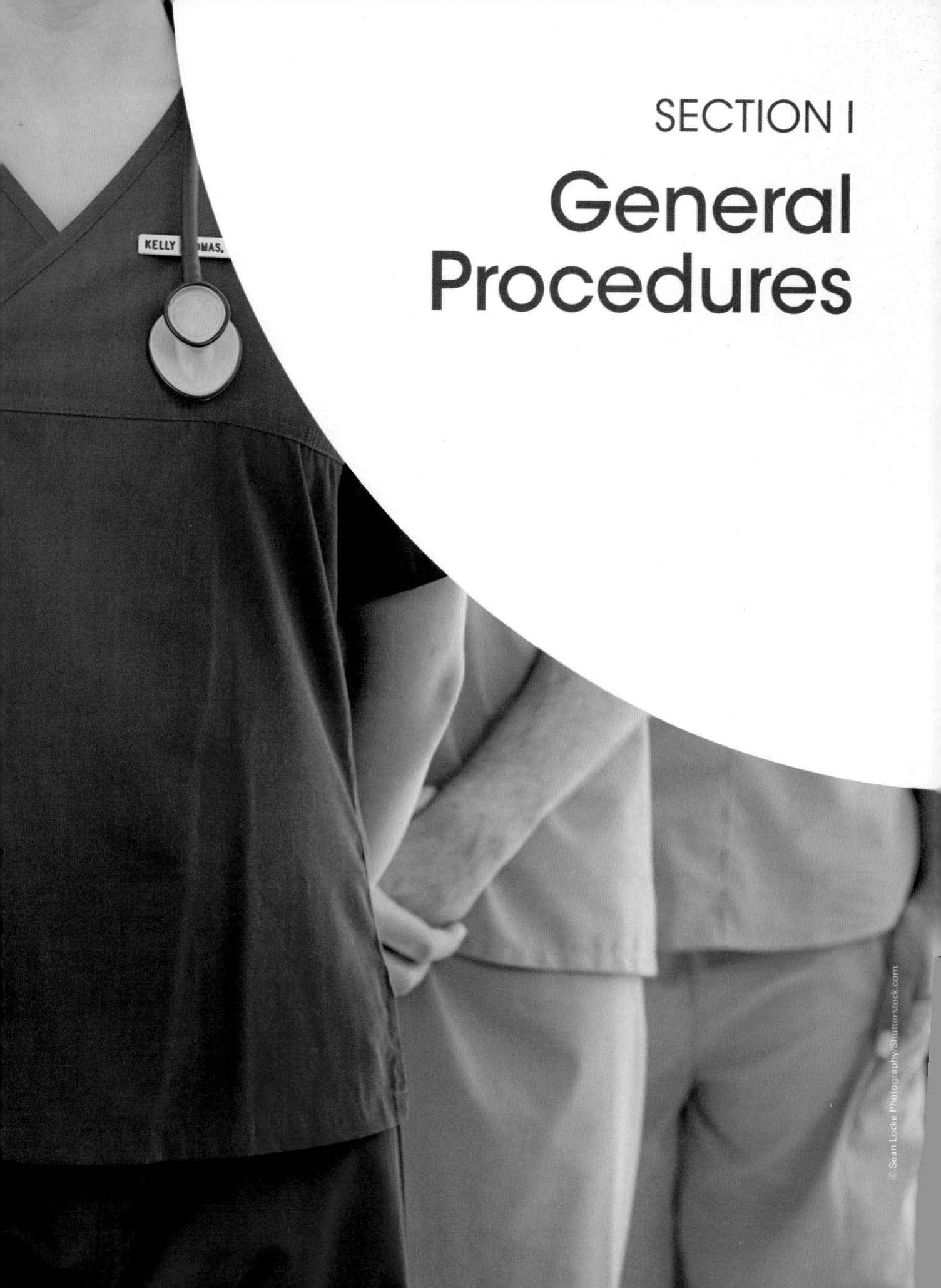

SECTION I
General Procedures

UNIT I
INTRODUCTION TO MEDICAL ASSISTING AND HEALTH PROFESSIONS

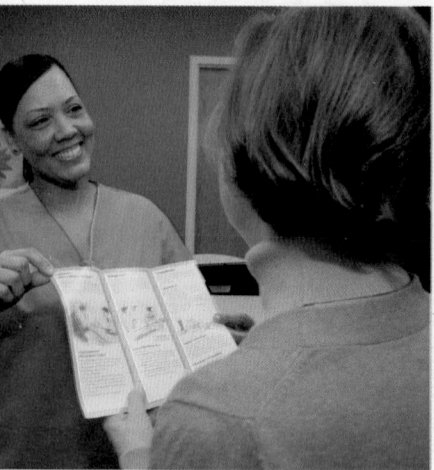 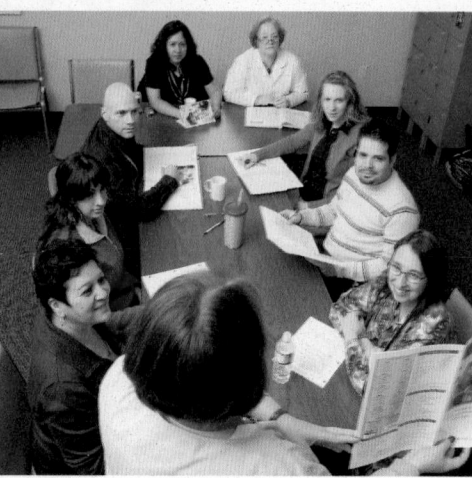 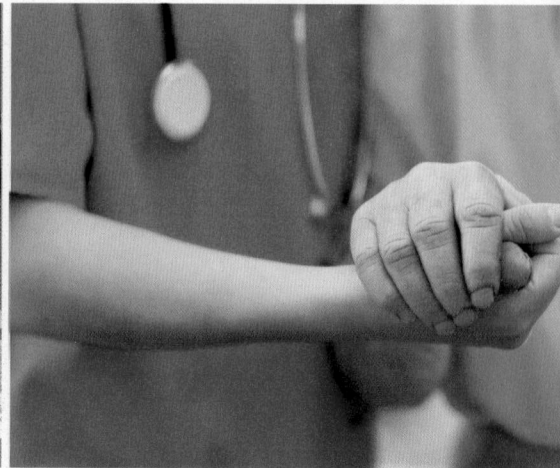

ATTRIBUTES OF PROFESSIONALISM

An essential attribute of a professional medical assistant is respect. Every person that enters your presence must be treated with respectful reverence. Patients, peers, and co-workers must all be held in high regard. Your willingness to show appreciation and consideration will facilitate a positive experience for all involved, and foster a true team atmosphere. On occasion, difficult patients will test the tolerance of even the most experienced medical assistant, because they seldom seem content with the care or services received. However, patients should never be treated with disinterest or in an unfriendly manner. You must always be pleasant and courteous. Seeking health care is a very personal experience. As a medical assistant, that means you must always respect the patient's information, resulting care, and documentation of that care, regardless of the circumstances.

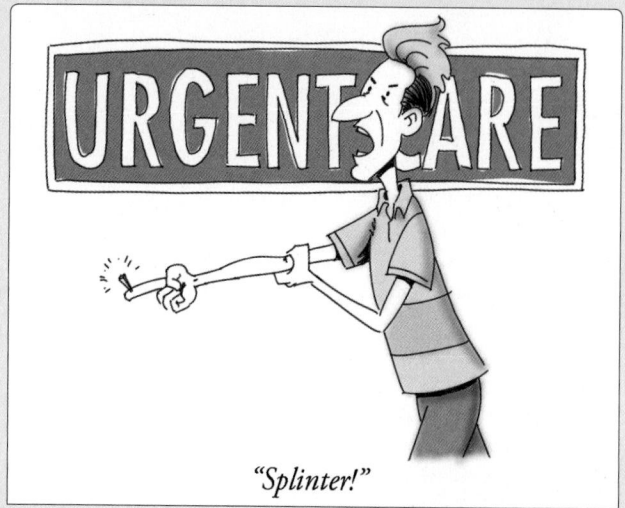

"Splinter!"

Listed below are a series of questions for you to ask yourself, to serve as a professionalism checklist. As you interact with patients and colleagues, these questions will help to guide you in the professional behavior that is expected every day from medical assistants.

Ask Yourself

COMMUNICATION

- ☐ Do I apply active listening skills?
- ☐ Do I display professionalism through written and verbal communication?
- ☐ Do I demonstrate appropriate nonverbal communication?
- ☐ Do I display appropriate body language?
- ☐ Does my knowledge allow me to speak easily with all members of the health care team?

PRESENTATION

- ☐ Am I dressed and groomed appropriately?
- ☐ Do I display a positive attitude?
- ☐ Do I display a calm, professional, and caring manner?

COMPETENCY

- ☐ Do I pay attention to detail?
- ☐ Do I ask questions if I am out of my comfort zone or do not have the experience to carry out tasks?
- ☐ Do I display sound judgment?
- ☐ Am I knowledgeable and accountable?

INITIATIVE

- ☐ Do I show initiative?
- ☐ Do I seek out opportunities to expand my knowledge base?
- ☐ Am I flexible and dependable?
- ☐ Do I implement time management principles to maintain effective office function?
- ☐ Do I assist co-workers when appropriate?

INTEGRITY

- ☐ Do I work within my scope of practice?
- ☐ Do I demonstrate respect for individual diversity?
- ☐ Do I immediately report any error I made?
- ☐ Do I do the "right thing" even when no one is observing?

CHAPTER 1

The Medical Assisting Profession

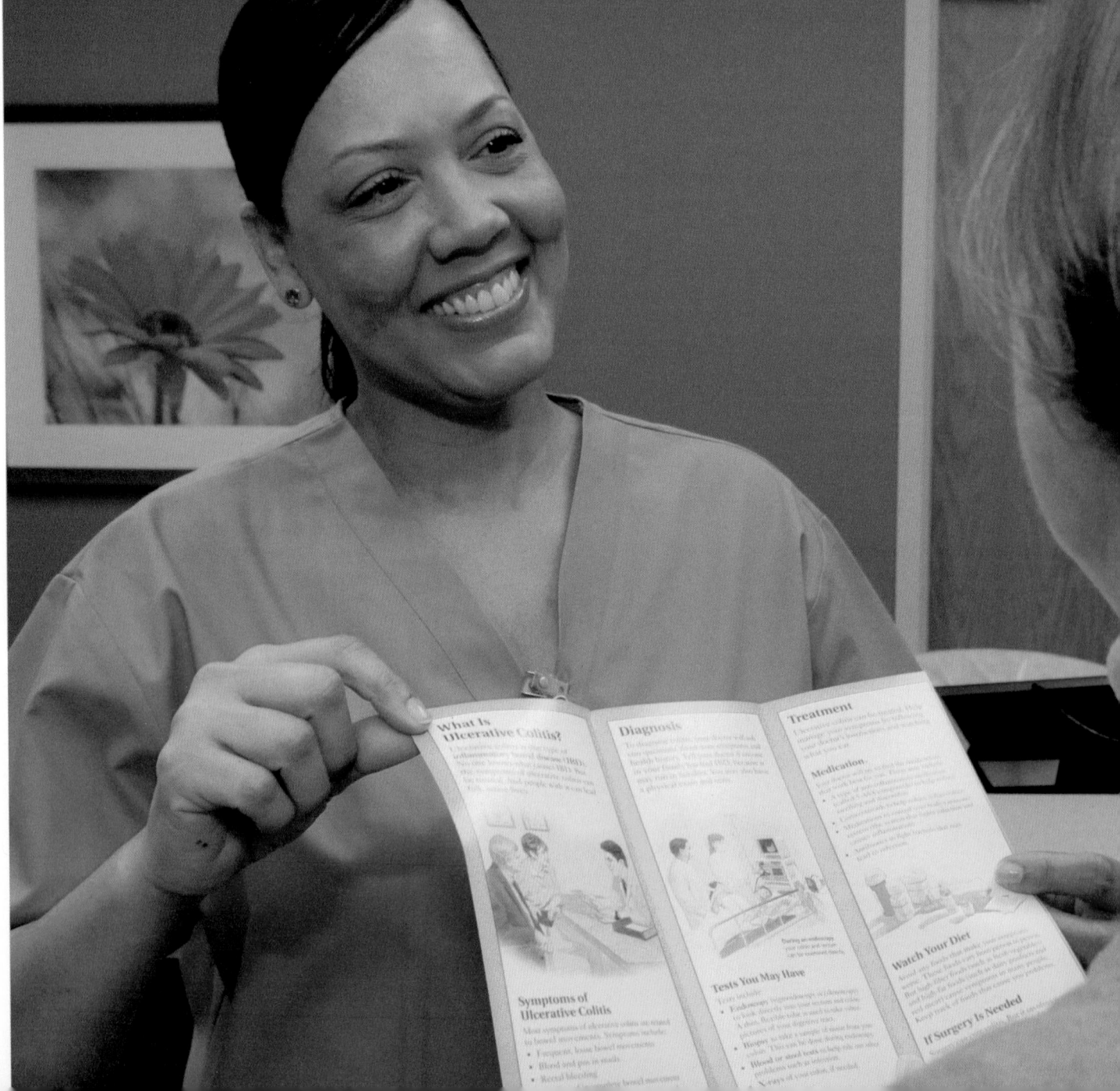

1. Define and spell the key terms as presented in the glossary.
2. Discuss the history of medical assisting.
3. Describe the practicum experience.
4. Recall two criteria for the selection of practicum sites.
5. Identify three benefits of the practicum to the student and the site.
6. Describe the profession of medical assisting and analyze its career opportunities in relationship to your interests.
7. Identify and discuss five attributes that are essential to a professional medical assistant's career.
8. Describe the American Association of Medical Assistants and discuss its major functions.
9. Discuss the role of the American Medical Technologists in the credentialing of medical assistants.
10. Explain the purpose of the National Healthcareer Association.
11. Explain accreditation, certification, and continuing education as they pertain to the professional medical assistant.
12. Differentiate the requirements for certification and recertification for each of the credentialing bodies.
13. Identify the importance of the accreditation process to an educational institution.
14. Recall at least two methods available to obtain recertification.
15. Compare the five means of obtaining continuing education units.
16. Differentiate among certification, licensure, and registration.
17. Identify the importance of understanding the scope of practice for the medical assistant.

KEY TERMS

accreditation

Affordable Care Act (ACA)

ambulatory care setting

associate's degree

attributes

bachelor's degree

certification

Certified Clinical Medical Assistant (CCMA [NHA])

Certified Medical Administrative Assistant (CMAA [NHA])

Certified Medical Assistants (CMAs [AAMA])

competency

compliance

credentialed

dexterity

diploma

disposition

empathy

externship

facilitate

improvise

internship

license

licensure

practicum

professionalism

proprietary

Registered Medical Assistant (RMA [AMT])

scope of practice

SCENARIO

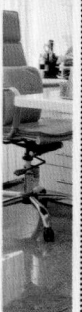

A group of high school freshmen have come to tour a medical assisting class and laboratory areas. The Program Director of Medical Assisting is showing the students around the department. The Program Director then takes them into the medical assisting laboratory, where senior medical assistant students are practicing their clinical skills. Each senior student pairs up with a high school freshman, and each pair talks about medical assisting, with the medical assistant students answering questions the others may have. The medical assistant students are in uniform as part of their preparation to go into various health care agencies to do their externship or practicum. The medical assistant students look professional, clean, fresh, and motivated. They tell the high school students about medical

continues

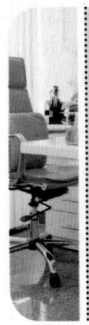

assisting and describe the personal and physical attributes desirable for those who want to become medical assistants. They explain the importance of these attributes, as well as what duties a professional medical assistant performs and what education is needed to pursue a career in medical assisting.

Throughout the question and answer discussions, the senior medical assistant students and the program director stress the importance of ethics, empathy, attitude, dependability, and teamwork as necessary attributes. Individuals seeking a career in medical assisting must develop and maintain these characteristics.

Chapter Portal

There are many fascinating aspects of the medical assisting profession. When a person pursues formal education to enter the world of medicine as a professional medical assistant, he or she may take on a new role in his or her family and community. In this new role, the medical assisting student can have a major, positive influence on the community-wide knowledge of health and the process for seeking medical care. This influence is just the beginning of the many highly rewarding aspects of becoming a medical assistant.

The medical assistant is defined by the American Association of Medical Assistants (AAMA) Board of Trustees as "A multi-skilled member of the health care team who performs administrative and clinical procedures under the supervision of licensed healthcare providers." According to the 2015 statistics released by the Bureau of Labor Statistics, the majority of medical assistants are employed in provider offices, with outpatient care centers following as the next largest employer. The list of licensed health care providers that can supervise medical assistants has expanded to include nurse practitioners, physician's assistants, podiatrists, chiropractors, and optometrists.

Medical assistants come from a variety of backgrounds and educational experiences. Due to the sophistication of the health care consumer and the complexity of delivering health care, employers are seeking medical assistants who are educated and are credentialed for employment in their practices.

There is an entire body of knowledge—such as anatomy and physiology, medical terminology, and practical clinical skills—that must be acquired in your studies to become a professional medical assistant. An equally important aspect of a medical assistant's career is **professionalism**. Professionalism combines your acquired knowledge and skills with the types of behavior that demonstrate your moral, ethical, and respectful attributes when interacting with patients and colleagues.

HISTORICAL PERSPECTIVE OF THE PROFESSION

There is a rich history of medical assisting and the medical assistants who enjoy the profession. Historically, medicine has included the role of the handmaiden. This person served to assist the provider in his daily tasks caring for an ill population. This role was essential, but undefined. The first recognition of this important aspect of health care was nursing. As time progressed, another vital role emerged—that of the medical assistant.

The last 100 years have brought an acceleration of medical technology that has impacted both the diagnosis and treatment of many disease processes as well as the maintenance of wellness. With advancing technology, the provider has increased the demands on the staff of the practice. The American Association of Medical Assistants defines medical assistants as "multiskilled members of the health care team who perform administrative and clinical procedures under the supervision of licensed health care providers." As the availability of testing and treatment has moved from a more acute-care setting to the provider's clinic, there has been an expanding role for the medical assistant in the delivery of care. The medical assistant must possess a wide array of skills including excellent communication skills, clinical skills that relate to patient care, and administrative skills that are required to manage the facility and the practice's finances. These skills are all part of the requirements for a professional medical assistant in today's market.

CAREER OPPORTUNITIES

Medical assistants have been described as health care's most versatile, multifaceted professionals.

According to the Bureau of Labor Statistics, there are well over half a million medical assisting jobs in the United States, with the job outlook expected to increase by 23% from 2014 to 2024. This significant growth in available employment highlights the vital role that medical assistants currently play in the provision of health care. There are multiple factors recognized as the driving force for this expanding role. The aging baby-boom population requires health maintenance, preventive care, and outpatient management of chronic illness. With the implementation of the **Affordable Care Act (ACA)**, millions of people that previously had no insurance coverage are now seeking health care. There was a reported shortage of health care providers prior to the ACA, and with expanded patient demand due to the law's implementation, the shortage has grown. To help fill the gap, providers have hired medical assistants to perform routine administrative and clinical duties. This allows professional provision of care to a practice's increased patient population.

That medical assistants possess a broad scope of knowledge and skills makes them ideal professionals for any **ambulatory care setting**. Indeed, because of such versatility, medical assistants find employment in a variety of settings: clinics, medical laboratories, insurance companies, government agencies, pharmaceutical companies, educational institutions, surgical centers, urgent-care facilities, and electrocardiography (ECG or EKG) departments in hospitals. Other career opportunities are available to the medical assistant. Some medical assistants work as phlebotomists, coding specialists, medical laboratory assistants, and medical administrative specialists. The broad application of the skills of a medical assistant is relevant to many aspects of a medical practice. This ensures the continued growth of responsibilities and opportunities for medical assisting.

EDUCATION OF THE MEDICAL ASSISTANT

Prior to the 1950s, medical assistants were trained on the job. Organizing professionally brought about the need for a formalized education that incorporated a standardized curriculum. Today, education of medical assistants takes place in community and junior colleges, as well as in **proprietary** schools. In 1997, in coordination with the National Board of Medical Examiners, educators, and practicing **Certified Medical Assistants (CMAs [AAMA])**, the AAMA developed the Medical Assistant Role Delineation Chart, now known as the Occupational Analysis of the CMA (AAMA). This analysis can be found on the AAMA website at www.aamantl.org. Entry-level competencies must be mastered by students in academic programs.

Instruction takes place in a variety of settings. A future medical assistant will be educated in the classroom and in the laboratory, allowing both an understanding of foundational knowledge and processes, as well as an opportunity to practice the hands-on skills required to master the responsibilities of the profession. An important new mode of education is online education. Some schools offer medical assistant courses online, and if the school is accredited many students who cannot or desire not to take traditional classroom courses can work toward becoming certified or registered through this method. Upon graduation from a medical assisting program, the student will receive a **diploma** or certificate of completion. If a student decides to pursue general education courses, it could take another year to complete an **associate's degree** (a total of 2 years) or longer for a **bachelor's degree**.

Courses in a Medical Assisting Program

Some of the administrative, general, and clinical content taught in a medical assisting program is listed in Table 1-1.

Practicum

Practicum, **externship**, and **internship** are all terms used to define the transition period between the classroom and actual employment. A practicum

TABLE 1-1

SOME TYPICAL ADMINISTRATIVE, GENERAL, AND CLINICAL CONTENT TAUGHT IN AN ACCREDITED MEDICAL ASSISTING PROGRAM

Administrative Content	Electronic medical records (EMRs) and electronic health records (EHRs)
	Document management
	Appointments and scheduling
	Insurance claims/coding
	Billing, collections, and patients' accounts
General Content	Anatomy and physiology
	Medical terminology
	Pathophysiology
	Law and ethics
	Patient education
Clinical Content	Infection control
	Disease prevention
	Pharmacology
	Temperature, pulse, respirations, and blood pressure
	Assisting the provider with physical exams
	Assisting the provider with minor surgery
	Drawing blood samples
	Medication Administration
	Urine and blood testing in the laboratory
	CPR (provider-level certification), first aid

is planned and supervised by a coordinator from the medical assisting program and the health care facility that agrees to become a partner in the education and employability of the student. The benefit of this practical training is to allow the student a safe environment to implement their knowledge and, if needed, return to the educational setting for reinforcement of skills or knowledge.

Practicum Sites. Sites for practicums are chosen carefully to ensure that a variety of experiences are available for the student. The sites should provide the student with adequate administrative, clinical, and general experiences. The staff at the various sites must be willing to make a commitment to the medical assistant's education by spending appropriate time observing and instructing the student (see Chapter 44 for more information on supervising student practicums).

Benefits of Practicum. The practicum experience is mutually beneficial to the student and staff at the health care facility that is providing the educational experiences. Students are able to apply classroom knowledge and skill in a real-world medical setting, while using the practicum experience to build a résumé and begin to establish a network of support through colleagues. As students progress in their skills and abilities, they become oriented to the practice. The practicum may be considered an extended interview for possible job placement.

Associate's and Bachelor's Degrees

The expanding role and applicable job openings for medical assistants have allowed a new focus on degrees in medical assisting. Both proprietary schools and more traditional educational institutions have added both associate's and bachelor's degrees in medical assisting to their curriculum.

The primary benefit of these degrees is positioning in the job market. With an expanded curriculum, the medical assistant is prepared with college-level classes that include college math, English, and psychology as well as more in-depth classes related to medical assisting. Employers are eager to hire candidates with a demonstrated commitment to education and to their profession. Movement up the career ladder in health care is assisted by educational credentials as well as job experience.

With the increase of allied health education programs in the United States ranging from the certificate level to degree levels, a new opportunity has been created for tenured medical assistants: that of instructor. Required credentials for instructors in each medical assisting program are outlined by the credentialing bodies of each educational organization.

ACCREDITATION OF MEDICAL ASSISTING PROGRAMS

Educational institutions seeking **accreditation** for a medical assisting program must develop the curricula to meet the *Standards and Guidelines* set by the Commission on Accreditation for Allied Health Education Programs (CAAHEP), or the standards set by the Accrediting Bureau of Health Education Schools (ABHES) to ensure the highest quality medical assistant education and employment preparedness.

CAAHEP

The Commission on Accreditation for Allied Health Education Programs (CAAHEP) is an accrediting body for medical assisting programs in private and public postsecondary institutions and programs that prepare individuals for entry into the profession.

A medical assisting program that is accredited by CAAHEP meets the standards as outlined in the *Standards and Guidelines for an Accredited Education Program for the Medical Assistant*. Standards are the minimum standards of quality used in accrediting programs that prepare individuals to enter the medical assisting profession.

On-site review teams evaluate the program's **compliance** with, or adherence to, the standards. All aspects of programs seeking accreditation status undergo scrutiny to ascertain the program's quality and to ensure continued compliance with the standards.

For more information, see the CAAHEP Web site at www.caahep.org.

ABHES

The Accrediting Bureau of Health Education Schools (ABHES) is the agency that also grants accreditation to medical assisting programs. ABHES is recognized by the United States Department of Education (USDE) as an accrediting agency of public and private schools and colleges that primarily offer health education. This includes medical assisting, medical laboratory technology, and surgical technology programs. Besides being recognized by the USDE, recognition for ABHES comes from the AAMA, American Medical Technologists (AMT), National League for Nursing Accrediting (NLNA), and National Board of Surgical Technology and Surgical Assisting (NBSTSA).

More information about ABHES can be obtained through the ABHES Web site at www.abhes.org.

ATTRIBUTES OF A MEDICAL ASSISTANT PROFESSIONAL

Medical assistants should strive to cultivate certain characteristics or personal qualities. These are the **attributes** that identify a true professional; when caring for patients, these qualities should be sincere. They will enable the patient to trust you, the caregiver. Figure 1-1 lists some of the questions you must ask yourself as you work to develop your professional attributes. As you interact with patients and colleagues, the questions listed in the figure will serve as guidelines for the

COMMUNICATION

- ☐ Do I apply active listening skills?
- ☐ Do I display professionalism through written and verbal communication?
- ☐ Do I demonstrate appropriate nonverbal communication?
- ☐ Do I explain to patients the rationale for performance of a procedure?
- ☐ Do I speak at each patient's level of understanding?
- ☐ Do I display appropriate body language?
- ☐ Do I respond honestly and diplomatically to my patients' concerns?
- ☐ Do I refrain from sharing my personal experiences?
- ☐ Do I include the patient's support system as indicated?
- ☐ Do I reassure patients of the accuracy of test results?
- ☐ Do I show sensitivity when communicating with patients regarding third party requirements?
- ☐ Does my knowledge allow me to speak easily with all members of the health care team?
- ☐ Do I accurately and concisely update the provider on any aspect of a patient's care?
- ☐ Do I utilize tactful communication skills with medical providers to ensure accurate code selection?

PRESENTATION

- ☐ Am I dressed and groomed appropriately?
- ☐ Do my actions attend to both the psychological and the physiological aspects of a patient's illness or condition?
- ☐ Am I courteous, patient, and respectful to patients?
- ☐ Do I display a positive attitude?
- ☐ Do I display a calm, professional, and caring manner?
- ☐ Do I demonstrate empathy to the patient?
- ☐ Do I show awareness of patients' concerns related to the procedure being performed?
- ☐ Do I show awareness of patients' concerns regarding a dietary change?
- ☐ Do I display sensitivity when managing appointments?

COMPETENCY

- ☐ Do I pay attention to detail?
- ☐ Do I ask questions if I am out of my comfort zone or do not have the experience to carry out tasks?
- ☐ Do I display sound judgment?

- ☐ Am I knowledgeable and accountable?
- ☐ Do I incorporate critical thinking skills in performing patient assessment and care?
- ☐ Do I recognize the implications for failure to comply with CDC regulations in health care settings?
- ☐ Do I demonstrate professionalism when discussing the patient's billing record?
- ☐ Do I display sensitivity when requesting payment for services rendered?
- ☐ Do I interact professionally with third party representatives?
- ☐ Do I recognize the physical and emotional effects on persons involved in an emergency situation?
- ☐ Do I demonstrate self-awareness in responding to an emergency situation?

INITIATIVE

- ☐ Do I show initiative?
- ☐ Have I developed a strategic plan to achieve my goals? Is my plan realistic?
- ☐ Do I seek out opportunities to expand my knowledge base?
- ☐ Am I flexible and dependable?
- ☐ Do I direct the patient to other resources when necessary or helpful, with the approval of the provider?
- ☐ Do I implement time management principles to maintain effective office function?
- ☐ Do I assist co-workers when appropriate?
- ☐ Do I make adaptations for patients with special needs?

INTEGRITY

- ☐ Do I demonstrate the principles of self-boundaries?
- ☐ Do I work within my scope of practice?
- ☐ Do I demonstrate respect for individual diversity?
- ☐ Do I demonstrate sensitivity to patient rights?
- ☐ Do I protect the integrity of the medical record?
- ☐ Do I recognize the impact personal ethics and morals have on the delivery of health care?
- ☐ Do I protect and maintain confidentiality?
- ☐ Do I immediately report any error I made?
- ☐ Do I report situations which are harmful or illegal?
- ☐ Do I maintain moral and ethical standards?
- ☐ Do I do the "right thing" even when no one is observing?

FIGURE 1-1 Medical assistants should reflect on these questions to ensure that they are embodying the characteristics and qualities of a true medical professional.

type of professional behavior that is expected from medical assistants. It is difficult to list all of the requirements for presenting the demeanor of a competent professional. Many of the aspects of professionalism are those that cannot be measured. Communication and competency can be monitored and evaluated to improve performance, but other aspects—such as presentation, initiative, and integrity—are harder to quantify. Being a professional incorporates all of these attributes. You should continue to reflect on these important aspects of professionalism as you increase your knowledge of anatomy and physiology, medical terminology, procedures, and other concrete aspects of the profession.

Communication

Communication

It is important that medical assistants learn to develop the ability to communicate well both verbally and nonverbally with patients, staff, and other professionals (see Chapter 4). Written communications must be clear and concise and reflect on the practice's professional reputation. Letters and other professional communications must utilize correct grammar, punctuation, and medical terminology.

Compliance with the provider's treatment plan is important for a positive outcome of patients' illnesses (Figure 1-2). Also, patients will feel more comfortable and less threatened in a medical clinic or ambulatory center that encourages staff to keep them informed. Consistent kindness and concern help patients develop trust in you.

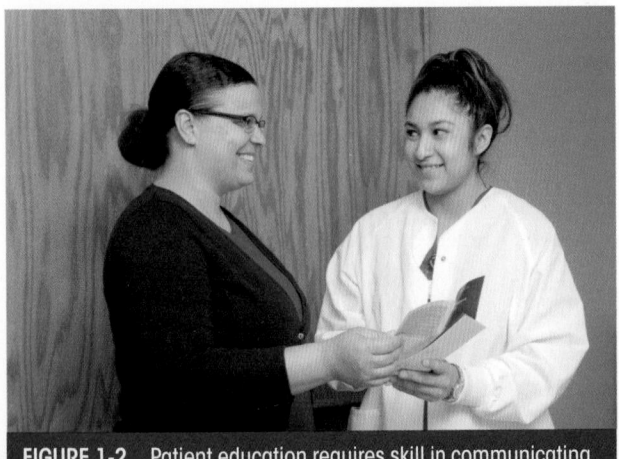

FIGURE 1-2 Patient education requires skill in communicating instructions to patients in language appropriate to their needs.

Presentation

Presentation

Presentation is the style or manner in which something is displayed. The professional medical assistant is required to present professionalism even when there is no conversation going on, no procedure being performed, and no documentation being recorded. Medical assistants should always be groomed and dressed appropriately in order to project a professional image. In addition to maintaining a professional appearance, medical assistants must also be able to communicate and interact with patients, family, and staff in an effective and constructive manner. Treating others with care and respect while displaying a positive attitude are equally important aspects of presenting a professional image.

Physical Attributes. Appearance is important in patients' perceptions of the delivery of their care. Imparting the look of a professional requires an appearance that is clean, fresh, and wholesome—in general, an appearance that reflects good health habits (Figure 1-3). Good personal hygiene practices (daily shower, deodorant), weight control, and healthy-looking skin, hair, teeth, and nails all contribute to a professional appearance. Rest, good

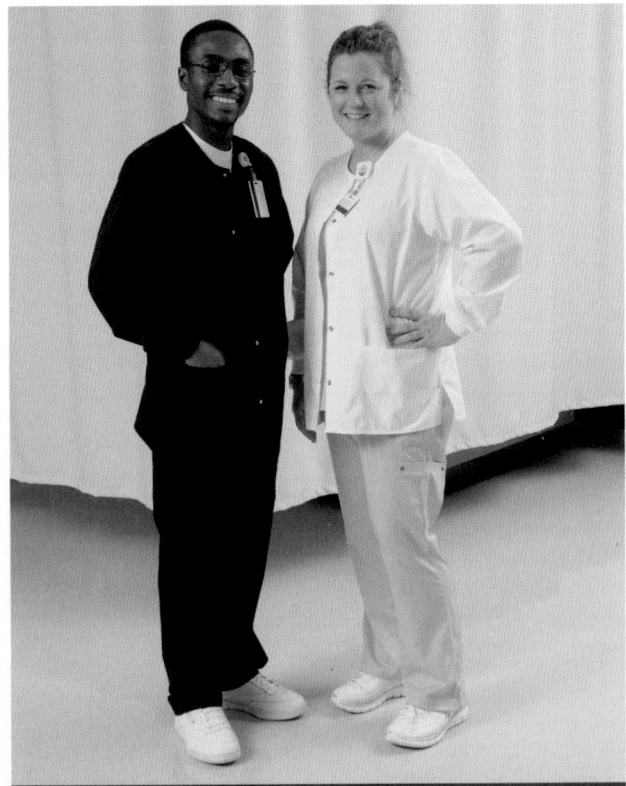

FIGURE 1-3 Medical assistants should always look very professional. Uniforms should always be crisp and clean.

nutrition, scheduled dental care, regular exercise, and recreation all promote good health. A smile can help alleviate some of the anxiety a patient may be experiencing. Your smile gives a pleasant and encouraging appearance to the patient.

Female medical assistants should wear only appropriate light daytime makeup. For the safety of both the professional and the patient, no necklaces or dangling earrings should be worn. The only jewelry worn should be single earposts or wedding rings. Hair should be neat. Fingernails should be short and manicured. Male medical assistants should be clean-shaven and have short hair. Colognes, perfumes, and aftershave should not be worn at work. Body piercings and tattoos should not be visible. There are a variety of cosmetic products manufactured specifically for the covering of visible tattoos. These cosmetics come in a variety of colors to match skin tone and are waterproof. Proper appearance instills confidence in your skills and abilities.

It is important to know and follow the appropriate dress code for your facility. The Centers for Disease Control and Prevention (CDC) recommends that artificial nails and nail extenders not be worn when caring for "high-risk" (intensive care, surgery, or dialysis) patients. Many ambulatory facilities have more stringent rules about artificial nails and extenders.

Patient care can place physical demands on medical assistants. Lifting and moving patients are often required, and the use of correct body mechanics will help minimize injuries to the back. Although every reasonable accommodation is made for medical assistants with physical challenges, it is important to be mobile without assistance because medical assistants move about throughout the day while performing tasks and procedures. It is frequently necessary to bend, stoop, kneel, and crouch, especially when filing and retrieving patients' records, as well as for other tasks. Most procedures require that medical assistants have the ability to hear and see well for the accurate completion of tasks (Figure 1-4). Listening to blood pressures, taking a medical history, observing patients, performing phlebotomy, and identifying microorganisms under a microscope are some of the routine tasks and procedures performed daily in a medical facility.

Manual **dexterity** is also needed for manipulating certain instruments, administering medications, and for entering data using a computer.

Empathy. To have **empathy** means to consider the patient's welfare and to be kind. It means stepping

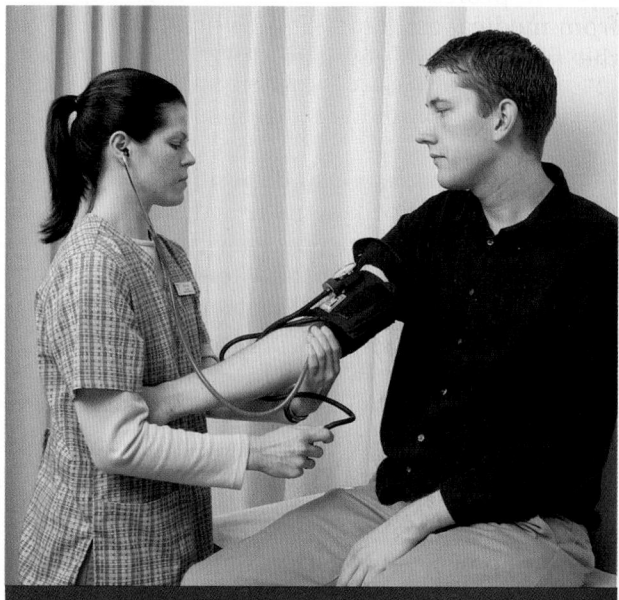

FIGURE 1-4 Measuring blood pressure is a task that requires the medical assistant to see and hear well.

into the patient's place, discovering what the patient is experiencing, and then recognizing and identifying with those feelings.

Medical assistants should treat patients as they themselves would want to be treated. A visit to the providers' clinic is often a time of fear and anxiety. Patients can feel vulnerable. Apprehension can be allayed tremendously when patients realize that their caregiver understands their feelings and desires to make their lives more pleasant and comfortable (Figure 1-5).

It is important to realize that patients' health problems can have a profound effect on you, the medical assistant. By maintaining a balanced outlook, medical assistants can safeguard themselves

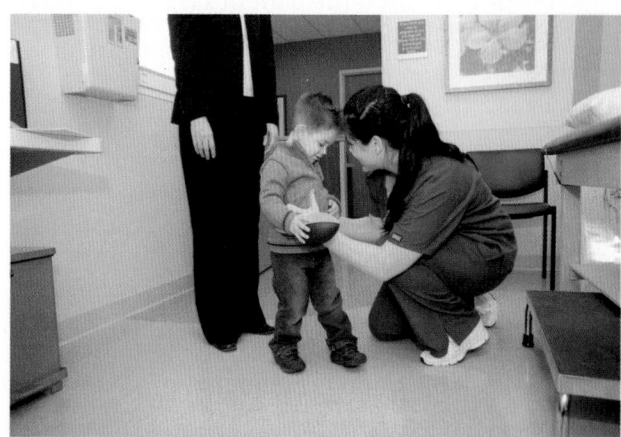

FIGURE 1-5 The medical assistant should have a friendly disposition and communicate empathy for the patient.

from becoming too emotionally involved with patients' problems. Empathy is extremely important in the health care profession; however, emotionalism can cloud one's judgment.

Attitude. A friendly, warm **disposition** and a sense of humor will help patients feel more at ease. A sincere affection for people can be conveyed by actions that **facilitate** open and honest communication. Your attitude should radiate genuine interest. Be sure that all contact with patients is positive.

An essential aspect of a good attitude is respect. Every person that enters the presence of a professional medical assistant must be treated with esteemed reverence. Patients, peers, co-workers, and other clients of the practice must be held in regard. A medical professional's willingness to show appreciation and consideration is an attitude that facilitates a positive experience for all involved. Seeking health care is a very personal experience. On the part of the medical assistant, it necessitates a respect for the patient's information, resulting care, and documentation of this care.

On occasion, difficult patients can test the tolerance level of the most experienced medical assistant because they seldom seem to be content with the care or services received. But no matter what the circumstances, patients should never be treated with disinterest or in an unfriendly manner. The medical assistant should always be pleasant and courteous.

Diversity

Patients should be treated equally, with no reservations about their disease, race, religion, economic status, or sexual orientation. As a member of the health care delivery team, the medical assistant needs to be cooperative and supportive of all other members, working with the team in an honest, open manner while keeping in mind the patient's right to privacy and confidentiality.

Competency

Competency

Competency is the ability to perform a set of skills on a reproducible basis. Competent medical assistants have knowledge of the reason, the methods, and the expected outcomes of the tasks they perform, and are able to execute them consistently. Competency is not just doing your job well. It is a commitment to keeping skills sharp and presentation professional.

Dependability. When providing for a patient's well-being, it is important to focus attention on activities in the office or clinic environment that will demonstrate that you are well organized, accurate, and responsive to patients' needs.

Being dependable means that the employer and coworkers rely on the medical assistant to be respectful of them, patients, and equipment and materials. Other members of the health care team will expect you to be accountable for the duties and responsibilities you undertake. A dependable person interacts with coworkers in a supportive manner, is punctual, and limits absences from work.

Flexibility. The ability to be adaptable is a trait that serves all professionals well. When caring for ill people, unexpected situations arise daily, and medical assistants must be able to respond to a variety of situations (many of them emergencies and unanticipated) without losing a sense of equilibrium. Finding solutions to problems and developing alternative action plans demonstrates flexibility. To **improvise**, or solve problems that arise either routinely or spontaneously, is a characteristic worth nurturing. Willingness to help with various aspects of the clinic offers opportunities to adjust to various situations. It shows your adaptability and willingness to respond to new circumstances.

Initiative

Initiative

The willingness and ability to work independently shows initiative. A person with initiative is observant, notices work that needs to be done, and then takes action to complete those tasks without being told to do them. Employers and coworkers must be able to count on one another to anticipate patients' needs and be attentive to work that needs to be accomplished. The successful medical assistant will be ready to pitch in and recognize when others need assistance. Teamwork and a positive work ethic are valuable characteristics.

By asking appropriate questions and seeking information that will improve performance, medical assistants will demonstrate that they have the foresight and the "get up and go" needed to complete the numerous and varied tasks of the ambulatory care environment.

Desire to Learn. A willingness to continually learn and grow is the mark of a true professional. With the growing use of technology in medicine, there is an ongoing necessity for constant learning. Medical assistants must be dedicated to high standards of performance, which can be accomplished by showing a desire to acquire information and by constantly updating their knowledge and skills. Keeping abreast of the latest diseases, treatments, procedures, and techniques can be achieved in a variety of ways, such as college courses, seminars, workshops, reading, and simply by being observant. The sharper the power of observation, the more the medical assistant will learn from the provider and co-workers.

The gaining and maintaining of competency through participation in continuing education is the responsibility of every medical assistant. Active involvement and membership in the medical assistant professional organizations allows students and CMAs (AAMA) and RMAs (AMT) to participate in meetings and events that can increase professional skills. This benefits medical assistant skills as well as future careers. Students can attend medical assisting meetings (usually free of charge), enjoy student discounts, and network at the meetings.

Integrity

Integrity

Another crucial attribute of professionalism is integrity. Being honest is just one of the hallmarks of integrity. Adherence to moral and ethical principles also describes those who have integrity. The application of integrity is one of the professional characteristics that is in high demand in the profession of medical assisting. Integrity applies to every aspect of patient care, beginning with the first encounter with a patient and continuing through the end of the patient's episode of care. Integrity is not a learned trait, but rather a core personal attribute that can be nurtured and honed to become the cornerstone of one's reputation in the medical field.

Accountability. Accountability is the willingness to accept responsibility. If you reflect upon the numerous aspects of the role of an allied health care provider, you will discover that responsibility plays a key role. The medical assistant is responsible for collecting data, maintaining accurate documentation, interacting with the financial record, planning, and patient teaching, just to name a few tasks. Accountability is demonstrating the highest level of integrity when accepting the responsibility for a patient's care and management of his or her confidential information.

Ethical Behavior. No discussion about personal attributes is complete without the mention of ethics. Ethics is a system of values each individual has that determines perceptions of right and wrong. Our life experiences mold this set of values, which is considered a personal code of ethics.

Medical ethics govern medical conduct or that behavior practiced as health care providers. These ethics involve relationships with patients, their families, fellow professionals, and society in general. Ethical behavior will have a positive impact on the profession of medical assisting and on the medical community as well.

By adhering to the medical assistants' Code of Ethics, we endeavor to elevate the profession to a position of dignity and respect. Medical assistants interact on a daily basis with patients and are entrusted with information about their medical and personal histories. Such information must, by law, be kept confidential. (A more in-depth discussion of ethics and the Code of Ethics can be found in Chapter 7.)

The personal qualities of empathy, professional attitude, dependability, initiative, integrity, accountability, flexibility, the desire to learn, a wholesome physical presence, the ability to communicate well, and ethical behavior are some of the characteristics that most professionals have and that medical assistants should strive to develop. When entering into the profession of medical assisting, it is important to learn more about these and other qualities and to begin to use and refine them. Skills and knowledge alone do not guarantee success. There are personal characteristics that must go along with them.

Professional attitudes, attributes, and values are important for beginning medical assistant students to understand. Students' behaviors can impact the public's opinion of both the provider and the medical assistant profession.

The public has a right to expect that the medical assistant will be competent to practice medical assisting in accordance with the medical assistants' Code of Ethics (see Chapter 7) and with the standards and guidelines set by their professional organizations (such as AMT, AAMA, and NHA).

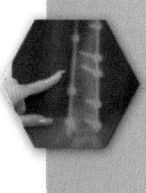

Critical Thinking

Of all the personal attributes that your text describes, which do you think is your most developed attribute? Give an example of that attribute that comes from your daily life.

AMERICAN ASSOCIATION OF MEDICAL ASSISTANTS (AAMA)

In the mid-1950s, there was a movement to form a national organization for medical assistants. The Kansas Medical Assistants Society met in Kansas City, Kansas, and accepted by vote the name American Association of Medical Assistants (AAMA) (see Figure 1-6). In 1956, this organization was supported by the American Medical Association by the passage of a resolution commending the objectives of the AAMA. By 1962, the AAMA had developed a sample certification exam, and in 1963, it offered the first certification. In order to continue to promote and gain recognition for this special set of medical assisting skills, with the collaboration of the American Medical Association, the AAMA began in 1966 to have influence over curriculum and accreditation of postsecondary levels of education. (See Chapter 46 for more information about credentialing for medical assisting.)

Certification

As the profession grew and developed, some states came to require special licensure or certification to perform certain tasks; in other states, other health professionals were challenged by the skill and broad spectrum of the medical assistant's abilities. To defend medical assistants whose right to practice clinical procedures was being challenged, the AAMA responded at their 1995 convention with the following policy:

> that any candidate for the AAMA Certification Examination be a graduate of a CAAHEP-accredited medical assisting program or a graduate of an ABHES-accredited program with one year of documented work experience. Anticipated benefits of the recommendation are to: (1) safeguard the quality of care to the consumer; (2) ensure the CMA's role in the rapidly evolving health care delivery system; and (3) continue to promote the identity and stature of the profession.

In order to sit for the CMA exam, a medical assistant must have not only completed an accredited program, they must also have a clean legal record. If a candidate for the exam has pled guilty to or been convicted of a felony, they generally are not permitted to take the CMA exam. There is a waiver that may be granted based on mitigating circumstances. A request must be submitted for waiver consideration.

Certified Medical Assistant. **Certification** is voluntary, not mandatory, for medical assistants to practice, although an increasing number of employers prefer (or even require) that their medical assistants be CMA (AAMA) certified. The examination measures professional knowledge at the job-entry level. Successful completion of the examination earns the individual the CMA (AAMA) credential (Figure 1-7). (For information on recertification, please see Chapter 46). The initials follow the individual's name. Conferring of the CMA (AAMA) status is referred to as being **credentialed**. The Certification Program of the Certifying Board of the American Association of Medical Assistants is accredited by the National Commission for Certifying Agencies (NCCA) as a result of demonstrating compliance with the *NCCA Standards for the Accreditation of Certification Programs.*

Continuing Education

The AAMA vigorously encourages continuing education for all medical assistants. This can be accomplished through various means such as educational meetings, seminars, workshops, conventions, and the AAMA's self-study publications, a series of study courses for continuing education credit.

Membership in the AAMA is trilevel: local, state, and national. Educational meetings are held regularly at local and state meetings and conventions. The annual AAMA national convention provides an

AMERICAN ASSOCIATION OF MEDICAL ASSISTANTS®

FIGURE 1-6 Logo of the AAMA, a professional organization founded in 1956.

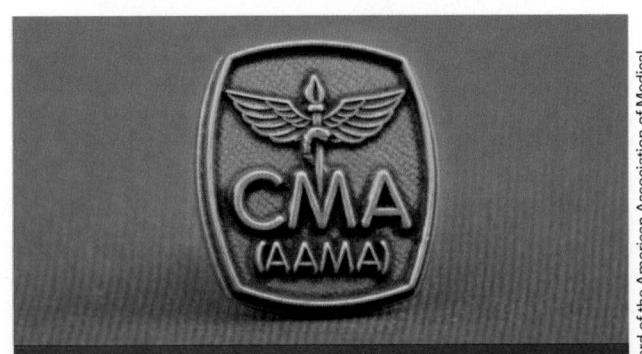

FIGURE 1-7 Certified medical assistant (CMA) pin awarded by the American Association of Medical Assistants on successful completion of the national certification examination.

excellent forum for attaining knowledge through its educational offerings and for networking with other medical assistants.

Continuing an education is a lifelong process and serves as testimony to a commitment to professionalism (see the AAMA Web site at www.aama-ntl.org).

AMERICAN MEDICAL TECHNOLOGISTS

Founded in 1939, the American Medical Technologists (AMT) is a national certification and professional membership association that represents 60,000 allied health care individuals. Its purpose is to certify and credential medical assistants, clinical laboratory personnel, allied health instructors, dental assistants, medical administrative specialists, and others. The AMT has its own bylaws, conventions, committees, state chapters, officers, and registration and certification examinations.

Registered Medical Assistant (RMA)

In 1972, the AMT established the certification examination for medical assistants. The designation of **Registered Medical Assistant (RMA [AMT])** is conferred on those individuals who successfully pass the examination (Figure 1-8).

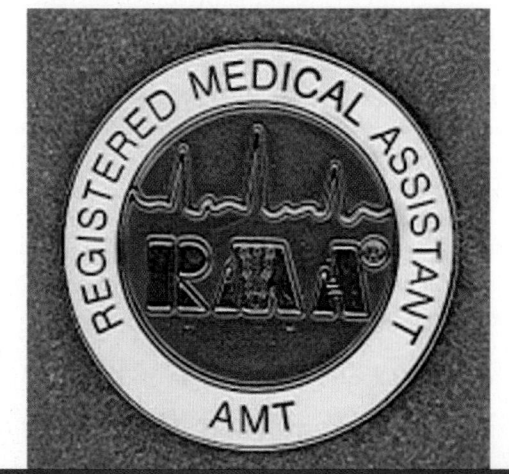

FIGURE 1-8A AMT Logo.

FIGURE 1-8B Registered Medical Assistant (RMA) pin.

The RMA certification examination includes general medical assisting topics, medical terminology, clinical medical assisting, medical law and ethics, human relations, administrative medical assisting, pharmacology, therapeutic modalities, laboratory procedures, electrocardiography, and first aid.

RMAs have been active in legislation to protect medical assistants, ensuring improvement in medical assistant education. American Medical Technologists advocate education and the evolution of professionalism in medical assisting.

Certified Medical Administrative Specialist (CMAS)

Another profession that the AMT certifies is the Medical Administrative Specialist (CMAS). Individuals who successfully pass the AMT certification examination are conferred with the credential of Certified Medical Administrative Specialist (CMAS). The CMAS exam is given in both computerized and paper and pencil formats.

The CMAS serves an important role in the hospital, clinic, or medical office. The CMAS is competent in a multitude of skills such as medical records management, coding and billing for insurance, practice finance management, information processing, and fundamental management practices. The CMAS also is familiar with the clinical and administrative concepts that are required to coordinate office functions in the health care setting.

Continuing Education

AMT encourages and promotes continuing education. The Certification Continuation Program (CCP) requires members to document activities that attest to their continued effort to carry the competencies needed to maintain certification. Proof of compliance is required every three years.

OTHER CERTIFICATION

National Healthcareer Association (NHA)

The National Healthcareer Association (NHA) is a certifying body for health care professionals (Figure 1-9). Its main goals are to certify and to offer continuing education course development, membership services for professionals, and a registry for certified professionals. The NHA offers

National
Healthcareer
Association®

FIGURE 1-9 Logo of the National Healthcareer Association.

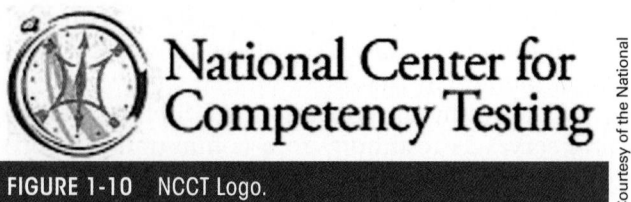

National Center for
Competency Testing

FIGURE 1-10 NCCT Logo.

certification for many allied health professions, including the **Certified Clinical Medical Assistant (CCMA [NHA])** and the **Certified Medical Administrative Assistant (CMAA [NHA])**.

National Center for Competency Testing (NCCT)

The National Center for Competency Testing (NCCT) (Figure 1-10) is an independent certifying body for many allied health professions, including Medical Assistant, Medical Office Assistant, and Phlebotomy Technician. There are two routes to qualify to sit for a certification exam with NCCT. These two routes are graduation from an approved educational program or qualifying work experience with the goal of validating competency.

National Certified Medical Assistant (NCMA). The NCMA certification exam is offered by the NCCT.

It measures job knowledge, skills and abilities in the front and back office, general medical clinic management duties, medical procedures, and pharmacology. To assure proficiency, this exam also tests knowledge of anatomy and physiology as well as medical terminology.

REGULATION OF HEALTH CARE PROVIDERS

One way health care providers can be regulated is through the process of credentialing. Credentialing recognizes health care providers who are professionally and technically competent. Recognition comes from professional associations, certifying agencies, and the state or federal government. Regulation ensures:

- The competence of health care providers
- A minimum standard of knowledge, training, and skill
- The limiting of the performance of certain procedures to a specific occupation

Licensure, certification, and registration are three kinds of regulations/credentialing (Table 1-2).

TABLE 1-2

COMPARISON OF REQUIREMENTS FOR CERTIFICATION, LICENSURE, AND REGISTRATION

	CERTIFICATION	LICENSURE	REGISTRATION
Practice Requirement	Voluntary	Mandatory	Voluntary
Conferred by	Nongovernmental agency or professional association If qualified and meets requirements Must pass national examination	Legislated by each state If qualified and meets requirements Must pass state examination	Professional association If qualified and meets requirements Listed on an official roster Passing examination not always required
How restrictive	Used by most professionals	Most restrictive	Least restrictive

Scope of Practice

Medical assisting is not licensed as a profession; however, some states require that medical assistants be graduates of an accredited medical assisting program and be certified to work as medical assistants.

Two examples of licensed professions are medicine and nursing. A licensing body regulates the activities of these professions by enacting laws that specify educational requirements and by defining the **scope of practice**. A **license** is conferred on an individual who successfully completes specialized educational requirements and successfully passes an examination administered by the state in which the individual resides. The state grants a license to that individual to practice medicine or nursing. Licensure is mandatory and forbids anyone who is not licensed from performing activities that are designated by that particular license. For example, the law states that the medical license allows diagnosing and prescribing treatment. If someone were to diagnose or prescribe without a medical license, that individual would be committing an illegal act and would be practicing medicine without a license, which is considered a felony.

There are state laws that govern the practice of medicine and nursing (medical practice acts, nursing practice acts), and many states have acts that give providers the right to delegate certain clinical procedures to qualified allied health professionals. Because medical assistants are not required to be licensed, they can become certified voluntarily. They are allowed to perform clinical procedures only under the supervision of the provider or other licensed health care professional who is granted that right and who delegates the specific clinical procedures to the medical assistants.

In some states, including California, Washington, and others, unlicensed health care providers are required to have authorization from the state to perform allergy testing and venipuncture and to give injections. A registration fee and mandatory training are required. In such circumstances, medical assistants or other health care providers would be breaking the law if they performed these procedures without registration and training. In some states, authorization is required for unlicensed health care providers to expose patients to X-rays. It is essential that you research your state's scope of practice for medical assistants.

There has been an effort by the U.S. Senate to introduce legislation that would require additional education and credentialing for health care professionals that provide radiologic imaging and radiation therapy. Initially introduced in 2007, the Consistency, Accuracy, Responsibility and Excellence in Medical Imaging or Radiation Therapy (CARE) bill was sent to the Subcommittee on Health in April 2013. Since that time, there has been no further action on the bill.

The AAMA supports legislation that would require specific educational and certification standards for individuals performing medical imaging. Medical assistants do not perform procedures for which they have not been educated and in which they are not proficient. The AAMA's Occupational Analysis for the CMA (AAMA) (which can be accessed at www.aama-nlt.org) and the AMT's Medical Assisting Task List (which can be accessed at www.americanmedtech.org) are excellent reference sources that identify the clinical, administrative, and general procedures medical assistants are educated to perform. However, because of the variability of state statutes, the medical assistant would be wise to check with the AAMA or AMT if in doubt about the legality of certain clinical procedures.

The AMT and the AAMA (the two leading organizations that certify medical assistants) agreed on a model state law outlining the medical assistant's scope of practice. Both the AMT and AAMA took from existing state laws regarding medical assistants' right to practice the most important aspects of these and developed the model. Both organizations agreed to require a medical assistant to graduate from an accredited medical assistant program and to obtain certification from AMT, AAMA, or other approved agencies that certify. A nonexclusive list of functions that a supervised medical assistant may perform was developed. The purpose of the model state legislation is to protect the medical assistant's right to practice. A copy of the model legislation is available at state medical assistant societies.

As the scope of medical assisting practice expands and diversifies, there are many questions regarding state-by-state legislation. Resources to answer these questions are available at www.aama-ntl.org.

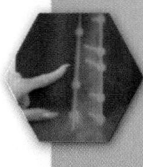

Critical Thinking

A medical assistant relates to a patient on the telephone that her symptoms are "probably the flu" and to "take over-the-counter cough syrup" for her cough. Is this an appropriate or inappropriate action for the medical assistant to take? Discuss your answer and explain why you came to your decision.

Refer to the scenario at the beginning of the chapter.

CASE STUDY REVIEW

1. If you were a freshman in high school and interested in medical assisting, would you like to have an opportunity to visit a program and tour the classroom and laboratories? Why or why not?

2. List three or four questions you might ask of the senior medical assistant students while you are touring the medical assisting department that would help to clarify what the profession is, the course requirements, etc.

Summary

- Progress has been made in the advancement of the profession of medical assisting since the first group of medical assistants gathered to become organized and formed the AAMA and the AMT.

- The total number of medical assistants in the work force is nearly 600,000, and employment opportunities continue to grow.

- The AAMA, AMT, and NHA continue to promote standards of excellence for their members, encouraging continuing education and awarding continuing education credits to members of AAMA, AMT, and NHA via various means.

- Becoming a professional is a gradual process and cannot be learned in its entirety from a textbook.

- The challenge of becoming a professional medical assistant will require open-mindedness and a desire for continued learning and education, certification and recertification of the professional credential, and professional involvement through organizational participation.

- As the scope of work done by medical assistants broadens and medical assistants seek and require formal education, the professional medical assistant will gain additional respect and be in even greater demand.

- Medical assistants must continuously pursue excellence, which is the hallmark of all professional behavior.

Study for Success

To reinforce your knowledge and skills of information presented in this chapter:

- Review the *Key Terms* and *Learning Outcomes*
- Consider the *Critical Thinking* features and *Case Studies* and discuss your conclusions
- Answer the questions in the *Certification Review*

CERTIFICATION REVIEW

1. Which of the following has resulted in an increase in employment opportunities for medical assistants?
   a. The volume of paperwork
   b. Managed care's emphasis on ambulatory care
   c. Baby boomers beginning to retire
   d. All of these

2. Which professional organization awards the CMAS designation?
   a. AAMA
   b. ABHES
   c. AMA
   d. AMT
   e. CAAHEP

3. Which of the following is the definition of ethics?
   a. A system of values each individual has that determines perceptions of right and wrong
   b. A code established by an agency that has nothing to do with the medical assistant's belief in right or wrong
   c. Making patients more comfortable
   d. Willingness to work as a team member
4. Which of the following describes accreditation?
   a. Meeting appropriate standards
   b. Obtaining the CMA (AAMA) or RMA (AMT) credential
   c. Being listed on an official roster
   d. Having a curriculum with courses that are unrestricted
   e. Sitting for an examination that proves mastery of a body of knowledge
5. Which of the following describes licensure?
   a. It is voluntary and up to the individual practitioner.
   b. It is unrestrictive in scope.
   c. It is conferred on an individual through a nongovernment agency.
   d. It is mandatory and legislated by states.
6. Medical assistants possess a skill set that is appropriate for which of the following settings?
   a. Provider's clinics
   b. Urgent care clinics
   c. Insurance companies
   d. Hospitals
   e. All of these
7. Benefits of a medical assistant practicum or externship include which of the following?
   a. Receiving a paycheck for experience gained
   b. Obtaining references for future employment
   c. Improving performance and knowledge
   d. Both b and c
8. Which of the following statements is true?
   a. Medical assisting is a licensed profession.
   b. Medical assistants must obtain an associate's degree.
   c. Medical assistants are governed by state laws.
   d. Medical assistants have mandatory certification.
   e. Medical assistants may perform any procedures that nurses can.
9. Which of the following is a true statement regarding the American Association of Medical Assistants (AAMA)?
   a. It provides certification for Registered Medical Assistant (RMA).
   b. It was the first national organization for medical assisting.
   c. It defined the occupation of medical assisting.
   d. Both b and c
10. Which of the following are attributes of the professional medical assistant?
    a. Communication skills
    b. Integrity
    c. Empathy
    d. Initiative
    e. All of these

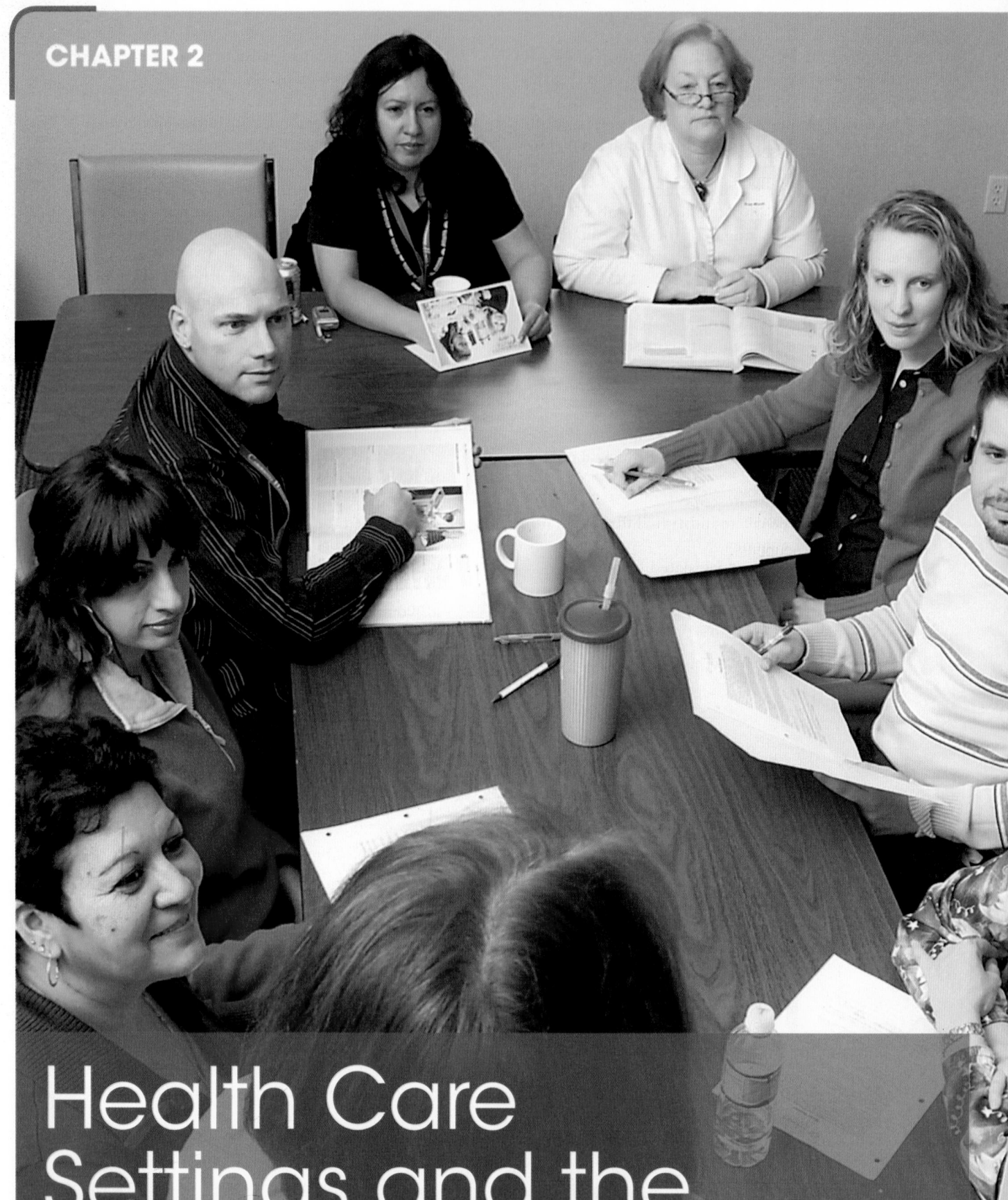

CHAPTER 2

Health Care Settings and the Health Care Team

1. Define and spell the key terms as presented in the glossary.
2. Critique the three primary medical management models.
3. Analyze the benefits and limitations of working in the different ambulatory health care settings.
4. Assess the role of managed care in the health care environment.
5. Compare the patient-centered medical home to accountable care organizations.
6. Describe the function of the health care team.
7. List and describe a minimum of 12 health care providers.
8. Research a minimum of three complementary health care specialists.
9. Compare a minimum of 12 allied health professionals.
10. Discuss the role of the medical assistant in ambulatory health care.
11. Critique complementary and alternative therapies and discuss their role in today's health care setting.
12. Comment on the value of the medical assistant to the health care team.

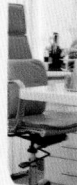

KEY TERMS

accountable care organization (ACO)

acupuncture

ambulatory care setting

complementary and alternative medicine (CAM)

health maintenance organization (HMO)

homeopathy

independent provider association (IPA)

integrative medicine

managed care operation

patient-centered medical home (PCMH)

preferred provider organization (PPO)

SCENARIO

You always had thought you wanted to be a medical assistant and work in a clinic where you would see a variety of patients. But after discussing this chapter in class, you are really intrigued with becoming a physical therapy assistant and want to investigate the profession further. What kind of research can you do to make certain you have chosen the right path? Consider working hours, rate of pay, patient contact, required schooling and attributes of professionalism, and job availability.

There are few professions in our society as rich and complex as the health care profession. Particularly in recent years, the health care environment has changed radically and continues to evolve as the profession seeks ways to provide quality care while containing costs. The Affordable Care Act that became law in March 2010 was created to address unsustainable health care spending, to enhance the "preventive" model of health care coverage, to reduce the high uninsured rate and health disparities across demographic lines, and to hopefully improve health outcomes for our nation's citizens.

Even before the Affordable Care Act was passed, the effort to curtail costs resulted in the rise of managed care, which, in turn, spawned a number of medical models such as **health maintenance organizations (HMOs)** and **preferred provider organizations (PPOs)**.

Many other types of networks and alliances are also being established as providers merge to give patients the best of care while controlling their costs. **Ambulatory care settings**, where services are

continues

provided on an outpatient basis, are the focus of this text, but note that outpatient care is provided via many and varied avenues. Hospitals more frequently provide outpatient care as it has become more common for patients to appear at the emergency department (ED) for routine ailments when they have nowhere else to go. Large retail stores such as Walmart, Target, and CVS have also entered the field of outpatient care through their walk-in clinics. These retail sites, commonly staffed by nurse practitioners, provide routine medical services for a set fee.

Just as the medical setting continues to evolve to meet new societal needs, health care technology is ever changing. Health care is a dynamic, stimulating industry that requires the medical assistant and other professionals to constantly develop new skills if they are to contribute to the team effort. The range of skills within the health care team is astonishing and includes providers in more than 30 specialties, an increasing number of nontraditional complementary/integrative practitioners, and more than 20 kinds of allied health professionals.

AMBULATORY HEALTH CARE SETTINGS

Although medical assistants work in a number of different environments, including laboratories and hospitals, most are employed in an ambulatory care setting such as a medical clinic (either a solo provider or group practice), an urgent or primary care center, or a managed care organization where they give outpatient care.

Often, the medical assistant chooses to work in one setting rather than another based on interests, personality, and work preferences. For instance, the individual practice may provide medical assistants with the opportunity to use their full array of skills, whereas in larger group practices, the work of the medical assistant is often more specialized in nature.

It is helpful if medical assistants recognize the three major and basic forms of medical practice management and how they affect salary, benefits, and liability issues (Figure 2-1).

Medical assistants employed in ambulatory care settings or medical clinics are likely to see three major forms of medical practice management or a combination of three: sole proprietorships, partnerships, and corporations.

Sole Proprietorships

In the past, many providers preferred a solo practice. A solo practice entitles the sole proprietor to hold exclusive right to all aspects of the medical practice or sole proprietorship, including profits and debts. If the business fails, the sole proprietor's personal property may also be attached. As a self-employed sole proprietor, health and dental insurance is a deductible expense. A sole proprietorship may employ other providers to participate in the practice. Any employed providers are entitled to any employee fringe benefits such as health insurance and paid vacation, also.

The sole proprietor sees and treats all patients. Although this type of arrangement is limited in the number of people it can serve, many patients feel secure in this kind of health care setting because they come to know and trust their provider, and they feel their health care is being managed in a personal way. The sole proprietor practice, however, can be an expensive arrangement, because one provider must undertake the costs of clinic space, equipment, and personnel. Today, the majority of solo providers are found in many of the nontraditional alternative or complementary medical practices.

Partnerships

When two or more providers join together under a legal agreement to share in the total business operations of the practice, a partnership is formed. Several providers who share a facility and practice medicine are often referred to as a group. Partners share income, expenses, debt, equipment, records, and personnel according to a predetermined agreement. Partners are liable for only their own actions but may be liable for the whole amount of the partnership debts.

Professional Corporations

Providers may form a corporation, usually referred to as a professional service corporation. The shareholders are considered employees of the corporation. A corporation allows income and tax advantages to all employees. A variety of fringe benefits can be offered to the employees, which may include pension; profit-sharing plans; medical expense reimbursement; and life, health, and disability insurance. These benefits are separate from salary. Another advantage is that professional employees of a corporation are liable only for their own acts, and personal property cannot be attached in litigation. A sole proprietor may incorporate if the practice is large enough.

FORMS OF MEDICAL PRACTICE MANAGEMENT

	Sole Proprietor	Partnership	Professional Corporation
Ease of Formation	Very Easy	Written agreement is helpful	Articles of Incorporation
Management	Owner	Often divided among partners	Board of Directors
Number of Owners	One	Unlimited	State law dictates
Owner Liability	Unlimited	Unlimited if general partner; investment is determined for limited partners	Limited to investment
Allocation of Income	100% to owner	Based on partnership agreement	Normally based on per share/per day rule
Retirement Plans	Any retirement plan	Any retirement plan; must be established by partnership; contributions are deductible by partner	Keogh plans not allowed; deductible at corporate level

FIGURE 2-1   Different forms of medical practice management.

Group Practices

Corporations or group practices are attractive arrangements where providers can share the costs of space, equipment, and personnel. The advantages of a group practice, however, are not solely economic; providers learn from and consult one another, and patients receive the benefit of this exchange of information and knowledge. Often, a group practice has more than one clinic, and some employees are asked to travel between sites to cut overhead. Group practices may be formed to offer specialized care, such as oncology or women's health care.

In many group practices, patients may request that they see the same provider for all appointments, although sometimes patients are assigned to the next available provider. For emergencies, group practices have the staff and flexibility to ensure that there is always a provider on call.

Many providers in small groups turn to large practice management firms, seeking to decrease the time spent managing the business side of their practice. These services often include coding, billing, collecting, or the complete financial management of a practice, and even human resource management. Such a plan is designed to allow providers and their medical assistants more time in patient care activities and less time in paper processing. The health maintenance organization (HMO) is one type of corporation in which providers often practice. Basically, providers are employees of the HMO and are paid by various methods; providers in the HMO usually serve as the primary care provider (PCP). In this situation, a referral from the PCP may be necessary before a patient can see a specialist or allied health professional.

Whatever form of management is chosen by providers, they are responsible for the employees that serve with them. (Refer to the discussion of *respondeat superior* in Chapter 6.) Employers and their medical assistants must have the kind of healthy working relationship where mutual trust and respect are apparent. The provider must understand the skill level of the medical assistant, and the medical assistant must feel secure enough to ask any necessary questions or admit any errors. Critical errors are often made when this trust does not exist between employer and employee. This causes a breakdown in the delivery of the best health care for patients.

Urgent Care Centers

Urgent care centers are usually private, for-profit centers that provide services for primary care, routine injuries and illnesses, and minor surgery. Sometimes laboratory services and a radiology department are located on the premises. The number of urgent care centers in the United States is estimated to be between 7,000 and 9,000, depending upon the inclusion of walk-in care clinics. Providers and other health care professionals in the center are often salaried employees, not owners who share in the profits, and some are associated with other medical facilities, sometimes even hospitals.

The pace in many urgent care centers is brisk, and typically a number of providers are working at one time. Patients are usually encouraged to make appointments, but drop-ins are accepted, so long as providers are available. Serious emergencies are still referred to the emergency department. As mentioned earlier, certain retail chain stores, including Walmart, Target, and CVS, have entered into this market. All over the country, there are walk-in urgent care chains such as Concentra and U.S. Healthworks providing patient care. According to the Urgent Care Association of America, an estimated 3 million patients visit these centers each week. About 25% of patients who patronize these locations have a primary care provider (PCP), but feel they can be seen quicker in this environment. It is also estimated that close to 25% of urgent care patients are uninsured and are required to pay cash for their services. Insurance may be accepted, but most of the centers do not accept Medicaid.

Because these centers often see a higher volume of patients during expanded hours (often 10 AM to 10 PM, 365 days of the year), usually for a lower cost than a hospital emergency department, urgent care centers have continued to grow in popularity. This increase in popularity is also partly due to patients who are used to doing their banking 24/7 seeking greater accessibility in their health care as well.

Managed Care Operations

Health maintenance organizations, or HMOs, are a common **managed care operation**. Originally, HMOs were designed to provide a full range of health care services under one roof. Today, the "HMO without walls" is more common and typically consists of a network of participating providers within a defined geographic area.

Originally, the HMO with walls was conceived to provide patients with comprehensive health care services at one facility. Today, as managed care and managed competition sweep through the health care industry, other arrangements include the preferred provider organization (PPO), where providers network to offer discounts to employers and other purchasers of health insurance, and the **independent provider association (IPA)**, the members of which agree to treat patients for an agreed-upon fee.

"Boutique" or "Concierge" Medical Practices

According to the American Academy of Family Physicians, there are now more than 12,000 "boutique" or "concierge" practices in the United States that are growing in popularity with both patients and providers. Providers who are discouraged by their shrinking insurance reimbursements and by managed care plans dictating what procedures and tests will be performed have turned to another avenue for providing health care. Patients who are disappointed in the quality of care received and frustrated by being bounced from one insurer to another as employers seek a cost reduction in their health care benefits are increasingly willing to pay the extra amount for the concierge care.

Concierge care generally offers patients the following services for a monthly or annual fee:

- Immediate access to their provider by phone 24 hours a day, 7 days a week
- Convenient and unhurried same-day appointments
- Unlimited email, fax, or phone consultation with the provider
- Home or work visits as needed
- Coordination of specialist referrals
- Friendly staff who understand each patient's unique health needs
- Free parking, luxury robes, shower facilities, and Internet access

There are two main types of concierge practices—retainer-based (concierge) and direct primary care (DPC). Neither of these have co-pays, deductibles, or co-insurance fees. About 80% of providers offering concierge service will accept insurance in their practice. DPCs do not accept insurance.

Patients who choose this type of service pay a set fee per year from $2,000 to $3,000 for one individual, and up to $5,000 to include a spouse or $6,000 to include children. Patients are expected

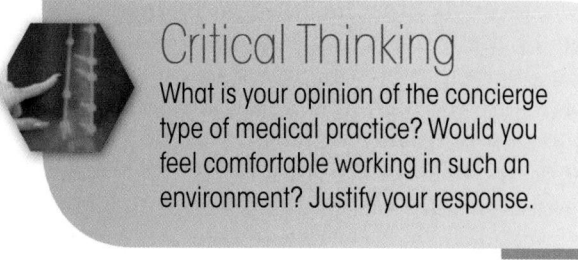

Critical Thinking

What is your opinion of the concierge type of medical practice? Would you feel comfortable working in such an environment? Justify your response.

to carry a major medical plan to cover referrals to specialists, hospitalization, and emergency care.

Legal

Ethical concerns have been raised regarding concierge services. Some say the "extra" services should be available to everyone; others believe the extra fees make the service very exclusive. There is concern that today's decreasing number of PCPs is only made worse when providers choose a concierge-type service over the traditional model of care, sometimes leaving as many as 2,000 patients to find a new PCP. There is speculation that concierge providers also hand-pick the healthiest patients for their service, leaving the sicker patients to be absorbed in traditional health care. Legal concerns surface also. For instance, those concierge providers who accept insurance run into issues with federal Medicare laws that prohibit charging recipients more than the allowable amount. They often turn to the DPC model of not accepting any type of insurance. Also, patients making a decision to embrace concierge medical care must realize that fees paid to these providers are not tax deductible as are fees paid to providers in the traditional model of health care.

Providers practicing in a concierge service report a greater satisfaction with their chosen profession, enjoy really getting to know their patients, and serve a few hundred patients rather than a few thousand as are seen in a traditional practice. Patients report satisfaction with receiving more time and personal care from a provider who determines the best options for maintaining their health.

Patient-Centered Medical Home (PCMH)

In the continuing effort to provide the best of medical care to the largest number of individuals, another model has surfaced. The **patient-centered medical home (PCMH)** is a model that listens to what patients want and seeks to provide better quality, experience, and cost. Presently more than 15% of PCP practices are recognized as PCMHs by the National Committee for Quality

Assurance (NCQA). To be recognized by NCQA, practices must meet rigid standards for addressing patient needs. These include the following:

- After-hours and online access to providers
- Long-term relationships established in team-based care
- Patients seen as partners in health and health care decision making
- Higher quality and experience of care
- Reduced emergency department and hospital care, reducing costs

PCMH transformation is not without difficulty, however. A long-term commitment is required of each team member and a significant financial investment is involved. The goals of PCMHs are admirable. These goals include the best possible care being given to patients and coordination with better prevention methods to reduce emergency department and hospital care. PCPs give "whole" person care at the first contact, and every person in the practice is respectful and responsive to patients' individual needs. It is hoped that all this will bring greater satisfaction to providers, making their PCMH medical practice more successful.

In the future, the hope is for PCMHs to expand to include a medical neighborhood of specialists and hospitals, with practitioners of behavioral health, mental health, public health, and worksite/retail clinics and pharmacies. The Department of Defense is transforming its primary care practices into NCQA PCMHs. The Department of Health and Human Services is assisting community health centers in becoming recognized. Congress is looking toward legislation to move Medicare into support of PCMHs nationwide with new payment systems. Currently, 37 states have public and private PCMHs recognized by NCQA.

The road to success for the PCHM model, however, is a bumpy one. Many providers balk at the detailed assessment of practice capabilities and processes required for NCQA certification. Measuring patients' experiences, the original and ongoing cost of PCMH recognition, and on-site patient surveys are problematic. Providers, already bogged down in the paperwork required for insurance reimbursement and patient record-keeping, resist the addition of any program that requires more paperwork and valuable time. Other providers argue that the goals of PCMH practices are no different from what the goals of every medical facility ought to be right now, even without the NCQA recognition.

Accountable Care Organization (ACO)

Another model for health care is known as the **accountable care organization (ACO)**, which was launched in 2012. The ACO is much like the PCMH practices in its goals. An ACO is a network of providers and hospitals that agree to manage all the health care needs for a group of patients. For example, under the Affordable Care Act, an ACO would agree to provide health care for a minimum of 5,000 Medicare beneficiaries for at least three years. ACOs are intended to reduce health care costs by creating savings incentives, offering bonuses to providers who keep costs down or meet certain benchmarks, focusing on prevention of illness, and carefully managing patients with chronic illnesses. ACOs are similar to HMOs, except that patients in ACOs can and often do receive treatment outside the network.

ACOs have similar problems as the PCMH model. In addition, there is often concern about who is in charge—hospitals, providers, or insurers? In most cases, the answer to that question depends upon where and how the ACO was organized. There is also the concern that in a rural area, the ACO might grow so large that all the providers in the region are involved, often eliminating choice for patients.

THE HEALTH CARE TEAM

In every kind of health care setting, the team concept is critical to the quality of patient care. A PCP is most likely the main source of health care for patients. From time to time, however, a specialist is sought or recommended. A number of different allied health professionals, including the medical assistant, supply additional health care as ordered by the provider. Increasingly, patients are looking outside traditional medicine for portions of their health care. The Centers for Disease Control and Prevention's (CDC) National Health Interview Survey revealed that 38% of adults in the United States use some form of CAM care. The percentage is higher for those persons 50 years and older. The survey also indicated greater use of **complementary and alternative medicine (CAM)** among women and individuals with higher education. In 2012, the World Health Organization (WHO) estimated that between 65% and 80% of the world's population relied on alternative medicine as their primary health care source. Most medical schools in the United States now have courses in CAM. Although CAM care is not always covered by medical insurance, traditional and nontraditional health care practices are nonetheless blending in many areas. Today, many practitioners recognize the benefits of merging the traditional with some of the nontraditional therapies found in complementary medicine; this is recognized as integrative medical care.

In whatever manner health care is sought, all members of the health care team must communicate with one another, sometimes in person and sometimes just through the medical history and record, to ensure quality patient care. The Patient Education box on page 28 discusses the role of the patient as a major member of the health care team.

The Title *Doctor*

The public is often confused by the title *doctor.* The term implies an earned academic degree of the highest level in a particular area of study. Physicians have earned the MD, or Doctor of Medicine, degree. Other medical degrees include the Doctor of Osteopathy (DO), Doctor of Dentistry (DDS), Doctor of Optometry (OD), Doctor of Podiatric Medicine (DPM), Doctor of Chiropractic (DC), and Doctor of Naturopathy (ND). In the medical field, the abbreviation *Dr.* is used and the title *doctor* is used to address these individuals qualified by education, training, and licensure to practice medicine.

In nonmedical disciplines, persons who have achieved a doctorate conferred by a college or university include the Doctor of Education (EdD), the Doctor of Philosophy (PhD), and the Doctor of Psychology (PSYD). All three have several areas of specialty and are referred to as *doctor.*

Health Care Professionals and Their Roles

Doctor of Medicine. A doctorate degree in medicine and a license to practice allows a person to diagnose and treat medical conditions. The doctor of medicine candidate attends four years of medical school after receiving a bachelor's degree. Newly graduated MDs enter into a residency program that consists of three to seven years of additional training and education depending on the specialty chosen. This residency comes under the direct supervision of senior medical doctor educators. Family practice, internal medicine, and pediatrics each require a three-year residency; general surgery requires a five-year residency. Some refer to the first year of residency as an internship; however, the American Medical Association (AMA) no longer uses this term. At this point, many medical doctors choose to be board certified, which is optional and voluntary. Certification assures the public that the doctor's knowledge, experience, and skills in a particular specialty area have been tested and he or she has been deemed qualified to provide care in that specialty. Doctors of medicine can be certified through 24 specialty medical boards and in 88 subspecialty fields. Table 2-1 gives a partial listing of these fields.

TABLE 2-1

SELECTED MEDICAL AND SURGICAL SPECIALTIES

SPECIALTIES	TITLE OF DOCTOR	DESCRIPTION
Allergy and Immunology	Allergist and Immunologist	Evaluates diseases/disorders of the immune system and problems related to asthma and allergy
Anesthesiology	Anesthesiologist	Evaluates sleep and pain control
Cardiology	Cardiologist	Evaluates and treats medical conditions of the heart
Dermatology	Dermatologist	Evaluates disorders/diseases of skin, hair, nails, and related tissues
Emergency Medicine	Emergency Medical Doctor	Evaluates and treats medical conditions that result from trauma or sudden illness; manages the emergency department
Family Medicine	Family Practitioner	Treats the whole family from infancy to death
General Surgery	Surgeon	Operates to repair or remove diseased or injured parts of the body
Colon and Rectal Surgery	Colorectal Surgeon	Operates to remove or repair diseased colon and rectal areas of the body
Neurological Surgery	Neurosurgeon	Treats conditions of the nervous systems, often through surgery
Plastic Surgery	Plastic Surgeon	Repairs and reconstructs physical defects; provides cosmetic enhancements
Thoracic Surgery	Thoracic Surgeon	Performs surgery on the respiratory system, chest, heart, and cardiovascular system
Internal Medicine	Internist	Provides comprehensive care, practices preventive care, and treats long-term and chronic conditions
Medical Genetics and Genomics	Geneticist	Provides information in medical and genetic pathology
Nuclear Medicine	Doctor of Nuclear Medicine	Evaluates molecular and metabolic conditions using radiopharmaceuticals
Obstetrics and Gynecology	Obstetrician and Gynecologist	Provides care to pregnant women, delivers babies, and treats disorders/diseases of the female reproductive system
Ophthalmology	Ophthalmologist	Provides comprehensive care of the eye and its structures and offers vision services
Orthopedic Surgery	Orthopedist	Examines, diagnoses, and treats diseases and injuries of the musculoskeletal system
Otolaryngology	Otolaryngologist	Treats diseases/disorders of the ears, nose, and throat
Pathology	Pathologist	Evaluates body tissues
Pediatrics	Pediatrician	Treats diseases/disorders of children and adolescents; monitors growth and development of children
Physical Medicine and Rehabilitation	Doctor of Physical Medicine and Rehabilitation	Evaluates pain, orders rehabilitation, and practices sports medicine
Preventative Medicine	Doctor	Encourages healthy living

continues

Table 2-1 continued

SPECIALTIES	TITLE OF DOCTOR	DESCRIPTION
Psychiatry and Neurology	Psychiatrist and Neurologist	Diagnoses and treats patients with mental, emotional, or behavioral disorders as well as disorders of the brain and central nervous system
Radiology	Radiologist	Interprets diagnostic images, performs special procedures, and manages radiological services
Urology	Urologist	Treats diseases/disorders of the urinary tract

Medical doctors must still obtain a license to practice medicine from the state or jurisdiction of the United States in which they are planning to practice. They apply for the permanent license after completing a series of examinations and completing a minimum number of years of graduate medical education. Medical doctors must continue to receive a certain number of continuing medical education (CME) requirements each year to ensure that their knowledge and skills are current. CME requirements vary by state, professional organizations, and hospital staff organizations. Medical assistants are often required to maintain their employer's CME records for easier reporting at the time of license renewal.

Doctor of Osteopathy. Osteopaths are generally recognized as equal to medical doctors in all respects. The Doctor of Osteopathy, or DO, is a fully qualified provider licensed to perform surgery and prescribe medication. The training and education are quite similar to that of the MD. Osteopathic medicine was established in 1874 by Dr. Andrew Taylor Still, who was one of the first practitioners to study the attributes of good health to better understand the process of disease. He identified the musculoskeletal system as a key element of health and encouraged preventive medicine, eating properly, and keeping fit. The education of an osteopath includes a four-year undergraduate degree plus four years of medical school. After graduation from medical school, a DO can choose to practice in any of the 18 American Osteopathic Association specialty areas, requiring from two to six years of additional training. Approximately 65% of all osteopaths practice in primary care areas such as family practice, pediatrics, obstetrics/gynecology, and internal medicine. DOs must pass a state licensure examination and maintain currency in their education. Most patients find little difference between an MD and a DO. However, doctors of osteopathy can incorporate osteopathic manipulative treatment (OMT) in their treatment of patients as deemed helpful.

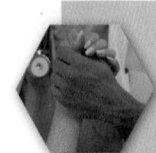

Patient Education

Continually remind your patients of the important role they play in their own health care. *Only your patients* know exactly what happens to their bodies and minds in any particular illness. *Only your patients* know if their pain is too much to bear. *Only your patients* know whether they will remain on any treatment regimen that has been established. *Only your patients* know if they are already embracing some alternative form of treatment. *Only your patients* know how much financial burden they can handle for health care. In initial interviews and preprovider preparations, ask your patients questions that encourage them to tell you what is happening, whether they are coping, and how their particular problem affects their daily lives. Listen to them carefully. Do not rush or second-guess their responses. Be mindful of the special needs of older adult patients and individuals for whom English is their second language. They are likely to be unfamiliar with taking a major role in their own health care. Always remember to be therapeutic and observe nonverbal cues. Empower your patients to be a member of their own health care team.

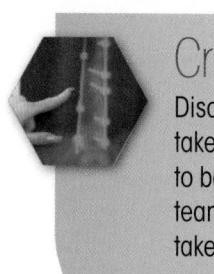
Integrative Medicine and Alternative Health Care Practitioners

Many **integrative medicine** and alternative health care practitioners also carry the title *doctor,* but they have a different training regimen than required for the MD or DO. The training is highly specialized and specific; when licensed, these professionals are allowed to diagnose and treat medical conditions.

As mentioned earlier, alternative therapies are increasingly being perceived as complements to traditional health care in a form of integrative medicine. In this text, three broad alternative therapy disciplines are identified: chiropractic, naturopathy, and Oriental medicine/acupuncture.

Doctor of Chiropractic.

Chiropractic is a branch of the healing arts that gives special attention to the physiological and biochemical aspects of the body's structure and it includes procedures for the adjustment and manipulation of the bones, joints, and adjacent tissues of the human body, particularly of the spinal column. Chiropractic is a nonsurgical science that also does not include pharmaceuticals.

The roots of chiropractic care can be traced back to the beginning of recorded time. Text from China and Greece written in 2700 BCE and 1500 BCE, respectively, mention spinal manipulation and maneuvering of the lower extremities to ease lower back pain. Daniel David Palmer founded the chiropractic profession in the United States in 1895. Throughout the twentieth century, doctors of chiropractic (DC) gained legal recognition and licensure in all 50 states.

Doctors of chiropractic complete four to five years of study at an accredited chiropractic college. The curriculum includes a minimum of 4,200 hours of classroom, laboratory, and clinical experience. About 555 hours are devoted to adjustive techniques and spinal analysis. This specialized education must be preceded by a minimum of 90 hours of undergraduate courses focusing on science. On successful completion of their education and training, doctors of chiropractic must also pass the national board examination and all examinations or licensure requirements identified by the particular state in which the individual wishes to practice.

Doctors of chiropractic frequently treat patients with neuromusculoskeletal conditions such as headaches, joint pain, neck pain, lower back pain, and sciatica. Chiropractors also treat patients with osteoarthritis, spinal disk conditions, carpal tunnel syndrome, tendonitis, sprains, and strains. Chiropractors also may treat a variety of other conditions such as allergies, asthma, and digestive disorders. There are obstacles to chiropractors in some areas, however, because states vary in what they authorize chiropractors to practice and may limit their ability to practice **homeopathy** or **acupuncture** or to dispense or sell dietary supplements.

Doctor of Naturopathy.

Naturopathy, often referred to as "natural medicine," is based on the belief that the cause of disease is violation of nature's laws. The goal of the naturopath is to remove the underlying causes of disease and to stimulate the body's natural healing processes. Naturopathic treatments may include fasting; adhering to natural food diets; taking vitamins and herbs; tissue minerals; counseling; homeopathic remedies; manipulation of the spine and extremities; massage; exercise; naturopathic hygienic remedies; acupuncture; and applications of water, heat, cold, air, sunlight, and electricity. Most of these treatment methods are used to detoxify the body and strengthen the immune system.

In the United States, a Doctor of Naturopathy (ND) or Doctor of Naturopathic Medicine (NMD) receives education, training, and credentials from a full-time naturopathy college. Full-time education includes two years of science courses and two years of clinical work. Naturopaths are currently licensed to practice in 16 states, the District of Columbia, four Canadian provinces, and Puerto Rico and the Virgin Islands. In many states, naturopaths practice independently and unlicensed, or they practice under the direction of a physician.

Oriental Medicine and Acupuncture.

Oriental medicine is a comprehensive system of health care with a history of more than 3,000 years. Oriental medicine includes acupuncture, Chinese herbology and bodywork, dietary therapy, and exercise based on traditional Oriental medicine principles. This form of health care is used extensively in Asia and is rapidly growing in popularity in the West.

Oriental medicine is based on an energetic model rather than the biochemical model of Western medicine. The ancient Chinese recognized a vital energy behind all life-forms and processes called *qi* (pronounced "chee"). Oriental healing practitioners believe that energy flows along specific pathways called *meridians*. Each pathway is associated with a particular physiological system and internal organ. Disease is the result of deficiency or imbalance of energy in the meridians and their associated physiological systems. Acupuncture points are specific sites along the meridians. Each point has a predictable effect on the vital energy passing through it. Modern science has measured the electrical charge at these points, corroborating the locations of the meridians. Traditional Oriental medicine uses an intricate system of pulse and tongue diagnosis, palpation of points and meridians, medical history, and other signs and symptoms to create a composite diagnosis. A treatment plan then is formulated to induce the body to a balanced state of health.

The WHO recognizes acupuncture and traditional Oriental medicine's ability to treat many common disorders, including the following:

- *Gastrointestinal disorders.* Food allergies, peptic ulcer, chronic diarrhea, constipation, indigestion, anorexia, gastritis
- *Urogenital disorders.* Stress incontinence, urinary tract infections, sexual dysfunction
- *Gynecological disorders.* Irregular, heavy, or painful menstruation; premenstrual syndrome (PMS); infertility
- *Respiratory disorders.* Emphysema, sinusitis, asthma, allergies, bronchitis
- *Neuromusculoskeletal disorders.* Arthritis; migraine headaches; neuralgia; insomnia; dizziness; low back, neck, and shoulder pain
- *Circulatory disorders.* Hypertension, angina pectoris, arteriosclerosis, anemia
- *Eye, ear, nose, and throat disorders.* Otitis media, sinusitis, sore throats
- *Emotional and psychological disorders.* Depression; anxiety; addictions to alcohol, nicotine, and drugs
- *Pain.* Elimination or control of pain for chronic and painful debilitating disorders

In the hands of a comprehensively trained acupuncturist, patients do not find acupuncture painful. Sterile, very fine, flexible needles about the diameter of a human hair are used in treatment. Practitioners may also recommend herbs, dietary changes, and exercise, together with lifestyle changes.

Training for acupuncture and Oriental medicine can be obtained in schools and colleges accredited by the Accreditation Commission for Acupuncture and Oriental Medicine. Applicants must have a bachelor's degree. Most of these specialized programs are three years, and on completion graduates are conferred with a master's degree in Acupuncture and Oriental Medicine (MAOM) or a master's degree in Acupuncture (MA) degree. Nearly all states regulate the practice of acupuncture and Oriental medicine, either through licensure or a ruling by the Board of Medical Examiners. In most cases passing a national certification examination or other testing procedure is required before licensure. Many doctors (MDs, DOs, DCs, and NDs) have become qualified to perform acupuncture and to use Oriental medicine in their practices through additional education and training.

Future of Integrative Medicine

There was a time when osteopaths and chiropractors were not accepted by the medical establishment and had difficulty with licensure. Naturopaths, acupuncturists, and Oriental medicine practitioners face similar challenges, and states vary greatly in their regulations of any form of alternative medicine and the scope of practice for each.

The road may be bumpy for CAM practitioners, but their numbers continue to increase. Managed care health plans are offering increased access to CAM practitioners, mostly because of the ability to expand patient choices at a lower cost. It is expected, however, that states will continue to wrestle with licensure and scope of practice issues for the increased numbers of well-educated and trained CAM practitioners.

Neither the growth in the number of CAM practitioners nor the laws and insurance practices that facilitate their access by patients likely would have occurred without broad public acceptance of alternative and complementary medicine. Americans seem quite willing to pay out-of-pocket expenses for alternative forms of treatment, such as massage therapy, aromatherapy, biofeedback, guided imagery, hydrotherapy, hypnotherapy, and homeopathy. Furthermore, many patients are seeking the more integrated form of medicine that occurs when primary care providers are willing to refer to a CAM practitioner and vice versa. Table 2-2 gives a brief description of a few alternative modalities that integrate fairly easily with traditional medical practices.

TABLE 2-2

SELECTED ALTERNATIVE MEDICINE MODALITIES

Ayurveda	5,000-year-old system of natural healing from India; three "energies" shape mind/body characteristic. A person's ideal state is determined and diet, herbs, aromatherapy, massage, music, and medication are used to reestablish harmony when there is illness.
Biofeedback	Biofeedback machines gauge internal bodily functions and help patients tune in to these functions and identify the triggers that evoke symptoms. Relaxation can be taught to relieve the symptoms.
Guided Imagery	Uses images or symbols to train the mind to create a definitive physiological or psychological effect; relieves stress and anxiety and reduces pain.
Homeopathy	Healing that claims highly diluted doses of certain substances can leave an energy imprint in the body and bring about a cure. Homeopathic remedies are made from naturally occurring plant, animal, or mineral substances and are manufactured by pharmaceutical companies under strict guidelines.
Hydrotherapy	Hydrotherapy uses the buoyancy, warmth, and effects of water and its turbulence to speed recovery after surgery and to reduce pain and stress, spasm, and discomfort. It is especially beneficial for work- or sports-related injuries and arthritis.
Hypnotherapy	Hypnotherapy facilitates communication between the right and left sides of the brain with the patient in a state of focused relaxation when the subconscious mind is open to suggestions. It is currently used to help people lose weight; stop smoking; reduce stress; and relieve pain, anxiety, and phobias.
Massage	Massage reduces stress, manages chronic pain, promotes relaxation, and increases circulation of the blood and lymph. Hand stroking on the body helps patients become more familiar with their pain.
Movement Therapies	A group of therapies that include movement to establish balance, enhance relaxation, correct posture, elevate the spirit, and invigorate the mind. Pilates, Tai Chi, and Feldenkrais are examples.

ALLIED HEALTH PROFESSIONALS AND THEIR ROLES

In the health care team, allied health professionals bring specific educational backgrounds and a broad array of skills to the medical environment. Medical assistants are allied health professionals with a very specific set of skills for ambulatory care.

The Role of the Medical Assistant

In the ambulatory care setting, a critical and most beneficial allied health professional is the medical assistant. The medical assistant, performing both administrative and clinical tasks under the direction of the provider, is an important link between patient and provider (Figure 2-2). The medical assistant serves in many capacities—receptionist, secretary, office manager, bookkeeper, insurance coder and biller, sometimes transcriptionist, patient educator, and clinical assistant. The latter requires the medical assistant to be able to administer injections, perform venipuncture, prepare patients for examinations, assist with examinations and special procedures, and perform

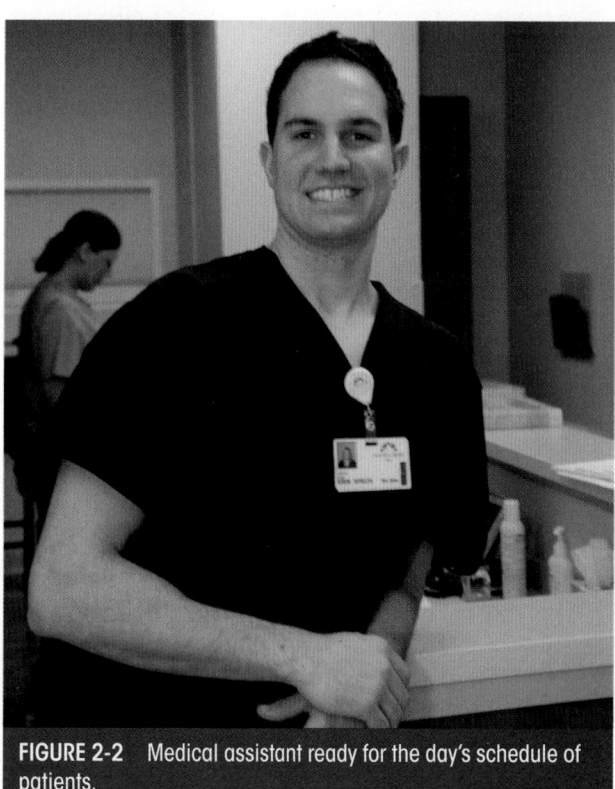

FIGURE 2-2 Medical assistant ready for the day's schedule of patients.

electrocardiography and various laboratory tests. Medical assistants screen and assess patient needs when scheduling appointments and tests. Although medical assistants have a broad range of responsibilities, it is critical that they perform only within the scope of their training, education, and personal capabilities and always function within ethical and legal boundaries and state statutes. To perform outside the scope of training is both illegal and unethical.

Legal　Presentation

Because medical assistants are often the patient's first contact with the facility and its providers, a positive attitude is important (see Chapter 1). They must be excellent communicators, both verbally and nonverbally, and project a professional image of themselves and their employer. Medical assistants who believe in their work, who are proud of their career, and who convey compassion and caring provide a positive experience for patients who are ill or in a great deal of discomfort.

Table 2-3 lists some of the allied health professionals recognized by the Commission on Accreditation of Allied Health Education Programs (CAAHEP) and the Accrediting Bureau of Health Education Schools (ABHES).

As a medical assistant, you may not work directly with all the identified allied health care professionals, but you likely will have contact with many of

TABLE 2-3

SELECTED ALLIED HEALTH PROFESSIONS

OCCUPATION	ABBREVIATION	JOB DESCRIPTION
Anesthesiologist Assistant	AA	Performs preoperative tasks; performs airway management and drug administration for induction and maintenance of anesthesia during surgery under direction of a licensed and qualified anesthesiologist
Athletic Trainer	AT	Provides a variety of services, including injury prevention, recognition, immediate care, treatment, and rehabilitation after athletic trauma
Clinical Laboratory Technician *Associate Degree*	CLT	Performs all routine tests in a medical laboratory and is able to discriminate and recognize factors that directly affect procedures and results. Works under direction of pathologist, provider medical technologist, or scientist
Diagnostic Medical Sonographer	DMS	Provides patient services using medical ultrasound under the supervision of a provider
Electroencelphalographic Technologist	EEG-T	Possesses the knowledge, attributes, and skills to obtain interpretable recordings of a patient's nervous system functions
Emergency Medical Technician—Paramedic	EMT-P	Recognizes, assesses, and manages medical emergencies of acutely ill or injured patients in prehospital care settings, working under the direction of a provider (often through radio communication)
Medical Assistant	MA	Functions under the supervision of licensed medical professionals and is competent in both administrative/office and clinical/laboratory procedures
Medical Illustrator	MI	Creates visual material designed to facilitate the recording and dissemination of medical, biological, and related knowledge through communication media
Occupational Therapist	OT	Educates and trains individuals in the application of purposeful, goal-oriented activity in the evaluation, diagnosis, and treatment of loss of ability to cope with the tasks of daily living and impairment caused by physical injury, illness, or emotional disorder; congenital or developmental disability; or the aging process
Ophthalmic Medical Technician or Technologist	OMT	Assists ophthalmologists to perform diagnostic and therapeutic procedures

continues

Table 2-3 continued

OCCUPATION	ABBREVIATION	JOB DESCRIPTION
Personal Fitness Trainer	PFT	Develops an activity plan for each individual that integrates a complete approach to fitness and wellness through exercise, strength training, and proper diet
Radiographer	RT(R)	Provides patient services using imaging modalities, as directed by providers qualified to order and perform radiologic procedures
Registered Health Information Administrator	RHIA	Manages health information systems consistent with the medical, administrative, ethical, and legal requirements of the health care delivery system
Registered Health Information Technician	RHIT	Possesses the technical knowledge and skills necessary to process, maintain, compile, and report patient data
Respiratory Therapist	RRT	Applies scientific knowledge and theory to practical clinical problems of respiratory care
Surgical Technologist	ST	Works as an integral member of the surgical team, which includes surgeons, anesthesiologists, registered nurses, and other surgical personnel delivering patient care and assuming appropriate responsibilities before, during, and after surgery

them by telephone and written or electronic communication. Knowledge of the roles these health professionals play enables you to interact more intelligently with all members of the health care team.

In addition to the professionals listed in Table 2-3, you may encounter some or all of the following health care professionals in daily patient care.

Health Unit Coordinator

Health unit coordinators (HUCs) perform non-clinical patient care tasks for the nursing unit of a hospital. General secretarial and clerical duties allow HUCs to maintain patients' charts, schedule tests, order supplies, screen new patients, and give directions to visitors. This profession requires a self-motivated, mature individual who can handle the stress and hectic pace of coordinating personnel and their duties at the nurses' station. Also called unit secretary, administrative specialist, ward clerk, or ward secretary, a health unit coordinator receives on-the-job training or completes a six-month to one-year certificate program.

Medical Laboratory Technologist

Medical laboratory technologists (MLTs) physically and chemically analyze, as well as culture, urine, blood, and other body fluids and tissues

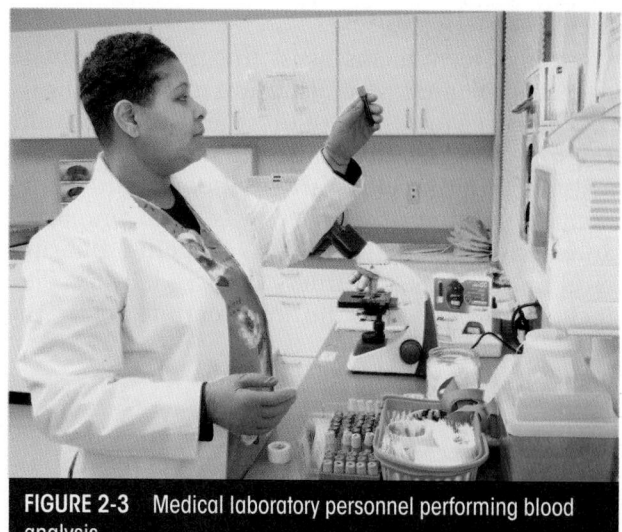

FIGURE 2-3 Medical laboratory personnel performing blood analysis.

(Figure 2-3). They work closely with specialists such as oncologists, pathologists, and hematologists. Knowledge of specimen collection, anatomy and physiology, biochemistry, laboratory equipment, asepsis, and quality control is essential. The American Society of Clinical Pathology (ASCP) is a professional organization that oversees credentialing and education in the medical laboratory professions.

Registered Dietitian

Registered dietitians (RDs) have specialized training in the nutritional care of groups and individuals and have successfully completed an examination conducted by the Commission on Dietetic Registration. Dietitians assist patients in regulating their diets. Although they are typically employed in hospitals and clinics, they can also be found working with the public in personal nutritional counseling. Education includes a bachelor's degree with a major in dietetics, food and nutrition, or food service systems management, in addition to completion of an approved internship.

Pharmacist

Pharmacists (RPh) are licensed by each state to prepare and dispense all types of medications as well as medical supplies related to medication administration. They can practice in hospitals, medical centers, and pharmacies. The minimum training for a pharmacist is a five-year bachelor's degree; some pharmacists pursue a Doctor of Pharmacy degree (PharmD), which is offered by major universities in the United States.

Pharmacy Technician

Pharmacy technicians assist the pharmacist with preparation and administration of medications; they also perform receptionist and billing duties (Figure 2-4). In hospitals, nursing homes, and assisted living facilities, their responsibilities may include reading patient charts and preparing and delivering medications to patients. Pharmacists must check all orders before delivery. The technician can copy the information about the

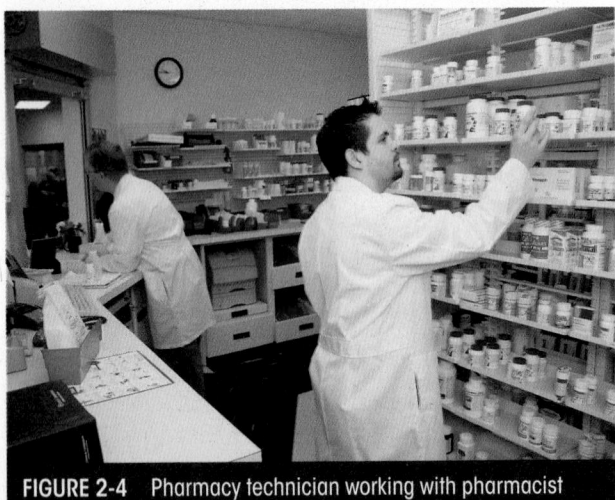

FIGURE 2-4 Pharmacy technician working with pharmacist preparing medications.

prescribed medication onto the patient's profile. Professional certification of pharmacy technicians varies from state to state and is administered by state pharmacy associations.

Phlebotomist

Phlebotomists are trained in the art of drawing blood for diagnostic laboratory testing. Phlebotomists are also referred to as laboratory liaison technicians. Phlebotomists may be nationally certified and are employed in medical clinics, hospitals, and laboratories. Training consists of one to two semesters in a community college program or on-the-job training.

Physical Therapist

Physical therapists (PTs) are licensed professionals who assist in the examination, testing, and treatment of physically disabled or challenged people. They also assist in physical rehabilitation of patients after an accident, injury, or serious illness, using special exercises, application of heat or cold, ultrasound therapy, and other techniques. Educational requirements for a PT are a minimum of a four-year bachelor's degree (bachelor of science) or a special certificate course after obtaining the bachelor of science in a related field. PTs must also successfully complete a state licensure examination.

Physical Therapy Assistant

Physical therapy assistants (PTAs) are trained to use and apply physical therapy procedures, such as exercise, and physical agents under the supervision of a physical therapist. The PTA has earned an associate of science degree from an accredited program and must pass a licensure or registry examination in selected states.

Nurse

Neither ABHES nor CAAHEP is responsible for nurse education or accreditation, but nurses are listed here as a major participant in health care. Nurses are licensed by the state in which they practice. Although nurses' education and training are oriented to bedside care, some may be employed in medical clinics as clinical assistants, especially in clinics where surgery is performed. Nurses play a number of roles on the health care team.

Registered Nurse. In the United States, registered nurses (RNs) are professionals who have completed, at a minimum, a two-year course of study at a state-approved school of nursing and have passed the National Council Licensure Examination (NCLEX-RN). Employment settings most often include hospitals, convalescent homes, clinics, and home health care.

Licensed Practical Nurse. A licensed practical nurse (LPN) is a professional trained in basic nursing techniques and direct patient care. LPNs practice under the direct supervision of an RN or provider and are employed in similar settings to RNs. Training includes completion of a state-approved program in practical nursing and successful completion of the National Council Licensure Examination (NCLEX-PN).

Nurse Practitioner. Sometimes referred to as an advanced registered nurse practitioner (ARNP), a nurse practitioner (NP) is an RN who, by advanced education (usually a master's degree) and clinical experience in a branch of nursing, has acquired expert knowledge in a specific medical specialty. Nurse practitioners are employed by providers in private practice or in clinics and sometimes practice independently, especially in rural areas. They have increased in numbers as the number of primary care providers continues to decrease. ARNPs may or may not be licensed to prescribe medications.

Physician Assistant

Physician assistants (PAs) receive formal education and training to provide diagnostic, therapeutic, and preventive health care services delegated by and under the supervision of providers and surgeons. PAs take medical histories, examine and treat patients, order and interpret laboratory tests and X-rays, and make diagnoses. They also treat minor injuries by suturing, splinting, and casting. PAs write progress notes, instruct and counsel patients, and order tests and therapy. In all 50 states, the District of Columbia, and Guam, PAs may prescribe certain medications. They can supervise technicians and medical assistants. PAs may be primary care providers in areas where the supervising physician is not present all the time but is always available for conferring as necessary and required by law. PAs, too, are growing in numbers.

Most PA programs are two years in length with the added requirement of at least two years of college and some health care experience. For licensure, all states require PAs to complete an accredited, formal education program and to pass the Physician Assistant National Certifying Examination administered by the National Commission on Certification of Physician Assistants (NCCPA). The examination is available only to graduates of an accredited PA education program. Upon successful completion of the examination, the credential "Physician Assistant–Certified" can be used.

THE VALUE OF THE MEDICAL ASSISTANT TO THE HEALTH CARE TEAM

Professional

With their broad range of competencies in both administrative and clinical areas, medical assistants are the most valued ambulatory health care team member. Medical assistants are the great communicators, serving as liaisons between provider and hospital staff and between provider and any number of allied and other health professionals. Because they often are the first providers to see or speak with patients, they undertake responsibility for directing, informing, and guiding patient care while establishing a professional and caring tone for the entire health care team. The value of a competent, professional, compassionate medical assistant is immeasurable in today's fast-paced and challenging health care environment.

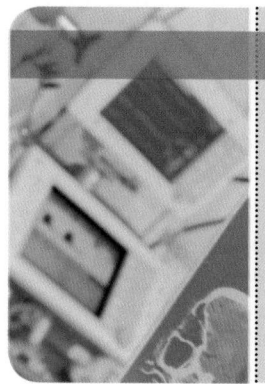

CASE STUDY 2-1

Refer to the scenario at the beginning of the chapter.

CASE STUDY REVIEW
1. Where will you research additional information on being a physical therapy assistant?
2. Compare the working hours, rate of pay, contact with patients, required schooling, and job availability to those of the medical assistant in your geographic location.
3. If other health professions discussed in the chapter are of special interest to you, answer the same questions. This review helps to clarify the position of the medical assistant for you.

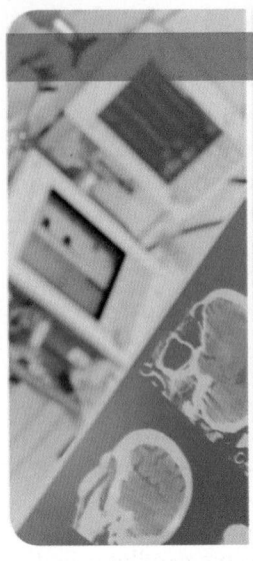

CASE STUDY 2-2

You are the medical assistant for a family-practice provider, Dr. Bill Claredon, who is close to retirement. He is much adored by all his patients, but he thinks any complementary therapies are outright quackery. Marjorie Johns, a patient with debilitating back pain, tells you she is seeing an acupuncturist and is taking less and less of her prescribed medications. You quietly mention this to Dr. Claredon before he enters the examination room to see Marjorie. He glares at you with disgust at the information and is quite agitated when he enters the examination room.

CASE STUDY REVIEW

1. Describe the discussion that you think might occur between Dr. Claredon and Marjorie.
2. If Marjorie is unhappy when she is ready to leave the facility, what professionalism skills can you use to help her?
3. As the medical assistant, what attributes of professionalism can be utilized to ease Dr. Claredon's concern and help bridge this gap for Marjorie?

Summary

- The health care environment is a dynamic service that changes rapidly in response to new technology and societal needs.
- Some form of managed care likely will dominate the health care industry for years to come.
- A strong health care team is critical in the health care setting, as primary care providers, specialists of all disciplines, complementary care practitioners, and allied and other health professionals collaborate on the best way to provide integrative medicine and quality patient care.
- The medical assistant is a vital link in the team and is responsible for a range of responsibilities, both clinical and administrative.

Study for Success

To reinforce your knowledge and skills of information presented in this chapter:

- Review the *Key Terms* and *Learning Outcomes*
- Consider the *Critical Thinking* features and *Case Studies* and discuss your conclusions
- Answer the questions in the *Certification Review*

CERTIFICATION REVIEW

1. Where are the majority of medical assistants employed?
   a. Hospitals
   b. Nursing facilities
   c. Ambulatory care settings
   d. Insurance companies
2. Which term best describes a health maintenance organization?
   a. Managed care operation
   b. Individual practice
   c. Sole proprietorship
   d. Hospital
   e. PCMH

3. With its emphasis on controlling costs, what will managed care likely affect the most?
   a. Only hospitals
   b. All health care settings
   c. Only providers in private practice
   d. Only patients
4. How is the health care team best described?
   a. It should exclude the patient as part of the team.
   b. It is only important in the hospital setting.
   c. It consists of physicians and nurses.
   d. It includes physicians, nurses, allied health care professionals, patients, and integrative medicine practitioners.
   e. It refers to only the PCP and the patient.

5. Which of the following statements best identifies integrative health care approaches?
   a. It is increasingly accepted as complementary to traditional health care.
   b. It is always covered by insurance.
   c. It is seldom approved for licensure.
   d. It is not important to understand.
6. When a medical assistant permitted by law to draw blood for diagnostic laboratory testing performs such a procedure, it is similar to those performed by which of the following?
   a. A health unit coordinator
   b. A health information technician
   c. A phlebotomist
   d. A respiratory therapist
   e. A nurse
7. Which of the following best describes a "boutique" or "concierge" medical practice?
   a. It is another form of managed care.
   b. It allows patients special privileges in their health care.
   c. It is covered by all major insurance plans.
   d. It does not require special fees for services.
8. Providers just establishing their practice often seek to work with another provider in the same field. When expenses and profits are shared, what is the name given to this form of management?
   a. HMO
   b. Corporation
   c. Sole proprietor
   d. Group or partnership
   e. Community care organization
9. Which of the following will the medical assistant *not* do in health care?
   a. Code and bill insurance, bookkeeping
   b. Diagnose and treat ailments
   c. Screen when making appointments
   d. Assist provider, perform clinical and laboratory procedures
10. What is an alternative approach to medicine that treats patients using thin, flexible needles called?
    a. Acupuncture
    b. Naturopathy
    c. Chiropractic
    d. Homeopathy
    e. Ayurveda

UNIT II
THE THERAPEUTIC APPROACH

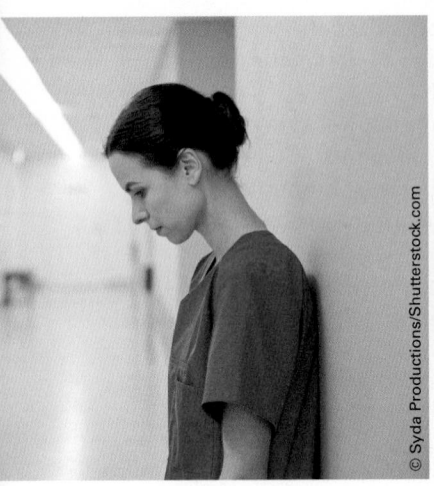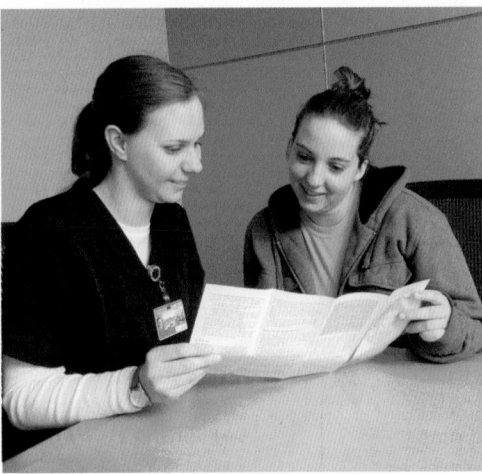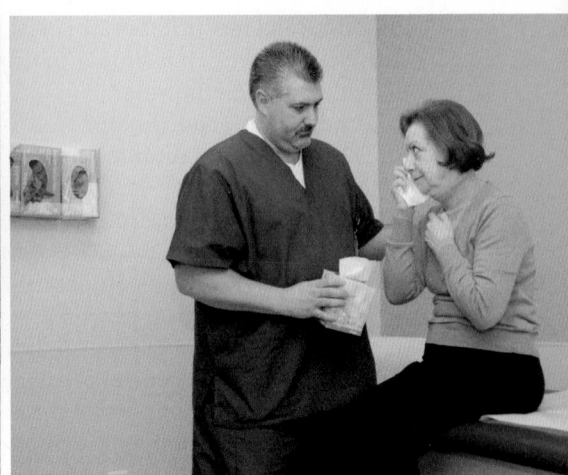

© Syda Productions/Shutterstock.com

ATTRIBUTES OF PROFESSIONALISM

The professional medical assistant is very aware of the importance of communication skills and strives to be therapeutic in all situations. Therapeutic communication requires clear communication of technical information in a manner that is empathetic to the patient's emotional state. It requires adherence to accepted social behavior and political correctness. It is also important to remember that nonverbal communication or body language can be an even stronger communicator than words. Body language generally communicates our true feelings and often we are not even aware of the messages we are sending. Because nonverbal communication can easily be misinterpreted, the professional medical assistant will look for agreement between verbal and nonverbal communication in order to send and receive a clear message.

Listening is often identified as the passive aspect of communication. However, if it is done well, listening is very active. Good listeners focus on the speaker, are attentive, and are aware of the nonverbal messages as well as the verbal information being shared. The professional medical assistant should have three listening goals: (1) to improve listening skills so that

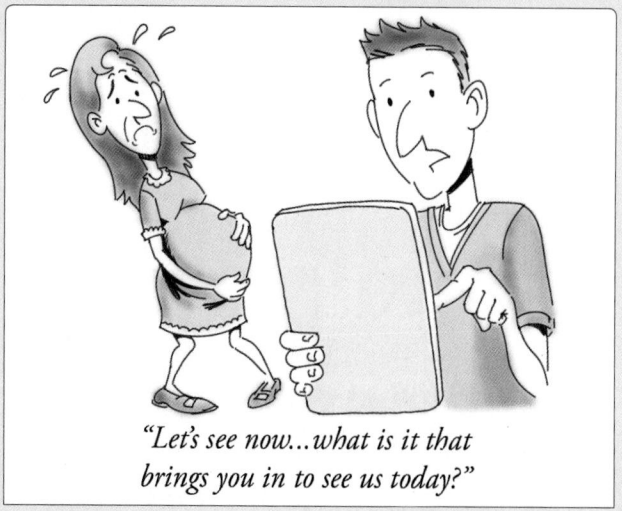

"Let's see now...what is it that brings you in to see us today?"

patients are heard accurately; (2) to listen for what is not being said or for information transmitted only by hints; and (3) to verify that the information was heard accurately.

Listed below are a series of questions for you to ask yourself, to serve as a professionalism checklist. As you interact with patients and colleagues, these questions will help to guide you in the professional behavior and therapeutic communication that is expected every day from medical assistants.

Ask Yourself

COMMUNICATION
- ☐ Do I apply active listening skills?
- ☐ Do I display professionalism through written and verbal communication?
- ☐ Do I demonstrate appropriate nonverbal communication?
- ☐ Do I speak at each patient's level of understanding?
- ☐ Do I display appropriate body language?
- ☐ Do I respond honestly and diplomatically to my patients' concerns?
- ☐ Do I refrain from sharing my personal experiences?
- ☐ Do I include the patient's support system as indicated?
- ☐ Does my knowledge allow me to speak easily with all members of the health care team?
- ☐ Do I accurately and concisely update the provider on any aspect of a patient's care?

PRESENTATION
- ☐ Am I courteous, patient, and respectful to patients?
- ☐ Do I display a positive attitude?
- ☐ Do I display a calm, professional, and caring manner?
- ☐ Do I demonstrate empathy to the patient?

COMPETENCY
- ☐ Do I pay attention to detail?
- ☐ Do I ask questions if I am out of my comfort zone or do not have the experience to carry out tasks?
- ☐ Do I display sound judgment?

INITIATIVE
- ☐ Do I show initiative?
- ☐ Have I developed a strategic plan to achieve my goals? Is my plan realistic?
- ☐ Am I flexible and dependable?
- ☐ Do I direct the patient to other resources when necessary or helpful, with the approval of the provider?
- ☐ Do I assist co-workers when appropriate?
- ☐ Do I make adaptations for patients with special needs?

INTEGRITY
- ☐ Do I demonstrate the principles of self-boundaries?
- ☐ Do I demonstrate respect for individual diversity?
- ☐ Do I demonstrate sensitivity to patient rights?
- ☐ Do I recognize the impact personal ethics and morals have on the delivery of health care?

Coping Skills for the Medical Assistant

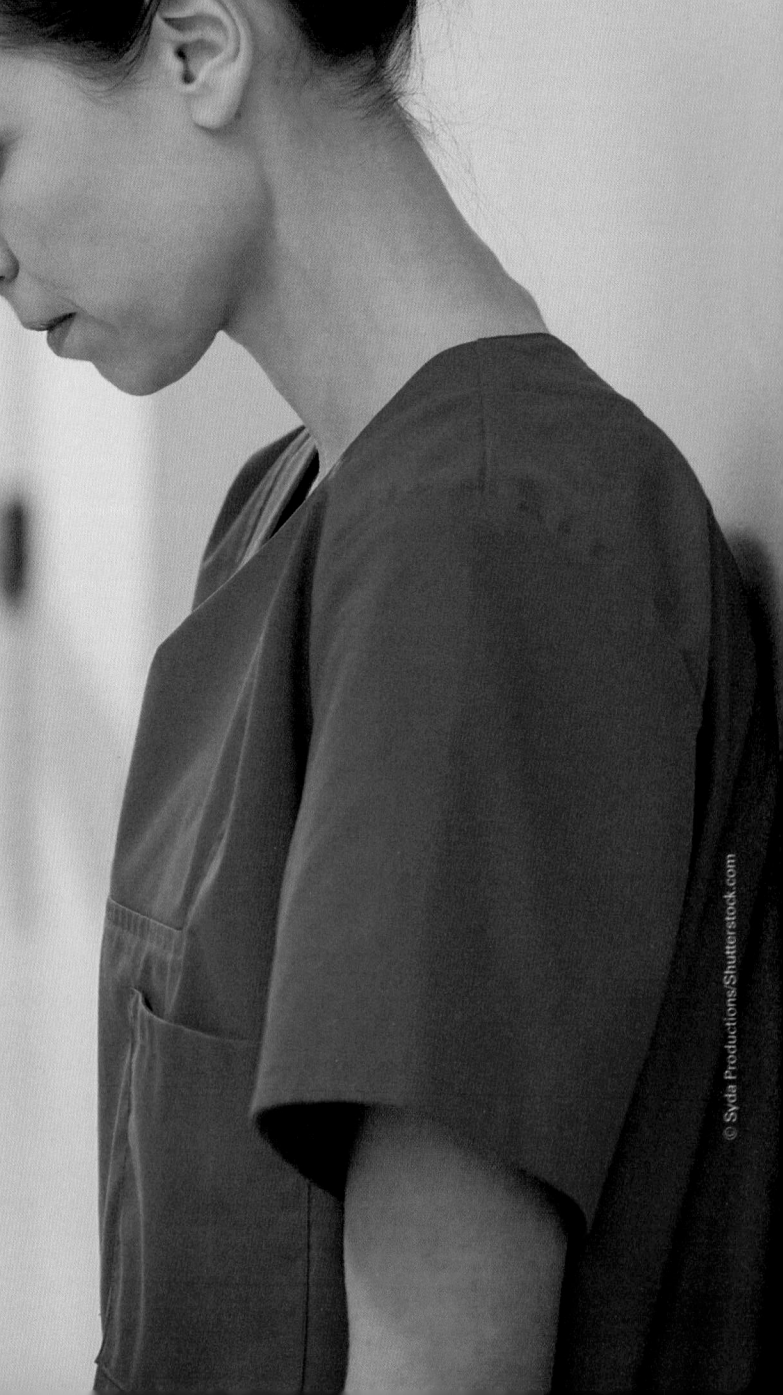

1. Define and spell the key terms as presented in the glossary.
2. Analyze the difference between stress and stressors.
3. Describe the three categories of stressors.
4. Discuss Hans Selye's General Adaptation Syndrome (GAS) theory.
5. Differentiate between short-duration and long-duration stress.
6. Analyze the body's response to stress as displayed by the sympathetic and parasympathetic nervous systems.
7. Summarize stress in the work environment and discuss ways to eliminate or cope with it.
8. Model ways a positive attitude may reduce the level and duration of stress.
9. Discuss physical illnesses and psychological symptoms of stress on the body.
10. Describe characteristics of prolonged stress.
11. Compare the four stages of burnout.
12. Identify persons most vulnerable to burnout.
13. Differentiate between long-range and short-range goals.

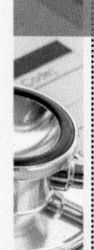

KEY TERMS

acute stress
burnout
chronic stress
episodic stress
goal

inner-directed people
long-range goals
outer-directed people
parasympathetic nervous
    system

self-actualization
short-range goals
stress
stressors
sympathetic nervous system

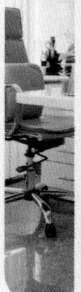

SCENARIO

At Inner City Health Care, there are four full-time medical assistants who collaborate to make the clinic run smoothly, both administratively and clinically. One day a month, though, clinic manager Marilyn Johnson, CMA (AAMA), is out of town, leaving Ellen Armstrong, CMAS (AMT), the administrative medical assistant, in charge of a busy reception area and an ever-ringing telephone.

On these days, Ellen pays close attention to details and is particularly careful to organize her work so that things run as they should. Implementation of time management principles helps ensure the clinic functions effectively. Although Ellen cannot anticipate every emergency, she does try to influence the situation rather than let events control her.

Chapter Portal

Even in the most well-managed ambulatory care setting, medical assistants and other health providers are likely to feel the effects of stress from time to time. They may be overworked on certain days, they may face difficult patient situations, and they may find that the administrative and paperwork load is getting ahead of them.

This chapter helps today's busy, multifaceted medical assistant pinpoint the symptoms of stress and provides ideas for coping with stress as it occurs. The better equipped the medical assistant is to confront and solve the sources of stress, the less likely stressors will become so overwhelming as to lead to burnout on the job. Goal setting, recognizing one's limitations and potentials, setting priorities, and keeping a balanced perspective can work together to reduce stress and enable the medical assistant to take pleasure in working with patients and colleagues.

WHAT IS STRESS?

The body's response to mental or emotional strain or tension is termed **stress**. Walter Cannon, a neurologist, is credited with first determining that both emotional and physical events act as **stressors** and that the body reacts in a similar way to either type of event. What constitutes stress is highly individual and depends to a great extent on personality type. Events that may be stressful to one person may be enjoyable to another. A delayed airplane flight may be very stressful to a person who worries about making another connection or missing a meeting. Another person will simply look for an alternative flight or notify the people that he was to meet and then take the time to enjoy a good book, experiencing little or no mental or physical change. The key is to learn how to manage stress so that it works for you rather than against you.

Adaptive behavior patterns we assume in response to real physical threats or emotional effects result in either eustress (positive feelings) or distress (negative feelings). Moving to a new city or receiving a promotion usually are perceived as positive events, whereas going through a divorce or losing a job are, conversely, perceived as negative events; however, each of these events can result in inducing stress in the body. These events are called stressors. Stressors can be divided into three categories:

1. *Frustrations.* Circumstances that prevent us from doing what we want to do
2. *Conflicts.* Incompatibility between two important things or objectives equally important to us
3. *Pressure.* Demands of schedule, workload, or expectations placed on us by ourselves or others

Complete the "How Stressed Are You????" exercise in Figure 3-1 to help assess your current stress level.

HOW STRESSED ARE YOU????

Answer each question with a 0, 1, 2, 3 or 4.

0 = never 1 = rarely 2 = sometimes 3 = often 4 = very often/always

Instructions for scoring follow the questions.

1. ____ My sleep is poor—delayed onset, wake early or not restful.
2. ____ I have headaches regularly (tension or migraine).
3. ____ I feel tense and anxious.
4. ____ I rarely have enough time to complete tasks.
5. ____ I experience frustration when trying to get things accomplished.
6. ____ I feel like escaping, I wish I were somewhere else.
7. ____ I feel like my schedule is controlled by outside factors or other people.
8. ____ I feel angry even for no reason.
9. ____ I feel overwhelmed by things that shouldn't be that hard.
10. ____ I eat more sugar and junk food than I want.
11. ____ I am not happy with the way I look.
12. ____ I have digestive difficulties (gas, cramping, irregularity).
13. ____ I feel like I want to cry, I am tearful more often than normal.
14. ____ I can't concentrate.
15. ____ I have constant colds/flu/infections.
16. ____ I feel isolated even when around others.
17. ____ I am forgetful, even important things slip my mind.
18. ____ I have pain in more than one place in my body.
19. ____ I feel irritable.
20. ____ I am unorganized and lose things.
21. ____ I have cold hands and/or feet.
22. ____ I am late for appointments or meetings.
23. ____ I have moist or sweaty hands.
24. ____ I talk rapidly.
25. ____ My heart pounds in my chest.

Scoring

Add all your points together. You can have a total of 100 points.

The higher the score, the greater your stress response.

Keep in mind that your symptoms may not be just stress related—it is important to see your doctor if you are not feeling well!

0–25: low	37–50: moderate-high	+ 65: VERY HIGH
26–36: low-moderate	50–65: high	

John Jordy, The Stress Clinic, LLC

FIGURE 3-1   Determining how well you handle stress will help identify personal strengths and weaknesses and point you toward the skills needed to be a successful health care professional. Complete the stress self-test.

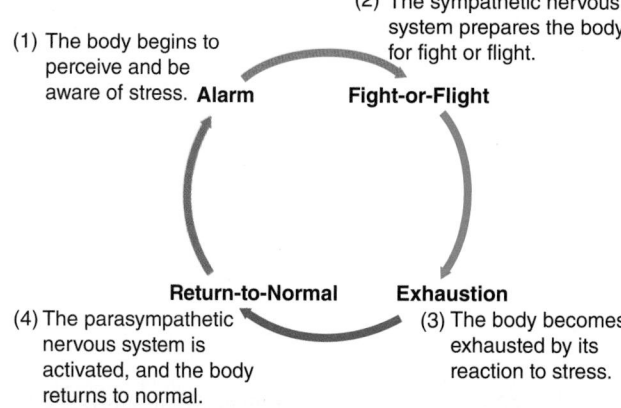

(1) The body begins to perceive and be aware of stress. **Alarm**

(2) The sympathetic nervous system prepares the body for fight or flight.

Fight-or-Flight

Return-to-Normal

(4) The parasympathetic nervous system is activated, and the body returns to normal.

Exhaustion

(3) The body becomes exhausted by its reaction to stress.

FIGURE 3-2 Hans Selye's General Adaptation Syndrome (GAS) theory proposes that four stages are involved in adapting to stress.

According to Hans Selye, who first conceived the theory of nonspecific reaction as stress, which is the body's response to any demand or stressor, the body does not differentiate between positively and negatively induced stress. It is only the level of the stress and its duration that affect the body. See Figure 3-2 illustrating Hans Selye's General Adaptation Syndrome cycle.

Types of Stress

Short-duration stress, sometimes termed **acute stress**, can be beneficial. Acute stress adds anticipation and a feeling of "being alive." For example, when we experience bungee jumping from a cliff, we experience acute stress. The short-lived adrenaline rush brings the world into sharper focus and enhances our lives. It helps us focus on details, achieve difficult goals, and perform at our best.

Competency When we have a last-minute rush in the clinic or are hurrying to get an assignment finished for school, we are experiencing short-duration stress. Short-duration stress is experienced when the telephone rings, the examination rooms are full, and the provider is called to the hospital for an emergency. Immediately, the body's stress mode is activated and adrenaline is produced, enabling you to make quick judgments and decisions, to be organized and efficient, and to accomplish tasks within minimal time limits. Recovery from acute stress occurs when the stress has been dealt with.

Acute stress that is experienced frequently or lasts longer in duration is termed **episodic stress**. Examples of episodic stress include taking on too many projects and placing unrealistic demands on

one's self, and then worrying needlessly. Individuals who are very competitive and demanding or referred to as "Type A" personalities may experience episodic stress. Episodic stress ceases from time to time or once the stress has been managed.

Chronic stress is an unhealthy form of stress. Often chronic stress is the result of events over which we have little control, such as long-term unemployment, dysfunctional relationships, or chronic illness. Long-duration stress that results from chronic stress can be life-threatening, leading the person to resort to violence, self-harm, or even suicide.

The Body's Response to Stress

The body's response to stress helps humans survive whatever fearful crisis they experience. The **sympathetic nervous system** prepares the body for "fight or flight" by signaling specific body systems.

Short term, these responses are not harmful, and the body's **parasympathetic nervous system** returns the body to normal after the stressor has been removed. Long-duration stress, over an extended period of time, can have harmful, even life-threatening results. For more information, see the "How Body Systems React to Stress" Quick Reference Guide.

Clinical responses to stress include emotional, physical, behavioral, and cognitive signs and symptoms, as described in Table 3-1. The more signs

TABLE 3-1

CLINICAL RESPONSES TO STRESS

CLINICAL RESPONSE	SIGNS AND SYMPTOMS
Emotional	Anxiety, worry, guilt, nervousness, anger, frustration, hostility, feeling overwhelmed, loneliness, isolation, mood swings, depression
Physical	Aches, pains, muscle spasms, dizziness, light-headedness, feeling faint, nausea, diarrhea, constipation, difficulty breathing, chest pain, palpitations, rapid pulse, belching, flatulence
Behavioral	Increased or decreased appetite, sleep disorders (insomnia, nightmares), nervous habits (fidgeting, feet tapping, nail biting, pacing, procrastinating or neglecting responsibilities), lies or excuses to cover up poor work
Cognitive	Difficulty concentrating, racing thoughts, forgetfulness, disorganization, confusion, difficulty making decisions or making poor judgments, decreased interest in appearance and punctuality

Body System	Fight-or-Flight Response	Response to Long-Duration Stress	Organ(s)
Nervous	Brain signals adrenal glands to release adrenaline and cortisol. This causes heart to beat faster, increasing blood pressure.	Depression, anxiety, stroke, degenerative neurological disorders such as Parkinson disease	Brain
Musculoskeletal	Large muscles and heart muscles dilate to increase blood flow.	Tension headaches, migraines, various musculoskeletal conditions	Muscles
Respiratory	Increased respiration rate supplies plenty of oxygen to the body.	Hyperventilation, panic attacks	Lungs
Cardiovascular	Increased heart rate and stronger contractions increase blood flow.	Inflammation in the coronary arteries, which may lead to heart attacks	Heart
Endocrine	Hypothalamus causes adrenal cortex to produce cortisol, and the adrenal medulla to produce epinephrine. The liver produces more glucose to provide increased energy.	Increased blood pressure and heart rate, increased glucose from glycogen in the liver, increased fatty acid in the blood, and decreased activity in the gastrointestinal (GI) tract	Glands
Gastrointestinal	Changes here increase glucose levels in the bloodstream.	Eating disorders, heartburn, acid reflux, butterflies, nausea or pain in stomach; diarrhea or constipation	Intestinal Tract

(continues)

Body System	Fight-or-Flight Response	Response to Long-Duration Stress	Organ(s)
Reproductive	Changes here may lead to reproductive dysfunction.	Males may experience impaired testosterone and sperm production, or impotence. Females may experience irregular menstrual cycles or painful periods, reduced sexual desire.	Male Female

and symptoms you notice, the closer you may be to stress overload. It is important to remember that many of these signs and symptoms can also be indicators of other psychological or medical problems.

FACTORS CAUSING STRESS IN THE WORK ENVIRONMENT

Stress in the work environment may come from many different sources, some of which you may control by making a few adjustments to resolve the stress. Conditions that cannot be changed may need to be accepted as a part of the job. Examples of work environment conditions that may cause stress include the following, but are not limited to these mentioned.

Overwhelming Situations

Initiative

Inability to control expectations, workload, and duties; feelings of frustration; and panic because of schedules can all result in feelings of powerlessness and not knowing where to start. Planning and prioritization can help to prevent panic and reduce stress when faced with the inevitable situation of too much work and too little time. A job that looks impossible can be broken down into elements that are manageable. Prioritization of the smaller elements and proceeding without wasting any time procrastinating usually results in getting the job finished in the allotted time, or at least with a minimum amount of stress. Requesting that you have a written job description can control powerlessness. You will then know your duties and responsibilities, and you will not experience sudden change when you least expect it. A job description will also help to avoid some of the instability resulting from a manager who is too sanguine (laid back) or manages from one crisis to another. If you know what your job entails, you can anticipate the events and take action to prevent a crisis.

Round Peg in Square Hole

Competency

Being a round peg in a square hole means not being emotionally suited or qualified for the position you hold. The only solution for this situation is changing jobs or obtaining training to become qualified for the requirements of the present job. Medical assistants can find themselves in emotional distress if a provider asks them to do tasks that they are not allowed to perform under the scope of their education and training. An example of this could be a medical assistant working for a provider who does outpatient surgery and expects the medical assistant to suture the incision after he or she has completed the major part of the procedure.

Traumatic Events on the Job

You may not be emotionally prepared for trauma involved in the job. Not every medical assistant can handle assisting with surgery or performing invasive procedures. A medical assistant finding himself or herself in this position could be proactive and seek a move from clinical to administrative duties or take steps to obtain another position having fewer traumatic events.

Physical Environment

Physical conditions such as noise, lighting, or some other types of stressors are frequently within the control of the worker. Additional lighting could be added or light shields could be used as suits the situation, and dressing in layers to accommodate temperature changes could mitigate the "too cold" stressor. The main point is not to sit back and become upset about situations over which you have some control. Take proactive steps to alleviate the stress-causing condition.

Management Style

Your manager's management style may cause uproar or instability in work demands. Talking to the manager might affect the situation, but it is highly unlikely. Obtaining a detailed job description; being able to say "no"; and utilizing goal-setting techniques, as discussed later in this chapter, are the best ways to reduce stress from this cause.

Difficult Coworkers

Integrity

Difficult people are all around us; in fact, you may be one to someone else. Maintaining a good interpersonal relationship with fellow employees is important to achieving a satisfying work experience and has a remarkable effect in reducing the problem of difficult people. Before a strong interpersonal relationship is established with others, a positive self-attitude is needed. The choices we make affect our positive attitude. Making positive decisions will affect the work environment, and hence the level and duration of stress experienced. Following are some choices we all make in our lives:

- To be respectful of others
- To be a diligent worker
- To be willing to learn

- To be honest
- To be willing to assume responsibility for one's actions
- To express appropriate humor
- To have an attitude of humility
- To be goal directed
- To understand Maslow's hierarchy of needs (see Chapter 4 for information related to Maslow's hierarchy of needs)

If you do all these things and still have difficult people in your work environment, develop a plan and take steps to have the least contact possible with those people. Taking proactive steps will in itself reduce stress.

Failure to Meet Needs

Certain job conditions do not permit achievement of Maslow's needs. Failure to meet our needs results in frustration, lack of job satisfaction, and ultimately burnout. Failure to meet needs can result from low salary, little opportunity for career growth, and discrimination in opportunities available and perceived distribution of assignments.

Job Instability

Job instability is an example of a stressor capable of causing worry. Worry is excessive concern about situations over which we have no direct control. Ensuring job stability is not directly within the medical assistant's control, but the medical assistant can be proactive in developing an employment plan and working toward its implementation. Taking these proactive steps to alleviate a potentially difficult situation over which you have no direct control will reduce worry and stress.

Technological Changes

Competency

Change, even good change, can cause stress. Implementation of a practice management (PM) system (see Chapter 10) into a medical facility is an excellent example of an event that will result in stress for almost all employees; they are divorcing themselves from the familiar and being asked to embrace the unknown. The resulting level and duration of stress would be dependent on the comfort level of each individual with computer technology. For some older employees it may create stress until they retire. The best way to avoid stress from technological change is to remain current with the tools of your profession through continued education programs.

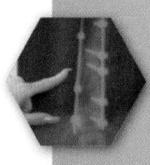

Critical Thinking

Practice in Time Management Analysis
List all of the tasks you do in a typical day. Beside each task write down how many minutes/hours you spend on each task. At the conclusion of the exercise, draw a histogram showing the percentage of each day spent on each task. This will quickly show where you spend most of your time. How could you save time? Develop a plan to reduce time spent in nonproductive, inessential activities.

Organization Size

Working in a large organization may lead to less understanding of the total job picture by the worker, resulting in less predictability and less control of the job to which the employee is assigned. This frequently results in feeling overwhelmed and frustrated. As the formalization and centralization of an organization increase, the stress experienced by an employee also increases. Downward delegation by management is the best approach to minimizing this problem.

Overspecialization

Overspecialization represents a limited practice exposure that isolates the employee from seeing the big picture and patient outcomes. This results in the employee receiving little or no satisfaction from his or her work, causing boredom, dissatisfaction and frustration.

WAYS TO REDUCE STRESS

Internal factors that influence your ability to handle stress include your nutritional status, overall health and fitness, and emotional well-being. There are numerous methods of reducing stress. A beginning place might be to review your diet and eating habits. Nutritious meals and snacks can boost the immune system, making it easier to cope with stress. Reducing the amount of caffeine and sugar in your diet has many health benefits. Alcohol, smoking, and drugs should be avoided.

Start an exercise regime. Exercising on a regular basis helps reduce the production of stress hormones and associated neurochemicals. Studies have found that exercise is a potent antidepressant, combats anxiety, and serves as a sleeping aid for many people. The amount of sleep and rest you get can determine your body's ability to respond to, and deal with, external stress-inducing factors. Sleep relaxes and refreshes the body and promotes clear thinking. Relaxation techniques such as meditation, yoga, deep breathing, aromatherapy and music are great stress relievers as well.

Goal Setting as a Stress Reliever

Do you direct your life, or do you allow others to influence and make decisions for you? **Outer-directed people** let events, other people, or environmental factors dictate their behavior. By contrast, **inner-directed people** decide for themselves what they want to do with their lives.

Studies prove that goal-oriented employees are more effective and assertive than are colleagues with no goals or future objectives. Recognizing the value of goal planning, many employers arrange planning sessions or seminars to encourage goal setting as a practical application for coping with stress and burnout and to develop career objectives. If your employer does not offer these outlets, seek your own seminars for goal setting. Such an activity not only "centers" you in your current employment, but also helps you clearly picture your future plans and hopes.

What is a **goal**? According to *Merriam-Webster's Collegiate Dictionary*, a goal is "the result or achievement toward which effort is directed." To reach a desired goal, a person must implement planning supported by a sincere desire to work hard. Skill in goal setting allows the medical assistant to clarify what must be accomplished and to develop a strategic plan to successfully achieve that goal.

A goal must be specific, challenging, realistic, attainable, and measurable. Specific goals are focused and have precise boundaries. A goal that is challenging creates enthusiasm and interest in achievement. Realistic goals are practical and beneficial both for the present and for future **self-actualization**, or fulfilling one's ultimate potential. An attainable goal refers to the fact that the goal is possible to fulfill. Measurable goals achieve some form of progress or success. By reflecting on the process, one is encouraged to establish additional goals.

Long-range goals are achievements that may take three to five years to accomplish. Long-range goals give direction and definition to our lives and serve to keep us "on track," so to speak. Much discipline, perseverance, determination, and hard work will be expended in accomplishing long-range goals. Some adjustment and readjustment to your goals may be necessary, however. The rewards of goal achievement include satisfaction, pride, a sense of accomplishment, and a job well done.

Short-range goals take apart long-range goals and reassemble the required activities into smaller, more manageable time segments. The time segments may be daily, weekly, monthly, quarterly, or yearly periods. Successfully completing a short-range goal encourages you to go on to the next goal and promotes a sense of achievement.

As a graduate and new employee, one of your long-range goals might be to become the clinic manager in the ambulatory care setting in which you are currently employed. You may wish to attain this goal within the next three to five years; by breaking it into three longer range goals and a series of short-range goals, you will be able to measure progress and feel a sense of accomplishment. Examples of long- and short-range goals might include:

Long-range goal 1:

- To become proficient in all clinical skills during the first year of employment.

Short-range goals necessary to achieve this:

- Practice accuracy and proficiency when performing tasks and skills.
- Practice efficiency by planning ahead for the equipment and supplies needed for each task performed.
- Evaluate your progress on a regular basis, and identify areas that need improvement.

Long-range goal 2:

- To add administrative tasks and skills to your routine during the second year of employment.

Short-range goals necessary to achieve this:

- Practice accuracy and proficiency when performing all administrative tasks and skills.
- Practice efficiency by planning ahead for the equipment and supplies needed for each task performed.
- Evaluate your progress on a regular basis, and identify areas that need improvement.

Long-range goal 3:

- To begin to focus on clinic management during the third year of employment.

Short-range goals necessary to achieve this:

- Develop a procedure manual for all clinical and administrative tasks and skills.
- Enroll in clinic management classes.
- Focus on team-building skills.

By the fourth year, you will be ready to move into the clinic manager position.

Long- and short-range goals work together to help make changes in our lives. Goals keep life interesting and give us something for which to strive. We can all reach goals successfully with some planning, hard work, discipline, and dedication.

EFFECT OF PROLONGED STRESS—BURNOUT

Burnout is a psychological term for the experience of long-term emotional, mental, and physical exhaustion accompanied by a diminished interest and motivation that affects job performance, health-related outcomes, and mental health issues. Burnout has four stages:

- *Honeymoon.* Love your job and have unrealistic expectations placed on you either by your manager or by yourself if you are a perfectionist; take work home and look for all the work you can get; cannot say "no" to accepting additional work.
- *Reality.* Begin to have doubts you can meet expectations; feel frustrated with your progress and work harder to meet expectations; begin to feel pulled in many directions; may not have a role model to follow and guidelines may not be established or defined.
- *Dissatisfaction.* Loss of enthusiasm; try to escape frustrations by binges of one sort or another: drinking, partying, shopping, or excessive eating or sexual activity; fatigue and exhaustion develop.
- *Sad state.* Depression, work seems pointless, lethargic with little energy, consider quitting, and look on yourself as a failure; represents full-blown burnout.

All of these stages are part of the process leading to burnout. The honeymoon stage might seem desirable, and it is pleasant; however, the seeds of the illness are present in the unrealistic expectations and the workaholic attitude of the employee. Unless these causes are eliminated, the progression to full burnout is ensured.

Burnout results in physical illnesses such as headaches, insomnia, allergies, cancer, acute indigestion, stomach ulcers, hypertension, blood clots, stroke, and immune system disorders. Psychologically, the body also is influenced by long-duration stress. Onsets of depression and anxiety, as well as eating problems resulting in weight loss or gain, are associated with the body's psychological response to stress. Anorexia and bulimia are common eating disorders attributed to long-duration stressful events. Long-duration stress can also affect our ability to think clearly, and objectivity may be impaired. Animal studies strongly suggest that maternal stress can also affect a fetus in later life. Physical symptoms of these emotional effects include alcohol abuse, drug abuse, cigarette smoking, obesity, depression, and lack of interest in or excessive sexual activity. A person in danger of burnout may also experience loss of energy and make poor exercise and nutritional choices, leading to a further cycle of medical problems and a more serious burnout condition.

Persons Most Vulnerable to Burnout

People with inadequate social support networks who are poorly nourished, sleep deprived, or physically ill have a reduced capacity to handle the pressures and stressors of everyday life and consequently are at greater risk of burnout. Some stressors are particularly associated with certain age groups or life stages. Persons facing life transitions such as children, adolescents, working parents, and older adults are vulnerable simply because of the increased stress associated with these transitional changes.

Personality type can have a role in susceptibility to burnout. When individuals with a high need to achieve do not reach their goals, they are apt to feel angry and frustrated and become negative toward their job. Failing to recognize these signs as symptoms of burnout, they may throw themselves even more fully into work-related goals. Unless there is some type of revitalization outside of the workplace, burnout occurs. Perfectionists try to do everything equally well without setting priorities; thus fatigue and exhaustion associated with burnout begin to set in after time.

Tips to Avoid Burnout

If you are stressed, or recognize that you are in one of the stages of burnout, you have reached a turning point. It is imperative that you make some changes in your relationship with your job. The following changes are appropriate and helpful in stress management or once you have entered the burnout stage:

- Make a concerted effort to say "no" when asked to assume additional work. Job scope creep is a leading factor in burnout.
- If you have more work than you can realistically accomplish, either prioritize it with the approval of your superior or delegate it within the limits of your authority.

- Change your work-related environment by creating variations. Modify your work routine slightly, rearrange your workstation to make it more personal, or change the computer desktop picture or screensaver to something you find pleasant that generates positive emotions.
- Evaluate the negative feelings you have regarding your job and attempt to replace them with more positive thoughts (i.e., instead of thinking the glass is half empty, think of the glass as half full).
- Try to look on work as a "fun" experience and an adventure.
- Establish some long- and short-term realistic goals and write them down along with a plan to make them happen.
- Develop strong social support networks by promoting friendships with coworkers; with family; or in outside religious, fraternal, or professional organizations. Occasionally going to lunch together with coworkers to laugh a little will promote a strong clinic support network and may help with that difficult person in your clinic life. Embark on a program of relaxation and meditation to reduce stress. Relaxation reduces muscle tension resulting from stress and can be achieved in a few minutes. Meditation requires about 20 minutes each day. Meditation affects body processes such as heart rate, blood pressure, metabolic rate, and brain activity and helps to obtain a feeling of "well-being."

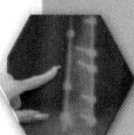

Critical Thinking

Self-Evaluation

- List several situations in your life that are stressful. Select the one that is most stressful.
- List as many things as possible about the situation that make it stressful to you.
- How would you change each of the things you have listed to make them less stressful?
- List the things you "could do" to effect the changes you listed.
- Rank the items in your "could do" list in terms of achievability.
- Select one or two of the items that are achievable and discuss them with a classmate. Now attempt to put them into practice for a week. Report back to your classmate on how effective these items were in reducing stress in your life.

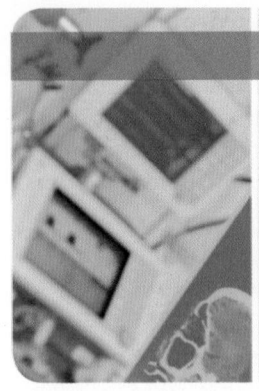

CASE STUDY 3-1

Refer to the scenario at the beginning of the chapter.

CASE STUDY REVIEW

1. What work can Ellen Armstrong, CMAS (AMT), organize the night before the clinic manager is out of town, leaving Ellen in charge of the reception area and the ever-ringing telephone the next day?
2. What professional skills should Ellen implement in this scenario?
3. How might Ellen relieve stress as the hectic day progresses?

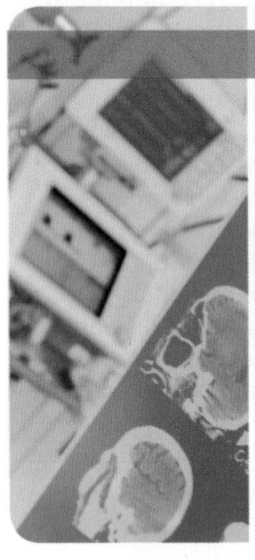

CASE STUDY 3-2

Ellen Armstrong, CMAS (AMT), has been employed for five years as an administrative medical assistant with Inner City Health Care. Ellen is a perfectionist and has pushed herself to achieve many of her short-and long-term goals. The clinic staff has become aware that Ellen does not have a sense of humor lately. She seems frustrated and irritable, and she is becoming critical of herself and others. Ellen has felt physically and emotionally exhausted, yet she continues to focus on her high standard of job performance; however, work is becoming a chore. At the end of the day, if everything has not been completed to her satisfaction, she feels like a failure.

CASE STUDY REVIEW

1. Do you think Ellen is stressed or experiencing burnout? On what do you base your conclusions?
2. What might Ellen do to differentiate these two conditions?
3. What changes might Ellen implement to resolve this problem?

Summary

- Stress is the body's response to mental and emotional strain or tension.
- Stressors are mental and emotional events that create stress and may be divided into three categories: frustrations, conflicts, and pressure.
- The four stages involved in adapting to stress according to the General Adaptation Syndrome cycle include alarm, fight-or-flight, exhaustion, and return-to-normal.
- Different kinds of stress include acute, episodic, and chronic stress.
- The sympathetic nervous system prepares the body for fight-or-flight. The parasympathetic nervous system returns the body to normal function. Long-duration stress can lead to harmful effects on the body, even life-threatening conditions.
- Clinical responses to stress include emotional, physical, behavioral, and cognitive signs and symptoms. The more signs and symptoms you notice, the closer you may be to stress overload. It is important to remember that many of these signs and symptoms can also be indicators of other psychological or medical problems.
- Stress in the work environment comes from many contributing factors, such as the physical environment, management style, difficult workers, failure to meet needs, job instability, technological changes, organization size, and overspecialization.
- Ways to reduce stress include reviewing your diet and eating habits. Nutritious meals and snacks boost the immune system, making it easier to cope with stress. Reduce caffeine and sugar, and avoid alcohol, smoking, and drugs. Exercise on a regular basis to strengthen the body and build core muscles. Sleep relaxes and refreshes the body and

continues

Summary *continued*

promotes clear thinking. Relaxation techniques such as meditation, yoga, deep breathing, aromatherapy, and music are great stress relievers.

- The benefits of goal setting are satisfaction, pride, a sense of accomplishment, and a job well done. Successfully completing short-range goals encourages you to go on to the next goal and promotes a sense of achievement. Long- and short-range goals work together to help make changes in our lives. Goals keep life interesting and give us purpose and something for which to strive.

- The four stages of burnout are honeymoon, reality, dissatisfaction, and sad state.

- Tips to reduce burnout include making a concerted effort to say "no" when asked to assume additional work; evaluating the negative feelings you have regarding your job and attempting to replace them with more positive thoughts; trying to look on work as a "fun" experience and an adventure; establishing some long- and short-term realistic goals and writing them down along with a plan to make them happen; developing strong social support networks by promoting friendships with co-workers, family, or in outside religious, fraternal, or professional organizations; and embarking on a program of relaxation and meditation to reduce stress.

Study for Success

To reinforce your knowledge and skills of information presented in this chapter:

- Review the *Key Terms* and *Learning Outcomes*
- Consider the *Critical Thinking* features and *Case Studies* and discuss your conclusions
- Answer the questions in the *Certification Review*

CERTIFICATION REVIEW

1. Which answer is *not* true about stress?
   a. It does not occur suddenly.
   b. It has physical and emotional effects on the body.
   c. It may be positive or negative in its effects on the body.
   d. It is the body's response to change.

2. How many stages occur in Hans Selye's General Adaptation Syndrome theory?
   a. 2 stages
   b. 3 stages
   c. 4 stages
   d. 5 stages
   e. 6 stages

3. Which is *not* a stage in the General Adaptation Syndrome?
   a. Fight-or-flight
   b. Exhaustion
   c. Burnout
   d. Alarm

4. Which of the following signs and symptoms is *not* associated with burnout?
   a. Physical illnesses such as headaches and insomnia
   b. Psychological influences such as anxiety and depression
   c. Feelings of accomplishment and pride in work
   d. Ability to think clearly and objectively
   e. Loss of energy; poor exercise and nutritional choices

5. The four stages of prolonged stress–burnout include which of the following?
   a. Honeymoon, reality, dissatisfaction, sad state
   b. Honeymoon, frustrations, conflicts, pressures
   c. Honeymoon, reality, conflicts, pressures
   d. Honeymoon, dissatisfactions, frustrations, pressures

6. Which response is *not* true of long-range goals?
   a. They may take 3 to 5 years to accomplish.
   b. They are divided into a series of short-range goals.
   c. They don't involve too much hard work.
   d. They may need to be adjusted and readjusted.
   e. They give direction and keep us on track.

7. The GAS theory proposes which order for its stages?
   a. Fight-or-flight, alarm, exhaustion, return-to-normal
   b. Exhaustion, alarm, fight-or-flight, return-to-normal
   c. Exhaustion, fight-or-flight, alarm, return-to-normal
   d. Alarm, fight-or-flight, exhaustion, return-to-normal

8. Stressors can be divided into which three categories?
   a. Frustrations, conflicts, pressure
   b. Pressure, anxiety, depression
   c. Conflicts, resolution, burnout
   d. Frustrations, conflicts, burnout
   e. Depression, burnout, suicide
9. Which of the following is *not* considered a sign and symptom of burnout?
   a. Anger
   b. Frustration
   c. Negativity
   d. Self-actualization

10. Which of the following is *not* true of the sympathetic nervous system?
    a. Returns the body to normal after the stressor has been removed
    b. Prepares the body for fight-or-flight
    c. Signals adrenal glands to produce adrenalin and cortisol
    d. Releases hormones into the bloodstream
    e. Causes stronger contractions of the heart muscle

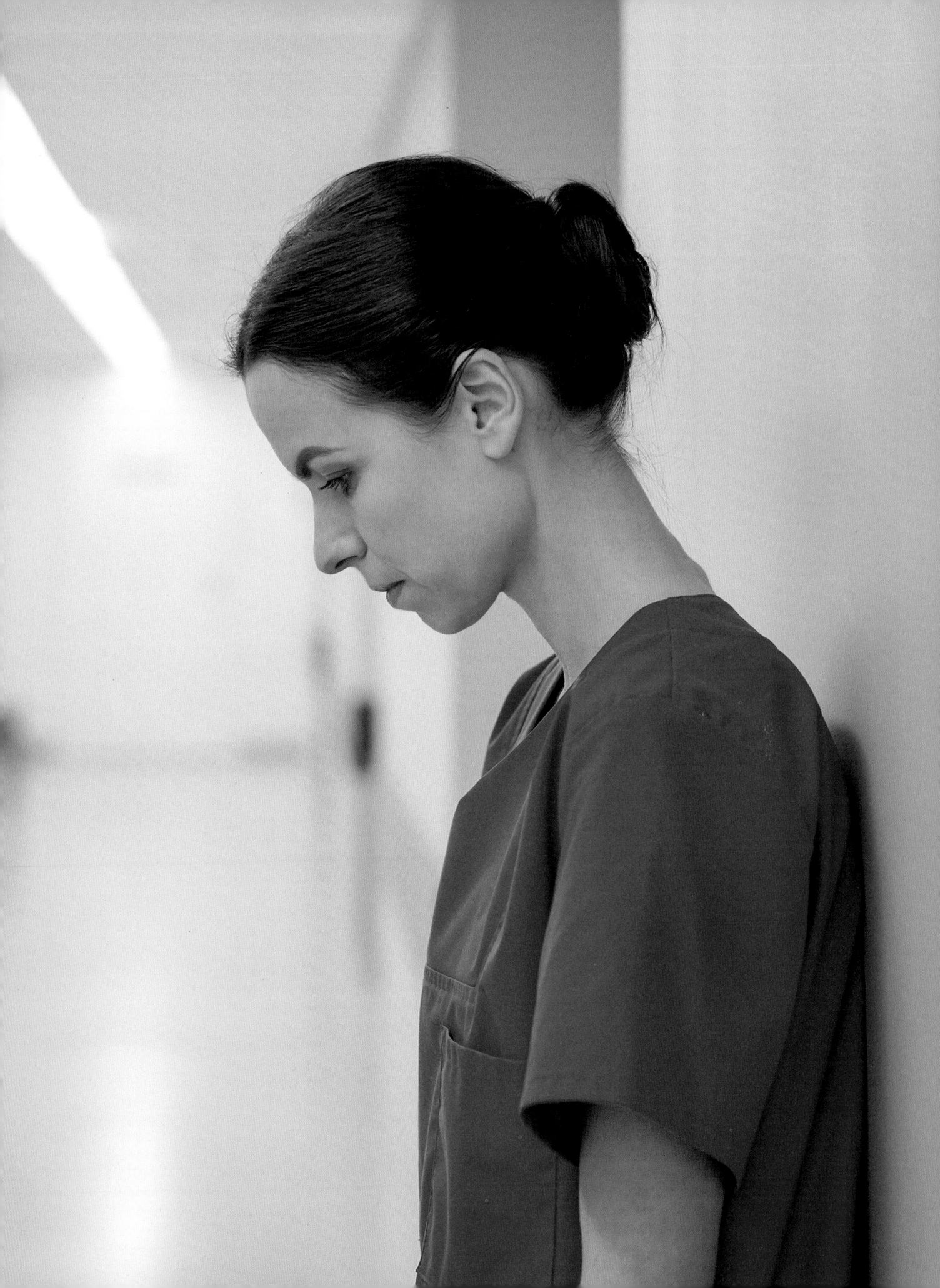

CHAPTER 4

Therapeutic Communication Skills

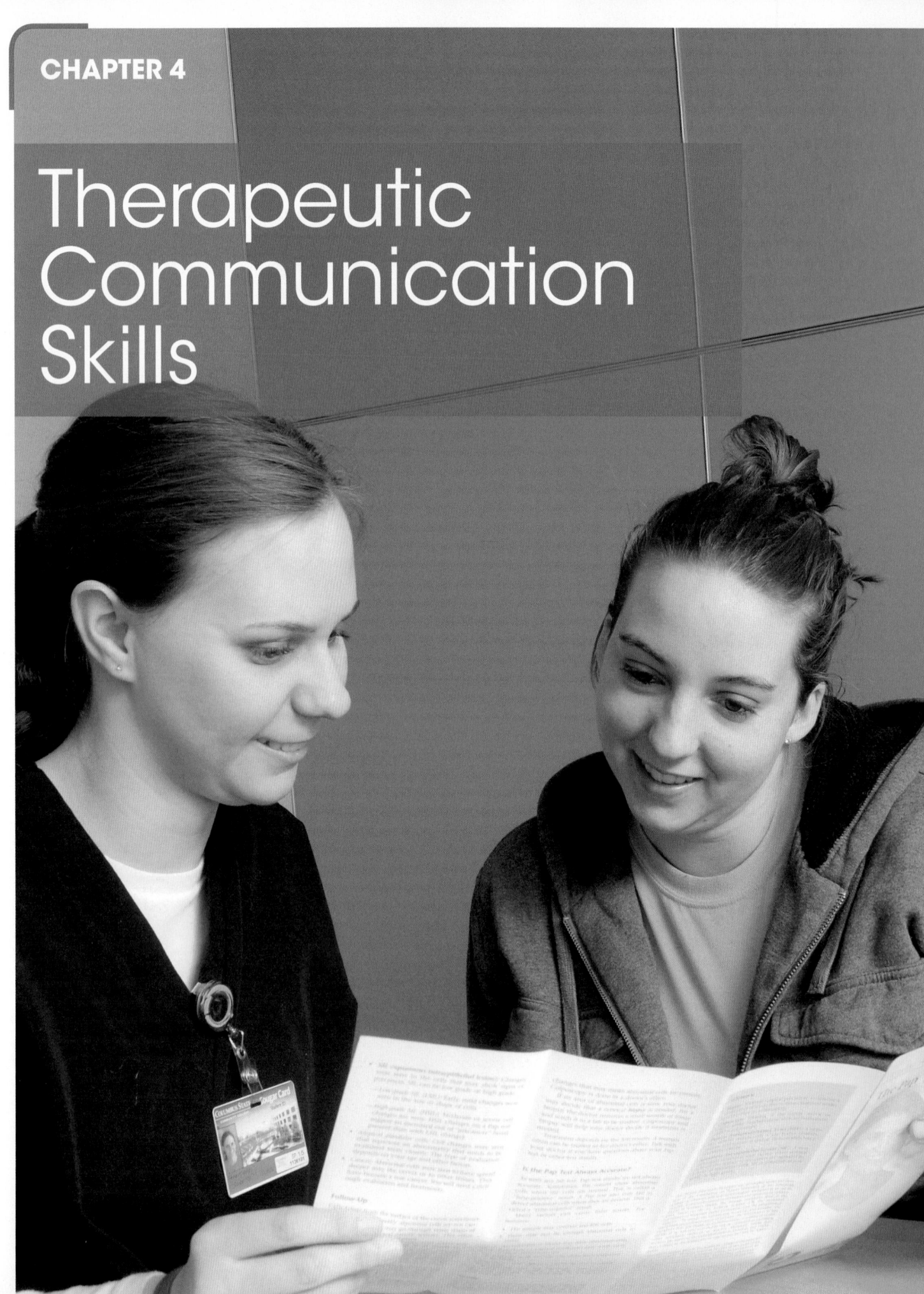

1. Define and spell the key terms as presented in the glossary.
2. Identify the importance of communication.
3. Describe the four basic elements of the communication cycle.
4. Explain the five modes or channels of communication most pertinent in our everyday exchanges.
5. Model the importance of active listening in therapeutic communication.
6. Recognize differences between the terms *verbal* and *nonverbal communication.*
7. Discuss the five Cs of communication and describe their effectiveness in the communication cycle.
8. Analyze the following body language or nonverbal communication behaviors: facial expressions, personal space, position, posture, gestures/mannerisms, and touch.
9. Explain congruency in communication.
10. Differentiate between low-context and high-context communication styles.
11. Discuss generalizations of cultural/religious effects on health care.
12. Summarize the use of Maslow's Hierarchy of Needs in therapeutic communication.
13. Recall at least three steps to building trust with culturally diverse patients.
14. Recognize eight significant roadblocks or barriers to therapeutic communication.
15. Analyze common defense mechanisms.
16. Contrast closed questions, open-ended questions, and indirect statements.
17. Differentiate between coaching and navigation in health care.

KEY TERMS

active listening	denial	prejudice
bias	displacement	projection
body language	encoding	rationalization
closed questions	Hierarchy of Needs	regression
clustering	high-context communication	repression
coach	indirect statements	roadblocks
compensation	kinesics	sublimation
congruency	low-context communication	suppression
culture	masking	therapeutic communication
decode	navigator	time focus
defense mechanisms	open-ended questions	undoing

SCENARIO

At Inner City Health Care, four medical assistants constantly interact with patients, allaying their concerns, scheduling their appointments, instructing them on medications, and helping them understand their insurance coverage. On this busy day, clinic manager Marilyn Johnson, CMA (AAMA), is arranging for a patient whom it has just been discovered needs an interpreter, wants to personally greet new patients Anna and Joseph Ortiz, but is also concerned about Ellen Armstrong, the administrative assistant who informed her this morning her brother is gravely

continues

ill in a neighboring state and she must take time off to be with him. Marilyn's warm manner and calm demeanor put everyone at ease.

Ellen is able to greet Martin Gordon, who has prostate cancer, and seems depressed and anxious. Setting aside their personal concerns, both Marilyn and Ellen try to create an environment where patients feel free to share their concerns and anxieties.

Ellen demonstrates therapeutic communication by acknowledging each patient as they arrive for appointments and puts them at ease by providing instructions. Medical assistants who project a warm and courteous presence while maintaining composure, even during difficult situations, and who ask the right questions in a nonthreatening manner will achieve therapeutic communication.

This scenario would be quite different if Marilyn were upset and angry that prior warning was not given of the need for an interpreter, she never has time to greet new patients to the practice, and Ellen is so upset by her brother's sudden illness that she accidently drops a call on hold and scowls at Martin Gordon and tells him to just take a seat.

Chapter Portal

Of all the tasks and skills required of the medical assistant in the ambulatory care setting, none is quite so important as communication. Communication is the foundation for every action taken by health care professionals in the care of their patients. Because medical assistants are often the liaison between patient and provider, it is critical to be aware of all the complexities of the communication process.

Every day, Marilyn, Ellen, and the two clinical medical assistants at Inner City Health Care face many communication challenges. This chapter describes effective communication principles, applies those principles to face-to-face communication, and describes the basic roadblocks to communication. The key word to all communication in the medical setting is therapeutic. In all conversations with patients, the more *therapeutic* the conversation, the more satisfied the patient will be with the care provided.

THERAPEUTIC COMMUNICATION DEFINED

Therapeutic communication differs from normal communication in that it introduces an element of empathy into what can be a traumatic or difficult experience for the patient. It imparts a feeling of comfort in the face of even the most frightening news about the patient's prognosis. The patient is made to feel validated and respected. Therapeutic communication uses specific and well-defined professional skills.

Therapeutic communication in the health care setting is the foundation of all patient care and is of the utmost importance. Communication must be in nontechnical language the patient can understand, delivered with feeling for the patient's emotional situation and state of mind, and yet it still must be technically accurate. The medical staff must be alert to the patient's state of stress and whether **defense mechanisms** have taken over to the extent that the patient has "tuned out" and is no longer communicating with the staff.

Patients seeking an ambulatory care service look for medical professionals with technical skills and a competent clinical staff capable of communicating with them. Questions frequently asked by individuals seeking a new provider and clinic include "Will the doctor talk with me so that I understand?" "Will the doctor listen to what I have to say?" and "Can I talk to the doctor honestly and openly?" The answer to all of these questions needs to be "yes."

THE COMMUNICATION CYCLE

All communication, whether social or therapeutic, involves two or more individuals participating in an exchange of information. The communication cycle involves sending and receiving messages even when not consciously aware of them.

Five basic elements are included in the communication cycle. They are (1) the sender, (2) the message, (3) the channel or mode of communication, (4) the receiver, and (5) feedback (Figure 4-1).

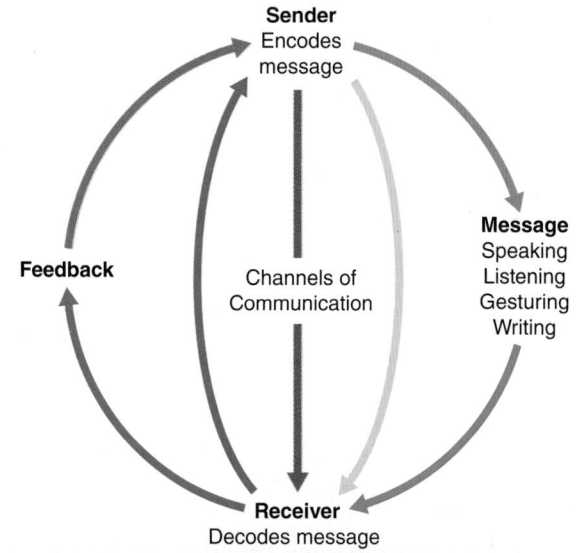

FIGURE 4-1 The communication cycle and modes or channels of communication.

The Sender

The sender begins the communication cycle by **encoding** or creating the message to be sent. Before creating the message, the sender must observe the receiver to determine as much as possible the complexity of the words to be used within the message, the receiver's ability to interpret the message, and the best channel by which to send the message. Encoding is an important step, and much care should be taken in formulating the message.

The Message

The message is the content being communicated. The message must be understood clearly by the receiver. Various levels of complexity in communication are used depending on the ability of the receiver to recognize and understand the words contained within the message. Children do not have the vocabulary base or the cognitive skills to communicate and understand at the same level as adults. Individuals with special needs will require special attention as well. The health of the receiver also must be considered. A patient who is distressed or is in pain may find it difficult to concentrate on the message. If the patient is of a different nationality or culture from the sender, verbal communication may require special skill. When visual or hearing acuity is impaired, this challenge must be surmounted.

The Channel or Mode of Communication

The three channels of communication, also called modes of communication, most pertinent in our everyday exchange are (1) speaking and listening, (2) gestures or body language, and (3) writing. These channels or modes are affected by our physical and mental development, our culture, our education and life experiences, our impressions from models and mentors, and how we feel about and accept ourselves as individuals. Each channel or mode of communication has its appropriate usage and must be considered when formulating the message.

The Receiver

The receiver is the recipient of the sender's message. The receiver must **decode**, or interpret, the meaning of the message. The primary sensory skill used in verbal communication is listening. It is hard work to concentrate and listen. When decoding the message, the receiver must be aware that not only the spoken word but the tone and pitch of the voice and the speed at which the words are spoken carry meaning and must be evaluated. Body language and how it is interpreted is a critical piece in face-to-face communication. The written word as a mode of communication (see Chapter 14) adds a dimension not realized in verbal communication—the ability to review the information or message being sent.

Feedback

Feedback takes place after the receiver has decoded the message sent by the sender. Feedback is the receiver's way of ensuring that the message that is understood is the same as the message that was sent. Feedback also provides an opportunity for the receiver to clarify any misunderstanding regarding the original message and to ask for additional information.

Listening Skills

A vital part of feedback in the communication cycle is listening. A good listener is alert to all aspects of the communication cycle—the verbal and nonverbal message, as well as verification of the message through appropriate feedback.

Active listening is one method used in therapeutic communication. In this technique, the received message is sent back to the sender, worded a little differently, for verification from the sender.

Sender: How can I possibly pay this fee when I have no insurance?

Receiver: You're worried about paying your bill?

The preceding example illustrates how the receiver is able to validate the sender's concerns at the same time the message is checked for accuracy. The door is then left open for a therapeutic response, such as:

Sender: Our bookkeeper will be glad to work out a payment plan with you that will fit your resources.

Active listening involves listening with a "third ear," that is, being aware of what the patient is *not* saying or picking up on hints to the real message by observing body language. The health care professional should have three listening goals:

- To improve listening skills sufficiently so that patients are heard accurately
- To listen either for what is *not* being said or for information transmitted only by hints
- To determine how accurately the message has been received

So many health professionals try to "fix" everything with a recommendation, a prescription, or even advice. Sometimes, none of those things is necessary. The patient simply needs someone to listen, to acknowledge the difficulty, and to remember that the patient is not helpless in finding a solution to the problem.

Skill in communication takes years of practice and frequent review. It will never become perfect; we can only hope that we will become better at it with each passing day.

VERBAL AND NONVERBAL COMMUNICATION

Communication

We communicate not only by what we say, but also by our tone of voice, body movements, and facial expressions. The following paragraphs present important aspects of verbal communication, the importance of listening skills, and nonverbal communication. The importance of maintaining consistency between verbal and nonverbal messages also is stressed.

Verbal Communication

Verbal communication takes place when the message is spoken. To be effective, it involves both speaking and listening. It is a two-way process. The purpose of verbal communication is to relay a message to one or more recipients. The majority of communication taking place in the health care community is verbal and has many purposes.

The Five Cs of Communication. Numerous authors, in and out of health care, have identified important pieces to communication. Some say there are seven components; others refer to six. For the purpose of this text, five components are identified. They are (1) complete, (2) clear, (3) concise, (4) coherent, and (5) courteous. These five Cs apply equally well in all health care professions.

Complete. The message must be complete, with all the necessary information given so that a patient is informed enough to take action. The medical assistant cannot expect the patient to be compliant if all the instructions are not given and understood.

Clear. The information given in the message must also be clear. Health care professionals must be able to articulate by using good diction and by enunciating each word distinctly. It is important to keep the ideas in the message to a minimum. The patient must be allowed time to process the message and verify its meaning. They should not have to read between the lines or make assumptions about the message.

Concise. A concise message is one that does not include any unnecessary information. It should be brief and to the point. Patients must not be overloaded with technical terms that may not be understood or that tend to distract them by diverting their attention away from the balance of the message.

Coherent. A coherent message is organized and logical in its progression. The coherent message does not ramble and does not jump from one subject to another. The patient should be able to follow the message easily. The medical assistant should always allow time to summarize detailed messages and use responding skills to verify that the patient fully understands the message.

Courteous. Courtesy is important in all aspects of communication. It takes only a moment to acknowledge a patient with a smile or by name. Be friendly, open, and respectful. There should be no hidden tones of disinterest. Remember to be courteous to colleagues in the clinic, also. Good working relationships and professionalism are always enhanced by simple courtesy.

When communicating within health care professions and to patients, keep in mind the following:

1. Good communication skills and following the five Cs are necessary in establishing rapport with co-workers and patients.

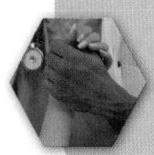
2. Patients feel respected and validated when called by their full name, such as Mary O'Keefe or Mrs. O'Keefe.

3. Patients should be encouraged to verbalize their concerns and to ask questions.

4. Patients should be given technical information (verbally and written) in a manner that they can understand.

5. Patients should have the opportunity to suggest and discuss any personal applications to their health care.

Nonverbal Communication

Verbal communication alone is not always adequate in conveying the message being sent. In most instances, more than one mode or channel of communication is used. Nonverbal communication, often referred to as **body language**, includes the unconscious body movements, gestures, and facial expressions that accompany speech. The study of body language is known as **kinesics**. Experts tell us that 70% of communication is nonverbal. The tone of voice communicates 23% of the message—only 7% of the message is actually communicated by the spoken word.

Nonverbal communication is the language we learn first. It is learned seemingly automatically when infants learn to return a smile or respond to touches on the cheek. Much of our body language is a learned behavior and is greatly influenced by the primary caregivers and the culture in which we are raised.

Feelings and emotions are communicated most often through nonverbal means. The body expresses its true repressed feelings using body language. Expressions and appearances communicate volumes of information. For instance, their appearance, attitude, and behavior sends messages about what health care professionals are thinking and feeling. Similarly, patients often convey their discomfort nonverbally before they verbalize a concern. Most of the negative messages we communicate are also expressed nonverbally and usually are unintentional (Figure 4-2).

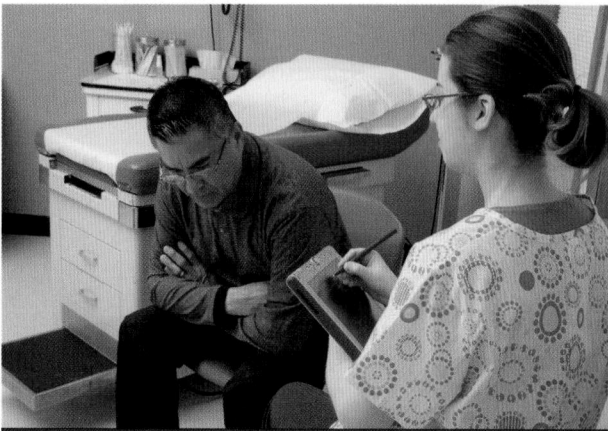

FIGURE 4-2 Body language can communicate more than spoken words.

Facial Expression. Facial expression is considered one of the most important observed nonverbal communicators. Each facet or aspect of the anatomy of the face sends a nonverbal message, most commonly through a smile or a frown.

Often expressions of joy and happiness or sorrow and grief are reflected through the eyes. The anatomy of the eyes does not change, but the movements of the structures surrounding the eyes enhance or magnify the message being communicated. Very brief or broken eye contact may express nervousness, shyness, or mistrust.

Children are told it is not polite to stare at people. It is acceptable to stare at animals in the zoo or art objects in the museum, but not at humans. Staring is dehumanizing and is often interpreted as an invasion of privacy.

The medical assistant must learn not to stare when patients present with ailments that make them "look" different. Patients such as these are individuals who have needs, who feel pain and discomfort, and who have decreased self-esteem and value. These feelings will only be amplified if the medical assistant and other health professionals are unable to "see" them as humans. A lack of eye contact may also be viewed as avoidance or disinterest in being involved.

The movements of the eyebrows indicate many nonverbal cues as well. Surprise, puzzlement, worry, amusement, and questioning are often nonverbal messages reflected by the position of the eyebrow. It may be difficult to "read" a patient's body language when they have lost their hair, even their eyebrows, during chemotherapy treatments. Wrinkling of the forehead sends similar messages.

Cultural influences affect customs and different forms of facial expressions. It is important to remember that there are many cross-cultural similarities in body language, but there are also many differences. For example, some cultures believe that prolonged eye contact is rude and an invasion of privacy, whereas others consider it a sign of intimacy. Some people stare at the floor when concentrating or thinking through a process. Other cultures avoid eye contact to display modesty, whereas others feel eye contact expresses hostility or aggression. It is important to understand the cultures of the patients treated in the facility in which you are employed.

Personal Space. Personal space is the distance at which we feel comfortable with others while communicating. In the classroom, for example, students claim their personal space the first day of class. The area is well defined by using books and papers, or by placing the arm, hand, or chair on boundary lines. When another invades the personal space, a shift in body position or the use of eye contact sends the message, "This is my area." Individuals may feel threatened when others invade their personal space without permission. Some examples of comfortable personal space for U.S. culture are as follows:

- Intimate: touching to 1½ feet
- Personal: 1½ to 4 feet
- Social: 4 to 12 feet (most often observed)
- Public: 12 to 15 feet

As with facial expressions, personal space is handled differently by various cultures. For example, there is no word for privacy in the Japanese language. Population numbers require crowding together publicly, as well as privately. Public crowding is often viewed as a sign of warmth and pleasant intimacy in Japan. In the private home, several generations may live together; however, each considers this space to be their own and resents intrusion into it.

Arabs like to touch their companions, to feel and to smell them. To deny a friend your breath is to be ashamed. When two Arabs talk to each other, they look each other in the eyes with great intensity. U.S. businessmen often end a business arrangement with a handshake; however, Native Americans view a handshake as an act of aggression or an offensive behavior. Each culture has its own distinct nonverbal communication cues.

It is beneficial to explain procedures that invade their space to patients before beginning the procedure so that it will not be perceived as threatening. This helps to empower the patient by involving the patient in the decision-making process and builds a sense of trust in the medical assistant.

Posture. Like personal space, posture is important to health care professionals. Posture relates to the position of the body or parts of the body. It is the manner in which we carry ourselves, or pose in situations. We tend to tighten up in threatening or unknown situations and to relax in nonthreatening environments. Those who study kinesics believe that a posture involves at least half the body, and that the position can last for nearly five minutes.

When the patient is seated with the arms and legs crossed, the message of closure or being opinionated may be relayed. In contrast, sitting in a chair relaxed with the hands clasped behind the head indicates an attitude of being open to suggestions. Slumped shoulders may signal depression, discouragement, or, in some cases, even pain.

Position. Position, the physical stance of two individuals while communicating, is a key factor to consider while communicating with the patient. Most provider–patient relationships use the face-to-face communication arrangement. When speaking with a patient, the provider or medical assistant will want to maintain a close but comfortable position, enabling observation of all cues being sent, both verbal and nonverbal (Figure 4-3).

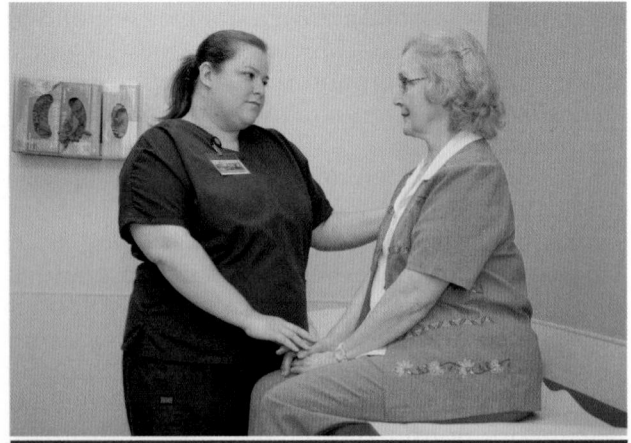

FIGURE 4-3 Positive posture and position encourage therapeutic communication.

Standing over a patient can convey a message of superiority, and too much distance between the two parties may be interpreted as avoidance or exclusivity. Generally, leaning toward the patient expresses warmth, caring, interest, acceptance, and trust. Moving away from the patient may be interpreted as dislike, disinterest, boredom, indifference, suspicion, or impatience.

Whenever possible, it is best to have a chair in the examination room and to have the patient seated comfortably in the chair to begin the communication cycle. The medical assistant or provider can sit on a stool that can be moved easily toward the patient. This arrangement aids the patient in feeling valued, listened to, and cared for as a fellow human being.

Gestures and Mannerisms. Various cultures denote different meanings to various gestures. If your patient is from another culture, never assume that gestures used hold the same meaning for the patient as they do for you. Most of us use gestures and mannerisms when we "talk" with our hands. This form of body language may be useful in enhancing the spoken word by emphasizing ideas, thus creating and holding the attention of others. Some common gestures and their possible meanings are as follows:

Finger-tapping	Impatience, nervousness
Shrugged shoulders	Indifference, discouragement
Rubbing the nose	Puzzlement
Whitened knuckles and clenched fists	Anger
Fidgeting	Nervousness

Touch. The medical assistant may perform many invasive tasks during the course of a clinic visit. Examples include taking vital signs or giving injections, both of which require touching the patient. Touch is a powerful tool that communicates what cannot be expressed in words. Its appropriateness in the patient–health professional relationship has well-defined boundaries and requires the use of good judgment on the part of the professional. Infants who are not touched, cuddled, and loved do not grow and develop as do those who receive these reassuring gestures. Touch is personal and is linked closely to personal space.

Diversity

Understanding touch as it relates to various cultures must also be considered. For example, Vietnamese, Cambodian, Hmong, and Thai families traditionally consider the head to be the site of the soul. During conversation and patient assessment, avoid touching the patient's head unless it is necessary for the examination. Southeast Asian patients may fear bodily intrusion; therefore, physical examination and treatment procedures should be explained carefully and completely before they are performed. The touch that communicates caring, sincerity, understanding, and reassurance is usually welcomed and considered to be a therapeutic response. Most patients will understand and accept the touching behavior as it relates to the medical setting; however, we must remember that not all patients are comfortable with touch. Whenever the patient is not comfortable with touch, explain the procedure fully, ask permission, and create as safe and reassuring an environment as possible.

Congruency in Communication

There must be **congruency** between the verbal and nonverbal communication. For example, shaking your head "no" while saying "yes" verbally sends a mixed message. In most cases, the nonverbal messages will be accepted as the intended message.

It is also important to remember that most nonverbal messages are sent in groups of various forms of body language. The grouping of nonverbal messages into statements or conclusions is known as **clustering**. **Masking** involves an attempt to conceal or repress the true feeling or message. The perceptive professional will be aware of all these messages. Perception as it relates to communication is the conscious awareness of one's own feelings and the feelings of others. To be most useful and therapeutic as health professionals, we must first explore our own feelings and appreciate and accept ourselves.

Learning to use perception involves the ability to sense another's attitudes, moods, and feelings. It takes practice and experience to develop and use this skill effectively. Being attentive to other professionals and observing their use of perception will yield insight into its usefulness and provide an example to emulate. A word of caution—the use of perception may easily be misinterpreted, especially when going with your feeling or assessment of what is happening regarding the patient. Always follow perceived assessments with verbal validation before assuming your perception of the circumstance is correct.

Nonverbal communication is easily misinterpreted. Careful observation for congruency between verbal and nonverbal communication, and clustering nonverbal cues being sent into nonverbal statements will strengthen your ability to interpret the message accurately.

INFLUENCE OF TECHNOLOGY ON COMMUNICATION

There will always be face-to-face and telephone conversations in the medical clinic, but clinics are also establishing secure portals to permit their patients access to their medical records. This approach permits the patient to schedule and review appointments, view laboratory reports, renew prescriptions, and communicate with medical personnel.

Social media has also created a niche in health care. Currently, it is being used for education, networking, goal setting, and receiving support (for example, weight loss, diabetes monitoring, and tracking personal progress). Health care providers use Facebook, Twitter, and YouTube to connect with patients and share information related to health issues through blogging. The Internet can be used to search for information related to health issues and treatment options. The CDC uses the number of searches on medical conditions, such as the flu and communicable diseases, as an indicator for epidemic warnings.

In some cases, satellite video and teleconferencing are being used to share information, receive education and training, or conduct meetings that include participants from various locations. Robots make rounds in the hospital setting and electronically communicate information regarding a patient's health. The patient can also see the provider on the robot's monitor and voice their concerns. (See Chapter 10 for more information related to the virtual medical clinic.) The major downside to using technology to communicate in the medical setting is security issues. Another disadvantage of technology is minimized interpersonal interaction. Chapter 10 discusses ways to ensure security at various levels and also presents ways to help the patient feel valued and included during interpersonal interactions via electronic means.

FACTORS AFFECTING THERAPEUTIC COMMUNICATION

Anything that interferes with the patient's ability to focus has a negative impact on therapeutic communication. The following paragraphs discuss significant barriers. The medical assistant must recognize that until these barriers are dealt with or minimized, therapeutic communication will be significantly affected.

Age Barriers

Professional medical assistants must understand human growth and development and be able to adapt their communications appropriately to any age group. Many scientists and researchers have studied human growth and development and have proposed guidelines for communication with patients during each stage. Erik Erikson (1902–1994) taught that each stage or phase is part of a continuum throughout the life cycle. The "Stages of Human Growth and Development" Quick Reference Guide lists Erikson's stages of human growth and development and identifies communication problems and suggested actions to be taken during each stage.

Economic Barriers

The influence of economics may reveal discomfort if the clinic staff and patients have a different perception about how billing is managed and when and how payment is expected. A discussion of billing and payment procedures at the first clinic visit or before a major procedure will be beneficial to all concerned parties.

Educational and Life Experience Barriers

Educational and life experiences will, in part, determine how patients react to their care. Patients with family members being treated for a chronic illness will have more knowledge and understanding of that illness in their own lives. Individuals who have already suffered a great deal of loss and grief in their lives may handle the information of a life-threatening illness more calmly than someone who has experienced little grief.

Bias and Prejudice Barriers

Personal preferences, biases, and prejudices will enter into many provider–patient relationships. Such biases affect the types of communication possible.

For therapeutic communication to take place, biases must be examined, a person's comfort level with each bias should be determined, and measures need to be taken to ensure that a hostile attitude is not present. **Bias** is defined as a slant toward a particular belief. **Prejudice** is defined as an opinion or judgment that is formed before all the facts are known; prejudice is a preconceived and unfavorable concept of some other person or group.

>> QUICK REFERENCE GUIDE

>> STAGES OF HUMAN GROWTH AND DEVELOPMENT

	Age Group	Communication Problem	Action Taken
	Infant 0–1 years Trust versus Mistrust	Total dependence on others for life support	• Respond to social smiles • Provide warm, friendly atmosphere • Consider safety issues • Wear colorful uniform
	Toddler 2–3 years Initiative versus Guilt	Limited vocabulary, fear of encounter with medical staff, separation anxiety if separated from caregiver	• Use child's own vocabulary and rephrase • Encourage and praise • Use simple commands • Allow child some control by permitting ambulation • Establish consistent clinic visit routine • Display a cordial relationship with parent to promote trust by child
	Preschooler 3–6 years Initiative versus Guilt	Unable to comprehend abstract ideas, cannot tolerate direct eye contact, creative imagination, short attention span, seeks control	• All of the above as appropriate • Physical contact at child's eye level if possible • Role play therapy (for example, give pretend injection to stuffed toy) • Allow control by permitting child to make as many choices as possible (for example, say, "Would you like to be measured to see how tall you are or weighed first?")
	School Age 6–11 years Industry versus Inferiority	Developing ability to comprehend, taking some ownership of health care, concern for privacy	• Include child in explanation of treatment and protocols using child's vocabulary • Encourage and praise • Make health care a teaching opportunity • Respect privacy of child
	Adolescent 12–18 years Identity versus Role Confusion	Increased comprehension, capable of abstract thought, may be fiercely independent, may use colloquial language, sexually maturing, concerned about confidentiality	• Actively listen, using patient's own language idioms as much as possible • Use abstract thought, but be alert to lack of understanding • Reassure that confidentiality will be protected, but state limits • Recognize peer pressure • Be aware of body image impacts

(continues)

	Age Group	Communication Problem	Action Taken
	Early Adulthood 19–40 years Intimacy versus Isolation	Greater comprehension and abstract thought capability, usually more in touch with reality than adolescents	• All of the items listed for adolescent • Provide health care options • Describe benefits and expectations of good health care
	Middle Adulthood 40–65 years Generativity versus Stagnation	Established socioeconomically, thinks of charities, concerns for succeeding generation	• Listen • Validate • Provide health care choices when appropriate
	Late Adulthood 65 years to death Integrity versus Despair	Anxious and stressed, hearing or vision impaired, slow to respond to inquiries, prone to omitting facts, overemphasis on somatic concerns, fear or embarrassed by loss of physical control, fear of being alone at death	• Be in proximity to patient and gently touch as appropriate • Speak slowly and clearly • Pace the encounter to match patient's tolerance • Be gentle and truthful

Common biases and prejudices in today's society include:

1. A preference for Western-style medicine
2. Choosing providers according to gender
3. Prejudice related to a person's sexual preference
4. Discrimination based on race or religion
5. Hostile attitudes toward people with different value systems than one's own
6. A belief that people who cannot afford health care should receive less care than someone who can pay for full services

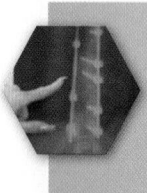

Critical Thinking

Define in your own words the terms *bias* and *prejudice*. Now identify one bias and one prejudice that you have. How will these impact your ability to respond therapeutically in the medical setting? What steps can you take to become more accepting of the uniqueness of others, thereby improving therapeutic communication?

Medical assistants must recognize such biases and prejudices so that their own culture with its biases does not prevent them from responding therapeutically in communications with all patients. Such recognition requires being aware of the differences among human beings and willingly accepting the uniqueness of each person.

ROADBLOCKS TO THERAPEUTIC COMMUNICATION

Being sensitive to patients' unique personalities and needs will enable the health care professional to avoid **roadblocks** to communication (see Table 4-1).

It must be the concern of each health care professional to facilitate communication by encouraging and enabling patients to express themselves honestly without fear. Roadblocks close therapeutic communication and prevent quality care of the total person.

Well-intentioned attempts to make the patient feel more comfortable can sometimes have negative effects on therapeutic communication. The following are some examples:

• Attempting to dispel the patient's anxiety by implying that there is not sufficient reason for it to exist is to completely devalue the

TABLE 4-1

ROADBLOCKS TO COMMUNICATION

ROADBLOCK	EXAMPLE
Reassuring clichés	"Don't worry about not having a job, Mr. McKay; you'll find another one really soon."
Moralizing/lecturing	"If you were smart, Mrs. Johnson, you'd lose 50 pounds and you wouldn't have such a problem with your diabetes and hypertension."
Requiring explanations	"Why would you not want to have chemotherapy, Mr. Gordon? Seeing your wife die of cancer should surely make you want to seek treatment."
Ridiculing/shaming	"Ha, ha, Mr. Gordon! It's not *prostrate* cancer—it's *prostate* cancer."
Defending/contradicting	"Mr. Marshal, I assure you the physician is *very busy.* He will not see you until he has finished with his other patients."
Shifting subjects	"Yes, Mrs. Jover, your work is very interesting, but I must ask you to sign this permission form to test for HIV."
Criticizing	"Mrs. O'Keefe, why in the world would you stay with an abusive husband?"
Threatening	"There is no way you will get rid of this cough if you do not stop smoking, Mr. Fowler."
Giving advice/approval	Often occurs when health care professional is doing more talking than listening or feels the need to control the patient's thoughts or actions. "If I were you…" or "You should…"
Stereotyping	A preconceived notion that all people are the same. Anytime you group races or individuals together and make a judgment about them without knowing them, you are stereotyping. Remarks about racial groups, sexual orientation, and gender are the most common stereotyping subjects.

patient's own feelings. Developing a sincere interpersonal relationship more readily helps the patient. The health care professional should remain neutral in regard to the patient's condition. He or she should remain empathetic, but nonjudgmental.

- Rejecting the patient's ideas or comments causes therapeutic interaction to cease and thwarts the patient's expression.

- Indicating accord with the patient by using statements such as "That's right" or "I agree" can result in the health care professional speaking for the patient and can sometimes unintentionally put the health care professional's conclusions in the patient's mind.

Defense Mechanisms as Barriers

Therapeutic communication becomes difficult if a patient is in a highly emotional state. A patient who is frightened, ashamed, guilty, or threatened often will resort to defense mechanisms as a means of avoiding injury to the ego. We all use defense mechanisms to some limited extent, but they become harmful when they result in a breakdown in therapeutic communication. Failure by the patient to face problems often results in inability to provide satisfactory treatment on the part of the health care professional. Recognizing common defense mechanisms enables the medical staff to minimize the triggering event and to communicate more effectively.

Defense mechanisms are defined as behaviors that are used to protect the ego from guilt, anxiety, or loss of esteem. Use of defense mechanisms is most often subconscious to the person using them. It is the body's way of seeking relief from uncomfortable or painful reality. A mentally healthy person uses defense mechanisms to put a problem on hold until sufficient time has passed to permit him or her to address it without unacceptable emotional pain. Excessive use of defense mechanisms or failure to address a problem even after sufficient time has elapsed may be a sign of mental health issues.

Defense mechanisms are usually readily apparent to the disaffected observer; however, they are difficult to analyze without knowledge of the motive behind the behavior. Study each defense mechanism presented in the "Defense Mechanisms" Quick Reference Guide.

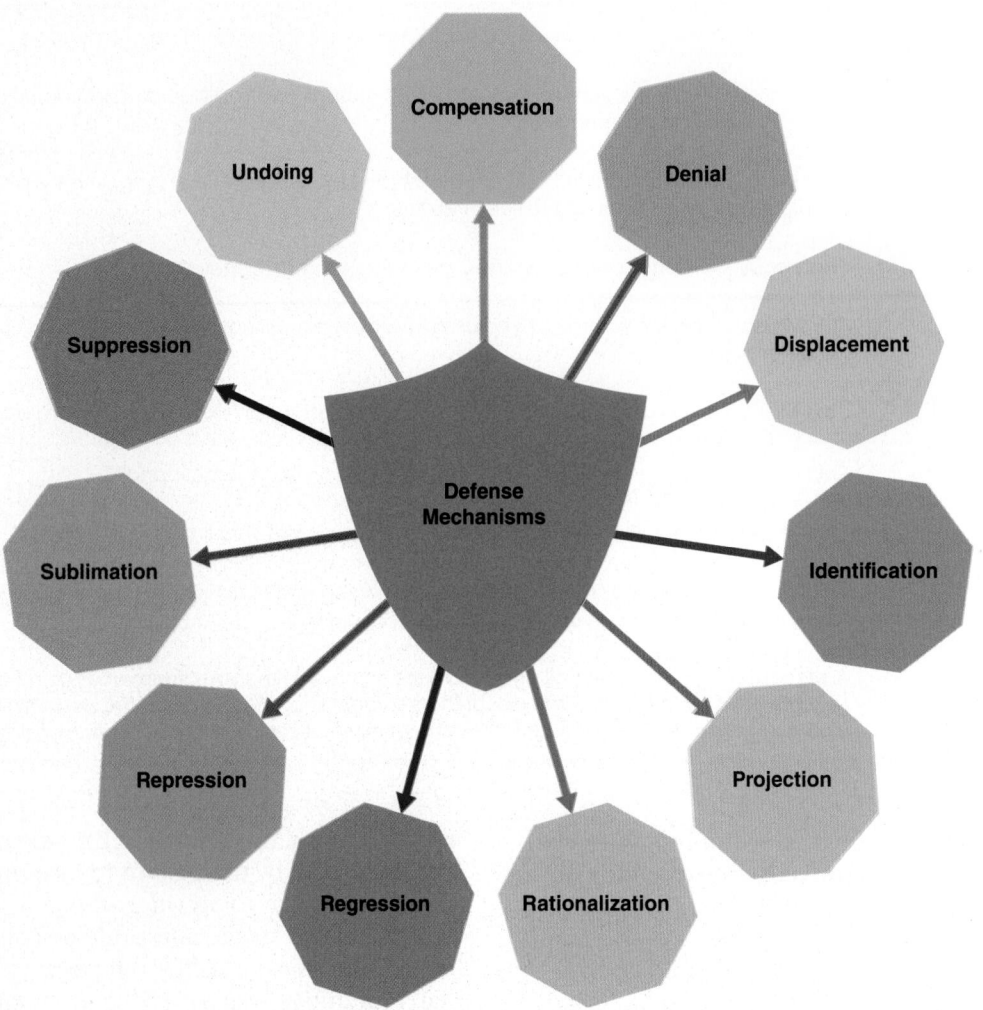

COMPENSATION

A conscious or subconscious overemphasizing of a characteristic to offset a real or imagined deficiency.

Example: A young boy whose physical stature keeps him from being a football star, so he compensates by achieving an academic award.

DENIAL

The refusal to accept painful information that is readily apparent to others. Careful attention to what the person is saying will reveal that he or she does not accept his or her situation and is not mentally conscious that it is happening.

Example: Often occurs when a person is diagnosed with a disease such as cancer or experiences the death of a close family member or associate.

(continues)

DISPLACEMENT

The subconscious transfer of unacceptable emotions, thoughts, or feelings from one's self to a more acceptable external substitute.

Example: A patient who is angry with the provider for some reason slams the door as he or she leaves the clinic.

IDENTIFICATION

An unconscioous defense mechanism in which a person assimilates or copies the identifying characteristics, traits, or actions of other persons or groups. Overuse of this defense mechanism denies the person the benefits and self-actualization of their own accomplishments.

PROJECTION

Attributing unacceptable desires, impulses, and thoughts falsely to others to avoid acknowledging they are actually the person's own experiences.

Example: A mother who abuses her child might accuse the medical assistant of being rough with the child while performing patient assessment to conceal her own feelings of wanting to throttle the child.

RATIONALIZATION

The mind's way of making unacceptable behavior or events acceptable by devising a rational reason in order to avoid embarrassment or guilt.

Example: A patient who tells the provider that he or she did not take his or her blood pressure medication because he or she did not have enough time before leaving for work.

REGRESSION

An attempt to withdraw from an unpleasant circumstance by retreating to an earlier, more secure stage of life. Usually occurs when a person feels powerless or desperate.

Examples: A toddler soiling himself after the arrival of a new baby sibling; An adult or child using a security blanket.

REPRESSION

The mind's way of defending itself from mental trauma by forgetting or wiping things out of the conscious memory.

Example: A child subconsciously forgetting to tell parents that he or she got into trouble at school.

SUBLIMATION

The channeling of a socially unacceptable behavior into a socially acceptable behavior.

Example: An overly aggressive person directed to play football to relieve aggression.

SUPPRESSION

The conscious or unconscious attempt to keep threatening material out of consciousness.

Example: The failure to remember a significant childhood event, such as the death of a grandmother.

UNDOING

Acting in ways designed to make amends or to cancel out inappropriate behavior.

Example: An abuser showering the abused person with gifts to compensate for unacceptable actions that took place in the past.

BARRIERS CAUSED BY CULTURAL AND RELIGIOUS DIVERSITY

Diversity

True therapeutic communication cannot take place without taking into consideration the cultural and religious background of the patient. **Culture** is a pattern of many concepts, beliefs, values, habits, skills, instruments, and art of a given group of people in a given period. Culture and religion influence the patient's communication context, caregiving expectations, time focus, and attitude toward Western medicine practiced in the United States. Table 4-2 presents characteristics that are typical of different cultural and religious groups.

TABLE 4-2

GENERALIZATION OF CULTURAL/RELIGIOUS EFFECTS ON HEALTH CARE

CULTURE OR RELIGION	MEDICAL CARE BACKGROUND	CAREGIVING STRUCTURE	COMMUNICATION TRAITS	TIME FOCUS*
Caucasian, Western Culture	**Western medicine,** rely on prescription medications, practice preventive medicine, may rely on folk medicine in some rural areas.	**Individual,** immediate family, close friends.	**Low context,** direct, eye contact expected, not adverse to therapeutic touching, may challenge medical opinions, basic English, speaks loudly.	**Future**
African American, Western Culture	**Western medicine,** rely on prescription medications, practice preventive medicine, may rely on folk medicine in some rural areas.	**Extended family,** relatives, close friends, neighbors, church family.	**Low context,** direct, eye contact expected, not adverse to therapeutic touching, may challenge medical opinions and can distrust medical personnel, basic English sometimes mixed with street language (Ebonics).	**Present/Future**
Black, African, or Caribbean Culture	**Mixture** of Western combined with spiritualism.	**Extended family,** relatives, close friends, neighbors, church family, tribal affiliation.	**Low context,** eye contact expected, highly emotional, basic English strongly mixed with local dialect.	**Present**
Asian Culture Asian, Indian, Chinese, Filipino, Japanese, Korean, Thai, Laotian, Vietnamese	**Mixture** of Western combined with Confucian principals, i.e., mind control of the body and maintaining a balance between natural forces and energy in the body, eating foods designated as having hot and cold properties to cure illness is common, mental illness is considered shameful and is denied.	**Immediate family,** opinions of family and particularly elders are important.	**High context,** indirect, avoid eye contact, show little emotion, avoid therapeutic touching, youth speak basic English, elders may speak little English, may agree with what is said even when they do not understand in order to avoid conflict or to avoid losing face, speak softly.	**Present/Past**
Native American, South Sea Island Cultures	**Mixture** of Western and folk medicine combined with importance of a balance between the forces of nature.	**Extended family,** relatives, close friends, neighbors, tribal affiliation.	**High context,** avoid eye contact, speak softly and slowly, basic English mixed with tribal dialects.	**Present**
Hispanic and Latino Cultures	**Mixture** of Western and folk medicine combined with a strong belief in intervention by God, eating foods designated as having hot and cold properties to cure illness is common.	**Extended family,** relatives, church family, collective community.	**High context,** be respectful and make direct eye contact, speak softly, some basic English, most speak Spanish.	**Present/Past**
Judaism	**Western medicine,** religion does not allow eating pork and requires kosher food.	Culturally dependent.	Culturally dependent.	**Future/Present**
Hinduism/ Buddhism	**Western medicine,** religions do not allow eating meat, modest regarding their body.	Culturally dependent.	Culturally dependent.	**Future/Present**
Islam	**Mixture** of Western combined with a strong belief in intervention by Allah, match gender of care-giver and patient, women may not be permitted to be examined by male medical professional, mental illness denied, do not ingest alcohol, believe complete rest is proper for all illnesses, do not eat pork.	**Immediate family,** opinions of family and particularly male head of household are important.	**High context,** touching between men and women is prohibited for strict believers, do not discuss sexual dysfunction, females do not make direct eye contact, will not discuss many taboo subjects (mental illness, birth defects, contraception, hospice), those from Middle East speak loudly to indicate the importance of what they are saying.	**Future/Present**
Christian Science	Most are unfamiliar with Western medicine, preferring to rely on prayer and spiritual intervention; accept clinical diagnosis, but attribute the causation to an underlying spiritual condition, healed by prayer; do not believe in drug therapy and may reject vaccination; each has freedom to seek modern medical treatment.	**Immediate family** and the use of Christian Science practitioners and nurses committed to a ministry of healing, but none have medical training or knowledge.	Christian Scientists could have any cultural background and hence communicate in the context of that culture; because of their lack of medical knowledge, the provider should clearly explain any procedures.	**Present/Future**

*The bold term represents the predominant focus.

Communication Context. Communication context can be one of two styles: low-context or high-context. **Low-context communication** uses few environmental idioms to convey an idea. It relies on explicit and highly detailed language. **High-context communication** relies on body language, reference to environmental objects, and culturally relevant phraseology to communicate an idea. Neither communication style is superior to the other. It is important, however, that both the speaker and the listener be cognizant of the style being used in the conversation. In the medical clinic, the medical assistant should be aware of communication content and attempt to utilize the style used by the patient to the extent that it is practical.

Persons having different communication styles can easily develop an incorrect impression of the other person. Low-context communication is direct and in your face, whereas high-context communication is indirect and seems to take forever to reach a conclusion. The high-context speaker is often thought of as mentally slow or uneducated, and the low-context speaker is thought of as being rude or arrogant. Conclusions based on communication style usually are preconceived misconceptions and should be considered at all times when health care professionals are working with patients.

Caregiving Expectations. Caregiving expectations refer to the arrangements for taking responsibility for medical requirements. Most persons from Western cultures are individualistic and take personal responsibility for their medical care, though children and older adults generally must rely on family or medical professionals for caregiving. However, many other cultures and religions do not share this individualistic philosophy, focusing more on the immediate or extended family for support. This can result in problems related to privacy requirements and patient compliance if a medical power of attorney has not been established.

Time Focus. The cultural background as well as the socioeconomic environment of the patient have considerable impact on time focus. **Time focus** relates to whether the patient's attitude toward life is focused on the future, present, or past. Time focus is usually related to culture and religion and is not necessarily related to current circumstances, though children, regardless of culture or religion, are present focused and older adults are more likely to be past focused.

Future time focus is found in persons whose physical needs have been met and who can sacrifice immediate gratification to achieve perceived greater future returns. Future-oriented persons are time conscious and plan out their daily lives in considerable detail. Persons from affluent Western cultures usually are future oriented.

Present time focus is found in persons who are less assured of being able to meet their physical needs. It is difficult to plan for the future when basic items in the hierarchy of needs have not been met. Punctuality usually is not important to present-focused persons, as they are immersed in the present and oblivious to time.

Past time focus is associated with persons from cultures having long-standing traditions. Tradition and past life experience become the central focus of their life.

Human Needs as Barriers

Human needs, such as those discussed in Maslow's Hierarchy of Needs, are barriers to effective therapeutic communication if they are not met. A patient who does not know where he or she will find food or shelter or who feels rejected and unloved will frequently make these needs first and of primary concern in their mind. It is nearly impossible to focus on communication regarding other concerns until these basic needs have been met. This section discusses human needs and how they can be addressed by the medical assistant or by referrals provided by health care professionals.

Maslow's Hierarchy of Needs. Abraham Maslow is considered the founder of humanistic psychology and is most well known for his **Hierarchy of Needs** (Figure 4-4). *Webster's Dictionary* defines *hierarchy* as "a group of persons or things arranged in order of rank, grade, class, etc." According to Maslow's theory, human needs are grouped into five levels. He

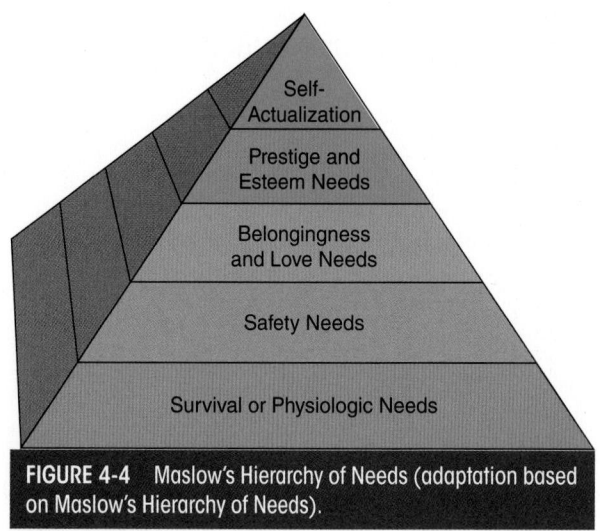

Self-Actualization

Prestige and Esteem Needs

Belongingness and Love Needs

Safety Needs

Survival or Physiologic Needs

FIGURE 4-4 Maslow's Hierarchy of Needs (adaptation based on Maslow's Hierarchy of Needs).

also theorized that each level of need must be satisfied before one can move on to the next level.

The needs in the first level include physiologic or survival needs. These needs include food, water, and air to breathe—homeostasis for the body. The second level includes needs of safety and security, that is, the need for security, stability, and protection. Everyone has the desire to be free from fear and anxiety. Safety needs also include the need for structure, law and order, and limits.

The third level involves belonging and love needs. This level of need involves both giving and receiving affection. Additional words that express our connectedness are *roots, origins, peers, friends, family, neighborhood, territory, clan, class*, and *gang*. We have a basic animal tendency to herd, flock, join, and belong.

The fourth level, prestige and esteem needs, comes from a basic need for a stable, healthy self-respect for ourselves and others. There is the desire for achievement, strength, and confidence. Also, there is the need for recognition, prestige, reputation, status, and even fame. Satisfaction of these needs leads to feelings of self-confidence and worth. The final level is self-actualization. In this stage, we are at our peak, doing what truly fits us. It is an achievement of potential.

Individuals may move back and forth from one need to another depending on circumstances. Understanding this hierarchy helps to assess a patient's needs. If the most basic of needs are not met, it is highly unlikely that a patient can be successful with any treatment protocol. Keeping this hierarchy in mind will help to facilitate therapeutic communication.

Patients with Special Needs

The Americans with Disabilities Act requires that health care facilities, both public and private, large and small, provide effective communication alternatives to patients with language and hearing loss or speech impairment. The provider can choose the communication method or device as long as it results in effective communication. The expense for this accommodation must be charged against the overhead of the clinic and may not be billed to the patient.

A language deficiency can be overcome by using an interpreter, employing a human translator, using a telephone or service translator, or using online translation systems with software applications such as Google Translate, Speak and Translate, FaceTime, or Skype. These applications can translate in real time with text or with voice recognition software. Current technology has the capability to translate some 100 languages. The main disadvantage of voice systems is that they require speaking slowly and have difficulty translating technical terminology. When a person-to-person interpreter has been considered to be the translation mode used in the clinic, a resource list of interpreters should be compiled. The Registry of Interpreters for Deaf, Inc. is an excellent resource (www.rid.org). Your local city or state registry of interpreters may also be useful. It is also important to document the mode of preferred communication within the patient's medical record.

Patients who are visually challenged may be able to understand the spoken language; however, their vocabulary may be limited because of their disability. Utilize large-print materials and assure adequate lighting in all patient areas. Always speak in a normal voice to the patient as you enter the examination room or before you touch them. Extra caution must be exercised to ensure that patients who are visually impaired understand the message you are attempting to transmit.

Challenges with mental cognition will be a deterrent to communication. Dementia or other types of mental impairment, or even a serious illness, may make communication difficult if not impossible. Communication should include the patient's legal guardian or caregiver. Even so, every attempt should be made to have the patient involved in the conversation so he or she is not frustrated and feeling powerless and overwhelmed by the situation.

Environmental Factors

Environmental factors such as noise or any visual commotion that causes a distraction for either the patient or the health care professional will be an extreme barrier to communication of any type. Your conversation with the patient should be

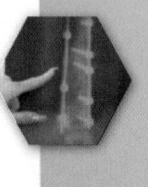

Critical Thinking

An established patient arrives 20 minutes early for his appointment. He is in obvious pain and discomfort and tells the administrative medical assistant, "I can't sleep, I can't eat, and I can't go to work today." Which of Maslow's stages most accurately describes this patient? What actions should the medical assistant take to assist this patient?

stopped until you can either move to a more suitable environment or the distraction has stopped. Physical barriers such as a computer screen or a desk between the patient and health care professional should be avoided. The medical professional should attempt to take a position close to the patient and at eye level, taking care not to invade his or her personal space. Always be vigilant to ensure there are no privacy issues violated.

Time Factors

Therapeutic communication requires time. Rushing a conversation with a patient and expecting effective conveyance of a message is unrealistic. The patient will listen but not retain your message if he or she is being rushed. The emotional state of the health care professional will be conveyed by body language in such circumstances.

ESTABLISHING MULTICULTURAL COMMUNICATION

Diversity

Multicultural communication is the ability to communicate effectively with individuals of other cultures while recognizing one's own personal cultural biases and prejudices and putting them aside.

Approximately one third of the population of the United States comes from a culture other than Caucasian, English-speaking, Judeo-Christian. Figure 4-5 illustrates the percentage of various cultures living in the United States.

Medical professionals working within a specific cultural community should seek further information relating to that particular culture. In many instances, health care professionals can develop rapport with their ethnically diverse patients by simply demonstrating an interest in their culture and background.

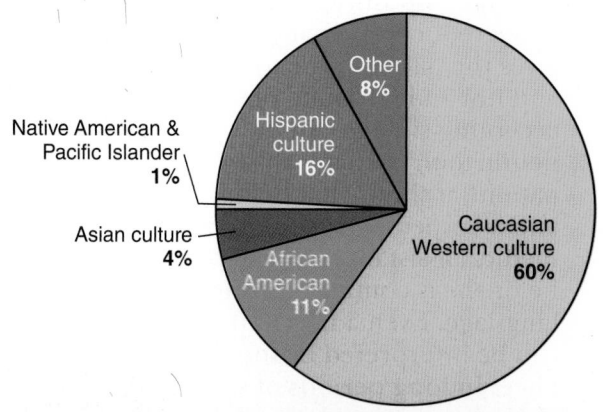

FIGURE 4-5 United States demographic make-up (2010 Census).

Before multicultural or any therapeutic communication can begin, the patient must first be willing to discuss his or her health care issues, listen to the professional's questions, and give honest answers to those questions. The patient must trust the professional. Several steps to building trust include:

- *Risk/trust.* It is essential for the helping professional to build an atmosphere of trust, making it easier for the patient to risk expressing feelings and attitudes about the problem. Trust has to be earned. Remember to promise no more than you can deliver, be honest, and carefully and thoroughly explain procedures and policies. Answer all questions truthfully and honestly.

- *Empathy.* Empathy is the ability to accept another's private world as if it were your own. Empathy communicates identification with and understanding of another's situation. It states, "I'm available to walk this road with you."

- *Respect.* Respect values another person and considers him or her as a special individual. It is important to respect the patient's personal space, to provide privacy, and to use his or her full name and title when appropriate.

- *Genuineness.* This means being real and honest with others. The health care professional must be able to communicate honestly with others, while being careful not to blame or condemn.

- *Active listening.* Active listening involves verbal and nonverbal clues that send the message you are completely involved in the communication. Sit facing the patient with no barriers, such as a desk, between you. Lean toward the patient slightly to convey genuine concern and interest. Establish and maintain appropriate eye contact to elicit interest and concern. Maintain an open, relaxed posture to establish a nonthreatening environment for the patient. Listen carefully to the words the patient uses to describe problems, and use those terms rather than medical terminology when discussing symptoms.

THERAPEUTIC COMMUNICATION IN ACTION

The following section identifies the proper communication techniques medical assistants should use as part of the most important communication function they perform: patient interview techniques.

Interview Techniques

Communication

All health professionals must be adept at interview techniques—knowing how to encourage the best communication between themselves and the patient. It is important to remember that an unequal relationship exists between the health professional and the patient. The health professional, whether it be the provider or the medical assistant, is in the power position and has a great deal of control over the patient. Therefore, it is important to equalize the relationship as much as possible.

Early in the interview, the patient must feel comfortable enough to risk being honest with the health professional. The health professional must build an atmosphere of trust by showing concern for the patient. A gentle touch and a warm, caring facial expression may be all that is necessary. Always be honest and genuine in your responses to patients. Be sympathetic and empathic and use responding skills such as sharing observations, validation and acknowledging, and paraphrasing to create an environment that is free of hypocrisy.

When the medical assistant is interviewing the patient for the presenting problem or chief complaint, it is important to listen with a "third" ear. Listen to what the patient is not saying but is apt to exhibit through nonverbal communication.

You might choose to share your observation of the nonverbal message with the patient, thus encouraging the patient to verbalize more freely. When concerns are shared, validate and acknowledge those concerns through statements such as "I can understand why you would be concerned." You can verify the communication by reflecting or paraphrasing what the patient has said. Reflecting focuses on the patient's emotional expression as well as observation of her body language. "You feel …" will often be used at the beginning of or within your response to the patient. Paraphrasing restates in the health professional's own words what the patient has said. The patient has opportunity to verify the accuracy of his message and that the professional understood the message as intended. Using words such as "You feel … because …" connects the two skills. For example, "You feel the back exercises are not working because you are still experiencing pain and discomfort."

When the health care professional is not sure of the meaning of the message communicated, clarifying skills are useful. Statements such as "I'm not sure I understand what you mean" or "Do you mean ...?" are examples of asking for clarification.

Knowing how to ask questions that help the patient express concerns takes practice and skill.

The answers to these questions are vital to patient care and for accuracy of the medical record. Three basic types of questions are used to elicit information.

Closed questions are useful when collecting information for the patient history. They can be answered with a simple yes or no and usually begin with *do, is,* or *are*. Examples include:

"Are you still taking your medication?"

"Do you have pain in your back now?"

You will also use **open-ended questions** with the patient. These questions encourage therapeutic communication because they encourage the patient to express more detail. Open-ended questions usually begin with *how, what,* or *could*. Examples include:

"What kind of help will you have at home during your recovery?"

"How are you coming along on this diet?"

Indirect statements will also prove helpful in facilitating therapeutic communication. An indirect statement will elicit a response from a patient without the patient feeling questioned. Such statements encourage verbalization and express interest in the patient from the health care professional. Examples include:

"Tell me what you've been doing since you retired."

"I'd like to know more about your exercise program."

Additional helpful approaches to establishing therapeutic communication include:

- *Silence.* Utilizing the absence of verbal communication gives the patient time to put his or her feelings and thoughts into words, regain composure, and continue talking. Silence reduces the pace of the encounter and gives the patient time to feel like a human and not an inanimate object. A positive and accepting silence can be a valuable therapeutic tool, particularly for a shy and quiet patient; it shows that he or she has worth and is respected by another person. The medical assistant needs to be alert to what he or she is communicating through body language. Even a momentary loss of interest can be interpreted by the patient as indifference. In long periods of silence, the medical assistant must not become bored or allow his or her attention to wander from the patient. The medical assistant should give a broad

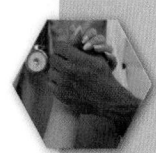

Patient Education

Education of a patient or caregiver should consist of the following fundamentals regardless of the subject:

- Do not attempt to educate the patient while he or she is emotionally upset or distressed. Under these conditions the individual will not be communicative; that is, he or she is listening but not hearing what is said. Make every effort to calm the patient. If necessary, reschedule another time for the educational session.
- Use multiple teaching methods, such as visual (including multimedia), verbal, and action, to convey the message. This approach ensures that your communication style will be versatile and meet the needs of the patient. Convey information in a clear, concise manner using context that is relevant to the patient.
- Limit the amount of material covered. If necessary, schedule additional sessions so that the patient is not overwhelmed.
- Communicate in simple words, avoiding medical terminology that may not be understood by the patient.

opening such as "Where would you like to begin" and avoid small talk. Let the use of silence encourage patients to express themselves.

- *Feedback.* Nodding "yes," saying "I understand" if you do, or just "uh hmm" are forms of feedback. Offer general leads and give encouragement to the patient to continue by using statements such as "Go on," "And then?" or "Tell me about it." Acknowledge the patient's right to his or her opinion, to make decisions, and to think for himself or herself. Seeking to make clear that which is not meaningful or that which is vague provides useful feedback. Attempt to verbalize what the patient has hinted at or suggested. Search for mutual understanding and for accord in the meaning of words.
- *Giving recognition.* Give recognition and acknowledge his or her presence through greeting the patient by name. When the patient makes an effort or accomplishes something, the medical assistant should acknowledge it and give encouragement.
- *Offering comfort.* Help the patient to be comfortable during the medical encounter by showing empathy with the patient's situation. Introduce yourself and explain what is about to happen or to be done to the patient. Make available the facts the patient needs to feel at ease and to make the encounter less stressful.

Refer to Chapter 22 for additional information related to patient interviewing.

PATIENT COACHING AND NAVIGATION

Primary care providers struggle to adequately cover every agenda item a patient may have within the 15-minute clinic visit. This is especially true for patients with chronic conditions. As a result, a paradigm shift away from a provider diagnosing and prescribing a treatment plan toward a collaborative approach where the patient and provider discuss options for health care has developed, utilizing both coaching and navigation. The primary objective of the **coach** is to educate patients regarding self-health management and to encourage patients to take a more active role in staying healthy. Each member of the health care team can integrate elements of coaching into their interactions with patients; however, at least one team member should be designated as a coach. It is the responsibility of the coach to help patients gain the knowledge, skills, tools, and confidence to become active participants in the management of their health care.

Health coaches may act as advocates or intermediaries in the patient–provider relationship by sharing relevant information with the provider and by motivating and encouraging the patient to follow provider protocols. The coach may also instruct the patient about diagnostic and therapeutic modalities and guide the patient in making informed choices about when, how, and where to use community health care resources. (See Chapter 11 for community resource information.)

Procedure

A **navigator** works in conjunction with the medical home health care team and assists with answering questions about care and medications, keeping the family informed and engaged in patient care, providing one-on-one education aimed at improving health, helping schedule appointments, and arranging community resources as needed. These resources may include home health care, skilled nursing facilities, and rehabilitation centers. The navigator can also help with transition care, including specialist to specialist, hospital to home, and hospital to skilled nursing or rehabilitation centers. Procedure 4-1 provides the steps to coach or navigate a patient regarding a collaborative approach to health care.

Integrity

Qualifications for the role of coach or navigator include being an excellent listener; having good communication skills; and utilizing planning, organization, and follow-up techniques. Medical assistants are prime candidates for this role due to their multifaceted professional education. They are ideally suited to provide linguistic and cultural coaching as well. Since scope of practice varies from state to state, you will want to check your state's regulations as they relate to coaching and navigation. Generally, medical assistants are not permitted to make medical assessments.

PROCEDURE 4-1

Coach or Navigate a Patient Regarding a Collaborative Approach to Health Care

Procedure

PURPOSE:

To educate patients regarding self-health management, to encourage patients to take a more active role in staying healthy, and to assist them in navigating the medical home health care team.

EQUIPMENT/SUPPLIES:

- Paper and pen
- Computer
- Information ordered by provider for coaching/navigation session

PROCEDURE STEPS:

1. Check your state's scope of practice regulations. RATIONALE: You must always ensure you are working within your scope of practice.

2. Develop a written plan (approved and included in the clinic's procedure manual) on who the coach/navigator will be and what information will be disseminated by the coach/navigator. RATIONALE: Communication skills and barriers, developmental life stages, and cultural and religious diversity issues should all be considered in the patient approach in order to foster a positive patient/provider relationship.

3. Introduce yourself by name and title, and identify the patient.

4. Provide a written copy of all instructions to the patient and review them verbally with the patient. RATIONALE: Ensures that all instructions are discussed.

5. Ask the patient to repeat instructions and answer any questions or concerns he or she may have regarding the instructions. Provide the office telephone number in case the patient has any additional questions. RATIONALE: Ensures clarification for all parties.

6. ***Demonstrate empathy, active listening, and respect for individual diversity*** throughout the session.

7. Document in the patient's medical record what information and instructions were given.

DOCUMENTATION:

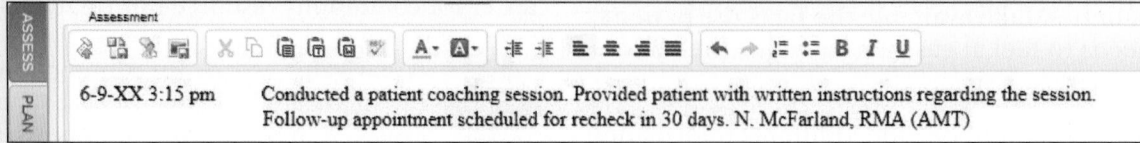

Assessment	
6-9-XX 3:15 pm	Conducted a patient coaching session. Provided patient with written instructions regarding the session. Follow-up appointment scheduled for recheck in 30 days. N. McFarland, RMA (AMT)

Courtesy of Harris CareTracker PM and EMR

When using a coach or a navigator, the benefits to the patient and the practice include:

- Helping patients navigate an increasingly complex health care system
- Reviewing progress since the last visit with the patient and the medical team
- Answering questions regarding medical instructions and processes
- Confirming that information is correct in the medical record
- Following up with the patient after a visit to the practice
- Strengthening patient satisfaction
- Motivating the patient to change behavior and to self-manage his or her health toward mutually agreed-on goals

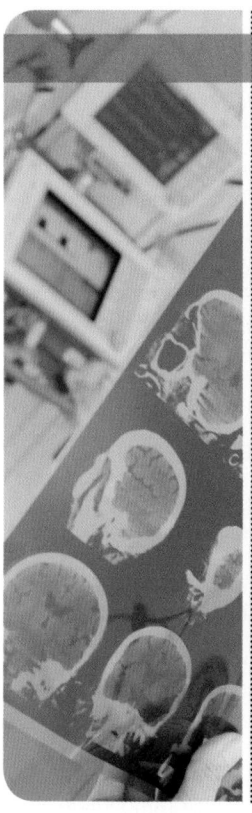

CASE STUDY 4-1

It is a very busy day at Inner City Health Care. Despite the three emergencies in the early afternoon and the full schedule of patients, everything is running smoothly with Dr. Lewis, and the entire staff, responding quickly but thoroughly to patient concerns.

At 4:00 PM another emergency patient arrives; at the same time, Jim Marshal, an architect in a downtown firm, comes in early for a routine appointment and demands to be seen immediately. Jim, a regular patient, has a history of being difficult and impatient; being a bit arrogant, he tends to put his needs first. However, Dr. Lewis is occupied with another patient. It is critical to treat the patient with the emergency as soon as possible, and Jim is half an hour early.

Ellen Armstrong, CMAS (AMT), the clinic's administrative medical assistant, calmly asks Mr. Marshal to please wait until his scheduled appointment time. When he threatens to leave, Ellen explains to Mr. Marshal that there are two patients ahead of him, but that the provider will see him at his scheduled appointment time.

CASE STUDY REVIEW

1. What communication roadblocks did medical assistant Ellen Armstrong avoid as she reacted to Jim Marshal's demands to see the provider?

2. With another student, role-play the scenario, with one student taking the role of patient and one student the role of the medical assistant. Identify roadblocks to communication imposed by the patient. How is the medical assistant using the five Cs of communication to deal with the situation?

3. Do you think the medical assistant reacted appropriately? What else could she have done? What should she *not* do in this situation?

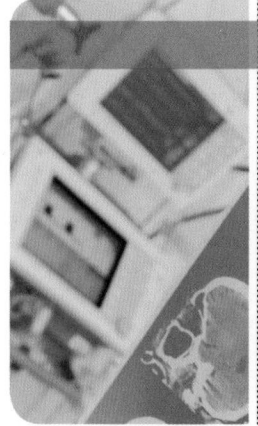

CASE STUDY 4-2

You have learned in this chapter that communication has not been successful until the communication cycle is complete. Consider the following scenario.

An 82-year-old woman with moderate dementia and a hearing impairment is brought to the surgeon's clinic for a follow-up appointment after hip replacement surgery. The woman's daughter, who is the patient's medical power of attorney, accompanies her. The goal of the appointment is to make certain the hip is healing nicely and to discuss precautions before the patient returns to her assisted-living apartment. Almost immediately, the conversation is directed toward the daughter because it is so much easier to explain to her what should be done.

continues

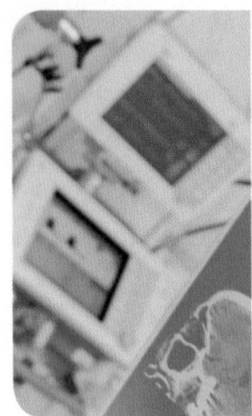

CASE STUDY 4-2 *continued*

CASE STUDY REVIEW

1. What might the staff do to help the patient understand the following?
   - Use the walker consistently.
   - Wear shoes that are leather, tennis-shoe type, or uniform style; consider Velcro closure as opposed to laces that have to be tied.
   - Do not walk your dog on a leash.
2. Should the patient be left out of the conversation? Should the daughter be included?
3. In cases such as these, is something other than verbal communication indicated?

Summary

- Therapeutic communication uses specific and well-defined professional skills. It is understandable to the patient, delivered with empathy, and technically accurate.

- Communication involves two or more individuals participating in an exchange of information. The communication cycle includes the sender, the message, the channel or mode of transmission, the receiver, and the feedback.

- Verbal communication involves speaking and listening while using the five Cs of communication.

- Nonverbal communication or body language includes the unconscious body movements, gestures, and facial expressions that accompany speech.

- To avoid miscommunication there must be congruency between the verbal and nonverbal communication.

- There will always be face-to-face and telephone conversations in the medical clinic; however, technology is rapidly breaking ground for the virtual medical clinic.

- The medical assistant must recognize that until the barriers affecting therapeutic communication are dealt with or at least minimized, therapeutic communication will be significantly impacted.

- Culture and religion influence the patient's communication context, caregiving expectations, time focus, and attitude toward Western medicine practiced in the United States.

- According to Maslow's Hierarchy of Needs, human needs are grouped into five levels and must be satisfied before one can move on to the next level.

- The Americans with Disabilities Act requires that all health care facilities provide effective communication alternatives to patients with language and hearing loss or speech impairment. Any expense incurred with the accommodation must be charged against the overhead of the clinic and may not be billed to the patient.

- Approximately one third of the population of the United States comes from a culture other than Caucasian, English-speaking, Judeo-Christian. Multicultural communication requires recognizing one's own personal cultural biases and prejudices and putting them aside to promote therapeutic communication.

- All health care professionals must be adept at interview techniques that build an atmosphere of trust by showing concern for the patient, being sympathetic and empathic, using appropriate responding skills, and asking questions in a nonthreatening manner.

- The primary objective of the coach is to educate patients regarding self-health management and to encourage patients to take a more active role in staying healthy. A navigator works in conjunction with the medical home health care team.

- Throughout this text you are reminded of the importance of effective communication techniques. Good communication takes practice. Use the techniques identified in this chapter with your family and with your peers. Watch for roadblocks, be aware of defense mechanisms, and remember the five Cs of communication.

To reinforce your knowledge and skills of information presented in this chapter:

- Review the *Key Terms* and *Learning Outcomes*
- Consider the *Critical Thinking* features and *Case Studies* and discuss your conclusions
- Answer the questions in the *Certification Review*

- Perform the *Procedure* using the *Competency Assessment Checklist* on the *Student Companion Website*

Procedure

CERTIFICATION REVIEW

1. Which of the following factors affect therapeutic communication?
   a. Gestures and mannerisms
   b. Posture
   c. Personal space
   d. Education and life experience

2. What does encoding mean in the cycle of communication?
   a. Deciphering a message
   b. Creating the message to be sent
   c. Sending the message
   d. Receiving the message
   e. Interpreting the message

3. What is true of body language?
   a. It is used to express feelings and emotions.
   b. It is not as important as verbal communication.
   c. It only makes up 7% of the message.
   d. It is only used in Eastern cultures.

4. What is a comfortable social space?
   a. Touching to 1½ feet
   b. 1½ feet to 4 feet
   c. 12 to 15 feet
   d. 5 to 16 feet
   e. 4 to 12 feet

5. Which of the following accurately describes a reassuring cliché?
   a. It is a way of calming down a patient.
   b. It is a means of rationalizing a decision.
   c. It is a roadblock to communication.
   d. It is always useful in daily communications.

6. Redirecting a socially unacceptable impulse into one that is socially acceptable is an example of which of these defense mechanisms?
   a. Sublimation
   b. Rationalization
   c. Projection
   d. Displacement
   e. Repression

7. Which of the following is true of open-ended questions?
   a. They usually require just a "yes" or "no" answer.
   b. They usually begin with *do, is,* or *are.*
   c. They elicit a response from a patient without the patient feeling questioned.
   d. They usually begin with *how, what,* or *could.*

8. Which statement is true of kinesics?
   a. It is the study of body language.
   b. It is the study of personal space.
   c. It is the study of touch.
   d. It is the study of congruency.
   e. It is the study of defense mechanisms.

9. Low-context communication relies on which of the following?
   a. Body language
   b. Reference to environmental objects
   c. Explicit and highly detailed language
   d. Culturally relevant phraseology

10. Which of the following describes defense mechanisms?
    a. They are a refusal to accept painful information that is readily available to others.
    b. They are the conscious or subconscious overemphasis of a characteristic to offset a real or imagined deficiency.
    c. They are behaviors used to protect the ego from guilt, anxiety, or loss of esteem.
    d. They are the mind's way of making unacceptable behavior or events acceptable by devising a rational reason.

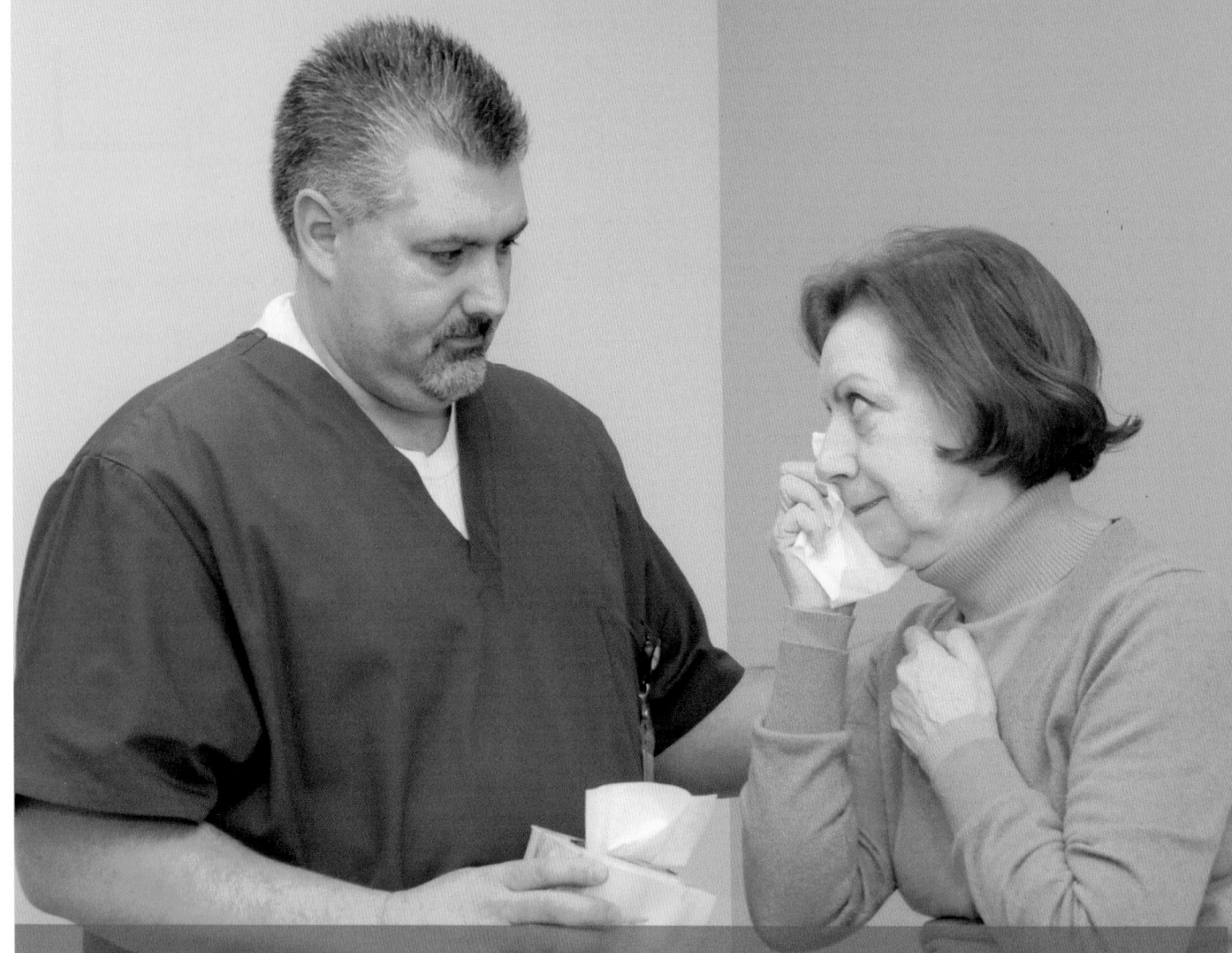

CHAPTER 5

The Therapeutic Approach to the Patient with a Life-Threatening Illness

1. Define and spell the key terms as presented in the glossary.
2. Recognize possible patient perspectives when facing a life-threatening illness.
3. Define "life-threatening" illness.
4. Critique the cultural manifestations of life-threatening illness.
5. Identify the strongest cultural influence in the life of a patient.
6. List at least four choices to be made when facing a life-threatening illness.
7. Analyze the different forms of health care directives.
8. Explain how a durable power of attorney for health care is used.
9. Discuss the range of psychological suffering that accompanies life-threatening illnesses.
10. Summarize additional concerns/fears when the life-threatening illness is cancer, AIDS, or end-stage renal disease.
11. Demonstrate the therapeutic response to persons with a life-threatening illness.
12. Summarize four questions to help patients verbalize their feelings in end-of-life communication.
13. Explain the five stages of grief and the meaning of the acronym TEAR.
14. Recall a number of challenges faced by the medical assistant when caring for people with life-threatening illnesses.

KEY TERMS

durable power of attorney for health care   palliative

health care directive

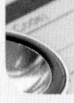

SCENARIO

You have seen the medical reports and agonize with your employer who must tell long-time patient Suzanne Markis when she comes in today that she has inoperable pancreatic cancer. When she arrives, you treat her as you normally would, making certain she suspects nothing from you. When she emerges from the provider's room, you make certain to meet her, take her arm, and ask if you can call someone for her. You do not present her with a bill or make another appointment at this time. You recognize that anything you say probably will not be remembered, so you focus entirely on this patient and her immediate needs. In a day or two, as instructed by your employer, you will telephone to make an appointment for Suzanne and anyone she might want present at her next visit with the provider so any questions can be answered.

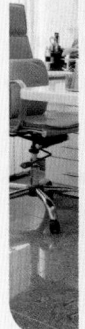

Chapter Portal

Everything you learned in Chapter 4 regarding therapeutic communication is heightened and considered more challenging when the patient has a life-threatening illness. If you were told today that your life will probably be shortened because of a serious illness, your perspective likely would change. What was important yesterday may mean little or nothing now. Something that meant nothing to you yesterday suddenly takes on great importance to you now. It is essential for the medical assistant to remember this difference in perspective and remember what is likely to be important to patients with a life-threatening illness.

continues

It also must be remembered that no two individuals respond to a life-threatening illness in the same way. Some respond with denial and act as if the information had never been shared with them. Others alter their lives radically and drastically change their priorities. Still others quietly continue their lives, changing little outwardly, but recognizing that their choices may now be limited (Figure 5-1).

LIFE-THREATENING ILLNESS

A life-threatening illness is not easily defined. Some use the word *terminal;* others refuse to use that word because they believe it removes any hope from the situation. Still others believe even the term *life-threatening* is too hopeless and prefer to use the term *life-altering;* however, a life-altering illness can quickly become life-threatening. Also, what one individual considers life-threatening may not be the same for another. For our purposes, life-threatening is used to imply a life that in all probability will be shortened because of a serious or debilitating illness or disease. It may be defined as death that is imminent; it may be defined in terms of a serious illness that a person will battle for many years but one that will ultimately shorten his or her life.

Cultural Perspective on Life-Threatening Illness

Diversity

Strong cultural manifestations will be seen during the treatment of a life-threatening illness and in anyone facing death. Culture is defined as how we live our lives, how we think, how we speak, and how we behave. Cultures can be accepting, denying, or even defying of death. Death can be considered either as the end of existence or as a transition to another state of being or consciousness. Death can be considered as profane or sacred. In some cultures, a life-threatening illness may be viewed or referred to as a "slow-motion" death because of degenerative diseases that often exhaust the resources and emotions of patients and their families.

Some cultures prefer that the life-threatening illness not be shared with the patient in the beginning, but with the family who helps to prepare the patient for the inevitable. A few cultures generally do not seek care for an illness until it is quite advanced; this practice can make pain management and treatment more difficult or impossible in some cases. Some cultures surround the person who is ill with great attention, never leaving the person alone. Other cultures view the illness as something that must be removed from the body, perhaps even believing that the individual has been given this illness because of some past sin or transgression.

Pain is viewed in the same manner. Some cultures believe it is to be endured quietly without complaint; others believe there is to be no pain, and family members will go to great lengths to have health care providers relieve the pain. When questioning a patient about the pain level, it must be within a cultural perspective. For example, cultures with an Asian influence are more likely to describe pain in general terms related to the imbalance of the body rather than in terms such as "piercing, intermittent, or throbbing" or "on a scale from 1 to 10."

Integrity

Skilled health care professionals will remember that the strongest influence in managing any life-threatening illness in the life of the patient is *not* the health care team; it is the family and those closest to the patient. Therefore, great care must be taken to determine and understand the patient's cultural perspective as much as possible, and the patient must be given great respect. Often, the cultural influence may contradict the standard of care preferred by the health care provider. It is better to understand the culture and work within that parameter than to deny it and continually work

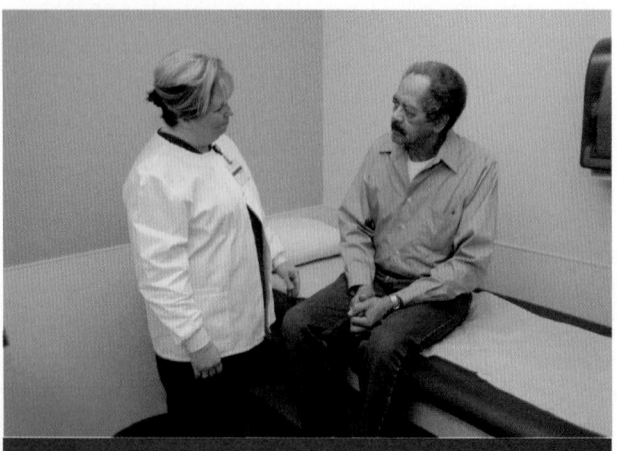

FIGURE 5-1 Establishing a caring and trusting relationship can help the patient come to terms with a life-threatening illness.

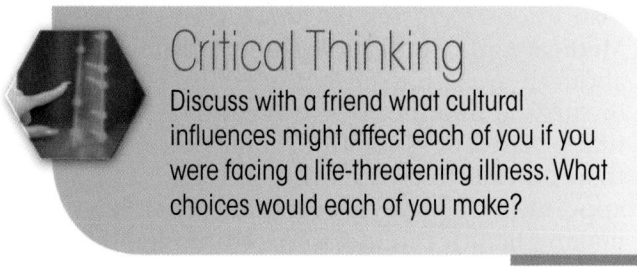

Critical Thinking

Discuss with a friend what cultural influences might affect each of you if you were facing a life-threatening illness. What choices would each of you make?

against the patient's belief system and the influence of family.

CHOICES IN LIFE-THREATENING ILLNESS

Many choices are available to a patient with a life-threatening illness, but there are also many decisions to be made. The urgency of the decisions will depend, in part, on possible life expectancy. Patients often want an answer to the question, "How long do I have?" Providers are unable to give a definitive answer; however, estimates may be given in terms of weeks, months, or even years. Patients may choose to make decisions that seem contrary to recommended medical intervention. Often, too, these decisions are clouded by a provider's desire and need to heal even in light of overwhelming odds.

Early in the process, it is a good idea for the provider to ask patients how they might like to be involved in the decision-making process. The question might be "How much do you want to know?" There is a fine line between overwhelming patients with information and providing them the information they need or want to make appropriate choices and necessary decisions.

Patients generally have the right to choose or to refuse treatment. Some rush into a treatment protocol only to discover later that their choices have brought them pain, disability, and expense far beyond what originally was assumed. Although it is the health care professional's goal to heal, if healing is not likely or possible, patients ought not to be "urged" into treatment protocols that are likely to be contrary to their personal wishes for the sake of treatment only.

In fact, those facing a life-threatening illness may make many different choices, and there are several schools of thought regarding those choices:

Legal

1. As stated earlier, patients may choose to forgo any treatment, including medications, transfusions, artificial hydration and feeding, respirators, surgery, chemotherapy, radiation, and dialysis.

2. The choice might be **palliative** care that focuses on quality of life while relieving symptoms of pain and suffering alongside of or instead of disease-focused treatment.

3. There is a growing group of individuals who consciously choose not to eat or drink anything by refusing all food and fluids for a more natural death. This choice is referred to as VSED (voluntarily stop eating and drinking) in medical circles.

4. Total sedation may be sought and is used when dying patients experience unbearable suffering and their bodies do not respond to other treatments. The medication causes unconsciousness and eventually death.

5. In an increasing number of states there is the option to seek aid in dying, usually through self-administration of medication prescribed by a physician.

Although health care professionals are generally less comfortable with some of these choices and death than they are with saving life, there are issues appropriate to consider with patients especially when facing life-threatening illness. Those issues include the following:

1. *Alternative methods of treatment should be discussed, as well as the outcome if no treatment is sought.* At some point, many patients will want to know *all* the treatment protocols that are feasible. This is a logical time to discuss any alternative or integrative medicine therapies that have shown success. Explanations should be made in language that the patient can understand. Illustrations and diagrams can be beneficial. Referrals might be made to integrative medicine practitioners, and patients are to be encouraged to discuss any chosen alternative therapies with their primary care provider. Sometimes treatment alternatives the patient may consider are not within the realm of recognized medical acceptability, but it is better to have that discussion than to ignore the possibility. Patients may also ask what happens if no treatment is chosen. This question can be difficult for health care providers who are anxious to provide some form of treatment for patients, but patients may have a number of reasons not to seek treatment. Remember the earlier statement indicating that family members and friends bring more influence to bear than does the health care professional.

2. *Discussion of pain management and treatment is essential.* The major fears patients have in facing life-threatening illness are pain, loss of self-image, and loss of independence. A frank discussion of pain control and how that can be accomplished can alleviate a fair amount of concern. Loss of self-image is devastating to many. To experience serious gain or loss of weight, loss of mobility, and the inability to perform daily tasks is seen by some as a fate worse than death. Providers will want to be ready to discuss loss of independence related to any life-threatening illness or to make a referral to someone who can be helpful. Patients have concerns such as wanting to know how long before the disease takes its toll, how long can they drive, what kind of care or assistance will be necessary, whether they can remain in their own home, and how long before they must have someone make decisions for them.

3. **Legal** *Health care directives such as a durable power of attorney for health care or health care proxy allows an individual to make decisions related to health care when the patient is no longer able to do so.* Such documents are increasingly important when a life-threatening illness is being faced. In the best of circumstances, these documents attempt to carry out the decisions the patient has already made regarding terminal conditions and whether to prolong life. Advances in medicine allow patients' lives to be sustained even when they are unlikely to recover from a persistent and vegetative state. The **health care directive** and the **durable power of attorney for health care** allow patients to make decisions before becoming incapacitated on whether life-prolonging medical or surgical procedures are to be continued, withheld, or withdrawn, as well as if or when artificial feeding and fluids are to be used or withheld. These documents can help providers and patients talk about dying and open the door to a positive, caring approach to death. The health care directive and the durable power of attorney for health care documents are legal in all 50 states. Although states may vary somewhat in the wording of these documents, they provide the same overall benefit to patients (see Chapter 6 for more information.) The federal government passed the Patient Self-Determination Act in 1990, which gives all patients receiving care in institutions receiving payments from Medicare and Medicaid written information about their right to accept or refuse medical or surgical treatment. The act also requires that patients be given information about their options to create living wills and to appoint someone to act on their behalf in making health care decisions (durable power of attorney for health care). Any documents of this nature that the patient has should be copied in the medical chart that goes with the patient when admitted to the hospital. Whenever the patient makes a change in such a document, the old document is to be replaced with the new one.

4. *Finances are to be considered.* If there is medical insurance, what will be covered? Who makes the decisions in a managed care environment? What family resources can or will be used? Finances are no one's favorite subject, especially for providers. However, such a discussion is important. Often, patients fear not being able to meet their financial obligations and leaving large debts to surviving family members almost as much as the life-threatening illness itself. As a medical assistant, you can help patients understand the parameters of their health insurance and any restrictions there might be on particular illnesses or treatments. Can medical insurance be canceled if the patient's employer pays a portion of the health insurance and the patient is no longer able to work? If there is a life insurance policy, help patients determine if any portion of the policy can be used for end-of-life expenses. Any services you can provide to the patient or family members in relieving the financial stress can bring great relief to everyone involved.

5. *Emotional needs of the patient and their family members are important.* Emotional support is vital when dealing with a life-threatening illness. Health care professionals will want to determine the source of that support for the patient. Can a support system be suggested for the patient and family members? For some patients and families, an individual giving spiritual guidance is seen as a member of the family and as a member of the health care team. For others, no spiritual influence is recognized or sought. For some life-threatening illnesses, there are support systems specifically related to the particular illness, for example, cancer support groups that offer coping strategies and management of personal struggles.

It is not the responsibility of health care professionals treating the individual with life-threatening illness to provide all these services, but a health care professional who suggests that patients and families address these issues is more closely in tune with a patient's power in the illness.

Life-threatening illnesses are *family* illnesses. There are primary (the person suffering from the illness) and secondary (family and friends) patients. Stress on a spouse or partner is enormous as they think about taking over the other person's role and as they try to deal with their own feelings. The stress on parents faced with the possible death of a child is especially devastating. Patients and their families and friends often feel angry. The situation is especially tragic if it might have been avoided (for example, a long-time smoker dying of lung cancer or a family member paralyzed in a crash caused by a drunk driver). There needs to be time for everyone to grieve. Depression is common among patients with life-threatening illnesses and their families. Warning signs should be reported to the provider. Remember that how patients live their last days are just as important as the numbers on the laboratory reports.

THE RANGE OF PSYCHOLOGICAL SUFFERING

The range of suffering associated with a life-threatening illness is extensive. Patients feel extreme distress. Anxiety and depression are common. At the time of diagnosis, patients' responses may include denial, numbness, and an inability to face the facts. Sadness, hopelessness, helplessness, and withdrawal often are exhibited.

The range of psychological suffering often leads to physical symptoms, such as tension, tachycardia, agitation, insomnia, anorexia, and panic attacks. The provider may be so intent on treating the physical ramifications of the illness that the psychological suffering is mostly ignored.

Relationships of individuals with a life-threatening illness often change. Close friends may feel uncomfortable with someone who is dying. Some fear touching or caressing the dying patient and become aloof and distant. However, new friendships can often be made if patients meet others with the same or similar life-threatening issues and help maintain each other's self-esteem. Relationships are important because they provide support and encouragement beyond any other source. Patients experience a loss of self-esteem when they are ill, are in pain, and have a body that is failing them. When self-image is lost, patients feel useless,

see themselves as burdens, and have difficulty accepting help from anyone. The psychological effect of this "loss of self" can even hasten death.

It is often helpful to encourage patients to set goals for themselves. These can be small goals such as walking around the block, eating all their dinner, or connecting with a friend. The goals may also be much larger, such as staying alive until a son graduates from college, or putting all financial matters in order for surviving family members. Personal goals give the patient something other than the illness to plan for and work toward.

Communication

Carefully listening to patients and seeking clues for what *may not* be said is essential for the medical assistant and support staff caring for patients. Putting yourself in their shoes and asking what would be helpful is often beneficial. Be ready with a list of community resources that may benefit patients at this time.

It is not the intention of this chapter to specifically identify the many life-threatening illnesses and their particular needs, but some of the more common life-threatening diseases include coronary artery disease (CAD), chronic obstructive pulmonary disease (COPD), Alzheimer disease, and diabetes. Three of the most common life-threatening illnesses are identified in the following sections along with some specific information.

PATIENTS WITH CANCER

The first reaction patients with cancer usually have is the fear of loss of life. More than any other disease, patients think, "Cancer equals death. I am going to die." Following this reaction, issues begin to differ for each person. A few may choose no treatment and allow life to take its course. Most, however, will wonder about what treatment to choose, how to make that choice, and how effective it will be. Many patients are empowered by taking a major role in the decision making related to their cancer. Research can be helpful in studying the many options that may be available in treatment. The facts are that many patients diagnosed with cancer will die, whereas others diagnosed will live many years after diagnosis and treatment.

The three most widely known treatments of cancer are surgery, radiation, and chemotherapy. Often, treatment is a combination of the three. Patients can experience serious side effects from both radiation and chemotherapy. In today's world, there are other treatment options as well. They include hormone therapy, stem cell or bone

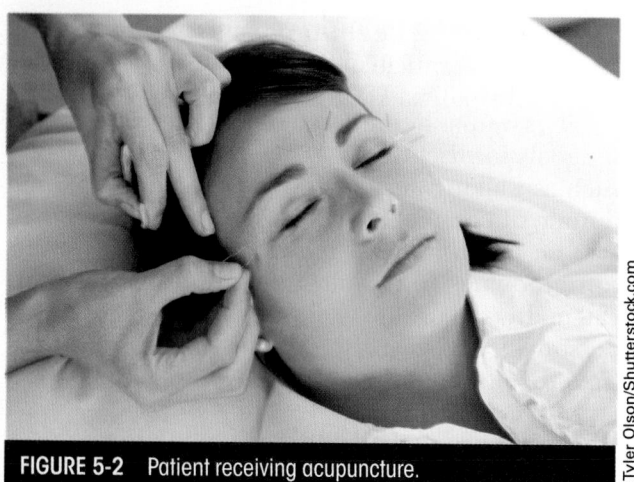

FIGURE 5-2 Patient receiving acupuncture.

marrow transplant, targeted therapy, and immunotherapy. Practitioners of complementary and integrative medicine have shown that many of their modalities can either enhance traditional treatment or ease their side effects. For instance, complementary practices that enhance the immune system give the body a stronger chance to overcome cancer cell growth. Meditation or acupuncture (Figure 5-2) can help ease the side effects for some patients. Loss of hair, nausea, vomiting, and pain are quite disconcerting to patients trying to cope, and they are relieved to find something that may be helpful. The American Cancer Society (http://www.cancer.org) has a number of resources for patients.

The most common signs and symptoms of advanced cancer are weakness, loss of appetite and weight, pain, nausea, constipation/diarrhea, sleepiness or confusion, and shortness of breath. Make certain patients understand your provider's willingness to relieve and treat these symptoms. Even when there is "nothing more to do" related to the cancer, there is still "much to do" to maintain comfort and to give patients the chance to do the things that are meaningful to them and their families.

PATIENTS WITH HIV/AIDS

Patients testing positive for human immunodeficiency virus (HIV) and those with acquired immune deficiency syndrome (AIDS) feel great stress from the infection, the disease, and the fear of other life-threatening illnesses. Some persons with HIV infection may have only a short time before the onset of AIDS; others may have a much longer period. AIDS is a disease that can have many periods of fairly good health and many periods of

serious near-death illnesses. Recent developments in the treatment of HIV infection and AIDS help patients to live much longer, but there is no cure and their lives are greatly compromised because of their suppressed immune system.

Complex criteria determine whether a patient's illness is identified as AIDS rather than HIV infection. Some providers prefer not to use the term *AIDS;* rather, they discuss the illness as early or later stage HIV infection. Many providers in the United States and around the world use the term *AIDS* when patients' CD4 counts (healthy T4 lymphocytes) decline to less than 200. (The average healthy individual will have D4 lymphocyte counts of 800 to 1,500.) Many developing countries in the world, however, are unable to measure CD4 counts. AIDS is then diagnosed by the symptoms and any immunodeficient illnesses the patients have. Using only a CD4 count for diagnosis can be quite discouraging for patients who monitor those counts quite closely. Also, a patient's CD4 count can decrease dramatically into the "AIDS zone" one time, and then increase in sufficient numbers to move the patient back into HIV infection another time. Other criteria that may identify an illness as AIDS are a particular type of opportunistic infection or tumor, an AIDS-related brain or lung illness, and severe body wasting. Allied health professionals will need to take the lead from their employers.

In the three decades since HIV was first diagnosed, the stigma attached to the illness has lessened only a little. In some cases, guilt develops over past behavior and lifestyles or the possibility of having transmitted the disease to others. Individuals with HIV infection may feel added strain if this is the first knowledge their families have of any high-risk behaviors they have that are associated with the transmission of the disease. When the disease is contracted by individuals who feel they are protected or safe from the disease, anger is paramount. HIV affects mostly individuals who are relatively young. Thus, they are not as likely to have substantial financial resources or permanent housing. Treating HIV is expensive, and many patients have little or no insurance coverage.

Patients with HIV may experience central nervous system involvement. Forgetfulness and poor concentration may be followed by psychomotor retardation, or the slowing of physical and mental responses, decreased alertness, apathy, withdrawal, and diminished interest in work. Some patients later experience confusion and progressive impairment of intellectual function or dementia. When HIV-infected patients contract other opportunistic diseases, those symptoms are experienced as well.

PATIENTS WITH END-STAGE RENAL DISEASE

Loss of kidney (renal) function leads to a serious illness known as end-stage renal disease (ESRD). When the kidneys fail completely, patients cannot live for long unless they receive dialysis or a kidney transplant. A successful kidney transplant relieves the person of kidney failure. However, there are not enough transplants for every person who needs one, and not all transplants are appropriate or successful. Dialysis is the process of artificially replacing the main functions of the kidneys—filtering blood to remove wastes (Figure 5-3). Choosing dialysis as a treatment plan can sustain life for years and is covered by Medicare, but it does have complications that burden patients and their caregivers.

Depending on age, a patient's general health, and other circumstances, some patients will opt not to have dialysis and to let death come from

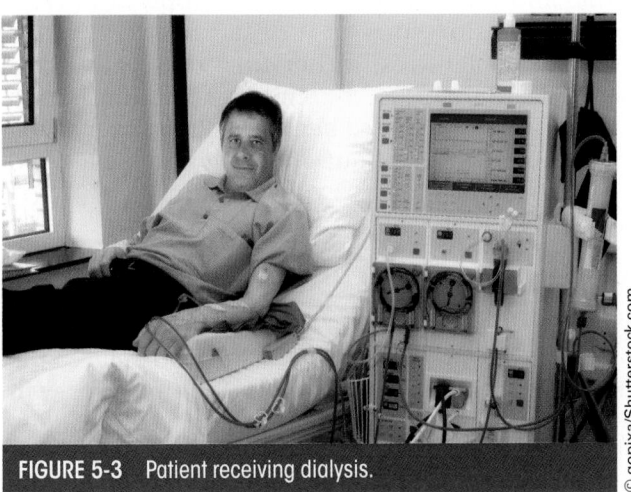

FIGURE 5-3 Patient receiving dialysis.

© gopixa/Shutterstock.com

kidney failure. The by-products of the body's chemistry accumulate in renal failure and cause an array of symptoms. Mild confusion and disorientation are common. Upsetting hallucinations or agitation can occur. Certain minerals concentrated in the blood can cause muscle twitching, tremors, and shakes. Some patients experience mild or severe itching. Appetite decreases early, and breathing can be rapid and shallow. Many patients with kidney failure pass little or no urine. Fluid overload results in edema, or swelling of the body, particularly of the legs and abdomen. Patients with some urine output may live for months even after stopping dialysis. People with no urine output are likely to die within a week or two. Patients will lose energy and become sleepy and lethargic. Typically, patients slip into a deeper sleep and gradually lose consciousness. Kidney failure has a reputation for being a gentle death.

THE THERAPEUTIC RESPONSE TO PATIENTS WITH LIFE-THREATENING ILLNESSES

Health care professionals will want to remember that when individuals face a danger such as a life-threatening illness, the brain's response of "flight or fight" kicks in before cognitive processes do. This means that patients often report hearing "nothing" after hearing the words "cancer" or some other feared diagnosis. Health care professionals who mostly focus on the cognitive data often miss a patient's reaction of surprise, shock, fear, and anger.

Presentation   Communication

For this reason, therapeutic health care professionals must carefully observe their patients' reactions. This is accomplished by being aware of the patient's displayed emotion and responding to it. Such a process is called empathy—putting yourself in the other person's shoes to imagine what her life is like under these circumstances. The therapeutic response then is to let your patients know you understand: "This has to be really difficult news to hear. I'm trying to imagine what this must be like for you." Then you assure patients that they have your support: "My team and I will help you every way we can through this process." Carrying out such a promise creates an openness in communication that is beneficial through the treatment of a life-threatening illness.

A word of caution here is to remind yourself that the tendency when caring for someone with a life-threatening illness is to care only for the patient's clinical needs, thus ignoring their very real needs as a human being whose life has been threatened to the core. Your compassion and empathy will go a long way in making life more meaningful and comfortable.

COMMUNICATION IN END-OF-LIFE CARE

Communication

There comes a time in a patient's life-threatening illness experience when a transition is made to end-of-life care. This may be when there are no further anticancer care options, and all treatment ceases. It may be when the antiviral medications so beneficial in the treatment of HIV are no longer effective. For patients with heart failure, it may be when the heart simply no longer functions properly. Either providers or their patients and family members may raise the issue of end-of-life care, but it can be an uncomfortable conversation either way. There is some research, however, that indicates that the majority of patients choose to have some control over the process.

Questions to help patients better verbalize their feelings might include the following:

- What is most important to you now that we have reached this stage?
- What are you hoping for?
- What plans, if any, have you made for this transition in your life?
- How can my team and I be of help?

The last question will help patients verbalize their wishes. Perhaps it is a discussion about comfort and lack of pain, not wanting to die on a machine in a vegetative state, or even donating organs after death. This stage is difficult at best for all involved, but following these guidelines fosters an atmosphere in which health care professionals will be remembered for their respectfulness, their attention to care and treatment, and their empathy.

THE STAGES OF GRIEF

Living with a life-threatening illness or making a transition to end-of-life care causes grief for both patients and family members. There are a number of different philosophies on grief and the stages patients are apt to experience when they know their lives are about to end, but none is so widely known as that of Dr. Elisabeth Kübler-Ross, who was one of the first to conduct research and determine possible stages of grief: denial, anger,

bargaining, depression, and acceptance. These stages are discussed in greater detail in the "Stages of Grief" Quick Reference Guide.

Dr. Kübler-Ross reminds health care professionals that while not all patients go through all five stages, some patients go through all five stages over and over again, each time with a little less stress. When moving through these stages multiple times, the grief and pain is most pronounced in the beginning, but gradually diminishes as grief is resolved. Others get stuck in one stage, usually denial. Grief and dying are very personal. No two patients will follow the same pattern. Family members also suffer grief and are often in different stages; therefore, it is often difficult for them to communicate and help each other.

Remember that grief work is exhausting. So much energy is spent in the grief process that it is often difficult to carry on day-to-day tasks. Any help that can be made available is appreciated.

The acronym TEAR is fairly popular and is often used to describe the grieving process. It has similarities to the five stages of grief:

T: To accept the reality of the loss

E: Experience the pain of the loss

A: Adjust to what was lost

R: Reinvest in a new reality

Although the five stages of grief and the TEAR stages discussed in this chapter are directed toward patients with life-threatening illnesses, remember that the family members and loved ones of patients also will experience grief. Both of these principles can be applied to any kind of serious loss that occurs in one's life—loss of a job, divorce, disaster, war, famine, loss of a limb or important body function, Alzheimer disease, loss of a friend, or even the death of a beloved pet. The stages of grief and the acronym TEAR can apply just as easily to these situations.

Dr. Kübler-Ross, in her final days before her own death in 2004, reminded her co-author to "Listen to the dying. They will tell you everything you need to know about when they are dying. And it is easy to miss."

THE CHALLENGE FOR THE MEDICAL ASSISTANT

Professional

As a medical assistant, you face the challenge of caring for people with life-threatening illnesses; you can comfort those who face great suffering and death. You will become a source of information

Stages of Grief

DENIAL

This is the stage where patients cannot believe that this is happening. They are likely to experience shock and dismay. If the grief is for the loss of a loved one, it is difficult for them to believe that the loved one is dead. If the grief is for themselves and some incident in their lives, they have a hard time accepting the reality of the loss. Words such as "I can't believe it is true" and "There must be some mistake" are common.

It is difficult to help someone in denial. You may be able to reaffirm the reality of the circumstances, but there is little you can do to move someone from the stage of denial.

ANGER

Patients express anger, sometimes openly and assertively. Other times, the anger is turned inward and is difficult to accurately express. Patients ask the question "Why?" and often need explanations of what is occurring. Anger is often expressed to others who have no idea what is happening in patients' lives.

When possible, this type of anger should be realized for what it is and never taken personally. Patients are angry at the event, not at you. Patients can be helped to express the anger in a realistic and nonhurtful manner.

BARGAINING

In this stage, patients bargain with God or a higher being and even their providers and express their desire to make a certain milestone in their lives. "If you can just get me through this current crisis so I can make it to my 40th wedding anniversary, I can accept what is happening." Goals can be very helpful to patients, and they can be encouraged to continue to set realistic goals during their grieving.

DEPRESSION

Patients who reach this stage are sad and sometimes quiet and withdrawn. There is a feeling that they have given up. They often prefer not to be around anyone. The depression can be and often is treated so that patients' grief is eased somewhat. This is true especially when patients remain in this stage for a very long time.

ACCEPTANCE

This is the time that patients accept the loss. If it is death that is being faced, they often feel they are ready. Everything is in place, and peace has been made with the prognosis. If a loss is being suffered, it is the time when patients begin to move on and make other plans for their lives and their future.

---

for patients and their support members. Be sensitive and respectful toward individuals who may be shunned by society. Examine your own beliefs, lifestyle, and biases so that you can be comfortable treating all patients, no matter what the illness is or how it was contracted.

As well as assisting your employer in providing the best possible medical care, you may be required to provide many nonmedical forms of assistance for patients suffering from life-threatening illnesses. You may need to make referrals to community-based agencies or service groups. Health departments, social workers, trained hospice volunteers, and AIDS and cancer volunteers may also be helpful to you, your patients, and their families.

The best therapeutic response to the patient with a life-threatening illness will build on the person's own culture and coping abilities, capitalize on strengths, maintain hope, and show continued care and concern. Patients may want up-to-date information on their disease; its causes, modes of transmission, and treatments available; and sources of care and social support. Honor their wishes. Be prepared to recommend support systems where patients can further discuss their feelings and express their concerns. Treat patients with concern and compassion and assure them everything will be done to provide continuity of care and relief from distress. Patients also may be encouraged to call on a spiritual advisor.

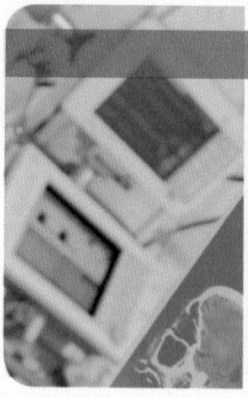

CASE STUDY 5-1

Refer to the scenario at the beginning of the chapter. As you prepare for the second visit of Suzanne Markis, you make a mental note of what kind of information you will have available.

CASE STUDY REVIEW

1. What paperwork might be necessary?
2. What questions might you have for Suzanne?
3. What might family members who may accompany Suzanne want to know?
4. As the medical assistant, how does your role differ from that of your employer?

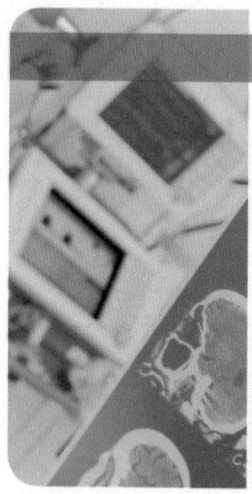

CASE STUDY 5-2

The extended family of Wong Lee is concerned about his illness and his care. Chronic obstructive pulmonary disease (COPD) has ravaged his body. He is on oxygen all the time now. He wants to remain at home to die; his family wants that, too. The family has been with him and has been involved in his care plan all along. However, you are uncertain of how much information to give to members of his extended family when they call.

CASE STUDY REVIEW

1. Are the questions that the extended family members raise intended to harm or help Mr. Lee?
2. Is there a durable power of attorney for health care in place?
3. Which, if any, of the family's desires are related to the culture?
4. What can you and your employer suggest to be of help to everyone involved?

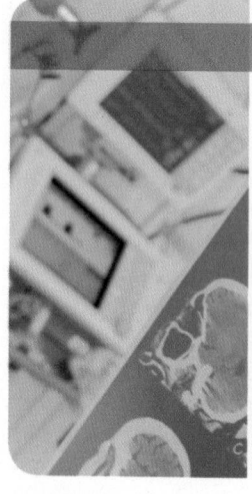

CASE STUDY 5-3

Jeff and Amy live in rural Tennessee. They are expecting their first baby and are excited beyond belief because they had so much trouble getting pregnant. You are the medical assistant for their family practice provider. Test results from their recent ultrasound have been returned to your clinic, and the news is not good. There appears to be some difficulty and one or more apparent birth defects in the developing fetus. You and your employer discuss possible resources.

CASE STUDY REVIEW

1. As the medical assistant, what is your first responsibility to these expectant parents?
2. Where might you look for possible resources?
3. Identify three to five possible resources.
4. If referral to a specialist is to be made, what role might you play in that referral?

Summary

- Note the differing expressions for "life-threatening" and recall the influence of cultural diversity on how an individual faces a serious or debilitating illness.

- Life-threatening illnesses create challenging and numerous options for decision making, such as type of treatment, if any; pain management; health care directives; financial concerns; and emotional needs of self and family.

- Grief and end-of-life decisions often result in anxiety, depression, sadness, helplessness, and withdrawal.

- Patients with ESRD, cancer, and AIDS will require special attention, understanding, and compassion.

- The best therapeutic response builds on a person's culture, coping abilities, and strengths. Recommend support systems and assure patients that everything will be done to provide continuity of care and relief from distress.

- Medical assistants will want to remember that when caring for patients with a life-threatening illness, having even the slightest fear of death can undermine the ability to respond professionally, with empathy and support.

- If you feel yourself losing the ability to be helpful, it is time to briefly step aside. This does not mean withdrawal from your position or refusal to care for your patients. It means that you do whatever is necessary so that your perspective is not lost.

- Take time to "fill up your psyche" and to give yourself a rest. If the ambulatory care setting has an abundance of patients with life-threatening illnesses, it may require that you spend some time in a support group of your own so that you are better able to cope.

- Never be afraid to feel sad or weep with your patients. It is better to sense their pain and, at times, feel the pain with them, than it is to be so clinically objective that you miss their true needs.

Study for Success

To reinforce your knowledge and skills of information presented in this chapter:

- Review the *Key Terms* and *Learning Outcomes*
- Consider the *Critical Thinking* features and *Case Studies* and discuss your conclusions
- Answer the questions in the *Certification Review*

CERTIFICATION REVIEW

1. When a practice treats patients with HIV/AIDS, cancer, or ESRD, what is it important for medical assistants to do?
   a. Warn other patients about the dangers of transmission
   b. Segregate these patient reception areas from other patient areas
   c. Be supportive and free of prejudice
   d. Deny any information to patients regarding the seriousness of the illness

2. What is characteristic of the Patient Self-Determination Act?
   a. It allows a patient to have a choice of providers.
   b. It ensures a patient's right to request a referral to another provider.
   c. It gives patients the right to formulate advance directives.
   d. It ensures that Medicare and/or Medicaid can help pay for treatment.
   e. It allows patients to choose their hospital care plan.

3. Who or what is the strongest influence on a patient with a life-threatening illness?
   a. The provider
   b. The hospital
   c. The patient
   d. The family

4. How is life-threatening illness best defined?
   a. A life shortened because of illness or disease
   b. An illness that is harmful but not dangerous
   c. An illness serious enough to require hospitalization
   d. An illness that makes palliative care improbable
   e. An illness that begins in childhood

5. How might a patient's culture affect his or her view of a life-threatening illness?
   a. It will have no impact on a patient's decisions.
   b. It can cause a patient to be accepting, denying, or even defiant of death.
   c. It will determine the type of care or pain medication used.
   d. It will dictate care outside the United States for treatment.
6. Which of the following statements is true regarding therapeutic communication with a patient with a life-threatening illness?
   a. It is no different than communicating with any patient.
   b. It comes naturally and requires no special skill.
   c. It is heightened and considered more challenging.
   d. It is left to nonmedical support staff.
   e. It often is unappreciated.
7. What is an appropriate therapeutic response to a patient with a life-threatening illness?
   a. I hope you'll feel better soon.
   b. You can conquer this; don't let it get you down.
   c. Everything will be fine once treatment begins.
   d. I'm having a hard time imagining how I might feel in your shoes.
8. What does a durable power of attorney for health care accomplish?
   a. It enables someone other than the patient to make only health care decisions.
   b. It enables someone other than the patient to make any decisions for the patient.
   c. It makes certain that patients' financial responsibilities are met.
   d. It makes certain an attorney's wishes are followed.
   e. It prevents hospitals from using experimental treatment.
9. Which stage of grief attempts to negotiate an event or experience?
   a. Acceptance
   b. Depression
   c. Denial
   d. Bargaining
10. What might effective pain management depend upon?
   a. The patient's wishes and needs
   b. The patient's loss of self-image
   c. Professional nursing criteria
   d. The patient's range of psychological suffering
   e. Insurance allowance for pain control

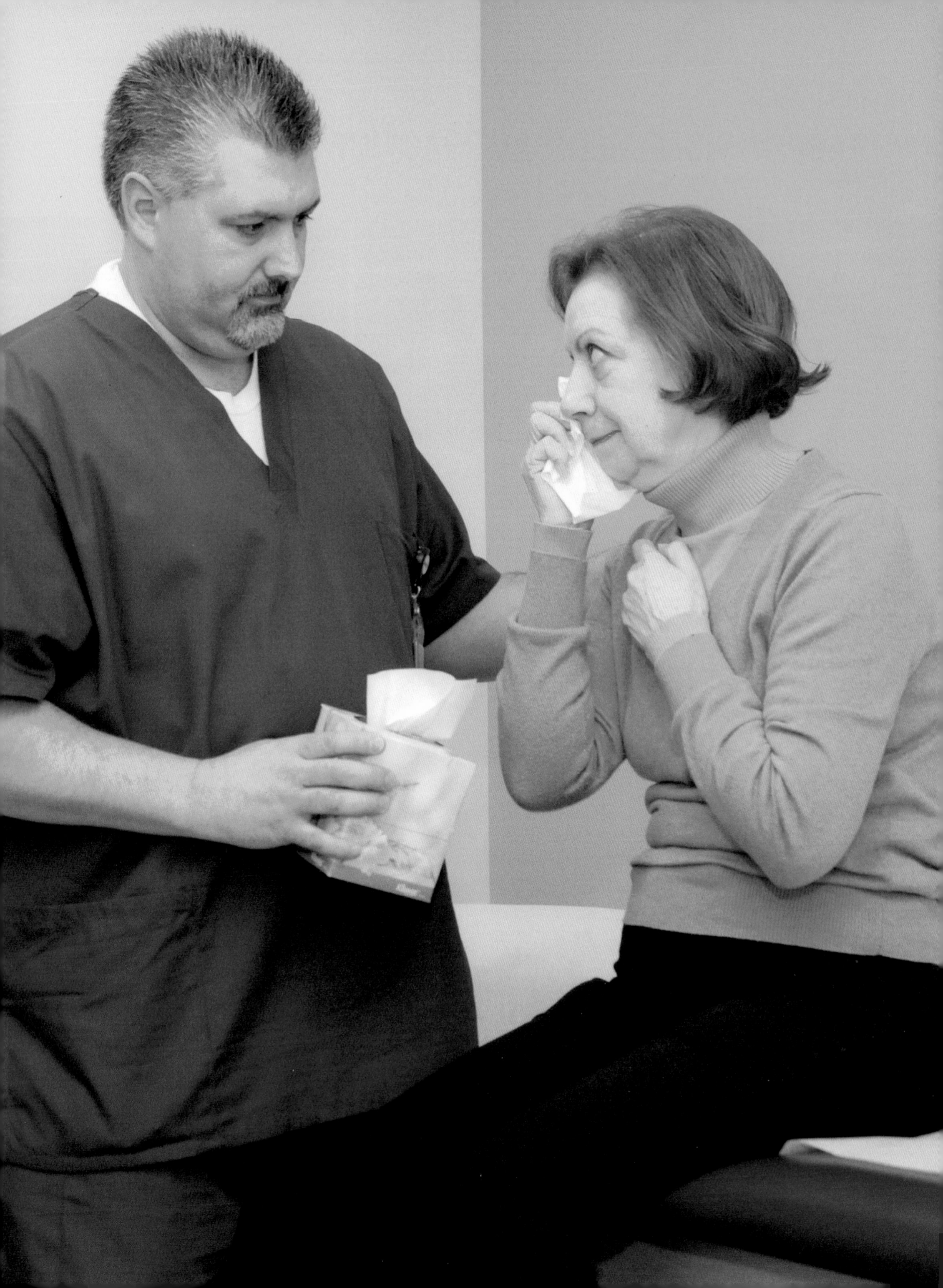

UNIT III
RESPONSIBLE MEDICAL PRACTICE

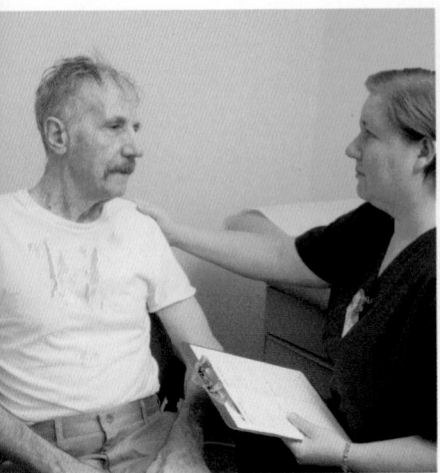
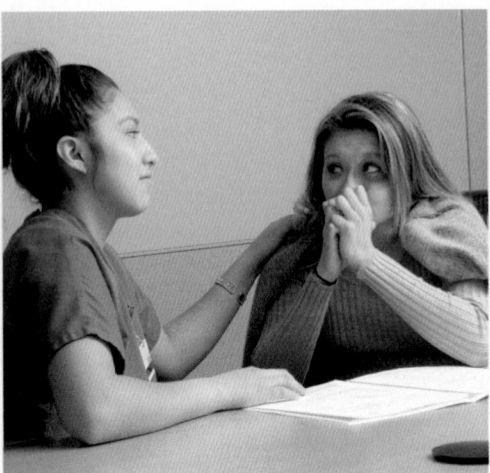
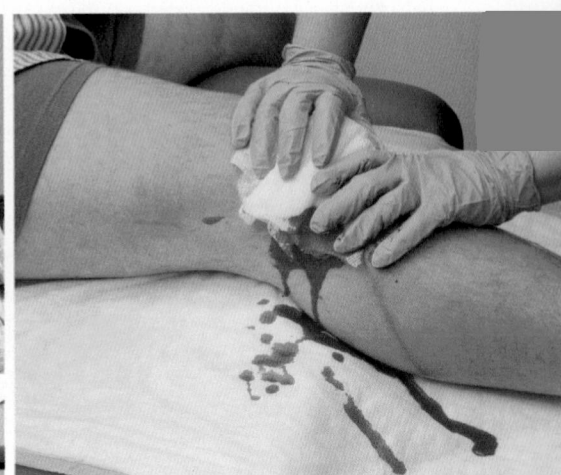

ATTRIBUTES OF PROFESSIONALISM

The professional medical assistant will understand the absolute necessity for abiding by all laws pertinent to outpatient care, and serving with the utmost moral integrity and absolute ethical behavior. Prior to entering into the profession, professional medical assistants must examine their prejudices and biases and realize that even when there is a difference of beliefs and personal ethics between the patient and the professional, bias can never enter into the care of that patient.

It is also imperative that the professional medical assistant maintain current first aid certification and understand how and when to give first aid both within the facility and when in public. You must never attempt to perform any procedure outside your scope of training, knowledge, and experience.

As a true professional medical assistant, you will maintain your personal integrity and practice within your personal ethical boundaries, always treating patients with compassion and understanding. In emergency circumstances, you will act appropriately,

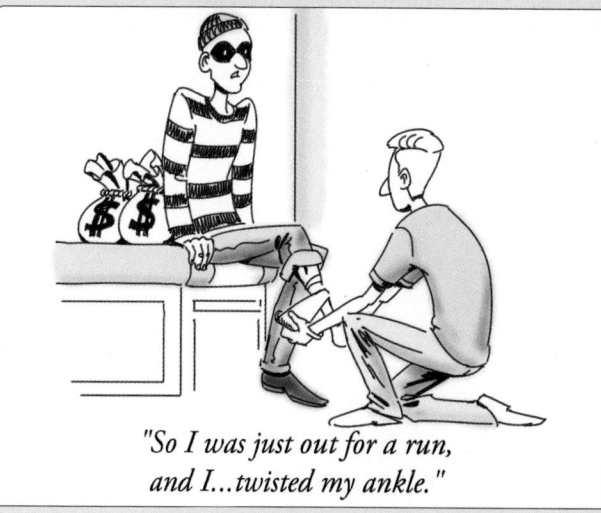

"So I was just out for a run, and I...twisted my ankle."

keeping in mind the patient's immediate safety and comfort, and understanding when additional assistance is needed.

Listed below are a series of questions to ask yourself and to serve as your professionalism checklist. As you interact with patients and colleagues, these questions will help to guide you in the professional behavior that is expected every day from medical assistants.

Ask Yourself

COMMUNICATION
- ☐ Do I apply active listening skills?
- ☐ Do I display professionalism through written and verbal communication?
- ☐ Do I demonstrate appropriate nonverbal communication?
- ☐ Do I display appropriate body language?
- ☐ Does my knowledge allow me to speak easily with all members of the health care team?

PRESENTATION
- ☐ Am I dressed and groomed appropriately?
- ☐ Do I display a positive attitude?
- ☐ Do I display a calm, professional, and caring manner?
- ☐ Do I demonstrate empathy to the patient?

COMPETENCY
- ☐ Do I pay attention to detail?
- ☐ Do I ask questions if I am out of my comfort zone or do not have the experience to carry out tasks?
- ☐ Do I display sound judgment?
- ☐ Am I knowledgeable and accountable?
- ☐ Do I recognize the physical and emotional effects on persons involved in an emergency situation?
- ☐ Do I demonstrate self-awareness in responding to an emergency situation?

INITIATIVE
- ☐ Do I show initiative?
- ☐ Have I developed a strategic plan to achieve my goals? Is my plan realistic?
- ☐ Do I seek out opportunities to expand my knowledge base?
- ☐ Am I flexible and dependable?

INTEGRITY
- ☐ Do I demonstrate the principles of self-boundaries?
- ☐ Do I work within my scope of practice?
- ☐ Do I demonstrate respect for individual diversity?
- ☐ Do I recognize the impact personal ethics and morals have on the delivery of health care?
- ☐ Do I protect and maintain confidentiality?
- ☐ Do I maintain moral and ethical standards?
- ☐ Do I do the "right thing" even when no one is observing?

CHAPTER 6

Legal Considerations

1. Define and spell the key terms as presented in the glossary.
2. Briefly describe the five sources of law, differentiating between civil and criminal law.
3. Recall at least seven of the nine administrative law acts important to the medical profession.
4. Outline the implications of HIPAA for the medical assistant.
5. Paraphrase administering, prescribing, and dispensing of controlled substances.
6. Describe the measures to take for disposal of controlled substances.
7. Discuss licensure renewal and revocation for physicians.
8. Follow established policies when initiating or terminating medical treatment.
9. List and characterize the four Ds of negligence.
10. Distinguish provider and medical assistant roles in terms of standard of care.
11. Identify three common torts that can occur in the outpatient care setting and what constitutes each one.
12. Discuss informed consent and classify types of minors.
13. Evaluate at least 10 practices to help in risk management.
14. Outline the necessary steps in civil litigation, including how and when subpoenas are used.
15. Recall special considerations for patients related to issues of confidentiality, the statute of limitations, and public duties.
16. Describe procedures to follow in reporting abuse.
17. Discuss Good Samaritan laws.
18. Recall maintenance of advance directives in the ambulatory care setting.

KEY TERMS

administer
administrative law
agents
alternative dispute resolution (ADR)
arbitration
civil law
common law
constitutional law
contract law
criminal law
defendant
deposition
discovery
dispense
durable power of attorney for health care
emancipated minors

expert witness
expressed consent
expressed contract
felony
Health Insurance Portability and Accountability Act (HIPAA)
implied consent
implied contract
incompetence
informed consent
interrogatory
intimate partner violence (IPV)
libel
litigation
malfeasance
malpractice
mature minors
mediation

medically indigent
minor
misdemeanor
misfeasance
negligence
noncompliant
nonfeasance
Patient Self-Determination Act (PSDA)
plaintiff
precedents
prescribe
risk management
slander
statutory law
subpoena
tort
tort law

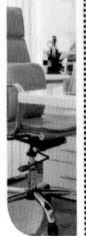

Marilyn, the clinic manager at Inner City Health Care, is reviewing some concerns in a staff meeting. Even though each employee is well aware of privacy, confidentiality, and the many ways their actions are legally binding, Marilyn notices occasional carelessness creeping into their busy activities. Marilyn has heard voices of staff from the hallway discussing confidential matters and notices the staff carrying on personal conversations in the presence of patients. As well as reviewing HIPAA compliance, Marilyn spends some time discussing the importance of focusing all attention on patients.

Chapter Portal

The law as it relates to health care has grown increasingly complex in the last decade. The agendas of federal and state governments include an investigation of quality health care, a desire to control health care costs (while hoping to ensure equitable access to health care), and an interest in protecting the patient. The Patient Protection and Affordable Care Act of 2010 further added to this complexity. Today's medical assistant must have knowledge of federal, state, and local laws related to health care. A full discussion of health law requires several volumes; therefore, the aim of this chapter is awareness of the law and its implications and establishment of sound practices and procedures to both safeguard patient rights and protect the health care professional.

SOURCES OF LAW

Legal

Law is a binding custom or ruling for conduct that is enforceable by an agency assigned that authority. Laws come from state statutes, common law, both civil and criminal laws, administrative law agencies, and contract and tort law. The highest authority in the United States is the U.S. Constitution. Adopted in 1787, this document provides the framework for the U.S. government. The Constitution includes 27 amendments, 10 of which are known as the Bill of Rights. This authority is sometimes referred to as **constitutional law**. The U.S. Constitution calls for three branches of the federal government:

- *Executive branch.* The president and vice president (elected by U.S. citizens), cabinet officers, and various other departments of the federal government.
- *Legislative branch.* Members of the U.S. Senate and the House of Representatives (elected by U.S. citizens) and the staffs of individual legislators and legislative committees.
- *Judicial branch.* The courts, including the U.S. Supreme Court, courts of appeals for the nine judicial regions, and district courts.

Laws enacted at the federal level are often referred to as acts or laws, or by a specific title. An example is Title XIX of Public Law, the Social Security Act, established in 1967 to provide health care for the **medically indigent**. This program is known as Medicaid. Federal law is the supreme law of the land.

Statutory Law

The body of laws made by states is known as **statutory law**. Constitutions in the 50 states identify the rights and responsibilities of their citizens and identify how their state is organized. States have a governor as the head and state legislatures (both elected by the state's citizens), as well as their own court systems with a number of levels. All powers that are not conferred specifically on the federal government are retained by the state, yet states vary widely in their interpretation of that power. State law cannot override the power of any laws defined in the U.S. Constitution or its amendments, although states often attempt to do so. State statutes commonly include practice acts for doctors and nurses. Some identify licensure or certification requirements for medical assistants, also. These practice acts broadly define the scope of practice for the profession as well as licensure and/or certification requirements.

Common Law

Common law is not so easily defined but is essential to understanding law in the United States. Common law was developed by judges in England and France over many centuries and was brought to the United States with the early settlers. Common law is often called judge-made law. The law consists of rulings made by judges who base their decisions on a combination of a number of factors: (1) individual decisions of a court, (2) interpretation of the U.S. Constitution or a particular state constitution, and (3) statutory law. These decisions become known as **precedents** and often lay down the foundation for subsequent legal rulings.

Criminal Law

Criminal law addresses wrongs committed against the welfare and safety of society as a whole. Criminal law affects relationships between individuals and between individuals and the government. Another term that might be used to describe a criminal act is *malfeasance*. **Malfeasance** is conduct that is illegal or contrary to an official's obligation. Criminal offenses generally are classified into the basic categories of a **felony** or a **misdemeanor** that are specifically defined in statutes.

Felonies are more serious crimes and include murder, larceny or thefts of large amounts of money, assault, and rape. Punishment for a felony is more serious than for a misdemeanor. A convicted felon cannot vote, hold public office, or own any weapons. Felonies often are divided into groups such as first degree (most serious), second degree, and third degree. Sentences are generally for longer than one year and are served in a penitentiary. Misdemeanors are considered lesser offenses and vary from state to state. Punishment may include probation or a time of service to the community, a fine, or a jail sentence in a city or county facility. Misdemeanors also can be divided into groups or classifications, such as A, B, or C class misdemeanors, denoting the seriousness of the crime (Class A is the most serious).

For a person to be found guilty of a crime, a judge or jury must prove the evidence against the individual "beyond a reasonable doubt." In a criminal case, charges are brought against an individual by the state with the intent of preventing any further harm to society. For example, a physician practicing medicine without a proper license may be subject to criminal action by the courts for endangering a patient's life.

Civil Law

Civil law affects relationships between individuals, corporations, government bodies, and other organizations. Terms that may be used in civil law are **misfeasance**, referring to a lawful act that is improperly or unlawfully executed, and **nonfeasance**, referring to the failure to perform an act, official duty, or legal requirement. The punishment for a civil wrong is usually monetary in nature. When a charge is brought against a **defendant** in a civil case, the goal is to reimburse the **plaintiff** or the person bringing charges with a monetary amount for suffering, pain, and any loss of wages. Another goal might be to make certain the defendant is prevented from engaging in similar behavior again. In civil law, cases need to show that a "preponderance of the evidence" is more than likely true against the defendant. The most common forms of civil law that directly affect the medical profession are administrative law, contract law, and **tort law**.

ADMINISTRATIVE LAW

Legal

Administrative law establishes agencies that are given power to specialize and enact regulations that have the force of law. The Internal Revenue Service is an example of an administrative agency that enacts tax laws and regulations. Health care professionals are bound by federal administrative law through the Medicare and Medicaid program rules administered by the Social Security Administration.

There are a number of other regulations in administrative law governing health professionals and their employees. It is important that medical assistants be informed of legislation and any federal or state regulations that are critical to patients and the medical profession. Identified here with a brief description are a number of administrative acts, some of which also are referred to in other chapters in this textbook.

Affordable Care Act and Patients' Bill of Rights

Congress passed the Affordable Care Act (ACA) and President Obama signed the act into law on March 23, 2010. In June 2012, the U.S. Supreme Court upheld the law as constitutional. Commonly referred to as Obamacare, the law has 10 titles or sections and includes the following provisions: (1) ending preexisting condition exclusions for children, (2) keeping young adults covered under parents' health care plans until age 26, (3) preventing insurers from cancelling coverage due to honest errors, (4) guaranteeing the right to appeal, (5) ending lifetime coverage limits, (6) reviewing premium increases, (7) maximizing services for premium dollars, (8) covering recommended preventive health care services, (9) allowing choice of primary care provider from a plan's network, and (10) removing insurance barriers to emergency services.

The ACA also provides for the Patients' Bill of Rights to make certain that patients receive all the benefits of the law. Today, health care providers, clinics, and hospitals provide a document outlining these benefits to their patients. Providers can vary in their approach, but must cover all the aspects of the 2010 law. Many of the documents also include a statement on the patient's responsibilities. See Chapter 7 for further discussion, and do a Web search for sample documentation.

The Civil Rights Act

Title VII of the Civil Rights Act of 1964 protects employees from discrimination. The act states that an employer with 15 or more employees must not discriminate in matters of employment related to age, sex, race, creed, marital status, national origin, color, or disabilities. (Some states are more restrictive in their laws and identify employers with 8 or more employees.)

Through the years, many additions have been made. They include such topics as voting rights, fair housing, and unlawful harassment in the workplace. The Genetic Information Nondiscrimination Act (GINA) was passed in 2008 and prohibits the use of genetic information in employment and health insurance decisions. This amendment was added in order to protect individuals from the misuse of genetic information brought about by the ever-increasing expansion and advances in the use of genetics in medicine.

The Equal Employment Opportunity Commission (EEOC) enforces Title VII and provides oversight of equal employment regulation and policies. The Departments of Labor, Health and Human Services, and the Treasury have responsibility for issuing regulations addressing the use of genetic information in health insurance. Although some health care settings have fewer than 15 or even 8 employees, it is best to follow state and federal guidelines on all matters of employment.

Currently, 22 states have laws banning employment discrimination because of sexual orientation. Those states are California, Colorado, Connecticut, Delaware, Hawaii, Illinois, Iowa, Maine, Maryland, Massachusetts, Minnesota, Nevada, New Hampshire, New Jersey, New Mexico, New York, Oregon, Rhode Island, Utah, Vermont, Washington, and Wisconsin. The District of Columbia, Guam, and Puerto Rico have passed similar legislation.

Harassment. Included in Title VII is an employee's protection from sexual harassment and a hostile work environment.

Harassment occurs when sexual favors are implied or requested by a supervisor in return for job advancement or special treatment on the job. Another form of harassment and a more common problem that may exist in the workplace is referred to as a hostile work environment. A hostile work environment exists when pervasive or severe sexual comments, jokes, or inappropriate touching create a workplace so negative that it interferes with an employee's work performance.

A written policy on sexual harassment detailing inappropriate behavior and stating specific steps to be taken to correct an inappropriate situation should be established. The policy will include (1) a statement that harassment is not tolerated, (2) a statement that an employee who feels harassed needs to bring the matter to the immediate attention of a person designated in the policy, (3) a statement about the confidentiality of any incidents and specific disciplinary action against the harasser, and (4) the procedure to follow when harassment occurs.

It is illegal for a supervisor or employer to ignore an employee's complaint. An employer or supervisor who does not take corrective action is liable. The EEOC guidelines make the employer strictly liable for the acts of supervisory employees, as well as for some acts of harassment by coworkers and clients (see Chapter 45).

Equal Pay Act of 1963

Ambulatory health care clinics may not have as much of an issue with this act as some other places of employment, but it is important to note. The Equal Pay Act (EPA) of 1963 protects men and women in the same place of business who perform substantially the same work with substantially equal skill, effort, and responsibility from sex-based wage discrimination. In other words, the starting salary for two medical assistants of the opposite sex is to be the same when they are performing essentially the same job with equal skill and experience under similar working conditions.

Federal Age Discrimination Act

The Federal Age Discrimination in Employment Act of 1967 protects certain individuals 40 years and older from discrimination based on their age in matters of employment, promotion, discharge, compensation, or privileges of employment. This act has become increasingly important as individuals are working longer and seeking employment in their later years. Age restriction may be applied *only* when required by law. For instance, servers of alcohol must be 21 years of age. Valid reasons to decline applicants for employment include (1) health issues that may interfere with the safe and efficient performance of the job, (2) unavailability for the work schedule of the particular job, (3) insufficient training or experience to perform the duties of the particular job, and (4) someone else is better qualified.

Americans with Disabilities Act

The Americans with Disabilities Act (ADA) of 1990 prohibits discrimination that prevents individuals who have physical or mental disabilities from accessing public services and accommodations, employment, and telecommunications. A disability implies that a physical or mental impairment substantially limits one or more of an individual's major life activities. ADA is identified in five titles. Title I, enforced by the EEOC, prohibits discrimination in employment (see Chapter 45 for further details). Essentially, Title I requires a potential employer to identify and prove that certain disabilities cannot be accommodated in performing the job requirements. Employers only have to provide reasonable accommodations rather than anything an employee demands or something that is extraordinarily expensive. Individuals who formerly abused drugs and alcohol and those who are undergoing rehabilitation also are covered by the ADA and cannot be denied employment because of their history of substance abuse.

Titles II, III, and IV mandate access to public services, public accommodations, and telecommunications for individuals with disabilities. The ADA protects persons with HIV infection or AIDS, making certain they cannot be refused treatment by health care professionals because of their health status. Generally speaking, health care professionals with HIV infection or AIDS cannot be kept from providing treatment either, unless that treatment could be found to be a significant risk to others. Title V covers a number of miscellaneous issues such as exclusions from the definition of *disability*, retaliation, insurance, and other issues. Again, the ADA applies to businesses with at least 15 employees, but some states have more stringent laws.

Of note is the 2008 amendment to the ADA, known as the Americans with Disabilities Act Amendments Act (ADAAA). In this act, Congress made it easier for individuals seeking protection under the ADA to establish their disability by broadening the scope of the term *disability*. Disability is now defined as a physical or mental impairment that substantially limits one or more major life activities. For example, individuals formerly denied protection from impairments caused by cancer, diabetes, and epilepsy can now be covered. For greater detail on the ADAAA, go to https://www.eeoc.gov and search for "ADAAA Fact Sheet."

Family and Medical Leave Act

The Family and Medical Leave Act (FMLA) of 1993 is important for large ambulatory care centers and hospitals. FMLA requires all public employers and any private employer of 50 or more employees to provide up to 12 weeks of job-protected, unpaid leave each year for the following reasons: (1) birth and care of the employee's child, or placement for adoption or foster care of a child; (2) care of an immediate family member who has a serious health condition; and (3) care of the employee's own serious health issue. Employees must have been employed for at least 12 months and have worked at least 1,250 hours in the 12 months preceding the beginning of the FMLA leave. Effective March 2015, the definition of spouse under FLMA covers employees in legal same-sex marriages, regardless of where they live.

Health Insurance Portability and Accountability Act

The **Health Insurance Portability and Accountability Act (HIPAA)** of 1996 required the Department of Health and Human Services to adopt national standards for electronic health care transactions. The law also required the adoption of privacy and security standards to protect an individual's identifiable health information. This mandate required greater protection of a patient's protected health information (PHI). The privacy of telephone conversations, all verbal exchanges, and all written data regarding a patient must be assured. The goal of HIPAA was also to assist in making health insurance more affordable and accessible to individuals by protecting health insurance coverage for workers and their families when they change or lose their jobs.

HIPAA law is identified in seven titles. They are summarized briefly as follows:

I. *Health insurance access, portability, and renewal.* Increases the portability of health insurance, allows continuance and transfer of insurance even with preexisting conditions, and prohibits discrimination based on health status.

II. *Preventing health care fraud and abuse.* Establishes a fraud and abuse system and spells out penalty if either event is documented; improves the Medicare program through establishing standards; establishes standards for electronic transmission of health information.

III. *Tax-related provisions.* Promotes the use of medical savings accounts (MSAs) to be used for medical expenses only. Deposits are tax-deductible for self-employed individuals who are able to draw on the accounts for medical expenses.

IV. *Group health plan requirements.* Identifies how group health care plans must provide for portability, access, and transferability of health insurance for their members.

V. *Revenue offsets.* Details how HIPAA changed the Internal Revenue Code to generate more revenue for HIPAA expenses.

VI. *General provisions.* Explains how coordination with Medicare-type plans must be carried out to prevent duplication of coverage.

VII. *Assuring portability.* Ensures employee coverage from one plan to another; written specifically for health insurance plans to ensure portability of coverage.

As of April 21, 2006, all covered health care entities were required to be in compliance of HIPAA's privacy regulations. Government and industry allocated billions of dollars to electronic medical records software and the transfer of the paper medical record to the digitized format through the Health Information Technology for Economic and Clinical Health (HITECH) Act. (See IV above.) Federal stimulus money approved in 2009 helped underwrite the cost to clinics or hospitals that serve Medicare and Medicaid patients when their electronic medical records software meets the required standards for sharing information between proprietary networks.

Occupational Safety and Health Act

Safety

The Occupational Safety and Health (OSH) Act of 1967 is a division of the U.S. Department of Labor. Its mission is to ensure that a workplace is safe and has a healthy environment. Penalties assessed by OSHA can be quite high for repeated and willful

violations. (OSH Act refers to the actual law, while OSHA refers to the administration or group of individuals who oversee and govern the law.) Among these guidelines are those that make certain all employees know what chemicals they are handling, know how to reduce any health risks from hazardous chemicals that are labeled 1 to 4 for severity, and have Safety Data Sheets (SDSs) listing every ingredient in the product. Other sections of this law protecting medical assistants and patients are detailed in additional chapters. They include the Clinical Lab Improvement Amendments of 1988 (CLIA) (see Chapter 37), the Bloodborne Pathogens Standard of July 1992 (see Chapter 21), and the Needlestick Prevention Amendment of 2001 (see Chapter 21).

Controlled Substances Act

The Controlled Substances Act of 1970 became effective in 1971. The act is administered by the Drug Enforcement Administration (DEA) under the auspices of the U.S. Department of Justice. The Controlled Substances Act lists controlled drugs in five schedules (I, II, III, IV, and V) according to their potential for abuse and dependence, with Schedule I having the greatest abuse potential and no accepted medical use in the United States. In the most recent years, there has been a move to either declassify or reclassify marijuana from its Schedule I listing—the highest potential for abuse. The Drug Policy Alliance of New York stresses scientific research that confirms marijuana's medical benefits and its wide margin of safety. Yet, the DEA and the National Institute on Drug Abuse (NIDA) continue to block any attempt to allow marijuana to be marked as a prescription medication. This issue is further complicated by the number of states that have legalized marijuana, against federal regulations.

The Controlled Substances Act and the U.S. Code of Federal Regulations regulate individuals who **administer**, **prescribe**, or **dispense** any drug listed in the five schedules. Any individual who administers, prescribes, or dispenses any controlled substance must be registered with the DEA. The DEA supplies a form for registration and mandates that renewal occur every 3 years.

A provider who prescribes only Schedules II, III, IV, and V controlled substances in the lawful course of professional practice is not required to keep separate records of those transactions. The majority of providers fall within this category. Providers who regularly administer controlled substances in Schedules II, III, IV, and V or who dispense controlled substances are required to keep specific records of each transaction.

For those providers who dispense or administer controlled substances, an inventory must be taken every 2 years of all stocks of any controlled substances on hand. The inventory must include (1) a list of the name, address, and DEA registration number of the provider; (2) the date and time of the inventory; and (3) the signatures of the individuals taking the inventory. This inventory must be kept at the location identified on the registration certificate for at least 2 years. All Schedule II drug records must be maintained separate from all other controlled substance records. These records must be made available for inspection and copying by duly authorized officials of the DEA. Some state requirements are even more restrictive than the federal requirements.

Any necessary disposal of controlled substances, usually occurring when they become outdated or when a medical practice is closed, requires specific action. The provider's DEA number and registration certificate should be returned to the DEA. Specific guidelines for destruction of the controlled substances will need to be obtained from the nearest divisional office for the DEA. Using the Internet, search using "Controlled Substances Act of 1970" for a listing of sites providing more information. You will find a listing of drugs in each of the five schedules. The listing changes from time to time as new drugs come on the market and are classified. (See Chapter 34 for additional details.)

Uniform Anatomical Gift Act

The Uniform Anatomical Gift Act of 1968 allows persons 18 years and older who are of sound mind to make a gift of all or any part of their body (1) to any hospital, surgeon, or physician; (2) to any accredited medical or dental school, college, or university; (3) to any organ bank or storage facility; and (4) to any specified individual for education, research, advancement of medical/dental science, therapy, or transplantation. The gift may be noted in a will or by signing, in the presence of two witnesses, a donor's card. Some states allow these statements on the driver's license. There is no cost to donors or their families for gifts of all

or part of the body, and there is a great need for organ donors in this country.

Regulation Z of the Consumer Protection Act

Regulation Z of the Consumer Protection Act of 1967, referred to as the Truth in Lending Act, requires that an agreement by providers and their patients for payment of medical bills in more than four installments must be in writing and must provide information on any finance charge (see Chapter 19). This act is enforced by the Federal Trade Commission. These guidelines are often seen in fee-for-service plans in prearrangements for surgery or prenatal care and delivery, because patients may not be able to pay the entire fee in one payment.

Medical Practice Acts

Each state has medical practice acts that regulate the practice of medicine with the intent of protecting its citizens from harm. These statutes govern licensure, standards of care, professional liability and negligence, confidentiality, and torts. Table 6-1 summarizes licensure, renewal, and revocation rules for medical doctors. Medical assistants sometimes are asked to maintain their employer's records of continuing education for license renewal and to process the renewal at the proper time. In some states, the renewal may be done online if the license is active and in good standing.

TABLE 6-1

LICENSURE, RENEWAL, AND REVOCATION FOR MEDICAL DOCTORS

LICENSURE	RENEWAL	REVOCATION
Completion of medical education	Payment of a fee	Conviction of a crime
Completion of internship	Documentation of continuing medical education (CME)	Unprofessional conduct
Passing the U.S. Medical Licensing Examination (USMLE)	CMEs might include appropriate medical reading, teaching health professionals, and attending conferences and workshops	Personal or professional incapacity

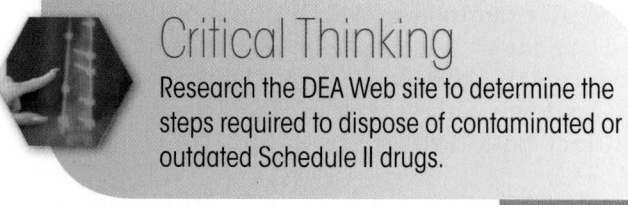

Critical Thinking

Research the DEA Web site to determine the steps required to dispose of contaminated or outdated Schedule II drugs.

PROCEDURE 6-1

Identifying a State's Legal Scope of Practice for Medical Assistants

Procedure

PURPOSE:

To determine a medical assistant's scope of practice in the state where employment will take place.

EQUIPMENT/SUPPLIES:

Computer and Internet access

PROCEDURE STEPS:

1. Research the scope of practice for medical assistants in the state assigned to you by your instructor (sources to consider include local AAMA, AMA, and state statutes). RATIONALE: Allows students to learn about various states' rules and regulations regarding scope of practice for medical assistants.

2. Report your findings for your particular state in a summary that can be shared with the class. RATIONALE: Informs students of as many states' regulations as possible.

3. From your assigned state's report, identify any skills learned in your education that you will not legally be able to perform. RATIONALE: Demonstrates any limitations placed on medical assistants by state.

States also may regulate personnel who are employed in the outpatient care setting. Generally, medical assistants perform their duties and responsibilities under the direct supervision of the physician or doctor, and therefore are governed by medical practice acts or the state board of medical examiners. Medical assistants employed and supervised by independent nurse practitioners are governed by the nurse practice acts and the state board of nursing. Other health professionals, such as chiropractors and naturopaths, may have separate practice acts as well. Medical assistants employed by these practitioners will need to be knowledgeable of those laws. Some states require that medical assistants be licensed or certified to perform any invasive procedures. Other states require additional education and training in radiology for the medical assistant to be able to take radiographs. Furthermore, there are still a few states so strict in their regulations that medical assistants mostly perform clerical functions and noninvasive clinical duties.

  Certainly, medical assistants desiring to use their skills must be aware of state regulations and always perform only within the scope of those regulations as well as their education and

Competency   Integrity   Procedure

professional preparation. Medical assistants will want to be as diligent as any other health professional about maintaining their certification, registration, and licensure and should monitor any legislation that pertains to licensure or certification (see Procedure 6-1).

CONTRACT LAW

The contractual nature of the provider–patient relationship necessitates a discussion of contracts, which are an important part of any medical practice. A contract is a binding agreement between two or more persons. A provider has a legal obligation, or duty, to care for a patient under the principles of **contract law**. The agreement must be between competent persons to do or not to do something lawful in exchange for a payment.

A contract exists when the patient arrives for treatment and the provider accepts the patient by providing treatment. An example of a valid contract occurs when a patient calls the office or clinic to make an appointment for an annual physical examination. Assuming both provider and patient are competent, and that the provider performs the lawful act of the physical examination and the patient pays a fee, all aspects of the contract exist.

There are two types of contracts: expressed and implied. An **expressed contract** can be written or verbal and specifically describes what each party in the contract will do. A written contract requires that all necessary aspects of the agreement be in writing. Examples of a written contract in the medical environment include a third party's agreement to pay a patient's bill, or the contract between a patient and the provider indicating a bill can be paid in four or more installments. An **implied contract** is indicated by actions, even silence, rather than by words. The majority of provider–patient contracts are implied contracts. It is not required that the contract be written to be enforceable as long as all points of the contract exist. An implied contract can exist either by the circumstances of the situation or by the law. When a patient reports a sore throat and the provider takes a swab for a throat culture to diagnose and treat the ailment, an implied contract exists by the circumstances. An implied contract by law exists when a patient goes into anaphylactic shock and the provider administers epinephrine to counteract shock symptoms. The law says that the provider did what the patient would have requested had there been an expressed contract.

For a contract to be valid and binding, the parties who enter into it must be competent; therefore, people who are mentally incompetent or legally insane, individuals under heavy drug or alcohol influences, infants, and some minors cannot enter into a binding contract.

Medical assistants are considered **agents** of the employers they serve, and as such must be cautious that their actions and words may become a binding contract for their employers. For example, to say that the provider can cure the patient may cause serious legal problems when, in fact, a cure may not be possible.

Termination of Contracts

A broken contract or breach of contract occurs when one of the parties does not meet contractual obligations. A provider is legally bound to treat a patient until:

- The patient discharges the provider
- The provider formally withdraws from patient care
- The patient no longer needs treatment and is formally discharged by the provider

Patient Discharges Provider. When the patient discharges the provider, a letter should be sent to the patient to confirm and document the termination of the contract. The notice is sent by certified mail with return receipt requested. Keep a copy of the letter in the patient's record (Figure 6-1).

Provider Formally Withdraws from the Case. To avoid any charges of abandonment, the provider should formally withdraw from the case when, for example, the patient becomes **noncompliant** or the provider feels the patient can no longer be served. Again, notice should be sent to the patient by certified mail with return receipt requested, and a copy of the notice should be filed in the patient's record (Figures 6-2 and 6-3).

The Patient No Longer Needs Treatment. Unless a formal discharge or withdrawal has occurred, a provider is obligated to care for a patient until the patient's condition no longer requires treatment.

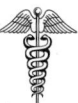

Inner City Health Care
8600 Main Street, Suite 200
River City, XY 01234

January 6, 20XX

CERTIFIED MAIL

Jim Marshal
76 Georgia Avenue
Millerton, XY 43912

Dear Mr. Marshal:

This will confirm our telephone conversation today in which you discharged me as your attending physician in your present illness. In my opinion your condition requires continued medical supervision by a physician. If you have not already done so, I suggest that you employ another physician without delay.

You may be assured that after receiving a written request from you, I will furnish the physician of your choice with information regarding the diagnosis and treatment which you have received from me.

Very truly yours,

Winston Lewis

Winston Lewis, DO
WL:ea

FIGURE 6-1 Letter confirming a physician's discharge by the patient.

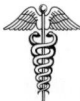

Inner City Health Care
8600 Main Street, Suite 200
River City, XY 01234

May 9, 20XX

CERTIFIED MAIL

Lenny Taylor
260 Second Street
River City, XY 01234

Dear Mr. Taylor:

You will recall that we discussed our professional relationship in my office on May 6, 20XX.

Your son, George Taylor, and Bruce Goldman, my medical assistant, were also present. As you know, the primary difficulty has been your failure to cooperate with the medical plan for your care.

While it is unfortunate that our relationship has reached this stage, I will no longer be able to serve as your physician. I will be available to you on an emergency basis only until June 10, 20XX. Meanwhile, you should immediately call or write the Medical Society, 123 Omega Drive, Carlton, MI 11666, Tel. 123-456-7899 and obtain a list of providers. Any delay could jeopardize your health, so please act quickly.

Your physical (and/or mental) problems include hypertensive heart disease, decreased kidney function, and arteriosclerosis. You could have additional medical problems that may also require professional care. Once you have found a new provider have him or her call my office. I will be happy to discuss your case with the provider assuming your care and will transfer a written summary of your case upon the receipt of a written request from you to do so.

Thank you for your anticipated cooperation and courtesy.

Very truly yours,

Winston Lewis

Winston Lewis, DO
WL:ea

FIGURE 6-2 Letter reiterating "for the record" the osteopath's decision to withdraw from the case discussed during a previous meeting with patient.

TORT LAW

A **tort** is a wrongful act, other than a breach of contract, resulting in injury to one person by another.

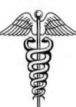

Inner City Health Care
8600 Main Street, Suite 200
River City, XY 01234

December 5, 20XX

CERTIFIED MAIL

Rhoda Au
41 Academy Road
River City, XY 01234

Dear Ms. Au:

I find it necessary to inform you that I am withdrawing further professional medical service to you because of your persistent refusal to follow my medical advice and treatment.

Because your condition requires medical attention, I suggest that you place yourself under the care of another provider without delay. If you so desire, I shall be available to attend you for a reasonable time after you have received this letter, but in no event later than January 7, 20XX. This should give you sufficient time to select someone from the many competent practitioners in this area.

You may be assured that, upon receiving your written request, I will make available to the provider of your choice your case history and information regarding the diagnosis and treatment that you have received from me.

Very truly yours,

Mark King

Mark King, MD
MK:ea

FIGURE 6-3 Letter notifying patient of provider's withdrawal from the case.

Standard of Care and Scope of Practice

Legal   Integrity

To better understand torts, we must consider the standard of care and the four Ds of negligence. All health care providers have the responsibility and duty to perform within their scope of training and to always do what any reasonable and prudent health care professional in the same specialty or general field of practice would do. That is what is expected of every provider when a contact is made by a patient. Failure to do what any reasonable and prudent health care professional would do in the same set of circumstances can be seen as a breach of the standard of care.

Negligence is defined as the failure to exercise the standard of care that a reasonable person would exercise in similar circumstances. Negligence occurs when someone experiences injury because of another's failure to live up to a required duty of care. This is a primary cause of malpractice suits. **Malpractice** is professional negligence or the failure of a medical professional to perform the duty required of the position, causing injury to another.

Four Ds of Negligence. The four elements of negligence, sometimes called the four Ds, are:

1. *Duty.* Duty of care
2. *Derelict.* Breach of the duty of care
3. *Direct cause.* A legally recognizable injury occurs as a result of the breach of duty of care
4. *Damage.* Wrongful activity must have caused the injury or harm that occurred

If an individual has knowledge, skill, or intelligence superior to that of a layperson, that individual's conduct must be consistent with that status. For instance, medical assistants are held to a high standard of care by virtue of their skills, knowledge, and intelligence. As professionals, medical assistants are required to have a standard minimum level of special knowledge and ability. This is what is known as duty of care.

Legal

The Medical Assistant's Role in Negligence. Throughout this text, you will be reminded again and again of the critical role played by the medical assistant in patient care. Always remember to treat *all* patients with dignity and respect. Medical assistants must be certain to recall the four Ds of negligence and the standard of care required of their profession at all times. The first rule is to remember to *always* practice within the scope of one's instruction and education. The second rule is to remember that each state is likely different in what is included in the medical assistants' scope of practice. Understanding and performing within that scope of practice is essential.

Medical assistants may commit a tort that can result in **litigation**. When it can be proven that the injury resulted from the medical assistant (or other health care professional) not meeting the standard of care governing their respective professions, then litigation is a possibility. If, however, the medical assistant (or other health care professional) commits a wrongful act but the patient experiences no injury or harm, then no tort exists. For example, if the medical assistant changes a wound dressing and breaks sterile technique, and

the patient suffers a severely infected wound, the medical assistant has committed a tort and can be held liable to any legal action taken. In contrast, if the medical assistant changes a wound dressing and breaks sterile technique, and the patient's wound does not become infected, no harm has occurred, and a tort does not exist. If a medical assistant fails to report to the provider an abnormal result on a blood test that prevents the provider from making an early diagnosis of a disease, the assistant's omission of an act has caused a breach in the standard of care.

Classification of Torts

There are two major classifications of torts: *intentional* and *negligent*. Intentional torts are deliberate acts of violation of another's rights. Negligent torts are not deliberate and are the result of omission and commission of an act. Malpractice is the unintentional tort of professional negligence; that is, a professional either failed to act in a reasonable and prudent manner and caused harm to the patient, or did what a reasonable and prudent person would not have done and in so doing caused harm to a patient.

There are two Latin terms that can be used to describe aspects of negligence. These are known as doctrines. *Res ipsa loquitur*, or "the thing speaks for itself," is the term used in cases that involve situations such as a nick made in the bladder when the surgeon is performing a hysterectomy. The negligence is obvious. The other doctrine, *respondeat superior*, or "let the master answer," expresses that providers are responsible for their employees' actions. If a medical assistant violates the standard of care, therein lies the basis for a suit of medical malpractice. For example, the medical assistant used the incorrect solution to clean the patient's wound and the patient sustained injuries to the wound. The provider-employer can be sued under the doctrine of *respondeat superior* because the provider-employer is responsible for the acts employees commit in the scope of their employment. The medical assistant also can be sued because individuals are responsible for their own actions.

Common Torts

Some common areas of negligence may result in torts when adherence to the standard of care has not been fulfilled. Specific examples of common torts that can occur in the office or clinic are *battery, defamation of character,* and *invasion of privacy.*

Battery. The basis of the tort of battery is unprivileged touching of one person by another. A patient must consent to being touched. When a procedure is to be performed on a patient, the patient must give consent in full knowledge of all the facts. It does not matter whether the procedure that constitutes the battery improves the patient's health. Patients have the right to withdraw consent at any time.

One example of battery is when a medical assistant insists on giving the patient an injection that was ordered for the patient even though the patient refuses the injection. Another example can be seen when a surgeon performs additional surgery beyond the original procedure (the surgeon performed a hysterectomy, for which consent was given, but is liable for battery for removing a suspicious looking abdominal nevus from the patient's abdomen without consent). It does not matter that the surgeon does not charge for the additional procedure. It also does not matter if the patient would have given consent if asked in advance.

Defamation of Character.

The tort of defamation of character consists of injury to another person's reputation, name, or character through spoken or written words for which damages can be recovered. Two kinds of defamation are libel and slander. **Libel** is false and malicious writing about another, such as in published materials, pictures, and media. An example can be seen when the medical assistant writes in the patient's record, "Mr. O'Keefe's wife and her negative attitude appear to be the cause of his ulcer." A copy of Mr. O'Keefe's records were later sent to a new provider, who reviewed the record and read the remarks quoted by the medical assistant.

Slander is false and malicious spoken words. Slander can be seen in the following comment directed by a patient to the provider, "Dr. Woo is incompetent. He should have his license revoked." The statement is overheard by the clinic administrative medical assistant and other patients waiting in the reception area.

For a tort of defamation of character (either libel or slander) to exist, a third party must see or hear the words and understand their meaning.

Integrity Presentation

Invasion of Privacy. Invasion of privacy is another kind of tort. It includes unauthorized publicity of patient information, medical records being released without the patient's knowledge and permission, and patients receiving unwanted publicity and exposure to public view. For example, if a minor unmarried girl has been examined for possible pregnancy, and the medical assistant telephones the girl's home and inadvertently gives the laboratory results to someone other than the patient, her privacy has been invaded. A second situation exists when persons other than those providing care and performing examinations and procedures (essential or nonessential personnel) are allowed to be present without the patient's consent. Yet another example of the patient's right to privacy being violated is when the patient is asked to walk from the examination room across the hall to a treatment room while wearing only a patient gown in full view of other patients and personnel.

Medical assistants and other health care professionals should:

- Close a door, pull a curtain, or provide a screen when looking at, handling, or examining the patient
- Expose only body parts necessary for treatment (drape the patient, exposing only the part that is being treated)
- Discuss the patient with no one except those individuals involved in the patient's care, and then discuss only those aspects of care that relate to the needs of the patient

It is not an invasion of privacy to disclose information required by a court order, subpoena, or statute to protect the public health and welfare, as in the reporting of violent crime.

INFORMED CONSENT

Documentation of **informed consent** becomes an important part of the patient care process. Every patient has a right to know and understand any procedure to be performed. The patient is to be told in language easily understood:

- The nature of any procedure and how it is to be performed
- Any possible risks involved, as well as expected outcomes of the procedure
- Any other methods of treatment and the risks they involve
- Risks if no treatment is given

It is the responsibility of the health care provider to make certain the patient understands. If an interpreter is necessary, the provider must procure one.

Often, consent forms will be signed if there is to be a surgical or invasive procedure performed. For specific samples of consent forms for medical treatment go to http://www.who.int and search "informed consent form templates." The medical assistant may be asked to witness the patient's signature and may be expected to follow through on any of the provider's instructions or explanations, but is not expected to explain the procedure to the patient. The signed consent form is kept with the medical record, and a copy also is given to the patient.

Increasingly, providers who perform invasive procedures on a regular basis (i.e., surgeons, dermatologists, etc.) use video to further explain the procedure(s) to be performed. Some formal consent forms ask patients to explain in their own words the procedure to be performed. The explanation given serves as a measure of the patient's understanding of the process.

Expressed Consent

When patients indicate to their providers they understand the process to take place, or when they are asked to sign an informed consent document, they are making an **expressed consent**. Expressed consent indicates that patients have directly communicated their consent to the provider either by a verbal "Yes, I consent," or by signing a consent form.

Implied Consent

Two circumstances related to consent are worth mentioning at this point. **Implied consent** occurs when there is a life-threatening emergency, or when the patient is unconscious or unable to respond. The provider, by law, is allowed to give treatment within his or her scope of practice without a signed consent. Implied consent also occurs in more subtle ways. For example, the patient who rolls up a shirtsleeve for the medical assistant to take a blood pressure reading is implying consent to the procedure by the action taken. Implied consent is generally understood from the facts and circumstances surrounding the treatment.

Consent and Legal Incompetence

Consent for treatment is not valid if the patient is legally incompetent to give consent. Legal **incompetence** means that a patient is found by a court to be insane, inadequate, or to not be an adult. In such instances, consent must be obtained from a parent, a legal guardian, or the court on behalf of the patient. Consent for treatment can be given only by the natural parent or legal guardian as determined by the court for a minor child. A **minor** is a person who has not reached the age

of majority (18–21 years old), depending on the laws of each state. Generally, a minor is considered unable to give effective consent for medical treatment; therefore, without proper consent from parents or guardians, medical professionals can be held liable for battery if medical treatment is given. Exceptions to this rule are in cases of emergency and for mature and emancipated minors. **Emancipated minors** are minors younger than 18 years who are free of parental care and are financially responsible, married, become parents, or join the armed forces. **Mature minors** are persons, usually younger than 18 years, who are able to understand and appreciate the nature and consequences of treatment despite their young age. Nearly every state allows minors to give consent for treatment for pregnancy, drug or alcohol addiction, and sexually transmitted disease. Some states have passed legislation that names minors as statutory adults at 14 years old for the purpose of receiving medical care. In these states, minors may consent and be protected by confidentiality and privacy even though their parents or legal guardians may still be financially responsible for their medical bills.

Questions related to the ability of minors and emancipated minors to give consent often must be determined on a case-by-case basis because state statutes vary. Placing a telephone call to the state attorney general's office can help clarify issues, questions, and concerns that involve consent and treatment of minors.

RISK MANAGEMENT

Practicing good **risk management** makes the medical assistant and the provider-employer less vulnerable to litigation.

Following are some ways to avoid incidents that may lead to litigation:

- Perform only within the scope of your training and education.
- Comply with all state and federal regulations and statutes.
- Keep the clinic safe and equipment in readiness.
- Never leave a patient unattended; if you must leave, pass the responsibility for the patient's care on to another individual.
- Keep all patient information confidential.
- Follow all policies and procedures established for the clinic.
- Document fully only facts; formally document withdrawing from a case and discharging patients.

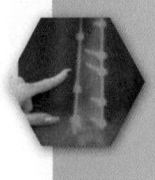

Identify the suggestions in the previous risk management list that are most likely not performed when the staff in the ambulatory care setting find themselves overworked, overwhelmed, and behind. What might be done to prevent carelessness brought on by such circumstances?

- Log telephone calls and return calls to patients within a reasonable time frame.
- Follow up on missed or canceled appointments.
- Never guarantee a cure or diagnosis, and never advise treatment without a provider's order.
- Secure informed consent as necessary.
- Do not criticize other practitioners.
- Explain any appointment delays.
- Be particularly watchful with patients who have special needs, such as the elderly, pediatric patients, and those with physical and emotional disabilities.
- Report any error that may have occurred to your employer.

Professional Liability Coverage

The vast number of legal concerns providers must attend to in the care of patients as well as all the many things that can go wrong demand that providers carry professional liability or malpractice insurance. Therefore, providers commonly carry professional liability insurance coverage in order to cover the costs of any litigation that may occur. In today's health care climate, there is a great deal of discussion regarding the cost of such insurance and the dollar amounts of awards being made to plaintiffs. While not recommended, some providers are doing without professional liability coverage and notifying their patients of such action. Others have chosen to limit their practice to procedures that are not high risk. For instance, a family practice provider may choose not to deliver babies because of the high cost of professional liability coverage for deliveries. Obstetrics, gynecology, and surgery professional liability coverage are among the highest.

Health care employees need their own professional liability coverage. While litigation activities may seek out the "highest-paid" individual to sue, employees can be and are sued quite regularly. Medical assistants can purchase professional liability coverage from the American Association of Medical Assistants (AAMA). Such insurance is designed to help protect personal assets from being taken in order to cover any judgment awarded the plaintiff.

CIVIL LITIGATION PROCESS

Legal

Despite all the best efforts of health care professionals and their employees, litigation can occur. Litigation is the process of taking a lawsuit or a criminal case through the courts. It is helpful to understand the steps taken for civil litigation to occur. The greatest amount of any litigation seen in the ambulatory care setting occurs when relationships between individuals break down for one reason or another. When this happens, the party, or plaintiff, bringing the action, usually a patient, seeks an attorney who agrees to bring the complaint to the courts. The provider, or defendant, is summoned to court. This summons or subpoena notifies the provider of the plaintiff's suit and allows the defendant to file an answer with the court.

Subpoenas

The **subpoena** is an order from the court naming the specific date, time, and reason to appear. A portion of a medical record or the entire medical record may be subpoenaed, the health care provider may be subpoenaed to testify in court, or both the medical record and the provider may be subpoenaed (*subpoena duces tecum*). The staff in the ambulatory care setting usually will have ample time to make certain the record is current and complete before its inclusion in court. Out of courtesy, a provider will notify patients whose records have been subpoenaed. If, for any reason, the patient does not want the record released, the provider must call for legal advice on how to respond to the subpoena.

Certain records, because of their sensitive nature, may require more than a subpoena to be released. These include records related to sexually transmitted diseases, including AIDS and HIV testing; mental health records; substance abuse records; and sexual assault records. For the courts to have access to these records, a *court order* is required in many states.

HIPAA law requires clinics to identify in written policies and procedures what information they will release regarding patients. Before patient information is released, the following must be identified: (1) the purpose or need for the information, (2) the nature or extent of the information to be released, (3) the date of the authorization, and (4) the signature(s) of the person(s) authorized to give consent. Release only what the subpoena or court order specifically requests rather than releasing the entire medical record. Many practitioners keep a patient's consent information in a specific section of the medical record for quick referral and to demonstrate HIPAA compliance.

The care taken with subpoenas and court orders for certain information is to ensure patients of confidentiality. The information in the medical record, including the information a patient shared with the provider and medical assistant, is private.

No patient information can be given to another person or entity (provider, patient's attorney, insurance carrier, or federal or state agency) without the expressed written consent of the patient. Care must be exercised at all times to ensure that the patient's right to confidentiality is not breached. For example, information given to unauthorized personnel associated with the provider's or clinic's practice in regard to the patient's condition, or financial status regarding payment of bills, violates the patient's right to confidentiality. Likewise, when discussing issues over the telephone that can be overheard by others, such as the patient's account being turned over to a collection agency, the patient's right to confidentiality has been violated.

Certain disclosures of information about a patient's conditions and suspected illnesses are required by law. Legally required disclosures are necessary when the public needs to know certain information for its safety and welfare. The disclosures supersede the patient's right to privacy and confidentiality (see the Reportable Diseases/Injuries discussion in the Public Duties section).

Discovery

In the litigation process, the period of **discovery** follows the subpoenas. This is the time in which both parties are allowed access to all the information and evidence related to the case. Rules of discovery vary from state to state but may include the following:

1. An **interrogatory** is a written set of questions that can come from either the plaintiff or the defendant and that must be answered, under oath, and within a specific time period.

2. A **deposition** is oral testimony taken with a court reporter present in a location agreed on by both parties. Both attorneys are usually present when depositions are taken.

Medical assistants may be asked to respond to an interrogatory or may be deposed by the plaintiff's attorney. The defendant's attorney will provide specific instructions in both situations. Because both are done under oath, honesty is an absolute. The medical assistant may be asked to refer to certain documents, recall specific information, or identify documentation in a medical record.

Expert Witnesses. Providers and members of their staff may be called to testify in court to the standard of care. In such a case, they are usually considered expert witnesses. An **expert witness** is one who has enough knowledge and experience in a field to be able to testify to what is the reasonable and expected standard of care. Expert witnesses are expected to tell what they know to be fact and are best counseled to use lay terms rather than complicated medical language. The goal is for jurors and judges to understand the nature of any medical information shared. Visual aids, charts, and computer simulations often are used to illustrate or clarify testimony given by expert witnesses.

Pretrial Conference

A pretrial conference is generally held close to the trial date to decide if there is just cause for the suit, to make certain that both parties are ready, and to determine if there might be an out-of-court settlement. If a trial seems imminent, **alternative dispute resolution (ADR)** may be suggested. ADR saves money, time, and adverse publicity that can come from a trial.

Mediation allows a neutral facilitator to help the two parties settle their differences and come to an acceptable solution. If no settlement is reached, the case can still look to the court for satisfaction. **Arbitration** allows the neutral party to settle the dispute. This arbitration can be binding or nonbinding. In binding arbitration, both parties agree at the outset to accept the neutral party's decision as final. In nonbinding arbitration, the case can look to the court for settlement.

Trial

A trial can be held before a judge or before a judge and a jury. When the trial begins, opening statements outlining the details of the case are made by both sides. The plaintiff's attorney calls witnesses

The Civil Litigation Process

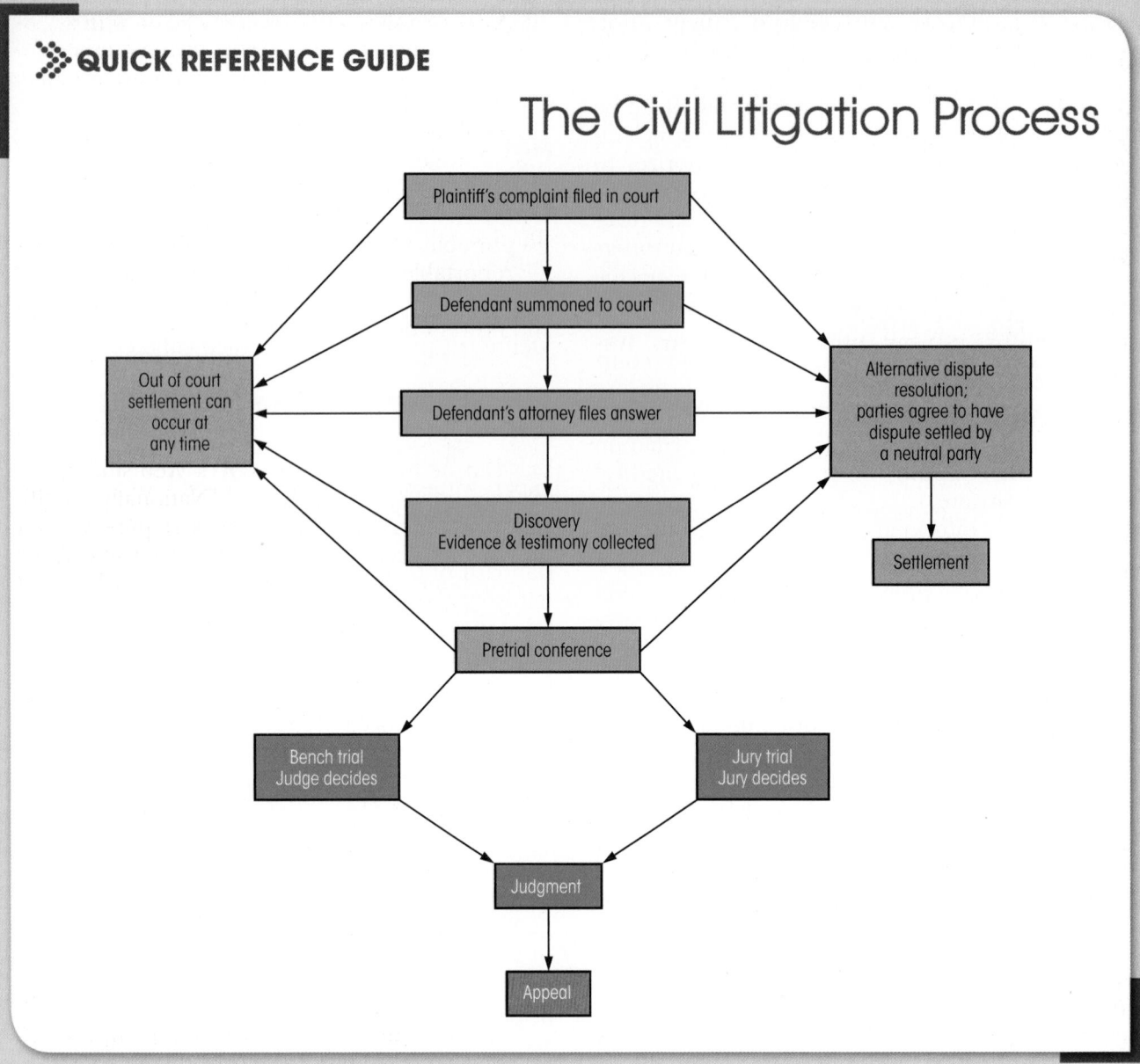

to produce evidence first. This is known as direct examination. In cross-examination, the defendant's attorney questions the witness. When the plaintiff's case is finished, the defendant presents the case in the same manner. When all the information has been presented, the case is turned over for judgment.

If the plaintiff's case is successful, the judge or jury may award a specific amount of money or damages. The judge will instruct the jury regarding the kinds of damages that can be considered in that state. A number of states have placed limits on monetary awards in malpractice cases, making it impossible to go above the maximum award allowed even when juries determine that the monetary award should be higher than allowed by the state. If the defendant's case is successful, the case is dismissed. After a court decision, the party that has lost the case can begin an appeal process. The appeal requests an opinion from higher courts that review cases usually on the basis of a faulty legal process or action.

See the "Civil Litigation Process" Quick Reference Guide for an outline of the civil case process.

STATUTE OF LIMITATIONS

No discussion of negligence, malpractice, or medical records is complete without a brief statement regarding the statute of limitations that will, in part, determine timelines for any litigation and how long medical records are kept. Statutes of limitations most commonly begin at the time a negligent act was committed, when the act was discovered, or when the care of the patient and the provider–patient relationship ended. Therefore, generally all records should be retained until after the statute has run out, usually 3 to 6 years. It is easy to understand why many providers choose to keep their records indefinitely, a plan made much easier with electronic files.

State and federal statutes set maximum time periods during which certain actions can be brought or rights enforced; there is a time limit for individuals to initiate legal action. The statute of limitations varies from one jurisdiction to another, and a lawsuit may not be brought after the statute of limitations has run. For example, in the Commonwealth of Massachusetts, the statute of limitations for an act of medical malpractice committed on an adult is 3 years. If harm to a patient resulted from a medical assistant administering the wrong dose of medication to a patient in Massachusetts, a lawsuit must be brought within 3 years from the time the medication error was made, with the 3 years commencing at the time the negligent act was committed.

PUBLIC DUTIES

Providers and their employees must comply with all federal, state, and local health care laws and regulations. When a good working relationship exists between providers and their employees, compliance to these regulations is less likely to be compromised. There are a number of public duties to be considered.

Reportable Diseases/Injuries

All medical providers have a duty to the public to report diseases and injuries that jeopardize public health and welfare. Transmittable or contagious diseases and/or injuries resulting from a knife or gunshot are examples; these must be reported to the appropriate authorities. This can be done without the patient's consent because it is required by law. When reporting, it is important to do so properly and according to the laws of the state in which one is employed. Knowledge of which

Legal

illnesses, injuries, and conditions to report, to whom to report, and the appropriate forms to submit is essential. Copies of all information must be kept for the clinic.

MedlinePlus, a Web site sponsored by the U.S. National Library of Medicine and the National Institutes of Health, has an excellent site connected to the Medline Encyclopedia titled "Reportable Diseases" that identifies guidelines for reportable diseases. Local, state, and national agencies such as the Centers for Disease Control and Prevention (CDC) require such diseases to be reported when diagnosed by providers or laboratories. States may vary in the diseases that require reporting, but their lists are likely to include the list of "Nationally Notifiable Infectious Diseases" that can be found on the CDC's Web site (go to www.cdc.gov and search for "Nationally Notifiable Conditions"). Some diseases require written reports. Others require reporting electronically or by telephone; they include rubeola (measles) and pertussis (whooping cough). Still others ask for only the number of cases to be reported. Such reporting is beneficial to society and all health care managers in tracking and preventing illness. The list changes as new diseases occur and are diagnosed.

Other generally required facts to report include births; deaths; childhood immunizations; rape; and abuse toward a child, elder, or intimate partner.

Some states have laws specific to the release of information relative to mental or psychological treatment, HIV testing, AIDS diagnosis and treatment, sexually transmitted diseases, and chemical substance abuse.

Procedure

Local or state health departments can provide lists of diseases and injuries to report and will also provide the appropriate forms (see Procedure 6-2).

Abuse

Legal

Child abuse, **intimate partner violence (IPV)**, and elder abuse are becoming more commonly known in today's society. As a result, patients experiencing such abuse may be seen in the ambulatory care setting. In all cases of abuse, medical records hold valuable information if a court procedure ensues. Careful documentation is critical. State laws are fairly specific and consistent in mandates to report child abuse, but laws related to elder abuse and domestic violence or intimate partner violence are not as detailed. In any case, the rights of the abused must be protected. (See Table 7-1 for a summary.)

Perform Compliance Reporting Based on Public Health Statutes

PURPOSE:

To report a communicable disease.

EQUIPMENT/SUPPLIES:

- Patient's medical record
- Local, state, and national guidelines for reporting communicable disease
- Computer and Internet access, telephone, and fax machine

PROCEDURE STEPS:

1. From the patient's medical record and/or provider's instructions, determine the disease to be reported. RATIONALE: Helps determine if local, state, or national reporting is necessary or all three are required.

2. Access the Medline Encyclopedia "Reportable Diseases" and the CDC's Web site to determine how the disease is to be reported. RATIONALE: Regulations may change; ensures the most recent guidelines.

3. Follow the instructions from the above sites to prepare the confidential report via telephone, fax, or written notice. RATIONALE: Makes certain proper protocol is followed.

4. Place a copy of the report in the patient's medical record. RATIONALE: Indicates completion of the reporting process.

Child Abuse. All 50 states and the District of Columbia mandate, or require, that health care professionals, teachers, social workers, and certain others who suspect child abuse report the incident to the proper authorities. Confidentiality in the provider–patient relationship does not exist when children are abused. If a person has a reason to suspect abuse and reports the abuse to the police and, in the case of child abuse, to the child protective agency, this individual is protected against liability as a result of making the report. Failure to report could result in criminal or civil penalties. Usually, the child protective unit of the state department of social services is called to investigate suspected cases of child abuse. Some injuries that are commonly seen in child abuse are bruises, welts, burns, fractures, and head injuries. Evidence of neglect, intimidation, or sexual abuse also may be seen.

If a suspicion of abuse exists, the provider should do the following:

- Treat the child's injuries.
- Send the child to the hospital for further treatment when necessary.
- Inform parents of the diagnosis and that it will be reported to the police and social services agency.

- Notify the child protective agency (keep phone number posted).
- Document all information.
- Provide court testimony if requested.

Elder Abuse. Elder abuse may consist of neglect, physical abuse, punishment, physical restraint, and/or abandonment. Examples are seen when elders are overmedicated or undermedicated, physically restrained, intimidated by shouting or profanity, sexually abused, neglected or abandoned, or in any other way have their rights and dignity violated. The person reporting the abuse is generally a health care professional who observes or suspects the abuse, and the reporting agency is most likely one of a social service or welfare nature. The majority of states have laws protecting vulnerable adults and the elderly from abuse.

Intimate Partner Violence (IPV). The term *domestic violence* has been changed to be more encompassing of an escalating problem. *Intimate partner violence (IPV)* is now used and refers to violence or abuse between a spouse or former spouse; boyfriend, girlfriend, or former boyfriend/girlfriend; and same-sex or heterosexual intimate partner or former same-sex or heterosexual intimate partner. The abuse may include physical or sexual violence, threats of the same, and psychological or emotional violence. Physical violence is a criminal act, and failure to report it is considered a misdemeanor in some states. Victims of IPV should be treated as soon as possible after the assault so that evidence can be preserved for legal purposes. Some forms of IPV are considered acceptable behavior in many cultures, even in the United States. Some cultures believe the woman is chattel, or property, of her spouse; that she has no rights or authority; and that she must submit to her husband's, brother's, or father's demands.

An individual who manages to come to the ambulatory care setting with signs of IPV is courageous and probably is extremely frightened as well, because reporting the violence may increase the risk for continued violence and even death in some instances.

Make certain that community resources are readily available for survivors of IPV, even if they choose to stay in the abusive situation. In many cases, the abused patient's options are so few that leaving is more frightening than staying in the abusive relationship. Do not pass judgment on these survivors; they desperately need understanding and compassion.

Professional

Your understanding and compassion are perhaps the only door through which they might feel comfortable enough to leave the abusive relationship.

Good Samaritan Laws

Legal

All 50 states have laws regarding the rendering of first aid by health care professionals at the scene of an accident or sudden injury. Good Samaritan laws, although not always clearly written, encourage health care professionals to provide medical care within the scope of their training without fear of being sued for negligence. In an emergency situation, medical assistants cannot be held liable should an injury result from some form of first aid rendered or from first aid they omitted to render as long as they acted in a reasonable way within the scope of their knowledge. Medical assistants and other health care professionals with skills in cardiopulmonary resuscitation (CPR) who are present when CPR is needed must perform the procedure on the victim or otherwise could be declared negligent. Emergencies that arise in the ambulatory care setting generally are not covered by Good Samaritan laws.

FRAUD

Unfortunately, illegal activities can and do take place in the health care environment. As a result, it is important to discuss how fraud may occur. Following is a list of the most common violations committed:

1. Billing for services not provided
2. Billing a noncovered service as if it is covered
3. Misrepresenting dates, locations, and providers of service
4. Incorrect reporting of diagnoses or procedures
5. Taking kickbacks and bribery
6. False or unnecessary issuance of prescription drugs, especially opioids

This list may seem obvious, but without appropriate checks and balances, an illegal act is often committed due to carelessness rather than malicious intent. Consider the following examples:

- The PCP is on maternity leave and the team's nurse practitioner fills in, but all charges are made at the PCP level of service.
- The PCP indicates a higher level of service during the appointment and/or indicates procedures the medical assistant observes to be inaccurate.
- The PCP misrepresents dates of services on a labor and industry case in order to assure payment of the claim.
- The PCP continues to issue opioid prescriptions without following proper procedures.

In a very large medical clinic or a hospital clinic, there likely is a quality assurance protocol in place. However, illegal matters should be reported to proper authorities. Billing fraud can be reported to the appropriate agency (e.g., Medicare/Medicaid or to the clinic's accountant). Providers who create these acts can be reported to the local branch of the American Medical Association and to the police. Employees must recall that not reporting illegal activities makes them an accessory to the crime.

ADVANCE DIRECTIVES

Medical assistants in the ambulatory care setting will be asked to attach advance directives or living wills to patients' medical records These directives are legal documents in which patients indicate their wishes in the case of a life-threatening illness or serious injury.

Health care providers in many states and cities have adopted the Physician Orders for Life-Sustaining Treatment (POLST) form. This form is to be completed by a health care provider based on the patient's preferences regarding the type of life-sustaining treatment wanted and medical indications. POLST is most often brightly colored (neon pink or green). To be valid, the form must be signed by the proper authority. Some states may use another name than POLST, but the intent is quite similar. POLST is appropriate for seriously ill individuals with life-threatening or terminal illnesses. Some providers believe that even with an advance directive in place, it is advisable to complete a POLST form. This form goes with the patient when he or she is moved between care settings. For those living at home, it is recommended that the form be posted on the refrigerator where emergency responders can locate it easily. For a current listing of states' development of POLST, go to www.polst.org and click on the "Programs in Your State" link. Such documents should always accompany patients to the hospital for any treatment or care. They may be updated from time to time, and patients can ask to rescind such a document at any time. Medical assistants must remember that these documents reflect the choices of their patients and are to be respected as such.

Living Wills/Advance Directives

Patients who desire to make known in advance their choices related to health care, especially when death is near, are likely to have living wills, advance directives, a health care proxy, or a POLST order. The title of such a document is largely determined by the state in which the document is made. These documents are necessary because advances in medicine allow medical professionals to sustain life even if the individual will not recover from a persistent vegetative state. Persons who prefer not to remain in that state can use the living will or advance directive to make decisions about life support and to direct others to implement their wishes in that regard. Such a document allows individuals to indicate to family and health care professionals whether life-prolonging medical or surgical procedures are to be continued, withheld, or withdrawn, and whether artificial feeding and fluids are to be used or withheld. The document allows individuals to make this decision before incapacitation.

To be valid, the proper and particular form, which is different in each state, must be used, and it must be lawfully executed. States vary in the number of witnesses required and whether a notary public is required for those signatures. The form goes into effect when provided to a patient's health care provider *and* when the patient is no longer capable of making health care decisions. Examples of incapacity include permanent unconsciousness, life-threatening illness in the latter stages, and inability to communicate. The U.S. Legal Forms Web site (http://USlegalforms.com) has samples of living wills for all 50 states and the District of Columbia under the heading "Living Will." A sample from each state is available without a fee.

Durable Power of Attorney for Health Care

Another document seen in the ambulatory care setting is the **durable power of attorney for health care** or designation of health care surrogate or health care proxy. This document allows a patient to name another person as the official spokesperson for that patient should he or she be unable to

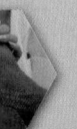

Patient Education

Legal

Because of the increased awareness of confidentiality as a result of HIPAA, medical assistants can be helpful by suggesting that any family member(s) who might be involved and need to know about the patient's care be indicated in the patient's medical record with a signed release from the patient. There have been examples recently of adult children of elder adults who were either not informed when their ailing parent was taken to emergency services in another state or were unable to get any information about their parent from a hospital or provider even though a durable power of attorney for health care was in place. If that directive does not go with the patient, no information can be given. For that reason, it is suggested that patients may want to keep a wallet card containing a notice of the advance directive, any appointed agent named, and any family member(s) who is allowed information.

make health care decisions. A basic durable power of attorney document allows another person to manage finances and personal matters; however, it takes a durable power of attorney for health care for that person to make medical decisions.

Every state has a slightly different version of their living will, advance directive, durable power of attorney for health care, or POLST. Most forms and specific information can be found on the Internet by keying in a particular state and the title of the document wanted. Also, the Web site for Compassion and Choices (http://www.compassionandchoices.org), located in Portland, Oregon, is quite helpful.

Patient Self-Determination Act

In 1991, the federal government passed the **Patient Self-Determination Act (PSDA)**, which applies to all health care institutions receiving payments from Medicare and Medicaid. PSDA requires that all adults receiving health care from these institutions be given the opportunity to provide information about their wishes in an advance directive.

Copies of advance directives are to be given to patients' providers so the documents can be transferred to a hospital or nursing facility as necessary. Any named agent should have a copy, and family members also may have a copy.

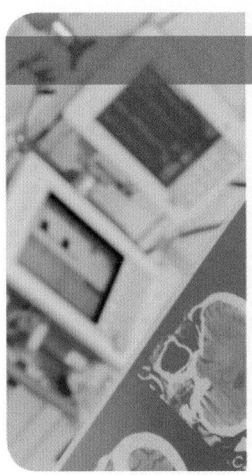

CASE STUDY 6-1

Refer to the scenario at the beginning of the chapter. You realize that any breach of confidentiality is a serious matter, whether intentional or accidental, and that the lack of professionalism can lead to such errors in judgment.

CASE STUDY REVIEW

1. What corrective measures can you suggest to decrease voices heard in the hallway or from examination rooms?
2. How can private patient information be kept private even among staff?
3. What suggestions do you make to keep personal conversations and interactions out of view and/or sound of patients?

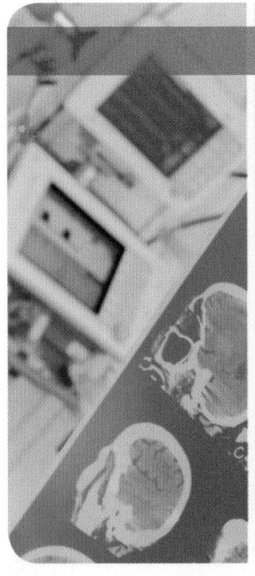

CASE STUDY 6-2

Three weeks ago, Dr. King treated a new patient, Boris Bolski, for lower back pain, which the patient believed was the result of consistent heavy lifting at his job. Medical assistant Joe Guerrero, CMA (AAMA), assisted Dr. King during the examination. Today, both Joe and Dr. King were served with subpoenas by Mr. Bolski's attorney. Mr. Bolski is alleging that unsafe conditions at his workplace caused severe strain on his back, and he is suing his employer for damages. Dr. King and Joe Guerrero were called as expert witnesses to a civil hearing; Joe, especially, is a bit nervous about this, because he has never been on the witness stand in court and is not sure what is expected of him.

CASE STUDY REVIEW

1. How will Mr. Bolski's medical record help Joe answer questions at the hearing?
2. What information should Joe gather so that he is prepared to testify?
3. As an expert witness, what might Joe be expected to communicate to the judge in this case?

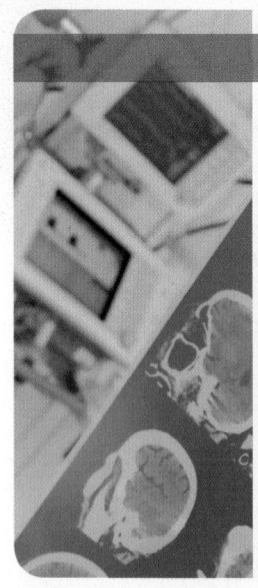

CASE STUDY 6-3

Wanda Hanson, RMA (AMT), is working on a part-time basis in Hudson, Florida, as an administrative medical assistant on the phone desk in the emergency department at Hudson Community Hospital when a frantic long-distance call is received. The caller is Larry Nelson from Cheyenne, Wyoming. He received a call from the nursing home where his 95-year-old mother is living informing him that she was taken by ambulance to your hospital. Larry wants to know if Muriel Nelson has arrived and what her condition is. Wanda is aware of a patient's right to privacy, confidentiality, and the HIPAA regulations. Wanda observed Mrs. Nelson arrive at the emergency department quite incoherent and confused.

CASE STUDY REVIEW

1. What can Wanda tell Mr. Nelson, especially after noting that no records were with the elderly Mrs. Nelson when she arrived at the hospital?
2. What information would Wanda need from Mr. Nelson before complying with his request?
3. How can Wanda put Mr. Nelson at ease? What can Wanda do to help?

Summary

- Today's medical professional must have a knowledge of all sources of law.

- Administrative law regulations include many components pertinent to outpatient care.

- Contract law will determine how patients are discharged, how providers withdraw from treatment, and necessary steps to take when patients no longer require treatment.

- Tort law, a wrongful act resulting in injury, dictates a professional's standard of care and scope of practice.

- Patients are more aware than ever of their rights, especially those of confidentiality and the right to privacy, consent, and records ownership. They are likely to seek redress when they perceive their rights have been violated.

- Consent, whether informed, expressed, implied, or written, is an essential part of the patient care process. Risk management procedures and a healthy relationship between all providers and patients as well as between medical assistants and patients, and respect for the patient's rights, reduces the likelihood of any malpractice litigation.

- An understanding of the statute of limitations and the civil litigation process is helpful when there is a lawsuit.

- Providers must fulfill all public duties and comply with reporting laws.

- Patients' advance directives and powers of attorney must be identified and followed.

- Sources of information regarding state and federal laws can be obtained from the state medical society, the provider's liability insurance company, the state medical assistant society, the state attorney general's office, the Internet, and/or the public library.

Study for Success

To reinforce your knowledge and skills of information presented in this chapter:

- Review the *Key Terms* and *Learning Outcomes*
- Consider the *Critical Thinking* features and *Case Studies* and discuss your conclusions
- Answer the questions in the *Certification Review*

Procedure

- Perform the *Procedures* using the *Competency Assessment Checklists* on the *Student Companion Website*

CERTIFICATION REVIEW

1. What type of contract most often exists between provider and patient?
   a. Expressed
   b. Implied
   c. Privileged
   d. Civil
2. Which administrative law act prohibits discrimination in employment and is enforced by the EEOC?
   a. Controlled Substances Act
   b. Federal Age Discrimination Act
   c. Americans with Disabilities Act
   d. Health Insurance Portability and Accountability Act
   e. Title VII of the Civil Rights Act
3. What stipulation was recently added/amended to the Family and Medical Leave Act?
   a. Unpaid leave to care for a family member with Alzheimer disease
   b. Changing eligibility requirements to a time of employment of 9 months and a minimum of 935 hours worked
   c. Changing definition of spouse to recognize legal same-sex marriages
   d. Eliminating military leave provisions
4. Occasionally, a provider will be sued for an employee's negligence, even though the provider is not guilty of any negligent act. This is done on the basis of what doctrine?
   a. *Res ipsa loquitur*
   b. *Respondeat superior*
   c. Proximate cause
   d. Employer–employee contracts
   e. Regulation Z of the Employee Protection Act
5. How do the courts interpret the standard of care expected of a provider?
   a. Perform within scope of training on a par with all other providers engaged in the same medical specialty anywhere
   b. Provide reasonable, attentive, diligent care comparable with other providers in the general field of practice
   c. Exercise skill as well as possible under the circumstances
   d. Match the national norm in performance

6. What is the purpose of advance directives?
   a. They allow patients to direct how their billing is to be handled.
   b. They encourage providers to render first aid in an emergency.
   c. They allow patients to determine their choices in life-threatening circumstances.
   d. Best expressed in the POLST form, they guarantee equal treatment under the law.
   e. They give the provider power of attorney to make health care decisions.
7. What are important characteristics of a subpoena?
   a. It is a court order requesting data, an appearance in court, or both.
   b. It is sufficient to enforce a release of any type of medical record or information.
   c. It may be ignored without consequences.
   d. It allows the person being served to select a specific date or time to appear.
8. What are the four Ds of negligence?
   a. Duty, danger, damage, disaster
   b. Derelict, direct cause, damage, danger
   c. Danger, direct cause, damage, disaster
   d. Duty, derelict, direct cause, damage
   e. Duty, despair, direct cause, damage
9. Which of the following statements is true of emancipated minors?
   a. They are 18 to 25 years in age but live with their parents.
   b. They are younger than 18, are considered adults, and can consent to treatment.
   c. They live on their own but are not self-supporting.
   d. They are not married and able to work only part time.
10. Which of the following statements best describes torts?
    a. They often include battery, defamation of character, and invasion of privacy.
    b. They are always intentional in nature.
    c. They are laws to make certain the standard of care has been fulfilled.
    d. They do not include malpractice.
    e. None of these

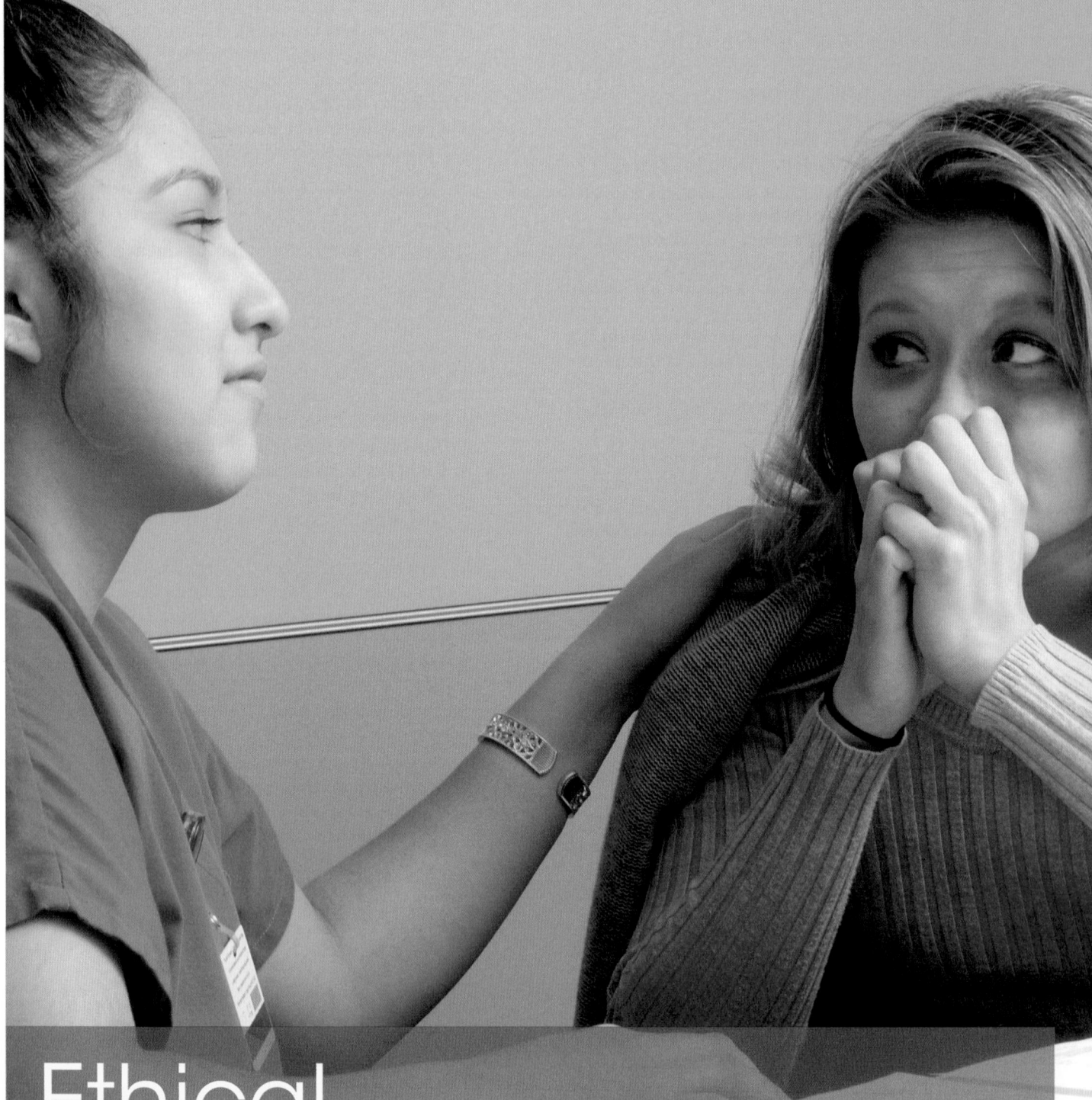

CHAPTER 7

Ethical Considerations

1. Define and spell the key terms as presented in the glossary.
2. Summarize reasons for codes of ethics.
3. Paraphrase the eight characteristics of principle-centered leadership.
4. Describe the five Ps of ethical power.
5. Implement the ethics check questions.
6. Relate the five principles of the AAMA code to patient care in the ambulatory care setting.
7. Discuss the role of ethical codes in ambulatory care.
8. Critique the ethical guidelines for health care providers, giving at least four examples.
9. Summarize professional rights and responsibilities for health care personnel.
10. Categorize the different types of abuse for those individuals at risk.
11. Restate the dilemmas encountered by the following bioethical issues: (a) allocation of scarce/limited medical resources, (b) health care as a right or a privilege, (c) HIV and AIDS, (d) reproductive issues, (e) abortion and fetal tissue research, (g) genetic engineering/manipulation, and (h) dying and death.

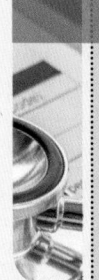

KEY TERMS

bioethics	genetic engineering	surrogates
cryopreservation	intimate partner violence (IPV)	tubal ligation
ethics	in vitro fertilization (IVF)	vasectomy
euthanasia	macroallocation	
female genital mutilation (FGM)	microallocation	

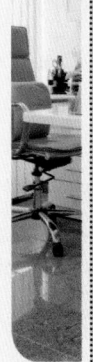

SCENARIO

Harley Navarro is a new medical assistant in a busy internist's clinic. He finished school a few months ago and is awaiting the date to take his exam to become a certified medical assistant. He is nervous and scared. All the other medical assistants are female and have many years of experience. Harley wants so much to be accepted and recognized for his skills. Today, however, he twice had a rough time taking a blood pressure reading. In fact, the provider was ready for one of Harley's patients before he was finished with the reading, and the provider stepped in to take the reading. Harley was embarrassed. His current patient is obese. His first attempt at getting a blood pressure reading failed. He gets a larger cuff for his second reading. His patient complains, however, that her arm is hurting about halfway through the reading. Harley hurries the process and takes a guess at the diastolic pressure figure, but he knows it is close.

Chapter Portal

It is impossible in today's world to function as a medical assistant without an awareness of the impact of ethics and bioethics on health care. Just as an understanding of the law and complying with the law are vital for the medical assistant, it is equally important to understand ethics and bioethics.

From Chapter 6, you have come to realize that there are many circumstances and situations that occur in health care that are guided and directed by state and federal laws. You, personally, are expected to be above reproach in all your actions in this regard. You must also work with your employer and other members of the health care team to ensure that each member of the staff functions within the law—protecting both patients and providers.

continues

Ethics plays a huge role in such an endeavor. To function ethically demands that you never function outside the law. Ethics, however, demands something more—ethics calls for honesty, trustworthiness, integrity, confidentiality, and fairness. To function ethically, you must know yourself well and understand weaknesses and any vulnerability that might prevent you from acting ethically.

The scenario described earlier is just one situation in which medical assistants may need to reflect on their actions and be sure that they are acting ethically and within the range of their skills. Medical assistants also need to recognize the warning signs that they, or some other staff member, may be about to breach a code of ethics. Often, this kind of breach occurs when one has, or seeks to have, too much power; when one attempts to take on too much authority; or when one has too little knowledge and experience and is afraid to ask for help. When a breach seems about to occur, the individuals involved should be encouraged to step back and review their actions and the likely consequences of those actions.

ETHICS

Traditionally, **ethics** is defined in terms of what is considered right or wrong. Sometimes ethics is referred to as *morals.* However, morals refer to personal choices of conduct, whereas ethics is more of a philosophy related to making judgments about right and wrong. Professional organizations often identify their ethics in codes, which provide a set of principles and guidelines.

The American Medical Association (AMA) has established such a code of ethics called the Principles of Medical Ethics. This code can be reviewed by accessing the AMA Web site (http://www.ama-assn.org). Also published every 2 years by the AMA is The Code of Medical Ethics Current Opinions with Annotations; this document provides up-to-date information on a number of ethical dilemmas. A number of other professional medical organizations have well-established ethical codes also. They include such professions as osteopaths, chiropractors, nurses, professional coders, and emergency medical technicians.

The American Association of Medical Assistants (AAMA) has a code of ethics and a creed shown in Figure 7-1. In addition, the AAMA Mission Statement, AAMA Medical Assistant Code of Ethics, and AAMA Medical Assistant Creed appear on the AAMA Web site (http://www.aama-ntl.org). Clicking on "About" and then selecting the "Overview" link will detail these statements for you.

AAMA CODE OF ETHICS

The Medical Assisting Code of Ethics of the AAMA sets forth principles of ethical and moral conduct as they relate to the medical profession and the particular practice of medical assisting.

Members of AAMA dedicated to the conscientious pursuit of their profession, and thus desiring to merit the high regard of the entire medical profession and the respect of the general public which they serve, do pledge themselves to strive always to:

A. Render service with full respect for the dignity of humanity.
B. Respect confidential information obtained through employment unless legally authorized or required by responsible performance of duty to divulge such information.
C. Uphold the honor and high principles of the profession and accept its disciplines.
D. Seek to continually improve the knowledge and skills of medical assistants for the benefit of patients and professional colleagues.
E. Participate in additional service activities aimed toward improving the health and well-being of the community.

CREED

The Medical Assisting Creed of the AAMA sets forth medical assisting statements of belief:
I believe in the principles and purposes of the profession of medical assisting.
I endeavor to be more effective.
I aspire to render greater service.
I protect the confidence entrusted to me.
I am dedicated to the care and well-being of all people.
I am loyal to my employer.
I am true to the ethics of my profession.
I am strengthened by compassion, courage and faith.

(A)   **(B)**

FIGURE 7-1   (A) American Association of Medical Assistants (AAMA) Code of Ethics. (B) AAMA Creed.

Reprinted with permission of the American Association of Medical Assistants

The American Hospital Association replaced its original Hospital Patient Bill of Rights with a brochure that informs patients about their rights and responsibilities while hospitalized. The brochure, "The Patient Care Partnership," is available in several languages and continues to be a standard for many hospitals. Similar statements have been adapted to the ambulatory health care setting as well. See Figure 7-2 for a simple generic sample. These codes give additional guidance for making ethical decisions, taking ethical action, and further identifying patient rights and responsibilities.

There are more than 50 different codes of ethics for professional organizations, and most are related to medicine and are designed to offer guidance and direction to health care professionals.

Seven ethical codes that pertain to the entire world are pertinent for review. They include such famous codes as the Declaration of Geneva, Declaration of Helsinki, and the International Code of Medical Ethics. A listing of these codes is found by searching the Internet for "World Medical Ethics Codes." Another fascinating Web site identifies the characteristics of traditional Chinese medical ethics when you use the Internet to search for "Chinese Medical Ethics." Chinese medical ethics emphasizes self-cultivation and personal ethics of practitioners rather than a strict organizational code of ethics.

Codes of ethics bring standards of moral and ethical behavior together in one place. They assist organizations and individuals in putting words to their expected behaviors and actions. There is a benefit to such codes when they become reminders to everyone regarding appropriate conduct. Codes also can have a limiting effect, however. For instance, if an organization does not have a code of ethics, that organization is not necessarily viewed as unethical. Further, having a code of ethics does not necessarily create an ethical organization, especially if the code is mostly ignored.

Integrity

Medical assistants and medical professionals are asked to balance personal and professional areas of their lives in the middle of constant pressure and crises. At the same time, the quality of one's personal life is going to be shown in the quality of his or her service to others in his or her professional life. To be effective in the medical profession, individuals need to demonstrate maturity in both personal and professional selves to create the utmost of ethical conduct and professionalism. To do so, it is helpful to discuss principle-centered leadership and the meaning of ethical power.

PATIENT BILL OF RIGHTS AND RESPONSIBILITIES FOR AMBULATORY CARE*

As a patient, you have the right to:

Be treated with courtesy and respect, with appreciation of your dignity and without discrimination at all times.

Participate in your healthcare by receiving a prompt and reasonable response to questions and requests, receiving information concerning diagnosis, course of treatment, alternatives, risks, and prognosis.

Access your medical record and receive a copy upon request. Seek a second opinion and to know who is providing your medical services.

Confidentiality at all times and your privacy protected.

An estimate of charges for medical care.

A reasonably clear and understandable itemized bill and to have the charges explained.

Refuse any treatment.

Have your advance directive on file.

Be informed of any medical treatment for purposes of experimental research and to give consent or refuse to participate.

As a patient, your responsibilities include the following:

You are expected to provide complete and accurate personal, health, and medical history information as required.

You are expected to ask questions when you do not understand information or instructions. You are responsible for outcomes if you do not follow your care plan.

You are expected to provide accurate information regarding health insurance coverage and pay any bills in a timely fashion.

You are expected to provide a copy of an advance directive if you have one.

You have the responsibility of keeping all scheduled appointments.

You are expected to treat all health care providers with courtesy and respect.

*Compilation of several clinics across the United States; prepared by Carol D. Tamparo. CMA (AAMA), PhD.

FIGURE 7-2 Patient bill of rights and Responsibilities for Ambulatory Care.

Principle-Centered Leadership

Stephen R. Covey, a very well-known author and leadership expert, has produced an audiobook that includes collections of three of his best-selling texts. It includes *The 7 Habits of Managers*, *Principle-Centered Leadership*, and *The 4 Imperatives of Great Leaders*. Covey's original work identified eight characteristics of principle-centered leaders because he understood that leaders who know themselves and understand their principles more easily abide by a code of ethics. Consider the following questions adapted from Covey's writings as guides to how you might perform ethically in a medical setting:

- *Are you continually learning?* Do you seek training, take classes, listen to others, and learn from your peers? Are you curious? Do you realize that developing new knowledge and skills is a lifelong endeavor?

- *Are you service oriented?* Do you see your life as a mission rather than a career? Are you generally a nurturing individual who seeks service in the medical field? Can you see yourself working alongside a co-worker and pulling together with that person toward a goal? Can you put yourself in the place of others?

- *Do you radiate positive energy?* Are you cheerful, pleasant, optimistic, and positive? Is your spirit hopeful? If it is, you carry a positive energy field that allows you to neutralize or sidestep a negative energy source. Do you see yourself as a peacemaker or one who can create harmony to undo negative energy?

- *Do you believe in other people?* Can you keep from labeling, stereotyping, or prejudging other people? Can you believe in the unseen potential of others? Can you keep from overreacting to negative behaviors and criticism? Can you put aside any grudges?

The final characteristics of principle-centered leaders Covey identifies are more personal. They can help you understand yourself and how you might make ethical decisions in the medical field:

- *Do you lead a balanced life?* Do you keep up with current affairs and events? Do you know what is happening in the medical field and how that affects you? Do you have at least one confidant with whom you can be transparent? Are you physically active within your limits of age and health? Do you enjoy yourself? Do you have a good sense of humor? Are you open to communication?

- *Do you see life as an adventure?* Are you able to rediscover persons each time you meet them? Are you interested in others? Do you listen well? Are you flexible and unflappable? Does your security come from within rather than from without?

- *Are you synergistic?* Synergy is what happens when the whole of something is greater than the sum of its parts. Do you know your weaknesses? Can you complement your weaknesses with the strengths of others on the team? Can you work hard to improve most situations? Are you trusting? Can you separate the person from the problem?

- *Do you exercise for self-renewal?* In this element, Mr. Covey identifies four dimensions of the human personality that need exercise: physical, mental, emotional, and spiritual dimensions. How do you keep your body in shape? How do you keep your mind alert? Do patience, unconditional love, and accepting responsibility for your own actions keep you emotionally healthy? Do you have a way to meditate, pray, or "draw away" for a period to "fill up your spirit"?

These questions and your responses to them can give you insight into your ability to function ethically and to be successful in the world of medicine.

Covey has another book entitled *The 8th Habit: From Effectiveness to Greatness* (now available in a summary version) that discusses how individuals can be more excited about their lives and their work when they reach beyond effectiveness toward fulfillment, contribution, and greatness. Individuals who feel fulfilled and excited about their work are more apt to perform ethically than those who do not.

Five Ps of Ethical Power

Another approach to how you might act in an ethical manner comes from Kenneth Blanchard and Norman Vincent Peale, who wrote a simple but powerful little book called *The Power of Ethical Management*. In it they discuss the "five Ps of ethical power." The five Ps are as follows:

1. *Purpose.* Understand your objective or your purpose. Your purpose may change from time to time, but it is something that requires you to behave in a way that makes you feel good about yourself.

2. *Pride.* Have pride in what you do. Feel good about yourself and your accomplishments. Nurture your self-esteem while remaining humble. Be proud to be a medical assistant.

3. *Patience.* It takes time to create an atmosphere in which your objective can be obtained. Strive to believe that no matter what happens,

everything is going to work out. Expect results from yourself and your work, but refrain from demanding it "now."

4. *Persistence.* To act in an ethical manner means to strive to act in that manner all the time, not just when you want to or it seems easy to do. Winston Churchill said, "Never, never, never, never give up!" That is what persistence is. If you make a mistake, admit it, correct it, learn from the mistake, and move on, but never give up. An individual who is truly aware of his or her personal ethical power is able to admit an error, does not compromise any procedure or any technique, and does not ever put the patient at risk, even if it means facing reprimand from a supervisor.

5. *Perspective.* Keep your life and your purpose in perspective. Find time each day to maintain balance in your life (perhaps looking again at the eight questions for principle-centered individuals). Plan some quiet time, some fun time, but certainly some reflective time. The constant pressure and the crises will become overwhelming without keeping perspective.

Ethics Check Questions

Finally, when there is uncertainty about a dilemma or there is little or no experience to draw from, those striving to act in an ethical manner can perform a simple test each time there is a question about ethics. This, too, comes from Blanchard and Peale. The questions to ask are:

1. *Is it legal?* Is it against the law or any company policy?

2. *Is it balanced?* Is this the best possible approach for all concerned? Does it promote a win–win situation?

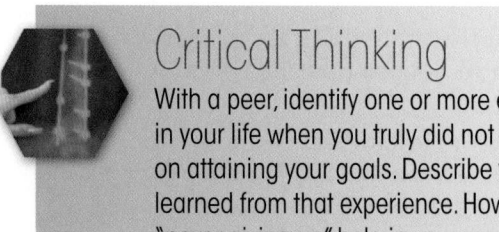

Critical Thinking

With a peer, identify one or more examples in your life when you truly did not give up on attaining your goals. Describe what you learned from that experience. How might "never giving up" help in your pursuit of a career?

3. *How will it make me feel about myself?* Will I feel good if my decision is published in a newspaper? Will my family and co-workers be proud of my decision?

These questions provide a simple yet profound guide that is easy to recall and to apply to almost any situation. They are used throughout the business world by managers and employees seeking to work and practice legally and ethically.

Ethics are not easy. Performing ethically is hard work. Being ethical means determining who you are and how you will act. Laws are more clearly defined than ethics, but acting in an unethical manner can cause as much pain and difficulty as can acting illegally. The ideas of Covey, Blanchard, and Peale give guidance, thoughts to ponder, and perhaps goals to reach. Keep them in mind both as you review the next section and as you enter into your career as a medical assistant.

KEYS TO THE AAMA CODE OF ETHICS

Professional

Medical assistants might consider the more salient points in the AAMA Code of Ethics (refer to Figure 7-1) and ask themselves the following questions:

A. *Render service with full respect for the dignity of humanity.*

- Will I respect every patient even if I do not approve of his or her morals or choices in health care?

- Will I honor each patient's request for information and explain unfamiliar procedures?

- Will I give my full attention to acknowledging the needs of every patient?

- Will I be able to accept people who are indigent, have physical and mental challenges, are infirm, have physical disfigurements, and who I simply do not like as equal and valid human beings with an equal right to service?

B. *Respect confidential information obtained through employment unless legally authorized or required by responsible performance of duty to divulge such information.*

- Will I refrain from needless comments to a colleague regarding a patient's problem?

- Will I refrain from discussing my day's encounters with patients with my family and friends?

- Will I always protect patients' medical information and records and everything included from unnecessary observation?
- Will I keep patients' names and the circumstances that bring them to my place of employment confidential?

C. *Uphold the honor and high principles of the profession and accept its disciplines.*

- Am I proud to serve as a medical assistant?
- Will I always perform within the scope of my profession, never exceeding the responsibility entrusted to me?
- Will I encourage others to enter the profession and always speak honorably of medical assistants?

D. *Seek to continually improve the knowledge and skills of medical assistants for the benefit of patients and professional colleagues.*

- Will I be willing to learn new skills, to update my skills, and seek improved methods for assisting the provider in the care of patients?
- Will I keep my credentials current and valid?
- Can I remember that I am a member of a group of broad-based health care professionals, and that my goal is to complement rather than to compete with that team?

E. *Participate in additional service activities aimed toward improving the health and well-being of the community.*

- Will I be able to serve in the community where I reside and work to further quality health care?
- Will I promote preventive medicine?
- Will I practice good health care management for myself and be a model for others to follow?

No matter how prepared, experienced, or principled one is in a chosen profession, there will still be times of great stress and concern about decisions made.

ETHICAL GUIDELINES FOR HEALTH CARE PROVIDERS

As stated earlier, it is fairly common for each professional group of medical practitioners to have its own code of ethics. The AMA's Principles of Medical Ethics and the "Current Opinions with Annotations of the Council on Ethical and Judicial Affairs" have been leaders in this field, but by no means are they the only codes. While the AMA Principles of Medical Ethics are identified in only nine principles, those principles are further identified in seven pages of specific policy issues. (Go to www.ama-assn.org and search "Medical Ethics.") The American Osteopathic Association has a Code of Ethics with 19 different sections. The American Chiropractic Association's Code of Ethics is identified in 14 sections. Other practitioners may consider their mission and policies to be their code of ethics. Some have no specific written code of ethics but rather call on their practitioners to refer to their culture as one based on ethics, mutual respect, and moral evaluation when ethical decisions are made. There are many similarities in these statements on ethics that are important for patients and medical employees. Only a few prominent statements are provided here.

Confidentiality

Legal

Providers must not reveal confidential information about patients without their consent unless the providers are otherwise required to do so by law. Confidentiality must be protected so that patients will feel comfortable and safe in revealing information about themselves that may be important to their health care. Extra caution must be taken to protect the confidentiality of any patient's data on a computer database. As few people as possible should have access to the computer data, and only authorized individuals should be permitted to add or alter data. Adequate security precautions must be used to protect information stored electronically. HIPAA has specific guidelines for computer privacy (see Chapters 10 and 13).

The following list contains examples of the kinds of reports that allow or require health professionals to report a confidence:

- A patient threatens another person and there is reason to believe that the threat may be carried out.
- Certain injuries and illnesses *must* be reported. These include injuries such as knife and gunshot wounds, wounds that may be from suspected abuse, communicable diseases, and sexually transmitted diseases.

- Information that may have been subpoenaed for testimony in a court of law.

When in doubt, it is always recommended that a provider have the patient's permission to reveal any confidential information.

Medical Records

Medical records and the information in them are the property of the provider and the patient. No information should be revealed without the patient's consent unless required by law. The record is confidential. Providers should not refuse to provide a copy of the record to another provider treating the patient so long as proper authorization has been received from the patient. Also, providers should supply a copy of the record or summary of its contents if a patient requests it. A record cannot be withheld because of an unpaid bill.

On a provider's retirement or death, or when a practice is sold, patients should be notified and given ample time to have their records transferred to another provider of their choice.

Professional Fees and Charges

Illegal or excessive fees should not be charged. Fees should be based on those customary to the locale and should reflect the difficulty of services and the quality of performance rendered. Fee splitting (a provider splits the fee with another provider for services rendered with or without the patient's knowledge) in any form is unethical. Providers may charge for missed appointments (if patients have first been notified of the practice) and may charge for multiple or complex insurance forms. Providers and their employees must be diligent to ensure that only the services actually rendered are charged or indicated on the insurance claim. Only what is documented in the patient's chart is to be billed.

There are a number of providers throughout the country who refuse any insurance payments and operate strictly on a cash-only basis. There are others who charge a yearly fee to care for a family, providing all services necessary at that flat fee. Providers, upset by the rules and regulations of insurance, find this method of payment creates a simpler form of medical practice. Providers and patients alike continue to discuss the ethics of such a move. Although providers may choose whom they wish to serve, the cash-only basis is difficult for low-income families and the poor, thereby creating an ethical dilemma.

Professional Rights and Responsibilities

As stated earlier, providers may choose whom to serve, but they may not refuse a patient on the basis of race, color, religion, national origin, or any other illegal discrimination. It is unethical for providers to deny treatment to HIV-infected individuals on that basis alone if they are qualified to treat the patient's condition. However, there are numerous instances of health care being denied to lesbian, gay, bisexual, and transgender (LGBT) individuals and those with AIDS throughout the country. Recently, lesbian mothers living in Michigan were denied care for their infant daughter because of their status. (Go to http://nwlc.org and search "Health Care Refusals" for a serious discussion of this issue.) Once a provider takes a case, the patient cannot be neglected or refused treatment unless official notice is given from the provider to withdraw from the case.

Patients have the right to know their diagnoses and the nature and purpose of their treatment and to have enough information to be able to make an informed choice about their treatment protocol. Providers should inform families of a patient's death and not delegate that responsibility to others.

Providers are expected to expose incompetent, corrupt, dishonest, and unethical conduct by other providers to the disciplinary board. It is unethical for any provider to treat patients while under the influence of alcohol, controlled substances, or any other chemical that impairs the provider's ability.

Providers who know they are HIV positive must refrain from any activity that would risk the transmission of the virus to others.

Any activity that might be regarded as a "conflict of interest" (for example, a provider holding stock in a pharmaceutical company and prescribing medications only from that company) is to be avoided. Financial interests are not to influence providers in prescribing medications, devices, or appliances.

Disaster Response and Emergency Preparedness

Medical professionals are essential at the time of any disaster, such as epidemics, floods, fires, weather-related disasters, and terrorist attacks. Care for the sick and injured is of primary concern when disaster strikes. Providers are encouraged to give their medical expertise not only to prepare for any type of disaster but to provide assistance when one occurs. Providers should consider seeking training in emergency preparedness and disaster response and lend their knowledge where it is most beneficial and effective in making certain that medical care is available during such events (see Chapter 8).

Treatment for a Culturally Diverse Clientele

Diversity

All providers are reminded to strive to provide the same quality of care to all their patients regardless of race or ethnicity. Providers must remember to eliminate biased behavior toward any group of patients deemed different from themselves. All patients have the right to participatory decision making with their providers based on mutual trust and understanding. Communication factors are to be considered and interpreters provided as necessary so that patients understand the medical information as well as any communication exchanged.

Diversity is to be encouraged in the medical profession and considered when hiring assistants. Ethnically diverse neighborhoods and clientele deserve an ethnically diverse group of medical professionals for their care. If it is not possible to employ an ethnically diverse group of medical professionals, then medical professionals who are keenly aware of and knowledgeable of the ethnic group served is of primary importance.

Care of the Poor

From the earliest history of medical treatment, care for the poor has been a concern and a goal for medical practitioners. Today that obligation is still mentioned in most ethical codes and discussions. All medical providers have a responsibility to ensure that the needs of the poor in their communities are met. Caring for the poor should be a regular part of every provider's practice and can be accomplished in a number of ways. Providers can be encouraged to take a certain number of patients on a reduced-cost basis or provide free services. Providers can volunteer their time and efforts to treat patients in reduced-cost, freestanding clinics that treat the poor or provide services to those in homeless shelters for battered and abused individuals. Providers can volunteer their time to

lobbying and being advocates for those without medical coverage.

Abuse

Legal

Abuse, first discussed in Chapter 6, usually is described as neglect, physical injury, emotional/psychological/mental injury, or sexual abuse. In child abuse, there also may be molestation, sexual exploitation, and incest. Elder abuse can come in the form of any other abuse, but financial abuse is included. Stalking and rape are also considered to be forms of abuse.

All 50 states have legislation defining child abuse and mandate who is responsible for reporting such abuse. The majority of states have enacted legislation regarding the abuse of elder adults 60 years of age or older. Intimate partner (or domestic) violence is a criminal offense in some states, but whether a state requires that **intimate partner violence (IPV)** be reported depends in part upon whether a weapon is used.

Stalking is the repeated act of spying upon, following, or making contact with an individual or appearing at an individual's residence or place of employment after being asked not to. It is a crime in some states. *Rape*, also a crime of violence, is forced sexual intercourse or penetration of a body orifice with the penis or some other object. Gang rape involves several individuals. Rape is a reportable criminal act.

Medical assistants must know if their state specifically names them as reporters for abuse. A discussion should be held with medical providers and employers regarding who, when, and how the abuse will be reported and documented. It is unethical for a medical assistant to fail to report abuse simply because an employer prefers "not to get too involved." For a clearer understanding of some of the factors that constitute abuse, review Table 7-1.

It is the responsibility of medical professionals and their employees to report all cases of suspected child abuse, to protect and care for the abused, and to treat the abuser (if known) as a victim also. This is not an easy task. Abuse is not easy to witness. Although there are specific laws regarding suspected child abuse, and in most states medical assistants are mandated to report abuse, the laws are vague or nonexistent for older adults or in cases of IPV. However, whatever form the abuse takes, it is best to treat all forms of abuse in the same manner by providing a safe environment for those abused and seeking treatment for the abused and the abuser.

TABLE 7-1

DESCRIPTIONS OF ABUSE

TYPE OF ABUSE	CHILD ABUSE	ELDER ABUSE	INTIMATE PARTNER VIOLENCE
Neglect	Failure to provide basic food, shelter, care; endangering health of child	Lack of attention that causes harm; withholding basic needs; abandonment; lack of help with hygiene or bathing	Not treating a partner with respect; not recognizing the human worth of an individual
Physical abuse	Causing burns, unusual or severe bruising, lacerations, fractures, injury to internal organs; usually obvious	Assault, beating, whipping, hitting, punching, pushing, pinching, force-feeding, shaking, rough handling during caregiving, causing bodily harm or severe mental stress	Intent to harm; hitting, pushing, grabbing, biting, punching, slapping, restraining, burning; use of a weapon or one's own strength to harm
Emotional/ psychological abuse	Causing harm to child's emotional and intellectual growth; not always obvious	Actions that dehumanize; social isolation, name calling, humiliating, insulting; threats to punish; yelling, screaming	Humiliating; controlling; isolating partner from friends/ family; denying personal support and encouragement
Sexual abuse	Using a child to engage in any sexual activity; abuse not always obvious	Sexual contact without permission; fondling, touching, kissing, rape, coerced nudity; spying while in bathroom	Sexual contact without permission; abusive sexual contact; sex with one who is unable to say "no"
Sexual exploitation	Pornography, prostitution; use of child's image in media; incest or sexual activity between family members	Showing an elderly person pornographic material; forcing the person to watch sex acts; forcing the elder to undress in presence of others	Forcing a partner to engage in sexual acts with others against that partner's will
Financial abuse	Refusal to provide the basics of adequate health care or clothing	Exploitation of an elder's resources; forging signature on documents; withholding or cashing funds received	Withholding funds or basic resources; monitoring to the penny funds spent for groceries or expenses of daily living

BIOETHICS

Bioethics brings the entire focus of ethics into the field of health care and into those ethical issues dealing with all aspects of life and death. Never before in the history of medical care has bioethics been such a topic of concern. In the past, most bioethical decisions were made by physicians and esteemed members of the medical or legal profession. However, advancing technology giving patients and consumers numerous choices regarding their health now has everyone taking a more active role in bioethics.

Medical assistants will encounter ethical and bioethical issues across a total life span. A few issues are identified for contemplation and discussion.

Infants

- Imperiled newborns (seriously disabled, deformed, often premature with low birth weight) who survive with modern technology incur soaring costs of expensive intervention not always covered by insurance.

Children

- When not well fed, housed, educated and clothed, children have great need for preventive, curative, and rehabilitative health care; proper inoculations against communicable diseases; and attention to any evidence of eating disorders.
- Obesity is a health concern that is often the result of poor food choices.
- Many children live in dysfunctional families where parents are absent, abuse substances, have mental health issues, or have very little time to spend with their children.

Adolescents

- The adolescent's need for independence, changing values, and desire for peer acceptance may lead to risky sexual behavior and drug and alcohol experimentation.

- Mental health issues often interfere with normal social development, yet mental health assessment and treatment are difficult to find.

- Adolescents as young as 14 to 18 years may seek treatment for substance abuse, birth control, and even abortion without parental consent.

Adults

- It can be difficult to balance full-time employment, parenting, housekeeping, and partnering and still take care of oneself.

- War, terrorism, and an overburdened military place stress on families. Many return from service with lifelong and debilitating injuries.

Senior Adults

- Older adults have the right to dignity and privacy that is often denied when they lose their independence.

- It is often difficult for new patients to find providers who take Medicare and Medicaid, leaving them without appropriate medical attention.

- Some older adults must still choose between food on their table and the purchase of prescribed medications.

- Dementia is a growing problem that is financially exhausting and heartbreaking.

- Even with advance directives, a dying patient's wishes may be ignored.

Issues of bioethics common to the medical community are the allocation of scarce or limited medical resources; whether health care is a right or privilege; reproductive issues such as contraception, assisted reproduction, abortion, and fetal tissue research; genetic engineering or manipulation; and the many choices surrounding life, dying, and death.

Guidelines for bioethical issues are even harder to define than are guidelines for ethics, because each of the bioethical issues calls for decisions that directly affect a person's life. In some instances, the bioethical issue requires a choice about who lives and requires defining quality of life. Such dilemmas are difficult, if not impossible, to approach from a neutral point of view, even though medical professionals should strive not to impose their own moral values on patients or co-workers.

ALLOCATION OF SCARCE OR LIMITED MEDICAL RESOURCES

One issue faced daily by health care workers is the allocation of limited medical resources, or what ultimately becomes rationing of health care. Even with the 2010 Affordable Care Act (ACA), medical resources are still not available to everyone. When the administrative medical assistant determines who receives the only available appointment in a day, when patients are turned away because they have no insurance or financial resources to pay for services, when Medicare and Medicaid patients are denied services because of low return from state and federal insurance programs, medical resources are being rationed and denied.

U.S. Census data from 2014 shows that the number of uninsured Americans declined by 8.8 million the first year the ACA took effect. That is down 13.3 percent from 2013. The Census Bureau reports, however, that those states choosing not to expand Medicaid will leave millions of poor Americans without access to affordable health care.

The ACA ended some issues of rationing. The act helps more children get health coverage, ends lifetime and most annual limits on care, allows young adults under age 26 to stay on their parent's health insurance, and gives some patients access to a number of recommended preventive services such as vaccinations, influenza and pneumonia shots, and blood pressure and diabetes screenings without co-payment or deductible costs. Other reforms are in process. Hispanic and non-Hispanic black children are still more likely to not have access to health care than are non-Hispanic white children. Of note, the average waiting time by new patients for a medical appointment is 18.5 days. Older patients, many of whom have both Medicare and supplemental health insurance, have difficulty finding providers who take new Medicare patients. Providers, who can choose whom to serve, increasingly are not taking any new patients because the Medicare return dollars are most often less than the costs incurred. This dilemma can be particularly problematic when older patients move from their homes and communities to be closer to their children.

Weightier decisions might include who gets the surgery, kidney transplant, or bone marrow transplant. These allocation and rationing decisions are being made and will continue to require dedication on the part of the health care team. Rationing of health care will continue to be an issue as politicians, health care providers, and consumers struggle to balance providing access to care with curtailing costs.

Decisions made by Congress, health systems agencies, and insurance companies are termed **macroallocation** of scarce medical resources. Decisions made individually by providers and members of the health care team at the local level are termed **microallocation** of scarce resources. No matter what the level, medical assistants will be involved.

Health Care: A Right or a Privilege?

Very close to the issue of allocation of limited medical resources is the question of whether basic health care is a right or a privilege. There are many countries in the world where health care is a privilege provided only to a few either because of the availability of health care or because of one's financial resources. However, even within the United States, where the best of health care is available, there are health care professionals whose personal ideologies often lead to discrimination and denial of basic health care.

For example, consider the following circumstances. How would you choose?

- *For the available kidney.* There is a perfect match for a young mother of two or a 45-year-old gentleman (a recovering addict) with numerous body piercings.

- *For the next available pediatric appointment.* A 16-year-old who needs an athletic physical or a troubled and combative 13-year-old whose only insurance is Medicaid.

- *For artificial insemination.* A single woman desiring a child of her own or a couple who have been trying to get pregnant for 3 years.

- *Referral to a mental health specialist.* A prominent businessman suffering from depression with symptoms of bipolar disorder or a mom receiving state aid and struggling with addiction.

It is often difficult to remain neutral and wait to make decisions until all the facts are known. One continuing area of discrimination surrounds the health care issue of AIDS and HIV.

HIV and AIDS

The general public's fear and wariness of AIDS (acquired immunodeficiency syndrome) continues

to cause bioethical issues. Patients who suspect they have HIV (human immunodeficiency virus) or AIDS should be tested for the virus. In fact, the CDC recommends that voluntary screening for HIV/AIDS become a routine part of medical care for all patients ages 13 to 64 years. Confidentiality must be safely guarded, however, because individuals with HIV/AIDS have been denied medical insurance, faced loss of employment and housing, and even suffered the loss of family members and friends. It is unethical to deny treatment to individuals because they test positive for HIV.

Although individuals with HIV/AIDS are to be protected, so must the public. Therefore, if providers suspect that an HIV-seropositive patient is infecting an unsuspecting individual, every attempt is to be made to protect the individual at risk. Health professionals will first encourage the infected person to cease any activity that endangers the other person. If the patient refuses to notify the person at risk, authorities can be contacted. Many states and cities have partner notification programs that will anonymously notify any person at risk, keeping the source confidential. The program informs him or her that it has been brought to their attention that he or she is a "person at risk" and provides free testing.

Reproductive Issues

Reproductive bioethical issues generally affect women more than men. A few are identified here. Most medical assistants will be faced with these issues at some time in their career, even if they are not employed in specialty clinics.

Female Genital Mutilation. The World Health Organization (WHO) reports that there are over 170,000 young girls and women in the United States who have been subjected to **female genital mutilation (FGM)**. FGM includes partial or complete removal of the clitoris (female circumcision); partial or total removal of the labia minora or labia majora; infibulation (narrowing the vaginal opening by creating a covering seal); and the pricking, piercing, or cauterizing of the genitals. These procedures are performed, in part, to enhance a man's sexual pleasure, but they destroy a woman's capacity for sexual pleasure and can cause serious infections. The practice can also cause recurring urinary tract infections, difficulties with menstruation, and pregnancy complications. FGM is illegal in this country, but can be seen in immigrants from countries such as some African, Asian, and Middle Eastern nations where it is regularly practiced.

Contraception. Birth control of any kind, other than *fertility awareness methods (FAM)* that require abstinence from sexual intercourse during ovulation, is still a taboo in some cultures and religions and becomes a bioethical dilemma. Many are opposed to any contraception that destroys a fertilized egg. Therefore, a thorough understanding of how a particular contraception works is essential for some patients.

The controversy gained attention when the RU-486 or mifepristone hormone drug became available for use in the United States in order to end an early pregnancy. In general, it can be used up to 63 days—9 weeks—after the first day of a woman's last period. Today, a primary issue is the availability of birth control to some women. In 2014, the U.S. Supreme Court ruled that employers (especially those that have a religious objection) can deny birth control as part of health insurance coverage available to their employees.

Sterilization. When permanent contraception is sought, sterilization has become the choice. It is not only used by those who simply wish to prevent pregnancy, but it may be practiced by those who prefer not to pass on a genetic anomaly. A **tubal ligation** for women and a **vasectomy** for men are considered permanent, even though there have been reversals. Some religious groups oppose permanent sterilization.

Assisted Reproduction. Assistance with reproduction is very common today. Artificial insemination, in vitro fertilization, and surrogacy are most commonly practiced.

For many individuals, *artificial insemination* is the only means by which they are able to conceive a child. Providers are called on to perform artificial insemination for couples and for women who want a child. If artificial insemination is performed, it is recommended that the signed consent of each party involved be obtained. It is also recommended that providers practicing artificial insemination by donor have several donors available for semen collection and that meticulous screening be performed before the insemination.

In vitro fertilization (IVF) is a process that has been shown to be very successful in the past decade. In IVF, the ovum is fertilized in a culture dish, allowed to grow, and then implanted into the uterus. This procedure can be used for women with blocked fallopian tubes or oviducts. Ethically, this procedure faces little controversy when a husband's sperm is used to fertilize his wife's ovum, which is then implanted into her uterus. Other procedures raise ethical concerns for some and are not addressed in law.

A woman can have a donor's egg fertilized by her husband's sperm for implantation. A woman can receive donor embryos (embryo adoption) from successfully completed IVF from two unrelated individuals. Couples who have successfully had a baby through IVF are sometimes willing to donate their additional embryos. A woman can carry an embryo created from a donor egg and donor sperm that will have no genetic relationship to her.

It is possible to screen for genetic flaws among embryos created by IVF; however, the latest medical research indicates that such analysis sometimes causes abnormalities.

Surrogacy is another method of assisted reproduction. Men have been used as **surrogates**, or substitutes, for decades with the practice of artificial insemination. Society still seems to have a more difficult time accepting surrogate mothers who are artificially inseminated by a donor and carry the fetus to term for another parent. Men sometimes seek surrogates who are able to provide them a child who represents half their genetic makeup. Women may choose a surrogate if they are unable to carry a pregnancy to term for medical or personal reasons. How should the rights of each individual in the arrangement and exchange be protected? For many of these issues, there is little protection or guidance under the law; therefore, health professionals are often required to make decisions on the basis of their personal belief systems.

Ethical questions are sometimes raised regarding assisted reproduction. Should artificial insemination and in vitro fertilization be performed for individuals who do not fit the "traditional" family model? Who will be a fit mother or father for a particular infant? Some religious faiths consider artificial insemination by donor to be the same as adultery. Who or what agency carefully protects the selection and screening process of donors and surrogates? How are donors selected? Is there a responsibility to make certain that individuals with the same father through artificial insemination by donor do not marry? Some fertility specialists recommend that a donor be chosen from a city far from where the potential mother lives and that formal adoption occur immediately when the infant is born. Some oppose in vitro fertilization because fertilized ova are destroyed if found to be genetically inappropriate. Others have great difficulty when embryos that are not implanted are often frozen for later use, but sometimes are abandoned and eventually destroyed.

Most assisted reproduction techniques were viewed as experimental and quite controversial just 25 years ago. Today, however, the procedures are widely practiced and available. Assisted reproduction is very costly and can create legal tangles for all involved if careful steps are not taken.

Abortion and Fetal Tissue Research

The issues associated with abortion and fetal tissue research will be with us for quite some time. Although the law as set forth in *Roe v. Wade* is specific on abortion guidelines, there is a continual challenge in the courts of its validity. A number of states have been successful in pressing for more restrictions regarding whether and how abortions might be performed in the second and third trimesters of pregnancy, and challenge the U.S. Supreme Court's decision in *Roe v. Wade*. However, the current law stipulates that a woman has a right to an abortion in the first trimester without interference from regulations in any state.

Medical professionals must decide whether to perform abortions within these legal parameters and under what circumstances. Providers cannot be forced to perform abortions, nor can any employee be forced to participate or assist in an abortion. Employees not wishing to participate in abortions are advised to seek employment where they are not performed.

Legal

The volatility of the issue is so strong that terrorism against some abortion clinics and their providers has made it difficult for a person wanting an abortion to receive one. Terrorism of any sort is illegal, but providers who perform abortions have been murdered, one even in a church during worship. Such terrorism points to the very passionate debate that is unlikely ever to find a common ground of agreement.

Many unanswered ethical questions related to abortion make the decision difficult for health care professionals. Should abortion be considered a form of birth control? If not, should birth control and abortion be readily available to all who seek it, regardless of age? Should insurance pay for birth control? Is it ethical to deny an abortion to a woman on welfare but provide one to a woman who has money for the procedure or whose insurance pays? Some question if *any* abortion should be legal. And, of course, the major unanswered question that must be considered by every individual is: When does life begin—at conception, when the brain begins to function, at quickening, or at birth?

The abortion issue raises the bioethical issue of fetal tissue research and transplantation. As early as the 1950s, fetal tissue research led to the development of polio and rubella vaccines. Today, fetal cells hold promise for medical research into a variety of diseases and medical conditions, including Alzheimer disease, Parkinson disease, spinal cord injury, diabetes, and multiple sclerosis. Some research indicates that fetal retinal transplants may be a successful treatment of macular degeneration, which is the leading cause of age-related blindness in the United States.

This issue is political as well as bioethical, and it changes with each major political shift in the government. About half of the states have laws regulating fetal research. Some ban research using aborted fetuses. Federal law prohibits the sale of fetal tissue and requires all federally funded fetal tissue research projects to comply with state and local laws. This issue came to light in 2015 when Planned Parenthood was accused of selling fetal tissue for profit by the Center for Medical Progress. Videos released by the Center for Medical Progress were edited, however, and Planned Parenthood can and does legally collect fees for the handling and processing of the fetal tissue. Fetal tissue research is not to be used to encourage women to have abortions; rather, the tissue would be available only after a decision had already been made regarding abortion.

While the debate related to the use of fetal tissues for research marches on, the door has opened for research using umbilical cord blood. The use of cord blood has met with little controversy. In 2005, President George W. Bush signed into legislation a federal program to collect and store cord blood and to expand the current bone marrow registry program to include cord blood. Stem cells in cord blood have shown to be beneficial. For example, they can help restore red blood cells in people with sickle cell anemia. When a small group of children newly diagnosed with type 1 diabetes were transfused with their own stored cord blood, they showed reduced severity of the disease.

Integrity

Medical assistants who work in fertility clinics must at all times respect the choices made by individuals seeking artificial insemination, IVF, or surrogacy. These procedures are truly private and very personal. Anyone who feels uncomfortable with such procedures is likely to be happier finding employment elsewhere.

Genetic Engineering/Manipulation

So much is possible today in the area of **genetic engineering** and new discoveries increasingly are being made. This biotechnology can be used in the diagnosis of disease, in the production of medicines, for forensic documentation (DNA used in solving crimes), and for research. Some reasons for continuing study in this area include determining if anything can be done to prevent or cure some 4,000 recognized genetic disorders and major diseases that have large genetic components. Few individuals would not like to see a cure for certain illnesses, but there is a fear among many that genetic engineering may lead to choices that should not be made. Deciding what should be done when the unborn is determined to have a severe birth defect, manipulating genes for a more perfect offspring, and discarding defective embryos are just a few of those concerns.

When countries move past the dilemma related to the use of embryonic stem cells, a number of significant medical advances might be made. Researchers may be able to create custom-made organs to replace those that are defective or diseased. Using small pieces of muscle and tissue from individuals, reproductive organs and nasal cartilage have been successfully grown and implanted. Although it might be a wonderful thing to create a new pancreas or a semisynthetic liver to replace an organ that is no longer performing its necessary function, the greater fear of some individuals is that of cloning.

Scientists already have cloned mice, sheep, rabbits, goats, pigs, and a dog. Where does cloning stop? Will human beings be cloned if science advances further into research with stem cells? Some countries with a different political arena than the one found in the United States are moving into this area. It is interesting to note, however, that in August 2005 the General Assembly of the United Nations voted to prohibit all forms of human cloning.

Dying and Death

The goal for all health professionals is to preserve and enhance life, thus making death an event contrary to the goals of health care. Yet, death cannot be avoided. How death is faced has both legal and ethical dimensions. Legally, individuals can make choices about their death and are often encouraged to do so by health care and legal professionals. When those wishes are indicated in documents such as advance directives and when health professionals disagree or refuse to honor those wishes, a legal problem arises. (Refer to Chapter 6.)

The legal aspect was made famous by the cases of Karen Ann Quinlan and Theresa (Terri) Schiavo. Both were young women, without any advance health care directives, whose deaths were caught in battles between family members, the medical staff, and the courts. Quinlan lived for

11 years in a vegetative state after much duress with health professionals and hospital staff who believed she should be kept on a respirator. The family members of Schiavo were in legal battles for 15 years before permission was received to remove her feeding tube; she died 14 days later. When there is conflict among family and those caring for someone near death, even a well-written and executed advance directive can be challenged. Then a legal dilemma becomes an ethical dilemma as well.

Legal

Patients continue to make decisions expressing their choices in death. Oregon was the first state to pass legislation allowing physicians to prescribe medications for patients to aid in their dying. The Oregon law was voted upon and passed on two separate occasions and was challenged by the U.S. Attorney General before the U.S. Supreme Court determined that the law could stand. Voters in the state of Washington approved similar legislation November 2008. Montana, Vermont, and California were recently added to the list. Several other states are struggling with issues to allow those who are dying a death with dignity. Many patients find comfort in a law that allows them the right to choose the time and place of their own death; however, the number of individuals who choose aid in dying still is small. Some make the choice, receive the medications from their physician, and then do not use the medication. Others receive the medication, find much relief in their choice, and do take the medication. There are still others who believe that any intervention that hastens death is criminal.

Religious Opposition to Assisted Dying. While much of society supports expanded options in dying, there is a large group that is opposed to any legislation that allows a patient to make certain decisions. There are religious groups that oppose *any* aid in dying, withholding food or hydration, and/or Do Not Resuscitate orders. Today, Catholic hospitals make up 10 of the 25 largest health care networks in America, and in many communities, the only hospital is a Catholic one. Catholic hospitals have long held to the tradition of not providing medical services that contradict Catholic religious principles and will not allow their providers (many not Catholic) to perform these services. For example, Catholic hospitals will not provide emergency abortion services to a woman with life-threatening pregnancy complications, and will also deny aid in dying to patients even in those states where such services are legal. This is a good example of a conflict between the law and ethics.

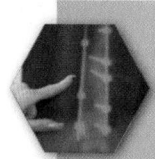

Critical Thinking

When there is conflict between what is legal and what might be considered by some to be unethical, how do you decide what action to take (see Procedure 7-1)? Could you work where abortions are legally performed? Could you deny a dying patient the right to carry out an advance directive if you did not believe in withholding food or hydration? While the law protects a woman seeking an abortion in the first trimester and allows patients to prepare very specific advance directives, what happens when the only health care source in the region does not allow either? Is this macro- or microallocation of limited resources?

someone else administers the life-ending medication. Neither is aid in dying assisted suicide. These individuals want to live, but are dying from some terminal illness, and prefer a death with dignity. Many of these patients are also receiving optimal end-of-life care in hospice. For the most up-to-date information, refer to your state's legislation.

Choices available to patients who are dying create the question "What is quality of life?" Although the answer to that question is different for everyone, it is a question often in conflict with today's medical technology that can, in many instances, keep a patient alive much longer than the patient might prefer. The benefits of advanced technology will continue to be weighed against what many consider the right to die with dignity and a minimum of medical intervention.

Hospice. *Hospice* is the term used to describe either a place of residence for those who are dying or an organization whose medical professionals and volunteers are in attendance of someone whose death is imminent. The main objective of hospice is to make patients comfortable and as free from pain as possible and to allow them dignity in their deaths.

The law is changing rapidly as additional states wrestle with the concept of aid in dying, but aid in dying is not **euthanasia**. The patient remains in complete control, unlike euthanasia where

---

> ## PROCEDURE 7-1
>
>
>
> ### Develop a Plan for Separation of Personal and Professional Ethics
>
> Procedure
>
> **PURPOSE:**
>
> To make a plan for circumstances when there is conflict between personal and professional ethics.
>
> **EQUIPMENT/SUPPLIES:**
>
> Paper, pen or computer
>
> **PROCEDURE SCENARIO:**
>
> A medical assistant who is also a lay Eucharistic minister (assists priest with mass and communion) must respond to a patient with end-stage pancreatic cancer requesting information regarding assisted death in Oregon.
>
> **PROCEDURE STEPS:**
>
> 1. Using the Internet or Oregon's state statute on assisted death, determine the steps necessary to make assistance in death legal. RATIONALE: It is important to know the steps in this legal process to determine if they are satisfied.
>
> 2. Given this scenario, answer the ethics check questions identified in the text, and determine if and how you might assist this patient. RATIONALE: Answering these questions helps to put the emotional aspect of the scenario in perspective.
>
> 3. If you *can participate*, explain how you will proceed. If you decide you *cannot participate*, explain how you will proceed. RATIONALE: These steps aid the medical assistant in choice of words necessary in an explanation to the patient and employer.
>
> 4. Record this process and the decision you made to be true to yourself, therapeutic to the patient, and professional in all aspects of your employment.

Cardiopulmonary resuscitation (CPR), intravenous therapy, and feeding tubes are discouraged. Death is treated as a natural end-of-life experience. Death is neither hastened nor prevented.

Hospice volunteers and their counselors indicate that although many patients may choose hospice, some family members may not be as comfortable in that choice. Family members may not be ready to let go of a loved one; also, they may be uncomfortable if the hospice service is in the home rather than the hospital or a hospice facility. The latter is related to how comfortable family members are in observing or being a part of the death process. The expense of hospice is often covered by medical insurance and is less expensive than inpatient hospital care.

Medical assistants may be involved with the hospice protocol when patients of their employers are referred to and become clients of hospice.

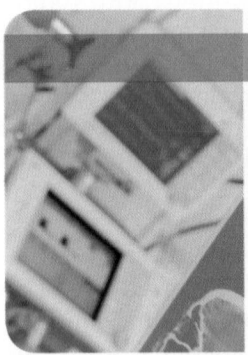

CASE STUDY 7-1

Refer to the scenario at the beginning of the chapter.

CASE STUDY REVIEW

1. If Harley's behavior does no harm to the patient, has he acted unethically? Illegally?
2. What might the office manager do if she senses Harley's lack of certainty?
3. Discuss the role of female and male medical assistants working together and how they might complement each other.

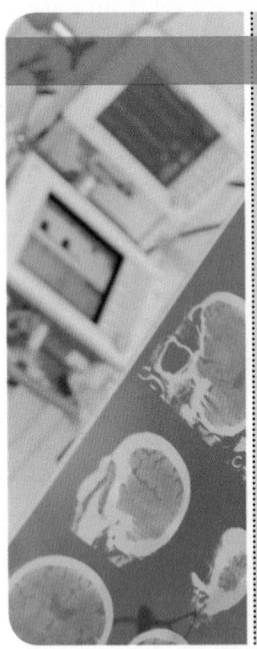

CASE STUDY 7-2

Lisa Chu is a medical assistant in the fertility clinic of a large metropolitan medical clinic and hospital. Lisa really likes her job and is delighted when parenthood is made possible for many of those seeking the clinic's advanced technology. The clinic also stores and maintains the unused frozen embryos that result from artificial insemination. She is a little alarmed when her provider-employer informs her that four of the embryos are to be destroyed. Her employer has been unable to contact the owners (now parents of more than one child from artificial insemination) for directions, and space for storage is limited. Lisa is instructed to destroy the embryos.

CASE STUDY REVIEW

1. Lisa is rather hesitant to comply with her employer's orders, so she does a little research. She discovers that most fertility clinics ask couples using **cryopreservation** to decide early in the process how to handle their excess embryos. The choices are to (1) discard the embryos, (2) donate anonymously to other infertile couples, and (3) donate to scientific research. What might Lisa do to influence the clinic's policy?
2. Can anything be done to ensure that couples do not abandon their embryos?
3. If embryos are given to other infertile couples, how is a decision made on who should have them?

Summary

- As medical technology continues to advance, a greater need for ethical guidelines is necessary.
- Providers and health care professionals at all levels must stay abreast of the issues and carefully consider all aspects before making any decision.
- Medical assistants must, however, keep the following legal and ethical guidelines in mind: (1) always practice within the law; (2) preserve the patient's confidentiality; (3) maintain meticulous records; (4) obtain informed, written consent; and (5) do not judge patients whose belief system differs from yours.

Study for Success

To reinforce your knowledge and skills of information presented in this chapter:

- Review the *Key Terms* and *Learning Outcomes*
- Consider the *Critical Thinking* features and *Case Studies* and discuss your conclusions
- Answer the questions in the *Certification Review*

- Perform the *Procedure* using the *Competency Assessment Checklists* on the *Student Companion Website*

Procedure

CERTIFICATION REVIEW

1. Typically, how has ethics been defined?
   a. It tells what is right and wrong.
   b. It determines whether an action is legal.
   c. It deals with what is the expedient thing to do.
   d. It is the best method for demonstrating professionalism in the workplace.

2. How is bioethics best explained?
   a. Biological reproduction is the main consideration.
   b. Bioethics is a new ethical dilemma.
   c. Bioethics is best explained in numerous codes of ethics.
   d. Bioethics focuses on ethical issues that deal with life and death issues.
   e. Bioethics always has to do with macro- and microallocation.

3. How is the AAMA Code of Ethics best identified?
   a. It applies only to patient rights.
   b. It is concerned with principles of ethical and moral conduct.
   c. It defines the duties the medical assistant can perform.
   d. It is intended for use by all providers.

4. When providers or medical assistants suspect child abuse, what should they do?
   a. Give the parent a warning
   b. Report it to the proper authorities
   c. Withdraw from treatment and refer elsewhere
   d. Give the child some hints on how to protect against abuse
   e. Omit the information from the electronic medical record

5. When a patient is HIV seropositive, what action should be taken?
   a. Make an immediate referral to an AIDS clinic
   b. Notify all possible unsuspecting individuals in contact with the patient
   c. Schedule appointments at the end of the day away from all other patients
   d. Protect their confidentiality while protecting any at risk

6. What does macroallocation of scarce medical resources imply?
   a. That the local health care team makes the decisions
   b. That Congress, health systems agencies, and insurance companies make the decisions
   c. That medical assistants will not be involved
   d. That patients will get the benefit of the best medical care
   e. That Medicaid patients will never be denied health care

7. Who authored the characteristics of principle-centered leaders?
   a. James R. Jones
   b. Stephen R. Covey
   c. Francis H. Ambrose
   d. Jason N. Diamond

8. What are the five Ps of ethical power?
   a. Personality, performance, purpose, pride, patience
   b. Purpose, patience, perfection, personality, procrastination
   c. Patience, purpose, pride, persistence, perspective
   d. Purpose, pride, patience, perfection, perspective
   e. Perfection, patience, perspective, personality, performance

9. Which of the following is true?
   a. A provider cannot choose whom to serve.
   b. It is unethical to charge for completing multiple and complex insurance claims.
   c. Providers and their employees cannot be forced to perform abortions.
   d. It is best to refer the poor and indigent to public health clinics.

10. When are you most likely to make ethical decisions correctly?
    a. When you do not need a clear picture of the situation.
    b. When you are emotional and passionate about the decision.
    c. When you have determined who you are and how you will act.
    d. When honesty and integrity do not influence a patient's care.
    e. When you remember to leave such decisions to your provider-employer.

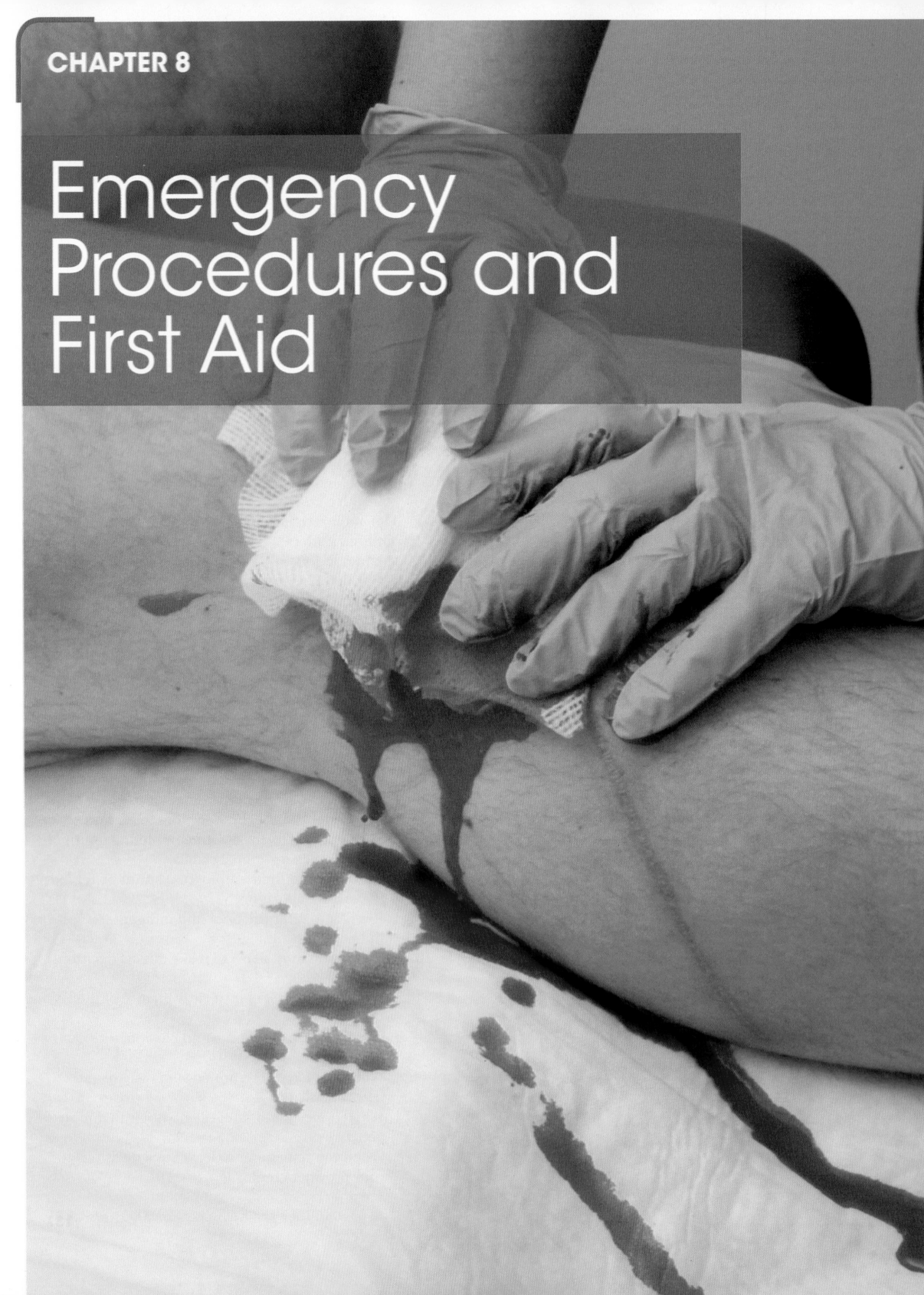

CHAPTER 8

Emergency Procedures and First Aid

1. Define and spell the key terms as presented in the glossary.
2. Recognize, prepare for, and respond to emergencies in the ambulatory care setting.
3. Outline basic principles of first aid and demonstrate first aid procedures.
4. Understand the legal and ethical considerations of providing emergency care.
5. Carry out appropriate interventions to prevent disease transmission considerations in emergency situations.
6. Perform the primary assessment in emergency situations.
7. Detect and care for different types of wounds.
8. Execute the basics of bandage application.
9. Discriminate among first-, second-, and third-degree burns.
10. Assess injuries to muscles, bones, and joints.
11. Summarize heat- and cold-related illnesses.
12. Explain how poisons may enter the body.
13. List the symptoms of a poisonous snake bite.
14. Recall six types of shock.
15. Detect a cerebral vascular accident.
16. Describe the signs and symptoms of a heart attack.
17. Identify potential role(s) of the medical assistant in emergency preparedness.

KEY TERMS

abrasion
anaphylactic
automated external defibrillator (AED)
avulsion
bandages
cardiogenic
cardiopulmonary resuscitation (CPR)
cardioversion
crash cart or tray
crepitation
diplopia
dislocations
dressings
electrocautery
emergency medical services (EMS)

explicit
first aid
fractures
Good Samaritan laws
hyperglycemia
hypoglycemia
hypothermia
hypovolemic
hypoxia
implicit
incision
ketoacidosis
laceration
myocardial infarction (MI)
neurogenic
normal saline
occlusion

puncture wound
rescue breathing
risk management
septic
shock
splints
sprain
Standard Precautions
status epilepticus
strain
syncope
triage
tonic-clonic phase
tourniquet
ulcers
universal emergency medical identification symbol
wounds

It has been a busy day at Inner City Health Care. The final patient is being seen. Just as Nancy McFarland, RMA (AMT), is closing the door to the lobby, Mr. Art Cochran enters holding his chest. He states, "Your clinic is closer than the hospital and I needed to see someone. My chest is hurting and I can't catch my breath."

Based on her knowledge and experience, Ms. McFarland is aware that that Mr. Cochran is exhibiting signs of a heart attack. She remains calm, immediately notifying the provider and instructing the front desk person to call 911. Ms. McFarland escorts Mr. Cochran to a treatment room, has him lie down, and immediately takes his vital signs. As Ms. McFarland is certified in cardiopulmonary resuscitation (CPR) and first aid, she begins to take the appropriate steps to make sure that the patient is safe and cared for prior to the arrival of emergency medical system (EMS) personnel. Per the standing orders for patients with chest pain, Mr. Cochran is given a full-strength aspirin to chew and oxygen is applied. Mr. Cochran is calm and his chest pain is easing just as the EMS team arrives. It is essential to activate the EMS system as soon as possible when an emergency presents itself in a nonacute care setting. Care is then relinquished to the EMS personnel to provide further intervention.

Chapter Portal

Although the ambulatory care setting is primarily designed to see patients under nonemergency conditions, occasionally a situation will arise that requires administration of emergency care. The medical assistant is often an essential team member during a crisis situation. For the medical assistant who may need to screen or assess the patient's condition, the first and most critical step in responding to an emergency is developing the skill to recognize when emergency measures should be taken.

Some emergencies can be treated in the clinic, while others cannot, and the medical assistant must know when to initiate the request for outside help. If the emergency occurs in the ambulatory care setting, the provider usually administers immediate care. It is possible, however, that the medical assistant may be the first emergency caregiver should the provider be out of the clinic. The medical assistant also may be called on to provide care in an emergency outside the clinic environment.

This chapter acquaints the medical assistant with types of emergency situations that may occur during the course of a routine day. This chapter is merely an introduction to emergency topics and does not substitute for first aid and cardiopulmonary resuscitation (CPR) instruction taught through the American Red Cross, the American Heart Association, the American Safety and Health Institute, or the National Safety Council. Medical assistants in CAAHEP- and ABHES-accredited programs must be certified to a provider level in CPR and must be taught by instructors who are certified to teach CPR. These hands-on classes are vital teaching tools, and all medical assistants should take them on a regular basis to continually update their skills.

RECOGNIZING AN EMERGENCY

An emergency is considered any instance in which an individual becomes suddenly ill and requires immediate attention. Most emergencies develop quickly and usually without warning. They can occur unexpectedly at any time to anyone. Some may be gradual, as seen with dehydration or slow blood loss, and become an emergency over time. As you mature in your career, you will begin to develop the ability to make quick determinations about the conditions of people around you. Your experiences in medicine will allow you to assess emergency situations simply by using your senses. By using your sense of sight, you will note an abnormal coloring of the skin, an expression of pain or discomfort,

or evidence of bleeding or bruising. Your sense of smell will help detect a wound that has become infected or identify the fruity breath that occurs when a patient's blood sugar is very high. Your sense of touch helps to assess a patient's pulse or the temperature of his skin. Your sense of hearing will help you recognize a wheeze or cough indicting respiratory distress. It is also essential to be acutely sensitive to any unusual behaviors such as screaming, crying, moaning, or staring blankly off in space.

In the ambulatory care setting, medical assistants may encounter a range of emergency situations requiring first aid techniques. **First aid** is designed to render immediate and temporary emergency care to persons injured or otherwise disabled before the arrival of a health care practitioner or transport to a hospital or other health care agency. Emergency situations can be minor or severe and can include:

- Choking and breathing crises
- Chest pain
- Bleeding
- Shock
- Stroke
- Poisoning
- Burns
- Wounds
- Sudden illnesses such as fainting/falling
- Illnesses related to heat and cold
- Fractures

Safety

Some of these situations will be life threatening; all will require immediate care. In either case, it is critical to remain calm, to follow the emergency policies and procedures established by the ambulatory care setting, and to be well versed in first aid and certified in CPR. The patient should not be further endangered.

Responding to an Emergency

Once it has been determined that an emergency exists, it is essential to act quickly. Before making any decisions about how to proceed, it is necessary to assess the nature of the situation. Does it include respiratory or circulatory failure, severe bleeding, burns, poisoning, or severe allergic reaction?

Sometimes, it is possible that more than one type of care must be administered. As a medical assistant approaches any situation, it is imperative to begin with the CAB assessment: Circulation, Airway, and Breathing. Based on this information, the next step is to assist the provider in assessing the patient's condition so that treatment can be prioritized. When an individual experiences more than one illness or injury, care must be given according to the severity of the situation. When two or more patients present with emergencies simultaneously, screening helps determine which patient is treated first. This process is known as **triage**. Table 8-1 lists the common ordering of screening situations.

To identify the nature of the emergency and respond effectively, it is critical that the patient's overall condition be taken into consideration, including vital signs. If the patient is conscious, ask for personal identification and identification of next of kin. Try to obtain information about symptoms being experienced to identify the problem. Always check for a **universal emergency medical identification symbol** (Figure 8-1) and accompanying identification card, which will describe any serious or life-threatening health problems that the patient has. Quickly observe the patient's general appearance, including skin color and size and dilation of pupils. Check pulse and blood pressure.

TABLE 8-1

EXAMPLES OF EMERGENCY CATEGORIES

FIRST PRIORITY	NEXT PRIORITY	LEAST PRIORITY
Burns on face	Second-degree burns not on the neck and face	Fractures (simple)
Airway and breathing problems	Major or multiple fractures	Minor injuries
Cardiac arrest	Back injuries	Sprains, strains
Severe bleeding that is uncontrolled	Severe eye injuries	Simple lacerations
Head injuries	Syncope	Dehydration without change in vital signs
Poisoning	Seizure	
Anaphylactic shock	Lacerations involving multiple tissue layers	
Stroke	Hyper- or hypoglycemia	
Open chest or abdominal wounds		

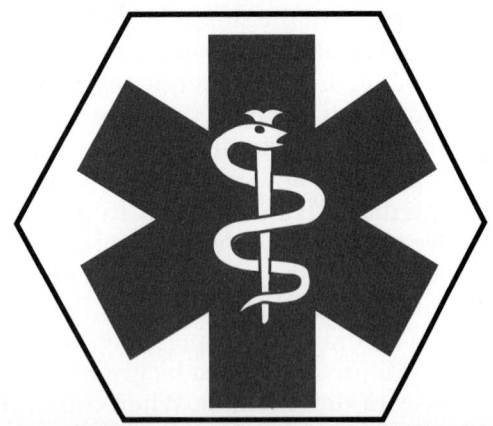

FIGURE 8-1 The universal emergency medical identification symbol.

 Patient confidentiality must be maintained during an emergency situation. Take care to be mindful of those around you when an emergency situation arises, as your voice when speaking to other health care providers may be overheard by other patients. Privacy must be maintained when faxing information to the emergency department. Be sure to verify the fax number and use a fax cover sheet. Always be cautious in keeping the patient's anonymity protected.

Primary Survey

A method for assessing life-threatening injuries is known as the primary survey. Previously, this sequence was known as the airway, breathing, circulation, disability, and expose and evaluate assessment (or ABCDE assessment). In 2015, the American Heart Association (AHA) changed its recommendations so as to initiate compressions first. See the "Primary Survey" Quick Reference Guide for more information on the current assessment guidelines.

Using the 911 or Emergency Medical Services System

The **emergency medical services (EMS)** system is a local network of police, fire, and medical personnel who are trained to respond to emergency situations.

This network is activated by dialing 911 in the United States. Even when preliminary emergency care is provided by the ambulatory care provider, the patient may still need to be transported to a hospital for follow-up care.

Good Samaritan Laws

 When delivering or assisting in delivering emergency care, the medical assistant may be concerned about professional liability. Most states have enacted **Good Samaritan laws**, which provide some degree of protection to the health care professional who offers first aid.

Most Good Samaritan laws provide some legal protection to those who provide emergency care to ill or injured persons on a voluntary basis. However, when medical assistants or any other individuals give care during an emergency, they must act as reasonable and prudent individuals and provide care only within the scope of their abilities. Remember that a primary principle of first aid is to prevent further injury.

Although Good Samaritan laws give some measure of protection against being sued for giving emergency aid, they generally protect *off-duty* health care professionals. Also, conditions of the law vary from state to state. As part of establishing emergency care guidelines, every ambulatory care setting should understand the **explicit** and **implicit** intent of the Good Samaritan law in its state (see Chapter 6 for more information on legal guidelines).

Blood, Body Fluids, and Disease Transmission

 When providing any care, including emergency care, medical assistants should always protect themselves and the patient from infectious disease transmission. Serious infectious diseases, such as hepatitis B (HBV), hepatitis C (HCV), and human immunodeficiency virus (HIV) infection, can be transmitted through blood and body fluids (see Chapter 21 for more detailed information).

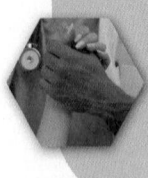

Patient Education

Alert patients to the importance of carrying the universal emergency medical identification symbol and its accompanying identification card if the patient has severe heart disease, diabetes, or other life-threatening illnesses or allergies.

⨠ QUICK REFERENCE GUIDE

⨠ **PRIMARY SURVEY**

Method of Assessment	Intervention	Considerations	Appropriate Action
(C) Circulation	Check carotid artery at the side of the neck below the ear.	If no pulse palpated, and if you are a trained CPR provider, initiate chest compressions.	Call for help and/or initiate 911 system. Obtain crash cart; an **automated external defibrillator (AED)** may be necessary (see Chapter 36). Initiate compressions
(A) Airway	Place face close to the patient's mouth and look, listen, and feel.	If breathing, support airway. If not breathing, first open the airway either by tilting the head and lifting the chin (Figure 8-2A) or by the jaw-thrust maneuver (see Figure 8-2B).	*CAUTION:* Do not attempt to tilt the head and lift the chin when the patient has a head, neck, or spinal cord injury.
(B) Breathing	Observe chest for rise and fall.	If no breath or only gasping, rescue breathing must be performed.	Ideally, breathing is checked simultaneously with circulation.
(D) Disability	Is the patient conscious? Responsive to questions? Pupils responsive?	Inform provider of findings. Work with provider to determine underlying causes.	Follow orders of provider to assist in delivery of care.

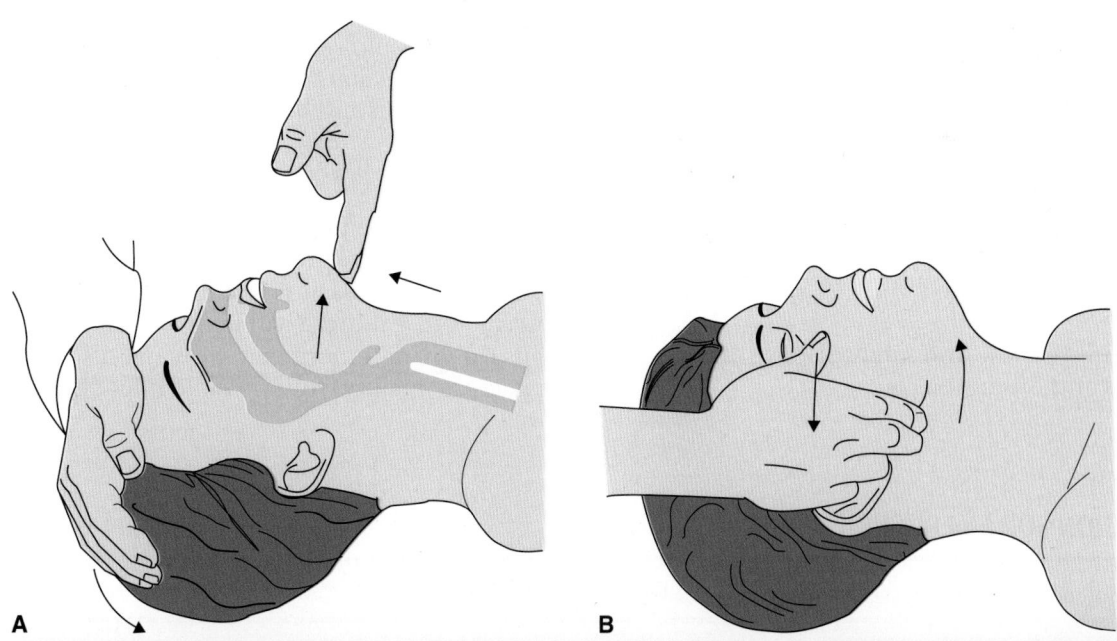

A **B**

FIGURE 8-2 If the individual is not breathing, first open the airway (A) by tilting the head and lifting the chin, for victim without head or neck trauma, or (B) by the jaw-thrust maneuver, for victim with cervical spine injury. This involves placing both thumbs on the patient's cheekbones and placing the index and middle fingers on both sides of the lower jaw.

(continues)

Method of Assessment	Intervention	Considerations	Appropriate Action
(E) Expose and Evaluate	Remove clothing. Obtain history from those accompanying the patient.	Monitor vital signs. Update provider with findings.	Initiate first aid if indicated. Never leave the patient unattended.

After performing the initial assessment:

- Continuously monitor all areas of the patient's progress and keep the provider informed until EMS arrives.
- Keep the patient warm and still.
- Legs may be elevated if no indication of spinal injury.

Always remember that a medical assistant must maintain current cardiopulmonary resuscitation certification for management of emergency situations.

By establishing and following strict guidelines, the risk for contracting or transmitting an infectious disease while providing emergency care is greatly reduced.

- Always wash hands thoroughly before (if possible) and after every procedure or use hand sanitizer.
- Use protective clothing and other protective equipment (gloves, gown, mask, goggles) during the procedure.
- Avoid contact with blood and body fluids, if possible.
- Do not touch nose, mouth, or eyes with gloved hands.
- Carefully handle and safely dispose of soiled gloves and other objects.

Refer to Chapter 21 for more information on standard precautions. **Standard Precautions** were issued by the Centers for Disease Control and Prevention (CDC) in 1996 and combine many of the basic principles of universal precautions with techniques known as body substance isolation. These precautions were reviewed and upheld in 2011 and represent the standard in infection control and are intended to protect both patients and health care professionals.

PREPARING FOR AN EMERGENCY

Emergencies are unexpected but can and should be anticipated and prepared for in the ambulatory care setting. The basic **risk management** techniques described in Table 8-2 will help medical personnel focus on giving emergency care and also will help protect the facility from possible litigation.

TABLE 8-2

PREPARATION FOR EMERGENCIES

TOOL	MEDICAL ASSISTANT'S ROLE
Policy and procedures manual	Participate in updates annually at the direction of the provider or office manager. Be aware of manual's location for ease of reference
Emergency phone numbers: • EMS (911) • Poison control (1-800-222-1222)	Post in designated locations Update as necessary

(continues)

Table 8-2 continued

TOOL	MEDICAL ASSISTANT'S ROLE
Maintain supply levels	Follow established inventory listings to maintain inventory
CPR certification (see Procedure 8-1)	Recertify biannually
Safe clinical environment	Wipe up spills to prevent falls Maintain clutter-free common areas Properly store medications
Crash cart or tray (see Figure 8-3)	Locate in accessible place Once the inventory is established by the provider, perform daily check for completeness, expiration dates, and functionality of equipment Remember that only the provider can order medications or treatment

PROCEDURE 8-1

Produce Up-to-Date Documentation of Provider/Professional Level CPR

Procedure

PURPOSE:

To provide evidence that one has mastered the knowledge of how to care for breathing and cardiac emergencies in adults, children, and infants.

EQUIPMENT/SUPPLIES:

Durable card provided by the training organization

PROCEDURE STEPS:

1. Attend and complete a professional level CPR training course through one of the approved organizations recognized for health care professionals, including medical assistants.
2. Photocopy your CPR card to present to your instructor and/or employer.
3. Keep the original documentation in your possession.

The Medical Crash Cart or Tray

Following is a brief list of some common supplies found on most crash carts and trays (see Table 8-3 for more information about medications found in a crash cart).

General supplies:

- Adhesive and hypoallergenic tape
- Alcohol wipes
- Bandage scissors
- Bandage material
- Blood pressure cuffs (standard, pediatric, large)
- **Tourniquet**
- Defibrillator/AED
- Dressing material
- Flashlight
- Gauze rolls
- Gloves
- Hot/cold packs
- Intravenous (IV) catheters in various sizes
- IV start pack
- IV tubing
- Needles and syringes for injection

- Glucose tabs or gel
- Penlight (with extra batteries)
- Personal protective equipment
- Stethoscope
- Syringes in 1-mL, 3-mL, and 20-mL sizes

Respiratory supplies:

- Airways of all sizes for nasal and oral use
- McGill forceps
- Ambu bag in infant, pediatric, and adult sizes
- Bulb syringe for suction
- Laryngoscope blades in various shapes and sizes
- Laryngoscope handles with batteries
- Nasal cannulas in infant, pediatric, and adult sizes
- 100% nonrebreather masks in infant, pediatric, and adult sizes
- Oxygen tank with Christmas tree adapter

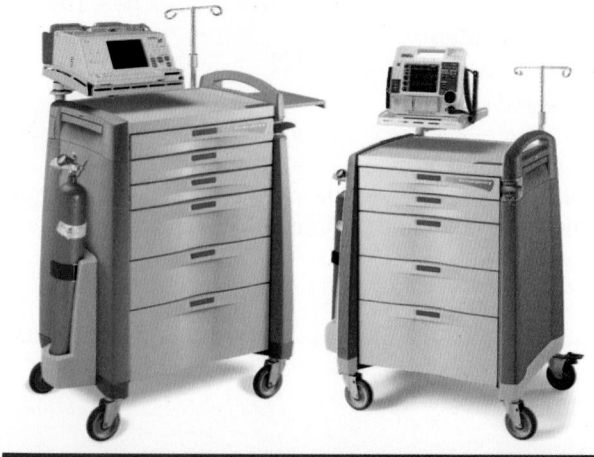

Courtesy of CAPSA SOLUTIONS

FIGURE 8-3 Medical crash carts.

Competency

This list represents many of the supplies to be found on a well-stocked **crash cart or tray**. The medical assistant should be familiar with the equipment and medication on the crash cart or tray. Mock codes simulating various emergency situations are helpful for preparing staff members for actual emergencies.

TABLE 8-3

EMERGENCY MEDICATIONS FOUND ON A CRASH CART

EMERGENCY MEDICATIONS	USES
Activated charcoal	Poisonings
Aspirin 325 mg	Fever, heart attack
Atropine	Slow heartbeat
Benadryl	IV for treatment of anaphylactic shock
$D_{50}W$	IV solution of dextrose in water (50%) for hypoglycemia
Dextrose	Insulin reaction
Diazepam*	Antianxiety
Diphenhydramine	Antihistamine
Dopamine	Increases blood pressure
Epinephrine	Constricts blood vessels, increases blood pressure
Glucagon	Insulin reaction
Insulin	Hyperglycemia
Lidocaine	IV for cardiac arrhythmia
Narcan	Reversal of narcotic overdose
Nitroglycerin tablets, patches	Chest pain from angina pectoris
Normal saline	IV access and delivery method for emergency drugs
Pepcid 20-mg vial	Treatment of anaphylactic shock
Phenobarbital*	Sedative
SoluMedrol	IV for treatment of anaphylactic shock
Verapamil	Hypertension, angina pectoris, irregular heartbeat, tachycardia
Xylocaine, Marcaine	Local anesthetics

*Controlled substance—must be kept in locked cabinet.

COMMON EMERGENCIES

Included in this discussion of common emergencies are shock, wounds, burns, musculoskeletal injuries, heat- and cold-related illnesses, poisoning, snake bite, sudden illness, cerebral vascular accident, and heart attack.

Shock

Procedure

When a severe injury or illness occurs, **shock** is likely to develop. Shock is progressive, and if not treated immediately, most types can be life threatening (see Procedure 8-2). Once shock reaches a certain point, it is irreversible. The "Shock" Quick Reference Guide provides detail on the physiology, signs and symptoms, and treatment of shock.

Types of Shock. Shock can be defined by categories or by the underlying cause. There are several categories of shock. Cardiogenic shock is due to decreased ability of the heart to function as a pump. Another category of shock caused by decreased venous return is hypovolemic shock. High cardiac output hypotension shock is caused by underlying factors such as sepsis. Other types of shock are anaphylactic, neurogenic, traumatic, and compression of the heart. Table 8-4 describes common types of shock seen in an ambulatory care setting.

PROCEDURE 8-2

Procedure

Perform First Aid Procedures for Shock

STANDARD PRECAUTIONS:

Handwashing   Gloves   Biohazard   Gown   Goggles & Mask

PURPOSE:

To support and monitor the patient in shock until EMS arrives.

EQUIPMENT/SUPPLIES:

- Pillow
- Blanket
- Sterile gloves (if hemorrhagic shock)
- Clean gloves
- Gown (if hemorrhagic shock)
- Mask (if hemorrhagic shock)
- Protective eyewear (if hemorrhagic shock)
- Sterile dressing material (if hemorrhagic shock)

PROCEDURE STEPS:

1. *Incorporating critical thinking skills when performing patient care*, notify the provider of the patient's condition immediately.
2. Activate EMS per the provider's orders.
3. Assist the patient into a reclining position. RATIONALE: This position minimizes pain and decreases stress on the body.
4. Elevate the patient's legs about 12 inches, unless you suspect head injury, spinal injuries, or broken bones involving the hips or legs. RATIONALE: This restores blood flow to the brain by decreasing the gravitational resistance.
5. As soon as possible, don clean gloves (sterile gloves if the cause of shock is hemorrhage and pressure to the wound is to be applied), and any other Personal Protective Equipment (PPE) that is appropriate.
6. Loosen any restrictive clothing or belts. RATIONALE: This allows adequate respiration.

(continues)

7. Check for pulse and respiration. If necessary, begin CPR after activating EMS or calling for assistance.

8. Control any external bleeding following steps in Procedure 8-3.

9. Assist the patient to maintain normal body temperature. Do not overheat. RATIONALE: A blanket over and under the patient can help avoid chilling.

10. ***Recognizing the physical and emotional effects on persons involved in an emergency situation***, reassure the patient.

11. Do not give the patient anything to eat or drink.

12. Ascertain that outside help has been called and stay with the patient until help arrives.

13. Obtain vital signs as soon as the patient is safely positioned. Repeat frequently, per provider's preference.

14. Assist with the transfer of care to EMS by sharing vital signs obtained.

15. If contact with blood or body fluids occurred, remove PPE and discard appropriately in biohazard waste container.

16. Wash hands.

17. Document the incident and care provided in the patient's chart.

DOCUMENTATION:

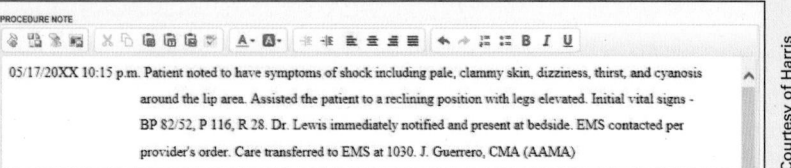

PROCEDURE NOTE

05/17/20XX 10:15 p.m. Patient noted to have symptoms of shock including pale, clammy skin, dizziness, thirst, and cyanosis around the lip area. Assisted the patient to a reclining position with legs elevated. Initial vital signs - BP 82/52, P 116, R 28. Dr. Lewis immediately notified and present at bedside. EMS contacted per provider's order. Care transferred to EMS at 1030. J. Guerrero, CMA (AAMA)

Courtesy of Harris CareTracker PM and EMR

TABLE 8-4

COMMON TYPES OF SHOCK WITH DESCRIPTIONS

TYPE OF SHOCK	DESCRIPTION
Cardiogenic	The cardiac muscle is unable to contract and adequately provide blood to the body. This can be caused by myocardial infarction, coronary artery disease, arrhythmias, or valve disease.
Hypovolemic	The body has lost blood or fluid volume to such an extent that there is not enough circulating volume to fill the ventricles. The heart attempts to compensate by increasing the heart rate.
Neurogenic	Injury or trauma to the nervous system causes loss of tone in the vessels, resulting in massive dilation of arterioles and venules. This results in a dramatic drop in blood pressure. This type of shock can be caused by brain or spinal cord injuries, general or spinal anesthesia, or pain and anxiety.
Anaphylactic	In this severe allergic reaction to substances such as drugs, blood products, contrast medium, insect or animal venom, or food products, chemicals are released that cause veins and arteries to vasodilate and decrease the amount of blood returning to the heart. Capillaries dilate and allow proteins and fluids to escape into the soft tissues, causing edema.
Septic	When overwhelming infection occurs in critically ill patients, chemicals are released into the bloodstream that cause vasodilatation and other organic products that are harmful to the organs and tissues. The vasodilation and decreased ability of the cells and tissues to utilize oxygen form the basis for this type of shock.
Respiratory	Trauma to the respiratory tract (trachea, lungs) causes a reduction of oxygen and carbon dioxide exchange. Body cells cannot receive enough oxygen.

Shock

>> PHYSIOLOGY

During shock, several things occur:

- The circulatory system is not providing an adequate blood supply to all parts of the body, causing a failure of normal functioning.

- The heart is unable to pump blood appropriately.

- Tissues don't receive adequate oxygenation (**hypoxia**).

- Blood flow shifts to critical organs (Figure 8-4).

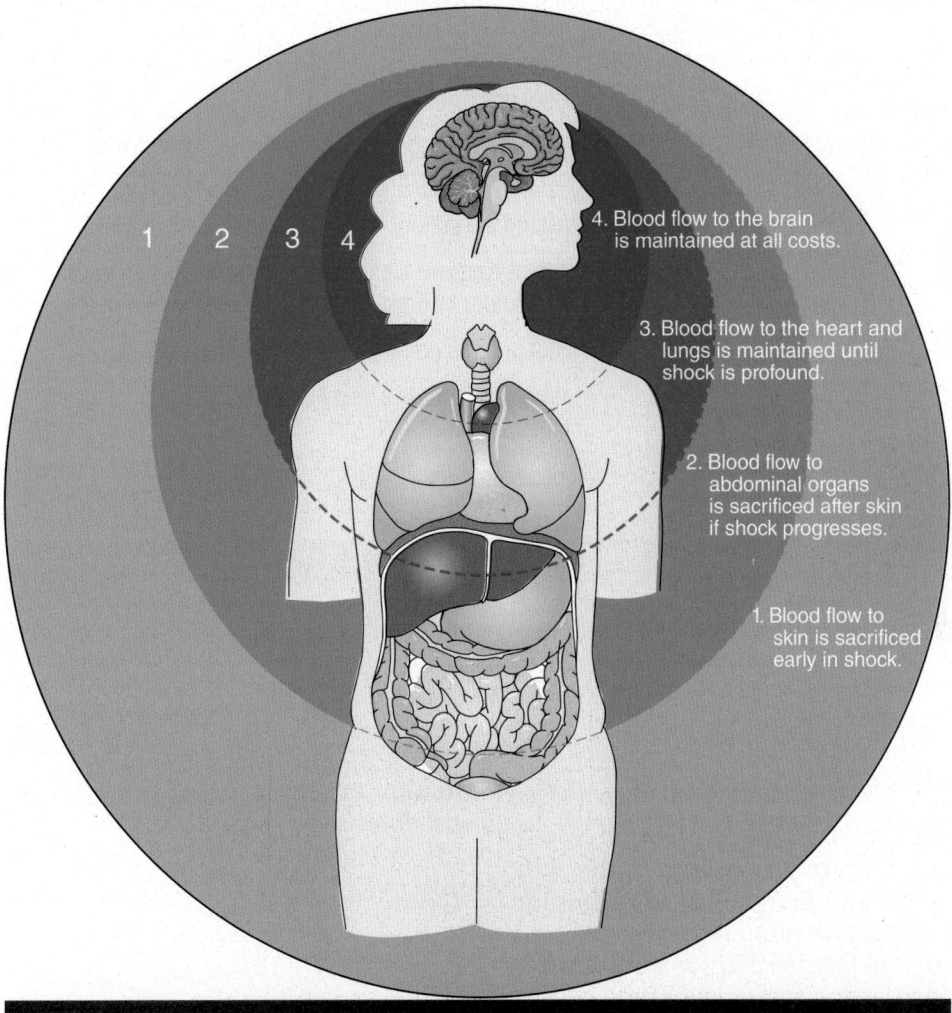

1   2   3   4

4. Blood flow to the brain is maintained at all costs.

3. Blood flow to the heart and lungs is maintained until shock is profound.

2. Blood flow to abdominal organs is sacrificed after skin if shock progresses.

1. Blood flow to skin is sacrificed early in shock.

FIGURE 8-4   When blood volume diminishes, as in cases of shock, the body tries to compromise by sacrificing blood supply to the less-significant organs in order to preserve blood for the vital organs such as the heart and brain.

(continues)

⨠ QUICK REFERENCE GUIDE

Signs and Symptoms	Treatment
Learn to recognize the signs and symptoms of shock:	*To care for a patient in shock (regardless of the type), follow these procedures:*

Signs and Symptoms

Learn to recognize the signs and symptoms of shock:

- Patient may be restless or feel irritable.
- Weakness, dizziness, thirst, or nausea may occur.
- Breathing may be shallow and rapid.
- Skin is cool, clammy, and pale.
- Pulse is weak and rapid.
- Blood pressure is low.
- Area around the lips, eyes, and fingernails may turn cyanotic (blue) from lack of oxygen.
- Confusion or sudden unconscious, or both.
- Dilated pupils and lackluster eyes are obvious.

Treatment

To care for a patient in shock (regardless of the type), follow these procedures:

- Activate EMS.
- Lay the patient down. This minimizes pain and decreases stress on the body.
- Loosen the patient's clothing.
- Check for an open airway.
- Check breathing.
- Control any external bleeding.
- Help the patient maintain normal body temperature. A blanket over and under the patient can help avoid chilling. Do not overheat.
- Reassure the patient.
- Elevate the patient's legs about 12 inches, unless you suspect head injury, spinal injuries, or broken bones involving the hips or legs.
- Do not give the patient anything to eat or drink.
- Ascertain that outside help has been called and stay with the patient until help arrives.
- Monitor vital signs.

Wounds

Typically, **wounds** are classified as open or closed. In a closed wound, there is no break in the skin; bruises, contusions, and hematomas are common closed wounds. An open wound represents a break in the skin and can be classified as an abrasion, avulsion, incision, laceration, or puncture wound. See Table 8-5 for more information on wound classifications.

A common procedure for treating a closed wound is to RICE or MICE it. It is generally thought that RICE is the preferred treatment for the first 24 to 48 hours. Once the signs of inflammation are gone, MICE is the more appropriate treatment.

Rice
- Rest
- Ice
- Compression
- Elevation

Mice
- Motion or Movement
- Ice
- Compression
- Elevation

Open Wounds.   Common types of open wounds are described in the "Types of Open Wounds" Quick Reference Guide.

TABLE 8-5

CLASSIFICATION OF WOUNDS

CLASSIFICATION	PHYSIOLOGY	INDICATIONS	CONSIDERATIONS
Open	The integrity of the skin has been interrupted. Types of open wounds include: • Incision • Laceration • Abrasion • Avulsion • Puncture • Gunshot wound • Burn • Ulcer	May constitute an emergency. Needs intervention, including: • Cleaning • Debriding • Suturing • Medicating • Dressing	Represents an opportunity for microorganisms to gain entry to the body and cause an infection. May involve heavy bleeding, which will need to be controlled, probably by suturing. A tetanus injection is indicated.
Closed	The skin remains intact. Types of closed wounds include: • Hematoma or bruise • Crush injury	Cold compresses to address pain and swelling: • Protect the skin from direct application of cold • Apply cold for 20 minutes, remove for 20 minutes for the first 24 hours Warm compresses after 24 hours: • Protect the skin from the source of heat • Apply heat for 20 minutes, remove for 20 minutes for the following 24 hours	May be dangerous and associated with internal bleeding. If the pain is severe and/or was caused by a high impact, call for help and keep the patient comfortable until help arrives. Watch for symptoms of shock. Monitor vital signs.

Use of Tourniquets in Emergency Care. There has been much discussion regarding the use of tourniquets to control bleeding in the recent past. Recommendations now include the application of a tourniquet to control bleeding with the following stipulations:

- A tourniquet should be applied only if direct pressure fails to control bleeding.
- The time of tourniquet application must be clearly indicated on the device.
- Control of bleeding should be assessed and a tourniquet should be replaced by a pressure dressing if bleeding can be controlled.
- A tourniquet that is at least 2 inches wide with a windlass, ratcheting device is recommended.

If the bleeding is controlled, direct pressure is still the best method to handle blood loss.

Dressings and Bandages. After the provider has treated an open wound, it is critical to dress and bandage it properly to curtail infection. Covering of the wound is accomplished by a series of **dressings** and **bandages**.

Typically, dressings are sterile gauze pads placed directly on the wound; they often have nonstick, sterile surfaces, but they are absorbent and will soak up blood and protect the wound from microorganisms. They are often made of a gauze-type material.

Bandages, which are nonsterile, are placed over the dressing. They hold the dressing in place and are made to conform to the area to be covered. Sometimes, as in a Band-Aid, the dressing and bandage are combined. Bandage materials are selected based on the location and type of wound to be covered. Kling is a type of flexible gauze that stretches and clings as it is applied. Roller bandages (sometimes called by their brand name, Ace Bandages), such as those made of elastic, can be placed over a dressing and used to help control bleeding or swelling. Recently, there has been a rise in the utilization of self-adherent elasticized wrap known as Coban.

	Open Wound	Description
	Incision	Wound caused by a sharp object, such as a knife or piece of glass. Incisions may need sutures. The wound must be cleaned with soap and water and a dressing applied.
	Laceration	Tears the body tissue and can be difficult to clean; therefore, care must be taken to avoid infection. If there is not severe bleeding, which in itself is a cleansing mechanism, these wounds may need to be soaked in antiseptic soap and water to remove debris. If there is severe bleeding, it must be controlled immediately (see Procedure 8-3). Lacerations with severe bleeding need suturing.
	Abrasion	A superficial scraping of the epidermis. Because nerve endings are involved, abrasions can be painful. However, they are not usually serious, unless they cover a large area of the body. Administer first aid by cleaning the area carefully with soap and water, apply an antiseptic ointment if prescribed by a provider, and cover with a dressing.
© Chaikom/Shutterstock.com	**Avulsion**	The skin is torn off and bleeding is profuse. Avulsion wounds often occur at exposed parts: fingers, toes, ear. First, control bleeding (see Procedure 8-3). Then clean the wound. If there is a skin flap, reposition it. Apply a dressing, then bandage as necessary. Note that pieces of the body may be torn away. If possible, save the body part, keep moist, and transport with the patient.
	Puncture wound	The skin is pierced and penetrated and there may be a deep wound while it appears insignificant. Usually, external bleeding is minimal, but the patient should be assessed for internal bleeding. Because a puncture wound is deep, the risk for infection is great and the patient should be advised to watch for signals of infection, such as pain, swelling, redness, throbbing, and warmth.

Some specific examples of open wounds include:

- Gunshot wounds, or ballistic trauma, which are caused by a projectile fired from a variety of firearms that inflicts damage to multiple structures. The entrance wound is usually smaller than the exit wound. Treatment is aimed at controlling bleeding, repairing damage, and preventing infection.

- Burns, which damage tissues from the skin downward into adjacent structures. Burns may be caused by direct heat, chemicals, electricity, sunlight, or radiation. Treatment varies based on the degree of injury.

- **Ulcers**, which are open cavities in the skin caused by tissue breakdown related to lack of oxygen supply to the tissues. This can be caused by vascular disease, inflammatory disorders, excessive fluid accumulation, or prolonged pressure. Treatment includes cleaning, debriding, and dressing, as well as resolution of the underlying cause.

Bandages and their applications can take many shapes and forms, depending on the type of injury and the injury site. In all cases, a bandage must be secure, but not constricting. Avoid too tight or too loose a wrap.

- Spiral bandages are useful for injuries to the arms or legs (Figure 8-5).
- A figure-eight bandage holds the dressing in place on a wound on the hand or wrist, knee, or ankle (Figure 8-6).

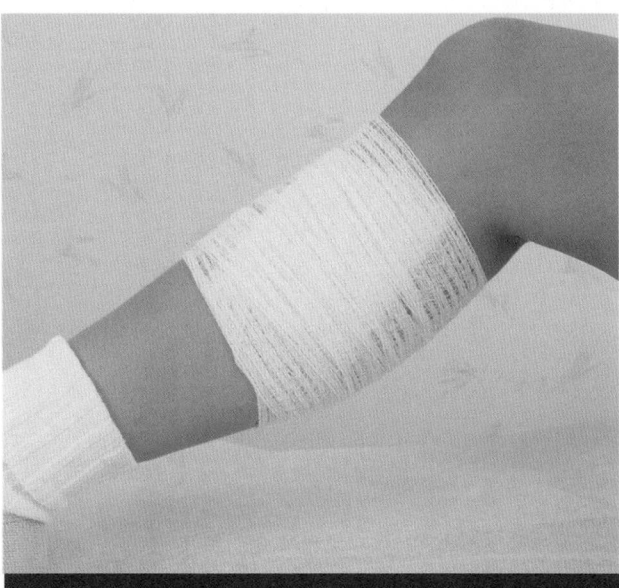

FIGURE 8-5 The spiral bandage is an option for arm and leg injuries.

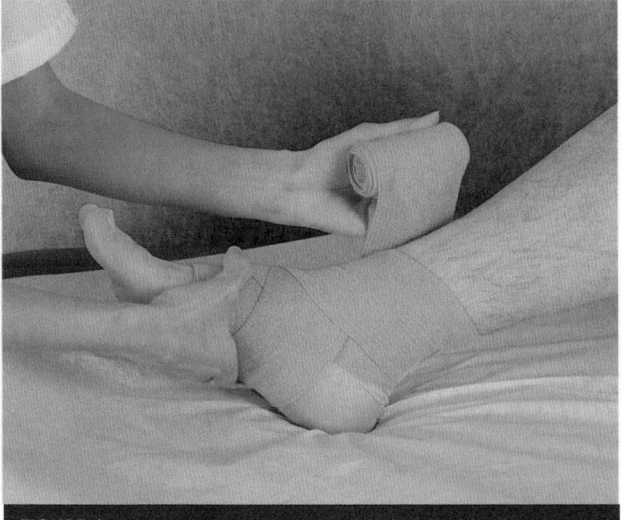

FIGURE 8-6 An elastic figure-eight bandage holds dressings in place or can be used for immobilization, as with an ankle sprain.

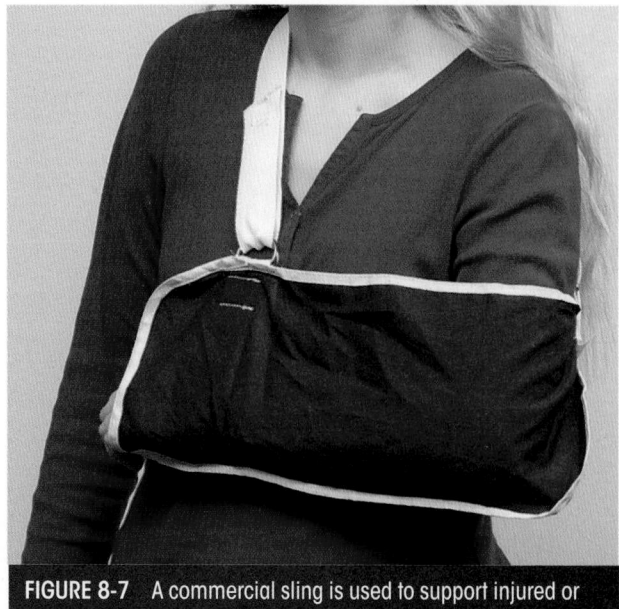

FIGURE 8-7 A commercial sling is used to support injured or fractured arms.

- Commercial arm slings are used to support injured or fractured arms (Figure 8-7). To apply, support the injured arm above and below the injury site while applying the sling.

Burns

Most burns are caused by heat, chemicals, explosions, and electricity. Critical burns can be life threatening and require immediate medical care. According to the American Red Cross, critical burns have the following characteristics:

- Involve breathing difficulty
- Cover more than one body part
- Involve the head, neck, hands, feet, or genitals
- The person sustaining the burn is a child or older adult (other than minor burns)

To distinguish critical from minor burns, it is important to understand the classifications of burns and what they mean (see the "Burn Classifications" Quick Reference Guide).

There is a formula for estimating the percentage of body surface areas that have been burned (see Figure 8-9). This formula is known as the rule of nines. In an adult, the head and each upper extremity are 9% each, the back of the trunk is 18%, as is the front (18%), each lower extremity is 18%, and the perineum is 1%.

PROCEDURE 8-3

Procedure

Perform First Aid Procedures for Bleeding

STANDARD PRECAUTIONS:

Handwashing   Gloves   Biohazard   Gown   Goggles & Mask

PURPOSE:

To control bleeding from an open wound.

EQUIPMENT/SUPPLIES:

- Sterile dressings
- Sterile gloves
- Mask and eye protection
- Gown
- Biohazard waste container

PROCEDURE STEPS:

1. Wash hands.
2. Assemble equipment and supplies.
3. Apply eye and mask protection and gown if splashing is likely to occur.
4. Put on sterile gloves.
5. Apply sterile dressing and press firmly (Figure 8-8A).
6. *Incorporate critical thinking skills when performing patient care.* If bleeding continues, elevate arm above heart level (Figure 8-8B). RATIONALE: Raising the arm above the heart level will slow the flow of blood because it is flowing against gravity.
7. If bleeding continues, press adjacent artery against bone (Figure 8-8C). Notify the provider if bleeding cannot be controlled, *demonstrating self-awareness in responding to an emergency situation.* RATIONALE: Pressing the adjacent artery against a bone provides solid pressure to help control bleeding.

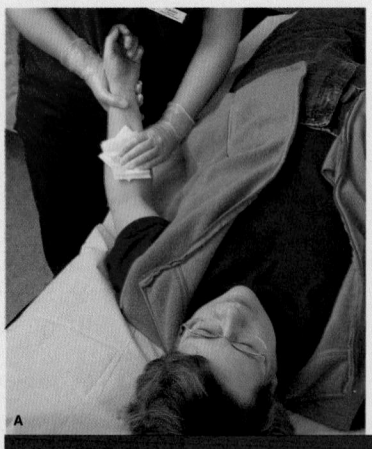 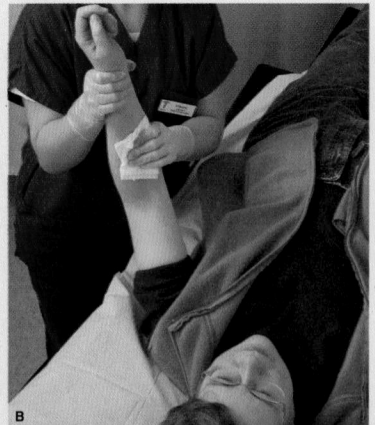 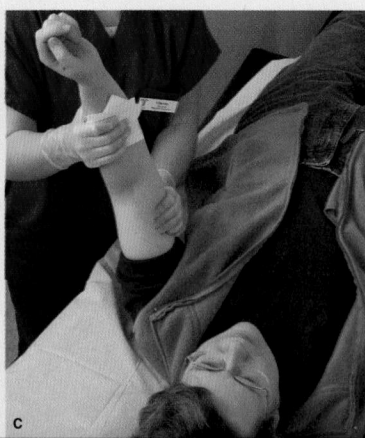

FIGURE 8-8 (A) Apply dressing and press firmly. (B) Elevate arm above heart level. (C) Press artery against bone.

(continues)

8. If bleeding still does not cease, notify the provider and continue to exert pressure on the wound with one hand while using your other hand to press the adjacent artery against bone.

9. Apply pressure bandage over the dressing.

10. Discard any waste in the appropriate container and prepare the patient for any follow-up procedure to be performed, such as suturing or stapling.

11. Remove gloves and dispose in biohazard container.

12. Wash hands.

13. Document procedure in patient's chart or electronic medical record.

CAUTION: If wound is large and bleeding is not controlled, the patient may go into hemorrhagic shock. Be prepared to call EMS immediately.

DOCUMENTATION:

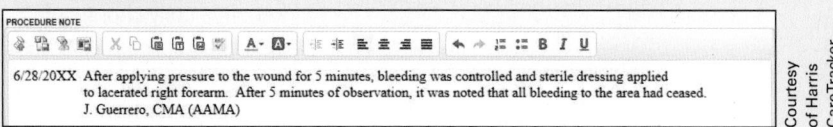

6/28/20XX After applying pressure to the wound for 5 minutes, bleeding was controlled and sterile dressing applied to lacerated right forearm. After 5 minutes of observation, it was noted that all bleeding to the area had ceased.
J. Guerrero, CMA (AAMA)

Courtesy of Harris CareTracker PM and EMR

In a child, the head, back, and front of the torso are 18% each, each upper extremity is 9%, each lower extremity is 13.5%, and the perineum is 1%.

Providers use the formula to determine the amount of body surface area that has been burned. Together with the depth of the burn, it helps the provider determine the percentage of the body that has been burned and the degree of burn. The severity of a burn can be determined and appropriate treatment given.

First Aid for Burns. First aid for burns is outlined in the Quick Reference Guide on page 155.

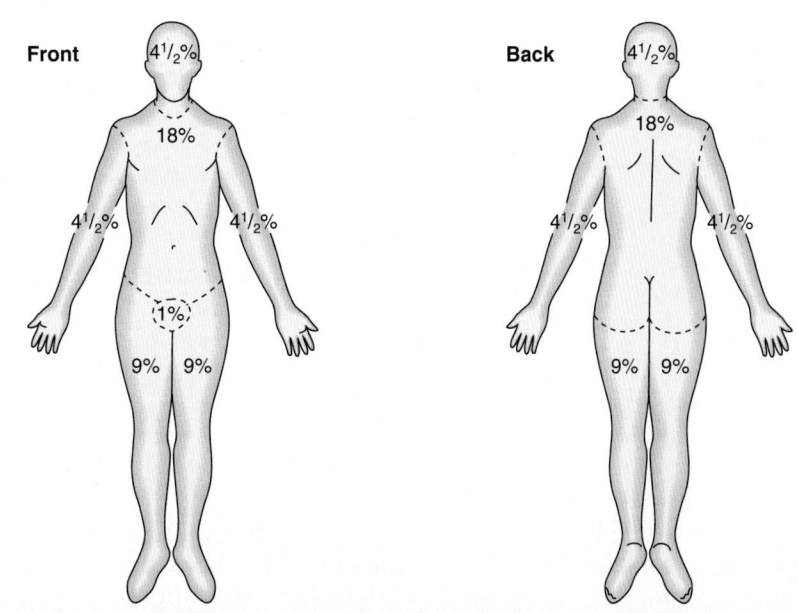

FIGURE 8-9 Diagram for use in calculating the extent of burns or other injuries in an adult.

BURN CLASSIFICATIONS

	Degree	Physiology	Considerations
© Chris Driscoll/Shutterstock.com	First degree	Superficial, involving only the top layer of the skin: • Red • Dry • Warm to the touch • Swollen • Painful • Heals quickly without scarring	Minor unless on face, hands, feet, groin or buttocks May be considered an emergency if area involved is large enough
© Photodiem/Shutterstock.com	Second degree	First layer of skin has been burned through and the underlying tissues are involved: • Skin is red • Blisters present • Painful May take a month to heal and scarring is likely	Do not break the blisters Requires daily change of dressing to prevent infection May be considered an emergency if located on face, hands, feet, groin or buttocks, or covers a large area of the body
Courtesy of the Phoenix Society of Burn Survivors, Inc.	Third degree	Affects or destroys all layers of tissue; fat, muscle, bone, nerve: • Tissues appear charred or brown, waxy and white, raised and leathery • Extremely painful • No pain if all nerves in the area destroyed Risk of shock and loss of large volumes of bodily fluid Extensive healing time required	Emergency treatment must be sought Elevate the body part that is affected if possible Do not remove clothing if sticking to the burn Remain calm and activate EMS

Types of Burns. Most burns are caused by heat; however, burns can also be caused by chemicals, electricity, and solar radiation.

Chemical Burns. Chemical burns can occur in the workplace or even in the home with "ordinary" household chemicals. To stop the burning process, you must remove the chemical from the skin. Have someone call EMS while you flush the skin or eyes with cool water. Remove any clothing contaminated by the chemicals unless they adhere to the skin. If clothing clings to the skin, it can be cut with scissors. Do not attempt to pull clothing away from a burned area.

Electrical Burns. Electrical burns can be caused by power lines, lightning, or faulty electrical equipment in the home or workplace. *It is important to remember never to go near a patient injured by electricity until you are sure the power has been shut off, because you could be injured.* If there is a downed line, call the power company and EMS.

A victim of an electricity burn may be suffering from two burns: one where the power entered the body, and one where it exited. Often, the burns themselves may be minor. Of more serious consequence are the possibilities of shock, breathing

⫸ FIRST AID FOR BURNS

First-Degree Burn Response Guide

Questions	Responses	Action to Take	Rationale
Is skin reddened without blisters? NO ⬇	YES ⇨	Submerge in cool **normal saline** ⇨ or water for 2 to 5 minutes.	Stops burning process.
Does area involve: • Hands? • Feet? • Genitals? • Face? NO ⬇	YES ⇨	Have patient come to clinic. ⇨	These are potential danger areas and require evaluation by the provider.
Is patient: • Elderly? • Very young? NO ⬇	YES ⇨	Have patient come to clinic. ⇨	These groups are susceptible to burn complications.
Consult provider.			Provider has final decision whether patient is seen.

Second-Degree Burn Response Guide

Questions	Responses	Action to Take	Rationale
Is skin reddened with blisters or splitting of the skin? NO ⬇	YES ⇨	Submerge in cool normal saline ⇨ or water for 10 to 15 minutes if skin is intact. Use compresses if skin is broken. Do not break blisters. Do not use anesthetic creams or sprays.	Stops burning process. If blisters are broken, the area is at greater risk for infection. Creams or spray may slow healing process and increase severity of a burn.
Does area involve: • Hands? • Feet? • Genitals? • Face? NO ⬇	YES ⇨	Have patient come to clinic or go ⇨ to the emergency department.	These are potentially dangerous areas and require medical attention.
Is the area involved larger than a child's hand? NO ⬇	YES ⇨	Have patient come to clinic or go ⇨ to the emergency department.	Burns of this size are susceptible to complications.

(continues)

Second-Degree Burn Response Guide

Questions	Responses	Action to Take	Rationale
Is patient experiencing trouble breathing? NO ⇩	YES ⇨	Patient should go to emergency ⇨ department.	There may be swelling of the airways because of heat and noxious fumes.
Consult provider.			Provider has final decision whether patient is seen.

Third-Degree Burn Response Guide

Questions	Responses	Action to Take	Rationale
Does skin appear gray, black, or charred? Can muscle, fat, or bone be seen in wound? NO ⇩	YES ⇨	Tell patient or family to call EMS ⇨ immediately. Do not apply cold; do not remove burned clothing from burn area.	This is a life-threatening emergency that requires prompt attention.
Is patient experiencing: • Pallor • Loss of consciousness? • Shivering? NO ⇩	YES ⇨	Patient in shock: ⇨ Tell family to call EMS and to: • Maintain airway • Maintain body temperature • Elevate feet if appropriate • Monitor breathing Patient may need oxygen and intravenous fluids while waiting for EMS to arrive.	Need to control shock caused by fluid loss.
Consult provider.			Provider has final decision whether patient is seen.

difficulties, and other injuries. CPR often is needed in this situation.

Solar Radiation. Most "sunburns," although not advisable or good for the skin, represent minor burns. If the patient has a severe burn, however, he or she should see a provider who will cover the burn area to reduce chance of infection and protect the patient against chill.

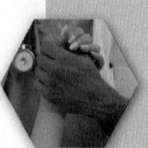

Patient Education

Some burns can be prevented. Advise patients who insist on sunbathing to protect themselves against harmful rays by using a sunscreen with 15 SPF or higher and avoiding the sun between 10 AM and 2 PM.

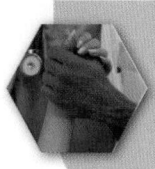

Patient Education

Advise patients not to run should their clothing catch on fire. They should fall to the ground or wrap themselves in a blanket or rug and roll on the ground to extinguish the flames. This method is known as "Stop, Drop, and Roll."

Musculoskeletal Injuries

Most injuries to muscles, bones, and joints are not life threatening, but they are painful and, if not properly treated, can be disabling. Some injuries, such as those to the spinal cord, can be quite serious and can result in paralysis. These injuries are not typically seen in the ambulatory care setting. See Table 8-6 for more information on types of musculoskeletal injuries.

Assessing Injuries to Muscles, Bones, and Joints. Sometimes it is difficult to determine the extent of an injury, especially in closed fractures. There are some assessment techniques to call on, however, to gauge the seriousness of an injury.

- Note the extent of bruising and swelling.
- Pain is a signal of injury.
- There may be noticeable deformity to the bone or joint.

TABLE 8-6

TYPES OF MUSCULOSKELETAL INJURIES

INJURY	DESCRIPTION	TREATMENT
Sprain	Injury to a joint that involves tearing of the ligaments; if minor, may heal quickly; if extensive, may require intervention Symptoms: • Rapid swelling • Discoloration at the site • Limited function	Seek medical assessment RICE or MICE as ordered by provider May require surgery Immobilize Protect from weight bearing as directed Pain management Physical therapy
Strain	Overuse or stretching of a muscle, tendon(s), or group of muscles	RICE or MICE as ordered by the provider Immobilize Protect from weight bearing as directed Pain management Physical therapy
Dislocation	Bone displaced from its normal location anatomically; usually occurs as a result of a wrenching motion	Requires urgent evaluation Radiologic imaging of affected area for diagnosis Relocation by trained professional or surgical intervention Immobilization Pain management Physical therapy
Fracture	Break or interruption of the integrity of the bone (see the "Types of Fractures" Quick Reference Guide for more information)	All fractures are emergent conditions and require urgent evaluation Radiologic imaging of affected area for diagnosis Medical intervention: setting, casting, or surgery to maintain approximation for healing Immobilization Pain management Physical therapy

	Type	Description
Transverse — Oblique —	Closed fracture (simple, complete)	Complete bone break in which there is no involvement with the skin surface: • Skin intact • Discoloration of the skin • Swelling • Pain • Deformity • Inability to move affected limb • **Crepitation** (grating sensation experienced or heard when bone fragments rub together)
	Open fracture (compound)	Skin integrity is interrupted. Bone protrudes though the skin surface, creating the possibility of infection.
	Incomplete or greenstick fracture	Fracture in which the bone has cracked, but the break is not all the way through; frequently seen in children.

(continues)

	Impacted fracture	Broken ends of the bone are jammed into each other.
	Comminuted fracture	More than one fracture line and several bone fragments are present.
	Spiral fracture	Fracture that occurs with a severe twisting action, causing the break to wind around the bone.

(continues)

	Depressed fracture	Fracture that occurs with severe head injuries in which a broken piece of skull is driven inward.
	Colles' fractures	Often caused by falling on an outstretched hand. Involves the distal end of radius and results in displacement, causing a bulge at the wrist.

- Use of the injured area is limited.
- Talk to the patient: What was the cause of the injury? What was the sound or sensation at the time of injury?

Caring for Muscle, Bone, and Joint Injuries. Most injuries to muscles, bones, and joints are treated in a similar way; some require motion, but most require rest, elevation of the injured part, immobilization, and the application of ice to the injury.

Procedure After calling EMS (always check for life-threatening symptoms, such as breathing difficulties; bleeding; or head, neck, or back injuries), it is important to immobilize the injured area if the patient must be moved. EMS personnel use a variety of **splints** to immobilize bones and joints. Some fractures must be treated in the hospital. Compound fractures and fractures with nerve or blood vessel involvement are some examples. Most often, a fracture can be treated with outpatient care. A splint and a cast may be applied to prevent movement and to hold the

fracture steady. Procedure 8-4 gives instructions for performing first aid procedures for fractures in the ambulatory care setting.

Critical Thinking

You are watching your son's regional championship baseball game and the runner from third base slides into home plate hands first. After the dust clears, it is evident that the player has sustained an injury. You are able to evaluate the player's condition and find bulging at the wrist with a definite bend in the distal arm. You work for an orthopedic office and have seen this type of injury before. What type of fracture do you suspect has occurred? What first aid measures can be implemented in a nonclinical setting?

Procedure

Performing First Aid Procedures for Fractures

STANDARD PRECAUTIONS:

Handwashing

PURPOSE:

To immobilize the area above and below the injured part of the arm in order to reduce pain, immobilize, and prevent further injury.

EQUIPMENT/SUPPLIES:

- Thin piece of rigid board; cardboard can be used if necessary
- Gauze roller bandage

PROCEDURE STEPS:

1. Wash hands.
2. Introduce yourself and identify the patient.
3. Carefully remove or cut away any clothing from the area of injury.
4. *Display a calm and professional manner* while observing the patient for swelling, bruising, difficulty moving the affected body part, pain, loss of strength, physical deformity, and symptoms of shock. *Incorporate critical thinking skills when performing patient assessment.*
5. It may be difficult to determine if the injury is a fracture, dislocation, sprain, or strain until radiologic films have been taken and interpreted by the provider. Until a diagnosis is made, treat the injury as a fracture.
6. Check the affected extremity for color, sensation, and movement.
7. If the fracture is open, apply sterile gloves and cover with a sterile gauze. Apply direct pressure around any bones. Do not attempt to force any protruding bone back into place.
8. If the fracture is closed, the injury will be immobilized by applying a splint. In order to apply the splint, follow these steps:
   a. Assist the patient into the position of greatest comfort with the least amount of movement of the affected area. RATIONALE: Not moving the extremity limits further damage to the soft tissues surrounding the fracture area.
   b. Without forcing movement, utilize a rigid splint to immobilize the extremity.
   c. The splint should be long enough to reach the joints above and below the injured area.
   d. Wrap the affected extremity with cast padding to protect from pressure and aid in comfort.
   e. Gently align the splint. Pad gaps between extremity and splint with gauze pads or other soft material. RATIONALE: Provides comfort for the patient.
   f. Secure splint to the injured extremity with an elastic bandage applied without undue pressure.
9. For a suspected fracture of a clavicle, apply a sling to support the arm and apply a wrap around the body to immobilize the arm and shoulder.

(continues)

10. For a suspected rib fracture, immobilize the rib area by applying wide pressure bandages around the area of injury.

11. Evaluate color, sensation, and movement of the affected area once the splint is applied and every 15 minutes thereafter while in your care.

12. Once the fracture area is immobilized, apply ice packs for comfort and management of swelling.

13. Elevate the area if possible.

14. Wash hands.

15. Accurately and concisely update the provider on the patient's care.

16. *Paying attention to detail*, document your findings and the procedures performed.

17. Check with the provider regarding pain medications that may be administered to the patient.

DOCUMENTATION:

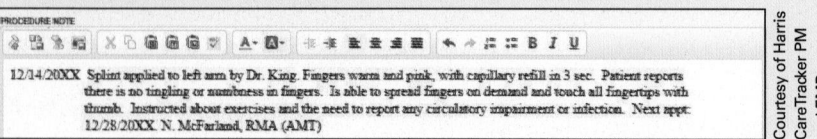

12/14/20XX Splint applied to left arm by Dr. King. Fingers warm and pink, with capillary refill in 3 sec. Patient reports there is no tingling or numbness in fingers. Is able to spread fingers on demand and touch all fingertips with thumb. Instructed about exercises and the need to report any circulatory impairment or infection. Next appt: 12/28/20XX. N. McFarland, RMA (AMT)

Courtesy of Harris CareTracker PM and EMR

Temperature-Related Illnesses

The condition of patients who have been subject to extreme heat and cold can deteriorate rapidly, and either a heat- or cold-related illness can result in death. Individuals especially vulnerable to extreme exposures include the very young and very old, individuals who work outdoors, and people who suffer from poor circulation. See Table 8-7 for more information on temperature-related illnesses.

Poisoning

Poisons can enter the body in four ways: ingestion, inhalation, absorption, and injection (see the "Four Routes of Poisoning" Quick Reference Guide for more information).

Some signs and symptoms of poisoning are dyspnea, nausea and vomiting, confusion, and convulsions. The Poison Control Center (1-800-222-1222) can advise if there is an antidote for the poison (if poison is known). For many years, the treatment of choice for ingested poison was to induce vomiting by using syrup of ipecac. This practice is no longer recommended. Activated charcoal given as soon as possible is the treatment of choice for ingested poison. It is quicker and more effective.

If a patient becomes unconscious, the provider will be concerned that the patient will vomit and aspirate vomitus into the lungs; therefore, the provider may insert a flexible tube into the larynx to alleviate that possibility.

In most poisoning cases, there are specific antidotes. They work either by reversing the effects of the poison or by interrupting the pathologic process.

On occasion, there is no specific treatment and treatment will be based on the management of symptoms. A ventilator may be needed if a patient has stopped breathing. Medications that control convulsions are available, and sedatives can be administered if the patient is disturbed and restless.

Whenever a patient calls regarding poisoning or there is a suspicion of poisoning, call the Poison Control Center (1-800-222-1222) or the local emergency number and ask for instructions. Telephone numbers of the poison control center should be posted in a familiar and accessible place.

The treatment for poisoning will vary according to the source of the poisoning and must be tailored to the specific incident. The provider will have advised staff regarding specific poisoning antidotes. Generally, do not give the patient anything to eat or drink; try to determine what poison the patient was exposed to and, if ingested, how much was taken; if the patient vomits, save some of the vomitus for analysis.

Insect Stings

The medical assistant in the ambulatory care setting is likely to receive calls every summer from patients who have been stung by insects, typically yellow jackets, hornets, honeybees, or wasps. In the nonallergic patient, the sting is likely to result in localized swelling, tenderness, and slight redness.

TABLE 8-7

TEMPERATURE-RELATED ILLNESS

COLD-RELATED ILLNESS

ILLNESS	SYMPTOMS	CAUSE	TREATMENT
Frostbite	Affects extremities Skin is discolored: • Frostnip: reddened (early) • Pale, yellow, gray, or bluish (later) Changes in sensation: • Prickling (early) • Numbness (later) Joint stiffening Hardening of the skin	Prolonged exposure to extreme cold	Protect the skin from further exposure to the cold Get out of the cold Slow rewarming of the skin (for frostnip) Seek emergency medical treatment (later stages) Pain management
Hypothermia	Shivering (early) Lack of coordination Slurred speech or mumbling Confusion Dizziness	Prolonged exposure to any environment cooler than body temperature	Remove person from cool environment Remove wet clothing Cover person with blankets Monitor vital signs (VS) Provide warm beverages Activate EMS

HEAT-RELATED ILLNESS

ILLNESS	SYMPTOMS	CAUSE	TREATMENT
Heat cramps	Large muscle group cramping Common in legs and abdomen Cramps are: • Painful • Involuntary • Brief • Intermittent • Self-limiting	Excessive body exposure or exercise in hot weather	Stop exercise Rest in a cool place Drink water Increase salt intake (mix ¼ to ½ tsp of salt in one quart water) Seek medical care if progresses to heat exhaustion
Heat exhaustion	Feeling of physical exhaustion Cold, clammy skin Profuse sweating Headache Generalized weakness Thirst Nausea and vomiting Confusion Loss of consciousness	Working or exercising in extreme heat	Get out of the heat immediately Apply cool, wet towels to the body or take a cool shower Slowly drink cool water If symptoms are not relieved in 15 minutes, seek emergency medical assistance
Heat stroke	Red, dry, hot skin Weak, thready, irregular pulse	Working or exercising in extreme heat	Activate EMS Apply cool, wet towels to body Stay with patient Monitor VS

	Route	Description
	Ingestion	Ingested poisons enter the body by swallowing. Swallowed poisons may include medications, plant material, household chemicals, contaminated foods, and drugs.
	Inhalation	Poisons are inhaled into the body in poorly ventilated areas where cleaning fluids, paints and chemical cleaners, or carbon monoxide may be present.
	Absorption	Poisons absorbed through the skin include plant materials such as poison oak or ivy, lawn care products such as chemical pesticides, and other chemical powders or liquids.
	Injection	Drug abuse is the most common cause of injected poisons. The stingers of insects inject poisons into the body and can be extremely dangerous and can lead to anaphylactic shock in allergic individuals.

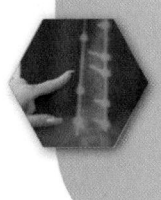
The provider will recommend that these localized symptoms be managed with a topical cream and oral antihistamines. Swelling can be significant and cause for serious concern if the sting occurred in a vulnerable area of the body such as the mouth or tongue. Swelling in these locations can be frightening and dangerous because it can impair breathing. An antihistamine, administered as soon as possible after the sting, may help to curtail symptoms somewhat. Treatment of insect stings in nonallergic individuals consists of removing the stinger by scraping it off with the edge of something rigid such as a credit card or a fingernail. Tweezers can cause more venom to be dispersed into the patient's body tissues, so this method should not be used. Wash the area with soap and water, apply a cold pack to the site, and watch for a possible severe reaction.

The individual who experiences an allergic reaction or hypersensitivity to a sting needs to be seen immediately, because in severe cases a sting may induce an anaphylactic reaction that can lead to death. If allergic, individuals who have been stung are likely to experience symptoms within a half hour of the incident. Symptoms are generalized throughout the body and may include hives, itching, and lightheadedness and may progress to difficulty breathing, faintness, and eventual loss of consciousness.

For individuals with known allergic reactions, the provider will prescribe epinephrine, which patients should carry with them and self-inject should they not be able to get immediate emergency care. EpiPen is an auto-injector device that delivers epinephrine. The patient should then seek immediate emergency treatment. For individuals who present at the ambulatory care setting with an apparent allergic reaction to a sting, the provider will prescribe epinephrine, an antihistamine, and corticosteroids if necessary.

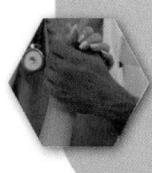

Patient Education

Remind patients who are parents of young children to remove any potential sources of poisoning from their homes or to keep such substances in locked cabinets. Also advise them to include the nearby poison control center in their list of emergency phone numbers. They should also keep activated charcoal on hand.

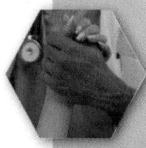

Patient Education

Snake Bite

Most snakes are not poisonous, and snakes usually will not strike unless provoked. Some poisonous snakes are rattlesnake, copper snake, cottonmouth water moccasin, and coral snake. Individuals who live in snake-inhabited areas, campers, hikers, and other outdoor lovers need to be mindful and cautious when outdoors. To avoid a possible snake bite, wear thick high boots, stay on the hiking path, do not reach down to pick up something from the ground unless you have a clear view around the area, and be careful on rocks (snakes like to live in or around piles of rocks).

Common signs and symptoms of a snake bite are rapid pulse, nausea and vomiting, severe pain, swelling, blood and fang marks at wound site, convulsions, thirst, and diaphoresis.

Emergency treatment consists of the following:

- Call for emergency help immediately.
- Wash wound with soap and water if possible.
- Immobilize body part and keep below heart level if possible.
- Cover wound with clean cool cloth.
- Monitor vital signs.
- Do not allow the victim to walk. Carry them or transport them by vehicle.

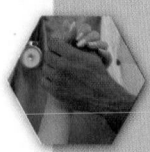

Patient Education

Advise all patients with known allergic reactions to be particularly careful when working or playing outdoors. Insects are not usually aggressive until their nests are approached; however, often these nests are not easy to detect, and an individual may approach one without being aware of its presence. Patients with allergies to insects should always wear shoes when outside; wear light-colored clothing, preferably with long sleeves and pant legs; look before taking a sip from a beverage when outdoors; and inspect lawn areas, shrubbery, and building walls periodically for evidence of stinging insect nests.

Attempt to allay patient apprehension and monitor vital signs while waiting for EMS personnel to arrive.

Sudden Illness

Sudden illness is, by definition, an unexpected occurrence. Although the cause of the illness may be unexplainable, it is important to respond sensibly and responsibly within the parameters of knowledge and resources.

Sudden illnesses include, but are not limited to, fainting, seizures, diabetic reaction, and hemorrhage (see Table 8-8).

TABLE 8-8

TYPES OF SUDDEN ILLNESS

TYPE OF ILLNESS	SYMPTOMS	CAUSE	TREATMENT
Fainting (**syncope**) (see Procedure 8-5)	May be preceded by: • Sweating • Weakness • Lightheadedness • Nausea • Disruption of sight • Ringing in the ears • Loss of consciousness	Most commonly, loss of adequate blood flow to the brain Other causes: • Emotional causes (vagal syncope) • Hypoglycemia • Severe pain • Hypotension • Dehydration • Hyperventilation	Gently lower patient into supine position Raise legs and feet above the level of the heart (if no spine or head injury) Treat the underlying causes Provide comfort measures such as loosening clothing and applying a cool cloth to the forehead Activate EMS for complex medical conditions
Seizures (see Procedure 8-6)	Absence (brief loss of consciousness) "Grand mal" or generalized tonic seizure: • Unconsciousness • Convulsions • Muscle rigidity Myoclonic seizure: • Sporadic (isolated) • Jerking movements Clonic seizure: • Repetitive • Jerking movements Tonic seizure: • Muscle stiffness • Rigidity Atonic seizure: • Loss of muscle tone	Normal brain functioning has been interrupted May be caused by: • Epilepsy • Fever • Diabetes • Infection • Brain injury	Care for the patient with medical understanding and compassion Do not restrain the patient Protect patient from self-injury: • Cushion the head • Clear the area of dangerous objects • Roll the patient onto his or her side to assist with managing fluids to prevent aspiration • Calm and comfort the patient Treat the underlying cause Activate EMS if patient is pregnant, diabetic, or injured **Do Not:** Attempt to stop the seizure even if the patient appears frightened and in pain Force anything between the patient's clenched teeth (the patient cannot swallow his or her tongue)

continues

Table 8-8 continued

TYPE OF ILLNESS	SYMPTOMS	CAUSE	TREATMENT
Diabetes (see Procedure 8-7) • Type 1 (insulin-dependent) • Type 2 non-insulin-dependent, which usually occurs in adults; in type 2, the body produces insulin in insufficient quantities)	**Hyperglycemia (ketoacidosis)**: Dry, flushed skin • Drowsiness • Dry mouth • Intense thirst • Nausea and/or vomiting • Air hunger • Fruity breath • Weak, rapid pulse • Dimmed vision • Blood glucose > 200 mg/dL Hypoglycemia: • Pale, moist skin • Excited behavior • Drooling • Hunger • Normal or shallow respirations • Full and pounding pulse • Double vision (**diplopia**) • Blood glucose < 40 to 70 mg/dL	The inability of the body to properly convert sugar from food into energy, resulting in hyperglycemia or hypoglcemia Sugar not able to be transported into cells due to a lack of the hormone insulin	Recognize the symptoms of hyperglycemia or hypoglycemia Check blood glucose level and patient vital signs Notify the provider of findings Treat the underlying issue: If **hypoglycemia** (low blood sugar), offer the patient a high sugar content drink or snack Be prepared to administer glucose as ordered by the provider If hyperglycemia (elevated blood sugar), the provider will order insulin Activate EMS if indicated. **Note:** Provider will assess the patient prior to release; notify provider once patient has returned to homeostasic vital signs and blood glucose level
Hemorrhage (external bleeding)	Bleeding from the capillaries, veins, and/or arteries due to damage to the skin and underlying structures • Venous bleeding (blood is dark red with a steady flow) • Arterial bleeding (blood is bright red and exits the body in a pumping or spurting manner) If not controlled, will lead to shock and death	Puncture or severing of capillaries, veins, and arteries from trauma or surgical intervention *Epistaxis.* Prolonged exposure to dry air, injury, high altitude, repeated nose blowing, hypertension, or use of anticoagulant medications that easily damage the delicate mucous membranes of the nose Vaginal bleeding due to miscarriage is a rare complication, but it is a leading cause of maternal complications Vaginal bleeding might also be caused by neoplasm or trauma	Apply direct pressure Treat the underlying cause of bleeding The provider may intervene with: • Suturing • **Electrocautery** (applying controlled heat to obtain hemostasis) • Pressure dressing application To treat epistaxis: • Elevate head • Pinch nostrils for 10 minutes • Tilt head forward to prevent swallowing or aspiration of blood • If bleeding not controlled in 20 minutes, active EMS • Assist provider with cauterization or insertion of gauze packing If bleeding is associated with trauma or head injury, activate EMS To treat vaginal bleeding: • Prepare the exam room for a pelvic exam • Provide a sterile tray setup that includes a speculum • Stand by to arrange transport to an acute care setting Activate EMS Monitor vital signs Provide shock prevention measures: • Spine position • Elevate legs • Maintain airway • Maintain body temperature • Keep patient npo

continues

Table 8-8 continued

TYPE OF ILLNESS	SYMPTOMS	CAUSE	TREATMENT
Internal bleeding	Bleeding from the capillaries, veins, and/or arteries internally Lack of visible blood flow after trauma or surgical intervention The following symptoms may occur: • Rapid and weak pulse • Low blood pressure • Shallow breathing • Cold and clammy skin • Dilated pupils • Dizziness • Faintness • Thirst • Restlessness • Feeling of anxiety • Pain • Fatigue • Swelling • Abdominal board-like stiffness	Trauma that damages any internal organ Damage to any artery or vein that causes bleeding Fractures, especially of long bones Ectopic pregnancy Postoperative bleeding Alcohol abuse that results in cirrhosis of the liver causing esophageal varices	Activate EMS Monitor vital signs Provide shock prevention measures: • Place in supine position • Elevate legs • Maintain airway • Maintain body temperature • Keep patient npo

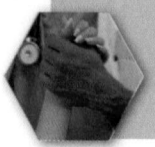

Patient Education

Advise the patient not to blow the nose for several hours after an epistaxis.

PROCEDURE 8-5

Procedure

First Aid Procedures for Syncope (Fainting Episode)

STANDARD PRECAUTIONS:

Handwashing

PURPOSE:

To provide protection from injury and administer first aid to a person experiencing a syncopal episode.

(continues)

EQUIPMENT/SUPPLIES:

- Pillows
- Blanket

PROCEDURE STEPS:

1. Be aware that if an individual that is conscious alerts you that he or she feels faint or dizzy, or when *incorporating critical thinking skills when performing patient assessment and care*, you note pallor and cool, clammy skin, syncope may be pending.
2. If the patient is conscious and still alert, assist him or her to a sitting position and help to bend forward, placing head between the knees until symptoms resolve.
3. If the patient has fainted or is no longer able to follow commands, position him or her on back and elevate legs. RATIONALE: This restores blood flow to the brain by decreasing gravitational resistance.
4. Loosen any restrictive clothing or belts. RATIONALE: This encourages adequate respiration.
5. Check for pulse and respiration. If necessary, begin CPR after activating EMS or calling for assistance.
6. Alert the provider to immediately assess the patient.
7. Obtain vital signs as soon as the patient is safely positioned. Repeat frequently, per provider's preference.
8. ***Recognizing the physical and emotional effects on persons involved in an emergency situation***, provide comfort measures to the patient, such as a blanket for warmth.
9. Document the incident and care provided in the patient's chart.

DOCUMENTATION:

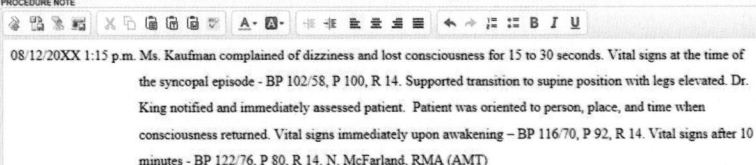

PROCEDURE NOTE

08/12/20XX 1:15 p.m. Ms. Kaufman complained of dizziness and lost consciousness for 15 to 30 seconds. Vital signs at the time of the syncopal episode - BP 102/58, P 100, R 14. Supported transition to supine position with legs elevated. Dr. King notified and immediately assessed patient. Patient was oriented to person, place, and time when consciousness returned. Vital signs immediately upon awakening – BP 116/70, P 92, R 14. Vital signs after 10 minutes - BP 122/76, P 80, R 14. N. McFarland, RMA (AMT)

Courtesy of Harris CareTracker PM and EMR

PROCEDURE 8-6

Perform First Aid Procedures for Seizures

Procedure

STANDARD PRECAUTIONS:

Handwashing Gloves Biohazard Gown Goggles & Mask

PURPOSE:

To appropriately manage a patient physically and ensure his or her safety during a seizure.

(continues)

EQUIPMENT/SUPPLIES:

- Pillow
- Clean gloves
- Appropriate PPE
- Biohazardous waste container
- Blanket

PROCEDURE STEPS:

1. ***Incorporate critical thinking skills when performing patient assessment and care.*** If the patient is standing or sitting at the onset of the seizure, gently ease him or her to a reclining position on the exam table or on the floor.

2. Turn the patient onto his or her side to manage oral secretions to avoid aspiration.

3. Assess patient's breathing. If needed, open the airway using the head tilt or jaw thrust maneuver.

4. Call for assistance and immediately notify the provider without leaving the patient's side. Accurately and concisely update the provider on any aspect of the patient's care.

5. Apply clean gloves as soon as possible once the patient is safely reclining.

6. Clear the immediate area around the patient to avoid injury during the **tonic-clonic phase** of the seizure.

7. Place a pillow under the patient's head for support. Manage clothing by removing glasses, loosening clothing, and loosening belts.

8. Time the seizure. Seizures usually resolve in 1 to 3 minutes. If the seizure lasts 30 minutes continuously or there are two or more seizures without a period of recovery, the patient may be in **status epilepticus**. Be prepared to activate EMS on the provider's order.

9. Cover the patient with a blanket for comfort once the seizure ends.

10. Stay with the patient. ***Recognize the physical and emotional effects on persons involved in an emergency situation.*** As he or she returns to consciousness, gently inform the patient of what has just occurred.

11. Obtain vital signs once the seizure has resolved. Continue to monitor vital signs frequently at an interval set by the provider's preferences.

12. Allow the patient to rest or sleep after the procedure.

13. Document the length of the seizure and any other relevant information in the patient's chart.

DOCUMENTATION:

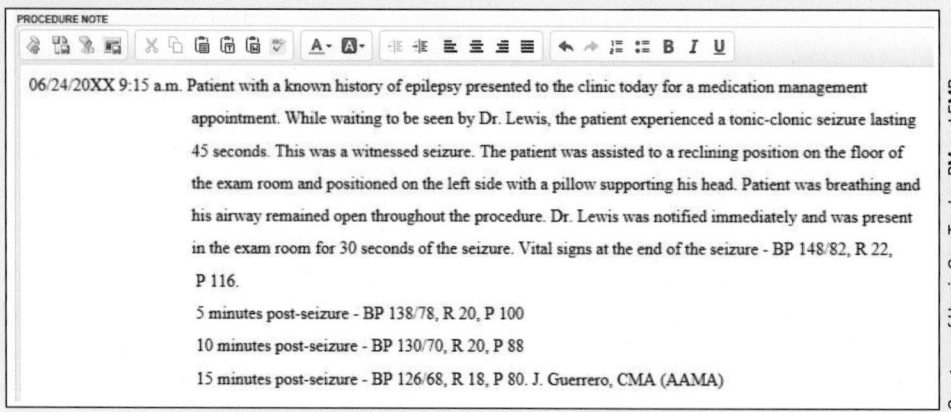

PROCEDURE NOTE

06/24/20XX 9:15 a.m. Patient with a known history of epilepsy presented to the clinic today for a medication management appointment. While waiting to be seen by Dr. Lewis, the patient experienced a tonic-clonic seizure lasting 45 seconds. This was a witnessed seizure. The patient was assisted to a reclining position on the floor of the exam room and positioned on the left side with a pillow supporting his head. Patient was breathing and his airway remained open throughout the procedure. Dr. Lewis was notified immediately and was present in the exam room for 30 seconds of the seizure. Vital signs at the end of the seizure - BP 148/82, R 22, P 116.

5 minutes post-seizure - BP 138/78, R 20, P 100

10 minutes post-seizure - BP 130/70, R 20, P 88

15 minutes post-seizure - BP 126/68, R 18, P 80. J. Guerrero, CMA (AAMA)

Courtesy of Harris CareTracker PM and EMR

PROCEDURE 8-7

Perform First Aid Procedures for Diabetic Emergencies

Procedure

STANDARD PRECAUTIONS:

Handwashing   Gloves   Biohazard

PURPOSE:

To appropriately assist a patient experiencing either hypoglycemia or hyperglycemia.

EQUIPMENT/SUPPLIES:

- Clean gloves
- Glucose analyzer
- Strips for glucose analyzer
- Sterile lancets

- Alcohol wipes
- 2-by-2 gauze
- Adhesive bandage
- Biohazard waste container

PROCEDURE STEPS:

1. When symptoms of hyperglycemia (ketoacidosis) or hypoglycemia are noted, have the patient sit or lie down. RATIONALE: This reduces the risk of a fall if loss of consciousness occurs.

2. Obtain vital signs.

3. Follow the provider's order for obtaining a blood glucose measurement and assemble the equipment needed to test blood glucose. ***Explain to the patient the rationale for performance of the procedure, showing awareness of the patient's concerns***.

4. Apply clean gloves and perform a blood glucose analysis, following steps in Procedure 43-4.

5. Notify the provider of findings and follow provider orders.

6. ***Incorporating critical thinking skills in performing patient assessment and care***, be prepared to offer the patient a drink that contains a high sugar content or a high sugar snack if the patient is hypoglycemic, with a blood sugar below 70 mg/dL.

7. ***Incorporating critical thinking skills in performing patient assessment and care***, be prepared to administer insulin per the provider's order if the patient is hyperglycemic, with a blood sugar above 200 mg/dL.

8. If at any time the patient loses consciousness, place her on her side, notify the provider, and prepare to activate EMS on provider's orders.

9. Document your findings and the procedures performed.

DOCUMENTATION:

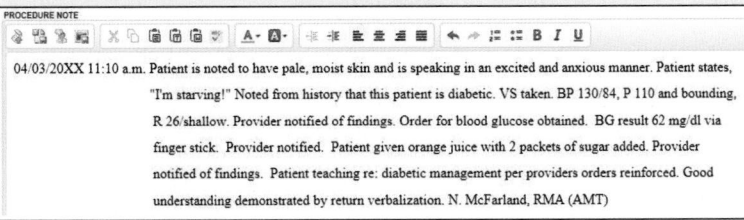

04/03/20XX 11:10 a.m. Patient is noted to have pale, moist skin and is speaking in an excited and anxious manner. Patient states, "I'm starving!" Noted from history that this patient is diabetic. VS taken. BP 130/84, P 110 and bounding, R 26/shallow. Provider notified of findings. Order for blood glucose obtained. BG result 62 mg/dl via finger stick. Provider notified. Patient given orange juice with 2 packets of sugar added. Provider notified of findings. Patient teaching re: diabetic management per providers orders reinforced. Good understanding demonstrated by return verbalization. N. McFarland, RMA (AMT)

Courtesy of Harris CareTracker PM and EMR

Vascular Events

Patients sometimes present in the outpatient setting with evolving vascular events that are true emergencies. Many patients may confuse what it means to suffer a stroke or heart attack because they are unclear regarding the anatomy involved, but public education has improved in recent years to encourage rapid recognition of symptoms and treatment plans to limit the damage caused by either of these physiologic vascular events. See Table 8-9 for more information in the symptoms, causes, and treatment of vascular events.

BREATHING EMERGENCIES AND CARDIAC ARREST

Breathing or respiratory emergencies occur for a variety of reasons, including choking, shock, allergies, and other illnesses or injuries such as drowning and electrical shock. When an individual stops breathing, artificial or rescue breathing must be given quickly, for without a constant supply of oxygen, brain damage or death will occur.

When the breathing problem is accompanied by cardiac arrest, the rescue breathing must be accompanied by chest compressions. This procedure is known as **cardiopulmonary resuscitation (CPR)**. Cardiac emergencies may occur in the medical clinic because of the large number of patients who have heart disease.

In order to graduate from a CAAHEP-accredited program, medical assistants must attain provider-level CPR certification and take first aid training courses. Frequent refresher courses and recertification in CPR are necessary.

TABLE 8-9

VASCULAR EVENTS

EVENT	SYMPTOMS	CAUSE	TREATMENT
Cerebral vascular accident (CVA) or stroke	Numbness in face and extremities on one side of the body Loss of vision Severe headache Confusion Slurred speech Nausea and vomiting Shortness of breath Difficulty swallowing Paralysis	Rupture or **occlusion** of vessel in the brain interrupting blood flow to brain cells, resulting in cellular death	Activate EMS Assist patient in lying down with head turned to side to manage oral fluids Provide comfort measures Maintain airway Allow no food or drink Monitor vital signs Follow provider's orders for medication administration
Myocardial infarction (MI) or heart attack	Chest tightness or pain Pain radiating down one or both arms Pain radiating to left shoulder or jaw Rapid, weak pulse Excessive perspiration Agitation Nausea Cold, clammy skin Women may have: • Abdominal discomfort • Burning sensation in chest • Discomfort or pain in lower chest or back • Sudden fatigue • Sweating • Breathlessness	Interruption in blood flow to the cardiac muscle, resulting in lack of oxygen to tissues and cell death	Activate EMS Obtain crash cart Follow provider's orders to apply oxygen and administer aspirin and other medications Attach to cardiac monitor Monitor vital signs Assist provider with **cardioversion** or defibrillation using an automated external defibrillator (AED) Begin CPR if indicated

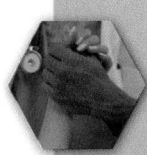

Patient Education

Lay Person CPR

- The person does not need to be certified.
- Chest compressions alone are sufficient.
- Patients are more likely to survive without brain damage with only chest compressions.
- Use 30 compressions per minute to keep blood moving to brain and heart.
- Drowning victims and smoke inhalation victims are the exception. Both need rescue breathing and CPR.

Rescue Breathing

Individuals in respiratory arrest require immediate emergency care. **Rescue breathing**, previously called mouth-to-mouth resuscitation, provides oxygen to the patient until emergency personnel arrive.

When performing rescue breathing procedures in the ambulatory care setting, it is recommended that resuscitation mouthpieces be used and that direct mouth-to-mouth (i.e., with no personal protective equipment) resuscitation never be used.

Cardiopulmonary Resuscitation

The combination of rescue breathing and chest compressions is known as CPR. Alone, CPR cannot save an individual from cardiac arrest—it represents preliminary care until advanced medical help is available to the heart attack victim.

In 2015, the American Heart Association (AHA) updated its emergency care guidelines for CPR and emergency cardiovascular care (ECC). (To review these guidelines, go to www.heart.org and search for "2015 CPR Guidelines.") The new guidelines recommend immediately beginning chest compressions rather than first opening the airway and beginning ventilations. A change in the ABC methodology to CAB was instituted in 2010 and remains the order for initiating CPR for the unresponsive patient. This change reflects the understanding that patients in cardiac arrest benefit from the return to blood flow as soon as possible. An emphasis has been placed on high-quality CPR, with chest compressions of adequate rate and depth, allowing complete chest recoil after each compression, minimizing interruptions in the compressions, and avoiding excessive ventilation.

Studies have found that if bystanders act as quickly as possible and begin CPR, many more victims could be saved. It was determined that CPR plus a shock with an AED (Figure 8-10) is the most effective immediate treatment for cardiac arrest. The AHA says that early recognition of the emergency, calling EMS, and performing immediate CPR can double or triple a victim's chances of surviving. Furthermore, the AHA says that CPR plus defibrillation (AED) started within 3 to 5 minutes of collapse can boost survival significantly. Lay rescuer AEDs are available in airports, sports facilities, airplanes, casinos, and many other locations. AEDs are becoming more readily available, are easy to use, and are very accurate. The current guidelines suggest that an AED be utilized immediately for a witnessed arrest.

The 2015 guidelines have changed the number of compressions per minute to between 100 and 120 from *at least* 100. The depth of compressions recommended is at least 2 inches. The look, listen, and feel method has been replaced by visually scanning the victim's chest for rise and fall for a period of time no longer than 10 seconds. AHA guidelines stress that compressions should begin immediately, prior to initiating rescue breathing. Table 8-10 summarizes the AHA's 2015 guidelines for CPR and defibrillation.

Immediate recognition and activation of the emergency response system once the health care provider identifies the adult victim who is unresponsive as having no breathing or no normal breathing (i.e., only gasping) is called for. Once no normal

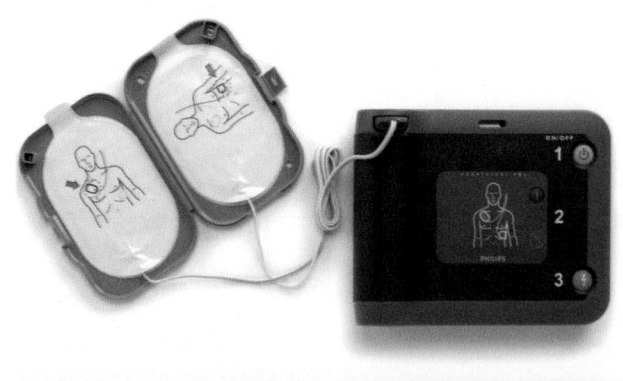

FIGURE 8-10 Automated external defibrillator.

Courtesy of Philips Healthcare

TABLE 8-10

SUMMARY OF THE AMERICAN HEART ASSOCIATION'S 2015 HIGH-QUALITY CPR GUIDELINES

COMPONENT	RECOMMENDATIONS		
Scene safety	Ensure the environment is safe for victim and rescuers.		
Recognition of cardiac arrest	Check for responsiveness No breathing or only gasping (no normal breathing) No definite pulse felt within 10 seconds (breathing and pulse check can be performed simultaneously within 10 seconds)		
Activation of EMS	**Adults and adolescents:** If you are alone and do not have a mobile phone, leave victim to activate EMS and obtain AED, and then begin CPR. If there is a second rescuer, send him or her to activate EMS and obtain the AED while you begin CPR.	**Infants and children, witnessed collapse:** Follow steps for adult and adolescent resuscitation. **Unwitnessed collapse:** Administer CPR for 2 minutes. Leave the victim to activate EMS and obtain the AED. Return to the child or infant to resume CPR, and use the AED as soon as it is available.	
CPR sequence	CAB		
Compression rate	100 to 120 per minute		
Compression depth	**Adult:** At least 2 inches (5 cm)	**Child:** At least ⅓ AP diameter About 2 inches (5 cm)	**Infant:** At least ⅓ AP diameter About 1½ inches (4 cm)
Hand placement	**Adult:** Two hands on the lower half of the sternum	**Child:** Two hands or one hand for small child on lower half of the sternum	**Infant:** Two fingers in the center of the chest (one rescuer) just below the nipple line Circle chest with hands and place two thumbs in the center of the chest, just above the nipple line (two rescuer).
Chest wall recoil	Allow complete recoil between compressions HCPs rotate compressors every 2 minutes		
Compression interruptions	Minimize interruptions in chest compressions Attempt to limit interruptions to < 10 seconds		
Airway	Head tilt–chin lift (HCP suspected trauma: jaw thrust)		
Compression-to-ventilation ratio (until advanced airway is placed)	**Adult:** 30:2, 1 or 2 rescuers	**Infants and Children:** 30:2 single rescuer 15:2 two rescuers	
Ventilations when rescuer untrained and not proficient	Compressions only		
Ventilations with advanced airway (HCP)	1 breath every 6 to 8 seconds (8 to 10 breaths/min) Asynchronous with chest compressions About 1 second per breath Visible chest rise		
Defibrillation	Attach and use AED as soon as available. Minimize interruptions in chest compressions before and after shock; resume CPR beginning with compressions immediately after each shock.		

AED, automated external defibrillator; AP, anterior-posterior; CPR, cardiopulmonary resuscitation; HCP, health care provider

*Excluding the newly born, in whom the cause of an arrest is nearly always asphyxia.

breathing has been identified, the provider then activates EMS and retrieves the AED (or sends someone to do so). Compressions should begin at this time.

More information is available from the following sources:

- American Heart Association (http://www.americanheart.org)
- American Red Cross (http://www.redcross.org)
- National Safety Council (http://www.nsc.org)
- National Institutes of Health (http://www.health.nih.gov)

Hands-Only CPR. The AHA recommends that if you witness an adult or teen suddenly collapse, call 911 and then push hard and fast in the center of the victim's chest. Further, the AHA recommends compression to the beat of the classic disco song *Stayin' Alive*. CPR can more than double a person's chances of survival, and *Stayin' Alive* has the right beat for hands-only CPR.

Once 911 has been called, you need to stay on the phone until the 911 dispatcher (operator) tells you to hang up. The dispatcher will obtain information about the type of emergency and your location. Try to be as specific as possible. This type of resuscitation is appropriate for "in the field" resuscitation in the absence of other trained personnel and emergency equipment.

SAFETY AND EMERGENCY PRACTICES

The Commission on Accreditation of Allied Health Programs (CAAHEP) believes allied health students should understand how to respond in an emergency situation, as health care professionals and citizens. Medical assistant programs accredited by CAAHEP have within their Standards and Guidelines a section requiring education regarding safety and emergency practices. Provider-level CPR and basic first aid are part of these requirements for graduation.

The Accrediting Bureau of Health Education Schools (ABHES) also has a requirement in its competencies under the heading of Medical Office Clinical Procedures.

Health professionals recognize an obligation to use their skills and knowledge in a disaster environment.

There are many kinds of mass disasters, natural and manmade. Some examples are floods, hurricanes, tornadoes, tsunamis, and earthquakes. Others are explosions, structural collapses (e.g., the 2011 Indiana State Fair stage collapse), transportation accidents, bioterrorism (see Chapter 21).

What would a large-scale disaster be like, and how could we respond? Disasters can threaten public health and safety; disrupt services (e.g., gas, water, electricity, transportation); destroy roads, bridges, homes, and other buildings; and make food and water unsafe or impossible to obtain. Law enforcement, fire departments, hospitals, and military all could be affected. There is a need for collaboration between disaster experts and health professionals to plan for emergencies.

What can medical assistants do to help? How could you use your skills without technology (i.e., if it were unavailable due to the disaster)? Some examples are assisting your neighbors at local shelters, using your first aid and CPR skills, helping out at a clinic, giving injections for mass immunizations, supporting overwhelmed providers, working with the American Red Cross, giving emotional support, and filling in at a hospital.

 In addition to mass disasters, medical assistants should be prepared to respond to emergency situations in the medical clinic or a home environment. Circumstances in which a patient goes into shock, an elderly family member has a fall, or a medical clinic needs to be evacuated for a fire are examples of such emergency situations.

Competency

Medical assisting curricula may include related courses to be certain that medical assisting graduates are prepared to help during emergency situations.

In 2002, President George W. Bush asked for teams of volunteers of medical and health professionals to contribute their skills during times of need in their communities. The Medical Reserve Corps (MRC) was established (http://www.medicalreservecorps.gov), and the teams of volunteers within the MRC work with Health and Human Services of the U.S. government and the American Red Cross. The MRC is community based. Its goal is to organize and use volunteers who want to donate their time and expertise to respond to emergencies and to promote healthy living throughout the year. The MRC supplements existing emergency and public health resources. Volunteers include providers, nurses, respiratory care therapists, massage therapists, pharmacists, dentists, and a wide array of allied health professionals such as medical assistants.

The MRC volunteer units are assigned to specific geographic areas. They work with and support county and state public health departments. The main office is in the surgeon general's office in Washington, D.C.

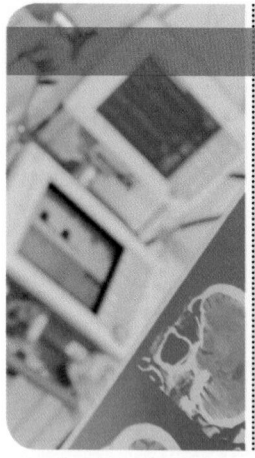

CASE STUDY 8-1

Refer to the scenario at the beginning of the chapter.

CASE STUDY REVIEW

1. Because Mr. Cochran is exhibiting symptoms of having a cardiac event, what are the first measures to be taken?
2. Why is it essential to activate EMS even though Mr. Cochran is being seen in an ambulatory care setting?
3. What questions should Nancy McFarland, RMA (AMT), ask Mr. Cochran?
4. What would be the next steps after assessing the patient if the chest pain continued and the patient lost consciousness prior to the arrival of EMS?

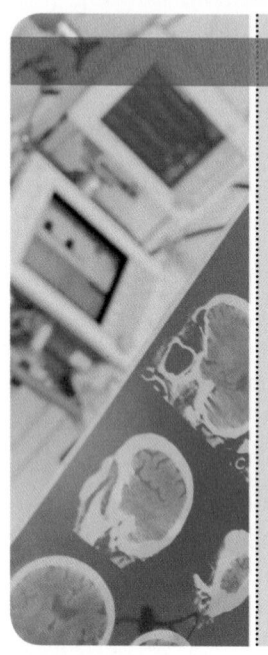

CASE STUDY 8-2

Carlette Jennings, a regular patient at Inner City Health Care, is walking her dog one morning and stops to rest on a grassy knoll, where she notices a wasp on her arm. She brushes it away, unthinking, and then realizes it has stung her. She receives two more stings and suddenly notices she is at a nest site. Carlette is now a half-hour walk from home but is not really concerned because she has never had an allergic reaction to a wasp sting. However, a few minutes after she resume walking, her palms become itchy, her ears start to burn, and she feels lightheaded. She is not having difficulty breathing. She is determined to get home and she does, at which point she notices she is covered with hives. She calls Inner City Health Care to ask whether she should come in.

CASE STUDY REVIEW

1. Joe Guerrero, CMA (AAMA), is screening calls the morning that Carlette is stung. What questions should he ask Carlette?
2. Because Carlette obviously is having a hypersensitive or an allergic reaction, she is advised to seek emergency care immediately. What first aid measures might be taken?
3. To prevent reactions to stings in the future, what patient teaching might be appropriate for Carlette?

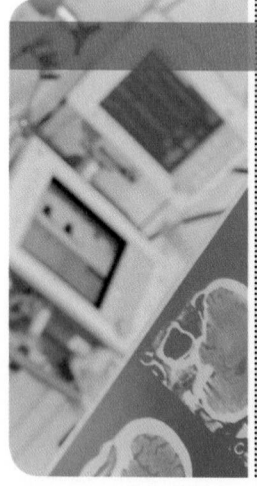

CASE STUDY 8-3

Bryan Mountjoy is a 32-year-old patient of Dr. Osborne. He has been working in the yard throughout the day, even though the temperature was over 100°F. Being so focused on the job at hand, Mr. Mountjoy has not taken in enough fluids over the course of the day. He calls out to his wife that he is feeling faint. She finds him with reddened, dry, hot skin; shallow, fast breathing; and a weak pulse. Mrs. Mountjoy calls the clinic seeking medical advice.

CASE STUDY REVIEW

1. What immediate questions should you ask Mrs. Mountjoy?
2. What would you advise Mrs. Mountjoy to do in order to receive the most appropriate level of care?
3. If Mrs. Mountjoy expresses panic, how could you help her to remain calm?

Summary

- It is crucial to be able to quickly recognize and begin intervention when an emergency occurs. These emergency situations may range from minor to severe.

- Appropriate action begins with assessment. This assessment begins with Circulation, Airway, and Breathing (CAB) as a priority.

- Response to emergencies depends on the ability to recognize an emergency immediately; being prepared to respond; knowledge of the EMS system and its activation; familiarity with the crash cart and the items that it contains; knowledge of the causes, symptoms, and treatment of the most common emergencies; CPR and AED training; and staff continuing education and certification in CPR.

- The professional medical assistant must be aware of the symptoms and treatment of common emergencies. Recognition of the various types of shock (cardiogenic, hypovolemic, neurogenic, anaphylactic, septic, and respiratory) allows early intervention to prevent an irreversible condition.

- Wounds are seen frequently in the clinic setting. Knowledge of how to provide first aid for closed and open wounds, how and when to apply a tourniquet, as well as the application of dressings are key components of the provision of first aid.

- Burns are classified as first-, second-, and third-degree burns. The physical presentation and treatment of each vary related to the degree of tissue injury.

- Orthopedic injuries include strains and sprains, as well as fractures. The goal of first aid practices is to immobilize the injured extremity to prevent further injury until radiologic evaluation and definitive treatment can be performed.

- Exposure to extreme heat or cold can be life threatening. Rapid initiation of first aid can prevent death, especially in the very young or older persons.

- Poisoning is a serious and potentially life-threatening emergency. Memorize the national Poison Control Center's phone number (1-800-222-1222).

- Other sudden illnesses such as fainting, seizures, hemorrhage, and diabetic reactions have a rapid onset and have interventions that are easy to implement. The awareness of the need to ensure the patient's safety and the knowledge of the actions that will resolve the underlying issue is the responsibility of all members of the health care team.

- Symptoms of CVA or stroke and myocardial infarction or heart attack indicate activation of EMS.

- Maintaining professional CPR certification will allow the medical assistant to recognized and initiate care for myocardial infarction.

Study for Success

To reinforce your knowledge and skills of information presented in this chapter:

- Review the *Key Terms* and *Learning Outcomes*

- Consider the *Critical Thinking* features and *Case Studies* and discuss your conclusions

- Answer the questions in the *Certification Review*

- Perform the *Procedures* using the *Competency Assessment Checklists* on the *Student Companion Website*

Procedure

CERTIFICATION REVIEW

1. Which of the following is true regarding Good Samaritan laws?
   a. They are designed to protect the public.
   b. They protect non–health care professionals.
   c. They require that all individuals providing assistance act within the scope of their knowledge and training.
   d. They protect health care professionals on the job.
2. Which of the following defines an avulsion?
   a. The skin is torn off and bleeding is profuse.
   b. There is superficial scraping of the dermis.
   c. It is a tear of the body tissue.
   d. It describes a surgical incision.
   e. All of these
3. First-degree burns are most accurately described by which of the following statements?
   a. They are the most serious burns and penetrate all layers of skin.
   b. They affect only the top layer of skin.
   c. They often leave scar tissue.
   d. They usually take more than a month to heal.
4. According to current AHA CPR guidelines, what is the order of steps for cardiopulmonary resuscitation?
   a. Airway, breathing, compressions
   b. Breathing, compressions, airway
   c. Compressions, airway, breathing
   d. Any of the steps can come first, as long as blood begins to circulate within 18 seconds
   e. None of these
5. A fracture in which the bone protrudes through the skin is called what?
   a. Greenstick fracture
   b. Compound fracture
   c. Depressed fracture
   d. Comminuted fracture
6. To control a nosebleed, it is important to take which of the following actions?
   a. Have the patient lie down
   b. Tilt the patient's head back
   c. Tilt the patient's head forward
   d. Call 911 immediately
   e. All of these
7. Which of the following is another name for a heart attack?
   a. Cerebral vascular accident
   b. Angina pectoris
   c. Myocardial infarction
   d. Stroke
8. Which of the following is the correct depth of compressions when administering CPR for adults?
   a. 1 inch
   b. 1.5 inches
   c. 2 inches
   d. 2.5 inches
   e. 3 inches
9. Exposure to extreme cold for prolonged periods can cause which of the following?
   a. Hypothermia
   b. Hyperthermia
   c. Frostbite
   d. Both a and c
10. Septic shock results from which of the following?
    a. A severe allergic reaction
    b. Overwhelming infection
    c. Trauma to the respiratory system
    d. Extreme loss of blood
    e. Hypothermia

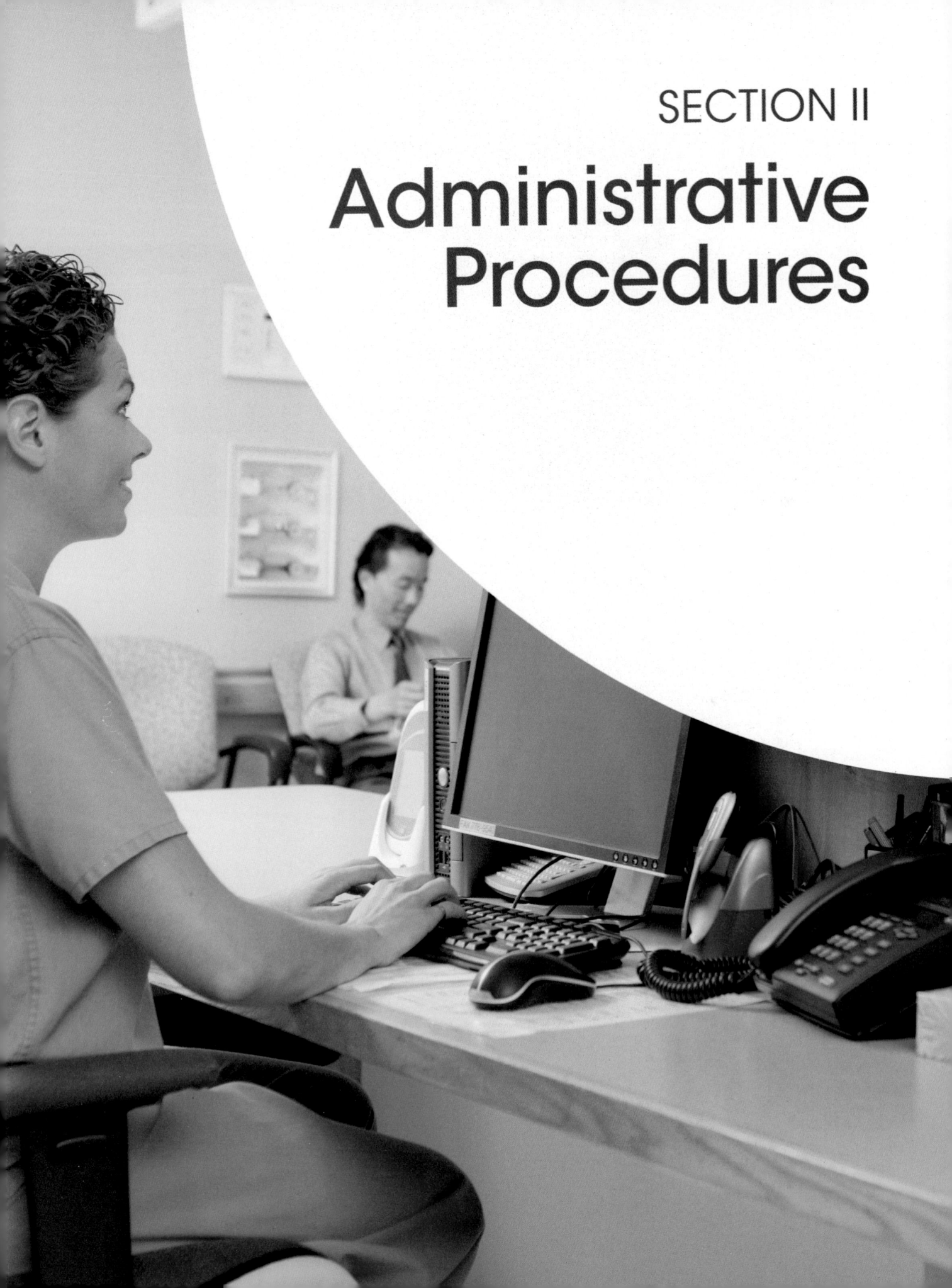

SECTION II
Administrative Procedures

UNIT IV
INTEGRATED ADMINISTRATIVE PROCEDURES

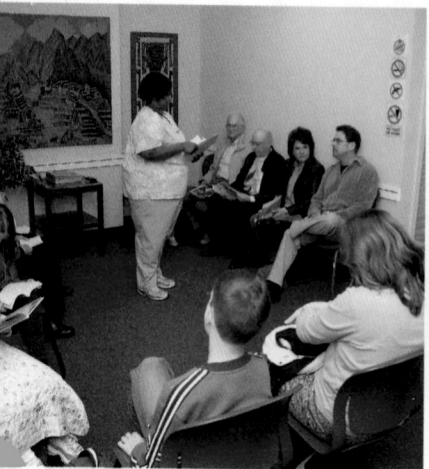
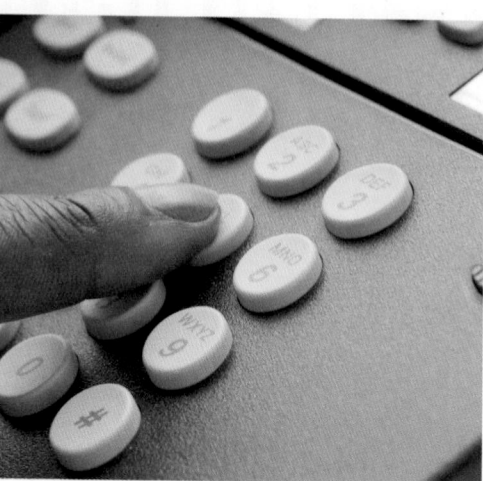
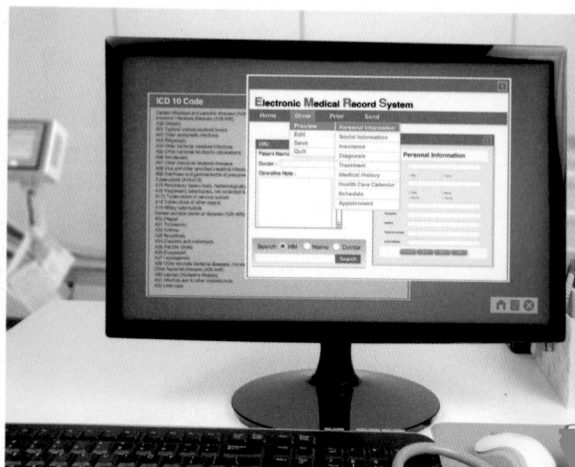

ATTRIBUTES OF PROFESSIONALISM

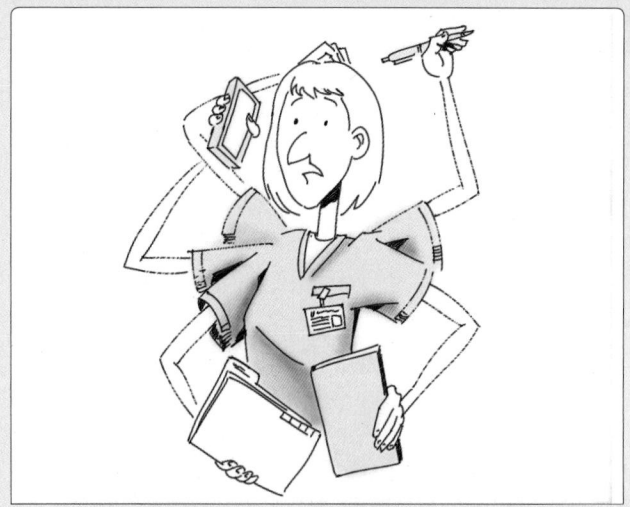

Medical assistants convey a great deal to patients through attitude and actions as well as empathy. A hurried or disinterested manner communicates that the patient is not a priority. Patients do not easily forget rude or insensitive staff. A hurried, disinterested manner toward patients is just as often the basis for legal action as is a negligent act.

The patient should always be made to feel worthy of attention. This validates his or her reason for calling. If you are scheduling a patient in the clinic and the phone rings, answer the call but excuse yourself first. Ask the caller to please hold for a moment. If you are on the telephone scheduling a patient and another patient walks in, acknowledge with a nod or signal that you will be right there—never let the person feel ignored. Today, patients have a variety of options for health care and tend to be much more consumer conscious of the treatment they receive.

Listed below are a series of questions for you to ask yourself, to serve as a professionalism checklist. As you interact with patients and colleagues, these questions will help to guide you in the professional behavior that is expected every day from medical assistants.

Ask Yourself

COMMUNICATION
- [ ] Do I apply active listening skills?
- [ ] Do I display professionalism through written and verbal communication?
- [ ] Do I explain to patients the rationale for performance of a procedure?
- [ ] Do I speak at each patient's level of understanding?
- [ ] Do I respond honestly and diplomatically to my patients' concerns?
- [ ] Does my knowledge allow me to speak easily with all members of the health care team?
- [ ] Do I accurately and concisely update the provider on any aspect of a patient's care?

PRESENTATION
- [ ] Am I courteous, patient, and respectful to patients?
- [ ] Do I display a positive attitude?
- [ ] Do I display a calm, professional, and caring manner?
- [ ] Do I demonstrate empathy to the patient?
- [ ] Do I display sensitivity when managing appointments?

COMPETENCY
- [ ] Do I pay attention to detail?
- [ ] Do I ask questions if I am out of my comfort zone or do not have the experience to carry out tasks?
- [ ] Do I display sound judgment?

- [ ] Am I knowledgeable and accountable?
- [ ] Do I recognize the physical and emotional effects on persons involved in an emergency situation?
- [ ] Do I demonstrate self-awareness in responding to an emergency situation?

INITIATIVE
- [ ] Do I show initiative?
- [ ] Am I flexible and dependable?
- [ ] Do I direct the patient to other resources when necessary or helpful, with the approval of the provider?
- [ ] Do I implement time management principles to maintain effective office functioning?
- [ ] Do I assist co-workers when appropriate?
- [ ] Do I make adaptations for patients with special needs?

INTEGRITY
- [ ] Do I work within my scope of practice?
- [ ] Do I demonstrate respect for individual diversity?
- [ ] Do I demonstrate sensitivity to patient rights?
- [ ] Do I protect the integrity of the medical record?
- [ ] Do I protect and maintain confidentiality?
- [ ] Do I immediately report any error I make?
- [ ] Do I do the "right thing" even when no one is observing?

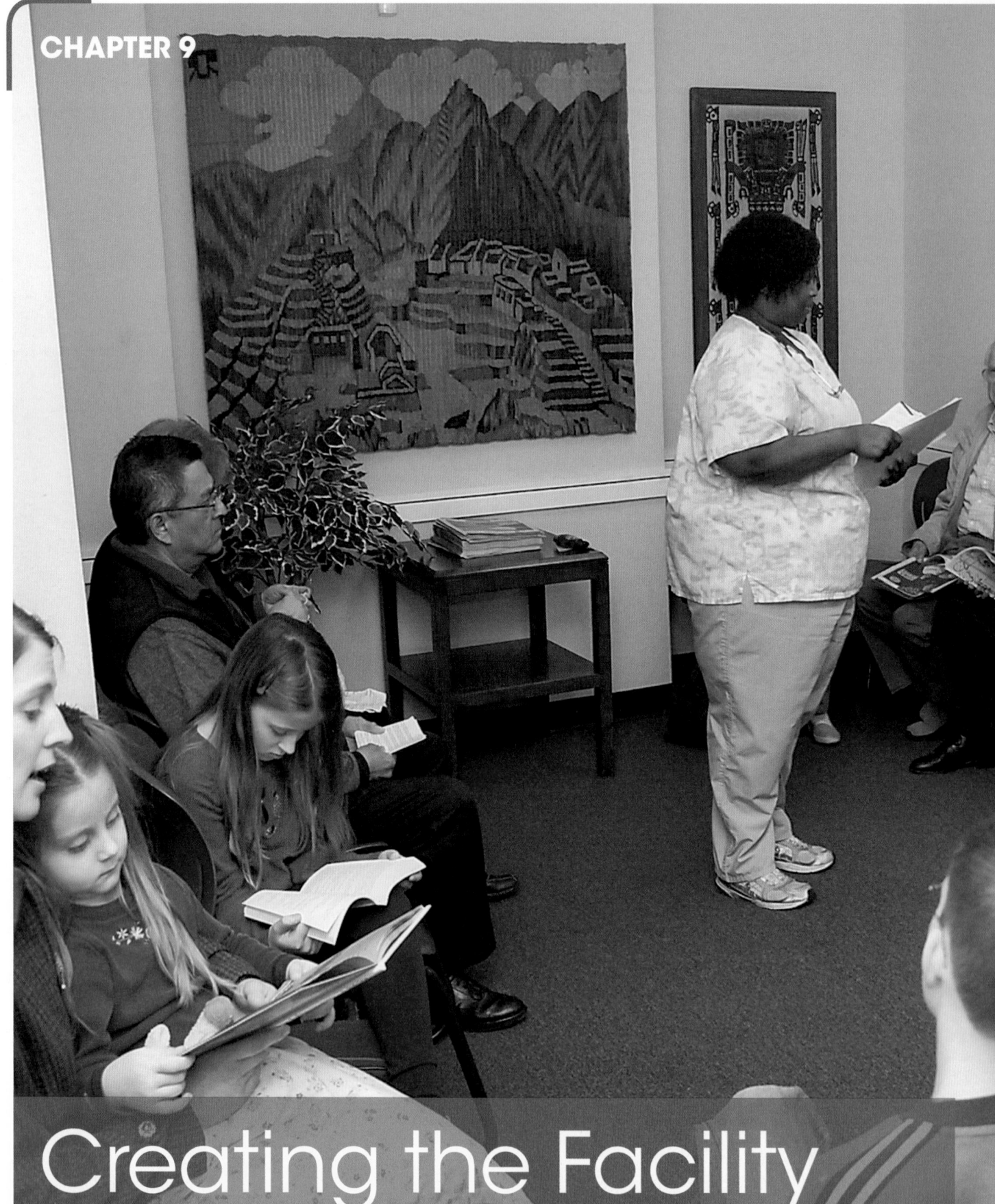

CHAPTER 9

Creating the Facility Environment

1. Define and spell the key terms as presented in the glossary.
2. Illustrate a comfortable, welcoming, and pleasing reception area.
3. Demonstrate important personality characteristics the receptionist should possess.
4. Determine cultural aspects to consider in the reception area.
5. Discuss the needs of children in the reception area.
6. Identify how the reception area can be used for educational purposes.
7. Explain the benefits of lighting, music, color, nature, and water in a facility.
8. Interpret the role of HIPAA in patient privacy and the facility environment.
9. Determine the number of patients a reception area should accommodate.
10. Recall essential elements of the Americans with Disabilities Act.
11. Evaluate the facility for safety and emergency preparedness.
12. Develop a personal and patient safety plan.
13. Explain the components of an evacuation plan for a provider's clinic.
14. Demonstrate proper use of a fire extinguisher.
15. Review steps to take in case of a natural disaster.
16. Outline the role of the medical assistant in emergency preparedness.
17. List at least three tasks to perform when opening and closing the facility.
18. Outline characteristics of future ambulatory and outpatient health care environments.

KEY TERMS

RACE
reception

SCENARIO

The design of any ambulatory setting often evolves as the needs of the clinic and patients change. At Inner City Health Care, a multiprovider family practice, the environment has always been warm and welcoming, which is particularly important because the providers see many children. However, the clinic was initially designed in the early 1980s, before the Americans with Disabilities Act (ADA) was passed by the U.S. Congress.

Once this act was passed in 1990, the clinic manager was aware of the need to comply with its mandates. In addition, the providers wanted to make all their patients, including those with disabilities, as comfortable as possible. Working with a local architect, changes were incorporated into the practice's existing space: A ramp was added outside, doorways were widened to provide wheelchair access, and new Braille signage was installed outside for patients with visual impairments. Although the changes were not without expense, the staff at Inner City Health Care willingly complied with the ADA not only because it is law but because it gave more patients better access.

More recently, while making certain the clinic protocol was in compliance with the Health Insurance Portability and Accountability Act of 1996 (HIPAA), the clinic staff took another look at the facility to ensure it was favorable in light of protecting patient confidentiality. They discovered that the reception area was seriously lacking in providing privacy and confidentiality for patient information and the entire clinic needed serious updating in many other aspects.

The environment of the medical facility contributes almost as much to a patient's well-being as does the medical attention given by providers and their medical assistants. The physical environment can foster a feeling that embraces and welcomes patients or, conversely, can cause them to feel alienated and intimidated. Numerous recent studies reveal that the physical environment of a clinic is linked to the comfort of both patient and staff. In fact, such "evidence-based design" can lead to reduced noise, improved lighting, better ventilation, and ergonomic designs with supportive work spaces and improved layout in medical clinics. These design changes make clinics safer, promote healing, lead to fewer errors on the part of staff, and reduce patients' pain and discomfort.

Dental providers have set a trend in the field of health care design. Dentists recognize that few individuals enjoy visiting the dentist and know that their patients expect to feel discomfort, pain, and extended-length procedures that are stressful. Dentists also realize that about one-fourth of the country's population refuses to see a dentist for any reason because of fear of pain and discomfort. In order to lessen patients' anxiety and to encourage patients to return on a regular basis for dental care, many dentists have turned to "spa-like" dental environments.

In this environment, patients can recline in heated chairs, are given blankets for their legs, can listen to soothing music, or may be given video headsets to watch their favorite television programs. The idea behind the entire spa-like environment is to make patients feel comfortable with their dental procedures and want to return.

Does this sound like the future of medical clinic design? Probably not, but careful observation and comparison will reveal an increasing number of medical clinics seeking to attract patients not only via high-quality medical care but also with attention to detail that creates an atmosphere conducive to comfort, confidentiality, safety, and healing. Medical providers understand that their best advertisement is a good word from patients who have had positive experiences during their medical care encounters. Closer attention to the clinic's environment and patients' personal needs might be more welcomed by patients who are not feeling well, suffering from a chronic illness, or facing a life-threatening disease.

Interior designers and experts who specialize in medical space planning advise all individuals involved in designing clinics and hospitals that patient comfort must be considered to be as important as the facility's functional utility and ease of maintenance.

CREATING A WELCOMING ENVIRONMENT

Presentation

In today's health care atmosphere, in which limited resources are being continually challenged and there are still individuals without sufficient resources to obtain proper medical care, creating a welcoming environment is essential. Creative and astute designers will tell you to consider the following concepts in fostering such an environment:

- Embrace warmth in design and in personnel
- Hide the health care's "scary" pieces from patients' view
- Create good acoustics
- Provide access to nature
- Promote health and healing
- Feed the soul

The creation of a health care facility involves many variables. Some are tangible elements, such as lighting, color choice, and furniture arrangement. Others are intangible and are expressed ways such as an administrative medical assistant's greeting and attitude toward patients. Important components of patient satisfaction are a warm and caring staff, comfortable surroundings, and the ability of patients and visitors to find their way around the medical clinic without getting lost. Convenience of access and privacy are essential. The ADA (see Chapter 6) also must be taken into account when creating any medical clinic environment by making provisions to accommodate patients who have physical challenges. HIPAA regulations (see Chapter 6) specify how a patient's privacy and confidentiality are to be protected and may also dictate medical clinic space planning. Finally, an environment that demonstrates attention to safety, the prevention of hazards, and effective response to emergency situations further enhances patient and even employee satisfaction. Together, all these elements help make an ambulatory setting the kind of environment where patients will feel comfortable and secure.

THE RECEPTION AREA

A **reception** area is just that—a place of reception. It should never be thought of as "the waiting room." The reception area is the area first viewed by the patient and this is the first opportunity to make the patient feel welcome, secure, and comfortable. First impressions are lasting. Adequate and comfortable seating, consideration for patients of all ages, proper lighting and ventilation, the use of color, noise reduction, and the influence of nature are all aspects to consider in creating the clinic environment and engaging the senses.

Space planners who specialize in medical clinics and hospitals and who have spent many hours analyzing patient flow indicate that the reception area should accommodate at least an hour's patients per provider plus a friend or relative who may accompany each patient. Another quick rule of thumb to use is 2.5 seats in the reception area for each examination room. Clinics where providers see patients without advance appointments will, of course, need a larger reception area.

Depending on the ambulatory care setting's clientele, consider the following items to help ease patients' time in any area where waiting is essential (e.g., pending laboratory results) and help take their minds off current medical problems: a table and chairs with a puzzle in progress, Internet access for busy patients attempting to work while waiting, an electronic Sudoku board, or a juice bar. Although these items are not appropriate in every setting, they certainly can be in some (refer to Case Study 9-2).

It is helpful if there is a place for patients to hang heavy coats or wet umbrellas. Accessories and artwork can easily add a special touch to a facility. Nature pictures elicit a more favorable response from patients than abstract art. Although fresh flowers might be a nice touch, they harbor microorganisms, and some patients are allergic to them. There is the tendency to use living plants in medical facilities, but silk plants and flowers also may be appropriate.

Even when the office or clinic is housed in an older building not originally constructed as a medical facility, much can be done to create an environment that enhances patient comfort. Remember to see things from the patient's point of view. If the facility is a maze of corridors where patients can easily get turned around, make certain that directions are clear and that directional signage is easily understood.

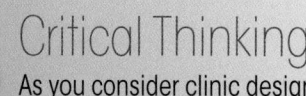

Critical Thinking

As you consider clinic design options, it is impossible to fully "expand your horizons" with just a few photos of incredible reception area designs in a textbook, but you can enhance your understanding of design possibilities by searching the Internet for "medical clinic reception designs." Select one or two that are particularly exciting to you. Why did you choose them? What was the particular appeal they held for you? Would you like to work in one (or both) of them? Justify your response.

It is worth the investment to have a professional designer who specializes in medical space planning look through the facility to make suggestions regarding color, artwork, and the general environment of the entire clinic. A designer considers the flow of patients, staff, and information; understands the focus and nature of the work of the clinic; and carefully designs the space to ensure all encounters enhance privacy and confidentiality, communication, and personal connection. What may seem like an unnecessary operational expense can result in greater satisfaction for all patients.

The Receptionist

Communication   Presentation

A receptionist who has a smile and genuinely friendly greeting for every patient, offers assistance, and carefully explains any waiting that might be necessary helps to create that desired reception environment. No matter how "rushed" the reception area may seem with patient activity and ringing telephones, the calm and reassuring attention of the receptionist helps set the stage for satisfied patients (Figure 9-1).

The receptionist must always keep a positive "We can help you" attitude, have a smile for each patient, and exude a genuine "We care about you" personality. This individual—who often has other duties as well—must be able to perform telephone prioritization, retrieve records, greet patients, present bills, make appointments, and log data into the computer, all the while remembering that each patient's comfort is of primary concern. All medical personnel, but especially the receptionist,

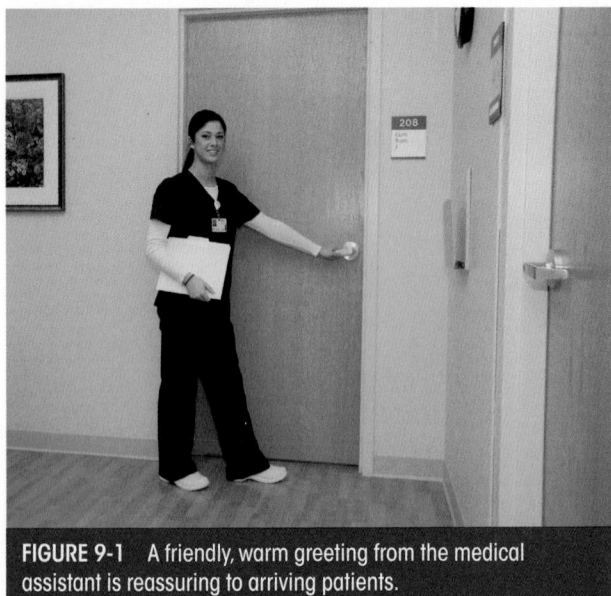

FIGURE 9-1 A friendly, warm greeting from the medical assistant is reassuring to arriving patients.

must genuinely like people and not react when patients are grumpy, irritable, or depressed and worried about an illness. Employees in the reception area of the clinic set the social climate for the interchange between patients and providers as well as the rest of the staff.

Patients who are very ill, injured, or upset should not have to wait in the reception area; rather, they should be shown to an examination room away from other patients where they can feel more comfortable. The receptionist may also have to help monitor children who may be intent on disrupting patients or whose parent is in the examination room.

Even with a number of administrative functions to accomplish, receptionists also are expected to maintain the tidiness of the reception area (even when the clinic closes for lunch). Magazines can be straightened, litter picked up, and surface counters attended to. Counters, table surfaces, and toys in medical clinics are among those most infested with microbes; therefore, they should be sanitized daily, or sometimes twice a day, especially when patients may have contagious diseases. Receptionists may be asked to remind patients that there are paper face masks in the reception area and instruct patients when they make their appointments to pick up a paper mask on arrival at the front door if they are experiencing a respiratory illness.

If there are unexpected delays in the provider's schedule, hopefully never more than 20 minutes, receptionists will notify patients of the delay tactfully and graciously and offer them the alternative of making other arrangements. The patient's time is as valuable as the provider's.

Cultural Considerations

Diversity

In consideration of cultural differences, there are some points to recall. Cultural sensitivity requires astute observation on the part of health care professionals. Keep in mind the following cultural views on health care:

- Middle Eastern and Latin cultures encourage closeness and touching, and individuals from these cultures may cluster themselves close together in the reception area.

- In general, no one likes to be touched by strangers. Cultural differences also impact the amount of space necessary for the reception area.

- In some cultures, patients are likely to bring several relatives with them to an appointment. This is especially common if the patient needs emotional support or a language interpreter. For example, Arabs, Jews, Mexicans, and Puerto Ricans tend to place greater emphasis on family care over self-care or professional care.

- Japanese patients often do not express feelings easily and expect health care professionals to make decisions about their health care, but are generally comfortable with physical closeness.

- Mexican patients believe that pain is to be endured and valued and rarely complain unless the pain keeps them from work.

Many people do not like to face other patients in the reception area and prefer anonymity. Culture aside, almost no one wants to be in close proximity to a stranger who appears to be contagious. Most are more comfortable in close quarters primarily with individuals of the same gender. Arabs may interact with health care professionals of only the same sex. While some patients are bothered by children, others find them to be a pleasant distraction. Adequate and comfortable seating affords patients their own space and respects these cultural preferences.

When Children are Patients

If the clinic treats children as patients or if children are apt to accompany adult patients, a children's area is especially helpful and appreciated. A special table and chairs for children, interactive toys (with emphasis on the interactive), and perhaps even a small television placed in a children's corner, can be provided. This area needs to be away from doors that swing or hazards on which children might be injured. A children's area should always be in sight of the administrative medical assistant or receptionist who may be charged with keeping order, especially if a parent must be seen unaccompanied by children in an examination room.

A pediatric facility that treats only children and youth might consider a particular theme for its design. Ocean murals and an aquarium are often used. Examination rooms may include examination tables designed to replicate a zoo animal. Staff in a pediatric clinic often wear bright-colored uniforms with animal prints, balloons, and similar motifs. The goal is to have much in the environment to keep children interested and enthused about their visit to the provider.

Education in the Reception Area

Many providers place appropriate educational materials for patients in the reception area. For example, new parents appreciate pamphlets related to raising children. If the provider is an ophthalmologist, the latest information on eye surgeries or new developments in contact lenses is likely to be seen in the reception area. It is also appropriate to have available in the reception area a patient information brochure that describes the services of the clinic, the function of medical staff members, measures to take in case of an emergency, and other issues that patients may need to consider (see Chapter 44 for more information on developing brochures for patient use). In some cases, the educational material may be presented in media form on a television screen.

CLINIC DESIGN AND ENVIRONMENT

Clinic environments are places where persons who are ill gather for support, diagnosis, treatment, and healing. There are a few very important factors that can make the environment more conducive to patient comfort. Some rooms in the facility, by their very nature, may cause patients to feel anxious. Recall the earlier recommendation to keep scary things out of sight. Consider a woman's discomfort when first seeing a gastroenterologist for a colonoscopy and viewing a large poster of the colonoscope on the wall. Reflect on a patient on an examination table who has on only a cloth or paper gown but must interact with the provider who is fully clothed, wearing a white lab coat and comfortably seated at a counter desk. The patient

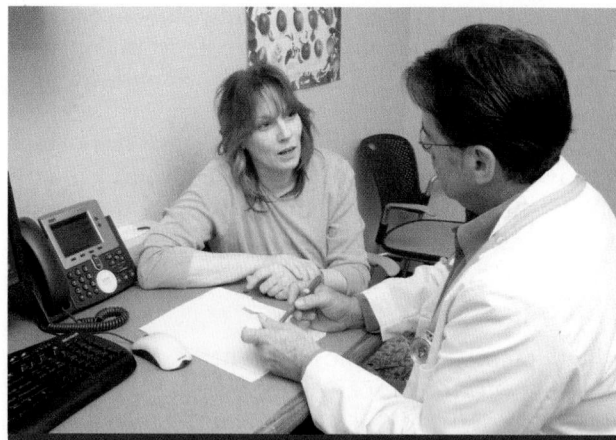

FIGURE 9-2 Patients are to be afforded as much dignity and empowerment as possible. Many patients feel more comfortable discussing conditions, treatments, or procedures face-to-face with the provider.

is at a disadvantage and may feel vulnerable in discussion and negotiation, contrary to the goal in medical care to empower the patient with as much control as possible (Figure 9-2).

Ventilation and Infection Control

The risk of contracting infectious diseases due to airborne and surface contamination is high in any medical facility; therefore, proper ventilation and effective infection control measures are essential. Many patients will find offensive the common odors that can be present in a medical facility, even when the odors are from necessary antiseptics. Proper ventilation can alleviate this issue. Although ventilation systems are often overlooked in medical clinics, appropriate air filters (usually HEPA), airflow direction, and air pressure are critical elements in reducing airborne infection and are to be considered in the heating and air conditioning design of the facility.

Diligent surface cleaning and the use of alcohol-based hand-rub dispensers that are easily accessible will encourage recommended hand washing and reduce contact contamination. All areas of a clinic are susceptible to contamination and diligence is necessary to curb transmission. As noted earlier, the reception area is one of the most contaminated areas of the clinic—countertops where patients likely check in, computer keyboards, telephone ear pieces, common pens used for writing—all are examples of where microorganisms often grow and multiply. Statistics show that the easier the access to the hand-rub dispensers and sinks for hand cleansing, the more likely they are to be used Many clinics also provide face masks and recommend they be used when a patient may have a respiratory infection.

Such measures described here are important in any clinic but absolutely essential when a majority of the provider's clientele have a depressed immune system.

Lighting

Many facilities pay close attention to lighting, use very few fluorescent lights, and allow natural light to penetrate the rooms as much as possible. The use of natural light and images of nature or nature itself in the form of a garden, plants, and so on has shown to be very beneficial to both patients and staff. Sunlight is known to boost serotonin, which helps to lessen pain and depression. The goal is to provide as much peace and relaxation as possible to reduce stress and promote healing. A poorly illuminated room also may suggest poor housekeeping, dusty baseboards, soiled carpets, or faded draperies. Lighting can be soft and inviting while providing proper illumination. Note that fluorescent lighting is not used in the

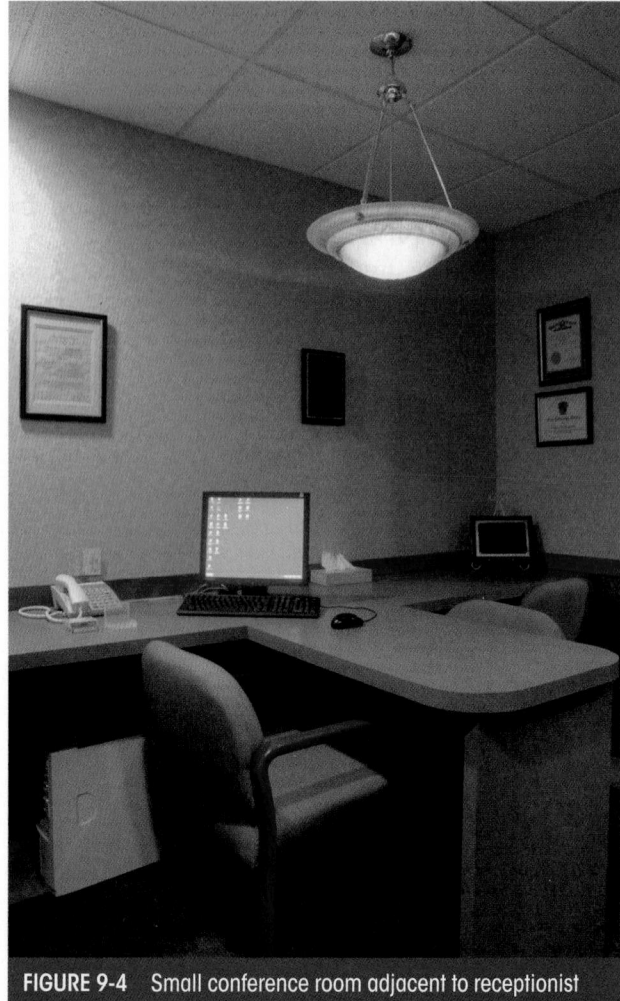

FIGURE 9-4 Small conference room adjacent to receptionist area where issues such as insurance coverage, financial arrangements, and surgical scheduling can be discussed.

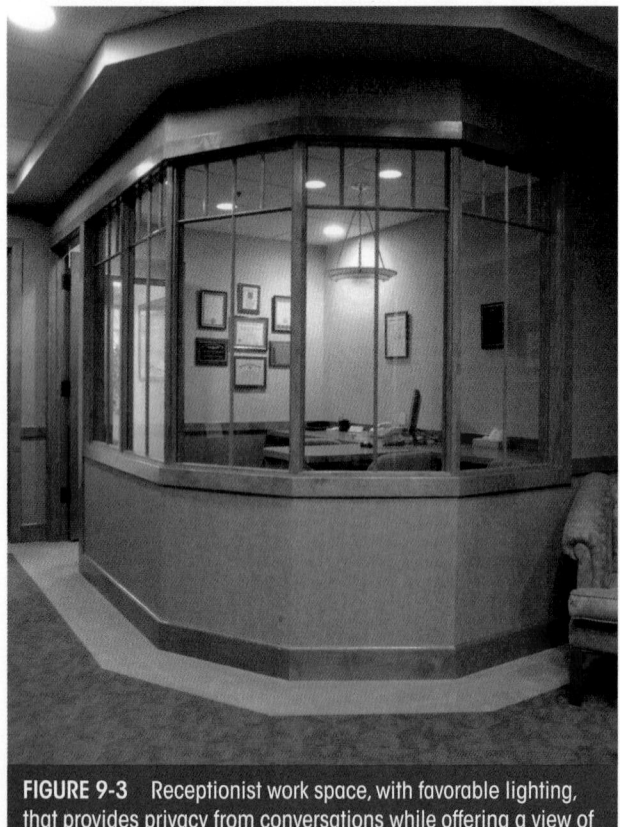

FIGURE 9-3 Receptionist work space, with favorable lighting, that provides privacy from conversations while offering a view of the entire reception area.

spaces shown in Figures 9-3 and 9-4. Ceiling can lights and lamps provide ample light for both the reception area and many of the work areas. Superior lighting in areas of any close examination, medication preparations, minor surgery, and so on helps to reduce the chance of errors.

Nature, Music, Water, and Color

Some clinics are designed with floor-to-ceiling windows throughout the clinic, especially in the reception area, that overlook a garden of plants, trees, and flowers as well as a waterfall or pool that attracts birds. A professionally maintained built-in aquarium can help to set a calming tone for clinic clientele. Other medical facilities are experimenting with the addition of music in their facilities. There is proof that certain melodious tunes and water sounds such as a babbling brook enhance healing. The use of these sounds

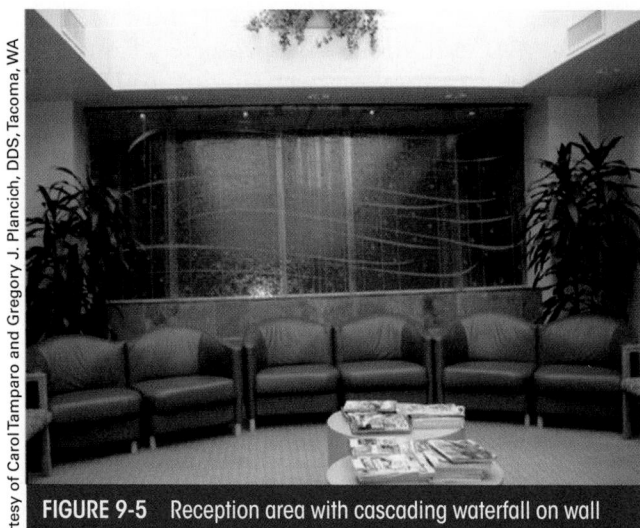

FIGURE 9-5 Reception area with cascading waterfall on wall behind chairs giving a peaceful and calming environment.

reduces the time-space experience of waiting and masks the noise of electronic medical technology and even voices that might otherwise be overheard. As well as reducing stress and anxiety and refreshing the minds of patients, visitors, and caregivers, such an environment emphasizes the facility's focus on compassion and caring. Figure 9-5 shows water cascading quietly down a wall.

Color can do much to establish a comfortable environment. Greens and blues are good in areas that require quiet and extended concentration. Cool colors cause individuals to underestimate time and make heavier items seem lighter, objects smaller, and rooms larger. Warm colors with high illumination cause increased alertness and an outward orientation. The elderly adult may have difficulty distinguishing pastels because of failing eyesight. Strongly contrasting patterns and extremely bright colors can be overwhelming and even intimidating or threatening to older adults. However, bright colors and designs are quite appropriate in a pediatric clinic.

Noise Reduction

Research has shown that patients and their families are more comfortable in surroundings that provide a quiet withdrawal from the hectic pace of the outside world. The use of sound-absorbing ceiling tiles and surfaces will help reduce clinic noise. A telephone system that produces a pleasing chime is preferred to the traditional shrill ring. Staff voices that are muted and pleasant are preferred; loud laughter and teasing are to be kept to the staff room and out of the hearing range of patients. Also appreciated are appropriate and current magazines and plants or pictures of nature. The fabric and texture of draperies, upholstery, and carpet should be pleasing, comfortable, and easy to maintain as well as assist in noise reduction.

LEGAL COMPLIANCE IN THE FACILITY

HIPAA

Legal

It is necessary to ensure HIPAA compliance for protecting patient information and privacy. With this in mind, HIPAA mandates certain building features. A reception window or desk should not make the patient feel closed off from the receptionist, yet it should provide privacy for the receptionist and total confidentiality for patients, while allowing a full view of the reception area. Figure 9-3 shows an efficient working space for the receptionist while still allowing visualization of the entire reception area. Figure 9-4 shows a small conference area in the same space that can be used when issues of privacy with a patient are particularly important. This space allows for discussion about insurance coverage, billing solutions, or patient education; voices cannot be heard in the remainder of the reception area.

To ensure HIPAA compliance, some clinics have the receptionist greet patients on their arrival and then direct them to a more private area where they are checked in, their insurance or payment plan is verified, and follow-up appointments are made. The telephones are located in this more private area so conversations with callers cannot be overheard in the reception area.

In the examination room, privacy is especially important to patients. Remember that privacy implies that the patient's conversation cannot be overheard in any other part of the facility. Studies have shown that when patients fear their voices can be overheard by others nearby, they will not respond to questioning as honestly as they would if their privacy were assured. In the examination room, provide space for patients to hang their undergarments and other clothes out of view. Always ask if a patient needs help in disrobing, and always knock before entering a room. A mirror is especially helpful for dressing after the examination—one placed appropriately and large enough so that it can be used by either a short person or someone much taller.

Americans with Disabilities Act

Legal

Accessibility, or making facilities and equipment available to all users, is a major consideration when creating the health care environment. The Americans with Disabilities Act (ADA) was passed by the U.S. Congress in 1990. The purpose of this act is to provide a clear and comprehensive national mandate to end discrimination against individuals with disabilities and to bring them into the economic and social mainstream of life. In addition to accessibility regulations identified in Titles II, III, and IV, this act also provides employment protection for persons with disabilities (Title I). ADA applies to businesses with 15 or more employees; however, some states have stricter legislation applying to businesses of only 8 or more employees. Even before the ADA became legislation, most health care facilities attempted to make their premises barrier free and accessible to patients with special needs. Although many ambulatory care settings will have less than 8 to 15 employees, accessibility for all patients in all settings is important. Refer to Chapter 6, "Legal Considerations," for a more complete discussion of the ADA and its latest requirements, including the Americans with Disabilities Act Amendments Act (ADAAA).

A professional designer not only can make suggestions regarding color, artwork, and the general environment of the clinic but also can provide advice on how the facility can be made accessible to people who have physical challenges. For example, all doors and hallways must accommodate a wheelchair. Likewise, a bathroom must accommodate individuals with special needs. Signage in Braille assists patients with visual disabilities (Figure 9-6). Elevators must be provided if the facility is on more than one level.

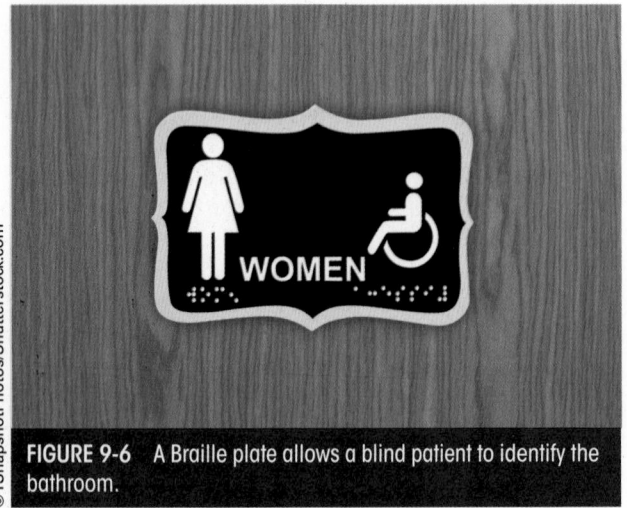

FIGURE 9-6   A Braille plate allows a blind patient to identify the bathroom.

At least one accessible entrance must comply with the ADA. It should be protected from the weather by a canopy or overhanging roof. Such entrances are to incorporate an accessible passenger loading zone. Ten percent of the total number of parking spaces at outpatient facilities must be accessible. (Visit the ADA Web site at http://www.ada.gov for more information.) Be mindful of patients whose impairments are not obvious—for example, individuals with impaired hearing or vision and individuals whose disability (temporary or permanent) may prevent them from doing certain physical activities.

SAFETY

Safety

Safety will always be paramount in any medical environment. Responsibility for a patient's safety begins the instant a patient enters the facility. Every staff member must be alert to any safety issue and be ready to offer assistance to patients at any time. Potential or current hazards are to be reported to a supervisor or provider in order to prevent or correct the hazard. On a regular basis, a safety inspection should be made of all areas of the facility. It is often best if one person is in charge of the inspection; some large clinics will have a designated safety officer. Even the smallest of clinics can maintain a checklist of safety features to be inspected on a regular basis. There are safety references throughout this text identified by the safety icon.

Creating a Safe Environment

Strict adherence to building ADA compliance identified earlier will greatly enhance a safe environment. Keep in mind that all areas must accommodate a wheelchair and provide for persons with special needs. Large multiclinic facilities often have attendants greet patients who arrive and need wheelchair assistance from their car to inside the facility. Other facilities provide parking attendants so that patients are not dropped off and left unattended while a family member parks the car.

In the facility itself, exit signs must be clearly indicated and easily seen. All restrooms should have safety bars and a pull cord that calls for special assistance when needed. The surface of all floors should be nonslippery, and all spills should be promptly cleaned and dried. A multiple-floor facility will need procedures for moving patients from one area to another or to the lower levels when elevators cannot be used. A regular inspection will check for any frayed or loose wires on equipment and uneven surfaces on floors or carpets so that immediate correction can be made.

Evacuation Procedures

Carefully identified procedures for evacuation are essential. Fire; hazardous chemical spills; power outages; earthquake; and threats of tornado, hurricane, or flood—all are examples that might necessitate evacuation of patients and all personnel. Large multiclinic facilities will have a written protocol and individuals assigned to particular areas to assist and manage in any evacuation. Smaller clinics will rely more heavily on providers and every employee for assistance. When the threat of any disaster is known, it is best to close the clinic facility for the period of the threat. Calls can be made to cancel appointments, and patients already in the facility may be directed to return home or to a designated public space prior to the event. When there is no advance warning, as in the case of earthquake or fire, clearly identified evacuation procedures are necessary.

Any necessary evacuation must include a check of every examination room, restroom, and procedure area. A wayfinding system should include easy-to-understand signs and numbers with clear directions to the exits. Special consideration is given to patients who need assistance or are in wheelchairs. Employees have the responsibility to assist patients and not leave the facility themselves until patients are safe. Any procedures that are underway, even minor surgery, must be stopped as soon as possible to facilitate the evacuation. It is important to turn off any oxygen or compressed gas systems. Never use elevators in a multistory building evacuation; always use the stairs. Close the door when an area is vacated.

Emergency Codes. There are some common emergency codes that can be helpful to understand. They are used primarily in hospitals and large ambulatory medical centers, but are applicable to any medical facility. Even though there are variations depending upon the facility, a few samples are identified as follows:

- *Code Red.* Fire emergency: Protect patients and staff from fire; it may be necessary to leave the facility.
- *Code Blue.* Adult medical emergency: Specialized personnel respond with necessary equipment.
- *Code Pink.* Infant/child abduction: Protect children and infants, block entrance and exit, notify authorities.

- *Code Gray.* Combative individual/assault: Respond to area, protect patients, notify authorities if necessary.
- *Code Green.* Bomb threat: Notify authorities of suspicious package, evacuate the building if advised.
- *Code Yellow.* Hazardous material spill: Identify unsafe exposure, safely evacuate area and protect others from exposure.
- *Code White.* Evacuation necessary: Move everyone out of the facility as quickly as possible.

Fire Safety

When there is a fire, evacuation must be considered unless the fire is quickly contained without threat to others. All employees must know where fire alarms are located and how they are activated; this is also true of fire extinguishers. Fire hazard has been decreased a great deal in medical facilities through the ban of smoking and smoking materials. Cracked or split electrical cords or plugs should be replaced, and electrical outlets should never be overloaded. If laundry is done within the facility, emptying the lint filter on the dryer after each use is a must.

Procedure

Periodically, all personnel should receive training on the use of a fire extinguisher for a small fire (see Procedure 9-1) and training for a planned evacuation when necessary. It is best remembered that fire prevention is the ultimate goal. However, if there is a fire, take the following emergency actions (**RACE**) if you are able to do so without putting yourself in danger and others are present to communicate the emergency and turn in the alarm:

- **Remove** patients and personnel from the immediate fire area if safe to do so.
- Activate the **alarm** at the fire alarm box and/or call 911. Notify other staff.
- **Contain** the fire and smoke by closing all doors to the fire area.
- **Extinguish** with proper fire extinguisher *only* if it is safe to do so, or **evacuate** as necessary.

Fire Extinguisher Safety. There are different types of fire extinguishers for different fires. The three most common are water, CO_2, and dry chemical types. A multipurpose dry chemical is suitable for fires most likely to be seen in outpatient care. Remember that all fire extinguishers should be checked periodically, usually monthly, to make certain pressure is at the appropriate level according to the manufacturer's suggestions. An extinguisher should be readily visible and not blocked by any furniture or doors. Make certain hoses and nozzles are free of insects and debris. The outside of the extinguisher should be clean and free of any oil or grease as well as any dents or signs of damage. Dry chemical extinguishers may need to be shaken monthly to prevent the powder from settling or packing. Pressure test the extinguisher periodically to ensure the cylinder is safe to use. Replace an extinguisher immediately after use. Local fire department personnel also check extinguishers and will do so in their regular facility inspections.

For more information on how to use a fire extinguisher, see the "Using a Fire Extinguisher" Quick Reference Guide.

PROCEDURE 9-1

Demonstrating Proper Use of a Fire Extinguisher

Procedure

PURPOSE:

To demonstrate the ability to operate a fire extinguisher or help another person operate the extinguisher and to describe the precise steps to take to prevent errors and delay in operation.

EQUIPMENT/SUPPLIES:

Fire extinguisher

PROCEDURE STEPS:

1. Determine the type of fire extinguisher(s) on the premises. RATIONALE: The type of extinguisher will determine the kind of fires it may be able to control.

2. Examine the cylinder and carefully read any instructions supplied from the manufacturer, *paying attention to detail.* RATIONALE: This gives a brief review of how to operate the equipment and tells you what kind of fires to use it on.

3. Determine if you are able to handle the weight of the extinguisher, *asking for assistance if you are unable to carry out the task.* RATIONALE: This will tell you if you can move forward or will have to ask another to manage the extinguisher.

4. If a fire is present, *be proactive* by calling 911 before you discharge the extinguisher. RATIONALE: You cannot tell how quickly a fire may get out of your control.

5. Check your nearest exit. If it is blocked, *display sound judgment* by evacuating without discharging the extinguisher. RATIONALE: Trying to fight a fire that threatens a safe exit is dangerous and can cost a life.

6. Break the seal and turn and pull the safety pin from the handle. RATIONALE: This step is necessary before you can use the extinguisher, as it unlocks the mechanism.

7. Aim the nozzle or hose at the base of the fire and squeeze the lever to discharge the extinguishing agent. RATIONALE: The base of the fire is its source and it is vital to stop the fire at the source.

8. Standing several feet back from the fire, sweep side to side to put out the flames. RATIONALE: A side to side motion helps to put out the fire.

9. If the fire does not respond after you have used up the fire extinguisher, *remain calm* and remove yourself to safety immediately. RATIONALE: Do not take a chance of being caught in a fire; allow the professionals to put the fire out.

10. If the area fills with smoke, *remain calm* and leave immediately. RATIONALE: Smoke can be more deadly than the fire and is often very toxic.

11. Replace the depleted fire extinguisher immediately. Never leave an empty extinguisher where someone might believe it is ready for use. RATIONALE: A fire extinguisher that is fully operational and ready for use is the only kind to have in any facility.

⋙ QUICK REFERENCE GUIDE

⋙ USING A FIRE EXTINGUISHER

1. ***Call for help before extinguishing a fire.*** A fire can quickly spread to dangerous levels. The typical extinguisher should never be used on anything but small contained fires that have just started. Remember that all fires produce smoke and carbon monoxide. Some fires also produce toxic gases that often form from burning nylon in carpeting, foam padding, and so on and can be fatal.

2. ***Are you strong enough to extinguish a fire?*** Some personnel will find any commercial extinguisher too heavy to handle or have difficulty exerting enough pressure to operate it.

3. ***Check for a clear exit for escape prior to using the extinguisher.*** If the exit is at all threatened, leave immediately.

4. ***Know which type of fire extinguisher to use.*** The most common classes of extinguishers are often characterized by the class of fire—A, B, or C—or the extinguisher type—APW, carbon dioxide (CO_2), or dry chemical (Figure 9-7A).

   - *APW.* An APW (air-pressured water) extinguisher has a silver casing and is suitable for Class A fires of cloth, wood, or paper. It weighs about 25 lbs and is 2 ft tall.

   - *Carbon dioxide.* A CO_2 extinguisher is filled with pressurized nonflammable CO_2 gas. It has a red casing and a horn or spout. It is suitable for flammable liquid (Class B) and electrical fires (Class C). It should not be used on Class A fires. Weight and size vary.

   - *Dry chemical.* A dry chemical extinguisher is mainly filled with monoammonium phosphate powder that is pressurized by nitrogen. It is also known as a DC fire extinguisher. It can be used either for Class B and C fires or for Class A, B, and C fires, and will be labeled as such. It has a red casing and can weigh between 5 and 20 lbs. The dry chemical fire extinguisher appropriate for Class A, B, and C fires is the most likely choice for the ambulatory care facility.

5. ***Ready the extinguisher.***
   - Break the seal and pull the safety pin or metal ring from the handle (Figure 9-7B).
   - Squeeze the lever to discharge the fire extinguishing agent.

   - Aim for the base of the fire and sweep back and forth (Figure 9-7C).

6. ***Remember PASS to help you use the extinguisher properly: pull, aim, squeeze, sweep.***

Refer to OSHA's Web site on evacuation plans and procedures. Go to http://www.osha.gov and search for "Extinguisher Basics" to find pictures, diagrams, and more details.

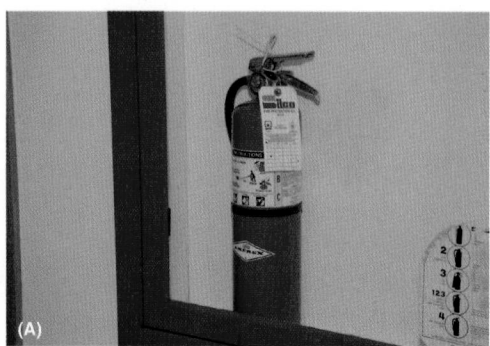

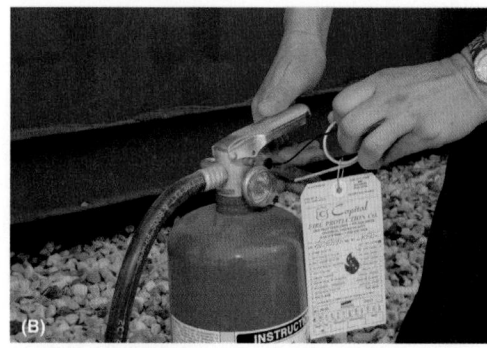

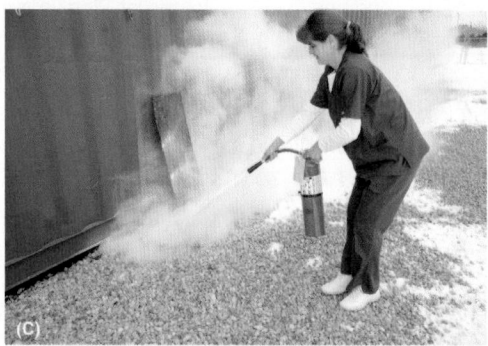

FIGURE 9-7 Operating a fire extinguisher. (A) Know the location of the fire extinguisher. (B) Pull the pin. (C) Point the hose at the base of the fire, squeeze the handle, and sweep from side to side.

Response to Natural Disaster or Emergency

Procedure

Disaster can strike quickly and without warning, causing evacuation of a home or any other building. It can also confine you to a building or home. Knowing what to do and being prepared is the best protection and is your responsibility (see Procedure 9-2). A very valuable resource can be found at https://www.dhs.gov by searching for "Prepare My Family for a Disaster." This information is prepared by Homeland Security and will direct you to a number of other useful sites that have free downloadable information. There are a number of hazards to consider: floods, tornadoes, hurricanes, thunderstorms, and lightning; winter storms and extreme cold; extreme heat; earthquakes, volcanoes, landslides, and debris flows (mudslides); tsunamis; fires and wildfires; hazardous materials incidents and household chemical emergencies; and nuclear power plant and terrorism (including explosions as well as biological, chemical, and nuclear and radiological hazards) emergencies.

PROCEDURE 9-2

Procedure

Developing a Personal and/or Employee Safety Plan in Case of a Disaster

PURPOSE:

In case of a disaster to develop a plan of action that promotes personal safety and can also be applied to both employees and patients in ambulatory care.

EQUIPMENT/SUPPLIES:

- Computer
- Clear plastic protector envelope for plan

PROCEDURE STEPS:

1. *Be proactive* by reviewing state and local recommendations for emergency preparedness. *Pay attention to detail.* RATIONALE: Some areas of the country are prone to particular natural disasters such as floods, tornados, or hurricanes. Your plan should be pertinent to your geographical area.

2. *Show initiative* by gathering family members or other employees together to discuss a disaster plan. RATIONALE: When those close to you are involved in the process, they are more likely to participate in the activity and understand the importance of the actions to be taken.

3. List supplies necessary for your supply kit. Be certain to include any special needs required in your supplies. Allow each person one personal item for the kit. Plan your needs for at least 3 days. RATIONALE: A detailed list of the supply kit items reminds you of what you will need to purchase, when items will expire or lose their usefulness, and what one item is most important to each individual.

4. Plan for evacuation. Where are the exits? Identify the safest route for exit. List the steps to take prior to evacuation. RATIONALE: Planning ahead makes it easier to function in a time of great stress. Who will be responsible for picking up the supply kit? A first aid kit? Who will turn off electricity, gas, water?

5. Determine a communication or contact plan to follow should you be separated from others during the disaster. Where will you meet? Name a "neutral" person or friend in another location who can be a telephone contact. RATIONALE: Following any disaster, the first concern is always for the well-being of your loved ones and those closest to you. Knowing how to reach one another will reduce this stress.

6. Schedule updates to the personal safety plan at least every quarter, *developing strategic plans to achieve your goals.* RATIONALE: This time frame allows for changes that may be necessary in the supply kit, reinforcing the safety protocol you have devised and the ability to make any other necessary changes.

7. Make certain everyone has a copy of the plan. Post a copy of your plan in a prominent place where it will be noticed regularly. RATIONALE: Unless everyone has a copy of the plan and it is posted where everyone is continually reminded of it, the plan loses its effectiveness.

While it is not the purpose of this chapter to detail responses to each of these disasters, there are some simple guidelines to keep in mind.

Every emergency plan will include information on what to do if there is no access to food, water, or electricity for some time. Most of these plans suggest creating kits to last, if necessary, for as long as two weeks but certainly never less than for 3 days. Kits can be assembled in storage bins or some other sturdy container, but should be readily accessible and regularly updated. Kits should be available for use at home, in a vehicle, and at a place of work.

In a disaster emergency it is important to pick two places for family members to meet, perhaps right outside the home or at a particular spot in the neighborhood. Decide how you will communicate with and reach others, especially family members you might be separated from during a disaster. Ask an out-of-town relative or friend to be your "family contact." It is often easier to make a long distance call than a local call. Know the location of your nearest shelter should you be required to evacuate. Make emergency phone numbers readily available to everyone. Teach everyone how to turn off the water, gas, and electricity. Keep necessary tools near gas and water shut-off valves. These safety tips are applicable to your workplace, too.

Sadly, the majority of households and places of employment do not have disaster kits. This is because it often takes a serious warning of a disaster or the experience of a disaster before individuals make the effort to prepare.

The Medical Assistant's Response to Disaster Preparedness

Competency

Because medical assistants are individuals with both administrative and clinical education, experience, and training and are able to perform emergency first aid and CPR, they can be very valuable to a community in a time of need. Individuals who respond to emergencies must not only have the skills necessary to attend to those in need, they must also be able to curb the stress they are likely to feel in order to function in a calm, yet "take control" manner. Anyone who responds in an emergency also is to be reminded of the "fallout" or "letdown" that follows a period of severe stress and/or intense care management. That is the time to have some rest to allow the body to function in a less stressful mode.

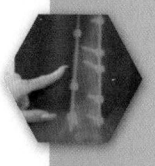
Critical Thinking

Visit the Web site indicated in this section to identify what you need to establish a disaster plan. What will you need to purchase for your supply kit for your home or car? What will be readily available to you or easy to procure? Identify special supplies you may want for any additional needs such as medications, pets, and so on. Estimate the cost of any purchases as well as any other action to be taken to establish a safety plan.

OPENING THE FACILITY

When the facility is opened in the morning, everything should be in readiness. The receptionist or administrative medical assistant, who arrives at least 20 minutes before the first patient, will make a visual check of each room to be certain it is prepared and ready for the day.

Rooms should be at a comfortable temperature, well organized, pleasantly illuminated, and spotless. The clinical medical assistant will check all necessary supplies and equipment for readiness. At all times, patient comfort and safety should be paramount.

A schedule of the day's activities is either printed for all personnel in the facility or available to all on the computer. It includes patients to be seen by the providers, meetings to be held that day, and any other information important in keeping the day's schedule running smoothly. As cancellations, no-shows, or added appointments are made, they can be changed and flagged in the schedule. If printed, this schedule can be posted in a place where staff can view it quickly, but it should never be visible to any patient. Patient charts for the day should be retrieved if not done so the prior evening. Facilities whose records are all electronic will sometimes print the latest laboratory results and information from the most recent visit to the facility for the provider to refer to when seeing the patient. The patient's information should be checked to make certain all information is up to date and accurate. The administrative medical assistant will check the answering service or machine for any telephone messages and follow up as necessary.

An effective way to check a room's readiness is to view yourself in the room as a patient. Ask yourself how you feel about being there, what mood the surroundings create for you, and whether you would feel welcome and comfortable as a patient.

CLOSING THE FACILITY

At the close of the day, each room should be checked to make certain all equipment is shut down and doors and windows are secured. Be sure that all materials of a sensitive nature are under lock and key. All file cabinets are to be closed and locked to ensure protection and confidentiality. Any drugs identified in the Controlled Substances Act list of narcotics and non-narcotics must be in a locked and secure cabinet and should also be checked when leaving the clinic. Petty cash kept on the premises must be locked in a safe container. It is best to ensure each room and area is in readiness for the next day. The day's receipts, plus a bank deposit slip, should be taken to the bank to be deposited or locked in a safe for a later deposit.

Local law enforcement officers can advise you on appropriate indoor and outdoor lighting, as well as any other security measures to take both during and after business hours.

Always contact the answering service to notify them that the clinic is closed and where and how the medical staff can be reached in an emergency.

THE FUTURE ENVIRONMENT FOR AMBULATORY CARE

Increasingly, outpatient care is claiming a larger percentage of the total health care volume than inpatient care. Outpatient/ambulatory care more often addresses chronic illness while inpatient care concentrates on acute illnesses. Moreover, there is a much greater emphasis upon preventive care and wellness than in previous decades. Much of this shift is attributed to the popularity of complementary and integrative medicine as well as the need to cut health care costs.

Another prediction is quite certain in outpatient care. The number of patients 85 years or older—who are most likely to require medical care for multiple chronic conditions—will greatly increase in the next few years. It is predicted that by 2020, almost 40% of a provider's time will be spent treating members of the population who are older adults. Although somewhat improved by the Affordable Care Act, the federal government still struggles with Medicare reimbursement policies, which do not adequately cover most costs incurred by providers when caring for this older population. Outpatient care centers will continue to struggle to provide facilities and services with environments conducive to the needs of this population.

To address this situation, the number of primary care providers willing to take new patients 65 years and older must increase. Patients will need to access their provider via convenient public transportation, take care of as many of their needs as possible in one day, and have prescriptions filled before returning home. The older population will need to navigate a wheelchair easily down corridors, into examination rooms, and into laboratories for assessment. Providers can be expected to spend additional time with older adults who will ask many questions and will be quite knowledgeable of their medical needs.

Members of the older adult's family will have an increasing presence in the care of their parents. Providers will want to give patients the opportunity for family members of their choosing to have access to their health information. HIPAA requires providers to have patients sign a release allowing their family members to be kept informed. Providers can expect family members of patients to want the very best for their loved ones, both medically and environmentally.

Discussions with older adults regarding their health care experiences reveal that their greatest frustration comes from the lack of clear instructions given by *all* health professionals, ranging from the administrative medical assistant to the primary provider. The most successful approaches to solving this dilemma include:

1. Providing clear and concise written instructions whenever possible in easy-to-read print

2. Creating an environment where movement from one department to another is not confusing

3. Making certain all patients fully understand their prescription instructions, directions for continuing care, and orders for additional tests

4. Identifying for patients under what circumstances they should report back to their primary provider for follow-up.

The goal of a medical facility and its staff should be not only to welcome and receive patients with a "we care for you" attitude but also to have patients leave the facility and staff with a sense of satisfaction related to the care received. As higher efficiency is demanded of providers and their staff members in order to reduce medical costs, thoughtful and attentive personalized care must not be forsaken.

Another prediction for the near future of health care is that the population will grow increasingly diverse. The influx of immigrants, especially in some border areas, places a great demand for bilingual providers and staff, and there is a need for health care availability in the neighborhoods where these individuals settle. These patients have many of the same needs as the older population and the four approaches above will need to be carefully adhered to.

Electronic mail (email) communication between patients and providers is now commonplace in many areas; however, patients are asked to give written permission for the transmission of information via email because privacy cannot always be guaranteed. Laboratory and radiological results can be viewed online, as can appointment reminders. Some providers offer treatment online when they understand a patient's medical history and needs. Providers may use a video chat tool such as Skype with a patient in order to discuss treatment protocols, order diagnostic services or medications, and/or schedule an in-clinic appointment.

At the same time, medical providers work diligently to decrease the number of medical errors made, and advancing technology creates new patterns of health care. Also, patients are becoming more astute consumers. These new consumers are better educated; they seek value and are comparison shoppers. They know that managed care has its limitations, and that providers can be wrong. These patients believe they know their own bodies better than anyone, and that quality of life is important. They know, too, that cost containment and the complexities of the health care system leave them vulnerable to medical difficulties if they do not take responsibility for themselves and their medical care.

Today's patients are exposed to numerous Internet sites and magazine articles that provide medical information 24 hours a day, 7 days a week. These patients arrive at their appointments with the ability to discuss potential diagnoses and treatment plans. Hopefully, the health care team welcomes this new partnership, even if health care professionals have to assist patients in weeding out some of the invalid medical information available. Providers will be continually challenged to make patients the center of their activities to provide a better experience while keeping costs reasonable.

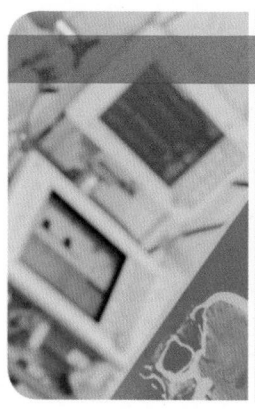

CASE STUDY 9-1

Refer to the scenario at the beginning of the chapter.

1. What is your first reaction to the environment in the medical facility described? Justify your response.
2. List as many solutions as you can to address the lack of privacy and confidentiality in the reception area. Begin with simple solutions and then move to the more complex ideas that surface in your planning.
3. How do you think patients will be affected by each of your solutions?
4. What other improvements might be considered when updating the clinic?

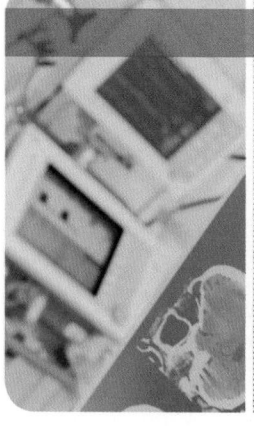

CASE STUDY 9-2

The eighth-floor orthopedic surgery department in a large metropolitan clinic has an interesting approach to patient dynamics. Providers and their assistants see patients for diagnosis and preparation for surgery. Patients often are seen in this department three to five times before and after their procedures. The staff involves their patients in the process to relieve any anxiety they might have.

Addison Burton approaches the reception desk, where he is immediately greeted and asked to wait a moment until the administrative medical assistant clears a previous patient. There is a huge box filled with slightly used tennis shoes that patients and staff are collecting for needy children and the homeless. Addison remembers he has a couple of pairs at home he could bring. After checking in, he is directed to a counter where coffee, tea, and water are available, as well as the

continues

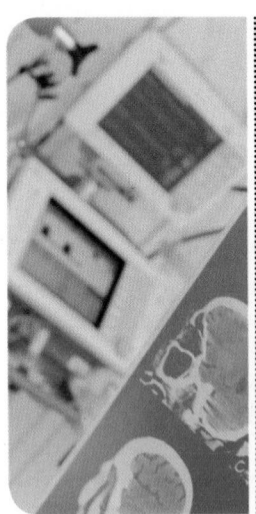

CASE STUDY 9-2 *continued*

daily newspapers. Addison can take a seat in a chair, on a couch at a window that allows him to put his feet and legs up, or at a table with chairs. The window seat gives a view of the city and a terrace garden four floors below. At the table there is an unusual puzzle being put together, and Addison takes a seat there. He is able to put four to five puzzle pieces together before being called for his appointment.

CASE STUDY REVIEW

1. When Jorja Anderson, CMA (AAMA), calls Mr. Burton to the examination room, what might the conversation be? Would this conversation help to dispel anxiety?
2. When the surgeon sees Mr. Burton for his hip problem, everyone has a good laugh—on the bottom of Addison's shoe is a puzzle piece. What kind of mood has been established for this visit?

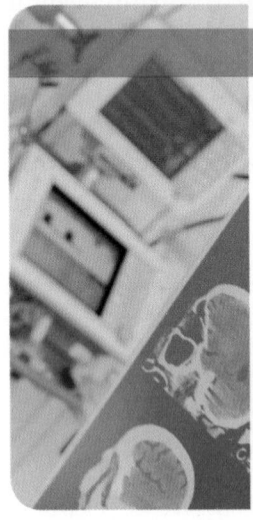

CASE STUDY 9-3

Even though she appears calm and collected on the outside, Abigail Johnson, who is about 75 years old, is quite nervous about having her annual physical. Clinical medical assistant Gwen Carr, CMA (AAMA), senses her patient's underlying tension and wants to do what she can to help Abigail relax. She knows that this patient has hypertension, suffers from occasional dizziness, and says she feels guilty about going off the diet that was designed to help manage both her high blood pressure and her diabetes. At this moment, Gwen is helping Abigail get ready to see Dr. King, her provider. She does not want to intrude on her patient's privacy but does want Abigail to relax a bit.

CASE STUDY REVIEW

1. What are some actions Gwen can take to ensure her patient's privacy?
2. In what ways can the physical environment itself become a calming influence for Abigail?
3. How will Gwen's sympathetic attitude affect her patient?

Summary

- Keep in mind that the environment in which patient care is given must promote health and healing rather than aggravate illness and feed anxiety.
- Evidence-based design will help create environments that provide effective, safe, and caring-centered facilities.
- The environment must be clean, fresh, cheerful, safe, and nonthreatening, with contemporary furnishings, appropriate colors, proper lighting, and soothing textures.
- Even if patients are not consciously aware of the message they are getting from the clinic design and environment, they are subconsciously receiving it. The clinic environment reveals things that might subconsciously undermine a patient's confidence in the provider and the health care team.
- Safety preparedness may not be obvious to patients, but its importance cannot be minimized. Every space in the facility with its appointed purpose must be designed and maintained to protect patient and employee safety, and every employee must be safety conscious every moment of the day.
- Opening and closing the facility involves a number of important steps to follow each day.
- The future of ambulatory/outpatient care will see greater demands than inpatient care. There will be increased care of people with chronic illness, an emphasis upon prevention and wellness, and cooperation with complementary or integrative therapies.

Study for Success

To reinforce your knowledge and skills of information presented in this chapter:

- Review the *Key Terms* and *Learning Outcomes*
- Consider the *Critical Thinking* features and *Case Studies* and discuss your conclusions
- Answer the questions in the *Certification Review*

Procedure

- Perform the *Procedures* using the *Competency Assessment Checklists* on the *Student Companion Website*

CERTIFICATION REVIEW

1. Which of the following is appropriate for the reception area of an ambulatory care setting?
   a. Heavily scented flowers
   b. Medical journals with graphic colored pictures
   c. Dim lighting
   d. Live or silk plants

2. What is one of the goals in treating patients?
   a. Give them as much control as possible
   b. Get them in and out as quickly as possible
   c. Remind them that there is little privacy in a medical clinic
   d. Make sure they arrive on time for their appointment
   e. A full waiting room to show the success of the providers

3. What is one design element to avoid in a medical clinic?
   a. A mirror for dressing
   b. The colors green and blue
   c. Extremely bright, contrasting patterns
   d. Accessories and artwork

4. What is the ADA's primary concern?
   a. Segregating individuals according to type of disability
   b. Providing access and opportunity for individuals with physical challenges
   c. Only the work environment
   d. Getting economic benefits for people with physical challenges
   e. Making certain employees have adequate salaries

5. In any medical facility, what is the receptionist's KEY responsibility?
   a. Do not keep the provider waiting
   b. Make sure all plants are watered
   c. Greet patients in a friendly, warm manner
   d. Be efficient, even if it means ignoring patient requests

6. Which of the following statements is accurate regarding a visual check of each examination room?
   a. It is the responsibility of weekly housekeeping.
   b. It is done when opening and closing the clinic.
   c. This is a task only of the administrative medical assistant.
   d. Whoever is the last one to leave the clinic performs this task.
   e. Security is assigned this task.

7. What do space planners recommend for the reception area?
   a. Three to four seats for each examination room
   b. Seats to accommodate 1.5 hours of patients
   c. 2.5 seats for each examination room
   d. Not bringing family members to appointments

8. The ADA requires that what percentage of the total number of parking spaces in outpatient facilities be reserved for individuals with disabilities?
   a. 5%
   b. 10%
   c. 12%
   d. 7%
   e. 4%

9. What challenges will the medical environment face in the future?
   a. Increasing numbers of pediatric patients
   b. Increasing numbers of older and more diverse patients
   c. Decreasing numbers of hospital patients
   d. Decreasing government compliance

10. Which of the following is an appropriate guideline for safety in a medical facility?
    a. Be able to use fire extinguishers and have an evacuation plan.
    b. Keep an employee at the door to assist patients with special needs.
    c. Provide good quality fluorescent lights to prevent falls.
    d. Enhance proper ventilation by opening windows and doors.
    e. Call 911 to assist with any evacuation necessary.

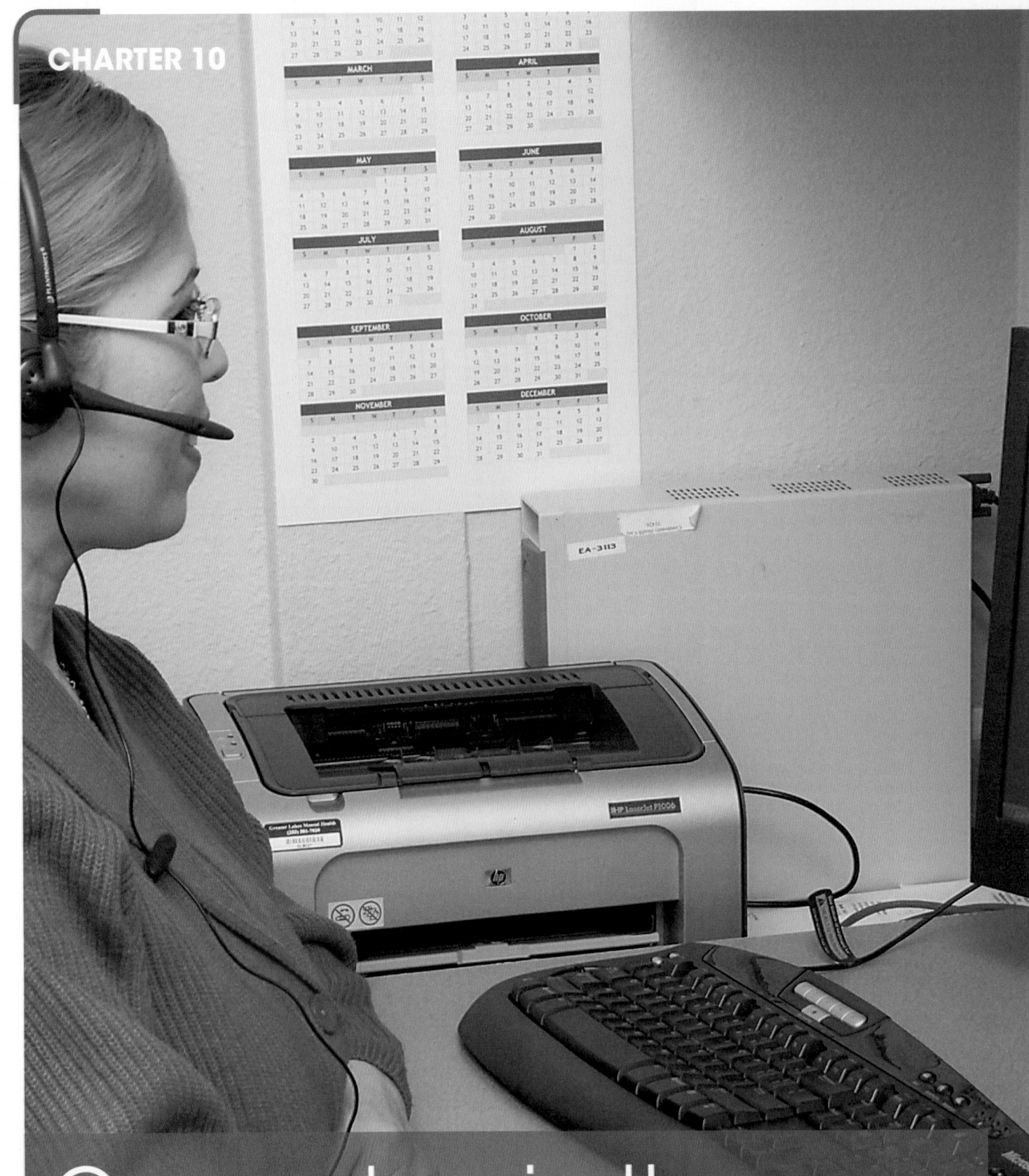

Computers in the Medical Clinic

1. Define and spell the key terms as presented in the glossary.
2. Identify the four main types of computers.
3. Describe the four fundamental elements of a computer system.
4. Differentiate four input devices and describe the function of each.
5. List three examples of data output devices.
6. Differentiate and discuss various types of storage devices and how they might be used in ambulatory care settings.
7. Discuss the use of flash technology and tape drives and describe how each might be used in ambulatory care settings.
8. Identify the difference between system and application software.
9. Analyze the importance of computer system documentation and how it is upgraded.
10. Differentiate the various network and connectivity technologies.
11. Analyze the principles and techniques of promoting network and computer security.
12. Discuss computer maintenance and defragmenting of the hard disc drive.
13. Differentiate between electronic health records (EHR), electronic medical records (EMR), and a practice management (PM) system.
14. Discuss principles of using electronic medical records (EMR).
15. Explain the importance of system backup.
16. Demonstrate design considerations when computerizing a medical clinic.
17. Analyze why ergonomics is important and recall at least five guidelines for setting up a computer workstation.
18. Identify guidelines for maintaining confidentiality for safeguarding personal health information (PHI) as well as electronic personal health information (ePHI) while keeping in mind HIPAA requirements.

KEY TERMS

central processing unit (CPU)

cloud computing

defragmentation

documentation

electronic health record (EHR)

electronic medical record (EMR)

ergonomics

Ethernet

firewall

hardware

input devices

Internet

license

memory

motherboard

networking

operating system (OS)

output devices

patches

phishing

practice management (PM)

program software

secure sockets layer (SSL)

server

surge protection

system backup

system software

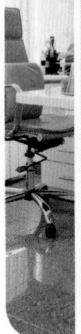

SCENARIO

Inner City Health Care, a multiprovider clinic in a large urban area, is considering a new practice management system. Clinic manager Marilyn Johnson, CMA (AAMA), has been working with the team investigating and determining specific areas of need. During meetings, Marilyn uses active listening skills and feedback techniques such as reflection, restatement, and clarification to be sure that each team member is heard and understood. The team has been charged with recommending the practice management system that best satisfies their clinic's specific needs while protecting the integrity of electronic protected health information (ePHI) and electronic medical records (EMR). All Health Insurance Portability and Accountability Act (HIPAA) security regulations must be incorporated, including the development of security audits and related policies and procedures that detect any unauthorized access to ePHI and EMR.

Chapter Portal

We interact with and rely on computers in almost all aspects of our personal lives and in the work environment. In the cars we drive, home appliances, entertainment systems, transactions with our credit or debit cards, bill paying, social networking, mobile phones, and a host of other applications, computers are at work. The medical clinic is no exception, and medical assistants will work with some form of computer whether in an administrative, a clinical, or a laboratory environment. A modern clinic could not effectively work without computers. This chapter will introduce the student to the basics of how a computer works, how it is used in the medical clinic, and some of the safeguards for maintaining confidentiality.

CATEGORIES OF COMPUTERS

Common computers can be grouped into four basic categories: supercomputers, mainframe computers, servers, and microcomputers. The following Quick Reference Guide gives the characteristics of each type of computer.

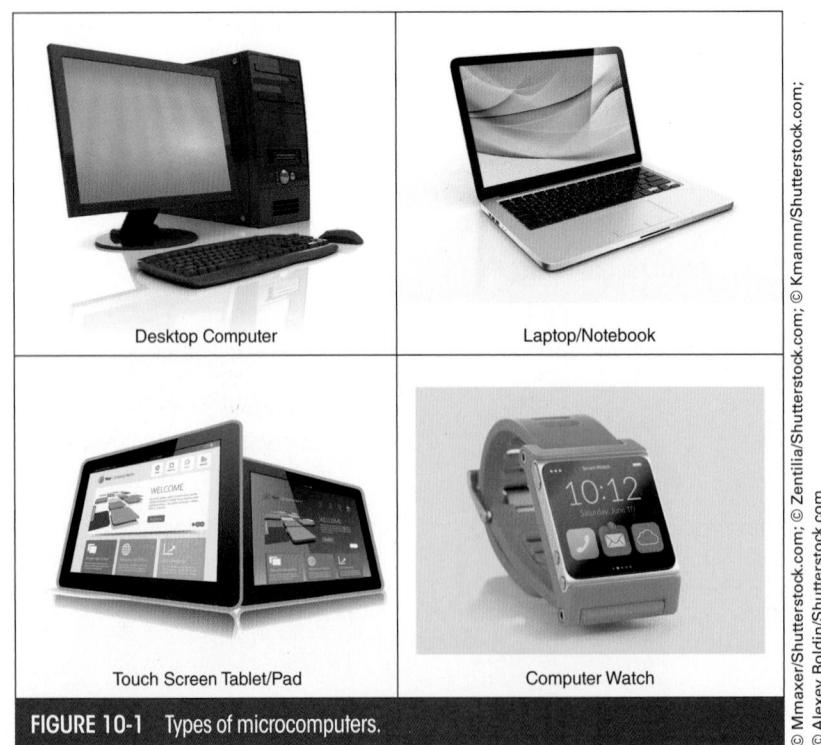

FIGURE 10-1   Types of microcomputers.

QUICK REFERENCE GUIDE

≫ TYPES OF COMPUTERS

CATEGORY	CAPABILITY	USE	EXAMPLE
Supercomputer	Very rapid processing speed through use of multiple processors connected in parallel Computer can fill a building	Space program, medical research, weather simulation, nuclear science, and computational intensive tasks	© Timofeev Vladimir/Shutterstock.com
Mainframe computer (enterprise computer)	Large computers capable of running multiple programs simultaneously Less powerful than supercomputers Computer will fill a large room Being replaced by minicomputers	Used by large businesses and governments for accounting and client information storage	© Scanrail 1/Shutterstock.com
Minicomputer	Smaller desk-size computer with slightly less speed and power than a mainframe computer	See mainframe computer	©iStock.com/Zern Liew
Server—specialized minicomputer designed to provide program and data storage for networked microcomputers	Massive data storage capability Racks of servers can fill large buildings and consume large amounts of electricity	Data and application program storage for multiple networked microcomputers	© datshock/Shutterstock.com
Microcomputer	Small but powerful personal computing devices designed for one user	Word processing, presentations, small databases, social networking, communication, controlling test, and manufacturing equipment	Personal computer, laptop, desktop, pads, tablet, notebook, smartphone, computer watch (see Figure 10-1)

BASIC COMPUTER ELEMENTS

All computer systems are composed of four fundamental elements (see the "Fundamental Elements of a Computer System" Quick Reference Guide). In addition to these basic elements, many support systems such as timekeeping devices, power supplies, and firewalls are part of a computer system.

Hardware

The components of a computer system that you can see, touch, or hear are referred to as **hardware**. Hardware consists of **input devices**, **output devices**, and the **central processing unit (CPU)**, as well as some firewalls and modems.

Data Storage Devices. Data storage devices are devices capable of permanently or temporarily storing digital data. Data storage device capacity is often referred to as **memory**. Together with computer speed, this area of the computer has seen the greatest improvement, with capability doubling every few years. Computers used by most of us today have no functional limitation for memory, with portable memory cartridges providing unlimited memory expansion. Data storage devices consist of read-only memory (ROM), random access memory (RAM), and data storage memory.

ROM and RAM Memory. The computer manufacturer permanently writes data or instructions into the memory on ROM chips, which are installed directly onto the **motherboard.** They contain instructions for operations such as booting the computer when the power is turned on. RAM memory is also in the form of chips and is also part of the motherboard. It provides the computer with registers in which to store in-process data. RAM memory is erased or "lost" when the computer is turned off or experiences a power failure. RAM memory is important to the user, in that a RAM capacity that is too small will cause the computer to run slow or not to run some program software.

Data Storage Memory. Data storage memory is nonvolatile, or permanent, and is not erased when the computer is turned off. It can be either read-only or read-write. Read-only data storage memory is used to store program software for loading onto the computer. CDs and DVDs have been used for this purpose, but Internet servers are increasingly used today. The following paragraphs describe several devices for providing data storage.

Mechanical Hard Disk Drive (HDD). HDDs are nonvolatile read-write storage devices consisting of a rotating metal disk coated with a magnetic material capable of locally being magnetized to store data as 0 or 1 depending on its magnetic state. The disk spins at 7,000 rpm and data is read by a head that hovers a few thousandths of an inch above the disk. The devices are subject to mechanical failure, resulting in potential loss of system software and data and should be backed up frequently. (See Cloud Storage and RAID storage for backup of data and system software.)

Solid State Drive (SSD). Solid state drives serve the same function as a mechanical hard drive, except that the data is stored on interconnected flash memory chips instead of on the surface of a metal disk with a magnetic coating. The flash memory chips are also nonvolatile and retain the data even when there is no power to them. They are less susceptible to rough treatment, although they have a limited read-write life. Except for heavy download users, however, the computer will usually become obsolete prior to the flash memory failing.

Optical Drives. Two types of optical drives are used in computers: compact disks (CDs) and digital video/versatile disks (DVDs). Currently, Internet storage and advances in flash technology are replacing optical drives.

CDs used in the computer environment are similar to those used to store music. They are used for storing both permanent and temporary records, as they have the capability to be used as read-only disks (CD-ROM), write disks (CD-R), and re-write disks (CD-RW). In addition to data storage, they are sometimes used to hold program software for installation on the computer; however, when Internet connection is available software programs are more likely downloaded directly from a server.

DVDs are identical to the DVDs used to view home movies. They look similar to CDs, except that the format for writing the data to DVDs is different, permitting storage of up to 26 times more data. Several formats for writing data are used at this time. For the system to function, it is important that the storage media, disk, and drive are of the same format.

USB Thumb Drive. Thumb drives utilize flash technology and are connected to the computer using a universal serial bus (USB 1.0, 2.0, or 3.0) port or higher performance USB serial port. The memory

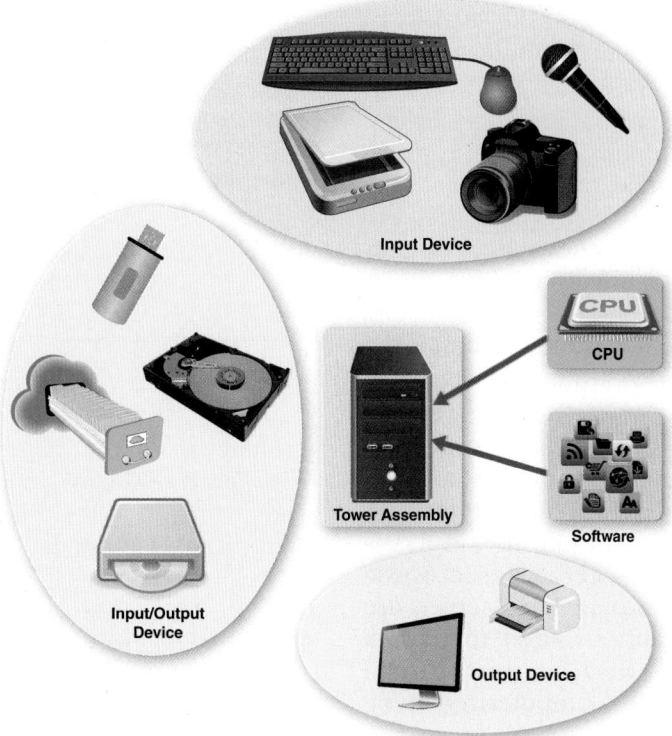

ELEMENT	FUNCTION	EXAMPLE
Input device	Device that translates analog data into a form useable by the computer microprocessor (CPU)	Keyboard, mouse, digital camera, touch screen, scanner, laboratory test equipment, server file, CD, magnetic tape
Central processing unit (CPU)	Performs mathematical computations, makes logic decisions, and controls computer functions in accord with instructions provided by system software; commonly referred to as the brain of the computer	Approximately 2-inch square microchip located on the motherboard
System software • Operating system (OS) • Program software • Driver software	Manages computer resources Instructions for specific task Instructions for support hardware	Windows 10, iOS Word, Excel, PhotoShop Printer or graphics driver
Output device	Device that displays or stores the results of operations performed on the input data by the CPU	Printer, monitor, data storage device, modem, fax machine

is nonvolatile and is slower and less reliable than the flash memory in a SSD drive. Thumb drives are about the size of a human thumb, and are useful for transferring data between computers that are not networked and for limited backup of data. (*NOTE*: Thumb drives from a nontrusted source should not be connected to a computer system as they can contain a virus that could compromise the security of the entire network or individual computer.)

Tape Drives. Tape drives are data storage devices capable of storing large amounts of data on replaceable reels of magnetic tape, much like a tape recorder but on a larger scale. Because they are much slower than many other storage devices, they are used when time is not usually too significant, such as in backing up a computer system (data, OS, and system software). The storage media cost is significantly less with this type of storage device.

Servers. **Servers** are not true data storage devices. They are pseudo-computers connected to massive hard drives. In many networked systems they become the storage devices for the user workstations. Servers may be located remote from workstations or even on the Internet. When servers are used, special protocols must be used to protect confidentiality of records, which are discussed in "Patient Confidentiality in the Computerized Medical Clinic," page 217.

Cloud Storage. Cloud storage involves storage of digital data using multiple servers in a physical facility that is frequently owned and managed by a hosting company, although it can be operated by the using organization. The servers are generally located at different locations to avoid catastrophic loss of data due to natural or man-made events. The Internet or a cable system provides the means for data transfer to the storage site. Cloud storage has many advantages over in-house data storage: Data is accessible from multiple sites, and the system requires little capital investment or technical resources by the using organization. The cloud can also host program software, freeing up computer capacity and capability requirements (see the "Cloud Computing" section on page 211).

Life Span of Stored Data. The life of stored data is dependent on the storage media, temperature and humidity, and whether the data are frequently retrieved. Assuming the media are stored under cool and dry conditions and data are infrequently retrieved, Table 10-1 provides a conservative

TABLE 10-1

LIFE SPAN OF STORED DATA

MEDIA	ESTIMATED LIFE SPAN
CD	2 to 5 years
Cloud storage	Indefinite
Flash drive	5 to 10 years
Floppy drive	10 to 20 years
Hard drive	3 to 5 years
Magnetic tape	10 to 20 years

Data Source: Storage Craft, www.storagecraft.com/blog/data-storage-lifespan/

estimate of data storage life for different media. The quality of the original media can also affect the storage life; do not go with the lowest price for storage media for important data.

RAID Storage. Redundant array of independent disks (RAID) storage is a storage system that can use any of the storage media described previously. Storage devices are combined in a redundant array so that should any one device fail, a new device can be installed without shutting down the system or losing data (hot swapping).

Documentation

Computer system **documentation** consists of the manuals and **licenses** that define how many computers can use the software, and how the programs operate. Manuals explain how to execute specific functions and give the specifications for hardware, such as the frequency of the internal clock, RAM, and hard drive available memory. Although documentation is more likely to be online, it may be printed format or provided on an optical disk that contains the program or OS.

Updates to program documentation are increasingly made available on the Web site of the company providing the program, together with **patches** for glitches discovered in the basic program. The system should always be backed up prior to installing updates and patches in case they cause problems. It is recommended that this work be done when supplier technical support is available. Third-party manuals defining

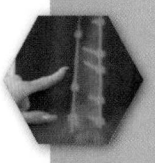

Critical Thinking

Your clinic has received legal notification requiring you to provide a list of all the software used in the practice and to show proof that all necessary licenses are current. You are successful in showing compliance, but clinic procedures were disrupted for days in meeting this court mandate. Prepare a clinic protocol designed to ensure that all software is legal and that unauthorized persons have not installed illegal software on any clinic computers.

how to use software are becoming increasingly popular and are frequently more user-friendly than documentation from the software supplier. All documentation—including licenses, recovery software, and program disks that come with the computer system; add-on hardware; and software—should be maintained in a safe location for the life of the equipment and software, and then disposed of when the system or software is phased out of use.

Hardware and Software Compatibility

The hardware drivers and **program software** of a computer system must be compatible with the **operating system (OS)**. Many program software applications share files with the operating system (OS); if there is a conflict with files having the same name, either the OS will not allow the applications program to load or it will not function properly. The documentation for most applications programs defines the versions of the operating system for which compatibility has been established and should always be checked before purchase of either a new applications program or a new version of the OS. Hardware driver requirements should also be checked for compatibility with the OS. The amount of RAM memory, CPU clock speed, and available drive storage space can affect whether a program will run satisfactorily.

Computer Networks

Networking is the electronic or optical connection of computers and peripheral equipment for the purpose of sharing information and resources.

Types of Networks. The most common networks encountered in the medical clinic are:

- Local area network (LAN)
- Wide area network (WAN)
- Internet

Both LAN and WAN are dedicated networks limited to connected computers operated by a single company, clinic, or hospital. They differ principally by the size of the geographic area covered. The LAN usually is limited to a single clinic or building, whereas the WAN covers a wider geographic area and may be linked by leased telephone lines, fiber optic cables, microwave links, or even radio. Each computer in the LAN or WAN usually has its own computing power, but it can also access other devices on the network subject to the permissions it has been allowed.

The **Internet** is a worldwide publicly accessible network of networks and computers. It differs from a LAN or WAN not only in sheer size but also in the manner of data transmission, called *protocols*. Data transmitted on the Internet are broken into packets, which are routed over different networks to the final destination, where they are reassembled for use by the client computer. If one network is inoperative the system chooses another. Data that are in transit are almost impossible to intercept, making them immune from most unauthorized users.

Connecting Networks. Connection to a network can be through either a hard-wired system or a wireless system. Hard-wired connections include standard telephone modem (dial-up), digital subscriber phone line (DSL), local area network, or through a modem using either copper wire or fiber optic cable. Wireless connections include WiFi, Bluetooth, satellite systems, and cellular technology.

Hard-Wired Connection. Hard-wired connections are often referred to as **Ethernet** connections. Connections can be made using a telephone line–type cable called a *crossover cable* between computers having an installed network interface controller. Most new computers have this feature. Hard-wired systems are capable of higher data transmission rates than wireless systems, but with advanced technology WiFi systems, the difference is not noticeable unless very large files are being transmitted.

WiFi Connection. WiFi can be used to connect computers directly or to connect a computer to the Internet. WiFi is a brand originally licensed by the Wi-Fi Alliance to describe the underlying technology of wireless local area networks (WLANs). It was developed to be used for mobile computing devices, such as laptops, but is increasingly used for more services, including Internet, voice over Internet protocol (VoIP) phone access, gaming, and basic connectivity of consumer electronics. It has a range of about 300 feet.

Because WiFi uses radio transmission, it is vulnerable to unauthorized users eavesdropping on the transmission. Measures to deter unauthorized users include:

- Suppressing the access point's (AP's) Service Set IDentifier (SSID), which is used by the AP to tell the world that it is online
- Allowing only computers with authorized media access control (MAC) addresses to join the network
- Using various encryption standards (WAP2, WAP, WEP)

WAP2 has the most sophisticated encryption and is almost totally secure. WAP encryption is the next best alternative, and WEP is better than nothing. If the eavesdropper has the ability to change his MAC address he can potentially join the network by forging his MAC to an authorized address that he determines by listening to network activity using a scanning device.

Bluetooth Connection. A technology called Bluetooth can be used to connect computers to a LAN. Bluetooth is the name given to a radio technology capable of transmitting signals over short distances (30-foot range). This means of connecting networks is primarily used to connect smartphones and microcomputers to each other and to a host computer. Because Bluetooth is a radio technology, it is vulnerable to eavesdropping, but because of the short range it is less vulnerable than WiFi. Most systems that are designed to hold personal data have built-in security in the form of a four or more digit alphanumeric personal identification number (PIN), much like the one used for an ATM at the local bank. Product owners should share PIN numbers only with trusted associates to ensure maintaining of security.

Systems Security

All systems connected to the Internet or to computers that are connected to the Internet are vulnerable to attack by hackers and require strong security measures. In the past, hackers limited their activities to those that would earn them notoriety, but that is no longer the case. Their motives have changed; they are now in it for the money. The nuisance-type attack on a computer system will always be a concern, and the theft of electronic records from a medical practice can be a virtual gold mine to a criminal hacker. Electronic theft of Social Security records of staff and patients can lead to identity theft. Theft of bank account and credit card information can result in untold consumer fraud, and compromised medical records may lead to medical insurance and reimbursement fraud.

Protection of sensitive data is a legal responsibility for any business that has such data in its computer system. The Federal Trade Commission takes enforcement actions against corporations or businesses that fail to provide adequate data security. Protection of a computer system from unauthorized access requires defense in depth. Protection can be broken into the following defenses:

- *Protocols and audits.* All medical facilities must have protocols in place to hold workers accountable for their actions while using electronic protected information (ePHI) and electronic medical records (EMR). Security audits should be randomly conducted using audit trails and audit logs that offer a back-end view of system use to ensure policies are being followed. The very knowledge that a user's actions are being recorded can act as a significant deterrent to prevent wrongdoers from committing malicious acts. The audits provide evidence of security incidents and breaches of patient privacy and help establish a culture of responsibility and accountability for patient health information (PHI). They also provide information for responding to patient privacy concerns regarding unauthorized access by family members, friends, or others. Audits are helpful in preemptively detecting new threats and intrusion attempts to the system and meeting regulatory requirements.
- *Operating system (OS).* Select an OS with the fewest flaws for hackers to use and always install the latest security fixes (patches). No OS is perfect, so diligence is the watchword.
- *Program software.* Program software has been the source of the greatest number of security vulnerabilities. As with the OS, always install security patches as they become available. Check on vulnerability ranking and select program software with the least detected

vulnerability if possible while meeting your application needs. Web browsers have the most security vulnerabilities because they are a popular gateway to access servers and spread malware.

- *Control of software downloads.* The greatest risk to computer security is the unauthorized installation of software by the computer operator. Downloaded software and data using thumb drives or from unknown Internet sites can introduce viruses and malware into the system, defeating the best **firewalls** and virus protection systems. All personnel should be made aware of this vulnerability. If possible, an information technology (IT) technician should be listed as administrator of all computers, and users should not be given authority to add software.

- *Firewall.* Protect the network with a firewall, which limits access to the system from outside.

- *Antivirus software.* Have an active, updated virus protection system.

- *Password.* Require passwords to gain access to sensitive medical and financial data. Passwords should be changed on a regular basis.

- *Training.* To avoid **phishing**, instruct personnel not to open email from unknown sources and not to go to Web sites received in an unsolicited fashion.

- *Inventory control.* Maintain strict inventory control of laptops, memory cards, and other portable devices that contain data. The best network security system in the world can be breached if a laptop is taken home and either is stolen or used with unprotected Internet access. Unknown to the user, the laptop can have programs downloaded that reveal passwords or provide a free ride into the secure system of the clinic network.

- *Data management.* Purge the system of inactive files containing sensitive data; archive or destroy them as necessary.

- *System backup.* **System backup** includes all clinic systems (data, OS, and program software) on a regular basis to permit restoration of the system in case of a catastrophic event.

- *Manual selection of WiFi access points.* Do not let the computer automatically search for and connect to the access point with the strongest signal. Hackers operate access points designed to gain access to your computer. If in doubt, check the address of the access point to be sure it represents a legitimate source or connect only to officially known access points.

- *Personal access points.* The personal access point, which is part of your network system, should be given a unique name that does not reflect the business name or the name of personnel. It should be security protected as previously described.

-
Integrity
Deactivate file sharing by your computer. Allowing files to be shared may be convenient for co-workers, but it leaves a wide open door for hackers.

- *Enable email encryption.* Enable the **secure sockets layer (SSL)** option for transmission of email by your email service provider.

Virus Protection Programs. Protection from viruses, worms, and malicious software (malware) is extremely important to prevent damage to files; unauthorized access to the files; and slowing, damage, or shutdown of the system. Viruses find their way onto a system principally through downloading materials and programs from the Internet, opening attachments from email files containing a virus, and unauthorized software. Antivirus software is one of the main defenses against computer viruses.

Antivirus software is a computer program that can be used to scan files to identify and eliminate computer viruses and malware. Most commercial antivirus software uses two different techniques to accomplish this:

- Examining files to look for known viruses by means of a virus dictionary
- Identifying suspicious behavior from any computer program that might indicate infection

In the virus dictionary approach, when the antivirus software examines a file, it refers to a dictionary of known viruses that have been identified by the author of the antivirus software. If part of the file matches a virus identified in the dictionary, the software will either delete the file or quarantine it, making it unable to spread. The program may also attempt to repair the file. The virus dictionary approach requires periodic online downloads to update the virus dictionary. The dictionary approach to detecting viruses is often insufficient due to the continual creation of new viruses.

Dictionary-based antivirus software typically examines files when the computer's operating system creates, opens, and closes them and when the files are sent or received as email. A known virus can be detected immediately upon receipt. The software can also typically be scheduled to examine all files on the user's hard disk on a regular basis.

The suspicious behavior approach attempts to monitor the behavior of all programs. If a program tries to write data to an executable program, this action is flagged as suspicious behavior, and the user is alerted and asked how to proceed.

Safety

Recognizing Secured Sites. Secure Internet sites are easily discernible by either a small padlock in the web browser window, not the Web site window itself, or by the site address (Figure 10-2). Secure sites utilize encryption and have an address beginning with *https://*. Sites that are not secure have an address beginning with *http://*, without the s.

Secure wireless sites can be identified by the same padlock next to the network name shown when your wireless device searches for a signal. When a padlock is shown, you will have to configure your device to connect to the hotspot. This is usually in the form of a password or passphrase.

Firewalls. Firewalls come in two varieties: hardware and software. Both types function in a similar fashion; namely, they establish a list of acceptable sites based on a profile the device develops of the users of the system. It will then allow these sites access to your computer. All other sites are blocked. Some firewalls limit the type of files that can be transmitted. Other firewalls cloak specific network channels, making them invisible to hackers trying to gain access to your computer. Still others monitor the content of incoming packets of data.

System Backup. Viruses, equipment failure or damage, and hacker attacks make system backup mandatory. System backup devices are basically data storage devices that store the entire contents (data, OS, and program software) of the nonportable computer memory so it can be recovered if a catastrophic system loss should occur. All clinic systems should use backup on a regularly scheduled basis. The frequency of the backup should be dependent on how much data the user can afford to lose. Magnetic tapes, optical drives, and flash drives are frequently used for this purpose. The backup is commonly done during hours when the system is not being used. Some system backup devices are automatic, requiring only that the tape or disk from the disk drive be changed in the morning and placed in safe storage. Current backup media should be stored in a secure off-site location. A backup system should be tested to ensure it is capable of restoring the computer to the initial state.

Power Outage, Electrical Surge, and Static Discharge Protection Devices. Protection devices must be an integral part of a medical clinic computer system. Computer systems should have an uninterruptible power supply, or battery backup, to prevent power outages from shutting down the system or destroying data. The power supply should also have a **surge protection** capability to prevent voltage surges on the utility line from damaging computer components. Static electricity can also be highly damaging to computers by transferring thousands of volts of electrical charge to components that are damaged by only a few hundred volts. This is the type of charge we all experience during dry weather when we get a shock from touching a grounded object and draw a spark. Synthetic clothing and walking on a synthetic fiber carpet can create static charges. To prevent damage from static discharge, grounding mats should be required at all workstations.

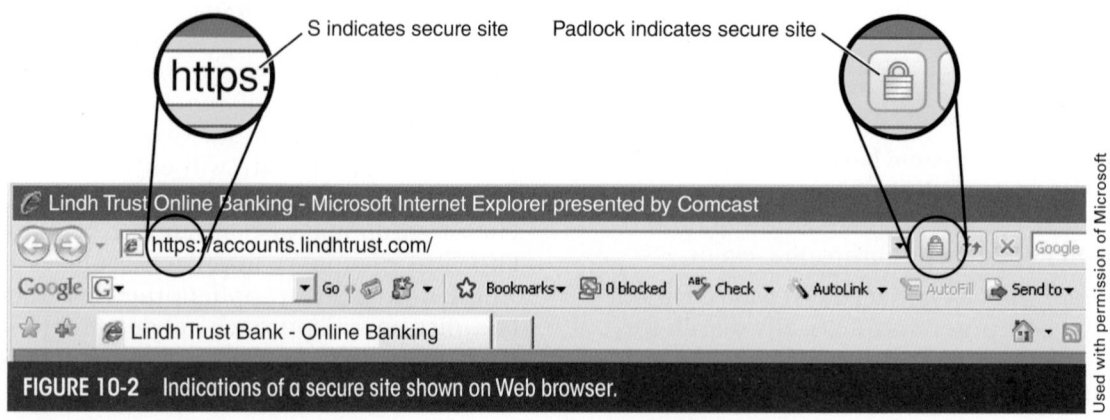

FIGURE 10-2 Indications of a secure site shown on Web browser.

CLOUD COMPUTING

While cloud storage was previously described in this chapter, **cloud computing** takes matters one step further, storing program software on servers at a hosting company so that software download is available on demand.

The cloud is like a computer rental agency where an order is placed for the applications (or apps) to be performed, such as keying in a document, or preparing graphics for a clinic bulletin board, scheduling appointments, coding procedures and billing insurance for services, and so on. The computing requirement is sent to the cloud and the app appears on the clinic monitor screen. Hardware and software updates, loading programs, or having to call the information technology (IT) person will be a thing of the past. It is all done in the cloud. The term *cloud* comes from the vision of cyberspace, where the Internet is represented by a cloud. In cloud computing, the cloud will provide all computing needs for a fixed service price on a pay-for-use basis. It will securely store data in a manner that all authorized persons in the clinic can access, and provide it as requested. This is not magic, of course; behind the service are computer resources and a management system, but the only user concerns will be availability on demand and reliability of the service. Cloud computing is made possible by the commoditization of apps, just like rental cars, airline flights, or utilities. Payment is required for only those services used. The main advantages of cloud computing are:

- Reduced cost resulting from reduction in IT personnel, hardware, software, and service hours
- Improvement in resource availability time, more secure data backup, and better disaster recovery

Some computing equipment will still be required in the medical clinic. A very basic computer and input devices capable of connecting to the Internet, as well as having a graphics capability to produce an image on the monitor, will still be necessary. A printer will still be required. Both the printer and the monitor will have to be selected to meet the requirements of the practice, just as is the case with current computing systems.

Data confidentiality will continue to be a concern to the medical community. Cloud computing services will not be without potential threats to data security, but by using encryption, virtual local area networks, and firewalls, the threats can be minimized. Multiplicity of geographical data storage can reduce the problem of data loss.

Cloud computing will be the development that makes worldwide electronic health records a reality. Electronic medical records that are accessible through a single facility or clinic using its servers are localized. Until those records are global, where anyone with authorization, regardless of their geographic location, can obtain access, electronic health records will not become a reality.

COMPUTER MAINTENANCE

Maintenance of computer systems is generally limited to cleaning the monitor screens, replacing printer ink or toner cartridges, and refilling paper trays. Other maintenance tasks that are within the capability of a computer-literate member of the health care team are file removal, disk **defragmentation**, and installation of security patches recommended by the supplier of the computer software. Defragmenting of the HDD is automatic in some OSs, and is not required with an SSD.

The HDD of a computer accumulates a host of old files ranging from old emails to obsolete programs and data files. If not removed, they use hard drive storage space and ultimately can slow the speed at which the computer stores and retrieves data. Simply right-clicking on the file with the mouse and then selecting Delete from the menu can remove these old files. After removing files, you should also empty the recycle bin. Be careful with this step, however, because once the recycle bin has been emptied, the files can no longer be recovered without extraordinary means.

When files are deleted from the hard drive, blank spaces are left on the disk. For the computer to save new files it must sort through these blank spaces. The defragmentation process removes the blank spaces similar to the way you move all the books on a shelf to one side so new books can be added to the empty side. Defragmentation is easily done using a disk defragmenter that is included with the OS. Defragmentation takes a significant amount of time and should be performed when the clinic is closed.

The medical assistant may have as one of his or her responsibilities establishing a service agreement for maintenance of computers on a periodic basis as well as any emergency repairs resulting from a major system failure. These agreements may also include personnel training and general technical support services. The medical assistant responsible for this contract should make certain that the vendor has signed the contracts required by the confidentiality protocols established by the medical clinic and that all removable data storage media have been removed and secured before hardware is taken to the service company's facility.

USE OF COMPUTERS IN THE MEDICAL CLINIC

Computers are an integral part of the medical clinic. According to 2013 CDC data, all of the hospitals and half of the clinic-based providers surveyed reported using an enhanced form of **practice management (PM)** software. PM software handles the day-to-day actions involved with a medical clinic using either an integrated piece of PM software or individual pieces of software that incorporate specific functions (Figure 10-3). Table 10-2 indicates the many tasks performed by computers.

Specialized software that ties together management of the entire practice is expensive, sometimes costing several hundred thousand dollars per application. Increased revenue resulting from improved productivity and reduction in the amount of undercoding or overcoding during the billing process have been found to more than justify the expenditure.

Electronic Records

Electronic records take two forms, **electronic health records (EHR)** and **electronic medical records (EMR)**. Both contain the same type of data, but differ in scope. EHR include all medical information from all providers and hospitals in a patient's medical universe, whereas EMR are limited to one provider, clinic, or hospital. Most records at the present time are EMR. As of 2013, CDC data showed that 78% of clinic-based providers and 60% of hospitals had adopted some form of EMR. Growth of EHR will take more time to develop and will be achieved only as the United States adopts a nationalized health care system. Such a system will allow digital health information to follow patients across the health care spectrum so that it will be available for all providers globally.

 Legal In order to satisfy legal requirements, practice management (PM) systems must demonstrate complete functionality by ensuring that the record is complete, accurate, secure, and compatible with all

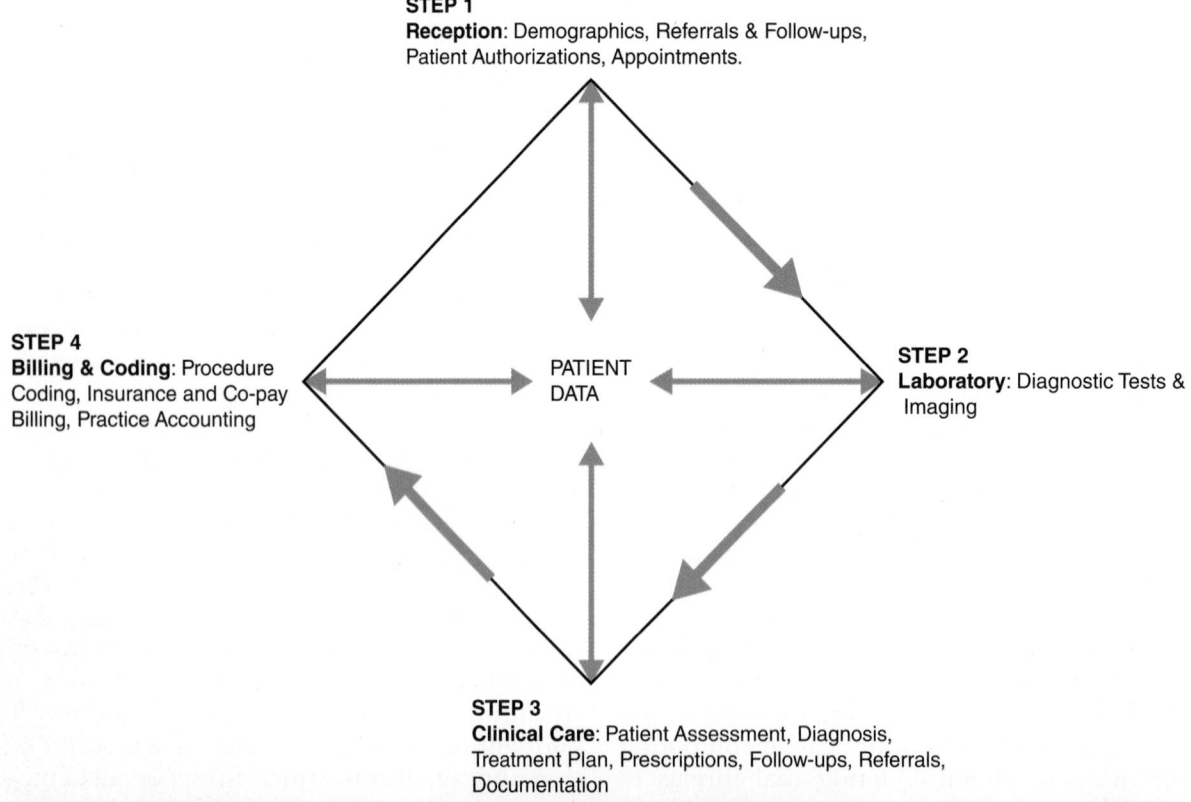

STEP 1
Reception: Demographics, Referrals & Follow-ups, Patient Authorizations, Appointments.

STEP 4
Billing & Coding: Procedure Coding, Insurance and Co-pay Billing, Practice Accounting

PATIENT DATA

STEP 2
Laboratory: Diagnostic Tests & Imaging

STEP 3
Clinical Care: Patient Assessment, Diagnosis, Treatment Plan, Prescriptions, Follow-ups, Referrals, Documentation

FIGURE 10-3 Practice management (PM) flow chart.

TABLE 10-2

THE USES OF COMPUTERS IN THE MEDICAL CLINIC

APPLICATION	TASKS
General clinic software	Patient demographics, appointment scheduling, email communication, provider referrals, follow-up directions, patient authorizations, insurance information, coding and billing procedures, accounts receivable data, accounts payable data, bank statements, monthly balance sheet (see Chapters 12 and 17)
Clinical and laboratory software	Patient assessment, diagnosis and treatment plans, follow-up lab tests and appointments, medications and e-prescriptions, scanning diagnostic tests, quality assurance data (see Chapters 22 and 24)
Administrative software	Clinic protocols, personnel data, staffing requirements, job descriptions, equipment inventory and maintenance, vendors and agreements, requests for equipment and facilities (see Chapter 44)

systems from which information about the patient is obtained. The system must meet the preliminary American Recovery and Reinvestment Act of 2009 (ARRA) certification requirements of the Certification Commission for Health Information Technology (CCHIT) (http://www.cchit.org).

The Virtual Medical Clinic

The revolution coming within the next 5 years is the virtual medical clinic, where patients will be treated remotely. The trend is being driven by value-based health care as part of the Affordable Care Act (ACA), in which providers, hospitals, and insurers are given financial incentives for keeping large groups of patients healthy. Prior to the enactment of the ACA, hospitals were paid when patients were hospitalized, under what is called fee for service. Health care providers are now eager to be proactive in treating anything from a cold or the flu to chronic illnesses. Insurers are providing 24/7 access to consultation by telephone, email, or Skype, with nurses providing assistance for minor illnesses and advice on when a provider should be involved. Many hospitals and large ambulatory care centers are adding urgent care options as a means of keeping down the costs of emergency care at hospital settings.

Providers are also taking advantage of wearable data-gathering platforms which remotely provide data on almost every chronic condition suffered by mankind. With this data in hand the provider can verify the patient's condition, prescribe medications, and advise the patient—all remotely, thereby increasing the productivity of the provider and reducing cost. The wearable sensors are FDA approved since they are a part of the treatment

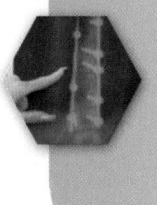
Critical Thinking
Your clinic has obtained new practice management software. List options you can think of for training clinic personnel to use the PM software effectively. Identify the pros and cons for each option.

loop. Some of the illnesses/conditions for which data links are being established include epilepsy, physiological stress, grand mal seizures, sleep disorders, diabetes, atrial fibrillation, and other cardiovascular disease issues. For all of the wearable sensors the computer plays a vital role.

Computers are also being used to identify illness outbreaks such as the flu or epidemics by sampling Internet search frequency for the disease. Recent trials show several weeks' advance warning of an outbreak in a given area.

DESIGN CONSIDERATIONS FOR A COMPUTERIZED MEDICAL CLINIC

Safety

Computerization of a medical clinic requires careful consideration of the computer system, software, and physical layout of the facility. If the change to a computerized system is well planned, with input sought from all affected personnel, and with time allotted for training, the experience will be less stressful for all concerned. Involving all clinic personnel in the design of the system is extremely important because it creates a feeling of ownership and garners more willing support during the disruptive changeover period.

Software Selection

The first step in selection of software is to choose a knowledgeable and trustworthy vendor. The vendor should not only understand computers and software but also the needs of the medical clinic. A reliable vendor should be able to assist in anticipating and allowing for future needs (at least 2 years' future needs) as the medical practice grows and new diagnostic tools are introduced.

The next and most important step in developing a plan for computerization of a medical clinic is determining what tasks will be computerized and preparing specifications that will become part of the contract with the vendor. This is done in conjunction with the vendor, by seeking input from staff, and by talking with other people in medical clinics similar to your facility. Software available for each of the tasks should be identified and evaluated, preferably by actually using the programs on a trial basis. The best program for each task should be identified, and the hardware requirements for each program should be defined. Keep in mind that the program should be selected with operational commonality with all of the other software taken into consideration. Programs with similar menus and appearance on the monitor screen make training personnel much easier. Packaged programs that perform multiple tasks are commonly available. The Microsoft Office suite is an example of a packaged program that includes word processing, spreadsheet, scheduling, email, and database programs with commonality in menus and procedures. Similar programs tailored to the medical clinic are available.

Hardware Selection

Once the memory capacity (RAM, hard drive data storage capacity), CPU speed, and input and output device requirements have been identified for the software, the next step is to determine whether you are going to network. The type of network selected will be based on data transmission speed requirements and facility considerations related to running cables and the distance between computers and output devices. The hardware selected should meet or exceed the identified minimum requirements and be name-brand equipment to ensure future availability of replacement parts. If possible, get a computer system with substantially more memory than required by the software, because inadequate memory or CPU speed may restrict the ability to use future software updates or improved programs. The CPU speed should be as fast as technology permits at the time you make your purchase. The computer should also have one or more USB 3.0 ports to allow faster connection speeds. The trend is toward using more memory and requiring greater CPU speed, especially if graphic programs will be used on your system. The more memory and CPU speed you can purchase, the longer your system will be viable without replacement of hardware. The size of the monitor and screen display resolution limit should be selected to be compatible with the type of work the computer is used to perform. These requirements are necessary to achieve image sharpness and avoid eyestrain of personnel. The computer control panel display settings should also be set to match the monitor display resolution limit. Resolution is usually expressed as pixels in the horizontal and vertical dimensions of the screen. Many inexpensive computer monitors have a resolution of 1280 × 1024 and this is adequate for most clinic work. Persons doing graphic design frequently use a monitor with a resolution of 3840 × 2160, and a resolution of 3280 × 2048 is used in medical diagnostic work. For reference purposes, the most common wide-screen HD television has a resolution of 1920 × 1080 and an ultra HD screen has a resolution of 3840 × 2160. If the monitor is to be used for diagnostic work, a much wider grayscale range is required so that it can render nearly every shade of gray; the latest medical monitors offer up to 4,096 shades of gray. Color display monitors should not be used for this purpose as they have a poor grayscale response.

Scheduling the Changeover

The installation of a computer system is disruptive to the clinic routine. Not only does it take time to install the hardware and load the software, but it takes time to transfer files and data. Personnel may be intimidated by the computer and must be well trained to avoid feeling overly threatened. The installation of hardware should be scheduled during a down period such as a long holiday or vacation period. It is best to introduce the new system while continuing to use the old system. Start by transferring files and data, then when the staff is comfortable with the system and their computer skills, make the changeover. If your staff does not accept ownership for the system and is not trained and comfortable with it, disaster is almost guaranteed. The process cannot be rushed, and short-term inefficiency must be accepted as a trade-off for the efficiency that will result from a computerized medical clinic.

ERGONOMICS

 Safety

Although **ergonomics** in the medical clinic is an important consideration even without computerization, specific problems must be addressed when changing over to a computerized clinic environment. Safety issues and concerns specific to the computer, if addressed, can be minimized or avoided.

Eyestrain

Eyestrain can be a problem associated with the use of computers. The computer monitor should be positioned to prevent excessive glare entering from windows or reflecting from interior lighting. Attachment of an antiglare screen to the monitor further reduces eyestrain by reducing remaining residual glare. Computer operators should take a 5-minute break each hour and focus on a distant object to prevent ocular accommodation and the headache and blurred vision associated with it. Using eye drops can minimize dry and itchy eyes. Figure 10-4 illustrates the proper positioning of the flat screen monitor to prevent glare from artificial lights in a room and incoming light from windows.

Cumulative Trauma Disorder

The most widely known injury associated with individuals routinely using a computer is carpal tunnel syndrome. It is attributed to repetitive wrist motion. It can be prevented or the onset delayed by using a special keyboard that conforms to the natural position of the hands or by using a conventional keyboard with wrist support, as show in Figure 10-5A and 10-5B.

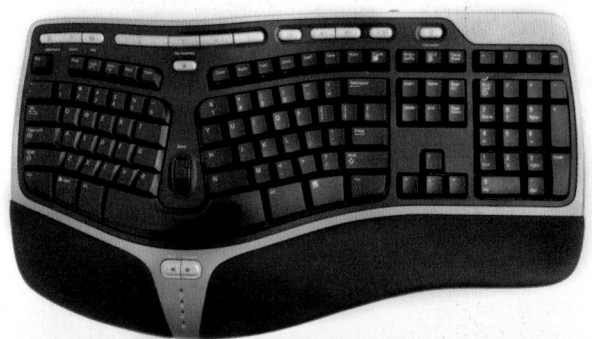
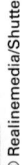

FIGURE 10-5A Ergonomic keyboard.

© Realinemedia/Shutterstock.com

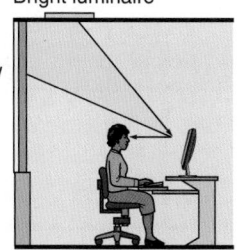
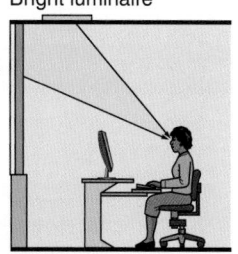

Poor location of flat screen monitor user

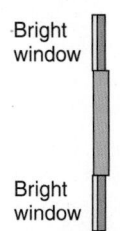
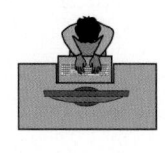

Good location of flat screen monitor user (sight line parallel to window)

FIGURE 10-4 Proper positioning of the flat screen monitor will prevent glare from incoming light from windows and artificial lights in the room.

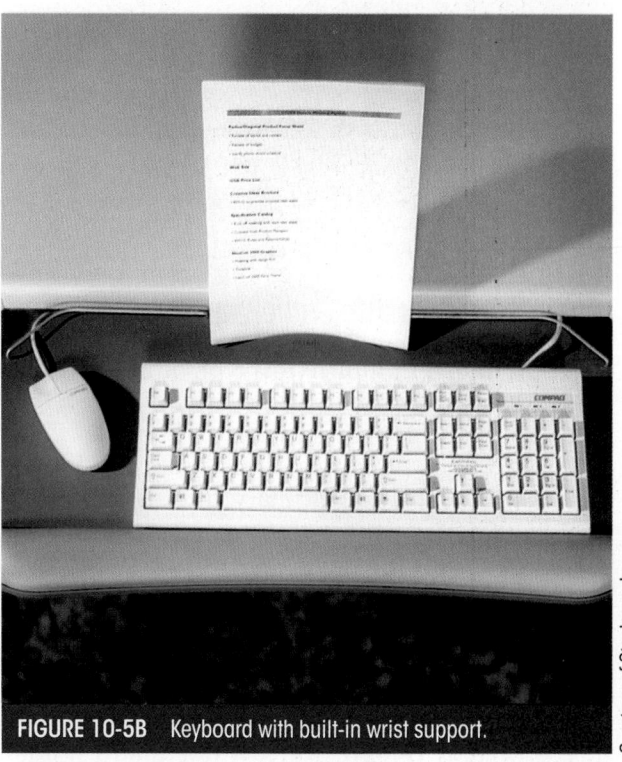

FIGURE 10-5B Keyboard with built-in wrist support.

Courtesy of Steelcase, Inc.

This diagram shows the recommended sitting posture for computer operators. The recommendation is based on establishing a posture that is comfortable while minimizing the risk of cumulative trauma injuries. Correct posture also minimizes operator fatigue and increases productivity.

• Distance to the screen should be adjusted so that the chin does not jut forward when the trunk is against the chair back.

• Top of the screen should be slightly below eye level. It should be squarely in front of the body to prevent twisting the body or the neck.

• The chair seat should not be so deep that the front edge is against the calve of the operator's leg, preventing the operator from supporting the back against the chair while in an erect position.

• The keyboard should be adjusted so that the forearms and hands are in alignment with minimal bending of the wrist to minimize cumulative trauma to the wrist. The forearms should angle downward slightly from the elbow to the keyboard. If the chair has armrests, they should be positioned so that the forearms do not touch while keyboarding.

• The chair adjustment should place the thighs level with or slightly above the knees to allow upper body weight to pass directly from the spine into the chair.

• The keyboard should be placed in front of the operator so that the elbows are in line with or slightly forward of the centerline of the body trunk.

• Feet should be in firm contact with the floor. A foot rest should be used if necessary. The foot space should be free from obstructions.

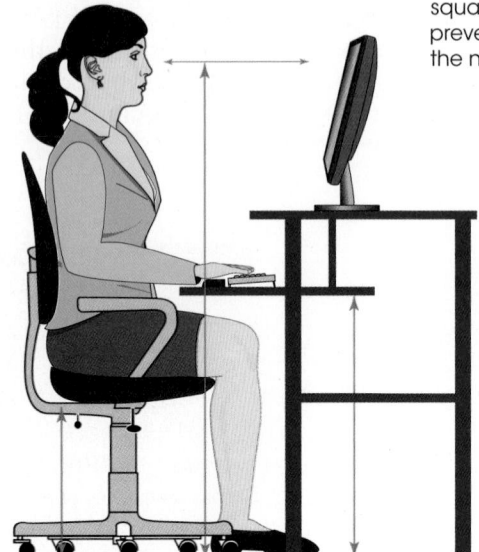

• High seat back with lumbar support is recommended to relieve spinal stress. Adjust the back to match the lumbar curve of the spine so that the chair supports some of the body weight. The spine should be as erect as possible to let it support a maximum amount of body weight to reduce fatigue.

FIGURE 10-6   Recommended computer operator position with ergonomic considerations.

Posture

Reports of back pain resulting from poor posture while using the computer are quite common. Carefully choosing and setting up computer equipment can minimize this type of injury. Computer operators should use a comfortable chair with lumbar support adjustment. A special chair with ergonomic features should be considered for individuals whose primary duty is keyboarding. Figure 10-6 shows the recommended computer operator position for proper posture to prevent back strain while operating a computer. The desktop should be 28 to 30 inches above the floor with an adjustable keyboard holder allowing adjustment for individual operator body size. A footrest may be helpful in further minimizing posture problems (Figure 10-7). A document holder

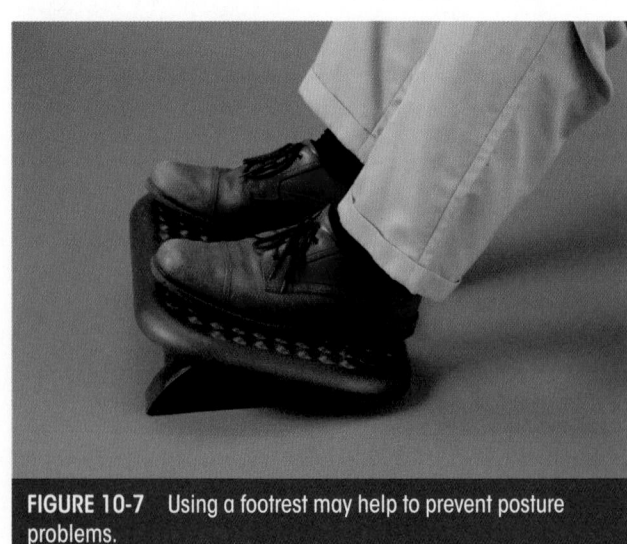

FIGURE 10-7   Using a footrest may help to prevent posture problems.

should be used to avoid excessive turning of the neck and looking downward (Figure 10-8). Operators who talk on the telephone while keyboarding or inputting data should use a headset telephone.

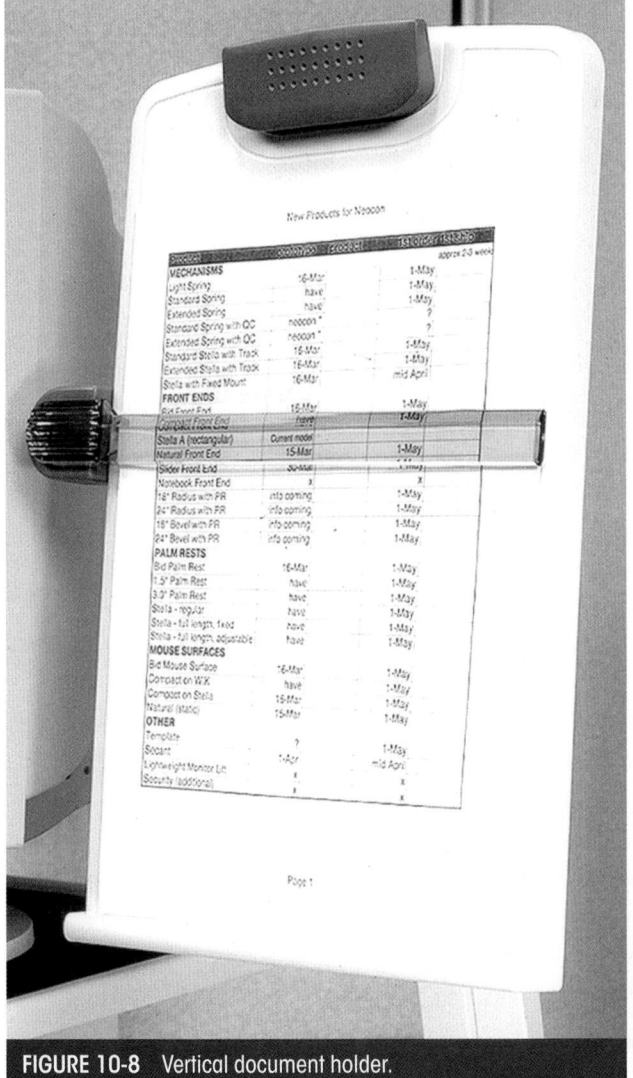

FIGURE 10-8 Vertical document holder.

Courtesy of Steelcase, Inc.

PATIENT CONFIDENTIALITY RELATED TO A COMPUTERIZED MEDICAL CLINIC

Legal

Integrity

The following guidelines are in compliance with HIPAA standards for safeguarding personal health information, and provide a starting point for maintaining confidentiality of patient information:

- Confirm the patient's identity by verifying at least two of the following: clinic number, date of birth, or photo ID prior to any discussion.
- Never discuss the patient's case with anyone without the patient's permission (including family and friends).
- Safeguard computer screens and never leave hard copies of forms or records where unauthorized persons may view or access them. Restrict access to electronic databases to designated staff.
- Destroy or archive outdated or unneeded records.
- Use only secure means to send patient records or test results (for example, use password protection, encryption, official mail) and always mark information confidential with directions to destroy if misdirected.
- When using vendors or an interpreter, ensure that confidentiality protocols are in place and persons have been trained.
- Have written confidentiality protocols and provide training for personnel.

The American Medical Association (AMA) supports the adoption of standards to protect individual confidential information. To review the AMA computer confidentiality guidelines, known as Opinion 5.07, go to www.ama-assn.org and search the term "Confidentiality: Computers."

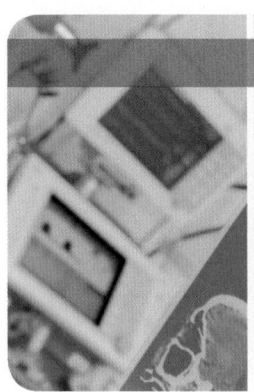

CASE STUDY 10-1

Refer to the scenario at the beginning of the chapter.

CASE STUDY REVIEW

1. How will Marilyn establish benchmarks or comparisons for computer needs?
2. Identify effective communication techniques used by Marilyn during team meetings to ensure everyone was heard and comments were understood.
3. What steps might Marilyn implement to ensure a smooth transition from a manual to a computerized system?

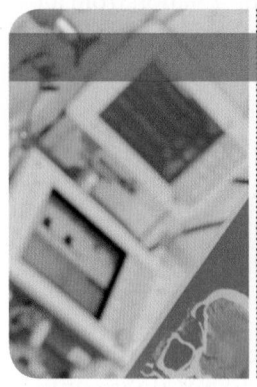

CASE STUDY 10-2

Marilyn Johnson, CMA (AAMA), who is employed by Inner City Health Care, has been given approval to computerize the clinic. Marilyn is also concerned about confidentiality issues involved with a computerized medical clinic.

CASE STUDY REVIEW

1. Identify the areas where confidentiality is most likely to be jeopardized.
2. Suggest possible solutions to protect confidentiality in each of these areas. Write a one-page summary and submit it to your instructor.

Summary

- All computer systems, from the largest supercomputer to the smallest microcomputer, consist of input devices, one or more CPUs, software, and output devices.

- The computer employs three types of memory for storing data: ROM, RAM, and data storage memory. Various forms of memory have different life spans and should be considered when archiving medical records.

- Computer software and elements of the computer system should be continually kept up to date with the latest updates and patches, and licenses and manuals should be safely filed for ready access. The system should be backed up prior to installing patches or new OS editions.

- When adding new program software or installing OS editions, compatibility with existing system software and hardware should be checked.

- Computers in the clinic may be networked using hard-wired, WiFi, or Bluetooth networks. WiFi is a wireless connection and requires security protocols to ensure confidentiality. Computers linked to the Internet should have firewalls and antivirus software loaded and kept up to date. All emails should be sent using encrypted transmission.

- Critical systems should be protected from electrical outages, surges, and static discharge.

- Computer usage in the medical clinic will typically be limited to patient demographics, scheduling, maintaining EMR, laboratory tests, billing and accounting, communication, and remote diagnosis and treatment of patients. These functions will be handled using stand-alone programs or using specialized practice management software.

- Introduction of computers or practice management software to a medical clinic requires careful planning. All personnel must be involved from the beginning to ensure the system will meet their needs and to develop ownership. Part of the planning must also take into consideration ergonomics and training of personnel.

Study for Success

To reinforce your knowledge and skills of information presented in this chapter:

- Review the *Key Terms* and *Learning Outcomes*
- Consider the *Critical Thinking* features and *Case Studies* and discuss your conclusions
- Answer the questions in the *Certification Review*

CERTIFICATION REVIEW

1. What is the best description of microcomputers?
   a. They are the fastest and most powerful computers.
   b. They handle large amounts of processing and challenge the capabilities of old mainframe systems.
   c. They are widely used in today's health care facilities.
   d. They are expensive and complex.

2. What is the best way to describe the CPU?
   a. It consists of electronic tablets with pointers, scanners, and touch screens.
   b. It is the brain of the computer system.
   c. It is often referred to as memory.
   d. It frequently is referred to as a computer program.
   e. It is also known as system software.

3. Which of the following is not considered a data output device?
   a. The monitor
   b. Printer
   c. Keystrokes, motion, and temperature
   d. Fax machine

4. What is the best definition of computer documentation?
   a. It performs a specific data processing function.
   b. It is a set of instructions that a computer follows to control computer hardware and to process data.
   c. It frequently is called the operating system (OS).
   d. It consists of the manuals and documents that define how programs or hardware operate.
   e. It is also known as a software driver.

5. Which of the following describes types of networks?
   a. Optical drives, compact disks, and digital video disks
   b. Flash drives, tape drives, optical drives, and digital video disks
   c. LANs, WANs, and Internet
   d. CDs, DVDs, and LANs

6. What is the best description of EMR?
   a. EMR are limited to one provider, clinic, or hospital.
   b. EMR include all medical information from all providers and hospitals in a patient's medical universe.
   c. EMR are used by only a handful of clinics and hospitals.
   d. EMR is a computer program that can be used to scan files to identify and eliminate computer malware.
   e. EMR are a type of CD used to store medical records.

7. What is the correct definition of ergonomics?
   a. Study of body language
   b. Granting of licenses to practice a profession
   c. Scientific study of work and space, including factors that influence worker productivity and that affect workers' health
   d. Reorganization of information on a hard disk to store files as continuous units rather than as small packets

8. The beginning point for a meaningful information security system is a comprehensive security policy that does what?
   a. Involves the use of LANs
   b. Adheres to HIPAA policies and procedures
   c. Ignores office policies and procedures
   d. Involves the use of WANs
   e. Applies phishing techniques

9. Which of the following is not an advantage of cloud computing?
   a. Cloud computing is made possible by WiFi connections
   b. Reduced costs in IT personnel
   c. Reduced hardware and software costs
   d. Important in secure data backup

10. Which of the following is not a guideline for compliance with HIPAA standards for safeguarding PHI and ePHI?
    a. Verify the patient's identity confirming two identifiers
    b. Never destroy outdated or unneeded records
    c. Never discuss PHI with others without patients' permission
    d. Have written confidentiality protocols
    e. Never leave hard copies of forms or records where unauthorized persons may view them

CHAPTER 11

Telecommunications

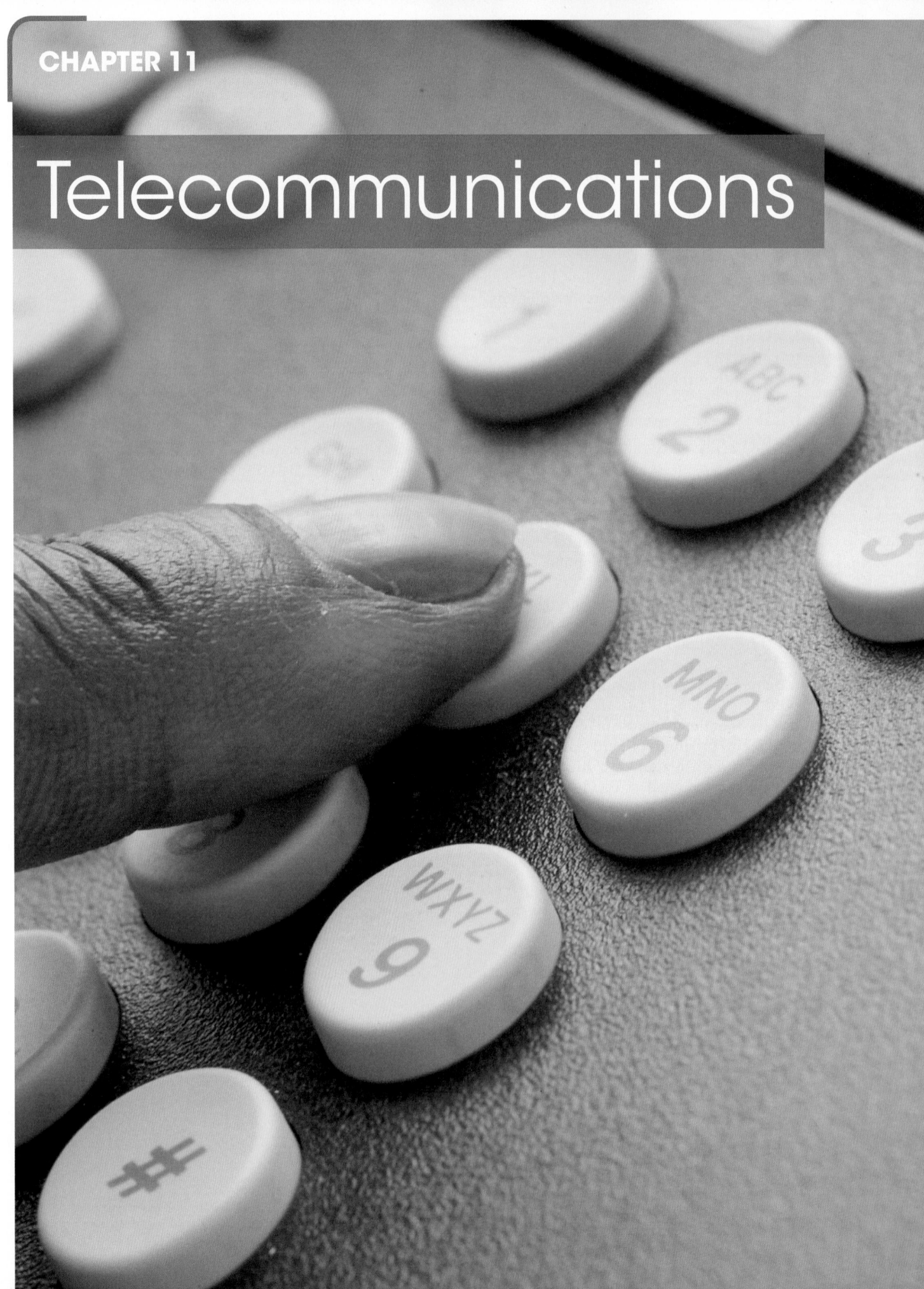

1. Define and spell the key terms as presented in the glossary.

2. Name at least three types of calls the medical assistant can take, and state the reasons why. Name three types of calls the medical assistant should refer to the provider, and state the reasons why.

3. Discuss proper screening techniques, including six questions that should be asked during the telephone screening.

4. Discuss how calls from angry individuals should be handled in a professional manner, and demonstrate steps to follow when this type of call is received.

5. State at least five common telephone courtesies.

6. Model the proper procedure for answering incoming calls and transferring calls.

7. Describe the information every message should contain.

8. Model the proper procedure for placing outgoing calls.

9. Discuss telephone documentation.

10. Discuss the impacts of HIPAA regulations on telecommunications, including identifying ways to ensure patient confidentiality when using the telephone.

11. Identify several security measures to consider before sending a fax containing confidential information.

12. Recall several risk management considerations to address before implementing email communications.

13. Discuss VoIP telecommunications.

14. Describe email encryption and its importance.

15. Discuss the purpose of the patient portal system, including how it increases efficiency and productivity in the clinic.

16. Name at least five tasks patients can accomplish with the use of a patient portal system.

17. Define telemedicine and describe at least two patient benefits.

KEY TERMS

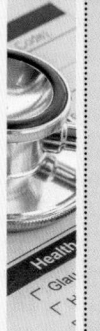

answering services	jargon
articulating	mHealth
automated routing unit (ARU)	modulated
buffer words	patient portal systems
electronic mail (email)	screening
encryption	smartphone
enunciation	telemedicine
fax (facsimile)	URLs (Uniform Resource Locators)
Good Samaritan laws	Voice over Internet Protocol (VoIP)

SCENARIO

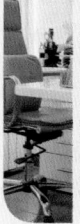

At Inner City Health Care, the telephone lines are rarely quiet. Yet administrative medical assistant Ellen Armstrong, CMAS (AMT), has learned to maintain her composure when she is responsible for managing incoming calls. Ellen has in her favor a naturally warm telephone manner, but she has had to cultivate other traits so that she can represent the practice in a professional manner, help patients and other callers feel at ease, and efficiently screen or refer calls as necessary.

continues

Chapter Portal

As in many clinic settings, the telephone is the lifeline of the ambulatory care setting. By means of telecommunication, which can also include fax, wireless technology, and email transmissions, patient appointments are scheduled, referrals made, critical information related, and the practice personality conveyed.

Medical assistants, more multiskilled than ever, have a wealth of knowledge to bring to telecommunications. Over the telephone, they welcome new patients, reassure current patients, collaborate with other organizations on patient care, and calmly and efficiently deal with emergencies. They will need to draw on their resource of administrative and clinical knowledge; they will also need to cultivate a telephone personality that is warm and accessible while also being efficient and organized.

In this chapter, medical assistants will come to understand the principles basic to successful telecommunications, whether initiating or answering calls; will learn the extent and limits of their authority as medical assistants; will discover how to prepare themselves for making or receiving calls; and will be introduced to telephone systems and new technologies.

BASIC TELEPHONE TECHNIQUES

Telephone answering techniques are rapidly changing in all clinics, even the smaller single-provider practices. The medical assistant responsible for answering the telephones previously was the first contact most people had with the practice, but today the first contact is usually with an automated phone system. Just as with a human answering the phone, first impressions are lasting. The program setup in the automatic phone system should be user friendly. It is not uncommon for a person unfamiliar with a menu-driven telephone system to be unable to find the menu that applies, and it is extremely frustrating if the person cannot find a way to connect with a human operator. An option to speak with an administrative medical assistant should always be offered. An automatic answering system should begin with a message instructing the caller what to do if the call is an emergency. In most locations, the caller is instructed to hang up and dial 911. After this should be a list of menus for such items as prescription refill, billing, scheduling an appointment, and so forth. If at all possible, the menu system should only be one level deep; for example, the billing selection should not lead to another menu for Medicare, HMO, or other finance categories.

Regardless of whether the automated system or a medical assistant makes first contact with the caller, at some point the medical assistant will speak with the caller. The impression the patient forms of the practice will depend on your telephone personality and how you answer incoming calls. To create a positive impression, answer the telephone by the end of the first ring and certainly within three rings. If your station has more than one incoming line, it may be necessary to interrupt a conversation to answer another call. Some guidelines to follow in this instance include:

- Excuse yourself to the first caller by saying, "Excuse me, another line is ringing. May I put you on hold for a moment?" This should be done only once, not repeatedly during the conversation.

- When, and not before, the first caller has given permission to be put on hold, answer the second call. Determine who is calling and the nature of the call. If it is not an emergency and permission is given, place the caller on hold. Never try to quickly resolve the second call before returning to the first call.

- Return to the first caller and thank the person for holding.

- Explore the possibility of an automated message after three rings to put the calls into a waiting queue with a message that you are on another line and will answer the next call momentarily.

Telephone Personality

Presentation

First impressions are usually conveyed through verbal and nonverbal communication (see Chapter 4 for a review of these communication modes.) In telephone communications, however, personality and attitudes are conveyed only through the tone in which words are spoken and the words themselves. Remember, callers are not an interruption of your work but the reason for your job. Even in a large practice, it is rare that someone just answers the telephone and has no other duties. No matter what other duties are pressing, the primary responsibility of every employee in a medical clinic is patient care; everything else is secondary. Whoever answers incoming calls should be prepared to give the caller their complete attention.

Use a voice that is pleasant and well **modulated** (i.e., one that varies in pitch and intensity) and conveys interest in the caller's needs. Hold the handpiece correctly, about 1 to 2 inches away from the mouth, and project your voice *at* the mouthpiece, not *over* it. The use of headsets permits the mouthpiece to be positioned appropriately and frees the hands to use the computer and input information easily.

Volume, enunciation, pronunciation, and speed all have a profound effect on how you sound to the person on the other end of the line.

- Volume should be the same as when speaking conversationally.

- **Enunciation** implies speaking your words clearly and **articulating** carefully.

- Pronunciation involves saying the words correctly.

- Speed should be at a normal rate, neither too fast nor too slow. Err on the side of speaking more slowly.

Posture, the way the body is carried, also affects the voice. If the body is slumped in a chair, the diaphragm (the muscle separating the abdominal and thoracic cavities) is compressed and breathing may be restricted. Using the headset speaker with the phone promotes good ergonomic position because it decreases neck and shoulder stress by allowing you to sit up straight (Figure 11-1). If you are less tired and tense, you can focus more easily on professional alertness, which comes across to the caller in the sound of your voice.

Being organized and prepared in advance for each telephone call enables the medical assistant to respond to each caller appropriately. A pleasant vocal impression can be delivered by taking a deep breath and putting on a smile before answering the call.

Competency

Medical assistants who enjoy their work and want to be of assistance to patients communicate enthusiasm. Enthusiasm conveys interest in the caller and projects a sincere, caring attitude that can be "heard" over the telephone (Figure 11-2). Though some callers will be upset, frightened, or even angry, the medical assistant must always be patient and in control. Some calls may be about life-threatening emergencies; medical assistants need to remain

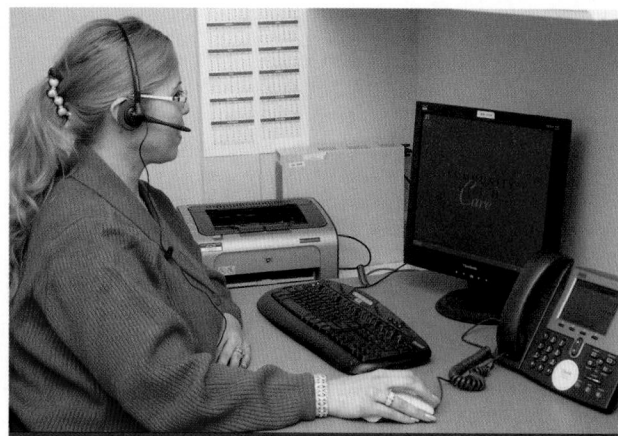

FIGURE 11-1 The headset-type telephone frees the medical assistant's hands to document and record while maintaining an ergonomic position.

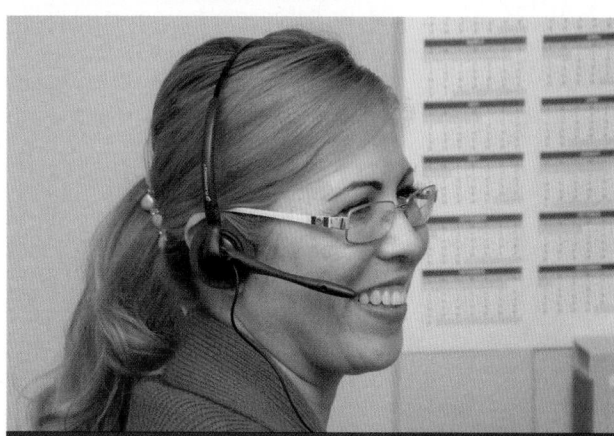

FIGURE 11-2 Tone of voice can put callers at ease during a telephone conversation.

calm to be of help to the caller, remembering their professional role as health care providers.

Professional Telephone Etiquette

Professional

Telephone etiquette, as with all good manners, simply involves treating others with consideration. Medical assistants have chosen a profession in which care and concern for others are paramount, so it is especially important to keep the patient's feelings in the forefront at all times. Basic telephone courtesies should be kept in mind when answering any professional call (see the "Telephone Courtesies" Quick Reference Guide).

⋙ QUICK REFERENCE GUIDE

⋙ TELEPHONE COURTESIES

Communication

- Always use callers' names and titles (e.g., Mrs. O'Keefe, Dr. King) during the course of a conversation when confidentiality is assured; this shows interest in them as individuals.
- Do not use technical terms if simpler ones will convey the information adequately. Using professional **jargon**, or terminology, is an easy trap to fall into because this terminology is used daily with co-workers. Jargon often confuses people outside the profession; the goal in communication is mutual understanding.
- Do not use slang or nonstandard terms in a business setting. Slang terms may have entirely different meanings to individuals from another generation or cultural background. However, patients may use slang when they communicate. It is important not to be offended by slang terms; also, be certain that patients who use slang understand any common medical terminology you may use.
- Say "good-bye" when closing the call, and allow the caller to hang up first.

Presentation

- The "hold" button on the telephone is often misused and should be used sparingly. Never put a caller on hold until you know who is calling and why. Never place an urgent or emergency call on hold. Never put a caller on hold without asking for and receiving permission to do so. No call should be left unattended for more than 20 to 30 seconds. If it is necessary to keep callers waiting longer, go back to the caller and give the option of continuing to hold or receiving a call back in a few minutes.
- Never eat or chew gum when talking on the telephone. This impedes enunciation and is distracting to the caller.

Competency

- Pay attention to what the caller is saying and how he or she sounds. Do not interrupt or finish sentences for slow talkers. The caller may have difficulty putting some thoughts into words, but give the person a chance to explain the problem or question. Listen with empathy for the caller. Also listen to what the tone of voice expresses.
- Do not attempt to work on other things while talking on the telephone.

Integrity

- Never talk to someone in the clinic while on an open line. This is confusing to the caller, and confidential information could be inadvertently overheard.

Initiative

- When it is necessary to get additional information and call back later, let the person know when to expect the call. If for some reason the information is not available when the time for the call back arrives, call anyway to let the person know when to expect another call.
- When taking a message for someone in the clinic, give the caller an idea of when to expect a return call. If the person will be out of the clinic for an extended period, see if someone else can help or if the caller would rather wait to hear from that specific individual. Avoid promising to have someone call back when you cannot control if or when this will happen.

Answering Incoming Calls

Most calls received in an ambulatory care setting are from patients or prospective patients, but some are from other providers or medical facilities. The remaining incoming calls are from family members, salespeople, and miscellaneous others. Personal calls should not be permitted in the medical clinic because the busy lines are intended for business. Occasional personal emergency calls are appropriate.

Preparing to Take Calls. Before answering incoming calls or making outgoing calls, medical assistants should devise a simple system to keep organized throughout the hectic day of telephone communications. If the reception desk is computerized, the first step is to boot up the computer and prepare ready access to the scheduling, patient demographics, and note screens. Figure 11-3 illustrates a scheduling screen from Harris CareTracker PM and EMR. If the reception desk is not computerized, collect materials such as message pads, the master schedule book, and prescription refill request forms. Regardless of whether the reception desk is computerized, a list of frequently used telephone numbers and clinic extensions and a supply of sharpened pencils and working pens are needed. A handy reference to practice protocols would be helpful, as would a supply of new patient registration forms, release

of information, and confidentiality information forms required by HIPAA.

Answering Calls. When answering incoming calls, the name of the facility should be clearly identified, as well as the name of the person with whom the caller is speaking. The name of the clinic is important because the caller wants to know the correct number has been reached. To avoid clipping off the clinic name, practice using **buffer words**. Buffer words are expendable words and may consist of introductory words, phrases, or statements such as "Good morning." They allow a caller to realize they have reached the desired number and to collect his or her thoughts.

Obtain the caller's full name and correct spelling, and ask if this is an emergency call. Ask for the caller's telephone number, street address, and date of birth (DOB). This information is necessary for retrieval of the caller's correct medical chart. Determine how you can be of assistance, and complete the call efficiently by following all established clinic protocols.

Screening Calls. One of the medical assistant's responsibilities is to screen incoming calls. The purpose of screening is twofold: (1) to be sure the caller talks to the person who will be most helpful (this is not necessarily the person asked for) and (2) to ensure the provider's time with calls is efficiently managed.

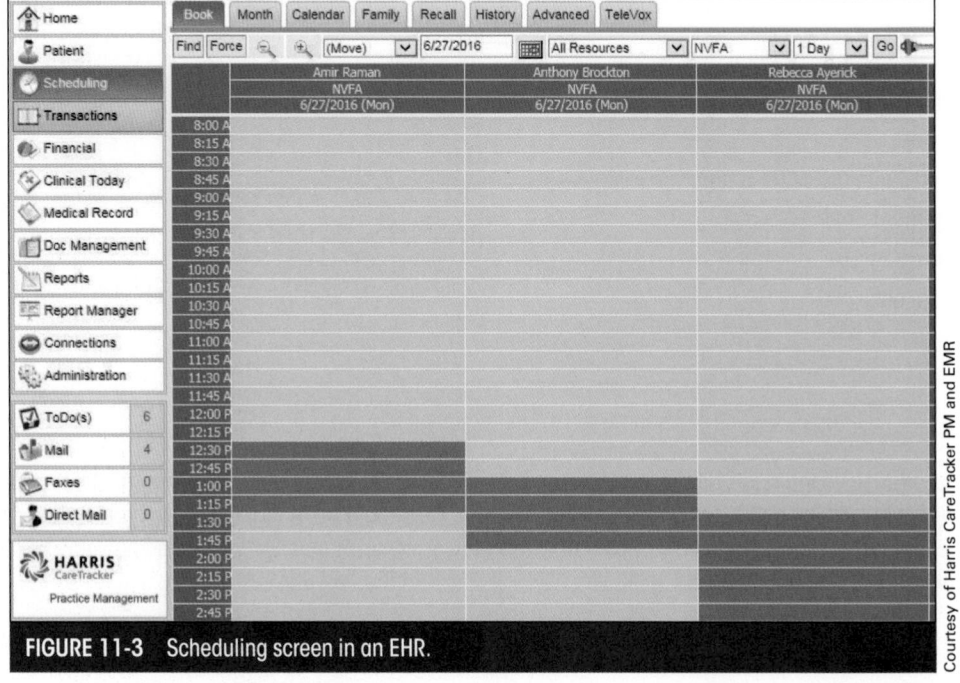

FIGURE 11-3 Scheduling screen in an EHR.

Courtesy of Harris CareTracker PM and EMR

Many people who call the clinic will ask to speak to the provider. Patients calling for appointments or with billing problems or insurance questions will sometimes ask to speak to their provider, assuming he or she is the person in charge, and therefore should answer any question or solve any problem. In most practices, this is not the case. Medical assistants and other administrative employees are equipped to deal with administrative functions; usually, providers are not involved in these procedures and sometimes may not be aware of administrative routines.

Screening Techniques. Screening is usually a simple process of asking the caller's name and the reason for the call. There are situations, however, that will require tactful persistence to get the information needed to properly direct the caller. Sometimes callers hesitate to give information because the questions are of a confidential and possibly even embarrassing nature.

Occasionally, a caller flatly refuses to give any information or will just say, "I'm a friend." If it is a patient who refuses to give information after gentle prodding, respect the patient's privacy and take a message. If you do not know who the caller is and you are unable to get any information, take the message and give it to the provider. If the provider does not know the person, he or she can decide whether to return the call. In any event, do not argue with the caller. Be polite and professional at all times. Procedure 11-1 provides steps for answering and screening calls.

Transferring a Call. During the screening process, calls may mistakenly be directed to someone who is unable to assist the caller adequately. This call will need to be transferred to someone with more expertise in a particular area. Guidelines that ensure successful transfer of calls include:

- Get the caller's full name, telephone number, and any other situation-associated information before attempting to transfer the call.

- Determine who would be the best person to assist with this situation.

PROCEDURE 11-1

Demonstrating Professional Telephone Techniques

PURPOSE:

To answer telephone calls professionally, acquiring all necessary information from the caller, documenting it correctly, and properly acting on it.

EQUIPMENT/SUPPLIES:

- Telephone
- Computer with message screen
- Appointment book
- Calendar
- Message pad
- Pen or pencil
- Notepad

PROCEDURE STEPS:

1. Be prepared. Have materials organized and computer with message screen up. *Implement time management principles by* answering the telephone promptly. The phone should not ring more than three times before it is answered. RATIONALE: Being ready for calls conveys professionalism and lets the caller know you are prepared to give him or her your full attention.

(continues)

2. Introduce the clinic and yourself by answering the call with the preferred clinic greeting, speaking directly into the mouthpiece. The mouthpiece should be 1 to 2 inches away from the mouth. Sample greeting: "Good morning. Inner City Health Care. Ellen speaking. How may I help you?" RATIONALE: Use a pleasant tone of voice to convey a warm greeting. Holding the phone correctly and speaking directly into the mouthpiece aid the caller in hearing your message clearly.

3. Ask the name of the caller as quickly as possible, and **use sound judgment** to determine whether this is an emergency call. RATIONALE: Using the caller's name personalizes the call and acknowledges that you heard the name correctly. If this is an emergency call, follow emergency protocols.

4. **Apply active listening skills.** You may need additional information to assist or direct the call appropriately. RATIONALE: This gives the caller a sense that you are listening attentively while eliciting additional facts and assures that information will be transmitted correctly.

5. Repeat information back to the caller, **using appropriate responses/feedback**. RATIONALE: This technique confirms that facts are complete and accurate. The caller also has an opportunity to hear the message and confirm that it is accurate or add something to modify or clarify the message.

6. Follow established written screening protocols for all telephone calls, **working within your scope of practice.** RATIONALE: Ensures that you understand your role in the health care practice and that all pertinent information is collected.

7. When using a multiline telephone as shown in Figure 11-4, it is helpful to keep a notepad by the telephone. When you answer the phone and have the caller's name, *pay attention to detail* and jot down the name, which line the caller is on, and some quick notes about the content of the call. At the end of your work shift, **protect and maintain confidentiality** by shredding all notepapers containing PHI. RATIONALE: Using this simple technique avoids problems if another line rings and you must put the first person on hold. Reviewing your notes allows you to accurately respond to the caller. PHI must be confidential, so disposing of notepapers properly is critical for adherence to HIPAA guidelines.

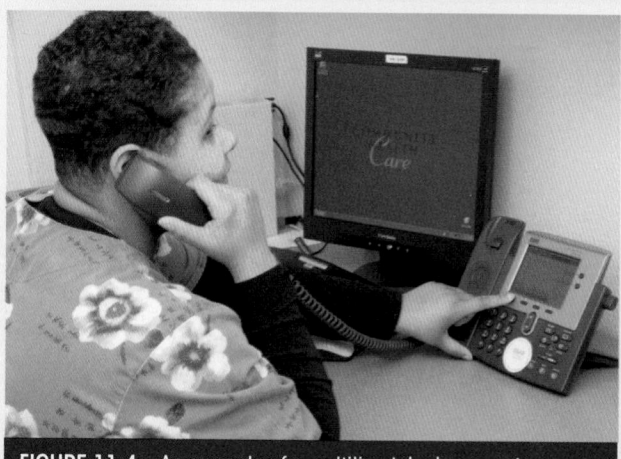

FIGURE 11-4 An example of a multiline telephone system.

8. Ask if the caller has any other questions. RATIONALE: This saves you and the caller time. It is frustrating to have to place a second call because you forgot to ask something. It also ties up the telephone lines and is not cost effective.

9. **End the call courteously.** Say "thank you" and "good-bye" (not "bye-bye"). Allow the caller to hang up before you disconnect. RATIONALE: Saying good-bye conveys professionalism and leaves the caller with a positive image of the clinic. Often callers think of questions just as they are ready to hang up. It is more time efficient to handle the questions immediately rather than having the caller make another call.

10. Document information and record any necessary actions. RATIONALE: This procedure is necessary for legal reasons. Remember that in a court of law, a deed not documented is a deed not done.

DOCUMENTATION:

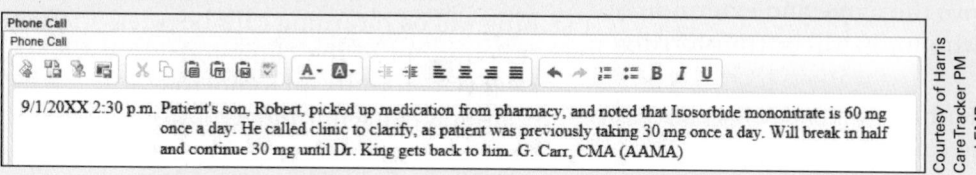

Phone Call
Phone Call

9/1/20XX 2:30 p.m. Patient's son, Robert, picked up medication from pharmacy, and noted that Isosorbide mononitrate is 60 mg once a day. He called clinic to clarify, as patient was previously taking 30 mg once a day. Will break in half and continue 30 mg until Dr. King gets back to him. G. Carr, CMA (AAMA)

Courtesy of Harris CareTracker PM and EMR

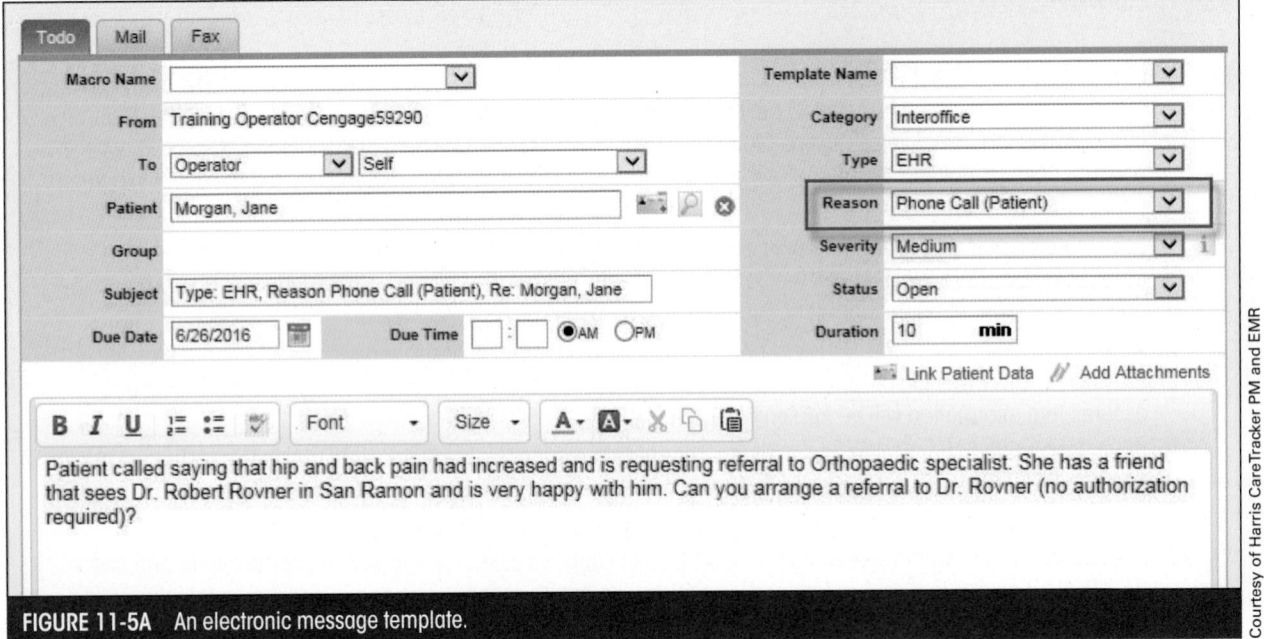

FIGURE 11-5A   An electronic message template.

Courtesy of Harris CareTracker PM and EMR

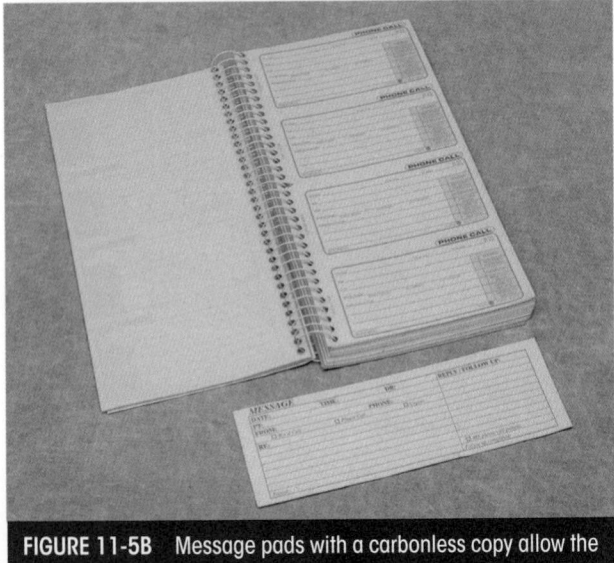

FIGURE 11-5B   Message pads with a carbonless copy allow the clinic to maintain a written record of all incoming calls.

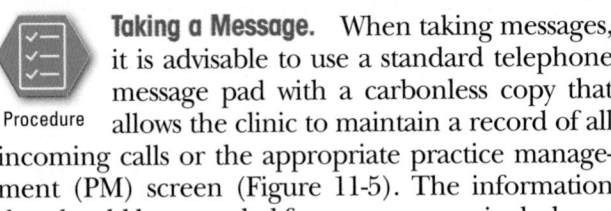
Procedure

Taking a Message.   When taking messages, it is advisable to use a standard telephone message pad with a carbonless copy that allows the clinic to maintain a record of all incoming calls or the appropriate practice management (PM) screen (Figure 11-5). The information that should be recorded for *every* message includes:

1. Date and time call is received
2. Who the call is for
3. Caller's name, telephone number, and DOB
4. When the caller can be reached
5. Nature and urgency of the call
6. Action to be taken (e.g., will call back, returned your call, please call back)
7. Message, if any
8. Your name or initials (in case there are questions)

Be sure to repeat the information back to the caller to verify that you have heard and copied it correctly. When taking a message, give callers an approximate time when they might expect to receive a call back if there is an established policy and all staff understand and follow that policy. ("Dr. King will be returning calls between 4:30 and 5:00." "Ellen is out of the clinic today, but I'll ask her to call you before 10 am tomorrow.")

Always attach a message from a patient to the patient's chart before placing the message on the provider's desk. The provider cannot discuss the patient's condition or answer questions without this

- Ask if you may place the caller on hold while you collect any pertinent data and make a call to confirm that the person best suited to assist is available.
- Return to the caller, thank him or her for holding, and give the name and extension of the person to whom you will be transferring the call.
- Follow your telephone system's procedure for transferring the call.
- Follow up to be sure the call transferred correctly.

information. Clinics using a PM system can send and receive messages via the computer and can have immediate access to the EMR. Procedure 11-2 identifies the steps and rationales in taking a telephone message.

Ending the Call. Ending the telephone call is as important as answering the call promptly. Bring the conversation to a courteous close and repeat any pertinent information back to the caller. ("Your appointment is scheduled for Friday, January 12, at 9 AM with Doctor King.") Pause just a moment to see if the caller has any additional questions. If not, say "Good-bye." Never use slang terms such as *bye-bye, see you later,* or *so long.* These terms do not reflect a positive professional image. You should always stay on the line until the caller hangs up. The caller might think of something else he or she wanted to ask or verify, and staying on the line gives the caller the opportunity to verbalize a thought rather than having to call back.

ROUTING CALLS IN THE MEDICAL CLINIC

The administrative medical assistant staffing the reception desk is responsible for greeting each patient, whether in person or via telephone, with a warm, friendly response. Incoming calls in the

---

PROCEDURE 11-2

Procedure

Documenting Telephone Messages Accurately

PURPOSE:

To record an accurate telephone message and follow up as required.

EQUIPMENT/SUPPLIES:

- Telephone
- Message pad
- Black ink pen
- Notepad
- Medical record if available
- Clock or watch

PROCEDURE STEPS:

1. Answer the telephone following the steps outlined in Procedure 11-1. RATIONALE: Being prepared and answering the phone promptly with the preferred clinic greeting prepares the medical assistant mentally to focus on the caller's needs. Using a pleasant tone of voice conveys a warm greeting.

2. Use a message pad, or document directly into the EMR. **Pay attention to detail** when requesting the following information:
   - Date and time call is received
   - Full name and correct spelling of person calling, and daytime and evening telephone numbers, including area code and extension when appropriate
   - Date of birth, clinic number, or social security number to verify correct patient
   - Who the call is for
   - The reason for the call
   - The action to be taken
   - The name or initials of the person taking the call

   RATIONALE: Complete and accurate information is necessary to respond to the caller's requests efficiently.

(continues)

3. Repeat the above information back to the caller. RATIONALE: Verifies that the information was recorded accurately and allows the caller to acknowledge that the message is correct.

4. If the call is from an established patient or concerns an established patient, pull the medical record/chart and attach the message to it before delivering the message to the intended individual. When using EMR save the message and forward it to the intended recipient. RATIONALE: Information about the patient is available should it be needed, and any required documentation can efficiently be made in the chart.

5. Maintain the old message book with all carbon copies intact. RATIONALE: Documents all telephone calls received by the clinic. This information could be useful in determining the need for additional telephone lines into the clinic.

DOCUMENTATION:

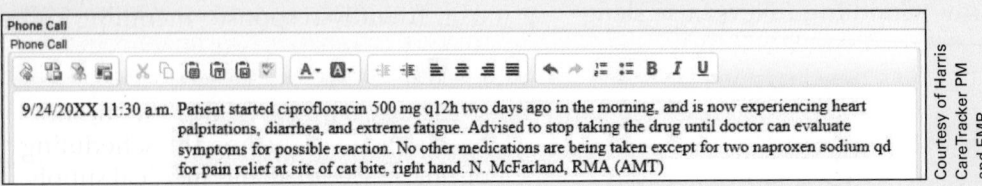

| Phone Call |
| Phone Call |

9/24/20XX 11:30 a.m. Patient started ciprofloxacin 500 mg q12h two days ago in the morning, and is now experiencing heart palpitations, diarrhea, and extreme fatigue. Advised to stop taking the drug until doctor can evaluate symptoms for possible reaction. No other medications are being taken except for two naproxen sodium qd for pain relief at site of cat bite, right hand. N. McFarland, RMA (AMT)

Courtesy of Harris CareTracker PM and EMR

medical clinic typically are routed by the administrative medical assistant according to subject and who can best respond. The administrative medical assistant, as well as clinical medical assistants, must always follow the provider-approved protocols when screening and responding to telephone calls. Table 11-1 illustrates examples of routing calls in the medical clinic.

Types of Calls the Medical Assistant Can Take

Keep in mind that, no matter how experienced, the medical assistant has definite limitations of authority and knowledge. Most calls can be handled by the knowledgeable medical assistant, but there are situations that only the provider should manage simply because the provider ultimately is responsible for what happens in the practice. Examples of calls the administrative or clinical medical assistant can take are as follows:

1. *Established patients.* When an established patient calls to set up an appointment, record the patient's name, daytime telephone number, and the reason for the appointment.

2. *New patients.* Require the same information for as the established patient plus some additional information, including:

   - Address
   - Age/DOB
   - Employer
   - Insurance carrier, HMO, Medicare, and any secondary insurance

TABLE 11-1

ROUTING CALLS IN THE MEDICAL CLINIC

ADMINISTRATIVE MEDICAL ASSISTANT	CLINICAL MEDICAL ASSISTANT	PROVIDER
Scheduling appointments	Scheduling tests and procedures	Other providers
Changing appointments	Prescription refills	STAT reports
Cancelling appointments	Progress reports	Provider's family
Fees and billing questions	Radiological and lab reports	Request for test results (positive)
Insurance questions	Patient referrals	
Information requests	Request for test results (negative)	
General questions about practice	Complaints about medical service	
Salespeople	Salespeople	

- Insurance ID numbers of subscriber or policy holder
- Name of insured (self, spouse, or parent)
- Name of referral source

This information serves as a source for the establishment of the chart and may lead to a discussion regarding payment of fees. Information for both new and established patients should be entered into the PM system or appointment book if not a computerized clinic.

3. *Scheduling appointments.* A major portion of telephone communications is spent scheduling patient appointments. (See Chapter 12 for detailed information on patient scheduling and rescheduling.)

4. *Scheduling patient tests.* Scheduling tests for patients can involve a great deal of coordination. Often appointment times need to be arranged among providers, the patient, and the facility where a test may be conducted.

5. *Billing questions.* Billing questions can be involved and complex, and medical assistants should be prepared to answer questions by retrieving information on the patient's insurance and billing status.

6. *Insurance information.* Calls will come from patients about insurance, as well as from insurance carriers and HMOs with questions about patients or their treatment. Prior to responding to insurance carrier requests for patient records, authenticate that the call is from the carrier using established clinic protocols and ensure that a signed release of information form is on file.

7. *Requests for prescription refills.* If a patient or family member is requesting that a prescription be refilled, medical assistants may take the call. However, they may not authorize a refill or tell the patient that a prescription will be refilled without the provider's approval. Most clinics ask that the patient call his or her refill requests directly into the pharmacy; the pharmacy then calls or faxes the provider's clinic for approval. Messages taken on these calls should be attached to the patient's chart or entered into the PM system and given to the provider for review and for permission to refill. When the provider approves the refill, the pharmacy may be called with an approval. Some practice protocols give authority to the CMA and RMA to refill standard medications with appropriate guidelines, for example, oral contraceptives or maintenance drugs, such as blood pressure medications, among others.

 Procedure 11-3 identifies the steps for calling a pharmacy to refill an authorized prescription.

8. *Receiving routine progress reports.* Frequently, providers will ask patients to report on their progress. If the patient is doing well, it is acceptable for the medical assistant to take that information on a message form or enter the message into the patient's EMR.

9. *General information about the practice.* People may call requesting information about hours, location, financial protocols, or areas of practice.

10. *Salespeople.* The medical clinic should have policies regarding the scheduling of pharmaceutical and medical supply representatives.

Today, many medical clinics take advantage of options offered through their computerized PM system when responding to telephone calls. The medical assistant will screen calls and forward messages to other personnel as "tasks." These tasks or messages can go back and forth between administrative and clinical medical assistants as necessary, or they may include the provider if his or her professional judgment is required to handle the call. An example of this screening procedure is as follows: (1) The administrative medical assistant answers a call from a patient wishing to have a prescription refilled. (2) The administrative medical assistant collects all of the pertinent information and sends a message to the clinical medical assistant. (3) When checking the patient's chart, the clinical medical assistant sees there are no additional refills authorized by the provider. (4) The clinical medical assistant forwards the pertinent information to the provider. (5) The provider, having complete access to the EMR of the patient, authorizes the refill, documents the order, and sends the notice to the clinical medical assistant. (6) The clinical medical assistant calls or sends a fax to the pharmacy to authorize the prescription refill.

Types of Calls Referred to the Provider

Providers have many demands on their time: surgeries, hospital rounds, patient appointments, documentation, and consultations with other providers, to name a few. Therefore, their time is extremely valuable, and misuse of time impacts the clinic in many ways. It is important to carefully screen calls going to providers to ensure that they receive only the calls that are necessary.

Procedure

Calling a Pharmacy to Refill an Authorized Prescription

PURPOSE:

To notify a pharmacy to refill an authorized prescription.

EQUIPMENT/SUPPLIES:

- Patient's chart
- Provider authorization to refill prescription
- Drug name, dosage, and instructions for when and how to take the medication
- Pharmacy name and telephone number
- Telephone

PROCEDURE STEPS:

1. Receive patient's request for a prescription refill. Follow appropriate telephone techniques. RATIONALE: Appropriate telephone techniques demonstrate consistent customer service.

2. Obtain the following information from the patient and include it on the message form or EMR message screen:
   - Patient's full name and correct spelling, and patient's DOB
   - Telephone number where the patient can be reached
   - Name of medication and how long patient has been taking it
   - Patient's symptoms and current health condition
   - If patient is a child, ask his or her weight
   - History of this condition (last clinic visit)
   - Treatments the patient has tried
   - Any known allergies
   - Pharmacy name, telephone number, and address if a chain

   RATIONALE: This information is needed by the provider for assessment as to whether a prescription will be refilled, if something else should be prescribed, or if the patient needs to be seen by the provider.

3. Attach the completed message to the patient's chart or EMR and give it to the provider. RATIONALE: The provider may wish to review the patient's history before refilling the prescription.

4. After the provider has responded, review comments in the chart by the provider. If the refill is authorized, call the patient's pharmacy with the refill information. Ask the pharmacy to repeat the information back to you. RATIONALE: Verifies the pharmacy has recorded the prescription accurately.

5. ***Paying attention to detail,*** document in the patient's chart the date and time the prescription was called to the pharmacy and the pharmacy address. Verify that the correct drug, dosage, and dosage instructions were provided to the pharmacy. RATIONALE: Provides accurate documentation in the patient's chart.

DOCUMENTATION:

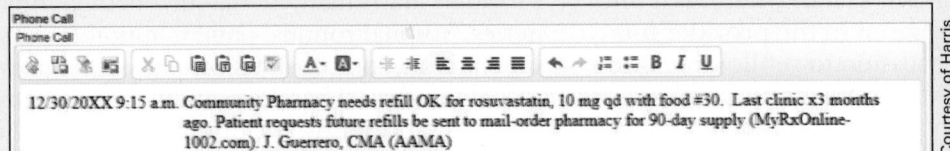

12/30/20XX 9:15 a.m. Community Pharmacy needs refill OK for rosuvastatin, 10 mg qd with food #30. Last clinic x3 months ago. Patient requests future refills be sent to mail-order pharmacy for 90-day supply (MyRxOnline-1002.com). J. Guerrero, CMA (AAMA)

Courtesy of Harris CareTracker PM and EMR

Examples of calls that should be referred to the provider include the following:

1. *Other providers.* When other providers call, always ask if they need to speak to the provider immediately or if they would like a call back. Be sure to ask if the call is regarding a specific patient; if so, attach a message to the chart.

2. *STAT reports.* In most cases the provider will only initiate STAT reports when the results are needed immediately.

3. *Provider's family.* Most providers will have an established protocol related to calls from family members. Family members generally do not call unless it is necessary, so in most cases their calls are put through directly.

Many other calls coming into the clinic may require the provider's professional judgment. Generally the majority of these calls can be handled with the PM system task/message feature. When the provider has a minute between patients, he or she can respond or provide specific instructions.

Special Consideration Calls

Competency

Answering the telephone in an ambulatory care setting places the medical assistant in contact with a variety of callers: those needing referrals to other facilities; emergency calls; and callers who may be angry, older, or speak English as a second language. As a professional, your goal is to treat every individual with courtesy and respect and to respond to their queries appropriately or to transfer the caller to another team member who can assist.

Initiative

Referral Calls to Other Facilities. If it is necessary to refer the caller to someone outside the clinic, such as to a laboratory or another provider, be sure to tell the caller:

- Why he or she should speak to someone else
- The telephone number to call (be sure to include the area code and extension)
- Who, specifically, to speak with at that number
- What information to have ready when he or she makes the call
- When to call
- If you would like a call back after the other contact is made

Legal

Emergency/Urgent Calls. The medical assistant must be careful when handling emergency or urgent calls to ensure that he or she works within the scope of his or her education and training. Donald A. Balassa, JD, MBS, Executive Director and Legal Counsel for the AAMA, states: "Procedures which constitute the practice of medicine, or which state law specifically delegates to licensed professionals to perform, may not be delegated to unlicensed professionals such as medical assistants." Therefore, prior to screening calls the medical assistant should always direct the caller to call 911 if the caller believes he or she may be experiencing a life-threatening emergency. Every attempt should be made to obtain the caller's name and telephone number before assisting with making the 911 call if it appears the person is confused or unable to dial for himself or herself.

Screening is the act of evaluating the urgency of a medical situation and prioritizing the call. Telephone screening is one of the most important functions for the person answering the telephone. Telephone screening requires skill and experience. An urgent condition is one that requires medical intervention that can be handled in a timely manner at an ambulatory care center.

To determine if a call is truly a medical emergency, keep a list of provider-approved questions near the telephone to assist in evaluating the situation. Standard screening questions can determine the nature of an emergency. Not all questions are appropriate to every call; suitable questions depend on the nature of the situation. Screening questions to ask may include:

- What happened?
- Who is the patient? (Ask name and age.)
- Is the patient breathing?
- Is there bleeding? How much? From where?
- Is the patient conscious?
- What is the patient's temperature?
- If the patient ingested something:
  - What did the patient take?
  - How much?
  - Are there poison or overdose instructions on the bottle?

Screening does not only pertain to emergency calls. Screening techniques can also help determine when a patient with symptoms should be seen by asking the caller questions such as:

- How long have you had the symptoms?
- Is there any fever?
- Are you taking any medications?

This information helps determine whether an appointment should be scheduled immediately or if it can wait a few days.

Legal

The practice should periodically review procedures for handling emergency/urgent calls. If a clinic situation involves a great deal of telephone screening, the staff should enroll in an advanced first-aid course. This will enable all participants to more accurately give instructions or to handle these calls if there is no provider in the clinic at that moment. In service training provided by the providers is a great tool to make telephone screening run smoothly. Remember, you should only render aid *within the areas of your training and expertise*. **Good Samaritan laws** do not cover paid employees, only uncompensated situations. All ambulatory settings should also post a list of numbers to be used in case of emergencies, such as the poison control telephone number.

Procedure

Angry Callers. Medical assistants will probably have occasion to speak with callers who are upset or angry. Although these calls eventually may need to be referred to the clinic manager or the provider, medical assistants need techniques for managing problem calls.

Competency

The first priority is to defuse the situation. This cannot be accomplished if you become upset or angry. As a professional, it is important to remain calm and in control at all times. Like most skills, defusing a difficult situation becomes easier with practice (see Procedure 11-4).

Older Adult Callers. Several issues may arise when dealing with older adult patients, such as impaired hearing, confusion, and an inability to understand procedures or technical information.

Do not assume that all older adults are senile or hard of hearing. This is a dangerous pitfall into which many people stumble.

If the individual has a hearing impairment, speak more slowly, more clearly, and a little louder

PROCEDURE 11-4

Handling Problem Calls

Procedure

PURPOSE:

To handle calls in a positive and professional manner while providing necessary comfort, empathy, and information to the caller to resolve the problem.

EQUIPMENT/SUPPLIES:

- Telephone
- Message pad
- Pen or pencil

PROCEDURE STEPS:

1. Answer the call as outlined in Procedure 11-1.
2. Remain calm and avoid becoming upset with an angry caller. Let the caller say what needs to be said without interruption (unless it is a medical emergency requiring immediate action). RATIONALE: Permits the caller to express concerns without having to repeat information or possibly forget something important.
3. Lower your voice both in pitch and volume. RATIONALE: Has a calming effect on an angry caller.
4. *Listen to and acknowledge* what the caller is upset about. Paraphrase information to verify that you have understood the problem. RATIONALE: Lets the caller know you are truly listening and have understood the problem.
5. *Be courteous, patient, and respectful.* Use the words "I understand" and show that you are interested in hearing the caller's concerns. RATIONALE: This does not necessarily mean you agree with the caller, but rather that you are willing to empathize and at least accept that, from a particular point of view, there is a reason to be upset.
6. Do not take the call personally. RATIONALE: It is the situation that made the caller angry; you have not done so.
7. Offer assistance. RATIONALE: Ask what you can do to help, and then follow through.

(continues)

8. Document the call accurately and properly. RATIONALE: Complete documentation promotes risk management and prevents lengthy litigation experiences.

9. When dealing with a frightened or hysterical caller, *display a calm, caring, and professional manner* by speaking in a soothing voice; use a slower, lower tone than normal. RATIONALE: This often has a calming effect on the caller.

10. If the call is an emergency, begin screening procedures as needed and *attend to any special needs of the patient.* RATIONALE: Have a list of screening questions at hand to refer to or instruct the caller to dial 911. Be sure you have the name and telephone number for follow-up.

11. Always have the caller repeat the instructions you provided. RATIONALE: People who are upset may not hear or comprehend much of what is said. Your instructions may deal with an emergency situation; thus it is important they are clearly understood.

12. Finalize and follow through on action to be taken, whether it is confirming emergency medical personnel are on the scene or scheduling an emergency appointment. RATIONALE: Ensures quality patient care.

13. Always report problem calls to the provider or clinic manager at once. RATIONALE: This will ensure appropriate action is taken, and it is important for risk management purposes.

DOCUMENTATION:

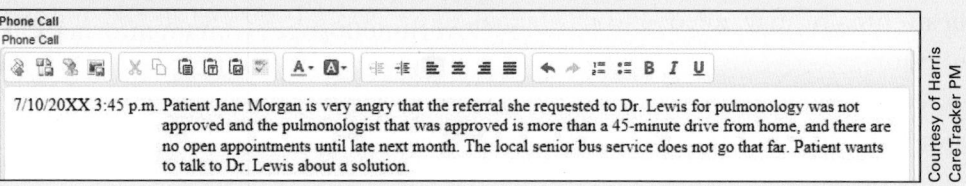

7/10/20XX 3:45 p.m. Patient Jane Morgan is very angry that the referral she requested to Dr. Lewis for pulmonology was not approved and the pulmonologist that was approved is more than a 45-minute drive from home, and there are no open appointments until late next month. The local senior bus service does not go that far. Patient wants to talk to Dr. Lewis about a solution.

Courtesy of Harris CareTracker PM and EMR

than normal. Do not shout. If you are uncertain that the person has heard everything, ask if there are any questions, or ask the person to repeat information back to you.

If the person has difficulty understanding you, simplify the information; ask frequently if there are any questions; and try to explain in simple, concrete terms. At times, if it is difficult to communicate with an older adult patient, someone from the patient's family should be given certain information. Discuss this option with the clinic manager or provider first, and be sure signed documentation is on file.

English as a second Language Callers. In any clinic, it is possible to have contact with many patients whose primary language is not English.

Diversity

It is extremely helpful to have at least one person in the clinic who is bilingual. For the nonbilingual medical assistant, certain techniques may help when communicating with all but totally non-English-speaking patients.

- A patient who does not *speak* fluent English may still *understand* as well as anyone. Do not assume that individuals with strong accents cannot understand you.

- Speak at a normal volume; raising the voice does not increase the other person's ability to comprehend.

- If the other person has difficulty understanding, speak more slowly. Avoid complicated words when simple ones will express the meaning just as well.

- Ask the person if clarification is needed. Be willing to review the information again.

- Be patient.

If these techniques are not successful, it is the responsibility of your provider-employer to supply an interpreter.

TELEPHONE DOCUMENTATION

Requests for medical information over the telephone should be discouraged. A provider or facility that needs the information to treat the patient usually places an emergency request. A call back verification procedure should be implemented for this type of request. Request the caller's name and telephone number, and state that you will call back with the necessary information. Then call back to verify the identity of the caller and provide or fax the information. It is important to follow this procedure

Patient Education

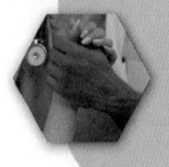

Patients who have difficulty with English may be confused by medical terms. Listen to the terms the patient uses and use those terms during conversation with the patient. Avoid using abbreviations without first explaining what they mean.

Diversity

during routine telephone interchanges that take place between facilities/provider clinics and laboratories seeking test results or consult findings.

Legal

All telephone requests for medical information should be documented either in a log reserved for that purpose or in the patient's medical record. This information is important to protect yourself and the medical practice in case of litigation. Documentation includes the following:

- Date of the request
- Name of the requestor
- The information requested
- Patient's name (and patient number)
- Name of the treating provider
- The information released
- To whom the call was referred (if applicable)

When a patient telephones the clinic to request prescription refills, is displeased with medical treatment, or expresses some form of a complaint, documentation of the call should always be recorded in the medical chart. Follow established clinic protocols when handling each and every telephone call. Document every call you have with a patient, including all pertinent information.

USING TELEPHONE DIRECTORIES

The medical assistant should have on hand in the clinic a variety of print and online telephone directories and be skilled in their use. The telephone directory contains an organized, accurate, and complete listing of the name, address, zip code, and area code with telephone number for most individuals with telephone service. Often, the pages within the directory are color-coded; residences are listed on white pages, business numbers on blue pages, and advertisements on yellow pages. The front pages of many directories contain other useful information such as:

- Information related to emergency and nonemergency numbers is provided.

- The Internet guide makes it easy to get online.
- An information guide and consumer tips provide a variety of free facts and answers about the things you want to buy and the services you need.
- Community pages provide attraction, event, and general-interest information unique to a particular geographic area. Often, maps are provided on these pages.
- Phone service pages answer questions you may have regarding your phone service.
- Government pages contain information about county, state, tribal, and federal government clinics, as well as information regarding public schools and voter registration.
- An index makes finding what you need easy.

While print telephone directories are still being published and distributed, it is becoming more popular to use Internet resources as the general public becomes more savvy with digital devices.

There are many types of online resources available, in the form of business directories, local listings, and search engines that will list web links for any key word or topics requested. This includes extensive information on local, state, and federal government sites, as well as a wealth of resources for finding people, places, events, and maps, beyond what the printed directory is able to offer.

Most medical centers and hospitals produce their own directory. These directories list important telephone numbers specific to that facility. Examples of information available within these directories include:

- Community education services
- Nurse counseling service/nurse line
- Main hospital/facility telephone number
- Automated operator
- TTY line for the hearing impaired
- Medical center departments
- Medical staff, including department and photo of providers and their names with credentials

Some of these publications list providers who no longer maintain their active/associate privileges at the facility. Often, a map of the facility is included within the front or back pages. Large facilities also may produce supplements to maintain current information.

Community Resources

Community resources are assets in a community that are available in the form of people, organizations, and locations that offer support and assistance to the needs of a certain population and improves quality of life. Often, there are patient needs that go beyond the capabilities of the clinic environment. In such situations, the clinic and its staff can provide guidance as a patient navigator and recommend, refer, or facilitate connecting the patient to the available resources that best meet their needs. In many cases, patients may be unaware that there are community resources that can aid them, as most are dealing with health related issues that may be new to them and their families.

It is a good idea to have community resources specific to the needs of the patients related to the clinic's speciality gathered and available for easy reference. Brochures, phone numbers of contacts,

and other useful information can be given out when needed. Representatives of service providers can provide materials, and some insurance carriers will have social or case workers that work with certain plans to assist the clinic with covered services and facilities from within a network. The Internet can provide a plethora of information on local resources and downloadable information or applications.

Examples of types of community resources for health care include adult day care, assisted living facilities, Alzheimer's support, cancer care, counseling services, crisis hot line, disability services, HIV/AIDS, home health agency and in-home treatment, hospice, medical equipment and supplies, mental health services, nursing homes, pain management, psychiatrists, senior citizens' services, Spanish/Hispanic services, substance abuse services, support groups, transportation, utilities assistance, veterans services, victims' services, and youth services.

Procedure

Procedures 11-5 and 11-6 provide direction on creating a list of community resources, and providing patient referrals to these community resources.

PROCEDURE 11-5

Procedure

Developing a Current List of Community Resources Related to Patient Health Care Needs

PURPOSE:

To use research tools to assemble a list of current community resources as a referral resource for patient health care needs.

EQUIPMENT/SUPPLIES:

- Internet access and search engine
- Telephone directory
- Hospital directory
- Pen or pencil
- Notepaper and binder

PROCEDURE STEPS:

1. Assemble research tools and equipment. Select three types of community resources discussed in the "Community Resources" section of this chapter. RATIONALE: Researching community resources will be based on the specialty practice and needs of the patients receiving services at the clinic. Select three of particular interest to you.

2. For each type of community resource selected, gather information and organize your data in a useful table for patient reference. Include name of resource; a brief description of the services or assets available; phone number, address, contact names if applicable; Website address; special instructions, if applicable; and other pertinent

(continues)

information. RATIONALE: Information given to patients should be accurate and as complete as possible to promote ease of use and compliance by the patient seeking services.

3. For each type of community resource selected, verify the information gathered and request further documentation and brochures, and ensure the resource is up to date with the latest data. RATIONALE: Services, location, and contacts often change and can become outdated. Periodically verifying and updating information will keep resources relevant for patients.

4. Create a binder for the clinic staff as a reference of the community resources researched. Organize the data in a Word table or Excel spreadsheet and print copies as a patient handout. RATIONALE: Community resources should be easily accessible for staff reference and made readily available to patients as the need arises.

PROCEDURE 11-6

Facilitating Referrals to Community Resources in the Role of a Patient Navigator

Procedure

PURPOSE:

To use a list of current community resources as a referral resource to facilitate referrals by guiding patients with information.

EQUIPMENT/SUPPLIES:

- Internet access and search engine
- Telephone directory
- Hospital directory
- Pen or pencil
- Referral sources from Procedure 11-5

PROCEDURE STEPS:

1. Using the referral sources from Procedure 11-5, offer the patient one of the resources by discussing services and assets, contact information, Web address, and other pertinent information gathered on the resource that is useful to the patient. RATIONALE: The patient or patient's family may need to be coached and advised when community resources are required. Assisting with contact information, other details, and feedback will help guide the patient where needed.

2. Verify the information with the patient, and then document the referral. Follow up in 48 hours by placing a call to the patient. RATIONALE: Documenting the referral in the patient record allows for follow-up with the patient, and offers a reminder to the staff of the resources given to the patient.

3. Print the referral information documented in the patient record to give to the patient.

PLACING OUTGOING CALLS

When making calls for the medical clinic, whether to patients, health care facilities, or other providers, know what information is needed and have it at hand before making the calls. For example:

- If arranging for a patient to receive care at another facility, have the patient's health

record and insurance information available. Determine provider instructions as to the diagnosis and type of care (specific tests, radiographs, and so on) that need to be ordered.

- If calling insurance companies for claim follow-up, gather copies of all claim forms and medical documentation so you can answer specific questions regarding each claim.

- If scheduling meetings or outside appointments for clinic providers, have their schedules in front of you.

Legal Arrange to make outgoing calls from a telephone in a location that is free of distractions. If the calls concern patients (whether about bills, insurance, or care), it is mandatory that the calls be made from a telephone where you cannot be overheard by other patients or people in the reception area.

Always choose a time when calls can be made without interruption. Do not make outgoing calls while covering incoming call responsibilities.

It is best to establish a routine for making various types of outgoing calls. Most clinics call the next day's patients to confirm appointments near the end of each day. Collection and insurance calls, as well as pharmacy callbacks, are usually done either before the clinic is open for patients in the morning, during the period from noon to 2 PM when the clinic is closed for lunch, or after the last patient has been seen.

PLACING LONG-DISTANCE CALLS

Most long-distance calls medical assistants make are likely to be direct dialing calls, that is, calls placed without the help of an operator. Many business phone packages used in the clinic will include free or low-cost long distance calling. There may be times when operator-assisted calls are necessary, although the use of these types of calls are less common. These can include:

- Person-to-person calls
- Conference calls
- International calls
- Collect calls

Conference calls may be local or long distance and are convenient for communicating or discussing information with several individuals at the same time. Each person involved in the conference call must be notified about specifics regarding the date and time, and any special instructions related to the call. Many clinics have conference call capabilities on their telephone or computer systems.

International direct distance dialing (IDDD) is available in many parts of the Unites States. Additional numbers or codes may preface the international access, country, and city codes when using IDDD. Station-to-station calls may be dialed following this sequence:

- Dial the international code 011
- Dial the country code
- Dial the city code
- Dial the local telephone number
- Press the pound sign (#) button if the telephone is touchtone

It may take up to 45 seconds after dialing any international code for the ringing to begin. The Internet posts frequent updates on international call procedures and country and city codes.

When making a long-distance call out of the area code, it is possible that a time zone change may occur (Figure 11-6). When scheduling the day's calls, it is important to keep in mind the location of the call and plan accordingly. Time zones in the United States include Pacific, Mountain, Central, and Eastern times and usually span a three-hour difference. If it is noon in New York, it is 11 AM in Illinois, 10 AM in Arizona, and 9 AM in Washington state.

Many conventional telephone companies, wireless services, and Internet providers are competing for long-distance business. Judging the offers and services of long-distance companies can be a complex task, but a wise choice can save a clinic hundreds of dollars a year or more in telephone charges. It is important to analyze the medical clinic's long-distance requirements and then make comparisons among several long-distance companies. Company representatives usually are more than willing to discuss their services in light of specific needs to help you comparison shop. The decision of which service to use will usually be made by the providers and the clinic manager with feedback from all employees.

LEGAL AND ETHICAL CONSIDERATIONS

Legal Two of the most important issues in the medical setting are patient confidentiality and the right to privacy. Respecting the confidentiality of all patient information

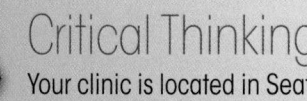
Critical Thinking
Your clinic is located in Seattle, WA, and you are calling Charleston, NC. What are some important considerations before placing the call?

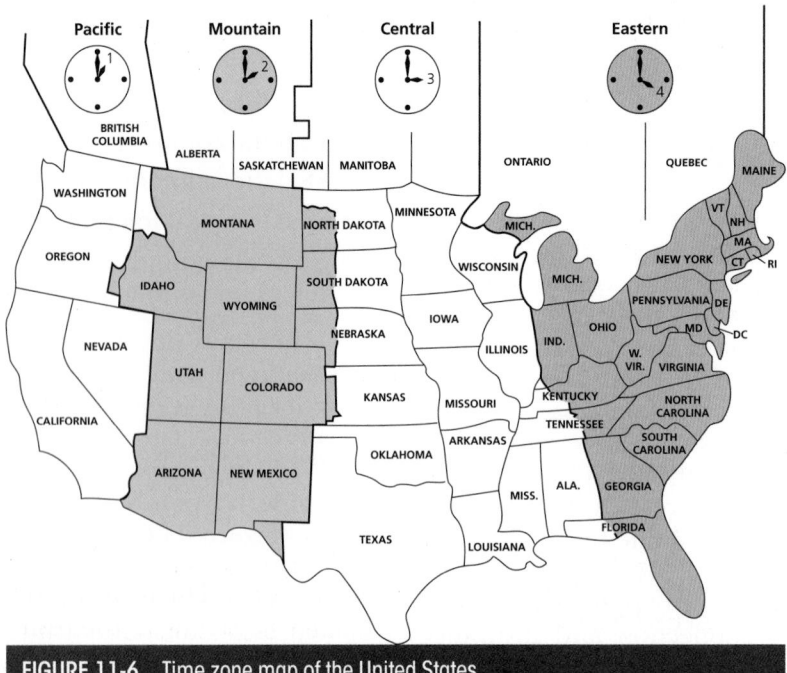

FIGURE 11-6 Time zone map of the United States.

is a legal and ethical obligation. No information about patients is to be discussed outside the clinic, with family or friends, or with other patients. All notes that may be jotted down on paper during telephone calls must be disposed of following clinic protocols. In most cases, this means shredding the notes. Violations of confidentiality leave you and your provider open to lawsuits. More importantly, they are violations of patient trust.

Integrity

When calling patients, whether to discuss treatment or finances, do so with respect for the patient's privacy at all times. The front desk is certainly not the place to make collection calls when other patients are in the reception room. Either make calls from another location or choose a time when other patients cannot overhear you. Always be aware of the surroundings and who may be able to overhear conversations.

There are many situations when individuals will call the clinic to discuss a patient. Parents, spouses, grandparents, other relatives, significant others, employers, and friends often will have questions about a patient's condition or finances. Usually these people are asking questions out of genuine concern and a desire to help. The information they request may seem harmless, but discussing anything about a patient can turn into an ethical and legal issue.

To ensure patient confidentiality and practice sensible risk management, never discuss a patient with:

- The patient's spouse or family, without specific permission and a signed release
- The patient's employer
- Insurance carriers, HMOs, or attorneys without a signed release
- Credit bureau/collection agencies (reporting a patient to a credit bureau or collection agency is a violation of confidentiality if medical information is disclosed)
- Other patients
- People outside the clinic (friends, family, acquaintances)

When necessary for medical or administrative reasons, you can discuss a patient with:

- Members of the clinic staff as necessary to the patient's care
- The patient's insurance carrier or HMO, if you have a signed release
- The patient's attorney (usually in accident or Workers' Compensation cases), if you have a signed release
- The patient's parent or legal guardian, except concerning issues of birth control, abortion, HIV, or sexually transmitted disease (check

the laws in each state regarding minors' right to privacy)

- Another health care provider (provider, laboratory, or hospital) that is providing care to the patient under orders from the patient's provider
- Referring provider's clinic

HIPAA GUIDELINES FOR TELEPHONE COMMUNICATIONS

The following guidelines should be followed when communicating information to patients by telephone:

- Determine whether the patient has requested confidential communications. Specific instructions should be provided to staff members on how to determine whether the patient has requested and been granted special conditions for keeping communications with the medical practice confidential.

- If the patient has not requested confidential communication, the patient should simply be called at the standard phone number contained in his or her records. If the patient has requested confidential communications and has provided an alternative telephone number, care should be taken to ensure that only the alternative number is called.

- The caller should identify himself or herself by name and say that he or she is an employee of the medical practice (use the complete official name of the practice).

- If the patient is not available, it is acceptable to leave a live or recorded message asking the patient to return the call. Leave the telephone number, and if the medical practice is returning a call made by the patient, it is acceptable to state this in the message that is left for the patient. However, it is important that the message does not contain any medical information or mention the purpose of the call. Never leave a message containing test results.

- When the patient is contacted, it is acceptable to discuss his or her medical information over the telephone. It is critical, however, that test results and other protected health information (PHI) *not* be given to anyone other than the patient or a person designated as the patient's representative.

AMERICANS WITH DISABILITIES ACT (ADA)

Safety

The ADA requires that communication procedures are available for persons with disabilities. Combined with HIPAA requirements, this presents a challenging situation in dealing with patients who are deaf or hearing impaired. The act requires that health care providers give effective communication alternatives using auxiliary aids and services that ensure that communication to people with hearing loss is equal to others without this disability. This includes patients as well as caregivers of patients, guardians, or spouses.

Alternative devices or services include interpreters for individuals with a language problem, assistive hearing devices, note takers for individuals who have difficulty writing, written materials, and so forth. The health care provider can choose the device as long as the result is effective communication. The patient who is deaf or hard of hearing should be consulted on which device he or she finds to be most effective. The cost of alternative devices or services cannot be billed to the patient. The expense must be charged against the overhead of the clinic or practice.

Telephone service for patients who are hearing impaired is required by the ADA. Many individuals who are hearing impaired, deaf, or speech impaired may use a teletype (TTY) or telecommunication device for the deaf (TDD). These devices transmit a keyed-in message via the telephone network just as a voice message would be sent if spoken. The recipient of the message reads the keyed-in message on the TTY's text display. A TTY or TDD device is required at both ends of the conversation in order to communicate. In addition, Internet chat capability that can replace TTY or TDD devices is readily available online.

TELEPHONE TECHNOLOGY

Though much of this chapter has been dedicated to the interpersonal nature of telephone communications, astute medical assistants will also investigate and become knowledgeable about the technology of telecommunications.

Ongoing advances in telecommunications have had a tremendous impact on how the staff of a medical clinic communicates both within the clinic and with patients, hospitals, and others outside the clinic. These advances include telephone systems with automated routing units, Voice over Internet Protocol (VoIP), electronic transmissions (fax and email), and cellular phones.

Automated Routing Units

Many hospitals and larger ambulatory care settings have **automated routing unit (ARU)** telephone systems to manage heavy telephone traffic. The system answers the call, and a recorded voice identifies departments or services the caller can access by pressing a specified number on the touch-tone telephone. If callers indicate they are having a medical emergency, the system can be programmed to immediately route calls to the medical assistant. This saves patients with immediate medical problems from waiting during busy telephone times.

Most automated telephone systems have electronic mailboxes so the caller can leave a message if the person they are calling is unavailable. In many ARU systems, selecting any of the numbered choices often gives the caller a second, third, or fourth menu of choices. If the caller does not select an option, the ARU will usually switch the call automatically to a live operator.

A disadvantage with ARU systems is that the recorded voice may be difficult to hear, especially for older adults or patients who are hearing impaired. Many patients may not understand the recorded options. Clinics with an ARU system should provide to all patients an information sheet explaining their options when calling the clinic and how to get through to the clinic quickly in an emergency.

Answering Services and Machines

One responsibility of the clinic manager/medical assistant is to ensure that patient calls are answered after clinic hours, both in the evenings and on weekends. Although in smaller ambulatory care settings it may not be possible to have staff on telephone duty 24 hours a day, nonetheless calls must be answered and messages taken. **Answering services**—typically staffed by a live operator—and answering machines are two methods of taking calls after hours.

Many ambulatory care centers favor answering services because a live operator is reassuring to patients and other callers. These services also can provide flexibility in routing calls and locating the provider for emergencies. Typically, fees for answering services are by the month or by the number of calls.

Answering machines are convenient but perhaps less reassuring for the caller. The machine must be checked frequently for messages should an emergency occur. Sometimes, the message may leave a telephone number where the provider can be reached, but this system is likely to be cumbersome, because too many nonemergency calls may be directed to the provider. If an answering machine is used, the message often contains a number, other than the provider's, that callers can use for emergencies. That call is answered by a live operator who then screens and refers the call appropriately.

Voice over Internet Protocol (VoIP) Telecommunications

Voice over Internet Protocol (VoIP) is a rapidly growing form of telecommunication. The biggest advantages to VoIP are price and flexibility. On the surface, a VoIP phone seems like a common landline telephone, but VoIP services convert a voice into a digital signal that travels over the Internet or a virtual private network. When calling a regular telephone number, the signal is converted to a regular phone signal before it reaches the destination. VoIP calls can be made directly from a computer, a special VoIP phone, or a traditional telephone connected to a special adapter wherever there is broadband connectivity.

Three different types of VoIP services are in common use:

- *Analog Telephone Adapter (ATA).* The ATA allows connection through a standard telephone using a computer or network connection. The ATA is an analog-to-digital converter. It takes the analog signal from a traditional phone and converts it into digital data for transmission over the network. VoIP providers usually bundle the ATAs free with their service.

- *IP Phone.* These specialized phones look just like normal telephones. They have an RJ-45 Ethernet connector in place of the standard RJ-11 telephone connectors. IP phones connect directly to the cable router with all the hardware and software included. Special WiFi phones allow making VoIP calls from any WiFi hotspot. These devices have all of the security problems associated with WiFi (see Chapter 10).

- *Computer to Computer.* This was the original VoIP form of telecommunication. Several companies offer free or very-low-cost software that can be used for this type of VoIP service. Aside from an Internet-connected computer with audio card, microphone, and speakers, nothing else is required. Except for a normal monthly ISP fee, there usually is no charge for computer to computer calls regardless of distance. This type of VoIP can be vulnerable to security problems depending on the security of the URL employed.

Most VoIP providers bundle call waiting, caller ID, three-way calling, repeat dial, return call, and call transfer with the service plan.

Some of the disadvantages of VoIP telecommunications are as follows:

- Most VoIP services do not work during power outages.
- Emergency services through 911 may not be available.
- Directory assistance/white page listings may not be available.

 VoIP Security. Small and medium-sized organizations are increasingly adopting VoIP technology. With the increased popularity of this technology, the likelihood of attacks by cyber criminals increases. A cybercriminal attack on a VoIP service could mean the criminal eavesdrops on conversations; interferes with audio streams; or disconnects, reroutes, or even answers other people's phone calls.

Safety

VoIP is part of the Internet and is susceptible to disruption of service and spam just as are other Internet services. A potentially more serious security problem with VoIP, however, is eavesdropping on sensitive conversations. Hackers can eavesdrop on unprotected media streams and intercept VoIP packets to obtain sensitive information by reassembling the packets into speech. One way for hackers to do this is through a man-in-the-middle attack, where a third party spoofs the unique hardware address (MAC address) of the two speaking parties, forcing the IP packets to flow through the hacker's system. Although eavesdropping is not just a risk for VoIP telecommunications, the nature of IP networks makes access to the phone conversations much easier. Eavesdroppers no longer need to physically put a tap into a phone line; they can simply gain access from a laptop connected to the network. A hacker breaking into a VoIP data stream has access to more calls than he or she would with a traditional telephone wiretap. As a result, the hacker has a much greater likelihood of getting useful information by tapping a VoIP data stream than from monitoring a traditional phone system. Another security compromise possible with VoIP is intercepting a genuine call to a bank and rerouting it to a bogus bank teller.

 The following are a few of the safeguards that can be used to provide in-depth protection to a VoIP system:

Safety

- Use dedicated VoIP phone instruments (having a digital certificate), not a *softphone*. A softphone uses software for making telephone calls over the Internet on a general purpose computer.
- Use a stateful packet inspection (SPI) firewall. This type of firewall technology ensures that all inbound packets are the result of an outbound request.
- Ensure that VoIP service providers have security in place for their internal systems.
- Update security patches for computer operating systems and VoIP software.
- Encrypt voice traffic.
- Use a virtual private network (VPN) to separate the data stream from the public Internet over which it travels. This is accomplished by connecting to a server that is set up to communicate with your device using an encrypted data flow. Any data that may be intercepted by a nearby hacker is rendered totally useless unless the encryption code is known. Most corporations use VPNs they operate, and VPN-for-hire firms are available to provide servers to small organizations and individuals. In the case of VPN-for-hire servers, the connection between your device and the Internet is secure; however, the connection between the server and your traffic's destination is not.

Facsimile (Fax) Machines

 Fax machines are common in ambulatory care settings as they are used to send reports, referrals, insurance approvals, and informal correspondence. A **fax** is a **facsimile** transmission sent over telephone lines from one fax machine to another or from a modem to a fax machine. A fax can be sent as easily as putting the document in the machine, similar to the way a document is put in a copy machine, and dialing the receiving telephone number. There are other issues involved in using the fax, especially when sending patient information. Several legal and confidentiality issues should be considered before sending any communications by fax. These include obtaining proper

Legal

records release authorization, using fax machines in secure and not publicly accessible areas only, using a cover sheet with a confidentiality warning, and confirmation of the receiving fax number, with a follow-up call to verify arrival at proper destination.

HIPAA requires all medical practices to implement technical measures to protect against unauthorized access to protected health information (PHI) when it is transmitted over electronic telecommunications networks. Two security measures must be addressed: the integrity of the information transmitted, and the vulnerability of the information to unauthorized use or disclosure.

When information is transmitted over public networks, static and other less benign problems can introduce errors into the information. The security rule requires the implementation of security measures to verify the integrity of the information that is transmitted.

Information transmitted over public networks may be intercepted and used by unauthorized users. In some cases, the interception can be deliberate to access sensitive information. In other instances, the interception may be the result of error by the person making the transmission. For example, a person sending a fax dials the wrong number and sends information to an unintended recipient.

The security rule requires implementation of a mechanism to encrypt PHI when appropriate. Encryption requires the cooperation of both parties to the transaction, and the encryption methods are specified in any agreement between the parties.

With the increasing use of electronic records, much of the information that was sent between medical facilities by fax is now being accessed through secure, digital means.

Each medical facility involved in a particular transaction will need to have access to the same system, and as electronic software becomes more wide-spread in use, this will be more easily possible. The required data are obtained faster and under more secure circumstances because they are contained in the EHR.

Additionally, if the medical record is not accessible between facilities, patients can now be given their records on digital media, such as a DVD or flash drive, containing documents, digital images, and other necessary data that can easily be taken to the next provider that needs to review this information. Even uploaded large files, such as images, can be shared between business associates using secure file sharing systems over the Internet.

Electronic Mail (email)

Electronic mail (email) involves the process of sending, receiving, storing, and forwarding messages in digital form over computer networks. Email is a non–real-time method of communication—it permits us to leave a message at our convenience and allows the recipients to read and respond at their convenience. Emails can be sent to multiple people at the same time, something a traditional telephone call does not allow. Keep in mind, however, that there is a professional email etiquette that must be adhered to. It is not acceptable to forward email messages without the permission of the original author, and caution must be taken to avoid sending information that is not appropriate in a professional setting.

Composing email is similar to composing any written communication. Just as a letter or memo has a particular format, the email transmission should also follow a format style. The subject line should be brief and clearly identify the content of the email body.

If your message is in response to another piece of email, your email software probably will preface the subject line with *Re:* (for "regarding"). If your email software does not do this, it would be polite to key in "RE:". If your message is time critical, starting with "URGENT" is appropriate. If you are referring to a previous email, you should explicitly quote that document to provide context.

If a message is to be sent to several parties, individual email messages may be sent to each, thereby protecting their privacy. In many instances, however, it is useful for parties involved in a group "conversation" to be aware of who the other participants are. In this case, all of the addresses may be included on the same email message. Sending a "bcc," or blind copy, also protects the privacy of your email because it does not show to whom else the message was sent.

The body of the message should contain short and clear sentences. In trying to be brief and to the point, however, it is important to not leave out important facts or information. Remember also that some email software only understands plain text. Italics, bold, and color changes should be used sparingly. Some software recognizes **URLs (Uniform Resource Locators)**, more commonly known as Web site addresses, in the text and makes them "live" so they can be clicked and opened. Because different software recognizes different parts of the address, if you include a URL in your email message, it is much safer to use the entire address, including the initial http://. See the following Quick Reference Guide for additional email etiquette.

The advantages of using email as a means of communication include:

- Asynchronous communication—both parties need not be available at the same time for communication to take place
- Providers and patients can prepare, leave, read, and respond to messages at times that are convenient
- Can be used to automate certain tasks such as sending out appointment reminders or normal reports of laboratory results
- Creates a documentation trail of interactions between provider and patient
- Some patients may be more forthcoming using email than in face-to-face discussion
- Reimbursement for time spent receiving and responding to clinical email may be billed under the Online Medical Evaluation section of the Current Procedural Terminology reference (see Chapter 17). Codes should be checked for changes and updates annually for these services. As of January 2016, modifiers have been introduced, to be used with CPT codes. The current CPT and Healthcare Common Procedure Coding System (HCPCS) codes that describe a telehealth service are generally the same codes that describe an encounter when the physician and patient are in the same location.
- Modifiers are being used to describe the technology used in a Telehealth encounter. One of these modifiers should be used to distinguish between an encounter that has taken place by telecommunication, as opposed to the provider and patient being at the same site. These modifiers are—GQ (Via Asynchronous Telecommunications systems) and—GT (Via Interactive Audio and Video Telecommunications systems).

The disadvantages of email communications include:

- Lack of real-time interaction and feedback
- Lack of body language or vocal inflection, which may lead to misunderstanding
- May not be suitable for time-sensitive material because determination of when the message will be delivered or read cannot be assessed

Safety

Encryption of Email. To prevent possible compromise of medical data when using email, **encryption** renders the transmission essentially secure. Encryption of email can be accomplished in several ways: The email service provider can employ TLS (transport layer security) protocol or its predecessor, SSL (Secure Socket Layer). The email will automatically be encrypted for transmission. The URL address will display the *https* prefix and a padlock icon when the email provider uses this protocol (see Figure 10-3). If the provider does not use this protocol, the sender can initiate encryption by obtaining and using a digital ID. Digital IDs, sometimes referred to as certificates, allow recipients to verify that an email was actually sent by the intended person. Because forging, hijacking email addresses, and even hackers intercepting email is common, a digital ID can be used to encrypt messages, hide their content, and protect the email as it reaches its destination.

If the e-mail service provider used in the clinic does not already provide Digital ID, follow the instructions provided by the service to turn on this feature, when available. At many businesses, the system administrator will provide and set up emails for office use with encrypted email. Most email service providers are working toward encrypting messages sent to and from servers. TLS is being adopted as the standard for secure email, and most of the well-known providers, such as Outlook, Google Mail, and Amazon, have already implemented this encryption technology, either TLS, SSL, or both.

Patient Portal Systems

Patient portal systems are secure online Web sites or applications combined with other software, such as an EMR, that allow patients to have convenient 24-hour access to interact and communicate with their health care providers. Because the patient uses a login and password, the portal environment is much more secure compared to using regular email. The area for communications is usually set up much like the standard email interface most people are now accustomed to, including buttons to compose (write), send, and read messages.

A patient portal system may be available as a stand-alone Web site, offered and administered as a service by vendors to health care providers. Other portals can be integrated directly into the existing Web site of the clinic or hospital, and yet others are application modules that can be added to the EMR. These patient portal systems are becoming more popular to use, as they offer the capacity to utilize patient health information in a secure manner via the Internet.

⫸ EMAIL ETIQUETTE

Most organizations implement etiquette rules for the following reasons:

- Professionalism: Using correct grammar, spelling, and language conveys a professional image.
- Efficiency: Email is a more effective means of communication.
- Protection from liability: Appropriate, business-like language in all email communications limits liability risks.

Remember that an email message is not delivered with body language. A great deal of human communication comes from nonverbal signals such as facial expressions and tone of voice. These cues help make the message clearer. The following etiquette rules promote professionalism, efficiency, and protection from liability:

- Use proper structure and layout. Use short paragraphs and blank lines between each paragraph. When making points, number or bullet each point. Keep it brief, but give pertinent details.
- Do not attach unnecessary files.
- When sending attachments is necessary, tell the recipient the format of the attachment. If a large attachment must be sent, call the recipient first to be sure his or her Internet service will accept it.
- Do not overuse the high priority option.
- Do not overuse Reply to All. Use this feature only when your message needs to be received by everyone. Do not copy a message or attachment without permission. You could be infringing on copyright laws.
- Use a meaningful subject. This helps the recipient focus immediately.
- As a courtesy to your recipient, include your name at the bottom of the message. The recipient may not know that the return address belongs to you.
- Do not write anything you would not say in public.
- Do not write in CAPITALS. If you write in capitals, it seems as if you are shouting.
- Do not send flame emails; that is, insulting messages designed to cause pain, as when someone "gets burned."

When confidential or privileged material is sent via email, it should include a disclaimer stating that any review, retransmission, dissemination, or other use of the material is prohibited. It should also state that if the message is received in error, the recipient should contact the sender and delete the material from the computer. See the example below:

This message is a privileged and confidential clinical communication intended solely for the person to whom it is addressed. If you are not the intended recipient, please be advised that any disseminating, copying, or distributing of this message is strictly prohibited. If you received this message in error, please forward it back to the sender.

Providers and patients are realizing the benefits of using a portal system in terms of increasing efficiency and productivity. Clinics are reporting reduced costs in mailing referrals, lab results, and other correspondence. Reduced phone calls to the clinic for routine requests and inquiries have also been realized. The ability for staff or providers to respond to patients at a time of convenience, and redirecting tasks as required to medical assistants, billing specialists, or other providers has its benefits. Below is a list of health information patients can view, as outlined by the Health IT Standards Committee at www.healthit.gov:

- Recent doctor visits
- Discharge summaries
- Medications
- Immunizations
- Allergies
- Lab results

In addition to exchanging email with the health care team, patients may also be able to do the following tasks in the portal:

- Request prescription refills
- Schedule nonurgent appointments
- Check benefits and coverage
- Update contact information
- Make payments

- Download and complete forms
- View educational materials

As is usually the case with similar technology, the patient portal system can have some drawbacks. The patient must provide information to the clinic so that a registration password, or token, can be issued. This will allow the patient to set up a secure login and password and create an account. Some patients can forget to follow through with the process upon arriving home from the clinic, and for others, having to track multiple family members, such as individual children, becomes difficult with so many logins. Another drawback comes for patients who have multiple providers. A person with a PCP and a few specialists due to complex health issues may very well have many portals that are not integrated, causing a disconnect with continuity of care. This is an area that may be addressed in the future, and become more standardized, especially with EMR modules.

One concern providers may have is that they will be overwhelmed with email messages, patients not adapting to the patient portal, or communication issues between patients and providers. Table 11-2 lists some common concerns, many of which are actually unfounded, based on studies done on the current patient portal systems in use today.

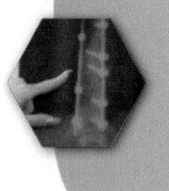

Critical Thinking

What legal and ethical issues should be considered when using email? How might the medical facility protect its employees and patients with regard to email use?

Patient portal systems also factor in where Meaningful Use is concerned. Meaningful Use encourages providers to switch from paper charts to electronic records. If a provider provides services to Medicare or Medicaid patients, that provider may be eligible to qualify for the Meaningful Use program. For providers that do not participate, Medicare penalites began in 2015. Medicare offers incentive payments for adopting electronic health records. These incentive payments are equal to 75% of Part B allowed charges up to an annual maximum. In contrast, those providers that do not comply will be penalized starting at 1% of their Part B Medicare reimbursements, increasing each year to the 5% maximum.

There are three stages to the implementation of the Meaningful Use program. In order to have met the 2014 requirements of the Centers

TABLE 11-2

COMMON CONCERNS WHEN USING PATIENT PORTAL SYSTEMS

CONCERN	FACTS
Providers will be flooded with email messages from patients.	Rather than being inundated with messages, providers report increased efficiency and appreciate being able to respond to patients at their convenience. Evaluation studies find that telephone volume decreases when secure messaging is introduced.
Patients may use messaging inappropriately.	Studies find that the communication content of patient messages tends to be appropriate, addressing non-urgent care issues. Best practice is to educate patients about when and how to use secure messaging.
Providers will be unable to bill time for communicating with patients on the portal and the practice will lose revenue.	Portal features have been found to provide cost savings by decreasing indirect and direct labor costs, such as mailing costs for lab results, online billing questions versus telephone, online appointment scheduling, and online appointment reminders.
Patients will be confused or upset by information contained with the EHR.	Best practices for displaying test results include providing a brief explanation and guidance for any follow-up along with the results.
Patients won't adapt to using a patient portal.	A majority of consumers favor using online tools to communicate with providers, obtain lab results online, and make appointments. Medical practices have had success in getting a wide range of patients—including the elderly, lower income, and those with chronic illnesses—to use a patient portal.

Source: HealthIT.gov

for Medicare and Medicaid Services (CMS) Electronic Health Record (EHR) for Meaningful Use, health care providers must have a patient portal installed. The requirements for how actively the provider and patients use the portal are dependent on which stage of the Meaningful Use program the provider is in.

Legal and Ethical Issues. When using email or communicating within a patient portal, it is important for providers and staff to remember that the same ethical responsibilities to patients must be adhered to as for other types of encounters. The same standard of professionalism must also be satisfied. Along with the convenience offered through digital communications come some risks. Fortunately, following specific guidelines can minimize risks to a level considered acceptable by many practices.

Legal

Patients who meet criteria for digital correspondence established by the practice should be identified, and an informed consent form should be signed by each patient desiring this mode of communication. The form may be part of the form used for handling release of PHI or may be part of the registration process for the patient portal. The form should provide instructions to the patient in the secure use of email, the security risks involved, and practice policies for communication. As discussed, a disclaimer absolving the practice in the event of patient noncompliance or technical failure in the system is recommended. The original signed form should be filed in the patient chart and a copy given to the patient for his or her records.

A procedure should be established to automatically respond to patients' email messages informing them they have been received. Patients should also be requested to respond to your messages acknowledging their receipt.

DOCUMENTATION

From: Elizabeth J. Parker
Sent: Tuesday, July 20, 20XX 8:55 am
To: Dr. King [King@doctor.com]
Subject: Prescription refill

Please call in a prescription refill for my thyroid medication. The pharmacy is Inner City Pharmacy and the phone number is 890-271-2600. The prescription number is RX6437350 and I have enough pills for three days

---

Telemedicine, Video Conferencing, and mHealth

The remote delivery of health care by means of telecommunications is referred to as **telemedicine**, also known as telehealth. Video conferencing is a method of having an interactive encounter with a patient in a remote location using two-way video and audio transmission. For patients, this means having access to medical professionals and services, no matter their geographic location, which offers them the potential to receive care that may not be available locally. Providers can now make virtual house calls, conduct consultations, and monitor ICU and emergency department patients, in cooperation with on-site staff. For patients with mobility issues, who are incarcerated, or who are otherwise unable to afford travel or to physically do so, the possibilities of expanding access to medical care through video conferencing are exciting.

In addition, providers using video conferencing have the opportunity to not only access expanded information and training, they also have the ability to collaborate with other professionals in the latest medical developments and techniques, or obtain assessments before moving forward with a patient care plan. The potential for professionals to improve quality of care, outcomes, and benefit to patients by sharing expertise and knowledge beyond the local hospital or clinic will eventually transform how health care is delivered.

mHealth, or m-health, stands for *mobile health*, a term that refers to the practice of medicine supported by mobile devices. The term *mHealth* is most commonly used when referencing the specific use of mobile devices, such as smart phones, tablets, and other portable devices, for health services. According to the analyst firm Berg Insight, the number of people monitored using mobile telecare systems in Europe and North America was about 450,000 at the end of 2015. Growing at a compound annual growth rate (CAGR) of 40%, this number is expected to reach almost 3.4 million by 2021. In addition, as smart phones and tablets continue to become commodities available around the world, especially in more poor regions or those just recently gaining access to the Internet, there will be more opportunities for much needed medical care and resources to reach these areas virtually by connecting patients and health care providers remotely.

An added benefit is the cost saving potential of telemedicine, for both providers and patients. A current challenge is getting insurance companies to adopt this technology and have a consistent reimbursement system for telemedicine options. Many are slow to adopt what is considered relatively new or unproven health care delivery methods. Medicare will consider reimbursement only for patients in rural areas or medically underserved areas, and then only for video conferencing. However, as the projected mass use of mHealth devices continues to grow worldwide, eventually insurance administrators will need to start integration of and payment for telemedicine services.

PROFESSIONALISM IN TELECOMMUNICATIONS

Professional

Professionalism in telecommunications is crucial in the medical clinic environment. The way in which the telephone is answered conveys either a message of a sincere desire to help or a message of interruption. Callers expect to have the phone answered in a professional manner and their concerns addressed promptly. Forwarding calls to someone else in the clinic who is more specialized in the topic of the caller's questions and following up to see that the situation was resolved provide evidence of a responsible attitude and of being a team player. One should always be courteous and diplomatic and work within the scope of one's education, training, ability, and legal boundaries.

Remember that personal telephone calls, other than emergency calls, should be avoided during working hours. When speaking with patients or other health care members, slang terms should not be used. Never eat or chew gum while answering the telephone. When completing a call, say "good-bye" and allow the caller to hang up before you do.

Additional attributes of professionalism include using appropriate guidelines when releasing information. Confidentiality guidelines must always be followed, with awareness of any ethical or legal responsibilities. Documentation is mandatory for follow-up care and for any legal implications. Continuing education is important to stay on the leading edge of new technologies being implemented in the area of telecommunications.

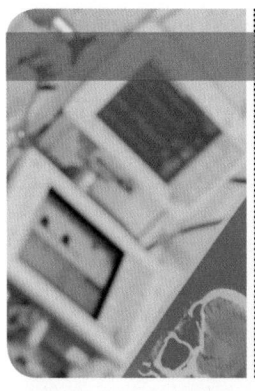

CASE STUDY 11-1

Refer to the scenario at the beginning of the chapter.

CASE STUDY REVIEW

1. Recall ways to maintain composure when handling and screening incoming telephone calls.
2. Describe the three types of VoIP services and identify safeguards that can be used to provide in-depth protection to a VoIP system.
3. Discuss HIPAA requirements related to fax machine use and PHI.
4. What is encryption, and how is it used with email communication?

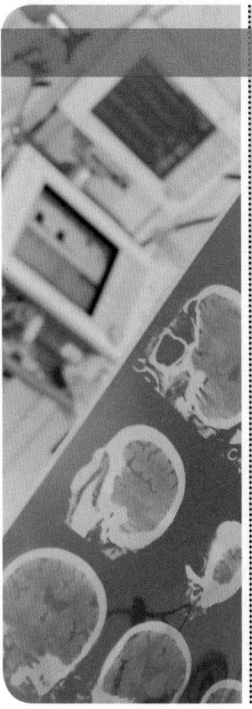

CASE STUDY 11-2

Nancy McFarland, RMA (AMT), a clinical medical assistant at Inner City Health Care, receives a telephone call from Claussen-Mason Laboratories requesting medical information about patient Juanita Hansen. Nancy is told by laboratory personnel that the information is needed to perform the tests scheduled by Dr. King. Wanda is not familiar with this request and asks if she can check the chart and return a call to the laboratory (callback verification procedure).

CASE STUDY REVIEW

1. What information will Nancy need from Claussen-Mason Laboratories?
2. What is the purpose of the callback verification procedure?
3. After the verification has been established, what should Nancy do?

DOCUMENTATION:

In the log reserved for telephone documentation, the following entry could be made based on Case Study 11–2.

PROCEDURE NOTE

A▾ Ⓐ▾   B *I* U

07/16/XX 4:00 p.m. Claussen-Mason Laboratories requested previous laboratory findings from Qwik Lab for Juanita Hansen, patient number 306-30-7840. Juanita is a patient of Dr. King. The information was released to Janet Bailey, employee of Claussen-Mason Laboratories, as directed by Dr. King. N. McFarland, RMA (AMT)

- By means of telecommunication, which can also include fax, wireless technology, and email transmissions, patient appointments are scheduled, referrals made, critical information related, and the practice personality conveyed.

- Medical assistants are to be prepared for incoming and outgoing calls.

- The medical assistant must be familiar with basic telephone techniques, project appropriate tone and personality, and maintain telephone etiquette and courtesies.

- Effective screening techniques must be used, so that each caller is directed to the area or individual best able to assist him or her. Screening promotes good use of time and resources for those receiving calls, by redirecting to those better able to handle the call, or by collecting further information so that a response can be obtained and addressed at a more appropriate time.

- Proper telephone techniques include transferring calls with the data necessary to follow through, and taking detailed messages, so that the respondent has complete information for returning the call.

- The medical assistant will take a variety of calls, and must know the proper responses or actions to take, as agreed to by the provider-employer or clinic manager. This facilitates routing of calls correctly and establishes a "put through" list of the types of calls to be referred to the provider immediately.

- The medical assistant will also handle special considerations calls, including placing calls to facilities outside the clinic, using clear and direct language; maintaining proper composure and action when receiving emergency phone calls; dealing with older adults or those that speak English as a second language; and defusing and assisting angry callers.

- Proper documentation of messages should be completed, and care must be taken with requestors of personal information. Basic data gathered should include name of the requestor, the information requested, patient's name (and patient daytime or mobile number), name of the treating provider, and the information released.

- The medical assistant must understand email use in the clinic, and the legal and ethical responsibilities for using it, adhering to the same standards as for other encounters.

Study for Success

To reinforce your knowledge and skills of information presented in this chapter:

- Review the *Key Terms* and *Learning Outcomes*

- Consider the *Critical Thinking* features and *Case Studies* and discuss your conclusions

- Answer the questions in the *Certification Review*

Procedure

- Perform the *Procedures* using the *Competency Assessment Checklists* on the *Student Companion Website*

CERTIFICATION REVIEW

1. How can the medical assistant create a positive first impression over the telephone?
   a. Using the hold button sparingly
   b. Being authoritative with the caller
   c. Not permitting the caller too much leeway to speak
   d. Working while talking on the telephone

2. What telephone personality techniques convey an effective telephone personality?
   a. Volume, enunciation, pronunciation, and control of speed
   b. Being assertive with the caller
   c. Not spending too much time talking
   d. Referring all calls to the provider
   e. Talking in a distracted manner

3. When transferring a telephone call, what guidelines will not ensure the successful transfer of the call?
   a. Determining who would be the best person to assist
   b. Following your telephone system's procedure for transferring the call
   c. Following up to be sure the call transferred correctly
   d. Getting the caller's name and telephone number is not necessary

4. How should the medical assistant handle a problem from an angry caller?
   a. Take it personally
   b. Listen calmly to the upset person
   c. Become upset to identify with the patient
   d. Ask emotionally charged questions to calm down the patient
   e. Put the caller on hold

5. What is the proper callback verification procedure?
   a. It should never be documented.
   b. It should always be documented.
   c. It should sometimes be documented.
   d. It is not appropriate in the ambulatory clinic setting.

6. What is an example of an inappropriate security measure when using the fax to send PHI?
   a. Have a signed form authorizing the release of PHI before releasing the information
   b. Faxed messages should only be sent to telecopiers that are located in a secure area
   c. A cover sheet containing warning of confidential information is not necessary when faxing
   d. Always recheck before sending the fax that the correct telephone number was selected and entered correctly
   e. After faxing, call the person who is receiving the fax and confirm that it was received

7. What is the definition of screening telephone calls?
   a. It is the act of evaluating the urgency of a medical situation and prioritizing the call.
   b. It is expressing oneself clearly and distinctly.
   c. It is using expendable words while answering the telephone.
   d. It is the ability to be objectively aware of and have insight into others' feelings, emotions, and behaviors.

8. When are TTY and TTD devices used in the clinic?
   a. By individuals with hearing and/or speech impairments
   b. When most individuals are placing long-distance calls
   c. When using smart phones
   d. When using facsimile machines
   e. Never

9. Which example does not apply to the use of clinical email to or from the patient?
   a. Clinical email to or from patients should be treated differently than telephone messages or letters
   b. Print and file the initial message and any reply to clinical email in the patient's chart
   c. Have a written agreement of understanding signed by all patients using clinical email
   d. Use clinical email protocols in the clinic procedure manual

10. How does the medical assistant provide privacy when making telephone collection calls?
    a. By ensuring no other patients can overhear details of the call
    b. By selecting a private location to place collection calls
    c. Collection calls made at the front desk during office hours are always acceptable
    d. Collection calls are always handled by a collection agency
    e. Both a and b

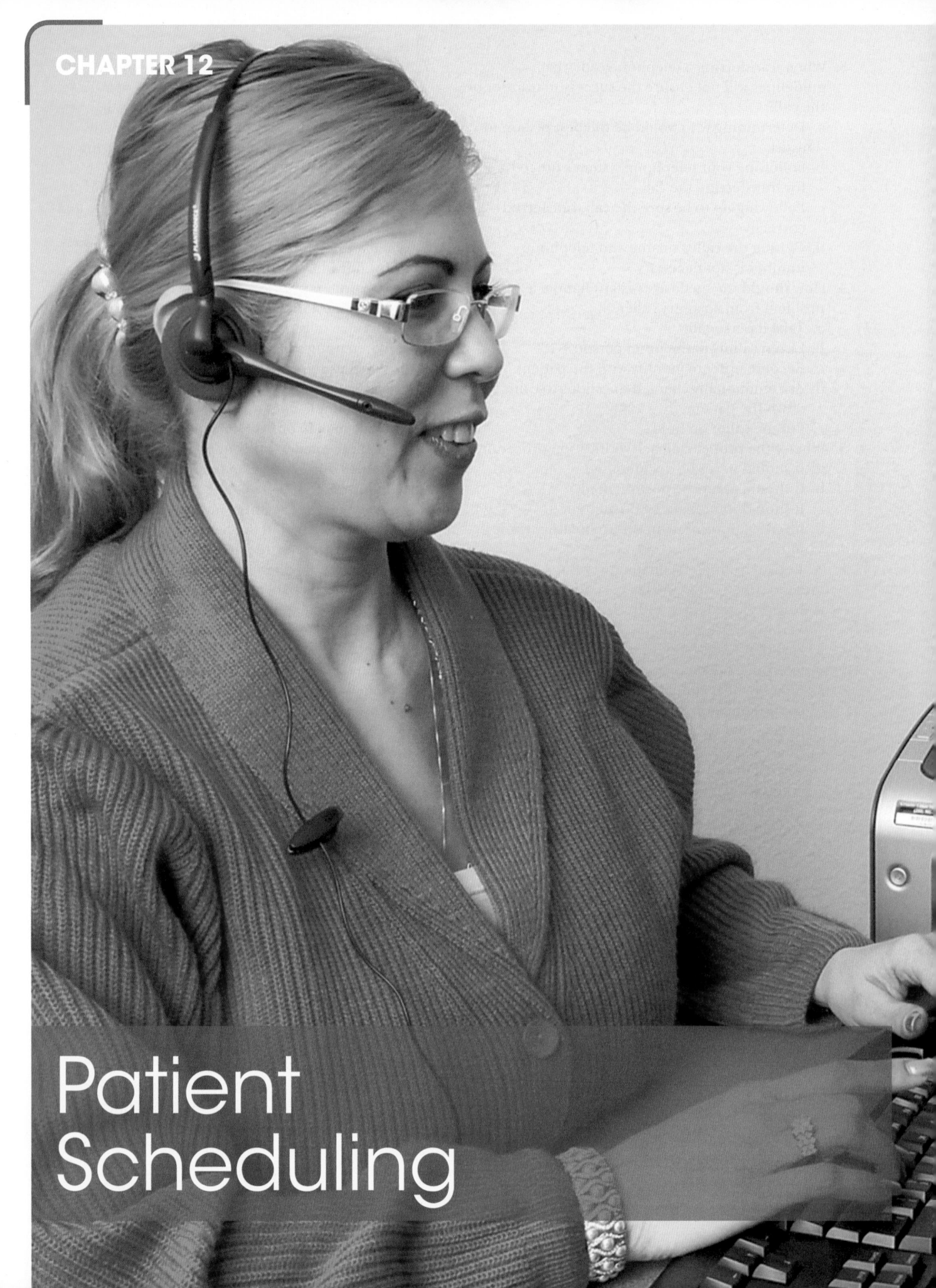

Patient Scheduling

1. Define and spell the key terms as presented in the glossary.
2. Identify pros and cons of six major scheduling systems.
3. Describe the guidelines in scheduling appointments.
4. Explain the importance of screening in scheduling patient appointments.
5. Review proper cancellation procedures and explain the legal necessity of documenting cancellations.
6. List and define three types of reminder systems.
7. Choose an appropriate appointment scheduling tool and describe its advantages.
8. Establish a matrix for the upcoming quarter for a provider.
9. Check in patients using a daily appointment sheet.
10. Schedule appointments using a manual system and an electronic system.
11. Schedule outpatient procedures and inpatient admissions.
12. Explain why there is a move toward online scheduling and DIY appointments using EMR and patient portals.

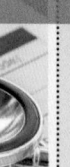

KEY TERMS

cluster scheduling

double booking

encryption technology

matrix

modified wave scheduling

practice-based scheduling

screening

stream scheduling

wave scheduling

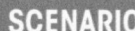

SCENARIO

At Inner City Urgent Care, medical assistant Walter Seals, CMA (AAMA), is responsible for efficient patient flow. Because Inner City is an urgent care center, patients are seen as walk-in appointments, on a first-come, first-served basis unless there is an emergency situation. Inner City also operates specialty care clinics, and these clinics require scheduled appointments. Walter has found that the clustering system is most efficient for these specialized care clinics, with certain days dedicated to certain procedures.

Because of the high volume of patients and the need to coordinate multiple provider schedules, Walter's job is not an easy one. However, Inner City is computerized, so paperwork is easy to generate as appointments are made, canceled, or rescheduled. And although Walter manages a smooth patient flow, he makes it a point to remain flexible to accommodate patient needs and keep stress to a minimum.

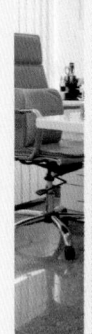

Chapter Portal

Patient scheduling has undergone many changes. A medical appointment is most often scheduled over the telephone or in person. Information technology allows appointment scheduling through secure online access using the clinic's Web site or patient portal system. However the appointment is made, the medical staff will need the patient's home telephone number and will want the number of the cellular phone that often accompanies the patient

continues

or is used in place of a landline telephone. In the case of online appointment requests, the patient's email address is necessary. If online appointment scheduling is available at the clinic, the medical assistant may ask if the patient has a computer and is willing to use the computer for online appointment scheduling.

Patient scheduling is an integral part of the daily workload for medical assistants, whether in large family practices, urgent care centers, or sole proprietor clinics. Scheduling becomes more complicated if providers are practicing in more than one location and traveling between them. Scheduling patients can be stressful, especially if the telephone rings constantly and the medical assistant is unable to provide patients a convenient appointment.

Although patient appointment scheduling may seem like a routine function, a smooth patient flow often determines the success of a day in the clinic. A variety of administrative skills are used in the performance of this vital function. By effectively scheduling patients to fit a particular practice, it is possible to make profitable use of provider and staff time.

In addition, efficient patient flow pleases the patient. A common patient complaint is the time spent waiting in the reception area or the examination room. Most patients appreciate a clinic that recognizes the value of their time. Accordingly, these patients do not hesitate to advertise their experience (good or bad) to friends and families—a fact of great significance to any medical setting.

In addition to the required administrative skills, medical assistants involved in scheduling patients must put into practice their best interpersonal and communication skills. Scheduling an appointment may be the first contact patients have with the medical facility. They remember and value the treatment they receive from the time of first contact. The personality of the clinic is always reflected in the treatment and respect given to patients.

Whether scheduling is done online, through a computerized system, or in the paper appointment book (rare these days), practitioners and their staff must remember the importance of that first impression and make it satisfying for patients.

TAILORING THE SCHEDULING SYSTEM

Competency

The patient population of each medical facility will determine the best method for scheduling appointments. A surgeon's clinic will have a much different flow of patients than a pediatrician's clinic. The key is to customize the system to best accommodate the practice. Primary goals in determining this should include:

- A smooth flow of patients with a minimal amount of waiting time
- Flexibility to accommodate acutely ill, STAT (or emergency) appointments, work-ins, cancellations, and no-shows

Medical providers may feel uncomfortable if their days are not busy with patients or they experience idle time. It is also true that patients want access to their medical providers when needed and prefer not to wait several days to be seen. There is no one perfect scheduling style, and some facilities may even be unable to identify their style of scheduling by name. One thing is certain, however; patients, providers, and their staff will know when scheduling is not working successfully.

SCHEDULING STYLES

There are a number of methods for patient scheduling. The best method for a practice is the one that effects good patient flow and proper utilization of staff and physical facilities and meets the needs of the provider(s). Traditionally, all scheduling was done by writing appointments in a book by hand. Increasingly, however, scheduling is done using computer software designed specifically for that purpose or using scheduling programs that are part of practice management (PM) software. Keep in mind that even the most sophisticated computerized system will fail if the scheduling style does not comfortably fit the predetermined and necessary patient flow.

It is important to note that some clinics may use terminology that makes a distinction between types of hours kept in a clinic. For instance, *patient hours* may be used to indicate the hours patients are seen by providers in the clinic. *Office hours* may indicate when the clinic is open. For example, a clinic may have office hours of Monday through Friday, 8 AM to 5 PM and be closed on Wednesday afternoons. However, patient hours are Monday mornings and afternoons, Tuesday afternoons, and Thursday and Friday mornings. Whenever the clinic does not have patient hours, the staff customarily will be at the clinic completing the many tasks of the practice.

Some clinics ask patients to sign in as they arrive. Some legal authorities believe that the only infallible way to prove patients have kept a medical appointment is to have them sign their name upon arrival and give the time. The Health Insurance Portability and Accountability Act (HIPAA) has ruled that patients can be asked to sign their name upon arrival as long they are not asked to provide any other personal information, such as address, telephone number, Social Security number, or clinic identification number. HIPAA has also ruled that patients cannot be forced to sign if they feel uncomfortable in doing so. A word of caution is important here. The patient's right to privacy ensures that patients do not see confidential information (such as the reason for the visit) of other patients. HIPAA regulations have caused facilities to be more cognizant of patients' rights to privacy and confidentiality.

If the setting and circumstances indicate that a sign-in sheet for patients is the most efficient means of checking in patients, forms can be purchased that meet the privacy and confidentiality expectations of patients.

Figure 12-1 illustrates a carbonized pack with perforations that allows a patient to sign in giving the necessary information. The patient is instructed to remove the top ticket, leaving the information on the bottom form only. The next person to sign in does not see the information of the previous patient. In cases where complete confidentiality is required, this type of ticket also has a number in the upper right-hand corner. The medical assistant can call the patient by number, instead of by name, in environments where this may be necessary.

Open Hours

In open hours scheduling, patients are seen throughout a particular time frame, for example, 9:00 AM to 11:00 AM or 1:00 PM to 3:00 PM. Patients are seen on a first-come, first-served basis. Many clinics frequently choose this method because they are able, by their nature, to maintain a steady flow of patients. A sign-in sheet is often helpful with open hours scheduling, because patients are seen on a first-come, first-served basis. It is important to remember that a sign-in sheet can never replace a warm, welcoming greeting from the administrative medical assistant to set the tone for care given that day.

Double Booking

When the **double booking** method is used, two or more patients are given a particular appointment time. This method is limited to a practice that can attend to more than one patient at a time. For instance, Maria Jover and Jim Marshal are both given a 9:30 AM appointment. Ms. Jover requires a complete checkup including lab tests, vitals, and provider visit. Mr. Marshal is being seen for suture removal. While the staff conducts the lab tests on Ms. Jover, the primary care provider can see Mr. Marshal. Obviously, this method requires a precise accounting for time, rooms, and adequate staff. A good rule to remember is that if patients consistently have to wait for staff to attend to them, double booking is not a wise choice of scheduling method.

Clustering

The **cluster scheduling** method involves grouping or categorizing similar types of visits or procedures on particular days or blocks of time. Cluster scheduling is sometimes referred to as *specialty scheduling*, or **practice-based scheduling**. It is popular in clinics where groups of patients require similar visit types and are scheduled during these predetermined times.

Examples would include an OB/GYN clinic, where all prenatal checks are scheduled so that two to three patients come in every 15 or 30 minutes. The medical assistant generally will handle the vitals sign, weight, and other pertinent information, and the provider can check in on patients and focus on those that turn out to not be routine, have problems, or are more complex cases that require attention.

Another example would be a day or time block set aside by surgeons for postoperative checks. Most of these follow-up visits involve making sure incision sites are clean and healing well, and that the patient is following all medication and therapy

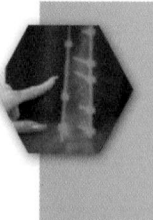

Critical Thinking

When a sign-in sheet is used for patients but the administrative medical assistant is assisting the other staff members when patients arrive, what can be done to create an atmosphere that welcomes patients and puts them at ease?

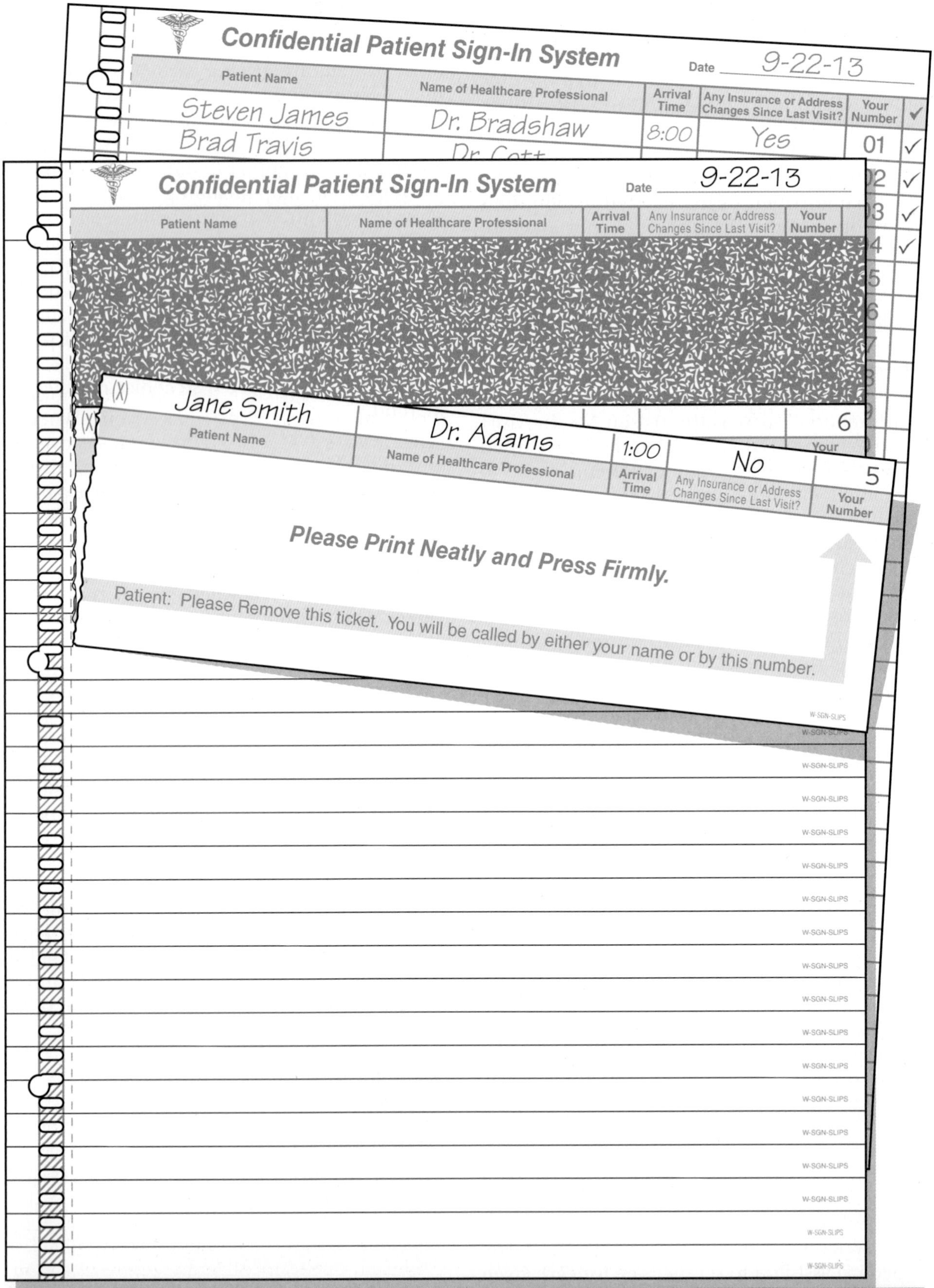

Confidential Patient Sign-In System   Date _____ 9-22-13 _____

Patient Name	Name of Healthcare Professional	Arrival Time	Any Insurance or Address Changes Since Last Visit?	Your Number	✔
Steven James	Dr. Bradshaw	8:00	Yes	01	✓
Brad Travis	Dr. Cott			02	✓
				03	✓
				04	✓

Confidential Patient Sign-In System   Date _____ 9-22-13 _____

Patient Name	Name of Healthcare Professional	Arrival Time	Any Insurance or Address Changes Since Last Visit?	Your Number
				6

(X) Jane Smith   Dr. Adams   1:00   No   5

| Patient Name | Name of Healthcare Professional | Arrival Time | Any Insurance or Address Changes Since Last Visit? | Your Number |

Please Print Neatly and Press Firmly.

Patient: Please Remove this ticket. You will be called by either your name or by this number.

W-SGN-SLIPS

FIGURE 12-1   Confidential patient sign-in system that offers privacy. A patient can be called by the number of the ticket or by name.

orders and progressing as expected. Again, these visits are normally quick and routine. Clustering allows a higher volume of patients to be seen comfortably. This can be very convenient for the patient, taking away long wait times for what might be a 5- or 10-minute post-op check.

There are many creative ways for certain specialties to utilize cluster scheduling. Having similar patients together also offers opportunities for patient education. Presenting videos or information sessions on particular procedures or conditions can optimize everyone's time. This could include initial visits for bariatric surgery, where patients will be evaluated and need to complete a battery of required assessments or meetings before surgery can be approved or scheduled.

It is important for the clinic to maintain an atmosphere of individualized care, and avoid an assembly-line feel. Staff, rooms, and resources will need to be carefully planned to keep the larger volume of patients flowing efficiently.

Wave Scheduling

Wave scheduling is another method that can be used effectively in medical facilities that have several procedure rooms and adequate personnel to staff them. Using the wave scheduling system, patients are scheduled only in the first half hour of each hour. For example, three patients may be given the time of 11 AM. Generally, the first one to arrive is seen first. If they all arrive on time, the one who is most ill is usually seen first, and there will be a waiting time for the other two patients. Depending on the practice, some administrative medical assistants will be instructed to schedule three patients at the top of the hour and another two or three patients at the bottom of the hour (e.g., 11:30 AM). Patients who do not understand this system of scheduling may become irritated if they discover that another patient has the same appointed time with the same provider. This method takes into account that there will be no-shows and late arrivals. It can also accommodate work-in appointments. However, it does require personnel who are able to prioritize patient problems precisely when establishing the appointments.

Modified Wave Scheduling

Modified wave scheduling is a variation of the wave method where patients are scheduled in "waves." In this method, two or three patients are scheduled at the beginning of each hour, followed by single appointments every 10 to 20 minutes the rest of the hour.

A variation of this method assesses major and minor problems. Major time-consuming problems are seen at the beginning of the hour (e.g., new patients). Minor problems are seen from 20 minutes past the hour to half past the hour (e.g., follow-ups, bandage changes, and other minor procedures), and walk-ins (e.g., a child with a 103°F temperature) are accommodated at the end of the hour. Again, good screening will determine the success of this method.

With both the clustering and wave methods, empty or unscheduled periods can be used to catch up on other responsibilities.

Stream Scheduling

Stream scheduling is perhaps the best known and most widely used scheduling system. When this system works as it should, there is a steady stream of patients at set appointment times throughout the workday. There could be, for example, a 30-minute appointment at 9:00 AM; a 15-minute appointment at 9:30 AM; and a 15-minute appointment at 9:45 AM. Each patient is assigned a specific time. This can best be accomplished by establishing realistic time guidelines for particular types of appointments, such as 45 minutes for consultations, 15 minutes for immunizations, and 30 minutes for hearing tests.

Online Scheduling

As technology advances in health care, so does the concept of self-scheduling patient appointments. New self-scheduling software that integrates with electronic health record software is available, and not just for smaller or specialized practices with small or no staff. Larger practices are realizing higher efficiency, decreased phone calls, and happier patients by allowing do-it-yourself (DIY) appointments.

In this age of people reserving tables at restaurants, hailing a taxi, or buying groceries right from their smart phones, the demand for self-scheduling of routine doctor appointments is more prevalent. Currently, many clinics are using *patient portals*, which may include either appointment requests or self-scheduling modules (see Chapter 11).

A patient portal is a secure Web site that provides a patient with 24-hour access to his or her health care information for a particular practice. Popular functions include communicating via email with the health care team, obtaining test results, requesting medication refills, and many other capabilities, such as requesting or scheduling appointments.

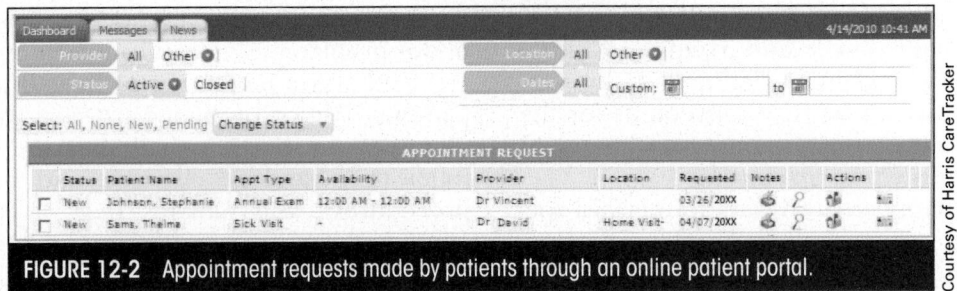

FIGURE 12-2 Appointment requests made by patients through an online patient portal.

Some portals will allow a patient to request an appointment, and a staff member will schedule it and send a confirmation back to the patient (Figure 12-2). Others enable the patient to select a date, or the next available date and time, and self-schedule an appointment.

Consider a recent survey by Accenture, a business services and consulting company, which shows 77% of patients think that the ability to book, change, or cancel appointments online is important. A rapid explosion in the use of digital solutions for DIY appointment scheduling will radically alter the U.S. health system marketplace over the next 5 years. Accenture research predicts that by the end of 2019, there will be 66% of U.S. health systems offering digital self-scheduling and 64% of patients will book appointments using digital tools. Nearly 38% of appointments will be self-scheduled, representing almost 986 million appointments.

ANALYZING PATIENT FLOW

When reviewing the current scheduling practice, a simple analysis can maximize a clinic's scheduling practices. This entails looking at appointment times, patient arrival times, the actual time a patient is seen, and the time a visit is completed. A simple grid chart can be produced for a given period, for example, 1 to 2 weeks (Figure 12-3). In addition, monitor and chart the number of no-shows and cancellations. An electronic scheduling system can automatically provide the detail necessary to analyze the effectiveness of patient scheduling. It has the capability of indicating the scheduled time for specific procedures, for each provider, and for each service given to the patient.

This analysis will provide a clear picture of patient flow and whether personnel are being used efficiently. The data will assist in estimating how many patients to schedule and realistic time frames for particular problems or procedures. If the staff is scheduling return patients every

PATIENT FLOW ANALYSIS

February 2, 20XX — Dr. King

Patient Name	Length of Appt.	Appt. Time	Time Seen	Time Out
Martin Gordon	15	10:20	10:22	10:45
Jason Jover	45	11:20	11:20	12:30
Nora Fowler	30	1:00	1:25	1:45
Jim Marshal	15	1:30	1:50	2:10
Herb Fowler	60	2:45	2:15	3:25

FIGURE 12-3 Patient flow analysis helps a practice determine realistic time frames for appointments.

15 minutes yet the analysis shows these visits average 24 minutes, then the scheduling method needs adjustment. This may mean either allowing more minutes for follow-up visits or building in slack time when no appointments are made.

Develop a simple list of commonly scheduled visits with time estimates for each. This procedural sheet will be particularly useful when training new employees or when temporary help is used for scheduling. A list of commonly scheduled visit types with set duration times can also be set up when using an electronic scheduling system (Figure 12-4).

Waiting Time

One of patients' frequently voiced frustrations with medical clinics is excessive waiting time. Obviously, emergencies and other unexpected

Appointment Type	Group	Duration	Active
Established Patient CPE	All	30	Y
Established Patient Sick	All	15	Y
Follow Up	All	15	Y
Lab	All	15	Y
MA Visit	All	15	Y
New Patient CPE	All	45	Y
New Patient Sick	All	45	Y
PAT	All	60	Y
Pap Smear	All	30	Y
Procedure	All	30	Y
X Ray	All	15	Y

Add New | Build Schedule | Show All

FIGURE 12-4 Most practices have a list of typical types of visits with time estimates.

interruptions cannot be anticipated. However, there are certain measures the medical assistant can take when attempting to keep the schedule on target. If patients are kept waiting, it is a good strategy to explain the reason for the delay and give patients an estimate of how long the delay will be. *Never* ignore the delay hoping patients will not notice; doing so may even increase perceived waiting time. Find ways to make patients comfortable while they wait; for example, provide an appropriate choice of reading materials (or in the case of children, activities). If a delay can be anticipated—for example, if the provider is called away for a baby delivery or surgery—attempt to contact patients before they leave home to reschedule the appointments.

If the delay is likely to be a half hour or longer, provide patients with options, for example:

1. Offer patients the opportunity to run an errand, having them return at a specified time.

2. Offer to reschedule appointments for another day, or later that day, or to see another provider in the practice if possible.

In any case, remember that good customer relations dictate your willingness to acknowledge the inconvenience to the patients, and do attempt to provide an acceptable solution. Remember also that some patients simply will not appreciate any efforts to apologize for a delay, in which case you must continue to act professionally toward them.

LEGAL ISSUES

Legal

Information provided in any patient scheduling system may be used for legal purposes. A case of malpractice or questions regarding a provider's availability may require a copy of the daily schedule. It might become necessary to identify how many times a particular patient was a no-show or canceled an appointment, never calling to reschedule. The appointment schedule could verify that a patient was seen and treated on a particular day, thus affirming the information in the patient's record. A patient sign-in sheet may serve this purpose, also.

All computerized systems provide a permanent record of patients seen, and any alterations to that schedule are saved and are shown when a printout is produced. If an appointment book is still used, the staff will have to make certain there is a permanent record or daily appointment sheet that indicates cancellations, work-ins, urgent care needs, and no-shows. Any changes to the daily appointment sheet are to be made in pen; therefore, there will be no question regarding accuracy.

Taking the time to accurately and consistently document all aspects of patient care makes a statement about the providers in the practice and their staff and reflects positively on the presumed quality of patient care.

INTERPERSONAL SKILLS

Presentation Communication

Scheduling appointments requires interpersonal skills. Medical assistants convey a great deal to patients through attitude and actions as well as empathy. A hurried or disinterested manner communicates that the patient is not a priority. Because patients are often distraught or anxious when making appointments, it is extremely important to reduce rather than increase anxiety. Also, the medical assistant who schedules appointments may be the first contact a patient has with the clinic; patients do not easily forget rude or insensitive staff. A hurried, disinterested manner toward patients is just as often the basis for legal action as is a negligent act.

If any form of online scheduling is used, be certain that it is user friendly, has a rapid response time of no more than 24 hours, and provides patients an option if the online scheduling proves unsatisfactory for any reason. Make certain that staff are ready for online scheduling and that those responsible for assignments and backups are carefully prepared. It is important that patients not be made to feel inadequate if they choose not to use online scheduling.

The patient should always be made to feel worthy of attention. This validates his or her reason for calling. If you are scheduling a patient in the clinic and the phone rings, answer the call but excuse yourself first. Ask the caller to please hold for a moment. If you are on the telephone scheduling a patient and another patient walks in, acknowledge with a nod or signal that you will be right there— never let the person feel ignored. Today, patients have a variety of options for health care and tend to be much more consumer conscious of the treatment they receive.

GUIDELINES FOR SCHEDULING APPOINTMENTS

Whether completed by manual methods or computer technology, the process of scheduling appointments for patients and other visitors to the clinic involves a number of variables, including (1) the urgency of the need for an appointment; (2) whether the patient is a referral from another provider; (3) recording methods for new and established patients; (4) implementation of check-in, cancellation, and rescheduling policies; (5) use of reminder systems; and (6) accommodating visits from medical supply and pharmaceutical company representatives.

Screening Calls

Urgent calls will need to be screened or assessed, before they can be scheduled. **Screening** calls is defined as the person making the appointment determining the actual urgency of that call and how the patient can best be scheduled. This requires both communication skills and medical knowledge, especially details specific to the clinic itself according to the practice specialty.

Appropriate questions will be asked to determine the actual urgency. Is the patient in immediate need of medical assistance? Is there any bleeding? If so, where? How profuse is the bleeding? Are there chest pains? How intense is the pain? Is the pain localized? How long have the symptoms been present? The medical assistant needs to determine whether this is a life-threatening matter, or whether the problem is urgent in the patient's eyes but not a medical emergency. Precise information

will help to determine the critical or noncritical nature of the call.

In screening the patient's urgency of care, be tactful in questioning and avoid making the patient feel that the need is insignificant. If questioning indicates this is a medical emergency, follow the policy for having the patient seen (whether it be an emergency appointment or referral to the emergency department). If referral to the emergency department or a call to 911 is necessary, make the call for the patient, being certain you have the correct address and telephone number available. Such a referral minimizes disruption to patients being seen in the ambulatory care setting. If it is determined that the best method in handling this emergency is to see the patient in the clinic, let scheduled patients know of the emergency and offer them the opportunity of rescheduling or waiting until the emergency has been resolved. A built-in slack time of 30 minutes in the morning and 30 minutes in the afternoon can provide some flexibility in last-minute emergency scheduling. If it is determined that the situation is not an emergency, work the patient into the schedule as the situation warrants and time allows, and make certain the patient is comfortable with the scheduled time. Be sure to leave the patient with the understanding that you have done your best to address the situation. (See Chapters 8 and 11 for more information on screening.)

Referral Appointments

One of the primary sources of patients for any provider is referrals from other providers. This is especially true in a managed care climate, where patients usually must have a referral from their primary care provider and where providers are part of an HMO network. It is important that these appointments be given special consideration and that referred patients are given an appointment as soon as possible.

Adequate information needs to be obtained to determine the urgency of scheduling. If the referring provider or clinic staff calls directly, the situation can be assessed at that time. However, if the referred patient calls, it is best to obtain necessary records and information from the referring provider's clinic to determine the urgency and appropriateness of an appointment. Often, the referring provider's clinic has initiated a referral authorization from the patient's insurance and this is forwarded to the appropriate provider. The patient also receives a notification that the referral was approved, and to which doctor. The notification may be sent to the patient by regular mail, a patient portal system, or other secure method.

If the patient does not know if a referral authorization has been obtained, or the authorization has not been received, it may be necessary to direct the patient to ask the referring provider for authorization. In some cases, the medical assistant will need to call the referring provider's clinic to obtain more information before an appointment is scheduled. Assure the patient that an appointment will be scheduled upon receipt of the authorization, and then follow up as required.

Recording Information

Patients can be sensitive to the amount of information they are required to provide to make an initial appointment. Keep the information as simple as possible and obtain only essential information. It should be tailored to fit the practice; for example, an obstetrician and a pediatrician will have different questions for the first-time patient.

When patients schedule an appointment online via the clinic's Web site, they are directed to a patient preregistration and health history that can be completed online prior to coming to the facility. The information provided in this format is often more detailed than what is obtained over the telephone. Nevertheless, the following basic items should be obtained from a new patient:

1. The patient's full legal name (with the correct spelling)
2. A daytime telephone number
3. The reason for the visit
4. The referring provider, and when relevant, if a referral authorization has been obtained
5. Date of birth
6. Type of insurance
7. Insurance identification and group numbers

In privacy, repeat this information back to the patient to ensure accuracy. The critical determination is whether the information is essential to the first contact or whether it can be obtained at the time of the visit.

An established patient, someone who has already been seen in the clinic, should be required to provide only the following information:

1. Full legal name
2. Chief complaint or reason for the visit
3. A daytime telephone number
4. If the patient has not been to the office in more than six months, or if it is the first quarter of the year, confirm whether address or insurance information have changed and update where needed.

When the information is recorded, print legibly and accurately if using a manual system and key in the information if using a computer system. Check for accuracy in either system. Record the appointment as soon as it is made—never rely on memory.

When scheduling an appointment time, ask the patient what day and time is most convenient and then make the appointment for the first available time stated. If possible, provide the patient with a choice of appointment times. Finally, confirm that the patient clearly understands the date and time of the appointment; be sure to repeat the date and time to ensure that both of you have recorded the same information. If the patient is making the appointment in person, provide an appointment reminder.

Scheduling an appointment for the clinic's available times for anyone with an extremely busy schedule can require a great deal of patience. If the patient requests a particular appointment that is not possible, courteously offer an explanation.

Many ambulatory care settings, especially those specializing in family practice and pediatrics, provide alternative hours for scheduling appointments. Having evening appointments at least one day a week or Saturday morning appointments can be helpful for individuals whose work schedule does not permit weekday appointments.

Appointment Matrix

Procedure

Before appointments can be scheduled, the times a provider is not available will need to be blocked out. This is called establishing the **matrix**. The matrix provides a current and accurate record of appointment times available for scheduling patient visits. Clinic hours are noted with times blocked when the facility is closed. Provider's schedules, vacations, holidays, hospital rounds, and any responsibilities that make providers unavailable for appointments are recorded. The matrix of the scheduling plan might include slots for patients who need to see only staff members for their appointment; therefore, times when they are unavailable are important to the matrix. Any evening or weekend appointment slots available also are noted (see Procedure 12-1).

Typically, when using an electronic system for scheduling, the program will search through a database of appointments, find an open appointment, and allocate an appointment time according to your instructions. These instructions can include finding an open appointment with a specific time length, on a specific day, or within a

PROCEDURE 12-1

Establishing the Appointment Matrix

Procedure

PURPOSE:

To have a current and accurate record of appointment times available for scheduling patient visits.

EQUIPMENT/SUPPLIES:

- Paper appointment scheduling system or computerized PM system
- Provider and staff schedule

PROCEDURE STEPS:

1. Block off times in the appointment scheduler when patients are not to be scheduled. Ideally, the whole year can be mapped out to avoid scheduling patients when the provider has other commitments or when the clinic is closed.

   a. In paper system, make an *X* through these time slots. This establishes the matrix.

   b. In a PM system, open the scheduling module and block the time slots patients are not to be scheduled by date and time.

   RATIONALE: Identifies visually when patients cannot be scheduled for an appointment.

2. Indicate all vacations, holidays, and other clinic closures as soon as they are known. It may be helpful to indicate absences that might affect patient scheduling; for example, the vascular laboratory technician is gone April 20–23, so no Doppler procedures will be scheduled. RATIONALE: Informs all staff members of absences from the facility and indicates when these members are not available to see patients.

3. *Paying attention to detail,* note all provider meetings, hospital rounds, appointments, conferences, vacations, and other prescheduled provider commitments. If the provider has routine items, such as a Medical Society meeting that is always held on the first Thursday of the month at 7:00 PM or daily hospital rounds at 8:00 AM, write these in. RATIONALE: Informs all staff members of prescheduled commitments when a provider is unavailable to see patients.

4. If the clinic has a scheduling system for certain examinations or procedures (e.g., all cast removals are done in the morning before 10:30 AM), these can be color coded with highlighters in a paper system. In a PM system, use the method specific to the software to assign either color, room assignment, or staff assignment for special procedures and equipment. By utilizing these methods, it is easily and quickly evident where particular types of appointments are available to be scheduled. RATIONALE: Allows all staff members to see at a glance where certain examinations or procedures can be scheduled. The color-coded highlighting helps prevent errors in establishing such specific times for certain procedures. The completed matrix provides proof of the completed task.

specified time frame. Once the appointment time is confirmed with the patient, patient data are keyed in, and the appointment is automatically scheduled.

Telephone Appointments

Procedure

More appointments are made by telephone than by any other method. Remember the guidelines for appointment scheduling and appropriate screening of all calls to determine urgency and need, and to follow your provider-employer's instructions regarding patient referrals for appointments. Make certain that you get all the necessary information from the patient when the appointment is made. Procedure 12-2 provides practice for telephone appointments. The professional manner in which telephone appointments are made for patients sets the tone for their satisfaction with the clinic, its providers, and their care.

Patient Check-In

Procedure

Records of patient appointments serve a legal purpose. Establishing a procedure for checking in appointments simplifies tracking the arrival of patients (see Procedure 12-3). This is particularly true in

Making an Appointment

Procedure

PURPOSE:

To schedule an appointment, entering information in the appointment schedule according to clinic policy.

EQUIPMENT/SUPPLIES:

- Telephone
- Paper appointment scheduling system or computerized scheduling PM system

PROCEDURE STEPS:

1. In a private and quiet location, answer the ringing telephone before the third ring. Identify the facility and yourself. RATIONALE: Assures the patient calling that he or she has the correct number; sets the tone for the conversation. The private location ensures that others will not hear any information said during the telephone call.

2. As the patient begins to speak, make notes on your personal log sheet of the patient's name and reason for the call. RATIONALE: Makes certain you are focusing on the call and will not have to ask the patient to repeat something you missed.

3. *Applying active listening skills*, determine whether the patient is new or established, the provider to be seen, and the reason for the appointment. RATIONALE: Provides necessary information to determine when the patient should be seen and how much time will likely be necessary.

4. *Discuss with the patient any special appointment needs*, and search your appointment schedule (using appointment book or the appointment search feature in the PM system) for an available time. RATIONALE: Tells the patient that his or her needs and the needs of the clinic are essential to this conversation.

5. Once that patient has agreed to an appropriate time, enter the patient's name in the schedule.

   a. In a paper system, enter last name first, followed by the first name, telephone number (home, work, or cell), and the chief complaint (reason for the visit).

   b. In a PM system, use the patient selection feature and select the patient to be scheduled. Select the date, time, and provider using the software, and enter the reason for visit where indicated.

   RATIONALE: Provides necessary information for staff to pull a record or to make a chart; chief complaint helps identify the length of time to allot for the appointment. The telephone number provides immediate information without having to pull the chart should there be a need to change the appointment.

6. Repeat the date and time for the appointment, using the patient's name. Provide any necessary instructions about coming to the facility. RATIONALE: Confirms the appointment date and time with the patient and gives information about how to get to the facility.

7. *End the call politely*, perhaps saying, "Thank you for calling. We will see you at 3:45 PM Monday. Good-bye."

8. Make certain you transferred all necessary information from your telephone log to the appropriate appointment schedule. Draw a diagonal line through your notes on the log. This indicates you have completed the task.

multiprovider settings where patients are attended by a number of staff before, or instead of, seeing the primary care provider.

As mentioned earlier, more than one method can be used to check in patients. A sign-in sheet might be used, especially in a facility with open hours scheduling. The administrative medical assistant can place a check mark (usually in red) by the patient's name in the appointment book or make an indication electronically in scheduling software (Figure 12-5).

The check-in procedure serves the additional purpose of alerting the staff when a patient has arrived and is available to be seen. Communication among the administrative medical assistants and the clinical medical assistants is important for a smooth patient flow and to save time for both patients and providers (Figure 12-6).

Procedure

PROCEDURE 12-3

Checking in Patients

PURPOSE:

To ensure the patient is given prompt and proper care; to meet legal safeguards for documentation.

EQUIPMENT/SUPPLIES:

- Patient chart
- Black ink pen
- Required forms
- Check-in list or appointment book
- Computerized scheduling PM system, if applicable

PROCEDURE STEPS:

1. The previous evening or before opening the ambulatory care setting, prepare a list of patients to be seen.

   a. In a paper system, either type the names of the patients and scheduled times with provider name and photocopy for each area of the clinic that requires it, or photocopy the page of the appointment book for reference purposes. Charts for patients are then pulled and prepared for visits.

   b. In a PM system, create a schedule or reference sheet using the appointment scheduler. Each PM system will have a feature for producing this sheet. Distribute the reference sheet to each area of the clinic that requires it. If charts are used in the clinic, they are pulled and prepared for visits.

   RATIONALE: Provides a patient list to use as a guide through the day's schedule; charts are ready before patient arrival. If the task is left to the last minute, it may not get done.

2. Check charts or electronic patient records to see that everything is up to date, **_paying attention to detail_**. Gather necessary letters, test results, and other data that will be needed during the patient's visit. RATIONALE: Ensures that providers and staff have all the necessary data before seeing a patient.

3. **_When patients arrive, acknowledge their presence._** If you cannot assist them immediately, gesture toward a chair; thank them for waiting as soon as you are available. RATIONALE: Patients feel welcomed, their time is valued, and their presence is noted.

4. Check in the patient and review vital information, such as address, telephone number, insurance, and reason for visit. Be certain to **_protect the patient's privacy_** by reviewing this information where doing so cannot be overheard by others. RATIONALE: Ensures that you have the latest personal information regarding your patient; provides patients with the privacy and confidentiality to which they are entitled.

5. Use a pen to check off the patient's name from the Reference Sheet if one is used for the permanent record. If the PM system has a check-in feature, input the patient's arrival. RATIONALE: Ensures that there is a permanent record of the patient's arrival in the facility for an appointment. Provides documentation for later referral if necessary.

6. Politely ask the patient to be seated and indicate the appropriate wait time, if any. RATIONALE: Provides direction to the patient and indicates how long a wait might be.

7. Following clinic policy, place the chart where it can be picked up to route the patient to the appropriate location for the visit. RATIONALE: The patient's chart is in readiness when the clinical medical assistant, laboratory personnel, or provider is ready for the patient.

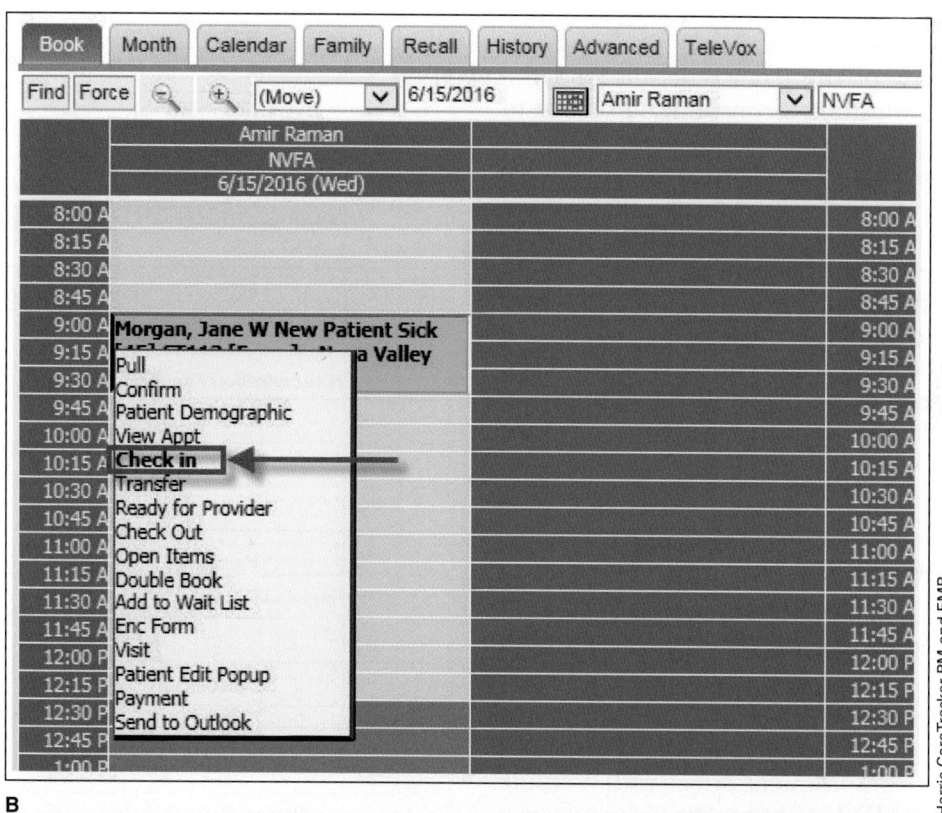

FIGURE 12-5 (A) Daily appointment worksheet (manual). (B) Checking in a patient using an electronic scheduling system.

Courtesy of Harris CareTracker PM and EMR

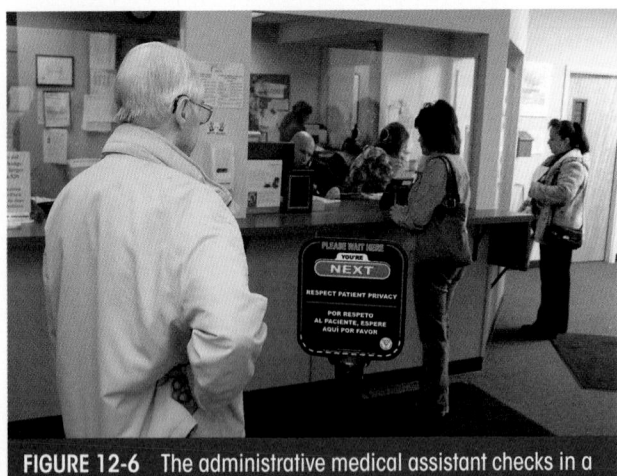
FIGURE 12-6 The administrative medical assistant checks in a patient and keeps the patient check-in list current.

complications and claim a provider was unavailable, the daily appointment sheet and chart would document the patient's failure to show.

Occasionally, patients do not arrive for an appointment because they simply forgot, or sometimes they come on the wrong day or at the wrong time. That can happen simply by human error or

Computer scheduling systems include a space to indicate when a patient arrives for an appointment. Some clinics use the printed activity schedule to check when patients arrive. Other clinics rely upon a copy of the day's schedule and the patient's chart indicating a consultation or visit to legally verify the patient's presence in the clinic.

Unfortunately, even the best of electronic systems may fail temporarily. In that case, the manual system is used as a backup. If the day's schedule has already been printed, it can be used to monitor the patient flow and to check in patients. It may also serve as adequate information for any work-in patients to be accommodated that day. However, for appointments to be made in the future, the administrative medical assistant may have to return a call to the patient when the computer is back up and running properly.

Patient Cancellation and Appointment Changes

Procedure

A permanent record of no-shows should be designated on the appointment sheet with a red *X* or some other distinctive mark. Cancellations should be marked through on the appointment sheet with a single red line (Figure 12-7A). Some facilities place a notation next to the patient's name. Computer scheduling will also provide an area to indicate no-shows and cancellations. No-shows and cancellations should always be noted in the patient's individual chart (Figure 12-7B). Again, it is imperative that the provider's care of the patient be thoroughly documented. Should a patient develop

MONDAY, NOVEMBER 23		Dr. King	Dr. Lewis
7	00		
	15		
	30		
	45		
8	00	Hospital	
	15		Surgery
	30	Rounds	
	45		
9	00	Abigail Johnson - Black	Lenore
	15	Diabetes Check/466-2964	McDonell
	30	Marge O„Keefe/CPE/296-7234	
	45		
10	00		Joseph Ortiz/New Pt./462-1121
	15		
	30	Nora Fowler/Back Pain/466-2234	Maria Tover/Stomach Problems/292-2104
	45		
11	00	Jim Marshal/CPE/763-2067	Maria Tover/Stomach Problems/292-2104
	15		
	30	Partners	Partners
	45		
12	00		
	15		
	30		
	45		
		Lunch Meeting	Lunch Meeting
1	00	Matt. Hanes/Consultation/763-3284	Boris Bolski/New Pt./466-8156

FIGURE 12-7A Multiprovider clinic where providers' commitments and no-shows are marked with a red *X* and cancellations are marked with a single red line.

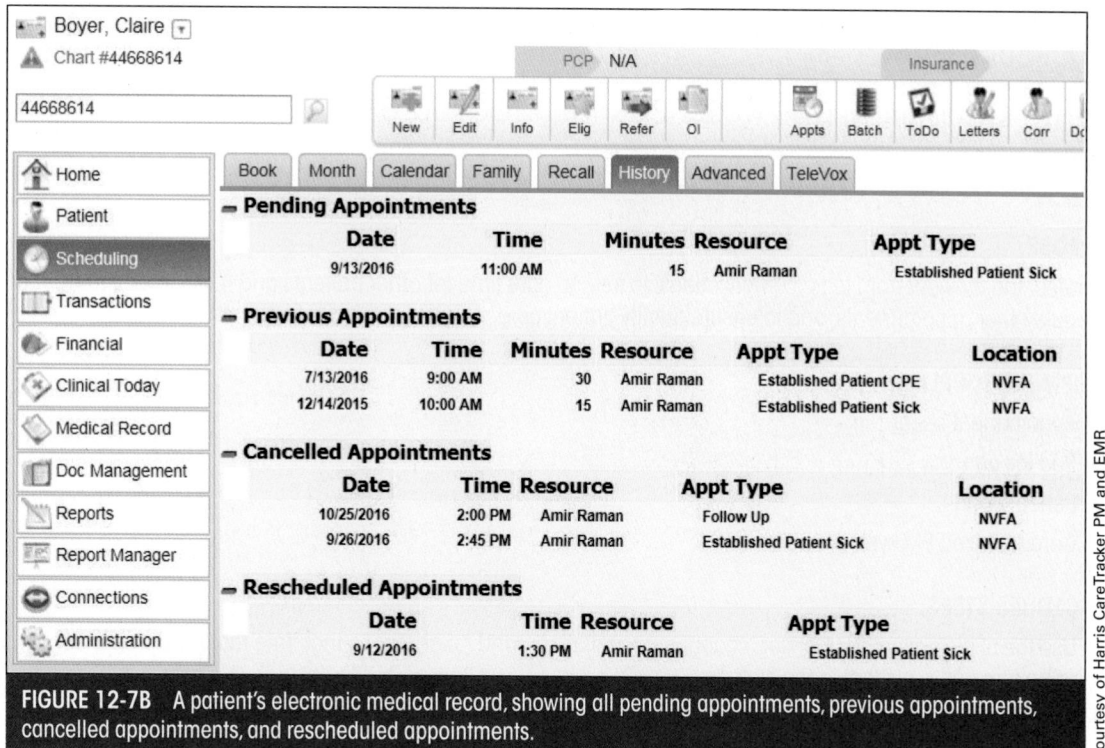

FIGURE 12-7B A patient's electronic medical record, showing all pending appointments, previous appointments, cancelled appointments, and rescheduled appointments.

Courtesy of Harris CareTracker PM and EMR

miscommunication. However, if one patient begins a pattern of getting the dates and times mixed up or forgets the appointment entirely, the primary care provider should be made aware of the fact. Sometimes, a pattern of missed and mixed-up appointments is a first sign that the patient may be experiencing memory loss and mental confusion.

Legal

Many clinics have established firm policies for multiple no-shows and cancellations. The general rule is that after three no-shows or cancellations in a row, the provider will review the records. For the provider to adequately treat a patient, the patient's cooperation is necessary. A no-show pattern may indicate that the patient is not truly committed to assisting in treatment. If a patient routinely cancels or does not show, the provider may write a letter terminating services and explaining why the provider is discontinuing care. This should be sent by certified mail, return receipt requested, to ensure that the patient received the notice (see Chapter 6 for more information on termination of services). Procedure 12-4 outlines the proper cancellation procedures.

Although software programs differ, cancellations are typically performed by deleting the patient's name from the time slot; if the appointment is to be rescheduled, the name is then keyed in to the appropriate time, usually the first time open for other appointments.

When canceling appointments by computer, be certain that the program maintains a list of canceled appointments including patient name, date, and time. This documentation is necessary for legal purposes. Also, be certain to record canceled appointments in the patients' charts.

Reminder Systems

When patients are reminded of their scheduled appointments, it results in a greater rate of fulfilled appointments. Give patients appointment card reminders when appointments are made at the medical facility. Those cards may easily be

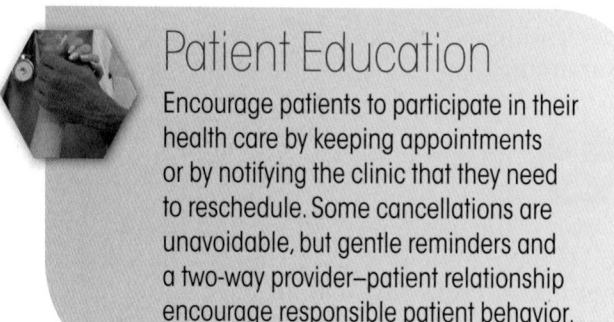

Patient Education

Encourage patients to participate in their health care by keeping appointments or by notifying the clinic that they need to reschedule. Some cancellations are unavoidable, but gentle reminders and a two-way provider–patient relationship encourage responsible patient behavior.

PROCEDURE 12-4

Cancelling and Rescheduling Procedures

Procedure

PURPOSE:

To protect the provider from legal complications; to free up care time for other patients and make open time evident to schedule other appointments; and to ensure quality patient care.

EQUIPMENT/SUPPLIES:

- Appointment sheet
- Red ink pen
- Patient chart
- Computerized PM system and/or EMR

PROCEDURE STEPS:

1. Use the clinic system for marking changes, cancellations, and no-shows so that time that is now open for other appointments is evident to the staff.

2. Indicate on the appointment sheet all appointments that were changed, canceled, or no-shows:

   a. *Changes.* In a paper system, note rescheduling in the appointment sheet margin and directly in the patient's chart; indicate new appointment time. In a PM system, use the appointment scheduler's feature to document changes to the patient's record. RATIONALE: Notifies all staff of a schedule change; documents same information in patient's chart or EMR.

   b. *Cancellations.* In a paper system, enter a note on both the appointment sheet and the patient's chart. Draw a single red line through canceled appointments. Date and initial cancellation in the patient chart. In a PM system, use the appointment scheduler's feature to cancel (and if applicable, reschedule) the appointment to document the cancellation in the patient's record. RATIONALE: Notifies staff of a schedule change; documents cancellation in patient's chart or EMR, thus identifying a change in the patient's plans. A cancellation may initiate a follow-up call from a staff member to determine the reason for the cancellation.

   c. *No-shows.* In a paper system, enter a note on both the appointment sheet and the patient's chart. Date and initial notations in the chart. No-shows can be indicated with a red *X* on the appointment sheet. In a PM system, use the appointment scheduler's feature to indicate a no-show to document the missed appointment in the patient's EMR. RATIONALE: Notifies the staff of a schedule change; documents the no-show in the patient's chart or EMR. Provides a reminder to a staff member to follow up on the reason for the no-show.

tucked in a wallet and forgotten, however. Many clinics notify patients the day before the appointment with a reminder via their choice for the communication—telephone, text message, or email.

Legal

Keep in mind that the reminder is confidential information and should not be left on a recording device without the patient's express permission to do so. (When initially seeing the patient, obtain a number where a personal message could be left.) Finally, reminders can be mailed. This would be most appropriate for patients who come in on a regular basis (e.g., once every 6 months).

Scheduling Pharmaceutical Representatives

Some medical facilities schedule time with representatives of pharmaceutical and medical supply companies. On the other hand, there are some medical clinics that refuse to see any pharmaceutical representatives. When representatives are seen, however, they can provide a valuable service to providers and staff, and with clear guidelines regarding when and how often representatives can visit, a working partnership can develop. Providers may set aside a specific time during the week to meet with these representatives; generally, a time allotment of 15 to 20 minutes is sufficient for these appointments. Some representatives try to establish a standard appointment once a month. If this is a representative your provider desires to see on a regular basis, that policy can be helpful to both the provider and the representative.

SCHEDULING SOFTWARE AND MATERIALS

No matter what materials and which methods are used, the proper tools will enable patient scheduling to be a smoothly functioning, easily documented process. Materials needed for scheduling should be customized to the ambulatory care setting. For instance, a smaller practice may prefer a manual method involving appointment books; a large urgent care–type setting will use a computer program for patient scheduling that may be part of a practice management (PM) software program.

Appointment Schedule

An appropriate appointment schedule system is essential to any medical practice in the ambulatory care setting. Each clinic has unique needs in its physical facility and for its staff. The physical arrangement of the scheduler, including the various combinations of time allotments, must be determined. Some have major headings for hours with minor spaces for 15-minute intervals, others have 10-minute intervals, and still others only hour intervals. An appointment sheet is necessary for both legal risk management and quality management purposes. Copies of the daily appointment sheet, also known as a *reference sheet*, are made available to the doctors, medical assistants, and any other staff members. Using the daily appointment sheet, it is easy to check in patients as they arrive and to indicate no-shows and cancellations. Indicating the check-in and checkout times can be useful for quality management purposes. More importantly, the daily appointment sheet enables all staff members to see the total scheme of the day's patient flow.

If a provider works between two clinics or a hospital and clinic, it is helpful to have this appointment schedule transferred to a handheld computer device for immediate referral. If a handheld computer is not used by the provider, reduce the dimensions of the appointment schedule sheet to pocket-size for the provider's easy access. Generally, if the provider makes hospital visits before coming to the clinic in the morning, this schedule is printed the previous evening before closing.

These daily appointment sheets can also be used to include other provider commitments such as meetings and visits from pharmaceutical representatives. Such a complete record of time ensures that no patient appointments will be booked when, in fact, the provider is not available.

Computer Scheduling Software

Even the smallest of medical facilities today will benefit from the use of information technology. Numerous software programs for the ambulatory care setting require only basic computer hardware that can save time for providers and their staff members. Other programs are more sophisticated and may require on-site technical support.

Some scheduling software programs will schedule resources, equipment, examination rooms, and specialty staff, as well as patients and providers. Some will show co-payments due, authorization expiration dates, and insurance expiration dates. They can select the next available appointment, search for appointments by provider, copy and paste appointments, and specify minimum time increments between appointments. The staff can view multiple schedules daily, weekly, monthly, or even yearly. Reminder notes can be created for both providers and patients.

Computerized scheduling systems that are a component of a complete practice management facility, including medical records, are able to indicate no-shows and cancellations in the system and the patient's chart at the same time. Facilities that are partially computerized will still want to indicate patients who do not keep their appointments on the daily worksheet and in the patients' medical records.

Online systems can handle prescription refill requests, patient–provider email messages, and laboratory results. Some will allow patients to update insurance data and complete registration forms. All of the online systems are done within the provider's Web site, which includes security measures and sophisticated **encryption technology**. Therefore, security is less of a concern.

With America's ongoing goal of giving patients increased access to their electronic health record (EHR) and Congress pushing to have prescriptions transferred electronically, electronic scheduling has become the "entry" to the entire field of computerized medical information. Employers in ambulatory care settings who make certain that patients understand computerized scheduling, who have put time and effort into determining the best program for their use, and who have trained their staff well will not be disappointed with the outcome. Whatever system is chosen, keep in mind that the patient's time, the staff's time, and the provider's time are extremely valuable. The goal is to manage that time as efficiently as possible.

INPATIENT AND OUTPATIENT ADMISSIONS PROCEDURES

Often, patients are scheduled for either outpatient or inpatient hospital admissions or for special procedures performed in another facility. These appointments are most likely made while the patient is present in the clinic and has just been seen by the provider. Have a calendar handy for visualization of the days discussed. If the patient has their agenda on hand, this is especially helpful. If not, the appointment may need to be scheduled at another time.

Outpatient procedures may include endoscopy examinations and specialized radiologic examinations such as Computerized tomography (CT), magnetic resonance imaging (MRI), mammography, and bone scans. If a patient prefers to make his or her own arrangements for a procedure, advise the patient the following information is necessary:

- Name, address, and telephone number of patient

- Name of provider ordering the procedure
- Name of the procedure and preoperative diagnosis
- Name of patient's insurance, ID number, and Social Security number

If required, follow up in a day or two to make certain the procedure has been scheduled (see Procedure 12-5). In addition, please be certain that the patient has been given and understands any special instructions that must be followed prior to the procedure. This might include, but is not limited to, fasting (no eating or drinking after midnight, or a specified time); withholding the consumption of certain medications (such as anything that can interfere with the anesthesia); having a spouse or loved one available to speak with the provider and staff; or not using lotions, oils, or powders prior to the procedure.

Generally, a real service is done for the patients and staff when the medical assistant schedules

---

PROCEDURE 12-5

Scheduling Inpatient and Outpatient Admissions and Procedures

PURPOSE:

To assist patients in scheduling inpatient and outpatient admissions and procedures ordered by the provider.

EQUIPMENT/SUPPLIES:

- Calendar
- Black ink pen
- Computerized PM system and/or EMR
- Telephones
- Referral slip
- Patient's calendar or schedule (helpful, but not critical)
- Provider requests/orders regarding procedures/admissions being scheduled

PROCEDURE STEPS:

1. In a private and quiet location, discuss with the patient the inpatient admission or outpatient procedure ordered by the provider. RATIONALE: Helps the patient identify the time necessary for this appointment and the reason for it.

2. If required, seek permission from the patient's insurance company for the procedure or admission. RATIONALE: Clearly identifies for the patient who is responsible for the bill and how it is to be paid.

3. Produce a large, easily read calendar and check to see if the patient has one also. RATIONALE: Visualization of the calendar is easier for determining available time for the appointment. Patient's calendar further identifies available days and times for the appointment(s).

(continues)

---

4. Place telephone call to the facility where the appointment is to be scheduled. Identify yourself, your provider, the clinic from where you are calling, and the reason for the call. RATIONALE: Alerts the receiver of the call that a provider's office is calling to schedule an appointment.

NOTE: The more familiar the medical assistant is with the specific procedure to be scheduled or a specific type of hospital admission, the easier it is to make certain the patient has all the information necessary. It can be helpful for medical assistants to discuss such arrangements with specialty clinics and hospitals.

5. ***Displaying sound judgment***, identify any urgency. Request the next available appointment for the particular type of appointment to be scheduled and provide the patient's diagnosis. Identify any time that is not possible for the patient. RATIONALE: Tells the receiver how quickly an appointment is to be made, for what reason, and if any dates or times are not possible.

6. As a time is suggested, confer with the patient for an immediate response.

7. Once the appointment has been scheduled, provide receiver pertinent information related to the patient (e.g., full name, insurance information, Social Security number, telephone number). RATIONALE: Provides essential information to secure the appointment for the proper patient.

8. Request any special instructions or advanced data necessary for the patient. RATIONALE: Helps to ensure that a smooth transition is made from the provider's clinic to the facility where the referral is made and provides the patient with any special instructions.

9. Complete a manual referral slip, or use the PM or EMR system to enter the referral for the patient; send or fax a copy to the referral facility. RATIONALE: Ensures that the patient, the referral facility, and the patient's chart have a copy of the reason for the appointment, any specific instructions, and the date and time of the appointment.

10. If an immediate hospital admission is to be made, ***attend to special needs of patient*** by providing him or her time on the telephone to call family members to make arrangements to receive personal items and any other arrangements necessitated by the appointment. RATIONALE: Provides patients a little time to notify family members and make necessary arrangements.

11. Place a reminder notice to yourself on the calendar or in a tickler file. RATIONALE: To check to make certain the appointment was completed and a report is received from the appointment facility.

12. Document the referral in the patient's chart. A copy of the referral slip and all pertinent data are to be included. Document in the chart when the appointment is completed and a report is received from the referral facility. Date and initial.

DOCUMENTATION:

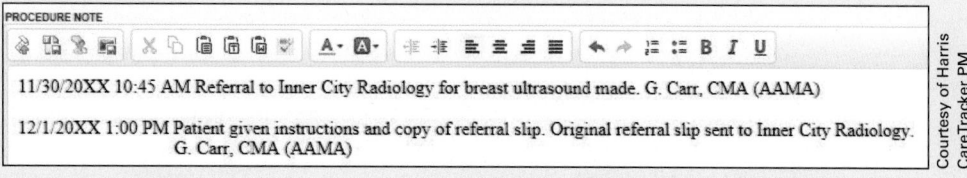

PROCEDURE NOTE

11/30/20XX 10:45 AM Referral to Inner City Radiology for breast ultrasound made. G. Carr, CMA (AAMA)

12/1/20XX 1:00 PM Patient given instructions and copy of referral slip. Original referral slip sent to Inner City Radiology. G. Carr, CMA (AAMA)

Courtesy of Harris CareTracker PM and EMR

the procedure. With the patient present, place a telephone call to the facility where procedures are to be performed. Identify yourself, your provider, and the clinic from which you are calling. Identify any urgency to the request and ask for the next available appointment. As dates and times are discussed, your patient is able to give an immediate response. Consider travel time for your patient and whether there is apt to be any uncomfortable pre-examination procedure that might make travel difficult. Be certain to advise the patient if someone is needed to provide transportation home after the procedure. Often, there is a paperwork follow-up that indicates the nature of the illness and the reason for the specialty examination. Your employer will tell you if a phone response to the examination is required, or if it is acceptable to wait for the written test results.

Once a date has been established, make certain the patient knows the correct date and time, as well as how to get to the place where the examination is to be performed. Inform the patient how and when he or she will receive test results.

Scheduling inpatient admissions to the hospital is similar. However, the provider may want the patient in the hospital as quickly as possible. Call the preferred or designated hospital. Expect to provide pertinent patient and insurance information required by the hospital. Assist the patient in determining whether it is permissible to return home for some personal belongings and to make home arrangements or whether admission is immediate. Some large facilities have a surgery scheduler to make all these arrangements. In primary care, the medical assistant will do this kind of scheduling.

When a surgery is being scheduled, the medical assistant must sometimes coordinate several entities. Arrangements must be coordinated with an assistant in the surgeon's clinic, with the hospital or outpatient surgery center where the surgery will be performed, and occasionally for scheduling specialty equipment and personnel to be available, as well as with the patient's schedule. If any one of these entities is not available at the time requested, the process needs to begin again and can become quite convoluted. If the scheduling of the surgery is especially complex, the medical assistant should consider obtaining the patient's scheduling preferences and limitations and letting the patient go home to be contacted later when all the parts are in place.

Be sensitive to the patient's needs at this time. Scheduling a specialty examination or a hospital admission is rarely a convenience. More likely it is a great inconvenience to the patient, even when necessary. Anything that makes the scheduling more accommodating or pleasant for the patient will help in creating a beneficial atmosphere for all involved.

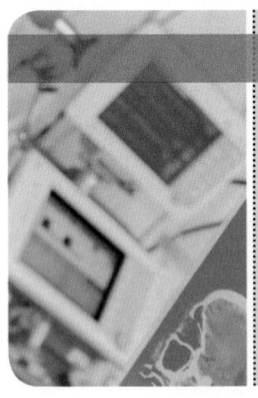

CASE STUDY 12-1

Refer to the scenario at the beginning of the chapter. It appears that this clinic has a smooth-flowing scheduling system and that Walter Seals has everything under control.

CASE STUDY REVIEW

1. What personal traits might Walter need to possess in order for this scenario to be true?
2. What factors, if any, might make the scheduling at Inner City Urgent Care work well?
3. If clients are seen on a first-come, first-served basis, how does the clustering system work if patients need to be referred to one of the specialty care clinics?

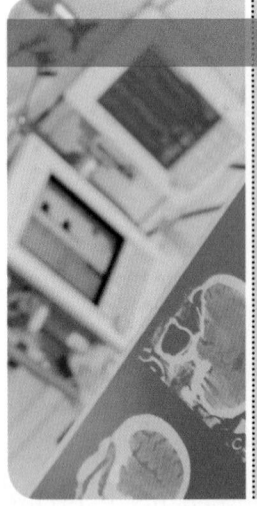

CASE STUDY 12-2

Rhoda Au has persistently canceled her appointments at Inner City Urgent Care. Although she always reschedules, she has canceled her last four appointments. Today, she did not call to cancel nor did she arrive for her fifth scheduled appointment. Walter Seals, CMA (AAMA), who is responsible for scheduling and patient flow, is concerned that Rhoda is canceling because she is afraid to come in for some reason. Rhoda has been a patient for a few years now, and she was always responsible about keeping her appointments.

CASE STUDY REVIEW

1. From the point of view of the urgent care center, why should Walter be concerned that Rhoda is canceling appointments? What action might be taken?
2. From the patient's point of view, why should Walter be concerned?
3. How should Walter record these cancellations and no-shows?

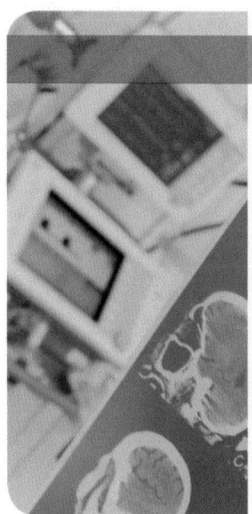

CASE STUDY 12-3

Nancy McFarland, RMA (AMT), is a clinical medical assistant at Inner City Health Care. In the past 3 weeks, Nancy has been doing phone screening, primarily because the clinic has been so busy and the providers believe screening calls will help. In fact, Nancy discovered that the administrative medical assistant is screening quite well, but that there does not seem to be sufficient appointment slots to meet the patient demand.

CASE STUDY REVIEW

1. What might be done to determine whether there is a better scheduling style to fit the current demands?
2. What happens when professional staff, providers, and patients view this medical facility as "too busy"?
3. What are some solutions that you can identify?

Summary

- Medical assistants involved in scheduling patients must put into practice their best interpersonal and communication skills. Scheduling an appointment may be the first contact patients have with the medical facility. They remember and value the treatment they receive from the time of first contact.

- Scheduling has undergone changes, and can be done in person, over the telephone, and using technology for online appointments.

- Scheduling can be stressful, especially when other office tasks are pressing at the front desk. The medical assistant must apply good organizational skills, a calm composure, and effective communication.

- Tailor the scheduling system to the needs of the type of practice, provider habits, and availability of equipment and staff with a focus on minimizing patient wait times. The ability to add unexpected visits for acute illness, add work-ins, and adjust for cancellations is important.

- The various scheduling styles include open hours, double booking techniques, clustering, wave scheduling, modified wave scheduling, stream scheduling, and online scheduling.

- The medical assistant must obtain key information required for scheduling, including the urgency of the need for an appointment and whether the patient is a referral from another provider; understand recording methods for new and established patients; implement check-in, cancellation, and rescheduling policies; use reminder systems; and coordinate visits from medical supply and pharmaceutical representatives.

- Use proper screening techniques to obtain basic information about new and established patients when scheduling appointments.

- The medical assistant must know how to use an appointment matrix, both in a manual and an electronic scheduling system, and apply this matrix to the needs of the practice and patients.

- Familiarize yourself with scheduling for inpatient and outpatient admissions procedures.

CERTIFICATION REVIEW

1. Which of the following is one of the legal guidelines for appointment scheduling?
   a. It should be recorded only in pencil.
   b. It should be current, accurate, and saved as documentation.
   c. It should be left on the front desk for patient viewing.
   d. It should be recorded only in red ink.

2. What is the definition of screening patient calls?
   a. It involves taking only emergencies.
   b. It is assessing the urgency of a call and need for appointment.
   c. It means sorting appointments by specialized procedure.
   d. It should only be performed by providers.
   e. Schedule the patient on a first-come, first-served basis.

3. How should representatives from medical supply and drug companies be scheduled?
   a. They should only be seen as a last resort.
   b. They should not be scheduled, but seen only if the provider has time.
   c. They can provide a valuable service and should be scheduled for short visits.
   d. They have complex information to communicate and need 1-hour appointments.

4. What is the definition of the double-booking method?
   a. It gives two or more patients the same appointment time.
   b. It keeps patients waiting unnecessarily.
   c. It is never the system of choice.
   d. It is purely for the provider's convenience.
   e. It is a way for the provider to see two patients at the same time.

5. What is a description of the stream method?
   a. It gives patients appointments as they walk in.
   b. It schedules appointments at set times throughout the workday.
   c. It only works in sole-proprietor clinics.
   d. It refers to streamlining paperwork for each appointment.

6. Why is it necessary to have daily appointment sheets?
   a. They indicate when providers and staff take lunch.
   b. They provide a permanent record for legal risk management and quality management.
   c. They are available only in computerized scheduling.
   d. They tell the staff which patient to see first.
   e. Both a and b

7. Why is analyzing patient flow important?
   a. It can maximize a clinic's scheduling practice.
   b. It often reveals why patient flow is not efficient.
   c. It may indicate a change in pattern for patient scheduling.
   d. All of these

8. What is the most important principle used in tailoring the scheduling system?
   a. Always schedule in ink.
   b. Schedule for the patient's convenience.
   c. Be flexible and sensitive.
   d. Referral patients are first.
   e. Double book the first appointment of the day.

9. What is the best way to approach a patient who must wait for an appointment?
   a. It is best to say nothing about the delay.
   b. Explain the delay and offer options when possible.
   c. Find ways to make the patient comfortable.
   d. Both b and c

10. Which of the following is true of scheduling outpatient procedures?
   a. It is best done by patients who understand their availability.
   b. It is coordinated and completed by the clinic's staff.
   c. It is an important way to enhance patient satisfaction.
   d. The patient cannot understand the urgency or the need for the procedure.
   e. Both b and c

ICD 10 Code

Certain infectious and parasitic diseases (A00
Intestinal infectious diseases (A00-A09)
A00 Cholera
A01 Typhoid and paratyphoid fevers
A02 Other salmonella infections
A03 Shigellosis
A04 Other bacterial intestinal infections
A05 Other bacterial foodborne intoxications
A06 Amoebiasis
A07 Other protozoal intestinal diseases
A08 Viral and other specified intestinal infectio
A09 Diarrhoea and gastroenteritis of presume
Tuberculosis (A15-A19)
A15 Respiratory tuberculosis, bacteriologically
A16 Respiratory tuberculosis, not confirmed ba
A17† Tuberculosis of nervous system
A18 Tuberculosis of other organs
A19 Miliary tuberculosis
Certain zoonotic bacterial diseases (A20-A28)
A20 Plague
A21 Tularaemia
A22 Anthrax
A23 Brucellosis
A24 Glanders and melioidosis
A25 Rat-bite fevers
A26 Erysipeloid
A27 Leptospirosis
A28 Other zoonotic bacterial diseases, not els
Other bacterial diseases (A30-A49)
A30 Leprosy [Hansen's disease]
A31 Infection due to other mycobacteria
A32 Listeriosis

Electronic Medical Record System

| Home | Show | Print | Send |

Preview	Personal Information
Edit	Social Information
Save	Insurance
Quit	Diagnosis
	Treatment
	Medical History
	Health Care Calendar
	Schedule
	Appointment

HN:

Patient Name

Doctor :

Operative Note :

Search ● HN ◯ Name ◯ Doctor

Search

Personal Information

☐ Male   ☐ Female

☐ Single   ☐ Married
☐ Widowes   ☐ Divorced

Occupation

Address

Telephone number

e-mail address

Previous   Done   Next   Exit

pandpstock001/Shutterstock.com

Medical Records
Management

1. Define and spell the key terms as presented in the glossary.
2. List the purpose of medical records.
3. Discuss the ownership of medical records.
4. State the reasons for accurately maintaining ambulatory care files.
5. Describe how and when information is released from the medical record.
6. State the pros and cons of the manual medical record and the electronic medical record.
7. Correct a medical record, manually and electronically.
8. Recall eight common supplies used in medical records management.
9. Identify the rules described under Basic Rules for Filing.
10. Describe the five steps commonly used when filing any documentation.
11. Name the two filing systems most often used in the clinic setting.
12. State the purpose of cross-referencing.
13. Recall four common documents kept in the patient's medical record.
14. Discuss storage and purging of medical records.
15. Describe electronic medical records and their usefulness to the clinic.
16. Discuss confidentiality and privacy as related to medical records.
17. Explain HIPAA security standards for electronic medical records.

KEY TERMS

accession record	problem-oriented medical record (POMR)
caption	purging
cross-reference	SOAP/SOAPER
indexing	source-oriented medical record (SOMR)
key unit	tickler file
meaningful use	unit
out guide	

SCENARIO

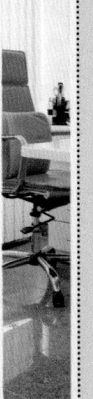

Consider a situation that might arise at multiprovider Inner City Health Care. Patient Juanita Hansen was seen on Tuesday morning by Dr. Lewis for acute stomach pain. She was given a thorough examination and sent for appropriate testing that afternoon. She was then scheduled to return to Inner City on Friday to see Dr. Lewis.

After she was seen Tuesday morning, Juanita received an upper and lower gastrointestinal series; the results were then sent to Dr. Lewis's clinic. However, Nancy McFarland, RMA (AMT), the medical assistant, attached the results to the wrong patient's file. Friday arrived and Juanita came back to Inner City for her appointment, anxious to know the results of her tests. Dr. Lewis reviewed Juanita's medical record and realized the patient's test results had not been filed correctly.

This left Dr. Lewis with an anxious patient. Nancy McFarland is off today, so the provider checks with the other medical assistants on duty. They have no knowledge of the test results. The act of not properly filing Juanita's test results causes undue stress for the provider, medical assistants, and patient.

Every medical facility generates a large amount of information. Business, insurance, personnel, and financial records must be maintained. Supplies and equipment records must be managed. Licensures and certifications must be current. Some records are kept for the life of the practice. The greatest bulk of information, however, comes from patient medical records. A vital function of any medical facility is the maintenance of patient records identifying the care given. Medical assistants, both administrative and clinical, will spend a fair amount of time managing patients' records. Medical records potentially record all medical data about an individual from birth until death.

Even in medical facilities where patient records are managed electronically, there are ample paper records to be stored and retrieved manually. A number of functions essential to proper records management are discussed in this chapter. A clear understanding of the proper methods used to manage the records in a medical facility is an important and necessary skill for medical assistants.

Chapter 10 defined electronic medical records (EMRs) as those coming from a single medical practice, hospital, or pharmacy. When EMRs from multiple sources are combined into one database for a patient, the term electronic health record (EHR) is used.

THE PURPOSE OF MEDICAL RECORDS

The primary purposes of medical records in the clinic are to:

1. Provide a base for managing patient care
2. Provide interoffice and intraoffice communication as necessary
3. Determine any patterns that surface to signal the provider of patient needs
4. Serve as a basis for legal information necessary to protect providers, staff, and patients
5. Provide clinical data for research

OWNERSHIP OF MEDICAL RECORDS

Legal

State statutes have ruled that medical records are the property of those who create them. The information within the medical record, however, belongs to the patient, and that information is always to be protected with the utmost privacy and confidentiality. Patients can be allowed access to their medical records, ask for notes or information to be added to their files, and request that certain information not be included in their files.

Integrity

Providers who include their patients in their medical record keeping foster trust and respect with their patients. For example, a provider who enters patient data into the electronic patient record while sitting at a computer monitor in the examination room beside the patient has the opportunity to explain that the information is entered now so there is no room for error in reporting or in the provider not accurately recalling the patient information if entered at a later time. Care should be taken when discussing sensitive information that may be of concern to the patient and requires strict confidentiality. For example, such diagnoses that involve psychiatric, infectious, or serious illness are areas where patients may feel that disclosure to certain entities, such as co-workers, employers, or even family members can be of concern. Respecting these concerns and taking the proper steps to assure the patient of their privacy is of utmost importance.

AUTHORIZATION TO RELEASE INFORMATION

Legal

It is recommended that before any information is released from the medical record, the patient be notified and written approval received. Medical facilities will have appropriate forms for such release of information. A sample release of information form is given in Chapter 22. The form should identify the reason for the release of information and what information is specifically requested. Only that information should be released. This does not include the release of information to a patient's chosen insurance carrier. A number of different methods exist to release that information. For some insurance carriers, the release is granted when the patient accepts the insurance coverage. For others, a yearly release form must be signed by the patient.

MANUAL OR ELECTRONIC MEDICAL RECORDS

Today's medical environment has a mixture of manual, or paper, medical records and the electronic form of medical records. Some medical providers continue to have difficulty with including the necessary information that is considered vital in documentation for further enhancing the transition to EMR. Key medical data have been either improperly documented or have been omitted from some patients' records, which can create numerous compliance and billing issues when corresponding with insurance companies. By becoming more specific in documentation, providers will ensure that all of a patient's data is included in the electronic record and further enhance the transition to EMR. During his presidency, President George W. Bush announced his Health Information Technology Plan, which included the goal of ensuring that most Americans would have electronic health records by 2014. Planned projects included transmitting X-rays and laboratory results electronically to providers for immediate analysis and standardizing electronic prescriptions, decreasing errors in patient care.

Consider the following advantages and disadvantages of both types of records:

MANUAL MEDICAL RECORD

ADVANTAGES	DISADVANTAGES
• Currently established and understood • Easier to protect confidentiality • No worry of computer malfunction	• Can be used by only one person at a time • Easily misplaced or misfiled • Equipment and storage space required • More susceptible to error

ELECTRONIC MEDICAL RECORD

ADVANTAGES	DISADVANTAGES
• Multiple users are possible • Not easily misplaced or misfiled • Errors less likely • Patterns and data more easily accessed • Quickly available in emergencies • Office storage space not required • Legible, organized patient documentation • Improved medication management • Improved quality of care	• Needs protection to prevent loss of data • Expensive to establish and maintain • May require on-site assistance • Can require up to 12 weeks for staff to prove productive after installation

In 2009, President Barack Obama signed the American Reinvestment and Recovery Act (ARRA). This law provides numerous incentives for providers and hospitals to make the transition to EMR. As mentioned in Chapter 11, **meaningful use** is a Centers for Medicare and Medicaid (CMS) program that awards incentives for using certified electronic health records (EHR) to improve patient care. To achieve meaningful use and avoid penalties, providers must follow a set of criteria that serve as a road map for effectively using an EHR. Meaningful use encourages providers to switch from paper charts to electronic records, improves efficiency, and will earn incentives for providers. Medicare reimbursement penalties for lack of participation began in 2015, and it is expected that other health insurance carriers will follow suit in the coming years in an effort to transition away from the use of paper records. For more information on meaningful use and its stages, go to http://www.healthit.gov and search for "Meaningful Use."

For the time being, not all clinics have fully computerized their medical records. Compliance issues may involve cost, labor, and time involved in transferring over data to an electronic medical record system. Although there are compelling reasons for providers to make the switch, the process has been slow, and will still require some time in the next decade to fully implement the changes.

No matter what stage of the transition a clinic is in, the management of the medical records must provide easy retrieval of information. All documentation must be complete and correct. Wording must be easily understood and grammatically correct. How corrections are made in the chart, how documents are removed from or added to the chart, and the format of the chart must be predetermined and understood by all users of the information.

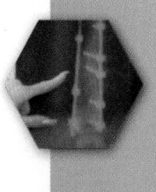

Critical Thinking

Your clinic is planning to implement an electronic medical records system. What steps must you take to ensure the transition goes smoothly? What factors should be considered when selecting an EMR system? How does the implementation of such a system affect overall patient care?

THE IMPORTANCE OF ACCURATE MEDICAL RECORDS

Accurate medical records are essential to patient care in any health care setting. One incorrect digit in a patient's Social Security number causes reimbursement problems. An incorrect address or telephone number or a misspelling of a name makes it difficult to contact patients about test results and prescription refills. Medical treatment documentation errors are even more disastrous and can cause serious medical problems for patients. Patient files are critical to the facility's smooth functioning and are important when referring the patient to outside specialists with whom the facility may need to coordinate care. Each treating primary care provider must be aware of tests, procedures, and diagnoses. Maintaining a conscientious record of patient care is also absolutely essential in controlling the costs of medical care.

Legal

Medical records management is also important because of the legal issues that every medical clinic and health care professional must face today. The standard in court is that if there is no record of any piece of information related to a patient and that patient's care and treatment, then it did not happen. The question to ask yourself about any piece of information is: "Does this relate to the patient's care, and should it be in the chart?" To be prepared in the event of medical litigation, you must document all medical treatment. No matter how competently a provider has performed treatment, if a written record cannot prove how and what was done, there is no basis for a defense in a court of law.

Creating Paper Charts and Electronic Records

Procedure

The patient's medical chart is prepared on or before the day of the patient's first visit to the medical facility. Paper charts require the assembly of appropriate file folders, divider pages labeled with identifying tabs, and a number of essential forms to be completed by the patient. Included forms provide demographic information, social and family medical history, previous surgeries, HIPAA guidelines, and release of information details. Often, paper charts include adhesive twin prong fasteners to ensure that sheets of paper are securely held within the chart. Electronic patient medical records are prepared in much the same manner with the exception being that all information is stored electronically. Patient information that is collected via the paper route will have to be scanned and entered into the record. The EMR will provide an orderly arrangement of patient information according to the particular software design or a predetermined plan selected by the providers and their staff. Procedure 13-1 provides guidance on creating a patient medical record.

PROCEDURE 13-1

Procedure

Establishing a Medical Chart or Record for a New Patient

PURPOSE:

To demonstrate an understanding of the principles for establishing a medical chart or record.

EQUIPMENT/SUPPLIES:
For Paper Charts

- File folder used in the facility (flip-up or book-style)
- Divider pages used in the facility (SOAP/SOAPER laboratory reports, HIPAA information sheets, and so forth)
- Adhesive twin prong fasteners for divider pages
- Twin hole punch for twin prong fasteners
- Selected tabs to identify folder and divider pages
- Demographic patient information completed before or at the first appointment

(continues)

For Electronic Charts

- Computer
- EHR program
- Demographic patient information completed before or at the first appointment

PROCEDURE STEPS:
For Paper Charts

1. Assemble all supplies at a desk or table. RATIONALE: Everything is in one place for efficient use.
2. Punch holes in the manila file folder and any necessary divider pages. RATIONALE: Creates holes for the twin prong fasteners.
3. Affix the adhesive twin prong fasteners. RATIONALE: Places fasteners as appropriate for material to be attached.
4. Assemble the divider pages dictated by the practice and the clinic policy in the proper location of the chart over the twin prong fasteners. RATIONALE: Ensures that items are placed in the same place as in all other charts in the facility.
5. Securely fasten twin prong fasteners over the divider pages. RATIONALE: Ensures that no pages will fall out of the chart.
6. Index and code the patient's name according to the filing system to be used (i.e., alphabetic, numeric, or color). RATIONALE: Determines where the chart will be placed.
7. Affix appropriately labeled tabs to the folder cut. RATIONALE: Prepares the chart for patient information.
8. Transfer demographic data in black ink pen or affix the demographic divider sheet to the inside front cover of the chart. RATIONALE: Identifying patient information is readily available inside the chart cover.
9. Affix HIPAA required information to the chart, after it has been read and signed by the patient, as determined by clinic policy. RATIONALE: Ensures that this task is not omitted.
10. Place prepared chart in proper location for pickup by the provider or clinical medical assistant. RATIONALE: Signals to all staff that the chart is ready for the patient's visit.

For Electronic Charts

1. Access EMR or PM system to be used and open a new patient record.
2. Enter demographic information provided by the patient.
3. Enter insurance information provided by the patient.
4. Review the information entered and confirm accuracy.
5. Save the patient's record and close out of it when complete.
6. Print and obtain HIPAA-required information after it has been read and signed by the patient, and file or scan to the EMR as determined by clinic policy.
7. Print documents and encounter form, or mark the daily appointment sheet for pickup by the provider or clinical medical assistant.

Correcting Medical Records

The medical record must be readable and accurate; however, errors do occur and may not be discovered immediately. Any corrections necessary to a paper medical record should be corrected using the following method: draw a single line using a red ink pen through the error, make the correction, write "Corr." or "Correction" above the area corrected, and indicate your initials and the current date. The red line through the information indicates the "error" portion of the report. The words "Corr." or "Correction" by the correction indicate the change. The date and initials identify when the correction was made and by whom. Obliterations should never occur. When the medical record becomes the center of attention in malpractice litigation, forensic experts will be able to tell if a record has been tampered with or if information or pages have been added later. When not properly done, altered records become a detriment to any provider's defense in court.

Errors discovered immediately after the fact in an electronic medical record are corrected

ADDENDUM

Pt requests referral to Dr. Robert Rovner for orthopedic evaluation.

FIGURE 13-1 Addendum added to electronic progress note.

differently. Each EMR has its own method of handling corrections and tracking them, often with a log that identifies the person making the correction, date, and time. In addition, it is customary for only certain staff members to be able to alter or correct medical records; therefore, access may be restricted for this purpose. Generally, a correction is made in an EMR using the Edit function, which does not change the original entry, but adds an addendum with the corrected information (Figure 13-1).

If a correction is necessary of any information after either a paper chart or an electronic chart has been sent to another provider or facility, make a copy of the corrected information and send it to the provider or facility as quickly as possible.

TYPES OF MEDICAL RECORDS

Whether patient charts are kept manually or electronically, there are common threads that run throughout medical records. How material is stored within records is important. The choice of method must be in accordance with how the information needs to be accessed and used for each individual clinic. No one method is best. In the examples that follow, arrangement of materials is also discussed.

Problem-Oriented Medical Record

The **problem-oriented medical record (POMR)** places in a prominent location vital identification data, immunizations, allergies, medications, and problems. The problems are identified by a number that corresponds to the charting relevant to that problem number, that is, bronchitis #1, broken wrist #2, and so forth. If the patient returns in 9 months with recurring bronchitis, the same number (#1) is used.

The patient chart is then further built by adding a numbered and titled section for each problem the patient experiences, for example, bronchitis #1, broken wrist #2. Figure 13-2 shows an example of a POMR.

Each problem is then followed with the **SOAP** approach for all progress notes:

S Subjective impressions

O Objective clinical evidence

A Assessment or diagnosis

P Plans for further studies, treatment, or management

Some medical facilities have added variations to the SOAP approach, creating **SOAPER** or the SOAPIE. These additional charting tools can be especially useful in providing additional information more specific to the practice and specialty requirements:

Added to SOAPER:

E Education for patient

R Response of patient to education and care given

Added to SOAPIE:

I Implementation of the plan (what was done)

E Evaluation, indicating whether care is effective, or results

This process makes the chart easier to review and helps in follow-up of all the patient's medical needs. The SOAP/SOAPER/SOAPIE approach also allows medical personnel to be aware of the patient's current medications. Starting and resolution dates for each problem also are noted on the tracking page. Figure 13-3 shows SOAP note documentation in a paper chart.

Internists, family practitioners, and pediatricians use the POMR system more commonly than do specialists because they see their patients for a variety of problems over a long span of time. It is commonly used in manual medical records as well as EMRs.

A number of medical supply companies produce various formats for POMR manual charts. There are flip-up folder styles and book-style folders with twin prong fasteners to hold paper documents in place. Divider pages may come with tabs that are preprinted to specific needs or have adhesive labels that can be printed on a printer exactly as you want them. Sometimes, the inside front and back covers are printed with information to be filled in. These areas are often used to provide essential personal information such as name, address, telephone numbers, insurance information, and responsible party. Over a period of time, however, because the information changes, entries on the inside cover are less desirable. A patient demographic form (see Chapter 22) can be attached to the inside cover. It can be updated annually and changed easily. In a prominent place, usually on the inside front cover, is the word *ALLERGIES*

Problem and Medication List

Patient Name: **DOB:**
Allergies: **Pharmacy #**

Date	Dx #	Chronic Problems	Dx #	Chronic Medications	Date		Refills
					Start	Date	
					Stop	Initials	
					Start	Date	
					Stop	Initials	
					Start	Date	
					Stop	Initials	
					Start	Date	
					Stop	Initials	
					Start	Date	
					Stop	Initials	
					Start	Date	
					Stop	Initials	
					Start	Date	
					Stop	Initials	
					Start	Date	
					Stop	Initials	
					Start	Date	
					Stop	Initials	
					Start	Date	
					Stop	Initials	

Preventive	Date	Date	Date	Date	Date	Date
History Update Every 2 Years						
Breast Exam (plus Self-Exam)						
Mammogram						
DEXA						
Diabetic Blood Sugar Monitoring						
Diabetic Foot Care						
Diabetic HbA1c						
Diabetic LDL						
Diabetic Retinal Exam						
Diabetic Proteinuria						
Fasting Glucose						
Lipid Panel						
Pap/Pelvic						
Prostate Exam, PSA						
Rectal Exam						
Sigmoid/Colonos						
Stool for Occult Blood						
Testicular Exam (plus Self-Exam)						

Immunizations						
Vaccination	Schedule	Date	Date	Date	Date
Hepatitis	As appropriate				
Influenza	At risk—q1y				
Pneumovax	At risk X 1				
Td Booster	PRN—q10y				

Education	Date	Date	Date	Date
Advanced Directives/ Power of Attorney				
Alcohol/Drug Use				
Birth Control/Menopause				
Diabetes				
Diet				
Exercise				
Smoking				
Stress				

FIGURE 13-2 A sample patient problem and medication list that also provides space for dates and details of preventive actions, patient education, and immunizations as well as for the patient's pharmacy phone number.

in big letters (often preprinted in red). Any allergies that patients have are listed here. Also prominently displayed should be any forms the patient has signed granting release of information, as well as any forms signed to comply with HIPAA regulations.

The problem list may be entered on a divider flap or on specially printed paper. Other dividers may be used for laboratory reports, progress notes, history and physicals, hospital admissions, and medications. Depending on the practice and the wishes of the provider, tab dividers are available for consultations, correspondence, insurance data, hospital notes, pathology reports, and electrocardiogram reports. The problem list is most likely the first divider used, followed by laboratory reports and progress notes, usually in the SOAP format.

SOAP is easily adapted to the EMR. There are a number of methods of indicating SOAP in the EMR. (See the example in Figure 13-4.) For a look at different models, use a computer search engine to key in "SOAP Charting in EMRs." You will be able to compare a number of examples.

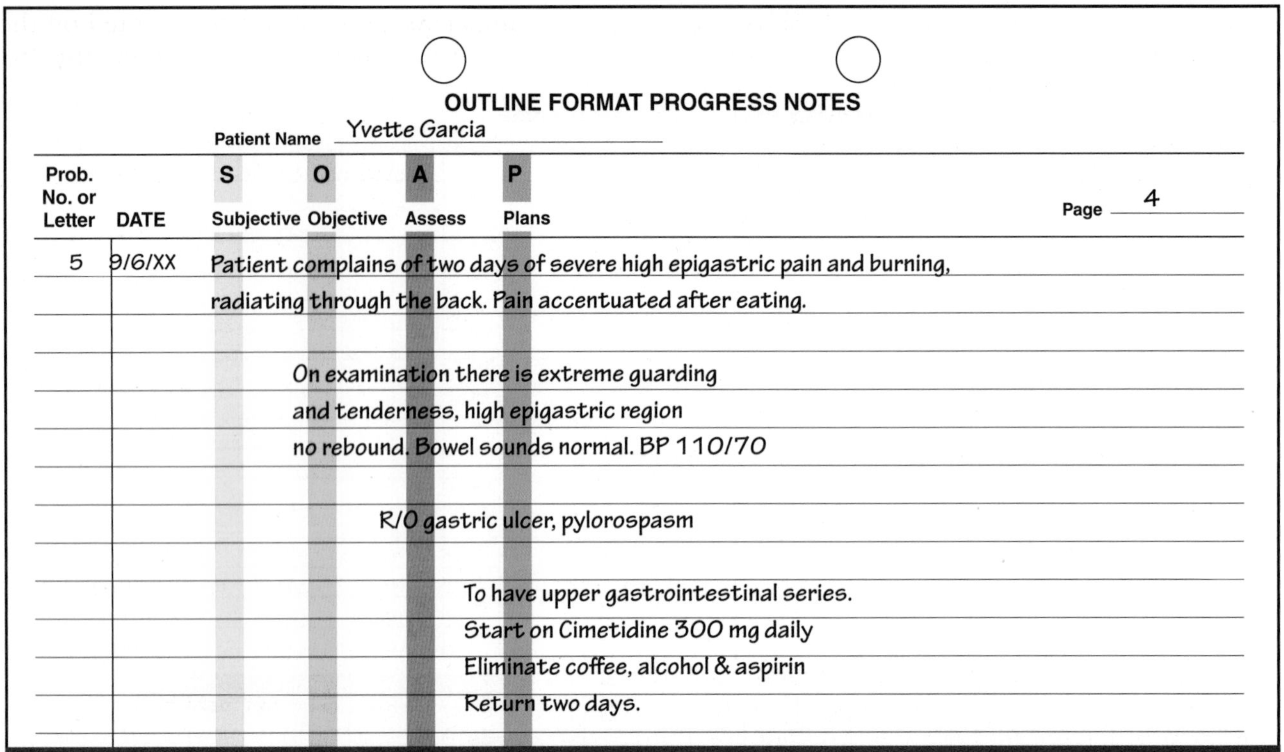

OUTLINE FORMAT PROGRESS NOTES

Patient Name **Yvette Garcia**

Prob. No. or Letter	DATE	**S** Subjective	**O** Objective	**A** Assess	**P** Plans
5	9/6/XX	Patient complains of two days of severe high epigastric pain and burning, radiating through the back. Pain accentuated after eating.			
			On examination there is extreme guarding and tenderness, high epigastric region no rebound. Bowel sounds normal. BP 110/70		
				R/O gastric ulcer, pylorospasm	
					To have upper gastrointestinal series. Start on Cimetidine 300 mg daily Eliminate coffee, alcohol & aspirin Return two days.

Page _____4_____

FIGURE 13-3 Example of SOAP progress note page in a paper chart.

Ms. Sabrina Katherine Lake   DOB 12/23/1977
01/29/XX

Subjective	Pt states, "I've been feeling very tired and weak for the past month," LMP 01-15-XX very heavy flow. Exam: 6 # Wt loss since last visit 12/19/XX.
Objective	BP 112/70, Hb 10.4, Hct 31%. Decrease in muscle strength, pale.
Assessment	R/O anemia.
Plan	CBC with diff sent to lab, return in 1 week.

FIGURE 13-4 An example of the SOAP method of charting in an electronic record.

Source-Oriented Medical Record

The manual **source-oriented medical record (SOMR)** groups information according to its source; for example, from laboratories, examinations, provider notes, consulting providers, and other sources. Facilities use this method because it makes different types of information quickly accessible. A fastener folder is used that contains several partitions with their own fasteners. This allows for a separate section for laboratory reports, pathology, progress notes, physical examinations, and correspondence to be filed chronologically within each section. In the SOMR system, many providers use the SOAP method to record their chart notes.

The organization of the SOMR is quite similar to that of the POMR chart with the one exception that the SOMR does not have the problem list. Also, the SOMR may continually add sheets of identifying information with appropriate sections in the chart rather than transferring any data. Many EMR software packages use either the POMR or the SOMR format and are easily adapted to a particular provider's practice.

Strict Chronological Arrangement

Using strict chronology, data are filed strictly with the most recently charted materials to the top of the folder. For instance, a patient is treated from 2008 to the present. To locate information recorded in 2009, it is necessary to flip through the chart until the material for the year 2009 is located. This method makes it difficult for a provider or medical assistant to quickly assess a patient's clinical picture. This type of arrangement may seem confusing, but it may fit a specialty clinic such as a dietitian, radiologist, or physical therapist where patients are usually seen on a short-term basis.

EQUIPMENT AND SUPPLIES

Three primary types of file cabinets are used in medical clinics where manual files are stored: vertical, lateral, and movable. For more information on the types of filing cabinets and filing supplies, see the "Filing Equipment and Supplies" Quick Reference Guide.

BASIC RULES FOR FILING

Regardless of the type of filing system used, alphabetizing is the key to organizing all files and charts. It is necessary to know more than just the alphabetic order of the letters *A* to *Z*. Thus, certain indexing rules have been developed by the Association of Medical Records Administrators (AMRA) to facilitate the alphabetic process in maintaining files in the medical clinic.

Indexing Units

There must be an organized method of identifying and separating items to be filed into small subunits. This is accomplished with the use of **indexing** units. A unit identifies each part of a name. In this process, each **unit** is identified according to unit 1 (the **key unit**), unit 2, unit 3, and so forth, with each segment of the filing label identified. This process can be applied to individual names, organizations, or clinics. Accepted filing rules describe how to assign unit numbers to each element.

Example: Annette Barbara Samuels

Unit 1	Samuels
Unit 2	Annette
Unit 3	Barbara

When working in a medical setting with patient charts, the patient's legal name is always used for the chart rather than a nickname or abbreviation. If the clinic has a practice of calling patients by preferred names, a note of name

preferences and nicknames may be noted on the chart. However, the filing label should use the proper name.

Example: The following items to be filed would be assigned units as illustrated:

| | Units Assigned | | |
	1	2	3
Cole Blanche Little	Little	Cole	Blanche
Wayne Lee Elder	Elder	Wayne	Lee
Kelso Medical Supply	Kelso	Medical	Supply

Filing Patient Charts

Rule 1. The names of individuals are assigned indexing units, respectively: last name (surname), first name, middle, and succeeding names.

| | Units Assigned | | |
	1	2	3
Jaime Renae Carrera	Carrera	Jaime	Renae
Lee Allen Au	Au	Lee	Allen
Bill Hugo Schwartz	Schwartz	Bill	Hugo

Rule 2. Names that include a single letter are indexed as the legal name and are placed before full names beginning with the same letter. "Nothing comes before something."

| | Units Assigned | | |
	1	2	3
J. Larson	Larson	J	—
James R. Larson	Larson	James	R

Rule 3. Foreign language prefixes are indexed as one unit with the unit that follows. Spacing, punctuation, and capitalization are ignored. Such prefixes include *d, da, de, de la, del, des, di, du, el, fitz, l, la, las, le, les, lu, m, mac, mc, o, saint, sainte, san, santa, sao, st, te, ten, ter, van, van de, van der,* and *von der* (*st, sainte,* and *saint* are indexed as written).

| | Units Assigned | | |
	1	2	3
Gerald Steven St. Simon	Stsimon	Gerald	Steven
Carol Louise del Rio	Delrio	Carol	Louise

Filing Equipment and Supplies

» TYPES OF FILING CABINETS

Vertical files (Figure 13-5)	Vertical files cabinets have pullout drawers where files are stored. Files are retrieved by lifting the appropriate file up and out. These are often used for business records and documents, and should include a locking device.
Open-shelf lateral files (Figure 13-6)	Records in open-shelf lateral file cabinets are retrieved by pulling them out laterally from the shelf. This type of cabinet is used most often with color-coded filing systems where visual inspection makes it possible to ensure files are kept in the proper order. Open-shelf lateral files are the most popular manual patient record system. It is necessary to be able to close and lock the open-shelf lateral files to protect confidentiality.
Movable file units	Movable file units allow easy access to large record systems and require less space than vertical or lateral files. These units may be electrically powered to move on floor tracks or may be physically moved with a handle mechanism. The movable shelving unit is electrically powered to open aisles for accessing files or to close aisles when those files do not need to be accessed. There are also movable file storage units that will automatically travel on a computer-controlled carousel track, moving files around until the required section reaches the operator.

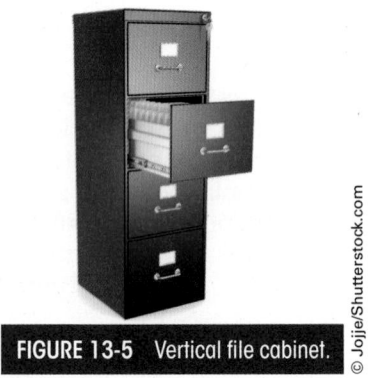

FIGURE 13-5 Vertical file cabinet.

© Jojie/Shutterstock.com

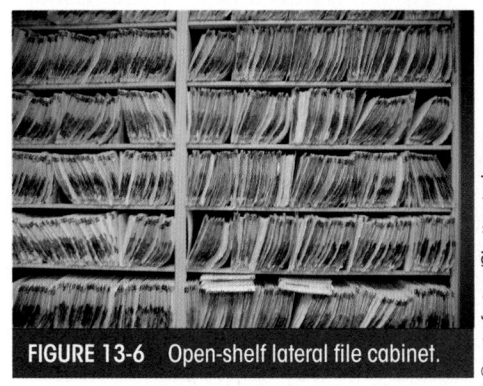

FIGURE 13-6 Open-shelf lateral file cabinet.

© peterfactors/Shutterstock.com

» FILING SUPPLIES

File folders 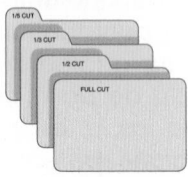	File folders are designed to use different types of labels. Extending along the top edge (the edge that will be visible when filing) are tabs that are cut in varying sizes and positions to allow for different methods of labeling. File folders should be constructed of good-quality card stock. If they are too light in weight, they will soon be bent, torn, and battered from use. They need to be sturdy enough for years of use.
Identification labels 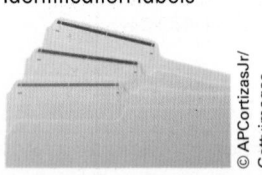 © APCortizasJr/ Gettyimages	A variety of labels are used to display the information required to select the correct name or number designation for a particular file. The identification label is adhered either along the top of the file folder (top tab) in vertical file cabinets or along the side of the file folder (side tab) in lateral file cabinets.

(continues)

| Guides and captions | Guides are used to separate file folders. Guides are somewhat larger than file folders and are of heavier stock. Guides are described by the position of the tab, designated according to its location. For instance, a tab located at the far left would be in the first position, the next one to the right would be in the second position, and so forth. Guides are used in vertical and lateral systems.

Captions are used to identify major sections of file folders by more manageable subunits (e.g., AA–AC, A, B, Office Supplies). Captions are marked on the tabs of the guides. These are denoted as single caption and double caption:

• *Single captions* contain just one letter, number, or unit:
  • A, B, C, D
• *Double captions* contain a double notation to denote a range of files:
  • Ab–Be, Co–Dy, Ho–Le |
|---|---|

Out guides	**Out guides**, or out sheets, are devices to help in tracking charts. An out guide is a piece of card stock or a plastic/paper sheet kept in place of the patient chart when the chart is removed from the filing storage.

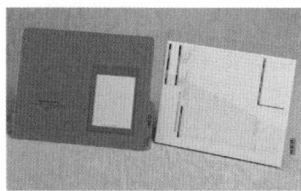

Rule 4. When titles are used, they are considered as separate indexing units. If the title appears with first and last names, the title is considered to be the last indexing unit. When dealing with patient charts, the first name always accompanies the title and last name.

	Units Assigned			
	1	2	3	4
Dr. Marlene Elaine Smith	Smith	Marlene	Elaine	Dr
Prof. Marcia Tai Lewis	Lewis	Marcia	Tai	Prof

Rule 5. Names that are hyphenated are considered as one unit.

	Units Assigned		
	1	2	3
Adele Marie Johnson-Smith	Johnson-smith	Adele	Marie
Ray Steven Reynolds-Martin	Reynolds-martin	Ray	Steven

Rule 6. When indexing names of married women, the name is indexed by the legal name. Remember that patient charts are legal documents, making this practice necessary (use cross-referencing as necessary).

	Units Assigned			
	1	2	3	4
Amy Sue Sung (Mrs. John)	Sung	Amy	Sue	Mrs John
Tami Jo Strizver (Mrs. Todd)	Strizver	Tami	Jo	Mrs Todd

Rule 7. Seniority and professional or academic degrees are the last indexing unit and are used only to distinguish identical names.

	Units Assigned			
	1	2	3	4
James Edward Brown, Jr.	Brown	James	Edward	Jr
James Edward Brown, Sr.	Brown	James	Edward	Sr

Rule 8. Mac and Mc are filed in their regular place alphabetically. Some clinics will provide a special guide for both Mac and Mc for ease in filing.

Mabbott
MacDonald
Mazziotti
McAffe

Rule 9. Numeric units are broken down such that numeric seniority terms are filed before alphabetic terms.

	Edward Lee Kletka, IV
BEFORE	Edward Lee Kletka, Jr.
	George Lee Curtis, II
BEFORE	George Lee Curtis, Sr.

Filing Identical Names

When names are identical, the address may be used to order files. The address is indexed by:

First	City
SECOND	STATE
Third	Street Name
FOURTH	**ADDRESS #**

Therefore, the following Acme Drug Supply files would be arranged from first to last as follows:

1. Acme Drug Supply, **839** *Kentucky Boulevard*, Crawford, MISSOURI

2. Acme Drug Supply, **683** *Wildflower Avenue*, Fairbanks, ALASKA

3. Acme Drug Supply, **1539** *Wildflower Avenue*, Fairbanks, ALASKA

4. Acme Drug Supply, **742** *Terminal Street West*, Fairbanks, ARIZONA

5. Acme Drug Supply, **731** *Terminal Street East*, New York, NEW YORK

Although this is the official indexing rule, most medical facilities prefer alternative methods for filing identical charts. The primary consideration here is that patient addresses often change frequently. Therefore, preferred methods include date of birth or Social Security number.

STEPS FOR FILING MEDICAL DOCUMENTATION IN PATIENT FILES

Before a discussion of the common filing systems, it is helpful to review procedural steps that accurately and efficiently process data sheets, laboratory requests, dictation, and so forth from the time they are generated to the time the file is returned to the medical records section. Efficiently following these steps will save considerable time in the clinic.

Inspect

Carefully inspect the report to identify the patient, subject, or file to whom the information belongs. Remove clips and staples. Make certain the information is complete.

Index

Use the indexing process to determine how the chart would be located, properly identifying indexing units and their order.

Code

Coding in medical records is the process of marking data to indicate how information is to be filed. If using a system other than a strict alphabetic system, determine the proper coding for the chart so it can be retrieved. Otherwise, identify the indexed units by underlining or highlighting. This makes refiling more effective and ensures that the item will always be filed in the same place. If a cross-reference is required, identify the cross-reference by double underlining and placing an *X* nearby. This chapter includes detailed information on coding and cross-referencing.

Sort

If there are a number of reports/documents to be filed, sort them into units according to the captions on the charts. This will eliminate wasted time in working back and forth through the alphabet or numbers.

File

The papers are placed in the proper charts and the charts returned to their proper place in the medical records section. Be alert to the labels and refile any information or charts that have been misfiled.

FILING TECHNIQUES AND COMMON FILING SYSTEMS

Three major filing systems are commonly used in the clinic setting: alphabetic, numeric, and subject. The alphabet is intrinsic to all methods, and the basic rules for filing, covered previously, are used in all systems.

Color coding is used a high percentage of the time in all three systems to minimize filing errors. Another system, geographic, is seldom used in the clinic unless there are multiple clinics. Even then, a form of color coding may be used.

Color Coding

Color coding is a technique often used in the three major filing systems. Numerous color-coding systems are available. Patient charts most often use an alphabetic system of color coding, although color coding can be used in numeric filing as well. There are a number of large suppliers that offer color systems and records management systems. Color coding may seem complicated at first, but once medical assistants understand the principles behind it and practice its application a number of times, the task becomes much easier, and there is immediate recognition if a chart is misfiled.

Color coding makes retrieval of files more efficient with the use of visible color differences that facilitate easier maintenance of the files. Color-coding filing systems also use an alphabetic system; after they are coded by color, that designation is used to order the files alphabetically.

Tab-Alpha System. The various forms of the Tab-Alpha system are designed primarily for filing systems in small clinics that use vertical files where all individual charts are clearly visible in one unit.

Each alphabetic letter is assigned a different color. Each folder has a color-coded label. Only full-cut folders are used:

- Colored labels are applied over the edge of the full cut for the first two letters of the key indexing unit (Winston, Paul Lewis: WI).
- A third white label is placed over the tab edge, which contains all of the indexing units (Winston, Paul Lewis).
- In addition, some clinics use a color-coded label to indicate the last year the patient was seen. This makes an efficient method for easily identifying active and inactive files.
- Any additional labels (e.g., allergies, last year seen, or industrial claim) are attached to the chart according to the clinic procedure.

Alpha-Z System. Forms of the Alpha-Z system are designed for use with either open lateral files or vertical drawer files (Figure 13-7A). Alphabetic letters are used as the primary guides. Breakdowns of alphabetic combinations are added as determined by the needs of a particular facility.

A combination of 13 colors is used in the Alpha-Z system with white letters on a solid colored background for the first half of the alphabet and white letters on a colored background with white stripes for the second half of the alphabet (Figure 13-7B).

The 13 colors used are shown in Figure 13-8. Folders have three labels:

- The first label contains the typed name, a color block, and the letter of the alphabet for the first letter of the first indexing unit:

  Winston, Lewis Paul YELLOW *W*

- The second and third labels are color-coded to correspond to the second and third letters of the first unit:

  ***I* on pink background and *N* on red-striped background**

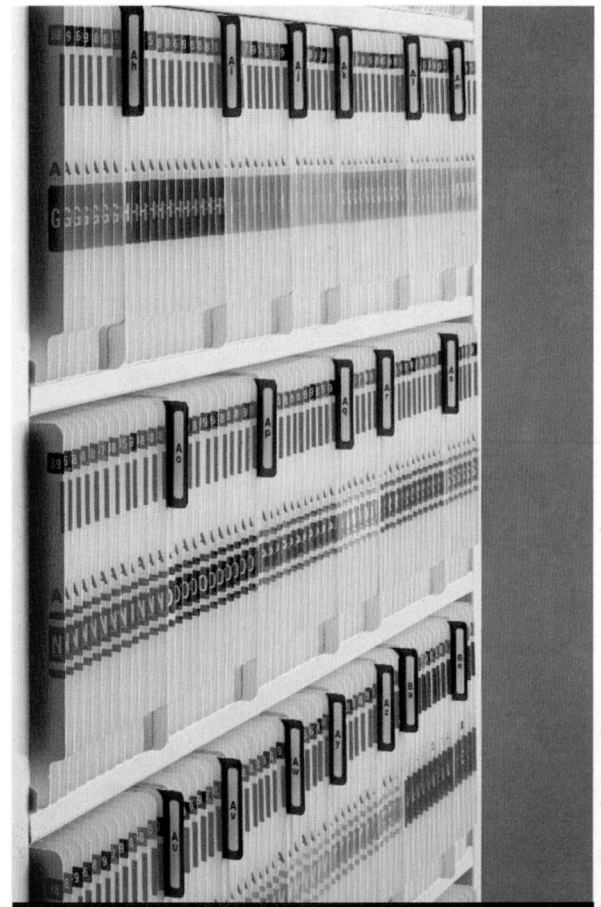

FIGURE 13-7A Color-coding filing system uses open-lateral shelving unit with color-coded files.

Courtesy Smead Manufacturing Company

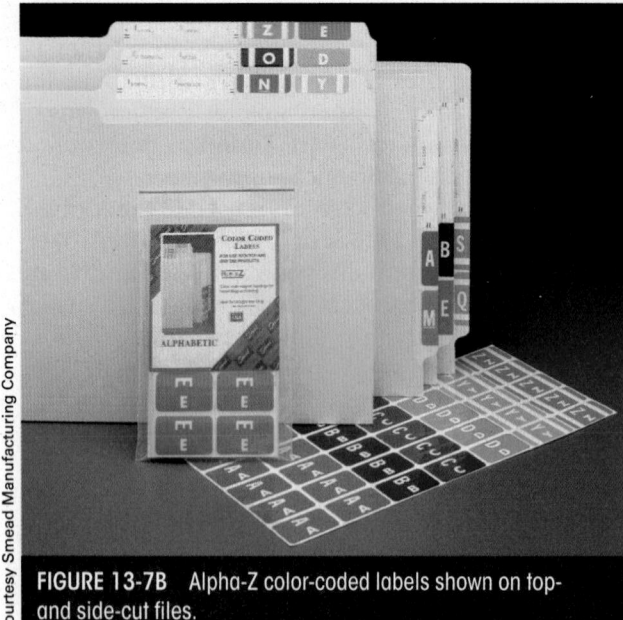

FIGURE 13-7B Alpha-Z color-coded labels shown on top- and side-cut files.

Courtesy Smead Manufacturing Company

White Letter Colored Background	White Letter Striped Colored Background	Color
A	N	Red
B	O	Dark Blue
C	P	Dark Green
D	Q	Light Blue
E	R	Purple
F	S	Orange
G	T	Gray
H	U	Dark Brown
I	V	Pink
J	W	Yellow
K	X	Light Brown
L	Y	Lavender
M	Z	Light Green

FIGURE 13-8 Thirteen colors are used in the Alpha-Z system.

Customized Color-Coding Systems. Many clinics use color systems to meet specific needs.

Colored File Folders by First Name. One method color codes the first letter of the first name. The folders then are filed alphabetically by last name.

Example: *A* is assigned red folders; *M* is assigned green folders; *S* is assigned blue folders

Annette Samuels	Red folder
Michael Taylor	Green folder
Susan Boyer	Blue folder

Many small medical clinics use this system and find it quite effective. In the multiprovider urgent care center, this would be quite time-consuming when locating files for patients of all providers.

Colored File Folders by Last Name. Another method using this system assigns colored folders according to the first letter of the last name. The folders are then filed alphabetically.

Example: *S* is assigned pink folders; *B* is assigned gray folders.

Bill Schwartz	Pink folder
Corey Boyer	Gray folder

This system makes it easy to spot folders that have been misfiled under an incorrect first letter, but it does not break it down further for misfiling within the first-letter guides.

Color-Coded Numbers. The color-coded number system is used in a numeric filing system and operates in the same way as alphabetic systems. Numbers from 0 to 9 are color coded. The appropriate colored numbers are then placed on the tabs of the patient's folder.

Alphabetic Filing

Procedure

Strict alphabetic filing is one of the simplest filing methods, as files are strictly maintained by assigning a label to each file. The first letter of that label (e.g., Jones, Invoices, or Pharmacies) is then used to alphabetize the files from A to Z. When a limited number of files are accessed, this is an acceptable method of maintaining records. Also note that every filing system will utilize the alphabet somewhere. Procedure 13-2 provides steps for manual filing with an alphabetic system.

Manual Filing with an Alphabetic System

PURPOSE:

To demonstrate an understanding of the principles of alphabetic filing.

EQUIPMENT/SUPPLIES:

- Documents to be filed
- Dividers with guides
- Miscellaneous number file section
- Alphabetic card file and cards
- Accession journal, if needed

PROCEDURE STEPS:

1. Inspect and index. RATIONALE: Ensures that the chart is ready for filing and determines the order in which the chart will be filed.

2. Sort the charts alphabetically. RATIONALE: Determines the order and placement of the record; allows for a second assessment for placement.

3. Create cross-reference files according to clinic policy.

4. File the charts appropriately.

5. Check the placement with the charts immediately before and after the chart being filed. RATIONALE: Makes certain the chart is filed in the correct location.

Numeric Filing

Numeric filing is organized by number rather than by letter. A key benefit of numeric filing is that it preserves patient confidentiality because the individual's name is not obviously apparent on the file folder. The numeric filing systems most often used in medical facilities are straight numeric and terminal digit.

Straight Numeric. Straight numeric filing places charts in exact chronological order according to assigned number. For example, records numbered 45023, 45024, and 45025 will be in consecutive order on a shelf. This is an easy system to learn and use; however, there are some disadvantages. The greater number of digits to recall, the greater the chance for error. Numbers transposition is common. Chart number 45024 can be misfiled as chart number 54024. The use of color with straight numeric can decrease misfiling.

Terminal Digit. In terminal digit filing, a six-digit number is most often used with a hyphen dividing three parts of two digits, for example, 85-32-07 and 86-32-07. Within these numbers, the primary units are the last two numbers; the middle digits are the secondary units; the first two numbers are the third and final units considered. In a terminal digit file, there are 100 primary sections from 00 to 99 to be considered. The medical assistant will consider the primary section first, match the record with the same group to the secondary set of digits next, and then file in numerical order by the third unit.

The advantage to this system is that files and numbers are equally distributed. Only every 100th new medical record will be filed in the same primary section. Filing using the straight numerical order of the first two numbers is simple to learn.

Middle Digit. In middle digit systems, the staff still files according to pairs of digits, but the pairs of digits are in different positions. The middle pair of digits is primary, the pair of digits to the left is secondary, and the pair of digits on the right is third.

The terminal digit and middle digit systems are most likely seen in hospitals and large multi-provider clinics.

Components of Numeric Filing.
Four essential components are used with a numeric system, whether it is a manual or computerized system.

Serially Numbered Dividers with Guides.
Consecutive numeric guides (5, 10, etc.; 50, 100, etc.) separate the individual file folders into smaller groups of files.

Miscellaneous (General) Numeric File Section.
This is reserved for records that have not been assigned numbers. Patients should automatically be assigned a number on the first visit. However, on occasion patients cannot be assigned a number initially. The miscellaneous section is generally in front of all the numeric folders for ease of locating items. Files in the miscellaneous section are filed alphabetically by patient name. This is the best place for the miscellaneous file(s) for two reasons:

1. They do not have to be moved each time a numbered file is added to the back of the order.
2. In a large system of files, retrieval from the front is quick and easy.

Alphabetic Card File.
This alphabetic file is necessary as a source to locate numeric files or records. A card contains name, address, and file number (or an *M* if located in the miscellaneous section); any **cross-reference** is here rather than in the numeric files.

The alphabetic card file in a manual system would be equivalent to the computerized record of the patient and whatever number is assigned to him or her in that computer record. If using a computerized system, the program generally will automatically cross-reference the number with the alphabetic list that was generated with the initial entry. If laboratory data on Leo M. McKay come into the clinic, there will need to be a method to know where to locate his chart to file the report, that is, the alphabetic listing.

With a manual system, the alphabetic file is kept in an index card fashion. This file will contain the complete name and address (and any other information denoted by the clinic policy, e.g., insurance and emergency numbers).

Noted with this information there needs to be either an *M* for miscellaneous (for those items not assigned a number) or an assigned number (Figures 13-9A and B).

If a cross-reference is required, prepare a cross-reference card and include an *X* next to the file number (or *M*) to indicate this is the cross-reference card and not the primary location (Figure 13-9C).

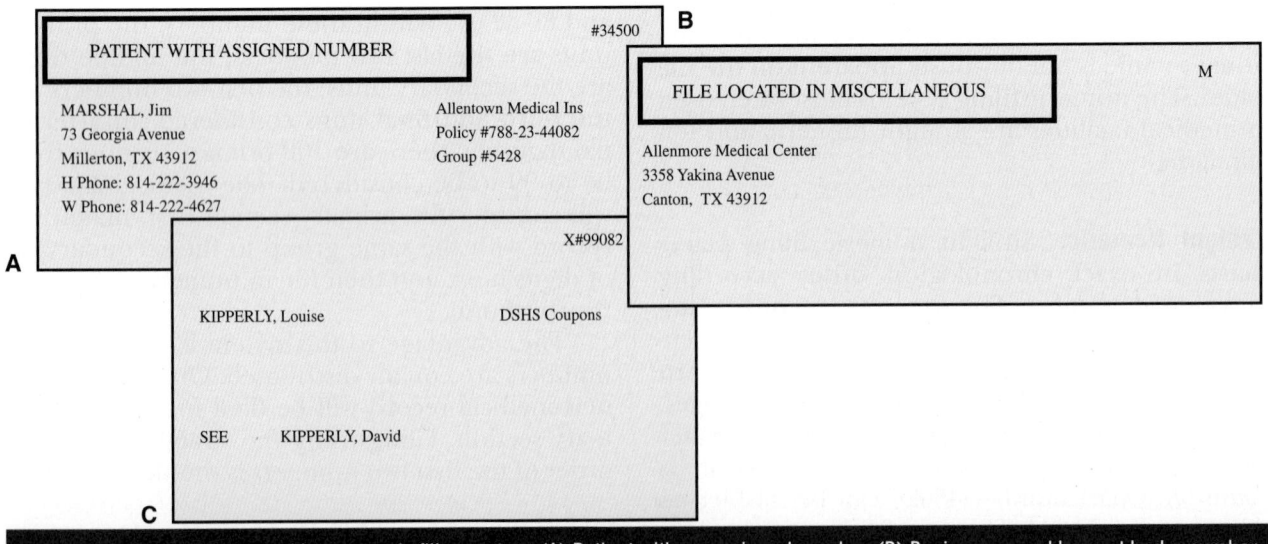

FIGURE 13-9 Card files used in a numeric filing system: (A) Patient with an assigned number. (B) Business record has not had a number assigned and is located in miscellaneous section. (C) Cross-reference card.

Accession Record. The **accession record** is a journal (or computer listing) where numbers are preassigned. Each new item to be assigned is written on the line next to the number (Figure 13-10). Each new entry for which a chart will be created must be assigned a number. A computerized system would have an accession record in its memory bank. Procedure 13-3 provides numeric filing steps.

Subject Filing

There are many reasons why material would be filed using a system of subjects in a medical clinic. If providers are doing research, they might wish to index research according to diseases. Subject files are convenient for locating frequently used services or for filing reference materials for patient needs. Insurance company information also might be filed by subject.

When using a subject filing system, scan the material to determine the subject or theme. As with color-coding and numeric filing, an alphabetic file is necessary. This can be either a subject list or an index card file listing the subjects. Also, as with numeric filing, all cross-reference cards are done only with alphabetic file listings.

Within the folders, material can be arranged either alphabetically or chronologically; keep in

---

PROCEDURE 13-3

Manual Filing with a Numeric System

PURPOSE:

To demonstrate an understanding of the principles of the numeric filing system.

EQUIPMENT/SUPPLIES:

- Documents to be filed
- Dividers with guides
- Miscellaneous numeric file section
- Alphabetic card file and cards
- Accession journal, if needed

PROCEDURE STEPS:

1. Inspect and index. RATIONALE: Ensures that the information is ready for filing and determines how the chart will be located.

2. Code for filing units. Check the alphabetic card file for each piece to see if the card has already been prepared. RATIONALE: Determines the number under which the chart will be filed.

3. Write the number in the upper right-hand corner if the piece has been assigned a number. RATIONALE: Tells you the number to be used in filing.

4. If no number is assigned (i.e., it has an *M* for miscellaneous), check the miscellaneous file. If a miscellaneous item is ready to be assigned a number, make a card and note the number in the right-hand corner of the card file, cross out the *M*, and make a chart file. RATIONALE: Tells you if a number should be prepared because of numerous items in the miscellaneous file, or if the piece to be filed should stay in the miscellaneous file.

5. If there is no card, make up an alphabetic card including a complete name and address, and then write either *M* or assign a number. RATIONALE: Ensures that there is always an alphabetic card with necessary demographic information and an assigned number or *M* for each piece of information and chart.

6. Cross-reference if necessary and file the card properly. You are then ready to file the document in the appropriate file folder/chart. RATIONALE: Ensures less likelihood of misfiling if necessary cross-references are prepared.

7. File in ascending order. RATIONALE: Establishes a pattern for filing.

ACCESSION LOG BOOK

#	File Name
800	CARRERA, Jaime
801	AU, Rhoda
802	TREMONT Drug Supply
803	
804	
805	
806	
807	

FIGURE 13-10 Accession record or log sequentially lists predetermined numbers to be used to assign to numeric records. The next number available in this system is 803.

mind the objective for maintaining the particular files. For instance, if using subject indexing for research projects providers have conducted, identify the subject category; then in the material, code an item for reference to that specific material. Procedure 13-4 provides subject filing steps.

Choosing a Filing System

To select a filing system, each facility must decide what the primary objectives are with respect to storage of patient files, business records, and research files. How will the charts be used primarily? Will information need to be tracked by others not familiar with the records? Often more than one filing system will be used, such as alphabetic filing for patient charts, a numeric system for research subjects, and a subject system for miscellaneous correspondence.

> ### PROCEDURE 13-4
>
> Procedure
>
> # Manual Filing with a Subject Filing System
>
> **PURPOSE:**
> To demonstrate an understanding of the principles of the subject filing system.
>
> **EQUIPMENT/SUPPLIES:**
> - Documents to be filed by subject
> - Subject index list or index card file listing subjects
> - Alphabetic card file and cards
>
> **PROCEDURE STEPS:**
> 1. Review the item to find the subject. RATIONALE: Checks the item for the main topic of information to determine where the piece will be filed.
> 2. Match the subject of the item with an appropriate category on the subject index list. RATIONALE: Saves you time so that you do not create an unnecessary subject index list.
> 3. If the item contains information that may pertain to more than one subject, decide on the proper cross-reference. RATIONALE: Ensures that any confusion will be checked with a cross-reference.
> 4. If the subject title is written on the material, underline it. RATIONALE: Readily identifies the subject used for filing.
> 5. If the subject title is not written on the item, write it clearly in the upper right-hand corner and underline (_____) it. RATIONALE: Indicates the subject used for filing; consistently places the subject in the expected place.
> 6. Use a wavy (＿＿＿) line for cross-referencing and an *X* as with alphabetic and numeric filing. RATIONALE: Clearly identifies any cross-referencing.
> 7. Underline the first indexing unit of the coded units. RATIONALE: Ensures the correct order for filing.

The number of documents to be filed is one primary determinant in selecting an alphabetic or numeric system. Alphabetic filing is quite manageable for many clinics. However, when the number of patients is quite large, a numeric system becomes practical because an infinite set of numbers is available. With the numeric system, there is only one of each assigned designation. However, with an alphabetic system, there are a number of common names (e.g., Smith, Jones, Adams, and Johnson) that can have many multiples requiring additional sorting to narrow the search for the correct chart. In addition, with multiple charts of the same last name, the chance for misfiling increases.

Legal

Confidentiality is another reason to select a numeric filing system. Confidentiality of charts is maintained more easily with numeric files because no name is visible on the outside of the chart. In addition, numerically referenced records can be used in research activities where random sampling and anonymity are required.

To make the medical facility HIPAA compliant when traditional paper-based or manual charts are used, you need to ensure that no patient-identifiable information is located on the outside of the chart. This includes the patient address or any other information that might be used to determine the identity of the patient, including Social Security number, birth date, or phone number. Any information that reveals a health condition or payment status also must be removed from the outside of the chart. Recall the earlier example of locked storage cabinets for manual files. Note that all file cabinets are to be closed and locked when no one is immediately present in the clinic; that includes lunch time when the staff may be eating in the staff lounge.

FILING PROCEDURES

By adhering to some common principles in medical records management, any filing system will be more effective and will enable the medical

assistant to store, identify, retrieve, and maintain medical records efficiently.

Cross-Referencing

In running an efficient medical facility, files must be stored for quick and accurate retrieval. If there is any doubt as to where a particular file would be located, cross-reference the file. Many clinics fail to take the extra time it requires to do this. However, with the growing number of foreign names, hyphenated names, and stepfamilies, it is well worth the effort. When the clinic receives a letter and a release of information form inquiring about medical facts on Mr. David Kipperly's four stepchildren who were involved in an accident, how will these files be located? If they are cross-referenced under the stepfather's name, this will be a relatively easy procedure. However, if the medical assistant is unfamiliar with the family (as in a larger urgent care center with a large volume of patients), this may become a time-consuming job. Another scenario might involve insurance information on Janet Morgan. A search of the records does not produce a file for any Janet Morgan. The reason for this is that Janet Morgan is married, and her chart has been filed under Janet Hill-Morgan. Time spent cross-referencing contributes to a more efficient method of retrieving information.

A cross-referencing system does not need to be elaborate. It is quite sufficient to use inserts with labels attached that are inserted in the appropriate place in the storage units. For instance, a plain piece of cardstock, rather than a file or chart, could be inserted for "Janet Morgan." This insert would simply have a label directing one to the location of the primary file.

The proper steps for cross-referencing, together with several examples where cross-referencing might be used, are discussed in the next section.

Steps for Cross-Referencing

1. Identify the primary filing label.
2. Make a proper file to be used as the primary location for all medical records.
3. Identify one (or more) alternatives where one might find the file.
4. For the alternative filings, make a cross-reference sheet, card, or dummy chart that lists the primary reference and refers back to the location of the primary file.

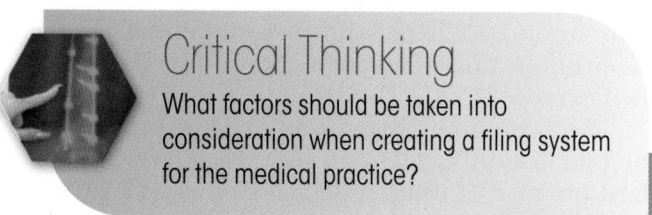

Critical Thinking

What factors should be taken into consideration when creating a filing system for the medical practice?

Example: The patient, Jaime Renae Carrera, has made it known to the clinic that most of his information received will refer to the name Renny Carrera, as this is his preference. The SEE reference will identify where the primary file is located.

PRIMARY FILE:	Carrera, Jaime Renae
X-REFERENCE FILE:	Carrera, Renny
	SEE Carrera, Jaime Renae

Rule 1. **Married Individuals.** When taking a spouse's name, the primary file would be the patient's legal name with the cross-reference listed under the spouse's.

PRIMARY FILE:	Au, Rhoda A. (Mrs.)
	Lee Au
X-REFERENCE FILE:	Au, Mrs. Lee
	SEE Au, Rhoda A. (Mrs.)

Rule 2. **Foreign Names.** The primary file would be located under the patient's legal name. It is important, therefore, that you identify the first, middle, and surname (last name) when the patient comes for the first visit. Unless people are familiar with a particular group of names, the first, middle, and surnames are often confused with one another. Again, your experience will teach you which cross-references should be set up.

PRIMARY FILE:	Sing, Yange Teah
X-REFERENCE FILE:	Yange, Sing Teah
	SEE Sing, Yange Teah
X-REFERENCE FILE:	Teah, Yange Sing
	SEE Sing, Yange Teah

Rule 3. **Hyphenated Names.** With the proliferation of hyphenated names, it is common for materials to be listed under different combinations of the hyphenated name. For instance, a married woman may have records under her maiden name, her husband's surname, and her hyphenated name. Therefore, it is necessary to make two cross-references.

PRIMARY FILE:	Krenshaw-Skiple, Rose Marie
X-REFERENCE FILE:	Skiple, Rose Marie
	SEE Krenshaw-Skiple, Rose Marie
X-REFERENCE FILE:	Krenshaw, Rose Marie
	SEE Krenshaw-Skiple, Rose Marie

Rule 4. **Multiple Listings.** A great deal of correspondence is received with multiple listings of names. At times, the medical clinic may receive correspondence from only one of the involved parties. Rather than keep a separate file for each, maintain a primary file as listed on the letter and then cross-reference file(s) for the individual names.

PRIMARY FILE:	Olsen, Piper, and Dillard Associates
X-REFERENCE FILE:	Piper, Richard C., M.D.
	SEE Olsen, Piper, and Dillard Associates
X-REFERENCE FILE:	Olsen, Francis William, M.D.
	SEE Olsen, Piper, and Dillard Associates
X-REFERENCE FILE:	Dillard, Thomas E., M.D.
	SEE Olsen, Piper, and Dillard Associates

Tickler Files

Sticky notes and writing notes on the calendar are popular methods of reminding clinic personnel to follow up with some required action. However, a well-organized, efficient clinic will maintain what is known as a **tickler file**, a method that serves as a reminder that some action needs to be taken at a date in the future.

Some systems have a calendar that pops up to allow reminders to be placed on the calendar. The computer system reminds you of the note when that particular day arrives. Some EMR systems have built-in reminders that automatically give a reminder for such things as annual physical examinations, monthly blood pressure checks, medication checks, and anything else that might be beneficial to both patient and provider. Some systems automatically pick up these reminders from the progress notes that are a part of the electronic medical record.

Most computer systems today have provisions for establishing ticklers on files. However, a standard practice of using index cards for tickler files is easy to maintain (Figure 13-11).

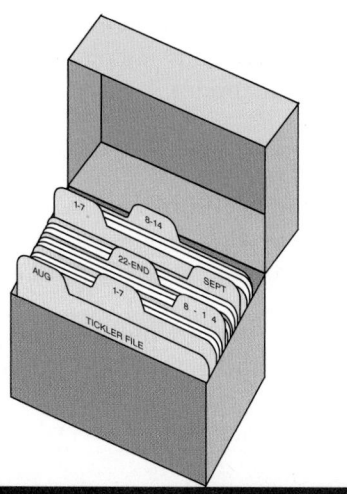

FIGURE 13-11 Tickler files should be reviewed daily or weekly to follow up on activities and actions that must be taken.

The tickler card should contain the following information:

- Patient name
- Tickler date (when action should be taken)
- Required action (e.g., schedule surgery or mail reminder)
- Additional relevant information (e.g., telephone number)

If action is to be taken with a patient or on behalf of the patient (e.g., scheduling a hospital admittance or sending a reminder of a checkup visit), place the information on the tickler card as soon as possible so this task is not forgotten.

When filing records, be sure to look for words such as *on _____ date we will*, *pending action*, or *follow-up*, indicating that some course of action needs to be taken.

It is important to remember that any tickler system, whether manual or computerized, is worthless if the reminder is not adhered to and appropriate action taken.

Release Marks

It is a good practice to use some type of release mark (date stamp, initials, check mark) on every item that is filed. Ideally, the provider should initial the document after it has been read. Then, if action is required by the medical assistant, a release mark is in a consistently identified place on every document. If no action is required after the provider has signed or initialed, place a release mark on the document. A release mark on every piece of information serves as an excellent quality-control measure.

Checkout System

Many clinics have developed dummy charts or files labeled "out sheets" or "out guides" for use when the chart is removed. Most of these guides are identified by an OUT label or metal holder, but they could be assigned a particular color; the key is that they stand out as different from the primary folders.

On the out guide, there should be a minimum of the following information:

- A record of when the chart was removed
- Where the chart can be located

Other information that is useful to note includes:

- Expected date of return
- Actual date the chart was returned
- Signature of the individual checking out the record
- Notation on what section of the chart file was borrowed, such as a laboratory report or specialty examination

Some clinics prefer to have *temporary folders* rather than just an out guide. There are also out guides with pockets to file data in the absence of a chart. This allows for data storage on a temporary basis until the primary file is returned. The data can then be filed permanently when the primary folder is returned. If these folders are of a different color or have a different type of tab/label, they can be spotted easily so the staff can track the temporary files to be sure they do not become permanent folders.

Locating Missing Files or Data

Misfiling can occur for a number of reasons. When this situation occurs, a specific procedure must be established to conduct a search for the missing information. By systematically searching, the missing data usually can be located. This systematic search can be aided by making a mental note of the particular items that commonly are misplaced, such as thin-paper laboratory reports, small laboratory slips, and look-alike names such as "Ward" filed under "Wart" or "Adam" filed under "Adams." Make a note of what was misfiled and where the information was located to more easily locate similar items in the future.

To locate missing pieces of information when the correct file is located but not the particular item within that file:

- Check all of the items within the file.
- Check other files with similar labels.

To locate missing files:

- Check the folders filed before and after the proper location of the misplaced file.
- Look at folders with similar labels.
- Check the provider's desk, the desk tray, and with other clinic personnel.
- If using a color-coding system, look for folders with the same coding as the misplaced file.
- If using a numeric system, look for possible transposition of combinations of numbers.
- Check for transposition of first and last names.
- Check for alternative spellings of names or look-alike names.

Misplaced files can be frustrating and time-consuming to locate. The best strategy is to check files for the proper filing order whenever returning or retrieving a file folder. When removing a file to answer a question, leave the file following it sticking out slightly to make its return easy and correct. Most importantly, when finished with a record, refile it immediately.

Filing Chart Data

Types of Reports. The patient's chart is the key source of information relating to treatment. A number of reports are kept in the chart, all serving to provide a total picture of patient care. Following are the most common documents that are part of the patient's medical record (see Chapter 15 for other documents).

Clinical Notes. Clinical notes include documentation such as the medical history, the physical examination, and the follow-up notes. They track the patient's course of treatment.

Correspondence. Filing of correspondence varies. Some file all types of correspondence together. Others file correspondence about the patient's treatment with the clinical notes.

Laboratory Reports. Included in laboratory reports are X-ray reports, CT scans, ultrasound reports, blood work, urinalysis, EEGs, ECGs, physical therapy–related reports, and pathology reports—information related to clinical data that assess the patient's condition.

Miscellaneous. The miscellaneous category includes insurance-related papers, requests for transfer of medical records, and personal notes from/to patients. In general, miscellaneous encompasses matters not related to direct treatment.

Retention and Purging

As information accumulates, it is necessary to maintain files by the process known as **purging**. Purging can involve several forms of action.

Record Purging. Record purging requires sorting through records and removing those not in active use. Each facility should establish a standard policy for control and processing of records.

 States have different time requirements for retention of various types of records that will take into account the statute of limitations (see Chapter 6). Table 13-1 lists general guidelines. As a way of controlling risk and practicing responsible risk management, many facilities choose to maintain large numbers of inactive files rather than to destroy any records. Check with the Medical Practice Act in your state to determine record-keeping requirements.

Active Files. Active files include records that need to be readily accessible for retrieval of information.

Inactive Files. Inactive files consist of records that need to be retained for possible retrieval of information. Files not currently being accessed for information would thus become inactive. Often, the type of practice dictates the relevant time period when files are determined to be inactive (generally 2 to 3 years).

Closed Files. Closed files are those that are no longer required. Again, patient files are retained for significantly longer periods of time because of litigation and research considerations, usually 3 to 6 years beyond the statute of limitations.

CORRESPONDENCE

Most clinics process a considerable amount of correspondence not directly related to patient care. Such items include employment applications, letters from/to pharmaceutical representatives, advertisements for medical supplies, magazine subscription information, and letters to/from other providers on a variety of subjects. This correspondence is processed using alphabetic filing rules. However, an additional step is necessary to determine whether the correspondence is incoming

TABLE 13-1

RECORDS FOR RETENTION

PATIENT INDEX FILES

These include appointment books or daily appointment sheets. They are kept for an indefinite period. They may be required for litigation or research.

CASE HISTORIES

The length of storage depends on state requirements and individual practice requirements. Product liability cases have deemed long-term storage of these records necessary (20+ years). The records of minors must be retained at least until the age of majority. The statute of limitations is a deciding factor as well, usually 3 to 6 years.

If records are to be destroyed because of the death of a provider or closure of a practice, the following procedure is required: Each patient should be notified of the circumstances and given the opportunity to have his or her records forwarded to another provider. After notification, the records must be retained for a "reasonable" period (determined by state regulations). A period of 3 to 6 months is generally determined to be a "reasonable" period. The records must be destroyed by burning or shredding to protect confidentiality.

LABORATORY AND X-RAY DATA

Originals should be retained permanently with the patient's case history.

PERSONAL/PROFESSIONAL RECORDS

Professional licenses should be stored permanently in a secure location.

OFFICE EQUIPMENT RECORDS

These records are generally kept until the warranties and depreciation are no longer valid. They should be kept in an easily accessible location if under maintenance contract.

INSURANCE RECORDS

Professional liability policies are kept permanently. Other policies are kept in active files while in force.

FINANCIAL RECORDS

Bank records are kept in active files for up to 3 years and then placed in inactive storage. Tax records must be retained permanently.

or outgoing. The correspondence must be filed under some aspect that will be distinctly identifiable; that is, what idea, subject, or name would most likely be thought of if someone wanted to retrieve that correspondence or file additional relevant correspondence.

Even when scanning documents for importing to the EMR, how to determine the category or subject for a document needs to be established. The digital version of the document can then be archived in the appropriate place within the record.

Filing Procedures for Correspondence

Once it is determined whether correspondence is incoming or outgoing, follow the basic rules for filing. In addition:

- Remove paper clips and staple items together.
- Inspect to see if the item is ready to be filed; that is, if appropriate action has been taken. If not, take care of copies and enclosures, and then place notes in the tickler file for future action before proceeding with the indexing.
- On incoming correspondence, be sure the letterhead is in direct relation to the letter.

Example: A personal letter written by a patient on hotel stationery—index the signature on the letter.

Example: When both the company name and the signature are important, index the company name. A letter from Preston Industries written by the company president—index Preston Industries, not the president's name, which may change.

Example: If there is no letterhead and you have determined the material is not relevant to a patient, index the name on the signature line. A letter received from Carlton Fiske, RPT, advising your clinic of services his firm has to offer your patients—index Fiske.

- On outgoing correspondence, look at the inside address and the reference line.

Example: A letter to the District Court regarding Karen Ritter, an employee who is summoned to jury duty—index Karen Ritter rather than District Court.

Example: If the correspondence is relevant to a patient, index the patient's name. A letter RE: Wayne Elder—index under Elder.

Example: If the correspondence is not relevant to a patient, look to the inside address for the indexing information. A letter inquiring about cost estimates for redecorating the clinic reception room—index the firm in the inside address, and cross-reference to the subject (redecorating clinic).

Example: When the inside address is relevant and contains both a company name and a person's name, index the company name. (This avoids the problem of personnel changes.) Cross-referencing would be done under the individual name. A letter to Marvin Fairchild, President of Brandex Pharmaceuticals—index Brandex Pharmaceuticals with a cross-reference for "Marvin Fairchild, President, SEE Brandex Pharmaceuticals."

Example: If the letter is personal, the name of the person to whom the letter is written would be used for indexing purposes. Dr. Lewis writes a letter to Dr. Whitney, one of his colleagues, asking if he plans to attend an upcoming conference—index Dr. Whitney.

- On incoming or outgoing correspondence, code the indexing units of the designated label. If the correspondence is being cross-referenced, be sure to note the cross-referencing unit and place the *X* in a visible place. You may find that the body of the letter contains an important name or subject.

- Create a miscellaneous folder for items that do not have enough in number to warrant an individual folder. Items in the miscellaneous folder are filed alphabetically first, and then identical items are filed with the most recent piece on top. An individual folder is then created when enough pieces accumulate on a particular item.

ELECTRONIC MEDICAL RECORDS

Total electronic automation in any medical facility is a major undertaking. It can be both frightening and exhilarating. Careful study of systems available, impact on providers and staff, time necessary for moving from manual to electronic files, and costs involved are measured against the benefits incurred.

With the government's mandate to have EMRs for most patients and Congress pushing to make all Medicare-covered prescriptions transferred electronically, EMRs are here to stay and one day will replace all paper/manual medical records. Evidence shows that fewer errors are created in EMRs because the "human element" is decreased. If all the data are entered correctly, the computer software "does all the thinking" to find the chart, store information appropriately, create reminder notices, check all medications for any contraindications, and flag any warning to providers, such as high cholesterol or blood pressure readings moving into the "alert" zone. The EMR will keep a record of all patient appointments and any missed appointments as well as any piece of information that might be found in a manual patient record. EMR software creates, stores, edits, and retrieves patient data. It has the added advantage of allowing more than one person to access a chart at the same time.

EMR software can be purchased as a single-computer application or as part of a larger "practice management" software package. Often, medical facilities start with one aspect of a practice management software package (usually not EMRs) and then gradually add the other pieces. EMRs are capable of the following:

- Create and print customized encounter forms and superbills
- View patient records of all provider encounters and laboratory results, transcription notes, radiologic images, and so forth
- Utilize predefined templates to make examination notes, procedures, review of systems, and postoperative checks quicker and more efficient
- Indicate or choose medications (from a predetermined list of those most prescribed), with specific instructions that can be electronically admitted into the chart and to the pharmacy
- Flag any drug interactions, contraindications, or allergies related to the patient
- Give providers pen units or small computers in which to enter data with a simple touch of the pen
- Provide providers and necessary staff members with immediate access to the patient record

- Be easily retrieved and never lost or misplaced
- Eliminate the manual coding and filing of medical charts
- Reduce the amount of phone tag retrieving necessary information from a paper file
- Create reminders for follow-up as necessary
- Provide a more efficient method of signing charts
- Can be emailed to a referring provider or easily printed, whether part of or the whole chart

EMRs require that providers use computers to open and view charts and write prescriptions. Progress notes can be created using clinical templates and a point-and-click form of entry. Commonly used clinical phrases can be dropped into the progress note with a push of a button. If providers prefer to dictate and have their notes transcribed, that can also be done. The transcribed and entered note will automatically update relevant information such as problem lists, vital signs, laboratory results, and so on. As voice recognition improves, it will become possible for the provider to speak the entries normally keyed into the system.

Confidentiality is often mentioned as a concern in EMRs, but with the ability to limit network access, system administrators can identify access and privileges according to the desired policy of the clinic. The EMR is fully recognized as a legal document, is able to track any changes made, and can be presented to a court of law. Because a standard part of any EMR installation is a system backup, you should never be without a medical chart even if the system goes down for a brief period.

Most medical assistants working in facilities that are fully computerized say they hardly remember how they could function any differently. They also report that moving from the manual to the electronic system can be frustrating at times, but it is worth the effort in the long run.

Archival Storage

Most providers preserve patient medical records for at least the life of their practice. This obviously is a space-consuming prospect, particularly in today's large practices. Computers help to solve this dilemma through EMRs. This not only eliminates the bulky storage problems encountered with traditional records, but records can be retrieved and viewed almost instantaneously on a computer screen.

One of the advantages of the EMR is the small amount of storage needed for all the patient charts; but remember that computer files, including patient charts, should have a backup system that stores the information in a secure place should there be a computer problem. Some systems provide for automatic backup every 30 minutes or less. Some systems include a second hard drive that stores data as they are being created or as often as determined by facility policy. With an effective and efficient backup system, no one on the clinic staff will ever be without a patient chart when it is needed.

Transfer of Data

EMRs are easily emailed in whole or in part. Computers also streamline transfer of records from one medical facility to another. Faxing is an everyday part of the medical clinic. Gone is the time when it took a provider days to obtain information vital to treating a patient. Within minutes, a patient's entire medical record can be sent electronically from one clinic to another. Scanners (optical character recognition) are devices that allow information to be converted to an image on the computer screen. For instance, a patient's entire medical record can be scanned by the device and then recreated as a computer file exactly as it was in paper form.

Confidentiality

Legal

Maintaining confidentiality is a major issue in using the computer and online devices for storage and transfer of medical information. Not enough emphasis can be placed on the confidentiality issue. Medical assistants employed in a medical facility will hear and see information that is completely private. It is never appropriate to discuss any of that information outside the clinic with any individual unless it is a person who needs that information for medical reasons. It is also unwise to discuss private information within the facility if it is not your concern, and especially if your voice might be overheard by someone waiting in an examination room, a patient using the restroom, or individuals in the reception area. An appropriate situation in which information can be shared is when giving the name, address, and Social Security number or clinic number to the radiology department that will be performing the X-rays ordered by the provider.

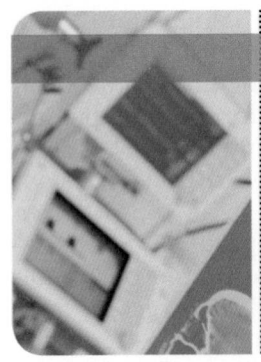

CASE STUDY 13-1

Refer to the scenario at the beginning of the chapter.

CASE STUDY REVIEW

1. Juanita Hansen is waiting in the clinic. Dr. Lewis and the staff are scrambling to find Juanita's test results. What can be done now to make certain Juanita has not made the trip unnecessarily?
2. Identify steps to be taken to prevent this situation from happening another time.

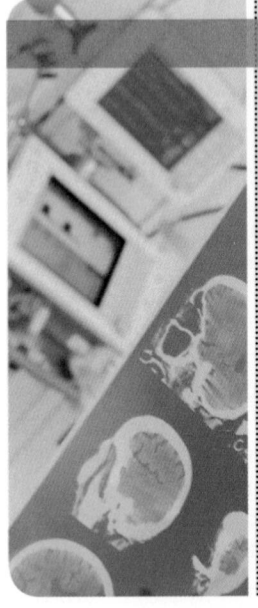

CASE STUDY 13-2

Ellen Armstrong, CMAS (AMT), administrative medical assistant at Inner City Health Care, has been chiefly responsible for managing this clinic's medical records. However, because Ellen is only a part-time employee, the clinic manager feels she needs to delegate some of the responsibility of maintaining all clinic files to Liz Corbin, CMA (AAMA), a medical assistant who also works part time. Ellen knows the system well and had a hand in designing an effective numeric filing method that both ensures patient confidentiality and satisfies the needs of Inner City and its large volume of patients. Now she is trying to orient Liz, who has little experience with the filing system, to the intricacies of medical records management.

CASE STUDY REVIEW

1. What is a good starting point for Liz Corbin's education in medical records management?
2. What are the basic procedures for filing any piece of documentation that Liz needs to learn?
3. Under the direction of the clinic manager, Inner City is gradually shifting to a computerized system for all operations. Eventually, patient files will be computerized. What can Ellen and Liz do to prepare for this eventuality?

Summary

- Records management plays an ever-increasing role in the clinic setting today. With the need for thorough and proper documentation, a majority of interactions on the patient's behalf are concerned with proper information processing.

- It is imperative that medical records be managed efficiently, and that the medical assistant possesses the skills required for sorting, filing, retrieving, and maintaining information effectively.

- Proper use of electronic medical records is necessary to ensure appropriate use of features to preserve documentation integrity and prevent fraud, waste, abuse, and improper payments.

- The medical assistant must understand the procedures for properly documenting, maintaining, updating, purging, correcting, and releasing medical information using both paper charts and EMR/PM systems.

- The medical assistant must be able to accurately create paper charts and electronic records for patient medical records.

- Types of medical records and information storage includes POMR and the SOAP note method, the SOMR method, and the chronological arrangement method.

- Basic rules for filing and applying the steps for filing medical documents include the procedural steps Inspect, Index, Code, Sort, and File.

- Medical assistants must be familiar with other filing techniques in addition to alphabetic, which can be used for patient or other types of organizational uses in a clinic setting. These include numeric filing, subject filing, cross-referencing, and tickler files.

- The medical assistant must be aware of proper archiving of medical records and backup systems for the EMR system.

CERTIFICATION REVIEW

1. What is the name of the process for maintaining order in files by separating active from inactive files?
   a. Indexing
   b. Coding
   c. Purging
   d. Alphabetizing
2. What is the name of the system used as a reminder of action to be taken on a certain date?
   a. Accession log
   b. Tickler file or reminder note
   c. Release mark
   d. Purging system
   e. Outguide
3. What is the name of the tool used to ensure that records are tracked when borrowed in order to maintain an accurate filing system?
   a. Release mark
   b. Out guide
   c. Alphabetic card file
   d. Cross-reference file
4. What answer describes the correct indexing for units 1, 2, 3, 4 in the name John Porter O'Keefe II?
   a. O'Keefe John Porter II
   b. John Porter O'Keefe II
   c. II O'Keefe John Porter
   d. The "II" would be disregarded
   e. John Porter O'Keefe
5. Of the four systems of filing, what is the best for every ambulatory care setting?
   a. The numeric system
   b. The color-coding system
   c. One customized to the needs of the clinic
   d. The alphabetic system
6. Who owns the medical record?
   a. The patients for whom the record is about
   b. Insurance carriers who help to pay medical costs
   c. The providers who create the record
   d. The insurance carrier
   e. Both a and c
7. What is the process for making corrections to the medical record?
   a. They are made by erasing the error and replacing it with the correction.
   b. They are made by placing a single line through the error and replacing it with the correction.
   c. They are never made to charts because of the legal nature of the information.
   d. They are made only by the provider.
8. Which of the following statements about EMRs is false?
   a. They are initially more expensive than paper medical records.
   b. They should be available to most Americans by 2020.
   c. They eliminate coding and filing of medical charts.
   d. They create reminders for follow-up as necessary.
   e. Solo practitioners are least likely to use EMRs.
9. When identical names are being indexed, which indexing system is preferred in a medical system?
   a. The address
   b. The telephone number
   c. The birth date or Social Security number
   d. A preassigned clinic number
10. What are the preferred steps for filing medical documentation?
    a. Code, index, sort, inspect, file
    b. Inspect, code, index, sort, file
    c. Sort, inspect, index, code, file
    d. Inspect, index, code, purge
    e. Inspect, index, code, sort, file

CHAPTER 14

Written Communications

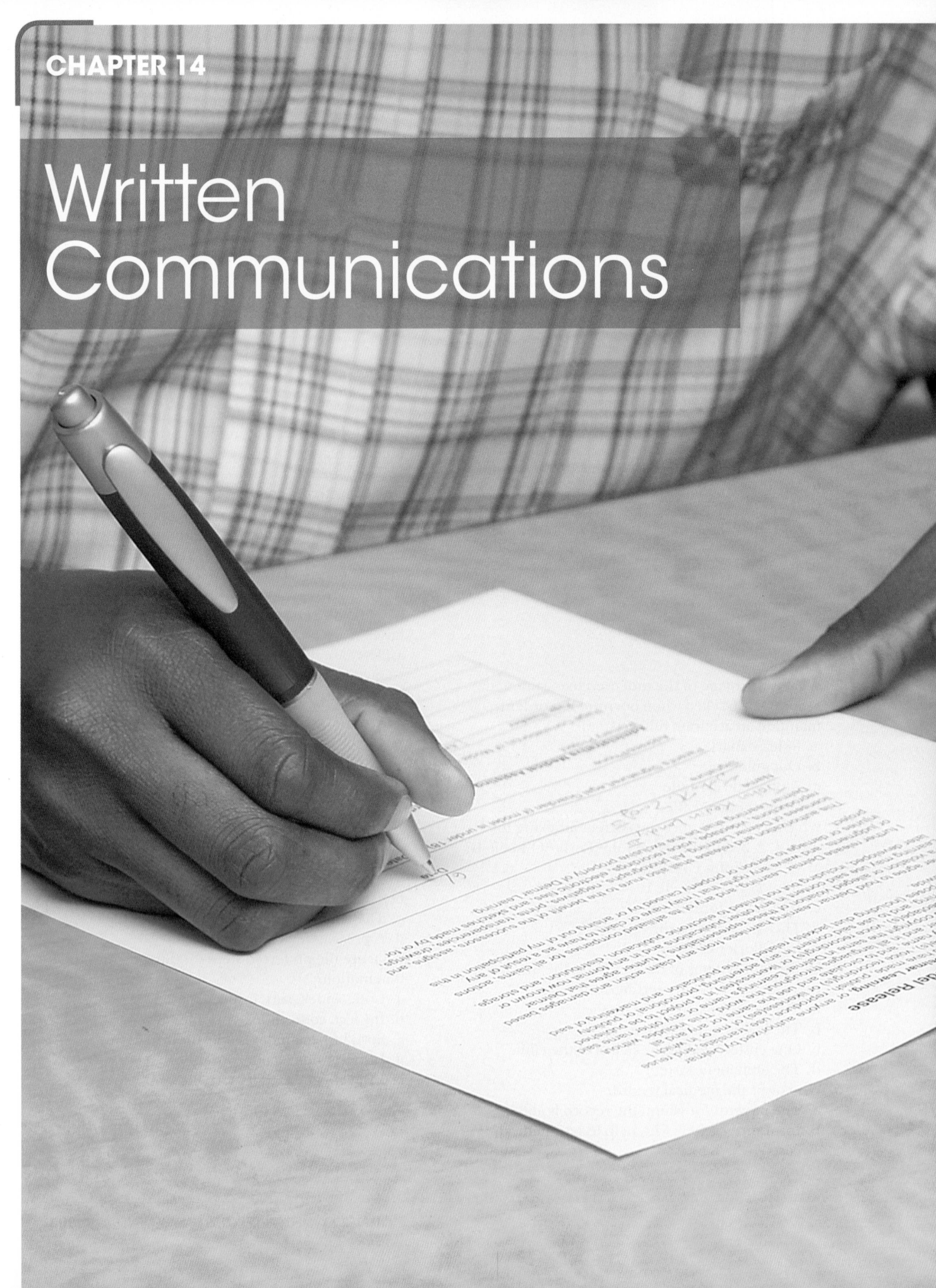

1. Define and spell the key terms as presented in the glossary.
2. Identify the role of the medical assistant in producing written communications.
3. List the four major letter styles.
4. Compose and key letters using appropriate components of a business letter.
5. Identify various types of form letters that may be written by the medical assistant.
6. Proofread a letter for grammar, spelling, and content.
7. Use proper proofreading marks to correct a document.
8. Describe the various classifications of mail and determine when each class should be used.
9. Address envelopes to satisfy postal regulations.
10. Discuss legal and ethical issues relating to written communications, as well as HIPAA regulations.

KEY TERMS

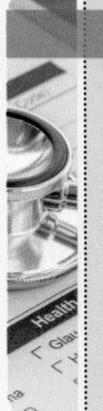

agenda	modified block letter, indented
blind copy	modified block letter, standard
bond paper	optical character recognition (OCR)
form letter	portfolio
full block letter	proofread
keyed	simplified letter
memorandum (memo)	watermark
minutes	ZIP+4

SCENARIO

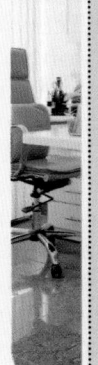

When they are produced with care, written communications can be a time-consuming part of the administrative medical assistant's day. This is why Marilyn Johnson, CMA (AAMA), the clinic manager at Inner City Health Care, has compiled a style manual for the multiprovider practice. Marilyn is clearly aware that professional appearing and worded letters send a positive message to all recipients. Yet, she wants to make correspondence writing and producing as efficient as possible; her style manual provides an easy-to-use resource for anyone in the clinic responsible for composing or sending written documents.

In her style manual, Marilyn has included examples of the "house" letter format, which is block style; a list of commonly used medical terms for easy spelling reference; answers to common questions staff have in regard to word usage; proofreader's marks; proper addressing procedures for envelopes and packages, depending on whether they are being sent by U.S. mail or by an alternative delivery method; and a quick list of the best ways to send various types of correspondence. Marilyn has also included a list of "Do Nots" to help her staff avoid mistakes in their written communications.

One of the key responsibilities of the administrative medical assistant is written communication. Letters to patients, to referring providers, to other health care organizations, and even interoffice correspondence should be thoughtfully composed, carefully produced according to the style selected by the clinic manager, and mailed and delivered in a way that is both time and cost efficient.

Written correspondence is important in conveying a professional image of the clinic and impacts public relations either positively or negatively. It must also be remembered that written documents provide a permanent or legal record in the event of any litigation and thus must be carefully and accurately worded.

In most clinics, medical assistants are responsible for creating many forms of written communications. Examples of these forms of communications include:

- Various types of letters, such as letters to order supplies and equipment, letters replying to various types of inquirie, collection letters, and promotional letters
- Memoranda and interoffice communications
- Referrals, consultation, and surgical report letters
- Written instructions for patients
- Meeting agendas and minutes
- Promotional brochures
- Policy and procedure documents

COMPOSING CORRESPONDENCE

The medical assistant must always remember that the quality of the correspondence reflects the standards of the medical clinic. It is important to also remember that there is a difference between social correspondence and business correspondence. Social correspondence tends to be lengthy and personal in nature, whereas business correspondence should be clear, concise, courteous, and accurate. It is best to keep business letters to one page in length whenever possible.

Writing Tips

Rosemary Fruehling, a writer and lecturer, states, "Business writing is good when it achieves the purpose the author intended." Practice and careful attention to detail are required to write effective business letters. Writing tips for consideration include:

- Follow the style and format determined by your provider-employer. Providers often prefer a professional, formal style of letter composition.
- Think about key points to be addressed in the letter and organize them before beginning composition. The first paragraph should identify what the letter is about and focus the reader's attention.
- Establish a tone of voice. Be personable and cordial in tone while remaining professional.
- Use only language that the reader will understand.
- Most sentences should be short and contain only one idea or thought.

Spelling

It is important that all correspondence contain no misspelled or incorrectly used words. When in doubt, always look the word up in a dictionary (Table 14-1). When checking spelling in a dictionary, develop the habit of reading the definition as well. This will help imprint the correct spelling and meaning of the word.

Be careful about relying on the spell check function of your computer; many medical words are not formatted into the computer. The computer does not recognize if you have used the wrong word, only that the word is spelled incorrectly. For example, the words *to, too,* and *two* may all be spelled correctly but may be misused within the sentence structure.

It may be helpful to develop a list of frequently misused words in an alphabetized notebook, card index, or special file on your computer (Table 14-2). Several computer word processing software packages contain English/medical spell check features. A new word that is not currently identified in the spell check or medical check package may be added to the program.

TABLE 14-1

FREQUENTLY MISSPELLED MEDICAL TERMS

abscess	malaise
aneurysm	ophthalmology
arrhythmia	palliative
calcaneus	parenteral
cirrhosis	pharynx
clavicle	pneumonia
curettage	pruritus
diarrhea	psychiatrist
hemorrhage	pyrexia
hemorrhoids	rheumatic
homeostasis	rhythm
humerus	roentgenology
ileum	sphygmomanometer
ilium	staphylococcus
ischemia	vesical
ischium	vesicle
larynx	

Proofreading

Before presenting any correspondence to the provider for signature or mailing, the document should be **proofread**. Proofreading is the process of reading the document and checking for accuracy. Accuracy involves checking to be sure that the correct grammar, spelling, punctuation, and capitalization have been used and that the message is clear and concise and presented in a logical organization.

Proofreading marks most commonly used are shown in Figure 14-1. Standard proofreading marks are symbols and short notations that are used to mark up documents indicating corrections and solutions to errors. Some proofreading tips that may be useful include:

- Proofread each document twice, once on the screen checking for obvious errors and then on a hard copy to be sure everything is accurate and makes sense.
- Prepare the document, set it aside, and proofread a third time later. Inaccuracies or errors may "jump" out in a later review.
- Do not proofread when tired.
- If the document is long, proofread in several short intervals.
- Read a long document to another person and have him or her check sentence structure and content accuracy.
- Use a card or ruler as a guide to maintain your place within the document.
- Use a piece of colored clear plastic over the document to rest your eyes. This is especially helpful when proofing a long document.

TABLE 14-2

FREQUENTLY MISUSED WORDS

advice	advise		hear	here	
affect	effect		hole	whole	
capital	capitol		knew	new	
coarse	course		know	no	
coma	comma		lean	lien	
command	commend		patience	patients	
complement	compliment		personal	personnel	
comprehensible	comprehensive		plain	plane	
council	counsel		precede	proceed	
conscience	conscious		principal	principle	
deposition	disposition		right	write	
device	devise		stationary	stationery	
elicit	illicit		taught	taut	
eligible	illegible		their	there	they are
elude	allude		to	too	two
ensure	insure	assure	vain	vein	
explicit	implicit		weak	week	
farther	further		weather	whether	
heal	heel		you	your	you are

∧	Insert	⌐	Move left
⸮	Delete	⌐	Move right
#	Insert space	⊓	Move up
⌒	Close up space	⊔	Move down
⸿	Delete and close up	⊐⌐	Center
⌗	Close up, but leave normal space	⌃	Insert comma
eq.#	Equal space between words	⌄	Insert apostrophe
‖	Align type vertically	:⎮	Insert colon
⸗	Align type horizontally	⊙	Insert period
Sp	Spell out (Wd or 5)	?⎮	Insert question mark
TR	Transpose letters words or	⸌⎮⸌	Insert quotation marks
BF	Boldface type	⌃	Insert semicolon
ROM	Roman type	=̂	Insert hyphen
ITAL	Italic type	⊥̸M	Insert em dash
CAP	Capital letter	⊥̸N	Insert en dash
LC	Lower case letter	⌃2	Subscript
SC	Small caps	⸮2	Superscript
STET	Let it stand	¶	Paragraph indent
WF	Wrong font	no ¶	No indent; run in
		⌐	Break; start new line

FIGURE 14-1 Common proofreader's marks.

Proofreading in the Cloud

When several persons are involved in preparing a complex document, proofreading involves one person reviewing and making changes and then sending it to the other author for their concurrence. If changes are made the cycle is repeated. The Cloud has changed the need for the back and forth transferring of a document from one author to another or between the author and an assistant. As of 2012, both Google apps and Microsoft Office 365 apps are available on the Cloud allowing composition of documents on a server that is available to multiple users having access via a password. The Microsoft Office 365 App allows sharing of documents by several users for modification and review, but not interactively. The Google documents sharing feature allows multiple users to change a document interactively during the same session. This makes the proofreading process much simpler and if combined with a conference call, simplifies obtaining agreement on changes to text.

COMPONENTS OF A BUSINESS LETTER

The following sections describe the components of most business letters. Procedure 14-1 provides steps for preparing and composing business correspondence. Figure 14-2 graphically illustrates the placement of business letter components, Table 14-3 provides guidelines for preventing errors in letter placement, and Figure 14-3 illustrates how placement can be altered to suit letter size.

PROCEDURE 14-1

Procedure

Preparing and Composing Business Correspondence Using All Components (Computerized Approach)

PURPOSE:

Prepare and compose a rough draft and final-copy letter using appropriate language and letter style to convey a clear and accurate message to the recipient.

EQUIPMENT/SUPPLIES:

- Computer, word processor and printer
- Printed letterhead and plain second sheet
- Dictionary
- Thesaurus
- Medical dictionary
- Style manual

PROCEDURE STEPS:

1. Organize key points to be addressed in a logical sequence. RATIONALE: To assist in writing an effective letter.

2. Go to Page Setup and set document margins, paper size and source, and layout. ***Paying attention to detail***, set the fonts to be used and paragraph parameters. Name and save the document. RATIONALE: Saves time and loss of formatting.

3. Compose a rough draft of the letter. With time and experience, these outlining steps may be eliminated before drafting the letter. RATIONALE: Business correspondence should be clear, concise, courteous, and accurate. A draft letter aids in checking that the letter is logical and achieves the intended purpose.

4. Use language that is easily understood. State the reason for the letter in the first paragraph and encourage action in the last paragraph. RATIONALE: For communication to take place, both parties must understand the message. The letter must be written so that the recipient understands the language and responds appropriately.

5. Read the draft for obvious errors in grammar, spelling, and punctuation. Use the appropriate reference material (dictionary, style manual, spell check, and so on) to check any inaccuracies. Read again for content. Is the message accurate, logical, and organized appropriately? Save the document again if any changes were made. Lay the letter aside and read it once more at a later time. RATIONALE: Reading several times allows you to concentrate on different elements of the letter. Errors may jump out when reading for the third time.

6. Choose the letter format that is customary to your clinic. Established templates saved on the computer or provided on computer software are time savers. RATIONALE: The letter style should be efficient to prepare and professional in appearance and content to represent the provider-employer in a professional manner.

7. Key in the date or use the computer's auto date feature on line 15 or two to three lines below the letterhead. RATIONALE: Using the component parts of a business letter ensures that the letter is professional in appearance and represents the provider-employer in a professional manner.

8. Key the recipient's name and address flush with the left margin beginning on line 20. RATIONALE: Using the component parts of a business letter ensures that the letter is professional in appearance and represents the provider-employer in a professional manner.

9. On the second line below the recipient's address, key the salutation flush with the left margin. Follow the salutation with a colon. RATIONALE: Using the component parts of a business letter ensures that the letter is professional in appearance and represents the provider-employer in a professional manner.

(continues)

10. Key the subject of the letter on the second line below the salutation flush with the left margin, if the subject line is being used. RATIONALE: Using the component parts of a business letter ensures that the letter is professional in appearance and represents the provider-employer in a professional manner.

11. Begin the body of the letter on the second line below the salutation or subject line. The body format will depend on the style of letter used. For example, if the full block format is used, paragraphs will begin flush with the left margin. Single space within paragraphs; double space between paragraphs. RATIONALE: Using the component parts of a business letter ensures that the letter is professional in appearance and represents the provider–employer in a professional manner.

12. Key the complimentary closure on the second line below the body of the letter. Capitalize only the first letter of the first word of the complimentary closure (e.g., Respectfully yours). RATIONALE: Using the component parts of a business letter ensures that the letter is professional in appearance and represents the provider-employer in a professional manner.

13. Key the signature four to six lines below the complimentary closing. RATIONALE: This ensures that the recipient will be able to determine who sent the letter.

14. If reference initials are used, key the initials two lines below the keyed signature (e.g., WL:jg). RATIONALE: Using the component parts of a business letter ensures that the letter is professional in appearance and represents the provider-employer in a professional manner.

15. Key the enclosure or copy notation one or two lines below the reference initials. RATIONALE: Using the component parts of a business letter ensures that the letter is professional in appearance and represents the provider-employer in a professional manner.

16. *Paying attention to detail,* proofread the document and make corrections as necessary. RATIONALE: All information contained in the letter must be accurate and written in a clear and concise manner with logical organization. The grammar, spelling, punctuation, and capitalization must be correct to ensure a professional appearance and represent the provider-employer in a positive manner.

17. Save the document again and print two copies. RATIONALE: The document is saved on the computer, and a copy for signature and mailing is produced. A hard copy for the file is also established.

18. Prepare the envelope. Place the envelope flap over the letter and attach it with a paper clip. RATIONALE: Prepare the envelope using U.S. postal regulations to ensure delivery in a timely manner. Proofread to be sure the address is accurate to ensure deliverability. By placing the envelope flap over the letter and attaching it with a paper clip, the two will not become separated.

19. Place the letter on the provider's desk for review and signature. RATIONALE: The provider's signature signifies the letter is accurate, sends the intended message, and represents the clinic in a professional manner.

20. File a copy of the letter in an appropriate filing system. RATIONALE: May be needed in the future for reference or as documentation.

Date Line

The date is usually **keyed** on line 15 or two to three lines below the letterhead. In keying, data are input by keystrokes on a computer. The date should be completely written out as January 15, 20XX, rather than 1/15/20XX. (If military style is used, the format would be 01 January 20XX.)

Inside Address

The inside address is keyed flush with the left margin. This address may be two, three, or four lines. Some rural areas only require two lines. If the letter is addressed to a provider, the credentials appear after the name. Do not type Dr. John Jones, M.D. (Both Dr. and M.D. are titles; use one or the other.)

Salutation

The salutation is keyed flush with the left margin on the second line below the inside address. A colon follows the salutation. The formal salutation should refer to the receiver of the letter using

1, 1.5, or 2"
Margin

1 line

4 lines

1 line

1 line

1 line

1 line

1 line

1 line

1 line

1 line

4 lines

1 line

1 line

Your Name
Street Address
City, State ZIP+4
Area Code and Phone
Email address

Date

SPECIAL NOTATIONS (e.g., **PERSONAL, CONFIDENTIAL, CERTIFIED MAIL**)

Recipient's Name
Company Name
Company Address

SUBJECT: (Subject of Letter, e.g., **RESIGNATION, PATIENT NAME ...**)

Dear (Recipient's Name):

SUBJECT: (Alternate location for SUBJECT LINE)

When using block format to write a business letter, all of the information is typed flush with the left margin. When using modified block or indented formats as shown here, your address block and date are five spaces to the right of the page center. The first line of each paragraph is indented 0.5 inch.

When more than three or four paragraphs are required, headings may be used for each paragraph to help the reader. The headings should be short and capture the key topic of that section of the letter. Headings should be **Boldfaced** or <u>Underlined</u> with the first letter of each word capitalized. Letters that have more than one page should have a heading on each continuation page that gives the name of the addressee, page number, and date.

After the body of the letter comes the closing, signature block, reference initials, enclosure information, and carbon copy information.

Sincerely yours,

Your Name
Your Title

YN/TN (Initials of writer and typist)

cc: (Names receiving copy)

FIGURE 14-2 Placement of business letter components.

title and last name (e.g., "Dear Mr. Marshal:"). If the receiver and sender know each other well, the receiver's first name may be used (e.g., "Dear Jim:").

TABLE 14-3

GUIDELINES FOR LETTER PLACEMENT

The following guidelines are helpful in preventing errors in placement:

1. An imaginary picture frame should surround the letter. Margins may be 1, 1.5, or 2 inches (see Figure 14-3).
2. The last line of the letter should end no less than 1 inch from the bottom of the page.
3. Do not divide the last word on a page.
4. A minimum of three lines should be keyed on the second page of a letter. When dividing a paragraph at the bottom of a page, keep a minimum of two lines on the bottom of the page and two lines at the top of the next page.
5. If using a computer to prepare letters, it is easy to make adjustments to create a professional letter.
6. Use single space within paragraphs.
7. Use double space between paragraphs.

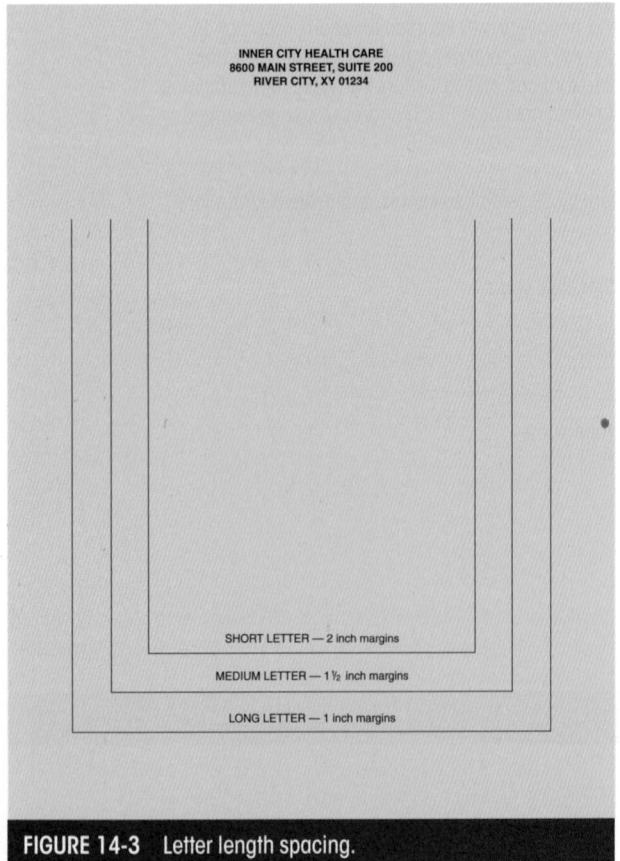

INNER CITY HEALTH CARE
8600 MAIN STREET, SUITE 200
RIVER CITY, XY 01234

SHORT LETTER — 2 inch margins

MEDIUM LETTER — 1 ½ inch margins

LONG LETTER — 1 inch margins

FIGURE 14-3 Letter length spacing.

Subject Line

If used, the subject line is keyed on the second line below the salutation starting at the left margin. This may begin flush with the left margin, indented five spaces, or centered. The patient's name or subject (meeting or topic) may be used on the subject line.

Body of Letter

The body of the letter should begin on the second line below the salutation unless a subject line is used that precedes two lines above the body. The body format will depend on the style of letter used. Paragraphs will begin flush with the left margin in full block letter style, or they may be indented five spaces when using the modified block letter style.

Complimentary Closing

The complimentary closure begins on the second line below the body of the letter. The closure depends on the formality of the letter. Only the first letter of the first word of the complimentary closure is uppercase.

The style used in the complimentary closure should correspond with the salutation (Table 14-4).

Keyed Signature

A keyed signature is a professional courtesy to the reader. Often, a letter is received in which the signature of the sender is not legible. The keyed signature should be at least four lines below the complimentary closing. This space may be lengthened to six lines if you are keying a short letter.

TABLE 14-4

RECOMMENDED COMPLIMENTARY CLOSINGS

LETTER STYLE	COMPLIMENTARY CLOSING
Formal	Respectfully yours or Respectfully
General	Very truly yours or Yours truly or Sincerely or Sincerely yours
Informal (used when reader and writer are on first-name basis)	Regards or Best wishes

Reference Initials

The reference initials used may only be those of the person named in the keyed signature if the same person composed and signed the letter. If reference initials are used, the name of the individual composing the letter should be in uppercase letters with the medical assistant's initials keyed in lowercase letters.

Example:

WL:jg or WL/jg

Enclosure Notation

The enclosure indication can be either one or two lines below the keyed reference initials.

The number of enclosures may be indicated using one of several methods:

- Enclosures
- Enc.
- 1 Enc.
- 2 Enclosures
- Enclosures (2)

Some enclosures should be identified specifically, for example, a check for $84. Enclosures also may be sent under separate cover. If this method is used, state that the enclosure is under separate cover. It may be written as: Enclosure under separate cover: Sarah Jones's medical record.

Copy Notation

If copies of the letter are to be sent to other parties, the copy notation should be one or two lines below the reference initials. The notation *c* (copy) or *pc* (photocopy) should be followed by the name of the person receiving the copy. When more than one person is to receive a copy of the original letter, key *c*: by the first name. Align the other names under the first person identified alphabetically or by rank.

Example:

---

c: Joseph Brown, MD

        John Smith, MD

A **blind copy** notation *bcc*: may be used to send copies of the letter to individuals without the recipient's knowledge. This message is only keyed on the copy of the individual receiving the blind copy. The use of blind copies has decreased and in some practices is no longer used.

Postscripts

Postscripts (abbreviated as P.S.) may be used to:

1. Express an afterthought
2. Identify a thought that has been intentionally deleted from the body of the letter
3. Make a strong significant point

Postscripts are keyed two spaces below reference initials and enclosures.

Continuation Page Heading

There are two methods used to begin the continuation page heading. There should be at least a 1-inch space at the top of each continuing page of the letter. Plain paper matching the color, weight, size, and quality of the letterhead should be used. The following are examples of appropriate continuation page headings.

Example:

(1 inch from top of page)

Jeremy Brown, MD   -2-   May 4, 20XX

or

Jeremy Brown, MD

Page 2

May 4, 20XX

LETTER STYLES

The administrative medical assistant may be responsible for creating a variety of letters that support the needs of the clinic. Word processing software has business letter and memo templates that are useful in creating these documents.

Communication

One efficient approach to letter composition is to create a **portfolio** or database of frequently used **form letters**. Individualize letters by using the current date and the receiver's name and mailing address. When a form letter is carefully composed and produced, it may not be perceived as a form letter by the recipient.

With the provider-employer's permission, the medical assistant may sign certain letters, including most form letters. Form letters that may be written by the medical assistant include:

- Letters to thank referring providers
- Letters emphasizing to patients criteria for care as directed by the provider
- Letters announcing new insurance or HMOs accepted

- Letters to order supplies or subscriptions
- Letters acknowledging speaking engagements
- Letters to announce vacation schedules or other clinic closures
- Letters to announce new staff
- Letters to remind patients of payment due or notification of collection procedures

Letters prepared for the provider's signature should be placed with an addressed envelope on the provider's desk for review and signature. Place the envelope flap over the letter and attach with a paper clip. Also include with the letter any enclosures for the provider's approval, as well as the patient file (if applicable for paper charts) if it will be needed for reference.

Four major styles of letters are used by medical and professional clinics:

1. Full block
2. Modified block, standard
3. Modified block, indented
4. Simplified

Full Block

The **full block letter** is the most time efficient for the clinic because the medical assistant does not have to use excessive motion to tab indentions or to place address, complimentary close, or keyed signature. When using the full block style, all lines begin flush with the left margin, and mixed punctuation is used (a colon is placed after the salutation and a comma after the complimentary closing). This style is suggested when desiring a contemporary-looking efficient letter.

Modified Block

In the **standard modified block** style letter, all lines begin at the left margin with the exception of the date line, complimentary closure, and keyed signature, which usually begin at the center position or five spaces to the right of center. Figure 14-4

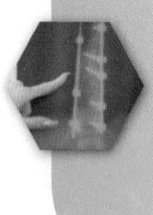

Critical Thinking

This text identifies spacing for short, medium-length, and long letters generated in medical clinics. What types of information or letters would be written using each type of length spacing?

illustrates a modified block style letter without indention.

The assistant may choose to use the **indented modified block** style letter. In this format, the first line of each paragraph may be indented five spaces. Figure 14-5 illustrates a modified block style letter with indented paragraphs.

Simplified

The **simplified letter** style omits the salutation and complimentary closure. All lines are keyed (input by keystroke) flush with the left margin. The subject line is keyed in capital letters three lines below the inside address. The body of the letter begins three lines below the subject line. The signature line is keyed in all capital letters four lines below the body of the letter. The Administrative Management Society recommends this style of letter. However, in medical clinics, this style is most often used when sending a form letter. Figure 14-6 illustrates a simplified style letter.

SUPPLIES FOR WRITTEN COMMUNICATION

Begin written communication at the computer workstation by checking to see that all supplies required to prepare the document are at hand. Check the computer settings and turn the printer on. Load the correct letter stock paper into the printer when the document is ready to be printed. The paper should be **bond**, of good quality, and at least 20 to 24 pound stock with a watermark. A **watermark** is legible when paper is held to the light. Choose a shade of white, cream, or gray bond paper.

Although colored paper may be more eye-catching, it does not display a professional image. Also, be sure that the paper stock is compatible with printers used in the clinic.

Letterhead

The letterhead style and design is usually chosen by the provider(s) and may include a specially designed logo for the practice. The provider/practice name, street address or post office box number, city, state, ZIP code, and telephone number with area code are usually printed on the letterhead. Many clinics also add their fax number and email address. Letterhead information may be placed at either side or in the center of the paper.

Second Sheets

When an order is placed for letterhead, the medical assistant should order additional plain paper

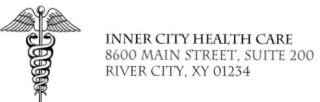

INNER CITY HEALTH CARE
8600 MAIN STREET, SUITE 200
RIVER CITY, XY 01234

January 12, 20XX (approximately 15th line)

Jeremy Brown, MD   (approximately 20th line)
111 S Main
Blossom, UT 10283-1120

Dear Dr. Brown:

SUBJECT: Blossom Medical Society Meeting

Thank you for inviting me to speak at the Blossom Medical Society Meeting June 15, 20XX. As requested, my topic will describe the use of MRI in assisting physicians to make a more accurate diagnosis without resorting to invasive procedures. The exact title of my speech will be sent by next Friday.

Please have your clinic manager send information regarding the number of participants expected, time of meeting, location, and any other details that will assist me in preparing my speech.

I will write or call if I have any additional questions.

Yours truly,

Winston Lewis, MD

Winston Lewis, MD

WL:ea

Enclosure: Handout on MRI

FIGURE 14-4 Sample standard modified block style letter; all elements start at left margin, except date, complimentary closing, and keyed signature.

of the same stock as the letterhead to be used for second page sheets. The number of sheets will vary from clinic to clinic. If providers normally dictate long letters, this must be taken into consideration when ordering quantities.

Printing Multipage Business Letters

Printing multipage business letters on letterhead stationery requires use of more than one tray in the printer, unless you want to collate the letterhead or hand feed it into the printer. The simplest procedure is to place the letterhead stationery into a tray other than the default tray. Then go to File, Page Setup, Paper Source, and from the menu that appears, specify the tray containing the letterhead stationery. The menu lets you choose the tray for the first page and the tray for the rest of the document. Make sure that the Apply To box is set for Whole Document.

Envelopes

The stock and quality of the envelopes should match the stationery used in the clinic. The address should be standardized so that it contains all delivery address elements. The correct name, city, state, and ZIP+4 codes must be used so that mail is processed efficiently and effectively.

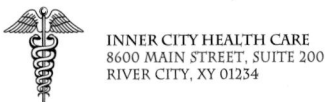

INNER CITY HEALTH CARE
8600 MAIN STREET, SUITE 200
RIVER CITY, XY 01234

January 12, 20XX (approximately 15th line)

Jeremy Brown, MD   (approximately 20th line)
111 S Main
Blossom, UT 10283-1120

Dear Dr. Brown:

Blossom Medical Society Meeting

Thank you for inviting me to speak at the Blossom Medical Society Meeting June 15, 20XX. As requested, my topic will describe the use of MRI in assisting physicians to make a more accurate diagnosis without resorting to invasive procedures. The exact title of my speech will be sent by next Friday.

Please have your clinic manager send information regarding the number of participants expected, time of meeting, location, and any other details that will assist me in preparing my speech.

I will write or call if I have any additional questions.

Yours truly,

Winston Lewis, MD

Winston Lewis, MD

WL:ea

Enclosure: Handout on MRI

FIGURE 14-5 Sample modified block style letter with indented paragraphs. This format is the same as the standard modified except that the subject line and paragraphs are not left-justified.

Example:

JEREMY BROWN MD

111 S MAIN

BLOSSOM UT 10283-1120

If Dr. Brown uses a post office box for the delivery of his mail, that address should be used. The postal service delivers to the last line before the city, state, and ZIP+4 code.

Example:

JEREMY BROWN MD

PO BOX 1453

BLOSSOM UT 10283-1120

Place the intended delivery address on the line immediately above the city, state, and ZIP+4 code. The other address may be placed on a separate line above the delivery line.

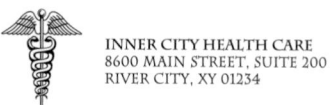

INNER CITY HEALTH CARE
8600 MAIN STREET, SUITE 200
RIVER CITY, XY 01234

January 12, 20XX (approximately 15th line)

Jeremy Brown, MD (approximately 20th line)
111 S Main
Blossom, UT 10283-1120

(triple-space)

SUBJECT: BLOSSOM MEDICAL SOCIETY MEETING

(triple-space)

Thank you for inviting me to speak at the Blossom Medical Society Meeting June 15, 20XX. As requested, my topic will describe the use of MRI in assisting physicians to make a more accurate diagnosis without resorting to invasive procedures. The exact title of my speech will be sent by next Friday.

Please have your clinic manager send information regarding the number of participants expected, time of meeting, location, and any other details that will assist me in preparing my speech.

I will write or call if I have any additional questions.

Winston Lewis, MD (4 line spaces)

WINSTON LEWIS, MD

WL:ea

Enclosure: Handout on MRI

FIGURE 14-6 The simplified style letter has no salutation or complimentary closing. The subject line and keyed signature are all upper case.

Example:

JEREMY BROWN MD
111 S MAIN
PO BOX 1453
BLOSSOM UT 10283-1120

This letter would be received at the post office box, not the street address.

General Standards for Addressing Envelopes. **Optical character recognition (OCR)** is a type of software that recognizes and decodes characters written on envelopes. The U.S. Postal Service uses OCR that recognizes various types of machine print, hand-print, and cursive styles. This automates the reading of most addresses on envelopes, although the Postal Service estimates that 30 million pieces of hand-written envelopes must still be decoded and delivered every day. The U.S. Postal Service suggests that the address on letter mail be machine-printed with a uniform left margin. It should be formatted in a manner that allows an OCR to recognize the information and find a match in its address files.

A scanner reads the ZIP code on the bottom line and prints a bar code in the lower right corner of the envelope. Envelopes that are handwritten cannot be read by the OCR. These letters must wait for more costly and slower manual sorting.

Procedure

To conform to standards, eliminate all punctuation in the envelope address with the exception of a hyphen in the ZIP+4 code. Leave a minimum of one space between the city name and two-character state abbreviations and the ZIP+4 code. The OCR can read a combination of uppercase and lowercase characters in addresses but prefers all uppercase characters (see Procedure 14-2).

Dark ink on a light background using uppercase letters is the suggested method in preparing a keyed address. There should be a uniform left margin on all lines of the address. An imaginary rectangle that extends ⅝ to 2¾ inches from the bottom of the envelope with 1 inch on each side should contain the address. The lower right edge should be kept free of any marks. This area will contain the bar code, whether it is preapplied or printed by an OCR. The bar code area is ⅝ inch from the bottom and 4½ inches from the right side of the envelope.

The U.S. Postal Service publishes several pamphlets and booklets that describe the format to be used when sending any mail. Check with the postal service regarding the latest publications. Service and deliverability will be improved if these standards are used.

Types of Envelopes. Number 6¾ and number 10 are the envelopes most often used. A window envelope may also be used, especially when mailing statements.

Number	Size
6¾	6½" long × 3" wide
10	9½" long × 4" wide
7	7½" long × 3" wide

See Figure 14-7 for an example of an envelope with the suggested zone sizes for OCR reading. The address on the statement need only be keyed once. The entire address is capitalized with no punctuation. Only one space should be used between the state abbreviation and the ZIP code. When this statement is folded with the address in view, it may be inserted into a window envelope. Make certain that the entire address is visible through the window.

PROCEDURE 14-2

Procedure

Addressing Envelopes According to U.S. Postal Regulations

PURPOSE:

To address envelopes according to U.S. Postal Service regulations to ensure timely delivery.

EQUIPMENT/SUPPLIES:

- Computer or word processor and printer with envelope tray
- Envelopes
- Address labels
- U.S. Postal Service Publication 221, *Addressing for Success*

PROCEDURE STEPS:

1. Insert the envelope in the printer and select the envelope format from the software program. When using a word processor or computer, labels may be used rather than printing directly on the envelope. The label is then adhered to the envelope. Many printers have an envelope tray and software that will transfer the address from the letter to the envelope. This feature is a time saver because you key the address only once. RATIONALE: U.S. postal regulations suggest that the address on letter mail should be machine printed, with a uniform left margin.

2. Visualize an imaginary rectangle on the envelope. The rectangle extends 5/8 inch to 2¾ inches from the bottom of the envelope, with 1 inch on each side. The address is placed within this rectangle (Figure 14-7). RATIONALE: U.S. postal regulations suggest that the address on letter mail should be machine printed, with a uniform left margin.

(continues)

3. Key the address in uppercase letters. Be sure to maintain a uniform left margin on all lines. Eliminate all punctuation in the address except the hyphen in the ZIP+4 code. RATIONALE: Leave a minimum of one space between the city name and the two-character state abbreviation and the ZIP+4 code. A scanner reads the ZIP+4 code on the bottom line and prints a bar code in the lower right corner of the envelope. The OCR prefers all uppercase characters.

4. If you are not using preprinted envelopes, key the return address in uppercase letters in the upper left corner of the envelope. Include the name on the first line; address on the second line; and city, state, and ZIP+4 code on the third line. RATIONALE: The return address should be printed in the upper left corner of the envelope should the letter need to be returned to the sender for any reason.

5. ***Paying attention to detail***, proofread the envelope and make corrections as necessary. RATIONALE: When all information is correct, processing will take place efficiently and correctly.

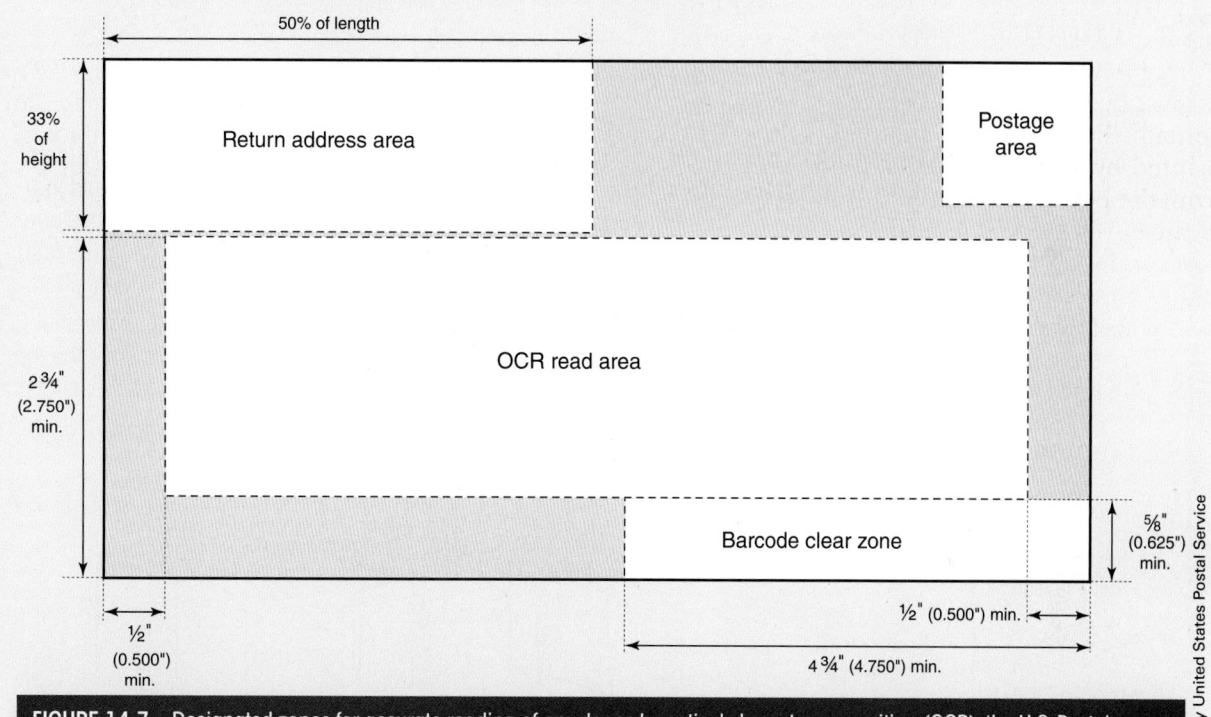

FIGURE 14-7 Designated zones for accurate reading of envelopes by optical character recognition (OCR), the U.S. Postal Service's computerized scanner.

Courtesy United States Postal Service

Procedure

To prepare envelopes for mailing, lay all envelopes facing upward in a row with the flaps displayed. Moisten all the envelopes with a sponge. With the dominant hand, seal the flap; with the nondominant hand, push the envelope aside while the next flap is closed. Procedure 14-3 illustrates letter folding and placement of envelopes for closure. The use of premoistened or peel-off strips helps speed up the process.

Mail Merge

Mail Merge lets you create form letters, envelopes, or mailing labels using data from a data source. You would use this feature to send mailings to your client base or to a list of prospects, among others. Mail Merge permits sending a form letter with envelopes to hundreds of recipients in a matter of minutes.

The client names and addresses are first stored in a Mail Merge data source, which can be a table or database such as Microsoft Excel. For Microsoft Word, a Mail Merge data source can be created by selecting Mail Merge in the Tools menu, selecting Mail Merge Helper, and following the instructions given in Helper. Almost all word processor programs let you carry out a Mail Merge with an external database. You will need to consult the program manual for details.

Folding Letters for Standard Envelopes

Procedure

PURPOSE:

To fold and insert letters into envelopes so that the letters fit properly in the envelopes.

EQUIPMENT/SUPPLIES:

- Letters to be mailed
- Number 6¾ envelope
- Number 10 envelope
- Window envelope

PROCEDURE STEPS:

1. To fit a standard-size letter into a number 6¾ envelope, fold the letter up from the bottom, leaving ¼ to ½ inch at the top, and crease it. Then fold the letter from the right edge about one third the width of the letter. Fold the left edge over to within ¼ to ½ inch of the right-edge crease. Insert the left creased edge first into the envelope (Figure 14-8A). RATIONALE: Ensures a proper fit of the letter into the envelope with a minimum of folds. The last crease made enters the envelope first. This enables the recipient to begin to read the letter with minimal effort.

2. To fit a standard-size letter into a number 10 envelope, fold the letter up about one third the length of the sheet and crease it. Then fold the top of the letter down to within ¼ to ½ inch of the bottom crease, and crease the top. Insert the top creased edge first into the envelope (Figure 14-8B). RATIONALE: Ensures a proper fit of the letter into

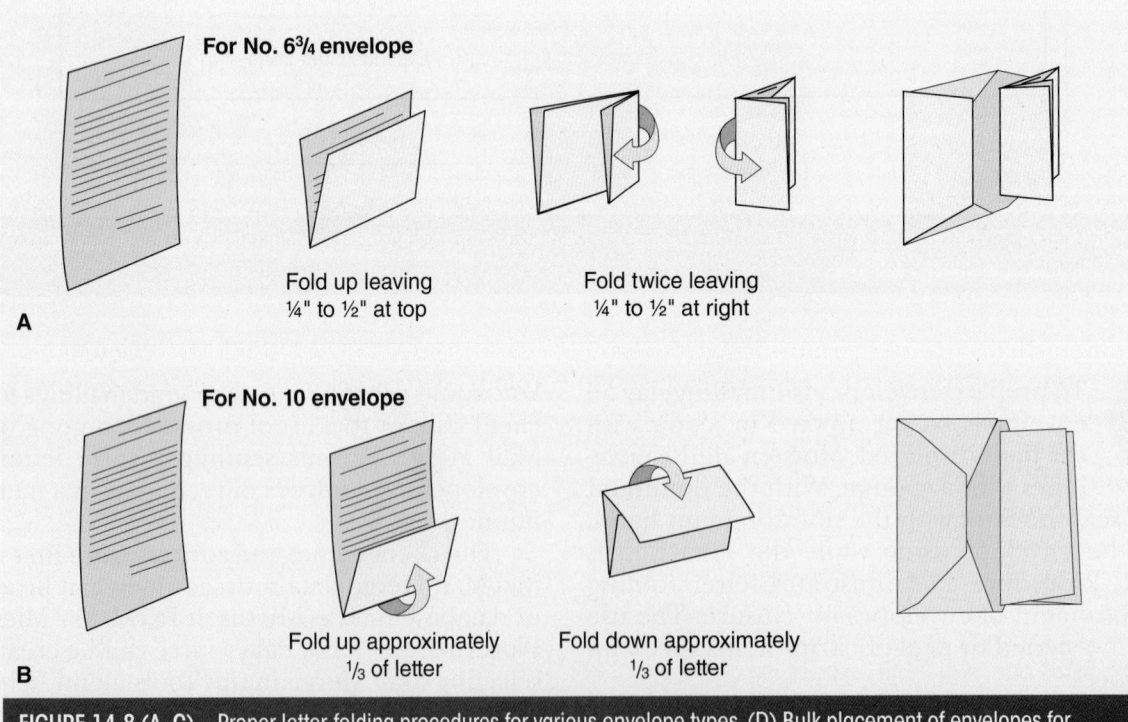

For No. 6³⁄₄ envelope

Fold up leaving
¼" to ½" at top

Fold twice leaving
¼" to ½" at right

A

For No. 10 envelope

Fold up approximately
¹⁄₃ of letter

Fold down approximately
¹⁄₃ of letter

B

FIGURE 14-8 (A–C) Proper letter-folding procedures for various envelope types. (D) Bulk placement of envelopes for moistening before closure.

(continues)

the envelope with a minimum of folds. The last crease made enters the envelope first. This enables the recipient to begin to read the letter with minimal effort.

3. To fit a standard-size letter into a window envelope, turn the letter over and fold the top of the letter up about one third the length of the page so that the address is facing you. Then fold the bottom of the letter back to the first crease. Insert the letter into the envelope bottom first (Figure 14-8C). **Paying attention to detail,** you should be able to read the entire address through the window. RATIONALE: Ensures that the entire address can be read through the window envelope and be delivered correctly.

4. Place envelopes as shown in Figure 14-8D to moisten before sealing. RATIONALE: Provides efficient method of sealing multiple letters for mailing.

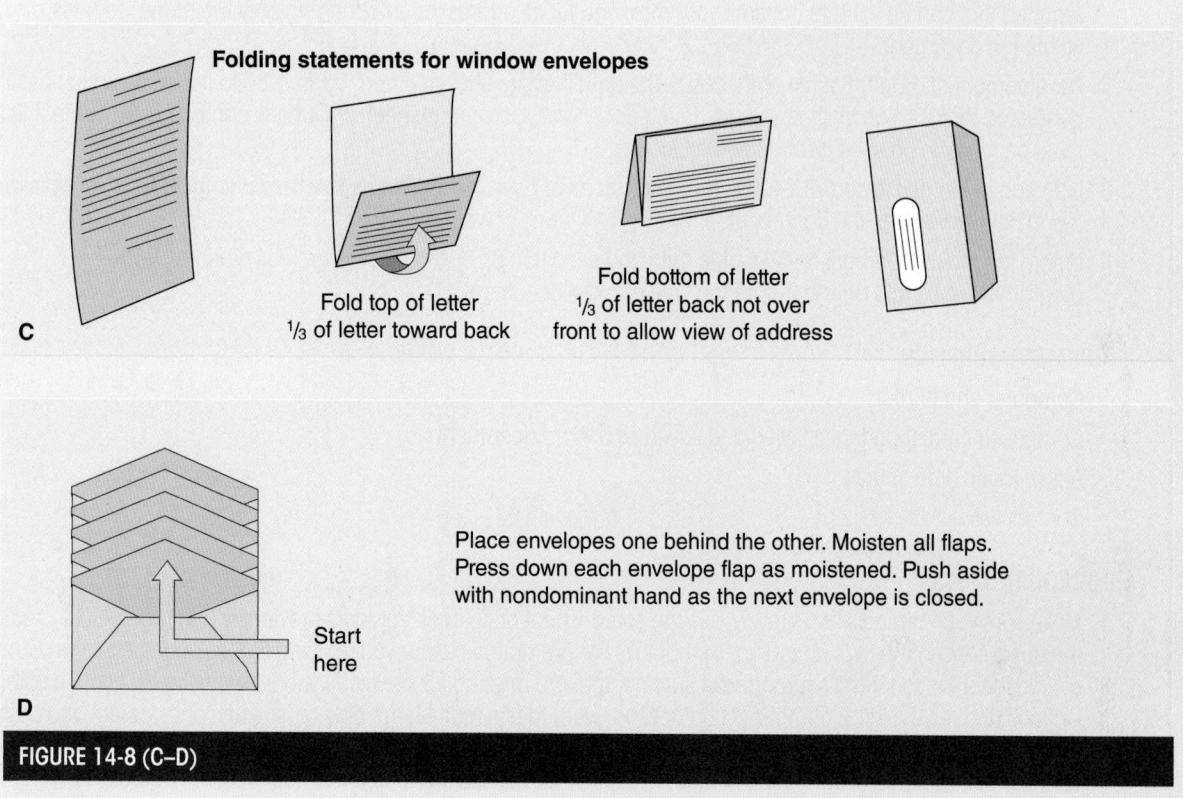

Folding statements for window envelopes

Fold top of letter
1/3 of letter toward back

Fold bottom of letter
1/3 of letter back not over
front to allow view of address

C

Place envelopes one behind the other. Moisten all flaps. Press down each envelope flap as moistened. Push aside with nondominant hand as the next envelope is closed.

Start here

D

FIGURE 14-8 (C–D)

Separate fields are suggested in the database for first name, last name, title, address, city, state, and postal code. To preclude time-consuming changes, three fields should be used for address, to accommodate clients with complex addresses. If a field is not required, leave it blank.

Procedure

The Mail Merge Helper will give you the choice of editing the main document. Compose the document you want to send, and for each field where you want a new name or address, select Insert Merge Field, and then select the name of the field you want to insert. You are now ready to print the form letters. Select Mail > Merge-Mail > Mail Merge Helper from the Tools menu and select Printer from the Merge To box.

Your printer should show the documents in the queue. Procedure 14-4 gives step-by-step instructions for using Mail Merge.

OTHER TYPES OF CORRESPONDENCE

Other specialized types of correspondence the medical assistant may be involved in preparing include memoranda, meeting agendas, and meeting minutes.

Memoranda

A type of interoffice correspondence is the **memorandum,** or **memo** for short. The use of memos permits messages to be sent quickly and without

PROCEDURE 14-4

Procedure

Creating a Mass Mailing Using Mail Merge

PURPOSE:

To create a mass mailing using the computer's Mail Merge Helper feature contained within Microsoft Word. The procedure consists of four steps:

1. Create a generic main document to be sent to different addressees. RATIONALE: A clear and concise document is required that can be used to transmit your message for all addresses by changing only the name, address, and title within the document.

2. Development of a Data Source. RATIONALE: The data that are changed from addressee to addressee must be generated for insertion by the program. Using either an Excel spreadsheet, or Outlook contacts, your contact list must be ready to be used during the Mail Merge.

3. Insertion of Merge Fields. RATIONALE: The program must have instruction as to where changeable or variable data are to be inserted into the document.

4. Merge the main document and variable data and send it to an output device such as a printer. RATIONALE: The program must be told how to output the final merged document.

EQUIPMENT/SUPPLIES:

- Computer and printer
- Composed correspondence keyed and saved as a Word document
- A developed data source
- Contact list

PROCEDURE STEPS:

1. Make sure your contacts list is ready. Use the spreadsheet or Outlook contacts previously prepared before creating the document so the Mail Merge goes smoothly. For example, whether you're using Outlook contacts or an Excel spreadsheet for your data source, make sure no data are missing for the fields you'll be pulling in. If you're using Outlook and have a large number of contacts but want to use Mail Merge only for specific ones, select and copy those contacts to a new folder. (To do this, select the contacts, right-click, choose Move and then Copy to Folder you create). Make sure you change the contact folder's properties so it will be shown as an email address book (right-click the new contacts folder, go to properties, and check Show This Folder as an Email Address Book).

2. Create a new blank document in Word.

3. Navigate to the Mailings tab.

4. Click Start Mail Merge and select your document type by selecting Letters.

5. Click Select Recipients and choose to create a new list, use an existing list, or choose from Outlook contacts.

    a. If you select Use an Existing List, you will be asked to browse to the file on your computer and then confirm the data table.

    b. If you select Choose from Outlook Contacts, you'll be asked to choose the Outlook contact folder and then add or remove recipients from the merge. Therefore, it is advised in step 1 to create a new contacts folder for your Mail Merge, so you will not have to scroll through all of your contacts in this small box.

6. Create the content for your document and insert the placeholders. When you get to the part where information is obtained and needs to be personalized from your data source, insert a placeholder with either the Insert Merge Field button or one of the two shortcuts Word offers for common fields: Address Block and Greeting Line.

(continues)

7. Use the Address Block shortcut. As the name suggests, Address Block creates a placeholder for a name and address, which is useful when creating letters, mailing labels, or envelopes. With both the Address Block and Greeting Line shortcuts, you'll be able to specify what gets inserted and preview what it will look like.

8. If the preview seems to be missing information, click Match Fields to tell Word where the data are for the missing fields. When the preview looks good, click OK, and Word will insert the address placeholder.

9. If applicable, insert other fields into your document. For other placeholders you might need, click on Insert Merge Field and select the field you want to insert at that point in the document.

10. Click Preview Results to preview the merge results after the document is finished and all fields are inserted.

11. If all looks good, click Finish & Merge and you can print individual documents, send them as email messages, or edit each individual document as needed.

12. Repeat this for other types of documents using Mail Merge. In addition to letters (which can be any sort of document), emails, envelopes, labels, or directories may be selected as the document type. Word also has a Step-by-Step Mail Merge Wizard (click the Mailings tab and then Start Mail Merge), which walks you through the process above.

labor-intensive preparation. The memo format may already be preformatted on your computer software. If not, it is easy to design your own memo format.

The side margins should be set for 1 inch. Begin to key the memo heading 2 inches from the top of the page (line 13). The heading includes the words *date, to, from,* and *subject,* which should be boldfaced and capitalized. The words should each be keyed on a separate line with a double space between each line. By setting a tab stop 10 spaces in from the left margin, you will be able to tab to each entry and clear the headings to add the appropriate information. Triple space after the entry for the subject heading.

The body of the memo may begin at the left margin or may be set 10 spaces in so that the text starts directly beneath the typed headings. No salutation is required in a memo. Figure 14-9 provides a sample memo.

Meeting Agendas

Most meetings operate by following *Robert's Rules of Order, Newly Revised* as their parliamentary authority. The outlined order of business is as follows:

- Reading and approval of the minutes
- Reports of officers, boards, and standing committees
- Reports of special committees (ad hoc)
- Special orders
- Unfinished business and general orders
- New business
- Date and time of next scheduled meeting

DATE: August 25, 20XX (key heading 2 inches from top of page, line 13)

TO: Staff of Inner City Health Care (embolden and capitalize headings and double space between them)

FROM: Marilyn Johnson, Clinic Manager

SUBJECT: Vacation Schedule (triple space after the subject)

Doctors Lewis & King will be on vacation January 1–15. Please do not schedule appointments during that time for either doctor. Clinic personnel should report to work as usual. During this two-week period, we will be preparing for the annual audit.

FIGURE 14-9 Sample memorandum.

The **agenda** lists the specific items that the group plans to discuss at the meeting under each of the above-mentioned divisions. The medical assistant preparing the agenda must determine the topics that are to be discussed. Copies of the agenda should be sent to each group member before the meeting date, and extra copies should be taken to the meeting for those who may have misplaced or forgotten to bring the agenda with them to the meeting. Figure 14-10 provides a sample meeting agenda.

Meeting Minutes

A written record of what transpired during a meeting is called the **minutes**. The minutes should record what business actions were taken during

AGENDA
STAFF MEETING
Tuesday, September 1, 20XX
Location–Conference Room

Reading and approval of last months' minutes
Reports
    Risk Management Committee
    Personnel
Unfinished business
    Purchase of new X-ray machine
New business
    Doctors Lewis & King vacation January 1–15
    Annual audit
Date and time for next meeting
Adjournment

FIGURE 14-10 Sample meeting agenda.

the meeting, who made each motion and what it was, who seconded the motion, any pertinent discussion, and whether the motion was passed. In the medical clinic, a designated person will take the minutes during a meeting, and then prepare the data for approval and documentation. In some cases, the clinic may rotate the responsibility of taking of minutes among staff members.

The first paragraph of the minutes should contain the following information:

- Kind of meeting (regular, special, emergency)
- Name of the group or association
- Date, time, and place of the meeting
- Who officiated at the meeting and names of members present and absent
- Whether the previous meeting minutes were read and approved

The body of the minutes should include a paragraph discussing each subject matter or each item listed on the agenda. All motions should be recorded including the exact wording of the motion, the name of the person making the motion, the person seconding the motion, and whether the motion passed or failed. If the meeting had a guest speaker, the speaker's name and title and the subject of the presentation may be included in the minutes.

The last paragraph should contain the next meeting date, time, and place and the time of adjournment for this meeting. The person recording the minutes should sign them, and a copy of all minutes

should be maintained in a notebook designated for that purpose. The minutes can also be scanned and saved to a hard drive or backup location. It is important that reliable backup is maintained, in two separate places, of all important documentation, especially if the originals are destroyed. Corporations are required to have regular meetings with recorded minutes for legal purposes. Figure 14-11 provides a sample of recorded minutes.

PROCESSING INCOMING AND OUTGOING MAIL

The management of written communications also involves developing procedures for sorting, distributing, and otherwise processing incoming mail. It also includes posting and shipping outgoing items by the most cost- and time-effective method.

Incoming Mail and Shipments

All mail should be sorted by type before opening. Incoming mail includes telegrams, faxes, certified or registered letters, personal letters, emails, checks from patients, insurance forms, invoices, medical journals, newspapers, magazines for the reception area, and advertisements regarding equipment and supplies.

Once it is categorized, incoming mail is directed to the appropriate personnel in the clinic. Checks from patients and invoices may be distributed to the bookkeeper, insurance forms to the insurance clerk, medical journals and advertisements can be placed on the provider's desk, and magazines and newspapers can be placed in the reception area.

Integrity

Personal or confidential letters should not be opened unless the medical assistant has been given this responsibility by the provider or clinic manager.

Use a letter opener to open all mail before taking out the contents and reading the document. After removing the contents:

- Stamp or write the date it was received in the clinic in the area of the document designated for this notation.
- If the address is not included on the letter, write the address on the letter, as identified on the envelope or on the bank check (if a patient is making a payment).
- When a colored reply envelope is sent with the statement to the patient, payments returned in these envelopes can speed up the sorting process.

```
STAFF MEETING MINUTES

      The monthly staff meeting of Inner City Health Care was held Tuesday, September 1,
20XX, in the conference room. The meeting was called to order by Marilyn Johnson,
Clinic Manager. Those members present included: Dr. Lewis, Dr. King, Walter Seals,
Nancy McFarland, Ellen Armstrong, Joe Guerrero, Gwen Carr, and Thomas Myers.
      The previous meeting's minutes were read and approved as published.
      Gwen Carr, CMA (AAMA), heading the Risk Management Committee, reported that
a thorough walk-through of the clinic had taken place to assess safety issues. It was
determined that the pull cords on the blinds could pose a potential hazard to small chil-
dren. Gwen made a motion that the blinds be upgraded with new vinyl louvered blinds
with the plastic rod-type louver adjuster. Nancy McFarland seconded the motion. After dis-
cussion, a unanimous vote was cast to replace the blinds at the earliest time possible.
      Walter Seals, Human Resource Manager, announced that he would be posting an
opening for a CMA (AAMA) to work in the lab. All staff personnel were asked to share infor-
mation about this opening with professionals who might be interested in working at
Inner City Health Care.
      Discussion was presented by Doctors Lewis & King regarding the purchase of a
new X-ray machine. A committee consisting of Nancy McFarland, Joe Guerrero, and
Thomas Myers was appointed to investigate the specific needs of the clinic and to
locate appropriate vendors. They will present their findings at the next scheduled staff
meeting.
      New business items include the fact that Doctors Lewis & King will be on vacation
January 1–15, 20XX. We are asked to not schedule appointments for them during that
time.
      Marilyn Johnson discussed preparations for the annual audit during the vacation
period of Doctors Lewis & King. She will provide a schedule and timeline at the next
staff meeting.
      The next scheduled meeting will be October 3 at 12:30 PM in the conference room.
      The meeting adjourned at 1:45 PM.

Ellen Armstrong
```

FIGURE 14-11 Sample meeting minutes.

- Look into the envelope to make certain that all contents have been removed.
- Attach the letter to the envelope with a paper clip, preferably on the left side.

Reply promptly to all requests, answering letters according to date of arrival; emergency situations need to be managed immediately.

Outgoing Mail and Shipments

Before placing postage on outgoing mail, weigh the item to be mailed, using a manual or electronic scale. A manual scale will read ounces. The assistant will then affix the appropriate postage, either stamps or postal meter. An electronic scale will automatically display the correct postage. If your clinic has a postal meter, this should be used to expedite mail. Metered mail does not have to be canceled or postmarked at the post office.

Procedure

A postage meter is leased or purchased from a manufacturing company recommended by the postal service. However, the postage meter must be taken to the

Critical Thinking

For the next week, practice sorting and prioritizing your personal incoming mail. If you live with others, ask permission to sort their mail and deliver it to them. Follow procedures outlined in this chapter. Write a paragraph about what you have learned by completing this exercise and how this experience might translate to a medical facility.

post office to purchase postage. The meter is locked for the amount of postage purchased. Clinics that send a large volume of mail may purchase a postage meter. Procedure 14-5 provides steps for preparing outgoing mail.

Postal Classes

The Postal Service provides a range of mail classes and pricing to accommodate most user needs. Visit http://www.usps.com and use the Calculate a Price tool to find prices for mailing various mailing pieces (envelopes, boxes, etc.) from one ZIP code to another.

Formats for Efficient Mail Processing

Certified and registered markings should be placed below the stamp or approximately nine lines from the right top edge of the envelope. *Personal* or *confidential* notation should be keyed in all caps three lines below the return address.

Adherence to other regulations will ensure accurate, timely delivery.

ZIP+4. ZIP+4 consists of the basic five ZIP code digits followed by a hyphen and four additional digits. The use of ZIP+4 will expedite the delivery of mail. If the envelope has been prepared properly to be read through OCR, the digits will be converted to a bar code. This piece of mail then goes to the bar code sorter, which rapidly sorts for the final destination.

Abbreviations. When addressing mail, use the abbreviations for states and U.S. possessions (Figure 14-12) and use official postal service abbreviations for street suffixes, directionals, and locators (Figure 14-13).

International Mail

Classes of international mail include letters and letter packages, postcards and postal cards,

---

PROCEDURE 14-5

Procedure

Preparing Outgoing Mail According to U.S. Postal Regulations

PURPOSE:

To prepare outgoing mail for expeditious delivery.

EQUIPMENT/SUPPLIES:

- Manual or electronic scale
- Postage meter or stamps
- Envelope or package to be mailed

PROCEDURE STEPS:

1. Sort the mail according to postal class. For example, all single-piece letters that weigh less than 11 ounces are included in first-class mail. Correspondence and statements are sent in this classification. RATIONALE: Sorting by postal class expedites processing at the post office.

2. Using the manual or electronic scale, weigh the item to be mailed. **Paying attention to detail**, if you are using a manual scale, read the weight in ounces and compute the amount of postage due. If you are using an electronic scale, the correct postage will be displayed on the scale. RATIONALE: Correct postage on each postal item is essential to ensure faster delivery service.

3. Using a postal meter or stamps, affix the appropriate postage to the piece to be mailed. Use of a postal meter expedites delivery of mail because metered mail does not have to be canceled or postmarked at the post office. RATIONALE: Correct postage on each postal item is essential to ensure faster delivery service.

4. Place the prepared mail in the area of the clinic designated for outgoing mail or deliver the mail to the post office according to clinic policy. RATIONALE: Ensures that all mail going out is centrally located and that the postal worker can pick up outgoing mail and deliver incoming mail efficiently.

AL	Alabama	NE	Nebraska
AK	Alaska	NV	Nevada
AS	American Samoa	NH	New Hampshire
AZ	Arizona	NJ	New Jersey
AR	Arkansas	NM	New Mexico
CA	California	NY	New York
CO	Colorado	NC	North Carolina
CT	Connecticut	ND	North Dakota
DE	Delaware	MP	No. Mariana Islands
DC	Dist. of Columbia	OH	Ohio
FL	Florida	OK	Oklahoma
GA	Georgia	OR	Oregon
GU	Guam	PA	Pennsylvania
HI	Hawaii	PR	Puerto Rico
ID	Idaho	RI	Rhode Island
IL	Illinois	SC	South Carolina
IN	Indiana	SD	South Dakota
IA	Iowa	TN	Tennessee
KS	Kansas	TX	Texas
KY	Kentucky	TT	Trust Territory
LA	Louisiana	UT	Utah
ME	Maine	VT	Vermont
MD	Maryland	VI	Virgin Islands, U.S.
MA	Massachusetts	VA	Virginia
MI	Michigan	WA	Washington
MN	Minnesota	WV	West Virginia
MS	Mississippi	WI	Wisconsin
MO	Missouri	WY	Wyoming
MT	Montana		

FIGURE 14-12 Abbreviations for states, territories, and the District of Columbia.

AVE	Avenue	PL	Place
BLVD	Boulevard	RD	Road
CT	Court	STA	Station
CTR	Center	ST	Street
CIR	Circle	TPKE	Turnpike
DR	Drive	VLY	Valley
EXPY	Expressway		
HTS	Heights	APT	Apartment
HWY	Highway	RM	Room
IS	Island	STE	Suite
JCT	Junction	PLZ	Plaza
LK	Lake		
LN	Lane	N	North
MTN	Mountain	E	East
PKY	Parkway	S	South
		W	West

FIGURE 14-13 Abbreviations for street suffixes, directionals, and locators.

aerograms (airmail letters), printed matter, direct sacks of printed matter, matter for people who are blind, small packets, and parcel post. Special services such as insurance, recorded delivery, registered mail, restricted delivery, return receipt, special delivery, cash on delivery mail, and certified mail are also available. For the most current information on rates and services, inquire at the local postal service.

LEGAL AND ETHICAL ISSUES

Legal

Written communication, no matter what form is used, must take into consideration legal and ethical issues. A copy of all written communication should be maintained in the patient medical record or in clinic files should it be needed at a later date.

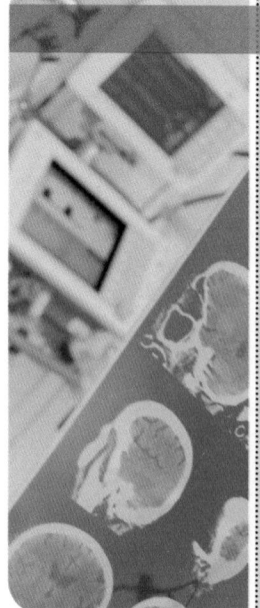

CASE STUDY 14-1

Refer to the scenario at the beginning of the chapter.

When she was assembling the style manual for all written communications generated by Inner City Health Care, clinic manager Marilyn Johnson wanted it to be as comprehensive as possible. Therefore, she gathered research over a period of months, noting problems the clinic had experienced in written communications, such as letters going out without the provider's signature. She became familiar with proofreading devices that would ensure letter-perfect correspondence. She also developed source materials on the different classes of mail and the services of the U.S. Postal Service.

CASE STUDY REVIEW

1. Marilyn is ready to outline the manual. Review the chapter information and create an outline indicating major topic headings for the Inner City Health Care style manual.

2. Because a few of the medical assistants are not comfortable with composing, what writing tips can Marilyn include to make them more confident?

3. Marilyn wants all letters to look alike. What information should she include to educate the manual users about the components of a standard letter?

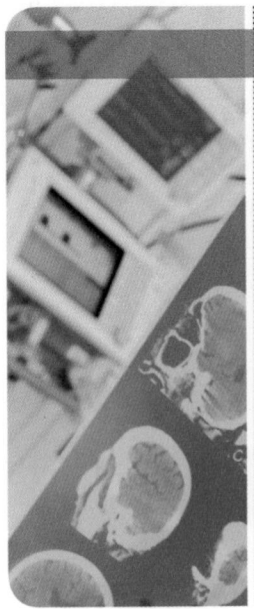

CASE STUDY 14-2

Inner City Health Care is considering adopting the use of clinical email because many of their patients have home computers and use email in their day-to-day communications. Clinic manager Marilyn Johnson is concerned about maintaining patient confidentiality and appropriate use of clinical email. She has decided to develop a written agreement of understanding and plans to ask each patient to sign the agreement before transmission of any clinical email is instituted. Marilyn also believes a privacy disclaimer could be of legal value to the clinic. Review Chapter 11's section on email etiquette for a sample disclaimer.

CASE STUDY REVIEW

1. Marilyn is developing the agreement of understanding. What are some key elements that should be included in the agreement?
2. Responding to patients using email correspondence is different than social communication. What are some guidelines for email correspondence that will be helpful to remember?
3. List several advantages and disadvantages to using email in the ambulatory health care setting.

Summary

- Written correspondence is important in conveying a professional image of the clinic and impacts the practice either positively or negatively.

- Written documents provide a permanent or legal record in the event of any litigation and thus must be carefully and accurately worded.

- The medical assistant must understand the components of a business letter and organizing the placement of these components in the proper order and spacing on a page.

- The medical assistant must be familiar with the various letter styles and properly setting up the components of each style.

- Medical assistants must know how to use Mail Merge for the creation of envelopes and mailing lists.

- Other types of correspondence include memoranda, meeting agendas, and taking meeting minutes.

- The medical assistant must know how to process incoming and outgoing mail, including types of postal mail classes.

Study for Success

To reinforce your knowledge and skills of information presented in this chapter:

- Review the *Key Terms* and *Learning Outcomes*

- Consider the *Critical Thinking* features and *Case Studies* and discuss your conclusions

- Answer the questions in the *Certification Review*

Procedure

- Perform the *Procedures* using the *Competency Assessment Checklists* on the *Student Companion Website*

CERTIFICATION REVIEW

1. How should you proofread a letter?
   a. Never read it against the document
   b. Always proof it only on the computer screen
   c. Read long documents a section at a time
   d. Always finish the job no matter how tired you may be

2. How can form letters be individualized?
   a. Form letters are never individualized
   b. By using the current date, receiver's name, and mailing address
   c. By limiting form letters to a select number of uses
   d. By using a letter style other than Simplified
   e. Form letters will be individualized if mailed first class only

3. Of the four major letter styles, which is the most contemporary?
   a. Full block
   b. Modified block, standard
   c. Modified block, indented
   d. Simplified

4. What form letters can the medical assistant sign for the provider?
   a. Letters to thank referring providers
   b. Letters to order supplies
   c. Letters to announce new staff
   d. None of these
   e. All of these

5. On what line is the subject line keyed?
   a. On line 15 or two to three lines below the letterhead
   b. On the second line below the inside address
   c. Four lines below the complimentary closing
   d. On the second line below the salutation

6. Which of the following is a guideline for letter placement?
   a. Use single line space within paragraphs.
   b. When dividing a paragraph at the bottom of a page, keep two lines on the bottom of the page and two lines at the top of the next page.
   c. A minimum of three lines should be keyed on the second page of a letter.
   d. None of these
   e. All of these

7. After removing the contents from incoming mail, what should you do?
   a. Stamp the date it was received in the clinic.
   b. Look in the envelope to make certain that all contents have been removed.
   c. If the address is not included on the letter, write it on the letter as it appeared on the envelope.
   d. All of these

8. Computer disks, film, video tapes, and books are sent in which postal class?
   a. Express
   b. First class
   c. Bulk rate
   d. Second class
   e. Media class

9. First-class mail is divided into which two subclasses?
   a. Automation and nonautomation
   b. Periodical and standard mail
   c. Standard A and standard B
   d. Bulk and parcel post mail

10. What is the most time efficient letter style for creating a variety of letters?
    a. Watermark
    b. Standard modified block
    c. Full block letter
    d. Indented modified block
    e. Simplified letter

CHAPTER 15

Medical Documents

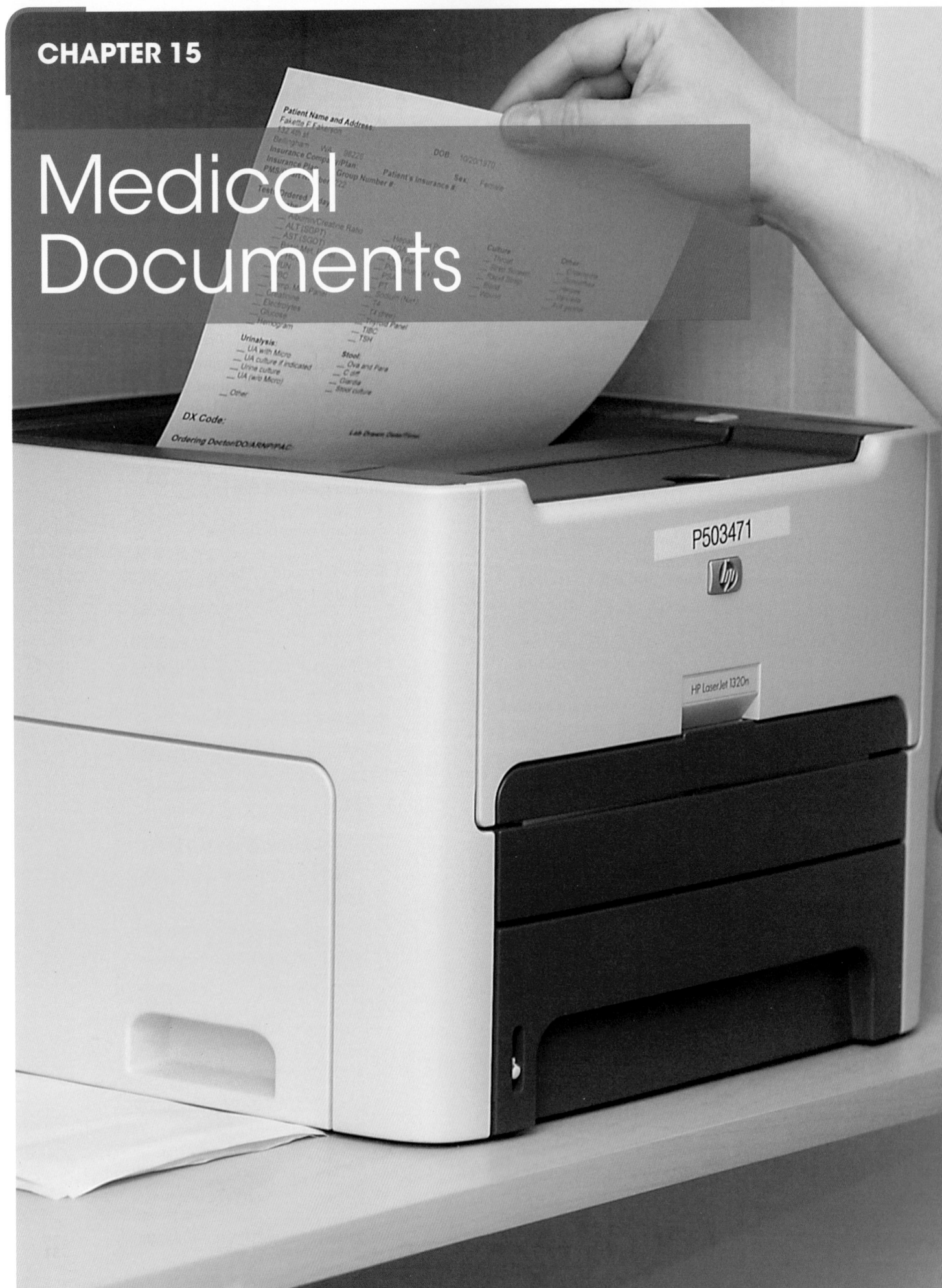

1. Define and spell the key terms as presented in the glossary.
2. Discuss the changing role of medical transcription.
3. Discuss the impact of electronic health records on medical transcription.
4. List a minimum of three reasons for justifying outsourcing medical transcription.
5. Discuss voice recognition software and its impact upon medical transcription.
6. List responsibilities of the medical transcriptionist serving as editor of medical documents.
7. Review the importance of quality assurance and risk management.
8. Describe the process of flagging and its significance.
9. Discuss what is meant by the term *authentication* and identify three ways it may be done related to medical reports.
10. State what is meant by *privileged* information.
11. Identify four ways the medical transcriptionist can be compliant with the Health Insurance Portability and Accountability Act (HIPAA).
12. Differentiate among chart notes, history and physical examination reports, radiology and imaging reports, operative reports, pathology reports, consultations, discharge summaries, autopsy reports, and correspondence.
13. Discuss turnaround time and its importance to medical records.

KEY TERMS

Association for Healthcare Documentation Integrity (AHDI)

auditor

autopsy report

certified medical transcriptionist (CMT)

chart notes

chief complaint (CC)

confidentiality agreement

consultation report

current reports

discharge summary (DS)

editor

electronic medical record (EMR)

flag

gross examination

Health Insurance Portability and Accountability Act (HIPAA)

history and physical examination (H&P) report

history of the present illness (HPI)

medical transcriptionist (MT)

microscopic examination

old report or aged report

operative report (OR)

outsourcing

pathology report

present problem (PP)

privileged

progress notes

quality assurance (QA)

radiology report

registered medical transcriptionist (RMT)

review of systems (ROS)

risk management

STAT report

turnaround time (TAT)

voice recognition software (VRS)

Chapter Portal

The development of new technology over the last few years is impacting medical facilities in a variety of ways. Computerized medical facilities have implemented electronic medical records (EMR), may use voice recognition software (VRS) and electronic signatures, or may outsource transcription to other areas of the United States or to foreign countries. These changes have a direct impact on the position medical transcriptionists (MT) once held in the medical environment. Today, the MT may be more involved with quality assurance (QA), risk management, and editing the completed document rather than transcribing written or dictated medical information.

THE CHANGING ROLE OF MEDICAL TRANSCRIPTION

Medical transcriptionists (MT), sometimes referred to as health care documentation specialists, listen to voice recordings dictated by health care providers and create medical records in the proper format for the type of document and according to the standards of the facility. MT may also review and edit medical documents created by speech recognition technology, to ensure accuracy between what was dictated and the document produced. An MT that does not actually type the document, but rather compares dictation to the text produced by the voice recognition software, and then edits the text where needed, may sometimes be called a dictation editor or a medical transcription editor.

Today's cost-conscious and rapidly changing economy along with new technology has brought about many changes to the MT profession. The following paragraphs discuss major changes impacting medical transcription today.

Electronic Medical Records

Clinics using **electronic medical records (EMR)** rather than paper-based medical records may delegate much of the MT's responsibility to other medical personnel. For example, the MA may record directly into the EMR the reason for the visit, medications the patient is currently taking, including over-the-counter and herbal products; height and weight; vital signs; and any observations. The provider, using the computer, has access to the entire patient medical record and may call up test results, various images, diagnoses, and treatment plans for verification or comparison. The provider may add to the EMR document by directly keying in chart notes or by dictating to a digital recording system or may use voice recognition software. The provider may complete and transmit prescriptions directly to a pharmacy or forward all or part of the medical record to a referring provider.

Each entry into the EMR is automatically date and time stamped, which facilitates documentation and tracking of patient care and outcomes. The EMR provides easy access to quickly locate accurate and readily usable information about the patient at the point of care. EMR are much more efficient in the clinical decision-making process than the old cumbersome paper-based patient records. EMR may be sent to all medical personnel involved in the care of a patient in a matter of seconds.

We have covered the process of changeover to a computerized system in the medical clinic in Chapter 10, but we have not covered the process of the physical transition from existing paper medical records to electronic health records. Two issues must be resolved: How much of the paper chart do we convert to a digital format and how do we make the majority of the existing clinical history available to the physician? Several options are available:

- *All patient charts are scanned into the EMR system.* This choice is the most attractive option, but it is also the most costly. Although the basic scanning can be performed by a relatively unskilled worker, a trained medical professional must file the data in the appropriate category of the new medical record so that it can be readily located by the medical provider.

- *Partial scanning of patient charts.* Charts are pulled for existing patients scheduled for the coming week and only the clinically pertinent information from the past three to six visits as identified by the medical provider are scanned and filed in the new system. This process is repeated until partial paper records for all patients are included in the EHR system. This approach requires that paper records be actively retained for a period before they are archived.
- *Do not scan any old information.* Develop an EHR record for all patients from a given date and have the old paper record for existing patients available for the medical provider for as long as the provider feels necessary. At some point the provider will no longer have a need for the paper record and it can be archived.

Some practices receive a lot of calls regarding patient questions or pharmacy requests. The summary page of the paper record can be scanned for all patients to establish an EHR that is useful in fulfilling these types of requests. One of the options for transitioning paper records can then be used to develop a more complete EHR for each patient.

The conversion of paper records to electronic records is most readily accomplished by scanning. It could be done using practice personnel; however, it is more cost effective for an outside firm that will come onsite to do the work. Care must be exercised to follow all HIPAA regulations. A trained medical professional will still be required to ensure that the records are filed appropriately in the EHR system.

The file system used in establishing an EHR system must be carefully thought out to ensure that the medical provider can easily retrieve data. The EHR program being used is a good place to begin in planning the details of the file system while tailoring it to the specific type of medical practice. Documentation of the file system and the conversion procedure is a first step to maintaining consistent nomenclature and data format throughout the conversion.

Outsourcing

Transcription is a task that is presently outsourced by many large clinics and hospitals. **Outsourcing** is the practice of contracting with a service outside the clinic or hospital to a company where the task can be accomplished at a lower cost and with a faster turnaround time. Outsourcing companies usually are located in countries where a source of English-speaking educated labor is present, the pay rate is low, and a stable business climate exists. Currently, outsourcing organizations are located in areas of the United States and Canada as well as offshore at companies primarily located in the United Kingdom, India, and the Philippines.

Today's medical clinics must keep a keen eye on the bottom line—cost. Some advantages given to support outsourcing of medical transcription include the following:

- Outsourcing transcription frees administrative and support personnel to complete tasks that often are delayed because of time crunch factors.
- Outsourcing companies are on the job 24/7 and 365 days of the year, so the medical clinic need not be concerned about vacation periods or sick leave. Someone is always on the job.
- Outsourcing companies focus on transcription without having to answer telephones, schedule appointments, or deal with any number of interruptions encountered in the medical clinic. Therefore, documents are more accurate, standardized, and completed with less turnaround time.
- Outsourcing transcription frees floor space (real estate) previously used to support a line item expense and converts it to a source of revenue.
- Outsourcing saves on costly employee benefits packages.

Digital dictation by the provider can be readily sent to the outsource organization that performs the transcription using the Internet, with the completed document returned in similar fashion. Some important considerations before outsourcing transcription include the following:

- Be sure the medical clinic and the transcription service are using compatible hardware and software.
- Investigate quality assurance, security, HIPAA, and confidentiality measures.
- Be cost conscious. Most transcription fees are calculated by the line, but it may be more cost effective to pay by the minute of recorded dictation time. A digital dictation system allows one to measure to the 10th or 100th of a minute.
- A transcription service that uses a digital dictation system should have a user-friendly method of tracking transcribed documents. The work should be able to be located in less than 3 minutes.

- When using a digital dictation system, a provider's dictation is available to the transcriptionist as soon as the provider hangs up the phone, allowing for no lost time, which equates to cost containment.

Outsourcing is rapidly eliminating the need for the traditional transcriptionist in medical facilities. This practice is in turn being replaced by the use of voice recognition software.

Voice Recognition Software

Voice recognition software (VRS), also known as speech recognition, automatic speech recognition (ASR), or natural language recognition software, converts voice to text using a computer. In essence, the software "translates" the sounds spoken into written words. This type of program has improved greatly in recent years, translating with little error. Specialized programs are capable of translating highly technical medical terminology.

The latest generation of VRS uses continuous speech technology, which allows the speaker to speak more naturally. All VRS systems require an enrollment process, during which a person sits at the computer and reads sample text out loud to help train the speech recognition software to understand the particular voice pattern. VRS integrates easily with Windows applications, including Microsoft Word, Outlook Express, Internet Explorer, and AOL Instant Messenger. Some VRS products are marketed that work with personal digital assistants (PDAs) and smartphones.

Medical Transcriptionist as Editor

With the use of EHR, outsourcing, or VRS methods of transcription, the MT professional is now serving as the **quality assurance (QA)** manager, responsible for **risk management**, and the **editor** or **auditor** of transcribed documents. A QA manager establishes a process that provides accurate, complete, consistent health care documentation in a timely manner. Figure 15-1 shows data flow for transcribed medical records produced using outsourcing and speech recognition software.

Editing is the process of reviewing the transcribed document for accuracy and clarity. It is important to remember that one must not change the dictator's style or meaning when editing. Common errors are

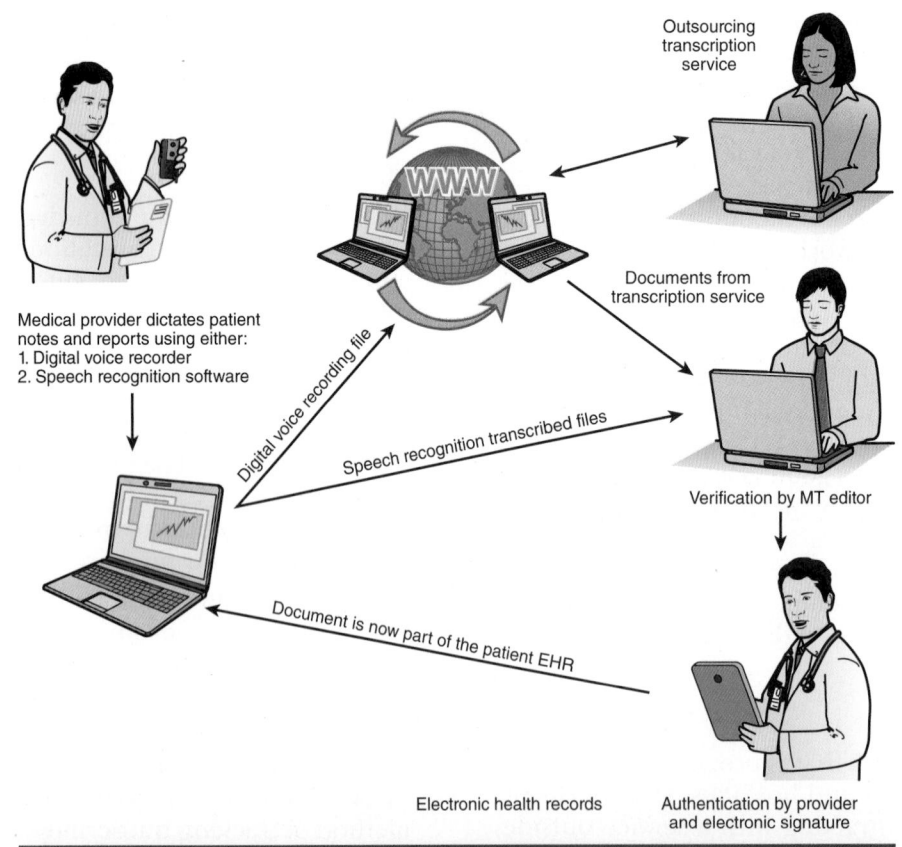

Outsourcing transcription service

Documents from transcription service

Medical provider dictates patient notes and reports using either:
1. Digital voice recorder
2. Speech recognition software

Digital voice recording file

Speech recognition transcribed files

Verification by MT editor

Document is now part of the patient EHR

Electronic health records

Authentication by provider and electronic signature

FIGURE 15-1 Data flow for transcribed medical records produced using outsourcing and speech recognition software.

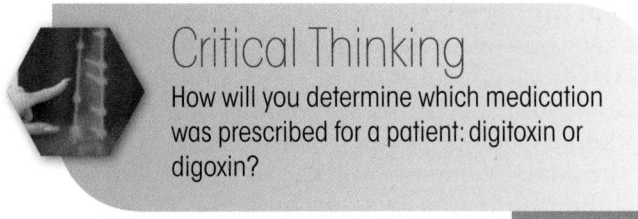

Critical Thinking

How will you determine which medication was prescribed for a patient: digitoxin or digoxin?

usually in sentence structure, punctuation, and spelling. They are easily changed without altering the dictator's style or meaning. Sound-alike words are another area where errors occur.

The **Association for Healthcare Documentation Integrity (AHDI)** recommends the following principles when reviewing a document:

- Compare the transcribed report against dictation. Do not just read the document.
- Use industry-specific standards for style, punctuation, and grammar (e.g., *The Book of Style for Medical Transcription*).
- Consider risk management issues.
- Third parties, such as the QA person, proofing a document should provide feedback to the transcriptionist. Although 100% accuracy is desired, accuracy of audited documents should not be less than 98%. Accuracy less than this figure requires corrective action.

If the MT encounters a term that cannot be interpreted or something new that cannot be referenced, the MT should **flag** that section of the document to alert the dictator that something needs to be corrected or resolved. The flagged message may indicate the provider is cut off, what the term sounds like, or the message is incomprehensible. Provide as much information as you can to assist the dictator in recalling the dictated area in question.

Flagging procedures vary from one facility to another and may depend upon the method used to transcribe documents. In large facilities using EHR, VRS, or outsourcing, the flagged documents may be referred directly to QA personnel. The notation may be incorporated into the computerized document using a color-code approach with a flag message. The correct information then can be added to the document and the color coding removed. In-house flagging may simply consist of a sticky note or a preprinted flag attachment.

Authentication

In most cases, the provider dictating the information will sign or authenticate the document. At times an attending provider or physician assistant will be responsible for dictating the material. The provider's signature on the document indicates that the information was accurate and complete at the time of dictation and as transcribed.

In today's technological world, electronic signatures have become common practice. The words *electronically signed by [provider's name]* underneath the signature are keyed to indicate an electronic signature. Electronic signatures may also be accomplished through:

- Use of alphanumeric computer key entries as identification
- Use of an electronic writing device
- Use of a biometric system

Legal Medicare and the Joint Commission guidelines require that the signature on medical reports, electronic or handwritten, be completed by the provider dictating the information and not delegated to anyone else. Federal law, state law, and Joint Commission accreditation standards all address the issue of electronic signatures.

CONFIDENTIALITY AND LEGAL ISSUES

Legal **Integrity** Confidentiality means treating the patient's medical information as private and not for publication. The patient has a right to privacy; therefore, medical information is **privileged**. Privileged information may only be communicated with the patient's permission or by court order. The MT must learn to follow the motto: *What you see here and what you hear here must stay here when you leave here.*

Health Insurance Portability and Accountability Act Regulations

Competency **Health Insurance Portability and Accountability Act (HIPAA)** regulations are government rules and procedures that have resulted from legislation designed to protect the confidentiality of patient information ranging from medical records to personal identification numbers that, if divulged, could result in identity theft.

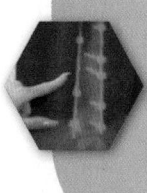

Critical Thinking

How would you go about designing a medical transcription workstation that was ergonomic and compliant with HIPAA regulations? Review Chapter 10.

The MT can meet most HIPAA regulations by adhering to the following simple rules:

- Do not divulge medical records you transcribe to anyone other than the dictator, your supervisor, or an authorized QA person. Files should not be discussed with the patient. Do not divulge files to an attorney or insurance representative without consulting with risk management personnel.

- Safeguard files in your possession. Take reasonable steps to keep files secure, such as keeping tapes and hard copy of reports in a locked file cabinet, using passwords for computer files, installing virus protection software, and using a firewall if appropriate. Do not carelessly carry files around on your person or in your car.

- Transmit files electronically only with the permission of your client or the dictating provider, and then agree on the proper procedures and protocols for transmission.

- Have a signed business associate agreement or similar document that defines the protocols you are expected to follow to protect patient confidentiality.

These general rules do not constitute legal advice; consult with appropriate legal counsel for specific questions.

Protocols

Protocols are the procedures your clinic has in place to ensure patient confidentiality. You are usually required to sign a **confidentiality agreement** stating that you will comply with the established procedures. Your contracts, together with the protocols, become a part of the institution's documentation demonstrating compliance with HIPAA regulations. The purpose of your signing a contract is to substantiate that you have received training and have been instructed in proper procedures to protect medical records.

From the MT's viewpoint, risk management involves protecting the confidentiality of the medical records and ensuring the accuracy of those records.

MTs are in an excellent position to assist the risk management officer, through their commitment to quality and their awareness of confidentiality procedures and possible medical errors indicated in the dictated data. Should a problem or error be detected that could be a risk management problem, the MT should immediately notify his or her superior, clinic manager, risk management officer, or the employer's or client's legal staff according to clinic policy.

You will recall from Chapter 7 that ethics are not laws but rather standards of conduct. These standards vary from state to state, so you should research your specific state's standards. The AHDI adopted a Code of Ethics (see the AHDI Web site for the AHDI Code of Ethics available at: http://www.ahdionline.org by searching for "Code of Ethics") for professional MTs.

Although, in certain cases, the MT can be held financially responsible for errors and omissions, the MT usually is under the jurisdiction of *respondeat superior*, meaning that the provider-director or clinic manager is responsible for the wrongful acts of the MT working under his or her supervision. This is not meant to imply that MTs should not protect themselves by instituting some personal risk management, such as carrying errors and omissions insurance. Insurance should be considered particularly if the MT is operating a home business and contracting transcription work.

Legal

Medical records are documents governed by laws and may be subpoenaed for review by various courts. The medical report may play a major role in substantiating injury or malpractice claims.

TYPES OF MEDICAL DOCUMENTS

Medical reports become part of the patient's permanent medical record and are vital to continued patient care. Other providers, attorneys, insurance companies, or the court may review the medical reports in part or in their entirety. Therefore, the medical report must be neat, accurate, and complete. *Neat* refers to a medical report that is legible and assembled to permit easy access to information as needed. *Accurate* means that the dictation has been transcribed as dictated, and *complete* indicates that the document has been dated correctly and signed or initialed by the dictator.

Complete documentation of medical reports is also important for payment or reimbursement of services for which the provider expects to be paid. The billing and diagnosis codes reported on the health insurance claim form must be supported by the documentation contained within the medical report.

A new trend in transcription is the integration of digital images directly into the transcribed record. The response to inputting digital images (photographs, scans, and radiographs) has been positive from both the local health care community and patients themselves. This is attributed to easier understanding of a picture by patients and more precise presentation using both pictures and written text to medical professionals.

The tools required for integrating digital images into word processing programs is already available to most MTs in their current Microsoft Word software packages. They only have to obtain the digital images from their provider-employer. If the transcribed record is included in the EHR, digital images can be attached, allowing other providers to view, enlarge, and manipulate the images at will.

The transcribed medical report may be formatted in a variety of styles similar to business correspondence. Common transcribed reports include:

1. Chart notes and progress notes
2. History and physical examination reports
3. Radiology reports
4. Operative reports
5. Pathology reports
6. Consultations
7. Discharge summaries
8. Autopsy reports
9. Correspondence

Hospitals and practices may require a specific format for reports different from those described in the following examples. A few helpful formatting rules are:

- Use section headings that clarify the report.
- Do not add sections left out by the dictator.
- Do not include unnecessary confidential information unless specifically instructed to do so.

- Note who dictated the report, if not the attending provider, and provide space for both to sign. The initials of the transcriptionist should be on the signature page.
- Use 1-inch margins all around, unless the document is to be filed in a chart that has a top opening, then use a 1.25-inch margin at the top only. If using sticky paper for chart notes, use 0.5-inch margins.
- Use paragraph format.

Chart Notes and Progress Notes

Chart notes, sometimes referred to as **progress notes**, are a concise description of the patient's encounter with the medical clinic. They are chronologically listed and may include in-person visits to the clinic and telephone and electronic mail (email) inquiries. Chart notes should be filed in the chart within 24 hours of the encounter. The present problem, the provider's physical findings, and the treatment plan should be identified within the chart note. Laboratory test results also may be included. The provider or clinic personnel may enter chart note information as informal handwritten notes, or keyed notes affixed to the appropriate space. All notes documented must include the date, time, and signature of the person entering the data along with his or her credential. This information is pertinent for follow-up questions or for litigation purposes. Figure 15-2 shows a sample chart/progress note in an EHR.

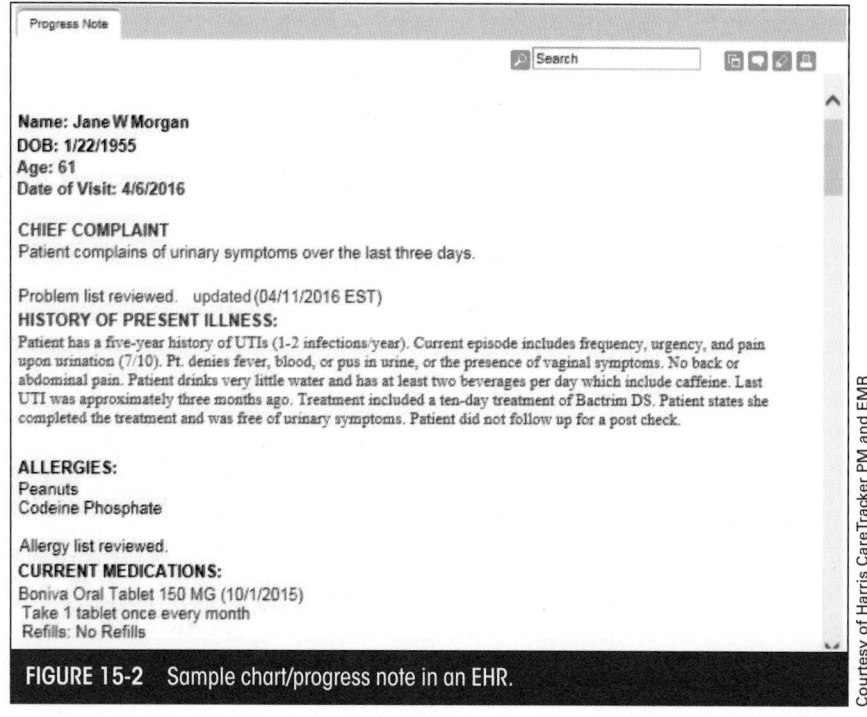

FIGURE 15-2 Sample chart/progress note in an EHR.

History and Physical Examination Reports

The **history and physical examination (H&P) report** documents information relating to the patient's main reason for treatment. The report is divided into two sections. The first is the history, which includes the **chief complaint (CC)** or **present problem (PP)**, a description of symptoms, problems, or conditions that brought the patient to the clinic; **history of the present illness (HPI)**, a chronological description of the development of the patient's illness; past medical and surgical history; family history; and social history.

The second section is the **review of systems (ROS)** and inquiry about the system directly related to the problems identified in the HPI. The provider determines the extent of the examination performed and documented based on the problems presented. The findings of the actual physical examination make up the documentation for the physical examination section of the report.

The Joint Commission accredits and regulates all policies and procedures of hospitals and provider's clinics owned by hospital organizations. The Joint Commission requires that hospitals provide H&P reports to be filed in patient charts within 24 hours of admission. Occasionally, the patient is seen in the provider's clinic and a decision is made to admit the patient to the hospital. In this case, the examination is performed in the clinic, but the report is dictated to the hospital that transcribes the document and files it within the patient's chart. The H&P format may also be used to document a patient's annual physical examination in the clinic. Figure 15-3 shows a sample H&P Report.

HISTORY AND PHYSICAL EXAMINATION

PATIENT: Donald Waite
CHART #: 97223

HISTORY: The patient is a 72-year-old male who was admitted because of intermittent, moderately severe chest pain starting from the substernal region radiating to the back and to the left arm and associated with a choking sensation. The pain lasted from minutes to half an hour and was relieved by two nitroglycerin tablets.

This condition has been going on for the last two weeks. The patient has known arteriosclerotic heart disease and since his discharge in July 20XX, has been doing reasonably well on Procardia, nitrates, Persantine, and digoxin.

PAST HISTORY: The patient had a pacemaker implantation for sick sinus syndrome four years ago. He has a history of angina and myocardial infarction. He also has essential hypertension.

His past surgical history includes an appendectomy and bilateral herniorrhaphies. He has no allergies.

The patient still works as a projectionist in a movie house. He does not smoke but drinks occasionally. He denies any history of diabetes, liver, or kidney disease. There is no evidence of claudication. There is dyspnea on exertion and fatigability. GI is negative; GU is negative.

PHYSICAL EXAMINATION: The patient is out of distress right now. He has been given two injections of Demerol. Blood pressure is 120/68, ventricular rate is 72 per minute, and respiratory rate is 20 per minute. Color is good. Skin is warm. Examination of the head shows that right lenticular opacity is greater than the left. Neck veins are flat. There are no bruits. Carotids are brisk, and there is no evidence of thyroid enlargement. The heart is regular with no S3 gallops. There is a systolic ejection murmur at the base III/VI. The lungs are clear. The abdomen shows surgical scars. Extremities have no edema. Pulses are 2+, and there is no calf tenderness.

IMPRESSION: Unstable angina secondary to coronary artery disease with obstructive and mixed pattern spasm on an affixed lesion. Status postpacemaker implantation and degenerative joint disease with cervical degenerative arthritis.

Review of the EKG shows nonspecific ST-T wave changes in II, III, and aVF and in the anterolateral leads. Chest X-ray showed cardiomegaly, and the enzymes are pending.

RECOMMENDATIONS: The patient should be hospitalized in the coronary care unit and monitored. The nifedipine should be increased up to 60 mg—slowly. Continue Persantine. Continue transderm nitro—increase to 10 mg/24 hr (0.4 mg/hr). Monitor the blood level. Consider angiogram when he is stabilized.

Electronically signed by Mark King, MD 11/3/20XX   5:37 PM

MK/jg
d: 11/2/XX
t: 11/2/XX

FIGURE 15-3 Sample history and physical examination report.

Radiology and Imaging Reports

A **radiology report** is a description of the findings and interpretations of the radiologist who studies the diagnostic procedure. Examples of radiology reports are X-ray studies, computed tomography (CT) scans, magnetic resonance image (MRI) scans, nuclear medicine procedures, and fluoroscopic studies. In some cases, a contrast medium is administered either orally or by injection before the procedure is performed. A scan is a procedure that requires the use of radioactive isotopes.

When dictating, the radiologist may switch from present to past tense; that is, the procedure was performed in the past tense, and the findings are given in the present tense.

Stereoscopy and tomography are technologies that view structures within the body in dimensions or layers. Computed tomography uses radiography with computers to visualize a slice of the body part. Sonograms and echograms are another imaging technology that uses high-frequency sound waves to compose a picture of an area of the body. Magnetic resonance imaging produces sectional images of the body without the use of radiology. New technologies create the need for understanding the imaging process and appropriate documentation of patient information.

When transcribing radiology or imaging reports, the date of service should be used rather than the date of dictation. Other details to be included within the report may include:

- Number and type of views taken
- Any special circumstances that could affect the examination
- Quality of the study (clear or blurry)
- Abnormal findings
- Normal findings
- Radiologist's impression, interpretation, diagnosis, and recommendations
- Signature of the radiologist

The report should be filed in the patient's chart within 4 to 8 hours of the procedure. Sufficient documentation must be in the report for the provider to use if he or she must prove that the study was medically necessary or if justification for reimbursement is required. Figure 15-4 shows an example of a radiology report.

Operative Reports

The **operative report (OR)** chronicles the details of a surgical procedure performed in a hospital,

MERCY MEDICAL CENTER
300 Main Street
Denver, CO 80201

RADIOLOGY #: 23445

PA & LATERAL CHEST   Date 10/07/XX

The pulmonary vessels are clearly outlined and are not distended. There are not any typical signs of redistribution. A few increased interstitial markings persist, but there are no typical acute Kerley B-lines. There may be a little residual pleural effusion at the costophrenic sinus and posterior gutters. Most of the pulmonary edema and effusion has otherwise cleared. The chest is not hyperexpanded. The thoracic vertebrae show spurring but no compression.

IMPRESSION:
1. No signs of elevated pulmonary venous pressure or frank failure at this time.
2. Residual pleural effusion is seen in the costophrenic sinus and posterior gutters, either residual or recent congestive failure.

BILATERAL MAMMOGRAMS   Date: 10/07/XX

Bilateral xeromammograms were obtained in both the mediolateral and craniocaudal projections. There is no previous exam for comparison. There is slight asymmetry of the ductal tissue in the lower outer quadrant of the right breast. There are no dominant masses, clusters of microcalcifications or pathologic skin changes identified.

IMPRESSION: Normal bilateral mammogram.

Electronically signed by
Renny Genray, MD 10/08/20XX 11:21 AM

JOHN DOE, M.D.   SMITH, HARRIET #123456-7
Dictated by: Renny Genray, M.D.
D&T: 10/07/XX | 10/07/XX | RG/mt
RADIOLOGY REPORT

FIGURE 15-4 Sample radiology report.

outpatient surgical center, or clinic. The surgeon or assistant dictates the OR immediately after the operation. The OR describes the surgical procedure, preoperative and postoperative diagnoses, and specimens removed. It sometimes includes a sponge count and instrument inventory, an estimate of blood loss, and the condition of the patient on leaving the operating room. The report should also include the name of the primary surgeon and any assistants. The type of anesthesia and name of the anesthesiologist should also be included in the report. Often the report will end with disposition or where the patient was transferred when he or she left the operating room and the condition of

PATIENT: Joseph Oritz

DATE: 6/25/XX

SURGEON: Raja Rao, MD

PREOPERATIVE DIAGNOSIS: Crohn's disease requiring central venous access for hyperalimentation.

POSTOPERATIVE DIAGNOSIS: Crohn's disease requiring central venous access for hyperalimentation.

OPERATION: Insertion of left-sided subclavian double-lumen central venous catheter.

ANESTHESIA: 1% lidocaine.

PROCEDURE: The patient was placed in the supine position with the neck extended to the right side. The left side of the chest was prepared and draped in the usual manner using Betadine solution. The subclavian vein on the left side was percutaneously and easily entered, and the guide wire was advanced into the superior vena cava. The double-lumen central venous catheter with VitaCuff was placed through the guide wire into the superior vena cava. Good blood flow was obtained. The catheter was sutured to the skin using 2-0 silk sutures and connected to IV solution.

A dry sterile dressing was applied.

The patient tolerated the procedure well.

Electronically signed by
Juan Esposito, MD 06/25/20XX
4:15 PM

JE/urs

d: 6/25/XX
t: 6/27/XX

FIGURE 15-5 *Sample operative report.*

PATHOLOGY REPORT

PATHOLOGY NO.: 792 304
DATE: 12/20/XX
CHART NO.: 56 84 20
NAME: Lee Allen Au   AGE: 15 Female
DEPARTMENT: Surgery   MD: Dr. Raja Rao

TISSUE: Appendix

HISTORY: Right Lower Quadrant Pain

CLINICAL DIAGNOSIS: RLQ Pain

PATHOLOGICAL REPORT: The specimen is labeled appendix and is received in formalin. The specimen consists of an appendix that measures $6 \times 1 \times 0.5$ cm in greatest dimension. The serosa surface has some white fibrinoid material attached to it and on a cross section. Some purulent fibrinous material can also be seen. Representative sections are submitted in 1 cassette.

DIAGNOSIS: Acute suppurative appendicitis with periappendicitis and mesoappendicitis.

Electronically signed by
Mark King, MD 12/20/20XX
2:22 PM

MK/gc

d: 12/20/XX
t: 12/20/XX

FIGURE 15-6 *Sample pathology report.*

the patient at the time of transfer. The authenticated report should be filed in the chart as soon as possible after surgery so that other staff members caring for the patient will have needed information. Figure 15-5 shows a sample OR.

Pathology Reports

A **pathology report** is generated to describe the **gross** and **microscopic examinations** performed on organs, lesions, tissue samples, or body fluid removed during a surgical procedure. In some cases, the pathologist examines the specimen before the patient is sutured to determine if a more extensive surgical procedure is required (e.g., in the case of malignant tumors).

Pathologists generally dictate the report in the present tense because they interpret the pathologic findings as they view the specimens. The report must be completed within 24 hours of receipt with a copy maintained by the laboratory and copies sent to each provider involved in the case. The original is maintained in the patient's chart. Figure 15-6 shows a sample pathology report.

Consultation

When one provider requests the services of another provider in the care and treatment of a patient, a **consultation report** is generated. The information may be disseminated in the form of a report or within the body of a letter. The contents of the consultation report/letter usually consist of all of the elements of an H&P with a focused history of the patient's illness and the body system directly related to the consultant's area of specialty. The consultant also includes within the report/letter the findings, supporting laboratory data, diagnosis, and suggested course of treatment. The report/letter usually ends with a comment from the consulting provider thanking the admitting provider for the referral. It should be filed in the patient's medical record within 24 hours of receipt. Figure 15-7 shows a sample consultation report.

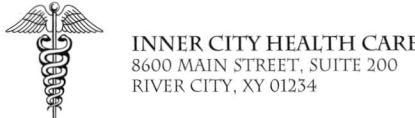

INNER CITY HEALTH CARE
8600 MAIN STREET, SUITE 200
RIVER CITY, XY 01234

January 4, 20XX

Margaret Holly, MD
Metroma Medical Center
900 Union Street, Suite 208
Metroma, MI 11666

RE: MARY O'KEEFE

Dear Dr. Holly:

Thank you for referring Mary O'Keefe to our clinic. She presented
today stating that she recently relocated to Clinton with her husband
and children to be closer to her parents. Mary has been experiencing
symptoms suggestive of pregnancy and is here for evaluation. Over the
past three weeks, she has noticed increased tenderness of her breasts,
fatigue, and a feeling of being bloated. A home pregnancy test was
positive.

Her past medical history is positive for the usual childhood diseases
and the births of two children, following normal pregnancies. She has a
negative past surgical history.

She has no allergies to medications and takes Tylenol for occasional
headaches. She is married and has two children, ages 3 years and 12
months. She is employed part-time in an insurance office. She does not
smoke or drink.

The family history is noncontributory.

On review of systems, her complaints are limited to those described
above. She has had no nausea or vomiting, and no change in bowel habits.
She has no dizziness, no fevers, and no urinary symptoms.

Physical examination revealed a 32-year-old white female in no acute
distress. HEENT normocephalic, atraumatic. PERRLA, EOMI. The thyroid
was not enlarged, and there was no cervical adenopathy. The lungs were
clear. The heart had a regular rate and rhythm. The abdomen was soft
and nontender. Bowel sounds were normal. The extremities revealed trace
ankle edema. The neurological examination was within normal limits.
Pelvic examination confirmed a gravid uterus, compatible with a very
early pregnancy.

An abdominal ultrasound has been ordered and a beta HCG was drawn.

I believe Mary is pregnant and I will put her on our OB regimen starting
with monthly visits. Thank you for your kind referral.

Sincerely,

Mark King, MD

Mark King, MD

MK/nf

FIGURE 15-7 Sample consultation report.

Discharge Summaries

The **discharge summary (DS)** documents the patient's history of hospital admissions. The DS includes the reason for hospital admission, a description of what transpired while the patient was in the hospital, the final diagnosis, follow-up instructions, discharge medications, patient's condition at discharge, and prognosis for recovery. If the patient is transferred to another facility such as a skilled nursing facility, the report is changed from DS to transfer summary. If the patient has expired during the stay, the report is usually called a death summary. The Joint Commission requires that the completed DS be filed in the patient's chart within 48 to 72 hours of discharge from the hospital. Figure 15-8 shows a sample DS.

Autopsy Reports

An **autopsy report** may also be called an autopsy protocol, a necropsy report, or a medical examiner report. Autopsies are performed to determine the cause of death or to ascertain and confirm presence of disease. It is important to understand that state law requires that autopsies be performed in certain situations. For example, an autopsy report is required when someone dies suddenly, when someone dies while unattended, or in the case of suspicion of crime.

When transcribing an autopsy report, more words should be spelled out and abbreviation use kept to a minimum because these records may be entered into a court of law and must be accurate and clearly understood. Many states require that military time be used when documenting the time a body arrives at the coroner's office. Temporary anatomic diagnoses should be placed in the medical report within 72 hours and in the completed report within 60 days. Figure 15-9 shows a sample autopsy report.

Correspondence

It is important for the MT to remember that all forms of medical correspondence also are considered medical documents and must be transcribed with the same care as any other medical

---

PATIENT: Kelly Cohen
CHART #: 29324

ADMITTED: 9/26/XX
DISCHARGED: 11/19/XX

HISTORY/LAB: This infant was born on 09/26/XX to a 30-year-old, gravida II, para 1 female, with a last menstrual period of 3/22/XX estimated date of confinement 2/29/XX. The mother had been observed regularly during her pregnancy. However, she did develop preterm labor necessitating early hospitalization. At that time, the mother was placed on antibiotics and dexamethasone and delivered at approximately 26 weeks' gestation. At the time of delivery, the membranes ruptured spontaneously and fluid was clear. The infant had an Apgar score of 5 and 8 at 1 and 5 minutes, respectively. The infant required intubation in the delivery room and was then transferred to the NICU. On admission, weight was 1,159 grams, length 38.5 cm, head circumference 25.5 cm, chest circumference 26 cm. Assessment was 26 weeks' gestation.

COURSE/CONDITION ON DISCHARGE/DISPOSITION: At the time of admission the infant had respiratory distress, was intubated, and required Survanta. The infant was placed on IV fluid and antibiotics, and appropriate blood work was done. During the hospitalization, the infant improved with regard to the respiratory distress. However, the infant developed bronchopulmonary dysplasia, hyperbilirubinemia, and apnea of prematurity. The infant was placed on the appropriate medications and improved steadily. Her weight increased gradually. During the hospitalization, the infant was evaluated by Dr. Lally of Ophthalmology who will follow up on an outpatient basis.

The infant was discharged home on 11/20/XX. She had a hearing test, eye examination as stated, and was going to receive home physical therapy three times a week. She was on Fer In Sol drops and was feeding on Neosure and breast milk. The overall prognosis was guarded to good.

FINAL DIAGNOSIS: Preterm, 26-week female infant, appropriate for gestational age, apnea of prematurity, anemia, respiratory distress syndrome, bronchopulmonary dysplasia, hyperbilirubinemia, and presumed sepsis.

Electronically signed by Amy M. Cox, MD 09/27/20XX   8:15 AM

AMC/nf

d: 11/20/XX
t: 11/20/XX

FIGURE 15-8 Sample discharge summary report.

AUTOPSY REPORT

Patient Name:	George Matthews
Hospital No.:	11509
Necropsy No.:	98-A-19
Admitting Physician:	Joe Abbott, M.C.
Pathologist:	Loraine Muir, M.D.
Date of Death:	04/05/20XX, 9 PM
Date of Autopsy:	04/06/20XX, 8 AM
Admitting Diagnosis:	Adenocarcinoma, maxilla.
Prosector:	Keith Johnson, P.A.

FINAL ANATOMIC DIAGNOSIS

1. Old fibrotic myocardial infarction of the anterior and septal walls of the left ventricle with anterior ventricular aneurysm, 4.5 × 3.0 cm.
2. Patchy old fibrotic myocardial infarction of the lateral and posterior septal walls of the left ventricle.
3. Probable recent ischemic changes, especially of the anterior and septal walls of the left ventricle.
4. Severe calcified atherosclerotic coronary vascular disease with up to 95% stenosis of the right coronary artery (RCA), up to 70% stenosis of the left anterior descending (LAD) coronary artery, and greater than 95% stenosis of the left circumflex coronary artery (LCCA).
5. Bilateral arterionephrosclerosis.
6. Atherosclerotic vascular disease, aorta, moderate to severe; circle of Willis, moderate.
7. Old infarct of right inner and inferior occipital lobe; small lacunar infarct, right caudate nucleus.
8. Bilateral pulmonary congestion, moderate.
9. Chronic passive congestion, liver, mild.
10. Simple cysts, right and left kidneys, up to 5.5 cm.
11. Diverticulum, 2.5 cm, duodenum.
12. Diverticulosis, sigmoid colon.
13. Status post partial left maxillectomy for adenocarcinoma, recent.

Electronically signed by Elizabeth M. Jones, MD 04/26/20XX   6:17 PM

EMJ:xx

D:04/26/XX
T:04/26/XX

FIGURE 15-9 Sample autopsy report.

report would. Review Chapter 14 for information regarding various styles and formats for business correspondence. Figure 15-10 shows a sample of medical correspondence.

TURNAROUND TIME AND PRODUCTIVITY

Specific time limits are often established for completion of medical reports. **Turnaround time (TAT)** indicates the specific time period in which a document is expected to be completed from the time it is received by the transcriptionist until it is returned to the provider to sign and made a part of the permanent medical record.

Turnaround times for hospital reports fall into three categories:

1. *STAT reports.* Should be completed within 2 to 4 hours.

2. *Current reports.* Should be completed within 24 hours or less.

3. *Old reports or aged reports.* DS reports are an example, except when the patient is being transferred to another facility. Old reports should be completed within 48 to 72 hours or less.

4. *When requesting copies of a medical record* the usual TAT is 7 to 10 business days.

Different facilities have different requirements; however, the transcriptionist or clinic personnel responsible for medical records should be aware that failure to meet deadlines could result in disciplinary or legal action. The reason for this stringent adherence to turnaround time is that STAT and current reports can influence timely treatment of the patient.

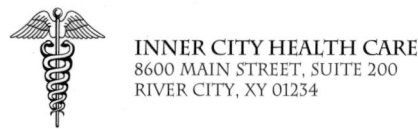

INNER CITY HEALTH CARE
8600 MAIN STREET, SUITE 200
RIVER CITY, XY 01234

January 4, 20XX

Susan Smith, Coordinator
Special Project Division
American Drug Company
90058 Northover Road
Welfond, PA 44578

Dear Ms. Smith:

It is my understanding that your department oversees the Aid for
Patients program, which provides Glucogenasin for indigent patients.
I am interested in learning more about this.

I have a 74-year-old female patient who would be greatly helped by this
medication. She suffers with hypertension, adult onset diabetes mellitus,
and moderate angina. Medication compliance has been a problem; however,
we feel that this new drug, with its q.d. dosage, will be easy for her
to deal with.

Any information you could forward would be appreciated.

Yours truly,

Winston Lewis, MD

Winston Lewis, MD

WL/tm

FIGURE 15-10 Sample medical correspondence.

Workload, as well as productivity of the transcriptionist, affects turnaround time. When workload is too great to meet turnaround times, the medical records administrator must be notified immediately. Once a job has been accepted, the transcriptionist or transcription service is legally bound to meet the schedule short of a major catastrophe of the type legally considered to be an "act of nature."

MEDICAL TRANSCRIPTION AS A CAREER

The medical transcription career has changed significantly in the United States. The career continues to evolve with the introduction of new technology and outsourcing. Most healthcare providers use either digital or analog dictating equipment to transmit dictation to medical transcriptionists. The Internet has grown to be a popular mode for transmitting documentation and allows for faster turnaround time. Speech recognition technology electronically translates sound into text and creates drafts of reports. The MT serve as QA managers, oversee risk management, and function as editors or auditors of medical documents. Medical transcriptionists are invisible, and yet invaluable, members of the patient care team.

MTs serving as editors enjoy detective work and are curious; if terminology is new to them, they use references to research and learn more. MTs must be self-disciplined, detail oriented, and independent, and usually they are perfectionists. They are dedicated to professional development and enthusiastically committed to learning. MTs possess integrity and understand the importance and legal implications of medical confidentiality.

Professionalism Related to Medical Transcription

Professional

Professionalism as related to medical transcription has many requirements. Following is advice on how to maintain a professional attitude.

- *Display a professional manner and image.* Working as an MT requires good hygiene practices and dress attire appropriate to the surroundings. The MT should always respect others and use good communication skills.

- *Demonstrate initiative and responsibility.* Demonstrating initiative means being to work early enough to organize and begin the workday at the appointed time. All deadlines must be met or changes approved.

- *Work as a member of the health care team.* The MT is a member of the health care team and as such must sign a business associate agreement and a confidentiality agreement. The MT should report incidents of confidentiality discrepancies and any perceived medical procedural errors to appropriate risk management personnel.

- *Prioritize and perform multiple tasks.* The MT must prioritize the documents to be edited to satisfy turnaround time and maintain productivity standards.

- *Adapt to change.* The MT must be flexible and willing to change. Technological advances require being open to new ways of handling medical documents. The MT's role and job description are changing to meet today's new demands.

- *Enhance skills through continuing education.* New technology, breakthroughs in medicine, and new medications are recognized daily as researchers explore ways in which to treat disease and increase longevity. The MT must remain current with new medical developments to maintain professionalism.

A qualified MT, described as one with a minimum of 2 years' experience in performing medical transcription in a variety of medical and surgical specialties, may wish to become a **certified medical transcriptionist (CMT)**, through a voluntary examination from the AHDI. Recent graduates, or MTs with less than 2 years' experience, may apply to become **registered medical transcriptionists (RMT)**. For additional information regarding AHDI credentialing, visit AHDI's Web site at: http://www.ahdionline.org.

Procedure

Transcribing Medical Referral Letters

PURPOSE:

To transcribe (type) medical referral letters using word processing software based on physician dictation.

EQUIPMENT/SUPPLIES:

- Computer and word processing software
- Source documents

PROCEDURE STEPS:

1. After setting up the transcription equipment and inserting the tape, open the word processing software.
2. Using the general formats for each document type, prepare and transcribe (type) the physician's dictation as shown on the source document. Use proper punctuation and grammar.
3. When complete, save the document.
4. Print the letter so the physician may sign it and turn in a copy to your instructor. Prepare a mailing envelope(s).
5. Close the word processor when done.

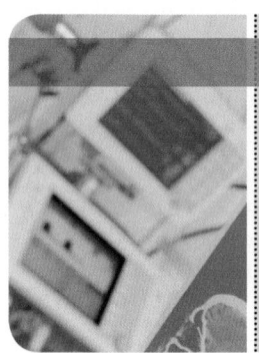

CASE STUDY 15-1

Refer to the scenario at the beginning of the chapter.

CASE STUDY REVIEW

1. List important issues Marilyn will want to consider before outsourcing medical transcription.
2. Using your favorite search engine, research outsourcing as well as VRS options. Write a summary of your findings and state your rationale for supporting either outsourcing, VRS, or keeping the transcription in-house.

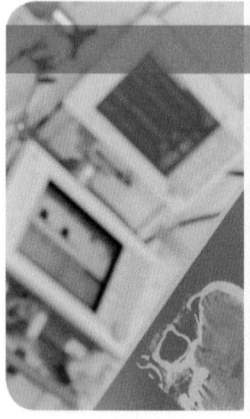

CASE STUDY 15-2

At Inner City Health Care, the MT has just transcribed the following content in a document: "This patient developed a persistent lesion on the inner aspect of the left upper lip. This lesion was at the junction of the vermilion and mucous membrane. A punch biopsy was obtained of this 1-cm lesion and was read as a probable verrucous squamous cell carcinoma of the lower lip."

CASE STUDY REVIEW

1. What inconsistencies, if any, do you find within this content?
2. What should the MT do to verify inconsistencies and inaccuracies?
3. How should these inconsistencies and inaccuracies be corrected?

Summary

- Medical documentation is a vital part of patient health care; without it, it is impossible to provide quality health care, to bill insurance carriers properly to ensure providers are reimbursed for services rendered, and to support and protect the provider should records be subpoenaed.

- The medical transcriptionist must keep all patient information strictly confidential and may be asked to sign a confidentiality agreement.

- Medical transcriptionists will continue to be medical language specialists, and are increasingly becoming editors as the use of voice recognition software becomes more prevalent.

- The medical assistant must understand the methods of accurately and confidentially converting paper records into digital documents in the EMR by scanning and then selecting the most useful information for use by the providers and staff.

- Medical document types include chart notes and progress notes, history and physical examination reports, radiology reports, operative reports, pathology reports, consultations, discharge summaries, autopsy reports, and correspondence.

- Proper formatting must be used for each medical document.

- Medical transcriptionists must have basic skills in transcribing or editing frequently used documents in a clinic.

Study for Success

To reinforce your knowledge and skills of information presented in this chapter:

- Review the *Key Terms* and *Learning Outcomes*
- Consider the *Critical Thinking* features and *Case Studies* and discuss your conclusions
- Answer the questions in the *Certification Review*

Procedure

- Perform the *Procedure* using the *Competency Assessment Checklists* on the *Student Companion Website*

CERTIFICATION REVIEW

1. What three factors influence the changing role of medical transcription?
   a. Cost
   b. Changing economy
   c. New technology
   d. All of these
2. What are examples of new technology used in medical transcription?
   a. EHR
   b. Outsourcing
   c. VRS
   d. Authentication
   e. All of these
3. Why does a medical transcriptionist place a flag within a medical document?
   a. The dictator made a mistake.
   b. The dictator could not be understood.
   c. The transcriptionist made an error.
   d. None of these.

4. What is the definition of authentication?
   a. Use of an electronic signature
   b. The information was accurate and complete at the time of dictation and as transcribed, and has been signed and dated by the dictating provider
   c. Use of a biometric system
   d. Use of an alphanumeric computer key entry as identification
   e. The typing was done by a medical transcriptionist
5. What would the medical transcriptionist do when there is a question that cannot be resolved?
   a. Guess at what is being dictated
   b. Edit the document and exclude what cannot be understood
   c. Flag the document
   d. Refuse to transcribe documents for that provider

6. What is the turnaround time for most STAT reports?
   a. Same as aged reports
   b. Current
   c. Within 2–4 hours
   d. Within 24 hours
   e. Both a and b
7. What is the definition of an H&P report?
   a. It is divided into a history section and the ROS section.
   b. It is sometimes referred to as a progress note.
   c. It describes gross and microscopic examinations.
   d. It documents the patient's history of hospital admission.
8. Which of the following is true of autopsy reports?
   a. They are also called narcolepsy reports.
   b. They determine cause of death, ascertain and confirm presence of disease.
   c. They should be brief and contain many abbreviations.
   d. They are always required to use military time.
   e. Temporary diagnoses should be placed within 24 hours.
9. In what time frame should chart notes be filed?
   a. 12 hours
   b. 24 hours
   c. 4–8 hours
   d. 48–72 hours
10. Which of the following statements is true regarding the CMT?
   a. It is a requirement.
   b. It is voluntary.
   c. It requires a minimum of 2 years' experience in a variety of specialties.
   d. Both b and c are correct.
   e. None of these

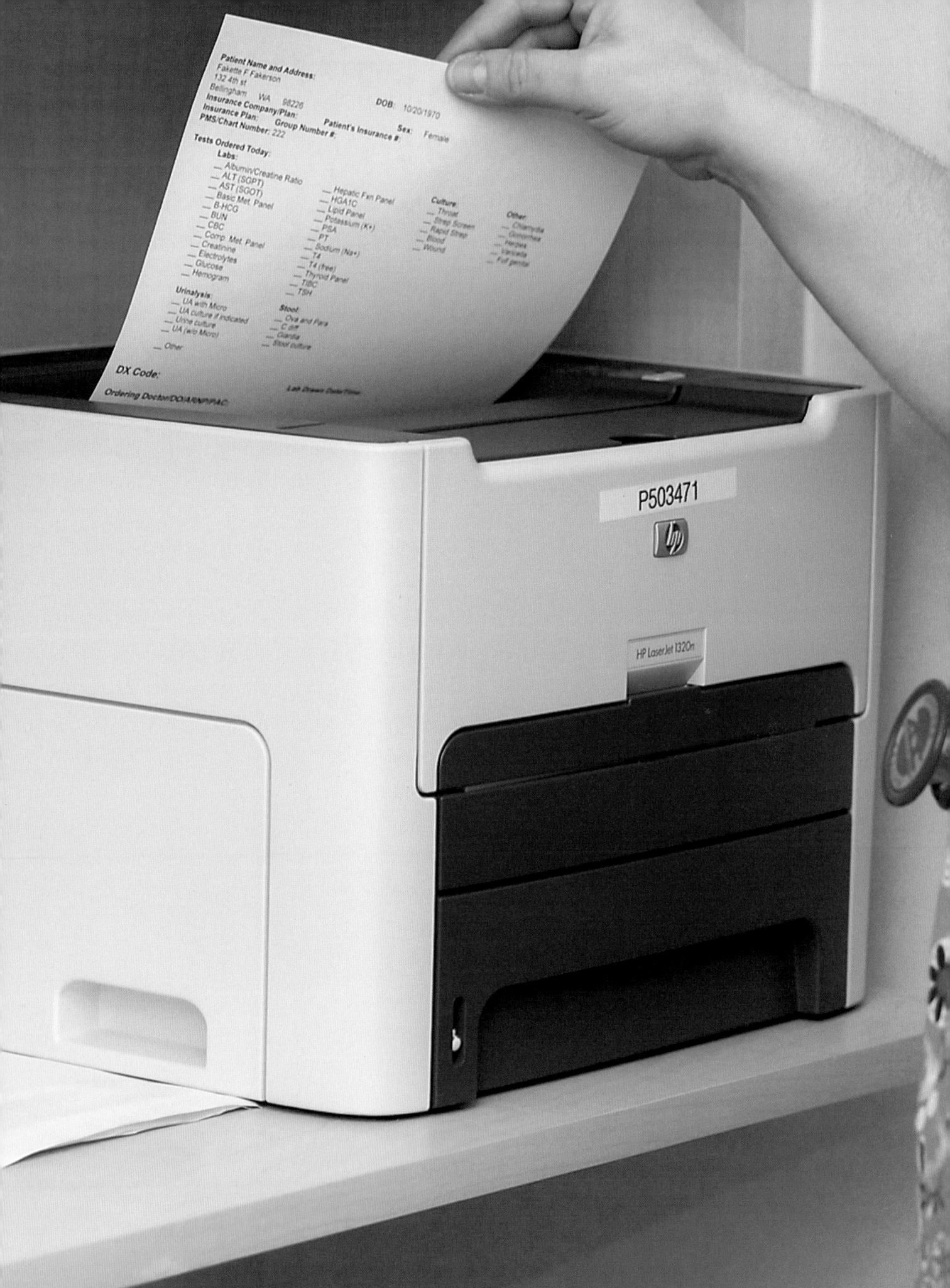

Patient Name and Address:
Fakette F Fakerson
132 4th st
Bellingham   WA   98226   DOB: 10/20/1970
Insurance Company/Plan: **Sex:**   Female
Insurance Plan: **Group Number #:**   **Patient's Insurance #:**
PMS/Chart Number: 222

Tests Ordered Today:
Labs:
— Albumin/Creatine Ratio
— ALT (SGPT)
— AST (SGOT)   — Hepatic Fxn Panel   **Culture:**   **Other:**
— Basic Met. Panel   — HGA1C   — Throat   — Chlamydia
— B-HCG   — Lipid Panel   — Strep Screen   — Gonorrhea
— BUN   — Potassium (K+)   — Rapid Strep   — Herpes
— CBC   — PSA   — Blood   — Varicella
— Comp. Met. Panel   — PT   — Wound   — Fxf genita
— Creatinine   — Sodium (Na+)
— Electrolytes   — T4
— Glucose   — T4 (free)
— Hemogram   — Thyroid Panel
                      — TIBC
Urinalysis: — TSH
— UA with Micro
— UA culture if indicated   **Stool:**
— Urine culture   — Ova and Para
— UA (w/o Micro)   — C diff
                      — Giardia
— Other   — Stool culture

DX Code: Lab Drawn Date/Time:

Ordering Doctor/DO/ARNP/PaC:

P503471

HP LaserJet 1320n

UNIT V
MANAGING FACILITY FINANCES

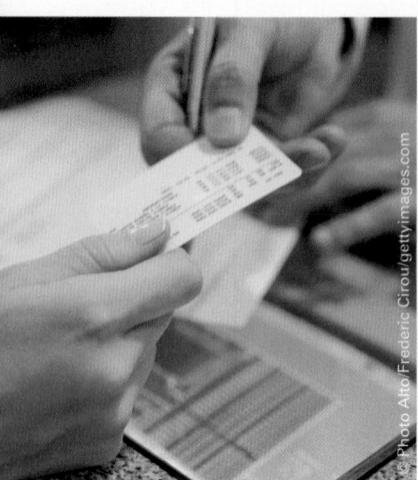
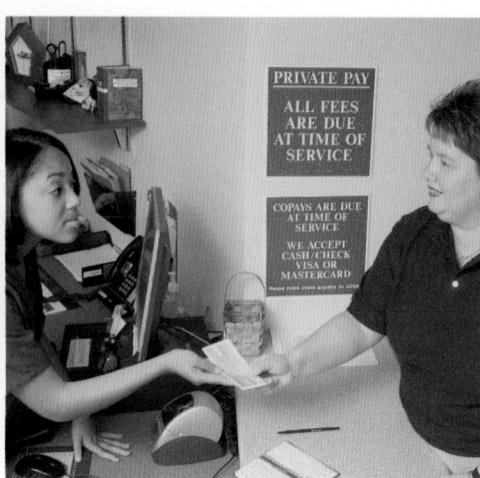
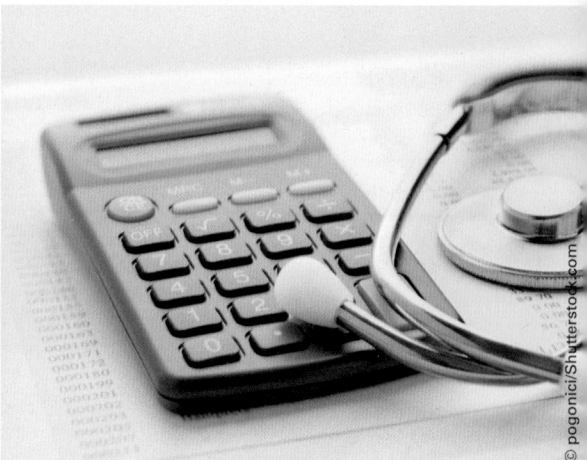

ATTRIBUTES OF PROFESSIONALISM

The administrative medical assistant often handles medical insurance billing and bookkeeping, especially when recording transactions from both patients and insurance plans. The medical assistant must be comfortable with handling money and following up for collections when necessary. Each patient must be respected, and not be stereotyped due to their type of insurance coverage, lack of coverage, or ability to pay.

It is not unusual for medical services to be provided at a discount, through negotiated contracts with insurance plans, courtesy adjustments for patients that need them, and other situations where collecting the full fee for service is not possible. The medical assistant must navigate patient questions regarding their insurance and accounts while maintaining a positive, professional, and respectful attitude. This promotes dignity for the patient and an atmosphere conducive to healing, which allows the patient to feel comfortable returning for follow-up care and health maintenance.

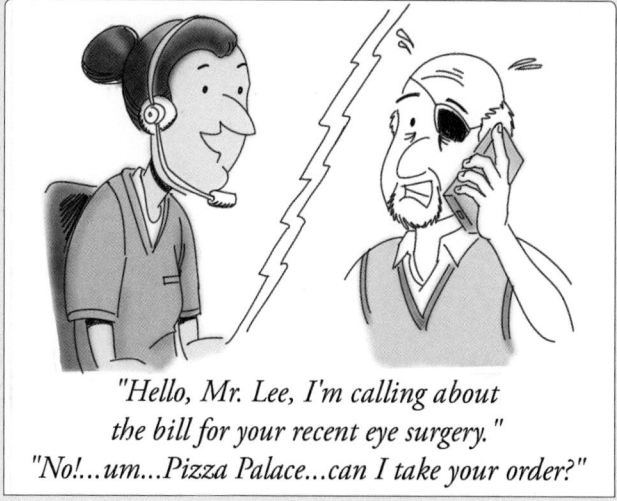

"Hello, Mr. Lee, I'm calling about the bill for your recent eye surgery."
"No!...um...Pizza Palace...can I take your order?"

Listed below are a series of questions for you to ask yourself, to serve as a professionalism checklist. As you interact with patients and colleagues, these questions will help to guide you in the professional behavior that is expected every day from medical assistants.

Ask Yourself

COMMUNICATION
- ☐ Do I display professionalism through written and verbal communication?
- ☐ Do I speak at each patient's level of understanding?
- ☐ Do I display appropriate body language?
- ☐ Do I respond honestly and diplomatically to my patients' concerns?
- ☐ Do I show sensitivity when communicating with patients regarding third party requirements?
- ☐ Does my knowledge allow me to speak easily with all members of the health care team?
- ☐ Do I utilize tactful communication skills with medical providers to ensure accurate code selection?

PRESENTATION
- ☐ Am I courteous, patient, and respectful to patients?
- ☐ Do I display a positive attitude?
- ☐ Do I display a calm, professional, and caring manner?
- ☐ Do I demonstrate empathy to the patient?
- ☐ Do I display sensitivity when managing appointments?

COMPETENCY
- ☐ Do I pay attention to detail?
- ☐ Do I ask questions if I am out of my comfort zone or do not have the experience to carry out tasks?

- ☐ Do I display sound judgment?
- ☐ Am I knowledgeable and accountable?
- ☐ Do I demonstrate professionalism when discussing the patient's billing record?
- ☐ Do I display sensitivity when requesting payment for services rendered?
- ☐ Do I interact professionally with third party representatives?

INITIATIVE
- ☐ Do I show initiative?
- ☐ Am I flexible and dependable?
- ☐ Do I direct the patient to other resources when necessary or helpful, with the approval of the provider?
- ☐ Do I implement time management principles to maintain effective office function?
- ☐ Do I assist co-workers when appropriate?

INTEGRITY
- ☐ Do I work within my scope of practice?
- ☐ Do I demonstrate sensitivity to patient rights?
- ☐ Do I protect the integrity of the medical record?
- ☐ Do I protect and maintain confidentiality?
- ☐ Do I immediately report any error I made?
- ☐ Do I do the "right thing" even when no one is observing?

Medical
Insurance

1. Define and spell the key terms as presented in the glossary.
2. Define the terminology necessary to understand and submit medical insurance claims.
3. List at least five examples of medical insurance coverage and discuss their differences.
4. Identify models of managed care.
5. Screen patients for insurance, verifying eligibility for managed care services.
6. Obtain managed care referrals, precertification, and preauthorization, including documentation.
7. Discuss workers' compensation as it applies to patients.
8. Discuss types of provider fee schedules.
9. Define diagnosis-related groups.
10. Discuss legal and ethical issues related to medical insurance and the provider's office.
11. Explore career opportunities in the insurance profession.
12. Describe procedures for implementing managed care and insurance plans.

KEY TERMS

abuse

adjustment

assignment of benefits

beneficiary

benefit period

birthday rule

capitation

Centers for Medicare and Medicaid Services (CMS)

co-insurance

coordination of benefits (COB)

co-payment

crossover claim

deductible

Defense Enrollment Eligible Reporting System (DEERS)

diagnosis-related groups (DRGs)

donut hole

exclusion

exclusive provider organization (EPO)

explanation of benefits (EOB)

fraud

health maintenance organization (HMO)

HIC number (HICN)

hospital outpatient prospective payment system (OPPS)

independent provider association (IPA)

integrated delivery system (IDS)

limiting charge

major medical insurance

managed care organization (MCO)

Medicare Part A

Medicare Part B

Medicare Part C

Medicare Part D

Medigap policy

personal injury protection (PIP)

point-of-service (POS) plan

preauthorization

preferred provider organization (PPO)

primary care provider (PCP)

referral

remittance advice (remit, RA)

resource-based relative value scale (RBRVS)

Self funded health care

subscriber

traditional indemnity insurance (FFS)

TRICARE

triple option plan

usual, customary, and reasonable (UCR)

Workers' Compensation insurance

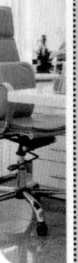

At Inner City Health Care, a multi provider clinic in a large city, medical assistant Ellen Armstrong, CMAS (AMT), is responsible for all patient billing procedures. Inner City participates in a number of insurance plans, so Ellen must stay abreast of policy changes regarding reimbursement, preauthorizations, and claims filing. She also tries to become acquainted with the conditions of each patient's insurance coverage and helps patients understand their responsibility, if any, for payment. Finally, Ellen holds periodic meetings with her assistants to update them; she continually stresses to them the importance of timeliness in filing claims and the need for absolute accuracy in diagnosis and procedure codes, which must always reflect services actually performed.

A n understanding of medical insurance and proper coding techniques is absolutely critical to the survival of the medical clinic. In recent years, much has changed in medical insurance coverage: more patients are choosing health maintenance organizations (HMOs) and other managed care options, and even traditional insurance carriers such as Blue Cross and Blue Shield are modifying their insurance plans to include some aspect of managed benefits.

In some ways, managed care coverage has simplified the patient's responsibility for payment, but it is more important than ever for the medical assistant to be accurate, timely, and conscientious in both filing insurance claim forms and understanding—and helping the patient to understand—the conditions of individual insurance policies.

The increasing complexity of health insurance today means that medical assistants must continually update their base of information. This chapter provides the groundwork for understanding the role of insurance, its terminology, and its various forms, and it gives the medical assistant the confidence to take responsibility for claim filing in the ambulatory care setting.

UNDERSTANDING THE ROLE OF HEALTH INSURANCE

Health insurance was designed to help individuals and families compensate for the high costs of medical care. Medical care consists of the diagnosis of diseases/disorders and the care and treatment provided by the health care team of professionals to individuals who are ill or injured. Medical care, which also includes preventive services, is designed to help individuals avoid health or injury problems and is termed *health care*.

Health care insurance is a contract between an individual policyholder and a third-party or government program that reimburses the medical provider or the policyholder for medically necessary treatment or preventive care covered by that specific health care provider.

There is much discussion today about changes in the health care insurance industry. Foremost is the goal that health care insurance should be available to all citizens of the United States. In the past, health insurance was usually tied to the employment package that covers the employee,

and possibly the spouse and dependent children. One problem with work-related coverage is that some part-time employees are not eligible for health insurance and thus often go uninsured. Another problem is if an employee takes a position elsewhere, medical benefits may not transfer equally. If a family member is ill with a preexisting condition such as cancer or diabetes mellitus, the new insurance policy may not cover that disease or condition for a fixed time period. This time-dependent limitation of coverage is known as an **exclusion**. If health insurance has previously been in effect for at least 18 months and any lapse in coverage between policies did not exceed 63 days, a preexisting condition cannot be given as a reason for exclusion. Some states have laws limiting the length of an exclusion period; otherwise it is at the discretion of the carrier. An exclusion also may include illnesses or conditions for injury specifically not covered by the policy.

The Patient Protection and Affordable Care Act (PPACA), signed into law by President Barack Obama in 2010, is intended to help resolve many of these concerns. The Act requires that all individuals who do not already have medical insurance coverage through a group plan with their employer or coverage through Medicare or Medicaid to purchase health coverage. There are many parts to the PPACA, which all together will be making many changes to our health insurance industry over the next 10 years. For example, as of January 2014, insurance companies were longer permitted to charge policyholders a preexisting condition a higher premium. It is also stated in the PPACA that by 2018, insurance plans are not to charge a co-payment if the office visit is for preventive medicine, such as well-women and well-child visits.

Another controversial aspect of health insurance is refusal to provide coverage for certain procedures because they have not been sufficiently proved to be effective. Although more insurance companies are beginning to cover procedures such as in vitro fertilization, there remain many other plans that do not agree. Because most insurance carriers will not extend coverage to experimental treatment, family and friends of patients often gather for fund-raising drives to ensure that medical costs are covered.

Not all insurance carriers cover the same exposures equally, and few carriers pay at the same rate. Similarly, carriers do not charge the same premiums to policyholders. Some insurance companies cover individuals, families, or employee groups through work or through groups such as the American Association of Retired Persons (AARP). Some premiums reflect the insured person's past medical history and the company's exposure in covering the person. Premiums may be less if the insured person selects a higher annual deductible. Other premiums represent the rate that a group is able to obtain based on the group's claim history.

MEDICAL INSURANCE TERMINOLOGY

Before discussing the types of insurance coverage, one must understand the language used by the insurance industry. The terminology is specific in meaning and has been tested in courts of law to further define its meanings.

Terminology Specific to Insurance Policies

A policy is an agreement between an insurance company or government program and the insured, or **beneficiary,** that is, the person covered under the terms of the policy. The insured may also be referred to as the **subscriber.** The insured person may include as beneficiaries a spouse and dependent minor children; others may be included if related by blood and dependent on the insured for more than 50% of their support. The insurance carrier pays a percentage (**co-insurance**) of the cost of the services covered under the policy in exchange for a monthly premium or charge. This premium is paid by the insured or the employer, or it is shared by both.

At the inception or beginning of the policy, the insured is given an identification card, which must be presented before receiving medical treatment. This card contains the insured person's name, identification number, group number, and any co-payment amount or restrictions for treatment. The back of the insurance card contains an address where claims should be submitted and telephone numbers needed to receive prior authorization for treatment when required.

Deductible. The language of the policy spells out the terms of the coverage. Usually there is an annual **deductible**, or an amount of money that the insured must pay out-of-pocket for medical services before the policy begins to pay. This deductible can range from $100 to $5,000, or an even greater amount, depending on the language of the policy. The deductible must be met each calendar year by medical charges that are incurred after the inception or anniversary date of the policy, usually at the beginning of each year.

For instance, if Boris Bolski went to the provider on January 22 and incurred $258 in charges but his policy did not go into effect until February 1, none of these charges would apply toward his deductible. If, however, he returned to the doctor on February 3 and incurred another $85 charge, that amount could be applied against his deductible.

Co-insurance. After application of the deductible to the submitted bills, the insurance policy pays a percentage of the remaining amount. This percentage or co-insurance can vary from 50% to 100% depending on the language in a specific policy. Most traditional plans pay 70% to 80%.

Co-payment. Some insurance policies, especially **health maintenance organizations (HMOs)** and other managed care policies, require the patient to make a payment of a specified amount, for instance, $20 or $50, at the time of treatment. This payment must be collected at the time of the office visit. Some policies have both a **co-payment** and a co-insurance clause. In addition, co-payment amounts may differ between a primary physician and a specialist. For example, the co-payment to the primary physician may be only $20 per office visit. However, when a patient visits a specialist, the co-payment may increase to $35. Co-payments may also be applied in the emergency room (ER) setting. Often, the ER co-payment is waived if the patient is admitted to the hospital. The co-payment may be possibly waived in other situations, such as when a patient is coming in for a follow-up visit after surgery for suture removal.

Preexisting Condition. Under the Affordable Care Act, health insurance companies cannot refuse to offer coverage or charge higher premiums because of a pre-existing condition. A pre-existing condition is a diagnosis the patient had before the date new health coverage begins. In addition, premiums cannot be higher based on gender. These rules went into effect for plans beginning on or after January 1, 2014.

The only exception to this rule is for any "grandfathered" individual health insurance plan that was purchased on or before March 23, 2010 that was not changed to reduce benefits or increase costs to the policyholder. If a patient has a grandfathered plan, they may not have some of the rights and protections other plans offer under the Affordable Care Act. The insurer must notify the patient if they have a grandfathered plan.

If a patient has a grandfathered plan, they may opt to switch to a plan that offers protections under the ACA during the annual open enrollment period. If the plan ends at any time during the year, a patient may switch at that time and purchase a plan outside of the open enrollment period.

As a medical assistant that works with insurance in the clinic, it is important to be aware of the protections that do not apply to grandfathered plans. These include coverage of preventative care, guarantee to appeal coverage decisions, protection of choice of doctors and access to emergency care, yearly limits on coverage, and coverage of a pre-existing condition. Protections that apply to all plans, including grandfathered individual plans do include no lifetime limits on coverage, and coverage for adult children up to age 26. As with any insurance plan, eligibility should be verified and plan details obtained as applicable to the clinic before services are rendered to the patient. In this manner, any non-covered services or out of pocket expenses can be discussed with the patient ahead of time.

Exclusions. Exclusions are noncovered services and are an important part of a policy. Some policies exclude services that are not medically necessary, such as cosmetic surgery, whereas other policies may allow these procedures with certain criteria that makes them medically necessary. An example might be repair of a deviated septum of the nose, due to frequent infections, snoring, and breathing problems. Other examples of exclusions or noncovered services might be preexisting conditions, dental services, chiropractic services, or routine eye examinations. Not every policy has the same exclusions.

Coordination of Benefits. Most health insurance policies have a clause that coordinates the benefits of one policy with those of another when a patient has dual coverage. Dual coverage, or having more than one policy, will put into effect this clause, named **coordination of benefits (COB)**.

Coordination of benefits rules follow a set of guidelines as put forth by the National Association of Health Insurance Commissioners (NAIC). The purpose of these guidelines is to avoid duplicate payment for medical services when there are two policies.

It is important to understand that COB is further determined by type of plan, whether the covered person is the insured or a dependent on the plan, and if there is Medicare and/or Medicaid, the rules are different.

Insurance carriers will use the following general guidelines:

- Group plans are those provided by an employer or other entity that are primary for the insured or subscriber. Group plans that do not have a COB clause will always be primary.

- Individual insurance, or those policies that are purchased by the insured and are not through an employer, normally pay benefits without regard to group policies. These policies might provide their own guidelines for dual insurance, and each needs to be verified.

- When dependent children have dual coverage (one policy per parent), determining the primary is done using the **birthday rule**. The plan of the parent whose birthday falls earliest in the year is the primary policy. Thus, if the father's birthday is October 17 and the mother's birthday is May 12, the mother's policy is primary. The year of the birth date is not relevant. If the parents have the same birthday, the policy in effect the longest is primary. For children of divorced parents who are covered under both parents' policies, the policy of the custodial parent usually is primary.

- Medicare and Medicaid have different guidelines which can be affected by the beneficiary being employed or retired, the size of the employer, and if the insured has certain diseases. These include end-stage renal disease and amyotrophic lateral sclerosis (ALS).

Whichever insurance is primary pays for covered services up to the maximum allowed under the plan, less the deductible and co-payment. The secondary insurance will coordinate the benefits and pay as appropriate, but the amount is never to exceed the total amount of the services. If the secondary insurance offers a COB, it will only consider the percentage paid as if it were primary.

Explanation of Benefits. The insurance carrier generates an **explanation of benefits (EOB)**, which is mailed to each patient (or may be obtained online). The EOB is a statement summarizing how the insurance carrier determined the reimbursement for services received by the patient. The backside of the EOB addresses questions frequently asked and defines the terms used within the EOB. The EOB is not to be considered a bill; it simply details information as to how the claim was processed by the insurance carrier. Figure 16-1 shows an example of an EOB.

Remittance Advice. The provider's office receives a **remittance advice** (**remit**, or **RA**) from the insurance carrier. The provider's RA summarizes all of the benefits paid to the provider within a particular period of time. The RA includes all of the patients covered by a specific insurance for that time period. The difference between the provider's charges and the amount paid by the insurance carrier may be billed to the patient. Figure 16-2 shows an example of a remittance advice.

Terminology Specific to Billing Insurance Carriers

There is specific terminology that one must understand when submitting insurance claims for medical benefits. Most clinics bill all appropriate insurance carriers to ascertain that the claim is made and the provider receives payment.

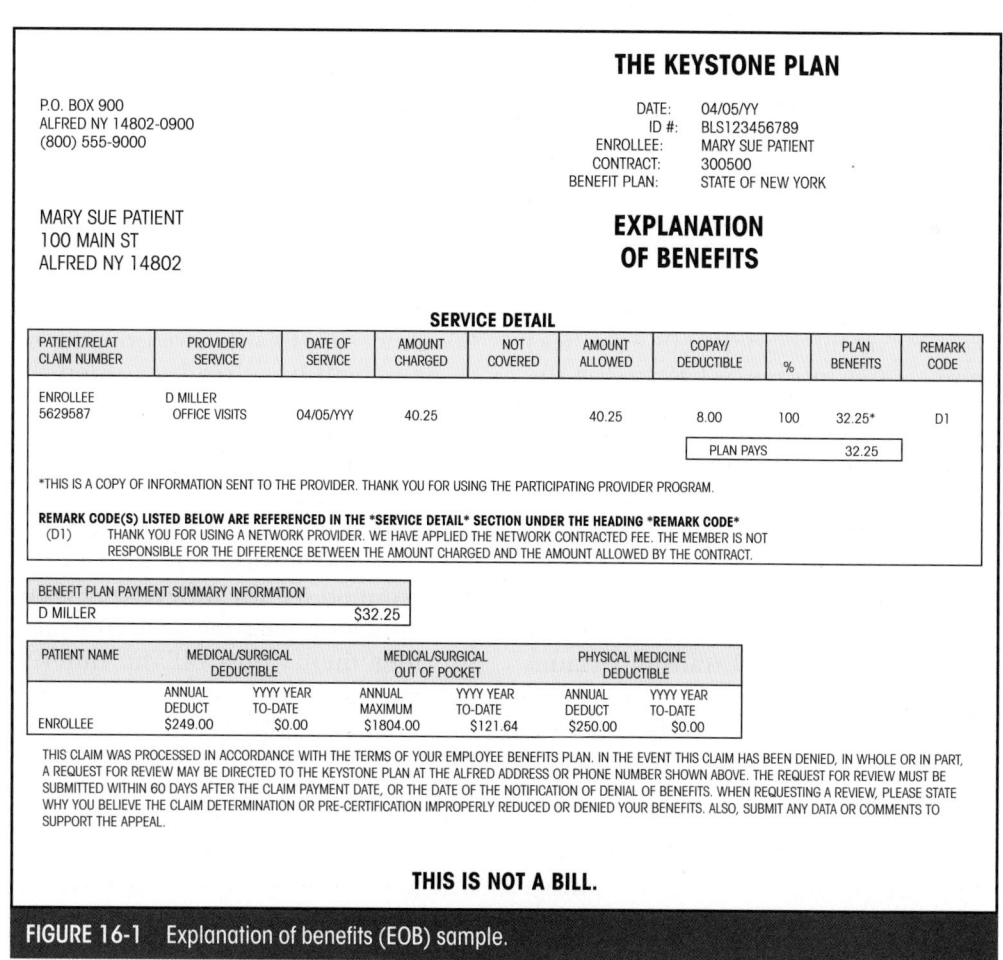

FIGURE 16-1 Explanation of benefits (EOB) sample.

ABC INSURANCE COMPANY
100 MAIN STREET
ALFRED NY 14802
1-800-555-1234

REMITTANCE ADVICE

DAVID MILLER, M.D.
101 NORTH STREET

ALFRED, NY 14802

PROVIDER #: 123456
PAGE #: 1 OF 1
DATE: 04/05/YY
CHECK/EFT #: 000235698

PERF PROV SERV DATE POS NOS PROC MODS BILLED ALLOWED DEDUCT COINS GRP/RC AMT PROV PD

NAME BAKER, JENNY HIC 235962541 ACNT BAKE1234567-01 ICN 1235626589651 ASG Y MOA MA01
236592ABC 0405 0405YY 11 1 99213 75.00 50.00 0.25 0.00 CO-42 15.00 50.00
PT RESP 10.31 CLAIM TOTALS 75.00 50.00 0.25 0.00 15.00

NET 50.00

TOTALS	# OF CLAIMS	BILLED AMT	ALLOWED AMT	DEDUCT AMT	COINS RC AMT	TOTAL AMT	PROV PD ADJ AMT	PROV AMT	CHECK AMT
	1	75.00	50.00	0.25	15.00	65.25	50.00	0.00	50.00

FIGURE 16-2 Remittance advice (single claim) sample.

Many policies require **preauthorization** before certain procedures or before a visit can be made to a specialist or a physical therapist. In these cases, the medical assistant must contact the insurance carrier with all of the diagnosis information and the proposed course of treatment. For instance, if a patient has a diagnosis of cholecystitis, preauthorization requires notification and approval before referring that patient to a surgeon for possible cholecystectomy. If this is not done, the surgery may not be covered.

A claim occurs when patients, having received treatment, wish to receive reimbursement under their insurance policies for charges for treatment. The patient (or the center's billing office) sends the claim to the insurance carrier for the amount of the treatment. This is done via a claim form, the most common of which is the CMS-1500 (02-12) (Figure 16-3). When this page opens, scroll down the page and click on Downloads: Intermediary-Carrier Directory. A PDF file listing all Medicare regional carriers will open.

The completed claim form is sent to the insurance carrier by mail, electronically, or through a holding system that batches and transmits claims at timed daily intervals. The most common and expeditious method for submitting claims is electronically. Depending on the policy language and the **assignment of benefits**, payment is sent either directly to the provider (known as direct payment) or to the patient/insured but payable to both the insured and the provider (known as indirect payment).

TYPES OF MEDICAL INSURANCE COVERAGE

In today's health care environment, medical assistants need to be aware of the different types of medical insurance policies.

Traditional Indemnity Insurance

Traditional indemnity insurance provides coverage on a fee-for-service basis (FFS). There is usually a deductible and a co-payment or co-insurance amount. The health care provider submits bills to the insurance carrier, and after any deductible has been met, the health care provider or the patient, if the patient has already satisfied the bill, is paid in agreement with the terms of the insurance policy. The patient may be responsible for fees in excess of the contracted amount if the health care provider is not a preferred or participating provider. In the case of a preferred or participating provider, the health care provider has agreed to a discounted fee for different types of procedures performed on patients insured by the carrier. The provider then writes off the difference, and the patient is not responsible for that amount.

Traditional indemnity insurance is sometimes marketed as having two types of coverage, depending on the policy. *Basic insurance* covers specific dollar amounts for provider's fees, hospital care, surgery, and anesthesia. Generally, it will not cover examinations to diagnose or treat fertility problems, but more carriers are covering

HEALTH INSURANCE CLAIM FORM

APPROVED BY NATIONAL UNIFORM CLAIM COMMITTEE (NUCC) 02/12

	PICA							PICA	

CARRIER

1. MEDICARE (Medicare#)   MEDICAID (Medicaid#)   TRICARE (ID#/DoD#)   CHAMPVA (Member ID#)   GROUP HEALTH PLAN (ID#)   FECA BLK LUNG (ID#)   OTHER (ID#)
1a. INSURED'S I.D. NUMBER   (For Program in Item 1)

2. PATIENT'S NAME (Last Name, First Name, Middle Initial)
3. PATIENT'S BIRTH DATE   MM   DD   YY   SEX   M □   F □
4. INSURED'S NAME (Last Name, First Name, Middle Initial)

5. PATIENT'S ADDRESS (No., Street)
6. PATIENT RELATIONSHIP TO INSURED   Self □ Spouse □ Child □ Other □
7. INSURED'S ADDRESS (No., Street)

CITY   STATE
8. RESERVED FOR NUCC USE
CITY   STATE

ZIP CODE   TELEPHONE (Include Area Code) ( )

ZIP CODE   TELEPHONE (Include Area Code) ( )

9. OTHER INSURED'S NAME (Last Name, First Name, Middle Initial)
10. IS PATIENT'S CONDITION RELATED TO:
11. INSURED'S POLICY GROUP OR FECA NUMBER

a. OTHER INSURED'S POLICY OR GROUP NUMBER
a. EMPLOYMENT? (Current or Previous)   YES □   NO □
a. INSURED'S DATE OF BIRTH   MM   DD   YY   SEX   M □   F □

b. RESERVED FOR NUCC USE
b. AUTO ACCIDENT?   YES □   NO □   PLACE (State)
b. OTHER CLAIM ID (Designated by NUCC)

c. RESERVED FOR NUCC USE
c. OTHER ACCIDENT?   YES □   NO □
c. INSURANCE PLAN NAME OR PROGRAM NAME

d. INSURANCE PLAN NAME OR PROGRAM NAME
10d. CLAIM CODES (Designated by NUCC)
d. IS THERE ANOTHER HEALTH BENEFIT PLAN?   YES □   NO □   *If yes*, complete items 9, 9a, and 9d.

READ BACK OF FORM BEFORE COMPLETING & SIGNING THIS FORM.
12. PATIENT'S OR AUTHORIZED PERSON'S SIGNATURE I authorize the release of any medical or other information necessary to process this claim. I also request payment of government benefits either to myself or to the party who accepts assignment below.

SIGNED _____   DATE _____

13. INSURED'S OR AUTHORIZED PERSON'S SIGNATURE I authorize payment of medical benefits to the undersigned physician or supplier for services described below.

SIGNED _____

PATIENT AND INSURED INFORMATION

14. DATE OF CURRENT ILLNESS, INJURY, or PREGNANCY (LMP)   MM   DD   YY   QUAL.
15. OTHER DATE   QUAL.   MM   DD   YY
16. DATES PATIENT UNABLE TO WORK IN CURRENT OCCUPATION   FROM   MM   DD   YY   TO   MM   DD   YY

17. NAME OF REFERRING PROVIDER OR OTHER SOURCE
17a.
17b. NPI
18. HOSPITALIZATION DATES RELATED TO CURRENT SERVICES   FROM   MM   DD   YY   TO   MM   DD   YY

19. ADDITIONAL CLAIM INFORMATION (Designated by NUCC)
20. OUTSIDE LAB?   YES □   NO □ $ CHARGES

21. DIAGNOSIS OR NATURE OF ILLNESS OR INJURY Relate A-L to service line below (24E)   ICD Ind.
A. ____ B. ____ C. ____ D. ____
E. ____ F. ____ G. ____ H. ____
I. ____ J. ____ K. ____ L. ____
22. RESUBMISSION CODE   ORIGINAL REF. NO.
23. PRIOR AUTHORIZATION NUMBER

24. A. DATE(S) OF SERVICE						B. PLACE OF SERVICE	C. EMG	D. PROCEDURES, SERVICES, OR SUPPLIES (Explain Unusual Circumstances) CPT/HCPCS MODIFIER	E. DIAGNOSIS POINTER	F. $ CHARGES	G. DAYS OR UNITS	H. EPSDT Family Plan	I. ID. QUAL.	J. RENDERING PROVIDER ID. #
From MM	DD	YY	To MM	DD	YY									
1													NPI	
2													NPI	
3													NPI	
4													NPI	
5													NPI	
6													NPI	

25. FEDERAL TAX I.D. NUMBER   SSN □ EIN □
26. PATIENT'S ACCOUNT NO.
27. ACCEPT ASSIGNMENT? (For govt. claims, see back)   YES □   NO □
28. TOTAL CHARGE $
29. AMOUNT PAID $
30. Rsvd for NUCC Use

31. SIGNATURE OF PHYSICIAN OR SUPPLIER INCLUDING DEGREES OR CREDENTIALS (I certify that the statements on the reverse apply to this bill and are made a part thereof.)

SIGNED _____   DATE _____

32. SERVICE FACILITY LOCATION INFORMATION
a. NPI   b.

33. BILLING PROVIDER INFO & PH # ( )
a. NPI   b.

PHYSICIAN OR SUPPLIER INFORMATION

NUCC Instruction Manual available at: www.nucc.org

FIGURE 16-3 CMS-1500 (02/12) claim form.

routine physical and preventive care. **Major medical insurance** covers catastrophic expenses resulting from illness or injury.

Some traditional indemnity insurance plans and most managed care insurance carriers require the patient to select a **primary care provider**, or **PCP**. The PCP becomes the first medical practitioner caring for the patient, is also known as the gatekeeper, and is responsible for making referrals for further treatment by specialists or for hospital admission. The insurance carrier frequently will refuse payment for treatments not referred by the PCP.

Blue Cross and Blue Shield (BCBS). Whereas many traditional policies are offered by commercial carriers, the "Blues" are the largest payer groups in the United States, with 36 independent and locally operated franchises. Originally, Blue Cross started as a prepaid hospital plan, and Blue Shield later was added to cover physician provider services. In the early 1980s, the two merged to become the BCBS Association. Independent franchises may be organized as not-for-profit or for-profit.

Today, BCBS offers coverage for large employer groups, small businesses, and individual plans. Additionally, BCBS also serves as a Medicare fiscal intermediary (FI), administering the Medicare program regionally throughout the United States, District of Columbia, Canada, Puerto Rico, and Jamaica. In the United States, a Medicare fiscal intermediary acts on behalf of the government to review reimbursement and coverage, and pays on approved claims.

A BCBS participating provider (PAR) chooses to sign a member contract and receives an incentive. PARs agree to accept the BCBS reimbursement as payment in full for covered services. BCBS agrees to reimburse providers directly and in a shorter turnaround time.

Each policyholder is given a card with the subscriber's name and a three-character letter prefix identification number. The letter prefix is important because it indicates under which BCBS plan the person is insured. This identification number must be included on each claim form submitted to BCBS; if it is not included, the claim will be denied.

Managed Care Insurance

Managed care insurance involves a **managed care organization (MCO)** that assumes the responsibility for the health care needs of a group of enrollees. The MCO can be a health care plan, hospital, provider group, or health system. The MCO contracts with an insurance carrier, or is itself the carrier, to take care of the medical needs of the enrolled group for a fixed fee per enrollee for a fixed period, usually a calendar year. This payment system is called capitation. If the medical costs exceed the fixed fee, the MCO/provider loses income; conversely, if the costs are less than the fixed fee, the MCO/provider makes a profit. An MCO relies on as large an enrollee base as possible to average the cost of medical care.

MCOs were established in an attempt to curb medical costs and provide for more efficient use of medical resources. Almost all MCOs use PCPs as case managers or utilization management services to control what medical resources are used for each patient and to strictly control treatment plans and discharge planning. This policy has led to disputes over quality of care, and many states have enacted laws requiring external quality reviews by independent organizations. The quality-control programs include government oversight, patient satisfaction surveys, review of grievances, measurement of the health status of the enrolled group, and reviews by accreditation agencies. Medicare has established measurable standards for MCOs through its Quality Improvement System for Managed Care (QISMC) program. The federal government requires providers to disclose incentive packages with MCOs to avoid conflicts of interest resulting in reduced level of care solely for the purpose of reducing costs or treatment, thus recognizing a profit at the expense of patient care.

Six models exist for managed care organizations:

1. *Exclusive provider organization (EPO).* Enrollees must obtain their medical services from a network of providers or health care facilities that are under exclusive contract to the EPO. The state insurance commissioner regulates EPOs.

2. *Integrated delivery system (IDS).* Enrollees obtain medical services from an affiliated group of service providers. The service providers consist of private practices and hospitals that share practice management and services to reduce overhead. An IDS may also be called one of the following: integrated service network, delivery system, horizontally integrated system, vertically integrated system or plan, health delivery network, or accountable health plan.

3. *Health maintenance organization (HMO).* Enrollees obtain medical services from a network of providers who agree to fixed fees for services but are not under exclusive contract to the insurance carrier.

4. *Point-of-service (POS) plan.* The enrollee has the freedom of obtaining medical services from an HMO provider or by self-referral to non-HMO providers. In the case of self-referral, the enrollee will have to pay greater deductibles and co-insurance charges.

5. *Preferred provider organization (PPO).* Enrollees obtain services from a network of providers and hospitals that have contracted their services at a discounted fee to an insurance company on a nonexclusive basis.

6. *Independent practice association (IPA).* Enrollees obtain medical services from an association of independent physician providers and other medical entities. Services are provided to MCOs either by capitation, flat fee, or a negotiated FFS schedule.

7. *Triple option plan.* Enrollees have the option of using the coverage as a traditional, HMO, or PPO health plan. This is also called a 3-in-1 plan.

Table 16-1 lists differences between traditional and managed care policies.

Health maintenance organizations, or HMOs, are probably the most familiar managed care organizations. Originally, HMOs were designed to provide a full range of health care services and preventative care. Some HMOs are referred to as "one-stop" medical care, as the providers, diagnostic imaging, laboratory, pharmacy, and other services are located under one roof. More recently, the HMO without walls has become more commonplace, which is typically a network of participating providers within a defined geographic area.

The Impact of Managed Care. The emergence of managed care in today's society provides new administrative and clinical challenges to members of the health care team as they struggle to provide the best health care while working within limitations often imposed by insurance carriers. Virtually all health care settings, whether they are individual or group practices, or urgent care centers, are experiencing the impact of managed care. Providers network and compete to serve patients better and more cost-efficiently.

Under managed care, critics charge, health care dollars have grown scarce, providers must strive to provide the same quality for reduced reimbursement, preapprovals must be obtained for many services, and some services may be denied because they are not considered cost-effective.

Clinically, managed care may set limits on services or length of services. Second opinions are encouraged and sometimes required. In some systems, the patient's PCP is considered the *gatekeeper*, approving and providing referrals to specialists and more costly procedures, surgery, and tests. Critics of managed care point out that restricting or denying services may lead to an increase in professional liability.

Administratively, paperwork and documentation have become increasingly important to ensure proper reimbursement. Although it is the patient's responsibility to understand the conditions of the insurance policy, these are often difficult to understand or interpret. The medical staff must be fully aware of when a preapproval or treatment plan is required, when a second opinion is necessary for reimbursement, and other clauses and restrictions that affect care and reimbursement for care.

Procedure

At the same time, although managed care is challenging even the most resilient of providers, the very real need to keep costs down has also generated considerable creativity and energy among the health care profession as providers seek to use technology more efficiently; as they collaborate on new, cost-effective delivery methods; and as everyone involved in health care—insurers, providers, and patients—works together to contain costs by emphasizing prevention and lifestyle changes. Procedure 16-1 provides the steps involved in applying managed care policies and procedures.

TABLE 16-1

DIFFERENCES BETWEEN TRADITIONAL AND MANAGED CARE POLICIES

TRADITIONAL PLANS	MANAGED CARE
Usually can go outside provider network	Usually must stay inside provider network
Co-insurance	Co-pay each visit
Annual deductible	No annual deductible
Illness or injury only	Preventive treatment, as well as illness and injury
Premium paid monthly to company by employer or subscriber	Premium paid monthly to company by employer or subscriber
Provider paid by fee for service	Provider paid by capitation

PROCEDURE 16-1

Applying Managed Care Policies and Procedures

PURPOSE:

To apply managed care policies and procedures that the provider or medical facility has partnership agreements with.

EQUIPMENT/SUPPLIES:

- Managed care contracts
- Managed care policies and procedures manuals
- Patient record
- Authorized forms from managed care organizations
- Clerical supplies

PROCEDURE STEPS:

1. Determine which managed care organization the patient has contracted with. RATIONALE: To ensure that the correct policies and procedures are applied to the correct organization.

2. Contact the insurance carrier(s) via telephone to:
   a. Verify the patient has insurance in effect and is eligible for benefits.
   b. Confirm any exclusions or noncovered services.
   c. Determine deductibles, co-payments, or any other out-of-pocket expenses that the patient is responsible for paying.
   d. Ask if preauthorization is required for referrals to specialists or for any procedures and/or services. RATIONALE: Ascertains that insurance is viable and what benefits and patient expenses are established within the contract.

3. Record the name, title, and telephone number and extension of the insurance person contacted. RATIONALE: Documents the name of the individual providing the information. If questions arise at a later date, a contact is readily available.

4. Collect any forms necessary to process the patient claims. RATIONALE: Submitting correct forms to the managed care organization expedites the process.

5. *Paying attention to detail*, document the information collected in the patient's medical record and on the Verification of Eligibility and Benefits form. RATIONALE: Provides a record of what has taken place.

6. *Show initiative* by attending seminars and workshops offered by managed care organizations or in-service training sessions. RATIONALE: Promotes obtaining up-to-date information regarding managed care policies and procedures.

Original Medicare

Medicare, also referred to as Original Medicare, was established in 1966, and is the largest medical insurance program in the United States. Most individuals 65 years and older, individuals with a disability that keeps them from working, and individuals with chronic kidney disease and amyotropic lateral sclerosis (ALS, also known as Lou Gehrig's disease) are eligible for Medicare.

Medicare coverage consists of Parts A, B, C, and D. Part A is the Medicare program for hospitalization and requires no monthly premiums. Parts B, C, and D require monthly premiums to be paid by the patient, with the amount depending upon income and specific plans selected. Medicare and Medicaid are administered by the **Centers for Medicare and Medicaid Services (CMS)** which is an agency within the U.S. Department of Health and Human Services.

An **HIC number (HICN)** is the identification number of a Medical beneficiary. Both CMS and the Railroad Retirement Board (RRB) issue

Medicare HIC numbers. The format of an HIC number issued by CMS is a Social Security number followed by an alpha or alphanumeric suffix. For patients with Railroad Retirement benefits, an alpha prefix precedes the Social Security number.

Medicare Part A.

Medicare Part A covers hospital admission and stay, home health care, and hospice care. It has a substantial deductible and a limit to the number of hospital days per stay and the total number of hospitalizations per year. Medicare Part A pays only a portion of a patient's hospital expenses, which are calculated on a **benefit period** basis. A benefit period begins with the first day of hospital stay and ends when the patient has been out of the hospital for 60 consecutive days. Many individuals subscribe to supplemental insurance (called Medigap policies) to cover the substantial deductible.

Individuals not yet 65 years old who already receive retirement benefits from Social Security, the Railroad Retirement Board, or disability are automatically enrolled in Part A and Part B. For all other qualified individuals, Medicare becomes effective the month of their 65th birthday. Three months before their 65th birthday, or the 24th month of disability, individuals are sent an initial enrollment package containing information about Medicare and a Medicare card. If both Medicare Parts A and B are desired, they simply sign the Medicare card and keep it in a safe place for use when needed. Figure 16-4 shows a sample Medicare card. Figure 16-5 is an example of the Railroad Retirement Board (RRB) card.

Medicare Part B.

Medicare Part B covers outpatient expenses that include providers' fees, physical therapy, laboratory tests, radiologic studies, ambulance services, and charges for durable medical equipment. Durable medical equipment (DME) charges are for items that can withstand repeated use, and are meant to serve only a medical purpose (meaning they are not needed in the absence of illness or injury). Such equipment includes such items as canes, crutches, walkers, commode chairs, and blood glucose monitors. Part B does not cover medications *except* certain diabetic testing supplies. Medicare Part B requires a monthly premium, which is adjusted annually and can be dependent on income level.

In 2016, the patient must pay an annual deductible of $166 before Medicare Part B will begin to pay its share of the bills. Medicare then reimburses 80% of the Medicare fee schedule for medical care and 100% for laboratory fees. Medicare's fee schedule was adopted in 1992 and is based on the **resource-based relative value scale (RBRVS).** The RBRVS was developed using values for each medical and surgical procedure based on work, practice, and malpractice expenses and is factored for regional differences.

Figure 16-6 shows how the Medicare worksheet would look if there were no exclusions or deductions.

Medical service providers can elect to accept Medicare fee schedules and become a participating provider (PAR), or they may accept assignment on a case-by-case basis as a nonparticipating provider (non-PAR). Medical providers, whether PAR or

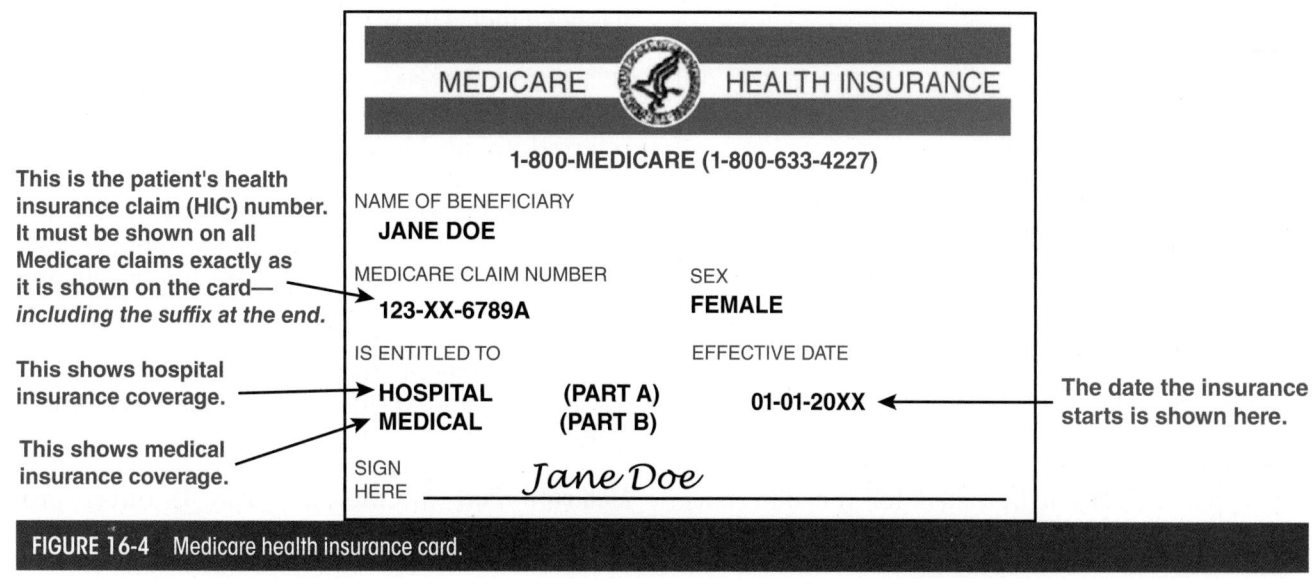

This is the patient's health insurance claim (HIC) number. It must be shown on all Medicare claims exactly as it is shown on the card—*including the suffix at the end.*

This shows hospital insurance coverage.

This shows medical insurance coverage.

The date the insurance starts is shown here.

MEDICARE   **HEALTH INSURANCE**

1-800-MEDICARE (1-800-633-4227)

NAME OF BENEFICIARY
JANE DOE

MEDICARE CLAIM NUMBER
123-XX-6789A

SEX
FEMALE

IS ENTITLED TO
HOSPITAL   (PART A)
MEDICAL   (PART B)

EFFECTIVE DATE
01-01-20XX

SIGN HERE   *Jane Doe*

FIGURE 16-4   Medicare health insurance card.

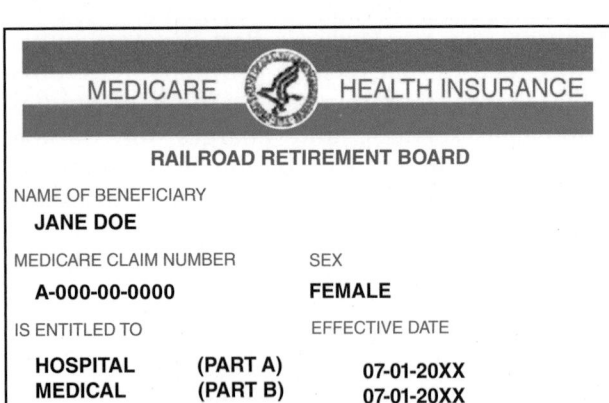

MEDICARE HEALTH INSURANCE

RAILROAD RETIREMENT BOARD

NAME OF BENEFICIARY
JANE DOE

MEDICARE CLAIM NUMBER   SEX
A-000-00-0000   **FEMALE**

IS ENTITLED TO   EFFECTIVE DATE

HOSPITAL   **(PART A)**   **07-01-20XX**
MEDICAL   **(PART B)**   **07-01-20XX**

SIGN HERE   *Jane Doe*

FIGURE 16-5   Railroad Retirement Board (RRB) Medicare health insurance card.

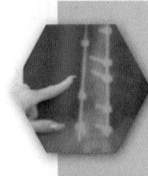

Critical Thinking

A Medicare patient has an office visit and is seen by a PAR provider. The allowed charge for the visit is $150. An insurance claim form is submitted to the local Medicare fiscal intermediary to apply against the deductible. At the next visit, the allowed charge is $125.00. This bill also is submitted to Medicare. How much of the bill will insurance pay after the deductible has been subtracted? How much does the patient owe?

Allowed Charges	
Office visit	$205.00
Return visit	+ 90.00
Total Charges	$295.00
Less deductible	−166.00
Subtotal	$129.00
Apply 80% co-insurance	x 80%
Insurance Payment	$103.20
Patient Owes	$25.80*

*In addition to the annual Medicare deductible, in this example, $166.00.

FIGURE 16-6   Sample Medicare worksheet with no exclusions or deductions.

non-PAR, are required to bill Medicare on behalf of the patient. The regional Medicare fiscal intermediary will file claims with supplemental insurers for PARs. This is called a **crossover claim**. Non-PARs must file claims directly to the supplemental plan. The patient cannot be billed for the difference between the participating provider's charges and the Medicare allowed fee. Providers can drop out of Medicare and enter into a contract with their Medicare patients that allows them to charge what they wish for services, but they must not bill Medicare for any services for the next 2 years, except in cases of emergency or urgent care.

In the example shown in Figure 16-7 the RBRVS allowed charge is applicable to both the participating and nonparticipating provider in computing the benefits Medicare pays to the provider. However, the non-PAR provider is limited to 95% of the RBRVS allowed charge in computing the amount of co-insurance. In addition, the non-PAR provider may only charge the patient up to 115% of the Medicare allowed amount. This is called the **limiting charge**. The difference between the limiting charge and the actual charge cannot be collected from the patient. The PAR provider must write off the difference between what the provider charges for the procedure and the Medicare allowed charge as a courtesy adjustment. This example assumes the yearly Medicare deductible has been met. The yearly deductible is the patient's responsibility to pay out of pocket.

Medicare Part C. **Medicare Part C** is commonly referred to as Medicare advantage plans. The plans are approved by Medicare and are run by private companies. Advantage plans provide Part A and Part B coverage and may also include Part D coverage. They may require a monthly premium and often have restrictions on approved providers and hospital facilities. Advantage plans have their own identification cards, provided to the patient, and verifying benefits and eligibility should be done for all plans.

Medicare Part D. **Medicare Part D** offers prescription drug coverage for everyone covered by Medicare. Part D requires a monthly premium

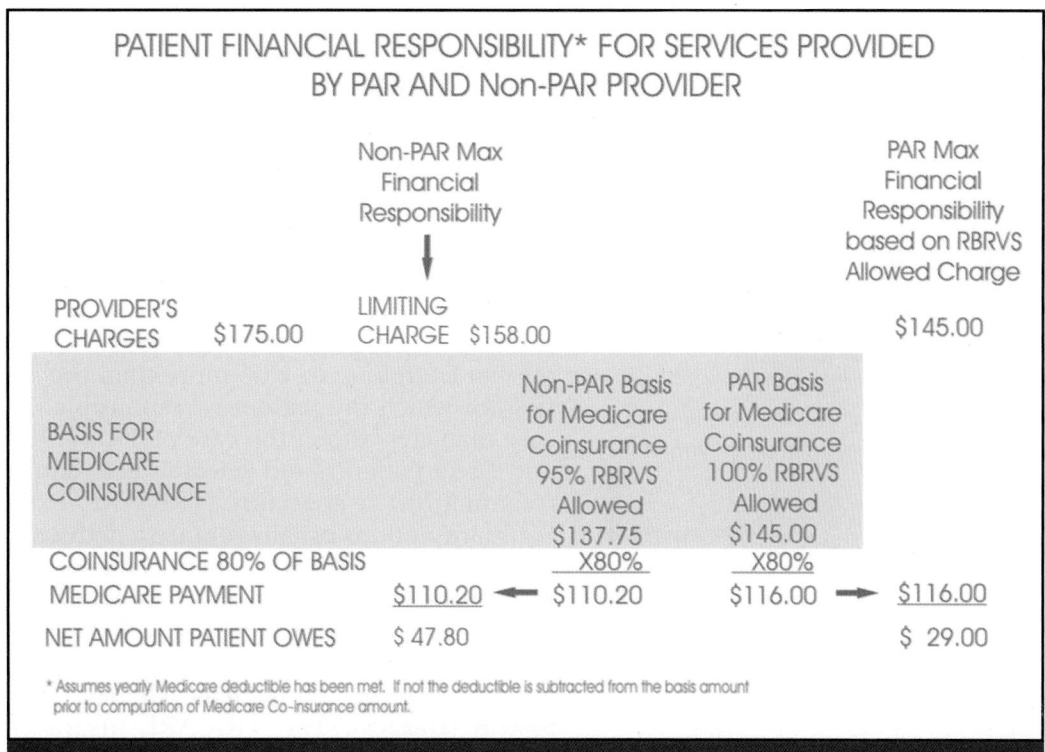

PATIENT FINANCIAL RESPONSIBILITY* FOR SERVICES PROVIDED
BY PAR AND Non-PAR PROVIDER

		Non-PAR Max Financial Responsibility ↓		PAR Max Financial Responsibility based on RBRVS Allowed Charge
PROVIDER'S CHARGES	$175.00	LIMITING CHARGE $158.00		$145.00
BASIS FOR MEDICARE COINSURANCE		Non-PAR Basis for Medicare Coinsurance 95% RBRVS Allowed $137.75	PAR Basis for Medicare Coinsurance 100% RBRVS Allowed $145.00	
COINSURANCE 80% OF BASIS		X80%	X80%	
MEDICARE PAYMENT		$110.20 ← $110.20	$116.00 →	$116.00
NET AMOUNT PATIENT OWES	$ 47.80			$ 29.00

* Assumes yearly Medicare deductible has been met. If not the deductible is subtracted from the basis amount
prior to computation of Medicare Co-insurance amount.

FIGURE 16-7   RBRVS allowed charge applicable to both the participating and the nonparticipating provider in computing the benefits Medicare pays to the provider.

that varies depending on the plan selected. In the case of advantage plans, the cost of Part D may be administered by private companies.

Part D prescription drug coverage plans have a unique feature called the **donut hole** or coverage gap. As of 2016, all plans provide coverage until the total drug costs reach $3310, then the patient is totally responsible for the next $3752 of drug costs. After that, the patient only pays a small co-payment for each prescription until the end of the calendar year. Drug coverage plans vary greatly. Selection should be based on convenience, cost, and drugs covered by the plan.

Medicare Supplemental Insurance

Medicare supplemental insurance is a secondary insurance that may cover Medicare deductibles, co-insurance requirements, and additional procedures not covered by Medicare. It is purchased by the patient through an insurance carrier or is provided as part of an employee retirement package. Supplemental **Medigap policies** are filed with the carrier by the Medicare regional carrier. The regional carrier is not required to file claims for employee retirement plan supplemental packages on behalf of the patient. Supplemental insurance frequently requires the patient to seek treatment

with specific providers and hospitals. Different programs have different coverage, which is dependent on the carrier and state requirements and should be determined when scheduling an appointment.

Medicaid Insurance

Medicaid insurance, also known as Title 19, or XIX, and Medi-Cal in California, was designed to assist those on public assistance, low income persons over the age of 65, the people with disabilities between the ages of 18 and 65, and those that

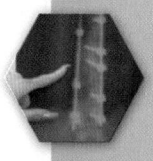

Critical Thinking

A patient has an office visit and is seen by a non-PAR provider whose office does not accept Medicare assignment. The charges are $175; however, the Medicare allowable amount is $125. A return office visit is charged at $100, with a Medicare allowable amount of $80. The $166 deductible has not yet been satisfied for the year. How much does the patient owe?

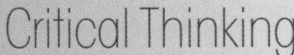
are blind. It is funded by the federal and state governments and is administered by each state's department of Supplemental Security Income (SSI). Pregnant single women with income below the poverty level; those who cannot work because of emotional, mental, or physical difficulties; and people who are on Aid to Families with Dependent Children may qualify for this program. Recipients have an identification card for the program. Not all providers accept Medicaid patients. When referring a patient to a specialist or another provider, it is wise to ascertain whether that provider accepts patients with Medicaid. A referral form prepared by the PCP or referring provider usually is required.

Because Medicaid is always secondary to any supplemental insurance, claims to Medicaid are considered only after all other insurance payments have been made. When a person has both Medicare and Medicaid, charges are submitted first to Medicare and last to Medicaid.

Legal

Because Medicare and Medicaid are federal programs, errors in billing could be construed as fraud, for which there are criminal penalties. It is therefore imperative that all billing practices conform to the legal requirements of these programs.

TRICARE

TRICARE, formerly the Civilian Health and Medical Program for Uniformed Services (CHAMPUS), is medical insurance for active duty, activated guard, reserves, and retired members of the military, and their families and survivors. Active duty, guard, and reserve service members are automatically enrolled in TRICARE Prime. Retirees and dependents must enroll in one of the three TRICARE options: Prime, Extra, or Standard (originally CHAMPUS). TRICARE Prime provides treatment mainly through military hospital facilities. TRICARE Extra provides care primarily through contracted civilian providers called *preferred providers*. TRICARE Standard provides care through traditional fee-for-service providers. Preferred providers receive a fee based on TRICARE Allowable Charges (TAC). Fee-for-service providers can charge up to 15% more than the TAC values, for which the patient is responsible. Primary care managers direct the care of TRICARE Prime and Extra patients, and referrals are required for treatment by a specialist. TRICARE Extra and Standard options usually require a deductible and co-payments. TRICARE patients are issued identification cards providing information on the type of plan in which they are enrolled. Qualifying subscribers must be listed in the Defense Department's **Defense Enrollment Eligible Reporting System (DEERS).** The TRICARE insurance program is managed by three regional centers in the United States and by a TRICARE overseas center.

Civilian Health and Medical Program of the Veterans Administration

Civilian Health and Medical Program of the Veterans Administration (CHAMPVA) is medical insurance for spouses and unmarried dependent children of a veteran with permanent total disability resulting from a service-related injury and for the surviving spouse and children of a veteran who died of a service-related disability. The patient has an identification card for the program. The program is administered by the Health Administration Center in Denver, Colorado.

Workers' Compensation Insurance

Workers' Compensation insurance is medical and paycheck insurance for workers who sustain injuries associated with their employment. In some instances, the insurance covers family members in the case of death of the worker. The employer usually pays the premium to the state or an insurance carrier designated by the state. Some large employers assume the insurance risk and are self-insured. Federal and state laws define minimum standards for Workers' Compensation programs. Workers' Compensation covers 100% of associated medical expenses. Claims are filed with the insurance carrier. Although most workers are insured under state programs, federal programs exist for the following specific groups:

- Office Workers' Compensation Programs (OWCP)
- Energy Workers' Occupational Illness Compensation Program
- Federal Black Lung Program
- Federal Employees' Compensation Act Program (FECA)
- Longshore and Harbor Workers' Compensation Program
- Mine Safety and Health Administration (MSHA)

Personal Injury Protection (PIP) Insurance

Personal injury protection (PIP) insurance is a component of automobile insurance that covers medical and hospital expenses due to a motor vehicle accident (MVA). It is often referred to as no-fault insurance because it pays out claims regardless of who is at fault in an accident. Other common terms are auto medical payment (AMP), Med Pay, and medical payments coverage. These terms are interchangeable and refer to the same no-fault insurance. Payments are based on the limits of the policy, and may pay for as much as 80% of expenses. PIP insurance covers the policyholder, but in some cases, may also extend to passengers and pedestrians involved in a car accident.

In addition to hospital and medical expenses, PIP may also cover lost wages as a result of a car accident, help pay costs of services, such as having someone take children to school, child care, or grocery shopping, and funeral expenses.

Coverage requirements vary by state; some require that drivers carry it, in others, it is optional. If a state requires PIP, there will be minimum coverage requirements. If not, the limits can be adjusted by what the policyholder chooses and can afford. Currently, the states that require PIP include Delaware, Florida, Hawaii, Kansas, Kentucky, Massachusetts, Michigan, Minnesota, New Jersey, New York, North Dakota, Oregon, Pennsylvania, and Utah.

PIP coverage is also required in Maryland, Texas, and Washington; however, a driver can sign a waiver and opt not to purchase the coverage. In this case, an exclusion agreement is signed, where the driver agrees to forego coverage, and affirms understanding that there is no personal injury protection and they will be liable for expenses sustained in a MVA as applicable.

Because PIP insurance regulations and requirements change, staying up to date on the topic and what is required in the state where you are located is a good idea.

Self-Funded Health Care

With **self-funded health care**, also known as **self-insurance**, the employer operates its own health plan, instead of purchasing a plan from an insurance carrier to cover employees. When operating a self-funded plan, the employer pays for the services of the insurance carrier to administrate the plan. Each self-insured plan differs in coverage and claim filing requirements. The plan administrator should be contacted before scheduling a patient appointment.

Medical Tourism Insurance

Medical tourism is an unusual option being added to conventional insurance plans in an effort to control rising health care costs. It consists of health-provider networks paying the insured client to go abroad for treatment at internationally accredited hospitals. This insurance option has several potential disadvantages that may outweigh the reduced costs. Safety of blood supplies for transfusions and tissue for bone grafts is questionable in some countries, long distance travel may be dangerous for some patients, and returning patients may find it difficult to obtain follow-up care due to providers' concerns about exposure to possible malpractice lawsuits. Medical tourism options are quite new to the industry. At this time, whether this will become the new wave in insurance or will disappear from the future of insurance is uncertain.

SCREENING FOR INSURANCE

It is the responsibility of the medical assistant to screen all new patients for their insurance. New patients should be asked to arrive 15 to 20 minutes earlier than their appointment time to complete a patient registration form. The form requests vital information that enables the medical office to contact the patient, process his or her billing and insurance claims, know who to contact in case of emergency, authorize payment of insurance benefits, and record method of payment. Commercial forms are available for purchase or can be designed by office management personnel for this purpose.

The medical assistant should review each section of the patient registration form to verify that all information is complete and legible. Many offices make a photocopy of the patient's driver's license and attach it to the registration form. This procedure helps in identifying the correct person through photo identification should it be necessary. It is important to verify the spelling of all patient names: first, middle, and last.

Ask the patient to show his or her health insurance card and verify the effective date and pertinent information. All medical offices should make a photocopy of both sides of the card to maintain in the patient's chart, or scan both sides of the card and upload to the patient's electronic medical record. In most cases, the back of the card contains information about any deductible, co-payment, and preapproval requirements, as well as the insurance company's name, address, and telephone number. It also shows any special claim submission instructions.

Each time a patient checks in, the medical assistant should ask questions to verify the following insurance information:

- Request DOB (date of birth) to establish correct patient.
- Confirm the patient's current address.
- Confirm the patient's insurance carrier and plan.
- Ask for the patient's insurance card and verify information and effective dates.
- Determine whether the insurance carrier covers the procedure.
- Determine that the patient's PCP is performing the procedure.

- Confirm whether a referral is required and whether an authorization number or authorization code is required. Confirm evidence of qualifying has been secured.
- Establish proof of eligibility (see Figure 16-8).

Procedure

When screening patients for insurance, it is important to understand the philosophy of the medical office. Some see patients regardless of ability to pay; responsible medical assistants will investigate all avenues for reimbursement first. Some situations include the patient who is eligible for Medicaid but has not yet applied, or the patient who has applied for Medicaid but has not yet received notification of qualification. Procedure 16-2 provides the steps for screening for insurance.

The medical assistant should investigate and verify that all avenues have been taken to achieve the proof of eligibility that the office needs to receive reimbursement from Medicaid. This may include calling the Medicaid office to verify eligibility or going online and printing a proof of eligibility directly from the Medicaid system. This electronic data exchange system is called an *envoy*. Proof of eligibility cards are distributed to recipients and are in effect for at least a year. However, the most common avenue to ensure that services will be reimbursed is not to see any patient who does not have proof of Medicaid coverage. Medicaid sends an eligibility Medical Assistance Identification (MAID) (medical coupon) to the patient the first day of each month. This coupon guarantees the ambulatory care center payment for the services provided. Unless it is an emergency, some offices will not schedule

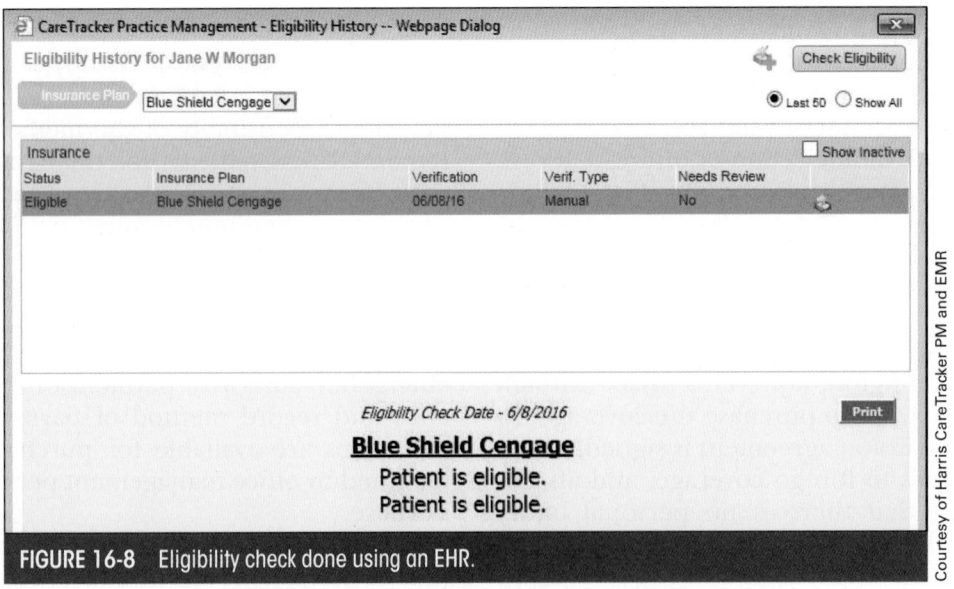

FIGURE 16-8 Eligibility check done using an EHR.

Courtesy of Harris CareTracker PM and EMR

PROCEDURE 16-2

Procedure

Screening for Insurance

PURPOSE:

To verify insurance coverage and obtain vital information required for processing and billing insurance claim forms.

EQUIPMENT/SUPPLIES:

- Patient registration forms
- Clipboard and black ink pen
- Patient's chart

PROCEDURE STEPS:

1. When scheduling the first appointment, ask the patient to bring his or her insurance card and to arrive 15 to 20 minutes before the appointment time to complete the patient registration form. RATIONALE: The insurance card is required to verify effective dates and pertinent information relative to insurance coverage. The registration form also requests vital information necessary for patient care and insurance billing.

2. When the patient turns in the completed registration form, review it immediately, **paying attention to detail,** to be sure that all information has been collected and is legible. RATIONALE: It is important that all requested information is included on the registration form and that the medical assistant can read it clearly when processing the insurance claim forms. If information is not provided on the claim form or is incorrect, the insurance carrier may deny the claim.

3. Ask the patient for his or her insurance card. Make a photocopy of both sides of the card to be maintained in the patient's chart, or scan the insurance card and upload to the patient's electronic medical record. RATIONALE: The insurance card provides vital information, including correct spelling of patient's name, insurance plan numbers, effective dates, telephone numbers to call regarding referrals and preauthorizations, and information about any deductible and co-payment.

4. Verify proof of eligibility for Medicaid patients. The patient should have his or her proof of eligibility card with him or her, or you may need to make a telephone call directly to Medicaid or use the online electronic data exchange system to determine proof of eligibility. RATIONALE: This information is required for Medicaid reimbursement.

5. Each time a patient checks in, whether established or new, the following information should be verified:

   - Address. Confirm the patient's current address and telephone number. RATIONALE: Patients may have moved and may not realize they had not reported the new address and telephone number to the office.

   - Verify insurance coverage. RATIONALE: This information is required for correct claims processing and billing procedures.

   - Using the copy of the insurance card, verify the information and effective dates. Also be sure that a photocopy of the card is maintained in the patient's chart. RATIONALE: This is a means of keeping insurance records current for billing purposes.

   - Determine whether the insurance carrier covers the procedure. RATIONALE: If the carrier does not cover the procedure, reimbursement will need to come from a third party or the patient.

   - Determine that the correct provider is performing the procedure. RATIONALE: This information is needed for reimbursement purposes.

   - Determine whether a referral is required and whether an authorization number or code is needed. RATIONALE: Reimbursement by the carrier cannot take place without the proper documentation and authorization number.

   - Confirm that evidence of qualifying has been secured. RATIONALE: Proof of eligibility must be verified for reimbursement from Medicaid.

Medicaid patients before the fifth of each month. This allows ample time for the beneficiary to receive the medical coupon. If the patient presents for an appointment without a medical coupon, and proof of eligibility cannot be determined elsewhere, it is common practice to have that patient reschedule the appointment. The exception is an emergency.

Medical assistants with responsibility for billing are vital to the success of a clinic. Billing the insurance carriers promptly, completing claim forms properly, billing patients as needed, and keeping track of aging accounts will do much to ensure a flow of adequate income. In all insurance matters, be available to patients with questions regarding their insurance or accounts because a friendly attitude helps patients feel positive about the care they receive and establishes a long-term relationship.

REFERRALS AND AUTHORIZATIONS

When a PCP refers a patient to a specialist, the term **referral** is used by managed care facilities. Referrals may be denied because of incomplete information contained on the referral form or because a medical necessity was not established. Referrals are generally categorized as one of three types:

- *Regular.* Usually takes 3 to 10 working days to review procedures and approve
- *Urgent.* Usually takes about 24 hours for approval
- *Stat.* May be approved via telephone after faxing the information to the utilization review department

The most common referral used by managed care plans is the regular referral. The member services department must be contacted to check the status of a referral. It is important to never tell the patient that the referral has been approved until you have obtained a hard copy of the *authorization* (a managed care term for approved referrals). Be sure to review the content of the referral carefully. The typical referral will contain important information regarding its limitations, such as:

- Number of authorized visits to the provider
- The type of services authorized
- Expiration date (i.e., most will last for only 90 days)

Preauthorizations and *precertifications* are terms used to determine whether a service or procedure is covered and if the insurance plan approves it as medically necessary. Preauthorization is required for some services, hospital admissions, inpatient and outpatient surgeries, and most elective procedures (Procedure 16-3). Once approved, an authorization number will be provided. The patient also receives a letter containing the authorization number and the approved services. The patient must present this letter to the specialist's office on the day the service is provided.

When questions arise regarding preauthorization, precertification, or referral procedures, the medical assistant should call the plan's contact number for specific information. Many offices

---

PROCEDURE 16-3

Obtaining Referrals and Authorizations

PURPOSE:

To ascertain coverage by the insurance carrier for specific medical services, hospital admissions, inpatient or outpatient surgeries, elective procedures, or when the PCP elects to refer the patient to another provider.

EQUIPMENT/SUPPLIES:

- Patient's medical chart and copy of his or her insurance card
- Name and telephone number of the contact person for the carrier
- Referral form
- Telephone/fax machine
- Pen/pencil

(continues)

> **PROCEDURE STEPS:**
>
> 1. Collect all necessary documents and equipment (patient's chart/record, insurance carrier's information and telephone number). RATIONALE: Allows for efficient use of time in acquiring the referral or authorization.
>
> 2. Determine the service or procedure requiring preauthorization. You will also need to know the name and telephone number of the specialist involved and the reason the request is being sought. RATIONALE: This information is required to complete the referral form to obtain authorization from the patient's insurance carrier.
>
> 3. Complete the referral form, being sure to include all pertinent information. RATIONALE: The request may be denied if all information has not been included.
>
> 4. Proofread the completed form, **paying attention to detail.** RATIONALE: Because of the importance of this step, accuracy is critical.
>
> 5. Fax or electronically send the completed form to the insurance carrier. RATIONALE: The completed form apprises the carrier of the patient's medical condition, requests preauthorization for treatment, requests a verification or authorization number, and confirms the treatment plan.
>
> 6. Maintain a completed copy of the referral form in the patient's chart. RATIONALE: The form can be accessed in the future should questions arise.

find it helpful to maintain a reference log regarding these requirements. Information to maintain includes:

- Name of the insurance plan
- Address and telephone number
- Name and telephone number of contact person or the person with whom you spoke
- Co-payment amount and deductible information
- Inpatient and outpatient surgery benefits
- Preauthorization requirements, second-opinion options
- Participating hospitals, radiology service providers, laboratories, and physicians

The authorization number and referral numbers are entered in Box 23 of the CMS-1500 form when billing for services.

DETERMINING FEE SCHEDULES

A provider charges for services using a variety of means for computing a fee schedule. Although all of the fee computation plans vary and give somewhat different results, they all have common elements. Note the following examples:

- *The overhead or practice expenses for the clinic or office.* This category includes rental of the physical building or office space and equipment; utilities; cost of medical supplies inventory; and salaries of nurses, medical assistants, bookkeepers, and other personnel who are paid on a salary or contract basis. It also includes cost of employee benefits such as retirement plans, sick leave, and vacation time.

- *The cost of medical malpractice insurance.* This cost is separated from the charge for general insurance, which is included in the preceding category, because of the significant portion of the fee attributed to this item and because it varies greatly for different types of services. Obstetric/gynecologic procedures are probably the greatest for the entire medical community, including surgical procedures.

- *Hourly rate for the services provided by the provider.* This rate varies depending on the skill and training required for the procedure, the cost of living in the area, and the rate charged by other providers in the area. (The law of supply and demand applies here as in any other economic arena.) Surgeons charge a greater rate than providers in general practice, rates are greater in a metropolitan area than in a rural area, and experience level commands greater rates.

All of these cost elements are derived on an hourly basis. The sum of the above elements combined with the time required is used to arrive at the fee schedule for a procedure or service.

The advent of insurance plans, Medicare, and managed care plans has resulted in specific formulas being developed and accepted by the different plans to establish a fee schedule acceptable to the carrier. Several of the fee schedule systems in common usage are discussed in the following sections.

All of them, however, incorporate the preceding three elements (practice expenses, malpractice expenses, and provider's experience).

Usual, Customary, and Reasonable Fees

The **usual, customary, and reasonable (UCR)** fee schedule is a fee system that defines allowable charges that will be accepted by insurance carriers. The actual rate may vary from one carrier to another, but the process is the same.

- Usual fee is the provider's average fee for a service or procedure. This fee is based on the economic analysis of the practice described earlier in this section.
- Customary fee is the average or range of fees within the geographic area that an insurance carrier will accept. It is frequently tied to a national average for a similar metropolitan or rural setting.
- Reasonable fee is the generally accepted fee for services or procedures that are extraordinarily difficult or complicated and require more time and effort by the provider.

An example of the operation of the UCR system is as follows. An insurance carrier operating on the UCR fee schedule may have determined a customary fee range for a new patient office visit with history taking and physical examination to be $140 to $225 for that region. If the amount billed by the provider were $160, the provider would be reimbursed for the service in full. Had the provider billed $250, the reimbursement would be $225, and the provider would have to write off the $25 nonallowed charge. The amount the provider would have to write off is often referred to as an **adjustment**. Providers who participate in UCR systems cannot bill the patient for the nonallowable charge.

Resource-Based Relative Value Scale (RBRVS)

Medicare has used the RBRVS since 1992. Under this system, a provider's services are reimbursed based on relative value units (RVUs). Each service, procedure, and medication is assigned a code compiled from the *Current Procedural Terminology* (CPT) manual issued by the American Medical Association for procedures and the *International Classification of Diseases, 10th Revision, Clinical Modification* (ICD-10-CM) manual

for diagnoses issued by the World Health Organization. Medicare then issues three RVUs for each code in the *Medicare Fee Schedule* (MFS) manual issued each year. The RVUs are for provider's work, practice expenses, and malpractice expenses. The practice expense is further differentiated based on location, that is, whether the work was done in a hospital (facility) or in a clinic or office (nonfacility). The nonfacility practice expense further differentiates between whether the nonfacility is transitioned or fully implemented. A geographic practice cost index (GPCI) related to the geographic area where the provider is located is issued for each RVU category. The GPCI is based on the ZIP code for the address of the practice or wherever the service is performed. The payment for service is then established from the sum of the geographically adjusted RVUs multiplied by a nationally uniform conversion factor for services.

The Formula for Calculating Payment Schedules

The American Medical Association provides a simplified table to assist with calculating the Medicare payment schedule. The Omnibus Budget Reconciliation Act of 1989 (OBRA 89) geographic adjustment provision requires all three components of the relative value for a service—physician work relative value units (RVUs), practice expense RVUs, and professional liability insurance (PLI) RVUs—to be adjusted by the corresponding GPCI for the locality. In effect, this provision increases the number of components in the payment schedule from three to the following six:

- Physician work RVUs
- Physician work GPCI
- Practice expense RVUs
- Practice expense GPCI
- PLI RVUs
- PLI GPCI

The general formula for calculating Medicare payment amounts for 2016 is shown in Table 16-2. The data to place into the formula changes annually, and can be obtained through the American Medical Association website (www.ama-assn.org) in the "Physician Resources" area.

The Medicare conversion factor is a scaling factor that converts the geographically adjusted

TABLE 16-2

MEDICARE FORMULA FOR PAYMENT OF SERVICES

	Work RVU1 × Work (GPCI)^2
+	Practice Expense (PE) RVU × PE GPCI
+	Malpractice (PLI) RVU × PLI GPCI
	= Total RVU
×	CY 2016 Conversion Factor of $35.8043 (Jan 1.–Dec. 31, 2016)
	= Medicare Payment

number of relative value units (RVUs) for each service in the Medicare physician payment schedule into a dollar payment amount. The initial Medicare conversion factor was set at $31.001 in 1992.

Budget Neutrality Adjustment (BNA) in the Medicare Fee Schedule

In 2009, Medicare changed its payment calculation in the Physician Fee Schedule. It moved the Budget Neutrality Factor from the Work RVU to the Conversion Factor.

The conversion factor decreased, but fees increased. This provided a 4-6% increase in E/M services. In previous years, applying the budget neutrality factor to the work RVU had the effect of decreasing payments more for services with high work RVU values.

Procedure

Clinics should review their third party contracts to be sure the BNA is not included in the calculation of fees. Contract amounts that are based on the Resource Based Relative Value Scale should be determined as a conversion factor multiplied by the total RVUs. If the fee is a percentage of Medicare, then the payer is including the BNA in the calculation and being paid less. Procedure 16-4

PROCEDURE 16-4

Computing the Medicare Fee Schedule

Procedure

PURPOSE:

To compute the Medicare allowable (MA) payment for services.

EQUIPMENT/SUPPLIES:

- CPT book
- Computer
- Calculator

PROCEDURE STEPS:

1. Using the *Current Procedural Terminology* (CPT) book, obtain the CPT code for the exact procedure or service for which a fee schedule is being computed. RATIONALE: Accurate code must be obtained to ensure correct billing.

2. Using the Medicare Fee Schedule, which is issued each year, determine the relative value units for (a) provider's time (work), (b) practice expense (PE), and (c) costs of malpractice insurance (MP) listed for the CPT code in step 1. These factors represent the relative amount of a fee allocated to each item.

3. Using the Medicare fee schedule, determine the geographic practice cost index (GPCI). This factor accounts for different cost of living values for urban versus rural and geographic locations in the United States.

4. Using the Medicare Fee Schedule, determine the relative value unit (RVU) conversion factor (CF). This factor converts RVU units to dollars based on an average for the entire United States.

5. Compute the Medicare allowable fee for the procedure or service using the equation supplied in Table 16-2.

provides steps for computing the Medicare allowable fee schedule.

Diagnosis-Related Groups

In order to consider a claim for accepted reimbursement, Medicare will carefully examine the **Diagnosis-Related Groups (DRGs)**. These designations are part of a reimbursement strategy that is designed to focus upon the diagnoses of the patient instead of the services rendered. They ensure that all given diagnoses are as specific as possible and also justify the length of a patient's stay in the hospital. This concept also brings together conditions that were known to be related to one another and could prove medical necessity, as well as validate the treatments given.

Hospital Inpatient Prospective Payment System

The inpatient prospective payment system (IPPS) is a reimbursement system for hospitals based on similar diagnosis-related groups (DRGs) of inpatients discharged. Rather than the traditional method of payment based on actual costs incurred in providing care, DRGs are based on an average cost for treatment of a patient's condition. The hospital is reimbursed for each discharge according to a predetermined rate for each DRG.

Hospital Outpatient Prospective Payment System

The **hospital outpatient prospective payment system (OPPS)** is a reimbursement system for hospital outpatients, certain Part B services furnished to hospital inpatients who have no Part A coverage, and partial hospitalization services furnished by community mental health centers. All services are classified into groups called Ambulatory Payment Classifications (APCs). Payments are established for each APC, and the hospital is reimbursed for each patient. Depending on the services provided, hospitals may be paid for more than one APC for an encounter.

Capitation

Capitation is a payment system used primarily by managed care organizations. A fixed dollar amount is reimbursed to the provider for patients enrolled during a specific period. The payment per patient is independent of services or procedures provided to a patient. To be financially responsible, this system requires enrollment of a large number of patients so that a few patients do not unduly skew an average cost. This type of system requires extensive practice of preventive medicine to be cost-effective.

LEGAL AND ETHICAL ISSUES

Most Medicare claims are now required to be submitted electronically, and private payers in growing numbers are also using electronic claims submission. In a computerized system, everything related to billing and reimbursement is computerized and transmitted electronically. If the office is participating in CMS's Electronic Data Interchange (EDI), it will be assigned a unique identifier number that constitutes its legal electronic signature. Be cautious with this electronic signature, because the office is responsible for any and all claims made with it. The Health Insurance Portability and Accountability Act (HIPAA) of 1996 (specifically title II, subtitle F) regulates the security and privacy of transmitted health care information. Review HIPAA's regulations in Chapters 11 and 15.

Integrity

The medical assistant faces legal and ethical issues related to insurance issues on a daily basis; therefore, it is important that each patient be treated equally and fairly. As mentioned in Chapter 4, it is critical that patients not be stereotyped, regardless of whether they have multiple insurance plans or are not covered by any insurance plan at all. Every patient must be cared for objectively, with respect, and in a professional manner.

Legal

Medical personnel are bound by law to maintain the confidentiality of all medical information and must be able to recognize information that is protected by privacy rules and understand how it is to be handled. Protected health information (PHI) may be considered individually identifiable health information. This includes information that describes the health status of an individual, including basic demographics and the use of medical services, as well as information that either identifies or can be used to identify an individual. Medical personnel must remember that informed consent is not consent to use and disclose personal information.

Insurance Fraud and Abuse

Competency Integrity

Insurance **fraud** and **abuse** may be involved in more than 10% of submitted medical claims according to the Insurance Information Institute. These estimates include both intentional as well as accidental coding and billing irregularities and, if detected and proved, such irregularities can result in legal action against the practice or clinic and personnel responsible for or having knowledge of the irregularities. Personnel involved in coding and billing should be alert for both accidental and intentional coding and billing irregularities and bring them to the attention of responsible managers. If no corrective action is taken, all personnel involved, including managers, are legally responsible to report the irregularities to the insurance carrier. Examples of fraudulent insurance activities include but are not limited to:

- Coding to a higher level of service to increase revenue (upcoding)
- Misrepresenting the diagnosis to justify payment
- Billing for services, equipment, or procedures that were never provided
- Unbundling service procedure codes
- Charging uninsured patients less than insured patients
- Receiving rebates or any type of compensation for referrals (kickbacks)

Insurance abuse involves activities that are inconsistent with accepted business practices. Some examples of abuse include but are not limited to:

- Charging for services that are not medically necessary
- Overcharging for services, equipment, or procedures
- Improper billing practices
- Violating participating provider agreements with insurance companies

Heavy penalties, including a $10,000 fine per claim form plus three times the fraudulent claim amount, may be sanctioned on individuals who knowingly and willfully misrepresent information submitted on insurance claim forms to gain greater payments or benefits.

To protect yourself and the medical practice from committing insurance fraud and abuse, you should begin by identifying risk areas based on errors in the past history of billing and insurance claims processing. Practice internal audits to monitor compliance with written protocols. Participate in seminars and in-service programs to keep current with coding and billing practices. Be sure to use only the current year's coding manuals to ensure accuracy. Code only what is documented in the medical record, and ask for clarification when needed.

An auditor should check claim forms, whether submitted electronically or by hard copy, to see that they are completed correctly. Include all pertinent dates and diagnostic and procedural coding information necessary for insurance payers to generate reimbursement. Auditors look specifically for any indicators of insurance fraud and abuse.

PROFESSIONAL CAREERS IN INSURANCE

Professional

To be successful in the health insurance specialist field, training and entry-level requirements are essential. An opportunity for employment in these specialties is greater for those with a college degree that includes course-work in medical terminology, anatomy and physiology, pharmacology, insurance and coding procedures, and communication skills.

Personal attributes that enhance employment possibilities as health insurance specialists include, but are not limited to, the following descriptions: self-motivated, works well independently, detail oriented, a critical thinker, ethical, maintains confidentiality, cooperative, reliable, and adaptable.

The following Internet links will help you explore a variety of health insurance specialist career opportunities.

- American Academy of Professional Coders (AAPC) at http://www.aapc.com
- American Health Information Management Association (AHIMA) at http://www.ahima.org
- American Medical Billing Association (AMBA) at http://www.ambanet.net
- Alliance of Claims Assistance Professionals (ACAP) at http://www.claims.org
- National Electronic Billers Alliance (NEBA) at http://www.nebazone.com

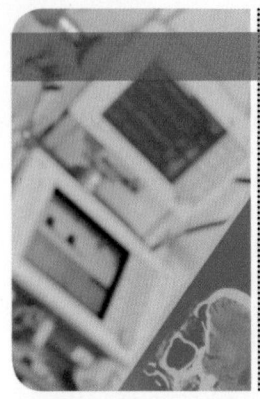

CASE STUDY 16-1

Refer to the scenario at the beginning of the chapter.

CASE STUDY REVIEW

1. Identify ways that Ellen Armstrong, CMAS (AMT), can stay abreast of policy changes regarding reimbursement.
2. List options for Ellen to take in order to be up to date with insurance coverage so that she can help patients understand their responsibility, if any, for payment.
3. Recall steps for screening patients for insurance. Why is this so important?

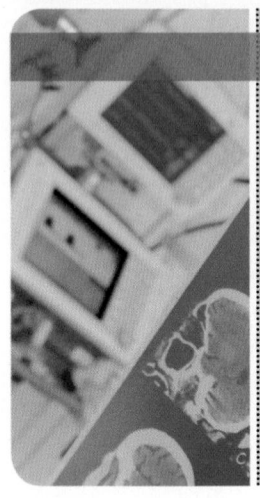

CASE STUDY 16-2

Ellen Armstrong, CMAS (AMT), is responsible for all patient insurance billing procedures. Ellen has the following information:

	Total Charges	Allowed Charges
Office visit	$150.00	$100.00
Return visit	$80.00	$75.00

Deductible has not been satisfied.

CASE STUDY REVIEW

1. Calculate the patient's correct billing if the provider accepts assignment.
2. Calculate the patient's correct billing if the provider does not accept assignment.

Summary

- An understanding of medical insurance terminology and various types of coverage is vital to a thriving clinic.
- The increasing complexity of health insurance today means that medical assistants must continually update their base of information.
- The Affordable Care Act has introduced a number of challenges, and as the number of Americans with coverage continues to grow, so will the need for a good understanding of medical billing and coding principles for medical assistants.
- Medical assistants must develop strong communication skills to explain insurance procedures to patients, and make contact with representatives to determine eligibility and verification of benefits.
- The medical assistant will need to be familiar with medical insurance terms and how these terms apply to the clinic, the policyholder, and impact on proper reimbursement. These terms include *beneficiary; policyholder; subscriber of a plan; deductibles; co-insurance and co-payments; exclusions and preexisting condition exclusions for grandfathered individual plans; coordination of benefits (COB), explanation of benefits (EOB), and remittance advice (RA) notices, preauthorization,* and *assignment of benefits.*
- Insurance plan types include traditional insurance, managed care insurance models (EPO, IDS, HMO, POS, PPO), Medicare (Parts A, B, C, and D) and Medicaid/Medi-Cal, Tricare, Workers' Compensation, and personal injury protection (PIP) insurance.
- Medical assistants must know screening techniques for insurance data and how to obtain referrals and precertifications as required by insurance plans.
- The medical assistant must be aware of legal and ethical issues as they relate to medical insurance in order for PHI to be protected, and minimize or eliminate unintentional insurance fraud and abuse.

Study for Success

To reinforce your knowledge and skills of information presented in this chapter:

- Review the *Key Terms* and *Learning Outcomes*
- Consider the *Critical Thinking* features and *Case Studies* and discuss your conclusions
- Answer the questions in the *Certification Review*

- Perform the *Procedures* using the *Competency Assessment Checklists* on the *Student Companion Website*

Procedure

CERTIFICATION REVIEW

1. Which of the following is the most common avenue to ensure that services will be reimbursed?
   a. Do not see any patient who does not have proof of Medicaid coverage.
   b. Complete an envoy.
   c. Go online and print a proof of eligibility directly from the system.
   d. Ask patients if they are covered.

2. What is the most common insurance claim form?
   a. UB04 form
   b. ICD-9-CM
   c. CMS-1500 (02-12) form
   d. Assignment of benefits
   e. ICD-10-CM

3. Which of the following statements is an accurate description of Medicare?
   a. It was created by Title 19 of the Social Security Act.
   b. It covers most persons age 65 years and older.
   c. It is designed to cover prescriptions.
   d. It is handled separately by each state.

4. If the RBRVS allowable is $150 and the deductible has not been met, Medicare will pay how much?
   a. $20
   b. $40
   c. $120
   d. 80% of RBRVS allowable after $166.00 deductible
   e. None of these

5. How many primary MCO models are in operation across the U.S.?
   a. Four
   b. Three
   c. Six
   d. Eight

6. Which of the following statements is an accurate description of Medicaid insurance?
   a. It is funded by the federal government and administered by each state's department of SSI.
   b. It requires a Medigap policy.
   c. It consists of Part A, Part B, Part C, and Part D.
   d. It requires PARs to accept assignment.
   e. All of these

7. Which of the following statements is an accurate description of BCBS?
   a. They are locally based in all 50 states in the United States.
   b. They operate like MCOs.
   c. They recognize Medicare Part B.
   d. They are part of CHAMPVA.

8. Which of the following statements is an accurate description of TRICARE?
   a. It is part of CHAMPVA.
   b. It is part of OWCP, MSHA, and FECA programs.
   c. It is a self funded plan.
   d. It was formerly the Civilian Health and Medical Program for Uniformed Services.
   e. It no longer exists.

9. Of the following, which is the best example of insurance abuse:
   a. Billing for services, equipment, or procedures that were never provided
   b. Charging for services that are not medically necessary
   c. Coding to a higher level of service to increase revenue
   d. Receiving rebates or any type of compensation for referrals

10. According to the birthday rule, which of the following is true?
    a. The father's insurance policy will always be the primary insurance plan.
    b. The policy with the later effective date will be the primary plan.
    c. The mother's policy will always be the primary insurance plan.
    d. The parent with the earlier DOB will carry the primary plan.
    e. The parent with the later DOB will carry the primary plan.

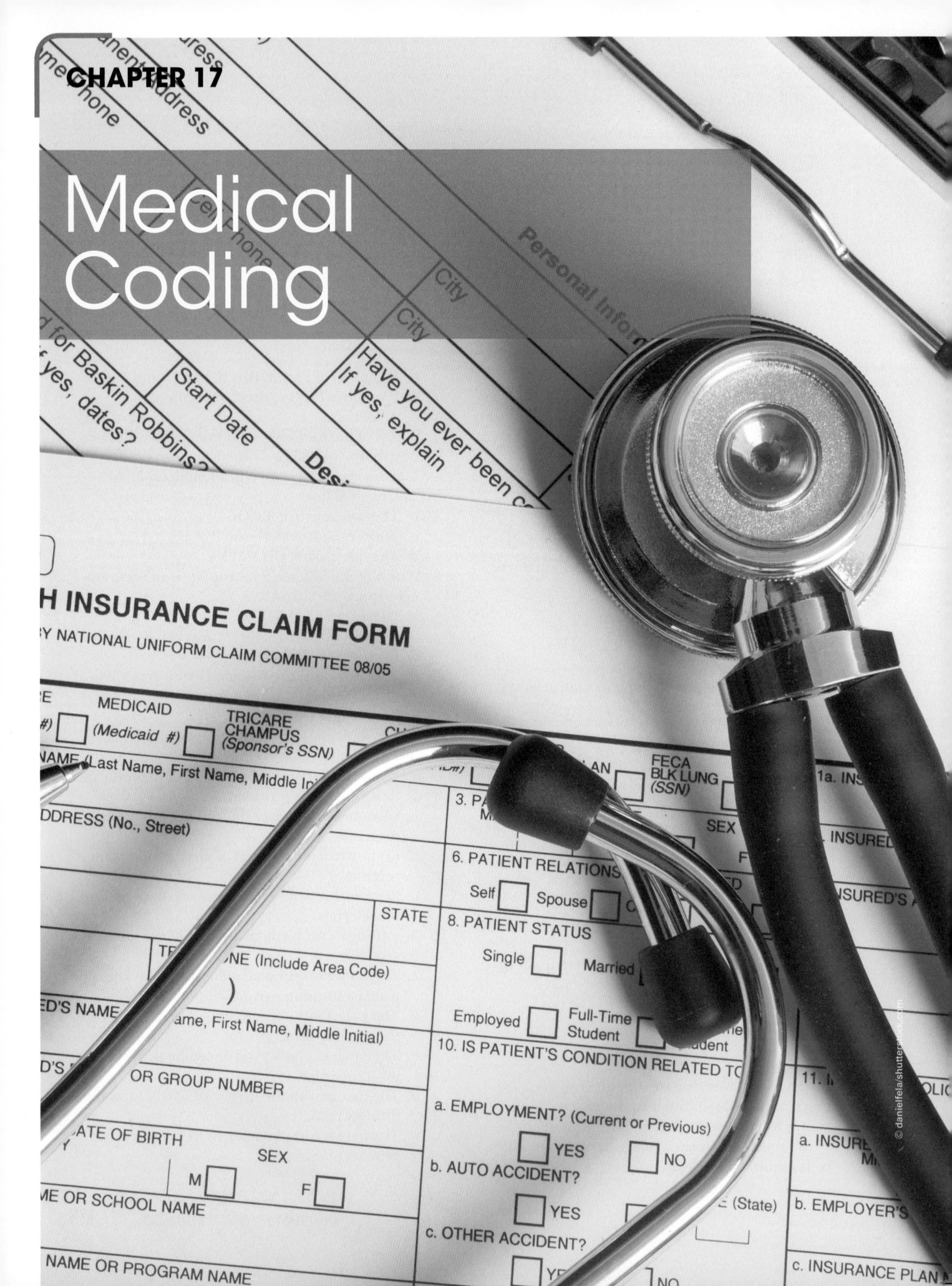

Medical Coding

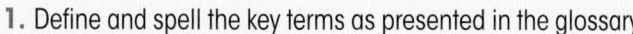

LEARNING OUTCOMES

1. Define and spell the key terms as presented in the glossary.
2. Define terminology necessary to understand and code medical insurance claim forms.
3. Describe how to use the most current procedural and diagnostic coding systems.
4. Code a sample claim form.
5. Apply third-party guidelines.
6. Recognize common errors in completing insurance claim forms.
7. Explain the difference between the CMS-1500 (02-12) and the UB-04 forms.
8. Compare processes for filing insurance claims both manually and electronically.
9. Discuss why claims follow-up is important to the ambulatory care setting.
10. Discuss legal and ethical issues related to coding and insurance claims processing.

KEY TERMS

assumptive coding

bundled codes

claim register

CMS-1500 (02-12)

Current Procedural Terminology (CPT®)

diagnosis

down-code

encounter form (superbill)

explanation of benefits (EOB)

Healthcare Common Procedure Coding System (HCPCS)

ICD-10-PCS

International Classification of Diseases, 9th Revision, Clinical Modification (ICD-9-CM)

International Classification of Diseases, 10th Revision, Clinical Modification (ICD-10-CM)

International Classification of Diseases, 10th Revision, Procedure Coding System (ICD-10-PCS)

medical necessity

modifiers

morbidity

mortality

nomenclature systems

point-of-service (POS) device

symbols

unbundling

Uniform Bill 04 (UB-04)

up-coding

SCENARIO

At Inner City Health Care, a multiprovider clinic in a large city, medical assistant Ellen Armstrong, CMAS (AMT), is responsible for all patient billing procedures, including insurance claim forms. Ellen stresses with her colleagues the fact that coding is the basis for information exchanged between the health care providers and various agencies that compile health care statistics as well as third-party payers for health care services rendered to patients. Understanding medical terminology, anatomy, physiology, and how to code medical procedures and diagnoses accurately is a must. Using the computer to complete insurance forms, while considering common errors that may lead to denial of a claim, and transmitting the claims electronically are reviewed during in-service meetings. Ellen emphasizes that accurate coding must always reflect services actually performed and documented within the patient's chart.

Coding is the basis for the information on the claim form. Medical coding is mandatory for the accurate transmission of procedures and diagnosis information between health care providers and various agencies that compile health care statistics and the insurance companies that act as third-party payers for health care services rendered to patients. To code accurately, the medical assistant must have a good understanding of medical terminology, especially of those medical specialties found in the ambulatory care setting.

The use of computers to generate the insurance claim form and to transmit the form to the third-party payer is commonplace today. Computers are able to compute and compare numbers only. Letters that are in a sequence, such as the alphabet, are able to be compared as to their relativity to each other. For instance, *A* comes before *B* in the alphabet, and thus, a computer can compare those two values. For that reason, all charges, patient accounts, insurances, diagnoses and procedures, and even various categories are assigned letters or numbers (alphanumeric). The letters/numbers assigned to diagnoses and procedures (services) are called insurance codes. People whose jobs are to check accuracy of insurance codes and assign billing parameters (such as code modifiers) are called medical coders. (See the "Professional Careers in Insurance" section at the end of Chapter 16 for more information.)

INSURANCE CODING SYSTEMS OVERVIEW

Coding is the application of alphanumeric characters selected from standard terms used to describe a condition, disease, or service in health care. Medical codes come from complex **nomenclature systems** comprised of a detailed organization of information based on body systems. Health care staff need to use their knowledge about medical terminology, anatomy and physiology, pathophysiology, and pharmacology when performing medical coding tasks.

Purpose of Coding

Coding is done in order to process demographic, insurance, and coded medical diagnoses and procedures in order to request reimbursement for services and supplies used in health care. The coded information is analyzed to improve quality of medical care through the development and use of quality indicators, which provides information for public health and safety. This includes processes to decrease outbreaks of contagious diseases.

Another use of coded information includes the identification of risk factors used to develop standards for treatment and prevention of diseases. In addition, the purpose of coding includes the improvement and development of new treatments, supplies, and medications and technology. Payers use coded data to determine that the appropriate level of services are provided for specific conditions in order to make payment determinations. Health care costs are controlled through the combination of medical codes and documentation guidelines which are necessary to justify medical necessity for the services provided to the patient.

Medical necessity is required to ensure that services or procedures for a specific diagnosis or specified frequency are in order for consideration for reimbursement by the patient's insurance covered benefits. This is directed by 42 CFR 405.500 1995. The provider of services is responsible for documenting that the service is necessary and is covered by the insurance plan.

The HIPAA Administrative Simplification Act provision of 1996 ruled that electronic transmission of health care data complies with legal standards. It mandated the use of standardized code sets for submission of health care data.

CODE SETS

The process of translating written or spoken description of diseases, injuries, medical procedures, services, and supplies into numeric or alphanumeric format is called *coding*. The following coding systems are used within the United States.

Current Procedural Terminology (CPT®)

The **Current Procedural Terminology (CPT)** system was developed by the American Medical Association (AMA) to convert commonly accepted descriptions of medical procedures into a five-digit numeric code with two-digit numeric **modifiers** when required. CPT guidelines instruct the coder to add more codes. **Symbols** are used to visually represent instructions. Modifiers are important because they can impact the charge that is associated with the code. This system is used to code medical procedures such as clinic visits, X-rays, laboratory tests, and professional fees for providers who have performed surgery. Each CPT code has a fee schedule which is used to request reimbursement.

The American Medical Association publishes the CPT manual annually. The first edition was published in 1966. The six sections of the CPT coding system include:

Evaluation and Management	99201 to 99499
Anesthesiology	00100 to 01999, 99100 to 99140
Surgery	10021 to 69990
Radiology (Including Nuclear Medicine and Diagnostic Ultrasound)	70010 to 79999
Pathology and Laboratory	80047 to 89398
Medicine (Except Anesthesiology)	90281 to 99199, 99500 to 99607

To determine the CPT code, turn to the Category I section of the CPT code book and select one of the sections that constitutes the general classification of the procedure being coded (e.g., Surgery, Radiology). Then select the name of the procedure or service that accurately identifies what you are looking for. Read all of the codes that are indented below the main code. Indented codes provide greater specificity. Do not select a CPT code that only approximately defines the service performed. If you cannot find a name that exactly defines the service provided, report the service using the appropriate unlisted code. Unlisted codes are found at the end of each subsection in the CPT code book, and are also listed within the guidelines that precede each of the main sections. Most unlisted CPT codes end in 99. When using an unlisted code, a special report must be submitted with an insurance claim form to avoid denial or rejection. A special report will contain the nature, extent, and need of the procedure performed. An example of a special report would be the provider's operative note. Unlisted codes should not be used if a Category III code is available. This section is found in the back of the code book and gives temporary codes for emerging technologies, services, and procedures.

Evaluation and Management. The Evaluation and Management section takes every possible combination of visits into consideration and assigns each its own number. For instance, Mary O'Keefe, a new patient, is seen for a period of 45 minutes during which the provider takes a detailed history, examines the patient, and makes a medical decision of moderate complexity. The CPT code for this visit (99204) is found by looking under Office and Other Outpatient Services, New Patient. In another instance, Abigail Johnson, an established patient, is seen in the hospital for several days. These visits (99231, 99232, or 99233) would be found under Hospital Services, Subsequent Hospital Care. Codes for any type of evaluation and management are found in this section. In many clinics, the provider determines the level or charge for visits; however, the medical assistant must be familiar with all of the codes to make certain that billings are correct and that codes match the provider's documentation.

Anesthesiology. The Anesthesiology section includes all codes for anesthesia required for any procedure (with the exception of local anesthesia). The codes listed begin with the head and continue down the body to the legs and feet, concluding with anesthesia for radiologic procedures. If you want to find the correct code for anesthesia during a total hip replacement (arthroplasty), you will find Anesthesia in the index, look for the subterm *hip*, and refer to the range of codes listed: 01200 to 01215. When you refer back to the Anesthesia section, you find:

01200 Anesthesia for all closed procedures involving hip joint

01202 Anesthesia for arthroscopic procedures of hip joint

01210 Anesthesia for open procedures involving hip joint; not otherwise specified

01212 hip disarticulation

01214 total hip arthroplasty

01215 revision of total hip arthroplasty

As you read through the codes, you see that the correct code is 01214. Please note that this CPT code represents only the services provided by the anesthesiologist, not the surgical procedure itself.

Surgery. The section on surgery divides the codes according to body system. It begins with the integumentary system, and continues through subsequent systems ending with the ocular and auditory systems. The codes are very specific in this section, and care must be taken at all times to ensure the selection of the correct code. For example, a simple laceration repair of the neck is found as:

12001 Simple repair of superficial wounds of scalp, neck, axillae, external genitalia, trunk and/or extremities (including hands and feet): 2.5 cm or less

12002 2.6 cm to 7.5 cm

12004 7.6 cm to 12.5 cm

12005 12.6 cm to 20.0 cm

12006 20.1 cm to 30.0 cm

12007 over 30.0 cm

Thus, the exact length of the laceration and complexity of the repair can be found and coded correctly on the claim form. However, the aforementioned code description illustrates three important points. First, the code selected must represent the site of the laceration. Second, the code must represent the correct level of complexity for the repair. Third, the code must specify the correct length of the repair. If the medical assistant selects a code that is off by even just one digit, there would be a delay in reimbursement. The insurance claim would have to be corrected and resubmitted to the insurance company.

Radiology. Coding in the Radiology section covers each procedure done and each specific alteration to the procedure. For instance:

75889 Hepatic venography, wedged or free, *with* hemodynamic evaluation, radiological supervision, and interpretation

75891 Hepatic venography, wedged or free, *without* hemodynamic evaluation, radiological supervision, and interpretation

Radiologic procedures are not often done in the provider's clinic, although they may be in larger urgent care centers. Occasionally, chest X-rays are done or, in an orthopedic specialty, many skeletal X-rays may be done. More often, though, radiologic studies are ordered by the provider through a local facility that bills the insurance company directly, using the **diagnosis** the provider has provided.

Pathology and Laboratory. The Pathology and Laboratory section includes every test and combination of laboratory tests that can be ordered, as well as a section on surgical pathologic evaluation. This latter section includes specimens sent for examination, such as Pap smears, analysis of biopsy tissue from surgical sites, and tissue typing. Following is an example of a laboratory procedure code for

hepatitis B that illustrates the complete selection of tests that may be ordered:

87340 Hepatitis B surface antigen (HBsAg)

86704 Hepatitis B core antibody (HBcAb); total

86705 IgM antibody

86706 Hepatitis B surface antibody (HBsAb)

87350 Hepatitis Be antigen (HBeAg)

86707 Hepatitis Be antibody (HBeAb)

Once again, it is very important that the code for the exact service be selected. The medical assistant should be aware of laboratory codes because when a laboratory test is ordered, the laboratory may call to clarify the order. If the coding is correct, the laboratory should have no questions.

For surgical pathologic evaluation, the codes are different. The level of examination (gross and microscopic) for the item determines the code. The provider usually determines these levels or the charge for these services based on the type of tissue obtained, and the reason for the service.

Medicine. The section of the CPT entitled Medicine includes codes for immunizations, injections, dialysis, allergen immunotherapy, and chemotherapy, as well as ophthalmologic, cardiovascular, pulmonary, and neurologic procedures, to name a few. Some of the procedures are considered invasive, although others are not. As in the earlier sections, there is a comprehensive breakdown of each procedure. For example:

Cardiography

93000 Electrocardiogram, routine ECG with at least 12 leads; with interpretation and report

93005 tracing only, without interpretation and report

93010 interpretation and report only

Chemotherapy Administration

96409 intravenous, push technique, single or initial substance/drug

96413 Chemotherapy administration, intravenous infusion technique; up to 1 hour, single or initial substance/drug

+96415 each additional hour (List separately in addition to code for primary procedure)

96416 initiation of prolonged chemotherapy infusion (more than 8 hours), requiring use of a portable or implantable pump

The plus symbol (+) before the CPT code indicates that the procedure is an add-on to a previously described procedure. For example, 96413 would be used to describe the service and the time administered up to 1 hour. Use +96415 for each additional 1 hour of administration.

Index. The final portion of the CPT code book is a comprehensive index listing every procedure alphabetically. The proper use of the CPT code book involves looking for the procedure in the index by its main term and then checking the number given to determine the precise code.

Category I codes found in the CPT have five numeric digits. This is the level of codes that are used the most to describe procedures and other professional services. Category II and Category III codes are made of four numeric digits and are followed by an alpha character. These codes would be used when no specific Category I code is available. Note that there are no decimal points in any of the codes. Each five-digit code stands for a specific procedure not duplicated elsewhere.

Modifiers. Occasionally, a service or procedure needs to be modified or altered in a certain way. In that case, there are two-digit numeric modifiers that can be applied to the five-digit CPT code. These modifiers can indicate unusual procedural services (–22), bilateral procedures (–50), multiple procedures (–51), two surgeons (–62), surgical team (–66), or repeat procedure by same provider (–76).

The modifiers are listed in the inside front cover of each of the CPT code books as well as Appendix A of the book to alert the coder to use modifiers available for that code. In addition, there are other modifiers of an alpha or alphanumeric nature that are also listed in the front of the CPT code book. These modifiers come from the HCPCS code book, and are commonly used with CPT codes. Review the following examples that illustrate the use of modifiers:

> Surgical arthroscopy of the right shoulder with rotator cuff repair: 29827-RT
>
> Bilateral otoplasty, protruding ear, with or without size reduction: 69300-50
>
> Blepharoplasty of the lower right eyelid; extensive herniated fat pad: 15821-E4

Procedure

See Procedure 17-1 for instructions on CPT coding.

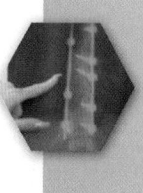

Critical Thinking

In which code book would you look to find the code for upper gastrointestinal endoscopy, simple primary examination (e.g., with small-diameter flexible endoscope) (separate procedure)? Which code did you select?

PROCEDURE 17–1

Coding with Current Procedural Terminology

Procedure

PURPOSE:

To convert commonly accepted descriptions of medical procedures (services) and visits of all types—clinic, hospital, nursing facility, home services—into a five-digit numeric code with two-digit numeric modifiers when required.

EQUIPMENT/SUPPLIES:

- CPT code book for the current year
- Copy of the encounter form and access to the patient's chart
- Pencil and paper

CASE SCENARIO:

Jane Smith, a new patient, is seen for 10 minutes, during which the provider takes a focused history and completes a problem-focused examination. A routine urinalysis, non-automated and without microscopy, is performed and a

(continues)

straightforward medical decision is made. Jane's preliminary diagnosis is painful urination. The urinalysis confirms a urinary tract infection. The provider writes her a prescription for an antibiotic and asks her to make an appointment in 10 days for another urinalysis to confirm the infection has cleared.

PROCEDURE STEPS:

1. Using the CPT code book, look in the Evaluation and Management section, Office or Other Outpatient Services, New Patient. Carefully read through the options until the code matching the described scenario has been found. RATIONALE: This section of the CPT code book provides codes used to report evaluation and management services provided in the provider's clinic or in an outpatient or other ambulatory care facility. You should have selected 99201.

2. Continue with the CPT code book, turn to the Index again, and look up Urinalysis, Routine. The code given is 81002. RATIONALE: This provides you with a code to investigate and determine its appropriateness.

3. Continue in the CPT code book and turn to the Pathology and Laboratory section. Follow the codes until you locate code 81002. When verifying the code, 81002 is an indented code and specifically states that the test is nonautomated, without microscopy. Be sure the description provided there matches what the provider has documented in the patient's chart. RATIONALE: To verify that the code is correct and matches documentation.

Healthcare Common Procedure Coding System (HCPCS)

Healthcare Common Procedure Coding System (HCPCS) was developed by Medicare as a supplement to the CPT system for procedures not defined with sufficient specificity. This system uses a five-digit alphanumeric code (one letter followed by four numbers) with an additional two-digit alphanumeric modifier if required. This code set includes supplies, durable medical equipment, and other medical services. Table 17-1 depicts the organization of the HCPCS codes.

Finding an HCPCS Code. Codes can be located by finding the main term or subterm in the alphabetical index. The name of the item, the type of service, the anatomical site, or abbreviation can also be used to look up the code. Modifiers are used to provide addition information about a service, item, or procedure. The code consists of a letter followed by four numbers. The Table of Drugs provides codes for the generic and brand names of drugs. Verify the code in the tabular list. You can also locate the code range and search the code that is needed.

International Classification of Diseases, Ninth Revision, Clinical Modification (ICD-9-CM)

The **International Classification of Diseases, 9th Revision, Clinical Modification (ICD-9-CM)** system was developed by the World Health Organization (WHO) in 1979 to classify all known diseases and disorders to assist in maintaining statistical records of **morbidity** (sickness) and **mortality** (death). Until October 2015, this system was used for both diagnostic coding (for all health care settings) and procedure coding (for inpatient services only). The ICD-9-CM code consists of a three-digit code (called a *category*) with one or two numeric digits following a decimal point. The ICD-9-CM coding manual was revised periodically and was updated yearly.

International Classification of Diseases, 10th Revision, Clinical Modification (ICD-10-CM)

The **International Classification of Diseases, 10th Revision, Clinical Modification (ICD-10-CM)** was developed by the World Health Organization in 1992. The official version is called the International Classification of Diseases (ICD-10). The WHO is responsible for revisions every 10 years. The United States implemented ICD-10-CM in October 2015 to replace ICD-9-CM. The National Center for Health Statistics is responsible for maintaining the diagnostic codes. The Centers for Medicare and Medicaid Services is responsible for maintaining the procedure codes for ICD-10-CM.

Revisions in ICD-10-CM from ICD-9-CM include the use of six and seven characters. In

TABLE 17-1

ORGANIZATION OF HCPCS CODES

CODE RANGE	DESCRIPTION
A0000 to A9999	Transportation services such as ambulance; medical and surgical supplies, including supplies for urinary incontinence, ostomy, respiratory, and dialysis; and radiopharmaceuticals
B4000 to B9999	Supplies, equipment, and nutritional products for enteral and parenteral nutrition
C1300 to C9899	New technology procedures, drugs, biologicals, radiopharmaceuticals, magnetic resonance angiography (MRA), and devices for outpatient hospitals to report
D Codes	Dental services—the ADA holds the copyright to D codes; they usually do not appear in the HCPCS manual
E0100 to C8002	Durable medical equipment (DME) for patient's activities of daily living, including crutches and oxygen equipment
G0008 to G9360	Procedures and services that may or may not have equivalent CPT codes, such as screening exams
H0001 to H2037	Mental health services, including treatment for alcohol and drug use
J0120 to J9999	Drugs that the patient does not self-administer
K00014 to K0900	DME for which there are no other HCPCS codes available, such as power wheelchairs
L0112 to L9900	Orthotics (devices that help to regain function) and prosthetics (replacement body parts), including cervical collars, lumbar support, artificial limbs, and male vacuum erection systems
M0064 to M0301	Codes represent an office visit for prescription drugs and miscellaneous therapies
P2028 to P9615	Pathology and laboratory services and blood products
Q0035 to Q9968	Temporary codes for drugs and supplies
R0070 to R0076	Transportation of portable diagnostic radiology equipment to provider locations
S0012 to S9999	Drugs, services, and supplies for Medicaid and other non-Medicare payers
T1000 to T5999	Medicaid services and supplies
V2020 to V564	Vision supplies, such as eyeglasses; hearing services and supplies; and speech language pathology services

Source: Centers for Medicare and Medicaid Services, www.cms.gov

addition, the codes have laterality and greater specificity. There were thousands of codes added from version ICD-9-CM. There are 1,943 new codes; 351 revised codes; and 313 deleted codes for the 2017 ICD-10-CM as published by CMS.

Revisions to the ICD-10-CM include codes that specify laterality such as the right arm or the left arm. Chapter 19, "Injury, Poisoning and Certain Other Consequences of External Causes (S00-T88)," has been expanded to include additional codes. There has been an increase of combination codes in which the code defines both a diagnoses and symptoms, reducing the need to record additional codes. The use of a sixth and seventh character contributes to greater specificity and validity for diseases, injuries, conditions, procedures, and so on. The official coding guidelines appear at the front of the coding manual as well as at the beginning of each chapter. In addition, there are two types of Excludes notes.

Tools used to convert ICD-9 to ICD-10 codes are called gem maps. These maps are published on the CMS Web site. It is important for many reasons to know how to convert the codes. One reason is to research and compare statistical data from the codes. Another reason is for claims resolution and processing of older claims. Because there are more codes in ICD-10, many of the codes do not directly convert from ICD-9.

The intent of the International Classification Disease system is to record morbidity and mortality. Morbidity is defined as conditions, injuries, or diseases that are not considered normal health. The physician documents changes in morbidity in the health record for each patient encounter. HIPAA mandates the recording of the various ICD-10-CM classifications as a standard in the electronic health care transactions for reporting purposes. Data generated from the reporting process are used to track diseases, injuries, and impairments in the population. Mortality means death.

There are 21 chapters in ICD-10-CM. Table 17-2 lists the code range and the description of each chapter.

ICD-10-CM uses conventions, instructional notes, punctuation marks, and abbreviations to help the coder select the appropriate code. Selecting the correct code is necessary in order for the code to be complete, correct, and accurate. The coding guidelines define the use of each convention. Examples include code also, code first, excludes 1, excludes 2, in diseases classified elsewhere, includes, not elsewhere classified (NEC), not otherwise specified (NOS), see, see also, and use additional codes. Examples of symbols include brackets, colon, parentheses, and a-point dash.

The coding guidelines are located at the beginning of the ICD-10-CM book as well as at the beginning of each chapter. The guidelines reference the appendices and sections. The coder must be familiar with these coding guidelines.

Procedure

See Procedure 17-2 for instructions on ICD-10-CM coding.

How to Find an ICD-10-CM Code. Using the main term, subterm, or synonym, search in the alphabetic index at the beginning of the code book. Find the code in the tabular section of the code book making sure to follow any instructions or directions described by symbols or coding guidelines.

ICD-10-PCS

ICD-10-PCS codes have seven alphanumeric characters. Each character has a specific meaning and/or value. The 16 sections of ICD-10-PCS include Medical and Surgical, Obstetrics, Placement, Administration, Measurement and Monitoring, Extracorporeal Assistance and Performance, Extracorporeal Therapies, Osteopathic, Other Procedures, Chiropractic, Imaging, Nuclear Medicine, Radiation Oncology, Physical Rehabilitation and Diagnostic Audiology, Mental Health, and Substance Abuse Treatment. These sections each have a number, which represents the first character of the PCS code. The remaining characters represent the following:

- The second place character represents the body system. There are 31 body systems that range from the central nervous system to the anatomical regions, lower extremities.

- The third place character represents the root operations. There are 31 root operations for the Medical Surgical section. Additional root operations are assigned for the other sections.

- The fourth place character represents the specific part of the body system on which the procedure is performed.

- The fifth place character for the Medical and Surgical codes is the approach used in the procedure. For example, an open approach means a cutting through of the skin or mucous membrane and any other body layers necessary to expose the site of the procedure.

- The sixth character indicates a device and specifies the device that remains after the procedure is completed. An example of one of the four types of devices is a cardiac pacemaker.

- The seventh character in the Medical Surgical section is a qualifier that has a unique value for an individual procedure.

TABLE 17-2

ICD-10-CM CODE RANGES AND DESCRIPTIONS

CODE RANGE	DESCRIPTION
A00 to B99	Certain infectious and parasitic diseases
C00 to D49	Neoplasms
D50 to D89	Diseases of the blood and blood-forming organs and certain disorders involving the immune mechanism
E00 to E89	Endocrine, nutritional, and metabolic diseases
F01 to F99	Mental, behavioral, and neurodevelopmental disorders
G00 to G99	Disease of the nervous system
H00 to H59	Diseases of the eye and adnexa
H60 to H95	Diseases of the ear and mastoid process
I00 to I99	Diseases of the circulatory system
J00 to J99	Diseases of the respiratory system
K00 to K95	Diseases of the digestive system
L00 to L99	Diseases of the skin and subcutaneous tissue
M00 to M99	Disease of the musculoskeletal system and connective tissue
N00 to N99	Diseases of the genitourinary system
O00 to O9A	Pregnancy, childbirth, and the puerperium
P00 to P96	Certain conditions originating in the perinatal period
Q00 to Q99	Congenital malformations, deformations, and chromosomal abnormalities
R00 to R99	Symptoms, signs, and abnormal clinical and laboratory findings, not elsewhere classified
S00 to T88	Injury and poisoning and certain other consequences of external causes
V00 to V99	External causes of morbidity
Z00 to Z99	Factors influencing health status and contact with health services

Source: Centers for Medicare and Medicaid Services, www.cms.gov

How to Use the ICD-10-PCS Code Book. Use the index at the beginning of the book. Using terms or general types of procedures, locate the correct PCS table which identifies the seven characters of the PCS code. Each code has a row that identifies the details of the procedure.

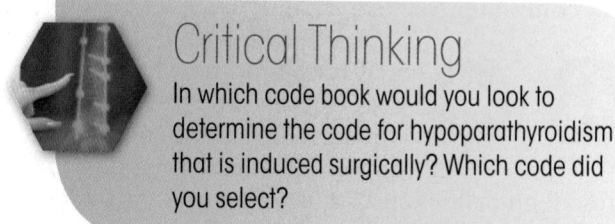

Critical Thinking

In which code book would you look to determine the code for hypoparathyroidism that is induced surgically? Which code did you select?

PROCEDURE 17–2

Procedure

Coding with International Classification of Diseases, 10th Revision, Clinical Modification

PURPOSE:

The ICD-10-CM code books provide a diagnostic coding system for the compilation and reporting of morbidity and mortality statistics for reimbursement purposes.

EQUIPMENT/SUPPLIES:

- ICD-10-CM code books for the current year
- Copy of the encounter form and access to the patient's chart
- Pencil and paper

CASE SCENARIO:

Mary O'Keefe, a new patient, presents at the clinic today reporting painful, frequent urination. She is seen for 10 minutes, during which time the provider takes a focused history and completes a problem-focused examination. A routine urinalysis, nonautomated and without microscopy, is performed and a straightforward medical decision is made. Mary's preliminary diagnosis is painful urination. The urinalysis confirms a urinary tract infection. The provider writes her a prescription for an antibiotic and asks her to make an appointment in 10 days for another urinalysis to confirm the infection has cleared.

PROCEDURE STEPS:

1. Using the ICD-10-CM code book, the alphanumeric Index to Diseases, look up the main symptom or condition that brought the patient to the facility or the specific diagnosis confirmed by test results. In this case, the laboratory results confirmed a urinary tract infection. Code N39.0. RATIONALE: Uses alphanumeric index choosing urinary tract infection.

2. Using the tabular section, look up code N39.0. Read through all of the N39 listings to determine the appropriate code having the highest level of specificity. RATIONALE: Establishes the most accurate code: urinary tract infection, site not specified.

MEDICAL CODING

Legal

When performing billing procedures, medical assistants and medical administrative staff are expected to adhere to ethical standards and legal practices. All diagnostic and procedural codes reported must be supported by documentation in the patient's chart. Understanding medical terminology, anatomy, pathology, pharmacology, and information about procedures is critical to coding accuracy and completeness.

Competency   Initiative

It is also important to maintain coding skills by attending continuing education activities that discuss changes in codes and present guidelines and regulatory requirements necessary for accurate coding and timely reimbursement

for services and supplies. Networking with other medical coders is another valuable method of staying current with what is happening in this profession. Organizations such as the American Health Information Management Association (AHIMA) and the American Academy of Professional Coders (AAPC) offer webinars, seminars, and online training sessions.

CODING ACCURACY

Accuracy and completeness in coding is vitally important. Imprecise coding affects how quickly the provider is reimbursed and the correct amount of the reimbursement. Codes must be appropriate to the documentation. Insurance carriers always **down-code** if documentation or codes are ambiguous and reimburse the provider for the lowest possible fee. Following are the three primary reasons why down-coding happens:

- The coding system used on the claim form does not match the coding system used by the insurance carrier. Failure to routinely update the charge master contributes to this problem. The carrier's computer will convert the submitted claim code to the closest recognized code. In most cases, the reimbursement amount will be less because each CPT code is assigned a fee schedule.

- If a Workers' Compensation claims examiner has to convert a CPT code to a relative value scale (RVS) code, the examiner will select the lowest-paying code. When billing Workers' Compensation, always use the RVS system used by that carrier and match the code to the best description of the CPT code.

- When attached documentation does not match the written description of the procedure, the reimbursement will always be the lowest-paying code that fits the written description. Denial of payment may occur due to a lack of documentation for medical necessity. As stated earlier, medical necessity is required to ensure that services or procedures for a specific diagnosis or specified frequency are in order for consideration for reimbursement by the patient's insurance covered benefits.

Up-coding, also known as *code creep, overcoding,* or *overbilling,* occurs when—to obtain greater reimbursements—the insurance carrier is deliberately billed for a higher rate service than what was performed. Computer software programs have been developed to detect this practice easily and are called scrubbers. Often, complete audits are performed to assess the extent of up-coding practices. Sanctions and penalties are imposed on offenders due to fraud and abuse allegations.

Assumptive coding is assigning a code before the diagnostic code is confirmed.

The Medicare program, in particular, uses CPT codes, which are **bundled codes**. A bundled code is a grouping of several services that are directly related to a specific procedure and are paid as one. For example, surgical dressings and reading test results may be bundled into evaluation and management codes. **Unbundling** refers to separating the components of a procedure and reporting them as billable codes with charges to increase reimbursement rates. This procedure may also be termed *fragmentation, exploding,* or *à la carte medicine.* This practice is considered fraud and may lead to audit, sanctions, and penalties.

The more accurate the coding on the claim form, the less chance there is for error, the more quickly the provider is reimbursed, and the better the chance that the provider's reimbursement will reflect the actual charge. Many insurance carriers keep a fee profile of each provider's charges. This profile reflects the amount of each charge for each service and can affect the provider's reimbursement for those services.

Do not guess when coding. The code becomes a permanent part of the patient's health record with the insurance carrier. If an incorrect code is used, that coded diagnosis will stay with that patient. This can be a difficult problem for insured persons if they change insurance carriers or if other health problems occur. Examples of protected diagnosis of health condition include HIV, AIDS, substance abuse, mental health conditions, and sickle cell anemia.

Consider a patient with hip pain. She has a history of ovarian cancer for which she has had radiology treatments. The hip pain is thought to be possible metastases from the original cancer site. When ruling out this possibility, the provider indicates the following code for the claim:

C79.89 Secondary malignant neoplasm of other specified sites: hip

When the pain is finally discovered to be arthritis and it is determined that the patient needs a hip replacement, the insurance carrier denies coverage for this operation for the following reason: The patient's condition is terminal, and the company does not want her to spend her last months having surgery and recovering from surgery when she is already in poor health. And, of course, there is the cost factor to consider in the eyes of the insurance carrier.

Incorrect coding can be a problem with ruling out a diagnosis. For instance, a patient presents many symptoms of peptic ulcer disease. Do not immediately code that patient as having that disease (which would be assumptive coding) until the diagnosis is confirmed. Instead, code the symptoms. When the tests come back and a specific diagnosis of peptic ulcer can be made, then code the disease as:

K27.7 chronic peptic ulcer, site unspecified, without hemorrhage or perforation

National Correct Coding Initiative (NCCI)

The Centers for Medicare and Medicaid Services (CMS) developed the National Correct Coding Initiative (NCCI) to promote national correct coding methodologies and to control improper coding leading to inappropriate payment in Part B claims. CMS developed its coding policies based on coding conventions defined in the AMA's CPT Manual, national and local policies and edits, coding guidelines developed by national societies, analysis of standard medical and surgical practices, and review of current coding practices.

CODING THE CLAIM FORM

For the insurance company to understand what is being billed, the claim form is completed by the medical assistant, administrative office staff, or billing clerk in the ambulatory care setting. The provider completes an **encounter form**, also known as a **superbill**, at the time of the visit. This encounter form (Figure 17-1) includes the date of service, the visit or consultation code, diagnoses for this visit, procedures done and laboratory tests ordered, and if necessary, the date the patient is to return. This information is then translated onto the claim form.

The **CMS-1500 (02-12)** is the claim form accepted by all insurance carriers (see Figure 16-3). This form is prepared using words and CPT codes

---

PLEASE RETURN THIS FORM TO RECEPTIONIST

NAME
Receipt No:

PLACE OF SERVICE:
( ) OFFICE
( ) COUNTY HOSPITAL
( ) COMMUNITY GENERAL HOSPITAL
( ) RETIREMENT INN NURSING HOME
( ) _____

DATE OF SERVICE _____

A. OFFICE VISITS - New Patient

Code	History	Exam	Dec.	Time
99201	Prob. Foc.	Prob. Foc.	Straight	10 min.
99202	Ex. Prob. Foc.	Ex. Prob. Foc.	Straight	20 min.
99203	Detail	Detail	Low	30 min.
99204	Comp.	Comp.	Mod.	45 min.
99205	Comp.	Comp.	High	60 min.

B. OFFICE VISIT - Established Patient

Code	History	Exam	Dec.	Time
99211	Minimal	Minimal	Minimal	5 min.
99212	Prob. Foc.	Prob. Foc.	Straight	10 min.
99213	Ex. Prob. Foc.	Ex. Prob. Foc.	Low	15 min.
99214	Detail	Detail	Mod.	25 min.
99215	Comp.	Comp.	High	40 min.

C. HOSPITAL CARE   Dx   Units
1. Initial Hospital Care (30 min) _____   99221
2. Subsequent Care   99231
3. Critical Care (30-74 min)   99291
4. Each additional 30 min.   99292
5. Discharge Services   99238
6. Emergency Room   99282

D. NURSING HOME CARE   Dx   Units

Initial Care - New Pt.
1 Expanded   99322
2 Detailed   99323

Subsequent Care - Estab. Pt.
3 Problem Focused   99307
4 Expanded   99308
5 Detailed   99309
6 Comprehensive   99310

E. PROCEDURES
1 Arthrocentesis, Small Jt.   20600
2 Colonoscopy   45378
3 EKG w/interpretation   93000
4 X-Ray Chest, PA/LAT   71020

F. LAB
1 Blood Sugar   82947
2 CDC w/differential   85031
3 Cholesterol   82465
4 Comp. Metabolic Panel   80053
5 ESR   85651
6 Hematocrit   85014
7 Mono Screen   86308
8 Pap Smear   88150
9 Potassium   84132
10 Preg. Test, Quantitative   84702
11 Routine Venipuncture   36415

F. Cont'd   Dx   Units
12 Strep Screen   87081
13 UA, Routine w/Micro   81000
14 UA, Routine w/o Micro   81002
15 Uric Acid   84550
16 VDRL   86592
17 Wet Prep   82710
18 _____

G. INJECTIONS
1 Influenza Virus Vaccine   90658
2 Pneumoccocal Vaccine   90772
3 Tetanus Toxoids   90703
4 Therapeutic Subcut/IM   90732
5 Vaccine Administration   90471
6 Vaccine - each additional   90472

H. MISCELLANEOUS
1 _____
2 _____

Mark diagnosis with
(1=Primary, 2=Secondary, 3=Tertiary)

DIAGNOSIS NOT LISTED BELOW _____

DIAGNOSIS	ICD-10-CM 1, 2, 3
Allergic rhinitis, unsp	J30.9
Anemia, unsp	D64.9
Anemia, iron deficiency, unsp	D50.9
Anemia, Vit. B12 deficiency, intrinsic factor	D51.0
Angina pectoris, other forms	I20.8
Abdominal pain, unsp	R10.9
Asthma, unsp, w/acute exacerbation	J45.901
Asthma, unsp, uncomplicated	J45.909
Atrial fibrillation, unsp	I48.91
Chest pain, other	R07.89
Bronchiolitis, acute, due to RSV	J21.0
Bronchitis, acute, unsp	J20.9
Bronchitis, NOS	J40
Cardiac arrest, cause unsp	I46.9
Cellulitis, unsp	L03.90
CI D/T, unsp occl/sten, unsp cereb art	I63.50
Contact dermatitis, NOS	L25.9
Contact dermatitis, irritant, due to solvents	L24.2
Convulsions, unsp	R56.9
COPD, unsp	J44.9
CVD, unsp, w/unsp sequelae	I69.90
Dehydration	E86.0

DIAGNOSIS	ICD-10-CM 1, 2, 3
Depress dis, mjr, sing ep, unsp	F32.9
Diab mell, Type 2, w/o comp	E11.9
Diab mell, Type 2, w/ hyperglycemia	E11.65
Dizziness and giddiness	R42
Drug rx, adv, meds bio sub, init enc	T50.995A
Dysuria	R30.0
Edema, unsp	R60.9
Fatigue, other	R53.83
Fever, unsp	R50.9
Gastritis, acute, w/o bleeding	K29.00
Gastroenteritis, other spec, noninf	K52.89
GERD, w/o esophagitis	K21.9
Heart failure, unsp	I50.9
Hepatitis A, w/o hepatic coma	B15.9
Hypercholesterolemia, pure	E78.0
Hypertension, essential (primary)	I10
Hypoglycemia, unsp	E16.2
Hypokalemia	E87.6
Impetigo, unsp	L01.00
Lymphadenitis, nonspec, unspec	I88.9
Mental d/o, uns, D/T kwn phys cond	F09
Mono, inf, unsp, w/o comp	B27.90

DIAGNOSIS	ICD-10-CM 1, 2, 3
Myocardial infarction, STE, unsp site	I21.3
Osteoarthritis, NOS	M19.90
Otitis externa, other infective, unsp ear	H60.399
Otitis media, NOS	H66.90
Peripheral vascular disease, unsp	I73.9
Pharyngitis, acute, unsp	J02.9
Pneumonia, unsp organism	J18.9
Prostate inflammatory disease, unsp	N41.9
Pulmonary heart disease, unsp	I27.9
Rash and other nonsp skin eruption	R21
Serous otitis media, chronic, unsp ear	H65.20
Sinusitis, acute, unsp	J01.90
Stomach and duodenum disease, unsp	K31.9
Tonsillitis, acute, unsp	J03.90
Upper respiratory infection, acute, unsp	J06.9
Urinary tract infection, unsp	N39.0
Urticaria, unsp	L50.9
Ventricular premature depolarization	I49.3
Viral agent, other, cause dis class elsew	B97.89
Weight loss, abnormal	R63.4

INNER CITY HEALTH CARE
8600 MAIN STREET, SUITE 200
RIVER CITY, XY 01234
PHONE No. (123) 456-7890
EIN# 00-1234560

□ W. LEWIS, M.D.   □ M. KING, M.D.
NPI# 9995010111   NPI# 9995020212

□ R. REYNOLDS, M.D.
NPI# 9995030313

ABN: I UNDERSTAND THAT MEDICARE PROBABLY WILL NOT COVER THE SERVICES LISTED BELOW

A. _____   B. _____   C. _____
Patient
Date _____ Signature _____

Doctor's Signature _____

RETURN: _____ Days _____ Weeks _____ Months _____

FIGURE 17-1   Encounter form.

for procedures performed and ICD-10-CM codes for diagnoses. Keep in mind that the codes must correlate; for instance, if a person had an ICD-10-CM diagnosis code of earache, otitis media, or H66.90, and the CPT procedure code indicated was 69090, ear piercing, the insurance company would question the claim and reject it for payment. The person completing the claim form must be *as precise as possible*. If the coding is wrong, the claim will be denied and the provider will not receive payment. Claims tracking investigates all coding errors and potential denial or delays in payment. Coding must correlate with the documentation note in the chart; otherwise, fraud is committed.

Coding the claim form is a precise way to communicate with the insurance carrier. Coding indicates the complexity of the visit using an evaluation and management CPT code, the diagnosis for the visit, and the specific procedures such as injections performed during the visit. This results in little confusion, and a minimum of additional communication is needed between the carrier and the provider's clinic because all information is contained in the codes.

For instance, Leo McKay, an established patient, is seen for an extended visit to determine the cause of his abdominal pain. Symptoms include diarrhea, fever, nausea, and anorexia. An abdominal ultrasound is ordered, as well as laboratory tests, and the results are unknown at the time of the insurance billing. The visit lasts 30 minutes and includes a full physical examination and a history of the present illness.

The CPT procedure coding for this visit is 99214, which reflects the examination and time spent with the patient, the history taken of this illness, and a medical decision of moderate complexity.

The ICD-10-CM diagnosis coding for abdominal pain is R10.9, for diarrhea R19.7, for nausea R11.0, and for anorexia R63.0. The claim form is submitted to the insurance carrier with these codes, and even though they are all symptoms, the claim will be paid because the visit and the tests ordered interrelate.

When the test results are known, they show a positive diagnosis of *Giardia lamblia*. The diagnosis code is changed to A07.1. Any further charges sent to the insurance carrier while Leo McKay is being treated for this problem are coded A07.1. The symptom codes from the first submission are dropped. *The Official ICD-10-CM Guidelines for Coding and Reporting* state that when signs and symptoms are integral to a definitive diagnosis, you are to code only for the definitive diagnosis.

Many electronic health records (EHR) use encoder programs (Figure 17-2), which are available online. Encoder programs are coding software programs that allow the user to locate CPT, ICD-10-CM, and HCPCS codes quickly using the computer. Many of the encoder programs permit the placement of bookmarks or notes for quick reference.

THIRD-PARTY PRIVACY, SECURITY, AND COMPLIANCE GUIDELINES

Legal   Integrity

Because patient information is easily accessed through medical charts, EHR, and the human factor, security and confidentiality measures must be in place in medical clinics. When patients schedule an appointment and are seen by the provider, they enter into a contract for specific services. The first party is the person receiving the contracted service. The second party

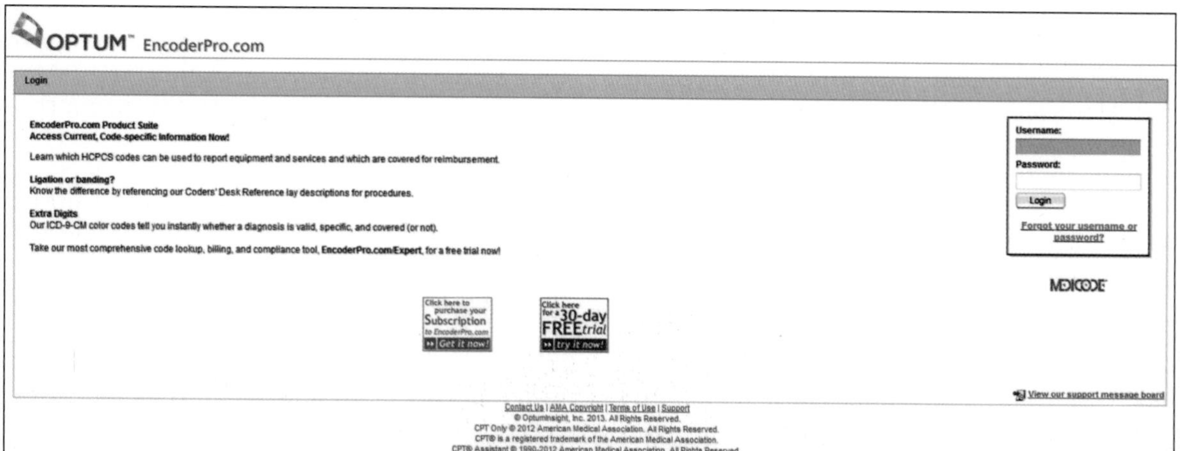

FIGURE 17-2 Encoder software.

is the person or organization providing the service. A third party is one that is not involved in the patient–provider relationship but rather with reimbursement procedures.

The patient has a right to expect that his or her health information will not be disseminated to others without written permission to do so. Confidentiality issues involve restricting the health information to only those individuals who need to know. Compliance with Health Insurance Portability and Accountability Act (HIPAA) of 1996 regulations is one way to safeguard protected health information (PHI). Chapters 11, 12, 13, 14, 15, and 17 of the HIPAA regulations all place emphasis on HIPAA as it relates to PHI.

Authorization to release necessary medical information to payers, such as insurance carriers, must be obtained from the patient, the parent, or the guardian *before* any information is released. A *breach of confidentiality* is the release of unauthorized PHI to a third party. One way to prevent this when processing insurance claims forms is to ask the patient, parent, or guardian to sign an authorization to release medical information statement *before* the claim form is completed. The CMS-1500 (02-12) form provides space for this signature in block 12.

Some medical clinics, especially those that send claim forms electronically, develop their own specialized authorization for release of medical information form. The customized form must contain the specific name of the insurance company and must be signed by the patient, parent, or guardian. This form is generally valid for 1 year. The insurance company may request a copy of the signed form. When completing the CMS-1500 (02-12), block 12 may contain the words *SIGNATURE ON FILE* or the abbreviation *SOF*. Practice management software typically tracks the signature dates.

Three authorization exceptions are allowed by the federal government. The first two exceptions apply to Medicaid and Workers' Compensation. In these instances, the patient becomes a third-party beneficiary in the contract between the health care provider and the government agency sponsoring the insurance program. Providers agree to accept the program's payment as payment in full, and the patient may be billed only if the payer does not cover services rendered or if the patient is ineligible for benefits. The third exception is related to hospital admission. The patient must sign a release of medical information *before* being seen by the provider or receiving treatment in a hospital.

 Most states have specific laws related to release of protected medical information regarding mental health services and federally assisted alcohol and drug abuse programs. Patients being screened for HIV infection or AIDS must sign an additional authorization statement *before* information may be released regarding their status. See Procedure 17-3 for specific steps involved in authorization to release PHI to third-party payers.

COMPLETING THE CMS-1500 (02-12)

In most clinics today, the CMS-1500 (02-12) form is completed using data from the patient's EHR. In the few cases in which the clinic does not use EHR, the paper encounter form is used by the billing specialist to complete the CMS-1500 (02-12) form. Each insurance carrier has its own thoughts on how the form is to be completed and no two companies agree entirely on the information required, the boxes checked, and the rationale about what information goes in which boxes.

With the transition to an increase in electronic claims submission and the HIPAA regulations, the National Uniform Claim Committee (NUCC) established a standardized data set for use in an electronic environment as well as with paper claim form standards. The NUCC continues to monitor how insurance carriers use the various claim form fields. Additional changes to the CMS-1500 (02-12) form may be required in the future as the NUCC works to create standardized national instructions for completing the form.

To illustrate the completion of a claim form, a fictitious insurance carrier will be used. Insurance carriers often change their rules and regulations for submitting claims. To avoid out-of-date material, we sent this claim for payment to How Much Insurance Company. Using the example given of Leo McKay in the coding section, the CMS-1500 (02-12) in Figure 17-3 shows the properly completed claim form.

Remember, many insurance carriers require some of the boxes to be filled in and others left blank. The billing person for the medical clinic needs to comply with the current requirements of the insurance carrier that is being billed. There is no right or wrong answer for every insurance carrier. If there is a question about billing, check with that carrier about its requirements. There are certain formatting guidelines for completing the claim form that will remain consistent, no matter which insurance company you are dealing with:

PROCEDURE 17-3

Procedure

Applying Third-Party Guidelines

PURPOSE:

To obtain written authorization to release necessary medical information to third-party payers.

EQUIPMENT/SUPPLIES:

- Patient chart
- CMS-1500 (02-12) claim form

PROCEDURE STEPS:

1. When the patient signs in at the reception desk, check his or her chart to ascertain whether an authorization to release medical information form has been signed and is currently valid. RATIONALE: PHI cannot be released without written authorization from the patient.

2. If there is no record of signature on file, have the patient sign block 12 of the CMS-1500 (02-12) claim form or the offices' customized authorization to release medical information form. RATIONALE: PHI cannot be released without written authorization from the patient.

1. MEDICARE	MEDICAID	TRICARE	CHAMPVA	GROUP HEALTH PLAN	FECA BLK LUNG	OTHER
(Medicare#)	(Medicaid#)	(ID#/DoD#)	(Member ID#)	(ID#)	(ID#)	(ID#)

2. PATIENT'S NAME (Last Name, First Name, Middle Initial)

3. PATIENT'S BIRTH DATE — MM | DD | YY — SEX M ☐ F ☐

5. PATIENT'S ADDRESS (No., Street)

6. PATIENT RELATIONSHIP TO INSURED — Self ☐ Spouse ☐ Child ☐ Other ☐

CITY — STATE

8. RESERVED FOR NUCC USE

ZIP CODE — TELEPHONE (Include Area Code) ( )

9. OTHER INSURED'S NAME (Last Name, First Name, Middle Initial)

10. IS PATIENT'S CONDITION RELATED TO:

a. OTHER INSURED'S POLICY OR GROUP NUMBER

a. EMPLOYMENT? (Current or Previous) — YES ☐ NO ☐

b. RESERVED FOR NUCC USE

b. AUTO ACCIDENT? — PLACE (State) — YES ☐ NO ☐

c. RESERVED FOR NUCC USE

c. OTHER ACCIDENT? — YES ☐ NO ☐

d. INSURANCE PLAN NAME OR PROGRAM NAME

10d. CLAIM CODES (Designated by NUCC)

READ BACK OF FORM BEFORE COMPLETING & SIGNING THIS FORM.

12. PATIENT'S OR AUTHORIZED PERSON'S SIGNATURE I authorize the release of any medical or other information necessary to process this claim. I also request payment of government benefits either to myself or to the party who accepts assignment below.

SIGNED _____ DATE _____

Courtesy of the Centers for Medicare & Medicaid Services, www.cms.gov

- The form must *always* be completed in black ink.
- The form must *always* be completed using all capital letters.
- The form must *never* contain any punctuation or symbols of any kind; only letters and numbers may be used.
- Any date entered on the form (DOS, DOB, etc.), must be in eight-digit format. For example, the DOB for our previously mentioned patient, Leo McKay, is April 1, 1963. Therefore, his DOB on the form should appear as 04011963. (Notice there are no hyphens or slashes.)

HEALTH INSURANCE CLAIM FORM

APPROVED BY NATIONAL UNIFORM CLAIM COMMITTEE (NUCC) 02/12

| | PICA | | | | | | | | | | | PICA | | |

1. MEDICARE ☐ (Medicare#) MEDICAID ☐ (Medicaid#) TRICARE ☐ (ID#/DoD#) CHAMPVA ☐ (Member ID#) GROUP HEALTH PLAN ☐ (ID#) FECA BLK LUNG ☐ (ID#) OTHER ☒ (ID#)

1a. INSURED'S I.D. NUMBER (For Program in Item 1)
555-55-555

2. PATIENT'S NAME (Last Name, First Name, Middle Initial)
MCKAY LEO M

3. PATIENT'S BIRTH DATE MM 04 DD 01 YY 1963 **SEX** M ☒ F ☐

4. INSURED'S NAME (Last Name, First Name, Middle Initial)
MCKAY, LEO M

5. PATIENT'S ADDRESS (No., Street)
123 W FIRST STREET

6. PATIENT RELATIONSHIP TO INSURED
Self ☒ Spouse ☐ Child ☐ Other ☐

7. INSURED'S ADDRESS (No., Street)
123 W FIRST STREET

CITY ANYWHERE   **STATE** XY

8. RESERVED FOR NUCC USE

CITY ANYWHERE   **STATE** XY

ZIP CODE 01234   **TELEPHONE** (Include Area Code) (123) 556-6189

ZIP CODE 01234   **TELEPHONE** (Include Area Code) (123) 556-6189

9. OTHER INSURED'S NAME (Last Name, First Name, Middle Initial)

10. IS PATIENT'S CONDITION RELATED TO:

11. INSURED'S POLICY GROUP OR FECA NUMBER
1122334

a. OTHER INSURED'S POLICY OR GROUP NUMBER

a. EMPLOYMENT? (Current or Previous) YES ☐ NO ☒

a. INSURED'S DATE OF BIRTH MM 04 DD 01 YY 1963 **SEX** M ☒ F ☐

b. RESERVED FOR NUCC USE

b. AUTO ACCIDENT? YES ☐ NO ☒ PLACE (State)

b. OTHER CLAIM ID (Designated by NUCC)

c. RESERVED FOR NUCC USE

c. OTHER ACCIDENT? YES ☐ NO ☒

c. INSURANCE PLAN NAME OR PROGRAM NAME

d. INSURANCE PLAN NAME OR PROGRAM NAME

10d. CLAIM CODES (Designated by NUCC)

d. IS THERE ANOTHER HEALTH BENEFIT PLAN? YES ☐ NO ☒ *If yes*, complete items 9, 9a, and 9d.

READ BACK OF FORM BEFORE COMPLETING & SIGNING THIS FORM.
12. PATIENT'S OR AUTHORIZED PERSON'S SIGNATURE I authorize the release of any medical or other information necessary to process this claim. I also request payment of government benefits either to myself or to the party who accepts assignment below.

SIGNED **SIGNATURE ON FILE**   DATE 01 14 20XX

13. INSURED'S OR AUTHORIZED PERSON'S SIGNATURE I authorize payment of medical benefits to the undersigned physician or supplier for services described below.

SIGNED **SIGNATURE ON FILE**

14. DATE OF CURRENT ILLNESS, INJURY, or PREGNANCY (LMP) MM 01 DD 10 YY 20XX QUAL.

15. OTHER DATE QUAL. MM DD YY

16. DATES PATIENT UNABLE TO WORK IN CURRENT OCCUPATION FROM MM DD YY TO MM DD YY

17. NAME OF REFERRING PROVIDER OR OTHER SOURCE

17a.
17b. NPI

18. HOSPITALIZATION DATES RELATED TO CURRENT SERVICES FROM MM DD YY TO MM DD YY

19. ADDITIONAL CLAIM INFORMATION (Designated by NUCC)

20. OUTSIDE LAB? YES ☐ NO ☐ $ CHARGES

21. DIAGNOSIS OR NATURE OF ILLNESS OR INJURY Relate A-L to service line below (24E)   ICD Ind. 10

A. R10.9   B. K52.89   C. R63.0   D.
E.   F.   G.   H.
I.   J.   K.   L.

22. RESUBMISSION CODE   ORIGINAL REF. NO.

23. PRIOR AUTHORIZATION NUMBER

24. A. DATE(S) OF SERVICE						B. PLACE OF SERVICE	C. EMG	D. PROCEDURES, SERVICES, OR SUPPLIES (Explain Unusual Circumstances) CPT/HCPCS MODIFIER	E. DIAGNOSIS POINTER	F. $ CHARGES	G. DAYS OR UNITS	H. EPSDT Family Plan	I. ID. QUAL.	J. RENDERING PROVIDER ID. #
From MM	DD	YY	To MM	DD	YY									
1	01	10	XX				3		99214	123	85 00	1		NPI	1543298760
2	01	10	XX				3		82270	12	13 00	1		NPI	1543298760
3														NPI	
4														NPI	
5														NPI	
6														NPI	

25. FEDERAL TAX I.D. NUMBER SSN ☐ EIN ☒
91-1234432

26. PATIENT'S ACCOUNT NO.
MCK111

27. ACCEPT ASSIGNMENT? (For govt. claims, see back) YES ☐ NO ☒

28. TOTAL CHARGE $ 98 00

29. AMOUNT PAID $

30. Rsvd for NUCC Use

31. SIGNATURE OF PHYSICIAN OR SUPPLIER INCLUDING DEGREES OR CREDENTIALS (I certify that the statements on the reverse apply to this bill and are made a part thereof.)

MARK KING MD   01 14 20XX
SIGNED   DATE

32. SERVICE FACILITY LOCATION INFORMATION

a. NPI   b.

33. BILLING PROVIDER INFO & PH # (123) 456-7890
INNER CITY HEALTH CARE
8600 MAIN STREET, SUITE 200
RIVER CITY, XY 01234

a. 36640210XX   b.

NUCC Instruction Manual available at: www.nucc.org   **PLEASE PRINT OR TYPE**   APPROVED OMB-0938-1197 FORM 1500 (02-12)

FIGURE 17-3 Completed CMS-1500 claim form.

Procedure

The CMS-1500 (02-12) claim form contains all of the identification information that the carrier needs to process or analyze the claim for payment. The new form is distinguishable from the old form in that the 1500 symbol and the date it was approved by the NUCC appear in the top left margin. When completing the PATIENT AND INSURED INFORMATION section, do not use commas to separate the last name, first name, and middle initial. Do not use periods within the name. Do not use commas, periods, or other punctuation in the address. When entering the nine-digit ZIP code, you may include the hyphen. This is the only exception to the punctuation rule. Do not use a hyphen or space as a separator within the telephone number. The top right-hand space, identified as CARRIER, provides space for the carrier's name and address be keyed in. Procedure 17-4 gives instructions for completing a Medicare claim form. Before completing claims for carriers other than Medicare, the medical assistant should verify with a carrier's representative exactly which blocks are required to be filled in for that particular carrier.

PROCEDURE 17–4

Procedure

Completing a Medicare CMS-1500 (02-12) Claim Form

PURPOSE:

To complete the CMS-1500 (02-12) insurance claim form for Medicare reimbursement.

EQUIPMENT/SUPPLIES:

- Patient information
- Patient account or ledger card
- Copy of patient's insurance card
- Insurance claim form
- Computer and printer

PROCEDURE STEPS:

1. The CARRIER section of the CMS-1500 (02-12) is in the upper portion of the form. Use the blank space at the top right of the section marked CARRIER to enter the name and address of the payer to whom this claim is being sent. The payer is the carrier, health plan, third-party administrator, or other payer who will handle the claim. The format for this information should be as follows:

   Key on line 4: first line—Name

   Key on line 5: second line—First line of address

   Key on line 6: third line—Second line of address

   Key on line 7: fourth line—City, state (2 letters) and zip code

   Do not use commas, periods, or other punctuation in the address. When entering a nine-digit ZIP code, you may include the hyphen. When printing page numbers on multiple-page claims (generally done by clearinghouses when converting the electronic claim form to the CMS 1500 claim form), print the page numbers in the CARRIER block on line 8 beginning at column 32. Page numbers are to be printed as Page XX of YY. RATIONALE: The claims processor must know who the claim is from.

2. The PATIENT AND INSURED INFORMATION section asks for specific information related to the patient and his or her health insurance plan. The following information is required for this section. Complete each block as directed. RATIONALE: These blocks must be accurately completed or the claim may be denied.

(continues)

HEALTH INSURANCE CLAIM FORM

APPROVED BY NATIONAL UNIFORM CLAIM COMMITTEE (NUCC) 02/12

PICA   PICA

CARRIER →

Courtesy of the Centers for Medicare & Medicaid Services, www.cms.gov

Block 1	Indicate the type of health insurance coverage applicable to this claim by placing an *X* in the Medicare box. Only one box can be marked.
Block 1a	Enter insured's ID number as shown on insured's ID card for the payer to whom the claim is being submitted. RATIONALE: The insured's ID number is the identification number of the person who holds the policy. This information identifies the patient to the payer. (For Medicare beneficiaries, this appears as a nine-digit number followed by a letter.)
Block 2	Enter the patient's full last name, first name, and middle initial in this block.
Block 3	Enter the patient's eight-digit birth date (MMDDYYYY). Enter an *X* in the correct box to indicate sex of the patient. Only one box can be marked. If gender is unknown, leave blank.
Block 4	Enter the insured's full last name, first name, and middle initial.
Block 5	Enter the patient's mailing address and telephone number.
Block 6	Enter an *X* in the correct box to indicate the patient's relationship to insured when block 4 has been completed. Only one box can be marked.
Block 7	Enter the insured's address and telephone number. If block 4 has been completed, then this field should also be completed.
Block 8	This is reserved for NUCC use. Leave blank.
Block 9	If block 11d is marked yes (to indicate that the patient carries a secondary insurance plan), complete fields 9 and 9a through 9d with the patient's secondary insurance information; otherwise, leave blank. When additional group health coverage exists, enter other insured's full last name, first name, and middle initial of the enrollee in another health plan if it is different from that shown in block 2.
Block 9a	Enter the policy or group number of the other insured. Do not use a hyphen or space as a separator within the policy or group number.
Block 9b	This is reserved for NUCC use. Leave blank.
Block 9c	This is reserved for NUCC use. Leave blank.
Block 9d	Enter the other insured's insurance plan or program name.
Blocks 10a to 10c	When appropriate, enter an *X* in the correct box to indicate whether one or more of the services described in block 24 are for a condition or injury that occurred on the job or as a result of an automobile or other accident. Only one box on each line can be marked. The two-letter state abbreviation must be shown if YES is marked in 10b. RATIONALE: Any item marked YES indicates there may be other applicable insurance coverage that would be primary.
Block 10d	Refer to the most current instructions from the applicable public or private payer regarding the use of this field.
Block 11	Enter the insured's policy or group number as it appears on the insured's health care ID card. If block 4 has been completed, then this field should also be completed.

(continues)

Block 11a   Enter the eight-digit date of birth (MMDDYYYY) of the insured and an *X* to indicate the sex of the insured. Only one box can be marked. If gender is unknown, leave blank.

Block 11b   This is the other claim ID designated by NUCC. Leave blank.

Block 11c   Enter the insurance plan or program name of the insured. (Some payers require an ID number of the primary insurer rather than the name in this field.)

Block 11d   When appropriate, enter an *X* in the correct box. If marked YES, complete blocks 9, 9a, and d. Only one box can be marked.

Block 12   Enter *Signature on File, SOF,* or legal signature. With a legal signature, enter the date signed in the proper eight-digit format. If there is no signature on file, leave blank or enter *No Signature on File.* RATIONALE: The patient's or authorized person's signature indicates there is an authorization on file for the release of any medical or other information necessary to process or adjudicate the claim.

Block 13   Enter *Signature on File, SOF,* or legal signature. If there is no signature on file, leave blank or enter *No Signature on File.* RATIONALE: The insured's or authorized person's signature indicates that there is a signature on file authorizing payment of medical benefits.

3. The PHYSICIAN OR SUPPLIER INFORMATION section must be accurately completed or the claim may be denied. This is the bottom section of the form under the bolded red line.

Block 14   Enter the eight-digit date of the first date of the present illness, injury, or pregnancy. For pregnancy, use the date of the last menstrual period (LMP) as the first date. Leave blank if unknown.

Block 15   Enter the first date the patient had the same or a similar illness. Enter the date in the eight-digit format. Previous pregnancies are not a similar illness. Leave blank if unknown.

(continues)

Block 16   If the patient is employed and is unable to work in his or her current occupation, an eight-digit date must be shown for the "from–to" dates that the patient is unable to work. RATIONALE: An entry in this field may indicate employment-related insurance coverage.

Block 17   Enter the name (first name, middle initial, last name) and credentials of the professional who referred, ordered, or supervised the service(s) or supply(ies) on the claim. Do not use periods or commas within the name. A hyphen can be used for hyphenated names.

Block 17a   The two-digit qualifier code is entered in the small box. Qualifiers are as follows:

0B	State License Number
1B	Blue Shield Provider Number
1C	Medicare Provider Number
1D	Medicaid Provider Number
1G	Provider UPIN Number
1H	CHAMPUS Identification Number
E1	Employer's Identification Number
G2	Provider Commercial Number
LU	Location Number
N5	Provider Plan Network Identification Number
SY	Social Security Number (the Social Security number may not be used for Medicare)
X5	State Industrial Accident Provider Number
ZZ	Provider Taxonomy

The other ID number of the referring, ordering, or supervising provider is reported in the larger space.

Block 17b   Enter the NPI number of the referring, ordering, or supervising provider. RATIONALE: The NPI number refers to the HIPAA National Provider Identifier number.

Block 18   Enter the inpatient eight-digit hospital admission date followed by the discharge date (if discharge has occurred). If not discharged, leave discharge date blank.

Block 19   Refer to the most current instruction from the applicable public or private payer regarding the use of this field.

Block 20   Complete this field when billing for purchased services. Enter an *X* in "YES" if the reported service(s) was performed by an entity other than the billing provider. If "YES," enter the purchased price under charges. RATIONALE: A "YES" indicates that an entity other than the entity billing for the service performed the purchased services. A "NO" indicates that no purchased services are included on the claim. Only one box can be marked.

Block 21   Enter the patient's diagnosis/condition. You may list up to 12 ICD diagnosis codes. Use the highest level of specificity. Do not provide a narrative description in this field.

Block 22   Enter the original reference number for resubmitted claims. Refer to the most current instruction from the applicable public or private payer regarding the use of this field. If it is not a resubmitted claim, leave this block blank.

(continues)

Block 23	Enter any of the following: prior authorization number, referral number, mammography precertification number, or CLIA number, as assigned by the payer for the current service. Do not enter hyphens or spaces within the number.
Block 24A	Enter date(s) of service, from and to. If there is one date of service only (such as a clinic visit), enter that date within the From blank as well as the To blank. Both the From and To areas must be completed in order to comply with proper completion rules.
Block 24B	Enter the appropriate two-digit code from the Place of Service Code list for each item used or service performed. Place of Service Codes are available at www.cms.hhs.gov/PlaceofServiceCodes /Downloads/POSDataBase.pdf.
Block 24C	This block was originally titled Type of Service and is no longer used. Check with the trading partner to determine if an emergency indicator is necessary. If required, enter *Y* for "YES" or leave blank if "NO." RATIONALE: The definition of emergency would be defined by either federal or state regulations or programs or payer contracts, or as defined in the electronic 837 Professional 4010A1 implementation guide.
Block 24D	Enter the CPT or HCPCS code(s) and modifier(s), if applicable, from the appropriate code set in effect on the date of service.
Block 24E	Enter the diagnosis code reference number as shown in block 21 to relate the date of service and the procedures performed to the primary diagnosis. When multiple services are performed, the primary reference number for each service should be listed first; other applicable services should follow. Enter the numbers left justified in the field. Do not use commas between the numbers.
Block 24F	Enter number right justified in the dollar area of the field. Do not use commas when reporting dollar amounts. Negative dollar amounts are not allowed. Dollar signs should not be entered. Enter 00 in the cents area if the amount is a whole number.
Block 24G	Enter the number of days or units. This field is most commonly used for multiple visits, units of supplies, anesthesia units or minutes, or oxygen volume. If only one service is performed, the numeral *1* must be entered. Enter numbers right justified in the field.
Block 24H	For Early and Periodic Screening, Diagnosis and Treatment-related services, enter the response as follows: If there is no requirement to report a reason code for EPDST, enter *Y* for "YES" if the service applies to EPDST. If "NO," leave blank.
Block 24I	Enter the qualifier identifying if the number is a non-NPI. The Other ID# of the rendering provider is reported in block 24J. The NUCC defines the same qualifiers as listed for Block 17a.
Block 24J	Enter the non-NPI ID number in the top portion of the field if applicable. Enter the NPI number of the service provider in the lower area of the field.
Block 25	Enter the provider of service or supplier federal tax ID or Social Security number. Enter an *X* in the appropriate box to indicate which number is being reported. Only one box can be marked. Do not enter hyphens with numbers. Enter numbers left justified in the field.
Block 26	Enter the patient's account number assigned by the provider of the service's or supplier's accounting system. Do not enter hyphens with numbers. Enter numbers left justified in the field.
Block 27	Enter an *X* in the correct box. Only one box can be marked.
Block 28	Enter total charges for the services (total of all charges in block 24F). Enter number right justified in the dollar area of the field. Do not use commas when reporting dollar amounts. Negative dollar amounts are not allowed. Dollar signs should not be entered. Enter 00 in the cents area if the amount is a whole number.

(continues)

Block 29	Enter the total amount the patient or other payers paid on the covered services only (such as a co-payment given on the date of service). Enter number right justified in the dollar area of the field. Do not use commas when reporting dollar amounts. Negative dollar amounts are not allowed. Dollar signs should not be entered. Enter 00 in the cents area if the amount is a whole number.
Block 30	This is reserved for NUCC use. Leave blank.
Block 31	Enter the legal signature of the practitioner or supplier, signature of the practitioner or supplier representative, *Signature on File*, or *SOF*. Enter the eight-digit date the form was signed. RATIONALE: The signature refers to the authorized or accountable person and the degree, credentials, or title.
Block 32	Enter the name, address, city, state, and ZIP code of the location where the services were rendered. Providers of service must identify the supplier's name, address, ZIP code, and NPI number when billing for purchased diagnostic tests. When more than one supplier is used, a separate claim form should be used to bill for each supplier. Follow the previously outlined format for entering address information.
Block 32a	Enter the NPI number of the service facility location.
Block 32b	Enter the two-digit qualifier identifying the non-NPI number followed by the ID number. Use the same qualifiers as listed in block 17a.
Block 33	Enter the provider's or supplier's billing name, address, ZIP code, and phone number. The phone number is to be entered in the area to the right of the field title. Follow the previously outlined format for entering address information.
Block 33a	Enter the NPI number of the billing provider.
Block 33b	Enter the two-digit qualifier identifying the non-NPI number followed by the ID number as listed in Block 17a.

Uniform Bill 04 Form

The NUCC has also updated the CMS-1450 claim form, also known as **Uniform Bill 04 (UB-04)**, to accommodate reporting the National Provider Identifier (NPI) number. The NPI, a requirement of HIPAA legislation, must be used by all HIPAA-covered entities. Figure 17-4 shows a sample of the UB-04 form.

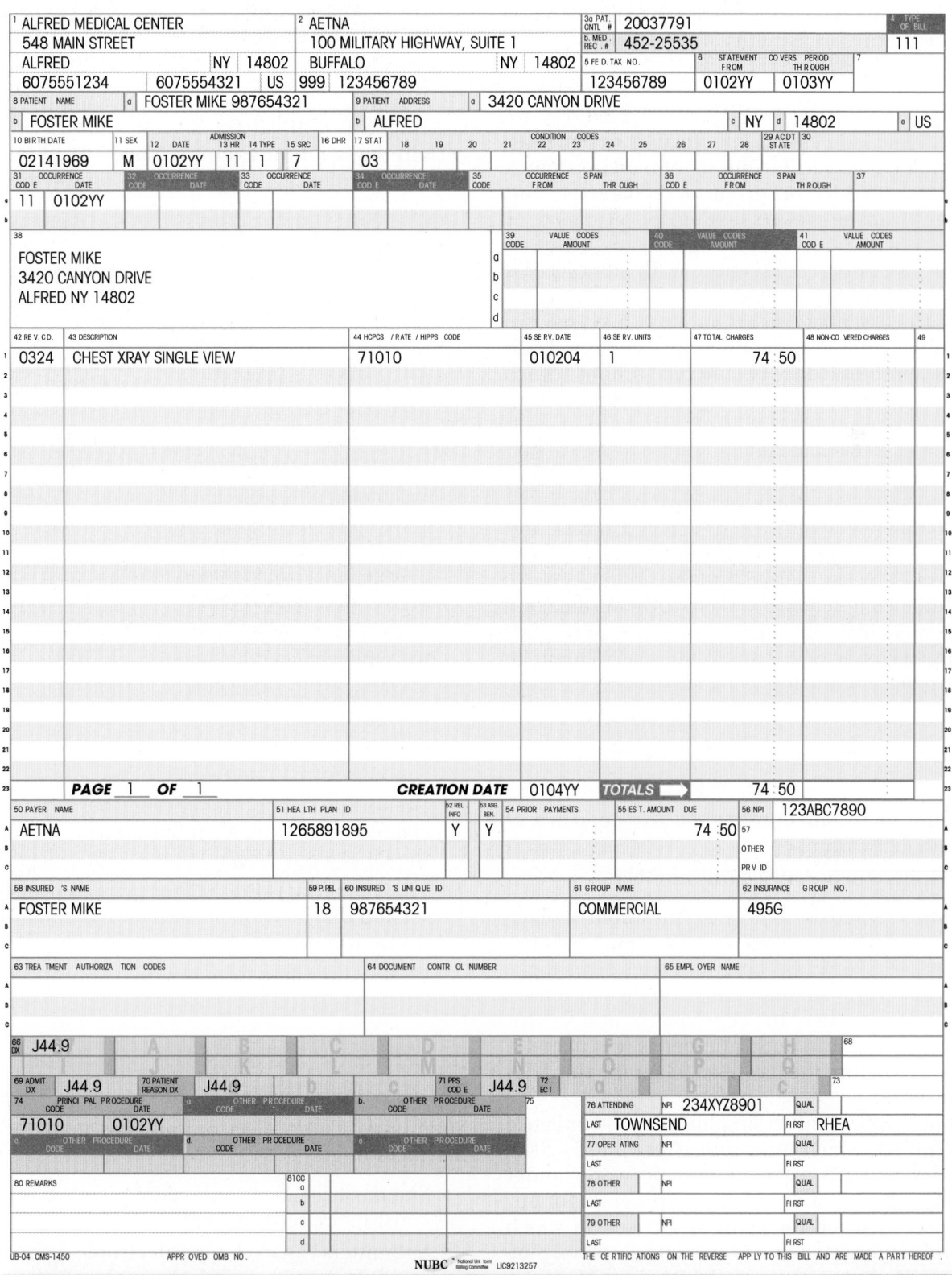

FIGURE 17-4 UB-04 claim containing sample patient data (with highlighted form locators that contain ICD and CPT codes).

The UB-04 form is the standard form used for inpatient admissions, outpatient and emergency department services and procedures, psychiatric facilities, drug and alcohol facilities, clinical and laboratory services, walk-in centers, nursing facilities, home health care agencies, hospice centers, and long-term care benefits under a health plan.

Using the Computer to Complete Forms

The CMS-1500 (02-12) claim form is designed to accommodate optical scanning of paper claims. A scanner is used to convert printed characters into text that can be viewed by the optical character reader (OCR). This technology greatly increases claims processing productivity, with some claims being paid within 7 to 10 days.

Practice management software may require data to be entered using uppercase and lowercase letters and other data be entered without regard to OCR guidelines. The computer program converts the data to the OCR format when the claim is printed or electronically transmitted to the carrier. Always use the software program's test pattern program to verify alignment of forms. Be sure the *X*s are completely within the designated boxes. You may need to check this alignment each time a new batch of claims is inserted into the printer.

While completing the claim form on the computer, remember not to interchange a zero (*0*) with the alpha character *o*. A substitute space should be used in place of the following keystrokes:

- Dollar sign or decimal in all charges or totals
- Decimal point in a diagnosis code number
- Dash in front of a procedure code modifier
- Parentheses surrounding the area code in a telephone number
- Hyphens in Social Security numbers

When a fee is expressed in whole dollars, always enter two zeros in the cent column. Birth dates should be entered using eight digits (MMDDYYYY). Two-digit code numbers are used for months (January 01, February 02, and so on). If the day of the month number is less than 10, add a zero before the day (e.g., 03 for the third day of the month).

The Administrative Simplification Compliance Act (ASCA), which went into effect July 5, 2005, specifies that no payment may be made under Part A or Part B of the Medicare program for any expenses incurred for items or services for which a claim is submitted in a nonelectronic form. Simply stated, paper claims submitted to Medicare will not be paid. Some exceptions to this rule can be found in the *Medlearn Matters* article MM3440 available at the CMS website (http://www.cms.gov by searching for "Medlearn Matters").

Common Errors in Completing Claim Forms

Once the claim form has been completed, it should be proofread for accuracy and to make certain that all information has been filled in correctly. The following list provides common errors:

- The patient name must match the name on the insurance card.
- Eliminate typographic errors. Check all numbers carefully to be sure they have not been transposed or entered incorrectly.
- Eliminate incorrect information. The name of the patient and the name of the policyholder must be the same (unless a wife is covered under a husband's insurance, a child under a parent's insurance, etc.).
- Verify that all blanks have been completed accurately. Specifically check that units of service are entered, hospital admission and discharge dates are included, and the procedure service date is provided.
- Verify that each procedure links correctly with the correct diagnosis (block 24E).
- Verify that the procedure was medically necessary.
- Include the patient's name and policy identification information on each page.
- Do not use staples when submitting paper claims because the form cannot feed through the OCR if it is defaced or creased.
- Verify that the printer alignment was properly set and that all claim information is contained within its proper field.
- Be sure the claim form is signed appropriately.

BENEFITS OF SUBMITTING CLAIMS ELECTRONICALLY

Submitting claims electronically has many benefits, including:

- Standardized electronic claim format ensures consistency, reducing errors.
- Submitters can exchange electronic data with multiple payers using the same data format.

- Supplies required (e.g., paper, postage) and administrative costs are reduced.
- Cash flow can be significantly improved because Medicare pays 14 days after receipt of complete and accurate electronically submitted claims (paper claims may take a minimum of 29 days to process).

MANAGING THE CLAIMS PROCESS

Once the claim form has been completed, a series of events take place. The medical assistant or administrative staff, who may have used a referral number generated by a point-of-service device, enters the claim into the office register (or practice management software) of submitted claims; the insurance carrier processes the claim; an explanation of benefits letter is sent to the insured person and the medical provider; and, if necessary, follow-up procedures are instituted if payment is not received from the carrier within a specified time period. Each of these events is discussed in detail in the following sections.

Documentation of Referrals

Many insurance plans require that a referral be preapproved by the plan before scheduling an appointment with someone other than the primary care provider. This is particularly true for managed care plans, especially HMOs. The medical assistant working in both the primary care facility and specialist facility must make sure that when an approval is required, the necessary authorization has been obtained and the referral number is recorded in the patient's file. The referral number must be submitted as part of the claim submitted to the carrier by the specialist. This piece of information would be entered in block 23 of the CMS-1500 (02-12).

Point-of-Service Device

An electronic device available to some health care providers is a **point-of-service (POS) device**. This device provides immediate and direct access to patient eligibility information and managed care functions through an electronic network connecting the medical clinic and the health plan's computer.

The POS device is a small card-swipe box similar in design and function to a credit card terminal (Figure 17-5). It allows medical clinic personnel to:

- Record a patient visit
- Check eligibility for patients in the health plan

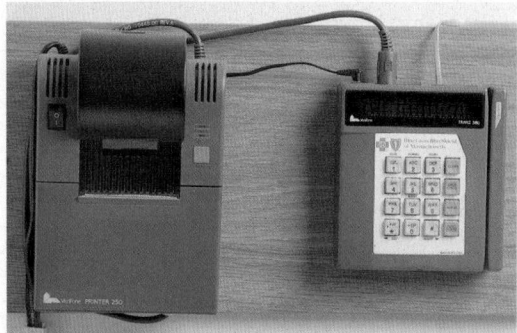

FIGURE 17-5 Point-of-service device. (Right) To enter information, the patient's insurance card is swiped through the machine, or the patient's identification number is entered on the keypad together with specific transaction code numbers. (Left) Responses from the plan's computer are printed directly in the medical office.

- Enter referrals for patients in managed care plans
- Verify referral information
- Check authorization status
- Enter inpatient authorization requests
- Enter outpatient authorization requests

After the necessary information is entered by the medical assistant, the POS device communicates with the health plan's computer system. The computer then returns an acknowledgment to the medical clinic confirming the transaction or giving an error message code. For example, when visits are recorded accurately, a reference number is generated that is used as the medical clinic's confirmation that the transaction is complete. On successful entry of a referral, a referral number is generated. Specialists may use this number on claims they submit for services they render under the referral.

Maintaining a Claims Registry or Claims Tracking System

When claim forms are sent to the appropriate insurance carrier, it is wise and necessary for the medical clinic personnel to keep a diary or register of submitted claims (Figure 17-6). This **claim register**, created with a spreadsheet or software, should include the patient's name, the insured's name if it is different from the patient's name, the dates of service for which the claim is being made, the amount of the claim, and the date the claim is submitted. When payment is received, the date of payment should be entered. When aging and

ACTION DATE	LAST NAME	FIRST NAME	INSURANCE COMPANY	ORIGINAL BILLING DATE	TOTAL CHARGES $	AMOUNT RECEIVED	STATUS / ACTION TAKEN
1/30/2008	McKay	Leo	Nationwide	1/30/2008	$ 88.00	$ -	Submitted
2/14/2008	Lovelace	Terry	World Health	9/24/2007	$ 128.00	$ -	Add'l data submitted
4/15/2008	Taxman	William	US Health	12/15/2007	$ 640.00	$ 640.00	Paid in full
5/1/2008	Fooler	April	Surprise Health	4/1/2007	$ 375.98	$ -	Collection
5/16/2008	Zonker	James	Gotcha Covered	4/3/2008	$ 236.00	$ 136.00	Patient billed $100.00
7/5/2008	Stripes	Stanley	Bangor Insurance				

FIGURE 17-6 Sample claim register.

reconciling accounts, the bookkeeper then can check the diary to note where the claim is in the process.

Following Up on Claims

Occasionally, claims are denied because the claim form was incomplete. However, if there is no payment from the carrier and no other notification after a period of 1 to 6 weeks, it is necessary to follow up on the claim. The claim register will enable the clinic to keep track of the progress of claims (Figure 17-6).

To follow up, a toll-free number is provided by most carriers. The necessary information to have on hand before making the call includes a copy of the claim form and the patient's name and insurance identification number. The carrier should be able to give the status of the claim. If payment is delayed, the carrier should be able to give the date when it can be expected. It is possible that payment was sent to the insured person, in which case a statement should be sent to the patient. If there is a problem with the claim, the medical assistant may need to investigate the cause of the error and submit a revised claim.

See Chapter 19 for information on billing and collection procedures.

THE INSURANCE CARRIER'S ROLE

The claims processor at the insurance carrier checks the codes to confirm that the procedures and accompanying diagnoses link properly with one another. The processor then analyzes the information to confirm that:

1. The coverage was in force at the time of treatment.
2. The provider has contracted with the insurance carrier.

3. There are no exclusions or restrictions on the policy for payment of the diagnosis, service, or procedure.
4. There are no preexisting condition restrictions.
5. The diagnosis and procedures done are reasonable and meet medical necessity.

The processor also checks to make sure that the billed amount falls within the usual, customary, and reasonable fee that the insurance carrier has developed for that specific procedure CPT code.

Explanation of Benefits Letter

On completion of the processing of the claim, the insurance company sends an **explanation of benefits (EOB)** letter to the insured person. Figure 16-1 shows a sample EOB. This form includes the dates; charges; amounts applied toward the deductible; amounts not covered either because of an exclusion or excess over the usual, customary, and reasonable charge; and the amount the company is paying for this claim. Some EOB letters even serve as a "bill" or "notice" in that they indicate the amount the insured must forward to the provider for payment of the account in full.

LEGAL AND ETHICAL ISSUES

Legal

Issues of insurance fraud and abuse must be understood before accurate codes can be assigned to medical procedures, services, and diagnosis of disease. See Chapter 16 for a complete discussion regarding insurance fraud and abuse.

The Omnibus Budget Reconciliation Acts of 1986 and 1987 state that providers can be assessed civil penalties if they "know of or should know that claims filed with Medicare or Medicaid on their behalf are not true and accurate representations of the items or services actually provided." This means that providers can be held responsible not only for negligent mistakes they make but also for mistakes made on their behalf by their medical assistants or administrative staff who complete insurance claim forms. The penalties assessed are usually in the form of a monetary fine and may also involve exclusion from Medicare and Medicaid programs for a specified period of time.

Compliance Programs

Compliance programs based on guidelines issued by the Office of the U.S. Inspector General are not mandatory; however, they help prevent violations that can be financially costly and that may carry criminal penalties for the provider and clinic personnel. Participation in a compliance program demonstrates that the practice is making a good-faith effort to submit claims appropriately and is considered equivalent to practicing preventative medicine. The following are basic elements of a compliance program:

1. Have a designated compliance officer.
2. Develop and use written standards and procedures for coding.
3. Develop a plan for communicating coding standards and procedures.
4. Train personnel in standards and procedures.
5. Conduct periodic audits.
6. Respond to detected violations and notify appropriate government agencies.
7. Make personnel aware that they have an ethical duty to report suspected or observed fraudulent or erroneous coding practices so that they can be corrected. Publicize and enforce disciplinary standards on coding violations.

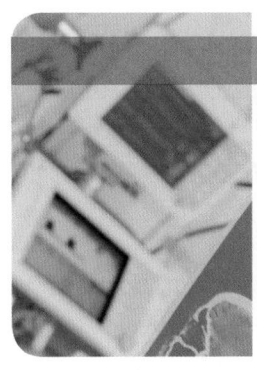

CASE STUDY 17-1

Refer to the scenario at the beginning of the chapter.

CASE STUDY REVIEW

1. Explain why coding accurately is important to health care providers and insurance companies that act as third-party payers for health care services rendered to patients.
2. List ways to ensure accurate coding.
3. Recall common errors in completing insurance claim forms.

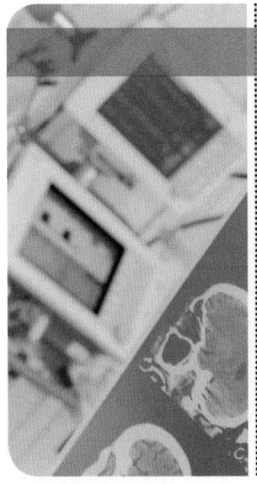

CASE STUDY 17-2

Leo McKay, an established patient at Inner City Health Care, schedules a visit, reporting nausea and severe abdominal pain. Dr. Winston Lewis spends 30 minutes taking a history and doing an examination. He suspects an ulcer and orders laboratory tests (complete blood count [CBC], guaiac, lipid panel, and urinalysis [UA]) to be done in the clinic and sends Mr. McKay for an upper GI series. Mr. McKay returns in 10 days to learn that the test results show a duodenal ulcer.

CASE STUDY REVIEW

1. What are the proper diagnosis codes for Mr. McKay?
2. What are the proper procedure codes for Mr. McKay?
3. In coding the claim form for Mr. McKay's visit, what ethical principle and legal principle should guide the medical assistant?

- Coding is the application of alphanumeric characters selected from standard terms used to describe a condition, disease, or service in health care.

- Coding is done in order to process demographic, insurance, and coded medical diagnoses and procedures in order to request reimbursement for services and supplies used in health care.

- The coding systems used within the United States include Current Procedural Terminology (CPT); Healthcare Common Procedure Coding System (HCPCS); International Classification of Diseases, 10th Revision, Clinical Modification (ICD-10-CM); and ICD-10-PCS.

- When performing billing procedures, medical assistants and medical administrative staff are expected to adhere to ethical standards and legal practices.

- Imprecise coding affects how quickly the provider is reimbursed and the correct amount of the reimbursement. Common types of coding errors and abuse include down-coding, up-coding, assumptive coding, and unbundling.

- The National Correct Coding Initiative (NCCI) promotes national correct coding methodologies.

- The claim form is completed by the medical assistant, administrative office staff, or billing clerk in the ambulatory care setting.

- Coding the claim form is a precise way to communicate with the insurance carrier. Coding indicates the complexity of the visit, the diagnosis for the visit, and the specific procedures performed.

- The CMS-1500 (02-12) is the claim form accepted by all insurance carriers.

- Security and confidentiality measures must be in place in medical clinics to protect patient information.

- Authorization to release necessary medical information to payers, such as insurance carriers, must be obtained from the patient, the parent, or the guardian before any information is released.

- The UB-04 form is the standard form used for inpatient admissions, outpatient and emergency department services and procedures, psychiatric facilities, drug and alcohol facilities, clinical and laboratory services, walk-in centers, nursing facilities, home health care agencies, hospice centers, and long-term care benefits under a health plan.

- Once the claim form has been completed, it should be proofread for accuracy and to make certain that all information has been filled in correctly.

- Once the claim form has been completed, the medical assistant or administrative staff enters the claim into the office register (or practice management software) of submitted claims and the insurance carrier processes the claim.

- The claims processor at the insurance carrier checks the codes to confirm that the procedures and accompanying diagnoses link properly with one another.

- Providers can be held responsible not only for negligent mistakes they make but also for mistakes made on their behalf by their medical assistants or administrative staff who complete insurance claim forms.

Study for Success

To reinforce your knowledge and skills of information presented in this chapter:

- Review the *Key Terms* and *Learning Outcomes*

- Consider the *Critical Thinking* features and *Case Studies* and discuss your conclusions

- Answer the questions in the *Certification Review*

Procedure

- Perform the *Procedures* using the *Competency Assessment Checklists* on the *Student Companion Website*

CERTIFICATION REVIEW

1. What is a description of CPT Codes?
   a. They are for diagnosis coding.
   b. They have five digits and may have two-digit modifiers.
   c. They have three-digit codes with a decimal point and one to two additional digits.
   d. They are updated semiannually.

2. What is the first reference that should be used when coding a diagnosis?
   a. CPT
   b. ICD-10-CM alphabetical index
   c. Z codes in ICD-10-CM
   d. V codes in ICD-10-CM
   e. HCPCS

3. What is an accurate description of Level II of HCPCS?
   a. It provides codes to enable the provider to report nonprovider services.
   b. It is the same as the regular CPT system.
   c. It is assigned by the fiscal intermediary.
   d. It uses the letter codes *W, X, Y* and *Z*.

4. What statement is true about ICD-10-CM codes?
   a. They were developed by the AMA as uniform descriptions of medical, surgical, and diagnostic services.
   b. They are divided into seven sections.
   c. They use modifiers.
   d. They code every disease, illness, condition, injury, and cause of injury known.
   e. They include codes for new and established patients.

5. Most insurance carriers accept which claim form?
   a. UB-04
   b. CMS-1500 (02-12)
   c. CPT
   d. HCFA-1450

6. What is the purpose of maintaining a claim tracking system?
   a. To anticipate claims to be sent to insurance companies for processing
   b. To check how many claims are sent to Medicare
   c. To monitor claims that have been sent to insurance companies for processing
   d. To help in aging accounts
   e. To record the amount of co-payments

7. What information is *NOT* included in the CARRIER section of the CMS-1500 (02-12) insurance claim form?
   a. The payer's name
   b. The patient's name
   c. The payer's address
   d. The payer's city, state, and ZIP code

8. What information is included in the PATIENT AND INSURED section of the CMS-1500 (02-12) insurance claim form?
   a. Health insurance plan
   b. Patient's name and address
   c. Insured's name and address
   d. NPI number of the billing provider
   e. Address and telephone number of the billing provider

9. Which of the following codes is an example of a CPT code?
   a. Irregular menstrual cycle, A99901
   b. Biopsy, soft tissue of neck, A98.5
   c. Dissection of the renal artery, A00.00
   d. Adenitis, lymph gland, except mesenteric, 99205

10. What unique billing form is used extensively by acute care facilities for processing inpatient and outpatient claims?
    a. UB-04
    b. CMS-1500 (02-12)
    c. CPT
    d. HCFA-1450
    e. Superbill

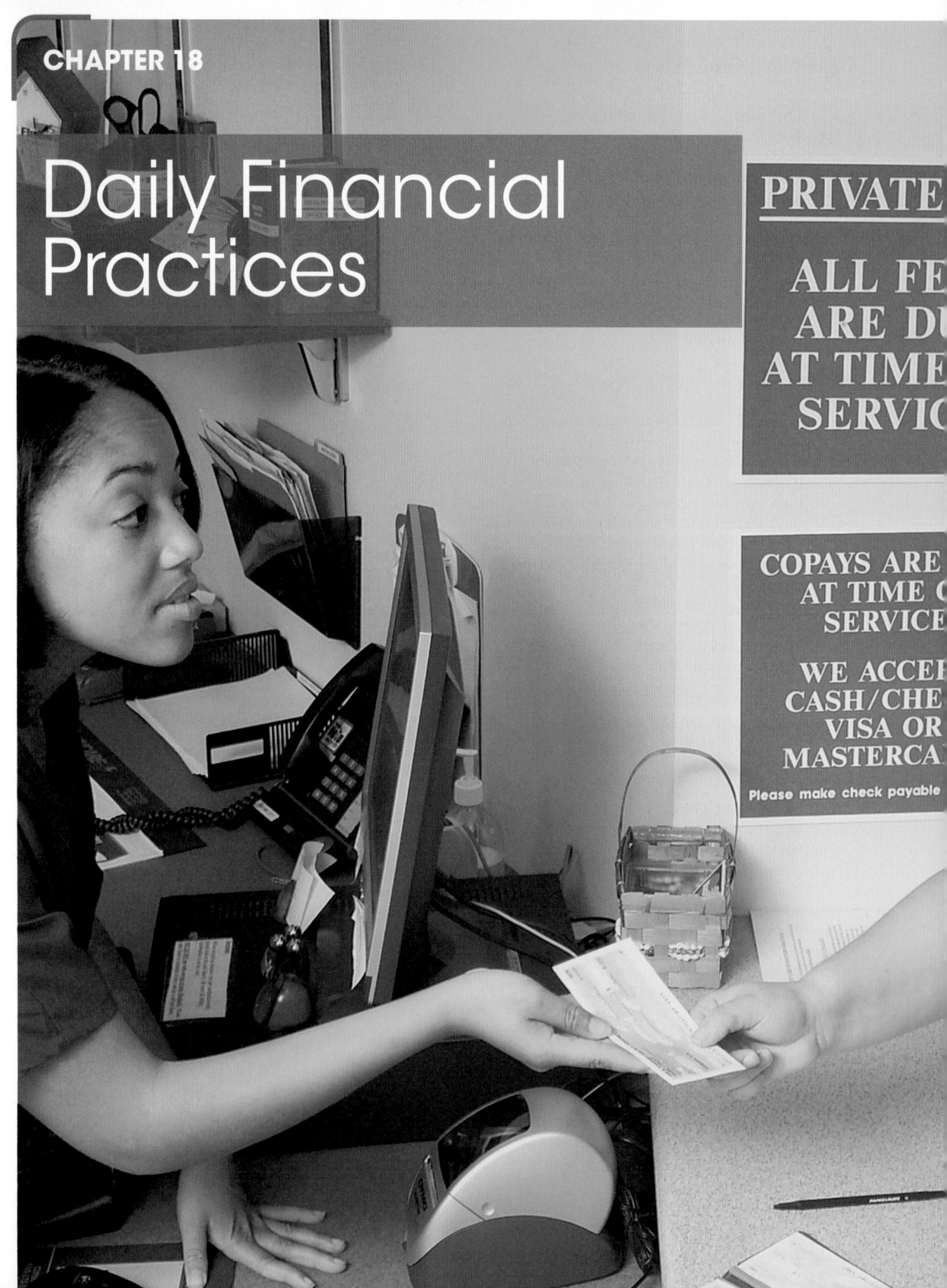

Daily Financial Practices

1. Define and spell the key terms as presented in the glossary.
2. Practice effective communication in regard to establishing patient fees.
3. Identify circumstances that require adjustment of fees and post accordingly.
4. Develop knowledge of various credit arrangements for patient fees.
5. Differentiate between bookkeeping and accounting.
6. Compare manual and computerized bookkeeping systems in ambulatory health care.
7. Describe the pegboard system.
8. State the advantages of computerized systems for financial practices.
9. List six good working habits for financial records.
10. Describe the encounter form.
11. Identify the parts of the patient account or ledger.
12. Discuss preparation of patient receipts.
13. Describe month-end activities.
14. Describe banking procedures, including types of accounts and services.
15. Show proficiency in preparing deposits and checks and reconciling accounts.
16. Explain the process of purchasing equipment and supplies for the ambulatory care setting.
17. Demonstrate proficiency in establishing and maintaining a petty cash system.

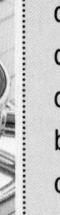

KEY TERMS

accounts payable	encounter form
accounts receivable	guarantor
adjustments	ledger
balance	money market savings account
cashier's check	notary
certified check	payee
credit	pegboard system
day sheet	petty cash
debit	posting
electronic check	remote deposit capture
electronic check conversion	voucher check

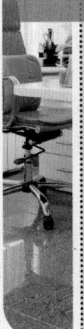

SCENARIO

At Inner City Health Care, many different types of patients are seen. Most have some kind of insurance, either a private or employer plan or an HMO plan; some are on Medicare; a few are on Medicaid; and occasionally a patient does not have any insurance or any financial resources to pay for treatment. Whoever schedules the first patient appointment also opens a courteous discussion with the patient about provider fees and the patient's anticipated method of payment. Initiating this discussion of fees at the beginning of the provider–patient relationship keeps patients informed of their responsibility for payment and helps the medical assistants at Inner City Health Care make any necessary credit arrangements with the patient before treatment begins.

C linic settings are primarily designed to serve the patient. However, without sound financial practices, patient care will suffer and the practice will not thrive and grow. The health care industry is complex and complicated. The impact of managed care and the many detailed insurance plans affect not only the way patients receive treatment, but the manner in which the ambulatory care center is administered from a financial point of view.

The discussion of fees is only a small part of the clinic setting's daily financial practices. Selecting an appropriate system for tracking patient accounts, overseeing banking procedures, managing the purchase of supplies, controlling patient accounts, and establishing a petty cash system all are important to the smooth functioning of the modern clinic.

PATIENT FEES

All providers receive education, training, and experience in diagnosing and treating the health issues of their patients. That is their major concern; therefore, the management of the business details usually becomes the responsibility of the medical assisting staff. This includes but is not limited to informing the patients about charges, collecting payments, making credit arrangements if necessary, and making certain that patients and their providers receive the full benefit of medical insurance. An attitude that anticipates that the majority of patients pay their medical bills in a timely and responsible manner is helpful in completing these tasks.

Helping Patients Who Cannot Pay

Communication Integrity

There are times when patients may have difficulty paying their bills. The economy is constantly changing, and with its fluctuations, individuals lose their jobs and often their medical insurance. The majority of today's employment force does not recall a time without medical insurance when patients expected to pay the total fee for medical services. These same patients may not fully comprehend what medical services cost. They likely do not understand the explanation of benefits (EOB) from their insurance reports. There is also a growing number of "working poor" in society, who may work two or more part-time jobs but never qualify for company insurance benefits and struggle daily to pay necessary bills. Some patients must decide whether to put food on the table or pay the provider. Emergencies can deplete an individual's financial resources as well. These are the times when the administrative medical assistant might make financial arrangements with patients allowing full payment for the services provided. Patients will appreciate the assistance,

and the administrative medical assistant can expect the patient to abide by the agreed plan. Such an agreement fosters a climate where patients are less likely to withdraw from any necessary medical treatment when their finances are low.

Determining Patient Fees

Providers place a value on their services. In today's managed care environment, the clinic has many different arrangements with patients, insurance carriers, and health maintenance organization (HMO) insurance contracts. Managed care contracts pay predetermined fees for specific procedures and services. Providers who practice in a concierge-type medical group collect an additional fee. This usually is a flat fee at the beginning of each year for the specialized service; many do not accept the insurance carrier's required co-payment. Patients who choose concierge medical services are willing to pay the additional fee and generally have the resources to do so. Provider fees for procedures, however, are billed and reimbursed according to standard insurance guidelines.

Discussion of Fees

The manner in which billing is done and fees are established varies depending on the type of medical facility, the needs of the practice, and the professional services rendered. Today, the fee for the visit is simply stated, and if a person does not have cash or a check, the option of credit or debit card payment is often provided. If a patient is a member of an HMO, the patient is expected to pay any established co-payment amount at the time of service.

Inherent to the total billing process is the necessity of informing patients of charges and exactly what portion of the bill they are expected to pay. Ideally, the patient should be told the approximate cost of the procedures at the start of treatment. For Medicare and Medicaid patients, a form officially known by Medicare as an Advanced Beneficiary Notification (ABN) or by Medicaid as a waiver is the only legal means a clinic has to collect payment on charges not allowed by Medicare or Medicaid (Figure 18-1). These forms are to be in writing, and should indicate the type of procedure(s), the total responsibility of the patient, and the reason why this payment is the patient's responsibility.

Charges for some routine visits may be submitted to an insurance carrier, and the clinic may not always know what portions are covered until information is received from the carrier. The facility may contract with numerous insurance plans, including private carriers, and participation in these plans determines the amount the patient owes. Many misunderstandings can be prevented and subsequent collection of delinquent accounts expedited when the clinic staff is well informed about insurance reimbursement and carefully explains fees to the patients.

Adjustment of Fees

Legal

Providers who accept assignment with Medicare and Medicaid are mandated to charge every patient the same amount for similar services rendered. If a professional courtesy is extended, then it is considered insurance fraud, because the clinic would be billing insurance an increased rate over what others are charged. Deductibles are to be collected from patients as part of their premium expectation. Unless you follow government guidelines for establishing when patients are financially unable to pay their portion of the bill, you cannot give discounts to patients for cash payments.

Adjustments may be made for patients with limited income. For example, for patients who recently lost a job or ran into unfortunate financial circumstances, the provider may write off a portion of the bill. This sum will be written off against the provider's income, and the patients do not pay that portion.

Adjustments also may occur with Medicare, Medicaid, Blue Cross/Blue Shield, and private health insurance patients. Providers who accept assignment in these programs agree to accept as payment in full what the insurer allows. For instance, a fee of $150 may be charged, but $95 is accepted as payment in full by the provider after deductibles and co-payments are satisfied. The

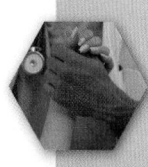

Patient Education

One way to easily provide information to patients regarding fees is to include in the clinic brochure policies regarding fees, insurance, co-payments, and how third-party payments are handled. If credit and debit cards are allowed, include that information as well.

remainder of the bill, $55, is written off so that the patient is not responsible for the nonallowed amount.

Communication

Medical assistants must be aware, however, of the pitfalls of adjusting or reducing fees. It is difficult to accept all hardship cases and still remain a viable practice. It is always a helpful resource to patients who cannot pay to be given the names and telephone numbers of local health care clinics that may be able to accept them as patients on a sliding scale or no-fee basis.

Refunds. On rare occasion, a refund will be necessary. It usually occurs when the insurance carrier pays more than anticipated, double pays for the same charges, or the patient paid and the insurance covered the charges. Notably, there are a few members of the older adult population who may still be a little uncomfortable with Medicare and are accustomed to paying for all their medical expenses out of pocket; therefore, they will pay their entire bill when the statement is received. When Medicare payments arrive, an overpayment is created. The financial transaction required is to prepare a check for the amount due to the patient and enter the transaction on the **day sheet** and patient account or ledger.

CREDIT ARRANGEMENTS

Communication

If the patient will need to pay a substantial out-of-pocket amount, it is beneficial to make the patient aware of this and discuss different credit arrangements that can be made. Many clinics will accept prearranged installment payments, usually without finance charges, to spread the cost of services over a preagreed period. This eases the financial burden on the patient and also makes it more likely that the balance due will be collected.

A. Notifier:

B. Patient Name: **C. Identification Number:**

Advance Beneficiary Notice of Noncoverage (ABN)

NOTE: If Medicare doesn't pay for **D.** _____ below, you may have to pay.
Medicare does not pay for everything, even some care that you or your health care provider have good reason to think you need. We expect Medicare may not pay for the **D.** _____ below.

D.	E. Reason Medicare May Not Pay:	F. Estimated Cost

WHAT YOU NEED TO DO NOW:

- Read this notice, so you can make an informed decision about your care.
- Ask us any questions that you may have after you finish reading.
- Choose an option below about whether to receive the **D.** _____ listed above.

Note: If you choose Option 1 or 2, we may help you to use any other insurance that you might have, but Medicare cannot require us to do this.

G. OPTIONS: Check only one box. We cannot choose a box for you.

☐ **OPTION 1.** I want the **D.** _____ listed above. You may ask to be paid now, but I also want Medicare billed for an official decision on payment, which is sent to me on a Medicare Summary Notice (MSN). I understand that if Medicare doesn't pay, I am responsible for payment, but **I can appeal to Medicare** by following the directions on the MSN. If Medicare does pay, you will refund any payments I made to you, less co-pays or deductibles.

☐ **OPTION 2.** I want the **D.** _____ listed above, but do not bill Medicare. You may ask to be paid now as I am responsible for payment. **I cannot appeal if Medicare is not billed**.

☐ **OPTION 3.** I don't want the **D.** _____ listed above. I understand with this choice I am **not** responsible for payment, and **I cannot appeal to see if Medicare would pay**.

H. Additional Information:

This notice gives our opinion, not an official Medicare decision. If you have other questions on this notice or Medicare billing, call **1-800-MEDICARE** (1-800-633-4227/**TTY:** 1-877-486-2048). Signing below means that you have received and understand this notice. You also receive a copy.

I. Signature:	J. Date:

According to the Paperwork Reduction Act of 1995, no persons are required to respond to a collection of information unless it displays a valid OMB control number. The valid OMB control number for this information collection is 0938-0566. The time required to complete this information collection is estimated to average 7 minutes per response, including the time to review instructions, search existing data resources, gather the data needed, and complete and review the information collection. If you have comments concerning the accuracy of the time estimate or suggestions for improving this form, please write to: CMS, 7500 Security Boulevard, Attn: PRA Reports Clearance Officer, Baltimore, Maryland 21244-1850.

Form CMS-R-131 (03/11)   Form Approved OMB No. 0938-0566

FIGURE 18-1   Advance Beneficiary Notice.

Payment Planning

Medical assistants can help patients plan for anticipated medical expenses (e.g., having a baby, surgery, extensive therapy). When patient and provider know in advance that there will be costly medical expenses, the medical assistant should review the patient's insurance coverage. It is helpful to prepare an estimate sheet, which will give the patient an idea of the cost of the medical services for the planned treatment. The estimate may also include the anticipated cost of anesthetist, consultants, and hospital charges.

Many clinics accept credit and debit cards as a means of payment. Remember, this service is strictly for the convenience of the patient, and providers cannot increase their charges for patients who wish to use these cards even though the provider is charged a fee for this service. Credit and debit cards are convenient and ensure payment; therefore, the practice may wish to encourage their use.

The one advantage to accepting credit/debit cards is that monies for fees charged usually are available within 24 hours. Also, the provider is relieved of the responsibility of collection. However, credit card companies do assess a fee for every charge made, which the clinic must pay.

Integrity

When a patient decides to use a credit or debit card, it is extremely important that confidentiality be maintained to the fullest extent possible. When writing a description of the services on the credit card receipt, the medical assistant should be as vague as possible to preserve patient confidentiality. For example, "medical services" is often used.

THE BOOKKEEPING FUNCTION

Daily financial management in the clinic is important to the functioning of the clinic, because it directly affects overall accounting and bookkeeping procedures. *Accounting* generates financial information for the ambulatory care setting and is defined as a system of monitoring the financial status of a facility and the specific results of its activities. Accounting provides financial information for decision making (see Chapter 20). *Bookkeeping*, the actual daily recording of the accounts or transactions of the business, is a major part of this accounting process. This chapter deals with daily bookkeeping (or recording) functions necessary to manage the income and expenses of an ambulatory care setting.

Managing Patient Accounts

Legal

All businesses must keep careful records of income and expenses for tax and legal purposes. One aspect of this recordkeeping in a medical practice is maintaining patient accounts. Because few patients are able to pay in full each time they are seen by the provider, it is necessary to maintain account records for each individual or family as opposed to simply keeping a record of cash received, as is done in many other types of business. The total amount of money owed to the medical facility by patients is known as **accounts receivable**; this must be carefully monitored to ensure that the provider is paid for services provided in a timely manner and that patients are properly credited for payments made.

There are various ways to track patients' balances. This chapter discusses the two most common methods:

- Computerized financial systems
- The **pegboard system** (also known as the write-it-once method)

Competency

Although the financial records of most practices are fully automated, many practices probably started with some sort of manual system (generally pegboard). Converting from manual to computerized recordkeeping seems cumbersome at the beginning, but it offers great versatility and reduces the need to record and re-record entries. A knowledgeable medical assistant will understand both the manual and computerized systems. In an emergency, when the computer system is down, or if the front desk staff needs to record payments quickly and batch them for input into the software later, modified use of a write-it-once daysheet accommodates this.

Pegboard System. A complete pegboard or write-it-once system consists of day sheets, ledger cards, **encounter forms** or charge slips, and receipt forms. The forms are designed to work together to simplify the task and to avoid mistakes in patient accounts. All forms have matching columns that align and are held in place on the pegboard when the system is in use (Figure 18-2). The forms are on NCR (no carbon required) paper, which permits entering of charges, credits, or adjustments, called **posting**, onto the day sheet, encounter form, or receipt and the patient's ledger simultaneously. The day sheet provides complete and up-to-date information about accounts receivable status at a glance. Also, a pegboard system is relatively inexpensive.

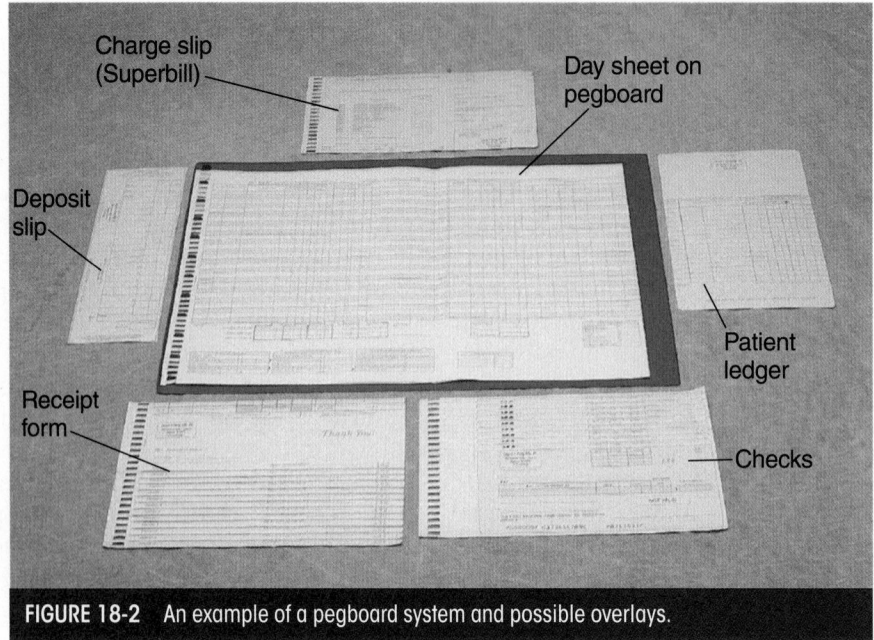

FIGURE 18-2 An example of a pegboard system and possible overlays.

Labels on figure: Charge slip (Superbill); Day sheet on pegboard; Deposit slip; Patient ledger; Receipt form; Checks

Computerized Financial Systems. The majority of medical facilities use computers for bookkeeping. A number of medical practice software packages are available on the market. These ready-made systems are available for both single or multiple-provider partnerships and large group practices. Occasionally, a consultant is hired to design a customized program, although this can be more expensive than purchasing mass-produced software.

The Importance of Good Working Habits in Financial Transactions. In managing the day-today finances of the clinic, always observe the following guidelines:

1. 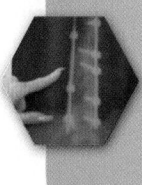 Always work with care and accuracy; it is extremely easy to transpose numbers (e.g., entering 23 instead of 32) or make other posting errors. A moment of carelessness can result in hours spent trying to find the mistake.

    Competency

2. The work must be kept current or it may become an overwhelming chore.
3. Double-check all entries made for accuracy.

In a manual bookkeeping system, follow these additional rules:

- Use a consistent ink color; black or blue is preferred.
- Form your numbers and letters carefully, using neat and clear writing.
- Align your columns carefully, preferably using paper with grid lines.

Critical Thinking

Discuss with another student the advantages and disadvantages of adopting a computer system that allows the practice to start with one component and add more components at a later time.

- Write small enough to stay within the columns.
- Be careful when placing or carrying decimal points.
- Double-check all math.
- If a mistake is found, draw one line through the error and write "Corr." or "Correction" above it. Red ink may be used in correcting errors on a paper copy.

RECORDING PATIENT TRANSACTIONS

The administrative medical assistant is largely responsible for recording patient transactions for the practice. Bookkeeping activities must be exact. Either they are right or they are wrong, and in any form of business, they have to be right to be correct and to be "in balance." In the pegboard or manual system, if an error is made during entry, it will carry through to all the other documents, thus compounding the error. In a computerized system, there is the old but true statement, "garbage in, garbage out." All entries must be correct; there is no room for just a "slight" mistake.

In one way or another, the forms and procedures discussed in the following sections are common elements to any system of bookkeeping for a medical practice.

Encounter Form

The encounter form (see Figure 17-1), also known as the charge slip, superbill, or multipurpose billing form, is used in both manual and computerized bookkeeping systems. It often is a two-part form that has the following functions:

1. Provides patients one copy with a record of account activity for the day (usually a pink form)
2. Provides a second copy that serves as the clinic's permanent copy of account activity (usually the original, white form)

The encounter forms can be custom designed to fit the particular practice, computer system, or pegboard. Often, the encounter form is attached to the patient's chart so that the provider is able to indicate the day's activities and charges; the provider can also use this form to indicate a requested return visit. The encounter form will typically include procedure and diagnosis codes. The most applicable procedure codes can be preselected and printed on the encounter form to fit the practice, with blank lines added for infrequently used procedures. Often, providers use the form to check the appropriate procedures and diagnoses while they are still with the patient in the examination room.

Encounter forms are designed to fit over the pegs of a pegboard system when a manual system is used. In a computerized system, an encounter form carrying the same information is prepared for the patient, printed, and attached to the patient chart. Some computer systems automatically match the correct charge to the procedure code identified. When a facility is totally automated (including medical records), the provider identifies patient procedures in the medical record on the computer. The computer software assigns appropriate codes and charges to create the encounter form, which can be printed for the patient at the completion of the service.

Patient Account or Ledger

The financial record of the patient is known as that patient's account. All the patient accounts with outstanding balances make up the accounts receivable. Patient accounts are recorded in an accounts receivable **ledger**. (Figure 18-3 illustrates a typewritten ledger.) The ledger, or record of services, lists payments and balances due. In family practice, each adult has his or her own ledger or account that carries insurance information, name of subscriber, and patient's relationship to the subscriber. A responsible party is identified for each minor or patient who does not have insurance, and that name also appears on the ledger. Charges for any members of the family seen in the clinic are entered on their own ledger. It is important that charges and credits be applied to the correct family member for insurance purposes and accurate bookkeeping practices.

In cases of divorced parents and blended families, the parent with physical custody of the child is considered to be the **guarantor** and the one responsible for payment if the child is not insured with a contracted insurance carrier or if there is any amount left over once the insurance has paid. This prevents the staff from having to interpret divorce decrees and parenting plan documents. This information should be clearly identified and discussed with the parent when appointments are made.

In the manual system of bookkeeping, ledger cards are used. They have a minimum of three columns for entering figures:

1. **Debit** column is on the left and is used for entering charges and a brief description of services, including a procedure code.
2. **Credit** column is to the right of the debit column and is used for entering payments.
3. **Balance** column is at the far right and is used to record the difference between the debit and credit columns and shows any amount due.

Most ledger cards have space for another column called **adjustments**, which are used to indicate any insurance payments, personal discounts or write-offs, or any other subtractions for the account that need to be recorded.

The adjustment column is a credit column; therefore, entries here normally reduce the balance due. When making an adjustment intended to increase the balance, a negative entry (in parentheses) is made to show that you reverse the function when you balance. (Add instead of subtract the amount.) For example, Edith Leonard had surgery, and because of a hardship, the provider agreed to reduce the fee by half of the balance remaining after insurance has paid. At the time of surgery, a charge of $2,500 is entered on her ledger and the day sheet. Today, payment is received from her

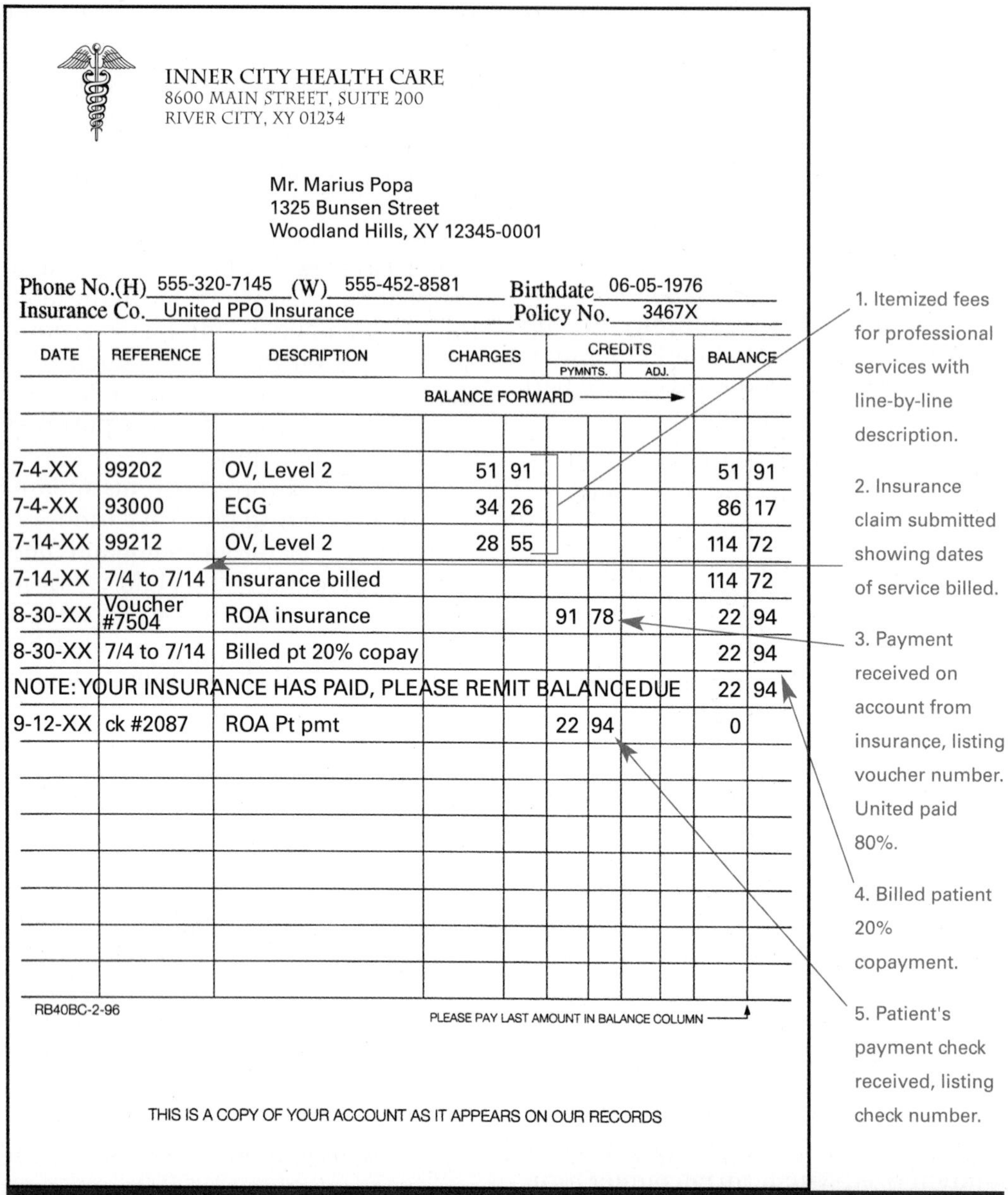

INNER CITY HEALTH CARE
8600 MAIN STREET, SUITE 200
RIVER CITY, XY 01234

Mr. Marius Popa
1325 Bunsen Street
Woodland Hills, XY 12345-0001

Phone No.(H)_555-320-7145_ (W)_555-452-8581_   Birthdate_06-05-1976_
Insurance Co._United PPO Insurance_   Policy No._3467X_

DATE	REFERENCE	DESCRIPTION	CHARGES	CREDITS PYMNTS.	CREDITS ADJ.	BALANCE
		BALANCE FORWARD →				
7-4-XX	99202	OV, Level 2	51 91			51 91
7-4-XX	93000	ECG	34 26			86 17
7-14-XX	99212	OV, Level 2	28 55			114 72
7-14-XX	7/4 to 7/14	Insurance billed				114 72
8-30-XX	Voucher #7504	ROA insurance		91 78		22 94
8-30-XX	7/4 to 7/14	Billed pt 20% copay				22 94
NOTE: YOUR INSURANCE HAS PAID, PLEASE REMIT BALANCE DUE						22 94
9-12-XX	ck #2087	ROA Pt pmt		22 94		0

RB40BC-2-96   PLEASE PAY LAST AMOUNT IN BALANCE COLUMN ──→

THIS IS A COPY OF YOUR ACCOUNT AS IT APPEARS ON OUR RECORDS

1. Itemized fees for professional services with line-by-line description.

2. Insurance claim submitted showing dates of service billed.

3. Payment received on account from insurance, listing voucher number. United paid 80%.

4. Billed patient 20% copayment.

5. Patient's payment check received, listing check number.

FIGURE 18-3 A manual patient ledger card illustrating posting of professional services, fees, payments, and balance due.

insurance company in the amount of $2,000, which would normally leave a balance of $500. However, because the provider agreed to write off half of that amount ($250), you enter $250 in the adjustment column when posting the insurance payment. That amount is subtracted from the previous balance to get the new total of $250.

The ledger is placed under the charge slip or encounter form in a pegboard system and aligned before posting. Never post any patient entry in this manual system without the patient's ledger in place. This prevents recording information on the day sheet while inadvertently omitting it from the JB patient's ledger. Procedure 18-1 identifies steps in recording/posting patient charges and adjustments.

In the computerized system, a patient's account or ledger can be printed with the same information by just entering the patient's name and usually an identification number. The computerized patient account ledger provides more room for helpful detail and is much faster to create than the manual paper ledger (Figure 18-4).

PROCEDURE 18-1

Procedure

Recording/Posting Patient Charges, Payments, and Adjustments

PURPOSE:

To record information including services rendered, fees charged, any adjustments made, and balances pertaining to a patient's clinic visit and patient's account.

EQUIPMENT/SUPPLIES:

- Calculator
- Patient's account or ledger
- Computerized PM System

PROCEDURE STEPS:

1. Check the patient's account before the patient's appointment to make certain it is current. The account will indicate any recent insurance payments, any amount received on the account, and any balance due. RATIONALE: Allows the medical assistant to focus entirely on the patient at arrival time and gives a current picture of the patient's account.

2. When the patient arrives, check for name, address, telephone numbers, and any changes regarding medical insurance. Make any changes in the PM system account for the patient, or on the ledger. RATIONALE: Ensures that information is current and up to date.

3. On the encounter form or superbill, complete any necessary items such as the date of service and the responsible party's name. RATIONALE: The encounter form allows the provider to indicate appropriate procedure and diagnosis codes.

4. When the provider completes the treatment or examination, he or she will check the procedures and diagnosis on the encounter form. RATIONALE: Provider marks the appropriate codes and signs the encounter form, indicating it is correct. The provider or licensed caregiver is the only one authorized to select the appropriate procedure codes.

5. When the patient returns to the front desk, refer to the provider's fee schedule, enter the charge next to each procedure, and calculate the total. If the procedure description is not indicated, one is to be provided. A description is necessary for each service. Check to see if the codes match the services provided. If they do not match, refer it back to the provider or licensed caregiver for correction. RATIONALE: Medical clinic staff and the patient can identify the charge to the particular service given and know that the coding and charges will match.

6. If using the manual pegboard system, post charges for today's services or procedures, any payments received, and adjustments applied, in the Charges, Payments, and Adjustment columns respectively. If using a PM system, open the module to post charges and open the patient's account. Post each service or procedure and any payments received and adjustments applied. Save the data to update the record. RATIONALE: Clearly indicates charges made and payments received, creating an updated account.

7. If any adjustment applies to the account, enter the amount in the adjustment column. If there is no adjustment column and the adjustment will *reduce* the bill, enter the amount in the payment column enclosed by parentheses. If the adjustment will *increase* the bill, place the amount in the charge column (no parentheses) with an explanation in the description column. In the *manual system,* the adjustment amount will be either added to or subtracted from the totaled figures. RATIONALE: Adjustment is shown as separate from basic charge so that the provider's fee profile is unaffected.

8. Using a manual system, determine current balance by adding credits and subtracting debits to the running balance and determine the amount in the current balance. Always use a calculator (one with a tape is recommended) to calculate and verify your mathematics. When using a PM system, the software will automatically calculate the

(continues)

balance. Verifying accuracy of the posting is integral for a properly updated balance. RATIONALE: Completes the recording of patient charges, payments, and adjustments.

9. If the posting includes a payment from the patient, place a restrictive endorsement on the check. RATIONALE: Ensures that the check can only be cashed by the authorized party.

10. In a manual pegboard system, enter the amount in the payment column. In the description column, identify as cash, check, or insurance payment. If payment is a check, enter the number of the check. When using a PM system, follow the guidelines for the payment posting module to indicate type of payment. RATIONALE: This information is necessary in making the bank deposit slip.

11. Place the cash or processed check in the appointed secure place awaiting deposit. RATIONALE: Keeps receivables together and ready for deposit.

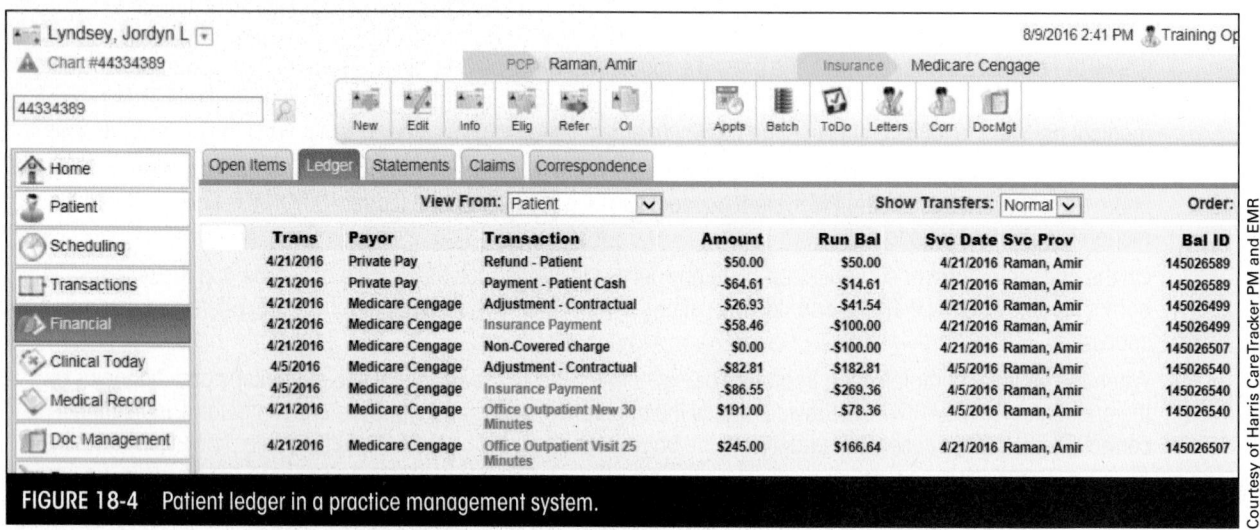

FIGURE 18-4 Patient ledger in a practice management system.

Procedure

See Table 18-1 for more information on the necessary components of a bookkeeping system including the day sheet and receipt forms. Procedure 18-2 describes the process for balancing a day sheet.

Month-End Activities

In the pegboard system, when the last day sheet for the month has been balanced, it is then necessary to verify that the month-end figures on the day sheet agree with patient accounts. Although this may be a time-consuming process in the manual system, it will find mistakes before they grow into major accounting or collection problems.

Reconciling the month-end sheet to the patient ledgers is accomplished by adding all the open balances on the ledgers and verifying that the total agrees with the end-of-month accounts receivable balance on the last day sheet of the month. When these figures agree, the accounts receivable balance is correct.

By following these procedures of "checks and balances," it is likely that all payments have been properly credited to patient accounts and deposited, and that all charges shown as outstanding on the day sheet agree with the outstanding balances of the individual patient accounts. If a payment is somehow misplaced, the deposits will not agree with the credits or with the patient ledgers, and an error will be revealed immediately. Not only does this catch errors, it also eliminates the possibility of loss of a check or undetected theft of funds, because when a mistake is caught immediately, the payer can stop payment on the missing check or credit or debit card slip and a new payment can be made.

TABLE 18-1

COMPONENTS OF THE BOOKKEEPING SYSTEM

COMPONENT	DESCRIPTION
Pegboard	A hard writing surface with a margin of "pegs" that hold documents in place while using the components of the system (superbill, ledger, receipts, etc.).
Encounter form	The encounter form, also known as the charge slip, superbill, or multipurpose billing form, is used in both manual and computerized systems. It provides the codes for the procedures performed and for which diagnoses during an encounter with the provider. The form serves as an itemized statement for insurance billing and a receipt for payments.
Ledger	The ledger, or record of services, lists payments and balances due from an individual patient, or the individuals of a family represented on a single ledger.
Day sheet	The pegboard write-it-once section is where individual transactions are posted for the day, using the ledger card and encounter form on top of the day sheet. The information in this section includes the date, patient name, description of transaction or service, charges, credits, and previous and current balances. At the bottom of the day sheet, transactions are totaled and balanced to be carried forward to the next day, or closed at the end of each month.
Receipt forms	Receipt forms used for payments on accounts usually are not customized with other than the name, address, and telephone number of the practice preprinted. The receipt form is used only when someone makes a payment on an account on a day when no services were rendered. It is not necessary to use a receipt form for payment received in the mail.

PROCEDURE 18-2

Balancing Day Sheets in a Manual System

Procedure

PURPOSE:
To verify that all entries to the day sheet are correct and that the totals balance.

EQUIPMENT/SUPPLIES:
- Day sheet
- Calculator

PROCEDURE STEPS:

1. *Column totals.* The first step in balancing a day sheet is to total columns A, B_1, B_2, C, and D, and enter the total for each column in the boxes marked Totals This Page. The column totals are then added to the figures entered in the Previous Page column boxes to arrive at the Month to Date totals, which provide the total charges, credits, and so forth entered from the first working day of the month to the present. RATIONALE: Establishes column totals.

2. *Proof of posting.* This box is used to verify that entries have been made correctly and that the column totals are accurate. *All figures entered here are taken from the "Totals This Page" column boxes.*

   a. Enter today's column D total, which shows the sum of all the previous balances entered when the transactions were posted.

   b. Added to this is the column A total of all charges for that day, to arrive at a subtotal. Enter the amount where indicated in the box.

(continues)

c. Because columns B_1 and B_2 are both credit columns that reduce balances, they are added together and entered in the box labeled Less Cols B_1 and B_2; the total of credits is subtracted from the subtotal. If all entries and addition are correct in the posting area, the result should equal the amount in column C and the transactions for that day are balanced. RATIONALE: Verifies entries have been made correctly and that the totals are accurate.

Overview: When an individual transaction is entered, the patient's previous balance (D) is added to the charges for the day (A). If there are any payments or adjustments made at that time, they are entered in the B columns and subtracted from the A + D amount to achieve the new balance (C). Because each transaction is actually D + A – B = C, the column totals of D + A – B will always equal the C total.

	D		A		B		C
	10	+	5	–	2	=	13
	2	+	7	–	1	=	8
Column Totals	12	+	12	–	3	=	21

3. *Accounts Receivable (A/R) Control.* This box simply adds the previous day's A/R balance to the current day's totals to include the current day's business and arrive at the new A/R total.

   a. The column A and column B totals are carried straight across from the Proof of Posting box to the corresponding blanks in the A/R Control box.

   b. Add the amount already entered in the Previous Day's Total space to the Column A amount to arrive at a subtotal.

   c. Subtract the amount carried over from the Less Columns B_1 and B_2 box to find the new A/R amount. RATIONALE: Determines new accounts receivable balance.

4. *A/R Proof* verifies, or proves, the A/R balance in the A/R Control box. *The figure entered on the first line of this box will not change during a calendar month* because it shows how much the A/R balance was on the first working day of the month. *All other figures entered will be taken from the Month-To-Date column boxes.*

   a. Enter the amount from column A (month-to-date) where shown.

   b. Add the column A amount to the A/R 1st of Month figure and enter the sum in the subtotal space.

   c. Enter the B_1 and B_2 month-to-date amounts and subtract from the subtotal. This amount goes in the Total A/R space.

   If all posting and addition are correct, the Total A/R amounts in the A/R Control and A/R Proof boxes will match and the day is balanced. RATIONALE: Verifies the accounts receivable balance in the accounts receivable control box.

5. *Deposit verification* involves totaling the columns in Section 2 and entering the sum of the columns in the space marked Total Deposit.

   NOTE: The Total Deposit and the Total of Payments Received in column B_1 should match. RATIONALE: Verifies deposit total.

6. *Business Analysis Summary.* If this section is used, total each column in the summary section.

   NOTE: If the Business Analysis Summary is used to break out charges by type or by provider, the sum of the columns should equal today's column A total. If it is used to credit payments to different providers, the sum of the columns will equal today's payment column.

   RATIONALE: The total deposit and the total of payments received in column B_1 should match to prove totals.

7. *After the day sheet is balanced,* there is one step remaining: the transfer of balances.

   a. Take out a new day sheet for the next day.

   b. Transfer the Month-To-Date column totals to the Previous Page columns boxes on the new sheet.

   c. Enter the Total A/R amount from the last day sheet in the Previous Day's Total space of the A/R Control box on the new day sheet.

   d. Enter the A/R 1st of Month Amount in the A/R Proof box on the new sheet. RATIONALE: Transfers balances to prepare a new day sheet for the next day's activities.

   The new day sheet is now ready for posting.

Computerized Patient Accounts

A practice management system offers many advantages in managing patient accounts. The program automatically creates an encounter form the day before the patient is seen or when the administrative medical assistant prints out the schedule. After the patient's examination, the program calculates the charges for the monthly billing statement (Figure 18-5). The management program also creates and updates the patient account, adds new names to the list of patients and to the daily log, and transfers data to produce insurance forms, statements, a list of checks received each day, and deposit slips. In addition, the program automatically ages accounts at each billing cycle and creates billing statements. As a result, when patient accounts are computerized, practice collections usually increase.

The computerized patient account contains personal information about each patient, including name, address, and telephone number; email address; the person responsible for payment; and all insurance carriers. The account also lists all previous clinic visits and the procedures, procedure codes, charges, payments, and adjustments for each visit. Most account management software can be customized to meet the special needs of the individual clinic.

As billing information is entered from the encounter forms, the computer automatically updates the account by adding a description of each procedure and procedure code and each diagnosis and diagnosis code. The computer software automatically posts the charges and calculates the balance after credits and adjustments are entered.

 Once charges and payments have been entered and the day has been closed, they are not easily removed or changed. This is an important software design because it ensures that monies are not removed from receivables credited to a previous month. This procedure would cause the practice year-end balance to be unresolved. Procedure 18-3 describes the steps for electronically processing patient credit balances and refunds.

Procedure

As useful and efficient as a computerized bookkeeping system can be, it is important to recognize that an inadequate manual system will not get better once computerized. Also, it takes time to move to a computerized system, train personnel, and enter existing patient data. Manual and computer systems may need to run concurrently for a month or two.

BANKING PROCEDURES

Understanding bank accounts and services, making deposits, preparing checks, and reconciling accounts are all a part of daily financial practices. Although many banking services are similar from one bank to another, it is a good idea for the medical assistant in charge of maintaining daily accounts to investigate the banking resources of the local community. In an effort to secure new business, many banks compete for customers by offering special services that can be of use to the medical practice.

Online Banking

Use of the Internet has changed banking and the services it provides. Online banking allows individuals to check account balances, transfer funds between accounts, pay bills electronically, check credit card balances, view images of checks and deposits, and download account information 24 hours a day, 7 days a week. Considerable time and expense can be saved with online banking, but remember that any online banking should be completed only through the use of secure and unique passwords granted to only those individuals deemed necessary.

Types of Accounts

Checking and savings accounts are the two primary types of accounts used in the medical practice.

Checking Accounts. The checking account is the primary account type the medical assistant will use in the clinic. Today, there are many variations on checking accounts. In the event that the medical assistant is responsible for establishing a new account, it is worthwhile to investigate features of different checking accounts both within the same bank and at competing banks.

Some features that may differ include:

- Interest paid
- Monthly fees
- Check charges
- Automated teller machine (ATM) access and fees
- After-hours deposit capabilities
- Initial deposit and balance requirements
- Overdraft protection
- Fees for checks

Napa Valley Family Associates

ACCOUNT #	38803-42539489	STATEMENT DATE	3/15/2014
LAST PAYMENT	$14.61	STATEMENT TOTAL	$266.64

Statement - Page 1

DATE OF SERVICE	PATIENT	DESCRIPTION OF SERVICES	PROCEDURE CODE	SERVICING PROVIDER	AMOUNT	PATIENT AMT DUE
3/10/2014	Lyndsey, Jordyn L (42539489)	Office Outpatient New 30 Minutes	99203	Raman, Amir	-$86.55	$21.64
		Per Your Insurance Company, Your Copay Has Not Been Paid In Full. The Balance Is Your Responsibility. Thank You.				
		Transaction 03/10/2014, Adjustment - Contractual			-$82.81	
		Transaction 03/10/2014, Charges			$191.00	
3/13/2014	Lyndsey, Jordyn L (42539489)	Office Outpatient Visit 25 Minutes	99214	Raman, Amir	$245.00	$245.00
		See Billing Note				
		Transaction 03/13/2014, Non-Covered charge			$0.00	

MAKE CHECKS PAYABLE TO: Napa Valley Family Associates

PLEASE PAY THIS AMOUNT	$266.64

TO ENSURE PROPER CREDIT, PLEASE DETACH AND RETURN BOTTOM PORTION WITH YOUR PAYMENT

···

Napa Valley Family Associates
101 Vine Street
Napa, CA 94558

707- 555-1212 Ext:

ACCOUNT #	38803-42539489	STATEMENT DATE	3/15/2014
AMOUNT ENCLOSED $		STATEMENT TOTAL	$266.64

☐ CHECK BOX AND ENTER ADDRESS OR INSURANCE CORRECTIONS ON THE REVERSE SIDE

☐ IF PAYING BY CREDIT CARD, FILL OUT THE INFORMATION ON THE REVERSE SIDE

ADDRESSEE:
JORDYN L LYNDSEY
PO BOX 84557
FAIRFIELD, CA 94533

REMIT TO:
NAPA VALLEY FAMILY ASSOCIATES
101 VINE STREET
NAPA, CA 94558

IF ANY OF THE INFORMATION HAS BEEN CHANGED SINCE YOUR LAST STATEMENT, PLEASE INDICATE...

ABOUT YOU:

YOUR NAME (Last, First, Middle Initial)	
ADDRESS	
CITY	STATE ZIP
TELEPHONE ( )	MARITAL STATUS ☐ Single ☐ Divorced ☐ Married ☐ Widowed
EMPLOYER'S NAME	TELEPHONE ( )
EMPLOYER'S ADDRESS	CITY STATE ZIP

IF PAYING BY CREDIT CARD, FILL OUT BELOW

☐ AMERICAN EXPRESS	☐ MASTERCARD ☐ VISA
CARD NUMBER	
CHARGE THIS AMOUNT	EXPIRATION DATE
SIGNATURE	CARDHOLDER NAME

ABOUT YOUR INSURANCE:

YOUR PRIMARY INSURANCE COMPANY'S NAME	EFFECTIVE DATE
PRIMARY INSURANCE COMPANY'S ADDRESS	PHONE
CITY	STATE ZIP
POLICYHOLDER'S ID NUMBER	GROUP PLAN NUMBER
YOUR SECONDARY INSURANCE COMPANY'S NAME	EFFECTIVE DATE
SECONDARY INSURANCE COMPANY'S ADDRESS	PHONE
CITY	STATE ZIP
POLICYHOLDER'S ID NUMBER	GROUP PLAN NUMBER

FIGURE 18-5 Computerized patient statement.

PROCEDURE 18-3

Procedure

Processing Credit Balances and Refunds Using a Computerized PM System

PURPOSE:

To post overpayment refunds to patient accounts with a credit balance.

EQUIPMENT/SUPPLIES:

Computer and PM system

PROCEDURE STEPS:

To post overpayment refunds to patient accounts with a credit balance.

1. Using your chosen PM system, navigate to the payment posting module and open the patient account.
2. Click on the line item for the date and procedure for which a refund shall be posted. *Hint:* If more than one service needs to be refunded, apply it to each separately. Check balances as you post to verify these are correct.
3. In the *Description* field, enter "Refund overpayment."
4. Enter the amount to be refunded. Save to apply the refund to the balance.
5. If applicable, apply a refund to the next service in the same manner.

- Special services extended free of charge such as **notary**, cashier's checks, traveler's checks, and online banking

When selecting an account, rather than choosing the account with the lowest fees, consider convenience, the relationship possible with a given bank, bank hours, number of bank locations, and other factors.

Savings Accounts. Savings accounts initially were distinguished from checking accounts because they paid interest on the money deposited. However, many checking accounts now pay interest as well. In either case, the interest is minimal on accounts that give immediate access to the deposit. **Money market savings accounts** often pay a higher rate of interest, although they may require a higher initial deposit and maintenance of a higher balance. Access to the account may require 24-hour turnaround time. Such accounts are useful when access to money is not needed frequently or when accumulating an amount necessary to invest for long-term goals.

Types of Checks

For the most part, the clinic setting uses a standard business check. However, for special purposes, it is useful to understand the other check types available:

- A **cashier's check** is occasionally used when a check must be guaranteed for the amount in which it is written. Because a cashier's check is the bank's own check drawn against the bank's accounts, the recipient has the assurance that the check will clear. Cashier's checks are obtained at the bank by paying the bank representative cash or sometimes a personal check for the amount of the cashier's check. It is important to understand, however, that not all facilities will accept a cashier's check. Be sure to check with the office manager about accepted policy.

- A **certified check** is the depositor's own check that the bank has "certified" with a date and signature to indicate that the check is good for the amount in which it is written.

- Money orders are available from a number of places, even online. The U.S. Postal Service and Western Union are common sites for the purchase of money orders. They are purchased with cash and are similar to cashier's checks. A few patients may use money orders to pay their bills.

- A **voucher check** is a type of check with a stub attached that can be used to indicate invoice dates, services provided, and so on. Some payroll checks are written on voucher checks.
- **Electronic checks** have become widely used in clinic settings. Although performing the same purpose as a paper check, electronic checks give the added convenience of faster processing, security, and guaranteed value.

Depositing Checks

Deposits are usually made daily because they serve as another proof of posting and because leaving large sums of money in the facility overnight is unwise. A rubber endorsement stamp from the bank should be used to immediately imprint the back of all checks received directly from patients and in the mail. Be sure all checks are stamped before depositing them. Scanning or photocopying all checks before deposit is one way to ensure accuracy, although with online banking images of deposited checks are available with the account statements.

Because the endorsement transfers rights to whoever holds the check, it is important to take certain precautions. A blank endorsement consists of a signature only (whether in pen or with a stamp) and presents a danger in that, if the check is lost or stolen, someone else could endorse the check below the signature and cash it. A restrictive endorsement should be used on all checks received in the clinic. Restrictive endorsements include the signature and the words *for deposit only* or *pay to the order of*. . . (include the name of bank and account number; in addition, all possible payees' names should be listed under the company name, with the clinic address). This restricts the use of the check should it be lost or stolen.

Deposits and Technology. Online banking affords many conveniences, and there are multiple ways to make deposits using technology. By using these methods, deposit preparation can be streamlined, speeding up receivables to account, and eliminating trips to the bank. Money is becoming more digital, and with the advent of online-only banks and money transfer apps, there are new ways to handle paper checks. Instead of using bank tellers or ATMs, making a deposit can be as easy as taking a picture of the front and back of endorsed checks and uploading images to the bank account. Two common deposit methods are remote deposit capture and electronic check conversion.

- **Remote deposit capture** is a process by which consumer and business check payments are deposited using a check scanner and PC at the clinic, or capturing images of endorsed checks via a smart phone and apps.
- **Electronic check conversion** is a process by which a paper check is used as a source of information. The check number, account number, and the number that identifies the financial institution are used to make a one-time electronic payment from the account. In effect, this is an electronic fund transfer, even though the check itself is not the method of payment. As such, the check is given back to the payer (even a blank check will suffice), but the check should not be used again for a different transaction. Businesses using this method are required to disclose to the payer that the check will be used for electronic transfer of funds.

Other methods of depositing or transferring money digitally would include direct deposit, pay-by-phone, bank pay, and person-to-person payments (various financial institutions have adopted proprietary names for person-to-person electronic fund transfer).

Cash on Hand

Most medical practices need to have cash available on a daily basis. If it is the practice to collect co-payments and any coinsurance at the time of service, some patients will pay in cash and need change. Cash usually is kept in a locked change drawer that contains up to $200 in small bills at the beginning of each day. Any time a patient pays cash for the service, a receipt is prepared. Receipts are prenumbered, thus monitoring loss or theft. Cash amounts paid by patients must also be noted in their account or ledger. The term *received on account (ROA) cash* is usually indicated in the

Critical Thinking

How does a practice management system save time, human resources, and increase efficiency in a clinical setting? Give three examples.

description column. If payment is made by check, follow the same procedure except the word *check* is used instead of *cash*.

At the end of each day, the cash drawer is balanced. The amount of cash received will be noted on the deposit slip as "currency." The remaining amount in the cash drawer will be the same as the beginning amount. Also, the day's cash received must match the cash control on the daily sheet. It is a good idea for only one person to handle the cash in the cash drawer; thus, it is not necessary for more than one person to balance the cash drawer at the end of the day. The cash drawer is not to be confused with petty cash, which is discussed later in this chapter. Petty cash is used to purchase small items such as postage, clinic refreshments, and so on. Checks are always written for major purchases, with the cash drawer used only to accommodate patient needs when payment is made in cash.

Most business accounts use deposit slips similar to the one shown in Figure 18-6. They are always completed in duplicate or a copy is made— one copy to accompany the deposit and one to be retained for clinic records. As shown, these deposit slips are longer than those generally used for personal accounts and have room for more entries and more information. If your manual day sheet has a built-in duplicate deposit slip, it will have been completed during posting.

Procedure

A computerized system of financial records can provide deposit slips that may be used. The same procedure is followed as previously discussed. Procedure 18-4 outlines the steps in preparing a deposit.

Accepting Checks

Competency

When accepting checks from patients and other individuals, take time to inspect the check. This may eliminate checks returned from the bank for various reasons:

- Inspect the check for correct date, amount, and signature.
- Do not accept a third-party check (a check written to the patient from another person or company) unless it is from the insurance carrier.

Procedure

- If a deposited check is returned marked *non-sufficient funds* (*NSF*), call the bank that returned it and verify availability of funds. If funds are available, immediately redeposit the check for processing. If the check is returned a second time marked

---

Inner City Health Care
8600 Main Street, Suite 201
River City, NY 01234
(123) 555-0326

DEPOSIT SLIP

_____ 20 __

First Bank
5411 Brown Rd.
River City, NY 01234

⑈1 22 01493 2⑈

Front

CURRENCY	
COIN	
CHECKS	
TOTAL FROM OTHER SIDE	
TOTAL	

List all items separately

Total
Enter on front side

Back

FIGURE 18-6 Sample deposit slip.

PROCEDURE 18-4

Procedure

Preparing a Deposit

PURPOSE:

To create a deposit slip for the day's receipts.

EQUIPMENT/SUPPLIES:

- New deposit slip
- Check endorsement stamp
- Calculator
- Cash and checks received for the day

PROCEDURE STEPS:

1. Separate all checks from currency (paper money). RATIONALE: Each must be entered as a separate total.

2. Count all currency to be deposited and enter the amount in the space provided. Gather bills facing the same direction in order (i.e., 50s, 20s, 10s, and so on). RATIONALE: Follows bank procedure.

3. Count all coins to be deposited and enter the amount in the space provided. Coins may need to be wrapped. RATIONALE: Follows bank procedure.

4. On the back of the deposit slip list each check separately. Include the patient name in the left-hand column and enter the amount of the check in the right-hand column. RATIONALE: Follows bank procedure.

5. Total the checks listed and copy the total on the front where it is indicated to place the total from the other side. RATIONALE: Follows bank procedure.

6. The sum of currency, coins, and checks should always equal the total in the Payments column on that day's day sheet. RATIONALE: Proof of accuracy.

7. Attach the top copy of the deposit slip to the deposit, leaving the carbon on the pad. RATIONALE: Provides the clinic and bank with a record of deposit.

8. Enter the date and amount of the deposit in the space provided on the checkbook stubs. RATIONALE: Keeps checkbook register current with money in account.

9. Add the amount of the deposit to the checkbook balance. RATIONALE: Keeps checkbook register current with money in account.

10. Deposit at the bank, either in person or at the night deposit. In either case, be sure a record of deposit is received (it will be mailed if the night deposit is used). It is not recommended that deposits be made through ATMs; currency should never be deposited in an ATM. RATIONALE: Proves bank processed the deposit as indicated.

NSF, it is necessary to perform two bookkeeping functions. First, deduct the amount from the checking account balance of the practice. Second, add the amount back into the amount due by the patient in his or her account balance by entering the amount in the paid column in parentheses and increase the balance by the same amount. Place a brief explanation in the description column. Follow the clinic procedure for notifying the patient that the check was returned. See Procedure 18-5.

Lost or Stolen Checks

In the event that a check is missing and is thought to be lost or stolen, report this to your bank immediately. In some cases, you may be advised to stop payment to prevent unauthorized cashing of the check. In other situations, the bank may place a warning on the account, advising bank representatives to be especially careful about checking signatures to detect any attempt at a forged signature.

PROCEDURE 18-5

Procedure

Recording a Nonsufficient Funds Check

PURPOSE:

To perform bookkeeping functions that keep accounts in proper balance.

EQUIPMENT/SUPPLIES:

- The practice's account balance
- Manual day sheet
- Manual ledger
- Nonsufficient funds (NSF) check

PROCEDURE STEPS:

1. Follow the clinic policy for notifying the patient of the returned check. RATIONALE: Policy may vary from clinic to clinic.

2. When the NSF check has been returned the second time, deduct the check amount from the account balance of the clinic. RATIONALE: The funds can no longer be counted as earnings received.

3. Add the amount of the NSF check back into the patient's ledger. Place the amount in parentheses in the paid column and increase the total by the same amount. In a manual system, the entry and math are performed by the medical assistant. RATIONALE: The amount is still owed by the patient, is not considered paid, and must be reflected in the amount due.

4. Place a brief explanation in the description of the column such as "NSF 12/09/20XX."

Writing and Recording Checks

Part of daily financial practices includes writing checks to pay bills (**accounts payable**), refunding overpayment, and replenishing petty cash. Writing the checks and paying the bills is usually done systematically. Chapter 20 discusses accounts payable and disbursement records in greater detail. It is important that checks be prepared either electronically or written legibly to avoid bank errors. Checks should be dated and must include the name of the **payee**. The amount of payment entered both in figures and in words should match exactly. If there is a discrepancy, the bank will not accept the check or may pay the incorrect amount. It is also advisable that the "memo" line indicates what the check is for and includes any account or invoice number for reference. Figure 18-7 shows a sample of a properly completed check.

Procedure

Rules for Preparing Checks. Follow these rules to ensure that checks are properly prepared and recorded (see Procedure 18-6).

- Confirm that the numeric and written amounts agree.
- Confirm that everything is spelled correctly.
- Follow clinic procedure for having the provider or office manager approve all expenditures and sign all outgoing checks.
- Determine that the check has been signed by an individual with signature privileges.
- Confirm that the check is payable to the correct payee and that the current date is used.

Chapter 20 provides information on electronic check writing.

Reconciling a Bank Statement

Each month the bank will send a statement for the checking account (Figure 18-8). With online banking, a bank statement can be accessed electronically at any time. It also can be printed and used similar to a standard printed bank statement. The statement will show the account

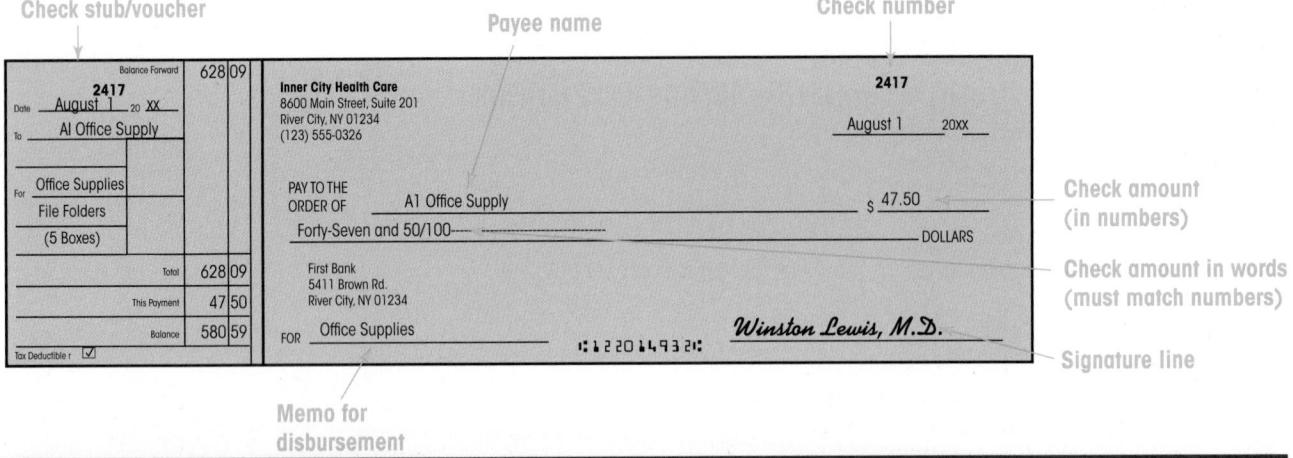

Check stub/voucher

Payee name

Check number

Check amount (in numbers)

Check amount in words (must match numbers)

Signature line

Memo for disbursement

FIGURE 18-7 Sample of properly completed check and check stub voucher.

PROCEDURE 18-6

Writing a Manual Check

Procedure

PURPOSE:

To write a check to pay for expenses incurred and provide proof of payment. (Never written a check before? Go to http://www.checkright.org for practice.)

EQUIPMENT/SUPPLIES:

- Checkbook and check register with balance of $7,298.35
- Pen with black ink
- Calculator

CHECKING WRITING EXERCISES:

Write checks for the following invoices using the current date:

1. $54.99 for case of printer paper to Landau Products
2. $450.00 for last month's janitorial services to MJB Services
3. $1,335.38 for clinical supplies to Redding Medical Supply House
4. $687.19 to Atlantic Electric for last month's heat and electricity
5. $350 to American Association of Medical Assistants for AAMA membership for the four medical assistants in the clinic

PROCEDURE STEPS:

1. Gather all invoices to be paid.
2. For the check register, use black ink:
   a. Enter check number 101 in the register if not preprinted.
   b. Enter the current date and year (usually in numbers, i.e., 02/14/20XX).
   c. Enter the individual or company the check is to be paid to: Landau Products.
   d. Enter the amount to be paid on the check: $54.99.

(continues)

e. Subtract check amount from the present balance. Total $7,243.36 appears as the available balance. RATIO-NALE: These steps ensure that the check register is not overlooked when writing a check and establishes a well-recognized routine.

3. To write the check, use black ink:

a. Enter check number 101 if not preprinted.

b. Enter the current date and year (usually written out, e.g., February 14, 20XX).

c. Enter the individual or company the check is to be paid to: Landau Products.

d. Enter the amount to be paid on the check: $54.99. Do not leave spaces between numbers or between the dollar sign and the first number. RATIONALE: This helps to prevent any tampering of the check by adding numbers.

e. Write out the amount to be paid by check (Fifty-four dollars and 99/100). Fill in any space left between the last number or word and draw a wiggly line over to the amount entered in numbers. RATIONALE: When the written amount and the number amount match, errors are prevented. The wiggly line makes it more difficult for anyone to tamper with the check.

f. Describe what the check is written for in the bottom left corner (Printer paper, case). RATIONALE: Explains the purpose of the check.

g. If you have check-writing authority in the clinic, sign the check with your name the same as indicated on the bank's records. If you do not have check-writing authority, hold this check and the others to give to the individual with that authority. RATIONALE: The person responsible can review the checks with the invoices to verify valid expenses.

4. Continue writing checks for items 2 through 5 in the Check Writing Exercises, being certain to number checks consecutively and to subtract each check. Submit checks and check register with final balance to your instructor for evaluation.

Front

Summary of Account Balance   Closing Date 1/15/XX

Account # 1257-164013   Ending Balance $8,347.62

Beginning Balance	$7,152.18
Total Deposits and Additions	$8,643.86
Total Withdrawals	$7,433.21
Service Charge	$ 15.24

Number	Date	Amount	Number	Date	Amount
201	12/18/XX	173.82	234	1/4/XX	96.31
223*	12/18/XX	44.12	235	1/4/XX	73.48
224	12/20/XX	586.00	236	1/6/XX	325.40
225	12/21/XX	24.15	237	1/7/XX	40.00
226	12/22/XX	33.90	238	1/8/XX	66.77
228*	12/23/XX	1250.00	241*	1/9/XX	15.55
229	12/24/XX	11.75	242	1/10/XX	12.45
230	12/24/XX	19.02	243	1/10/XX	4441.25
231	1/2/XX	43.80	244	1/10/XX	64.55
232	1/3/XX	39.00			
233	1/4/XX	71.50			

*Denotes gap in check sequence

Date	Deposit Amount	Date	Deposit Amount
18-Dec	361.75	4-Jan	825.00
19-Dec	586.00	5-Jan	1286.71
20-Dec	918.21	7-Jan	608.00
21-Dec	201.00	8-Jan	811.15
2-Jan	475.00	9-Jan	1092.68
3-Jan	1478.36		

Back

1. Enter Ending Balance from the front of this statement

$ 8,347.62

2. Enter deposits not shown on this statement

$ 3,162.50

3. Subtotal (add 1 & 2)

$ 11,510.12

4. List outstanding checks or other withdrawals here

Check #	Amount
222	37.89
227	161.15
239	11.50
240	92.12
245	835.17
246	21.75
247	586.00

5. Total outstanding checks

$ 1,745.58

Balance (subtract #5 from #3)

$ 9,764.54

This should equal your checkbook balance

FIGURE 18-8 Sample bank statement with check reconciliation.

balance according to the bank's records, a listing of all checks that have cleared the bank, deposits received by the bank, and any service charges deducted from the account. It is necessary to reconcile the entries in the checkbook against this statement to be sure there are no errors either in the checkbook or in the bank's records. Your bank statement is another means of ensuring that the accounts receivable is accurate for the previous month. If you use an accounting software package, this will also have a computerized option for reconciling.

Procedure

Procedure 18-7 details the steps involved in reconciling the statement.

PURCHASING SUPPLIES AND EQUIPMENT

It is important to ensure proper control over purchasing of supplies and equipment for several reasons:

1. To avoid purchase of unnecessary items
2. To avoid duplication of items purchased
3. To provide a system for payment of only those items properly ordered and received

To accomplish these things, you should follow the first rule of purchasing: nothing is ordered or paid for without a purchase order or purchase order number. A copy of the purchase order is sent to the supplier and a copy is retained by the

---

PROCEDURE 18-7

Procedure

Reconciling a Bank Statement

PURPOSE:

To verify that the balance listed in the checkbook agrees with the balance shown by the bank.

EQUIPMENT/SUPPLIES:

- Checkbook
- Bank statement
- Calculator

PROCEDURE STEPS:

1. Make sure the balance in the checkbook is current (all deposits and checks entered have been added or subtracted). RATIONALE: Ensures totals are accurate.
2. If a service charge is listed on the statement, subtract that amount from the last balance listed in the checkbook. RATIONALE: Reconciles current balance.
3. In the checkbook, check off each check listed on the statement and verify the amount against the check stub. RATIONALE: Verifies accuracy.
4. In the checkbook, check off each deposit listed on the statement. RATIONALE: Verifies accuracy.
5. The back of the statement contains a worksheet to be used for balancing.
6. Copy the ending balance from the front of the statement to the area indicated on the back.
7. Go through the check stubs and list on the back of the statement in the area provided any checks that have not cleared and any deposits that were not shown as received on the statement.
8. Total the checks not cleared on the statement worksheet.
9. Total the deposits not credited on the worksheet.
10. Add together the statement balance and the total of deposits not credited.
11. Subtract the total of checks not cleared. This amount should agree with the balance in the checkbook. If so, the checkbook is balanced and the statement should be filed in the appropriate place. RATIONALE: Following procedure steps 5 through 11 completes verification of accuracy.

clinic for verification of shipment and payment of invoice.

Preparing a Purchase Order

Purchase order forms are available from office supply companies or can be ordered from a printer and customized to the needs of the clinic setting. As an alternative to ordering preprinted purchase order forms, the clinic staff may choose to create their own forms using Microsoft Excel software. This enables the clinic to have electronic access to the form with embedded formulas. Figure 18-9 shows a typical purchase order form properly completed, which is reviewed here section by section.

The purchase order form can vary greatly; some have more or less information. The form shown in Figure 18-9 contains the usual information required. The important thing is that the purchase order is used consistently.

- *Date.* The day the purchase order is created.
- *Purchase order number.* A preprinted number that is used on invoices and statements from the supplier and on the check used to pay the invoice. It is also important for tracking the status of the order. In smaller practices, the purchase order number may simply be the name of the person ordering with the date the order was placed immediately following.
- *Bill to address.* This is generally used when items are to be shipped to an address different from the address where the supplier will send the bill for goods or services.
- *Ship to address.* When items are to be sent by supplier, this must always be completed.
- *Vendor information.* The name and address of the supplier where the purchase order is to be sent.
- *Req. by* ("Requested by"). States which individual or department has requested the item(s).

PURCHASE ORDER

NO. 1742

Date:

Bill To:

Inner City Health Care
8600 Main Street, Suite 201
River City, NY 01234
(123) 555-0326

Ship To:

Inner City Health Care
8600 Main Street, Suite 201
River City, NY 01234
(123) 555-0326

Vendor:

AZ Medical Supply
4721 E. Camelback Rd.
Phoenix, AZ 85252
(602) 555-3246

REQ BY	BUYER	TERMS
Ellen Armstrong	Marilyn Johnson	Net 30

QTY	ITEM	UNITS	DESCRIPTION	UNIT PR	TOTAL
10	427A	Box	Surgical gloves - Sz 7	9.20	92.00
1	327DC	Case	2" gauze pads	60.30	60.30
5	1943C	Box	Tongue depressors	5.80	29.00
15	7433	Ea	Examination table paper (roll)	10.50	159.50

SUBTOTAL		338.80
TAX		28.80
FREIGHT		Prepaid
BAL DUE		376.60

FIGURE 18-9 Purchase order form.

- *Buyer.* States the individual in the clinic who is authorized to issue a purchase order.
- *Terms.* Agreement between buyer and seller as to when payment is due.
- *Qty.* Quantity of item being ordered (number of units).
- *Item.* Vendor's catalogue part or item number.
- *Units.* How the item is sold—individually (ea.), by the box, case, or dozen. Many suppliers will not split units (i.e., will not sell less than a full case).
- *Description.* Brief description of item (helps as a cross-check for the vendor in the event that an item number is entered incorrectly).
- *Unit price.* How much *one* unit (ea., box, case, dozen) costs.
- *Total.* Cost of one unit multiplied by the number of units being ordered.
- *Discount.* If any discount is allowed for quick and early payment, it is noted here. For instance, there might be a 10% discount for paying within 10 days. The discount amount is entered before the Total column is summed.
- *Subtotal.* Sum of the Total column.
- *Tax.* Sales tax required by the state.
- *Freight.* How much the customer must pay to have the order delivered (not always applicable).
- *Bal. Due.* The sum of the subtotal, tax, and freight charges; this is how much the clinic will be billed.

Verifying Goods Received

Proper purchasing procedure does not stop with the completion and mailing of the purchase order. When goods are received, it is necessary to verify that the correct items and quantities were shipped by the vendor. Chapter 20 discusses accounts payable.

PETTY CASH

Petty cash is money kept in the clinic for minor, routine, or unexpected expenses such as postage-due mail or coffee supplies. Keep petty cash totally separate from the cash drawer that is used to make change for patients paying their co-payment. Keeping this cash on hand eliminates the necessity of the provider or office manager having to sign checks for such items. Petty cash is not used to pay bills or make large routine purchases.

The amount of cash on hand for this purpose is small, usually $75 to $100, and is usually kept in small denominations. However, records must be as carefully maintained as for any other financial transactions and balanced each day before closing.

Establishing a Petty Cash Fund

If your clinic does not already have a petty cash fund or if you are in a new practice that has not yet established a fund, determine how much the fund should be and write a check to "Cash" for that amount. The amount should be enough to cover several days of incidental expenses.

Tracking, Balancing, and Replenishing Petty Cash

Tracking. Keep a supply of petty cash vouchers on hand to track how petty cash is used. When money is taken from petty cash, a voucher must always be completed and the receipt from the purchase attached. Vouchers and receipts are kept in the petty cash box with the money until the fund is replenished. Figure 18-10 shows an example of a petty cash form used to track funds.

Procedure

Balancing and Replenishing. When the fund gets low, write another check to "Cash" to bring it back up to the original amount. To determine the amount of the check, it is necessary to first balance the account. After the account is balanced, list how funds were spent in such a way that the bookkeeper can disburse the check properly.

Procedure 18-8 outlines the steps involved in establishing and maintaining a petty cash account.

DOCUMENTATION

Financial records of patients are to be kept separate from the patients medical charts. Except for the attachment of the encounter form or superbill at the time of the visit, they rarely are seen together. Often, only the patient's medical record is necessary for documentation; other times, only the financial information is necessary. This policy also serves as a reminder that the care given to patients has nothing to do with their ability to pay.

Petty Cash Voucher

Ref:				Date _____
Details				
Acct No.	Account Name	Total		Received (dollar amount) $ _____
				For: _____
				_____
				_____
	Total			Approved By Received By

FIGURE 18-10 Petty cash voucher.

PROCEDURE 18-8

Procedure

Establishing and Maintaining a Petty Cash Fund

PURPOSE:

To establish and maintain a petty cash fund for incidental expenses, making certain that receipts match the difference between the beginning and ending balance of the fund.

EQUIPMENT/SUPPLIES:

- Petty cash box with cash balance
- Vouchers
- Calculator

PETTY CASH EXERCISES:

1. Write a check to "Cash" for $100 to be taken to the bank.
2. Vouchers are made for the following incidentals:
   a. $20 to staff employee to purchase coffee supplies. Actual amount for supplies is $13.87; employee returns $6.13 cash
   b. $2.24 for postage due to postal employee
   c. $3.18 to postal employee for guaranteed forwarding address
   d. $35.00 to Shannon's Pizza delivery for staff meeting lunch

PROCEDURE STEPS:

Establish the Fund:

1. Cash the check for $100 and receive the money in denominations of 1s, 5s, 10s, and 20s. Place the cash in the cash box at the clinic. RATIONALE: The amount establishes petty cash and provides bills for the incidental purchases.

(continues)

2. When cash is needed for an incidental expense, such as postage due, prepare a voucher for the amount needed. No cash is taken from the fund without a voucher. RATIONALE: The written voucher indicates what the money is used for.

3. After the purchase, attach the receipt for the purchase to the voucher. RATIONALE: This step provides proof of the purchase.

Balance Petty Cash Fund:

1. After the activity identified in the Petty Cash Exercises, count the money remaining in the box. RATIONALE: Verifies the amount of cash remaining in petty cash.

2. Total the amounts of all vouchers in the petty cash box. RATIONALE: Determines amount of expenditures.

3. Subtract the amount of receipts from the original amount in petty cash. This should equal the amount of cash remaining in the box. RATIONALE: Proves that the amount of expenditures deducted from the beginning amount equals the amount left in the box.

4. When the cash has been balanced against the receipts, write a check *only for the amount that was used.* RATIONALE: Brings dollar amount back to original petty cash amount.

Petty Cash Check Disbursement:

1. Sort all vouchers by account.

2. On a sheet of paper list the accounts involved.

3. Total vouchers for each account and record individual totals on the list.

4. Copy this list with its totals on the memo portion of the stub for the check written to replenish petty cash.

5. File the list with the vouchers and receipts attached, after noting the check number on the list.

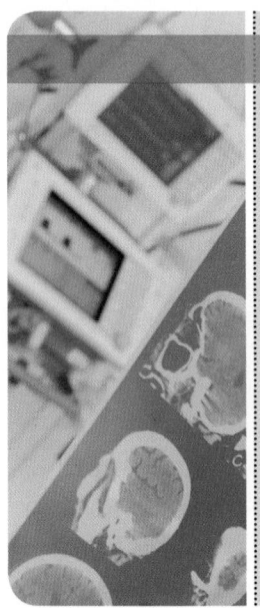

CASE STUDY 18-1

Refer to the scenario at the beginning of the chapter. As you consider the discussion of patient fees, determine what steps to take in the following situations.

CASE STUDY REVIEW

1. The clinic's patient has been diagnosed with non-Hodgkin's lymphoma (diffuse large B-cell lymphoma) in stage 3. Surgery and aggressive chemotherapy are in process. The patient has Medicare and a small Medigap policy. You know there are expenses coming soon that neither insurance will cover. What can you suggest?

2. This patient has been with the clinic for 11 years and was covered most of the time by excellent private insurance. The circumstances have changed, however. Today the patient works part time, has only Medicaid insurance, and has very few private funds. The provider's diagnosis is severe depression, and the provider instructs the patient to make two appointments weekly until the medication prescribed begins to make a significant difference in this patient's life. You know there are severe limitations to reimbursement from the state regarding this diagnosis. What steps will you take?

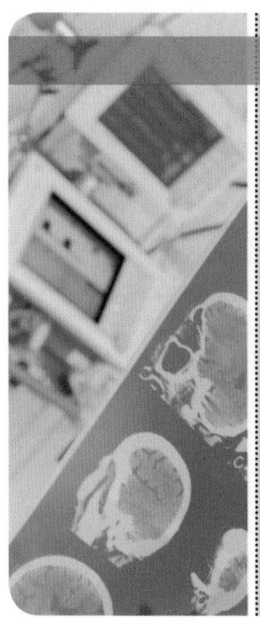

CASE STUDY 18-2

Joann Crier has completed her 3-month probation period with Inner City Health Care. She is doing quite well and has demonstrated skill in accurate financial documentation. She has been asked to take over reconciling the monthly bank statements and managing all the accounts payable, including getting the checks ready for the provider's signature. She has difficulty, however, completing these tasks until after hours when the clinic is closed and quiet. Clinic manager Marilyn Johnson, CMA (AAMA), has told her that it must be done within normal working hours unless special permission is granted.

CASE STUDY REVIEW

1. What suggestions can you make to Joann to allow her to complete these tasks during normal working hours?
2. What impact does the time of day, day(s) of the month, or place where the tasks are completed have on your suggestions?
3. Are there any circumstances you can identify when overtime might be warranted to allow Joann to complete the tasks after hours?

Summary

- The daily financial responsibilities of a medical clinic include patient bookkeeping, purchasing supplies and equipment, and petty cash.
- Proficiency in these functions is integral for a solvent practice that has the proper income, resources, and supplies available to provide appropriate patient care, and a healthy business in which to provide services, including a well-stocked and equipped clinic.
- The medical assistant must be familiar with using a system to post and track income data, as well as other types of financial transactions required by the practice.
- Clinics may use a pegboard system as a comprehensive manual system for tracking these data. Computerized bookkeeping offers many advantages related to speed, high accuracy, and elimination of some routine tasks while providing the same important financial data.
- Accurate and scrupulous maintenance of the accounts payable system ensures that bills are paid on time and those payments are properly documented for tax purposes.
- Practicing maximum accuracy in all bookkeeping functions is vital for the medical clinic.
- All charges and receipts must be recorded immediately.
- It is best practice for medical clinic personnel to make deposits of checks and currency the same day they are received.
- The medical assistant must always verify and recheck totals of all deposits and expenditures.
- Medical clinic personnel must stay current with all checking account duties such as account reconciliation.
- Medical clinic personnel must be prompt with all accounts payable.
- The medical assistant will likely be expected to maintain a petty cash fund and the clinic cash drawer for small daily cash transactions.

CERTIFICATION REVIEW

1. Which of the following is an accurate description of the debit column of a ledger?
   a. It is the column to the right of the balance column.
   b. It is the column on the left; used to enter charges, procedure codes, and description of services.
   c. It is the column at the far right that records the difference between the debit and credit columns.
   d. It is the column that indicates the patient's debt to the practice.

2. Which of the following statements regarding the use of debit/credit cards by patients to pay for services in ambulatory care settings is accurate?
   a. It is never done.
   b. It is unethical.
   c. It is sure to compromise the integrity of the clinic.
   d. It is a financial arrangement increasingly being used.
   e. It is done because most people carry no cash.

3. What is the purpose of the first section of the manual day sheet?
   a. To record deposits
   b. For business analysis
   c. To post individual transactions
   d. To total transactions

4. Which method is identified as a good working habit for financial transactions?
   a. Double-checking all entries for accuracy
   b. Keeping the bookkeeping tasks current and up to date
   c. Allowing the computer to create all the entries
   d. Managing the accounts on a weekly basis
   e. Both a and b

5. Which of the following statements is an accurate description of petty cash?
   a. It is necessary to give patients change when they pay in cash.
   b. It is used by the provider when taking a colleague to lunch.
   c. It pays for routine and unexpected minor expenses of the clinic.
   d. It comes from the provider's personal account.

6. Which of the following is true regarding encounter forms?
   a. They can be ordered to fit the practice.
   b. They provide a separate ledger for each patient household.
   c. They list common services provided, procedural code, and diagnosis code.
   d. They should be destroyed after processing.
   e. Both a and c

7. Which of the following is an accurate description of receipts?
   a. They are used for payments on accounts.
   b. They are not given unless services are rendered the same day.
   c. They are mailed to patients when payment is made by mail.
   d. They are unnecessary, especially in the computerized system.

8. When preparing checks from patients, it is important to:
   a. Inspect for correct date, amount, and signature
   b. Immediately stamp with a restrictive endorsement
   c. Automatically accept third-party checks
   d. Both a and b
   e. None of these

9. What is the name for a check with an attached stub for recording information?
   a. Certified check
   b. Cashier's check
   c. Voucher check
   d. Money order

10. Why is it important to ensure proper control over purchasing of supplies and equipment?
   a. To avoid purchase of unnecessary items
   b. To avoid duplication of items purchased
   c. To provide a system for payment of only those items properly ordered and received
   d. All of these
   e. None of these

Billing and Collections

1. Define and spell the key terms as presented in the glossary.
2. Analyze the importance of billing and collections to the clinic.
3. Describe the advantages of billing at least the co-payment and co-insurance at time of service.
4. Describe the impact of the Truth-In-Lending Act as it applies to collections.
5. Compare computerized billing and manual billing.
6. Recall the components of a complete statement.
7. Differentiate between monthly and cycle billing.
8. Explain the process of aging accounts.
9. Describe the importance of a courteous manner in telephone collections.
10. State legal and ethical guidelines for telephone collections.
11. Describe the impact of the Fair Debt Collection Practice Act as it applies to collections.
12. Describe the process of sending a series of collection letters.
13. List points to consider when using a collection agency.
14. Recall three special collections problems encountered in the clinic.
15. Explain how the statute of limitations impacts the medical assistant's practice.
16. Discuss the merits of a professional attitude in collections.

KEY TERMS

accounts receivable ratio

collection ratio

Fair Debt Collection Practice Act (FDCPA)

probate court

statute of limitations

Truth-in-Lending Act

SCENARIO

At Inner City Health Care, patient billing is typically done at time of service, and a charge slip noting date, description of charges, and fees is given to the patient on leaving the clinic. Clinic policy states that, if possible, patients should pay their part of the fee, or their co-pay, at time of service. Marilyn Johnson, CMA (AAMA), the clinic manager, has found that this is the most efficient way to ensure timely payment and eliminates the need to mail a separate statement. However, the clinic is flexible, and if the patient cannot pay all or part of the charge at the visit, Marilyn works out a payment schedule that is acceptable to both the clinic and the patient.

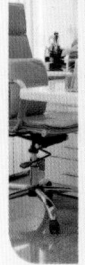

Chapter Portal

In the clinic, patient billing is a critical administrative function that helps to maintain a healthy, viable practice. Timeliness is essential in billing, because the clinic depends on its accounts receivable to pay its bills in a responsible manner. Billing need not be a complex activity, but it must be completely accurate. In the few clinics still using pegboard accounting, billing and collection procedures are done manually, often using the patient's ledger as the basis for the statement. When the facility is computerized, patient bills and collection notices are computer generated.

The best method of patient billing and collections is a method that is customized to the practice and that regards the patient as a consumer who should be respected. Patients appreciate knowing in advance what charges and fees they are expected to pay.

BILLING PROCEDURES

The clinic's cash flow and collection process are dependent on up-to-date and accurate billing techniques. The financial status of the practice is reflected in monthly financial statements indicating unpaid patient balances, which, if they persist, are reviewed for appropriate action, including possible referral to a collection agency. Copies of all billing forms will be retained in the patient account record.

Timeliness and accuracy have a significant influence on prompt payment and how soon collection of the patient account will be finalized. In other words, billing performance can be measured by the time it takes to generate and submit a complete statement, that is, a statement with full documentation. If a facility is experiencing problems generating patient bills, a billing timeliness analysis worksheet can be constructed to identify internal delays that affect how quickly an account is billed, and thus paid. By focusing on inefficiencies in the revenue cycle, processes may be identified that need to be streamlined. For example, the date of service and insurance verification, the date the bill was generated, and the date the bill was submitted to the patient or third party can determine the efficiency of the billing process.

A billing efficiency report is another instrument that may be used to monitor the efficiency of the billing process. This report lists the previous month's billing backlog, which is added to the number of new accounts. The number of processed accounts is then subtracted. The weekly number of accounts that were rebilled also is noted, and the amount of time billing personnel spent on billing accounts is recorded. Production efficiency is calculated from these data. Inherent to this system is the careful monitoring of follow-up bills, including whether they were paid, whether the insurance paid, and an assessment of the patient's responsibility for payment.

CREDIT AND COLLECTION POLICIES

It is important that patients understand the billing policy and are educated about their accounts, how they are paid, and what their responsibility is toward payment. This is most easily accomplished in a patient information brochure (see Chapter 44) identifying all aspects of the medical practice, including how bills are paid. The clinic staff also must have a well-defined policy related to patient billing and collecting.

Competency

Even uncomplicated patient billing should be done according to credit and collection policies established by the provider-employers of the clinic. Having a formalized policy makes decision making easier and gives the medical assistant or office manager responsible for billing and collections authority to act. For example, some questions the providers and office manager may want to address include:

- When will payment be due from the patient?
- What kind of payment arrangements can be made if the patient does not pay at time of service?
- Will the patient be responsible for obtaining referrals, and if so, how will patients who did not obtain one prior to the visit be handled?
- At what point should a patient be reminded of an overdue bill?
- How is the reminder initially managed: by telephone, a note on the statement, or a letter?
- At what point will a patient bill be considered delinquent?
- Will a collection agency be used? Who decides?
- If exceptions to the policy are to be made, who makes these exceptions and what steps are taken?

By answering these and other questions, a straightforward credit and collection policy can be devised that is a guide to both patients and the medical assistant in charge of billing.

PAYMENT AT TIME OF SERVICE

Procedure

Communication

The best opportunity for collection is at the time of service. This process begins with the medical assistant who schedules

Patient Education

Patients appreciate knowing their responsibility in terms of payment. Whoever schedules the first appointment with a new patient should diplomatically inform the patient of clinic policy on payment of fees. If the patient anticipates a problem in paying promptly, a schedule can be established that is agreeable to both parties.

appointments. Make certain all patients have the information they need. After determining the urgency and reason for the appointment, collecting information regarding a chief complaint, and assigning a time for the appointment, it is appropriate to discuss the financial concerns of patients (Procedure 19-1). Patients may be shy in asking certain questions, but they have questions about most of the following issues:

- Whether the providers contract with their insurance carrier
- How payment is made if insurance does not cover certain procedures
- Whether they can be billed for co-payments and coinsurance
- How payment is made for services if they have no insurance
- An approximate cost of a particular service

PROCEDURE 19-1

Procedure

Explaining Fees in the First Telephone Interview

PURPOSE:

To establish rapport with patients, to discuss providers' fees, and to identify the patient's responsibility before the first visit.

EQUIPMENT/SUPPLIES:

- Provider's fee schedule
- Appointment schedule
- Telephone

PROCEDURE STEPS:

1. Place the providers' fee schedule and the appointment schedule close to the telephone. RATIONALE: Prepared clinic staff do not have to search for something vital to the phone conversation.

2. Answer the phone before the third ring. *Identify the name of the clinic and yourself.* RATIONALE: The person calling feels attended to and knows the call has been correctly placed.

3. *Acknowledge the patient* and offer assistance; for example, a comment such as "How can I help you?" RATIONALE: Sets the tone for the patient to continue with the request.

4. After the patient is identified as a new patient and the nature of the visit is determined appropriate, discuss possible dates for the appointment. A statement such as, "Our next available appointment is Thursday at 11:30 AM. Can you make it then?" is a good way to begin.

5. Tell the patient that you will be discussing clinic policies briefly now and will mail the patient information brochure before the appointment. RATIONALE: The patient brochure details some of the information discussed in the telephone conversation and further verifies the clinic's policies.

6. Ask about medical insurance. If the patient is insured, get the identification number, the name of the subscriber, the employer, and a telephone number of the insurance carrier if possible. RATIONALE: This allows you to check for any preauthorization required and for the currency of the plan.

7. Explain that the clinic policy requires any co-payment and co-insurance to be paid at the time of the visit. RATIONALE: Establishes patient's financial responsibility immediately.

8. Check to see if the patient has transportation and knows how to get to the clinic, and provide directions if necessary. RATIONALE: Ensures that there is no confusion about location and accessibility.

9. Request that the patient arrive about 15 minutes before the appointment to complete some forms. RATIONALE: Ensures that the patient has time to complete information and can ask any questions that might occur.

10. After closing the telephone interview, promptly mail the patient information brochure.

Do not tell a patient, "We do not take your insurance." It is much better to make a statement such as, "Our providers do not contract with that insurance. However, we can work with you on a fee-for-service basis and help make finances workable for you." The atmosphere has now been created to ensure prompt collection and increased cash flow for the practice. To accommodate patients, clinics now increasingly accept debit and credit card payments. Remember, also, that if your facility does use a sign-in method as patients arrive, then the all-important personal contact may be missed. With that missed opportunity also goes the opportunity to discuss finances.

Most insurance contracts require the provider to bill the insurance company *before* billing the patient, except for the co-payment. It is critical to abide by each contract to protect the provider. If the patient is a member of a health maintenance organization (HMO) and the clinic is a participating provider, it is bound to the terms of that agreement. If not restricted by the insurance contract, be certain to explain to the patient at the time of service that any payment owed will be adjusted according to the patient's insurance and the terms of that policy. Also remember that all patients must be treated the same and charged the same for services.

With the knowledge of what portion of the fee can be collected at the time of service, the medical assistant says to the patient prior to leaving the facility, "The fee for your services today is $85. Will you be paying by cash, check, or credit/debit card?" When the policy for collecting fees is shared when the appointment is made, patients are not surprised by this approach. Allow the patient to be the next person to speak in response to the question asked. If for some reason a fee cannot be immediately paid, the patient will respond by asking what kind of arrangements might be made. Even if financial arrangements are necessary, the discussion of the day's fee for the service is in process.

TRUTH-IN-LENDING ACT

In those situations where a payment schedule is arranged, clinic policy will dictate if any interest is charged. Although it is not illegal to charge interest on patient accounts, many providers still prefer not to assign any interest on installment payments or past-due accounts.

Competency For installment payments (such as prenatal care or surgery), medical assistants need to be aware of the conditions of the **Truth-in-Lending Act**, Regulation Z of the Consumer Protection Act of 1968 (see Chapter 6). If there is bilateral agreement between providers and their patients for payment of medical services in more than four installments, that agreement must be in writing and must provide information on any finance charges. The information must be in writing even if there are no finance charges made (Figure 19-1). The patient is given the original copy of the disclosure statement; a second copy is kept in the clinic.

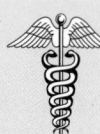

INNER CITY HEALTH CARE
8600 Main Street, Suite 200
River City, XY 01234
(123) 456-7890

FEDERAL TRUTH-IN-LENDING STATEMENT
For Professional Services

Patient _____ Cari R. Jacobson _____

Address _____ 913 Swanson Street _____

_____ River City, XY 61820 _____

Parent _____

1. Cost of services rendered	$1,500.00
2. Down Payment	225.00
3. Unpaid Balance	1,275.00
4. Amount Financed	1,275.00
5. Finance Charge	-0-
6. Annual Percentage Rate of Finance Charge	-0-
7. Total of Payments (4 + 5 above)	1,275.00
8. Total Amount After Payments	1,500.00

Total payment due is payable to Dr. Winston Lewis at above address in 5 monthly installments of $ 255. The first installment is payable on August 1, 20XX, and each subsequent payment is due on the same day of each consecutive month until paid in full.

07-24-XX
Date of Agreement

_____
Signature of Patient;
Parent if Patient is Minor

FIGURE 19-1 Truth-in-Lending Act document showing installment and interest agreement.

COMPONENTS OF A COMPLETE STATEMENT

Once a patient has been accepted for treatment, it is important to maintain accurate and timely records of his or her account and payment history. That information is just as vital to the healthy management of the practice as the patient's medical record. Invoice patient services promptly according to the clinic policy, send statements regularly, and make certain they are complete and accurate. Statements to patients must be professional looking, neat, inclusive of all services and charges, and easily understood. Procedure and diagnosis codes are necessary for insurance and reimbursement, but they usually mean nothing to patients. Make certain patients can understand the terminology used to explain the procedures they received.

Billing occurs in a number of different ways, with the computer-generated statement the most widely used. As mentioned in Chapter 18, an encounter form may be used as the statement, especially if payment is made at the time of the service (Figure 19-2). Typewritten statements will likely use the continuous-form billing statement that is printed on a roll with perforated edges for separation. Photocopied statements are often used with a pegboard system. The ledger cards are coordinated with the same-size copy paper. These photocopied ledgers are placed in a window envelope so that the address on the ledger card shows through the window.

If the statement is to be mailed, an enclosed self-addressed envelope is appreciated by the patient and may result in a faster turnaround of payment. Stamp the words *Address Service Requested* on the envelope just below the return address. When this statement is stamped on the envelope, a valuable tool in collections is available at minimum cost. If the statement cannot be delivered as addressed (the patient has moved or "skipped" and has left no forwarding address), the post office researches this information and returns the envelope to you with a yellow sticker providing the new address and any other updated information. If the patient has ordered that mail be forwarded, the post office will forward the statement to the patient and send the medical facility a form with the new address. There is a fee for this service.

DATE	PATIENT	SERVICE CODE	FEES CHARGED	CREDITS: PAID	CREDITS: ADJ.	BALANCE DUE		PREVIOUS BALANCE	NAME	RECEIPT NO.

THIS IS YOUR RECEIPT
AND/OR A STATEMENT OF YOUR ACCOUNT TO DATE

OFFICE VISITS AND PROCEDURES

99211	EST PT - MINIMAL OV	1				HOSPITAL VISIT	14		
99212	EST PT - BRIEF OV	2				EMERGENCY	15		
99213	EST PT - INTERMEDIATE OV	3				CONSULTATION	16		
99214	EST PT - EXTENDED OV	4			93000	EKG	17		
99215	EST PT - COMPREHENSIVE OV	5			93224	ELECTROCARDIOGRAPHIC MONITORING	18		
99201	NEW PT - BRIEF OV	6			93307	ECHOCARDIOGRAPHY	19		
99202	NEW PT - INTERMEDIATE OV	7			85025	CBC	20		
99203	NEW PT - EXTENDED OV	8			81000	URINALYSIS WITH MICROSCOPY	21		
99204	NEW PT - COMPLEX OV	9			36415	ROUTINE VENIPUNCTURE	22		
99205	NEW PT - COMPREHENSIVE OV	10			71020	RADIOLOGY EXAM-CHEST-2 VIEWS	23		
99238	HOSPITAL DISCHARGE	11			30300	REMOVE FOR. BODY-INTRANASAL	24		
99025	NEW PT - SURGERY PROC. PRIMARY	12					25		
	NURSING HOME VISIT	13					26		

AUTHORIZATION TO RELEASE INFORMATION: I HEREBY AUTHORIZE THE UNDERSIGNED PHYSICIAN TO RELEASE ANY INFORMATION ACQUIRED IN THE COURSE OF MY EXAMINATION OR TREATMENT.
SIGNED (PATIENT, OR PARENT IF MINOR) ______ DATE ______

PLACE OF SERVICE ☐ OFFICE ☐ OTHER ______
DIAGNOSIS OR SYMPTOMS ______
DOCTOR'S SIGNATURE ______

PATIENTS NAME ☐ M ☐ F
ADDRESS
CITY STATE ZIP
RELATIONSHIP BIRTHDATE
SUBSCRIBER OR POLICY HOLDER
☐ MEDICARE ☐ MEDICAID ☐ BLUE SHIELD ☐ 65-SP.
INSURANCE CARRIER
AGREEMENT #
GROUP #

D - OTHER SERVICES

NEXT APPOINTMENT AT AM PM
RETURN ______ DAYS ______ WEEKS ______ MONTHS

INNER CITY HEALTH CARE
8600 MAIN STREET, SUITE 200
RIVER CITY, XY 01234
(123) 456-7890

03626

FIGURE 19-2 The sample encounter form (charge slip) is a multipurpose form used to document information for insurance claims as well as to provide the patient with a receipt and documentation of procedures, diagnoses, and fees. It can be used as the patient's first bill.

A well-prepared patient statement should contain not only information for the patient but information needed to process medical insurance claims as well. The following information should be included (see Procedure 19-2):

- Patient's name and address
- Patient's insurance carrier and identification number
- Date and place of service
- Description of service and fee for each service
- Accurate procedure and diagnosis codes for insurance processing (see Chapters 16 and 17)
- Provider's signature and identification code or National Provider Identifier (NPI)

- Clinic name, address, telephone number, fax number, and Web site when applicable

Computerized Statements

By far the most common statements are computer generated. Typically, the medical assistant keys the computer command to search the patient database for outstanding balances and directs the computer to print statements.

Financial management software will age accounts (see the "Aging Accounts" section) and can generate collection letters that have been specifically designed for the practice, allowing the medical assistant to key in the appropriate specific information.

All provider orders, prescriptions, recommendations, and a copy of the visit and health summary can be waiting for the patient at the time of

---

PROCEDURE 19-2

Preparing Itemized Patient Accounts for Billing

PURPOSE:

To notify patients of the fees for services rendered and collect on those accounts.

EQUIPMENT/SUPPLIES:

- Computer
- Calculator
- Electronic patient account or ledger cards
- Billing statement forms

PROCEDURE STEPS:

1. Gather all accounts and ledgers with outstanding balances. RATIONALE: Everything in one place saves time and energy.

2. Separate any accounts that are labeled as overdue. RATIONALE: Individual decisions on these accounts are necessary before taking action.

3. *Paying attention to detail,* and for each account, perform the following:

   a. Verify the name and address of the patient and the person responsible for payment.

   b. Place current date on the statement.

   c. Scan the account information for any possible errors.

   d. Itemize the procedures in terms patients understand and indicate charges.

   e. Identify and subtract any payments (co-payment, co-insurance, down payment) that have been made.

   f. Verify the unpaid balance that is carried forward and is due.

4. Discuss with the clinic manager any action to be taken on past-due accounts. Follow through with those instructions. RATIONALE: More than one person is involved in the collection process.

5. Place statements in envelopes and mail. RATIONALE: Ensures timely delivery of statements.

checkout, if desired. With a single key entry, an electronic invoice is generated with appropriate diagnostic and procedural codes already applied. If insurance is to be billed, the claim is automatically placed in the insurance queue to be uploaded electronically to third-party payers.

Any payments made can be posted electronically and statements can then be printed for the patient. The collection portion of the financial management software keeps up with the daily billing tasks.

MONTHLY AND CYCLE BILLING

The billing schedule is often determined by the size of the medical practice. Monthly billing is a system in which all accounts are billed at the same time each month. In a smaller clinic, monthly billing may be the most efficient method. Cycle billing staggers bills during the month and is a flexible system for larger practices.

Monthly Billing

In a monthly billing system, one or two days of each month are devoted to billing and mailing all statements. Typically, statements should leave the clinic no later than the 25th of the month to be received by the first of the following month. The major disadvantage of monthly billing is that a medical assistant may neglect other activities during this time-consuming period. To avoid these problems, billing statements may be prepared intermittently over a one- or two-week period and stored until the mailing date. To avoid confusion caused by delays in mailing, a message to "Disregard if payment has already been made" should be printed on the form. Patients become annoyed and the practice appears disorganized if a statement arrives several days after payment has been made.

Cycle Billing

In a cycle billing system, all accounts usually are divided alphabetically into groups, with each group billed at a different time. In this way, administrative personnel with numerous bills to process each month will be able to handle them in a more efficient manner. Statements are prepared on the same schedule each month. They can be mailed as they are completed, or held and mailed at one time. A typical cycle billing schedule is shown in Figure 19-3. The system can be varied to suit the needs of the individual practice.

PAST-DUE ACCOUNTS

As efficient and effective as the billing process may be, there will still be collections on some accounts.

Sample of Cycle Billing

1. Divide the alphabet into four sections: A to F, G to L, M to R, S to Z.
2. Prepare statements for patients whose last names begin with A through F on Wednesday and mail them on Thursday of Week 1.
3. Prepare statements for patients whose last names begin with G through L on Wednesday and mail them on Thursday of Week 2.
4. Prepare statements for patients whose last names begin with M through R on Wednesday and mail them on Thursday of Week 3.
5. Prepare statements for patients whose last names begin with S through Z on Wednesday and mail them on Thursday of Week 4.

FIGURE 19-3 Typical schedule for cycle billing system.

The most common reasons for past-due accounts include:

- *Inability to pay.* People may have financial hardships from time to time (see Chapter 18).
- *Negligence.* People may forget to make a payment because they have been away or dealing with a family emergency.
- *Unwillingness to pay.* When a patient complains about a charge or refuses to pay, it may have nothing to do with finances. Often, they are dissatisfied with the care or treatment they have received. These patients should be referred to the provider or office manager for immediate attention.
- *Third-party payers.* Past-due accounts may result because of inaccurate or insufficient insurance information. Claims can be rejected because of many varied reasons, and time limits must be observed.
- *Minors.* Minors who are not legally emancipated may seek and receive treatment, but they are not responsible for paying the bill (see Chapter 6). If the medical practice treats minors who are not emancipated, a clinic policy should determine how these minors pay for their services. Emancipated minors are responsible for their bills. Many facilities ask for cash at the time of the service.

COLLECTION PROCESS

The process of collecting delinquent accounts begins with first establishing how much has been owed and for how long.

Ideally, collection of accounts receivable should be prompt and conducted in a timely fashion. Management consultants recommend collecting at least a portion of the fees at the time of service and that a **collection ratio** of 90% or better should be maintained. Another important factor is the **accounts receivable ratio**, which measures the speed with which outstanding accounts are paid. The desirable accounts receivable ratio is less than 2 months for collection of accounts receivable.

Collection Ratio

A collection ratio is a method used to gauge the effectiveness of the clinic's billing practices. This ratio shows the status of collections and the possible losses in the medical facility. It is a good idea to obtain the ratio monthly, quarterly, and yearly. Typically, the collection ratio is calculated by dividing the total collections by the net charges (gross or total charges minus any adjustments). This yields a percentage that is referred to as the collection ratio. See the following example:

$$\frac{\text{Total Amount Collected This Month}}{\text{Total Monthly Charges Minus Adjustments}} = \text{Monthly Collection Ratio}$$

$$\frac{\$34,650}{\$44,928} = .7712 \text{ or } 77\%$$

In this sample, you can determine that more time and energy needs to be spent in collecting accounts. The practice is losing almost 25% of its income potential. Not only is the income potential being lost but also the ability to invest that income is lost, making the potential loss even greater.

Accounts Receivable Ratio

An accounts receivable ratio indicates how quickly outstanding accounts are paid. It can also be a measure of how effective the collections are. To calculate the accounts receivable ratio, divide the current accounts receivable balance by the average monthly gross charges. This yields the typical turnaround for collecting accounts receivable. See the following example:

$$\frac{\text{Current Accounts Receivable}}{\text{Average Monthly Gross Charges}} = \text{Accounts Receivable Ratio}$$

$$\frac{\$145,048}{\$44,928} = 3.2$$

Because the goal of the accounts receivable ratio is payment in less than 2 months, you can quickly observe that this practice is over 1 month behind in collections. Chapter 20 gives additional information on accounts receivable and collection ratios.

The longer a practice delays attempting to collect delinquent accounts, the less chance there is of receiving payment. Statistics show that the value of the dollar decreases rapidly in the collection process. That is, the more time and energy put into collections, the less value received in return. You may manage to collect the full amount due, but when you consider the time and expense involved, it may not have been worth the effort and expense. Therefore, the value of the debt to be received after successful collection must be considered when determining how aggressive to be in debt collections.

AGING ACCOUNTS

Account aging is a method of identifying how long an account has been overdue. This means that past-due accounts are identified according to the length of time they have been unpaid. When using a pegboard bookkeeping system, color-coded strips are attached to the ledger cards to show the age of an account, or the cards can be stored behind a color-coded divider in a separate file labeled "Unpaid." For example, a red strip might be used for accounts 1 month overdue, a blue strip for accounts 2 months overdue, and other colors for additional months overdue. A written code such as "OD3/2/23" should be written on the ledger card to indicate when the overdue notice was mailed, meaning "Overdue notice No. 3 mailed on February 23."

Depending on the type of patient served, different aging systems are used. In a computerized billing system, the accounts are automatically aged, and the aging schedule or process is shown on the computerized ledger.

Computerized Aging

Aging accounts using a computer software system is simple. Before printing billing statements, the medical assistant keys the appropriate commands to age the accounts. The program can age accounts according to several criteria: for example, by past due balance, zero balance, or credit balance accounts. Accounts can also be aged by government agency category or by insurance carrier. All Medicare or Medicaid accounts might be aged separately from other accounts. Sorting out Medicare and Medicaid accounts may also be done when computing the accounts receivable ratio and the collection ratio.

The computer can also generate and print an accounts receivable report showing each overdue account, the balance overdue, and a breakdown showing how long the account has been overdue. This breakdown is usually divided into accounts 0 to 30 days overdue, 31 to 60 days overdue, 61 to 90 days overdue, and 90 days or more overdue. Additional reports can be generated from the accounts receivable report. For example, the clinic staff may wish to print a report showing accounts that have been delinquent for more than 90 days or accounts that are delinquent by more than a certain dollar amount.

COLLECTION TECHNIQUES

Clinic settings use both telephone and written communications in their collection techniques. Although both have some measure of effectiveness, some practices prefer to call the patient with a past-due account before officially initiating collection proceedings. The patient may have misplaced the statement, forgotten a payment, or been away on an extended vacation; a quick telephone call can often resolve the situation without the time and expense involved in collections. Also, the patient usually appreciates the courtesy and personal approach.

Many patients work part or full time, which sometimes makes telephone calls difficult to complete. It is often beneficial for providers to ask the office manager or the medical assistant in charge of collections to work 2 or more hours one evening a week for the purpose of making collection telephone calls. Calls are more likely to be answered in the time period from 5 PM to 8 PM than during the middle of the day. Figure 19-4 shows a sample collections policy.

Billing Insurance Carriers

Many patients have some form of medical insurance (see Chapter 16). Make it a practice to send each computer claim within 2 days or less of the patient account data being entered into the computer. Batches of claims to insurance carriers should be forwarded at the end of each day. In the era of electronic claims processing, much time is saved in not having to prepare hard copies of the forms for mailing. Electronic claims transmission (ECT; also known as electronic medical claims, or EMC, and electronic

SAMPLE COLLECTION POLICY SCHEDULE

- Encounter form (if used) given to patient at time of visit.
- Itemized statement sent no later than the end of that month.
- Itemized statement with overdue notice no later than the end of the second month.
- Telephone call reminding the patient of the bill. "We've sent two statements and we haven't received payment. Do you need more information from us?" Offer help at this point in establishing a payment schedule, and seek to get a commitment from the patient.
- If a financial schedule is to be established, prepare it and mail to the patient within a day of the phone conversation. Follow up on that commitment within 15 days. The follow-up message may be a thank you for sending the first payment. Carefully monitor payments and their timeliness.
- If no payment schedule is made by the patient, send a letter stating the amount due before the account is past due three months. Discuss with office manager and/or physician regarding the merit of continued collection at this time.
- If collections are to continue, notify the patient one more time of his or her responsibility and ask for payment.
- If no payment is received, send a letter stating that "Your account has been turned over to a collection agency" if outside collectors are used. Make no more phone calls.*

*Some physicians send a letter of discharge to patients at this time via certified mail. (See Chapter 6.)

FIGURE 19-4 Sample collection policy.

claims submission, or ECS) dictates that the practice's computer system must be able to communicate with the insurance carrier's computer. This paperless process yields fewer errors than the manual process because ECT software includes some built-in checks to determine any invalid codes, sex or age conflicts, and correct procedure and diagnostic code linkages to the services provided. Insurance claims sent via the paper route will take more time to process, and the turnaround time for payment is also longer. Most claim departments of insurance carriers and government agencies have large numbers of employees with varying levels of experience. Payment can be delayed because of an overburdened claim department, a form that has been lost in transit, a misfiled form, an inexperienced employee, or numerous other reasons.

The medical assistant should maintain an up-to-date claims register or insurance-pending report and take firm control of the practice's collection procedures to ensure that claims are paid promptly.

This claims register or insurance-pending report may be a part of the computerized billing system. If so, the printout will show how much the practice charged insurance carriers and how much was received. This clearly shows which carriers are slower than others and where other problems might arise. For any claim pending more than 45 days, it is a good idea to make a call to the carrier to find out whether the claim has been received, where it is in the process, and whether the clinic staff might have done something to delay the process. Such phone calls can become carefully cultivated personal contacts with insurance representatives to pave the way for cooperation in the future.

In clinics where the medical assistant files claims for patients, a follow-up collection policy is important to maintain strong cash flow. When carriers do not pay in full or question or deny a claim, the medical assistant should determine the nature of the problem and rebill or appeal the decision, whichever action is appropriate.

Telephone Collections

Presentation

The medical assistant is likely to use the telephone for collection procedures. Telephoning is often an effective measure because a patient may respond to a call more than to a bill received in the mail.

A successful telephone collection call is enhanced by keeping to the facts and being tactful, pleasant, and diplomatic. When making calls to patients regarding past-due accounts, there are some things to keep in mind to maintain the desired relationship with patients. Always remain courteous and respectful. Do not treat patients with suspicion or threats. Remember, the health profession is dedicated to helping people; avoid antagonizing patients.

Most people do not let their bills become past due on purpose or out of spite. Keep this in mind when making calls. Work with patients to encourage and enable them to pay any fees they owe.

Legal   Integrity

Certain legal rules and ethical guidelines govern telephone collections:

- When making collection calls, callers must identify themselves and ascertain that they are talking to the person who is responsible for the account.

- A collection call could be embarrassing to the patient; therefore, it should not be made to the patient's place of employment.

- In most states, a debtor may be contacted only between 8 AM and 9 PM.

- Do not make telephone calls at odd hours or make repeated calls to the debtor's friends, employers, or relatives.

- If a contact must be made to the debtor's place of business, do not reveal to any third party the nature of the call. Patients have a right to confidentiality and privacy.

- Do not threaten to turn the person's account over to collection agencies.

When collecting by telephone, it is helpful to keep complete, accurate records of the process indicating who said what and how much was promised as payment. If after 2 weeks nothing has been resolved as a result of the calls, then another course of action may be the solution, especially for large sums of money owed. Collection letters may be necessary.

Fair Debt Collection Practices Act. Violating rules regarding harassment makes the caller vulnerable to charges under the **Fair Debt Collection Practices Act (FDCPA)**. According to the guidelines set by the FDCPA, which is overseen by the Federal Trade Commission (FTC), debt collectors are not allowed to use their positions to collect a debt using any manner of work performance that is found to be abusive, deceptive, or unethical. The collectors must abide by certain guidelines, such as not calling a debtor at work without written consent and keeping calls to debtors between the hours of 8 AM and 9 PM. Under the FDCPA, debts that are created by medical expenses are a type of debt that can be sent to collection agencies and subsequently collected upon. The collectors are strictly prohibited from using profane language or any language that indicates a threat (such as wage or tax refund garnishment). It is very important that the administrative medical assistant abide by such guidelines as given within the FDCPA.

Collection Letters

Collection letters are sent to encourage patients to pay overdue balances. After two statements are mailed to patients and the charge slip or encounter form has brought no response, the clinic begins sending collection letters.

Lack of payment from a patient may not be considered serious until after 60 days. When the patient fails to respond to the encounter form, to the statement, or to a 60-day statement with an "Overdue" remark, a series of collection letters begins. One typical collection letter series is shown in Figures 19-5A through Figure 19-5C. Collection letters and notes are kept separate from a patient's chart.

USE OF AN OUTSIDE COLLECTION AGENCY

Occasionally, the clinic turns over highly delinquent accounts to an outside collection agency. Discretion is always advised here, however, because the fees to be collected may not justify the expense of collection. For unpaid accounts with large balances, however, this is often a viable solution.

One service provided by a collection agency is an intercept letter. For a nominal fee, this letter may be sent from the agency as the last resort before the account is turned over to collection. This communication alerts patients to the fact that if a response is not received, their account will go to collection. This often is the only action needed for the patient to pay the outstanding bill. Another service of a credit bureau or collection agency is to provide credit ratings of patients at the provider's request. Providers who pay for this service are able to monitor patients' ability to pay their bills, as well as to trace a "skip," someone who leaves with an outstanding bill and no forwarding address.

When selecting a collection agency, be certain to hire one that is compatible with the medical practice's philosophy. Questions that might be asked of potential collection agencies include the following:

- Does the agency handle only medical and dental accounts?
- What methods are used to make collections?
- Is the agency fee a flat charge per account or a percentage of the account recovered?
- How promptly does the agency settle accounts?
- Will the agency supply a list of satisfied customers or references?
- What ability does the medical practice have to end the agency's collection efforts?

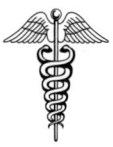

INNER CITY HEALTH CARE
8600 MAIN STREET, SUITE 200
RIVER CITY, XY 01234

June 14, 20XX

Mr. John O'Keefe
12 Gravers Lane
Northborough, XY 12345

Dear Mr. O'Keefe:

Your account with our clinic is three months past due, and you have not responded to our previous requests for payment. Please pay your balance of $852 at this time, or contact us with a plan for payment.

Please call me at (123) 456-7890 if you have a question about your account or a plan for payment. Otherwise, we expect your payment immediately.

Sincerely,

Marilyn Johnson
Clinic Manager

A

FIGURE 19-5 Sample collection letters. (A) First letter.
(continues)

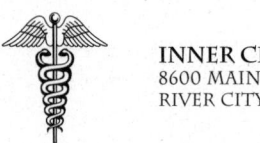

INNER CITY HEALTH CARE
8600 MAIN STREET, SUITE 200
RIVER CITY, XY 01234

July 15, 20XX

Mr. John O'Keefe
12 Gravers Lane
Northborough, XY 12345

Dear Mr. O'Keefe:

Your son, Chris, was seriously ill in March
when he was seen by Dr. King. Dr. King
used her experience and education to
treat Chris, believing you would pay your
account within a reasonable amount of time.

Four months have passed and you have still
not remitted the $852 outstanding balance
on your account. We cannot continue to keep
your unpaid account on our books. If you
are experiencing financial difficulties,
please call the clinic at (123) 456-7890
so we can arrange a payment schedule
that is agreeable to both of us.

Sincerely,

Marilyn Johnson
Clinic Manager

B

INNER CITY HEALTH CARE
8600 MAIN STREET, SUITE 200
RIVER CITY, XY 01234

August 17, 20XX

CERTIFIED MAIL

Mr. John O'Keefe
12 Gravers Lane
Northborough, XY 12345

Dear Mr. O'Keefe:

This is our final attempt to collect your
account of $852, which is five months past
due. You have not responded to all our
previous letters [or letters and phone calls],
so we have no alternative but to turn over
your account to a collection company.

Your account is being assigned to Ambler
Medical Collection Service, which will pursue
whatever legal means is necessary to collect
this debt. If you contact me at (123) 456-7890
within seven days, we can prevent
the account from this assignment and
resolve the balance.

Sincerely,

Marilyn Johnson
Clinic Manager

C

FIGURE 19-5 *(continued)* (B) Second letter. (C) Third letter.

Once a collection agency has been selected, carefully follow their instructions about any contact patients make with the medical clinic regarding their account as well as any other guidelines in their contract with the practice. Keep a record of accounts given to the agency, as well as their rate of return. Hopefully, the agency will be able to motivate patients to pay for the health care services they have received while still maintaining the practice's good reputation and increasing your profit margin. Medical collections let your patients know that the practice is serious about collecting past-due accounts.

Procedure

There is often a question about how payments from collection agencies are posted. This is one purpose of the adjustment column. Place the amount received in the adjustment column because it is a subtraction from the amount due. If there is no adjustment column, put the amount in the charge column and put red parentheses around it or circle in red so the amount is actually subtracted from the balance. The remaining balance after collections are paid is written off (Procedure 19-3).

USE OF SMALL CLAIMS COURT

Legal

In certain circumstances, a clinic's manager may consider bringing a case to small claims court. Typically, small claims courts handle cases that involve only limited amounts of debt (these vary from state to state), they usually do not permit representation by an attorney, and they are generally efficient and streamlined in their proceedings. Nonetheless, preparing for small claims courts and taking time to appear will require a certain investment of staff. It is important to note that if the court finds in the clinic's favor,

---

PROCEDURE 19-3

Procedure

Posting/Recording Collection Agency Adjustments

PURPOSE:
To keep track of financial adjustments.

EQUIPMENT/SUPPLIES:
- Manual bookkeeping system or computerized system
- Patient's account
- Black and red ink pens for use in manual bookkeeping system
- Computerized PM system

PROCEDURE STEPS:

1. If using a manual system, use the daily schedule of services/charges in front of you (the manual daily sheet), enter amount received from the collection agency on a patient's account and a note such as "Payment from ABC Collection Agency" in the explanation section. If using a PM system, use the payment posting module and locate the patient record. RATIONALE: Indicates funds received on a collection contract.

2. Record the amount received and the explanation in the patient's account as well.

   a. Using a manual system, post the amount received by subtracting from the account balance. Use the adjustment column to write off the balance amount. This should zero out the account.

   b. In a PM system, post the amount received to the patient account from the collection agency, and adjust the balance to zero out the account. RATIONALE: Clearly indicates what portion of the account the patient has paid and the amount that is not collectible. In a manual system, the difference between the amount collected and amount paid by the collection agency (including the agency's fee) is entered as a negative adjustment. In a PM system, this is tracked within the software. At the end of the year, totals can be obtained for the practice's income tax preparation.

the clinic still must collect the money from the defendant. An account assigned to a collection agency cannot be addressed in small claims court.

SPECIAL COLLECTION SITUATIONS

In patient billing and collections, a number of special situations may arise.

Bankruptcy

If a patient has declared bankruptcy, statements may no longer be sent nor may any attempts be made to collect delinquent accounts. A patient declaring bankruptcy usually does so under Chapter 7 or Chapter 13 bankruptcy law. In a Chapter 7 bankruptcy, a patient declares bankruptcy to all debtors and is allowed to clear all debts and start fresh. The medical clinic should file a proof-of-claim form and provide a copy of the patient's outstanding account to the bankruptcy court. In a Chapter 13 bankruptcy, also known as a "wage-earner's bankruptcy," patients (wage-earners) are protected from bill collectors and are allowed to pay their bills over a specified time. The court determines a monthly amount that the debtor can pay, collects that sum, and parcels it out to the creditors over a period as long as five years. The clinic must file a claim as directed by the debtor's attorney to collect any fees outstanding. Because a provider's fee is an unsecured debt, it is one of the last to be paid. Bankruptcy laws are federal and are subject to the Federal Wage Garnishment Law regarding attaching property to satisfy debt.

Estates

Collection of fees when a patient has died must be directed to the executor of the estate or the one responsible for overseeing the estate. Some general guidelines to follow include:

- Show courtesy by not sending a statement in the first week or so after a death.
- Prepare an itemized statement of the deceased patient's account. (In some cases, a special form is required for this.)
- Mail the account information via certified mail with a return receipt requested to the administrator of the estate. The name can be obtained by calling the probate department of the superior court.
- If there is no known or identified administrator, send a copy of the itemized statement to the "Estate of (name of patient)" at the patient's last known address. Often, a family member has assumed the responsibility for paying the patient's account balances.
- If unsure of how to proceed, contact the clinic's attorney or the clerk of the **probate court** for advice.

Tracing "Skips"

Legal   Integrity

A "skip" is a patient with an unpaid bill who has apparently moved with no forwarding address. If a statement is returned to your clinic marked "no forwarding address," first determine if any internal errors were made in addressing the envelope. If the address is determined to be correct, the medical assistant may try to call the patient at the telephone number on the patient ledger; it is possible that the patient has retained the same number, or there may be a new number given. If the medical assistant is unable to secure a telephone number, the facility needs to decide whether to pursue the unpaid debt. This will depend on clinic policy and the amount that is owed. If it is decided to pursue an unpaid account, it can be turned over to a collection agency. If the medical assistant attempts to trace the skip by calling employers or relatives, it is important not to violate any laws in doing so and to maintain the patient's confidentiality.

STATUTE OF LIMITATIONS

Legal

A **statute of limitations** is a statute that defines the period in which legal action may take place. When applying this concept to collections, the time period is usually defined by the class into which the account falls. These include open book accounts, which may have periodic charges against them; written contracts; and single-entry accounts, which have only one charge against them. The time period in which legal action must take place against any of these accounts varies from state to state. If an unpaid account is more than 3 years old, it is wise to investigate the statute of limitations in your state before spending time and effort in collections. (For state-by-state information on the statute of limitations on debts, see www.creditinfocenter .com, under "Debts.")

MAINTAIN A PROFESSIONAL ATTITUDE

Presentation

Collecting past-due accounts is one of the most difficult tasks delegated to medical assistants. Not everyone is able to perform this task. Placing calls can be discouraging, especially if the results seem less than anticipated. Not all accounts can be collected. Identify these accounts early, write them off, and save the medical practice time and money. Keep any bias and your emotions out of the process. Rely only on your information, the aged account, and the realization that the clinic policy is well thought out and provides a win–win solution for both the patient and the provider as much as possible. When dealing with a "true deadbeat" who has no intention of paying the bill, be proud of your provider's attention to that patient's need, but discuss with the provider the possibility of discharging the patient. Staff may need additional training and education from time to time to update skills on patient service and how to maintain goodwill during the collection process.

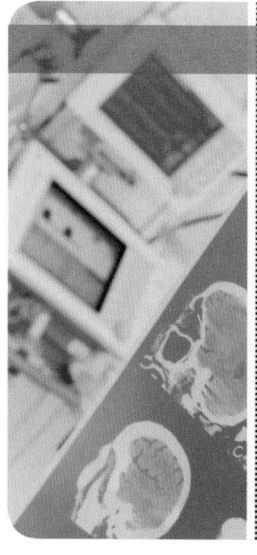

CASE STUDY 19-1

Refer to the scenario at the beginning of the chapter. For patient accounts more than 60 days overdue, Inner City Health Care begins a series of collection proceedings to attempt to collect the monies. Initially, they place a telephone call to the patient to determine whether a billing problem might be present that can be clarified over the telephone. If they cannot reach the patient or the patient does not respond to the call, then collections begin. Marilyn has assigned this function of the billing process to Ellen Armstrong, CMAS (AMT), because Ellen has a warm telephone manner and is good with patients.

CASE STUDY REVIEW

1. Why is Ellen's telephone manner important in the collection process?
2. In addition to telephone collections, what patient letters might Ellen send?
3. Ellen has come across an account that is delinquent and discovers that the patient has declared bankruptcy. What can Ellen do now?

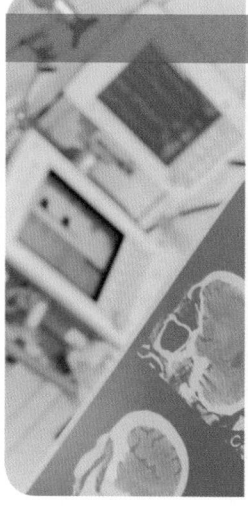

CASE STUDY 19-2

Morgan Bryant is the custodial parent and single mother of her 5-year-old son Custer, who has been a patient of Inner City Pediatric Clinic since his birth. Custer's father's insurance covered his medical expenses. During a separation and the resulting divorce, the medical bills continued to go to Custer's father. Morgan comes to the reception desk to discuss the collection letter she received. Her parenting plan requires her former husband to provide medical coverage for their son. However, it appears he canceled his policy coverage on his son 4 months ago and Morgan did not know this until she received the letter. Morgan is in tears.

CASE STUDY REVIEW

1. What is the first step the administrative medical assistant should take?
2. Is there anything the clinic staff might have done differently in collecting this account?
3. What might be done for Morgan now? Are any resources available to Morgan?

- The cash flow and collection process are dependent on up-to-date and accurate billing techniques.

- The financial status of the practice is reflected in monthly statements indicating unpaid patient balances, which will need to be reviewed regularly for appropriate action, including possible referral to a collection agency.

- Timeliness and accuracy have a significant influence on prompt payment and how soon collection of the patient account will be finalized.

- Understanding the formal credit and collections protocols of the clinic in order to educate patients of their financial responsibilities, thereby promoting cooperation and compliance from patients when collecting payments, is the responsibility of the medical assistant.

- Co-payments and other payments should be collected at the time of service.

- Medical assistants must have knowledge of the insurance plans accepted by the clinic, and alert patients when benefits are being used out of network, or are noncovered benefits.

- The medical assistant should discuss services not covered by the insurance plan with the patient, and payment plans that may be available to the patient if needed.

- The medical assistant should have knowledge of solutions and resources for uninsured or underinsured patients, including payment plans, when available.

- The medical assistant must be familiar with the Truth-in-Lending Act, Regulation Z of the Consumer Protection Act of 1967, as it applies to credit and collections in the clinic.

- The medical assistant is responsible for gathering data on collection ratios and account receivable ratios to target and achieve goals that keep outstanding balances to a minimum, and cash flow at a maximum.

- Medical personnel must use proper collection techniques, both by telephone and by letter, following the guidelines of the Fair Debt Collections Practices Act.

- Special collection resources can be used when needed, including small claims court, billing estates and contacting a probate court, and tracing skips properly, within the law.

- You must be aware of state laws regarding the statue of limitations for collection outstanding balances, and of bankruptcy laws for Chapter 7 and Chapter 13, the two most common types.

Study for Success

To reinforce your knowledge and skills of information presented in this chapter:

- Review the *Key Terms* and *Learning Outcomes*

- Consider the *Case Studies* and discuss your conclusions

- Answer the questions in the *Certification Review*

- Perform the *Procedures* using the *Competency Assessment Checklists* on the *Student Companion Website*

Procedure

CERTIFICATION REVIEW

1. Which of the following is true of the Truth-In-Lending Act?
   a. It is designed to place limits on the amount of debt for which consumers are liable.
   b. It is also known as the statute of limitations.
   c. It is also known as Regulation Z.
   d. It does not apply to medical facilities.

2. Which of the following is an accurate description of cycle billing?
   a. It is completed every fourth month.
   b. It is done only by computer.
   c. It is completed by the 25th of the month.
   d. It is a system in which accounts are divided into sections for billing purposes.
   e. It is done on a daily basis.

3. What is one of the most common reasons why patient bills go unpaid?
   a. Inability to pay because of financial hardship
   b. Patients consider the cost of medical care too high
   c. Patients think their insurance should cover all medical bills
   d. Patients think providers make too much money

4. What is the definition of aging accounts?
   a. It is a process of identifying overdue patient accounts.
   b. It describes patients who have a long-term relationship with the ambulatory care center.
   c. It describes older adult patients with Medicare.
   d. It applies to accounts considered inactive.
   e. It is the date the account is paid in full.

5. What happens when an unpaid account goes to small claims court?
   a. The medical clinic must engage an attorney representative.
   b. The medical clinic is still responsible for collecting even if the court finds in its favor.
   c. There is no need to show up at court.
   d. A large sum of money must be at issue.

6. Which of the following is true of a collection ratio?
   a. It shows status of collections and possible losses.
   b. It divides the current accounts receivable by the average monthly gross charges.
   c. It should be 90% or better.
   d. It is the amount of cash collected each day.
   e. Both a and c

7. What is a claims register?
   a. It identifies how many past-due claims have been collected.
   b. It may also be called the insurance-pending report.
   c. It is maintained by each insurance carrier for the provider.
   d. It is a tickler file that maintains all patients' insurance information.

8. Which statement below is true about using the telephone to help collect money from patients?
   a. Calls are best made after 8 PM when patients are home.
   b. Collections must abide by the Fair Debt Collection Practice Act.
   c. Collections are usually successful after numerous calls at the patient's place of employment.
   d. The collections process will require overtime pay for the medical clinic staff.
   e. Telephone collections are not an effective tool.

9. What is the definition of a "skip"?
   a. The time period when legal action cannot be taken
   b. An estate involved in probate
   c. One who moves without a forwarding address and leaves an unpaid bill
   d. One who has paid a portion of a debt

10. Which of the following is true regarding using a collection agency for patient accounts?
    a. It is better if the agency handles only medical and dental accounts.
    b. It creates a bad feeling between patients and providers.
    c. It cannot possibly do as good a job as the medical clinic staff.
    d. The agency seldom describes its methods for collections.
    e. The agency is used to collect highly delinquent accounts.

Accounting Practices

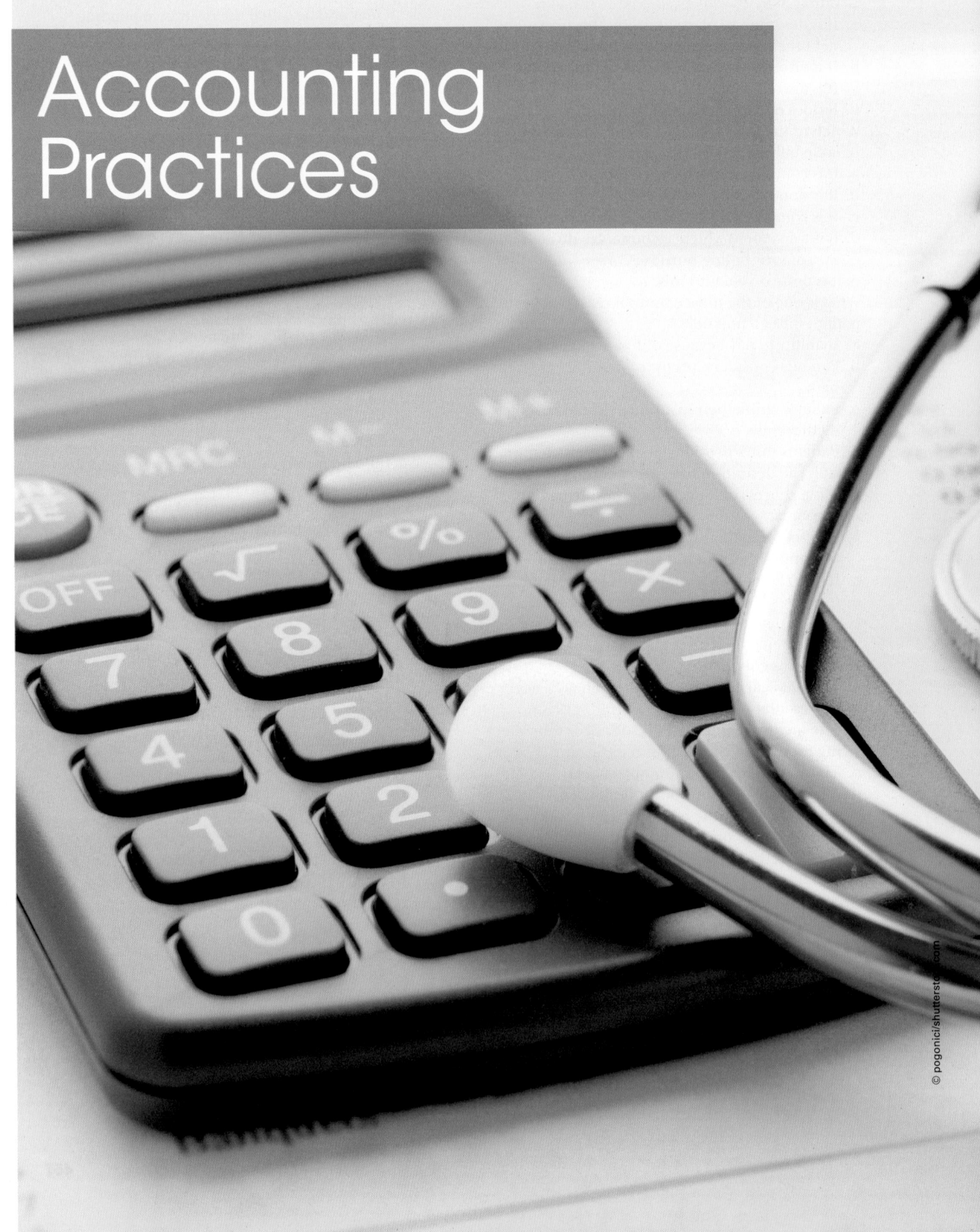

1. Define and spell the key terms as presented in the glossary.
2. Explain basic bookkeeping computations.
3. Explain the purpose and range of the accounting function in the clinic.
4. Describe the four different types of bookkeeping and accounting systems.
5. Recall the importance of the day-end summary and the accounts receivable trial balance.
6. Compare and contrast financial, managerial, and cost accounting.
7. Explain the use and validity of the income statement and the balance sheet.
8. Recall three useful financial ratios and explain them in detail.
9. Identify the proper steps in accounts payable management.
10. Discuss the impact of utilization review on reimbursement.
11. Discuss legal and ethical guidelines in accounting practices.

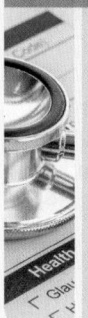

KEY TERMS

accounting	check register	income statement
accounts payable	collection ratio	liability
accounts receivable (A/R) ratio	cost accounting	managerial accounting
accrual basis	cost analysis	owner's equity
assets	cost ratio	trial balance
balance sheet	financial accounting	utilization review (UR)
cash basis	fixed cost	variable cost

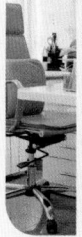

SCENARIO

When Mark King, one of the owners at Inner City Health Care, and clinic manager Marilyn Johnson, CMA (AAMA), decided to add a new medical assistant to the staff, they first reviewed the financial records for the previous year. Although the volume of work in the center generated the need for an additional employee, King and Johnson had to be sure it was financially feasible. In addition to past records, they also had to make some projections for the upcoming year; with certain new managed care fees, they had to be sure that anticipated revenues would be sufficient to sustain the salary of a new employee.

Chapter Portal

Medical financial management in the private practice setting is vitally important in the daily functioning of the medical clinic business. It directly affects overall bookkeeping and accounting procedures. Accounting generates financial information for the clinic and is defined as a system of monitoring the financial status of a facility and the specific results of its activities. It provides financial information for decision making.

Previous chapters have included the topics of proper daily bookkeeping financial practices (see Chapter 18), the accurate coding and the specific processing of insurance forms (see Chapters 16 and 17), and the efficient management of collecting on accounts (see Chapter 19). All of these functions are essential to obtaining maximum reimbursement and creating profitability for the practice.

This chapter ties many of these elements together and creates a total picture of their interdependence. Each element is critical to accurate accounting practices in the medical clinic.

BOOKKEEPING AND ACCOUNTING SYSTEMS

Medical practices use a variety of methods to monitor their financial accounts and the total financial operations of the business. Although some clinics still use the single-entry bookkeeping and pegboard systems, the majority prefer double-entry or computerized systems, or a combination.

Financial records should provide the following information at all times:

- Amount earned in a given period
- Amount collected in a given period
- Amount owed in a given period
- Where the expenses were incurred in a given period

The financial records can show these data as often as you like, usually on a monthly, quarterly, or yearly basis. Comparisons can be made with similar periods. Analysis of the financial data can help to determine if some services are not profitable, whether the practice is experiencing healthy growth, or why a loss might be realized. The accounts receivable and accounts payable data are vital to this information.

Single-Entry System

The single-entry system has been used in medical practices for many years. This includes a daily journal or log, patients' statements or accounts, ledgers, checks, and disbursement (expenditure) records. Information is first recorded in the journal, which provides a chronological record of financial transactions. Information from the journal is then transferred to the ledger through the process of posting. All amounts entered in the journal must be posted to the accounts kept in the ledger to summarize the results. This system has been used because of its simplicity and inexpensive nature. However, it is difficult to find errors because there are no internal controls, and financial analysis information is inadequate.

Pegboard System

As discussed in Chapter 18, the pegboard, or "write-it-once," system is easier to use than the single-entry system and has greater internal controls. The pegboard system provides control over collections, payments, and charges. It uses NCR (no carbon required) forms that are layered or shingled on pegs on the left of the board so that both income and disbursement entries need to be written only once. Many pegboard systems include a charge slip (or encounter form), which simplifies third-party payment processing for both the medical practice and the patients. The charge slip is used to record the input needed during the patient's visit, while serving as the patient's receipt for services performed and fees charged. An advantage of the pegboard system is its accuracy, because data are entered at the time of service and not recopied, so fewer errors can creep in.

Double-Entry System

The double-entry system is based on the fact that each transaction has two aspects, that is, a dual effect on the accounting elements. This system is based on the accounting principle that assets equal liabilities plus owner's equity.

$$\text{Assets} = \text{Liabilities} + \text{Owner's Equity}$$

Assets are the properties owned by the business (supplies, equipment, accounts receivable, and so on). **Liabilities** include what is owed to creditors. **Owner's equity** is the amount by which the business assets exceed the business liabilities. Net worth, proprietorship, and capital are often used as synonyms for owner's equity.

The double-entry system requires that the two aspects involved in every transaction be recorded on each side of the equation and that the two sides always be in balance. Although this accounting system requires time and skill, it provides a comprehensive financial picture and has built-in accuracy controls. It is orderly, fairly simple, flexible, and accurate, making it impossible for certain types of errors to remain undetected for long. For example, if one aspect of a transaction is properly recorded but the other aspect is overlooked, the records are out of balance. This occurrence may be easily discovered and subsequently corrected.

Practice Management System

The majority of medical practices rely on accounting software packages to prepare financial records, such as ledgers and reports, and to retrieve patient information. An increasing number of practices are using financial management software that is part of a practice management (PM) system. PM is a system of computerizing the entire facility and likely includes:

- Patient information data and scheduling
- Interface with electronic medical records (EMR) and electronic health records (EHR)

- Insurance coding and billing; processing claims electronically
- Management and human resources; payroll, purchases, personnel records
- Bookkeeping and accounting; generation of financial records including business income and expenses

A computerized accounting system is most likely to be based on the principles of either the pegboard (write-it-once) or a double-entry bookkeeping system, or a combination of both.

A computer financial system can be customized to meet the needs of the practice. Most large multi-speciality clinics have a computer system designed particularly for their needs. A PM system has the capability of including the most common procedure and diagnostic codes within a database to be recalled when completing insurance claim forms. The software will assist in matching the charges with the appropriate diagnosis codes.

A PM system has the flexibility of assigning codes in other categories to indicate whether a bill has been paid with cash, with a check, or by a third-party payer. Codes may also be assigned to identify the place of service and the professional performing the service. This facilitates the tracking of payments and also allows for the analysis of specific sources that generate income for the practice. Adjustments to reflect discounts or reduced fees may also be entered into the computer. The software is used in the preparation of billing statements, insurance forms, collection letters, and a number of financial ratios and statements to assist in monitoring the practice's financial stability.

Computer and Billing Service Bureaus

An option for clinics that choose not to purchase accounting software or a PM system in their practice is to use a computer service bureau for billing purposes and the creation of many financial records. In this case, the clinic provides the data, and the bureau provides basic billing and accounting services, furnishing financial statements, completed insurance forms, payroll materials, and checks.

Service bureaus handle accounts from the medical facilities in one of three ways:

1. Through the clinic's own computer terminal, online sharing occurs where the clinic is tied directly to the bureau's mainframe computer
2. Through online servicing, by which the clinic has its own terminal that allows direct communication with the service bureau's computer
3. Through off-line batch processing, where the medical assistant or bookkeeper sends daily batches of data to the bureau to process

Legal

Many facilities, however, prefer to have their own computerized financial or PM system because outsourcing computer services can compromise patient confidentiality and limit control over computer usage. A proper contract should be negotiated and signed with any computer and billing service bureau to ensure confidentiality, HIPAA compliance, and strict privacy of all patient information.

DAY-END SUMMARY

The financial summary at the end of the day is a helpful tool for a quick financial analysis. Computer accounting systems automatically create the day-end summaries in the form of reports. Pegboard systems require the administrative medical assistant to total the summaries that are shown at the bottom of the day sheet.

The first section of the day sheet identifies all the financial transactions of the day. The second section includes the month-to-date totals. This is where today's totals are added to the month-to-date totals; this must be in perfect balance. The third section identifies the year-to-date accounts, which includes all accounts to obtain the year-to-date total. A deposit slip included with most systems enables the assistant to verify the cash receipts with the checks received. This is helpful in preparing the day's bank deposit.

Integrity

When the totals do not balance at the end of the day, the medical assistant must begin the search for errors.

Tips for Finding Errors

Some tips for finding errors are as follows:

- Check the addition of each column, both horizontally and vertically. If a calculator is used, check the tape for entry errors.
- Compute the difference in the totals that are out of balance. Search the day sheet and patient accounts for that exact amount.
- If the amount of the error is divisible by 9, there may be an error in transposition of numbers.
- If the amount of the error is divisible by 2, the amount may have been posted in the wrong column.

- Check your entries when manually carrying forward previous balances. It is quite easy to carry forward an incorrect amount or to place numbers incorrectly. For example, the number $750 might be carried forward as $75.

Anyone who has worked with a manual pegboard system can report horror stories of chasing errors around for several days before finding them. It might be one error in one patient's account that creates the havoc. Also, a search for an error can continue at great length even as the assistant keeps seeing and missing the error. Set the problem aside for a bit, or even a day if you are not pressed with month-end billing deadlines. Have another person check for you. Often that individual sees the error in just a few minutes.

Errors in an electronic financial system can create almost as much havoc but often can be caught earlier. If all data are entered accurately and kept up to date, an error that occurs when keying in certain data will create a warning notice that indicates the data are incorrect. Computers do not automatically update all information when fees for services are changed, reimbursement adjustments are changed, salaries are increased, or new data from the laboratory or clinical area are determined. Any time there is a person who is entering data into the system, errors can occur. All medical professionals entering any data into the system must be reminded not to rush through the process and to carefully check for accuracy.

ACCOUNTS RECEIVABLE TRIAL BALANCE

Competency

Before preparing monthly statements, a **trial balance** should be done on the accounts receivable in either a pegboard system or a computer system. The trial balance is created by totaling debit balances and credit balances to confirm that total debits equal total credits. The trial balance will indicate any problem between the daily journal and the ledger. Use the following steps to create the trial balance:

1. Pull all patient accounts that have a balance.
2. Total the balance of those accounts.
3. Create an accounts receivable total.
   a. Enter the accounts receivable at the first of the month.
   b. Add the total charges for the month and subtotal.
   c. Subtract the total payments for the month and subtotal.
   d. Subtract the total adjustments for the month.
   e. The final total is the accounts receivable at the end of the month.

Procedure

This final total, the end of the month accounts receivable, must be the same as the figure received when adding all the patient account balances. If they match, the accounts are then in balance. If they do not balance, the error must be found (see Procedure 20-1).

ACCOUNTS PAYABLE

Accounts payable are an unwritten promise to pay a supplier for property or merchandise purchased on credit or for a service rendered. Accounts payable are the most common liability or financial obligation in the clinic setting. These include expenses such as medical and office supplies, salaries, equipment, and services. Payments for these expenses are made by check to ensure complete, accurate records of all money received and disbursed.

Supplies and equipment purchased usually come with a packing slip that describes the items purchased and their cost. An invoice may also be enclosed that serves as a bill for the items ordered; however, another invoice is sent to the business later as well. Take time to note on the invoice whether there is a discount for early payment. Some financial managers suggest attaching the invoice and packing slip to the purchase order. File in your tickler file or reminder file on the computer so that payment is made in a timely fashion to receive any discount. Some vendors prefer that payment not be made until a statement (or request for payment) is received from them. This is particularly the case if the practice uses that vendor more than once a month. When the statement arrives, check the invoice for accuracy before sending payment. Prepare the check for the accounts payable as appropriate, either monthly or as necessary to receive a discount (see Chapter 18). Write the check number on the invoice, as well as the amount paid, and place in a file for accounts paid according to the practice's filing system.

Disbursement Records

Computerized accounts payable systems track the disbursements and post to appropriate established accounts similar to a manual system.

Procedure

Preparing Accounts Receivable Trial Balance

PURPOSE:

To prepare a trial balance in order to determine if there is any problem between the daily journal and the ledger or patient accounts.

EQUIPMENT/SUPPLIES:

- Patient accounts
- Calculator

PROCEDURE STEPS:

1. Pull all patient accounts that have a balance due. RATIONALE: Provides only amount due information.

2. Enter the balance of those accounts into the calculator.

3. Add the balances and total. (A calculator with tape can make it quicker to check for errors.) RATIONALE: Gives you the total amount due to date.

4. Create an accounts receivable total:

   a. Enter the accounts receivable total from the first of the month into the calculator.

   b. Add total charges for this month and subtotal.

   c. Total the amount of all payments received this month.

   d. Subtract the total of payments from subtotal of b above and subtotal.

   e. Total the amount of the month's adjustments and subtract from the subtotal in d above.

   f. This total is the accounts receivable amount. RATIONALE: The end-of-the month accounts receivable total (f) above must match the total in step 3. If these totals do not match, an error has been made. If they do match, the trial balance is in order.

Computer accounts payable systems have a **check register** that records all checks written and categorizes them into separate columns, such as rent, insurance, office supplies, utilities, and so forth. These categories can be designed to be as general or detailed as preferred. The computer system also can create entries for bank deposits and payroll records.

The computer software has a check-writing file that presents checks on the screen. The information necessary to complete the check is entered at the keyboard; the computer stores it and prints out the check. Printing the checks can be done individually or by batch if several bills are being paid. The amount is automatically subtracted from the account's balance. The computer system also can recall data that need to be entered on the checks each time there is a payment. For example, the name of the company where most supplies are purchased can be recalled from the database; thus the assistant does not have to key in that information again. This feature is a particular timesaver when payroll checks are prepared (see Chapter 44).

The manual or pegboard system uses a check register page to record checks written. The check is aligned on the pegboard over the check register before completion. The pegboard checks have an NCR transfer strip that copies the date, the payee, the check number, and the amount to the check register. Pegboard checks can be designed so that the address is entered beneath the payee line and mailed in a window envelope. This check register has a number of columns to categorize expenses. All entries are totaled on the check register when completed, and these totals are carried forward. A balanced check register provides a way to verify the bank statement when it arrives. The check register can also be used for bank deposits and for payroll records.

THE ACCOUNTING FUNCTION

Accounting is a system of monitoring the financial status of a facility and the financial results of its activities. Accounting may be divided into two major categories: financial and managerial. **Financial accounting** provides information primarily for entities external to the organization such as the government. In contrast, **managerial accounting** generates financial information that can enable more efficient internal management. **Cost accounting** helps to determine what it costs the clinic to perform particular services and is an integral part of managerial accounting. A hospital cost report for Medicare is essentially a part of financial accounting because the report is generated for an external user—the Centers for Medicare and Medicaid Services (CMS), which administers the Medicare program. However, it is also a part of cost accounting because a cost report on Medicare will show what it costs to care for patients on Medicare.

COST ANALYSIS

An important aspect of the practice is **cost analysis**. The purpose of the analysis is to determine the costs of each service. There are two factors to consider: fixed costs and variable costs.

Fixed Costs

Fixed costs are costs that do not vary in total as the number of patients varies. For example, the annual depreciation cost of the equipment is fixed because it will remain the same regardless of the number of patients who use it.

Variable Costs

Variable costs are those that vary in direct proportion to patient volume, such as clinical supplies and laboratory procedures. Average costs to treat patients decline because of fixed costs, not variable costs. The greater the volume, the more widely the fixed costs are spread and the less cost any one unit is responsible for.

Patient cost factors include administrative costs, such as the cost of billing and collections, personnel costs for clinic staff providing patient care, equipment costs, and costs for clinical supplies. The provider cost will include costs for interpreting tests, diagnosing illnesses, and maintaining professional liability insurance.

Calculating and reviewing costs provide the clinic with data to set fees, market the practice, determine profit, and monitor the practice's performance.

FINANCIAL RECORDS

Indicators of the financial status of the medical facility include financial statements that reflect the daily operations of the business. These records comprise an accounting information system that is maintained for numerous reasons, one of which is to provide source data for use in the preparation of various reports. Two financial statements common to the clinic are the income/expense statement and the balance sheet.

Income Statement

Figure 20-1 shows a sample **income statement**, the most commonly generated year-end report. The sample shows the profit and expenses for a given month. The income statement shows the cumulative profit and total expenses by reporting patient income, outside revenue sources, and overhead expenses such as office and medical expenses. Provider's compensation and benefits and employees' compensation, benefits, and withholding taxes can be itemized as well.

Balance Sheet

Sometimes called the statement of financial condition or statement of financial position, the **balance sheet** is an itemized statement of the assets, liabilities, and owner's equity of a medical facility as of a specified date. Its purpose is to provide information regarding the status of these basic accounting elements.

The balance sheet is made possible through the double-entry system of accounting because every transaction is recorded by two sets of entries made in a ledger or journal. Increases in assets are recorded as debits; decreases are recorded as credits. Increases in liabilities and owner's equity are recorded as credits; decreases are recorded as debits.

Debit and credit entries to one or more accounts make up the system. In any recording, the total dollar amount of the debit entries must equal the total dollar amount of the credit entries. Each ledger or journal entry should have the following elements:

1. Date of transaction
2. Journal or ledger account names involved
3. Dollar amount of the charges
4. Brief explanation of the transaction

USEFUL FINANCIAL DATA

A business must determine how and when it will report income earned. There are two systems for doing this. The **accrual basis** reports income at the time charges are generated. This is used mainly in commercial environments. The **cash basis** is most often used in medical practices. In the cash basis, income is recognized when money is collected.

A few financial ratios can help evaluate how the practice is doing. Data from the current year and the previous year's financial statements can be converted into ratios to highlight different financial characteristics. However, ratios should always be viewed in relation to the total financial picture.

**INNER CITY HEALTH CARE
INCOME STATEMENT**

	Month of , 20XX	Year-to-Date	Budget for Year	Overhead Percentages
A. Revenue:				
1. Office #1	$	$	$	
2. Office #2	$	$	$	
B. Total Revenue:	$	$	$	100%
C. Expenses:				
1. Non–provider (staff) salaries—gross	$	$	$	%
2. Staff fringes:				
– Payroll taxes	$	$	$	
– Empl. benefits	$	$	$	
– Empl. seminars	$	$	$	
– Uniforms	$	$	$	
– Retirement plan	$	$	$	
	$	$	$	%
3. Occupancy costs:				
– Rent—Off. #1	$	$	$	
– Rent—Off. #2	$	$	$	
– Property taxes	$	$	$	
– Insurance	$	$	$	
– Utilities	$	$	$	
– Janitor/Grounds	$	$	$	
	$	$	$	%
4. Medical expenses:				
– Medications	$	$	$	
– Supplies	$	$	$	
– Lab fees	$	$	$	
	$	$	$	%
5. Office expenses:				
– Office supplies	$	$	$	
– Postage	$	$	$	
– Telephone	$	$	$	
	$	$	$	%
6. Malpractice ins.	$	$	$	%
7. Professional expenses:				
– Auto expenses (Providers')	$	$	$	
– Dues/subscriptions	$	$	$	
– Books and videos	$	$	$	
– Dues/memberships	$	$	$	
– Entertainment	$	$	$	
– Professional development	$	$	$	
– Travel	$	$	$	
	$	$	$	%

FIGURE 20-1 A sample income statement that can show profit and expenses for 1 month.

(continues)

	Month of , 20XX	Year-to- Date	Budget for Year	Overhead Percentages
8. Equipment costs:				
– Depreciation/amortization	$	$	$	
– Rent	$	$	$	
– Service/maintenance	$	$	$	
– Interest (if on equipment purchase loans)	$	$	$	
	$	$	$	%
9. Marketing expenses:				
– Advertising	$	$	$	
– Other fees	$	$	$	
	$	$	$	%
10. Professional expenses:				
– Accounting	$	$	$	
– Legal	$	$	$	
– Consulting	$	$	$	
– Ret. Plan Admin.	$	$	$	
	$	$	$	%
11.				
12.				
13.				
14.				
D. Total Non–Provider Expenses:	$	$	$	%
E. Operating New Income Before Provider's Costs (B minus C)	$	$	$	%
F. Associate Provider's Costs:				
– Salaries—gross:	$	$	$	
– Benefits	$	$	$	
–	$	$	$	
–	$	$	$	
G. Total Non–Owner Provider's Costs	$	$	$	%
H. New Income Available to Owner– Providers (E minus G)	$	$	$	%
I. Owner–Providers' Costs:				
1. Salaries—gross:				
–Dr. A	$	$	$	
–Dr. B	$	$	$	
2. Bonuses—gross:				
–Dr. A	$	$	$	
–Dr. B	$	$	$	
3. Retirement contributions:				
–Dr. A	$	$	$	
–Dr. B	$	$	$	
4. "Semi-personal" expenses:				
–Dr. A	$	$	$	
–Dr. B	$	$	$	
J. Total Owner–Providers' Costs	$	$	$	
K. Net Income (H minus J)	$	$	$	

FIGURE 20-1 (*continued*)

Ratios are not difficult to calculate, but they can be time consuming when using a manual system. They are quick to create in a computer system because all the data are readily available, already totaled, and sometimes created automatically. It is helpful to understand the concept, however, and not rely too heavily on computer-generated reports. Data that have been entered incorrectly at some point will be reflected in reports generated. The user of accounting software must train

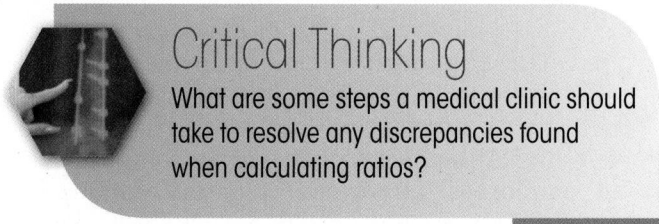

Critical Thinking

What are some steps a medical clinic should take to resolve any discrepancies found when calculating ratios?

his or her mind to think about the sensibility of the report.

Although two of these ratios were discussed in Chapter 19, some elaboration is in order in the context of this chapter.

Accounts Receivable Ratio

The **accounts receivable (A/R) ratio** formula measures the speed at which outstanding accounts are paid. The accounts receivable ratio provides a picture of the state of collections and probable losses. The longer an account is past due, the less the likelihood is of successfully making the collection.

$$\frac{\text{Total Accounts Receivable}}{\text{Monthly Receipts}} = \text{Turnaround Time}$$

Example:

$$\frac{\$120,000}{\$60,000} = 2 \text{ Months Turnaround Time for Payment on an Account}$$

The goal of an efficient billing and collecting policy should be a turnaround time of 2 months or less.

Collection Ratio

The **collection ratio** shows the percentage of outstanding debt collected. The goal should be a 90% collection ratio. Total receipts divided by total charges gives the unadjusted collection ratio, but adjustments may include federal and state insurance programs (Medicare and Medicaid, Workers' Compensation), managed care adjustments, and any other adjustments as directed by the provider.

Total Receipts	= $40,000
+ Managed Care Adjustments	$3,000
+ Medicare Adjustments	$2,000
TOTAL	$45,000
Total Charges	$52,000

$$\frac{\text{Total Receipts } \$45,000}{\text{Total Charges } \$52,000} = 86.5\% \text{ Collection Ratio after Adjustments}$$

Cost Ratio

The **cost ratio** formula shows the cost of a procedure or service and can help in determining, for instance, the cost effectiveness of maintaining a laboratory in the clinic setting. The ratio is:

$$\frac{\text{Total Expenses}}{\text{Total Number of Procedures for 1 Month}}$$

$$\frac{\text{Total Laboratory Expenses for September}}{\text{Total Number of Procedures Performed for September}}$$

$$\frac{\$48,000}{240} = \$200 \text{ per Procedure}$$

A conclusion might be reached that the laboratory is too costly because each procedure is not billed at $200.

LEGAL AND ETHICAL GUIDELINES

Legal

It is hoped that a careful hiring process (see Chapter 45) results in the best employees whose credentials, ethics, and personal actions are above reproach. However, embezzlement does occur in medical practices, partly because of the way in which the financial aspect of the practice is designed and managed. To decrease the opportunity for embezzlement:

- The accountant and the managing provider(s) should conduct regular and irregular audits of the practice accounts. Seek an accountant who is available at any time, not just when it is time to report wages or compute the yearly taxes. The accountant also becomes a valuable asset to the practice in providing essential information to the clinic staff.

- Separate duties among several employees. Consider having one employee open the mail and post checks received. A second employee handles all the cash transactions and prepares the deposit slips. A third employee might order the supplies and prepare all the checks. Many providers choose to sign the checks; however, this is also a task that can be assigned to the office manager.

- Only one person should use the signature stamp; better yet, consider not using a signature stamp at all.
- The signature card on file at the bank must include the names of each individual authorized to sign the checks.
- Seek employees whose personal honesty sets a good example for everyone.

Providers who demonstrate the same personal honesty and integrity expected of their staff are less likely to be victims of embezzlement.

Bonding

There is another recommended step to take. To protect the practice from embezzlement or other financial loss, providers can purchase fidelity bonds. These bonds reimburse the practice for any monetary loss caused by the practice's employees. There are three types of bonds to consider, and it is reasonable to have more than one type. These bonds include:

1. Position-schedule bonds, which cover the position rather than a specific individual. For instance, the bookkeeper, office manager, and receptionist might be covered.
2. Blanket-position bonds, which cover all employees. If the staff members often share duties, cover for one another when there are absences, or work really well together as a team during busy periods, this type of bond might be most beneficial.
3. Personal bonds, which are designed to cover specific individuals by name and generally require a personal background investigation. This type of bond may give the most assurance.

Bonding not only protects the providers and the practice, but it assures employees that they are covered by a bond should there be a problem with the finances during their shift. Bonding service companies will require implementation of certain procedures and security measures as outlined in their contracts. Costs depend on risk levels, but they are well worth the protection.

Payroll

Competency

The administrative medical assistant is likely to be involved in making certain the W-4 form, the Employee's Withholding Allowance Certificate, is completed by all employees. However, salary calculations, withholding taxes, and Social Security calculations are the responsibility of the office manager or, may be outsourced to a payroll service. Payroll tasks usually are assigned to the clinic manager or a service because of the privacy of salary issues, Social Security numbers, and confidentiality of the employees' tax information. Manual systems for managing payroll are available, but the most efficient systems are computerized. The financial management of the payroll responsibilities in the clinic is detailed in Chapter 44.

Utilization Review

In the present health care climate, in which there are many managed care plans, more attention has been focused on how the billing and financial management process should proceed. Because of the influence of governmental mandates in the practice of medicine and because of the growth of the **utilization review (UR)** industry, more accurate record-keeping and documentation in all facets of the clinic have become necessary. There are numerous UR Arms throughout the country. These companies aggressively sell their services to employers and to insurance carriers. UR is actually a review of the patient service required before the actual service may be performed. If the reviewer determines that the procedure or treatment is not needed, then it will not be approved or covered under the patient's insurance plan. Policies that once permitted medical decisions to be made solely by the provider often are now made by other health professionals who are employed by UR Arms. Some clinics may find it beneficial to have one medical assistant whose main responsibility is to present procedures to UR for acceptance or denial. Because of the increasing concern for quality of health care at low cost, more providers also are realizing that they need more documentation of both medical and financial information with more accessible means for retrieval.

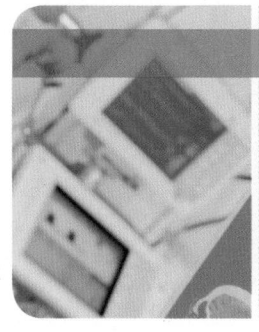

CASE STUDY 20-1

Refer to the scenario at the beginning of the chapter.

CASE STUDY REVIEW

1. Identify the financial records most likely reviewed by Mark King and Marilyn Johnson.
2. What information will be considered when projecting future income?
3. Identify other concerns to consider when hiring an additional medical assistant.

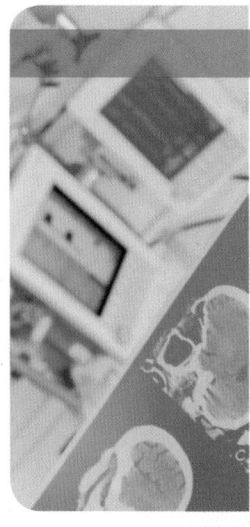

CASE STUDY 20-2

Richard Saxton is a newly licensed acupuncturist who has been in practice for less than a year. He is renting space for his procedures and services with an established doctor of osteopathy. Richard is using a simple pegboard system, makes his own appointments, and collects for most procedures at the time services are rendered unless the patients have medical insurance covering acupuncture. Richard has done fairly well, likes working in the environment the facility offers, and is beginning to show some profit. He would like to purchase a new table, chair, and stool for his acupuncture room.

CASE STUDY REVIEW

1. What facts might Richard want to consider before making the purchases?
2. Consider the variable costs versus the fixed costs of the practice of acupuncture. (You may need to do a little research to determine supplies and other factors.)
3. What information will his pegboard system give him?

Summary

- Accounting is the process of recording financial transactions, including storage, retrieval, report generation for summaries, sorting, and evaluation of clinic information.

- This information serves as a system of monitoring the financial status of a clinic and the specific results of its activities. It provides financial information for decision making at many levels. These functions are essential to obtaining maximum reimbursement and creating profitability for the practice.

- The various methods a clinic may use for accounting and monitoring financial accounts include the single-entry system, the pegboard system, the double-entry system, a practice management (PM) software system, and billing services and bureaus.

- The medical assistant must know how to run a financial analysis by using summary tools in a computer accounting system or manual pegboard systems, including preparing a deposit slip at the end of each day.

- Accuracy is necessary; the medical assistant will use various techniques to find and correct errors should they occur.

- The medical assistant must run and check the trial balance on account receivables before monthly statements are produced. It should be confirmed that total debits equal total credits by producing a final total at the end of each month. This ensures accuracy and that accounts are in balance.

- Collection techniques must be properly used, both by telephone and by letter, following the guidelines of the Fair Debt Collections Practices Act.

- Cost analysis methods include fixed costs and variable costs in order to collect data used to set fees, market the practice, evaluate profits, and monitor the clinic's performance.

- The accounts receivable ratio and cost ratio formulas provide a picture of collections and losses, as well as aiding in the determination of the cost effectiveness of equipment, insurance participation, and other clinic considerations.

CERTIFICATION REVIEW

1. What is a tip for finding an error of a transposed number in financial reports?
   a. The error is divisible by 4
   b. The error is divisible by 2
   c. The error is divisible by 9
   d. None of these

2. What is an example of a fixed cost?
   a. Salaries
   b. Cost of supplies
   c. Depreciation of equipment
   d. Cost of treating patients
   e. The monthly utility bill

3. What is the name for the itemized statement of the financial position of a business?
   a. Income statement
   b. Balance sheet
   c. Trial balance
   d. Collection ratio

4. What is the purpose of a check register?
   a. It records all checks and categorizes them into separate columns.
   b. It is used when taking cash from patients.
   c. It is an accounts receivable record.
   d. Both a and c
   e. None of these, it is not necessary.

5. What is the purpose of utilization review?
   a. It looks at the utility of all personnel.
   b. It examines how useful the ambulatory care center is to patients.
   c. It is a review of a procedure before it is performed to determine if it is necessary.
   d. It only affects hospitals.

6. Assets include which of the following?
   a. Equipment and supplies on hand
   b. Building or property
   c. Accounts receivable
   d. All of these
   e. None of these

7. What is a computer billing and service bureau?
   a. It is the service you hire to care for the clinic computer system.
   b. It may compromise patient confidentiality.
   c. It can function through linkage of computers, online servicing, or off-line batch processing.
   d. Both b and c

8. What is true of the collection ratio in a medical facility where the total receipts including any adjustments are $83,500 and the total charges equal $97,750?
   a. It would be great at 94%.
   b. It would be quite good at 88%.
   c. It shows a fair return at 85%.
   d. It shows a modest return at 75%.
   e. None of these

9. When can money be saved with accounts payable?
   a. When bills are paid promptly
   b. When discounts are realized
   c. When supplies are not purchased in bulk
   d. Both a and b

10. Which of the following is true of bonding?
    a. It binds providers to the safe caretaking of their patients.
    b. It protects medical clinic staff and providers if embezzlement occurs.
    c. It can be purchased in three different types.
    d. It is not very costly to the business.
    e. Both b and c

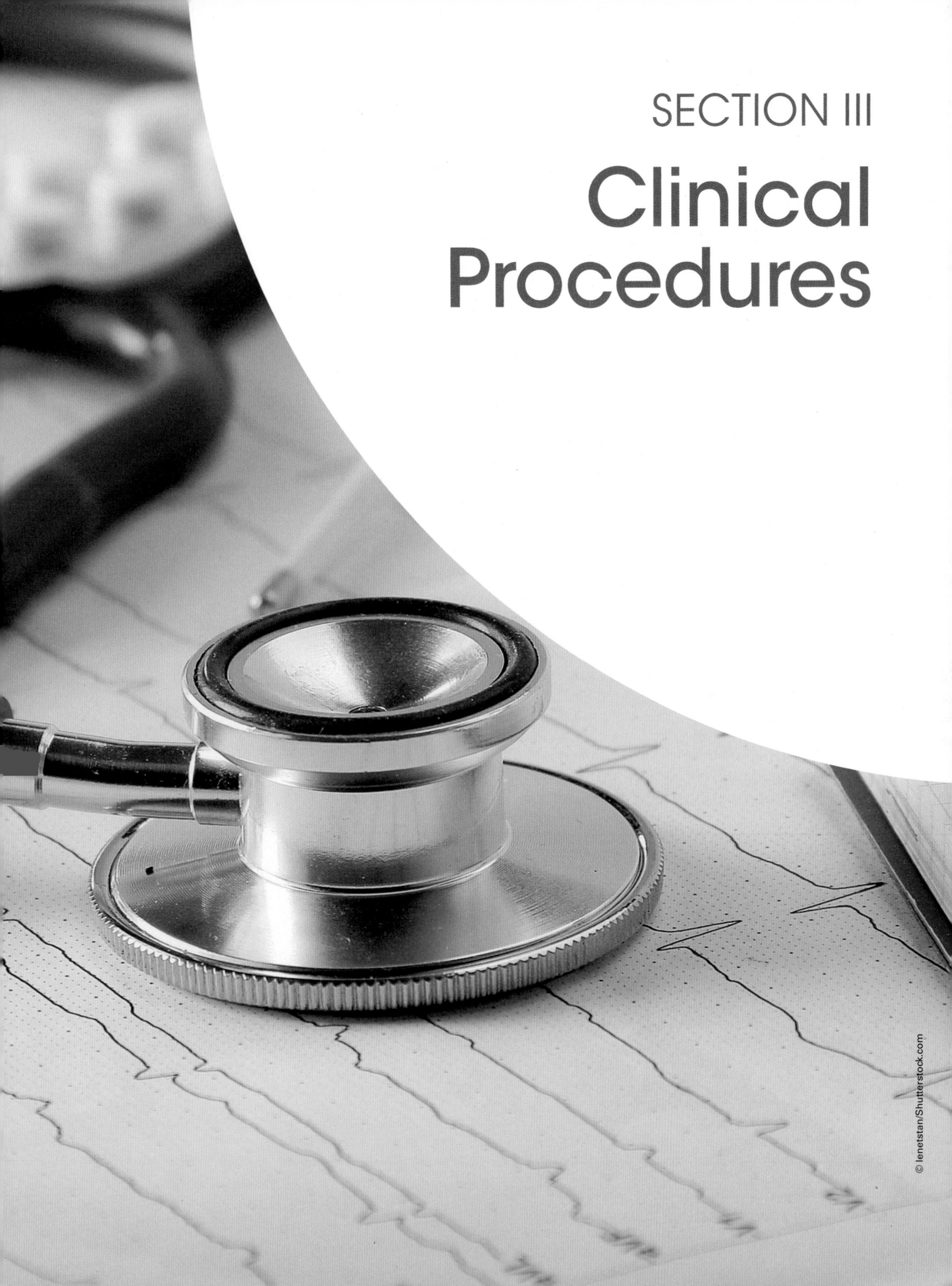

SECTION III

Clinical Procedures

UNIT VI
INTEGRATED CLINICAL PROCEDURES

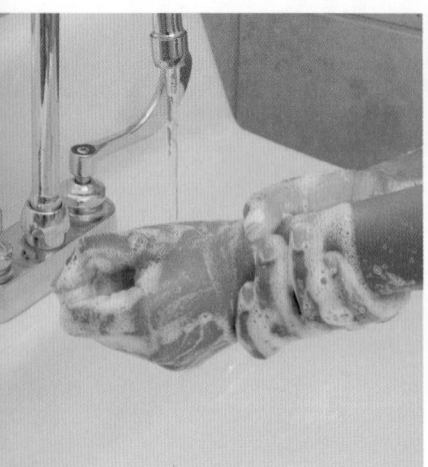
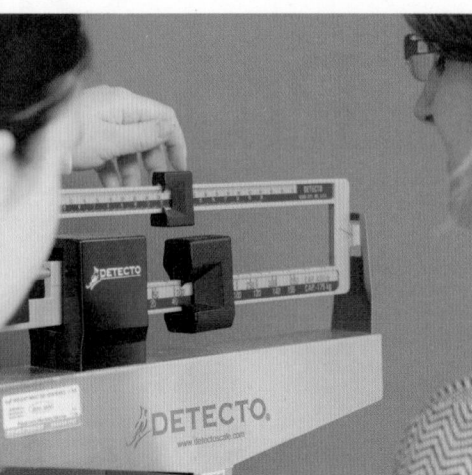
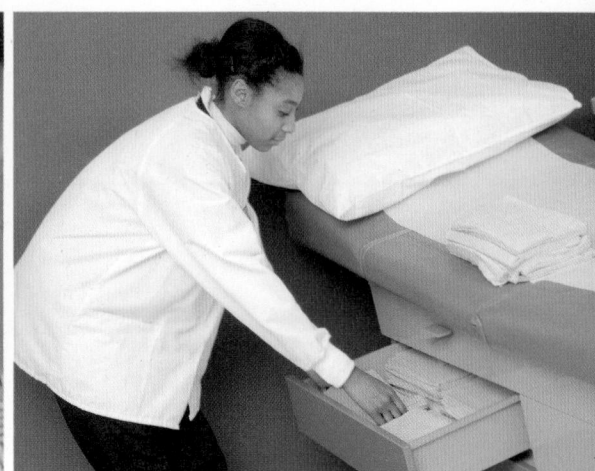

ATTRIBUTES OF PROFESSIONALISM

As a medical assistant who will come into contact with the patient on multiple levels, from taking the history to assisting with invasive procedures, a sense of accountability and sound judgement are qualities that are essential to the provision of quality care. Understanding the cycle of infection and the transmission of disease allows the medical assistant to behave in a manner that protects the patient and themselves.

Establishing trust and rapport with the patient are essential for appropriate delivery of care. A sense of confidence and skilled questioning will allow the medial assistant to elicit and record a concise medical history. This information will aid the provider in planning care for the optimal health of the patient. Skill is also required when obtaining vital signs and other critical data relating to a patient's medical profile. Accuracy in obtaining these mensurations are a part of the responsibilities of the professional medical assistant.

Assisting the provider to complete a patient's physical exam is another area of responsibility for the medical assistant. The medical assistant can aid in keeping the patient relaxed and cooperative, as well as assisting the provider to move easily from the assessment of one body system to another. Therefore,

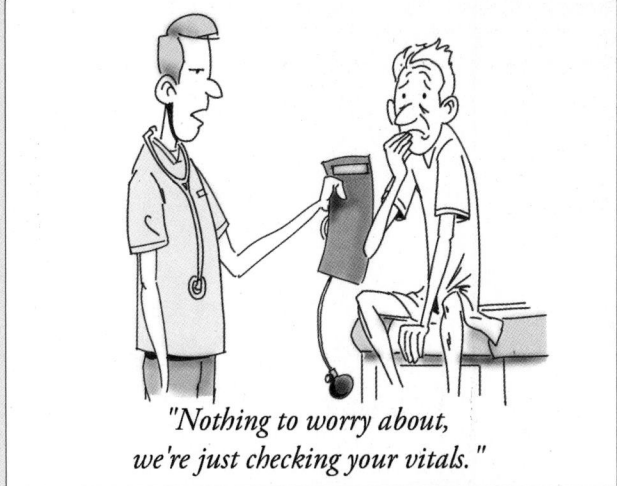

"Nothing to worry about, we're just checking your vitals."

it is important that the medical assistant pay close attention, stay present and aware, and anticipate the patient and provider's needs during this essential part of the visit.

Listed below are a series of questions for you to ask yourself, to serve as a professionalism checklist. As you interact with patients and colleagues, these questions will help to guide you in the professional behavior and therapeutic communication that is expected every day from medical assistants.

Ask Yourself

COMMUNICATION
- ☐ Do I apply active listening skills?
- ☐ Do I explain to patients the rationale for performance of a procedure?
- ☐ Do I speak at each patient's level of understanding?
- ☐ Do I display appropriate body language?
- ☐ Do I respond honestly and diplomatically to my patients' concerns?
- ☐ Do I refrain from sharing my personal experiences?
- ☐ Do I include the patient's support system as indicated?
- ☐ Do I accurately and concisely update the provider on any aspect of a patient's care?

PRESENTATION
- ☐ Am I dressed and groomed appropriately?
- ☐ Am I courteous, patient, and respectful to patients?
- ☐ Do I display a positive attitude?
- ☐ Do I display a calm, professional, and caring manner?
- ☐ Do I demonstrate empathy to the patient?
- ☐ Do I show awareness of a patient's concerns related to the procedure being performed?

COMPETENCY
- ☐ Do I pay attention to detail?
- ☐ Do I ask questions if I am out of my comfort zone or do not have the experience to carry out tasks?
- ☐ Do I display sound judgment?
- ☐ Am I knowledgeable and accountable?
- ☐ Do I incorporate critical thinking skills in performing patient assessment and care?

INITIATIVE
- ☐ Am I flexible and dependable?
- ☐ Do I direct the patient to other resources when necessary or helpful, with the approval of the provider?
- ☐ Do I assist co-workers when appropriate?
- ☐ Do I make adaptations for patients with special needs?

INTEGRITY
- ☐ Do I demonstrate the principles of self-boundaries?
- ☐ Do I work within my scope of practice?
- ☐ Do I demonstrate respect for individual diversity?
- ☐ Do I demonstrate sensitivity to patient rights?
- ☐ Do I protect the integrity of the medical record?
- ☐ Do I protect and maintain confidentiality?
- ☐ Do I immediately report any error I made?
- ☐ Do I report situations which are harmful or illegal?

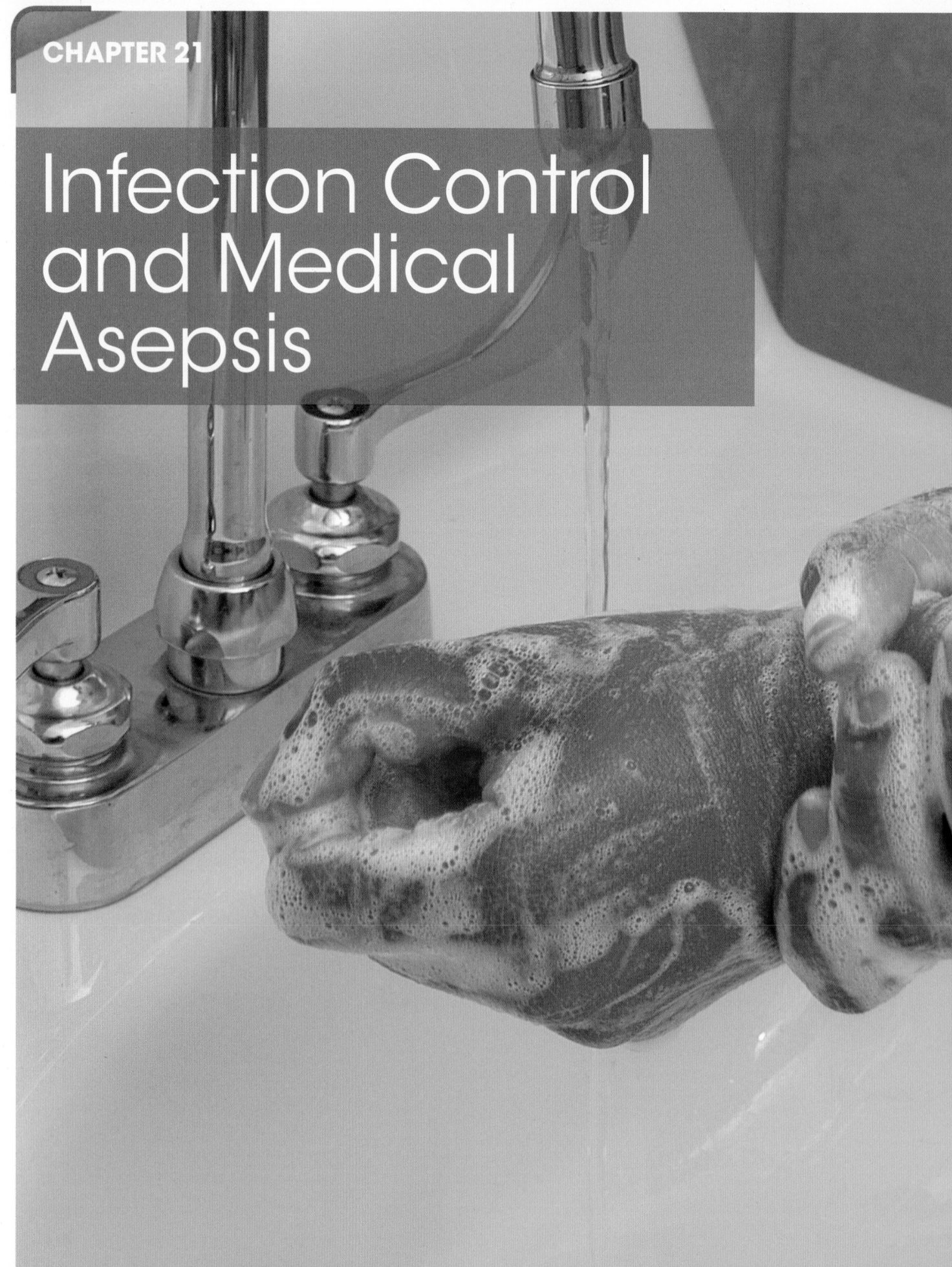

CHAPTER 21

Infection Control and Medical Asepsis

LEARNING OUTCOMES

1. Define and spell the key terms as presented in the glossary.
2. Identify and state the critical importance of infection control in the ambulatory care setting.
3. Outline the six stages in the infection cycle.
4. Cite the five classifications of infectious microorganisms.
5. Recall and elaborate on the four phases the immune system uses to defend against infectious disease.
6. Recite the four stages of infectious diseases.
7. Discuss at least five infectious diseases, their agents of transmission, and their symptoms.
8. Compare the routes of transmission of AIDS and hepatitis B and C and discuss the risk for infection from needlestick.
9. Identify the purpose of Standard Precautions and give six examples of ways health care providers should practice Standard Precautions.
10. Differentiate among the three types of Transmission-Based Precautions, defining what they are and how they are applied.
11. Characterize eight types of body fluids and give an example of each.
12. Identify appropriate personal protective equipment for potentially infectious situations.
13. State five situations in which exposure to a patient's blood can occur, and discuss why Standard Precautions are important.
14. Describe proper disposal of infectious waste.
15. Identify the role of the Centers for Disease Control regulations in health care settings.
16. Recognize human fluids that may contain HIV, HBV, and HCV.
17. Explain medical asepsis.
18. Define bioterrorism and describe five agents that could be used in a bioterrorism attack.

KEY TERMS

acquired immunodeficiency syndrome (AIDS)
aerobic
airborne transmission
amoebic dysentery
anaerobic
antibodies
aseptic
bacilli
barriers
bloodborne pathogen
carrier
caustic
cell-mediated immunity
chlamydiae
cocci
communicable

Contact Precautions
contact transmission
contracting
coryza
debris
declination form
droplet transmission
epidemic
epidemiology
excoriated
excretions
fomites
genotypes
gross contamination
helminths
human immunodeficiency virus (HIV)

humoral immunity
immune system
immunoglobulins
immunomodulators
immunosuppressed
infection control
infectious agents
inflammatory response
intracellular
isolation
isolation categories
lymphadenopathy
malaise
malaria
medical asepsis
microorganisms
morbidity

continues

473

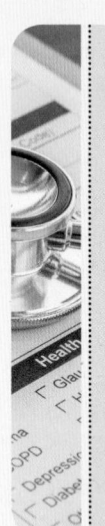

Key Terms, *continued*

mortality	pruritus	sputum
normal flora	regulated waste	Standard Precautions
nosocomial	resistance	Transmission-Based Precautions
one-handed technique	rickettsiae	
opportunistic infections	secretions	trichomoniasis
	severe acute respiratory syndrome (SARS)	ultrasonic cleaner
palliative		Universal Precautions
parenteral	sharps	vaccines
pathogens	solvent	vector
protozoa	spill kits	virulence

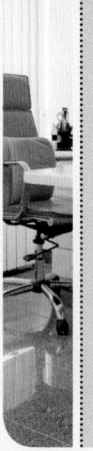

SCENARIO

Gwen Carr, CMA (AAMA), is a clinical medical assistant at Inner City Health Care. It is flu season again. Each provider at the clinic sees 25 to 30 patients a day and a large majority of them are complaining of symptoms of the flu. Gwen knows that because of the number of patients with influenza seen in the clinic and in order to protect the noninfected patients, it is imperative that she adhere to infection control precautions for all patient-care activities as well as aerosol-generating procedures, such as sputum collection and treatments that deliver medications using a nebulizer. She organizes a staff meeting to make sure that all staff members are aware of their role in preventing the spread of infection in the health care setting. Front desk staff, medical records staff, and business office personnel are all included in this meeting. Gwen provides information from the CDC that recommends immunization with the influenza vaccine, implementation of cough etiquette, and management of ill staff members. She spends extra time focusing on the importance of handwashing and the use of hand sanitizer to limit the spread of this virus. She has the approval of the providers to offer masks to persons who are coughing. By implementing these precautions, Gwen limits the risk of health care–associated infection.

Chapter Portal

nfectious diseases have plagued humans since the beginning of time. Recent scientific advances have changed our thoughts and behaviors regarding infectious disease. Advances such as antibiotic therapy and vaccination have significantly reduced risks for mortality from some previously fatal or debilitating infectious diseases. Infectious diseases that once were highly feared because of their likelihood of causing premature death are now preventable or treatable. Removing the deadly impact of many of these common diseases has allowed the public to forget the **virulence** and destructive potential of epidemics of infectious disease. The presence of **acquired immunodeficiency syndrome (AIDS)** as an incurable and fatal infectious disease (although people are living with HIV and AIDS for many years), as well as **severe acute respiratory syndrome (SARS)**, West Nile virus, avian flu, hepatitis C virus (HCV), and others, have caused the world to realize the enduring impact of pathogens on the human race.

Although these medical advances have reduced the incidence of **mortality** and **morbidity** from infectious diseases, humans must never underestimate the potential of resurgent infectious diseases. Tuberculosis is one of the leading causes of death in the history of humankind, yet was drastically reduced with the discovery of antituberculosis drugs. Today, however, the tuberculosis organism may have developed a resistance to our only line of defense. Medical assistants must pay close attention to the prevention of infectious diseases.

This chapter addresses the principles of the process of infection and control measures for use in ambulatory care settings. Because medical assistants deal directly with patients and other health care professionals, stringent adherence to the principles can greatly reduce transmission, or spread, of infectious disease. Continuous reliance on infection control measures ensures a clinical environment that is as safe as possible for employees, patients, and families. When infection control principles are not followed, infectious diseases may be transmitted to self, co-workers, or patients. The goals of infection control are to limit the presence of **infectious agents**, to create barriers against transmission, and to decrease the risk to others for contracting infectious diseases. These goals can be achieved through medical asepsis and sterilization, by observation of all Standard Precautions and Transmission-Based Precautions set forth by the CDC, and by following Occupational Safety and Health Administration (OSHA) guidelines.

IMPACT OF INFECTIOUS DISEASES

Since the discovery of the germ theory by Louis Pasteur and Robert Koch in the nineteenth century, we have seen dramatic changes in global mortality and morbidity statistics from infectious diseases. Many scientists devoted their professional lives to the quest for the prevention and cure of infectious diseases, which were the main cause of death in earlier centuries. In developed countries, deaths from diseases such as tuberculosis, pneumonia, and smallpox have been significantly reduced because of pharmacologic agents such as antibiotics and **vaccines**. Antibiotic agents were widely introduced during World War II, reducing deaths from traumatic wound infections. Edward Jenner is credited with the discovery of the first vaccine to protect against the deadly disease smallpox. Because of the vaccine, smallpox is considered to have been eradicated worldwide.

Epidemiology is the science that studies the history, causes, and patterns of infectious diseases. This field of medicine is credited to a Japanese bacteriologist in the late nineteenth century who recognized the connection between bubonic plague and rat infestation. Recent epidemiological studies have traced infectious diseases such as AIDS from the beginning of the epidemic. The future of studies in infectious diseases will focus on increasing the pharmacologic (medications) war against infectious diseases.

Reliance only on treatment of infectious disease does not address the crucial step in halting the spread of infectious diseases, that is, of prevention, or **infection control**. Emerging issues related to infectious diseases involve microorganisms that are resistant to present technology, **bloodborne pathogen** transmission, increased **immunosuppressed** populations, and global access to infection control and treatment. Developed countries become accustomed to anti-infective medications, clean water, and laws that protect the public from infectious agents found in food and other consumables. These safety measures may not be present in other countries where political or economic factors limit access to infection control measures.

In the future, drug-resistant infectious diseases will require greater emphasis on prevention because there may never be a safe and universally effective drug for all infectious diseases.

Diversity   Competency

Study of the history of infectious diseases allows us to realize the impact these diseases have on the lifestyles of people in various cultures. Infectious diseases such as AIDS and other sexually transmitted diseases have differing levels of social and cultural impact. Medical assistants should be aware of facts regarding the infectious process of specific diseases to reduce cultural isolation for the patient and to dispel myths regarding infectious diseases (see Chapter 5).

THE PROCESS OF INFECTION

Infectious diseases are caused by pathogenic microorganisms that are capable of causing disease. **Microorganisms** are microscopic living creatures capable of reproduction and transmission in specific circumstances. **Pathogens** are microorganisms that can cause infectious disease. Although all pathogens are capable of causing disease, not all microorganisms cause disease. Many microorganisms are necessary for human, animal, and plant life survival. In the absence of microorganisms, life would not be possible. The term **normal flora** is used to recognize the beneficial role of microorganisms in certain parts of the body, in which microorganisms normally occupy space and use nutrients, thus retarding the potential of pathogenic growth in that specific body area.

A fundamental concept in the study of infectious disease is that similar steps or phases occur in all infectious diseases; however, each specific microorganism causes unique characteristics and alterations in the process of infection. Medical assistants must apply the theoretical process of infectious disease growth and transmission to relate to specific pathogens. The goal is to reduce transmission and incidence of infectious diseases in patients, employees, and families.

Growth Requirements for Microorganisms

For microorganisms to survive and thrive, a suitable environment must be available to them. Following is a list of growth requirements for microorganisms:

- *Oxygen.* An **aerobic** microorganism needs oxygen to live; most pathogenic microorganisms need oxygen to survive: for example, *streptococcus* as in a "strep" throat.
- *Lack of or no oxygen.* An **anaerobic** microorganism needs little or no oxygen to live; two examples are tetanus and gas gangrene.
- *Moisture.* Microorganisms grow well in a moist environment; the body provides moisture.
- *Nutrition.* The body supplies plenty of nutrients.
- *Temperature.* The body's temperature of approximately 98.6°F is an optimum temperature for growth of microorganisms.
- *Darkness.* The body's cavities and organs provide darkness.
- *Time.* A single cell of bacteria can grow to approximately 150,000 cells within 6 hours.
- *Neutral or slightly alkaline pH.* The body's fluids are neutral when in a healthy state.

Through an understanding of the optimum requirements for microorganisms to grow and multiply, elimination of any or all of the factors helps keep microorganisms from growing and causing infection.

INFECTION CYCLE

For infectious diseases to spread, several necessary steps must occur. These steps, or stages, are known as the *infection cycle.* Each stage or step in the infectious process must occur for the spread of infection to take place. Infection control is based on the fact that the transmission of infectious diseases will be prevented when any of the levels in the cycle are broken or interrupted (see the "Breaking the Infection Cycle" Quick Reference Guide). The steps are:

1. Infectious agent
2. Reservoir
3. Portal of exit
4. Means of transmission
5. Portal of entry
6. Susceptible host

Infectious Agents

The cycle of infection begins with an organism that has the potential to cause illness. Infectious agents are microorganisms that can be grouped into six classifications: viruses, bacteria, fungi, **chlamydiae**, **protozoa**, and rickettsiae. Some sources include a seventh classification, helminths. For an infection to occur, an infectious agent or microorganism must be present. When infectious diseases are identified according to the specific disease-causing microorganism, the disease may be prevented with the use of anti-infective drugs or infection control practices. Each of these classifications of infectious microorganisms will be explored.

Viruses. Viruses are pathogens that require a living cell for reproduction and activity (Figure 21-1). These microorganisms are considered intracellular parasites, because they must live inside cells to multiply. They do so by altering particles of genetic material, such as DNA (deoxyribonucleic acid) or RNA (ribonucleic acid). Because viruses live inside cells, they are protected against agents such as chemical disinfectants and antibiotics. To survive, viruses have a notable characteristic of being able to change specific characteristics over time. For instance, viruses can adapt to their environment so they remain resistant to efforts to limit their growth. Viral infections have only a few pharmacologic treatment agents, and usually these agents are **palliative** because they only relieve symptoms of the disease instead of curing the infection. Some viral infections can be prevented by vaccination (Table 21-1). Figures 21-2A and B show the CDC's recommended adult immunization schedules.

It is particularly important for the professional medical assistant to understand the different types of hepatitis, the mode of transmission, vaccination recommendations, and symptoms in order to protect themselves and the patients under their care. The CDC Web site provides a wealth of information

BREAKING THE INFECTION CYCLE

The following graphic identifies the interventions that health care workers may use to break the chain of infection transmission.

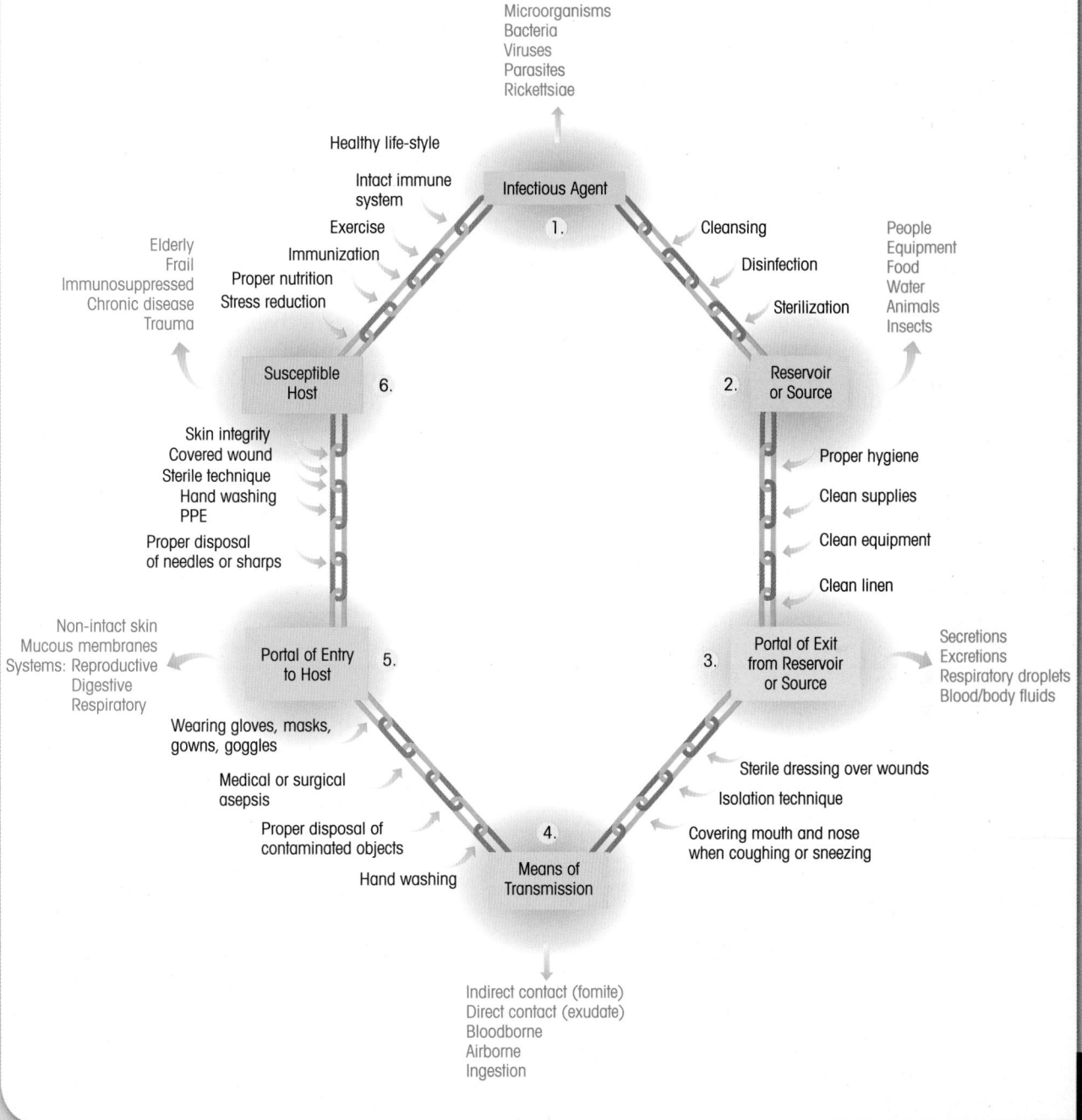

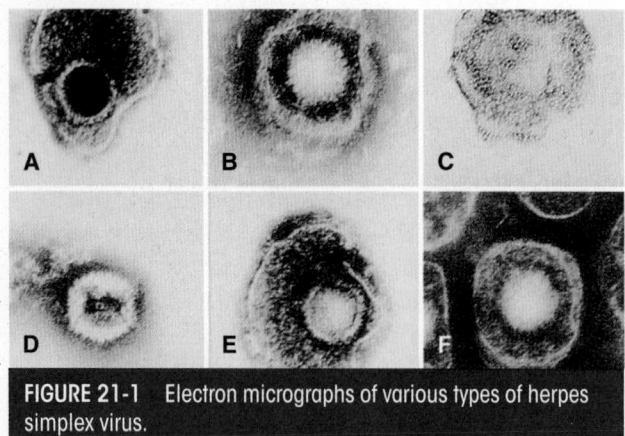

FIGURE 21-1 Electron micrographs of various types of herpes simplex virus.

about hepatitis A, B, and C. To access this information, go to www.cdc.gov and search for "The ABCs of hepatitis."

Bacteria. Bacteria are single-celled microorganisms that live in tissues rather than in body cells and are identified by characteristic shapes,

or morphology. Bacteria may also be grouped according to ability to accept laboratory staining agents. Gram-negative bacteria stain visibly red under the microscope, whereas gram-positive bacteria stain purple. Bacteria that do not accept stain are considered spores, which are bacteria with a covering that protects them from many chemical disinfectants and higher levels of heat. The three classifications of bacteria are **cocci** (sphere or dot shaped), **bacilli** (rod shaped), and spirilla (spiral shaped). Bacteria are either pathogenic or nonpathogenic. Nonpathogenic bacteria normally reside on the skin of humans and in mucous membrane areas of the body. These are known as *normal flora*. There are 10 times more bacterial cells in your body than human cells according to Carolyn Bohach, a microbiologist at the University of Idaho (UI). These nonpathogenic bacteria assist in digestion, immunity, and even brain function. Nonpathogenic bacteria use nutrients and occupy space, competing with the pathogenic bacteria. When nonpathogenic bacteria are reduced, the opportunity exists for pathogenic organisms to

TABLE 21-1

COMMON VIRAL DISEASES

DISEASE/AGENT	TYPE OF INFECTION AND SITE	VACCINE AVAILABILITY
Herpes groups		
Herpes simplex virus 1 (HSV-1) (Figure 21-1)	Cold sores/keratitis	No
Herpes simplex virus 2 (HSV-2) (Figure 21-1)	Genital herpes	No
Herpes zoster	Shingles (neurons)	Yes
Rubeola	Measles	Yes
Rubella	German measles	Yes
Poliovirus	Poliomyelitis	Yes
Influenza (ABC)	Flu, pneumonia	Yes
Human papillomavirus	Genital warts, cervical cancer	Yes
Hepatitis (A, B, C, D, E)	Liver	A, B only
Epstein-Barr	Infectious mononucleosis	No
Varicella zoster	Chickenpox (skin)	Yes
Respiratory syncytial virus	Respiratory system	No

Recommended Adult Immunization Schedule—United States - 2016

Note: These recommendations must be read with the footnotes that follow containing number of doses, intervals between doses, and other important information.

Figure 1. Recommended immunization schedule for adults aged 19 years or older, by vaccine and age group[1]

VACCINE ▼ / AGE GROUP ▶	19-21 years	22-26 years	27-49 years	50-59 years	60-64 years	≥ 65 years
Influenza*[,2]	1 dose annually					
Tetanus, diphtheria, pertussis (Td/Tdap)*[,3]	Substitute Tdap for Td once, then Td booster every 10 yrs					
Varicella*[4]	2 doses					
Human papillomavirus (HPV) Female*[,5]	3 doses	3 doses				
Human papillomavirus (HPV) Male*[,5]	3 doses	3 doses				
Zoster[6]					1 dose	1 dose
Measles, mumps, rubella (MMR)*[,7]	1 or 2 doses depending on indication					
Pneumococcal 13-valent conjugate (PCV13)*[,8]	1 or 2 doses depending on indication					1 dose
Pneumococcal 23-valent polysaccharide (PPSV23)[8]	1 or 2 doses depending on indication					1 dose
Hepatitis A*[,9]	2 or 3 doses depending on vaccine					
Hepatitis B*[,10]	3 doses					
Meningococcal 4-valent conjugate (MenACWY) or polysaccharide (MPSV4)*[,11]	1 or more doses depending on indication					
Meningococcal B (MenB)[11]	2 or 3 doses depending on vaccine					
Haemophilus influenzae type b (Hib)*[,12]	1 or 3 doses depending on indication					

*Covered by the Vaccine Injury Compensation Program

- Recommended for all persons who meet the age requirement, lack documentation of vaccination, or lack evidence of past infection; zoster vaccine is recommended regardless of past episode of zoster
- Recommended for persons with a risk factor (medical, occupational, lifestyle, or other indication)
- No recommendation

Report all clinically significant postvaccination reactions to the Vaccine Adverse Event Reporting System (VAERS). Reporting forms and instructions on filing a VAERS report are available at www.vaers.hhs.gov or by telephone, 800-822-7967.

Information on how to file a Vaccine Injury Compensation Program claim is available at www.hrsa.gov/vaccinecompensation or by telephone, 800-338-2382. To file a claim for vaccine injury, contact the U.S. Court of Federal Claims, 717 Madison Place, N.W., Washington, D.C. 20005; telephone, 202-357-6400.

Additional information about the vaccines in this schedule, extent of available data, and contraindications for vaccination is also available at www.cdc.gov/vaccines or from the CDC-INFO Contact Center at 800-CDC-INFO (800-232-4636) in English and Spanish, 8:00 a.m. - 8:00 p.m. Eastern Time, Monday - Friday, excluding holidays.

Use of trade names and commercial sources is for identification only and does not imply endorsement by the U.S. Department of Health and Human Services.

The recommendations in this schedule were approved by the Centers for Disease Control and Prevention's (CDC) Advisory Committee on Immunization Practices (ACIP), the American Academy of Family Physicians (AAFP), the America College of Physicians (ACP), the American College of Obstetricians and Gynecologists (ACOG) and the American College of Nurse-Midwives (ACNM).

FIGURE 21-2A Recommended adult immunization schedule, by vaccine and age group.

Figure 2. Vaccines that might be indicated for adults aged 19 years or older based on medical and other indications[1]

VACCINE ▼ / INDICATION ▶	Pregnancy	Immuno-compromising conditions (excluding HIV infection) [4,6,7,8,13]	HIV infection CD4+ count (cells/µL) [4,6,7,8,13] <200	HIV infection CD4+ count (cells/µL) [4,6,7,8,13] ≥200	Men who have sex with men (MSM)	Kidney failure, end-stage renal disease, on hemodialysis	Heart disease, chronic lung disease, chronic alcoholism	Asplenia and persistent complement component deficiencies [8,11,12]	Chronic liver disease	Diabetes	Healthcare personnel
Influenza*[2]	1 dose annually										
Tetanus, diphtheria, pertussis (Td/Tdap)*[3]	1 dose Tdap each pregnancy	Substitute Tdap for Td once, then Td booster every 10 yrs									
Varicella*[4]	Contraindicated	Contraindicated	Contraindicated	2 doses							
Human papillomavirus (HPV) Female*[5]		3 doses through age 26 yrs	3 doses through age 26 yrs		3 doses through age 26 yrs						
Human papillomavirus (HPV) Male*[5]		3 doses through age 26 yrs	3 doses through age 26 yrs		3 doses through age 21 yrs						
Zoster[6]	Contraindicated	Contraindicated	Contraindicated		1 dose						
Measles, mumps, rubella (MMR)*[7]	Contraindicated	Contraindicated	Contraindicated		1 or 2 doses depending on indication						
Pneumococcal 13-valent conjugate (PCV13)*[8]						1 dose					
Pneumococcal polysaccharide (PPSV23)[8]					1, 2, or 3 doses depending on indication						
Hepatitis A*[9]					2 or 3 doses depending on vaccine						
Hepatitis B*[10]					3 doses						
Meningococcal 4-valent conjugate (MenACWY) or polysaccharide (MPSV4)*[11]					1 or more doses depending on indication						
Meningococcal B (MenB)[11]					2 or 3 doses depending on vaccine						
Haemophilus influenzae type b (Hib)*[12]		3 doses post-HSCT recipients only			1 dose						

*Covered by the Vaccine Injury Compensation Program

Legend:
- Recommended for all persons who meet the age requirement, lack documentation of vaccination, or lack evidence of past infection; zoster vaccine is recommended regardless of past episode of zoster
- Recommended for persons with a risk factor (medical, occupational, lifestyle, or other indication)
- No recommendation
- Contraindicated

These schedules indicate the recommended age groups and medical indications for which administration of currently licensed vaccines is commonly recommended for adults aged ≥19 years, as of February 2016. For all vaccines being recommended on the Adult Immunization Schedule: a vaccine series does not need to be restarted, regardless of the time that has elapsed between doses. Licensed combination vaccines may be used whenever any components of the combination are indicated and when the vaccine's other components are not contraindicated. For detailed recommendations on all vaccines, including those used primarily for travelers or that are issued during the year, consult the manufacturers' package inserts and the complete statements from the Advisory Committee on Immunization Practices (www.cdc.gov/vaccines/hcp/acip-recs/index.html). Use of trade names and commercial sources is for identification only and does not imply endorsement by the U.S. Department of Health and Human Services.

U.S. Department of Health and Human Services
Centers for Disease Control and Prevention
CDC

FIGURE 21-2B Recommended adult immunization schedule, by vaccine and medical and other indications.

take over and cause infectious disease. A common cause of the reduction of nonpathogenic microorganisms is the use of antibiotic drugs. Examples of some bacterial infectious agents or pathogens are listed in Table 21-2 and shown in Figure 21-3.

Fungi. Fungi are microorganisms that may be unicellular (single cell) or multicellular (many cells). Mushrooms and molds are examples of fungi that are nonpathogenic. Pathogenic fungi cause athlete's foot, ringworm (Figure 21-4), and candida infections. Other pathogenic fungi include histoplasmosis and toxoplasmosis, which are fungal infections spread through the air from infected fowl and bird waste.

Protozoa. Protozoa are single-celled organisms whose name means "first animals" (Figure 21-5). They are found in every type of environment that exists on the earth from soil to the deepest part of the ocean. Some protozoa are a part of the normal flora in mammals, but there is a small number that cause disease in humans. Some examples are *Plasmodium*, the parasite that causes **malaria**; *Entamoeba histolytica*, which causes **amoebic dysentery**; and Trichomonas vaginalis, which causes **trichomoniasis**.

Chlamydiae. Chlamydiae are a unique group of bacteria that cannot exist outside of the host cell (**intracellular**). This type of bacteria is as small or smaller than many viruses. They survive outside the cell only in their infectious form. It is at this point in the life cycle that they are vulnerable to antibiotics. There are only three species of chlamydiae that can infect humans. *Chlamydia trachomatis* causes an eye disease, trachoma, and also infects the reproductive tract as a sexually transmitted disease. *Chlamydia pneumonia* causes a form of pneumonia. The third species is *Chlamydia psittaci*, which causes psittacosis, also known as parrot fever.

TABLE 21-2

EXAMPLES OF INFECTIOUS BACTERIAL DISEASES

DISEASE	INFECTIOUS AGENT	MODE OF TRANSMISSION
Anthrax	*Bacillus anthracis*	Inhalation
Chlamydia (sexually transmitted infection)	*Chlamydia trachomatis*	Sexual contact
Clostridial myonecrosis (gas gangrene)	Species of gram-positive clostridia	Wound entry
Escherichia coli	Gram-negative bacilli	Ingestion, wound entry
Gonorrhea (sexually transmitted disease)	*Neisseria gonorrhoeae*	Sexual contact
Legionnaire disease (pneumonia)	*Legionella pneumophila*	Inhalation
Nosocomial (hospital-acquired) infection	Gram-negative bacteria	Normal flora transmitted during illness/procedures; opportunistic pathogens transmitted during debilitated condition
Pneumococci	*Streptococcus pneumoniae*	Respiratory (inhalation)
Staphylococcal infection (abscesses, food poisoning, urinary tract infections)	*Staphylococci*	Direct contact, ingestion, inhalation, blood-borne, vectors (animals)
Streptococcal infection (strep throat, otitis media, pneumonia)	Hemolytic *streptococci* (usually beta-hemolytic group A)	Inhalation
Syphilis (sexually transmitted disease)	*Treponema pallidum*	Sexual contact
Tetanus (lockjaw)	*Clostridium tetani*	Wound entry
Typhoid fever (enteric fever)	*Salmonella typhi*	Fecal–oral

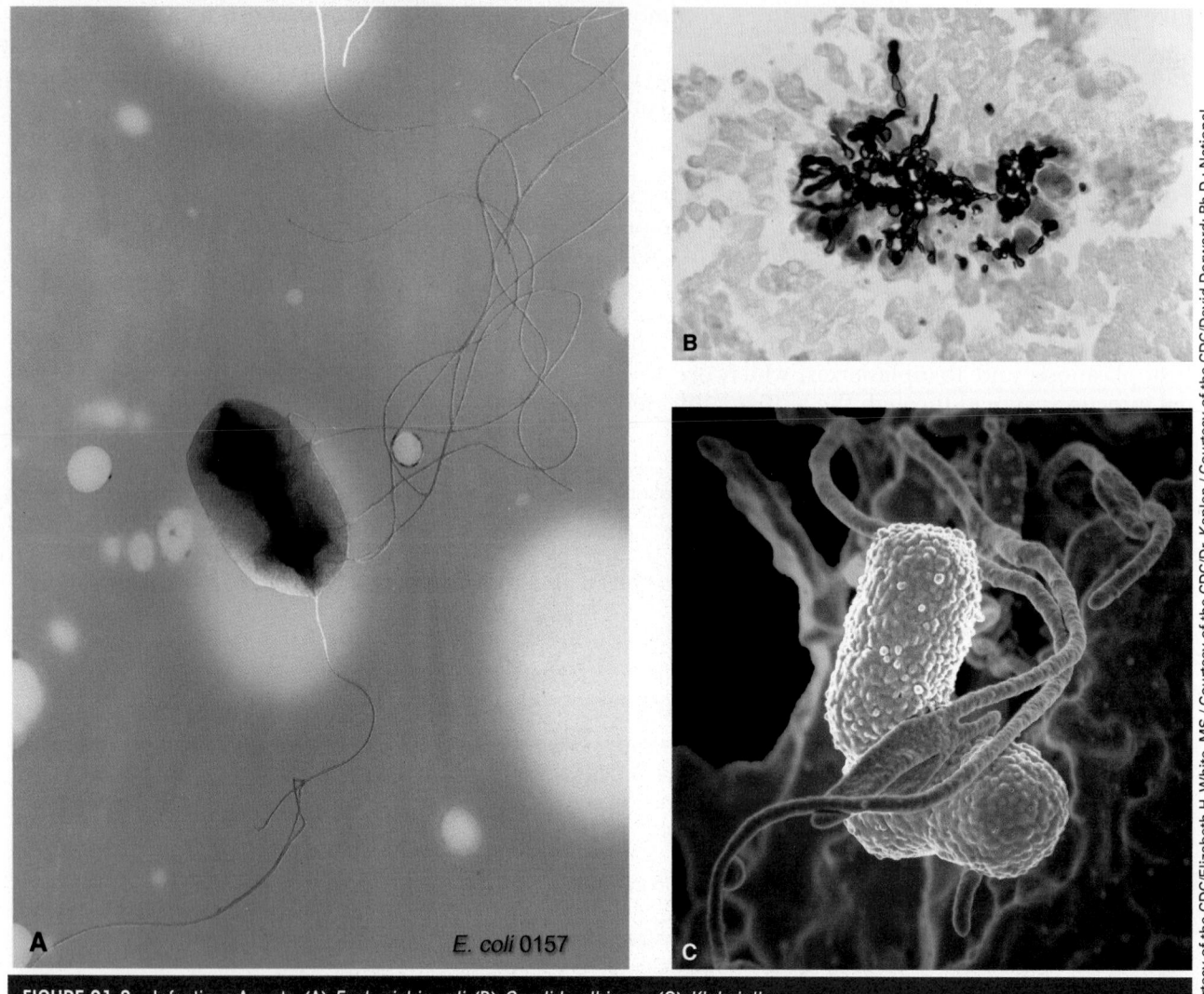

Courtesy of the CDC/Elizabeth H. White, MS / Courtesy of the CDC/Dr. Kaplan / Courtesy of the CDC/David Dorward; Ph.D.; National Institute of Allergy and Infectious Diseases (NIAID)

FIGURE 21-3 Infectious Agents. (A) *Escherichia coli.* (B) *Candida albicans.* (C) *Klebsiella.*

Rickettsiae. **Rickettsiae** are intracellular parasitic, small nonmotile bacteria. They are larger than viruses and can be seen under conventional microscopes after staining procedures. These microorganisms are susceptible to antibiotic therapy. Examples of rickettsial infections include typhus (transmitted by the body louse); Lyme disease (transmitted by ticks); and Rocky Mountain spotted fever (transmitted by ticks). Characteristic of rickettsial infections is a skin rash caused by the rickettsia invading the small blood vessels. This appears on the skin as a small hemorrhagic rash.

Prions. Prions are abnormal pathogenic agents. Unlike other infectious agents, prions are not living organisms. Prions are transmissible, but unlike bacteria or viruses, prions must be ingested. These agents exist as abnormally folded proteins that are found most abundantly in brain tissue. In humans, they result in diseases of the brain that are degenerative and fatal. Examples of such diseases are bovine spongiform encephalopathy (BSE), or mad cow disease, and Creutzfeldt-Jakob disease (CJD).

Helminths. **Helminths** is a category that consists of parasitic worms. There are subgroups within the category that include flat and round worms. Unlike other pathogens (viruses, bacteria, protozoa, and fungi), helminths do not multiply within their hosts. Worms grow, metamorphosize, mature, and then produce offspring that exit from the host to infect new hosts. Helminths grow more slowly than other types of infectious agents and may initially go unnoticed by the host. However, infection with some organisms in this group can result in serious illness and even death. A large percentage of the

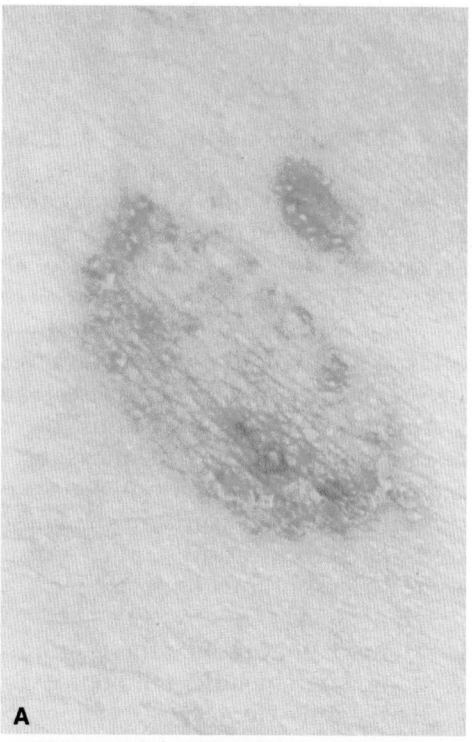

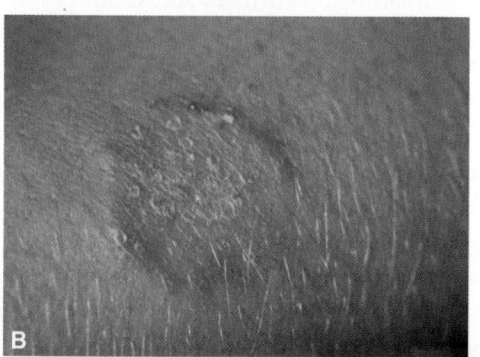

FIGURE 21-4 Ringworm can affect any area of the skin. (A) Back. (B) Arm.

Courtesy of the CDC/Dr. Lucille K. Georg / Courtesy of the CDC/Dr. Lucille K. Georg

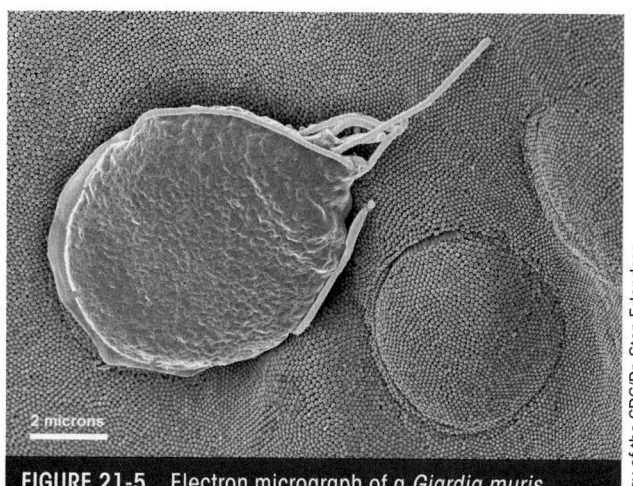

FIGURE 21-5 Electron micrograph of a *Giardia muris* protozoan adhering itself to an intestinal epithelial cell.

Courtesy of the CDC/Dr. Stan Erlandsen

world's population is infected with one or more of these soil-transmitted helminths. About 700 million people worldwide are infected with hookworm.

Reservoir

The second stage in the infection cycle is the reservoir or location of the infectious agent. The reservoir is the source of a pathogen. Reservoirs are people, equipment, supplies, water, food, and animals or insects (known as vectors). Methods of infection control in the reservoir stage include hand washing, environmental hygiene, disinfection, sterilization, and maintenance of employee health standards, such as annual tuberculosis skin testing and seasonal vaccines.

Portal of Exit

Although the infectious agent is housed or living in the reservoir, it must leave the reservoir in order to infect another person. The portal of exit is the method by which an infectious agent leaves the reservoir. Microorganisms may leave the human body with normally occurring body fluids, such as **excretions**, **secretions**, skin cells, respiratory droplets, blood, or any body fluid. The portal of exit may be continuous, such as with respiratory droplets, or dependent on the body fluid exiting the body under unusual circumstances, such as when blood leaves the body during a surgical procedure or phlebotomy. The portals of exit in humans are the respiratory, genitourinary, gastrointestinal, integumentary, and transplacental routes.

Safety

Standard Precautions and **Contact Precautions** are infection control methods based on the knowledge that infectious diseases exiting the body can be spread to others. These precautions attempt to control the spread of infectious diseases as infectious agents leave or exit the reservoir.

Modes of Transmission

The modes of transmission are specific ways in which microorganisms travel from one place (reservoir) to another (susceptible host). Transmission depends on the characteristics of the microorganisms. There are several modes of transmission.

Direct **contact transmission** occurs when there is physical contact between an infected person, or their body fluids, and a susceptible person that results in a transfer of microorganisms. This mode of transmission usually occurs between members of the same household or among close friends and family, as this type of transmission requires close contact with an infected individual. Examples of direct contact include:

- Touching an infected individual, especially touching body fluids
- Kissing, sexual contact, contact with oral secretions, or contact with body lesions

Indirect contact transmission occurs when there are microorganisms living on a surface that a susceptible person comes into contact with. Some organisms can survive for extended periods of time outside of a host. These are usually found on frequently touched surfaces such as doorknobs, tables, washroom surfaces, medical instruments, computer keyboards, clothing, uniforms, lab coats, and children's toys. These surfaces are referred to as **fomites**.

Droplet transmission delivers organisms via the air. Technically, droplet transmission is a form of contact transmission. Talking, coughing, and sneezing deliver microorganisms that can travel over a short distance. When these droplets come into contact with a susceptible host's eyes, nose, or mouth, the microorganism has found a route of entry. Droplets can also be generated during medical procedures such as nebulizer treatments, oral and endotracheal suctioning, or bronchoscopy.

Airborne transmission occurs when microorganisms are suspended in the air for long periods of time. Only organisms that can survive outside of the host for extended periods and are resistant to drying are a hazard for this mode of transmission. The upper and lower respiratory tracts are the portal of entry for this type of microorganism.

In the fecal–oral mode of transmission, pathogens enter the susceptible host by ingestion of contaminated food or water. These microorganisms multiply rapidly in the digestive tract and are shed in fecal material. To break this infection cycle, there must be adequate sanitation measures in place. An infected person working in the food industry is at risk for contaminating food that they come into contact with if basic sanitation guidelines are not followed stringently. Important measures include:

- Frequent hand washing, especially following washroom use
- Public awareness of the importance of hand washing and proper food handling
- Sanitation practices that include disinfection of frequently touched surfaces

- Following proper food storage techniques
- Cooking food to adequate internal temperatures

Vector transmission involves animals and insects that are capable of transmitting diseases. Well-known vectors include mice, ticks, fleas, rats, and dogs. Vectors allow diseases to be transmitted over a wide area due to the mobility of the animal or insect. The most common vector for disease worldwide is the mosquito. Typically, disease is spread by a bite from the vector; however, feces from the vector can spread certain diseases as well. Vectors can also transmit disease just by contacting food or a susceptible host's skin, as vectors can carry microorganisms on their outer surfaces.

Infection control measures in the ambulatory care area specifically address the transmission stage of the process of infection.

Safety

Methods that reduce the transmission of pathogens include adherence to Standard and Contact Precautions, hand washing, sanitization, disinfection, and sterilization. Methods of infection control are used in health care, food handling, water and sewage processing, humanitarian aid work, and child care.

Portal of Entry

Once an organism has found a useful mode of transmission, the next step in the infection cycle is to enter a susceptible host. Common entrance sites to the human body include nonintact skin, mucous membranes, and systems of the body exposed to the external environment, such as the respiratory, gastrointestinal, and reproductive systems. Breathing in airborne microorganisms allows infectious diseases to be spread to the lungs. Eating or drinking contaminated water is a cause of gastrointestinal infectious diseases. Sexually transmitted diseases spread through vaginal, oral, and anal intercourse. Care of patients with infectious diseases includes careful consideration of infection control to limit further spread of the microorganism. Methods such as correct wound care, Transmission-Based Precautions, and **aseptic** technique limit the transmission of infectious microorganisms. The portals of exit and entry need not be the same for infection to be transmitted.

Susceptible Host

The complex relationship between the potential host and the infective agent may or may not result in infection. The person who has come into contact with the microorganism may already have immunity or have the ability to resist colonization. Those without these abilities are considered a susceptible host and can develop a clinical disease. Some can become asymptomatically infected with the microorganism and become a carrier of the disease without ever actually being ill. Resistance to infection relies on several factors such as age, immune integrity, underlying disease, and situations such as surgery when the body's first line of defense is interrupted and the body is bombarded by microorganisms via various pathways of entry. The susceptibility of a person depends on several factors, including:

1. Number and specific type of pathogen
2. Duration of exposure to the pathogen
3. General physical condition
4. Psychological health status
5. Occupation or lifestyle environment
6. Presence of underlying diseases or conditions
7. Youth or advanced age (young and old at greater risk)

The goal of infection control at this stage in the infection cycle is to identify patients at risk for susceptibility, treat their underlying conditions if possible, and isolate them from those reservoirs that could be hazardous to the susceptible person.

Hospitalized patients are at risk for contracting a **nosocomial** infection, or health care–associated infections (HAI). These infections are caused by a wide variety of organisms. Some of these organisms are common viruses, bacteria, and fungi. Others are more resistant to intervention. In recent years, many strides have been made to limit the risk to those seeking health care. Strict adherence to infection prevention guidelines is the key to limiting patient risk. It is the responsibility of health care providers to maintain surveillance and gather information about HAIs. These data must be reported appropriately to various agencies on the local, state, and federal levels.

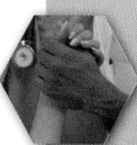

Patient Education

Drug-Resistant Bacteria

Antibiotic resistance occurs because bacteria can change their characteristics, thus reducing or eliminating the effectiveness of antibiotics. The resistant microorganisms survive, multiply, and cause a longer illness, necessitating more visits to the provider and more powerful and expensive antibiotics. Death can result from resistant bacteria. The number of antibiotic-resistant bacteria has increased significantly in the past 10 years. For example:

- MRSA (methicillin-resistant *Staphylococcus aureus*)
- Tuberculosis
- VRE (vancomycin-resistant *Enterococcus*)
- PRSP (penicillin-resistant *Streptococcus pneumonia*)
- XDR-TB (extensively drug-resistant TB)

These and other infectious diseases are becoming more resistant to standard antibiotic treatment. Drug options are increasingly limited, are expensive, or simply do not exist. An example of drug-resistant bacteria, mentioned above is the extensively drug-resistant tuberculosis (XDR-TB) bacteria. These bacteria are resistant to almost all antibiotics used to treat TB, including the two best first-line antibiotics, the second-line antibiotics, and at least one of three injectable antibiotics. Because XDR-TB is resistant to several antibiotics, providers are left with much less effective treatment options that frequently have worse treatment outcomes.

In order to prevent the development of other drug resistant pathogens, it is important to educate patients with the following key information:

- Antibiotics should be prescribed by a licensed provider and should be taken only when prescribed to treat a bacterial infection.
- Antibiotics should be taken exactly as directed for the entire course.
- Do not demand antibiotics from your provider. They do not cure a viral infection.

In your role as a patient advocate, it is your responsibility to assure that you are aware of infection control practices, use personal protective equipment appropriately, and observe Standard Precautions at all times. Infection prevention is the role of every health care provider. It protects those you care for, your peers, and you from exposure to pathogens. Remember that hand washing is the primary tool in prevention of infection!

Key recommendations from the CDC to control the risk of HAIs in the ambulatory care setting include:

- Developing and maintaining infection prevention programs
- Providing sufficient supplies to allow all staff to adhere to Standard Precautions
- Selecting a lead employee to maintain current training in infection prevention and appointing him or her to lead regular training sessions with other staff
- Ensuring that someone with current training is on staff during all clinic hours that include interaction with patients
- Developing a written policy and procedures that address infection control in your particular care setting and adhering to them rigorously

A number of different pathogens are present in the hospital and other health care settings, and as new patients arrive, new pathogens are introduced to the facility. Some health care staff become carriers of these microorganisms. The emergence of resistant bacteria is rapidly occurring worldwide. The crisis of antibiotic resistance has been attributed to the misuse and overuse of these medications. Pharmaceutical companies have not been aggressive in developing new medications due to reduced economic incentives and increasing regulatory requirements.

Since antibiotics were discovered by Alexander Fleming in 1928, antibiotic therapy has saved millions of lives. However, the overuse of antibiotics has led to the severe health care issue of antibiotic-resistant bacteria. Common antibiotic-resistant organisms that are found in the health care setting include methicillin-resistant *Staphylococcus aureus* (MRSA), vancomycin-resistant *enterococcus* (VRE), and extensively drug-resistant tuberculosis (XDR-TB). These organisms have become a major public health problem, and research demonstrates that they affect certain populations disproportionately. Those most vulnerable are

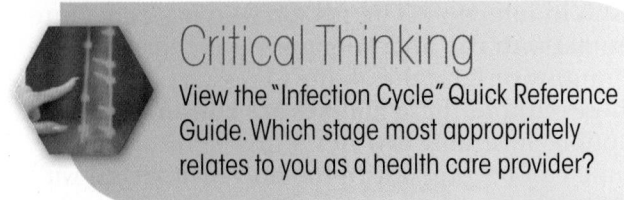

Critical Thinking

View the "Infection Cycle" Quick Reference Guide. Which stage most appropriately relates to you as a health care provider?

people receiving health care in an ambulatory or inpatient care setting. It is essential that health care providers do all that is in their power to break the infection cycle so as to protect those in their care.

THE BODY'S DEFENSE MECHANISMS FOR FIGHTING INFECTION AND DISEASE

The Body's Natural Barriers

The body has many natural barriers and defenses in place to help us avoid exposure to pathogens and infection. These barriers can be categorized under physical/mechanical, chemical, and cellular factors.

Physical barriers are the first line of defense. The skin and associated accessories, such as hair and nails, form an anatomical barrier from pathogens. Physical/mechanical factors include eyelashes and eyebrows, cilia (tiny hairs in the respiratory tract), and barriers such as eyelids and intact skin/mucous membranes. Mucous membranes are found in the lining of the mouth, nose, and eyelids, and they function to trap and fight invasion by microorganisms.

Chemical barriers include tears, sweat, mucus, saliva, gastrointestinal secretions, and vaginal secretions. Tears contain active enzymes that attack bacteria. Inhaled pathogens are trapped in the mucus secreted by the respiratory tract. This mucus contains enzymes that serve as antibiotics to protect the body from bacterial infection. Inside the gastrointestinal tract, there are various protective devices. The stomach contains strong acid that serves the dual purposes of digesting food and killing pathogens. Bile and pancreatic secretions also have anti-infective properties. The bladder is protected from infection by the mucous membrane lining of the urethra, and the normal acidic environment of the vagina protects from most infections.

Cellular barriers are also called body defenses and consist of white blood cells, which defend against infection in tissues in many ways; the bloodstream; and the lymphatic system. Cellular defenses are explained in more detail in the following two sections.

Inflammatory Response

Inflammation is the body's natural way of responding when invaded by a pathogen or physical trauma. Inflammation is a nonspecific response, meaning that it can occur with any threat to the body, not just in reaction to a particular pathogen. Inflammation can occur regardless of whether it is caused by an agent that is pathogenic, a trauma, a foreign body, or extremes in temperature. If a pathogen is present, the body goes through a distinct process in an attempt to destroy and eliminate the pathogenic microorganisms and their by-products and, if that is not possible, to restrict the amount of damage done.

The cardinal signs of inflammation are redness, heat, swelling, and pain. These symptoms may be slight, almost unnoticed, or quite evident. Remember, inflammation is a natural response and does not necessarily indicate infection. The two should not be confused. Inflammation can occur without infection, but infection does not occur without inflammation.

The steps in the inflammatory process are:

- Blood flow increases to the affected area and the vessels in this area become more permeable, allowing fluid and white blood cells to transfer in and out of the vessel.

- Plasma moves into the tissue causing swelling and pain due to pressure on nerve endings.

- White blood cells move into injured tissue to fight infection, and phagocytes destroy invading pathogens. This occurs within the first several hours after exposure to the pathogen. The bone marrow "turns on" and an increased number of specific white blood cells are released into the bloodstream.

After destruction of the pathogen, tissue repair can begin. If the **inflammatory response** is not effective, the specific immune response is necessary.

Indications that an inflammatory process is inadequate are: (1) the accumulation of purulent matter (pus) in the area (due to destroyed pathogens, white blood cells, and body cells); (2) lymph node enlargement (swollen glands); and (3) septicemia, which may result because pathogens have spread to the bloodstream.

Immediate antibiotic therapy is indicated in these circumstances because of the inadequacy of the inflammatory response.

The Immune System and Immunity

To fight infectious diseases, our bodies are equipped with several effective physical and chemical **barriers** such as the skin; mucous membranes; body excretions and secretions; and a complex, highly specific **immune system**. The immune system's purpose is to protect against pathogens and abnormal cell growth. The system is composed of various cells that collectively recognize, subdue, attack, and eliminate pathogens. The human immune system is very complicated and is comprised of numerous pathways that allow the body to defend against attacks.

The two types of immune responses include cell-mediated immunity and humoral immunity; they work interdependently inside the human body to nullify threats from the environment. **Cell-mediated immunity** is usually involved in attacks against viruses, fungi, organ transplants, or cancer cells. The process of cell-mediated immunity begins with the mobilization of various immune cells. Therefore, it is also termed cellular immunity. A group of "attack cells" is produced in the bone marrow and matured in the thymus gland. Known as T cells or T lymphocytes, these cells are members of the white blood cell family. These cells keep the body safe and secure from pathogens and foreign particles. T cells are the core of cell-mediated immunity, but there are innumerable and varied cell types that have specific assignments in the army that defends the body.

Humoral immunity is known as the antibody-mediated system because it deals with immune system structures called antibodies. This type of immunity is a result of the stimulation of B lymphocytes and plasma cells to produce antibodies. Antibodies are proteins that are produced by the immune system when the body detects harmful substances called antigens. Humoral immunity consists of two responses: primary and secondary. During primary immune response, an antigen is encountered by the susceptible host for the very first time. B cells are then activated and multiply. When this first exposure occurs, it may take a prolonged period of time for adequate numbers of cells to be produced. With a secondary exposure, there is already the "pattern" for response and the B cells can be produced much more quickly. Vaccination induces a primary immune response. This allows a more effective secondary response when a body is exposed to a known pathogen. This is known as passive immunity.

Generally, both types of immune responses occur in four phases:

1. *Recognition of the invader.* The immune system is equipped with cells that identify agents, pathogens, and abnormal cell growth as foreign substances. Macrophages and helper T cells recognize foreign invaders, whether they are pathogens, cancer cells, or transplanted tissues.

2. *Growth of defenses, which allows for multiplication of helper T cells and B cells.* After foreign substance recognition, the immune system alerts T and B cells to multiply and move to the site of the foreign substance. In cell-mediated immunity, activation of helper T cells means that the T cells are specifically oriented to a unique antigen, a substance such as bacteria the body recognizes as foreign. Activated T cells divide, forming memory T cells and killer T cells. In humoral immunity, activated B cells are antigen specific and divide into memory B cells and plasma cells.

3. *Attack against the infection.* Cell-mediated immunity uses killer T cells and macrophages to phagocytize, or engulf and destroy the pathogens. Humoral plasma cells have the ability to produce specific **antibodies** that lock on to specific antigens, which prevents the disease-producing characteristics of the pathogen from forming. These antibodies are called **immunoglobulins** and they render the pathogen unable to reproduce or continue growth.

4. *Slowdown of the immune response after death of the infectious agent.* After the death of the foreign substance, the immune response is halted. T and B cells return to normal levels, and in the case of humoral immunity, the presence of antibody production causes the immune system to resist the specific infectious pathogen in future contacts with the pathogen.

Susceptibility to some infectious diseases is closely linked to the person's unique resistance, or immunity. Immunity is the ability of the body to resist specific pathogens and their toxins. **Resistance** occurs after an exposure to a pathogen, which is the antigen–antibody reaction. These natural body defenses to fight infectious disease occur gradually and over time as pathogens and other foreign substances such as antigens enter the human body. When the antigen enters the body, the immune system recognizes the antigen as foreign and attempts to contain and subdue the foreign invader. Specific chemical antibodies to the antigen are produced by B cells, which attempt to prevent the antigen from further growth. After the completion of the stages of that infectious disease, the body retains the ability to produce antibodies in response to that specific microorganism or antigen. Therefore, immunity can last for some length of time, possibly to provide lifetime protection against specific infectious microorganisms. Several forms of immunity can occur in response to specific antigens:

- Naturally acquired active immunity results from contracting an infectious agent and experiencing either an acute or subclinical infectious disease. This immunity is usually permanent.
- Artificially acquired active immunity is achieved after administration of vaccines. This immunity is semipermanent to permanent.
- Naturally, congenitally acquired passive immunity occurs when antibodies pass to a fetus from the mother, providing short-term immunity for the newborn. This immunity is temporary.
- Artificially acquired passive immunity may be achieved through administration of ready-made antibodies, such as gamma globulin, used to treat or prevent infectious diseases. This immunity is temporary.

Our defenses against diseases can be categorized as specific and nonspecific. Specific defenses include those things that protect us against a specific pathogen, whereas nonspecific defenses are not so particular. Some examples of specific defenses are:

- *Vaccines/immunizations.* Designed for a specific pathogen
- *Antibodies.* Created against a specific pathogen
- *Active immunities.* Created against a specific pathogen
- *Globulin.* Antibodies for exposure to a specific pathogen

Some examples of nonspecific defenses are:

- *Tears.* Contain chemical harmful to a variety of pathogens
- *Skin.* Creates a barrier against many different pathogens
- *Saliva.* Contains chemicals harmful to a variety of pathogens
- *Species resistance.* Being human protects us from many diseases to which other animals are susceptible

Immunization. Immunizing individuals against specific infectious diseases provides immunity with active or passive vaccines. Vaccines have extended the life span of Americans by more than 30 years and reduced mortality from infectious disease significantly. Globally, vaccination saves 2 to 3 million lives per year. A child born in the United States has the opportunity to be immunized against 17 serious diseases and conditions according to the U.S. Department of Health and Human Services (HHS). HHS developed the 2010 National Vaccine Plan to provide guidelines for the U.S. vaccine and immunization schedule for the next 10 years. These are the overarching goals:

1. Develop new and improved vaccines
2. Enhance the vaccine safety system
3. Support communications to enhance informed vaccine decision making
4. Ensure a stable supply of, access to, and better use of recommended vaccines in the United States
5. Increase global prevention of death and disease through safe and effective vaccination

Several factors influence vaccination compliance rates, such as access to health care, cost of vaccinations, and irregularity or confusion in maintaining young children on the recommended schedule. There are pockets within large cities of significant numbers of underimmunized children. According to the Office of Minority Health, African Americans and Hispanics, across the age continuum, have a lower immunization rate than non-Hispanic whites. An outbreak could cause an **epidemic** of diseases that are preventable with vaccines (see Chapter 26). The Department of Health and Human Services has created a plan to address this issue. It is called the HHS Action Plan to Reduce Racial and Ethnic Health Disparities.

Legal

An antivaccination movement has influenced compliance with recommended immunization schedules since 1998 when a small study linked autism to vaccines, although there has been subsequent research that disputes those findings. Even though all states have immunization requirements for school admission, there is a significant number of parents and caregivers who are resisting the mandated childhood immunizations. These groups want state laws changed and feel that they, as parents and caregivers, should be allowed to decide if they want their children immunized.

Exemptions from mandated immunizations are allowed in all states if there are medical reasons. Some states will exempt children for religious reasons and some on philosophical grounds.

In general, children would more likely suffer greater complications associated with childhood diseases than from the immunizations given to prevent them. Because most of the vaccinations are administered in ambulatory health care settings, medical assistants may have the responsibility to administer, document, and monitor immunizations (see Chapter 26).

There are various classifications of vaccines, depending on the method of immune stimulation:

1. *Live attenuated (changed) pathogens.* These pathogens stimulate the body's own antibody production. However, the patient does not contract the infectious disease (or only a mild or subclinical case) because the pathogen has been altered in some mechanical or chemical means by the manufacturer. Examples of live attenuated pathogens include measles and varicella.

2. *Pathogenic toxins.* Some pathogens produce toxins (poisonous substances) that can stimulate antibody production. Examples of toxin vaccines include tetanus and diphtheria.

3. *Killed pathogens.* Inactivated pathogens stimulate antibody production; however, several vaccines may be required to provide sustained protection. Examples include pertussis, rabies, and poliomyelitis.

STAGES OF INFECTIOUS DISEASES

Depending on the specific pathogen causing an infectious disease, several stages occur from the time of exposure until full recovery and the absence of infection. These stages are often predictable and offer guidelines for patient education and treatment opportunities.

Incubation Stage

The incubation stage is the interval of time between exposure to a pathogenic microorganism and the first appearance of signs and symptoms of the disease. Some infectious diseases have short incubation stages, whereas other infections have lengthy stages, lasting for years. If an exposure to an infectious agent occurs, the patient will manifest (reveal in an obvious way) the disease if the patient's immune system cannot contain the agent. If therapeutic medications are available, it can help to prevent disease progression. Not all infectious agents are treatable or preventable.

Prodromal Stage

The prodromal stage is the initial stage of the disease. There may be signs and symptoms but full-blown illness is not present. It is characterized by common, general complaints of illness, such as **malaise** and fever. It is the interval between the earliest symptoms and the appearance of fever or rash that suggest an impending disease process is occurring.

Acute Stage

This stage is also known as the invasive phase or the period of illness. Disease processes reach their peak during the acute stage. Symptoms are fully developed and can often be differentiated from other specific symptoms. In this stage the host is experiencing full mobilization of the immune system. Treatment modalities are useful to reduce patient discomfort, to reduce possibilities of debilitation and adverse effects, and to promote healing and recovery.

The inflammatory process is the body's natural defensive reaction to the invasion by a foreign substance such as a pathogen, and it is in this acute state that the response is evident.

Acme

This is the peak stage of the disease symptoms. Resolution of the infection depends on the activity of the immune system, intervention by medical science, or the self-limiting aspect of the disease.

Declining Stage

Patient symptoms begin to subside or wane during the declining stage. The infectious disease remains, however, though the patient will demonstrate improving levels of health. It is often during the declining phase of an illness, when patients begin to feel better, that they prematurely discontinue taking the antibiotic that may have been prescribed. This premature discontinuance can result in microorganisms becoming resistant to antibiotics. It is important to educate patients in the proper use of antibiotics.

Convalescent Stage

Recovery and recuperation from the effects of a specific infectious disease are called the convalescent stage. The patient regains strength and stamina. The overall goal of this stage is returning the patient to as close as possible the original state of health.

Sequelae

If the body cannot fully repair the damage from the infectious disease, the pathological conditions that result are referred to as sequelae. Examples of sequelae of untreated strep throat include rheumatic fever, meningitis, and tonsillitis.

DISEASE TRANSMISSION

When providing patients with health care, medical assistants run the risk for **contracting**, or acquiring, an infection from pathogens that are causing patients' illnesses. Such pathogens are viruses, bacteria, fungi, and others that can be found in patients' blood and body fluids. In medical clinics, ambulatory care centers, and hospitals, many ill patients are seen every day. Pathogens can be easily transmitted to another person if care is not taken to prevent such an occurrence.

Consistent use and adherence to infection control measures significantly reduce the risk for disease transmission. The CDC recommends that health care providers consider each patient to be potentially infectious for AIDS, hepatitis B and C, and other bloodborne pathogens and that they routinely and conscientiously apply the techniques of Standard Precautions as a means of infection control.

Infectious diseases are caused by unique infectious agents, are characterized by various symptoms, are transmitted by differing means, and have unique treatments and prognoses. Medical assistants must recognize the unique characteristics of specific infectious diseases to prevent their transmission and help patients suffering from these infections. Table 21-3 classifies several common infectious diseases by critical components. When patients have contracted an infectious disease or are exposed to the risk for transmission, patient education plays an important role in infection control. Although a family member may have an infectious disease, proper training and education may protect other family members and close contacts.

Medical assistants are in a unique position of educating patients and the public about disease control. These measures become even more important with increased numbers of drug-resistant pathogens. All health care professionals must consistently and diligently use every infection control measure available, as well as teach our patients to do the same.

Initiative

TABLE 21-3

EXAMPLES OF INFECTIOUS DISEASES

DISEASE	AGENT	TRANSMISSION	SYMPTOMS	DIAGNOSIS	TREATMENT	COMMENTS	PATIENT EDUCATION
Acquired immuno-deficiency syndrome (AIDS)	Human immunode-ficiency virus (HIV)	• Bloodborne • Sexual contact • Intrauterine • Lactation	Opportunistic infections, **lymphade-nopathy**, fatigue, malaise, fever	CD4 T-cell level less than 200/mm³; Viral count Chest X-ray CBC	Palliative care and treatment for **opportunistic infections**, antiviral drugs	World Health Organization global statistics estimate that 39.9 million adults and children are living with HIV/AIDS (2014)	• Careful infection control and asepsis to reduce contact with pathogens that cause opportunistic infections. • Use of latex condoms in conjunction with effective spermicide. • Support groups/education.
Food-borne illnesses	Bacteria or viruses (i.e., staphylo-cocci, clostridium, botulinum, *E. coli,* shigella)	• Ingestion of contami-nated food or water	Nausea, stomach pain, vomiting, bloody diarrhea, dehydration, respiratory failure, death	Culture of feces, vomitus, or suspected food or water	Fluid balance restoration, medications, emergency treatment as required	Report outbreaks to local authorities; especially dangerous in children and older adults; undercooked meat as well as vegetables and fruits washed in dirty water can carry *E. coli.*	• Teach proper food handling. • Carefully wash hands before handling all food. • Report to provider all signs of dehydration. • Gastroenteritis usually communicable via feces for up to 7 weeks after exposure.
Impetigo	*Streptococcus*	• Direct contact with moist discharge from the lesions	Vesicles become pustular, rupture, and form crusts; **pruritus**	Culture of discharge	Antibiotics po or IV if severe; local antibiotic ointment	Good hygiene is necessary to help prevent transmission; gloves should be worn when cleaning lesions; expose lesions to air to help dry; can be fatal if not treated properly	• Good hygiene necessary to help prevent transmission. • Can be fatal to newborns if not treated promptly. • Wear gloves when direct contact with the patient or his or her environment is possible.
Influenza	Influenza viruses A, B, or C, *Haemophilus* (bacteria)	• Inhalation • Aerosolized • Mucous droplets	Acute upper/lower respiratory infection, severe cough, fever, malaise, sore throat, **coryza**	Tissue culture of nasal or pharyn-geal secretions	Palliative therapy, active immunization (annual vaccine recommended for persons at risk [older adults, heart patients] for complications from infection)	Report cases to local health authority; may be fatal in older adults and children; may cause meningitis; may easily become epidemic; 80% of elderly who contract the flu die	• Bed rest for 2-3 days after fever declines. • Force fluids. • Report signs of secondary infections (pneumonia, otitis media). • Vaccine available. • Practice cough etiquette.

continues

Table 21-3 continued

DISEASE	AGENT	TRANSMISSION	SYMPTOMS	DIAGNOSIS	TREATMENT	COMMENTS	PATIENT EDUCATION
Lyme disease	Bacteria (*Borrelia burgdorferi*)	• Transmitted by the bite of infected tick	Rash, flu-like symptoms, headache, fatigue, joint pain	Presence of symptoms; laboratory tests may be inconclusive, taking 6 weeks or more for antibodies to appear in the blood; erythrocyte sedimentation rate; total serum; Ig M level; aspartate aminotransferase level	Antibiotics, po or IV	The tick is so small and bite so mild, patients may not realize they were bitten for a few days to weeks later; bacteria spread to other sites, causing symptoms to heart, joints, and nervous system; arthritis develops and may become chronic	• Use insect repellant. • Remove tick promptly (save for laboratory testing if possible). • Wear pants tucked into socks when in wooded areas or where ticks are present. • Complete recovery usually occurs if treated with antibiotics. • Disease has exacerbations and remissions.
Meningitis	Bacteria* (more severe; *Neisseria meningitidis* is one type) Virus	• Bacterial through exchange of respiratory and throat secretions (coughing, sneezing, shared drinking glasses, bottles, cans, cigarettes)	High fever, severe headache, stiff neck, nausea, rash, vomiting, confusion, sleepiness, seizures	Culture and sensitivity of cerebrospinal fluid	Appropriate antibiotics; vaccine available for the bacteria responsible for 75% of the disease (vaccine lasts 3 to 5 years)	Rare but potentially fatal disease; there are two forms of meningitis: 1. inflammation of brain and spinal cord and 2. meningococcemia (infection in the blood); bacterial meningitis is contagious but not spread by casual contact or by breathing the air where an infected person is present; leading cause of meningitis in older children and young adults; cases have doubled since 1991	1. Meningitis usually peaks in late winter and early spring and can be mistaken for the flu. 2. High-risk persons are college students living in dorms, immunosuppressed individuals, and persons traveling to areas of world where meningitis is prevalent (these people should get vaccine). 3. The CDC can advise travelers about areas for which they recommend the vaccine be given.

continues

Table 21-3 continued

DISEASE	AGENT	TRANSMISSION	SYMPTOMS	DIAGNOSIS	TREATMENT	COMMENTS	PATIENT EDUCATION
Methicillin-resistant *Staphylococcus aureus* infections** (MRSA skin infections)	Bacteria (*Staphylococcus aureus*—"staph") commonly found on skin and in nose of healthy persons	• Direct skin-to-skin contact (for example, shaking hands, wrestling, other direct skin contact) • Shared towels or shared athletic equipment • Bacteria gain entrance to the body through any break in the skin	Pus-filled boils, pimples, and rashes; same symptoms as other "staph" infections	Culture and sensitivity of discharge from infected site; blood and other body fluids can be tested by culture and sensitivity	Good wound and skin care; keep area clean and dry; wear gloves and wash hands after caring for site; antibiotics, but MRSA is resistant to many common antibiotics	In the past, MRSA was primarily seen in hospitalized patients; now, MRSA is seen in healthy younger people; these infections commonly are not acquired in a hospital but rather in the community; children in day care, athletes, prisoners, IV drug users, and men who have sex with men are at higher risk; can cause surgical wound infections, septicemia, pneumonia; use Standard Precautions	1. Regular hand washing helps prevent acquiring and spreading staph, including MRSA. 2. Keep open sores and breaks in the skin covered until healed. 3. Avoid contact with other person's wounds or dressings. Avoid sharing towels, toothbrushes, washcloths, razors. 4. Keep skin healthy to help avoid staph on skin surface from causing an infection in nonintact skin and tissues. 5. Take all doses of antibiotic prescribed and do not share it with another person.
Pertussis*	*Bordetella* pertussis (bacteria)	• Direct contact with discharge from respiratory mucous membrane	Primarily seen in the pediatric population; severe coughing, whooping, and vomiting; apnea, pneumonia, seizures	Presence of whooping-type cough; nasal pharyngeal culture PCR (polymer chain reaction) in patients younger than 11 years; serology in patients older than 11 years	DPT vaccine prevents disease; antibiotics may be given for secondary infection of pneumonia	High rate of morbidity and mortality in many countries; incidence in United States has increased steadily since the 1980s; in the United States, epidemics occur every 3 to 5 years; increase seen in adolescents and adults	1. Highly contagious. 2. Adolescents and adults become susceptible when immunity wanes. 3. Practice cough hygiene.****

continues

Table 21-3 continued

DISEASE	AGENT	TRANSMISSION	SYMPTOMS	DIAGNOSIS	TREATMENT	COMMENTS	PATIENT EDUCATION
Pneumonia	Bacteria,**** viruses, ***** fungi, protozoa, rickettsia, aspirations of chemicals and dust	• Cough, sneeze, droplets in air	Cough with sputum, chills, fever, chest pain, dyspnea, fatigue	Chest X-ray, blood culture, sputum culture, CBC	Antibiotics if bacterial, treatment of symptoms if viral, oxygen therapy, bed rest	Elderly, immunosuppressed, and patients with chronic illness are more susceptible; vaccine available; practice cough hygiene	1. Get vaccine. 2. Practice proper respiratory hygiene (cover nose and mouth when coughing or sneezing). 3. Use tissues to contain secretions and expectorations; dispose of used tissues in nearest waste receptacle. 4. If no tissues available, cover nose and mouth with bend of the elbow. 5. Practice proper hand hygiene.
Rubella (German measles)	Virus	• Spread by contact with infected person through coughing and sneezing	Rash, fever for 2 to 3 days, lymph node enlargement in head and neck	Rubella titer; presence of rubella antibodies in blood	None other than treatment of symptoms; pain and fever medications as needed; treat for shock; practice cough etiquette	Rubella vaccine can prevent disease; part of the MMR vaccine; birth defects if a pregnant woman acquires rubella (deafness, mental retardation, liver and spleen damage to fetus)	1. The following individuals should get the MMR vaccine: college students or any student beyond high school, people employed in a medical facility, people who travel internationally, people who are passengers on a cruise ship, and females of childbearing age. 2. Vaccine not given during pregnancy.

continues

Table 21-3 continued

DISEASE	AGENT	TRANSMISSION	SYMPTOMS	DIAGNOSIS	TREATMENT	COMMENTS	PATIENT EDUCATION
Toxic shock syndrome (TSS)	*Staphylococcus aureus, Streptococcus*	• Associated with use of tampons and intravaginal contraceptive devices • Can occur postoperationally with staphylococcal wound infections	Sudden onset of fever, chills, vomiting, muscle aches, and rash; progresses rapidly to hypotension and multisystem breakdown, shock, and death	Presence of symptoms, vaginal culture; CBC, blood culture	IV fluids and antibiotics; management of respiratory disease, renal impairment, gastrointestinal problems	CDS says TSS could be stopped if use of vaginal tampons ceases; menstruating women, women using barrier contraceptives, and persons with postoperative *Staphylococcus* infections are at risk	1. A woman who has had TSS is at risk for recurrence and should not use tampons at all. 2. Women should wash hands carefully before inserting a tampon. 3. Tampon should be changed every 6 to 8 hours.
Tuberculosis (TB)*	*Mycobacterium tuberculosis* bacillus	• Inhalation of contaminated airborne mucous droplets • Possibly ingestion	Productive cough, fatigue, fever, weight loss (behavioral changes, anorexia). night sweats	Sputum culture for *M. tuberculosis*, Mantoux skin test (PPD), chest X-ray, pleural needle biopsy	Antituberculosis agents, Airborne Transmission–based precautions until drug agents started	Increase in incidence of TB, especially among persons with AIDS and the homeless; may become drug resistant; health care professionals should have annual skin testing; report outbreaks	1. Encourage hand washing, proper sputum tissue disposal. 2. Promote compliance with medications. 3. Encourage close contacts to have skin tests. 4. Encourage a well-balanced diet. 5. Practice cough etiquette.
Vancomycin-resistant *Enterococcus* (VRE)**	Bacteria (enterococci) normally found in intestines and female genital tract	• Direct contact with blood, urine, feces • Indirect contact with contaminated surfaces and from health care worker's hands	VRE can cause infections seen as septicemia, neonatal, and urinary disorders, otitis media	Culture and sensitivity of stool, urine, and/or blood	Antibiotics other than vancomycin	Spread directly by contact with feces, urine, or blood; spread indirectly from hands of health care workers or on contaminated surfaces; Standard Precautions used when caring for patients	1. Wash hands thoroughly after using toilet and before touching food. 2. Wear gloves if handling body fluids containing VRE.

continues

Table 21-3 continued

DISEASE	AGENT	TRANSMISSION	SYMPTOMS	DIAGNOSIS	TREATMENT	COMMENTS	PATIENT EDUCATION
Varicella (chicken-pox)	Varicella-zoster virus	• Direct and indirect contact with respiratory droplets	Sudden-onset fever, malaise, maculopap-ularvesicular skin rash	Vesicular fluid tissue culture during first 3 days after eruption; serology: increased antibodies 2 weeks after rash; lesion appearance characteristic of varicella	Acyclovir helpful to reduce severity of disease; zoster immunoglobulin (ZIG) for high-risk persons only within 96 hours of exposure; palliative therapy	Vaccine (varicella virus vaccine live) available in United States for children older than 12 months	1. Communicable 1 to 2 days before rash until lesions crust. 2. Avoid scratching lesions to prevent secondary infection and scarring. 3. Benadryl and calamine lotion can be used for itch. 4. Acetaminophen can be used for fever. 5. Practice cough etiquette.
West Nile virus	Virus	• Infected mosquito	Central nervous system; fever, headache, coma, convulsions, paralysis; 80% of people infected show no signs or symptoms	West Nile virus IgM capture, PRNT (plague reduction neutralization test)	None—supportive only; if hospitalized, IV fluids, ventilator	Potentially serious illness; may have permanent neurologic effects	1. Use insect repellent with DEET. 2. Wear long sleeves and pants when outside, especially at dawn and dusk. 3. Get rid of mosquito breeding sites by emptying standing water in flower pots, buckets, and barrels. 4. Keep children's pools empty and on their sides when not in use. 5. A small number of cases are spread through blood transfusions, organ transplants, intrauterine, and breast feeding.

* Resurgent disease: Case rates of recent years have reversed and are now increasing.

** Emerging disease: Have become recognized in recent years.

*** Although meningitis can be bacterial or viral, the information in this table applies to bacterial meningitis because it is the more severe of the two.

**** Bacteria and viruses are the two main causes of pneumonia. Of the two, bacterial is more serious.

HUMAN IMMUNODEFICIENCY VIRUS AND HEPATITIS B AND C

A great deal of attention has been focused on the **human immunodeficiency virus (HIV)** that causes AIDS, and yet there remains no cure for the disease, although great advances have been made. With the focus on AIDS, other potentially life-threatening and fatal illnesses may seem less dangerous. In reality, hepatitis B and C are examples of other diseases that place health care providers at great risk for serious illness or death. Acute viral hepatitis deserves close attention.

HIV and AIDS

Acquired immunodeficiency syndrome (AIDS) is caused by the bloodborne virus HIV. The viral infection directly affects the immune response. HIV is responsible for T cell destruction; T cells are the white blood cells that provide immunity.

HIV is carried in semen, blood, and other body fluids, and the virus can penetrate mucous membranes. Once HIV is inside the body, the reduced number of helper T cells leaves the patient vulnerable to a wide range of infections and malignancies. The infections that the patient contracts can be devastating. When people are positive for HIV infection, their T-cell counts must be regularly and closely monitored, and they must live their lives with careful consideration toward preventing opportunistic infections. If their T-cell count decreases to less than 200, they are considered to have AIDS. There is no curative treatment of HIV infections, but antiviral drugs such as lamivudine, azidothymidine, zidovudine, stavudine, and others are used to slow cell processes and weaken cell protein, which is important in the virus's reproduction. Many people are living for many years with HIV and AIDS. See the "Facts about HIV and AIDS" Quick Reference Guide for more information.

Acute Viral Hepatitis Diseases

In any of the acute viral hepatitis diseases, the liver becomes inflamed, and hepatic cells can be destroyed. Healthy persons can regenerate cells, but older adult patients usually cannot. There are several types of viral hepatitis: hepatitis A (HAV), hepatitis B (HBV), hepatitis C (HCV), hepatitis D (HDV), hepatitis E (HEV), and others. HAV, HBV, and HCV are the more common viruses; HDV and HEV are less common (Table 21-4).

Despite the similarities among HIV, HBV, and HCV, the risk for contracting HBV and HCV is greater than for contracting HIV. (For more information on HBV prevention, go to www.osha.gov and search for "Hepatitis B vaccination.") Statistics provided by the CDC indicate that the risk of contracting HBV from a cut or needlestick exposure ranges from 6% to 30%. HCV carries a risk of infection from a single needlestick at 18%. The risk of contracting HIV from a cut or needlestick exposure is only 0.3%. The hepatitis B virus can survive outside the body for up to 7 days and still be capable of producing an infection. HIV does not survive outside the body for more than a few hours even in high concentrations.

Medical assistants and all other health care providers must understand the importance of protecting themselves from the viruses that cause AIDS, HBV, HCV, and other pathogenic microorganisms. Through strict adherence to safety precautions and routine infectious disease control measures such as those found in **medical asepsis**, the risk for contracting an infectious disease can be minimized.

There is no vaccine to prevent HCV and no treatment after an exposure to prevent infection. Neither immunoglobulin nor antiviral drugs are recommended as a preventative measure. Once infected, HCV is a chronic disease, and patients carry the virus for the remainder of their lives. The virus is spread through blood and body fluids, sharing needles, IV drug use, needlesticks or sharps exposure, or from mother to baby during delivery. HCV patients may be at risk for infection with HAV, HBV, and/or HIV. Patients with HCV should be vaccinated for HAV and HBV. Infection control practices (Standard Precautions) are necessary to prevent infection with HCV through blood and body fluids. Patients exposed to HCV should be tested for HCV antibodies and liver enzyme levels as soon as possible after exposure and again in 4 to 6 months. Medication known as **immunomodulators** (i.e., that have the ability to change immune responses) are used to treat some patients who have chronic HCV. Historically, two drugs were used to treat HCV, a long-acting type of interferon (pegylated interferon or Peg-IFN) and ribavirin. Medications have evolved to treat the six specific **genotypes** of the virus. The next evolution of treatment includes the use of drugs known as protease inhibitors for people with HCV genotype 1. These drugs interact with the virus and prevent it from reproducing. Sofosbuvir, a once-daily pill, was approved by the FDA in 2013 to treat HCV genotypes 1, 2, 3, and 4. Genotype-based treatment continues today with front-line medications

FACTS ABOUT HIV AND AIDS

SIGNS AND SYMPTOMS*

EARLY (weeks to months after exposure):

- Flu-like illness
- Swollen lymph nodes
- Persistent fevers

LATE (years after exposure):

- Night sweats
- Prolonged diarrhea
- Unexplained weight loss
- Purple bumps on skin or inside mouth and nose
- Chronic fatigue
- Swollen lymph nodes
- Recurrent respiratory infections

TRANSMISSION

HIV is spread by:

- Vaginal sex
- Oral sex
- Anal sex
- Sharing needles to inject drugs, body piercing or tattooing
- Contaminated blood products (rare)
- Infected mother to newborn

HIV *cannot* be spread by:

- Shaking hands
- A social kiss
- Cups
- Animals
- Hugging
- Swimming pools
- Toilet seats
- Food
- Insects
- Coughing Infected

COMPLICATIONS/CONSEQUENCES

GENERAL

- Currently no cure available; most people eventually die of the disease (most live about 10 years after infection)
- Spread to other sex partners and persons sharing needles

PREGNANCY

- HIV can be passed to unborn children from infected mother during pregnancy or childbirth
- Infected mother may infect infant through breast milk (rare)

PREVENTION

- Always use latex condoms during oral, vaginal, and anal sex. Latex condoms, when used consistently and correctly, are highly effective in preventing the transmission of HIV, the virus that causes AIDS.
- Use a latex barrier (dental dam or condom cut in half) on a vagina or anus for oral sex.
- Limit or avoid use of drugs and alcohol.
- Do not share drug needles, cotton, or cookers.
- Do not share needles for tattooing or body piercing.
- Limit the number of sex partners.
- Tests are available to detect antibodies for HIV through providers, STD clinics, and HIV counseling and testing sites.
- Notify sex and needle-sharing partners immediately if HIV infected.

TREATMENT

- No treatment or medication available to cure HIV/AIDS.
- Early diagnosis and treatment can prolong life for years.
- Medications and treatments available to keep immune system working.
- Antiviral drugs slow cell processes and weaken cell protein.
- Medications available to treat AIDS-related illnesses.
- Medications available for HIV-infected pregnant women to greatly reduce the chance of passing infection to newborn.
- Experimental drug trials are testing new medications.

*NOTE: These symptoms are not specific for HIV and may have other causes. Most persons with HIV have no symptoms at all for several years.

TABLE 21-4

HEPATITIS VIRUSES A TO C

	A	B	C
Causative Agents	• Hepatitis A virus (HAV) • Fecal–oral; person to person	• Hepatitis B virus (HBV) • Blood; sexual contact; perinatal; breast milk; drug use (sharing needles); tattooing and body piercing	• Hepatitis C virus (HCV) • Blood or body fluids; intravenous drug use; mother to fetus; tattoo and body piercing; needle exchange
Risk Groups	• Household/sexual contact with infected persons • International travelers • Men having sex with men • Drug users	• Injection drug users • Household/sexual contact with infected persons • Infants born to infected mothers • Health care workers • Multiple sex partners	• Recipients of blood transfusions or organ transplants before 1992 • People sharing needles • People exposed to blood and blood products • HBV- and HIV-infected persons
Incubation Period	• 15 to 50 days	• 45 to 160 days	• 14 to 180 days
Infectious Period	• Usually less than 2 months	• Before symptoms appear; lifetime if carrier	• Before symptoms appear; lifetime if carrier
Diagnostic Tests	• IgM anti-HAV	• HBsAg • HBeAg	• Anti-HCV • Serum ALT increased 10× • HCVRNA
Symptoms	• Flu-like • Jaundice • Dark yellow urine • Light-colored stools • Anorexia • Fatigue	• Flu-like • May have jaundice • Dark yellow urine • Light-colored stools • Malaise	• 80% have no symptoms • Flu-like • Jaundice • Anorexia
Prevention	• Hepatitis A vaccine (entire series) • Standard Precautions • Enteric precautions • Good personal hygiene, sanitization • Immunoglobulin (for short term)	• Hepatitis B vaccine (entire series) • Standard Precautions • Reduce risk behaviors • Good personal hygiene, sanitization • Immunoglobulin (for short term)	• Standard Precautions • Reduce risk behaviors • No vaccine
Treatment	• Immunoglobulin within 2 weeks of exposure	• Immunoglobulin (HBIg) • Alpha-interferon • Lamivudine	• Alpha-interferon • Ribavirin (Virazole)
Prognosis	• Rarely fatal • Not a carrier	• No cure • May become a carrier • Liver cancer may develop	• 85% or fewer have chronic infection • Chronic liver disease or cancer develop in 70%

ALT, alanine aminotransferase; HBeAg, hepatitis Be antigen; HBIg, hepatitis B immunoglobulin; HBsAg, hepatitis B surface antigen

released in 2015 that specifically treat genotype 3 (daclatasvir; brand name Daklinza) and genotype 4 (ombitasvir/paritaprevir/ritonavir; brand name Technivie). These great advances have increased cure rates, shortened treatment times, and introduced therapy that consists exclusively of oral medications.

REPORTING INFECTIOUS DISEASE

Procedure

Certain infectious diseases must be reported to the state and county health departments (see Procedure 21-1). The CDC requires that the information be reported to them from these local departments. This helps the CDC control the spread of infection. Each state health department has forms for reportable diseases. Each disease has an identification number from the health department, and together with the appropriate form, the information is sent to the state health department and then to the CDC. Table 21-5 lists some of the more common diseases that must be reported to the CDC's Notifiable Disease Surveillance System. Disease reports can be sent via computer to the appropriate agencies, which will reply with orders for tests and procedures as well as follow-up orders.

TABLE 21-5

PARTIAL LISTING OF DISEASES THAT MUST BE REPORTED TO THE CDC

AIDS	Poliomyelitis
Anthrax	Rabies (animal and human)
Botulism	Rheumatic fever
Cholera	Rocky Mountain spotted fever
Diphtheria	Rubella
Encephalitis	Salmonella
Giardiasis	Streptococcal toxic-shock syndrome
Gonorrhea	Streptococcus pneumonia
Hepatitis A, B, C	Syphilis
HIV	Tetanus
Legionellosis	Toxic shock syndrome
Lyme disease	Tuberculosis
Malaria	Typhoid fever
Measles	Varicella
Meningitis	Yellow fever
Pertussis	

PROCEDURE 21-1

Procedure

Report Confirmed or Suspected Disease, Microorganism, Infection or Condition to the Appropriate Agency

PURPOSE:

Reporting of cases of communicable disease is important in the evaluation and planning of disease control and prevention programs, to assure appropriate medical therapy, and in the detection of common-source outbreaks. (*Note:* This procedure will vary slightly depending on state laws.)

EQUIPMENT/SUPPLIES:

- List of reportable diseases
- Confirmed laboratory report or request of the provider for suspicion of reportable disease, infection, microorganism, or condition
- Reporting phone number, fax number, or Web site
- Case report form specific to reportable conditions

PROCEDURE STEPS:

1. Refer to your state's listing of reportable conditions. Refer to the policy and procedure manual in your clinic for the list or do an internet search for your state's Department of Public Health.

(continues)

2. Check the guidelines regarding the timeliness of reporting certain diseases, infections, or conditions. Some diagnoses require immediate reporting, some within seven days, within a month, or six months of diagnosis. This guideline relates to a single case of or a group of cases.

3. If the condition must be reported immediately, phone the report to the number listed.

4. If the condition must be reported within seven days, most states have a Web site through which an electronic notification form can be submitted. Or, a form can be downloaded, printed, completed, and mailed to the address listed on the site or noted in the policy and procedure manual. Alternately, the form may be completed and faxed to the number listed on the Web site or in the clinic's policy and procedure manual.

5. Record the report in the patient's record or in a disclosure log according to the guidelines set by your provider or by the clinic's policy and procedure. *Note:* This type of governmentally mandated disclosure is allowable under HIPAA guidelines.

DOCUMENTATION:

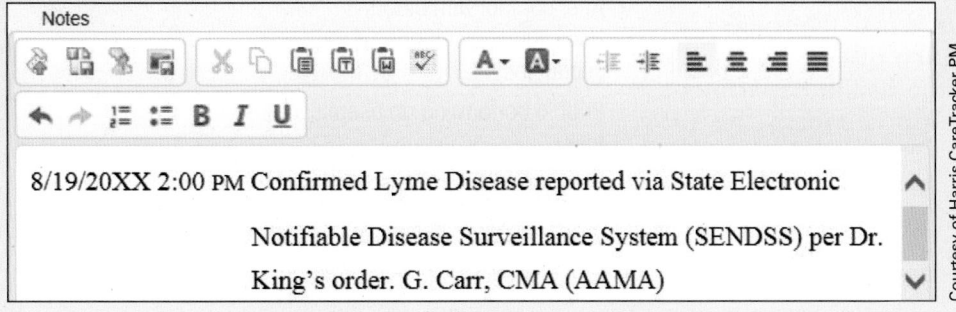

8/19/20XX 2:00 PM Confirmed Lyme Disease reported via State Electronic

Notifiable Disease Surveillance System (SENDSS) per Dr.

King's order. G. Carr, CMA (AAMA)

Courtesy of Harris CareTracker PM and EMR

STANDARD PRECAUTIONS

The CDC spent several years researching, improving, and developing recommendations to protect health care providers, patients, and their visitors from infectious diseases. This intensive period of research resulted in Standard Precautions, a set of infection control guidelines that are now used by all health care professionals for all patients. According to the CDC, Standard Precautions are "designed to reduce the risk of transmission of microorganisms from both recognized and unrecognized sources of infection in hospitals." They apply to:

1. Blood
2. All body fluids, secretions, and excretions regardless of whether they contain visible blood
3. Nonintact skin
4. Mucous membranes

To be effective, Standard Precautions must be practiced conscientiously at all times. Although Standard Precautions include many criteria specific to inpatient settings such as hospitals and skilled nursing facilities, they are absolutely applicable to any medical facility, including ambulatory care settings, where medical assistants are more likely to work.

See the "Standard Precautions" Quick Reference Guide for more information.

Latex Sensitivity

Health care providers should be aware that some people, including professionals and patients, can be allergic to latex products. Some personal protective equipment (PPE) is made from latex; medical and surgical products also are often made from this product.

The allergic reaction can be a localized one such as dermatitis or a more severe systemic reaction such as anaphylaxis (see Chapter 8), a form of shock marked by vascular collapse, respiratory failure, hypotension, arrhythmia, and laryngeal edema. Vinyl gloves can be worn in place of latex for hypersensitive individuals. Any person with an allergy to latex should wear a bracelet or other form of identification indicating this fact because, in any emergency, medical personnel wear latex gloves (see Chapter 8).

≫ STANDARD PRECAUTIONS

Category	Appropriate Use	Key Concepts	Methods
Hand Hygiene **Handwashing**	Before donning PPE After touching blood, body fluids, excretions, secretions, and contaminated items whether or not gloves are worn	Perform hand washing: • Before touching a patient even if gloves are to be worn • Immediately after gloves are removed • Before exiting the patient care area after having touched the patient or his or her immediate environment • After contact with blood, body fluids, excretions, or secretions • Prior to performing an aseptic task • Between tasks and procedures on the same patient to avoid cross-contamination between body sites	For directions on hand washing, see Procedure 21-5 For directions on applying alcohol-based hand sanitizer, see Procedure 21-6
Gloving **Gloves**	Apply clean nonsterile gloves that fit appropriately when contact with blood or potentially infectious materials, mucous membranes, nonintact skin, or potentially contaminated intact skin could occur	Remove gloves after contact with patient or his or her environment, using proper technique to prevent hand contamination Gloves must be changed between patients Never wash gloves for the purpose of reuse Don gloves last when using PPE	For directions on glove removal, see Procedure 21-2
Mouth, nose, and eye protection **Goggles & Mask**	Use PPE to protect mucous membranes of the eyes, nose, and mouth during procedures and patient care activities that are likely to spray or splash blood or body fluids, secretions, or excretions	Personal eyeglasses and contact lenses are *not* considered adequate eye protection Select mask, goggles, face shield, and combinations based on anticipated need for the activity to be performed If an N-95 or higher respiration is utilized, it must be fit-tested annually according to OSHA requirements	For directions on removal of face mask or respirator, see Procedure 21-3

(continues)

Category	Appropriate Use	Key Concepts	Methods
Gowning Gown	Wear a gown that is appropriate to the task based on anticipated exposure to contaminated materials	The gown is worn to protect skin and prevent soiling or contamination of clothing Do not wear the same gown for the care of more than one patient Remove gown and perform hand hygiene before leaving the patient environment Don gown first before other PPE components	For directions on gown removal, see Procedure 21-3
Handling of devices	If equipment is contaminated with blood, body fluids, excretions, or secretions, it must be handled in a manner that prevents exposure to skin, mucous membranes, contamination of clothing, and transfer of microorganisms to other patients or environments	Reusable equipment must not be returned to use for another patient until it has been cleaned and reprocessed Single-use devices must be properly discarded	Clean and disinfect all surfaces that are likely to be contaminated with pathogens Include surfaces that are close to the patient (e.g., exam table) Include frequently touched surfaces in the patient care area (e.g., doorknobs) Include other surfaces (e.g., waiting room furniture)
Handling of laundry	Handle, transport, and process linen to avoid contamination of air, surfaces, and persons		

Transmission-Based Precautions

When the CDC was in the process of developing new guidelines for isolation precautions in hospitals, the agency arrived at what it terms two tiers of precautions. The first tier is called Standard Precautions, discussed earlier, which was designed for all patients regardless of their diagnosis or presumed infection status. The second tier of precautions is intended for patients diagnosed with or suspected of having specific highly transmissible diseases. These are known as Transmission-Based Precautions.

Transmission-Based Precautions reduce the risk for airborne, droplet, and contact transmission of pathogens and are always to be used *in addition to* Standard Precautions.

Table 21-6 provides specific information on these three Transmission-Based Precautions. Remember that these precautions are for specific categories of patients and are to be used in addition to Standard Precautions, which are used for all patients.

TABLE 21-6

TRANSMISSION-BASED PRECAUTIONS

TYPE OF PRECAUTION	APPROPRIATE USE	KEY CONCEPTS	METHODS
Contact Precautions	Apply to patients with any of the following: • Signs of active infection such as diarrhea, rash, respiratory symptoms, draining wounds, or skin lesions • Presence of stool incontinence • Ostomy tubes • Drains for body fluids	Prioritize placement of patients in exam room if they have any of the symptoms listed Perform hand hygiene before touching the patient and applying gloves PPE use: • Don gloves when touching patient or items in his or her environment • Don a gown if substantial contact with the patient or his or her environment is anticipated • Perform hand hygiene after removal of PPE • Clean/disinfect exam room immediately after use • Instruct patients with known or suspected infectious diarrhea to use a designated bathroom and clean/disinfect the area prior to use by other individuals	*(NOTE:* Use soap and water if hands are visibly soiled with infectious material or after caring for a patient with infectious diarrhea)
Droplet Precautions	Use with known or suspected infection with pathogen that can be transmitted via droplet route; for example: • Respiratory viruses (influenza, parainfluenza, adenovirus, respiratory syncytial virus) • Bordella pertusis • For the first 24 hours of therapy: *Neisseria meningitides,* group A strep	Place the patient in an exam room with the door closed If an exam room is not available, provide a mask to the patient and place them as far away from waiting patients as possible PPE use: • Facemask should be donned upon entering patient's room • If substantial spraying of respiratory secretions is anticipated, gown, gloves, and goggles should be worn • Perform hand hygiene before touching the patient and after contact with respiratory secretions and contaminated objects • Clean/disinfect exam room and equipment after use	*(NOTE:* Use soap and water if hands are visibly soiled with infectious material)

continues

Table 21-6 continued

TYPE OF PRECAUTION	APPROPRIATE USE	KEY CONCEPTS	METHODS
Airborne Precautions	Apply to patients known or suspected to be infected with a pathogen that can be transmitted via the airborne route; for example: • Tuberculosis • Measles • Chickenpox • Herpes zoster	Have patients enter through a separate entrance to the facility (if available) Have patients avoid reception and registration area, if possible Place the patient immediately into an airborne infection isolation room (AIIR) If an AIIR is not available: • Provide a face mask to the patient and place in an exam room with the door closed • Instruct the patient that the face mask must remain in place while in the exam room • The face mask must be changed if it becomes wet • Initiate protocol to transfer patient to a health care facility that has the recommended infection control capacity to properly manage the patient • PPE use: • Wear a fit-tested N-95 or higher level disposable respiratory, if available, when caring for the patient • If substantial spraying of respiratory secretions is anticipated, don gown and gloves, and goggles or face shield • Perform hand hygiene after touching the patient or items in his or her environment • Instruct patient to wear mask when exiting the exam room and to avoid close contact with other people in the waiting area • Teach and enforce respiratory hygiene and cough etiquette • Once the patient exits, the exam room should remain vacant for at least one hour • If staff must enter the room prior to the elapsing of one hour, a respirator must be worn	(*NOTE:* The respiratory must be donned upon entry to the room and removed immediately after exiting the room) (*NOTE:* Use soap and water if hands are visibly soiled with infectious material)

continues

Table 21-6 continued

TYPE OF PRECAUTION	APPROPRIATE USE	KEY CONCEPTS	METHODS
Respiratory hygiene and cough etiquette	Applies to any person that is demonstrating signs and symptoms of a respiratory illness, including cough, congestion, rhinorrhea, or increased production of respiratory secretions	All persons with signs and symptoms of a respiratory infection will be instructed to: • Cover the mouth and nose with a tissue when coughing or sneezing • Dispose of tissue in the nearest waste receptacle • Perform hand hygiene after contact with respiratory secretions and contaminated objects/materials	If aware of risk prior to patient arrival: • Have patient arrive at a time when patient volume is low • Have patient enter and exit via a separate entrance from other patients • If the purpose of the visit is nonurgent, suggest a reschedule for after symptoms resolve • Instruct patient to don face mask upon entry • Place patient in exam room and close door as soon as possible If unaware of risk prior to arrival: • Provide face masks to all persons that are coughing and/or have symptoms of a respiratory infection • Place the patient in an exam room and close door as soon as possible • If room not available, instruct patient to sit as far away from other patients as possible • Family or friends that have accompanied a patient and are demonstrating signs and symptoms of a respiratory infection must be instructed to wait outside the facility

Blood and Body Fluids

In all infection control efforts, it is important to understand what is meant by blood and body fluids. Specifically, they are described as the blood, secretions, and excretions of a patient. Examples of blood and body fluids and some of the areas in which medical assistants may become exposed to them are:

Blood:

- Specimens drawn during venipuncture
- Open wounds or lesions of any kind
- Epistaxes, or nosebleeds
- Vaginal bleeding, including menses (menstruation), lochia (discharge after childbirth), and hemorrhage
- Feces and vomit or other body fluids with or without visible blood

Vaginal secretions:

- Physiologic leukorrhea (normal vaginal discharge)
- Vaginitis with discharge

Cerebrospinal fluid:

- Fluid aspirated, or withdrawn, during a lumbar puncture (spinal tap)
- Leakage of fluid due to trauma to the brain or spinal cord (through ear, nose)

Synovial fluid:

- Fluid aspirated during arthroscopic procedures

Pleural fluid:

- Fluid aspirated during thoracentesis, a surgical puncture of the thoracic cavity
- Fluid leakage caused by chest trauma

Pericardial fluid:

- Fluid around the heart exposed during cardiac surgery or caused by cardiac trauma

Peritoneal fluid:

- Fluid exposed during abdominal surgery (least likely fluid with which medical assistant will come into contact), but exposure can occur during a paracentesis

Semen:

- Seminal fluid as a laboratory specimen for sperm count in examination for fertility level

Amniotic fluid:

- Fluid aspirated during amniocentesis, a surgical puncture of the amniotic sac
- Vaginal leakage during pregnancy, labor, and delivery

Breast milk (possibility exists)

Sputum:

- Material coughed up and expectorated from the respiratory tract

Saliva:

- Oral mucous gland fluid in mouth during oral/dental procedures

Any other body fluid visibly contaminated with blood

Thus far, only blood and blood products, semen, vaginal secretions, and possibly breast milk have been directly linked to transmission of HIV; the virus is not spread casually or through close family contacts. There is not yet a vaccine to protect individuals from HIV.

HBV has been found in blood and blood products, vaginal secretions, semen, and saliva. Infection can spread through close family contacts, kissing, sexual contacts, intrauterinely, and during delivery. An infant may become a chronic **carrier**, one who has no symptoms but can transmit disease. If there has been exposure to the virus, a prompt injection of immunoglobulin, an antibody, will help provide protection from the virus. An HBV vaccine is available, and the series of three injections usually immunizes an individual from an attack of hepatitis B for approximately 18 years.

Some states require health care providers and allied health students to be immunized before employment and before admission into a health program in an educational institution. Also, many states require infants to be routinely immunized with the HBV vaccine.

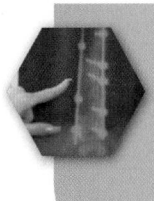

Critical Thinking

Give eight examples of body fluids considered to be biohazardous substances. Explain under what circumstances medical assistants could become exposed to blood and body fluids.

Personal Protective Equipment

Procedure

Standard and **Transmission-Based Precautions** all make use of barriers or personal protective equipment (PPE). The barriers consist of gloves, mask, gown, and goggles/face shield. Gloves reduce the risk for contamination to hands but do not prevent needles or other sharp instruments from penetrating the skin (Figure 21-6). For direction on how to apply and remove PPE, see Procedures 21-2 and 21-3.

Masks and protective eyewear reduce the contamination risk to mucous membranes of the eyes, nose, and mouth. Gowns protect clothing from contamination. Barriers or PPE are used in various combinations depending on the procedure or treatment being performed on patients. As a medical assistant, you may be exposed to infected blood and body fluids and must wear PPE.

Needlestick

One reason for exposure to blood is accidentally sticking oneself with a dirty (used) needle after performing invasive procedures such as injections, venipuncture, and attempted venipuncture. A needle should be considered contaminated if it has entered the skin of a patient, regardless of the reason. In the past, needlesticks were common because of the practice of needle recapping. Contaminated (used) needles should never be recapped, broken off, removed from syringes, or

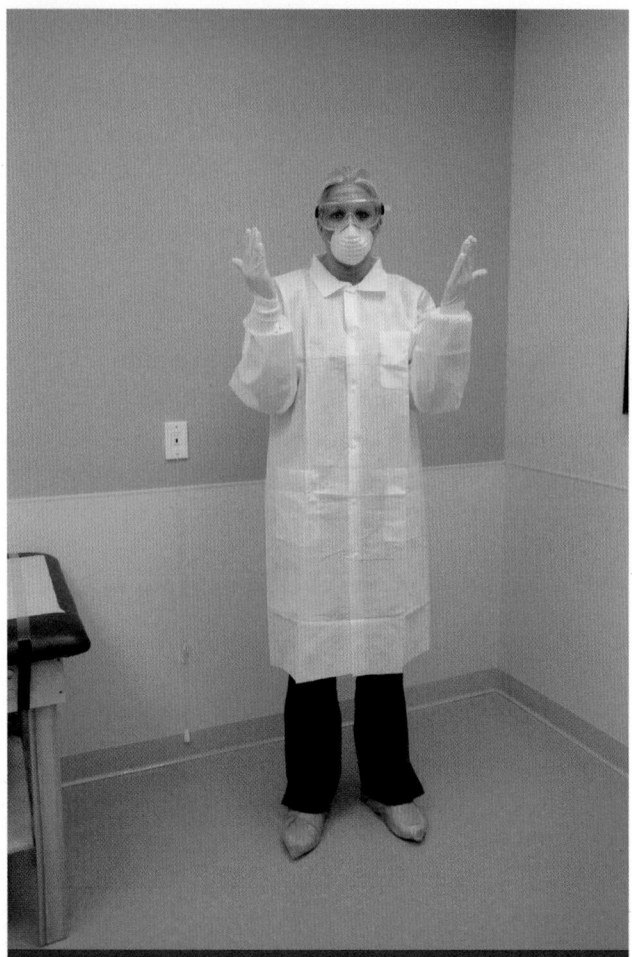

FIGURE 21-6 Medical assistant wearing personal protective equipment: goggles, mask, gown, latex gloves.

PROCEDURE 21-2

Procedure

Removing Contaminated Gloves

STANDARD PRECAUTIONS:

Handwashing   Gloves   Biohazard

PURPOSE:

To carefully remove and dispose of contaminated gloves to contain exposure.

EQUIPMENT/SUPPLIES:

- Biohazard waste container

(continues)

PROCEDURE STEPS:

1. Throughout this procedure, the hands should be held away from the body and the fingertips pointed downward.

2. If you are right hand dominant, remove the left glove first by carefully grasping the outside surface of the cuff with the right hand. If you're left hand dominant, reverse the procedure and begin by removing the right glove first (Figures 21-7A and B). RATIONALE: Holding the hands away from the body will further prevent exposure to biological contaminants.

3. Turn the used left glove inside out and hold it in the right gloved hand. Be careful not to touch your bare left hand on the contaminated right glove (Figures 21-7C through 21-7E). RATIONALE: Turning the glove inside out helps isolate the biological contaminants.

4. Continue to hold the removed left glove in the right hand while you insert two fingers of your left hand between your arm and the inside cuff of the right. Be careful not to touch any of the contaminated portions of the right glove (Figure 21-7F).

5. Turn the right, dirty glove inside out over the left. One glove is inside the other and you can handle the gloves because the dirty, contaminated area is inside the gloves (Figures 21-7G and H). RATIONALE: Both gloves are inverted with the biological contaminates isolated.

6. Dispose of the inverted gloves into a biological waste receptacle. RATIONALE: All biological waste should be placed into a red biohazard bag.

7. Wash hands thoroughly. RATIONALE: Immediate washing of hands is an additional precaution.

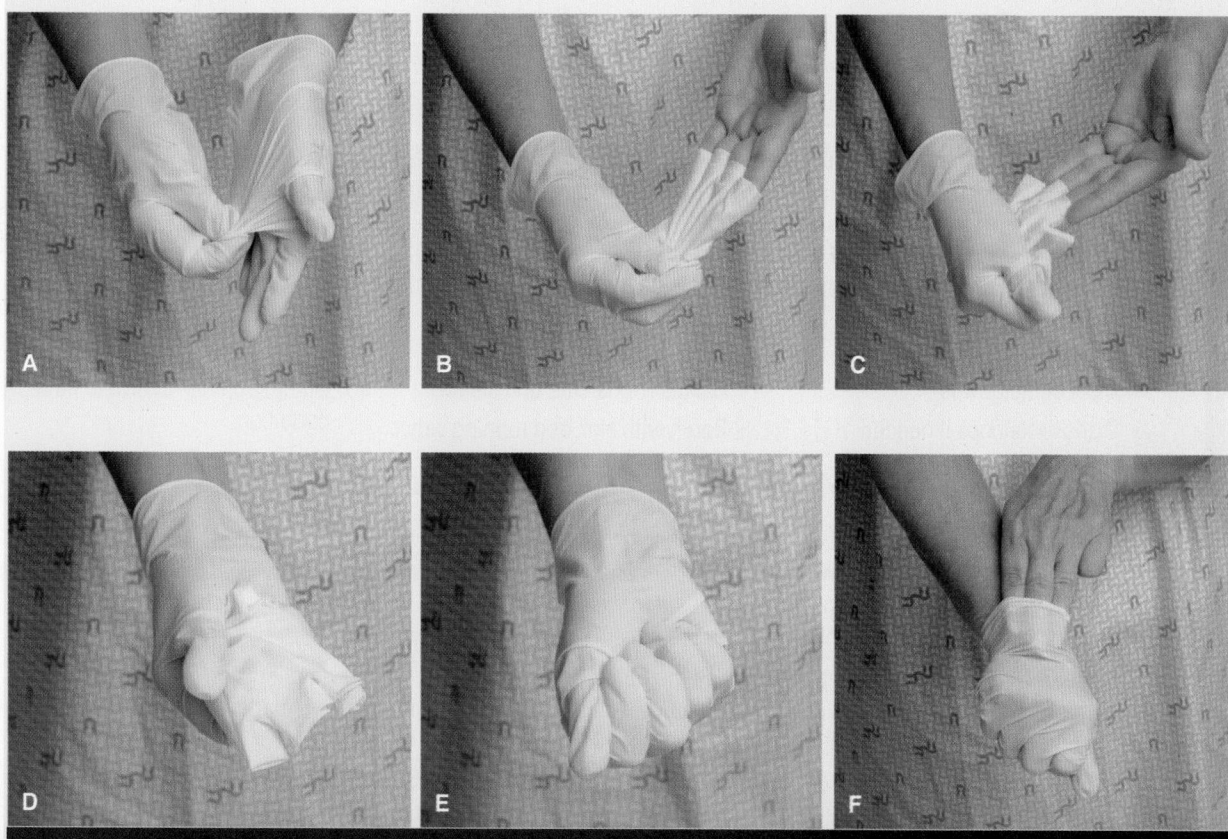

FIGURE 21-7 (A) Grasp the palm of the used glove with the right hand. (B) Begin removing the first glove. (C) Glove is turned inside out as it is being removed. Take care not to touch bare skin on the contaminated glove. (D) Inverted glove is completely removed into the contaminated glove. (E) Contain the inverted glove completely in the gloved hand. (F) Insert three fingers of the ungloved hand inside the back of the contaminated glove and turn it inside out over the other.

(continues)

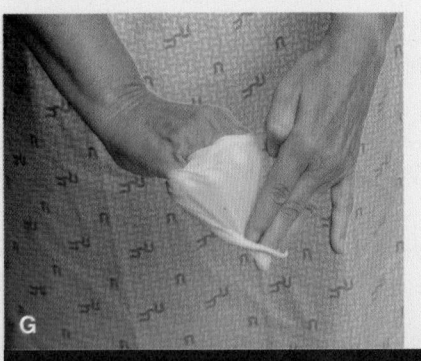
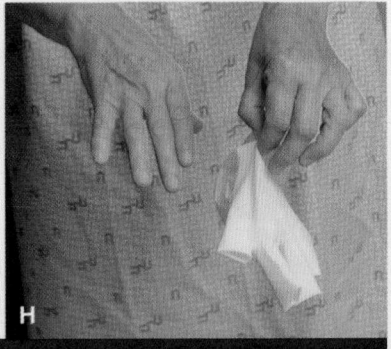

FIGURE 21-7 (G) Invert the second glove over the first. (H) One glove is now inside the other.

PROCEDURE 21-3

Donning and Proper Removal of Gown, Mask, Gloves, and Cap (Isolation Technique)

Procedure

STANDARD PRECAUTIONS:

Gown   Goggles & Mask

PURPOSE:

To provide barriers for medical assistant to be protected from airborne, contact, or droplet infectious diseases.

EQUIPMENT/SUPPLIES:

- Disposable gowns
- Disposable caps if needed
- Disposable masks
- Gloves (nonsterile and sterile)
- Room with sink and running water
- Paper towels
- Other supplies relative to patient's condition

PROCEDURE STEPS:

1. ***Paying attention to detail***, review provider orders and agency protocols relative to the type of isolation precautions. RATIONALE: Provides for patient comfort and decreases the spread of microorganisms. Limits the number of personnel coming into the patient's room and the patient's exposure to microorganisms.

2. Place appropriate isolation supplies outside the patient's room and note type of isolation sign on the door (e.g., airborne, droplet, or contact). RATIONALE: Ensures staff follows isolation protocol and alerts visitors to check with the nurses' station before entering the room.

3. Remove jewelry, laboratory coat, and other items not necessary in providing patient care. RATIONALE: Decreases the spread of microorganisms.

4. Wash hands and don disposable clothing:

   a. Begin with an impervious, disposable gown. Hold the gown in front of the body and place arms through the sleeves (Figure 21-8A). Tie the gown securely at the back of the neck and waist and pull the sleeves down securely to the wrists (Figures 21-8B and 21-8C). When applied appropriately, the gown should cover outer garments completely.

(continues)

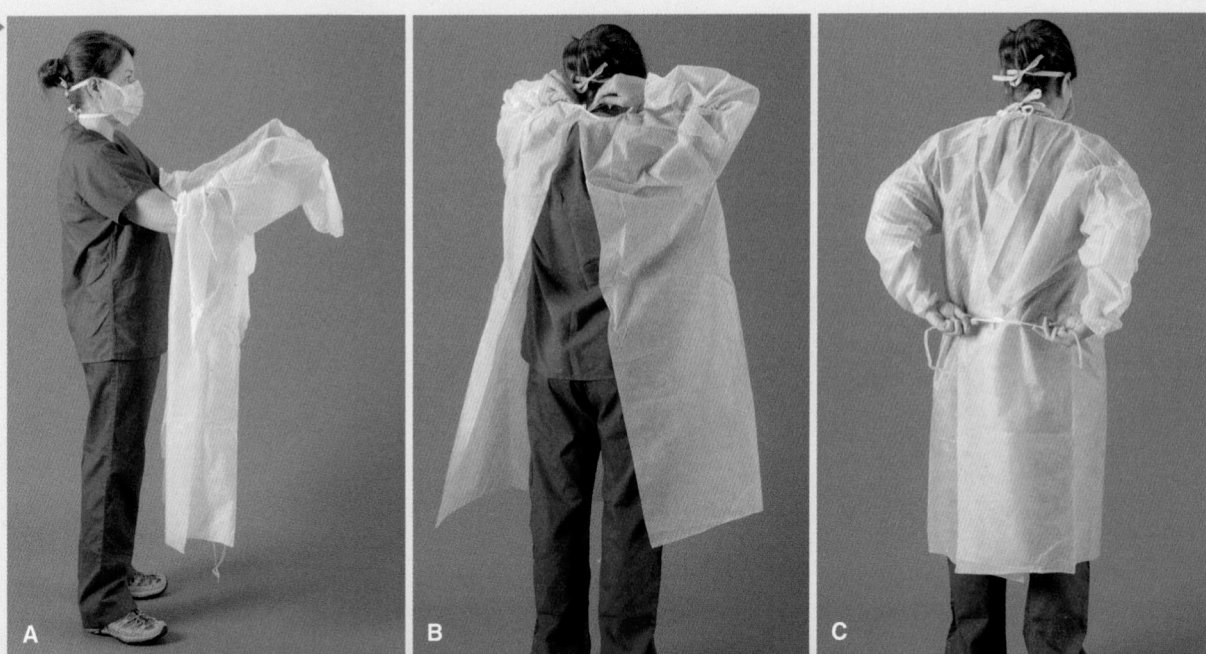

FIGURE 21-8 (A) Medical assistant has put on a mask and is donning the gown, pulling on the sleeves. (B) The neck of the gown is tied first and (C) the back of the gown, last.

   b. Apply cap and cover hair and ears completely.

   c. Apply a mask or respirator.

      i. Apply the mask to cover the mouth and nose completely. Adjust to ensure a snug fit.

      ii. To apply a respirator, stretch the elastic band and place the respiratory over the mouth and nose, covering completely. Release the elastic band over the back of the head and adjust for comfort and a secure seal around nose and mouth. Squeeze the metal band on the bridge of the nose to secure.

   d. If splashing is anticipated, apply goggles or utilize a face shield.

   e. Don nonsterile gloves and pull up and over the cuffs of the gown to create a seal.

   RATIONALE: Disposable garments act as a barrier in preventing the transmission of microorganisms from medical assistant to patient and protect the medical assistant from contact with pathogens.

5. Enter patient's room with all gathered supplies. RATIONALE: Prevents trips into and out of the patient's room and keeps supplies clean.

6. Once you leave the patient's room, remove and dispose of your contaminated gloves, following proper procedure.

7. Wash and dry your hands.

8. Remove your goggles or face shield by handling the earpieces. Place in a designated container to sanitize

9. Untie the neckties of the gown (Figure 21-9A).

10. Slip the fingers of your left hand inside the cuff of the right arm and pull the gown over your right hand, being particularly careful not to touch the outside of the gown (Figure 21-9B).

11. Using your covered right hand, pull the gown down over the left hand (Figure 21-9C). Then pull the gown down off your arms, holding the gown away from you as you do so (Figure 21-9D). Roll the gown into a ball, containing the contaminated side of the gown inside.

(continues)

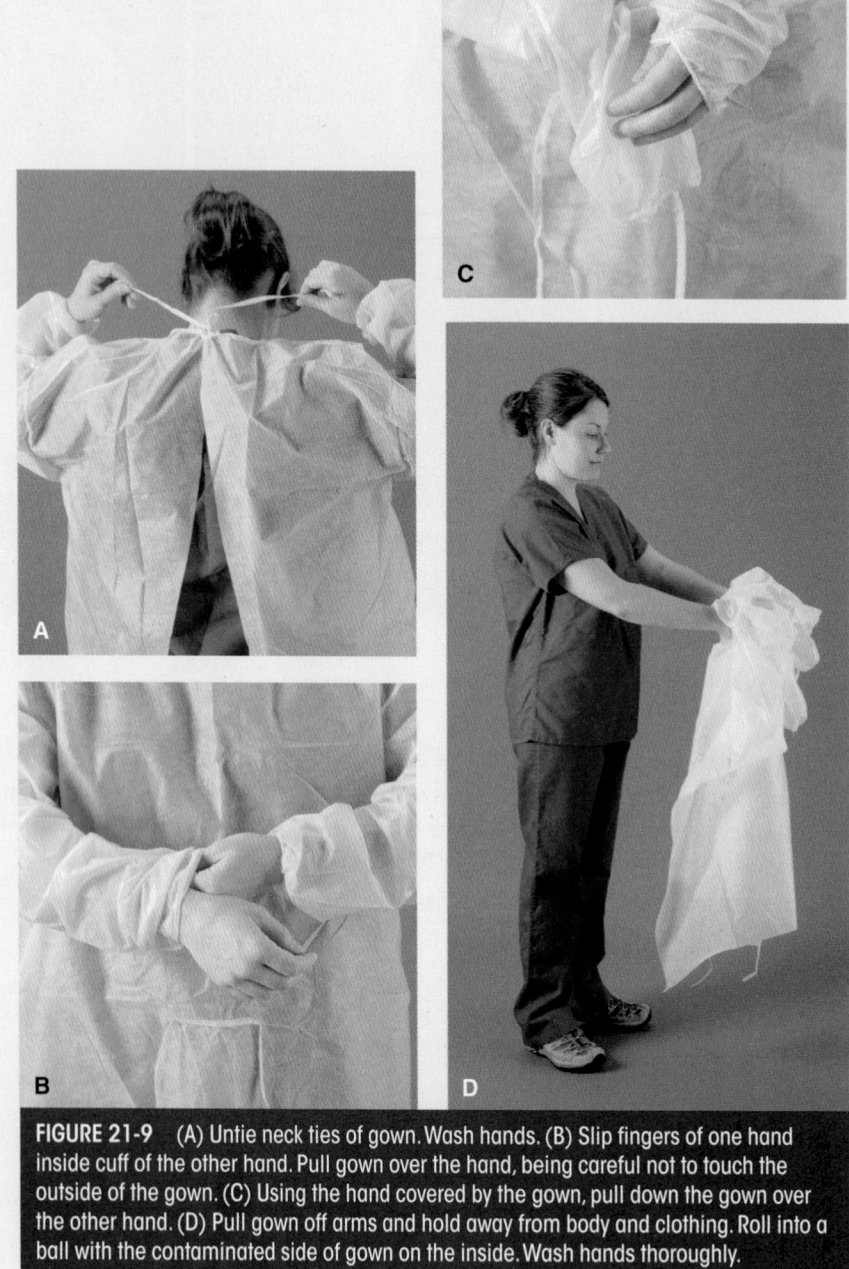

FIGURE 21-9 (A) Untie neck ties of gown. Wash hands. (B) Slip fingers of one hand inside cuff of the other hand. Pull gown over the hand, being careful not to touch the outside of the gown. (C) Using the hand covered by the gown, pull down the gown over the other hand. (D) Pull gown off arms and hold away from body and clothing. Roll into a ball with the contaminated side of gown on the inside. Wash hands thoroughly.

12. Remove the cap and discard. Remove the mask by pulling the elastic band up and away from the back of the head, touching only the elastic band.

13. Don another pair of gloves and disinfect any counter area that may have come in contact with items from the exam room.

14. Wash hands thoroughly before documenting patient care in the patient's medical record.

manipulated by hand in any way. They are disposed of in the approved puncture-proof container designated for **sharps** (Figure 21-10). The disposal container for sharps must be in the closest proximity as practical to the area where sharps are used. If a needle is used and an appropriate disposal container is not nearby ("point-of-use disposal"), the **one-handed technique** of recapping may be used (Figure 21-11), but only in this circumstance (i.e., no appropriate container nearby). Desirable characteristics of safety devices include:

- The device is needleless.
- The safety feature is built into the device.
- The device works passively (i.e., requires no activation by the user). If user activation is necessary, the safety feature can be engaged with a single-handed technique, allowing the worker's hands to remain behind the exposed sharp.
- The user can easily tell whether the safety feature has been activated. Some safety features have a sound, such as a click, indicating that the feature is engaged.
- The safety feature cannot be deactivated and remains protective through disposal.
- If the device uses needles, it performs reliably with all needle sizes.
- The device is easy to use and practical.
- The device is safe and effective in patient care.

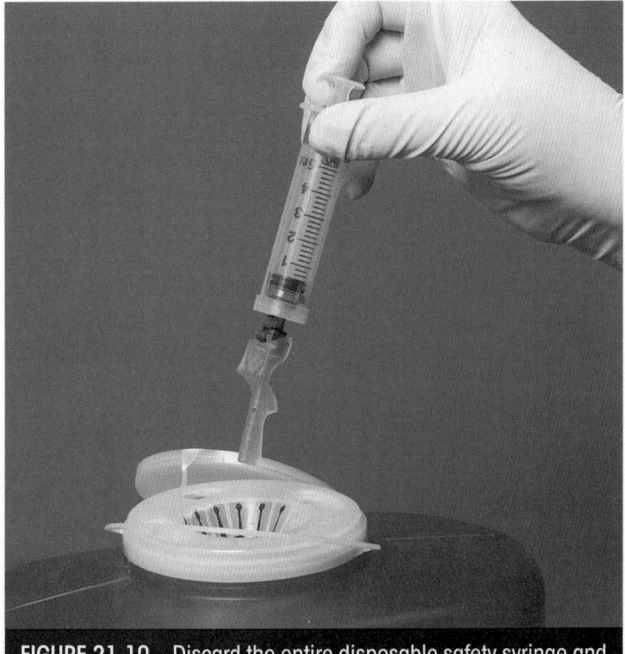

FIGURE 21-10 Discard the entire disposable safety syringe and needle into the biohazard puncture-proof sharps container.

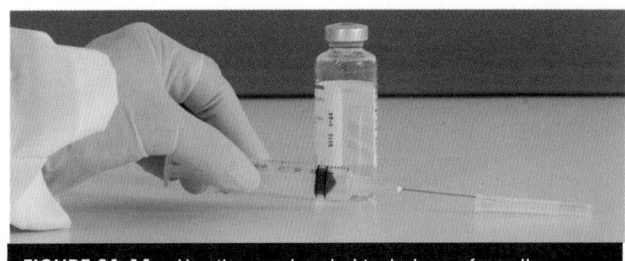

FIGURE 21-11 Use the one-handed technique of needle recapping to replace the sheath on the needle.

Additional information regarding specific procedures to follow should an accidental needlestick occur, as well as other safety procedures included in the OSHA and Clinical Laboratory Improvement Amendments (CLIA) rules and regulations, can be found later in this chapter and in Chapter 37.

Disposal of Infectious Waste

Infectious waste (contaminated items) is any item that has come in contact with patient blood or body fluids. These items must be handled with gloves and disposed of by placing them in the appropriate biohazard containers that are provided by an agency with which your employer has contracted (Figure 21-12). Infectious waste is either incinerated (burned) or subjected to sterilization by autoclave to render it harmless before it is disposed of in a sanitary landfill. For local rules and regulations of how to dispose of sharps and biohazard/infectious waste, contact your local department of health. Staff there can refer you to companies that specialize in the proper disposal of infectious waste and sharps. These companies follow strict state and federal regulations and can provide your clinic with containers, labels, and instructions. They will often work out a schedule for pickups, such as daily, weekly, monthly, or "on-call." Charges will usually be based on the amount of infectious waste that requires disposal.

Federal Organizations and Infection Control

The CDC is responsible for studying pathogens and diseases in an effort to prevent their spread. A division of the U.S. Public Health Department, the CDC has issued a number of guidelines over the last 25 years that have enabled health care professionals to practice responsible infection control. As diseases evolve and as new diseases are introduced into our society, the CDC revises and

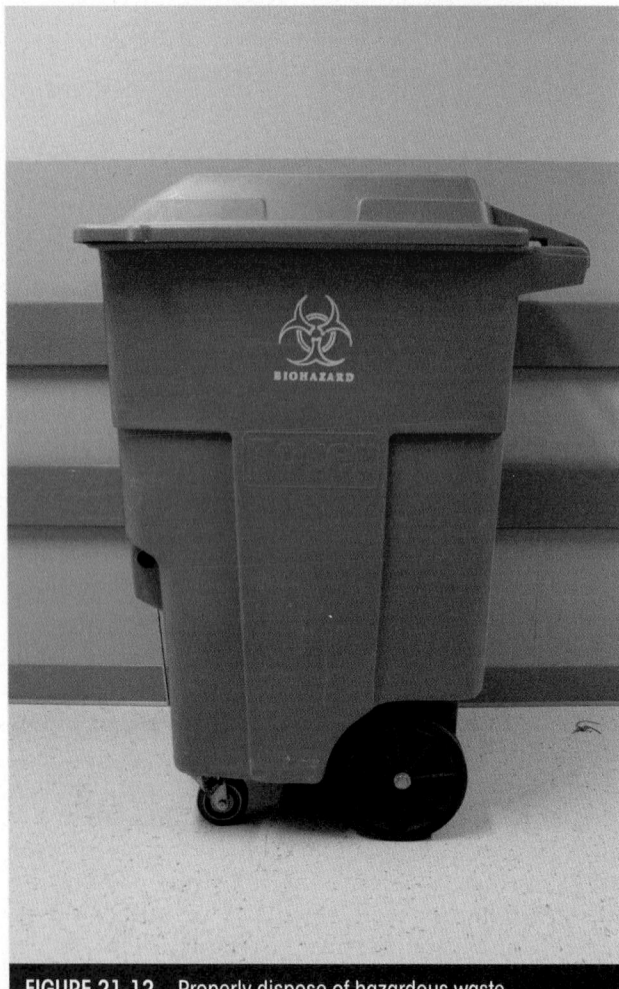

FIGURE 21-12 Properly dispose of hazardous waste.

updates existing guidelines or issues new control measures to contain the spread of infection.

In 1970, the CDC developed a system of seven **isolation categories** for patients with known infectious diseases. This category system included strict **isolation**, respiratory isolation, protective isolation, enteric precautions, wound and skin precautions, discharge precautions, and blood precautions.

In 1985, the agency released a set of guidelines known as Universal Blood and Body Fluid Precautions, or simply **Universal Precautions**. These infection control practices were written in response to the increase in AIDS and HBV, both bloodborne diseases, and other infectious diseases as well.

Beginning in 1991, the CDC infection control guidelines were reviewed and subsequently revised. In 1996, a new set of guidelines was released. Standard Precautions reflect improved recommendations intended to protect all health care providers, patients, and their visitors from a wide range of **communicable** diseases. At the same time that the CDC issued the new Standard Precautions, the organization also released a second tier of precautions called Transmission-Based Precautions. These are intended to be used in addition to Standard Precautions when caring for patients with known specific infectious diseases.

In 2007, the CDC published the *Guideline for Isolation Precautions: Preventing Transmission of Infectious Agents in Healthcare Settings* to update and expand upon the 1996 guidelines. The new guidelines were implemented to address the shift of health care from primarily acute care settings, the emergence of new pathogens (e.g., MRSA), the addition of respiratory hygiene/cough etiquette and safe injection practices, and other aspects of the changing health care delivery environment. This document added a set of prevention measures called Protective Environment that outline methods to prevent HAIs.

The 2007 guidelines specifically address transmission risks associated with each type of health care setting. There are different needs identified based on the location in which care is delivered. Hospitals, intensive care units, burn units, pediatrics, nonacute health care settings, long-term care, ambulatory care, and home care are addressed based on the unique needs of each. Focus is placed on the fundamental elements needed to prevent transmission of infectious agents in each of the above health care settings. Initially, administrative measures are to be enacted to make sure the system of care delivery recognizes the importance of disrupting the infection cycle in order to protect patients. Further guidelines are outlined based on the role of the health care provider.

Hand hygiene is recognized as the single most important practice to reduce the transmission of infectious agents in health care settings. Personal protective equipment (PPE) selection is also addressed item by item.

The 2007 guidelines also address precautions to prevent transmission of infectious agents. Several additions were made to the recommendations for Standard Precautions. Three areas of practice that were added are respiratory hygiene/cough etiquette, safe injection practices, and the use of masks for the insertion of catheters or injection of material into spinal or epidural spaces via lumbar puncture procedures.

The CDC strives to maintain the health and safety of the community, as well as patients and health care providers. It is the CDC's mission to continue educating, researching, and promoting healthy behaviors.

OSHA REGULATIONS

Safety Competency

The Occupational Safety and Health Administration (OSHA) has a mission of saving lives, preventing injuries, and protecting the health of America's workers. OSHA establishes guidelines and standards to promote worker safety and health. It is the responsibility of employers to obtain all applicable OSHA standards and fulfill the requirements outlined.

The Bloodborne Pathogen Standard

In March 1992, OSHA's *Bloodborne Pathogen Standard* became effective. Its primary objective was reducing occupational-related cases of HIV and HBV infections among health care workers. This standard was updated in 2011.

The standard covers all employees who can be "reasonably anticipated" to come into contact, as a result of performing their job duties, with blood and other potentially infectious materials. The *Bloodborne Pathogen Standard* seeks to limit exposure to bloodborne pathogens. An important aspect of this standard is an exposure control plan. This requires employers to identify tasks and procedures where occupational exposure to blood occurs. This plan must be accessible to employees and available to OSHA. Key to this exposure control plan are methods of compliance that mandate the use of Universal Precautions treating all body fluids/materials as if they were infectious. The mandate stipulates that employers provide, at no cost to employees, the full components of PPE and access to facilities for hand hygiene. It also includes the requirement for a written schedule outlining the cleaning, decontamination, and other cleansing for items that routinely come into contact with blood or body fluids. Hepatitis B vaccination is required to be made available to all employees who have occupational exposure to blood within 10 days of hire. There must also be postexposure evaluation and follow-up for all employees. For more information, please go to https://www.osha.gov and search for "Bloodborne Pathogen Standard."

OSHA published the *Model Plans and Programs for the OSHA Bloodborne Pathogens and Hazard Communications Standards* in 2003. This detailed booklet can be found at www.osha.gov. The publication contains model exposure control plans, model documents, and general guidance for meeting OSHA standards in this important area. These guidelines apply to students with potential for exposure to chemicals, blood, and other potentially infective material.

Methods of Compliance to Prevent Exposure. There are several major strategies mandated by OSHA for the prevention of exposure to bloodborne pathogens and other potentially infective material.

1. *Universal Precautions.* These are procedures that must be followed by staff when caring for a patient thought to be host to a pathogenic microorganism. This method extends beyond Standard Precautions and includes the use of PPEs to provide a barrier to prevent the mode of transmission of the pathogen. It includes the selection of appropriate PPEs; appropriate cleaning and disposal of potentially contaminated surgical equipment, needles, and laundry; and disposal of contaminated waste.

2. *Engineering and work practice controls.* Engineering controls and work practice controls consist of the physical equipment and mechanical devices an employer provides in an attempt to safeguard and minimize employee exposure. A common example of an engineering control is a sharps disposal container (Figure 21-13). Others are mechanical pipettes, fume hoods, splash guards, and eyewash stations (Figure 21-14). If and when occupational exposure continues after the engineering controls are in place, PPE must be used. Hand washing facilities or appropriate antiseptic hand cleanser (when hand washing facilities are not accessible) must be readily available.

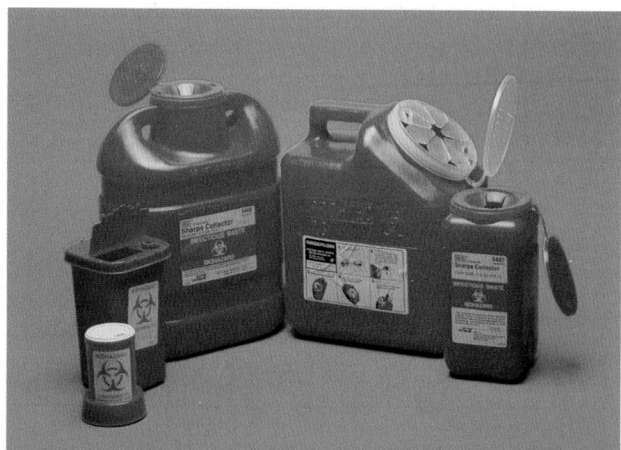

FIGURE 21-13 Various sizes of puncture-proof sharps containers. These and other biohazard waste containers are autoclaved when full and sent out to a biohazard agency for safe disposal.

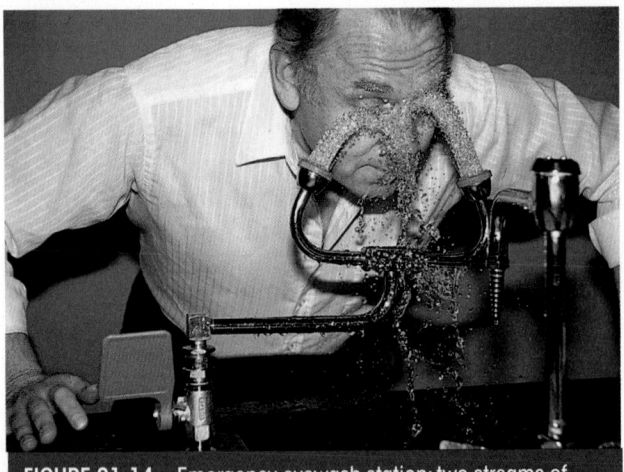

FIGURE 21-14 Emergency eyewash station: two streams of water or saline wash both eyes simultaneously and continuously.

3. *Personal protective equipment* (*PPE*). The employer must be certain that PPE is available and accessible and must provide an alternative type of glove if an employee is allergic to those originally provided (see the "Latex Sensitivity" section earlier in this chapter). Cleaning, laundering, and disposing of PPE are the responsibility of the employer, and the employee does not incur any expense for them.

   All PPE must be removed before the employee leaves the work site and placed in an appropriate container that is supplied by the employer. Figure 21-15 shows PPE.

4. *Cleanliness of work areas.* The employer must maintain a work site that is clean and sanitary and have a written schedule for cleaning and decontaminating the work area after contact with blood and other potentially infectious material. **Spill kits** must be readily accessible (Figure 21-16).

   Broken glass is placed in a sharps container after using cardboard or a dust pan and brush to remove it.

   Laundry that is contaminated is handled with gloves and placed in a labeled container. If the laundry is damp or wet, gloves and other appropriate PPE must be worn, and the damp or wet laundry must be placed in a plastic bag(s) to prevent blood or other potentially infectious material from leaking through it. PPE cannot be laundered at home. All other Standard Precautions must be adhered to.

5. *Hepatitis B vaccine.* HBV vaccine must be made available free of charge to every employee, full time, part time, or temporary, within 10 days of work assignment (Figure 21-17). This refers to employees who have the potential for occupational exposure, and who can "reasonably" be expected to have skin, eye, mucous membrane, or **parenteral** contact with blood or other potentially infectious material. The vaccine is given in three doses over a 6-month period and is used to protect the employee from infection with HBV. It is an intramuscular injection with an approximate 96% rate of effectiveness.

   An employee has the right to decline taking the vaccine but must sign a **declination form**. There is the option to reconsider receiving the vaccine at a later time.

6. *Follow-up after exposure.* An accidental exposure is broadly defined as one in which blood, blood-contaminated body fluids, or body fluids or tissues to which Standard Precautions apply are introduced into a mucous surface; into nonintact skin; or into the conjunctiva via a needlestick, skin cut, or direct splash. If an incident exposes an employee to any of these, the employer must make available a confidential medical evaluation in which the following are documented:

   - The circumstances surrounding the event
   - The route or routes of exposure
   - The identification of the person who was the source of the exposure

   The following procedure describes the steps to take following an exposure incident:

   - Immediately wash exposed area with soap and warm water.
   - If mouth area is exposed, rinse with water or mouthwash.
   - If eyes are exposed, flush with large amounts of warm water.
   - Report incident to a supervisor immediately for documentation.

   In addition, OSHA requires the following information:

   - The exposed employee must be tested for HBV, HCV, and HIV only if consent is given. An employee may refuse or may have blood drawn and stored for 90 days, at which time the choice can be made whether to have the blood tested.

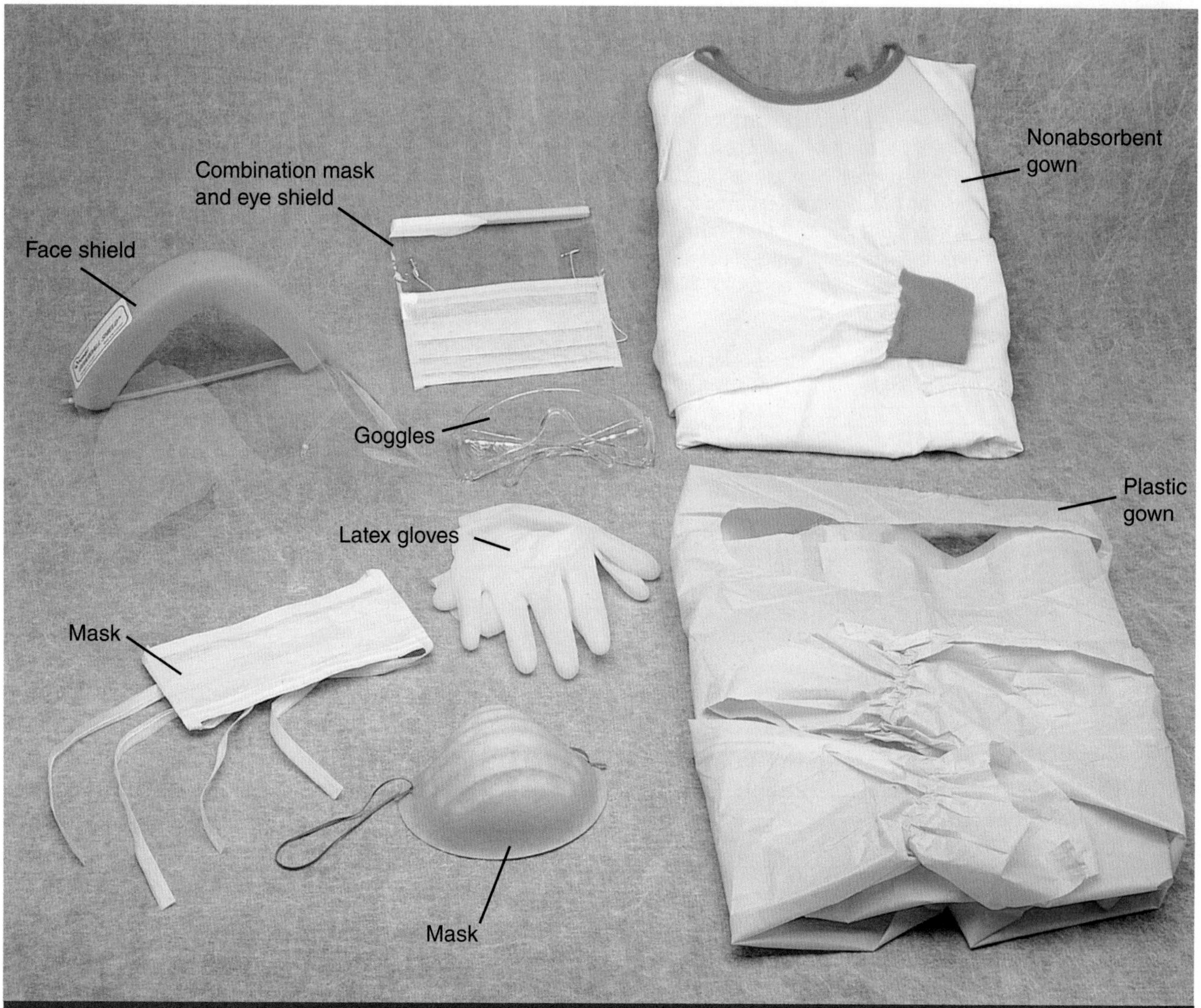

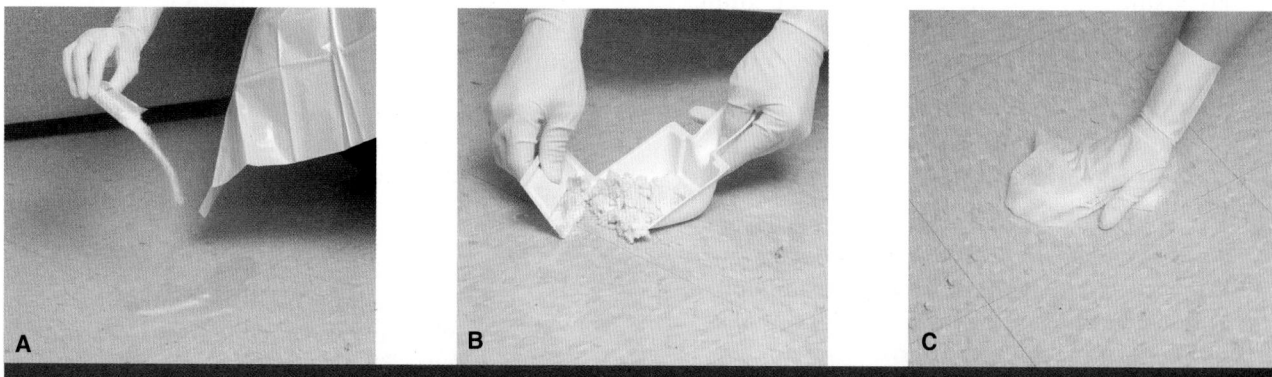

FIGURE 21-15 Personal protective equipment.

Face shield

Combination mask
and eye shield

Nonabsorbent
gown

Goggles

Plastic
gown

Latex gloves

Mask

Mask

FIGURE 21-16 (A) Sprinkle coagulating powder over spill wearing protective clothing and gloves. (B) Scoop up spill with scoop from kit. (C) The spill area is then cleaned with a 10% bleach solution.

SAMPLE

Hepatitis B Employee Vaccination Form

MEMO: To all employees with occupational exposure to blood or other infectious materials on an average of one or more times per month. OSHA and the CDC have identified the potential exposure of health care workers to hepatitis B virus (HBV) in the course of performing their duties in this office. For the protection of our employees, we are offering prescreening testing and the HBV vaccination with follow-up evaluation to all employees who are exposed to blood or other potentially infectious materials on an average of one or more times per month. *In accordance with recommended OSHA guidelines, this vaccine and testing will be offered at no cost to the employee.* You have the ability to decide whether or not you want the testing and/or vaccine.

At the bottom of this memo, you may indicate your choice. Please return this memo with your signature and date to your immediate supervisor.

[ ]   I want to receive the prescreening (optional)
[ ]   I want to receive the vaccine and follow-up evaluation testing
[ ]   I *do not* want the vaccine and testing and have read the following statement:

I understand that due to my occupational exposure to blood or other potentially infectious materials I may be at risk of acquiring hepatitis B virus (HBV) infection. I have been given the opportunity to be vaccinated with hepatitis B vaccine at no charge to myself. However, I decline hepatitis B vaccination at this time. I understand that by declining this vaccine I continue to be at risk of acquiring hepatitis B, a serious disease. If in the future I continue to have occupational exposure to blood or other potentially infectious materials and I want to be vaccinated with hepatitis B vaccine, I can receive the vaccination series at no charge to me.

_____   _____
NAME   DATE

_____   _____
SIGNATURE   SS#

PRESCREENING DATE _____   RESULTS _____

DATE OF VACCINATIONS _____

DATE OF FOLLOW-UP EVALUATION _____

RESULTS _____

NOTES:

Courtesy of POL Consultants, Inc., 2 Russ Farm Way, Delanco, NJ 08075, 856-824-0800

FIGURE 21-17 Sample hepatitis B employee vaccination form provides employee information regarding hepatitis B vaccine and space to sign indicating whether employee declines vaccine.

- The source individual's blood, if permission is granted (Figure 21-17), is tested for HBV, HCV, and HIV and the employee shall know the results (unless protected by the law).

- The employee is offered prophylaxis, gamma globulin, or HB vaccine after the exposure to HBV or HIV according to the current recommendation of the U.S. Public Health Service.

- The employee is counseled regarding precautions to take to avoid possible transmission and is provided information on potential illnesses for which to be alert.

- An OSHA 301 form must be filed (Figure 21-18).

7. *Medical records.* Medical records of an employee who has suffered an occupational exposure must be kept for the length of employment plus 30 years, and confidentiality must be guaranteed.

 Procedure

The following information is to be included in the employee's record: name and Social Security number, HB vaccination status with dates, results of any examinations or tests, a copy of the health care provider's written opinion, and a copy of the information that was provided to the health care provider (see Procedure 21-4).

The records must be available to the employee, OSHA, and anyone with the written consent of the employee, but *not* the employer.

PROCEDURE 21-4

Participate in a Mock Exposure Event with Documentation of Specific Steps

Procedure

PURPOSE:

To provide documentation required by OSHA in the event an employee becomes injured or is exposed to blood or body fluids. A post-exposure plan must be followed, and an incident report must be filled out.

EQUIPMENT/SUPPLIES:

- OSHA's form 301 (Injury and Illness Report)
- Pen

PROCEDURE STEPS:

1. Report the incident to a supervisor immediately.
2. Access a copy of OSHA form 301.
3. Complete the section regarding employee information.
4. Complete the section regarding the physician or other health care personnel.
5. Complete the section regarding information about the incident, including when the incident occurred, the nature of the injury or illness, and whether the employee died.
6. Submit form according to OSHA guidelines.
7. A copy of the incident report form must be kept on file by the employer.

OSHA's Form 301
Injury and Illness Incident Report

Attention: This form contains information relating to employee health and must be used in a manner that protects the confidentiality of employees to the extent possible while the information is being used for occupational safety and health purposes.

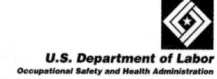

U.S. Department of Labor
Occupational Safety and Health Administration

Form approved OMB no. 1218-0176

This *Injury and Illness Incident Report* is one of the first forms you must fill out when a recordable work-related injury or illness has occurred. Together with the *Log of Work-Related Injuries and Illnesses* and the accompanying *Summary*, these forms help the employer and OSHA develop a picture of the extent and severity of work-related incidents.

Within 7 calendar days after you receive information that a recordable work-related injury or illness has occurred, you must fill out this form or an equivalent. Some state workers' compensation, insurance, or other reports may be acceptable substitutes. To be considered an equivalent form, any substitute must contain all the information asked for on this form.

According to Public Law 91-596 and 29 CFR 1904, OSHA's recordkeeping rule, you must keep this form on file for 5 years following the year to which it pertains.

If you need additional copies of this form, you may photocopy and use as many as you need.

Completed by _____

Title _____

Phone (_____)_____-_____ Date ___/___/___

Information about the employee

1) Full name _____

2) Street _____

City _____ State _____ ZIP _____

3) Date of birth ___/___/___
4) Date hired ___/___/___
5) ☐ Male
   ☐ Female

Information about the physician or other health care professional

6) Name of physician or other health care professional _____

7) If treatment was given away from the worksite, where was it given?

Facility _____

Street _____

City _____ State _____ ZIP _____

8) Was employee treated in an emergency room?
   ☐ Yes
   ☐ No

9) Was employee hospitalized overnight as an in-patient?
   ☐ Yes
   ☐ No

Information about the case

10) Case number from the Log _____ (*Transfer the case number from the Log after you record the case.*)

11) Date of injury or illness ___/___/___

12) Time employee began work _____ AM / PM

13) Time of event _____ AM / PM ☐ Check if time cannot be determined

14) **What was the employee doing just before the incident occurred?** Describe the activity, as well as the tools, equipment, or material the employee was using. Be specific. *Examples:* "climbing a ladder while carrying roofing materials"; "spraying chlorine from hand sprayer"; "daily computer key-entry."

15) **What happened?** Tell us how the injury occurred. *Examples:* "When ladder slipped on wet floor, worker fell 20 feet"; "Worker was sprayed with chlorine when gasket broke during replacement"; "Worker developed soreness in wrist over time."

16) **What was the injury or illness?** Tell us the part of the body that was affected and how it was affected; be more specific than "hurt," "pain," or sore." *Examples:* "strained back"; "chemical burn, hand"; "carpal tunnel syndrome."

17) **What object or substance directly harmed the employee?** *Examples:* "concrete floor"; "chlorine"; "radial arm saw." *If this question does not apply to the incident, leave it blank.*

18) **If the employee died, when did death occur?** Date of death ___/___/___

Public reporting burden for this collection of information is estimated to average 22 minutes per response, including time for reviewing instructions, searching existing data sources, gathering and maintaining the data needed, and completing and reviewing the collection of information. Persons are not required to respond to the collection of information unless it displays a current valid OMB control number. If you have any comments about this estimate or any other aspects of this data collection, including suggestions for reducing this burden, contact: US Department of Labor, OSHA Office of Statistical Analysis, Room N-3644, 200 Constitution Avenue, NW, Washington, DC 20210. Do not send the completed forms to this office.

FIGURE 21-18 OSHA's Injury and Illness incident report.

United States Department of Labor, Occupational Safety and Health Administration. www.osha.gov.

≫ TRAINING COMPONENTS OF THE BLOODBORNE PATHOGEN STANDARD

Scope and Application

- The standard applies to all occupational exposure to blood and other potentially infectious materials (OPIM), and includes part-time employees, designated first aiders, and mental health workers as well as exposed medical personnel.

- OPIM includes semen, vaginal secretions, cerebrospinal fluid, synovial fluid, pericardial fluid, peritoneal fluid, amniotic fluid, saliva in dental procedures, any body fluid that is contaminated with blood, and all body fluids in situations where it is difficult or impossible to differentiate between body fluids. It also includes any unfixed tissue or organ. Tissue or cell cultures that contain HIV or HBV are also included.

Methods of Compliance

- *General.* Universal Precautions are to be observed to prevent contact with blood or OPIM.

- Engineering and work practice controls are to be implemented to eliminate exposure.

- Personal protective equipment is to be utilized.

- Housekeeping.

Universal Precautions

- *All* human blood and OPIM are considered to be infectious.

- The *same* precautions must be taken with *all* blood and OPIM.

Engineering Controls

- Whenever feasible, engineering controls (devices that isolate or remove health hazards from the workplace) must be the primary method used to control exposure.

- Examples include needleless IVs, self-sheathing needles, sharps disposal containers, covered centrifuge buckets, aerosol-free tubes, and leak-proof containers.

- Engineering controls must be examined, maintained, and replaced on a regular schedule.

- Handwashing facilities must be readily accessible to all employees.

- If provision of handwashing facilities is not feasible, the employer must provide appropriate antiseptic hand cleaner with cloth or paper towels or antiseptic towelettes. Hands must be washed as soon as is feasible.

- Engineering controls must be evaluated and documented on a regular basis.

Sharps Containers

- Readily accessible and as close as practical to work area.

- Puncture-resistant.

- Labeled or color-coded.

- Leak-proof.

- Closeable.

- *Routinely replaced* so there is no overflow.

Work Practice Controls

- Hand washing should be performed following glove removal.

- No recapping, breaking, or bending of needles.

- No eating, drinking, smoking, or applying lip products or handling contacts in work areas where there is a reasonable likelihood of exposure.

- No storage of food or drink where blood or OPIM are stored.

- Minimize splashing, splattering of blood, and OPIM.

- All procedures involving blood or OPIM must be performed in a manner to limit splashing, spraying, spattering, and generating droplets of these substances.

- No mouth pipetting may be done.

- Specimens must be transported in leak-proof, labeled containers. They must be placed in a secondary container if outside contamination of primary container occurs.

- If the outside of the container becomes contaminated or if the container is punctured, it must be placed inside a secondary container.

- Equipment must be decontaminated prior to servicing or shipping. Areas that cannot be decontaminated must be labeled.

Personal Protective Equipment (PPE)

- Includes eye protection, gloves, gowns, laboratory coats, resuscitation equipment.

- Must be readily accessible and employers must require their use.

- Must be stored at work site.

- Provided at no cost to the employee.

- The employer must clean, launder, and dispose of PPE at no cost to the employee.

- PPE must be removed before leaving the work area.

- Worn PPE must be placed in appropriate containers for storage, washing, decontamination, or disposal.

(continues)

Eye Protection

- Eye protection is required whenever there is potential for splashing, spraying, or splattering to the eyes or ocular mucous membranes.

- If necessary, use eye protection in conjunction with a mask or use a chin-length face shield.

- Prescription glasses may be fitted with solid sideshields.

- Decontamination procedures must be developed.

Gloves

- Must be worn whenever hands have contact with blood, OPIM, mucous membranes, nonintact skin, or contaminated surfaces/items, or when performing vascular access procedures (phlebotomy).

- Type required:
  ○ Vinyl or latex for general use.
  ○ Alternatives must be available if employee has allergic reactions (i.e., powderless).
  ○ Utility gloves for surface disinfection.
  ○ Puncture-resistant when handling sharps (e.g., central supply).

- Single-use gloves shall be removed and replaced when they are torn or punctured, or when their ability to function as a barrier is compromised.

- Single-use gloves must not be washed or decontaminated for reuse.

- Gloves may not be required for routine phlebotomy based on employer policy.

- Gloves must be available for all employees that wish to use them for phlebotomy.

- Gloves must be worn for phlebotomy if the employee has cuts, scratches, or other nonintact skin.

Masks

- Masks in combination with eye protection devices must be worn when splashes, spray, spatter, droplets of blood, or OPIM may be generated and eye, nose, or mouth contamination can be anticipated.

Gown, Aprons, and Other Protective Clothing

- Must be worn whenever splashing or splattering to skin or clothing may occur.

- Type required depends on exposure. Prevention of contamination of skin and clothes is the key.

- Examples:
  ○ Low-level exposure: lab coats.
  ○ Moderate-level exposure: fluid-resistant gown.

- ○ High-level exposure: fluid-proof apron, head and foot covering.

- *NOTE*: If PPE is considered protective clothing, then the *employer must* launder it.

- If a garment is penetrated by blood or OPIM, the garment shall be immediately removed.

Housekeeping

- There must be a written schedule for cleaning and disinfection.

- Contaminated equipment and surfaces must be cleaned as soon as feasible for obvious contamination or at the end of the work shift if no contamination has occurred.

- Protective coverings may be used over equipment.

- Broken glassware that is potentially contaminated must not be picked up directly with hands. It must be cleaned up using mechanical means, such as a brush and dustpan, tongs, or forceps.

Regulated Waste Containers (nonsharp)
Must be:
  ○ Closeable.
  ○ Puncture resistant.
  ○ Leak-proof.
  ○ Labeled or color-coded.
  ○ Placed in secondary container if outside of container is contaminated.
  ○ Easily accessible to personnel.
  ○ Maintained upright during use.
  ○ Replaced routinely and not overfilled.
  ○ Closed immediately prior to removal or replacement.

- Reusable containers are not to be opened, emptied, or cleaned manually or in any other manner that would expose employees to percutaneous injury.

Laundry

- Handle as little as possible.

- Bag at location of use.

- Label or color-code.

- Transport in bags that prevent soak-through or leakage.

- Employees must wear gloves and other appropriate PPE when in contact with contaminated laundry.

Laundry Facility

- Two options:
  1. Standard precautions for all laundry (alternative color coding allowed if recognized).

(continues)

2. Precautions only for contaminated laundry (must be red bags or have biohazard labels).

- Laundry personnel must use PPE and have a sharps container accessible.

Hepatitis B Vaccination

- Made available within 10 days to all employees with occupational exposure.
- No cost to employees and at a reasonable time and place
- Participation in a prescreening program must not be a prerequisite for receiving a hepatitis B vaccination.
- May be required for students to be admitted to college health program as well as for externship.
- Routine boosters must be made available by the employer.
- Given in accordance with U.S. Public Health Service guidelines.
- Employees must first be evaluated by a health care professional.
- The health care professional gives a written opinion.
- If the vaccine is refused, the employee signs a declination form.
- Vaccine must be available at a future date if initially refused.

Postexposure Follow-Up

- Document exposure incident.
- Identify source individual (if possible).
- Attempt to test source if consent obtained.
- Provide results to exposed employee.

Labels

- Biohazard symbol and word *Biohazard* must be visible.
- Labels must include the biohazard image.
- Fluorescent orange/orange-red with contrasting letters may also be used.
- Red bags/containers may be substituted for labels.
- Labels required on:
  ◦ Regulated waste.
  ◦ Refrigerators/freezers with blood or OPIM.
  ◦ Transport/storage containers.
  ◦ Contaminated equipment.

Information and Training

- Required for all employees with occupational exposure.
- Training required initially, annually, and if there are new procedures.
- Training material must be appropriate for literacy and education level of each employee.

- Training must be interactive and allow for questions and answers.

Training Components

- Explanation of bloodborne standard.
- Epidemiology and symptoms of bloodborne disease.
- Modes of HIV/HBV transmission.
- Explanation of exposure control plan.
- Explanation of the appropriate methods for recognizing tasks and other activities that may involve exposure to blood or OPIM.
- Explanation of engineering and work practice controls.
- How to select the proper PPE.
- How to decontaminate equipment, surfaces, and so on.
- Information about the hepatitis B vaccine.
- Postexposure follow-up procedures.
- Label/color-code system.
- Opportunity for interactive questions and answers.

Medical Records

- Records must be kept for each employee with occupational exposure and include:
  ◦ A copy of the employee's vaccination status and date.
  ◦ A copy of postexposure follow-up evaluation procedures.
  ◦ A copy of the employee's hepatitis B vaccination status, including the dates of vaccinations and any medical records relative to the employee's ability to receive the vaccination.
  ◦ Health care professional's written opinions.
- Confidentiality must be maintained.
- Records must be maintained for 30 years plus the duration of employment.

Training Records

- Records are kept for three years from date of training and include:
  ◦ Date of training.
  ◦ Summary of contents of training program.
  ◦ Name and qualifications of trainer.
  ◦ Name and job title of all persons attending.
- Records must be maintained for 3 years from the date on which training occurred.

Exposure Control Plan Components

- A written plan for each workplace with occupational exposure.

(continues)

- Written policies/procedures for complying with the standard.
- A cohesive document or a guiding document referencing existing policies/procedures.

Exposure Control Plan

- A list of job classifications for which occupational exposure control occurs (e.g., medical assistant, clinical laboratory scientist, dental hygienist).
- A list of tasks during which exposure occurs (e.g., medical assistant performing venipuncture).
- Methods/policies/procedures for compliance.
- Procedures for sharps disposal.
- Disinfection policies/procedures.
- Procedures for selection of PPE.
- Regulated waste disposal procedures.
- Laundry procedures.
- Hepatitis B vaccination procedures.
- Postexposure follow-up procedures.
- Training procedures.
- Plan must be accessible to employees and be updated annually.

Employee Responsibilities

- Go through training and cooperate.
- Obey policies.
- Use Universal Precaution techniques.
- Use PPE.
- Use safe work practices.
- Use engineering controls.
- Report unsafe work conditions to employer.
- Maintain clean work areas.

Cooperation between employer and employees regarding the Bloodborne Pathogen Standard will facilitate understanding of the law, thereby benefiting all persons who are exposed to HIV, HBV, HCV, and OPIM by minimizing the risk of exposure to the pathogens.

Meeting the OSHA standards is not optional, and failure to comply can result in a fine that may total $10,000 for each employee.

To obtain copies of the Bloodborne Pathogen Standard, contact OSHA at 800-321-6742 or www.osha.gov.

Courtesy of the Occupational Safety and Health Administration, U.S. Department of Labor.

Hazard Communication for Blood. The employer is required to label containers of **regulated waste**, refrigerators, freezers, and other containers that are used to keep or transport blood or other potentially infectious material with warning labels that are orange or orange-red and have the biohazard symbol affixed to them. The labeling serves to warn employees of the hazard possibility of container contents (Figure 21-19).

Information and Training for Employees. Employers must ensure the presence of and maintain documentation that employees take part in training sessions during working hours at no cost to employees. The initial session must be provided when occupational exposure may occur and annually thereafter. If employee tasks and job description change, training must take place at that time.

Training components are listed in the "Training Components of the Bloodborne Pathogen Standard" Quick Reference Guide. Documentation of training sessions must be available and kept for 3 years.

BIOHAZARD LABELS

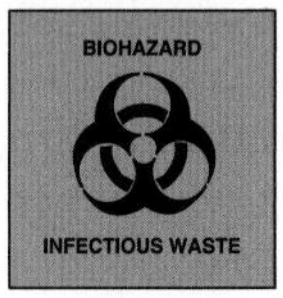

Containers that hold biohazardous materials must be properly labeled. Biohazardous materials include blood and body fluids as well as garments, gloves, masks, needles, gauze, wipes, aprons, and so on that may be contaminated with blood or other potentially contaminated body fluids. Labels shall be used to identify the presence of an actual or potential biological hazard.

CONSIDERATIONS:

- Labels shall be fluorescent orange or orange-red, with lettering or symbols in a contrasting color.
- Labels should be affixed onto or as close as feasible to the container by adhesive, string, wire, or other method.
- Red bags or red containers may be substituted for labels.
- If blood or control serum is stored in a refrigerator, the refrigerator shall be marked with a biohazard label.
- If blood is stored in a refrigerator for transport or same-day shipment, it does not need to be labeled but should be put in containment bags.

FIGURE 21-19 Biohazard labels alert employees to biohazardous materials, such as blood, body fluids, and other potentially infectious material.

PRINCIPLES OF INFECTION CONTROL

By understanding the dependent nature of the infection cycle, which holds that each step in the process must occur for infectious disease to occur, medical assistants can apply principles of infection control to eliminate or reduce the transmission of infectious microorganisms in the health care setting. Conscious and continual reliance on infection control is a professional standard and protects employees, patients, families, and the public from contracting infectious diseases. There are two general types of infection control: medical asepsis and surgical asepsis. Each is indicated in specific circumstances and each is achieved by the various techniques that are described in this chapter and in Chapter 30.

MEDICAL ASEPSIS

Medical asepsis includes the use of practices such as hand washing, general cleaning and disinfecting of contaminated surfaces, and adherence to Standard and Transmission-Based Precautions. These measures are aimed at destroying pathologic organisms. These techniques are used to decrease the risk for transmission to others. Objects should be medically aseptic if they are to be used in procedures that affect the external body or if they will enter a usually contaminated body part, such as the mouth. Many things, such as our hands, cannot be sterilized or even disinfected, but they can be rendered clean of **gross contamination** and most pathogens by simple hand washing. Many items, such as stethoscopes or sphygmomanometers, do not need to be sterile to be used on a variety of patients. These items do not enter into the body or into sterile areas of the body. These items should, however, be either cleaned or disinfected routinely. Sphygmomanometers and stethoscopes are used continuously throughout the day on different patients. Patients with hypertension, postsurgery patients, and patients having physical examinations routinely have their blood pressure monitored. Both pieces of equipment contact patients' skin, clothing, or both, making the blood pressure equipment an indirect source of pathogens. Alcohol-based wipes or a simplified method of detergent cleaning should be used regularly to decontaminate blood pressure equipment. Medical asepsis also involves environmental hygiene measures such as equipment cleaning and disinfection procedures.

Some specific examples of appropriate use of medical asepsis include:

- Wash hands before and after handling equipment and supplies, on arrival and before leaving, and before and after working with each patient, even when gloves are worn.
- Handle all specimens as if they were contaminated.
- Use disposable equipment whenever possible and dispose of it properly in a biohazard waste container. All equipment is contaminated after patient use.
- Use PPE as outlined in Standard Precautions and wash hands after removal of any PPE, including gloves.
- Keep contaminated equipment and supplies away from clothing to prevent transmission of pathogens to self and others.
- Place dressing materials, gauze, cotton balls, and any other damp or wet contaminated absorbable material in a waterproof bag before disposal in the biohazard waste container.
- Any break in the medical assistant's skin should be covered with a sterile dressing.
- Items that fall to the floor are contaminated. Either discard or wash and then disinfect them before using.
- If uncertain whether equipment or supplies are clean or sterile, consider them contaminated. Clean or sterilize them before use.

Hand Washing

There have been tremendous advances in the last two centuries in the overall hygiene of the human race. This has added to the quality and duration of our lives on earth. General cleanliness has assisted with the eradication of widespread infection outbreaks and epidemics. Hand washing continues to be the most important aspect of all of the infectious control procedures. Proper hand washing removes gross contamination and reduces pathogens that could be transmitted by direct or indirect contact to others. Because hand washing is frequently required, the use of a good lotion is advised to reduce the possibility of skin breaks caused by dryness. Infectious diseases continue to present serious challenges. One of the biggest concerns is the spread of HIV, HBV, and HCV. In May 2007, the WHO issued nine patient safety solution recommendations. The Joint Commission has adopted the nine recommendations.

The ninth patient safety solution is entitled "Improved Hand Hygiene to Prevent Healthcare Associated Infection (HAI)." The WHO and the Joint Commission say, "Effective hand hygiene is the primary measure for avoiding this problem."

The WHO's measures were reevaluated in 2011, and it was recognized that the biggest challenge to implementation of these solutions is access to the available information. Some of the barriers identified were difficulty finding the solutions on the WHO's Web site, limited translations to other languages, and implementation strategies that are aimed at governments instead of health care practitioners in the field. Efforts to overcome these barriers are currently being implemented.

Procedure

The CDC recommends washing hands with soap and water as the best way to reduce the number of microbes on them in most situations. (Procedure 21-5 describes hand washing for medical asepsis.) When soap and water are not available, the CDC advises using an alcohol-based hand sanitizer that contains at least 60% alcohol (see Procedure 21-6). Hand sanitizers must contain 60% to 95 % alcohol to be most effective. It must be noted that alcohol-based hand sanitizers can inactivate many types of microbes very effectively when used correctly, though people may not use a large enough volume of the sanitizer or may wipe it off before it has dried. Also, while these sanitizers reduce the number of microbes on the hands, they do not eliminate all types of bacteria. Research has indicated that washing hands with soap and water more effectively removes or inactivates dangerous microbes such as *Cryptosporidium*, norovirus, and *Clostridium difficile*.

When decontaminating hands with an alcohol-based hand rub, apply to the palm of one hand and rub hands together, covering all surfaces of the hands and fingers, including the palms; back of hands; fingertips; and between fingers, wrists, and thumbs until hands are dry. Do not wipe hand

PROCEDURE 21-5

Procedure

Medical Asepsis Hand Wash (Hand Hygiene)

STANDARD PRECAUTIONS:

Handwashing

PURPOSE:

To reduce pathogens on the hands and wrists, thereby decreasing direct and indirect transmission of infectious micro-organisms. Average duration is 1 minute before beginning to work with patients, 15 seconds (CDC hand hygiene recommendation) following each patient contact.

EQUIPMENT/SUPPLIES:

- Sink (preferably with foot-operated controls)
- Soap (preferably liquid soap in foot-operated container; bar soap discouraged)
- Water-based antibacterial lotion
- Disposable paper towels
- Nail stick or brush

PROCEDURE STEPS:

1. To ensure that no microorganisms are being harbored on your hands, remove all jewelry (a plain wedding band is the only acceptable jewelry). Push watch up on arm or remove. RATIONALE: Jewelry harbors microorganisms on the hands.

2. Ensure that nails are clipped short. RATIONALE: Longer nails have been proven to harbor larger colony counts of microorganisms. Check your employer's policy on artificial nails, nail extenders, and nail polish. If they are not

(continues)

allowed, employ the following processes: If you have artificial nails or acrylic overlays, or nail extenders, have them professionally removed. RATIONALE: The CDC recommends that health care workers not wear artificial nails or extenders when having direct contact with patients. Remove nail polish. RATIONALE: Chipped nail polish supports the growth of a larger number of microorganisms.

3. Roll sleeves to above the elbow. RATIONALE: Clothing harbors microorganisms and can be a vector in the transmission of disease.

4. Prepare disposable paper towel (if using pull-down dispenser, prepare the amount of paper towel necessary for drying hands after wash; if using folded towels, have accessible). RATIONALE: After the hand washing, you may not touch any contaminated surface, such as the handle on a paper-towel dispenser or the water faucets.

5. Never allow your clothing to touch the sink; never touch the inside of the sink with your hands. RATIONALE: The sink is considered contaminated at all times. (*NOTE:* Sinks must be sanitized and disinfected at the end of each day.)

6. Turn on the faucet with a dry paper towel (Figure 21-20A). Discard paper towel after adjusting water temperature to lukewarm. RATIONALE: Lukewarm water is best for hand washing because excessively hot water may overdry the skin and cause cracking, thereby interrupting the caregiver's first line of defense.

7. Wet hands and apply soap using a circular motion and friction; rub into a lather (Figure 21-20B). RATIONALE: This initial hand wash is to remove visible soil and some microorganisms.

8. Interlace fingers to clean between them (Figure 21-20C). Rub vigorously to remove microorganisms.

9. If this is the first hand washing of the day, use an orange stick or brush to clean any dirt and microorganisms from under the fingernails (Figures 21-20D and E). RATIONALE: Nails harbor microorganisms. Even with trimmed nails, this step must be performed on a daily basis.

10. Rinse hands with hands pointed down and lower than elbows (Figure 21-20F). RATIONALE: When hands are held lower than elbows, pathogens and contaminated water run off the hands and not up on the forearms.

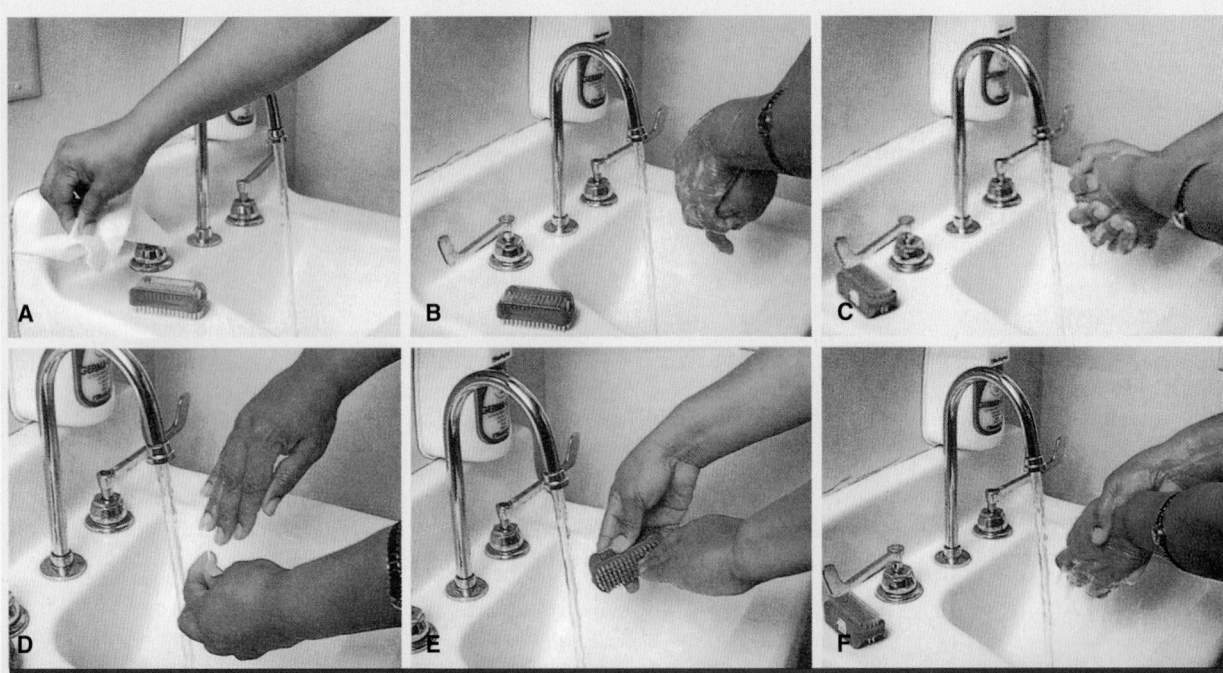

FIGURE 21-20 (A) Prepare towels for use. Turn on the faucet and adjust water to a lukewarm temperature. (B) Wet hands. Let water flow downward off hands and fingertips. (C) Use a circular motion to create friction and wash the palms and back of hands. Interlace the fingers to clean between them. (D) Use an orange stick to clean under fingernails. (E) A hand brush may also be used to clean under fingernails. (F) Rinse hands thoroughly, letting the water flow downward off your hands and fingertips.

(continues)

11. Repeat soap application and lather; interlace fingers well; wash with vigorous, circular motions all parts of hands including wrists; wash for at least 1 minute or longer depending on degree of contamination. RATIONALE: Appropriate length of hand washing is required to provide enough friction to remove soil and microorganisms.

12. Rinse well, keeping hands pointed downward. RATIONALE: Rinsing removes microorganisms, contaminated water, and soap from the hands.

13. If this is the first hand washing of the day, repeat the procedure again, making sure to use sufficient friction around the wrist, arms, and hands. Rinse hands, arms, and wrists as before. Dry hands and wrists using a blotting motion. Do not touch towel dispenser after hand washing. If the sink is not foot operated, use a clean disposable towel to turn off water faucet. RATIONALE: Touching the towel dispenser contaminates the hands. Blotting the hands dry reduces drying of the skin. Turning the faucet off with paper towel prevents recontamination from the dirty faucet.

14. Discard paper towel in waste container. Do not leave contaminated towels for repeated use. *NOTE:* Repeat hand washing procedure before and after each patient contact, procedure, or meal. RATIONALE: Hand washing must be performed on a regular and frequent basis to ensure the reduction of microorganisms transmitted by hands.

15. Use a paper towel to pump the appropriate amount of water-based antibacterial lotion onto the palm and apply to hands to prevent chapped, **excoriated** skin. If skin is excoriated, the medical assistant may not be able to work because of breaks in the skin or may have to wear gloves during any patient contact.

16. Repeat appropriate handwashing throughout the day on a frequent basis to ensure the reduction of microorganism transmission.

PROCEDURE 21-6

Correct Use of Alcohol-Based Hand Rubs (ABHR)

PURPOSE:

To avoid transmission of pathogens via the hands of health care personnel.

EQUIPMENT/SUPPLIES:

- Alcohol-based hand rub containing 60% to 90% alcohol

PROCEDURE STEPS:

1. Prior to using ABHR, ensure that hands are free from gross contamination such as any visible biologic material. RATIONALE: ABHR are ineffective when used in the presence of biologic material that is visible on the hands.

2. Dispense 2 to 3 mL into the palm of your hand. RATIONALE: The health care provider must use enough ABHR to cover all the surfaces of both hands.

3. The ABHR must be applied in the following manner:
   a. Palms rubbed together
   b. Right palm over the dorsal aspect of the left hand and vice versa
   c. Palm to palm with fingers interlaced
   d. Backs of fingers to opposing palms with fingers interlocked
   e. Rotational rubbing of left thumb clasped in right palm and vice versa
   f. Rotational rubbing, backward and forward, with clasped fingers of right hand in the left palm and vice versa
      RATIONALE: All surfaces and aspects of the hand must be covered with the ABHR to assure contact with any microorganisms present.

4. Hands should be rubbed together for at least 30 seconds until the hands are dry. RATIONALE: The antimicrobial activity of the ABHR is assured if the application is allowed to dry.

sanitizer off—it must be allowed to dry. The use of alcohol-based hand sanitizers *does not* replace a solid practice of health care providers washing hands using traditional soap and water.

The World Health Organization (WHO) has published the *Hand Hygiene Technical Reference Manual*. This document clearly outlines "My five moments for hand hygiene." These are logical, practical, and useful guidelines for hand hygiene (Table 21-7).

Antimicrobial wipes *cannot* be used as a substitute for an alcohol-based hand rub. Wearing gloves is *not* a substitute for hand decontamination. Artificial fingernails or nail extenders cannot be worn when in direct contact with patients at high risk. Natural nails should be kept less than ¼ inch long.

Sanitization

Sanitization (washing) of instruments and equipment rids them of gross contamination and blood, body fluids, tissue, and other contaminated **debris**. Enzymatic detergent especially designed for medical instruments and a soft scrub brush are used to remove all contaminates from surfaces, crevices, hinges, and serrations. Use of enzymatic detergents will help break down the proteins found in body fluids and tissues. Water temperature should be warm but not hot. Heat coagulates protein, making it more difficult to remove. A critical component to promoting effective sanitization is to complete the procedure as soon as possible after contamination so that tissue or body fluids do not have the opportunity to dry on the instruments. Dried debris are more difficult to remove and may require much scrubbing. Instruments may be left to soak in disinfectant solution or water with a **solvent** if sanitization cannot be performed immediately after use (Figure 21-21).

To avoid the risk for punctures or cuts from sharp instruments during sanitization, heavy-duty gloves should be worn. Some facilities use an **ultrasonic cleaner** (Figure 21-22). It uses high-frequency sound waves and agitates the instruments (sanitizes them) before sterilizing them. Goggles are worn to protect eyes from splashing of contaminated debris during the scrubbing procedure. A plastic apron provides protection from splashing of clothing (see Chapter 30). Hot water may be used for rinsing to remove all residue and aid in the drying process. Check instruments to ensure they are in working condition. Drying thoroughly will prevent damage from rust or water spots.

Larger items such as instrument trays or Mayo stands, stools, chairs, examination tables, and lamps should also have a decontaminating sanitization process with thorough washing, rinsing, and drying.

TABLE 21-7

RECOMMENDATIONS FOR HAND HYGIENE*

THE FIVE MOMENTS	CONSENSUS RECOMMENDATIONS
1. Before touching a patient	• Before and after touching the patient
2. Before clean/aseptic procedure	• Before handling an invasive device for patient care, regardless of whether gloves are used • If moving from a contaminated body site to another body site during care of the same patient
3. After body fluid exposure risk	• After contact with body fluids or excretions, mucous membrane, nonintact skin, or wound dressing • If moving from a contaminated body site to another body site during care of the same patient • After removing sterile or nonsterile gloves
4. After touching a patient	• Before and after touching the patient • After removing sterile or nonsterile gloves
5. After touching a patient's surroundings	• After contact with inanimate surfaces and objects (including medical equipment) in the immediate vicinity of the patient • After removing sterile or nonsterile gloves

*Overview of the 2009 *WHO Guidelines on Hand Hygiene in Health Care*

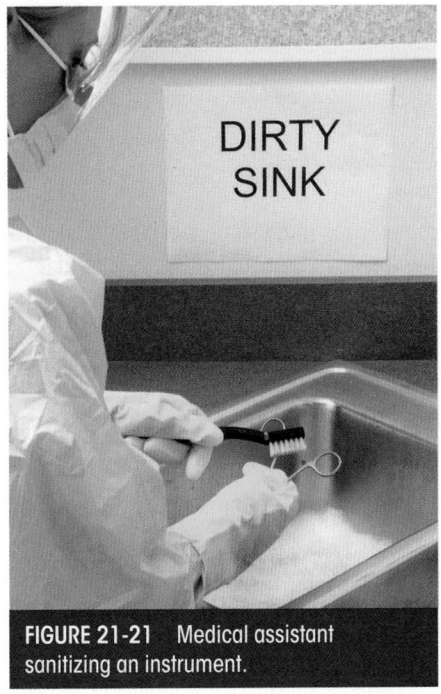

FIGURE 21-21 Medical assistant sanitizing an instrument.

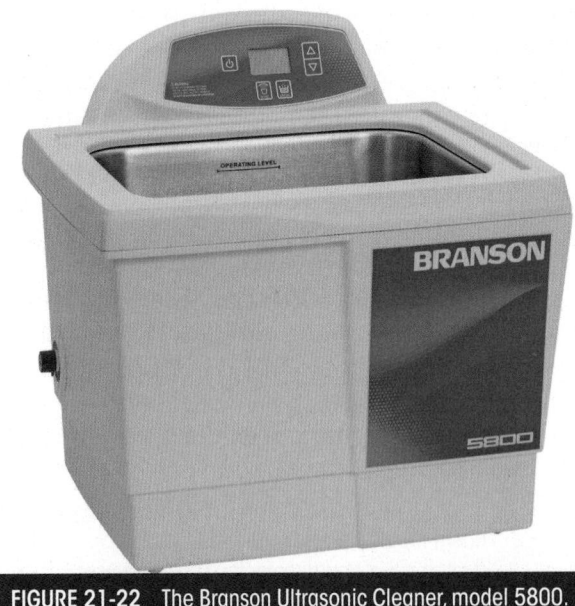

FIGURE 21-22 The Branson Ultrasonic Cleaner, model 5800.

Courtesy of Branson Ultrasonics Corporation

See Procedure 21-7 for instrument sanitization. Gloves contaminated with blood and body fluids should be removed carefully to contain the contamination.

Procedure 21-2 describes how to remove contaminated gloves, thereby preventing further exposure to biohazard substances.

PROCEDURE 21-7

Sanitization of Instruments

Procedure

STANDARD PRECAUTIONS:

Gloves   Biohazard   Goggles & Mask

PURPOSE:

To properly clean contaminated instruments to remove tissue and debris.

EQUIPMENT/SUPPLIES:

- Sink (or ultrasonic cleaner: follow manufacturer's instructions)
- Sanitizing agent (low-sudsing detergent, approved chemical disinfectant, or blood solvent)
- Brush
- Disposable paper towels
- Plastic apron
- Disposable gloves, heavy-duty if cleaning sharps

(continues)

- Goggles
- Biohazard waste container

PROCEDURE STEPS:

1. Wear heavy-duty gloves, goggles, and apron. RATIONALE: Contaminated instruments pose a blood and body fluid precaution as indicated by OSHA standards. Disposable gloves must always be worn to sanitize instruments. Wear heavy-duty gloves if cleaning sharp instruments. Goggles are worn to protect eyes from splashing of contaminated debris during the scrubbing procedure. A plastic apron provides protection from splashing of clothing.

2. As soon as possible after a procedure in which an instrument is contaminated, rinse the instrument in water and disinfectant solution; rinse again under running water. RATIONALE: Rinsing contaminated instruments as soon as possible after use removes debris and tissue that could quickly dry onto the instrument, making sanitization more difficult.

3. If contaminated instrument must be carried from one place to another for sanitization, place the instrument in a basin labeled Biohazard. RATIONALE: Do not carry contaminated instruments in your hands. Biohazard basins must be sanitized and disinfected daily according to procedures for Standard Precautions.

4. Scrub each instrument well with detergent and water; scrub under running water, and be sure to scrub inside any edges, serrations, and all surfaces. RATIONALE: Thorough scrubbing removes tissue and debris from all areas of the contaminated instrument. If all tissue is not removed with scrubbing, the instrument may not be sterilized during the sterilization procedures.

5. Rinse well with hot water. RATIONALE: Tissue and debris, as well as detergent, must be completely removed. Hot water will help remove all residue and aid in the drying process, and rust and water spots will be avoided.

6. After they are rinsed, place instruments on muslin or a disposable paper towel until all instruments have been scrubbed and rinsed. RATIONALE: Often more than one instrument is sanitized; do not place sanitized instrument in the bottom of the sink or on a countertop without a disposable paper towel or muslin towel.

7. Dry instruments with muslin or disposable paper towels. RATIONALE: Wet instruments may rust or corrode. Check instruments to ensure they are in working condition.

8. Remove gloves and wash hands.

Disinfection

Disinfection, a third procedure used in medical asepsis practices, consists of various chemicals that can be used to destroy many pathogenic microorganisms but not necessarily their spores. Disinfection chemicals are used on inanimate objects. Because of their **caustic** nature, these chemicals can irritate the skin and mucous membranes. Chemicals are used to disinfect items or equipment made from materials that could be damaged by heat or that are too large to fit into an autoclave, for example, stethoscopes, percussion hammers, examination tables, and Mayo trays and stands. These and other items that are chemically disinfected are used during *external* physical examination or procedures.

Boiling water (temperature 212°F) is considered a form of disinfection because it will kill some forms of microorganisms. It is important to note that this method *cannot* be considered a sterilization technique because the temperature is not high enough to kill the hepatitis virus, tuberculosis bacteria, or microbial spores. Boiling instruments is an archaic method of disinfection and is rarely used in today's medical settings.

Before chemical disinfection, articles must first be thoroughly sanitized and dried. Of special note are stainless steel gynecologic and proctologic examination instruments. These instruments are not sanitized with other instruments because of the risk for transmission of sexually transmitted diseases (STDs). They are sterilized in the autoclave after sanitization to eliminate transmission of microorganisms.

Chemical disinfectant solutions must be carefully prepared and used according to the manufacturer's instructions to ensure effective disinfectant properties. Medical clinics should use the disinfectant solution that best meets the needs of the ambulatory care setting as to the quantity of instruments to be disinfected, cost, preparation requirements, storage needs, and handling procedures. When choosing a chemical disinfectant solution, pay close attention to the manufacturer's report of the chemical disinfectant properties of the product. Some solutions are effective against a wide spectrum of microorganisms, whereas other solutions may be selective for certain common microorganisms. When chemically disinfecting, items must first be thoroughly sanitized and dried. Any debris or water left on the item being chemically treated will affect the chemical solution, thereby decreasing its effectiveness and compromising the disinfecting process.

For surfaces such as countertops, the least expensive and most readily available chemical is a 1:10 solution of ordinary household bleach (sodium hypochlorite). However, besides the obvious disadvantage of bleaching clothing, bleach is not easily rinsed, and it is effective only if the solution is mixed fresh daily. Nevertheless, its effectiveness is so highly respected that many medical laboratories depend almost entirely on bleach to chemically kill pathogens on countertops.

In summary, medical asepsis includes procedures for which all medical assistants must be responsible and qualified to incorporate into daily work practices. The responsibility for maintaining medical asepsis is the combined goal of the clinic staff and providers.

Sterilization

Instrument care includes sterilization. This is the most important part of infection control in any clinic or treatment facility (Table 21-8). One of the cardinal rules of infection control is "Do not disinfect when you can sterilize." The process of sterilization kills all microorganisms that are present on the surfaces and the working parts of instruments. Effectiveness of any sterilization process relies on several factors. Conditions must be present to effectively destroy living organisms. The design and operation of the equipment and the combination of temperature and sterilant must be effective to kill pathogens. Any devices or instruments that are to be sterilized must be sanitized first to reduce any biologic material that is present.

The CDC advocates the use of several sterilization methods. Those methods most commonly found in an ambulatory care setting are:

- *Steam.* Autoclaves are a common tool utilized in the ambulatory care setting. These devices utilize steam under pressure to deliver moist heat at a high temperature to kill all microorganisms by coagulating and changing the cellular proteins. There are strict guidelines that must be followed regarding the wrapping of instruments and the temperature (250 to 270°F), time (4 to 30 minutes based on temperature), and pressure (27 to 28 pounds of pressure) that are required to ensure 100% sterilization.

- *Liquid chemical sterilization.* This method is used to sterilize delicate or heat-sensitive devices that can be immersed. A germicidal solution and complete immersion for a prescribed period of time result in the death of microorganisms. There are a number of liquid chemicals that are commonly used. These include peracetic acid, glutaraldehyde, hydrogen peroxide, ortho-phthalaldehyde, and combinations thereof. There is a risk to health care providers who come into contact with these chemicals. Precautions should be taken to limit exposure to these hazardous materials. There are devices that are closed-processing systems that limit exposure to the liquid chemicals.

TABLE 21-8

MAXIMUM PROCESS FOR INFECTION CONTROL

MAXIMUM PROCESS	STETHOSCOPE	CHAIR	EAR SPECULUM	VAGINAL SPECULUM	FIBER OPTIC ENDOSCOPE	SURGICAL INSTRUMENT	SKIN
Sanitization	X	X	X	X	X	X	X
Chemical disinfection by wiping	X	X	X				
Chemical disinfection by soaking			X				
Sterilization					X	X	

BIOTERRORISM

Bioterrorism is the use of biologic weapons (pathogenic microorganisms) to create fear in people. A bioterrorism attack is the deliberate release of biologic agents (weapons) such as bacteria, viruses, and toxins to cause death or illness in people, plants, or animals (see Table 21-9). The agents can spread through the air, food, and water. Terrorists can easily obtain and use biologic agents. The agents can be very difficult to detect and difficult to protect against. They have no odor, are invisible, have no taste, and can be spread quietly. Only small amounts are needed to kill or cause serious illness to hundreds of thousands of people. The agents can be put into food and/or water, absorbed through or injected into the skin, and dispensed as aerosols. Some resultant diseases can be treated with pharmaceutical agents such as antibiotics and antitoxins.

TABLE 21-9

EXAMPLE OF AGENTS THAT COULD BE USED IN A BIOTERRORISM ATTACK

DISEASE	AGENT	TRANSMISSION	VACCINE AVAILABLE?	TREATMENT
Anthrax	Bacterium	Inhalation Not spread person to person	Yes, but not readily available	Antibiotics
Botulism (severe food poisoning)	Toxin	Toxin in food Not spread person to person	Antitoxin (state, local health departments, and CDC have)	Antitoxin should be given as soon as disease is suspected
Brucellosis	Bacteria (*Brucella*)	Ingestion Inhalation Entrance via skin/mucous membranes	None	Antibiotics
Cholera	Bacteria (*Vibrio cholerae*)	Ingestion	Two oral vaccines: Dukoral and ShanChol Not available in the United States Administration must be prequalified by WHO	Replacement of fluid and electrolytes Antibiotics
Ebola	Virus Four identified Ebola virus species that infect humans: • *Zaire* • *ebolavirus* • *Sudan ebolavirus* • *Taï forest* • *ebolavirus* • *Bundibugyo ebolavirus*	Direct contact with blood or body fluids, contaminated objects	None	Replacement of fluid and electrolytes Oxygen therapy Treatment of secondary infections
Escherichia coli (*E. coli*)	Bacteria (multiple strains)	Ingestion	None	Replacement of fluid and electrolytes Antidiarrheal medications Antibiotics (for some strains)

continues

Table 21-9 continued

DISEASE	AGENT	TRANSMISSION	VACCINE AVAILABLE?	TREATMENT
Q fever	Bacteria (*Coxiella burnetii*)	Inhalation	None	Antibiotics
Ricin (from the castor bean)	Toxin	Inhalation Ingestion Contact with open wounds	None	Treatment of symptoms
Salmonella	Bacteria Two species: • *Salmonella enterica* • *Salmonella bongori*	Ingestion	None	Antidiarrheal medications Antibiotics
Smallpox	Virus	Skin eruptions occur on arms, legs, feet, and face Virus settles in the nose and throat and spreads when infected person coughs, talks, or sneezes Can spread through ventilation systems, and contaminated clothes and bedding Highly contagious	Routine vaccination ended in 1972 Enough vaccine is stockpiled to immunize all U.S. citizens in the event of an emergency	FDA has approved a new smallpox vaccine that will be used in the event of a bioterrorism attack
Typhoid fever	Bacterium (*Salmonella typhi*)	Ingestion	Yes, commonly administered prior to traveling to typhoid-infected countries	Antibiotics

Education plays a vital role in raising awareness and increasing health care professionals' knowledge to aid them in being better prepared for threats to public health. Protection against the agents should be started early. PPE and high-efficiency particulate air (HEPA) filters will filter most biologic agents from the air. Antibiotics given even before the agent is identified help protect people, as do vaccines.

The Food and Drug Administration (FDA) has approved a new smallpox vaccine. The FDA said it is intended to inoculate people who are at high risk for exposure to smallpox, a highly contagious disease. The FDA said the vaccine could be used to protect people during a bioterrorism attack. There is no FDA-approved treatment for smallpox.

According to the CDC, the threat that biologic agents will be used is more likely now than it has been throughout history. The WHO, the CDC, the Department of Homeland Security, and state and local public health departments are excellent resources for more information about bioterrorism (see Chapter 8).

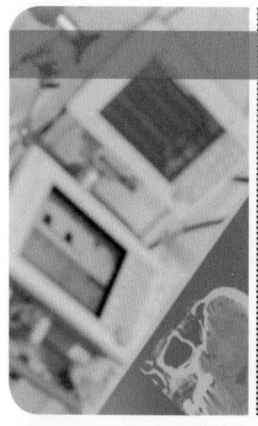

CASE STUDY 21-1

Refer to the scenario at the beginning of the chapter.

CASE STUDY REVIEW

1. Explain the importance of including the entire staff at the health care provider's clinic in the educational activity regarding infection control.
2. Make a list of Web sites that provide important information that is updated regularly on the current best practices for health care–associated infections and infection control.
3. What are some of the implications for failure to comply with CDC regulations in the health care setting?

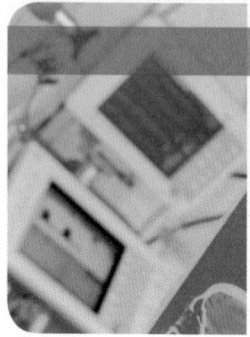

CASE STUDY 21-2

Your provider has asked you to take the lead in educating the staff on a monthly basis regarding cleaning and proper care of the instruments commonly used in the practice. Identify the appropriate care and methods of preventing the spread of pathogens and prepare one update that is appropriate for a general medicine practice.

CASE STUDY REVIEW

1. How often should this information be updated? Explain.

Summary

- Effective infection control measures are the first defense against the transmission of infectious diseases in the ambulatory care setting.

- Reliance on Standard and Transmission-Based Precautions, protective barriers, and basic principles of disinfection promotes professional and responsible clinical care for patients.

- When the processes of infection control are applied to all clinical procedures, the infection cycle may be broken by many varied means. Remember that an infectious disease will not spread to another person if the cycle is sufficiently broken at any stage.

- Infectious diseases spread and accidents occur through lack of education and carelessness.

- Medical assistants must understand the importance of the regulations and guidelines set forth by the federal government and follow through by helping employers and fellow employees implement them.

- The health and safety of patients and health care workers can be protected; the spread of infectious diseases can be kept under control; and the risk for contracting a serious infectious disease such as HIV, HBV, or HCV will be greatly minimized when health care professionals follow federal guidelines.

- Every medical clinic and ambulatory care setting must, by law, have clearly written and readily available manuals containing information about Standard Precautions and OSHA standards for the safe handling, storage, and disposal of blood, body fluids, and chemicals.

- Through consistent use of Standard Precautions and adherence to OSHA laws, health care providers can acquire the behaviors and techniques needed to safeguard themselves and their patients.

- It is necessary for medical assistants and all other health care providers to keep abreast of government mandates, as there are frequent changes in the law.

- All members of the health care team have a responsibility to protect their patients and themselves from infectious diseases.

- The medical assistant is an important part of the overall protection picture.

- The professional medical assistant must stay informed of changes in the practice of infection control.

Study for Success

To reinforce your knowledge and skills of information presented in this chapter:

- Review the *Key Terms* and *Learning Outcomes*
- Consider the *Critical Thinking* features and *Case Studies* and discuss your conclusions

Procedure

- Answer the questions in the *Certification Review*
- Perform the *Procedures* using the *Competency Assessment Checklists* on the *Student Companion Website*

CERTIFICATION REVIEW

1. Which governmental agency issued Standard Precautions?
   a. Health and Human Services
   b. Centers for Disease Control and Prevention
   c. Food and Drug Administration
   d. Occupational Safety and Health Administration

2. Which of the following is the primary concern of the Bloodborne Pathogen Standard?
   a. Reducing the transmission of HIV, HBV, and HCV infections
   b. Protecting the employer from lawsuits
   c. Regulating the use of personal protective equipment
   d. Taking blood samples from patients
   e. Protecting patients from needlesticks

3. The location of the infectious agent in the infection cycle is known as which of the following?
   a. Reservoir
   b. Portal of exit
   c. Portal of entry
   d. Means of transmission

4. The stage in infectious disease in which symptoms are vague and undifferentiated is called what?
   a. Incubation
   b. Prodromal
   c. Acute
   d. Onset of disease
   e. Convalescent

5. There are several types of infectious organisms. Which of the following are considered pathogens?
   a. Fomite
   b. Virus
   c. Bacteria
   d. Both b and c

6. Which of the following lists the correct order for the stages of infection?
   a. Prodromal, incubation, acute, declining, convalescent
   b. Incubation, prodromal, acute, declining, convalescent
   c. Acute, incubation, prodromal, convalescent, declining
   d. Declining, convalescent, acute, prodromal, incubation
   e. Acute, prodromal, incubation, convalescent, declining

7. Sneezing, coughing, and talking can produce which type of disease transmission?
   a. Contact
   b. Airborne
   c. Droplet
   d. Standard

8. Use of hand washing along with cleaning and disinfecting contaminated surfaces is known as what?
   a. Surgical asepsis
   b. Medical asepsis
   c. Sterilization
   d. Sanitization
   e. All of these

9. The CDC quotes the risk of infection with HIV from a single needlestick as what?
   a. 3%   c. 0.3%
   b. 30%   d. 10%

10. A cut on a healthy provider's finger would be considered which of the following stages in the infection cycle?
    a. Susceptible host
    b. Infectious agent
    c. Portal of entry
    d. Pathogen
    e. All of these

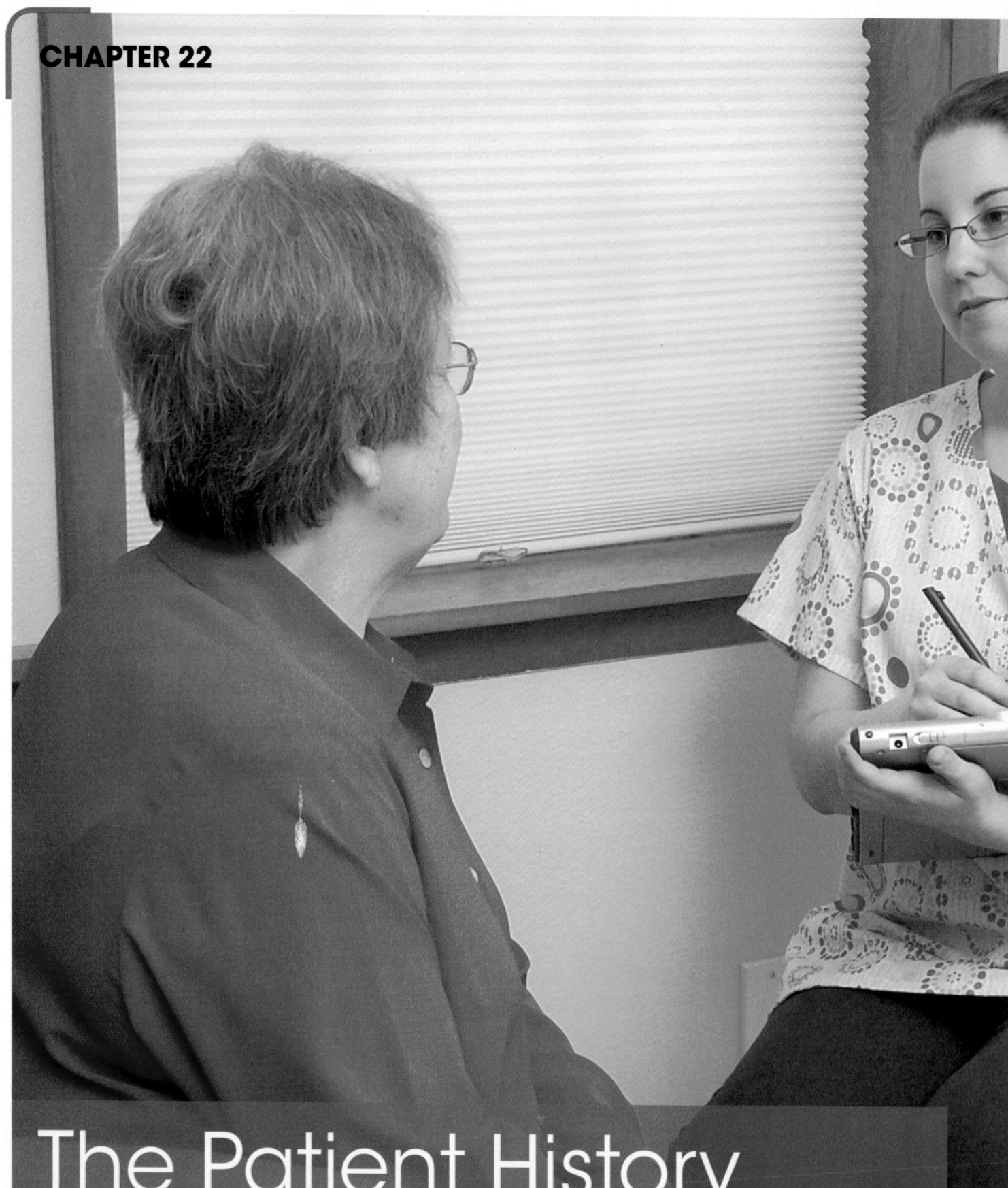

CHAPTER 22

The Patient History and Documentation

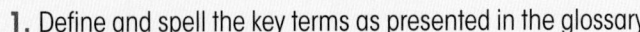

1. Define and spell the key terms as presented in the glossary.
2. Clarify the purpose of the medical history.
3. Recognize three tasks to complete prior to a patient's appointment.
4. Describe the four nonmedical information forms to be signed by patients.
5. Explain the medical assistant's general approach to the patient intake interview.
6. Identify at least four circumstances to address in displaying cultural awareness.
7. Formulate a strategy for communicating across the life span with patients.
8. List the components of the medical health history and their documentation.
9. Obtain a medical history from a patient.
10. Clarify the function and meaning of SOAP/SOAPER and CHEDDAR charting.
11. Discuss the characteristics of the patient's chief complaint and the present illness.
12. Compare and contrast the patient's medical, family, and social histories.
13. Explain the rationale for including adult immunizations in health histories.
14. Summarize how the review of systems is obtained and documented.
15. State five reasons the medical record is important.
16. Identify three areas of concern regarding HIPAA compliance and the patient's chart.
17. Recall the rules for charting and documenting in the patient's chart.
18. Compare/contrast SOMR and POMR.
19. State the advantages of electronic medical records.
20. Identify common charting abbreviations.
21. Describe the organization of a medical record.

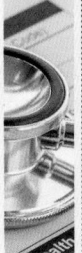

KEY TERMS

allergies	objective
CHEDDAR	problem-oriented medical record (POMR)
chief complaint (CC)	
clinical diagnosis	SOAP/SOAPIE/SOAPER/SOAPIER
DARP	source-oriented medical record (SOMR)
narrative charting	subjective

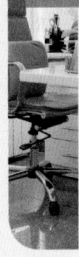

SCENARIO

When clinical medical assistant Joe Guerrero, CMA (AAMA), of Inner City Health Care takes a patient history, he typically uses a form custom designed for the clinic. Joe uses the form as a guideline to be sure he gathers all pertinent information. However, he has learned that he must tailor his questions to the patient and sometimes will rearrange the order of the questions if necessary. Although Joe is adept at gathering specific and necessary patient information, he also is aware of patient concerns and sensitivities and adapts his approach to accomplish the task while making the patient feel at ease.

A patient's medical record and all information in it, including the medical history, are key to competent medical care. Ideally, from the first encounter with the patient to any subsequent visits, all information regarding a patient's medical care is kept in one location—with the primary care provider.

The record created for all new patients will include a number of vital pieces of information. Established patients will have information updated upon each visit. Essential components of a complete medical record include present and past medical history, family and social history, chief complaints or problems, medications, allergies, laboratory results, summaries from other practitioners seen, and a host of other data related to the patient's health. A patient's record will also include demographic data, next of kin and their contact information, and current insurance details.

Often, a family practice or internal medicine clinic will have a new patient complete an extensive questionnaire that serves as the basis for the medical history. These questionnaires can be purchased with commonly asked questions relating to a patient's family as well as his or her social and medical history, or they can be created and customized by the practice, and they may be unique according to specialty. The questionnaire can be accessed via the clinic Web site; attached to an email to patients; or mailed to a patient's home address so that questions can be answered prior to the scheduled appointment, in the quiet environment of their homes, where they likely have access to the information requested. When patients are called the day before their appointment, they can be reminded to complete the questionnaire and to bring it with them to the appointment.

The role of the medical assistant in taking the patient history is to be as thorough as possible. It is important to obtain complete information that results in informed medical treatment and care.

The patient medical record is a collection of confidential patient information. Remember that even among the medical team, information is shared only if a team member is directly involved in a patient's care. Should a patient's medical record be introduced in court, it becomes a legal record of care given. It is always essential that charting in the record be accurate, clear, concise, and complete.

THE PURPOSE OF THE MEDICAL HISTORY

The medical history initiates the pathway for care. The information documented gives all providers that a patient might encounter a first glimpse at that patient's medical needs. Key components of the patient history are the chief complaint; history of the present illness; and the family, social, and medical history. The family history reveals conditions that the patient may be at risk of by listing medical events, diseases, and hereditary conditions. Aspects of a patient's personal life that have the potential to be clinically significant are included in the social history. Use of controlled substances, use of alcohol and tobacco, occupation, sexual preference, diet, and exercise are some pieces of information that are included in a social history. A patient's medical history reviews major illnesses, surgical procedures, hospitalizations, medications prescribed, allergies, and mental health issues. Documentation of this information is important for the provider in order to render care in an efficient and organized manner. It is considered a best practice to provide the patient history forms to the patient and/or his or her family for completion prior to the visit in order to use the appointment time most efficiently.

Legal

In addition, medical histories provide a base for statistical analysis for research, insurance data, and reporting infectious diseases to the health department. The health history and chart notes are a legal record of patient treatment. This is especially important if the patient makes an injury claim against another party or if the patient makes a malpractice claim against the provider. If the records in the chart are precise and correct, the chart becomes a good defense; however, if the charting or documentation is sloppy or incomplete, the entire record may be questioned as insufficient. The best policy is to document everything concerning patient care. See Chapter 13 for information on medical records management.

PREPARING FOR THE PATIENT

Before the patient's visit and obtaining the medical history, perform the following:

1. Make certain the examination room is clean, tidy, and ready for the patient.
2. Check to see that all necessary supplies are available according to the provider's preferences.
3. Review the patient's chart. Note the age, any possible need for assistance, and identified reason for the appointment.

When everything is ready, go to the reception area for the patient. It is preferable to call the patient's full name (John Nichols or Mr. Nichols) unless the patient previously requested the use of the first name or a nickname. Speak clearly and plainly, making certain that your patient will be able to hear. When the patient stands, quickly determine if assistance is necessary. (The physical assessment has begun.) If assistance is warranted, make that offer and accompany the patient to the examination room, remembering later to note in the chart the details of the assistance required. A friendly greeting is appreciated and helpful; a greeting such as, "How are you today?" may not be appropriate. Patients in the medical clinic generally are not feeling well and take that question seriously. Also, the reception area is not the appropriate place for the patient to begin sharing his or her medical issues. The following comments may be acceptable: "Did you have any trouble finding parking?" or "I really like the colors in the shirt you are wearing. They remind me of summer."

Communication

Once in the examination room with the door closed, seat the patient comfortably and sit face-to-face with the patient to begin the interview. Use the provided medical history forms as a basis for review of the patient's health history. Ask open-ended questions to explore areas of the history that might need more information for the provider. Find ways to build rapport with the patient, and speak directly and professionally. Maintain eye contact and respond positively, saying, "I see" or "Okay" as a way of establishing trust. Be sure to listen carefully and ask questions when clarification is needed. Give the patient time to answer your questions. Allowing uninterrupted time to express concerns enables your patient to be more open and complete.

A CROSS-CULTURAL MODEL

Diversity

It is important to understand that every patient interview is a cross-cultural one. Health and illness are inseparable from social and cultural beliefs. Who patients are—their background, their belief system, their family orientation, and their cultural heritage—influences their choices in health care. Providers and patients have different concerns and anticipations and view the gathering of the patient history and the personal visit differently. The medical assistant conducting the interview who is aware of these perspectives will keep the following in mind:

- *Patient's chief concern.* The illness. The personal and social significance and the problems created by the illness are important to the patient.
- *Provider's chief concern.* Disease. The provider is concerned with the malfunctioning and maladaptation of biologic and psychologic processes.
- *Patient's idea of treatment success.* A cure, if possible, is the patient's top desired outcome. However, being able to successfully manage an illness and its problems might be the best that can be hoped for.
- *Provider's idea of treatment success.* Successfully managing treatments, medications, and procedures to control disease problems.

The medical assistant may find it helpful to ask certain questions of patients to help him or her understand cultural influences, for example:

1. Do you have ideas about the cause of your problem?
2. When do you think it started?
3. What effect does it have on you?
4. What are your concerns about this problem?
5. What kind of treatment do you expect?

These questions respect the patient's perceptions while providing helpful information to the provider.

Integrity

Cross-cultural encounters can lead to significant ethical dilemmas when informed consent is required for a major test, procedure, or operation; when the truth about a terminal diagnosis is discussed; and when attitudes toward the role of the provider and the medical system arise in the context of a patient's mistrust. Recognition of a lack of understanding is key to successful care of the patient. The professional medical assistant plays a significant role in recognizing sociocultural differences such as spiritual beliefs, language barriers, and illiteracy, and making the provider aware if these exist.

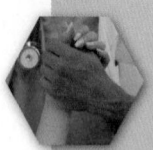
PATIENT INFORMATION FORMS

A number of important forms are created in the medical setting at the time of the first appointment.

Demographic Data Form

The demographic data form registers the patient's full name, address, mailing address if different, home and work telephone numbers, cell phone numbers, date of birth, a portion of the Social Security number, all insurance information, the person to be contacted in case of emergency, and a release of information signature.

Financial Information Form

Some facilities include the financial information form to be signed. This form contains information on the financial policy of the practice, including billing, insurance billing, co-payment billing, and any finance charges added to monthly billings.

Treatment Consent

It is a well-established principle that before treating a patient, a physician or other health care provider must obtain the consent of that patient. Treatment consent differs from informed consent. Consent to care or treatment serves as a blanket agreement to be seen by a provider; to be assessed; and to allow routine, minimally invasive procedures to be performed in the usual course of a medical office visit. Informed consent requires a conversation between the patient and the provider prior to an invasive procedure. Informed consent grants permission for procedures with knowledge of the possible consequences after a discussion of risks and benefits.

These forms may be combined to include the patient demographics, and the financial and treatment consent as illustrated in Figure 22-1.

Privacy Information Form

Since April 2004, the Health Insurance Portability and Accountability Act (HIPAA) privacy rule limited the circumstances in which individuals' protected health information (PHI) could be used or disclosed. It also required medical providers to give notice of their privacy practices to all patients. The notice must describe patients' rights, the facility's practices related to PHI, and where and how to file a complaint if patients feel their rights have been violated. Health care providers must make a good faith effort to obtain written acknowledgment from patients that the privacy notice was received. The privacy notice has a number of components and can be lengthy. Many facilities have printed their notice in a brochure format. Details of the privacy rule can be found on the Centers for Disease Control and Prevention Web site at www.cdc.gov by searching for "HIPAA Privacy Rule." Many varieties of privacy notices can be viewed online by searching for "HIPAA Privacy Notices."

There are civil penalties if a medical facility fails to comply with the privacy rule and criminal penalties if a person knowingly obtains or discloses PHI in violation of the HIPAA guidelines.

Release of Information Form

New patients may be asked to complete a release of information form (Figure 22-2) that is often created in the clinic. This form is sent to patients' former providers to obtain past medical records and in some cases can be used to

Patient Registration Form

Patient's Last Name	First (legal name)	First (Preferred name)	Middle Name
SMITH	JAMES	JIM	M

Address (Number, Street, Apt #)		City	State	Zip Code
2455 E. Front, Apt. 205		Napa	CA	94558

Mail will be sent to the address listed above, unless patient indicates a different address (leave blank if same as above)

Send mail to Address (Number, Street, Apt #)		City	State	Zip Code

Phone Options	Phone Number	Okay to leave detailed message	Call this number (circle one)
Home	(707) 221 - 4040	Yes _×_ No _____	(1st) 2nd 3rd choice
Cell	( ) -	Yes ____ No _____	1st 2nd 3rd choice
Work	(877) 833 - 7777	Yes ____ No _×_	1st (2nd) 3rd choice

Would you like to communicate by Email	Yes _×_ No __	Email Address	Jmsmith@email.com

Date of Birth	Gender	Last 4 digits Social Security Number
2/23/1965	Female ____ Male _×_	9009

Marital Status (*circle one*)	What is your preferred language / secondary language
(Single) / Married / Divorced / Widow / Partner	English

Race (*circle one*)	Ethnicity (*circle one*)
African American-Black / Asian / Bi-Multi-racial / Pacific Islander-Hawaiian / (Caucasian–White) / Native American Eskimo Aleut / Decline to state / Other	Hispanic-Latino / Non-Hispanic-Latino / Other

Religion		Organ Donor	Yes _____	No _____

Are you new to our practice	Who referred you to our practice	Who is your Primary Care Physician
Yes _×_ No _____	David Dodgin	Rebecca Ayerick

Additional Notes	No call after 8 pm

Emergency Contact

Emergency Contact's Name	Relationship to patient	Phone
Joan Smith	Mother	(510) 478 - 5151

On-Line Patient Portal Communication via Email

On-Line communication is used for non-urgent message/requests only. NVFHA uses secure technology to protect the privacy and confidentiality of your personal information. Only you, your physician, and authorized staff can read your message.

What is your preferred method of communication	Phone _×_ Letter _____ Patient Portal _____

Insurance Information

Subscriber (Insurance Holder) Name	Date of Birth	Relationship to patient	Subscriber Phone Numeber
James M. Smith	2/23/1965	Self	(707) 221 - 4040

Health Plan Information	Primary Health Plan	Secondary Health Plan
Health Plan Name	Blue Shield Cengage	
Health Plan Address	PO Box 32245, Los Angeles, CA, 90002	
Group Number	BCBS987	
Subscriber Number	BCBS987	

Elig Date From	1/1/2010	Copay	$ 25.00

Patient Employer Information

Employer Name & Address (Number, Street, Apt #, City, State, Zip Code)	Employer Phone Number
River Rock Casino, 3250 Highway 128, Geyersville, CA 95441	(877) 833 - 7777

Occupation	IT Support	Start Date	8/25/2009

Assignment of Benefits • Financial Agreement

I hereby give lifetime authorization for payment of insurance benefits to be made directly to Napa Valley Family Health Assoc., and any assisting physicians, for services rendered. I understand that I am financially resposible for all charges whether or not they are covered by insurance. In the event of default, I agree to pay all costs of collection, and reasonable attorney's fees. I hereby authorize this healthcare provider to release all information necessary to secure the the payment of benefits.

I further agree that a photocopy of this agreement shall be as vaild as the original.

Date: __XX/XX/20XX__   Your Signature: _____ *James M. Smith* _____

Method of Payment: ❑ Cash   ❑ Check   ❑ Credit Card

FIGURE 22-1 Sample patient demographic form.

AUTHORIZATION FOR RELEASE OF INFORMATION

Section A: Must be completed for all authorizations.

I hereby authorize the use or disclosure of my individually identifiable health information as described below.

I understand that this authorization is voluntary. I understand that if the organization authorized to receive the information is not a health plan or health care provider, the released information may no longer be protected by federal privacy regulations.

Patient name: _Hilda F. Goodman_   ID Number: _4309_

Identity of person/ organization disclosing protected health information

Persons/organizations providing information:
Practon Medical Group, Inc
4567 Broad Avenue
Woodland Hills, XY 12345-4700

Persons/organizations receiving information:
Jennifer P. Lee, MD
400 North M Street
Anytown, XY 54098-1235

Identity of those authorized to use protected health information

Specific description of information [including from and to date(s)]:
Complete medical records from 4-22-XX to 9-15-XX

Specific description of information to be used or disclosed with dates

Section B: Must be completed only if a health plan or a heath care provider has requested the authorization.

Purpose for disclosure

1. The health plan or health care provider must complete the following:
   a. What is the purpose of the use or disclosure?____Patient relocating to another city____

   b. Will the health plan or health care provider requesting the authorization receive financial or in-kind compensation in exchange for using or disclosing the health information described above? Yes__ No _X_

2. The patient or the patient's representative must read and initial the following statements:
   a. I understand that my health care and the payment for my health care will not be affected if I do not sign this form.

   Initials: __hfg__

   b. I understand that I may see and copy the information described on this form if I ask for it, and that I get a copy of this form after I sign it.

   Initials: __hfg__

Section C: Must be completed for all authorizations.

The patient or the patient's representative must read and initial the following statements:

Expiration date

1. I understand that this authorization will expire on _12_ / _31_ / _20XX_ (DD/MM/YR).

   Initials: __hfg__

Individual's right to revoke this authorization in writing

2. I understand that I may revoke this authorization at any time by notifying the providing organization in writing, but if I do not it will not have any effect on any actions they took before they received the revocation.

   Initials: __hfg__

Rediclosure conditions

3. I understand that any disclosure of information carries with it the potential for an unauthorized rediclosure and the information may not be protected by federal confidentiality rules.

   Initials: __hfg__

Individual's signature

_____Hilda F. Goodman_____   _____September 15, 20XX_____
Signature of patient or patient's representative   **Date**
(Form MUST be completed before signing)

Date of signature

Printed name of patient's representative:_____

Relationship to the patient:_____

YOU MAY REFUSE TO SIGN THIS AUTHORIZATION
You may not use this form to release information for treatment or payment except
when the information to be released is psychotherapy notes or certain research information.

FIGURE 22-2 Authorization for release of medical information.

allow sharing of information with family members at the request of the patient.

Under most managed care insurance policies, patients have one primary care provider (women may also have an obstetrician/gynecologist) who coordinates the patient's health care.

Medical History Form

The medical health history form can be as short as one page (8½ inches × 11 inches) or as long and detailed as six to eight pages.

The best form is neither too long nor too complicated. Patients may feel overwhelmed with a long form and may not finish it, stating they cannot remember all the information. A form that is simple and brief can provide adequate information in many instances. Some patients find a history form intimidating. It is often easier for these patients to talk directly with the medical assistant or the provider about the history, feeling a one-to-one exchange is more personal and private.

Many samples of health history forms can be viewed on the Internet. Facilities often utilize a patient portal to allow online completion, or for the form to be printed for manual completion. Again, patients are encouraged to complete this form prior to arrival for their first appointment. Depending on the ambulatory care setting, this form can be tailored to include vaccines and immunizations, usage of recreational drugs, exercise and diet regimens, accident information (especially if patient was hurt on the job), and any other information suited to the provider's specialty. Health history forms can be printed in other languages, such as Spanish.

ELECTRONIC HEALTH HISTORY

Health care facilities may use electronic health histories as a part of the patient's health record. These can be of two types: patient generated and provider generated. In patient-generated health histories, the patient responds via a patient portal to various questions and then reviews information with the medical assistant for completeness at the time of the visit. Patients who do not have access to or do not want to use the electronic health history should be given the option of answering the questions face-to-face. When using a provider-generated health history, the medical assistant completes the information on the screen during the patient interview. These programs are user friendly and save time for both the patient and medical assistant. The medical assistant should remember to interact with the patient by looking up from the computer from time to time during the entry of information (Figure 22-3). It is easy to forget to look at patients as you ask questions and enter the information. This habit can make the patient feel disconnected from the process.

THE PATIENT INTAKE INTERVIEW

Interacting with the Patient

Communication

Presentation

When the medical assistant takes the medical history, the first responsibility is to put the patient at ease. A comfort level

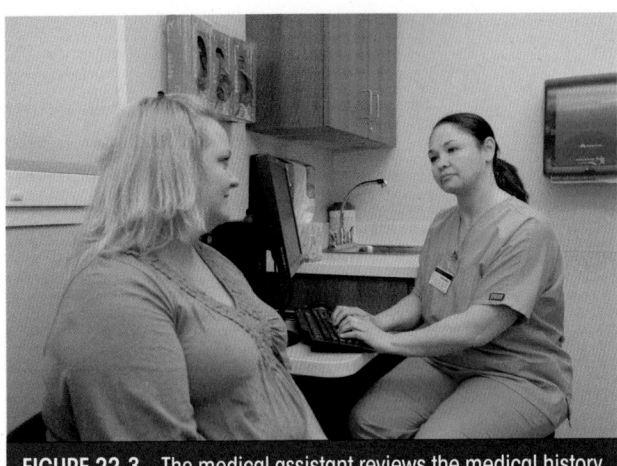
FIGURE 22-3 The medical assistant reviews the medical history with a patient while still maintaining eye contact.

must be developed as the medical assistant guides the conversation, keeps it on track, and obtains the most information for the provider. Allowing the conversation to wander, talking about other people, or letting the patient tell anecdotes does not help to complete the history. Also, refrain from sharing your own experiences with a particular diagnosis or set of symptoms. Explaining a term or concept that the patient does not understand is helpful. The medical assistant must remain professional and not be embarrassed or made uncomfortable by the patient's answers regarding illnesses, actions, or personal choices.

If the patient is already an established patient but has not seen the provider for several months or longer, update the medical history by asking if any illnesses have occurred in the time elapsed, if any new medications have been added by other providers, if any new allergies to any medications or other substances have occurred, and what the reaction was to each. Document the chief complaint for the current visit. The **chief complaint (CC)** is the problem that brings the patient to the provider. Sometimes patients bring several problems to discuss.

Depending on the appointment schedule for the day, this may be difficult to accomplish. If there is time in the schedule, every effort should be made to accommodate patients. However, the medical assistant notes the chief complaint before the provider sees the patient to ensure the main problem is addressed. Use of the electronic medical record (EMR) makes the patient intake process much easier. The data can be entered during the communication exchange between the medical assistant and the patient. Some settings allow the patient to see the data as they are entered.

Displaying Cultural Awareness

Diversity   Integrity

Remembering a cross-cultural model, the medical assistant begins the encounter with the patient aware that cultural differences and other problems may inhibit communication. Any number of situations may arise that the medical assistant must be prepared to address. The medical assistant will overcome major obstacles if it is known in advance the patient does not speak English as a first language, is hearing impaired and requires an interpreter, is from a culture in which the female patient does not disrobe for a male provider, or has a mental disorder that makes communication difficult.

If there is a language difficulty, the medical assistant may be required to arrange for an interpreter. There are language interpreters in most locales; especially in large urban areas, an interpreter might be found for nearly any language. A list of medical interpreter resources can be found at http://xculture.org by searching for "Medical Interpreter Services Resource Guide." If the patient is receiving medical care through Medicaid, special arrangements can be made for an interpreter through the state agency administering the program. Often the patient will bring a family member to interpret; however, if the matter is personal, the patient may not want to reveal personal matters with the family member present and may prefer an outside, objective interpreter. If the interpreter comes to the clinic as a contractor, a business associate contract should be completed to comply with HIPAA regulations. The contract is not necessary for a family member, a volunteer, or a clinic employee serving as an interpreter.

The medical assistant will direct their attention toward and listen attentively to the patient. The patient may be uneasy talking to the provider and may be more comfortable telling the medical assistant about problems. Medical assistants can play an important part in the medical practice by listening and communicating with both the patient and the provider.

Being Sensitive to Patient Needs

Professional

Some patients are frightened, hostile, or depressed. It is important to be open to nonverbal and verbal communication in answer to questions. Some patients react positively to a hand placed gently on the forearm; it calms and reassures them. Others have a negative response, pulling away from any such contact. The professional medical assistant uses nonverbal cues, such as eye contact and facial expressions, in determining the appropriate level of physical contact. Maintaining a professional boundary with the patient is essential. Boundaries respect the patient's needs for privacy, nurturing, validation, and separation (see Chapter 4 for additional information).

The medical assistant will know when to touch the patient appropriately, always with permission either expressed or implied. If the medical assistant tells the patient a blood pressure reading is next and reaches for the patient's arm and the patient extends an arm, permission to take the reading is implied. If, however, the patient pulls away and states no blood pressure is to be taken, permission is not given, and the reading must not be done at that time. Do not proceed at this time against the patient's wishes. The appropriate course of action is to chart "patient refused."

Attempting to get information from a reluctant patient can be difficult and requires patience and understanding. If the patient is hesitant to discuss a problem, it is better not to press for information. Pressing for information may make the patient become defensive or angry and can impair communication altogether. Make your provider aware of the patient behaviors that you observe so that he or she may be prepared to interact with the patient.

A patient may come to the clinic upset and crying. Care must be taken to attend to the emotional needs of this patient. Allowing the patient time to vent and giving choices will allow the patient to feel more in control. Sometimes, just taking a few moments to sit with such patients until they feel more settled is enough to calm them and enable the history-taking interview to proceed.

Creating a collaborative patient–provider relationship is the basis for effective treatment. There are multiple reasons for a patient's reluctance to communicate such as fear, denial, or hopelessness. Uncommunicative patients require special questioning techniques. Gentle encouragement, tentative guesswork, explanations of your reasons for seeking information, and reinforcement of your commitment to confidentiality are tools to utilize in this situation. If a relative has accompanied the patient to the appointment, it may be appropriate initially to have the relative present with the patient. In this way, the patient has a familiar face in the unfamiliar, often frightening, clinic. It is always the patient's decision whether anyone else is to be in the room. If the patient seems hesitant to answer with the relative present, it is perfectly acceptable to politely excuse the family member from the exam room to facilitate more open responses.

Approaching Sensitive Topics

Communication

Some of the most sensitive topics addressed in the health history include the use of alcohol, recreational drugs or chemicals, smoking, dietary habits, obesity, and sexual practices. An honest reporting on these topics can be important to the patient's well-being and treatment. Consider:

- Assuring the patient that the environment is private and free from distractions.
- Asking these questions in the later stages of the interview after rapport has been established.
- Using casual, direct eye contact without staring; this demonstrates the importance of the topic to the patient and your lack of embarrassment.
- Posing questions in a matter-of-fact tone.
- Adopting a nonjudgmental demeanor.
- Using the communication technique of "normalizing" when appropriate (e.g., "Some high school students drink alcohol/use drugs/engage in sexual relationships on a regular basis. Does this happen at your school? With you?").
- Assuring the patient that the information is an essential part of planning care and that all answers will be kept confidential.

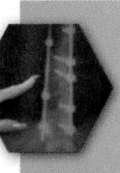

Critical Thinking

With two others in your class, role play a scenario where one person is the patient, another is the medical assistant, and the third is an observer. A social history is being taken. As the medical assistant, you ask the patient about the use of any recreational drugs or chemicals. The patient responds, "Yes." What additional questions will you ask the patient? What will you include in the medical record?

If the medical assistant can enhance communication with the patient, communication between the provider and the patient will be more effective.

COMMUNICATION ACROSS THE LIFE SPAN

Keep in mind your patient's age when communicating and seeking information for the medical history. See the "Communication Across the Life Span" Quick Reference Guide for more details.

Chapters 26 and 28 have helpful suggestions for communicating with children and with older adults.

⠶ QUICK REFERENCE GUIDE

≫ COMMUNICATION ACROSS THE LIFE SPAN

Professional

≫ GENERAL CONSIDERATIONS AT ALL AGES

- Observe verbal and nonverbal cues
- Take time to establish rapport
- Give the patient/parents your full attention
- Speak directly and clearly
- Frequently check with the patient/family for understanding
- Have the patient/parents demonstrate understanding of any instructions by asking for return verbalization

- Address the patient as a whole person, not just as a diagnosis
- Maintain eye contact with the patient
- Select and maintain an appropriate environment for communication
- Remind patients that all communication is confidential
- Keep a goal of building a relationship consistently at the forefront of each interaction
- Make sure the pace of communication matches the patient's cognitive level
- Offer reassurance during communication at all age levels
- Demonstrate empathy

(continues)

Age Group	Developmental Stages	Communication Considerations
Children 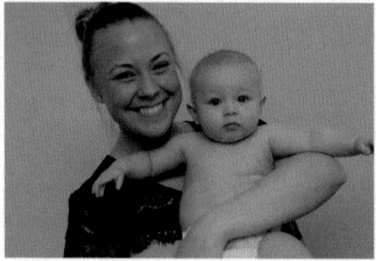	**Erikson's psychosocial theory** • Trust vs. mistrust (infancy) • Autonomy vs. shame and doubt (early childhood) • Initiative vs. guilt (ages 3 to 5 years) • Industry (competence) vs. inferiority (ages 5 to 12 years) **Freud's psychosexual theory** • Oral stage: birth to 18 months • Anal stage: 18 months to three years • Phallic stage: 3 years to 7 to 8 years • Latency stage: 7 to 8 years to puberty **Piaget's cognitive theory** • Sensorimotor stage (birth to 2 years) • Preoperational stage (2 to 7 years) • Concrete operational stage (7 to 11 years) • Formal operational stage (11 years and over)	• Consider the stage of development and utilize your knowledge of this stage when communicating with the patient/parent. • Remember that each child is different with different needs. • Speak to the child using words and delivery appropriate to the child's developmental stage. • Move slowly and announce touch prior to touching the child. • Use your imagination, tapping into the inner child all of us have to find creative ways to communicate. • Involve the child as much as possible in communication about his or her health. • Address the child using his or her name.
Adolescents 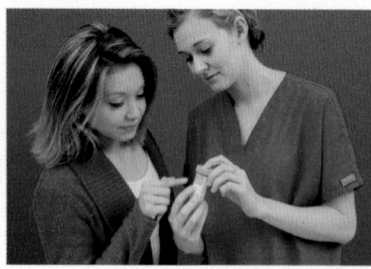	**Stages of adolescence** • Early (approximately 11 to 14 years old) • Middle (approximately 15 to 17 years old) • Late (approximately 18 to 21 years old) **Aspects of adolescent development** • Physical: puberty • Emotional: establishing independence, autonomy, conflict resolution	• Consider the stage of development and utilize your knowledge of this stage when communicating with the patient/parent. • Respect the older adolescent's private personal information that might be solely between the patient and the provider. • Support and accept the patient's self-concept. • Treat the patient with dignity and respect. • Independence from parents and authority is important. Allow this as appropriate.

(continues)

Age Group	Developmental Stages	Communication Considerations
	• Intellectual: increasing ability to reflect on long-term consequences of decisions and increased capacity to solve complex problems • Social: building relationships beyond the nuclear family **Erikson's psychosocial theory** • Identity vs. role confusion (ages 12 to 18 years) **Freud's psychosexual theory** • Genital stage: puberty to adulthood	• Communicate at the level of the patient's understanding and check in frequently to see if there are questions. • Carefully observe for signs of depression such as withdrawn affect, tearfulness, slowed thinking, speaking or body movements, and irritability.
Adults 	**Erikson's psychosocial theory** • Intimacy vs. isolation (ages 18 to 40 years) • Generativity vs. stagnation (ages 40 to 65 years) **Jung's theory** • Youth (puberty to 35 or 40 years) • Middle life (40 to 60 years)	• Consider the stage of development and utilize your knowledge of this stage when communicating with the patient. • Treat the patient with dignity and respect. • Recall that adults have had experiences with health care in the past that might be positive or negative. • Respect the adult's lifestyle choices.
Older Adults 	**Erikson's psychosocial theory** • Ego integrity vs. despair (ages 65 and older) **Jung's theory** • Old age (60 years and older)	• Consider the stage of development and utilize your knowledge of this stage when communicating with the patient. • Adapt communication to accommodate and sensory deficits (i.e., vision or hearing changes). • Avoid the stereotypical treatment of the older adult (e.g., people are not weak and sick). • Consider that fear of mortality is common in this age group. • Allow extra time to share information. • Stick to one topic at a time. • Write down patient instructions.

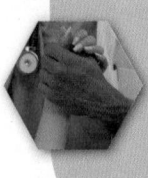
THE MEDICAL HEALTH HISTORY

The patient's medical health history contains the following components:

- Personal data from the demographic form
- Chief complaint as noted at each visit by the medical assistant
- Present illness
  - Medications
  - Allergies
  - Other providers or alternative therapy practitioners being seen
- Medical history
- Family history
- Social and occupational history
- Review of systems by physician or provider

SOAP/SOAPI/SOAPIER/SOAPER AND CHEDDAR

The **SOAP/SOAPI/SOAPER/SOAPIER** method of charting was introduced in Chapter 13. SOAP charting is very common (Figure 22-4); SOAPER, SOAPI, or SOAPIER is increasing in popularity and is often used in clinics attached to teaching and research hospitals. **CHEDDAR** is another approach to charting that may be used. These charting methods encourage more comprehensive charting and make evaluating and managing the levels of service easier to document.

SOAP/SOAPI/SOAPER/SOAPIER stands for the following:

S Subjective data; patient's complaint in his or her own words

O Objective, observable, measurable findings

A Assessment; probable diagnosis based on subjective and objective factors

P Plan for treatment, medications, instructions, return visit information

I Implementation, or how the actions were carried out

E Education for the patient

R Response of patient to education and care given or Revision of the plan

---

NAME: Dennis Finchhatten
DOB: 1/22/1949
AGE: 67
VISIT DATE: 4/4/2016

SUBJECTIVE:
"I feel pretty good since my last visit. I haven't been dizzy or had that annoying headache."

OBJECTIVE:
B/P: 148/66 rt arm sitting, P: 72, R: 16, T: 98.4° F

ASSESSMENT:
Vital signs within normal limits.

PLAN:
Reinforce patient education regarding antihypertensive medications.

FIGURE 22-4   Sample of a SOAP follow-up visit note.

Courtesy of Harris CareTracker PM and EMR

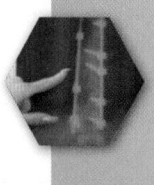
CHEDDAR charting encourages greater detail to SOAP/SOAPER. CHEDDAR stands for the following:

C Chief complaint, presenting problems, subjective information

H History, social and physical, of presenting problem; contributing data

E Examination; body systems reviewed

D Details of problem(s) and complaint(s)

D Drugs and dosages; list of current medications, dosages, frequency

A Assessment; diagnostic evaluation, further testing, medications

R Return visit, if applicable

The medical assistant and the primary care provider in attendance to the patient both contribute to the completeness of the medical history using SOAP/SOAPER and CHEDDAR.

Components of the Medical History

As previously mentioned, there are several components that make up a patient's medical history. For more information on each component, please see the "Components of the Medical History" Quick Reference Guide.

Each piece of the patient's medical history documents integral parts of the patient's health. If any part is lacking, the current understanding of the patient's health is not complete.

Procedure 22-1 gives the steps for taking a medical history.

Procedure

THE PATIENT RECORD AND ITS IMPORTANCE

Legal

The patient's record is a collection of confidential information that concerns the patient, care given to the patient, patient progress, and laboratory and other diagnostic test results that have been completed. If paper charting is used, this information is secured in a file folder or binder. The EMR is housed on a secure server and is viewed at the PC or Mac workstation. It is used for a variety of purposes, but primarily the record provides a foundation for planning patient care and making decisions about patient care. Other purposes for a medical record include using it as a basis for communication among caregivers, for statistical analysis in research, and for reporting infectious diseases to the health department. It is also a legal document and belongs to the provider or the agency at which the provider is employed. Chapters 6 and 13 discuss legal guidelines and medical records. Because it is a legal document, the medical record can be used to determine if patient care has been given according to the standards of care that the law recognizes; therefore, it must be complete, concise, accurate, and understandable. Many important items of information must be placed in the patient record and the medical assistant will be one of the professionals making chart entries.

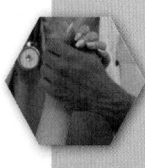

QUICK REFERENCE GUIDE

COMPONENTS OF THE MEDICAL HISTORY

Component	Details and Considerations
Chief complaint (CC); the specific reason that the patient came to see the provider	Keep in mind that the chief complaint needs to be descriptive and specific. • A **subjective** complaint is from the patient's perspective. Quote their exact words. • An **objective** complaint is from the perspective of the observer.

EHR Sample

Subjective Complaint

Courtesy of Harris CareTracker PM and EMR

Objective Complaint

Courtesy of Harris CareTracker PM and EMR

(continues)

Component

History of present illness (HPI): expanded information about the chief complaint

Details and Considerations

- *Location.* The anatomical area where the symptom is located.
- *Radiation.* Identifying how large an area the symptom covers.
- *Quality.* Describes the characteristic of the symptom.
- *Severity/character.* How bothersome is it? How much does it interfere with daily living? When the symptom is pain, patients may be asked to identify the pain on a scale of 1 to 10, with 10 being the most severe.
- *Associated symptoms.* Allows the patient to describe what other minor symptoms accompany the chief complaint.
- *Aggravating factors and alleviating factors.* Describes what makes the symptoms worse and what makes the symptoms decrease; this includes things that the patient has already done to treat the problem and if any medications have been taken for the symptoms.
- *Setting and timing.* When the symptoms started and what the patient was doing at symptom onset.

Use the patient's own words (subjective) when recording this information.

Additional questions that might be included at the request of the provider:
- Are you allergic to anything?
- Are there any other problems you are experiencing at this time?
- What medications are you taking? (Be sure to include over-the-counter medications, vitamins, and herbal supplements.)

EHR Sample

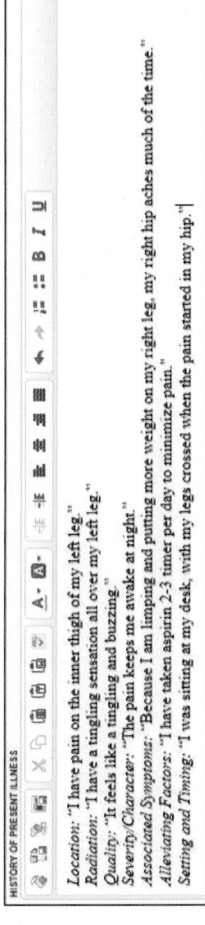

HISTORY OF PRESENT ILLNESS

Location: "I have pain on the inner thigh of my left leg."
Radiation: "I have a tingling sensation all over my left leg."
Quality: "It feels like a tingling and buzzing."
Severity/Character: "The pain keeps me awake at night."
Associated Symptoms: "Because I am limping and putting more weight on my right leg, my right hip aches much of the time."
Alleviating Factors: "I have taken aspirin 2-3 times per day to minimize pain."
Setting and Timing: "I was sitting at my desk, with my legs crossed when the pain started in my hip."

Courtesy of Harris CareTracker PM and EMR

(continues)

Component

Medical history (MH); includes all the patient's health problems, major illnesses, and surgeries and all current medications with dosages (if not included in history of present illness above)

Details and Considerations

Medications have side effects and contraindications that can affect patients.

Allergies (abnormal reaction to an ordinarily harmless substance) to medications can be serious and need to be noted in a readily visible part of the chart.

The information needs to be updated at least annually.

Update immunizations for adults at this time.

Childhood immunizations are regularly checked in pediatric examinations.

Questions that might be included at the request of the provider:
- Have you had any allergic reactions to environmental factors, medications, or foods since your last visit?
- Are you up to date with your immunizations? (For adults: tetanus, flu, pneumonia, HPV, shingles, hepatitis, and meningitis; for children: hepatitis A and B, rotavirus, DPT, flu, pneumonia, polio, MMR, chicken pox, meningitis, and HPV.)

EHR Sample

| History | Patient History | Sensitive Info | Family History | Advance Dir | Attachments | Log | Preview |

Reviewed +/- Clear All

☑ Medication List Reviewed   ☑ Past Medical History Reviewed
☑ Allergy List Reviewed   ☐ Social History Reviewed
☑ Problem List Reviewed   ☐ Family History Reviewed
☐ Denies significant past history.   ☐ No recent change in medical history.

GENERAL MEDICAL HISTORY +/- Clear All

Y N Alcoholism		Y N Depression	Y N Kidney Infections
☑ Y N Allergies/Hayfever		Y N DM Type 1	Y N Kidney stone
Y N Anemia		Y N DM Type 2	Y N Migraine
Y N Anxiety		Y N Epilepsy	Y N Multiple Sclerosis
Y N Asthma		Y N Fracture	Y N Obesity
Y N Atrial Fibrillation		Y N Gastric ulcer	Y N Old MI
Y N Blood Transfusions		Y N Gastrointestinal Disease	Y N Osteoarthritis
Y N CAD		Y N GERD	Y N Osteoporosis
Y N Cancer		Y N Gestational Diabetes	Y N Pneumonia
Y N Cardiac Pacer		Y N Glaucoma	Y N Progressive Neurological Disorder
Y N Cardiovascular Disease		Y N Heart Murmur	Y N Pulmonary Disease
Y N CHF		Y N Hepatitis	Y N Rheumatic Fever
Y N Cirrhosis		Y N High Cholesterol	Y N Rheumatoid Arthritis
Y N Colitis		Y N Hyperlipidemia	Y N STD
Y N COPD		Y N Hypertension	Y N Terminal Illness
Y N CRF		Y N Hyperthyroidism	Y N Thyroid Disease
Y N Crohn's disease		Y N Hypothyroidism	Y N TIA
Y N CVA		☑ Y N Joint Pain	Y N Tuberculosis

HOSPITALIZATIONS

a. Tonsillectomy at age 3. Doesn't know which hospital.
b. No other hospitalizations.

Courtesy of Harris CareTracker PM and EMR

(continues)

Component

Details and Considerations

Family history (FH): explores medical problems of siblings, parents, and grandparents; the provider is alerted to hereditary and familial diseases and disorders

The family history can provide clues to the patient's present condition.

Present ages of siblings, parents, and grandparents or causes of their death and age at time of death are noted.

Be aware of cultural differences when discussing family history.

Ask open-ended questions such as:
- How is your mother's health?
- Can you describe the health of your sisters and brothers?

EHR Sample

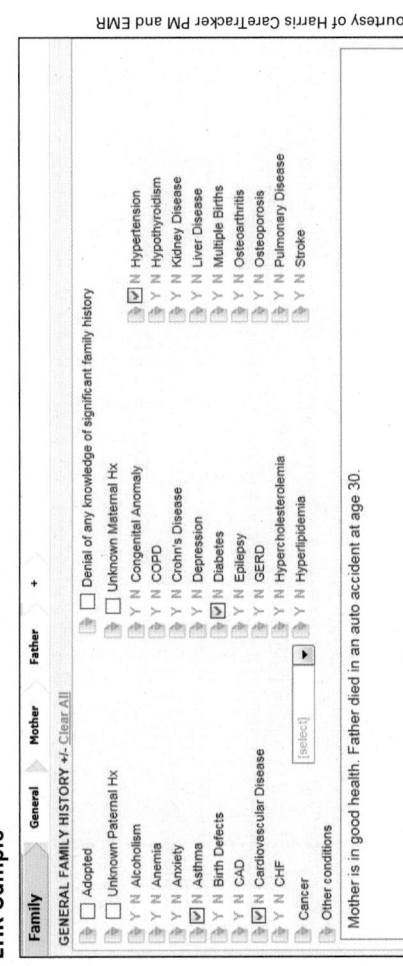

Courtesy of Harris CareTracker PM and EMR

Social history (SH): includes spouse/partner status; sexual habits; occupation; hobbies; and use of alcohol, tobacco, and recreational drugs or other chemical substances

Patients may not want to answer questions pertaining to sexual history.

Ask if discussing sexual activity with the provider would make the patient more comfortable.
- Do you feel comfortable answering a few questions about your sexual history now?
- If you would be more comfortable, you can discuss these sensitive subjects with the provider only.

(continues)

(continues)

(continues)

Component

Include those lifestyles and behaviors that may put the patient at greater risk for injury or disease than would normally be found from factors in the family history and medical history

Details and Considerations

The adolescent patient may refuse to answer questions of a sexual matter or may provide false answers if the parent or caregiver is present. It may be best to ask the parent or caregiver to leave the room at the completion of the health history so that you can ask the patient if there is anything else to note in the sexual history.

- Could I ask you, Mom, to leave us for a few minutes? If you will take a seat in the waiting area, I will come and get you in a few minutes.

Be alert for cues that demonstrate the patient's desire for knowledge on sexual matters, such as questions or requests for written information.

- Do you have any questions or can I provide any information about the sexual aspects of your life that I can answer for you?

It may be necessary to inquire about the patient's home environment. Be attentive for clues that signal the necessity of performing an in-depth home environment assessment.

- Can you describe your living situation to me?
- What kind of things make you scared when you are at home?

Be attentive to poor hygiene, frequent infections, smoke inhalation, burns, malnutrition, and falls (especially in older adults).

- I notice that you have a burn on your arm. How did that happen?

EHR Sample

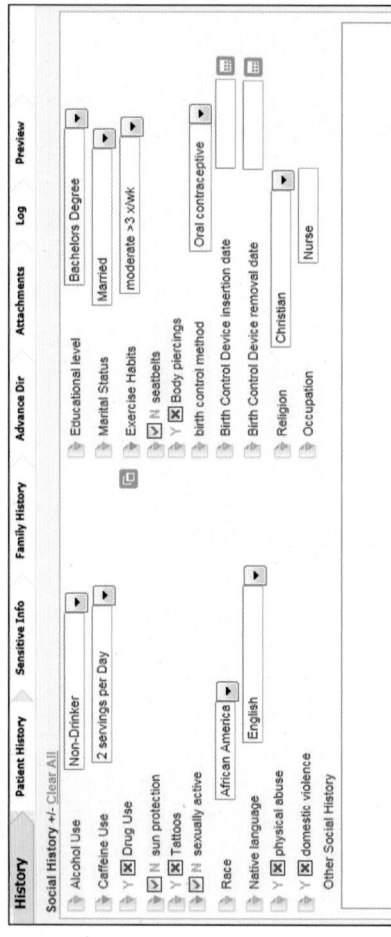

Courtesy of Harris CareTracker PM and EMR

(continues)

Component

Review of symptoms (ROS); performed

in conjunction with the physical examination, helps elicit information that is essential to the diagnosis of disease

Details and Considerations

Extent of ROS is determined by the nature of the visit.

ROS will be more extensive for a first visit and more focused for an established patient with a simple chief complaint.

The provider usually begins with an overall assessment and proceeds to check each body system in an organized manner, for example:

- Integumentary
- Ear, nose, throat
- Neurologic
- Endocrine
- Cardiovascular/vascular
- Respiratory
- Hematologic/lymphatic
- Gastrointestinal
- Genitourinary
- Musculoskeletal system

See Table 22-1 for more details.

The provider may order laboratory tests based on the review of symptoms and the probable diagnosis. These results, together with the history, examination, and patient symptoms, help to determine a **clinical diagnosis** (diagnosis made on the basis of medical signs and patient-reported symptoms).

EHR Sample

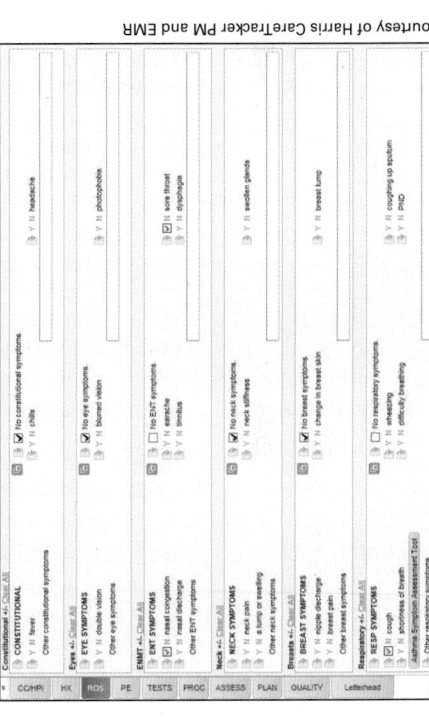

Courtesy of Harris CareTracker PM and EMR

TABLE 22-1

REVIEW OF SYSTEMS

General	Patient's perception of general state of health at the present time; difference from usual state; vitality and energy levels
Neurological	Headache, change in balance, change in coordination, loss of movement, change in sensory perception/feeling in an extremity, change in speech, change in smell, fainting, loss of memory, tremors, involuntary movement, loss of consciousness, seizures, weakness, head injury, disorientation, dizziness
Psychological	Irritability, nervousness, tension, increased stress, difficulty concentrating, mood changes, suicidal thoughts, depression
Integumentary	Rashes, itching, changes in skin pigmentation, black and blue marks, change in color or size of mole, sores, lumps, change in skin texture, odors, excessive sweating, acne, loss of hair, excessive growth of hair or growth of hair in unusual locations, change in nails, amount of time spent in the sun
Eyes	Blurry vision, visual acuity, glasses, contact lenses, sensitivity to light, excessive tearing, night blindness, double vision, drainage, bloodshot, pain, blind spots, flashing lights, halos around objects, glaucoma, cataracts
Ears	Hearing deficits, hearing aid, pain, discharge, lightheadedness, ringing in the ears, earaches, infection
Nose and sinuses	Frequent colds, discharge, itching, hay fever, postnasal drip, stuffiness, sinus pain, polyps, obstruction, nosebleed, change in sense of smell
Mouth	Toothache, tooth abscess, dentures, bleeding/swollen gums, difficulty chewing, sore tongue, change in taste, lesions, change in salivation, bad breath
Throat/neck	Hoarseness, change in voice, frequent sore throats, difficulty swallowing, pain/stiffness, enlarged thyroid
Respiratory	Shortness of breath, shortness of breath on exertion, phlegm, cough, sneezing, wheezing, coughing up blood, frequent upper respiratory tract infections, pneumonia, emphysema, asthma, tuberculosis
Cardiovascular	Shortness of breath that wakes patient up in the night, chest pain, heart murmur, palpitations, fainting, sleep on pillows to breathe better, swelling, cold hands/feet, leg cramps, myocardial infarction, hypertension, valvular disease, pain in calf with walking, varicose veins, inflammation of a vein, blood clot in leg, anemia
Breasts	Pain, tenderness, discharge, lumps, change in size, dimpling
Gastrointestinal	Change in appetite, nausea, vomiting, diarrhea, constipation, usual bowel habits, black and tarry stools, vomiting blood, change in stool color, excessive gas, belching, regurgitation or heartburn, difficulty swallowing, abdominal pain, jaundice, hemorrhoids, hepatitis, peptic ulcers, gallstones
Urinary	Change in urine color, voiding habits, painful urination, hesitancy, urgency, frequency, excessive urination at night, increased urine volume, dribbling, loss in force of stream, bed-wetting, change in urine volume, incontinence, pain in lower abdomen, kidney stones, urinary tract infections
Musculoskeletal	Joint stiffness, muscle pain, back pain, limitation of movement, redness, swelling, weakness, bony deformity, broken bones, dislocations, sprains, gout, arthritis, osteoporosis, herniated disc
Female reproductive	Vaginal discharge, change in libido, infertility, sterility, pain during intercourse, menses (last menstrual period, age period started, regularity, duration, amount of bleeding, premenstrual symptoms, intermenstrual bleeding, painful periods), menopause (age of onset, duration, symptoms, bleeding), obstetrical (number of pregnancies, number of miscarriages/abortions, number of children, type of delivery, complications), type of birth control, estrogen therapy

(continues)

Table 22-1 continued

Male reproductive	Change in libido, infertility, sterility, impotence, pain during intercourse, age at onset of puberty, testicular pain, penile discharge, erections, emissions, hernias, enlarged prostate, type of birth control
Nutrition	Present weight, usual weight, food intolerances, food likes, food dislikes, where meals are eaten
Endocrine	Bulging eyes; fatigue; change in size of head, hands, or feet; weight change; heat/cold intolerances; excessive sweating; increased thirst; increased hunger; change in body hair distribution; swelling in the anterior neck; diabetes mellitus
Lymph nodes	Enlarged, tenderness
Hematological	Easy bruising/bleeding, anemia, sickle cell anemia, blood type

PROCEDURE 22-1

Taking a Medical History

Procedure

PURPOSE:

To obtain a medical history from a patient new to the ambulatory care setting.

EQUIPMENT/SUPPLIES:

- Patient history forms
- Clipboard
- Pen

PROCEDURE STEPS:

1. Introduce yourself to the new patient. Confirm identity of the patient using two identifiers and escort to the examination room or private area.

2. *Use gentle eye contact and positive body language* to ensure a welcoming and warm interaction with the patient. RATIONALE: Puts patient at ease.

3. *Explain the purpose and importance of obtaining the patient information, speaking at the patient's level of understanding.* Ask the questions on the form, trying to get as much information as possible without letting the patient wander from the subject.

4. If using a paper document to record the medical history, use dark blue or black ink to fill in the information.

5. Ask the patient the questions on the facility's patient history screening tool.

6. Encourage the patient to provide comprehensive information while keeping the patient on topic.

7. Ask each question clearly, and clarify that the patient understands what is being asked. Confirm the patient's answers as necessary.

8. Ask about allergies and activities that could affect health, such as smoking or alcohol use.

9. Be specific when documenting the information, providing frequency, amount, or duration of activities.

10. Recheck the medical history form to be sure all parts are complete. *Pay attention to detail.* Note any additional information provided by patient. Make sure numbers, dates, spelling, and other information are accurate and legible. RATIONALE: Ensures that all components of the medical history have been completed.

(continues)

11. Electronic records are automatically dated and stamped with the name of the user entering the information. If using a paper record, date and sign the document, adding all credentials after your name.

DOCUMENTATION:

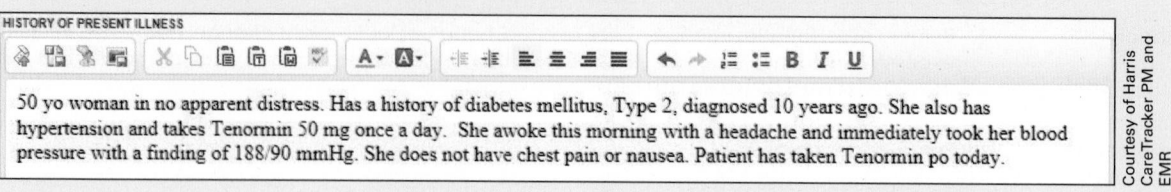

HISTORY OF PRESENT ILLNESS

50 yo woman in no apparent distress. Has a history of diabetes mellitus, Type 2, diagnosed 10 years ago. She also has hypertension and takes Tenormin 50 mg once a day. She awoke this morning with a headache and immediately took her blood pressure with a finding of 188/90 mmHg. She does not have chest pain or nausea. Patient has taken Tenormin po today.

Courtesy of Harris CareTracker PM and EMR

HIPAA Compliance

HIPAA regulations focus on three vulnerable areas with respect to medical records and the patient's chart:

- Paper record storage and computer/server areas
- Fax machines
- Workstations

A patient's paper chart must be stored in secure and locked areas. It is important that only those persons with need for access to charts have a key to the storage area. Locks should be changed periodically to ensure security. Sprinkler and fire detection systems should be installed and tested annually to protect paper records. Patients will respect and appreciate all procedures and policies to keep their history and medical records confidential and protected from harm.

Protection of the patient's EMR means that computer workstation terminals should have directional screen filters if they are located in areas where unauthorized individuals may view the screen. Automated screen time-out features should be installed to protect information from passersby. If the clinic connects to the Internet, telecommuters, or hospital networks, a commercial-grade network firewall should be installed, tested, and maintained to ensure security. Antivirus software should be in place and updated regularly. Review Chapters 10, 13, and 14 for additional HIPAA regulations.

Unintentional human, software, and telecommunication carrier code errors contribute to the security problem. Most records are currently scanned and sent via secure email accounts; however, you may have some exposure to fax machines in more rural areas or in smaller practices with older providers. Some key fax security measures include remembering that faxes are easily misdirected or intercepted by individuals for whom access was neither intended nor authorized, only authorized personnel should have access to the fax machine area, and patient information should be faxed only with assurance that the same security is afforded where the fax is being sent.

Contents of Medical Records

Each patient has his or her own medical record. All patients' records hold standard information. In addition to the patient information forms previously mentioned, other important components of the record include:

- Informed consent forms
- Physical examination outcomes
- Laboratory and diagnostic test results
- The provider's diagnosis and plan of treatment
- Surgical reports
- Progress reports
- Follow-up care
- Telephone calls related to care
- Discharge summary
- Other communications (from other providers, laboratories, or agencies)
- Patient records from other providers
- Medication history

Continuity of Care Record

The Continuity of Care Record (CCR) was developed by a number of medical groups, including the American Academy of Family Physicians and the American Academy of Pediatrics. The CCR is a standard for the creation of electronic summaries of patient health. Its aim is to improve the quality of health care and to reduce medical errors by making current information readily available to physicians. The CCR includes patient and provider information, insurance data, patient's health status, recent care given, recommendations for future care, and reason for referral or transfer. The patient's health status includes allergies, medications, immunizations, vital signs, pertinent laboratory results, and recent procedures and diagnoses. An expanded CCR likely includes any advance directives the patient might have. During a time when many referrals take place, especially in managed care, or when patients are transferred from a hospital setting to an assisted living environment where care is likely provided by someone other than the current primary care provider, such a record is most beneficial.

The CCR is likely to be completed by providers, nurses, medical assistants, and ancillary personnel such as social workers and physical therapists, among others. It can include outpatient, community-based, and inpatient services. It should be EMR compatible, as well as human readable, and can be transferred through a number of electronic formats. At all times, however, the CCR is to be protected and is designed to enhance patient confidentiality.

METHODS OF CHARTING/DOCUMENTATION

There are two primary ways to maintain chart notes. These methods can be used in both paper and electronic records. They are:

- Source-oriented medical records
- Problem-oriented medical records (review Chapter 13 for additional details)

Source-Oriented Medical Records

The **source-oriented medical record (SOMR)** consists of a chronologic set of notes for each visit beginning with the patient's first visit (Figure 22-5). This form of charting makes it difficult to follow or track a specific patient problem as each member of the health care team may make notations on a separate document or in a separate area of the chart. The caregiver must search through the record to locate information about a particular patient problem.

The example of handwritten chart notes in Figure 22-6 shows the complete history taken at the time of examination, including the present

Leo McKay
Date of Birth 01/22/1949
Office visit 04/01/20XX

This 57-year-old patient is seen after a several year absence because of abdominal pain which began approximately 2 weeks ago with progressively worsening abdominal pain. He has stopped eating to see if pain would improve, which it did not. Finally yesterday he stopped taking fluids as well. Until this episode, he was drinking several beers daily and smoking approximately 2 ppd.

Weight is 192. BP 152/88 rt. arm sitting P 78 R 18 T 97.6. He is a well-developed, moderately obese male in moderate distress. Abdomen is tense with some guarding at RUQ.

Abdominal pain - pt needs barium swallow, CBC, Chem 7 and UA. To restrict diet to clear liquids until seen in 2 days, omeprazole 20 mg every day.
JW/tlm

FIGURE 22-5 Sample of dictated and transcribed provider's chart note.

illness (if any), the medical history, allergies, family history, habits (social history), and ROS. The physical examination follows with each area noted. Impressions, changes in medications, and plan finish the examination notes.

The most traditional form of charting is narrative charting. **Narrative charting** is a chronologic account in paragraphs describing client status, procedures, interventions and treatments, and client's response. This method is the most flexible and usable in any setting.

Problem-Oriented Medical Records

Another method of keeping chart notes is the **problem-oriented medical record (POMR)**. A problem is defined as anything that causes concern to the patient or to the caregiver, including physical abnormalities, psychological disturbance, and socioeconomic problems. The master problem list usually includes active, inactive, temporary, and potential problems. This method is used extensively today, especially by clinics and any medical practice where more than one provider may see the patient (see Chapter 13). This method calls for a list of problems to be made, dated, and assigned numbers. When a patient is seen, the problems are identified by number throughout the record. This system makes it easier to follow the patient's progress.

The POMR has four major components:

- *The database.* The patient's medical history, results from laboratory and other diagnostic

Leo McKay 01/22/1949
04/01/XX 3:15 pm abdominal pain X 3 weeks
WT 192 BP 152/88 rt. arm sitting T 97.6 P78 R18
Pt complaining severe abdominal pain for 2 wks getting
progressively worse. Describes as burning, pressure.
Past Med. Hist. chronic Peptic Ulcer Disease
                    quit smoking 3 yr ago – now back to 2 ppd
Allergies–penicillin–hives 1950s
Family Hist   noncontributory
Habits   smokes 2 ppd
                  beer–several daily
ROS
HEENT noncontributory–PERRLA OU correct to 20/20
        CR–clear, no rales, ronchi; murmurs
        GI–some guarding. No masses, tenderness lower
        abdomen. No nausea, vomiting, diarrhea
        GU–clear
PE alert; oriented to time & place
    HEENT–pupils nat teeth
    fundi   thyroid   } Ø
    carotids
    chest–clear
    heart–no murmurs or enlargement
    abdomen–Ø masses
    rectal–soft brown stool in vault
    extremities–neg.
    neuro–reg.
    skin–clear
Impression–Chronic Peptic Ulcer Disease
              Hypertension, mild
Plan–Lab–CBC, Chem 7, UA, barium swallow
Rx–Omeprazole 20 mg every day
Return 3 days
M. Woo, MD 04/01/20XX

FIGURE 22-6 Sample of provider's handwritten chart note.

tests, and results of physical examinations are the core of the record.

- *The problem list.* Each problem is listed individually and assigned a number and dated.
- *The diagnostic and treatment plan.* This component addresses the laboratory and other diagnostic tests completed and the provider's plan for treating the patient.
- *Progress notes.* These notes are entered on every problem initially recorded. Documentation is done chronologically and includes the patient's complaints, problems, condition, treatment, and responses to treatment and care given.

The SOAP/SOAPER and CHEDDAR methods of charting can be used in either the source-oriented or the problem-oriented medical record.

Providers may dictate their notes to be typed by a medical transcriptionist and then filed in the chart (see Figure 22-5). These notes may follow the form seen in the handwritten chart note as shown in Figure 22-6.

DARP Charting. This charting method is further along the continuum away from straight narrative-chronologic. The POMR style progress note usually follows the **DARP** format:

D *Data* gathered are related to an issue to be focused upon.

A *Assessment* of the data (not the patient) with additional information not related by the flow sheet.

R *Response* to the need brought into focus during the assessment of available data.

P *Plan* for continuing care following the intervention.

ELECTRONIC MEDICAL RECORD (EMR)

The EMR can be viewed as simply a different mode of documenting and saving information related to a patient's care—digital storage versus paper storage. Most practitioners making the transition from paper to electronic records, however, seek a more efficient method for documenting patient care. Because EMR are mandated by the Affordable Care Act (ACA) and must have been implemented by 2015 in order to receive full Medicaid/Medicare reimbursement, paper medical records are seen increasingly less in the delivery of health care in all settings. EMR are available 24 hours per day and can be accessed by the provider from an outside location when necessary. More than one person can view the EMR at the same time. Storage of the EMR is much more efficient than the storage of paper records and much more accessible from a variety of locations when housed on a secure server. Errors are less likely in EMR because of the lack of handwritten data. Medication errors are lessened when prescriptions are electronically transmitted to the patient's pharmacy, and there is no confusion over the provider's instructions related to the medication or dosage. EMR have the capability of "flagging" information or queries to providers to ensure accuracy and completeness.

Figure 22-7 shows a sample EMR. Keep in mind the standard accepted rules for charting in both

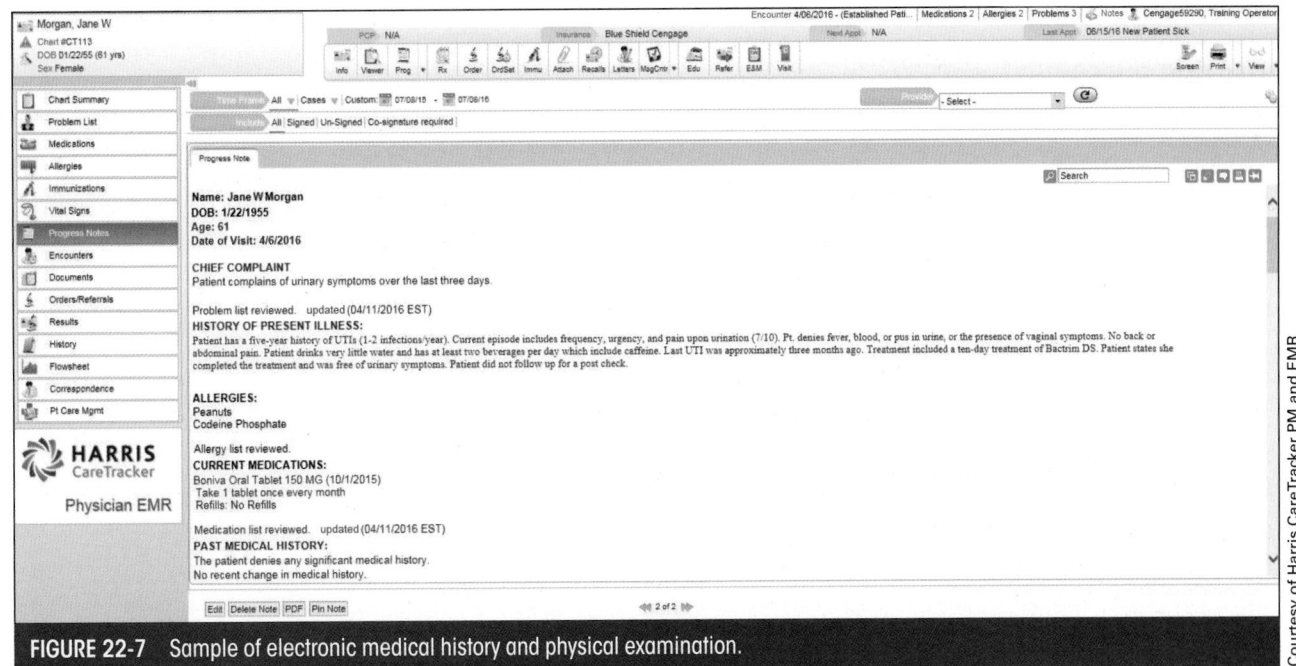

FIGURE 22-7 Sample of electronic medical history and physical examination.

the paper medical record and the EMR. Many of the rules are pertinent to both types of records.

RULES OF CHARTING

Charting is required for each medication, treatment/procedure, or provider and medical assistant action. Accounts of the patient's condition and activities must be charted in a clear and meaningful way. Information charted in the patient's record must be accurate, clear, complete, timely, and properly entered. There is a saying, "If it is not charted, it was not done." Some basic charting rules are given in Tables 22-2 and 22-3.

There are things that the professional medical assistant must avoid when documenting. Only chart the facts, such as what the patient tells you and what you observe. It is not the role of the professional medical assistant to draw conclusions. Avoid criticism, sarcasm, slurs, use of humor, and profanity. Do not remove parts of a paper chart system in order to chart elsewhere. It is also not advised to chart for others or to allow others to chart for you. If an incident occurs while the patient is under your care or during his or her clinic visit, this report does not belong in the patient's chart. Refer to the your institution's policy and procedure manual for how to document an incident and where to store or submit the documentation.

Abbreviations Used in Charting

Abbreviations are used extensively in charting to document information. Some are used as a shorthand to save time and space, whereas other abbreviations are used to give an exact meaning to a finding. For instance, the abbreviation *N&V* indicates "nausea and vomiting" without having to write out the entire expression. Table 22-4 lists commonly used abbreviation. (See Appendix A for a more comprehensive list of abbreviations.)

Although the use of abbreviations in medical charts is common, remember that there is an increasing expectation that the medical chart should be understandable to any person reading it, especially if it is required in any legal matter. The Joint Commission's *Journal on Quality and Patient Safety* reports that it is best not to use abbreviations when charting medications. As a result, there is an official "do not use" list, as well as a list of potential abbreviations that are under consideration for exclusion (see Table 22-5). The Joint Commission report states that the most common abbreviation resulting in medication error is *qd* rather than *every day or once daily*. The report also noted that medication errors are more likely made during prescribing and are related to improper dose or quantity. Therefore, keep abbreviations to a minimum and use only standard abbreviations. Be prepared to provide any attorney with a list of commonly used and accepted abbreviations in your medical practice. The Joint Commission posts a listing of prohibited abbreviations on their Web site (www.jointcommission.org) to further satisfy the goal of patient safety.

TABLE 22-2

CHARTING RULES

PAPER RECORDS	ELECTRONIC RECORDS
Identify the patient and make sure the paperwork matches the identified patient.	Identify the patient and make sure that the open EMR matches the identified patient.
Use appropriate forms.	Record in the appropriate application.
Always write legibly in black or blue ink.	Keyboard accurately and appropriately.
Document accurately, completely, and objectively.	Document accurately, completely, and objectively.
Use standard abbreviations.	Use standard abbreviations.
Use correct spelling and grammar.	Use correct spelling and grammar.
After charting, sign with first initial, last name, and title.	Type personal or electronic signature after each chart activity.
Include date and time.	Include date and time.
Keep records in chronologic order.	Keep records in chronologic order.
Leave no space between chart entry and first initial and last name handwritten.	Leave no empty spaces between chart notes and electronic signature.
Do not erase or obliterate any entry.	Do not erase or delete any entry.
Use only universally accepted abbreviations or avoid them all together.	Use only universally accepted abbreviations or avoid them all together.
If an error is discovered, draw a single line through the mistake and write the correct information above it.	Errors made at the moment of entry are corrected as usual. Errors discovered later require a new document identifying the error, correction, date, and signature of the person making the correction. This document is added to the original document with a note. EMR software programs have variable time lockouts to prevent tampering with the chart.
Never leave a chart unattended in an area that allows those without a need to know access to the contents.	Always close and password protect electronic medical records when they are not in active use.

TABLE 22-3

CHARTING RULES THAT APPLY TO BOTH PAPER AND ELECTRONIC CHARTING

Leave no blank lines in the chart. Enter your data in the next available line.

Ditto marks may not be used.

Use only standard abbreviations that have been determined to be not easily misinterpreted. See abbreviations common to medical charting in Table 22-4.

Avoid medical terminology unless you are absolutely certain of spelling and definition. Legal authorities advise keeping medical terminology to a minimum. The record must be understandable to the patient and to any authorized user.

Confirm the patient's name is on every page.

Use present tense. Never use future tense, such as "patient to be given a tetanus shot"; instead, wait until the injection is given, then chart the event.

Never chart for another person; chart only what you know, not what someone else has told you.

Describe events and behaviors; do not label them. "Patient was really angry" does not describe the event as well as "Patient yelled and threw the pencil on the counter."

Be as specific as you can. Charting "Patient complained of shoulder pain" is not as clear as "Patient complains of right shoulder pain when reaching overhead."

TABLE 22-4

ABBREVIATIONS COMMON TO MEDICAL CHARTING

ac	before meals	OPD	outpatient department
ad lib	at liberty	OR	operating room
BP or B/P	blood pressure	NVD	nausea, vomiting, and diarrhea
b.i.d.	twice a day	P	pulse
c̄	with	PERRLA	pupils equal, round, reactive to light and accommodation
CBC	complete blood count	po	by mouth
CC	chief complaint	prn	as needed
C/O	complaint of	PT	physical therapy
CPE	complete physical examination	R	respiration
DC or D/C	discontinue or discharge	R/O	rule out
D&C	dilation and curettage	ROM	range of motion
dx	diagnosis	ROS	review of systems
ECG, EKG	electrocardiogram	s̄	without
EEG	electroencephalogram	SOAP	subjective, objective, assessment, plan
ER	emergency room	SOB	short of breath
GI	gastrointestinal	T	temperature
GU	genitourinary	T&A	tonsillectomy and adenoidectomy
GYN	gynecology	t.i.d.	three times a day
HEENT	head, eyes, ears, nose, and throat	UA	urinalysis
H&P	history and physical	UCHD	usual childhood diseases
I&D	incision and drainage	URI	upper respiratory infection
IM	intramuscular	UTI	urinary tract infection
mg	milligram	x̄	without
mL	milliliter	WNL	within normal limits
MI	myocardial infarction	XR	X-ray
npo	nothing by mouth	Δ	change
N&V	nausea and vomiting		

TABLE 22-5

THE JOINT COMMISSION'S 2015 OFFICIAL "DO NOT USE" LIST

DO NOT USE	POTENTIAL PROBLEM	USE INSTEAD
U, u (unit)	Mistaken for "0" (zero), the number "4" (four) or "cc"	Write "unit"
IU (International Unit)	Mistaken for IV (intravenous) or the number 10 (ten)	Write "International Unit"
Q.D., QD, q.d., qd (daily)	Mistaken for each other	Write "daily"
Q.O.D., QOD, q.o.d., qod (every other day)	Period after the Q mistaken for "I" and the "O" mistaken for "I"	Write "every other day"
Trailing zero (X.0 mg)*	Decimal point is missed	Write "X mg"
Lack of leading zero (.X mg)		Write "0.X mg"
MS	Can mean morphine sulfate or magnesium sulfate	Write "morphine sulfate"
MSO_4 and $MgSO_4$	Confused for one another	Write "magnesium sulfate"

NOTE: Taken from JCAHO "Do Not Use" List.

Source: https://www.jointcommission.org/facts_about_do_not_use_list

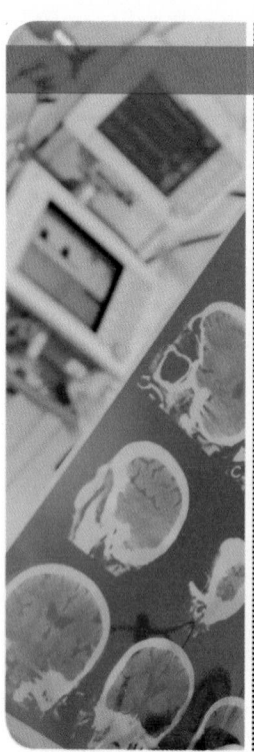

CASE STUDY 22-1

Refer to the scenario at the beginning of the chapter.

Barinda Edwards, a patient of Inner City Health Care, has finally convinced her teenage son to make an appointment for a physical. Travis Edwards is 17 years old, outgoing, fun loving, and apparently healthy. But Barinda is concerned that he may be engaging in harmful social activities and hopes that by seeing Dr. Winston Lewis, Travis may discover ways to protect himself and his health. Travis agreed to the appointment but is adamant that his mother not accompany him. At the ambulatory care setting, it is decided that Travis might be more forthcoming with a male medical assistant, so Joe Guerrero is scheduled to take Travis's medical history before Dr. Lewis does an ROS.

CASE STUDY REVIEW

1. When Joe Guerrero first sits down with Travis to take the history, he notices that Travis is ill at ease and nervous. What can Joe do to reassure Travis that his privacy will be protected?

2. When Joe attempts to take the social history, Travis seems evasive about answering Joe's questions and finally admits that he doesn't want his mother, Barinda, to know about his social activities. What is Joe's best response?

3. By the end of the interview, it becomes apparent that Travis may be engaging in some behaviors that put him at high risk for contracting the human immunodeficiency virus. How can Joe provide Travis with guidance without alienating him?

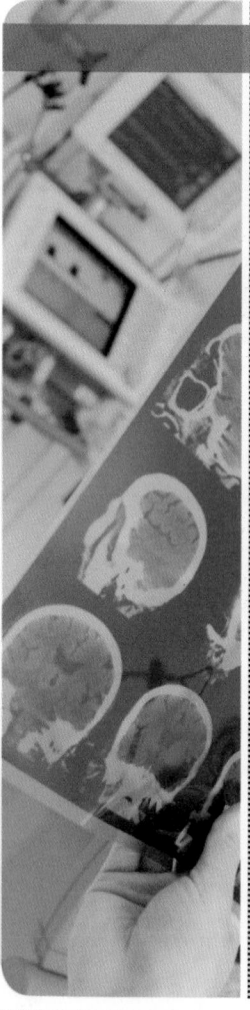

CASE STUDY 22-2

Arthur Cochran is a 58-year-old patient who lives at 45 W. Smith Avenue, River City, XY 01234. His date of birth is July 8, 1954. His phone number is 410-667-1870. He is a Baltimore city fire fighter and has been for 21 years. He has union medical insurance, and Blue Cross/Blue Shield (BC/BS) is his carrier. His number is 211-67-87-56. He also carries major medical, and his policy is Diagnostic #4. He has been referred by the fire department practitioner, Dr. Alan Byers. Mr. Cochran's complaint is severe "gripping" pain in the anterior mid-chest sometimes radiating to the abdomen, neck, and both arms. Pain seems to occur with strenuous exercise and when walking uphill. Pain usually lasts 20 minutes with each episode. Pain does "ease up" when he ceases activity. Mr. Cochran states his episodes have occurred while he was shaving, while climbing stairs at work, after a heavy meal, and during sexual intercourse. One episode last week was accompanied by dizziness, nausea, and fatigue. The episodes have been going on now once or twice a month for 5 months. Mr. Cochran's history is essentially noncontributory. It is questionable whether this is due to good health or the fact that the patient has not had a physical examination for 8 years. Surgeries include tonsillectomy and adenoidectomy (T&A) in 1958, and appendectomy in 1964. He had a fractured rib, left side, in 1984 due to a fire-fighting incident. Usual childhood diseases. Hospitalized for observation, 1962, Sinai Hospital, for an unusually long episode of bronchitis. Social history shows that the patient is a pump operator on the job with much heavy exertion. Smokes 1½ to 2 packs of cigarettes per day and is a moderate drinker. He has a weight problem off and on and tends to eat too much while on duty. Lives in a one-story home. Hobbies include carpentry and music. Some family problems and tension exist as both of his children are in adolescence. Patient describes himself as "fun loving" with a "quick temper" and worries about meeting financial needs of the family. He is in a position to retire from active duty but states he could not tolerate the boredom.

Family history shows both parents deceased—mother of heart attack, age 59, and father of unknown cause at age 49. Has two siblings, one brother with history of hypertension and one sister living and in good health. Has two children both living and well. Family history otherwise negative.

Physical examination revealed a well-nourished, well-developed male in no acute distress at this time. Patient does seem a bit anxious about this examination. T. 98.6, P. 94, R. 24, BP 175/104.

(continues)

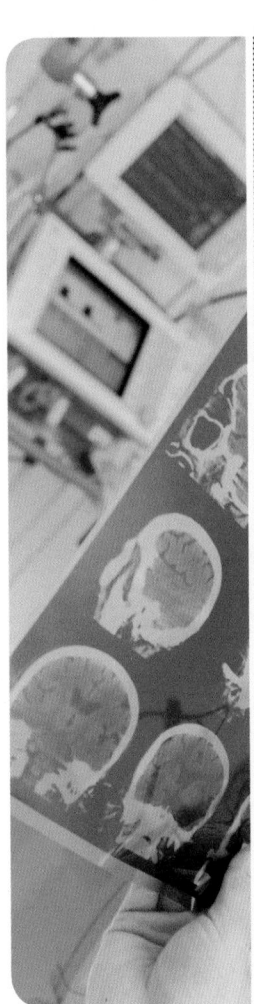

CASE STUDY 22-2 *continued*

Ht. 69 inches, Wt. 198 pounds. HEAD, EYES, EARS, NOSE, THROAT—normal. NECK—supple. Trachea in midline. CHEST—normal in contour. Calcium deposit on left sixth rib probably due to history of fracture. HEART—after careful examination with the patient recumbent and the scope placed lightly on the chest wall near the apex, a left atrial sound was heard (presystolic gallop). ABDOMEN—negative. EXTREMITIES—negative. GENITALIA—negative. SKIN—negative. NEUROLOGIC—negative. Laboratory tests performed show a hemoglobin of 11.0 gms. Awaiting results of serum cholesterol, calcium, phosphorus, and blood urea nitrogen. Chest radiograph essentially negative. EKG report showed atrial sounds occurring presystolically with long P-R intervals. DIAGNOSIS: (1) angina pectoris; (2) anemia; (3) hypertension. TREATMENT: Nitroglycerin tabs, sublingually as needed. To return to clinic in 2 weeks to follow medication effects. In consultation with patient, the patient was advised to control physical activity and quantity of food intake. Avoid extreme cold, 8 hours of sleep/night. Avoid emotional upsets. Attempt four meals/day. Low-fat 1,600-calorie diet. No smoking, moderate alcohol intake.

CASE STUDY REVIEW

1. Identify the following parts of the case study above and extract from the case study the portion that matches the appropriate medical history component.
   - Personal data
   - Chief complaint
   - Present illness
   - Medical history
   - Family history
   - Social history
   - Review of systems
2. Using appropriate terminology and abbreviations, make a charting entry for Mr. Cochran by using the SOAPER method of charting.

Summary

- It is important to ensure that the environment is prepared prior to the patient's arrival so that taking the patient history occurs in a private area by a medical assistant who is focused on this patient interaction.
- The patient's medical history and the information that appears in the medical chart form the basis for any and all treatment given to a patient.
- Information must be provided to and collected from the patient in order to appropriately provide care. Forms used for this purpose include demographics, financial and privacy information, and medical history.
- An efficient and effective medical chart tells the patient's story.
- Cultural diversity must be taken into consideration when obtaining the medical history in order to know how to appropriately respect a patient's cultural beliefs.
- Sensitivity to the patient's needs and delicate topics will result in a more accurate history.
- It is critical that all information be accurate, documented appropriately, and complete in every way.
- Taking the medical history, maintaining the patient's chart, and documenting information are major tasks for medical assistants.
- There are a variety of methods for charting/documentation. These may include SOAP, CHEDDAR, narrative, DARP, and others.
- There are several parts to the medical health history. They include the chief complaint (CC), medical history, family history, social history, and review of symptoms (ROS).
- Increased use of the EMR makes charting easier and quicker for clinic staff personnel and providers. Benefits include accuracy and accessibility.

CERTIFICATION REVIEW

1. Which of the following is the medical assistant's best course of action if the patient has difficulty with English?
   a. Make the appointment for the patient and obtain the services of an interpreter to be present
   b. Set the appointment after contact is made with the interpreter
   c. Speak more loudly so the patient will understand
   d. All of these

2. Of the following questions, which is the most helpful to ask a returning patient?
   a. Are you feeling bad today?
   b. Didn't you get better with the treatment prescribed last visit?
   c. Have you noticed any changes in your condition since your last visit?
   d. Do you realize you have gained 6 pounds since your visit last week?
   e. Have you read and understood our HIPAA policy?

3. What is the best course of action when the patient reports not feeling well?
   a. Mark the chief complaint as "patient not feeling well"
   b. Ask helpful questions to help the patient express specific problems or symptoms
   c. Pin down the symptoms by guessing what the problem could be
   d. Let the provider work with the patient

4. Which of the following is true about source-oriented medical records?
   a. They are chronologic notes beginning with the patient's first visit.
   b. They have four major components.
   c. They are the best for finding information quickly.
   d. They are best when many providers see the patient.
   e. They are the same as problem-oriented medical records.

5. Data that include the patient's name, address, telephone numbers, birth date, Social Security number, insurance information, and person to contact in an emergency are considered which of the following?
   a. Demographic data
   b. CCR of patient information
   c. Social history
   d. None of these

6. Which of the following is true about the chief complaint?
   a. It is often referred to as the CC in the chart.
   b. It is a statement of objective findings made by the staff.
   c. It is subjective data as expressed by the patient.
   d. It is determined by the provider after the physical exam.
   e. Both a and c

7. Interviewing patients for their medical history requires which of the following?
   a. Special credentials such as CMA or RMA
   b. Cross-cultural interviewing and communication skills
   c. Computer skills in medical note taking
   d. A major portion of the receptionist's time and energy

8. Which of the following statements about the CCR is accurate?
   a. It was created by medical groups, including the American Academy of Family Physicians and the American Academy of Pediatrics.
   b. It was developed to reduce errors and ensure certain information is shared among providers.
   c. It was meant to include input from all health care providers, nurses, and medical assistants.
   d. Both b and c
   e. All of these

9. Which of the following is true about progress notes?
   a. They include medical history and results of laboratory tests.
   b. They are the provider's plan for treating the patient.
   c. They include the CC, problems, conditions, treatment, and responses to care.
   d. Both a and c

10. Subjective, objective, assessment, and plan charting is sometimes referred to as which of the following?
   a. SOAP
   b. POMR
   c. SOMR
   d. CCRP
   e. SOAPER

CHAPTER 23

Vital Signs and Measurements

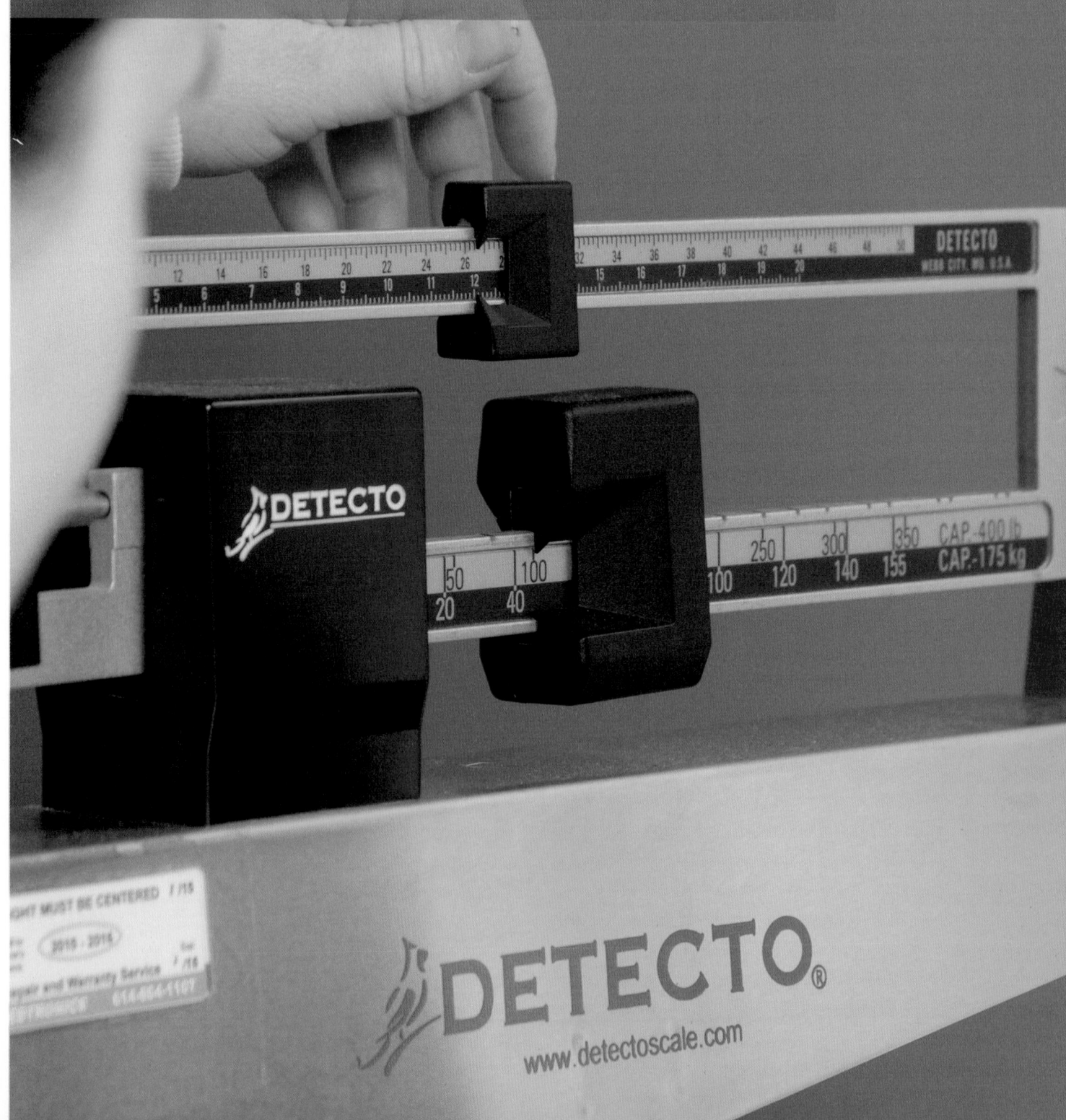

1. Define and spell the key terms as presented in the glossary.
2. Explain normal and abnormal temperatures, including factors affecting temperature.
3. Identify and explain the procedures for using, caring for, and storing the various types of thermometers.
4. Discuss the World Health Organization's initiative to phase out mercury thermometers and other mercury-containing equipment.
5. List the locations and procedure for obtaining pulse rates.
6. Detail the procedure for obtaining respiration rates.
7. Identify and describe normal and abnormal pulse and respiratory rates and the factors affecting each.
8. Describe the appropriate equipment and procedure for obtaining a blood pressure measurement.
9. Identify normal and abnormal blood pressure, including factors affecting blood pressure.
10. Recite the procedures for obtaining height, weight, and chest measurements of adults.
11. Accurately record measurements on the patient's chart or electronic medical record.
12. Explain two reasons a professional individual shows responsibility by learning about the dangers of mercury.

KEY TERMS

afebrile	febrile	orthopnea
apical	frenulum	peripheral
apnea	hyperpnea	pulse oximeter
arrhythmias	hypertension	pyrexia
atherosclerosis	hyperventilation	rales
baseline	hypotension	rhonchi
bradycardia	hypoventilation	stertorous
bradypnea	idiopathic	stridor
Cheyne–Stokes	increments	systole
diastole	lumen	tachycardia
dyspnea	manometer	tachypnea
eupnea	meniscus	wheezes

SCENARIO

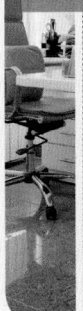

At Inner City Health Care, clinical medical assistant Joe Guerrero, CMA (AAMA), assists providers in taking patients' vital signs. One of his favorite patients is Doris Hougland, a friendly woman in her 70s who always has a kind disposition despite her financial and medical difficulties. Doris is overweight and has hypertension, so her blood pressure is monitored on a regular basis to be certain that it is under control. In reviewing Doris's chart, Joe notices that her blood pressure has been quite stable for the last few visits. He also checks her weight and notices that Doris is slowly losing weight. Doris's chart, with its history of blood pressure and other measurements, informs Joe's perspective and is a helpful record when evaluating the progress Doris has made since she became a patient 3 years ago.

One of the most important and commonly performed tasks of a medical assistant is obtaining and recording patient vital signs and body measurements. Vital signs include temperature, pulse, respiration, and blood pressure, abbreviated TPR B/P. They are indicative of the general health and well-being of a patient and, with regular monitoring, may measure patient response to treatment. The clinical measurements, in total or in part, are an important component of each patient visit. Height and weight measurements, although not considered vital signs, are often a routine part of a patient visit.

Patients will exhibit vital sign readings that are uniquely their own. As a result, baseline assessments of vital signs are usually obtained during the patient's initial visit. These baseline results are used as a reference point for future readings, differentiating between what is normal and abnormal for the patient.

Safety   Professional

Two important habits must be developed by the medical assistant before taking a patient's vital signs: aseptic technique in the form of hand washing, and recognition and correction of factors that may influence results of vital signs. Proper hand washing before taking vital signs will assist in preventing cross-contamination of patients. Refer to the discussion on Standard Precautions and medical asepsis in Chapter 21. It is important to understand that components of the set of vital signs, such as respirations, pulse, and blood pressure, vary from moment to moment and are influenced by a number of factors such as movement and positioning. Emotions influence vital signs as well. Anxiety can increase heart rate, for example. Explaining procedures allowing the patient the opportunity to relax to ease apprehension is also an essential role of the professional medical assistant.

THE IMPORTANCE OF ACCURACY

Vital signs may be altered by many factors. Medical assistants must recognize and correct factors that may produce inaccurate results. For example, patients may exhibit anxiety over potential test results or findings of the provider. They may be angry or may have rushed into the clinic. A patient may have had something to eat or drink before the visit or may have had a long wait in the reception area. Patient apprehension and mood must always be considered by the medical assistant, because these factors can affect vital signs. The medical assistant may be required to take vital signs more than once during a clinic visit to ascertain a **baseline** and obtain an impression of overall well-being of the patient. Body measurements such as weight may be influenced by what the patient is wearing or the pocket contents; height may be influenced by the patient's shoes or posture while being measured.

Accurately obtaining and recording vital signs is necessary because treatment plans may be developed based on the patient's condition as reflected by vital signs. Variations can indicate a new disease process or the patient's response to treatment. They may also indicate the patient's compliance with a treatment plan.

Competency

Although taking vital signs is a task commonly performed by the medical assistant, it is never to be approached casually, and it should never be rushed

or incompletely performed. Concentration and attention to proper procedure will help ensure accurate measurements and quality patient care. The following text discusses procedures used to measure the vital signs of children and adults. Procedures used for infant examinations are discussed in Chapter 26.

TEMPERATURE

Body temperature is maintained and regulated by two processes functioning in conjunction with one another: heat production and heat loss.

Body heat is produced by the actions of voluntary and involuntary muscles. As the muscles move, they use energy, which produces heat. Cellular metabolic activities, such as the process of breaking down food sugars into simpler components (catabolism), are another source of heat.

The body loses heat by a combination of five processes:

1. *Convection*. The process by which heat is lost through the skin by being transferred from the skin by air currents flowing across it, such as a fan used on a hot day for cooling purposes.

2. *Conduction*. The transfer of heat from within the body to the surface of the skin and then to surrounding cooler objects touching the skin, such as clothing.

3. *Radiation.* Body heat lost from the surface of the skin to a cooler environment, much like a cool room becoming warm when occupied by many people.

4. *Evaporation.* A heat-loss mechanism that uses heat absorption through vaporization of perspiration.

5. *Elimination.* Heat that is lost through the normal functioning of the intestinal, urinary, and respiratory tracts.

The delicate balance between heat production and heat loss is maintained by the hypothalamus in the brain. The hypothalamus monitors blood temperature and will trigger either the heat loss or the heat production mechanism with as little as 0.04°F change in blood temperature.

Body temperature is measured in degrees and is influenced by several factors, including:

- An increase in temperature may result from a bacterial infection, increased physical activity or food intake, exposure to heat, pregnancy, drugs that increase metabolism, stress and severe emotional reactions, and age. Age becomes a factor in that infants have an average body temperature that is 1 to 2 degrees higher than adults.

- Decrease in temperature may result from viral infections, decreased muscular activity, fasting, exposure to cold, drugs that decrease metabolic activities, and age. Age in this instance refers to older adults, in that older adults have decreased metabolic activity resulting in a decrease in body temperature.

- Another factor that can increase or decrease body temperature is time of day. During sleep and early morning, the temperature is at its lowest, whereas later in the day, with muscular and metabolic activity, the temperature increases.

Because of the many factors influencing body temperature and the uniqueness of individuals, there is no "normal" temperature. The medical assistant must think of temperatures in terms of the "average," which for an adult is 98.6°F (37.0°C).

Terms Used to Describe Body Temperature

The following terms are used to describe body temperature:

- *Afebrile.* Absence of fever
- *Febrile.* Fever is present

- *Fever.* Body temperature increased beyond normal range; **pyrexia** is another term for fever
- *Onset.* Time when fever begins
- *Lysis.* Body temperature gradually returns to normal after a period of fever
- *Crisis.* Body temperature decreases suddenly to baseline levels; the patient may perspire profusely (diaphoresis)
- *Intermittent.* A fluctuating fever that returns to or below baseline, then increases again
- *Remittent.* A fluctuating fever that does not return to the baseline temperature; it fluctuates but remains increased
- *Continuous.* A fever that remains above the baseline; it does not fluctuate but remains fairly constant

Figure 23-1 depicts types of fever.

Phaseout of Mercury Thermometers and Other Mercury-Containing Equipment

Glass mercury thermometers have been used for decades and have been common in health care agencies as well as the home. In recent years, concerns have arisen about mercury toxicity when mercury thermometers or other equipment containing mercury break and spill mercury into the environment.

This can create a mercury vapor in the indoor air, which is a serious problem. The mercury also can cause environmental damage if it enters lakes and rivers, where it can contaminate fish, which are part of the food chain. Even small amounts of mercury can do great harm. The fetus is at risk because its developing nervous system is susceptible to mercury toxicity if a pregnant woman eats fish contaminated with mercury. When thermometers break or are disposed of improperly, the mercury can enter the atmosphere, especially if the mercury waste is burned in an incinerator.

Safety

Even small mercury spills should be cleaned up as soon as possible. Becton-Dickinson, a thermometer manufacturer, makes the following recommendations for cleaning up a broken thermometer:

- Pick up the mercury with an eyedropper or scoop up the beads of mercury with a piece of heavy paper (cardboard, index card, or playing card).
- Place mercury, the dropper, heavy paper, and any broken glass in a plastic resealable

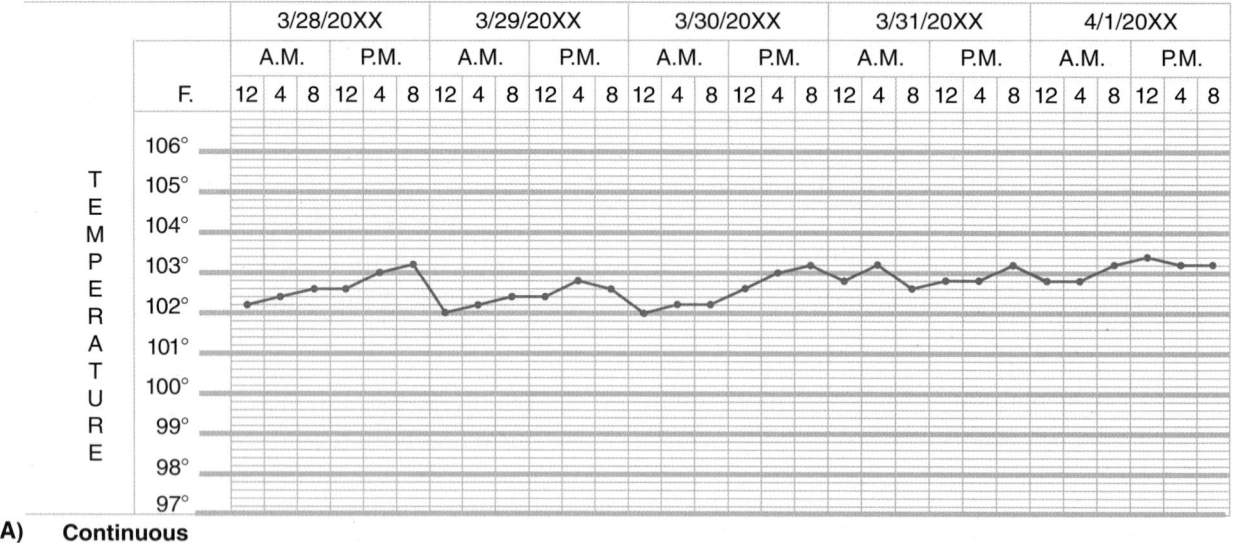

(A)   Continuous

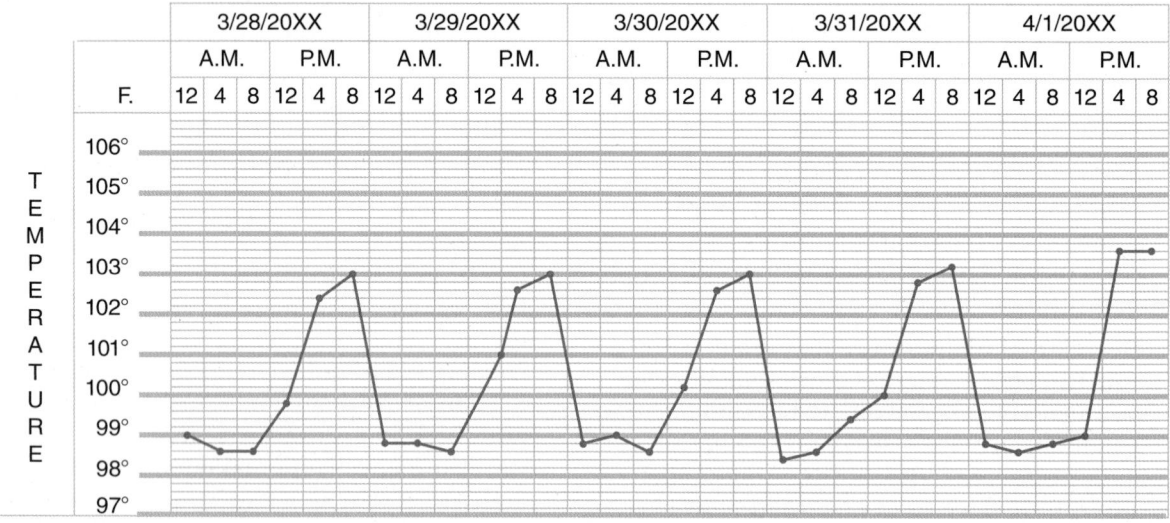

(B)   Intermittent

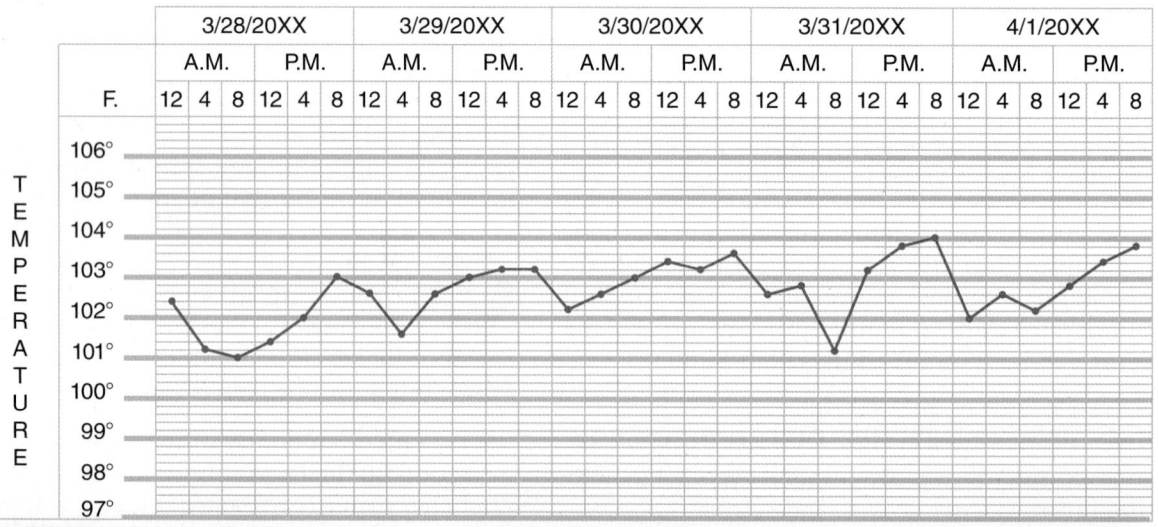

(C)   Remittent

FIGURE 23-1 Types of fevers. (A) Continuous—remains above baseline. Does not fluctuate. (B) Intermittent—a fluctuating fever. Returns to or below baseline, then rises again. (C) Remittent—a fluctuating fever but does not return to baseline temperature. Remains elevated, but fluctuates.

bag. Place this bag into two more resealable bags, zipping each within the other, finishing up with the contents bagged three times. Place this into a wide-mouth, sealable plastic container.

- Call the local health department for the nearest mercury disposal location. If no disposal location is available, dispose of the container according to local and state regulations. The health department can inform you regarding how to obtain the information.

- Leave windows open for about 2 days to ensure complete ventilation.

These recommendations can be applied to mercury spillage caused by other mercury-containing equipment. To follow is the list of "do nots":

- Do not use household cleaning products. Combinations of some cleansers with mercury can release toxic gases.

- Do not use a broom or brush to clean up mercury; it will only spread it around.

- Do not use a vacuum cleaner or shop vacuum. The mercury vapor escapes into the air and increases exposure to individuals in the area.

The World Health Organization and Health Care without Harm joined forces in 2013 to launch an initiative called Mercury-Free Healthcare to call for the phaseout of mercury fever thermometers and blood pressure devices containing mercury. The risk of mercury and mercury-containing compounds is well known to be potentially damaging to the brain and neurologic systems, especially in infants and children. Mercury can also damage the kidneys and the digestive system. Due to these risks and to the evolution of other methods of obtaining temperature and blood pressure, devices that contain mercury should not be utilized in a health care setting.

Types of Thermometers

The following are types of thermometers available for use in the ambulatory care setting:

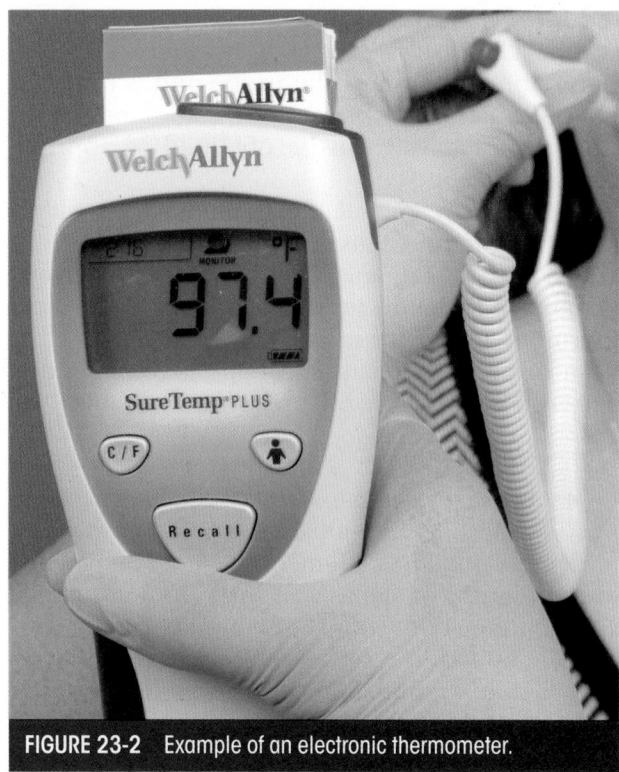

FIGURE 23-2 Example of an electronic thermometer.

- Disposable strips
- Electronic/digital (oral or rectal)
- Tympanic or aural
- Temporal artery

Disposable Thermometers. Disposable thermometers are individually wrapped strips with heat-sensitive dots that change color to indicate temperature. They are used once and then discarded. There are strips for use on the forehead and others for oral use. Although strips are easy to use and prevent patient cross-contamination, accuracy is questionable.

Electronic and Digital Thermometers. Electronic thermometers are widely used, handheld, battery-operated or plug-in units that have easy-to-read electronic display screens to indicate results (Figure 23-2). Electronic thermometers in Fahrenheit or Celsius scales are available. Probes are attached and are color-coded blue for oral and

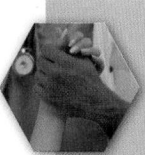

Patient Education

Teach patients the importance of replacing mercury thermometers with an alternative such as digital, disposable, or aural (tympanic) thermometers. The risk for mercury poisoning is great if a mercury thermometer (or other mercury-containing item) is broken and the mercury escapes into the environment.

red for rectal. The probes have disposable plastic covers. The plastic cover acts as a barrier to prevent contamination of the probe and is replaced for each patient to prevent cross-contamination. An accurate result can be obtained in approximately 10 seconds.

Inexpensive digital thermometers are widely available for home use (Figure 23-3). They are quick, easy to use, and accurate. Encourage your patients to switch to these from the mercury glass thermometers. These lightweight thermometers do not require recharging; their small imbedded batteries last for years but are not replaceable.

Procedure

Tympanic or Aural Thermometers. The use of tympanic thermometers is common as they are fast, provide no discomfort to the patient, can be used on patients over 6 months of age as well as adults, and usually are accurate. They consist of a handheld unit with a probe tip that is inserted into the ear securely to make a seal (Figure 23-4). Disposable tips are used to prevent cross-contamination. With the tympanic method of measuring body temperature, the procedure is complete in a few seconds. An aural or tympanic thermometer measures the patient's temperature by measuring the infrared waves produced by the tympanic membrane and displays the temperature in less than 2 to 3 seconds on a digital screen. The tympanic membrane and the hypothalamus of the brain share the same blood supply, so an accurate measurement of the body temperature can be obtained. Procedure 23-1 gives steps for obtaining an aural temperature using a tympanic thermometer.

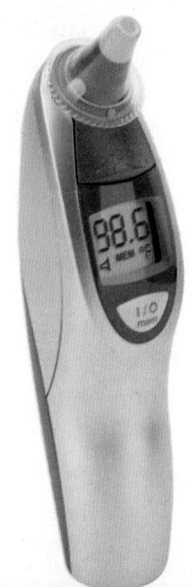

FIGURE 23-4 Thermo-scan tympanic thermometer.

Courtesy of Welch-Allyn

The greatest benefits of the tympanic thermometer are that it gives nearly instant results; it does not come into contact with mucous membranes, thereby minimizing cross contamination; it uses a site that is readily accessible; it is not affected by the patient smoking or drinking hot or cold liquids; it does not require that the patient be conscious; and it is an easy instrument to use. The unit is battery operated and uses a disposable probe cover or ear speculum.

The tympanic thermometer is comfortable for the patient, is nonthreatening to infants and children, and can be used when other methods are inappropriate. It is the thermometer of choice for pediatric patients older than 6 months. However, providers have found that inaccurate readings can result if patients have impacted cerumen in the ear of which they may be unaware. Also, if the patient has otitis media, a middle ear infection, the reading tends to be inaccurate and the procedure is painful.

Drawbacks to the tympanic thermometer have been demonstrated in pediatric patients with ear conditions such as otitis media. An inaccurate recording can result because fluid buildup in the inner ear limits infrared wave transmission.

Temporal Artery Thermometers. A noninvasive thermometer known as a temporal artery thermometer, or TA thermometer, has been developed and is currently in use. Studies performed at Harvard Medical School and the Hospital for Sick Children found the TA thermometer to be more accurate

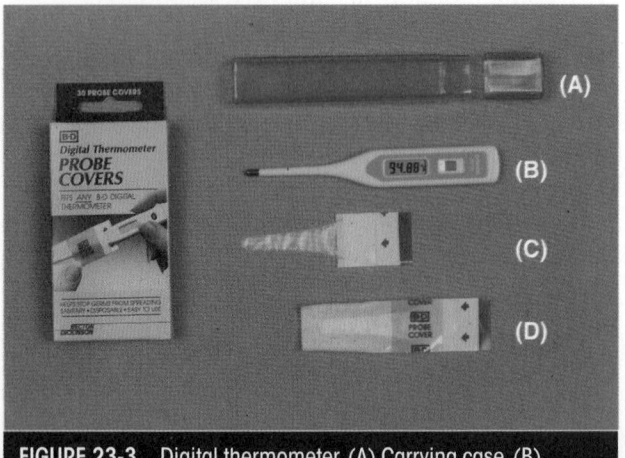

FIGURE 23-3 Digital thermometer. (A) Carrying case. (B) Digital thermometer. (C) Probe cover without backing. (D) Probe cover with backing.

Procedure

Measuring an Aural Temperature Using a Tympanic Thermometer

STANDARD PRECAUTIONS:

Handwashing

PURPOSE:

To obtain an aural temperature using a tympanic thermometer.

EQUIPMENT/SUPPLIES:

- Tympanic thermometer (see Figure 23-4)
- Probe covers or ear speculum
- Waste container

PROCEDURE STEPS:

1. Wash hands following Standard Precautions.
2. ***Paying attention to detail***, assemble equipment.
3. Introduce yourself to the patient. Identify the patient.
4. ***Explain the rationale for performance of the procedure, speaking at the patient's level of understanding.*** RATIONALE: This will help gain the patient's cooperation and consent.
5. Place cover on thermometer (Figure 23-5).

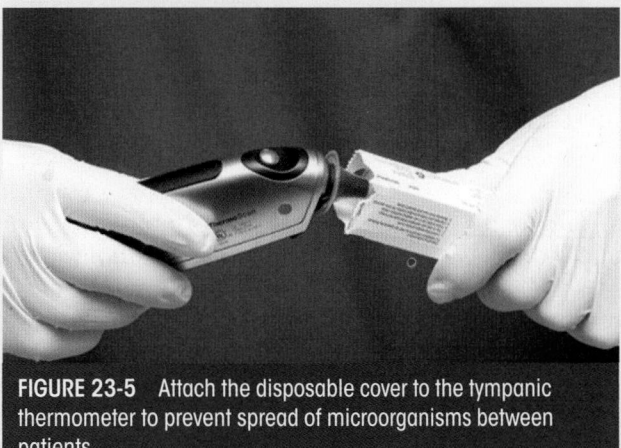

FIGURE 23-5 Attach the disposable cover to the tympanic thermometer to prevent spread of microorganisms between patients.

6. Gently straighten ear canal up and back for adults and place probe into ear canal to seal the area and activate the system (Figure 23-6). RATIONALE: Air leaks will occur if the ear canal is not sealed.
7. Wait until the temperature is displayed on the screen.
8. Remove probe from the ear.

(continues)

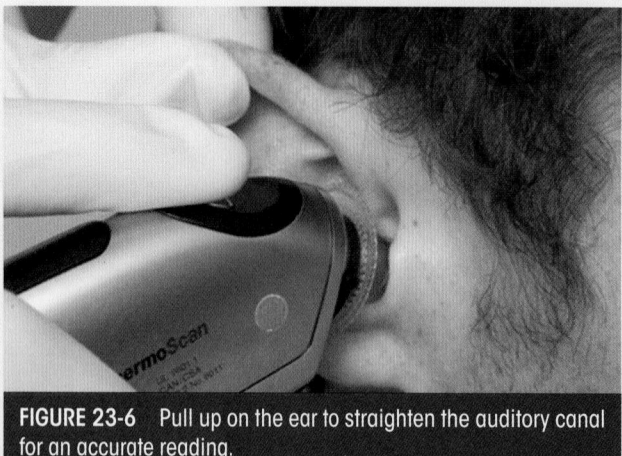

FIGURE 23-6 Pull up on the ear to straighten the auditory canal for an accurate reading.

9. Discard cover into waste container by pressing the release button.

10. Wash hands.

11. Replace thermometer in its storage area.

12. Record temperature in patient's chart or electronic medical record, indicating tympanic measurement (Tym).

DOCUMENTATION:

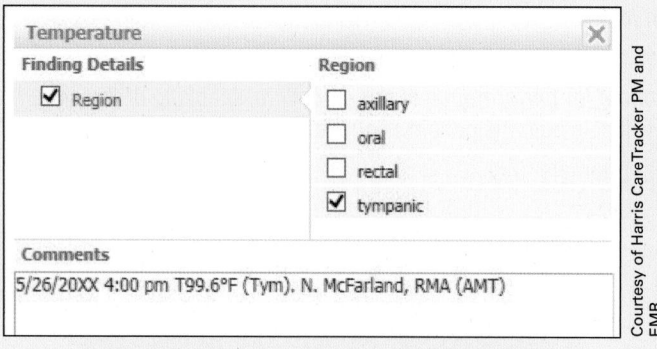

than the aural (tympanic) and rectal thermometers. It is used on adults and children.

Procedure

The temporal artery is a major blood vessel in the head. The thermometer measures the temperature of the skin surface over the temporal artery. The thermometer has a probe that contains a sensor. When the TA thermometer is slid straight across the forehead (midline forehead), the infrared heat from the artery is picked up by the sensor (Figure 23-7). Software accurately determines and displays the temperature. The TA thermometer can also be used behind the ear lobe (if the forehead is wet with perspiration). See Procedure 23-2. There are many advantages to the TA thermometer: It can be used for patients of all ages; it is accurate, painless, fast, convenient, safe, comfortable, and noninvasive; and it can be cleaned with an alcohol wipe between patients.

Some considerations should be kept in mind when using a TA thermometer. If there is perspiration on the forehead, an inaccurate measurement could occur. Other sites that can be used are the femoral, axillary, and behind the ear. Scanning too rapidly can cause a false reading, as can a hat or hair covering the forehead. The TA thermometer must be the same temperature as the room in which it is used. It cannot be stored in the sun or in a room where air-conditioned air has been blowing on the thermometer.

Procedure

Oral Temperatures. To use an oral strip for taking a temperature, make certain that the package is not damaged, then

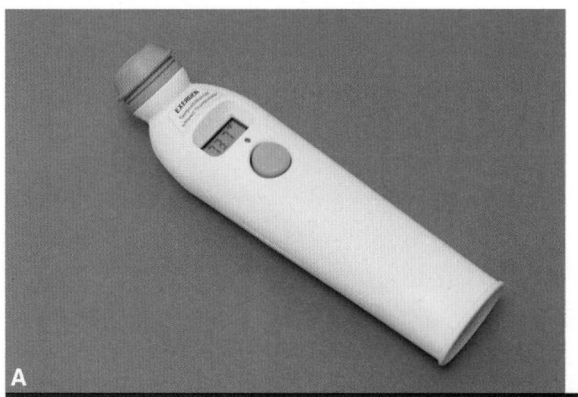
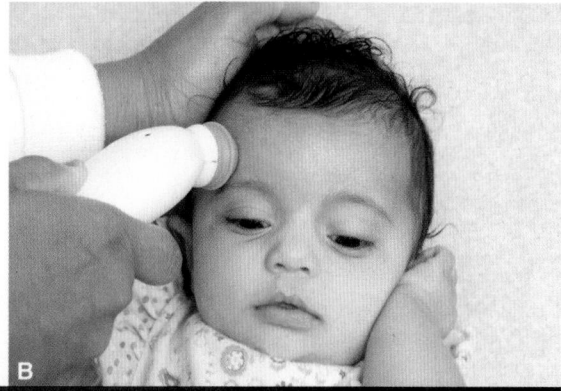

FIGURE 23-7 Using a temporal artery thermometer. (A) Temporal artery thermometer. (B) Slide thermometer across forehead.

PROCEDURE 23-2

Procedure

Measuring a Temperature Using a Temporal Artery (TA) Thermometer

STANDARD PRECAUTIONS:

Handwashing

PURPOSE:

To obtain a temporal artery temperature using a temporal artery (TA) thermometer.

EQUIPMENT/SUPPLIES:

- Temporal artery thermometer
- Alcohol wipes, probe cap or cover, or sheath

PROCEDURE STEPS:

1. Wash hands and follow Standard Precautions.
2. ***Paying attention to detail***, assemble equipment. Clean probe with alcohol or attach a probe. RATIONALE: The lens of the thermometer must be clean to work properly.
3. Introduce yourself to the patient. Identify the patient. RATIONALE: To be certain you have the correct patient.
4. ***Explain the rationale for performance of the procedure, speaking at the patient's level of understanding.*** RATIONALE: Gain patient's cooperation and permission.
5. Remove perspiration from forehead, remove hat, push back hair from forehead. RATIONALE: False readings can occur from moisture (perspiration) on forehead cooling the skin or from a hat or hair covering forehead, raising the temperature.
6. Hold the probe flush against the skin in the center of patient's forehead (Figure 23-8). RATIONALE: Probe must be centered properly for accurate reading over area.
7. Press the "scan" button and hold while sliding the thermometer slowly across the forehead to the temple area hair line. There will be a tapping or clicking sound that will stop when the temperature has been reached.

(continues)

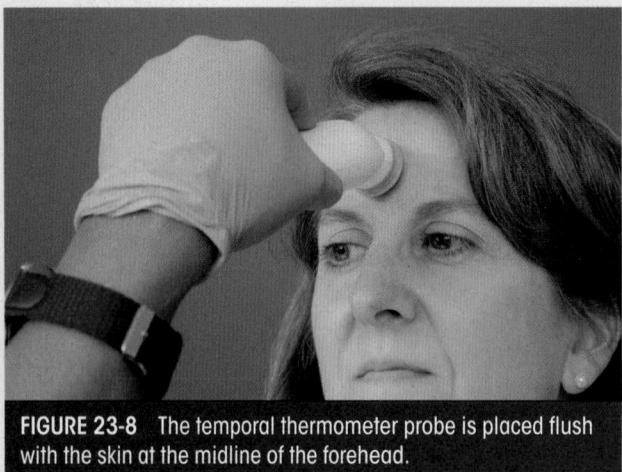

FIGURE 23-8 The temporal thermometer probe is placed flush with the skin at the midline of the forehead.

8. Release the button and remove the thermometer from the forehead.

9. Read the display for temperature measurement.

10. Turn upside down and wipe probe with alcohol wipe. Let dry. Return to holder. RATIONALE: TA thermometer must be dry to work effectively.

11. Wash hands.

12. Accurately record temperature in patient's chart or electronic medical record, indicating TA temperature.

PRECAUTIONS:

Check the manufacturer's manual. Some models cannot be used when oxygen is being used or when in close proximity to aerosols.

DOCUMENTATION:

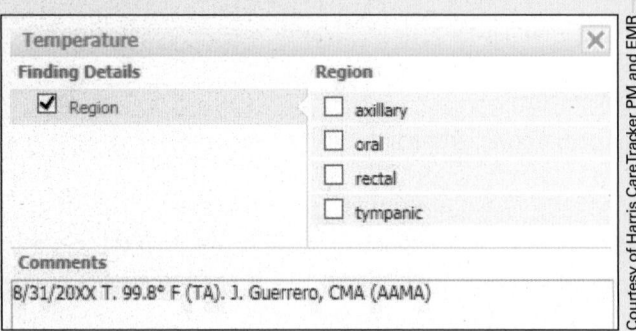

Courtesy of Harris CareTracker PM and EMR

peel it back to reveal the strip. Insert the strip into the patient's mouth. After the appropriate time interval has elapsed, remove the thermometer. The dots that have changed color are read using the scale located on the strip. Although convenient to use, accuracy is not always ensured with the strips, so these strips may not be the best choice for clinical use. The procedure for obtaining an oral temperature with an electronic thermometer is quick, easy, and accurate (Procedure 23-3). Some electronic thermometers are stored on a recharging base. When removed from the base, they are turned on and ready for use. A disposable cover is placed over the probe, and the probe is placed in the patient's mouth. When temperature measurement is complete, the thermometer beeps and the temperature is displayed on the screen. The probe cover is ejected into a biohazard container without touching the container, and the unit is returned to the base.

PROCEDURE 23-3

Procedure

Measuring an Oral Temperature Using an Electronic Thermometer

STANDARD PRECAUTIONS:

Handwashing

Biohazard

PURPOSE:

To obtain an oral temperature.

EQUIPMENT/SUPPLIES:

- Electronic thermometer
- Probe covers
- Biohazard waste container

PROCEDURE STEPS:

1. Wash hands and follow Standard Precautions.
2. *Paying attention to detail*, assemble equipment.
3. Introduce yourself to the patient. Identify patient.
4. Position the patient in a comfortable position.
5. Inquire if the patient has ingested hot or cold drinks or food or has been smoking within the previous half hour. RATIONALE: Ingesting hot or cold substances or smoking can result in an arbitrary increase or decrease in temperature results.
6. Being courteous and respectful to the patient, *explain the rationale for performance of the procedure, speaking at the patient's level of understanding*. RATIONALE: To obtain patient cooperation and consent.
7. Select the correct probe for an oral temperature.
8. Cover with the correct probe cover (Figure 23-9). RATIONALE: To prevent microorganism cross-contamination.
9. Insert the probe on either side of the frenulum (Figure 23-10). RATIONALE: Under the center of the tongue is the **frenulum**, which impedes placement in this area.
10. Instruct patient to close mouth without placing teeth on thermometer. RATIONALE: To prevent room air from interfering with the temperature inside the mouth.
11. Leave in place until the "beep" is heard.
12. Remove the thermometer probe.
13. Read the results on the digital display window.
14. Discard probe cover in biohazard waste container.
15. Replace electronic thermometer in the base holder, if required for recharging.
16. Wash hands.
17. Record temperature in patient's chart or electronic medical record.

(continues)

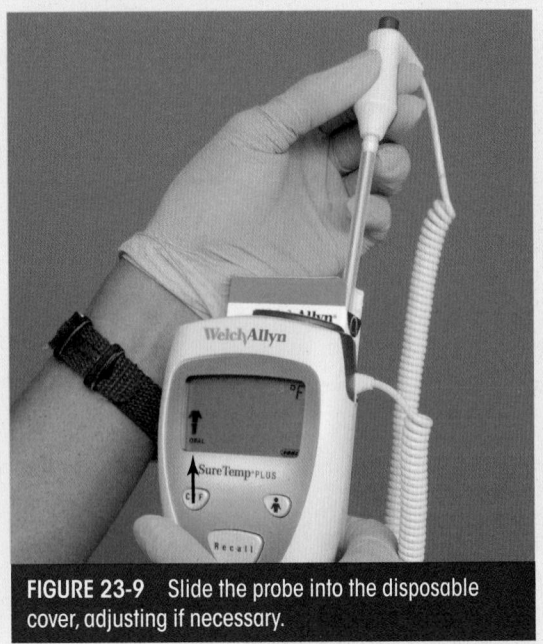

FIGURE 23-9 Slide the probe into the disposable cover, adjusting if necessary.

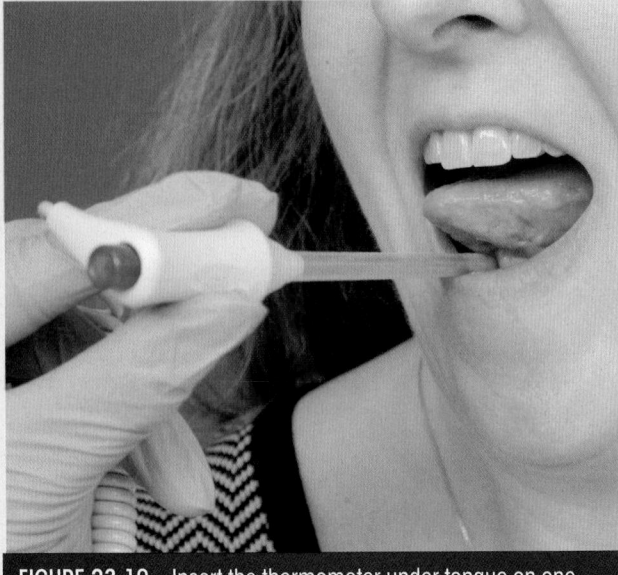

FIGURE 23-10 Insert the thermometer under tongue on one side or the other of the frenulum.

DOCUMENTATION:

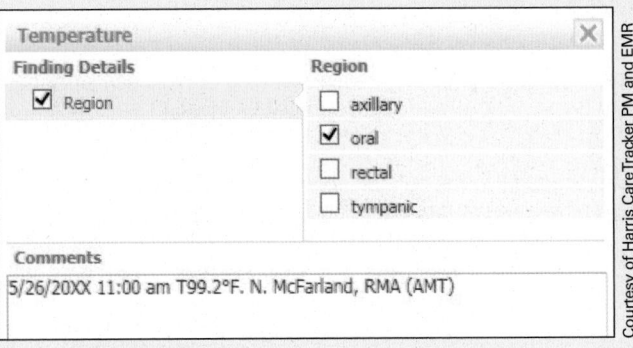

Courtesy of Harris CareTracker PM and EMR

The temperature is then recorded in the patient's chart. Always read and follow the manufacturer's directions for use and care of a digital unit.

Rectal and Axillary Temperatures. In the past, rectal and axillary methods for obtaining a temperature were widely used for infants, young children, and patients who were unable to undergo or uncooperative with oral temperature measurement. The new technologies—tympanic, temporal artery, and electronic and digital thermometers—have simplified temperature measurement. These thermometers are safe, are readily accepted by patients, greatly reduce microorganism transmission, are accurate, give a rapid reading, and are widely used in health care settings, including ambulatory care. The steps for obtaining rectal and axillary temperature measurements are included in Procedures 24-4 and 24-5.

For more information on normal temperature ranges and factors that influence a patient's temperature, see the "Vital Signs" Quick Reference Guide later in the chapter.

PROCEDURE 23-4

Procedure

Measuring a Rectal Temperature Using a Digital Thermometer

STANDARD PRECAUTIONS:

Handwashing

Gloves

Biohazard

PURPOSE:

To obtain a rectal temperature using a digital thermometer.

EQUIPMENT/SUPPLIES:

- Digital thermometer with red probe (rectal)
- Probe cover
- Lubricating jelly on a 4 × 4 gauze or in packet
- Gloves
- Biohazard waste container

PROCEDURE STEPS:

1. Wash hands and don gloves following Standard Precautions.
2. *Paying attention to detail*, assemble equipment.
3. Introduce yourself to the patient. Identify patient.
4. *Explain the rationale for performance of the procedure to patient, speaking at the patient's level of understanding*. RATIONALE: Ensures understanding and gains patient cooperation and consent.
5. Remove patient's clothing from the waist down, *protecting patient's personal boundaries*; drape as necessary. RATIONALE: Maintains patient's modesty, privacy, and warmth.
6. Position patient in Sims' position. If the patient is an infant, raise his or her legs as when changing a diaper.
7. Place probe cover on red probe (rectal). RATIONALE: To prevent microorganism cross-contamination when obtaining oral or rectal temperatures. The red probe indicates rectal thermometer.
8. Lubricate probe with lubricating jelly. RATIONALE: Easier insertion of thermometer for the safety and comfort of the patient.
9. Spread buttocks and gently insert thermometer into the rectum past the sphincter (1½ inches) for adult or ½ to 1 inch for an infant.
10. Hold buttocks together while holding the thermometer. Do not let go of thermometer. RATIONALE: Holding buttocks together prevents air leaks and inaccurate recording. Holding onto thermometer ensures patient safety.
11. Hold in place until the "beep" is heard.
12. Read results on digital display window.
13. Remove from rectum.
14. Discard probe cover into biohazard waste container by pushing the release button.
15. Replace thermometer on holder base.
16. Remove gloves, discard in biohazard waste container, and wash hands.

(continues)

17. Offer tissue to patient to wipe anus. Assist patient in dressing and position as necessary, ***attending to any special needs of the patient.***

18. Accurately record temperature in patient's chart or electronic medical record, indicating a rectal temperature (R).

DOCUMENTATION:

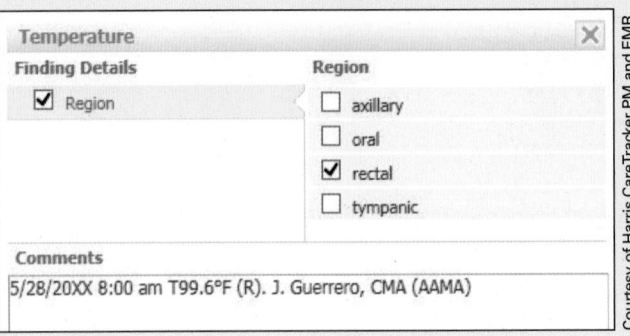

Courtesy of Harris CareTracker PM and EMR

Temperature		✕
Finding Details	**Region**	
☑ Region	☐ axillary	
	☐ oral	
	☑ rectal	
	☐ tympanic	
Comments		
5/28/20XX 8:00 am T99.6°F (R). J. Guerrero, CMA (AAMA)		

PROCEDURE 23-5

Procedure

Measuring an Axillary Temperature

STANDARD PRECAUTIONS:

Handwashing

PURPOSE:

To obtain an axillary temperature using a digital thermometer.

EQUIPMENT/SUPPLIES:

- Digital thermometer
- Sheath
- Towelettes
- Paper towels

PROCEDURE STEPS:

1. Wash hands following Standard Precautions.
2. ***Paying attention to detail***, assemble equipment; place sheath on thermometer.
3. Introduce yourself to the patient. Identify patient.
4. ***Explain rationale for performance of the procedure, speaking at the patient's level of understanding.*** RATIONALE: This elicits patient cooperation and consent.
5. Ask patient to remove clothing to provide access to axilla.
6. Cover patient with gown as necessary to maintain patient modesty and warmth.
7. Wipe axillary area with dry towel or towelette to remove moisture. RATIONALE: Moisture in the axilla will cause inaccurate reading.

(continues)

8. Place thermometer in axilla (Figure 23-11).

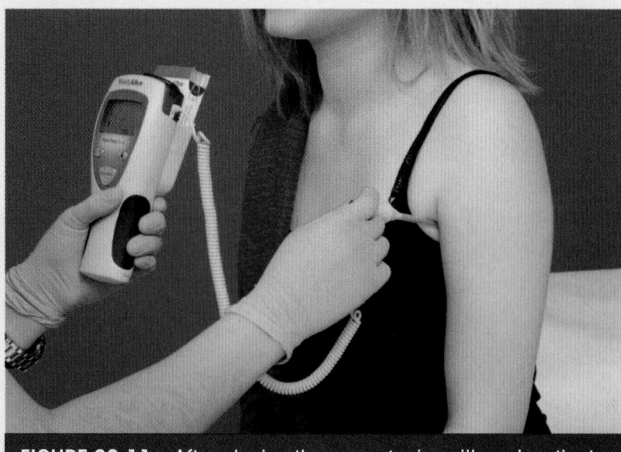

FIGURE 23-11 After placing thermometer in axilla, ask patient to fold arm against chest or abdomen.

9. Ask patient to fold arm against chest or abdomen.

10. Hold in place until the "beep" is heard.

11. Carefully remove from the axillary area.

12. Eject probe cover and appropriately discard.

13. Read temperature in the digital window.

14. Replace thermometer on holder base.

15. Wash hands.

16. Accurately, record temperature in patient's chart or electronic medical record, indicating axillary temperature (A).

DOCUMENTATION:

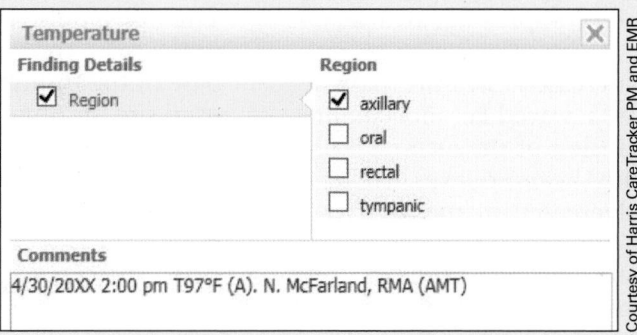

Courtesy of Harris CareTracker PM and EMR

Recording Temperature

Temperature may be taken on each visit to the provider's clinic to obtain a baseline for the patient. When recording the temperature in the patient's electronic medical record, the scale used for the results must be designated F for Fahrenheit and C for Celsius. The Fahrenheit scale is used almost exclusively in the United States. The route used must be labeled as well; methods other than oral must be labeled according to the route used because there is a difference in the measurement. Use R for rectal, A for axillary, Tym for tympanic, and TA for temporal artery.

Temperatures are recorded as shown:

Oral	T 98.6°F
Rectal	T 99.6° (R) F
Axillary	T 97.6° (Ax) F
Tympanic	T 98.6° (Tym) F
Temporal artery	T 99.4° (TA) F

When a facility uses a tympanic thermometer exclusively, the route is known and therefore does not have to be labeled.

Competency

The medical assistant must read all manufacturer's instructions before using any digital, tympanic, or temporal artery thermometer. Each may have a slight difference in operating procedure.

Cleaning and Storage of Thermometers

Digital, electronic, tympanic, and temporal artery thermometers are cleaned according to the manufacturer's directions. The covers protect the probes from contamination. Each type of thermometer has a storage case or a wall-mounted base made especially for storing the unit. Disinfect these types of thermometers by wiping with a mild disinfectant as instructed by the manufacturer.

PULSE

The pulse rate consists of two phases of the heart action and can be felt when compressing an artery. As the heart contracts, it increases pressure on the arterial walls. The increased pressure passes through the arteries in a wave-like movement resulting in a slight expansion of the arterial wall (contraction). When the heart relaxes (relaxation), the pressure is decreased in the arteries, resulting in the wall returning to its previous position. One contraction and one relaxation of the heart together is equal to one heart cycle or heartbeat. The pulse and heartbeat rate are usually identical in healthy individuals.

PULSE SITES

The pulse can be felt in areas of the body where an artery is close to the surface and to an underlying solid structure such as a bone. Common pulse sites include the apical, radial, carotid, temporal, brachial, femoral, popliteal, and dorsalis pedis arteries (Figure 23-12). Although the radial, brachial, and carotid arteries are the most frequently

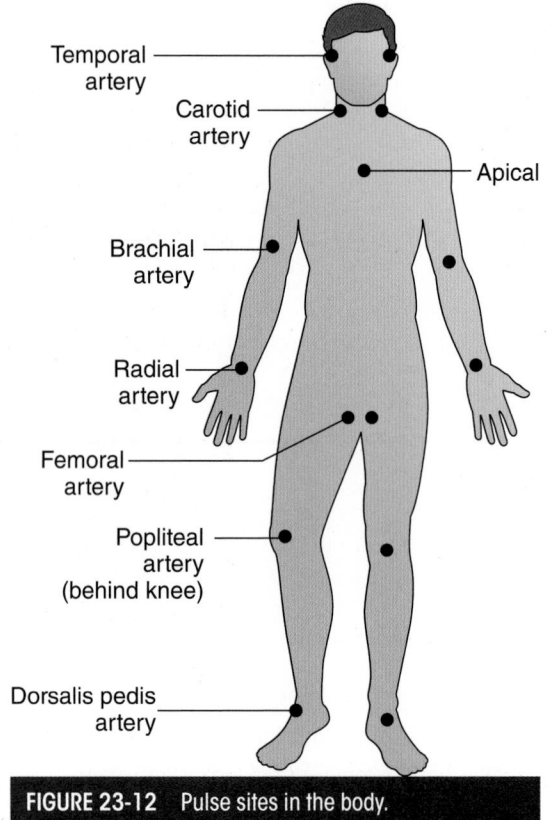

FIGURE 23-12 Pulse sites in the body.

used sites for pulse rates, it is important to recognize pulse beats because circulation may be monitored by palpating the other sites. Pulse sites are also used when necessary as pressure points for controlling severe bleeding.

- The *radial* pulse is located at the thumb side of the wrist approximately 1 inch above the base of the thumb. This is the most commonly used site for obtaining a pulse rate.

- The *carotid* pulse, used during emergency situations and when performing cardiopulmonary resuscitation (CPR), is found between the larynx and sternocleidomastoid muscle in the front side of the neck on either side of the trachea. When measuring the pulse at the carotid site, compress only one side at a time.

- The *brachial* pulse is found in the inner aspect of the elbow called the antecubital space. This pulse site is the most commonly used site to obtain blood pressure measurements.

- The *temporal* pulse is located at the temple area of the head. It is rarely used to obtain a pulse rate but may be used to monitor circulation, control bleeding from the head and scalp, and take a temporal artery temperature.

- The *femoral* pulse is located in the groin area. It is a deep artery and must be compressed firmly to be felt.

- The *popliteal* pulse is located at the back of the knee. The patient must be in a supine position with the knee flexed for it to be felt because the artery is deep within the knee. This artery is used for leg blood pressure measurements and to monitor circulation.

- The *dorsalis pedis* pulse is felt on the top of the foot slightly to the side of midline next to the extensor ligament of the great toe, between the first and second metatarsal bones. It is commonly used to monitor lower limb circulation.

- **Apical** pulse is found at the apex of the heart, located at the fifth intercostal space left side, midclavicular line, that is, between the fifth and sixth ribs perpendicular to the middle of the clavicle, left of the sternum. A stethoscope is required to obtain an apical pulse. Apical pulse is used for cardiac patients and patients with an arrhythmia, and to obtain infant pulse rates because they are difficult to obtain by the usual methods. The provider may want you to take an apical pulse for certain conditions or when the patient is taking specific medications (see Chapter 36).

Measuring and Evaluating a Pulse

When measuring a pulse rate, other characteristics besides the rate are noted, such as rhythm, volume of pulse, and condition of the arterial wall.

The rate is the number of pulsations or beats felt in 1 minute. The pulse is counted for 30 seconds and then the number is doubled. Or with practice, the pulse may be counted for 15 seconds and multiplied by four. When any pulse rate abnormalities or arrhythmias are felt, take the pulse for 1 full minute, note the frequency of the abnormality, record the abnormality, and alert the provider.

Rhythm of the pulse refers to the time between pulsations and regularity of the beat. Normal rhythm occurs when the beats are felt at regular intervals. In abnormal rhythms, **arrhythmias**, the interval between pulsations is altered by either an increased or decreased time span. Arrhythmias must be noted and reported because they may indicate heart disease.

The volume of the pulse refers to the strength of the beat that is felt. The pulsations may feel full, strong, hard, soft, thready, or weak. A pulse may have a regular rate and yet have a variation in intensity or volume. Volume should be noted and reported.

The condition of the arterial wall can be felt as the pulse is taken. The normal artery feels soft and elastic. The abnormal artery may feel hard, knotty, wiry, or a combination of these. These should be noted and reported because they may indicate cardiac disease.

For more information on normal pulse rates and factors that influence a patient's pulse rate, see the "Vital Signs" Quick Reference Guide later in the chapter.

Pulse Abnormalities

Abnormalities may occur in the rate, rhythm, and feel of the arterial wall. Common pulse rate abnormalities include **bradycardia**, a pulse rate less than 60 beats per minute, and **tachycardia**, a pulse rate greater than 100 beats per minute. Common arrhythmias include a pulsation felt before expected, which is called a premature contraction, and sinus arrhythmia. An occasional premature contraction can occur in response to stress, caffeine, nicotine, alcohol, or lack of sleep. Sinus arrhythmia may occur during respiration and can be found in some children and young adults. The rate increases with inspiration and decreases with expiration. It usually does not require treatment.

Recording Pulse Rates

Procedure

Pulse rates are normally recorded after the temperature; for example: T 98.6°F P 72 regular. Any unusual findings should be recorded and reported to the provider; for example, P 72 irregular × 2 minutes. Procedure 23-6 describes measuring a radial pulse, and Procedure 23-7 describes measuring an apical pulse.

RESPIRATION

The function of respiration is the exchange of the gases oxygen and carbon dioxide. External respiration occurs when oxygen is drawn into the lungs when breathing in and carbon dioxide is expelled from the lungs when breathing out. Internal respiration occurs when oxygen is used by the cells for cellular function. Carbon dioxide is a by-product of cellular function and is expelled via exhalation as a waste product. Respiration is an involuntary act controlled by a very specific part of the brain, the medulla oblongata. The medulla oblongata measures blood levels of carbon dioxide and triggers a respiration when the level of carbon dioxide

Procedure

Measuring a Radial Pulse

STANDARD PRECAUTIONS:

Handwashing

PURPOSE:

To obtain a radial pulse rate.

EQUIPMENT/SUPPLIES:

- Watch with second hand

PROCEDURE STEPS:

1. Wash hands.
2. Introduce yourself to the patient. Identify patient.
3. ***Explain rationale for performance of the procedure, speaking at the patient's level of understanding.***
   RATIONALE: Ensures patient cooperation and consent.
4. Position patient with the wrist resting either on a table or on lap.
5. Locate the radial pulse (found at the base of the patient's thumb on the dorsal aspect of the wrist) with the pads of your first three fingers (Figure 23-13). Do not use your thumb; it has its own pulse and could result in an inaccurate reading.

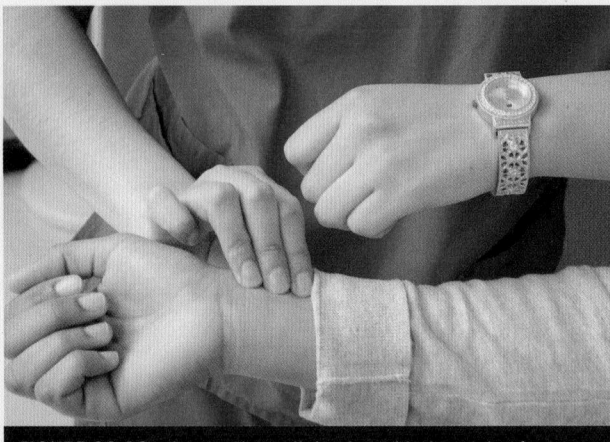

FIGURE 23-13 Locate the radial pulse with the pads of your first three fingers.

6. Gently compress the radial artery enough to feel the pulse.
7. Count the pulsations for 1 full minute using a watch with a second hand or a digital readout. Counting for a full minute allows for the most accuracy. However, with practice, counting for 30 seconds and multiplying the pulsations by two or counting for 15 seconds and multiplying by four to obtain the beats per minute is allowed as long as the pulse is regular.
8. Note any irregularities in rhythm, volume, and condition of artery.
9. Wash hands.
10. Accurately record pulse in patient chart or electronic medical record after the temperature, noting any irregularities.

(continues)

DOCUMENTATION:

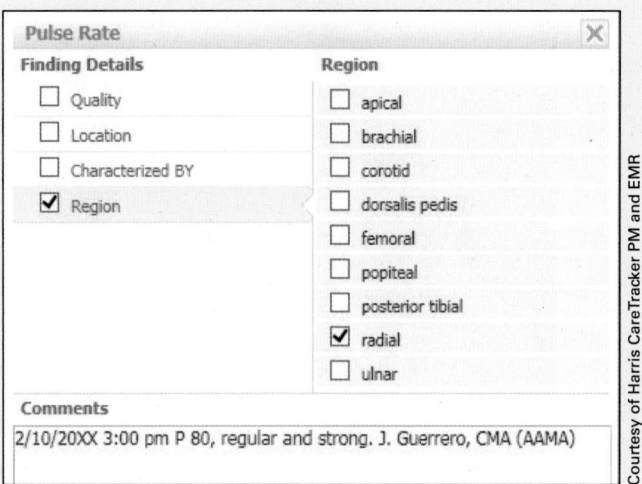

Pulse Rate

Finding Details	Region
☐ Quality	☐ apical
☐ Location	☐ brachial
☐ Characterized BY	☐ corotid
☑ Region	☐ dorsalis pedis
	☐ femoral
	☐ popiteal
	☐ posterior tibial
	☑ radial
	☐ ulnar

Comments

2/10/20XX 3:00 pm P 80, regular and strong. J. Guerrero, CMA (AAMA)

Courtesy of Harris CareTracker PM and EMR

PROCEDURE 23-7

Procedure

Taking an Apical Pulse

STANDARD PRECAUTIONS:

Handwashing

PURPOSE:

To obtain an apical pulse rate.

EQUIPMENT/SUPPLIES:

- Stethoscope
- Watch with second hand
- Alcohol wipes

PROCEDURE STEPS:

1. Wash hands.
2. ***Paying attention to detail***, assemble equipment.
3. Wipe stethoscope earpiece with alcohol wipes.
4. Introduce yourself to the patient. Identify patient.
5. ***Explain the rationale for performance of the procedure, speaking at the patient's level of understanding***.
   RATIONALE: Ensures patient cooperation and consent.
6. Assist patient in disrobing, removing clothing from the waist up, while protecting patient's personal boundaries.
7. Provide a gown or drape for patient modesty and warmth.
8. Position the patient in a supine position. RATIONALE: Easier access to apex of heart.
9. Locate the fifth intercostal space, midclavicular, left of sternum (Figure 23-14). RATIONALE: Location of apex of heart.

(continues)

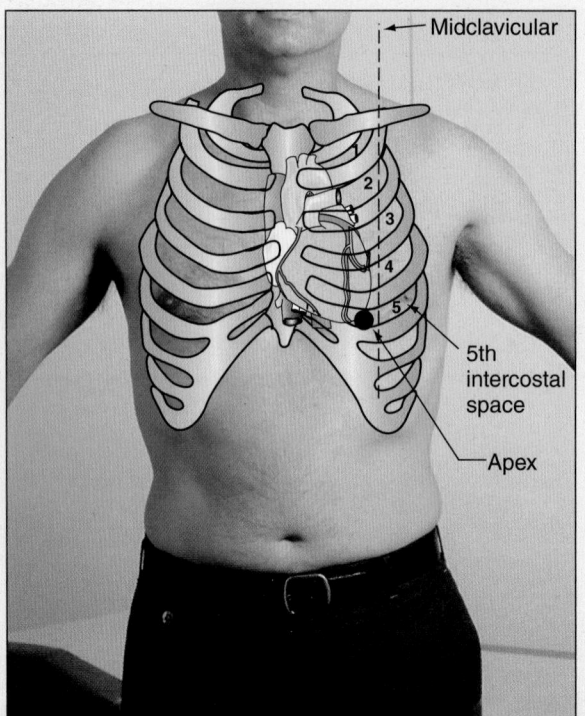

Midclavicular

2
3
4
5

5th
intercostal
space

Apex

FIGURE 23-14   Locate the apical pulse by counting intercostal spaces. Locate the fifth intercostal space.

10. Place stethoscope on the site and listen for the lub-dub sound of the heart.

11. Count the pulse for 1 minute; each lub-dub equals one pulse. Note any additional heart sounds or arrhythmias. NOTE: An apical pulse is normally counted for a full minute.

12. Assist the patient to sit up and dress, ***attending to any special needs of the patient***.

13. Wash hands.

14. Wipe earpieces, diaphragm, and tubing of stethoscope.

15. Accurately record pulse in patient chart or electronic medical record with the designation of apical pulse (AP) to denote method of obtaining the pulse and note any arrhythmias.

NOTE: Apical pulse and radial pulse are frequently taken simultaneously, with the radial pulse taken by another individual. Both pulse rates should be identical. A discrepancy may indicate a cardiac problem.

DOCUMENTATION:

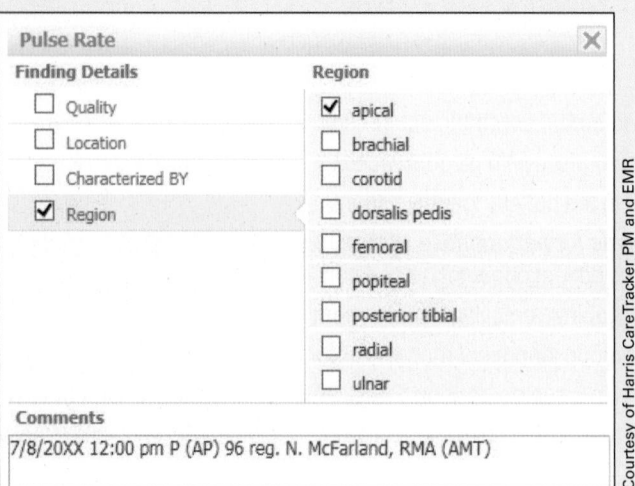

Courtesy of Harris CareTracker PM and EMR

Pulse Rate	✕
Finding Details	**Region**
☐ Quality	☑ apical
☐ Location	☐ brachial
☐ Characterized BY	☐ corotid
☑ Region	☐ dorsalis pedis
	☐ femoral
	☐ popiteal
	☐ posterior tibial
	☐ radial
	☐ ulnar
Comments	
7/8/20XX 12:00 pm P (AP) 96 reg. N. McFarland, RMA (AMT)	

increases. Although it is an involuntary act, respiration may be altered by holding the breath or when hyperventilation occurs. One inspiration (inhalation; drawing in of air) and one expiration (exhalation; expelling air) together equals one respiration.

Abnormalities in the characteristics of respiration, such as rate, rhythm, and depth, are noted when measuring respiration.

Respiratory rhythm refers to the pattern of breathing. It can vary with age, with adults having a regular pattern, but infants having an irregular pattern. Rhythm may be altered by laughing and sighing. The medical term for normal respiration is **eupnea**.

Depth of respiration is the amount of air that is inspired and expired with each respiration. In the resting state, the amount should be consistent. Depth is noted by watching the degree of rise and fall of the chest wall when measuring respiration rate.

Respiration Rate

Procedure

Respiratory rate is measured by counting breaths for 30 seconds and doubling the amount. Or with practice, respirations can be counted for 15 seconds and multiplied by four. This will give the number of respirations per minute. It is important that patients not be aware you are measuring their respirations. The best technique requires a good memory. While watching the second hand on your watch, count the pulse rate for 30 seconds. For the next 30 seconds count the respiratory rate. The rate may change if the patient knows he or she is being counted. Procedure 23-8 gives steps for measuring respiration rate.

For more information on normal respiration rates and factors that influence a patient's respiration rate, see the "Vital Signs" Quick Reference Guide later in the chapter.

PROCEDURE 23-8

Procedure

Measuring the Respiration Rate

STANDARD PRECAUTIONS:

Handwashing

NOTE: The respiration rate is normally taken immediately before or after the pulse rate. It should be taken without patient knowledge because respiration can voluntarily be altered. While counting respirations, it is best to continue grasping the wrist as if still taking the pulse. This procedure will assist in preventing alteration of breathing by the patient.

PURPOSE:
To obtain an accurate respiratory rate.

EQUIPMENT/SUPPLIES:
Watch with second hand

PROCEDURE STEPS:

1. Wash hands.
2. Introduce yourself to the patient. Identify the patient.
3. Position patient in a comfortable position.
4. Watch the rise and fall of the chest wall for 1 minute, or while holding the patient's arm, place it across the chest and feel for the rise and fall of the chest wall. Alternatively, place a hand on the patient's shoulder and feel and watch for the rise and fall of the chest wall. With practice, counting respirations for 30 seconds and multiplying by two or counting for 15 seconds and multiplying by four is allowable as long as the respiratory rate is regular.

(continues)

5. Note depth, rhythm, and breath sounds while counting.

6. Wash hands.

7. Accurately, record the respiration rate in the patient's chart or electronic medical record, noting any irregularities and sounds.

DOCUMENTATION:

Respiratory Rate		✕
Finding Details	**Quality**	
☑ Quality	☐ apnea (during sleep only)	
☐ Characterized BY	☐ bradypnea (<12/min)	
	☑ normal range (12-20/min)	
	☐ tachypnea (>20/min)	
Comments		
8/7/20XX 2:00 pm R 16. Rate and rhythm regular. J. Guerrero, CMA (AAMA)		

Courtesy of Harris CareTracker PM and EMR

Abnormalities

Abnormalities of respiration may be found in the rate, depth, rhythm, and sounds of respiration. Some respiration rate abnormalities include apnea, tachypnea, bradypnea, and Cheyne–Stokes. Sleep apnea and narcolepsy are considered sleep disorders and involve the respiratory system.

Apnea is the complete absence of breathing. It may result from a reduction in stimuli to the respiratory center of the brain. Apnea will occur when the breath is voluntarily held and in Cheyne–Stokes respiration. It can be a serious symptom of other conditions of the cardiovascular and renal systems. It also can result from a head injury such as a concussion.

Tachypnea is a respiratory rate greater than 20 respirations per minute. It may be caused by illness or emotional events or be transient in a newborn. Excessive loss of carbon dioxide may occur if tachypnea is prolonged; there is a potential for this to lead to more serious problems.

Bradypnea is a decrease in the number of respirations to less than 12 breaths per minute and is commonly seen during sleep or because of certain diseases.

Cheyne–Stokes is a breathing pattern that is rhythmic waxing and waning of the depth of respiration due to diseases affecting the respiratory centers such as brain damage or heart failure. The patient breathes deeply for several breaths and then breathes only slightly or stops breathing all together. This pattern of deep breaths and then absent breaths occurs over and over. The duration of these cycles are ordinarily 30 seconds to 2 minutes with 5 to 30 seconds of apnea.

Orthopnea is a respiratory condition of severe **dyspnea** (labored breathing). Breathing is difficult in any position *other* than sitting erect or standing. This condition may be seen in patients with heart failure, angina pectoris, asthma, pulmonary edema, emphysema, pneumonia, and spasmodic coughing. Patients who experience orthopnea must be examined in a sitting position. Other positions will cause discomfort and may not be possible.

Abnormalities in the depth of respiration are divided into shallow abnormalities, such as hypoventilation, and deep abnormalities, such as hyperpnea and hyperventilation.

Hypoventilation occurs when respiration is decreased in rate and shallow in depth. It may result from a depression of nervous stimuli of the respiratory center in the brain due to use of opioid medication or trauma, for example.

Hyperpnea is respiration that is increased in both depth and rate. It is commonly seen with activities such as physical exercise. It can also be associated with pain, respiratory diseases, cardiac diseases, hysteria, and use of certain drugs.

Hyperventilation is a type of breathing in which the amount of oxygen drawn in during inspiration is greatly increased, resulting in a decrease in the amount of blood carbon dioxide. Hyperventilation may be associated with asthma, pulmonary embolism or edema, and acute anxiety. The patient can be treated by reducing the amount of oxygen inhaled during an inspiration. The patient may be instructed to hold one nostril closed while breathing or may be instructed to breathe into a paper bag. Either procedure will reduce the amount of inspired oxygen and bring the oxygen and carbon dioxide blood levels back to within normal range.

Sleep Apnea.   Airflow during respiration that stops for more than 10 seconds is considered to be sleep apnea. The periods of apnea cause carbon dioxide to accumulate in the blood and oxygen to be depleted. For these reasons, sleep apnea can be dangerous. Oxygen depletion to the brain can cause memory impairment, cognitive changes, and daytime sleepiness. If the condition goes untreated, sleep apnea can result in cardiac arrhythmias, congestive heart failure, cerebral vascular accident (CVA), hypertension, and death.

Sleep apnea is associated with airway obstruction. The soft palate (especially in males who are overweight and who snore) can collapse while the patient is asleep. The result is apnea. The patient usually awakens from sleep enough to resume breathing.

Sleep apnea is diagnosed by sleep laboratory studies when apnea is observed while the patient is sleeping.

Treatment of sleep apnea commonly consists of continuous positive airway pressure (CPAP), which puts pressure on the airway while the patient sleeps. A mask is placed over the patient's face to keep the airway open. This prevents sleep apnea. There are other methods available to treat sleep apnea. A surgical procedure can be performed to remove parts of the soft palate and uvula. There are also dental appliances that reposition the lower jaw and tongue. One of the first recommendations for treatment is usually lifestyle changes. These include weight loss, smoking cessation, and alcohol avoidance.

Narcolepsy.   Narcolepsy is another type of sleep disorder that causes excessive sleepiness and frequent daytime sleep attacks. The patient can become paralyzed from the sleep, being unable to move, but can still breathe. The cause may be genetic. It is possible that this is an autoimmune disorder. Most commonly, symptoms first appear in 15- to 30-year-olds.

The diagnosis is made by ruling out sleep apnea (through sleep studies) and by the history of repeated episodes of daytime sleeping for a few seconds to half an hour. An EEG, an EKG, a sleep study, and genetic testing for the narcolepsy gene are all components of testing for narcolepsy. The disorder is not under the patient's control.

Breath Sounds.   The presence or absence of breath sounds can be indicative of respiratory problems. Sounds should be listened for and noted when taking the patient's respiratory rate.

Rales (pronounced "rahls") are crackling or rattling sounds heard during inspiration and expiration when the lung passageways contain secretions. The provider uses a stethoscope to auscultate or listen for rales, which are associated with some lung diseases. Rhonchi are sounds similar to snoring, usually produced by a rattle in the throat. These are also heard by auscultation.

Rhonchi are low-pitched sounds that are present during inspiration and expiration continuously. Their sound resembles snoring when auscultated through a stethoscope. Their presence indicates obstruction or the presence of secretions in conditions such as pneumonia, chronic obstructive pulmonary disease (COPD), or bronchitis.

Wheezes are high-pitched musical sounds heard on expiration. They can be the result of an obstruction in the bronchi and bronchioles of the lungs. Wheezes are commonly associated with asthma and emphysema, a chronic pulmonary disease characterized by dilated and damaged alveoli.

Stridor is a crowing sound heard on inspiration as a result of an obstruction of the upper airway. It is associated with laryngitis, a foreign body obstruction, and croup in children.

Stertorous respiration is described as a snoring sound with labored breathing. The sound usually is created by partial obstruction of the upper airway.

To hear examples of some of these respiratory sounds, go to http://www.easyauscultation .com.

BLOOD PRESSURE

Blood pressure assesses cardiovascular function by measuring the force of blood exerted on **peripheral** arteries during the cardiac cycle or heartbeat. The measurement consists of two components. The first is the force exerted on the arterial walls during cardiac contraction and is called **systole**. The second is the force exerted during cardiac relaxation and is called **diastole**. They represent the highest (systole) and lowest (diastole) amount of pressure exerted during the cardiac cycle. Blood pressure is recorded as a fraction, with the systolic measurement written, followed by a slash, and then the diastolic measurement.

systole/diastole or 118/68

Blood pressure may be affected by many factors, including blood volume, peripheral resistance, vessel elasticity, condition of the muscle of the heart, genetics, diet and weight, activity, and emotional state.

- Blood volume is the amount of blood in the vessels. An increased volume of blood increases blood pressure, whereas a decrease in blood volume decreases blood pressure, as in the case of a hemorrhage or severe dehydration.

- Peripheral resistance is the resistance to blood flow within the arteries. The resistance is in direct relation to the **lumen** or channel within the arteries. The smaller the lumen, the more pressure is needed to push blood through. The reverse is also true: The larger the lumen, the less resistance and less pressure are needed to push the blood through. The size of the lumen can become smaller from deposits of fatty cholesterol (plaque), resulting in an increase in blood pressure.

- Vessel elasticity refers to the ability of arteries to expand and contract to provide a steady flow of blood. As a person ages, elasticity of the vessels is reduced. **Atherosclerosis**, a disease in which plaque builds up inside your arteries, can cause an increase in arterial wall resistance, resulting in an increase in blood pressure.

- The condition of the heart muscle is extremely important to blood flow and blood pressure. A strong heart muscle provides a forceful pump resulting in efficient blood flow and normal blood pressure. A weak heart muscle results in an inefficient pumping action of the heart leading to a decrease in blood pressure and blood flow (see Chapter 36).

- Uncontrolled hypertension, over time, is responsible for changes in the heart's structure, vessels that supply the heart muscle, and electrical conduction system of the heart. These changes can lead to life-threatening conditions such as arrhythmias and congestive heart failure.

The viscosity of the blood also is a factor in blood pressure. Viscosity is the property of a fluid that offers resistance to flow. If the blood's viscosity is increased, it becomes thicker. Imagine holding a bottle of thin syrup upside down over your pancakes. The thin syrup comes out of the bottle quite readily. Now imagine holding a bottle of thick molasses over the pancakes. Being very viscous, the molasses is thicker and much more difficult to pour. So it is with viscous blood; it is thicker and requires a lot more work for the heart muscle to move it through the vessels, thus increasing the pressure inside the walls of the arteries. In fact, it may be so viscous that it might not be able to reach the tiniest capillaries of the kidneys, eyes, and other areas without substantial increase in blood pressure.

Equipment for Measuring Blood Pressure

Blood pressure is measured by the auscultatory method using a sphygmomanometer and a stethoscope (Figure 23-15). Listening carefully is the key to obtaining an accurate blood pressure measurement.

Three types of sphygmomanometers are commonly used in the ambulatory care setting: mercury, aneroid, and electronic (digital) manometers (Figures 23-16 through 23-18).

Mercury sphygmomanometers are being phased out with other mercury-containing medical equipment such as mercury thermometers and are rarely seen in health care settings. Aneroid and electronic blood pressure measuring devices are more commonly used. Few medical facilities continue to use mercury sphygmomanometers due to phasing them out in agreement with the Environmental Protection Agency (EPA), but the process has been slower than the phasing out of mercury thermometers; therefore, information about mercury sphygmomanometers is provided in this chapter.

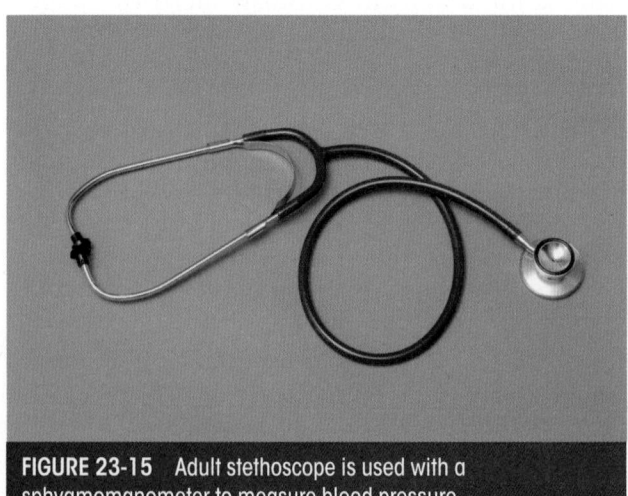

FIGURE 23-15 Adult stethoscope is used with a sphygmomanometer to measure blood pressure.

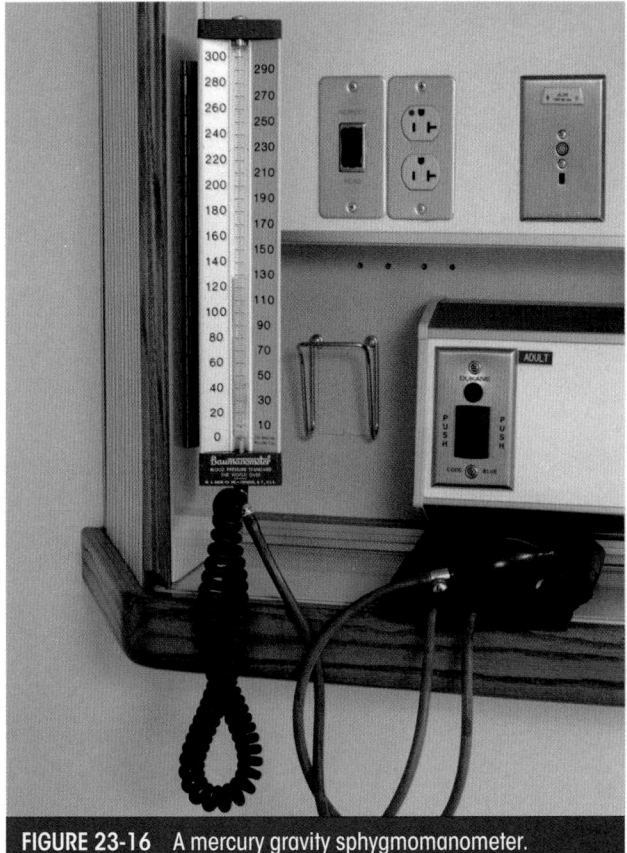

FIGURE 23-16 A mercury gravity sphygmomanometer.

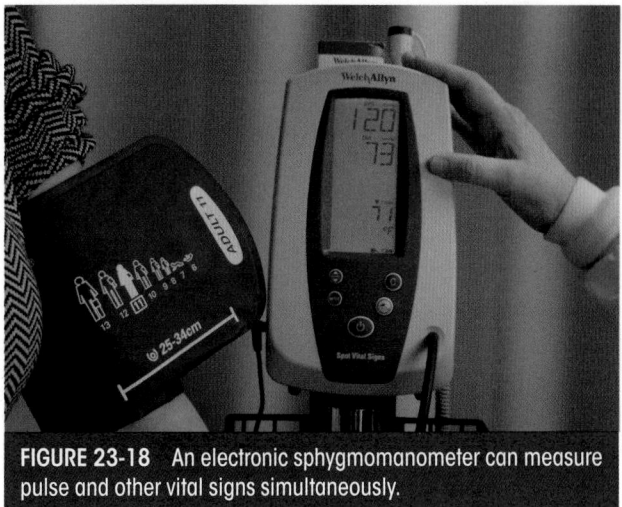

FIGURE 23-18 An electronic sphygmomanometer can measure pulse and other vital signs simultaneously.

The mercury **manometer** consists of a cuff containing a rubber bladder attached by rubber tubing to a glass column of mercury. Blood pressure is read at the **meniscus** of the mercury as it descends the column. The meniscus is the curve seen at the top of a liquid in response to its container. Mercury manometers are the most accurate method of blood pressure measurement and are considered the standard because blood pressure is measured in millimeters of mercury, but they are rarely found in health care settings in the United States. Although the most accurate, mercury manometers do have disadvantages: They are not as portable as aneroid manometers, and there is always the danger of a mercury spill that could cause health and environmental problems should the glass column break. Mercury manometers need to be cleaned and checked regularly for accuracy by a professional technician. Care in handling and storage is important to prevent air bubbles and dirt from forming in the column and to prevent breaking the glass containing the mercury.

The aneroid manometer is a cuff containing a rubber bladder attached to a dial. Blood pressure is read at the point of the needle descending the dial. Aneroid manometers need to be calibrated regularly because they do not maintain calibration easily. Care in handling and storage will decrease the loss of calibration. Although not as accurate as a mercury manometer, aneroid manometers are easily portable and there is no danger of a mercury spill.

An electronic sphygmomanometer is automatic and registers blood pressure in digital form on a screen (Figure 23-18). No stethoscope is needed. Once the cuff is secured on the patient's upper arm, the medical assistant pushes a button

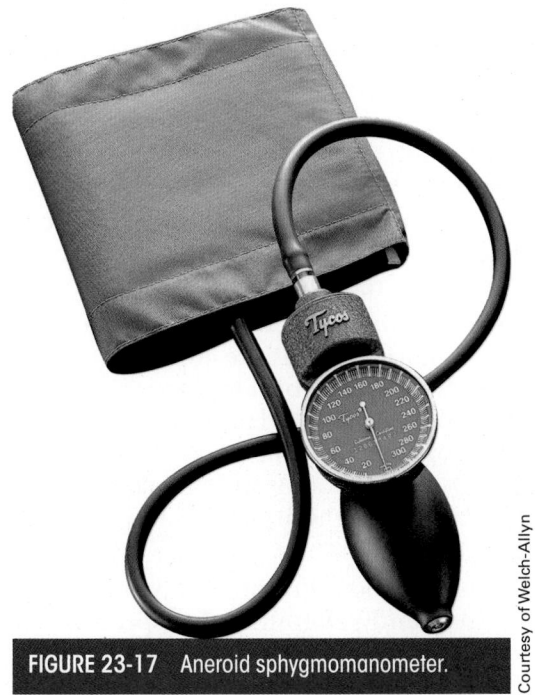

FIGURE 23-17 Aneroid sphygmomanometer.

Courtesy of Welch-Allyn

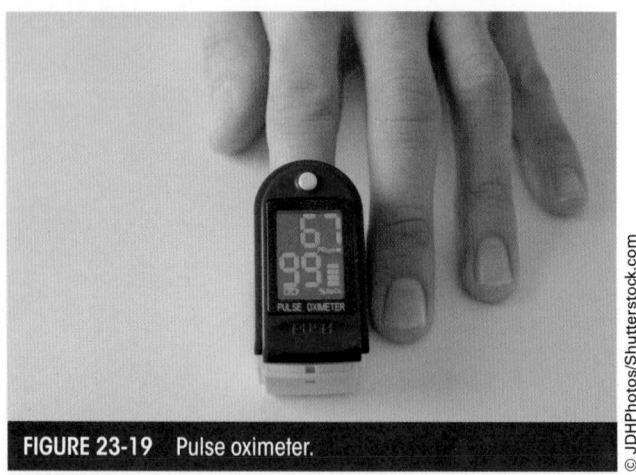

FIGURE 23-19 Pulse oximeter.

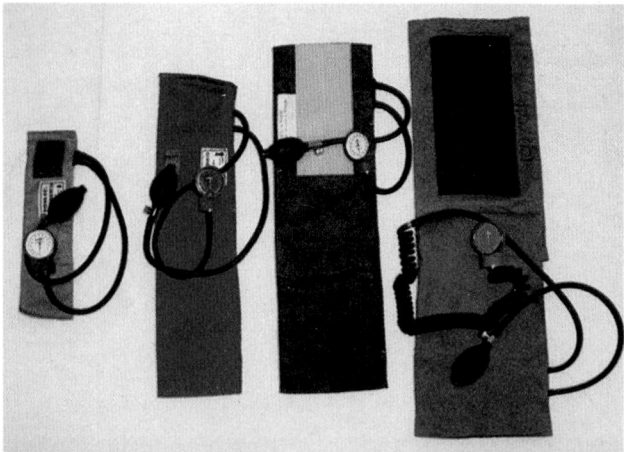

FIGURE 23-20 Blood pressure cuffs in sizes to fit the arm of a small child to the thigh of an adult. It is important to have the correct size to obtain an accurate reading.

and the cuff inflates; the medical assistant then releases the pressure slowly. The result is visible on the screen (e.g., 124/75). In addition to providing a blood pressure reading, the unit can automatically measure pulse rate and other vital signs.

A **pulse oximeter** (Figure 23-19) is a noninvasive method for measuring the amount of oxygen that is saturating the hemoglobin molecules contained in a red blood cell. Most pulse oximeters also provide an audible signal for the pulse and display a calculated heart rate. The measurement automatically appears on the screen when the device is attached to the patient. In order to obtain an accurate reading, the oximeter must be placed on an area that has good blood flow and can be held still. Usually, a finger is chosen for pulse oximetry. However, there are sensors specially designed for use on the earlobe or forehead.

Cuff sizes for manometers range from the smallest pediatric cuff to the largest adult obese and thigh cuff (Figure 23-20). The appropriate cuff size is necessary to obtain an accurate blood pressure measurement. A cuff that is too small will give an artificially high blood pressure reading, whereas a cuff that is too large will give an artificially low reading. The selection of the cuff size depends on the size of the arm, not the age of the patient. Due to the size of the arm, it may be necessary to use an adult-size cuff on a child or a pediatric-size cuff on an adult. Adult cuffs should have a width that covers one third to one half the circumference of the arm. The length of the bladder should cover approximately 80% of the arm (about twice the size of the width). The cuff for a child should cover two thirds of the upper arm. The American Heart Association recommends if there has been a weight loss or gain of 10 pounds, then the cuff size should be reassessed for the appropriate size.

Measuring Blood Pressure

The sounds heard during blood pressure measurement are named the Korotkoff sounds. The cause of the sounds is not known. They may be a result of distention of the vessels or the sound of the blood passing through the vessels. In either case, Korotkoff sounds have five distinct phases. Not all phases are heard easily, especially by beginners.

- *Phase I.* Begins with the first sound heard when deflating the cuff. It is a sharp tapping sound. Note this first sound, as this will be the *systolic reading* of the blood pressure.

- *Phase II.* This sound is the result of more blood passing through the vessels as the cuff is deflated. The sound is that of a soft swishing.

- *Phase III.* More blood continues to pass through the vessels as the cuff is deflated. The sound is a rhythmic tapping. If blood pressure measurements are not carefully followed and Phases I and II are missed, Phase III may erroneously be reported as the systolic pressure.

- *Phase IV.* Blood is now passing through the vessels fairly easily as the cuff is deflated. The sounds heard will be a muffling and fading of the tapping sounds. This phase may be used to record the diastolic pressure in children and in those patients where a tapping sound is heard throughout the deflation until the gauge reaches zero.

- *Phase V.* Blood is flowing freely at this time; consequently, all sounds disappear. The disappearance of sounds is noted and recorded as the *diastolic pressure.*

When measuring blood pressure, keep two things in mind: patient comfort and accuracy.

Auscultatory gap is heard in some patients. It is a time, usually between Phases I and II or III, when all sounds disappear. Within 20 to 30 mm Hg, or 20 to 30 **increments** on the aneroid manometer, the sounds reappear. If the procedures are not followed carefully, the auscultatory gap is easily missed, and the blood pressure measurement is incorrect in that systolic and diastolic readings may be in error according to the length of the gap (Table 23-1).

Pulse pressure is the difference between the systolic and diastolic measurements. It is important because it is a better predictor of clinical outcome than either systolic or diastolic pressure alone. An elevated pulse pressure causes more arterial damage and indicates more workload on the left ventricle. The normal range for pulse pressure is 30 to 50 mm Hg. The difference should be no more than one third of the systolic reading. For example, if the blood pressure is 120/80, a normal pulse pressure should be 120 minus 80, or 40. One third of the systolic reading of 120 is 40, and 40 mm Hg pulse pressure is within the normal range.

For more information on normal blood pressure readings and factors that influence a patient's blood pressure, see the "Vital Signs" Quick Reference Guide later in the chapter.

Recording Blood Pressure Measurement

The blood pressure is recorded on the patient chart or electronic medical record in a fraction format. The position of the patient (sitting or lying down) may be noted. The arm used is also noted, particularly if the blood pressure was taken in both arms.

Example:

$$120/80, \circledR \text{ arm, supine or } \frac{120}{80} \circledR \text{ arm, supine}$$

For children and patients whose blood pressure can still be heard to zero, the beginning of Korotkoff phase IV and zero both are recorded.

Example:

$$120/70/0 \text{ or } \frac{\frac{120}{70}}{0}$$

Procedure

Procedure 23-9 outlines the procedure for measuring blood pressure.

TABLE 23-1

ERRORS IN BLOOD PRESSURE MEASUREMENT PROCEDURES

ERRORS IN MEASURING BLOOD PRESSURE MUST BE AVOIDED. COMMON ERRORS INCLUDE:

1. Improper cuff size.

2. The arm is not at heart level. Do not hold the arm up or let the patient hold up the arm. Pressure is increased when this is done. It is essential that the arm be at the correct level and supported so that there is minimal muscle tension to obtain a correct reading.

3. Cuff is not completely deflated before use or after palpatory method, resulting in a higher pressure measurement.

4. Deflation of the cuff is faster than 2 to 4 mm Hg per heartbeat or 20 to 30 increments on the aneroid. Sounds are missed if this happens.

5. Reinflating the cuff during the procedure without allowing the arm to rest for 1 to 2 minutes.

6. Patient is not relaxed and comfortable. An anxious, apprehensive patient will have a reading that is higher than the actual blood pressure.

7. Improper cuff placement. Cuff is too loose, too tight, or not positioned correctly over the brachial artery.

8. Defective equipment in which there are air leaks in the bladder or valve, the mercury column is dirty, or air bubbles are present. Mercury and aneroid sphygmomanometers are not calibrated at zero.

9. Measuring blood pressure with thumb on the head of the stethoscope.

All of these errors are easily corrected by following careful procedure and by having the manometers calibrated and cleaned according to a regular maintenance schedule.

PROCEDURE 23-9

Procedure

Measuring Blood Pressure

STANDARD PRECAUTIONS:

Handwashing

PURPOSE:

To measure blood pressure.

EQUIPMENT/SUPPLIES:

- Stethoscope
- Sphygmomanometer
- Alcohol wipes
- Blood pressure cuff of suitable size

PROCEDURE STEPS:

1. Wash hands.
2. ***Paying attention to detail***, assemble equipment, making sure that cuff size is correct. RATIONALE: Inappropriate cuff size will result in inaccurate measurement.
3. Clean earpieces of stethoscope with alcohol wipe.
4. Introduce yourself to the patient. Identify patient.
5. ***Explain the rationale for performance of the procedure, speaking at the patient's level of understanding***. RATIONALE: May be the first instance blood pressure is measured; to allay anxiety and ensure cooperation and consent.
6. Position patient comfortably; feet flat on the floor, arm resting at heart level on the lap or a table. RATIONALE: Crossed legs may arbitrarily increase blood pressure; arm above heart level may result in inaccurate reading.
7. Bare the upper arm. If clothing is restricting, have patient remove it. RATIONALE: Tight clothing on the arm can produce inaccurate results. Right arm is used for consistency, but if one arm measures a higher reading, then that arm is used consistently to measure the blood pressure.
8. Select the appropriate cuff based on the diameter of the patient's upper arm.
9. Position the patient so that the brachial artery is at the level of the heart and the arm is supported so that there is not additional muscular tension.
10. Palpate brachial artery.
11. Securely center the bladder of the cuff over the brachial artery above the bend of the elbow. RATIONALE: Be sure that the lower edge of the cuff is at least 1 inch above the antecubital fossa so that the bell of the stethoscope does not touch the cuff or extraneous sounds may be heard. Be certain the needle on the gauge is at zero prior to inflating the cuff.
12. Locate and palpate the radial pulse and smoothly inflate cuff until the pulse is no longer felt. Note the number.
13. Quickly deflate the cuff and allow the arm to rest for about a minute. Calculate the peak inflation level by adding 30 mm Hg to the number where the pulse was no longer palpated. RATIONALE: This ensures that an auscultatory gap is not missed.
14. Make sure cuff is completely deflated.

(continues)

15. Position the stethoscope over the brachial artery and hold in position with the fingers only.

16. Inflate the cuff smoothly and quickly to the peak inflation level plus 30 mm Hg (Figure 23-21).

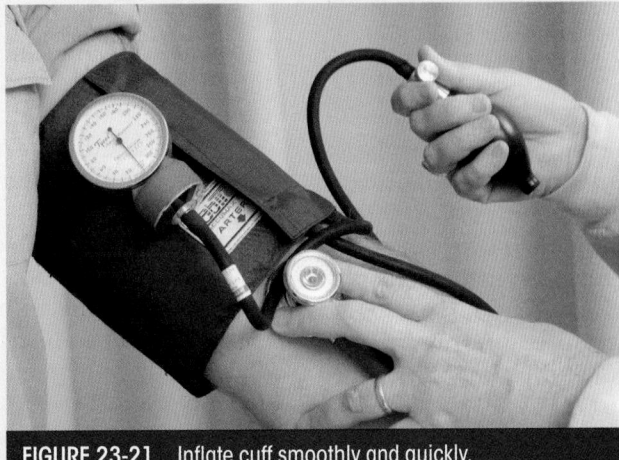

FIGURE 23-21   Inflate cuff smoothly and quickly.

17. Deflate the cuff at a rate of 2 to 4 mm Hg per heartbeat. RATIONALE: No matter how experienced you become, accurate blood pressure readings cannot be obtained if the cuff deflation is greater than 2 to 4 mm Hg per heartbeat.

18. Listen for Korotkoff phase I and note when it appears. This will be the systolic value reported.

19. Continue deflation, noting the Korotkoff phases.

20. Note when all sounds disappear, which is Korotkoff Phase V. This will be the diastolic value reported.

21. Continue deflating the cuff at the same rate for at least another 10 mm Hg after sounds have disappeared. RATIONALE: To avoid mistaking the auscultatory gap for the diastolic reading.

22. Deflate the cuff quickly.

23. Remove the cuff.

24. Clean the earpieces and diaphragm of the stethoscope with alcohol wipes.

25. Wash hands.

26. Accurately record blood pressure in the patient's chart or electronic medical record.

NOTE: On a patient's initial visit and in patients with hypertension, the provider may want the blood pressure taken in both arms. There is normally a slight variation in pressure between the arms. If it is necessary to repeat the procedure, wait approximately 5 minutes before doing so.

DOCUMENTATION:

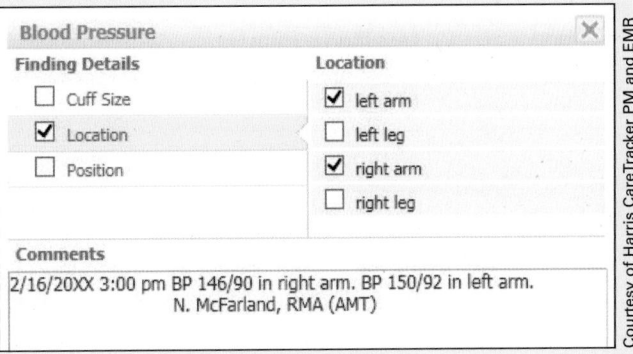

Courtesy of Harris CareTracker PM and EMR

Normal Blood Pressure Readings

Normal blood pressure is low at birth and gradually increases with age until adulthood, at which point it should remain fairly constant. Blood pressure measurements are taken during yearly physical examinations beginning at age 3.

Blood Pressure Abnormalities

There are only two possible blood pressure abnormalities: hypertension (blood pressure that is consistently above normal) and hypotension (blood pressure that is consistently below normal and patients are unable to perform their normal activities without dizziness and extreme fatigue). It is essential that any blood pressure abnormalities be reported to the provider in a timely manner.

Blood pressure measurement, as well as other vital signs, vary over the age continuum. An excellent reference for variations in children from birth to age 15 years can be found at http://www.pedscases.com by searching for "Vital Signs Reference Chart."

Hypertension. There are two primary types of **hypertension**: primary and secondary hypertension. Primary hypertension (also known as essential or **idiopathic** hypertension) is described as elevated blood pressure that is noticed over a period of time and most often is asymptomatic. There are no underlying disease processes that can be identified, even though there are lifestyle factors that influence this type of hypertension. These factors, which are modifiable, are obesity, diet, lack of exercise, smoking, and the consumption of alcohol.

One in three Americans adults has a blood pressure above 140/90 mm Hg. Several opinions were published in 2016 regarding treatment of essential hypertension. The *Journal of the American Medical Association* advises treatment at 140/90 for adults from ages 30 to 59, but starting only at 150/90 mm Hg for people 60 and older. The American Heart Association recommendations starting with lifestyle changes and then medication if necessary beginning at 140/90 mm Hg until age 80, then at 150/90 mm Hg (Table 23-2).

Secondary hypertension is the result of some underlying problem, such as renal disease, pregnancy, endocrine imbalances, obesity, arteriosclerosis, or atherosclerosis. The most common cause of secondary hypertension is cardiovascular disease in the arteries supplying the kidneys. Once the underlying problem is removed, blood pressure returns to normal or near normal. Secondary hypertension can be successfully treated.

Hypertension can become a medical emergency if it is uncontrolled and pressures rise to higher than 180 mm Hg systolic or higher than 110 mm Hg diastolic. This is considered hypertensive urgency. Diastolic pressure above 120 mm Hg is a hypertensive crisis. For either of these situations, the American Heart Association recommends seeking emergency medical treatment. Potential results of this elevated blood pressure may be severe and include stroke, heart attack, kidney failure, and damage to arteries in all areas of the body.

"White coat hypertension" is not related to an underlying disease process. It is caused by anxiety

TABLE 23-2

BLOOD PRESSURE CATEGORIES

SYSTOLIC		DIASTOLIC	AMERICAN HEART ASSOCIATION BLOOD PRESSURE CATEGORY
Less than 120 mm Hg	and	Less than 80 mm Hg	Normal
120 to 139 mm Hg	or	80 to 89 mm Hg	Prehypertension
140 to 159 mm Hg	or	90 to 99 mm Hg	High blood pressure (hypertension) stage 1
160 mm Hg or higher	or	100 mm Hg or higher	High blood pressure (hypertension) stage 2
Higher than 180 mm Hg	or	110 mm Hg or higher	Hypertensive crisis (emergency care needed)

Source: Adapted from American Heart Association guidelines, www.heart.org.

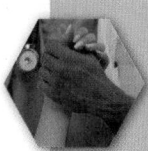

Patient Education

Hypertension is at epidemic proportions in the United States, and many patients are not treated because they do not know that they have the problem. This is known as the "silent epidemic" because most people do not experience symptoms over a span of years. However, untreated or poorly treated hypertension over time can damage the heart, cause myocardial infarction, cause a stroke (cerebrovascular accident), or lead to kidney failure.

There are several nondrug ways to reduce blood pressure, even for people who have inherited hypertensive tendencies. With the provider's advice, there are steps to take, including eating plenty of produce, grains, and low-fat dairy foods; cutting back on salt; stopping smoking; exercising regularly; maintaining a healthy weight; limiting alcohol intake; and reducing stress. It is easy to see that these recommendations all are lifestyle changes. They can significantly reduce blood pressure if practiced daily. Blood pressure must be monitored regularly by the provider.

or fear when blood pressure measurements are taken by a health care provider.

Hypotension. Hypotension is blood pressure persistently less than normal, usually less than 90/60, although this may be normal for some healthy adults. **Hypotension** is defined as a blood pressure so low that the patient is unable to maintain normal function. It is usually a result of various shock-like conditions such as hemorrhage, traumatic or emotional shock, central nervous system disorders, or chronic wasting diseases. With successful treatment of the underlying problems, the blood pressure usually is in the range of normal readings.

Orthostatic hypotension, sometimes called postural hypotension, occurs when a person rapidly changes position from supine to standing or stands in one position for too long. Alternatively, it can be a side effect of certain medications. In this instance, blood pressure has momentarily decreased, and the person experiences vertigo (dizziness) and may have blurred vision. These symptoms usually last only a few seconds, just long enough for the blood pressure to return to normal. Care should be taken when helping patients to an upright position from a supine position because orthostatic hypotension can lead to syncope (fainting) and injury from falling.

HEIGHT AND WEIGHT

Although not considered a vital sign, height and weight are routinely measured if warranted by the age and the physical condition of the patient. Many providers prefer that height and weight be measured as part of a yearly physical examination and otherwise may vary the frequency of patient height and weight measurements. Height and weight are normally measured simultaneously.

For children, height and weight are typically measured during each provider visit. The height of adults may be obtained on the initial visit only and weight taken on all visits. An adolescent or young adult may have height measured more frequently to plot body changes. Because older adult patients tend to lose the cushioning between vertebrae through osteoporosis as part of aging, they may need to have their height measured more frequently to check the stage of any degeneration.

Safety

Older adult patients require special attention by the medical assistant when measuring height and weight. It is especially important to assist older patients both on and off the scale, because the scale platform is movable, and older patients may lose their balance and fall if unassisted. A stand-alone walker can be placed over the scale platform to aid in stabilizing the patient.

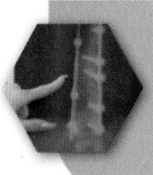

Critical Thinking

Discuss the normal vital signs differences expected between an infant and an adult. Why do they occur?

Height

To measure a patient's height, a scale with a measuring bar is necessary (Figure 23-22A). A paper towel is placed on the scale because the patient's shoes should be removed for accurate measuring. The patient is asked to step on the scale and face

>> QUICK REFERENCE GUIDE

>> VITAL SIGNS

TEMPERATURE

Method	Normal Range
Oral	0 to 2 years: not recommended
	3 to 10 years: 95.9°F to 99.5°F
	11 to 65 years: 97.6°F to 99.6°F
	>65 years: 96.4°F to 98.5°F
Axillary/Temporal Artery	0 to 2 years: 94.5°F to 99.1°F
	3 to 10 years: 96.6°F to 98°F
	11 to 65 years: 95.3°F to 98.4°F
	>65 years: 96°F to 97.4°F
Aural	0 to 2 years: 97.5°F to 100.4°F
	3 to 10 years: 97.0°F to 100.0°F
	11 to 65 years: 96.6°F to 99.7°F
	>65 years: 96.4°F to 99.5°F
Rectal	0 to 2 years: 97.9°F to 100.4°F
	3 to 10 years: 97.9°F to 100.4°F
	11 to 65 years: 97.1°F to 99.2°F

Factors That Influence Temperature

Increased Temperature	Decreased Temperature
Metabolism	Female hormones after menses
Female hormones prior to menses	Hypothyroidism
Hyperthyroidism	Addison disease
Environmental factors such as shower, sauna, or hot weather	Drug/alcohol abuse
Physical activity	Kidney failure
Pregnancy	Liver failure
Medications that increase metabolism	Shock
Emotional reactions	Cancer
Age—infants have a higher core temperature than adults	Viral infections
Bacterial infections	Medications that decrease metabolic activity
	Environmental factors such as immersion in cool water or freezing temperatures
	Sleep
	Age—older adults have a lower metabolic rate and therefore a lower core temperature

(continues)

PULSE

Age	Normal Range
Birth	120 to 170 beats per minute
Infants	100 to 150 beats per minute
Children • 1 year	120 to 160 beats per minute
• 2 years	80 to 140 beats per minute
• 3 years	70 to 120 beats per minute
• 7 to 14 years	50 to 90 beats per minute
Adults	60 to 100 beats per minute

Factors That Influence Pulse Rate

Increased Pulse Rate	Decreased Pulse Rate
Physical exertion	Rest and sleep
Females have a slightly higher rate than males	Beta blocker and digitalis medications
Age—increased in infancy and childhood as well as older age	Hypothyroidism
Elevated body temperature such as fever	Decreased body temperature (hypothermia)
Pain	Fitness level—very fit patients have a lower heart rate
Emotional upset or excitement	
Lower than normal blood pressure	
Stimulant medications	
Stress	
Fight or flight response	
Hyperthyroidism	
Dehydration	

RESPIRATION RATE

Age	Normal Range
Newborns	30 to 60 respirations per minute
Infants	24 to 40 respirations per minute
Children (1 to 7 years)	22 to 34 respirations per minute
Adults and Children > 8 years	14 to 20 respirations per minute

(continues)

Factors That Influence Respiration Rate

Increased Respiration Rate	Decreased Respiration Rate
Decreased blood pressure	Increased blood pressure
Increased body temperature (fever)	Decreased body temperature (hypothermia)
Pain	Resting and sleeping
Decreased levels of oxygen in blood	Decreased levels of carbon dioxide in blood
Exercise	Use of opioid pain medications
Allergic reactions	
Stress	
Fight of flight response	
Emotions such as distress, fear, and excitement	

BLOOD PRESSURE

Age	Normal Range
Newborn	65 to 85 mm Hg systolic; 45 to 55 mm Hg diastolic
Infant	70 to 100 mm Hg systolic; 50 to 65 mm Hg diastolic
1 to 3 years	90 to 105 mm Hg systolic; 55 to 70 mm Hg diastolic
3 to 6 years	95 to 110 mm Hg diastolic; 60 to 75 mm Hg systolic
6 to 12 years	100 to 120 mm Hg systolic; 60 to 75 mm Hg diastolic
12 to 20 years	110 to 135 mm Hg systolic; 65 to 85 mm Hg diastolic
Adult	Less than 120/80 mm Hg (less than 120 systolic AND less than 80 diastolic)

Factors That Influence Blood Pressure

Increased Blood Pressure	Decreased Blood Pressure
Obesity	Antihypertensive medications
Smoking	Diuretic medications
Increased salt intake	Rest and sleep
Older age	Shock
Inactivity—less physically fit	Bleeding
Stress	Physical fitness
Alcohol consumption	Heart failure
Hyperthyriodism	Dehydration
Family history	Younger ages
Emotions such as fear, anxiety, or excitement	Hypothyroidism
Kidney disease	
Sleep apnea	
Exercise or other physical activity	
Vascular disease	

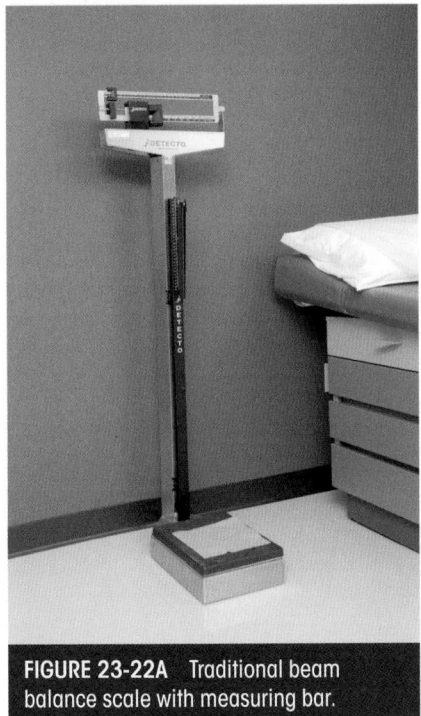

FIGURE 23-22A Traditional beam balance scale with measuring bar.

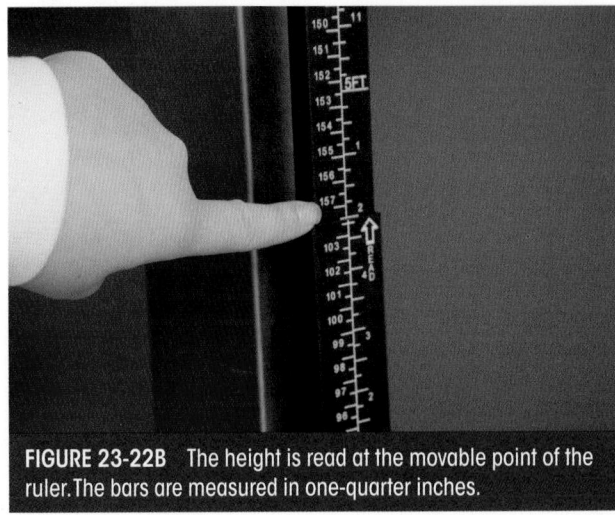

FIGURE 23-22B The height is read at the movable point of the ruler. The bars are measured in one-quarter inches.

away from the measuring bar. Assist the patient onto the scale; the scale platform is movable and the patient could fall.

There are two reasons for having the patient's back to the scale. When the measuring bar is lifted, it could cause face or eye injuries if the patient were facing the bar. Lifting the measuring bar prior to the patient stepping on the scale can also lead to eye and face injuries in that the patient could inadvertently walk into the bar. Another reason to have the patient's back to the scale is if the patient does not look straight ahead, the head is not level, which could result in a less-than-accurate measurement.

Procedure After the patient is on the platform, the measuring bar is placed firmly on the patient's head, and the line between where the solid bar and sliding bar meet is read. The bars are measured in quarter inches (Figure 23-22B). Children's heights are recorded in inches, whereas adults are recorded in feet and inches. Conversion from inches to feet is accomplished by taking the number of inches and dividing by 12. Procedure 23-10 gives steps for measuring height.

Weight

Provider preference and patient health dictate the frequency of measuring an adult's weight. Some providers require the patient's weight to be measured on each visit, whereas others do not if there are no health problems that require weight monitoring. Some health conditions that do require weight monitoring include obesity, eating disorders, hormone disorders such as diabetes and thyroid malfunction, hypertension, pregnancy, cancer, and some digestive disorders.

Integrity When measuring the weight of a patient, the medical assistant must maintain the patient's privacy. Most people are conscious of their weight and may become embarrassed if the measurement is taken where others may see and hear. Privacy is important and often overlooked. The medical assistant must also be careful of comments regarding a patient's weight, particularly with the obese patient and with those being treated for eating disorders (see Chapter 33). Encouragement for weight loss for the dieting patient is beneficial but must be done in privacy. Other comments are inappropriate.

Occasionally, a patient will be instructed by the provider to monitor weight at home. It is important for the patient to understand the necessity of weighing at the same time each day using the same scale. Weight may vary significantly throughout the day. A normal routine is to measure weight before breakfast.

Before an accurate weight can be obtained, the scale must be calibrated. The point of the balance beam must be floating in the center when no weight is applied to the scale. Some scales are equipped with a screw at the end that can be turned slightly until the beam is in the correct floating position. Once it is centered, it is calibrated and ready for use (Figure 23-24).

PROCEDURE 23-10

Procedure

Measuring Adult Height

STANDARD PRECAUTIONS:

Handwashing

PURPOSE:

To obtain the height of the patient.

EQUIPMENT/SUPPLIES:

- Scale with measuring bar
- Paper towels

PROCEDURE STEPS:

1. Wash hands.
2. Introduce yourself. Identify patient.
3. ***Explain the rationale for performance of the procedure, speaking at the patient's level of understanding***, to ensure understanding and cooperation.
4. Instruct patient to remove shoes and to stand on the paper towel on the scale with back against scale, looking straight ahead. RATIONALE: Back against scale aids patient safety.
5. ***Considering any special needs of the patient***, assist the patient onto the scale. RATIONALE: Scale platform is movable, and patient may become unsteady and lose balance and fall.
6. Lower measuring bar until firmly resting on top of head (Figure 23-23).

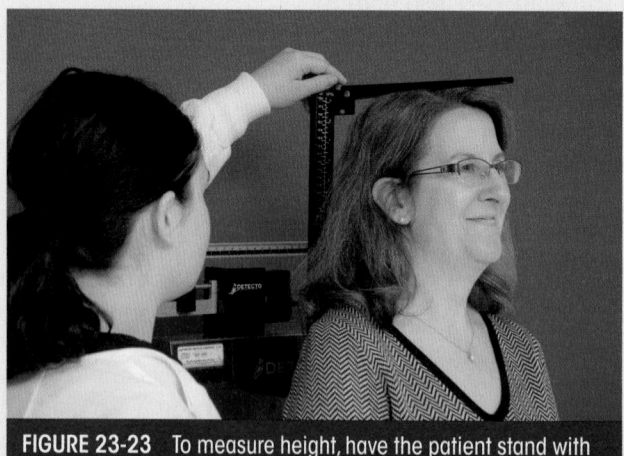

FIGURE 23-23 To measure height, have the patient stand with back against scale and keep head level.

7. Assist patient's stepping off of scale. Allow patient to sit and help with shoes if necessary.
8. ***Paying attention to detail***, read line where measurement falls.
9. Lower measuring bar to its original position.

(continues)

10. Wash hands.

11. Accurately record height in patient's chart or electronic medical record.

DOCUMENTATION:

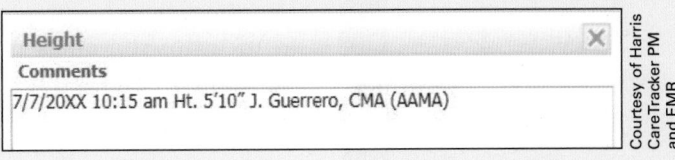

Height	✕
Comments	
7/7/20XX 10:15 am Ht. 5'10" J. Guerrero, CMA (AAMA)	

Courtesy of Harris CareTracker PM and EMR

An eye-level digital scale with measuring bar measures height in the same way on the measuring bar of the digital scale as it is on the balance beam measuring bar. Weight measurement is quicker, easier, and usually safer taken on the digital scale. The scale platform is stationary, and the patient is assisted as needed onto the scale; the digital reading is ready in a few seconds (Figure 23-25).

The patient can wear normal indoor clothing, rather than disrobing, for weight measurement. Heavy coats or other outerwear should be removed. Heavy objects, such as keys and pocket change, as well as purses, should not be held during the procedure. A chair or counter should be provided to place these objects on while the procedure is being performed. Shoes should be removed. Procedure 23-11 gives steps for measuring adult weight.

Occasionally, as in the case of medication dosage, the medical assistant is required to convert pound weight into kilogram weight.

1 kilogram = 2.2 pounds

To convert pounds to kilograms:
Take the number of pounds and divide by 2.2

Example:

130 pounds divided by 2.2 = 59.09 kg

To convert from kilograms to pounds:
Take the number of kilograms and multiply by 2.2

Example:

50 kilograms multiplied by 2.2 = 110 pounds

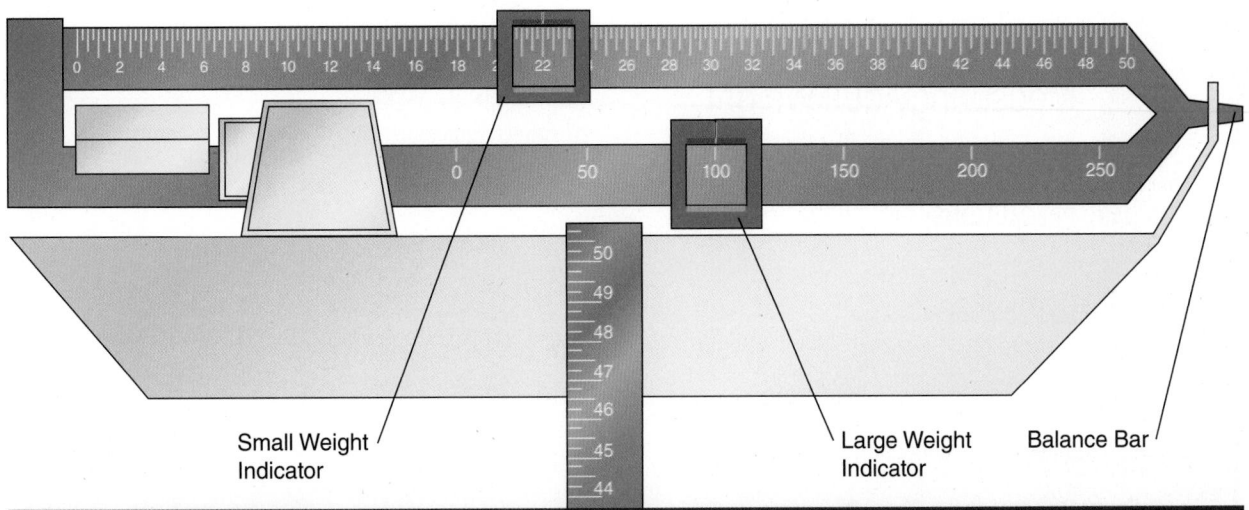

Small Weight Indicator

Large Weight Indicator

Balance Bar

FIGURE 23-24 The upper bar indicates small pound weights (from 0 to 50 lb). The weight shown on the lower bar is measured in 50-lb increments. The lower measurement is added to the upper bar amount that is shown. The upper bar shows 22 lb; the lower bar shows 100 lb. Upper bar 22 lb plus lower bar 100 lb equals total weight 122 lb.

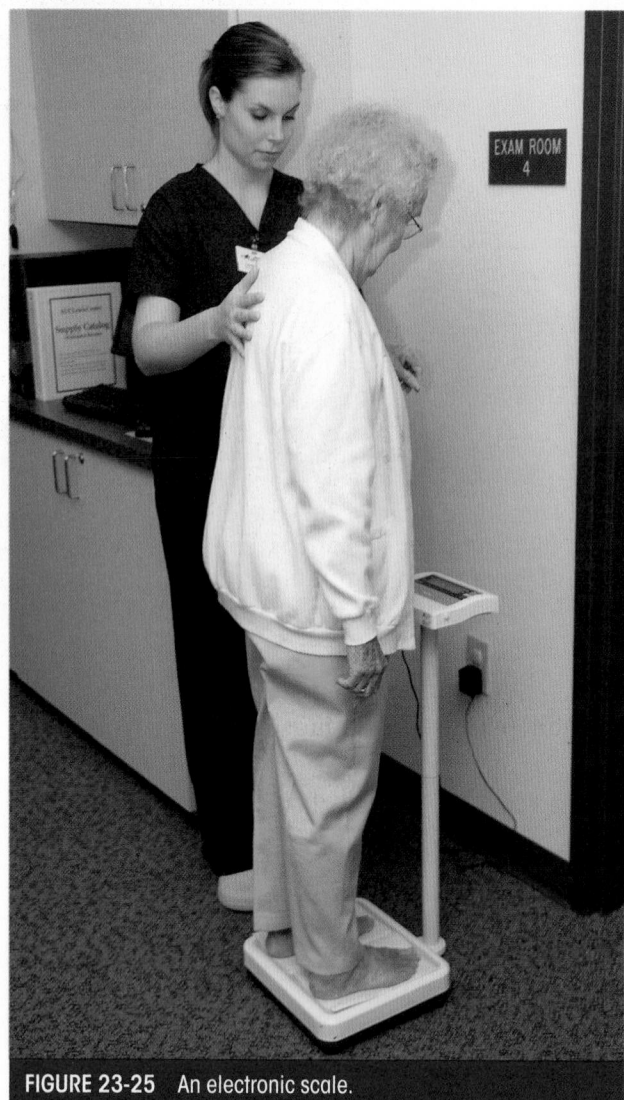

FIGURE 23-25 An electronic scale.

Significance of Weight

The careful monitoring of a patient's weight may provide an insight into metabolic, nutritional, and emotional problems.

MEASURING CHEST CIRCUMFERENCE

Occasionally, the medical assistant is instructed to measure the chest of an adult. This procedure may be done on patients with emphysema and as a requirement for insurance and truck driver licenses. Two measurements are taken, one on the deepest inspiration and one on the deepest expiration. A comparison is then made to ascertain chest capacity. To perform the procedure, ask the patient to disrobe from the waist up. Place a tape measure around the chest at nipple level. Instruct the patient to inhale deeply while you measure, then ask the patient to exhale completely while you take the second measurement. Record the results as inspiration number and expiration number (see Chapter 29).

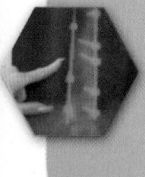

Critical Thinking

Discuss the methods the medical assistant may use to obtain patient cooperation when taking vital signs. Describe and demonstrate the appropriate charting procedure for normal vital sign results.

PROCEDURE 23-11

Measuring Adult Weight

Procedure

STANDARD PRECAUTIONS:

Handwashing

PURPOSE:
To obtain the weight of the patient.

EQUIPMENT/SUPPLIES:
- Balance beam or digital scale
- Paper towels

(continues)

PROCEDURE STEPS:

1. Wash hands.

2. Introduce yourself. Identify patient.

3. ***Explain the rationale for performance of the procedure, speaking at the patient's level of understanding,*** to ensure understanding and cooperation.

4. Place a paper towel on scale. RATIONALE: Paper towel protects patient's feet from microorganisms.

5. Instruct the patient to place heavy objects on the area provided, including heavy objects that may be in pockets such as change or car keys.

6. Zero balance beam or digital scale.

7. ***Considering any special needs of the patient,*** instruct the patient to remove shoes, jacket, and heavy sweater and step on the scale. Assist patient to the center of the scale. RATIONALE: The scale platform is movable, and the patient may become unsteady, lose balance, and fall. The platform on the digital scale is stationary, but assist the patient onto the scale platform and read the digital reading. If using a balance beam scale, continue with steps 8 through 14.

8. For balance beam scales, move the lower weight bar (measured in 50-pound increments) to the estimated number (the patient may be asked for approximate weight).

9. Slowly slide the upper bar until the balance beam point is centered (Figure 23-26).

10. Read the weight by adding the upper bar measurement to the lower bar measurement (see Figure 23-24). If using a digital scale, simply read and remember the number.

11. ***Considering any special needs of the patient***, assist the patient in stepping off the scale.

12. Provide a chair for the patient to sit and put on shoes. Return objects to the patient.

13. If using a balance beam scale, return the weights to zero.

14. Wash hands.

15. Accurately record weight in patient's chart or electronic medical record.

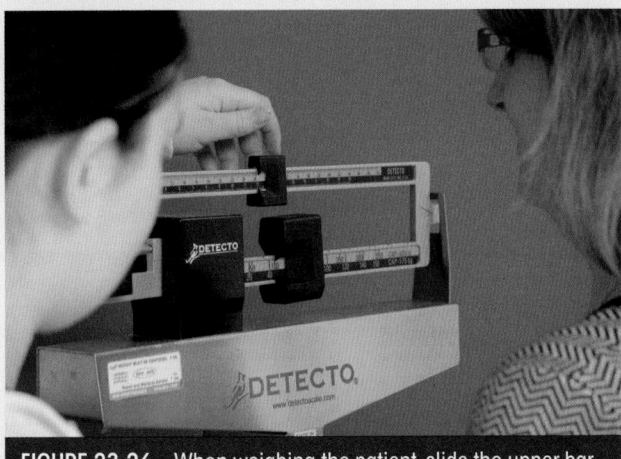

FIGURE 23-26 When weighing the patient, slide the upper bar until the balance beam point is centered.

DOCUMENTATION:

Weight	✕
Comments	
5/2/20XX 3:00 pm Wt. 142 lbs. N. McFarland, RMA (AMT)	

Courtesy of Harris CareTracker PM and EMR

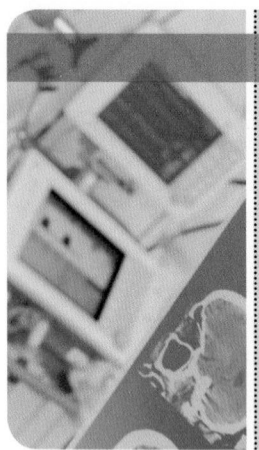

CASE STUDY 23-1

Refer to the scenario at the beginning of the chapter.

CASE STUDY REVIEW

1. There are three different kinds of sphygmomanometers. Give advantages and disadvantages of each.
2. When Joe weighs Mrs. Johnson, he notices from her record that she has lost 10 pounds in 6 months. What questions will Joe ask her about her weight loss?
3. Height and weight measurements are important for many reasons. What do you consider the most important of the many reasons? What do you consider the least important reason? Why?

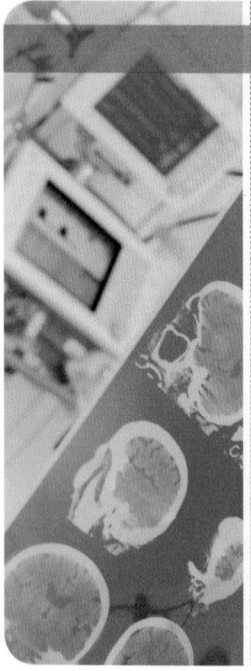

CASE STUDY 23-2

Herb Fowler, a regular patient of Dr. Lewis at Inner City Health Care, is an African American man in his 50s. He has smoked for many years and only recently has thought about quitting smoking because of a chronic cough. Herb is significantly overweight but is having a hard time making the decision to give up smoking *and* change his diet. Although his blood pressure has been stable for the last few years, Nancy McFarland, RMA (AMT), is concerned when she takes Herb's vital signs during his most recent checkup. His weight is slightly up, and his blood pressure has jumped from 140/90 to 156/100.

CASE STUDY REVIEW

1. Is a blood pressure reading of 156/100 a cause for concern? Should Nancy take a second reading?
2. In addition to alerting the provider to the change in Mr. Fowler's blood pressure and weight, Nancy feels she may be able to provide advice to the patient (with provider permission). How can Nancy use her communication and medical assisting knowledge to counsel Mr. Fowler on lifestyle changes?
3. To follow up, Nancy reviews her knowledge of hypertension and discusses the four types with the provider. What are the four kinds of hypertension and what are their characteristics?

Summary

- Throughout life, a patient will undergo various measurements to ascertain growth, development, and general health and well-being.
- The normal range for each of these measurements will vary according to the stage of life of the patient at the time of examination.
- The measurement of a patient's temperature is an indicator of overall wellness. Increased temperature or fever can indicate the body's response to a pathogen.
- There are many methods for measuring temperature that include various devices and areas of the body that serve as a site for taking that reading.
- Normal pulse rates for different ages are measured by palpating arteries in locations where they are close to the surface of the body.
- The pulse reflects the function of the heart and perfusion of the tissues distant from the heat.
- Respiration is important to maintain the balance of oxygen and carbon dioxide in the blood. Respirations are counted to assess adequate function of this body system.

Summary *continued*

- Variations in blood pressure occur across the life span. Blood pressure readings are noted in systolic and diastolic numbers that reflect the pressure inside the arteries during contraction and relaxation of the cardiac muscle.

- Height, weight, and chest circumference are measured to monitor growth in the younger patient and overall wellness in the older patient.

Study for Success

To reinforce your knowledge and skills of information presented in this chapter:

- Review the *Key Terms* and *Learning Outcomes*

- Consider the *Critical Thinking* features and *Case Studies* and discuss your conclusions

- Answer the questions in the *Certification Review*

- Perform the *Procedures* using the *Competency Assessment Checklists* on the *Student Companion Website*

Procedure

CERTIFICATION REVIEW

1. Which type of thermometer measures the temperature of the skin surface over the temporal artery?
   a. Aural
   b. TA
   c. Tympanic
   d. Axillary

2. Which artery is commonly used for taking a patient's pulse?
   a. Carotid
   b. Brachial
   c. Radial
   d. Popliteal
   e. Femoral

3. A blood pressure cuff that is too small for the patient's arm will have what effect?
   a. It will have no effect on the result.
   b. It will give an arbitrarily low result.
   c. It will give an arbitrarily high result.
   d. It will have an effect on certain patients only.

4. What term is used to indicate a pulse rate significantly above the average?
   a. Bradycardia
   b. Tachycardia
   c. Arrhythmia
   d. Sinus rhythm
   e. Dysrhythmia

5. The absence of respiratory activity is known as what?
   a. Eupnea
   b. Apnea
   c. Hyperpnea
   d. Dyspnea

6. What is the medical term for fever?
   a. Pyrexia
   b. Febrile
   c. Afebrile
   d. Both a and b
   e. None of these

7. Which of the following statements best describes wheezing?
   a. It is a normal breath sound.
   b. It is a clicking or rattling sound heard on inspiration.
   c. It is a high-pitched musical sound heard upon expiration.
   d. It is a sound sustained continuously during both inspiration and expiration.

8. Weight is an important measurement to be recorded during a patient assessment. Weight should be recorded in pounds or kilograms. In order to change pounds to kilograms, which of the following statements is true?
   a. Multiply by 2.2
   b. Divide by 2.2
   c. Add 2.2 to the total pounds
   d. Use a metric scale and reweigh the patient
   e. Allow the practitioner to calculate the weight in kilograms

9. Which of the following blood pressure results indicates hypertension?
   a. 110/60   c. 122/86
   b. 148/92   d. 128/78

10. Which of the following affects eupnea or normal respiratory rate?
    a. Stress
    b. Exertion
    c. Disease
    d. Anxiety or fear
    e. All of these

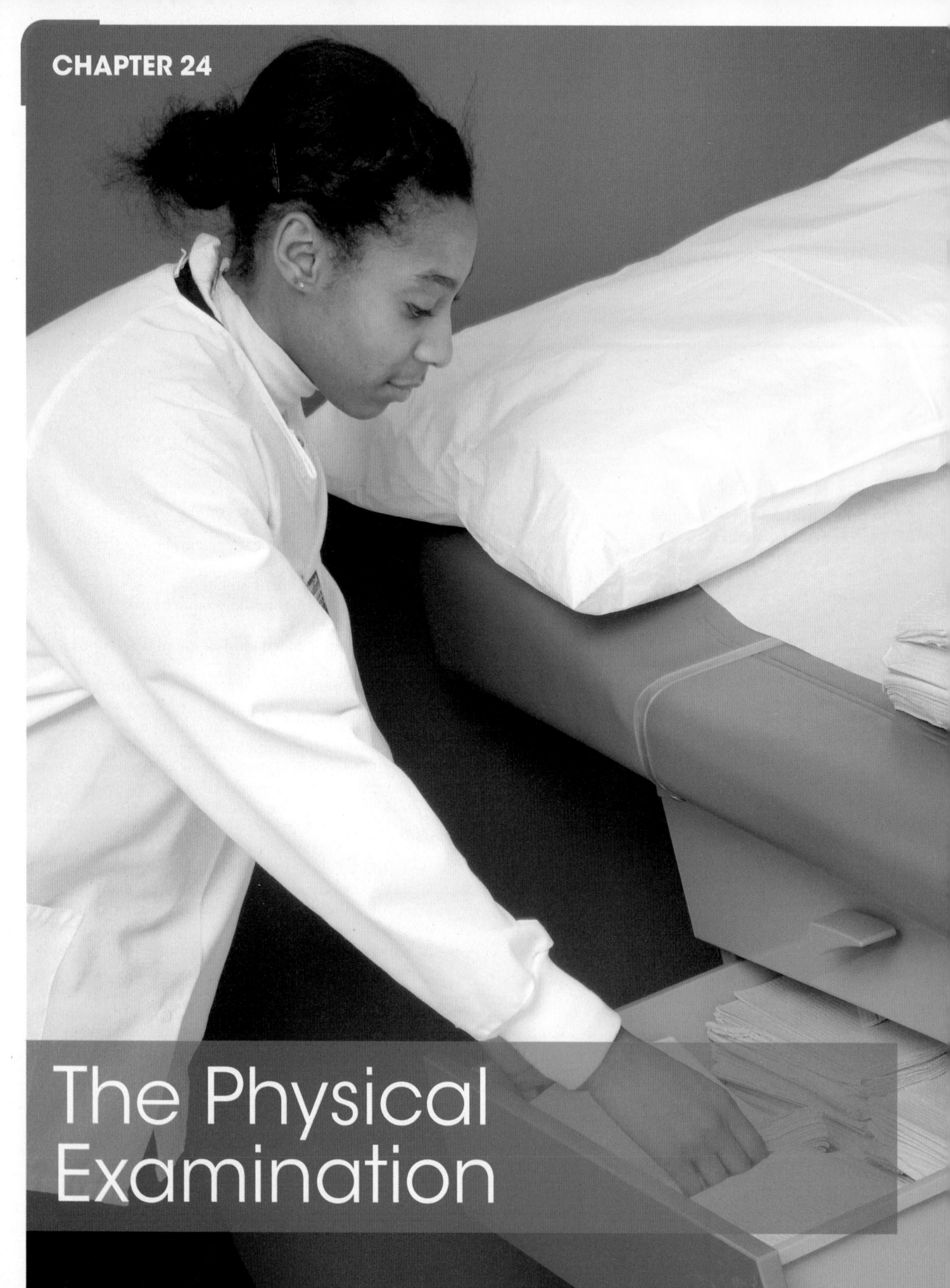

The Physical Examination

1. Define and spell the key terms as presented in the glossary.
2. Identify the six methods used in physical examinations.
3. List and describe seven positions used for physical examinations.
4. Discuss the purpose of draping and demonstrate appropriate draping for each position.
5. Recognize at least 10 instruments and supplies used for examination of various parts of the body.
6. Identify eight basic components of a physical examination.
7. Describe the sequence followed during a physical examination.
8. Recall method of examination, instrument used, and position for examination of at least eight body parts.

KEY TERMS

ataxia	labyrinthitis	scleroderma
auscultation	lithotomy	Sims'
bruits	mensuration	supine
catheterization	pallor	symmetry
cyanosis	palpation	tinnitus
dorsal recumbent	percussion	Trendelenburg
fenestrated drape	proctologic	vertigo
Fowler's	prone	vitiligo
jaundice	pyorrhea	

SCENARIO

At the multiprovider Inner City Health Care facility, five providers are employed on a rotating basis, with two or three working at any one time. Clinical medical assistants Gwen Carr, CMA (AAMA), and Thomas Myers, CCMA (NHA), have developed a clear understanding of what each provider prefers in both room and patient preparation. Gwen and Thomas also coordinate with each other and with clinic manager Marilyn Johnson, CMA (AAMA), to ensure patient comfort. Depending on the patient and the type of examination, Gwen will often assist with patient preparation when the patient is female and Thomas will assist when the patient is male.

Chapter Portal

Physical examinations are performed to obtain a picture of the health and well-being of the patient. An initial examination will provide a baseline reference for future examinations. The examination follows a standard routine, usually starting at the head and following through the entire body, including all major organs and body systems. Although the sequence of events for the physical examination is relatively standard, variations occur according to provider preference, type of practice, and patient's chief complaint. Diagnostic procedures such as laboratory tests and X-rays may be ordered or performed in the facility or sent to an outside laboratory. At the conclusion of the physical examination, the provider will have an impression of the patient's general health, a diagnosis if possible, and treatment plans. The provider uses information from three major sources to aid in making a diagnosis: the health history, the physical examination, and laboratory tests and diagnostic procedures.

continues

The role of the medical assistant throughout the physical examination greatly depends on the provider. Some providers delegate many duties to the medical assistant, whereas others require little assistance. Commonly performed clinical medical assisting duties related to physical examinations can be divided into two categories: patient preparation and room preparation. Patient preparation includes patient instruction and setting expectations, positioning, draping, vital signs, specimen collection such as urine and blood, and electrocardiogram (ECG). Room preparation includes assembling the appropriate instruments and equipment for the provider and ensuring patient privacy and comfort.

Integrity

When patients arrive for their appointments, the medical assistant maintains a professional and caring manner and will consider confidentiality to be of utmost importance. From the time the patient arrives until the patient leaves, there are multiple occasions to protect patient confidentiality. A patient's medical history, personal finances, and insurance matters must be handled privately, out of the hearing range of others. Pertinent personal information that you may elicit from the patient that will be helpful to the provider during his or her examination also must be kept private. When the patient is undergoing testing such as electrocardiology that requires the patient to undress in preparation for the examination, care must be taken to avoid violating the patient's right to privacy. Respecting the dignity of all patients by protecting their privacy and confidentiality is a sign of a professional who is aware of patient rights.

Additional medical assisting duties include supporting the patient, setting up instruments for examination, handing the provider instruments and equipment as required, and taking notes to be entered into the electronic medical record (EMR). Documentation of findings is often a key role for the medical assistant. Throughout and after the examination, the medical assistant adheres to the principles of medical asepsis and Standard Precautions as required by the Occupational Safety and Health Administration (OSHA).

Professional

Establishing a sense of trust and rapport with the patient from the time of the first interaction through the taking of the patient history eases the process of the physical exam. Presenting oneself as a professional by being courteous, patient, and respectful allows the patient to be comfortable in his or her surroundings while sharing health details. Obtaining accurate vital signs and easing the process of physical exams are the result of attending to both the psychologic and physiologic needs of the patient. The effective medical assistant establishes an efficient but flexible routine that provides for the needs of both the patient and the provider.

METHODS OF EXAMINATION

There are six methods used by the provider to examine the body. They include observation or inspection, palpation, percussion, auscultation, mensuration, and manipulation. The provider uses all in total or in part, depending on the type of examination being performed.

Observation or Inspection

Observation or inspection is the process of obtaining physical information by observing the patient. Inspection is perhaps the most important tool of examination and is the thorough and unhurried visualization of the patient. Many diagnoses may be made from the data collected by a skilled practitioner simply using the sense of sight.

General inspection includes taking in the body as a whole. The general health, posture, body movements, skin, mannerisms, and care in grooming are noted. Closer observation focuses on body **symmetry** (correspondence in shape and size of body parts located on opposite sides of the body)

and contour. Local inspection is the focus on a specific body area, for example, the skin. Deformities and skin rashes are observed. Skin color is noted (Figure 24-1).

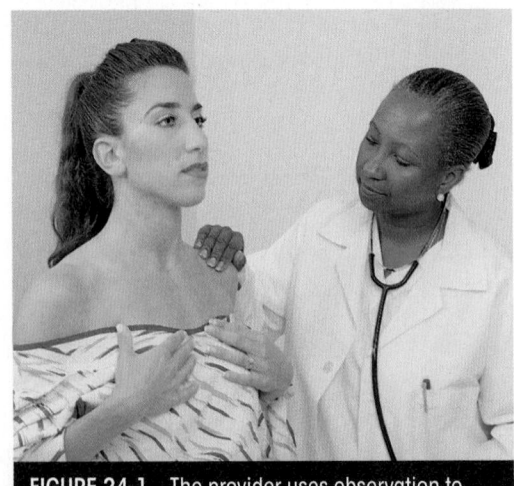

FIGURE 24-1 The provider uses observation to inspect the body for signs of disease.

Inspection is usually thought of as using the unaided eye. However, there are many instruments that aid in the examination of various body parts. Some examples are the otoscope to examine the health of the ears and the ophthalmoscope for observation of the inner structures of the eye.

Palpation

Integrity

Palpation is an examination of the body using touch and is often used to help verify observations. A body part or organ is palpated for size and condition. This examination technique is especially useful in evaluating the anatomy of the abdomen. For example, abdominal masses may be felt through the abdominal wall. Skin texture, moisture, and temperature are best evaluated by touching the patient. The contour of limbs, rigidity, and position of bones and joints may be felt. Palpation may be performed with the use of fingertips, one or both hands, or the palm of the hand (Figure 24-2). Palpation is utilized by the professional medical assistant within his or her scope of practice. Pulse is measured using palpation. The rate, rhythm, and quality of a pulse are all vital components that must be documented in the patient chart.

Percussion

Percussion is the process of eliciting sounds from the body by tapping with either a percussion hammer or fingers. The vibrations and sounds from

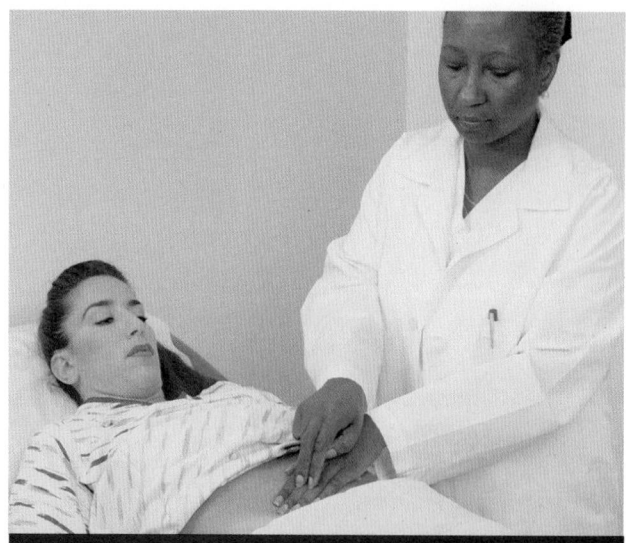

FIGURE 24-3 Percussion involves tapping on body parts and listening to sounds coming from body organs.

underlying organs and cavities can be felt and heard. Using this method can determine the presence of air or solid material in the organ or cavity being checked. Healthy structures that are dense, such as the liver, produce a dull sound. Hollow structures such as the lungs should produce a more hollow sound. There are two methods used to perform percussion. The direct method is performed by tapping directly on the surface of the skin. The indirect method is performed by placing a finger or hand on the surface of the skin and tapping the hand (Figure 24-3).

Auscultation

Auscultation is the process of listening directly to body sounds, normally with a stethoscope. The provider listens for lung and heart sounds such as murmurs, rales, or **bruits**, which generally are abnormal sounds heard on auscultation of an organ or vessel such as a vein or an artery. The abdomen is examined for bowel sounds that include the rumbling and gurgles of normal bowel activity, the sounds that occur with peristalsis (Figure 24-4). Blood pressure is one of the vital signs that are collected by the medical assistant as a part of collecting information. Auscultation using a stethoscope determines the blood pressure reading that is documented in a patient's chart.

Mensuration

The **mensuration** method of examination uses the process of measuring. The measurements of height and weight, the length of a limb, and the

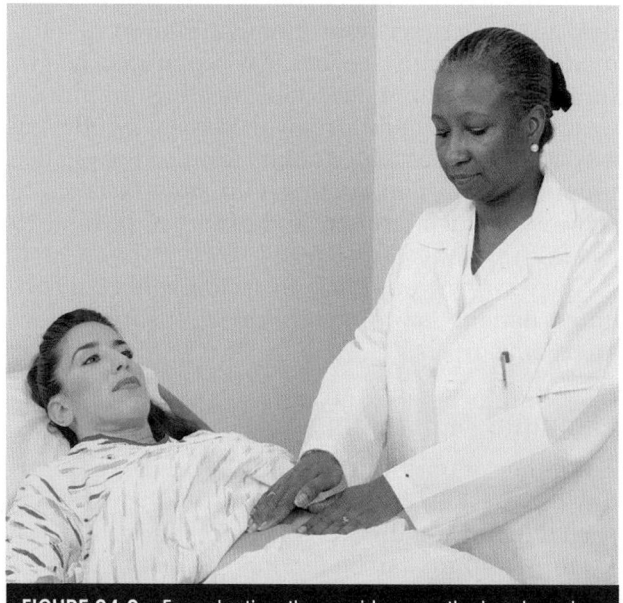

FIGURE 24-2 For palpation, the provider uses the hands and fingers to feel various body parts.

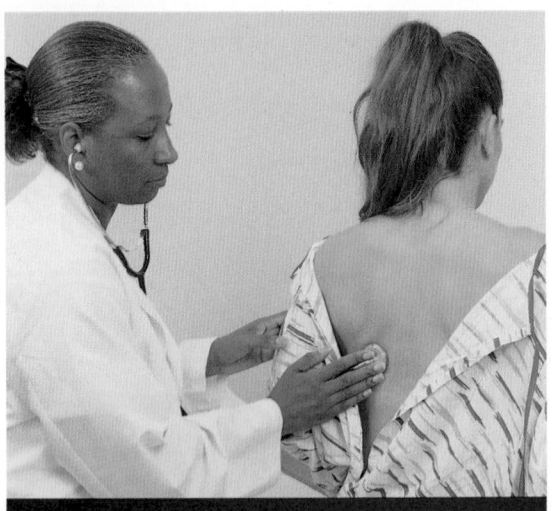

FIGURE 24-4 The provider is using a stethoscope to listen to heart and lung sounds. This is known as auscultation.

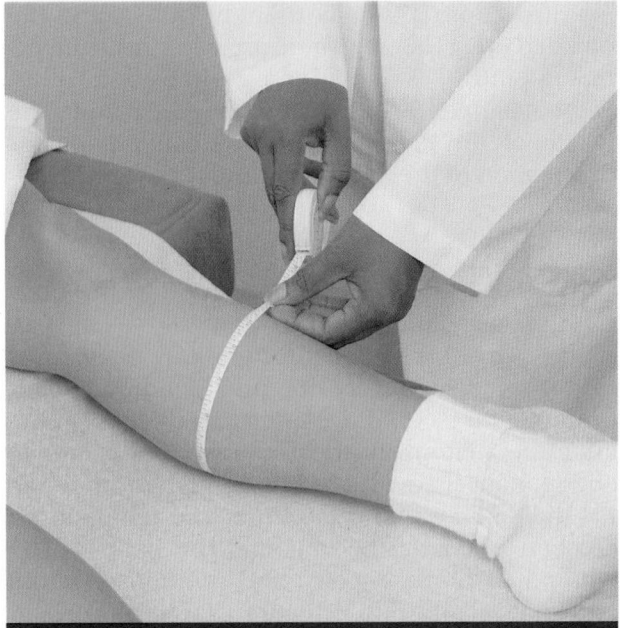

FIGURE 24-5 A tape measure may be used to measure the circumference of the calf of the patient's leg or other body part. This method of physical examination is known as mensuration.

amount of flexion and extension of an extremity are all forms of mensuration (Figure 24-5). Measurements of chest and infant head circumference are also forms of mensuration. In most instances, a tape measure is used to perform mensuration of an infant's head or circumference of a body part.

Manipulation

Manipulation checks the amount of flexion and extension of a joint by applying forceful passive movement on the joint. Range of motion of some joints may be checked using this method.

POSITIONING AND DRAPING

Safety

Physical examinations require patients to be placed in various positions. Each position is designed to make examination of a particular area of the body easier and more efficient. The medical assistant may assist patients in undressing and will provide the appropriate drape and gown. The medical assistant also instructs patients about the appropriate position required for the examination and may assist patients into position by providing support and guidance. Always provide for patient safety.

Presentation   Diversity

Demonstrating awareness of the need to protect modesty, prevent embarrassment, and provide comfort from chills is essential and is the key to proper draping of the patient. If patients are capable of helping themselves, the medical assistant should leave the room while patients

undress and put on a gown. In order to understand the cultural diversity that might be present with your patients, it is important to ask appropriate questions as they pertain to undressing for the physical exam. If patients are disoriented or extremely ill, the medical assistant must stay in the room; patient privacy can be provided by discreetly removing clothing and covering patients as quickly as possible. When the patient is a child, encourage the parent's participation whenever appropriate. Children develop modesty at an early age and may be embarrassed by sitting on the examination table wearing only underwear. Respect a child's right to privacy by offering a gown or drape. Older adults will need assistance with undressing and draping. Care must be taken to provide as much modesty and privacy as possible as you assist patients of all ages.

Never turn your back on seriously ill or disoriented patients or young children. Ensure patient safety at all times.

Examination Positions

A number of positions may be required of patients during the physical examination. The position used depends on the type of examination. The following positions can be used:

1. Supine (horizontal recumbent)
2. Dorsal recumbent

Position	Description	When It Is Used
Supine	Assumed when lying flat facing up.	Examination of the anterior surface of the body from head to toe.
Dorsal recumbent	Patients lie on their back (dorsal) face up, legs separated, knees flexed with feet flat on the table. This is the most comfortable position for patients with back and abdominal problems.	For rectal, genital, head, neck, and chest examinations, as well as abdominal palpation. It can also be used for urinary **catheterization**. Preteen and early teen girls requiring a pelvic examination may be placed in this position and will require careful instructions and procedure explanations. The patient is covered with a drape that is diamond shaped. One edge of the diamond can be lifted to examine the genitalia without exposing the rest of the body.
Lithotomy	To place patients in this position, assist them to lie on their back similar to the dorsal recumbent position except the buttocks should be as close to the bottom edge of the table as possible, and feet are placed in stirrups attached to the foot of the table. At the conclusion of the examination, patients should slide toward the head of the table before getting up from this position. Patients with special needs, such as older adults and those physically challenged, as with severe arthritis, may not be able to assume this position. If this is the case, assist patient into the Sims' position or modified dorsal position.	The lithotomy position is used for genital and pelvic examinations; it can also be used for urinary catheterization.
Fowler's • Semi-Fowler's 45° angle • High-Fowler's 90° angle	Patients sit with the back of the examination table raised to either 45 degrees (semi-Fowler's) or 90 degrees (high-Fowler's).	For patients having cardiovascular or respiratory problems to facilitate their breathing, and for examination of the upper body and head.

(continues)

Position	Description	When It Is Used
Proctologic	This position requires the use of a proctologic examination table. The patient is instructed to undress from the waist down and to kneel on the knee board of the table. The patient then bends at the hips and rests the chest on the table. The head is supported by a head board. The table is then turned to elevate the buttocks. A triangular, diamond-shaped, or **fenestrated drape** covers the patient from the shoulders to the knees.	For proctologic examinations.
Prone	The patient is instructed to lie face down on the table with head turned to side; arms may be placed above the head or along the side of the body. The drape must cover from the mid-chest area to the legs.	When examining the posterior aspect of the body, including the back or spine and legs.
Sims'	The patient is instructed to lie on the left side; the left arm and shoulder may be drawn back behind the body. The left knee is slightly flexed to support the body, and the right knee is flexed sharply. A small pillow is provided for placement under the patient's head. A pillow may also be placed between the patient's legs if it will not interfere with the examination being performed. The drape should be large enough to cover the patient from the shoulders to the knees (triangle or diamond shape to expose rectum).	For vaginal or rectal examination, for obtaining a rectal temperature, for a sigmoidoscopy, or for administering an enema.
Trendelenburg	The head of the table should tilt downward toward the floor and the feet should point upward toward the ceiling.	This position can be used for two reasons. The first is to aid a person who is in shock. By lowering the head and elevating the legs, blood flow from the major vessels in the lower extremities will, by gravity, flow upward toward the brain and major organs. This may help to increase blood pressure enough to sustain the patient until taken to the emergency department (see Chapter 8). The other reason for the Trendelenburg position is to elevate and incline the legs so that the abdomen and pelvic organs are pushed up toward the chest by gravity, making visibility and maneuverability easier for the provider doing either abdominal or pelvic surgery.

3. Lithotomy

4. Fowler's

5. Proctologic

6. Prone

7. Sims'

8. Trendelenburg

For more information on these positions, see the "Examination Positions" Quick Reference Guide.

EQUIPMENT AND SUPPLIES FOR THE PHYSICAL EXAMINATION

Equipment and supplies used for physical examinations should be properly cleaned and ready for the provider's use (see Chapters 21 and 30 for proper cleaning and care of instruments). Please see the "Common Instruments and Supplies" Quick Reference Guide for the instruments and supplies that are commonly used during the physical examination. Actual equipment and supplies needed vary with the provider and with the type of examination. Figure 24-6 shows some common instruments that may be used in the physical examination. (See Chapter 29 for instruments used in specialty examinations.) The medical assistant is responsible for room preparation prior to a physical examination. Equipment must be in working order (e.g., bulbs for scopes, good room lighting) and the room properly stocked with gowns, drapes, and other supplies such as gloves,

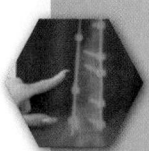

Critical Thinking

Describe a type of examination that may be performed while the patient is placed in each of the following positions: (1) lithotomy, (2) Sims', (3) Trendelenburg, and (4) supine. Decide in what position you should place a patient and what manner of draping you would use for a Pap smear, examining a patient with shortness of breath, obtaining a rectal temperature, and an examination of the spine.

Consider how to attend to both the psychologic and the physiologic aspects of a patient's anxiety related to positioning for each exam. How might you speak to a patient's level of understanding when describing positioning?

an antibacterial hand washing product, a biohazard container, and any other materials needed to comply with Standard Precautions, such as a sharps container. In addition, the medical assistant is responsible for patient preparation. Urine, blood samples, and an ECG may be performed (if requested by the provider). Vital signs and height and weight will be measured. Signed consent forms, if needed, should be in the patient's record. If the patient needs help undressing and putting on a gown, the medical assistant provides assistance. Patient data can be documented immediately using the computer to electronically record all of the information (vital signs, height and weight, known allergies, any medications the patient is taking) (Figure 24-7). Results of tests and the ECG usually are available within 24 hours and can be accessed in the patient EMR. Ensure patient confidentiality throughout the examination and documentation.

BASIC COMPONENTS OF A PHYSICAL EXAMINATION

The physical examination of the patient begins as soon as the patient enters the clinic. The provider uses information from the health history, physical examination, and laboratory tests to aid in making a diagnosis. Although the physical examination is performed by the provider, it is important for the medical assistant to be aware of the various examination components and the significance of each as an indicator of patient well-being.

Patient Appearance

Diversity Integrity

General appearance and actions are noted as the patient is received by the medical assistant and during the patient history (see Chapter 22). Skin color is checked and general grooming, ease of conversation, and answers to questions are noted. Be aware of cultural differences while assisting with a physical examination. Some patients of other cultures may appear to you to be unclean in their appearance, have an unpleasant body order, have poor hygiene, or otherwise appear to be different from your culture. In some cultures, a daily bath is considered unnecessary, and body odor is not considered offensive. Regard your patient in a nonjudgmental way, taking into account the other's cultural beliefs. The medical assistant should be alert to a patient with abnormal skin color, confusion or disorientation, or difficulty in movement. Such a patient may have a serious

⟫ COMMON INSTRUMENTS AND SUPPLIES NEEDED FOR A PHYSICAL EXAMINATION

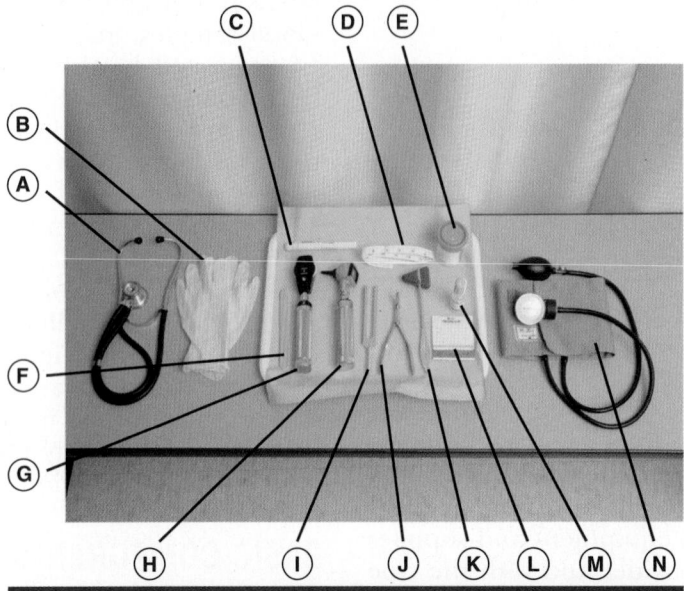

FIGURE 24-6 Instruments and supplies used in the physical examination.

	Name of Instrument
A	Stethoscope
B	Latex gloves
C	Penlight
D	Flexible tape measure
E	Urine specimen container
F	Tongue depressor
G	Ophthalmoscope
H	Otoscope
I	Tuning fork
J	Metal nasal speculum
K	Percussion hammer
L	Guaiac/occult blood slide
M	Guaiac/occult blood slide developer
N	Sphygmomanometer

The following equipment may also be used during the physical exam: Balance beam, digital scale, or electronic scale; patient gown; drape; thermometer; alcohol wipes; examination lights; cotton balls; safety pins; lubricant; emesis basin; gauze sponges; specimen bottles/slide-request forms; and biohazard and regular waste containers

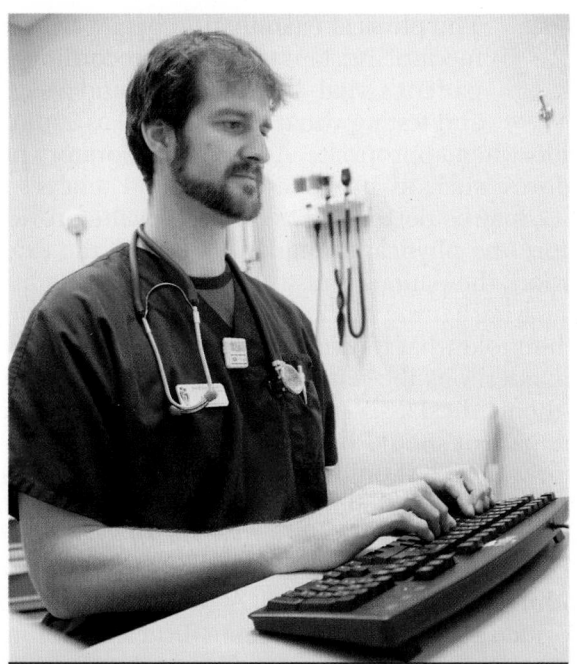

FIGURE 24-7 The medical assistant is able to document patient data in his or her electronic medical record immediately as it is obtained during the examination.

problem and should be placed in an examination room and the provider contacted immediately.

The following aspects of the patient's health are evaluated by the provider through the method of physical examination known as observation.

Gait

Gait pertains to the manner or style of walking. The patient may have a limp, walk with feet wide apart, appear to be dragging one leg, or have difficulty maintaining balance. The provider observes the patient's gait by instructing the patient to walk on a designated straight line. Abnormal gait can include **ataxia**, an uncoordinated wide-based walk; steppage, in which the leg stepping forward is raised high enough to raise the toes off the ground; drag-to, in which the feet are dragged forward rather than lifted and moved; and spastic, in which the legs are held stiffly together and the feet are slightly dragged forward. Each of these gaits can indicate a disease process or health problem associated with poor neurologic functioning.

Stature

The height of the patient is measured. The provider looks for height, trunk, and limb proportion. Stature is the natural height of a person in an upright position.

Posture

Because normal posture is erect with the head held up, a patient in pain may exhibit postural differences. The spine might be in a fixed position, or there may be limited motion in an extremity. The provider observes spine movement and alignment as the patient performs prescribed movements. Abnormalities can include kyphosis (humpback), which may be seen in older adult patients, particularly women with osteoporosis; lordosis, abnormal curvature of the lumbar area; and scoliosis, curvature of the upper spine.

Body Movements

Body movements may be either voluntary or involuntary. Voluntary body movements are those movements intended to be made by the patient. Involuntary body movements are movements not controlled by the patient. Tremors are a form of involuntary movement that may be seen in the mouth, fingers, hands, arms, and legs of a patient. Tremors can indicate a neurologic health problem. Involuntary body movements usually are easily observed.

Speech

Quality and regularity of speech is often one of the first aspects that the provider notices during a physical exam. The patient's speech may indicate abnormal conditions. Abnormalities include aphonia, a loss of voice usually because of laryngitis, but which may have other causes; aphasia, the inability to express oneself through speech or writing, which may indicate brain injury or disease; and dysphasia, an inability to use appropriate speech patterns, such as using words in the wrong order. This may indicate a brain lesion or disorder.

Breath Odors

Breath odors may be detected when speaking with the patient or when obtaining vital signs. A sweet fruity odor may indicate acidosis. This may result from diabetes mellitus, starvation, or renal disease. A musty odor may indicate liver disease, and an ammonia odor may indicate uremia.

Poor oral hygiene results in gingivitis (gum disease), caries (cavities), tooth loss, and foul breath odors. Gum disease and caries encourage the growth of microorganisms in the mouth and throat. Because of the vascularity of the oral cavity, microorganisms can enter into the circulatory system and travel to the heart, causing endocarditis. Maintaining good oral health is necessary for general health and well-being. Regular dental check-ups, cleaning, and daily flossing promote good health.

Weight

Various published charts contain guidelines for normal weight established by height and age. Overweight and underweight are defined as being above or below the published charts. Obesity and underweight are discussed in Chapters 23 and 33. Edema, which is excessive accumulation of fluids in the body tissues, causes weight gain. To test for edema, the provider presses a finger against the skin of the patient in an area over a bony prominence such as the ankle. If edema is present, pitting will be evident when the finger is removed. Fat tissue will not remain indented when pressed.

Skin and Appendages

Skin problems include abnormal skin color such as redness, pallor, cyanosis, jaundice, and vitiligo. **Pallor** is defined as lack of color or paleness often seen with anemia; **cyanosis** is a slightly blue or gray discoloration of the skin, often seen in patients with respiratory or cardiac problems; **jaundice** is a yellowing of the skin, often caused by obstructed bile ducts or liver disease; and **vitiligo** is characterized by white patches on the skin, observed against normal pigmentation. Other skin conditions are lesions, ulcers, bruises, and cancer. Skin texture may be smooth, rough, and scaly and have loss of elasticity. These findings may indicate health problems or excessive exposure to the sun. The nails can also indicate some forms of health problems. Infections, either local or systemic, may be observed in nails that are brittle, grooved, or lined. The appearance of the fingertips can be indicators of disorders as seen in clubbing, which may indicate congenital heart disease, and spooning, which may be seen in severe iron-deficiency anemias. Abnormal hair distribution, as in facial hair on a female patient, may indicate hormonal changes.

THE PHYSICAL EXAMINATION SEQUENCE

A sequence is followed for a physical examination, although provider preference and the patient's chief complaint can produce a variation to the sequence.

Communication

The physical examination begins with the medical assistant taking and recording the patient's vital signs, height, and weight, and testing visual acuity as well as auditory ability when appropriate. Additional laboratory procedures, such as urinalysis and blood analysis or ECG, may be performed as directed by the provider before the physical examination. Before the examination, the patient is instructed to empty the bladder, saving a urine specimen for analysis. The patient is then told what to expect during the examination. Any questions the patient has should be answered by the medical assistant or referred to the provider. The patient should be instructed about undressing (a private area should be provided for undressing). The medical assistant should be explicit as to what clothing is to be removed and what can be left on. If a complete physical examination is required, all clothing should be removed. A gown and drape are provided for the patient. The medical assistant may leave the room while the patient undresses unless the patient asks for help or is unable to manage alone. It is appropriate to knock before reentering the room.

Legal

When the provider is examining a patient, it is customary for the medical assistant to remain in the room for the patient's comfort, to assist the provider, and as a deterrent to potential lawsuits.

The medical assistant places the instruments for the examination on the counter or Mayo stand, according to provider preference, but usually in order of use. When lamps are used for the examination, the medical assistant may turn them on and have them ready for the provider. Make sure that the light is not directed into the patient's eyes. When the patient is comfortably positioned on the examination table, inform the provider that the patient is ready. Normally, the physical examination starts at the head and proceeds downward. Table 24-1 gives a detailed review of the components of the physical examination.

Head

The patient is in a sitting position for this examination. The face is checked for puffiness, especially around the eyes. Facial skin is checked for **scleroderma**, a tight and atrophied skin. The older adult patient may have fatty patches that appear raised and yellowish on the eyelids. The face, hair, and scalp are checked for scars, lumps, hair loss, or other lesions. The head and neck are palpated for painful areas, lumps, and swelling.

TABLE 24-1

COMPONENTS OF THE PHYSICAL EXAMINATION

BODY PART	APPROPRIATE POSITION(S)	EQUIPMENT AND/OR INSTRUMENTS NEEDED	METHOD OF EXAM	PROVIDER'S FINDINGS — NORMAL	PROVIDER'S FINDINGS — ABNORMAL
General appearance	Standing	Patient gown Drape	Inspection	Patient is cooperative; good hygiene, good skin color, ease of gait	Uncooperative, behavior inappropriate, unkempt appearance
Height and weight	Standing	Balance beam, digital scale, or electronic scale	Inspection	Weight and height appropriate for age	Shorter or taller than normal range stature; obesity or underweight
Vital signs	Sitting	Stethoscope Sphygmomanometer Thermometer Watch with second hand Biohazard waste container	Inspection Auscultation	Afebrile; blood pressure less than 140 mm Hg systolic or 90 mm Hg diastolic; pulse >60 and <100 beats per minute; respirations >12 and <20 breaths per minute (or age appropriate; see Chapter 23)	Temperature above 100°F; blood pressure elevated above 140 mm Hg systolic or 90 mm Hg diastolic; respirations <12 or >20 breaths per minute
Skin	Supine Prone	Flashlight	Inspection Palpation	Good color, warm to touch; no lesions such as warts, moles, abscesses, rashes	Jaundice, cyanosis, pallor, redness, flakiness of skin, lesions, rashes
Head and neck	Supine semi-Fowler's Seated on edge of table	Light source	Inspection Palpation	Symmetry of head; hair not dry or oily and distributed evenly; scalp free of lesions and not dry; no lymph node enlargement	Asymmetry of head; alopecia; dry, flaky scalp; swelling, lumps, or pain in head or neck
Eyes	Supine semi-Fowler's Seated on edge of table	Ophthalmoscope Snellen eye chart Ishihara plates Pen light	Inspection Mensuration	Snellen test shows accurate visual acuity; able to identify Ishihara color plates; no tearing; equal pupillary reactions to light; retina pink and blood vessels healthy; no bulging of eyeballs	Poor visual and color ability; dull-appearing eyes; drainage; unequal pupils; clouded lens; unequal pupillary reaction; tortuous, unhealthy retinal blood vessels; bulging eyeballs
Ears	Supine semi-Fowler's Seated on edge of table	Otoscope Tuning fork Audiometer	Inspection Percussion	Cerumen not impacted on tympanic membrane; tympanic membrane gray and intact; no discharge or pain; able to hear tuning fork or audiometer	Impacted cerumen: red, bulging tympanic membrane; discharge (pus or blood); inability to hear sound from tuning fork; poor auditory ability when checked with audiometer
Nose	Supine semi-Fowler's Seated on edge of table	Nasal speculum Flashlight Aromatic substance such as alcohol, coffee, cinnamon	Inspection	Mucous membranes moist and pink; able to detect specific odors; septum straight; nostrils equal in size; no abnormal discharge; no lesions	Dry, red, swollen mucous membranes; unable to detect specific odors; deviated septum; nostrils flaring; discharge, polyps noted

continues

Table 24-1 continued

BODY PART	APPROPRIATE POSITION(S)	EQUIPMENT AND/OR INSTRUMENTS NEEDED	METHOD OF EXAM	PROVIDER'S FINDINGS NORMAL	PROVIDER'S FINDINGS ABNORMAL
Mouth and throat	Supine semi-Fowler's Seated on edge of table	Gloves Flashlight or pen light Tongue depressor Sterile cotton-tipped applicator specimen collection tip (culturette) Emesis basin (in case of gagging) Biohazard waste container	Inspection	Gag reflex present; mucous membranes moist and pink; teeth intact, pink tongue; tonsils nonswollen, pink	No gag reflex; tongue rough; pallor of mucous membranes; dental caries; swollen tonsils
Arms and hands	Supine semi-Fowler's Seated on edge of table	Reflex hammer	Inspection Palpation Percussion	Good muscle tone; appropriate reflex reaction; normal range of motion; nails pink, smooth; ability to squeeze provider's hands with equal strength; normal reflexes	Poor muscle tone; lack of reflex reaction; poor range of motion; nails cyanotic; brittle, ridged nails; abnormal reflexes
Chest and lungs	Supine semi-Fowler's Seated on edge of table	Stethoscope Tape measure	Inspection Palpation Auscultation Mensuration Percussion	Axillary lymph nodes not palpable; lungs clear; no cough; ribs nontender; symmetrical chest wall; respirations and heart rate normal; normal chest sounds	Enlarged axillary lymph nodes; asymmetry of chest wall; respiration and heart rate abnormal; abnormal chest sounds
Heart	Supine semi-Fowler's Seated on edge of table	Stethoscope Sphygmomanometer Electrocardiogram (ECG)	Auscultation Palpation Mensuration	Normal heart function per ECG; regular rhythm, rate of heart sounds; no murmurs; blood pressure normal range; pulse points good quality	Abnormal heart function per ECG; irregularity of rhythm, rate; murmurs; blood pressure outside normal range; poor pulse quality
Breasts	Supine		Inspection Palpation	No lumps, tenderness, swelling, or thickening; no sores or lesions; no bleeding or discharge from nipples; no lymph node swelling in axilla; no dimpling or "orange peel" appearance	Lumps, tenderness, swelling, thickening; sores or lesions; bleeding or discharge from nipple; lymph node enlargement in axilla; "orange peel" appearance to breast tissue; dimpling of skin
Abdomen	Supine	Stethoscope Measuring tape	Inspection Palpation Auscultation Mensuration Percussion	Liver, spleen not palpable; symmetry to abdomen; no abnormal bowel sounds; no abnormal sounds from organs in abdomen; abdomen soft; no abdominal or inguinal hernias	Liver, spleen enlarged; asymmetric abdomen; increased or decreased bowel sounds; unusual sounds elicited from percussion of abdominal organs; abdominal distention; ascites; presence of abdominal, umbilical, or inguinal hernia

continues

Table 24-1 continued

BODY PART	APPROPRIATE POSITION(S)	EQUIPMENT AND/OR INSTRUMENTS NEEDED	METHOD OF EXAM	NORMAL	ABNORMAL
Female genitalia and rectum	Lithotomy Dorsal recumbent Sims'	Gloves Vaginal speculum Examination light Speculum Slides for occult blood (Hemoccult) Lubricating jelly Glass slide and fixative or ThinPrep Pap Kit Cervical spatula and cytobrush Biohazard waste container	Inspection Palpation	External genitalia without lesions, sores, ulcerations; vaginal mucosa pink and without discharge; nontender ovaries; cervix smooth, noneroded, noninflamed; good muscle tone in perineal floor and rectum; negative stool for occult blood; nonpalpable lymph nodes in groin	Lesions, sores, ulcerations; discharge from vagina, cervix; painful ovaries; cervix ulcerated, inflamed; poor muscle tone in perineal floor and rectum; prolapse of uterus or bladder into vagina; hemorrhoids; positive Hemoccult; enlarged inguinal lymph nodes
Male genitalia and rectum	Supine Standing	Gloves Lubricating jelly Slides for occult blood (Hemoccult) Biohazard waste container	Inspection Palpation	Penis -skin tone without cyanosis, no discharge; no lesions, sores, ulcers; testicles firm, nontender, and movable; rectal sphincter taut; prostate smooth upon palpation; nonpalpable lymph nodes in groin; stool negative for occult blood	Discharge from penis; ulcers, sores, other types of lesions; testicles tender, swollen; relaxed anal sphincter; hemorrhoids; positive Hemoccult slide; enlarged prostate; enlarged lymph nodes in groin; stool positive for occult blood
Legs and feet	Supine Prone	Tape measure	Inspection Mensuration Palpation	Normal muscle tone and range of motion; no edema; pulses normal; no varicosities; toenails smooth; no signs of fungus or other infection; calves equal in size	Muscle weakness; poor range of motion; edema; diminished pulse; varicose veins; toenails ridged, infected; unequal calf measurements
Neurologic examination	Supine	Percussion hammer Safety pin Cotton ball Alcohol wipes	Percussion Inspection	Normal reflexes; oriented to time and place; appropriate responses; normal responses to sensation; alert; steady gait; no vertigo or syncope	All reflexes disoriented; inappropriate responses; dulled response to pain and sensation; lethargic; unsteady gait; poor coordination; vertigo; syncope

Eyes

The appearance of the eyes is examined. The pupils of the eyes are checked for light and accommodation. When a penlight or flashlight is placed in front of the pupil, the pupil will constrict. The other pupil should constrict equally. The provider notes whether pupils are equal and react to light and accommodation (abbreviated as PERRLA). Pupils that do not constrict and return to normal equally may indicate a problem in the brain. The external eye area is examined for rashes, infection and lesions, and deformity and asymmetry. The sclera and conjunctiva are examined for any abnormalities. Any discolorations, redness, discharge, or lesions are noted. An evaluation of physical fields is a part of the eye exam. A Snellen chart is utilized to assess visual acuity (see Chapter 29).

The provider uses an ophthalmoscope to view the blood vessels of the retina. This is done by turning out the lights in the room, which allows the patient's pupils to dilate. The patient is instructed to look straight ahead while the provider looks into the eye. Retinal changes may indicate disease such as hypertension. The sclera are checked for jaundice.

Ears

An otoscope is used by the provider to examine the ears. The external ear is checked for redness in the ear canal and buildup of cerumen. A healthy tympanic membrane has a pearly gray appearance. A red appearance to the tympanic membrane may indicate infection in the middle ear, known as otitis media. **Vertigo** (dizziness) may indicate that the patient has an inner ear infection (**labyrinthitis**). **Tinnitus** (ringing in the ears) may indicate inner ear problems. Other symptoms of ear problems include pain, discharge, and deafness. The tuning fork is used in testing the sensations of hearing, including bone conduction and air conduction.

Nose

The nasal cavity is visualized by the provider with the use of a nasal speculum and flashlight. Clear drainage from the nose is normal. If the nasal discharge is any other color—white, yellow, green, pink, red, or black—that indicates processes that are outside normal limits (Table 24-2). Other abnormalities may include obstruction because of a deviated septum. Polyps and ulcerations may be found in the nasal cavity. Epistaxis, or nosebleed, may be seen when the capillaries rupture on the surface of the nasal mucosa.

Mouth and Throat

The provider uses a tongue blade or depressor and a light source. The teeth and gums are checked for dental hygiene conditions such as caries and

TABLE 24-2

WHAT THE COLOR OF MUCUS MEANS

COLOR	DESCRIPTION
Clear	This is normal. Mucus is mostly comprised of water, with proteins, antibodies, and dissolved salts, and it is being constantly produced by the nasal tissues.
White	This indicates congestion. The swollen tissues in the nose are slowing the flow of mucus, causing it to lose moisture and become thick and cloudy. White mucus may be a sign of a cold or nasal infection.
Yellow	This indicates that a cold or infection is progressing. Infection-combating cells may be rushing to the site of the microbial infection, including white blood cells. Once exhausted, the white blood cells are carried off, giving mucus a yellow color.
Green	This indicates that the immune system is fighting off the infection. The mucus is thick with dead white blood cells.
Pink or red	This indicates blood. The nasal tissue has become broken, possibly because it is dry or irritated, or it has suffered a trauma.
Brown	This could also indicate blood, but it is more likely due to something that was inhaled, such as dirt.
Black	For nonsmokers, this could indicate a serious fungal infection. This type of infection usually occurs in patients with compromised immune systems.

the gums are checked for signs of **pyorrhea** (discharge of pus from the gums around the teeth). If the tonsils are present, they are checked for signs of infection, such as redness or white pockets of pus. The floor of the mouth is examined both visually and by palpation for indications of swollen glands and ulcerations.

Neck

The provider palpates the neck, looking for swollen lymph nodes. The thyroid gland is palpated anteriorly and posteriorly for size, symmetry, and texture. The patient is asked to swallow several times while the provider feels the thyroid gland. A small glass of water may be given to the patient to aid in swallowing. Range of motion is checked by having the patient turn the head in each direction, and flex and extend neck. Care must be taken with older adult patients. The patient should be instructed to move the head slowly to avoid syncope.

Chest

The symmetry of the chest is observed, both anteriorly and posteriorly. Chest measurement may have been performed before the examination. The chest of a patient with emphysema will appear barrel-like in shape. While the patient is sitting, the provider listens for abnormal breath sounds in the lungs with a stethoscope. The patient may be instructed to take several deep breaths during this process.

 Carefully monitor the patient, particularly the older adult patient, because deep breathing may cause dizziness. The provider is listening for abnormal lung sounds. The provider may examine the lungs by percussion. Heart sounds will be auscultated both anteriorly and posteriorly.

Breast

The patient is placed in a supine position and instructed to place the hand behind the head on the side on which the examination is taking place. The provider examines the breast for masses by using a circular motion, starting at the outer edge of the breast and working toward the center. The nipple is gently squeezed to see if there is any discharge. The patient is then instructed to change arm positions so that the other breast can be examined. With the patient in a sitting position, the provider observes the breasts for symmetry. Female patients should be instructed on the procedure for performing monthly breast self-examination. This may be an embarrassing procedure for the female patient. Maintain as much patient modesty as possible by carefully draping and giving emotional support (see Chapter 25 for more detailed information on breast examination and breast self-examination).

Abdomen

The patient is placed in a dorsal recumbent or supine position with the arms at the sides for examination of the abdomen. The drape is lowered to just above the pubic hair. The female patient wears a gown open in the front that can be pulled to the sides while still covering the breasts. The abdomen is examined by palpation, percussion, and auscultation. Following the quadrants of the abdomen, the provider gently palpates the organs in each quadrant, working from side to side. The provider feels for organ size and location, as well as the presence of masses; percusses the abdomen, listening for sounds from abdominal organs; uses the stethoscope to listen for abdominal sounds; and visually inspects the abdominal area for changes in skin color, scars, or other abnormalities. The contour of the abdomen may be flat or slightly convex. The presence of hernias is checked in both the supine and the standing positions. Patients with abdominal disorders may give a history of dyspepsia, dysphagia or excessive flatulence, nausea, vomiting, bloating, and pain.

Genitals

Refer to Chapters 25 and 27 for more detailed information about genitalia examinations. Care must be taken to protect all patients' modesty and privacy.

Female Genitals. The patient is placed in the lithotomy position. The provider examines both the external genitalia and the reproductive organs. The rectum may be examined and a Hemoccult test done at the conclusion of the pelvic examination. (See Chapters 29 and 43 for information regarding the Hemoccult slide test.) After the examination, the patient is instructed to slide toward the head of the table and may be allowed to sit up slowly. Sitting up quickly may cause orthostatic hypotension and dizziness.

Male Genitals. The provider begins the examination by inspecting and retracting the foreskin of the penis if the patient is uncircumcised. The glans penis is inspected for discharge and redness. The penis and scrotum are palpated for possible tenderness and masses. Because of the seriousness of testicular cancer, the patient will be instructed, usually by the provider, on the procedure for performing monthly testicular examinations (see Chapter 27).

Rectum

The provider may examine the rectum as a part of the male and female genital examination. The patient may be placed in the Sims' position. The provider performs a manual examination. The prostate gland is examined by digital rectal palpation. The provider inserts the gloved index finger into the rectum and palpates the prostate gland for any masses or swelling (see Chapter 27).

Reflexes

The patient's reflexes in both the supine and sitting positions are observed by the provider. A percussion hammer is used. While sitting with the arm flexed, the elbow is lightly tapped to elicit movement from the biceps. The patellar or knee-jerk reflex is tested by tapping the area just below the patella at the knee. The Achilles reflex or ankle-jerk is tested by tapping the Achilles tendon. The Babinski reflex is tested on the sole of a relaxed foot (the great toe will flex) with the patient in a supine position. Reflexes determine the integrity of the neurologic system.

Procedure

Procedure 24-1 outlines the steps in assisting with the physical examination.

PROCEDURE 24-1

Procedure

Assisting with a Complete Physical Examination

STANDARD PRECAUTIONS:

Handwashing   Gloves   Biohazard

PURPOSE:

To assist the provider with a complete physical examination.

EQUIPMENT/SUPPLIES:

- Gloves
- Patient gown
- Drape
- Thermometer
- Stethoscope
- Sphygmomanometer
- Alcohol wipes
- Examination light
- Otoscope
- Tuning fork
- Ophthalmoscope
- Penlight

- Nasal speculum
- Tongue depressor
- Reflex hammer
- Tape measure
- Cotton balls
- Safety pins
- Gloves
- Tissues
- Lubricant
- Emesis basin
- Gauze sponges
- Specimen container(s)

(For specific examinations, there may be other equipment required such as vaginal speculum, ECG machine, audiometer, etc.)

(continues)

PROCEDURE STEPS:

Assisting with a Complete Physical Examination

1. Wash hands. Adhere to Standard Precautions.
2. *Paying attention to detail*, assemble equipment.
3. Introduce yourself. Greet and identify patient.
4. *Explain rationale for performance of the procedure to patient, speaking at the patient's level of understanding*. RATIONALE: To set expectations, obtain patient cooperation, allay apprehension, and gain consent.
5. *Incorporating critical thinking skills when performing patient care*, place instruments in easily accessible sequence for provider use. RATIONALE: Efficient use of time and space.
6. *Using active listening skills*, obtain/update medical history with patient (see Chapter 22 for obtaining patient history). RATIONALE: To ensure complete history has been obtained and is current. This will guide various aspects of the provider's exam and will key the medical assistant to assemble certain equipment to be utilized during the physical exam.
7. Take patient vital signs, test visual acuity, and check hearing ability.
8. Instruct patient to provide a urine specimen (see Chapter 41 for using collection procedures).
9. Obtain all required blood samples (see Chapters 39 and 40 for blood specimen collection procedures).
10. Provide patient with appropriate gown and drape.
11. If assistance is needed, assist patient to disrobe completely while *protecting patient's personal boundaries*; explain where the opening for the gown is to be placed. RATIONALE: To assist patient in maintaining modesty, privacy, and warmth.
12. Perform electrocardiogram (ECG) if directed by provider (see Chapter 36 for ECG procedure).
13. *Attending to any personal needs of the patient*, assist patient in sitting at the end of the table; drape patient across lap and legs. RATIONALE: Always drape patient to maintain modesty.
14. Inform provider when patient is ready.
15. When the provider arrives, *display a calm, professional, and caring manner*, and remain by the patient ready to assist the patient and provider.
16. Maintain a quiet atmosphere to enhance the ability of the provider in listening to heart and lung sounds. RATIONALE: Quiet is necessary to hear heart and chest sounds accurately.
17. *Paying attention to detail*, hand the provider instruments as required for various examinations (some providers do not require the medical assistant to hand the instruments). This might include general examinations of the head, throat, eye, ear, neck, and chest. This might also include specialty examinations such as breast, male and female genitalia, and rectal.
18. Assist in positioning the patient in the optimal position such as supine for abdomen or extremities, or prone so that an assessment of the posterior body can be conducted.
19. *Paying attention to detail*, stand by to assist the provider as needed, or to record findings as instructed by the provider.
20. On completion of the examination, assist patient to sitting position and allow patient to sit at the end of the table for a few minutes. RATIONALE: Allows patient to recover from potential dizziness.
21. Ensure patient stability (check color of skin, pulse) before allowing patient to stand up. RATIONALE: Prevents the patient from fainting due to orthostatic hypotension.
22. Assist patient with dressing; provide privacy.
23. Provide the patient with any written instructions as instructed by the provider.
24. Escort patient to provider's office for discussion of examination results.

(continues)

25. Don disposable gloves and clean and decontaminate the room by first disposing of the gown and drape in the appropriate receptacle.

26. Dispose of contaminated disposable materials in biohazard waste container. RATIONALE: Prevents microorganism cross-contamination of bloodborne pathogens and other potentially infectious materials (OPIM).

27. Disinfect counters and examination table with a solution of 10% bleach. RATIONALE: Prevents microorganism cross-contamination by blood and OPIM.

28. Remove gloves and discard in biohazard waste container. RATIONALE: Prevents microorganism cross-contamination by blood and OPIM.

29. Wash hands.

30. Replace table paper and equipment in preparation for the next patient.

31. Accurately enter any notes or patient instructions in patient's chart or electronic medical record per provider orders.

32. Document the procedure, as well as any test results or provider's notes into the patient's medical record.

DOCUMENTATION:

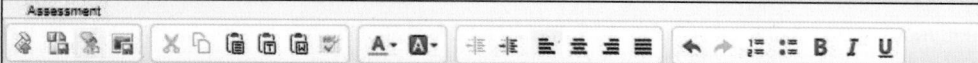

Assessment

11/8/20XX 3:15 pm T 98.2, P 84, R 16, BP 124/76. Complete physical examination performed by Dr. King. Urinalysis negative, Hemoccult slide negative. Venipuncture performed and specimens sent to laboratory for complete blood count and electrolytes. Electrocardiogram completed. Patient given instructions and appointment made for a colonoscopy. Says she understands the preparation for the colonoscopy. T. Myers, CCMA (NHA)

Courtesy of Harris CareTracker PM and EMR

AFTER THE EXAMINATION

Professional Once the examination has been completed, the patient is instructed to dress. The patient should be given privacy while dressing. Assist the patient as needed. Do not remain in the room to clean it while the patient is dressing. Remain in the room if the patient requires assistance. Further instructions regarding other testing procedures and treatment plans will be given by the provider. Be specific with instructions to patients regarding what they should do after they are completely dressed.

Once the examination is finished and the patient has left the examination room, the equipment and supplies (including the examination table) should be sanitized, disinfected, and sterilized as appropriate.

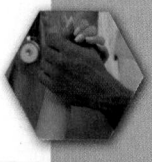

Patient Education

From the time the patient arrives until the time the patient leaves, including throughout the physical examination, there are many opportunities for patient education. Written instructions should be given when necessary, and provider information should be clarified if needed (Figure 24-8).

Opportunities for teaching the patient how to adopt a healthy lifestyle are abundant. Regular exercise; not smoking; weight control; limiting alcohol consumption; and using stress reduction techniques such as meditation, yoga, massage therapy, and so forth all help to decrease blood pressure and reduce the risk for heart attack, stroke, and other illnesses.

Weight Management: Overcoming Your Barriers

You may have many reasons why you're not ready to lose weight. You may not feel you have the time or the skills. You may be afraid of losing weight and gaining it back again. Well, you can lose weight. And you can keep the weight off, if you make changes slowly and stick with them. Consider that you may never find the perfect time to lose weight. Decide that the right time to be healthier is now.

Common Barriers

Barrier 1: **I don't want to deny myself.**	Barrier 2: **I lost weight before but I gained it right back.**	Barrier 3: **I don't have the time to be active.**
Barrier Buster: **You don't have to! Moderation is the key.**	Barrier Buster: **Make this time different.**	Barrier Buster: **It takes just a few minutes a day!**
• Watch portion sizes and know when you're eating more than one serving. • Ask for a doggy bag. • Have just one. • Choose lower-fat and lower-calorie versions of your favorites.	• List what worked and didn't work last time and what you can try this time. • Choose changes that you are willing to stick with. • Work exercise into your weight-loss plan.	• Be active with a pet or the kids. • Block off activity time in your schedule. • Borrow some time that you usually spend watching TV.

Feel Good About Yourself

Do you eat more because you feel bad about yourself, then feel even worse as you gain weight? This is a "vicious cycle." Breaking this cycle is not easy. You may need group support or counseling. Always remember that you are a valuable person, no matter what size or shape you are.

Do you have a health problem? If so, don't use it as an excuse for not losing weight. Ask your doctor, dietitian, or other health care provider about methods to lose weight that are safe for you.

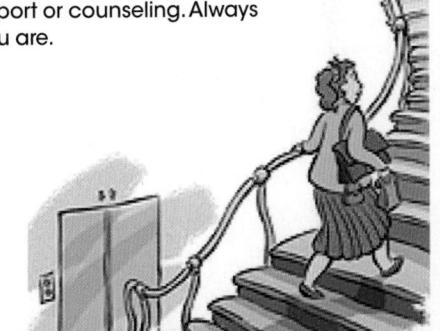

Courtesy of Harris CareTracker PM and EMR

FIGURE 24-8 Patient education forms can be printed from electronic medical records software and given to the patient right in the exam room.

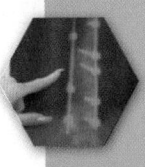

Critical Thinking

At the conclusion of the physical examination, the provider will have an impression of the patient's general health. What specific information can the provider obtain from the examination? From what sources other than the physical examination does the provider gain information to help in making a diagnosis? What types of information can the medical assistant accurately and concisely share with the provider to aid in the diagnosis?

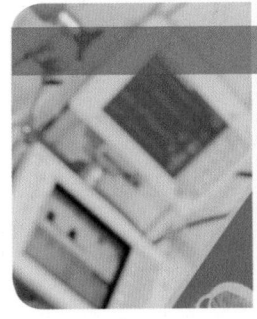

CASE STUDY 24-1

Refer to the scenario at the beginning of the chapter.

CASE STUDY REVIEW

1. Why do Gwen and Thomas prepare and assist for physical exams with patients of their own gender?
2. What are some examples of cultures where medical staff of the opposite gender are not allowed to be alone with or to examine the patient?

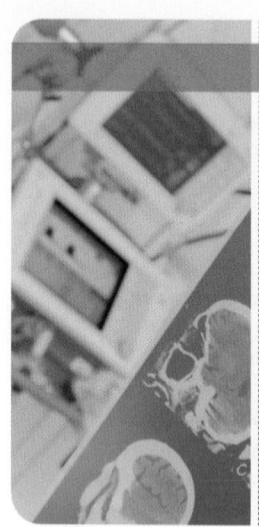

CASE STUDY 24-2

At Inner City Health Care, clinical medical assistant Gwen Carr, CMA (AAMA), is helping Liz Corbin, a part-time administrative/clinical medical assistant, to learn to prepare the examination room and patients for the physical examination. In addition to alerting Liz to provider preferences, Gwen wants to be sure that Liz has a solid understanding of the methods of examination, positions and draping, and the components of the physical examination.

CASE STUDY REVIEW

1. In reviewing with Liz the methods of examination used by the providers, what six primary methods would Gwen have Liz describe?
2. What patient positions would Liz need to know?
3. Gwen asks Liz to recall the various examination components and their significance. How should Liz respond?

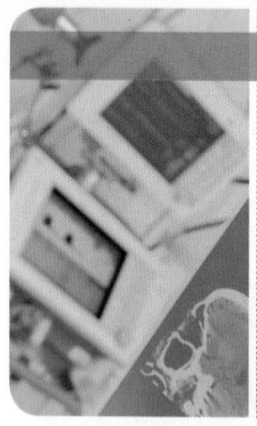

CASE STUDY 24-3

Mrs. Mason, a 72-year-old somewhat frail woman with arthritis and hypertensive heart disease, has an appointment today for a complete physical examination. It will include a basic physical examination and an examination of the pelvis because she has had bright red vaginal spotting.

CASE STUDY REVIEW

1. Discuss positions and draping for the physical examination, including pelvic examination for this patient.
2. Discuss any special safety needs for Mrs. Mason.
3. What additional supplies and equipment should be available for the provider?

Summary

- A complete physical examination will be performed during the patient's initial visit. Findings at this examination, both normal and abnormal, provide a baseline for future examinations.

- The role of the medical assistant throughout the examination is to assemble the necessary instruments and to hand them to the provider when requested.

- The medical assistant will also prepare the patient and obtain specimens as required by the examination and provider.

- Responsibilities to the patient include explanations and careful positioning; protecting modesty by careful draping; and, most important, providing comfort, emotional support, and safety. Knowledge of positions related to various examinations such as prone, supine, Fowler's, Sims' and Trendelenburg will assist the provider and support the patient throughout the examination.

- Components of the physical exam begin with overall examination and proceed to detailed examination of the systems of the body.

- At the conclusion of the examination, the medical assistant's role is to clean and restock the examination room as needed for the next patient.

CERTIFICATION REVIEW

1. Which of the following methods of examination is the process of listening directly to body sounds?
   a. Percussion
   b. Auditory
   c. Auscultation
   d. The direct method

2. The supine position is also known as which of the following positions?
   a. Horizontal recumbent
   b. Dorsal recumbent
   c. Knee-chest
   d. Sims'
   e. Fowler's

3. During the physical examination, ataxia might be observed. *Ataxia* is a term that relates to which of the following?
   a. Stature
   b. Posture
   c. Body movement
   d. Speech

4. When the patient asks a question of the medical assistant, what is the best course of action?
   a. Refer all questions to the provider
   b. Refer all questions to the clinic manager
   c. Try to answer all questions, even if uncertain
   d. Answer questions that relate to the scope of practice of the medical assistant and refer others to the provider
   e. Ask the patient to please hold all questions until the examination is complete

5. When the abdomen is being examined, what position is the most appropriate for the patient?
   a. Supine
   b. Prone
   c. Fowler's
   d. Sims'

6. A physical exam is usually conducted in which order?
   a. Caudal to cephalad
   b. Cephalad to caudal
   c. Medial to distal
   d. Distal to medial
   e. Proximal to distal

7. Which of the following is a common supply used during a neurologic exam?
   a. A cotton ball
   b. A safety pin
   c. A reflex hammer
   d. All of these

8. An annual GYN exam and Pap smear are conducted in which position?
   a. Dorsal recumbent
   b. Prone
   c. Lithotomy
   d. Fowler's
   e. Trendelenburg

9. An important method of assessment in which the practitioner observes the patient's appearance, gait, behavior, etc., is which of the following?
   a. Palpation
   b. Percussion
   c. Auscultation
   d. Inspection

10. Which supply is commonly utilized during the examination of the abdomen?
    a. Drape
    b. Stethoscope
    c. Otoscope
    d. Reflex hammer
    e. Both a and b

UNIT VII
ASSISTING WITH SPECIALTY EXAMINATIONS AND PROCEDURES

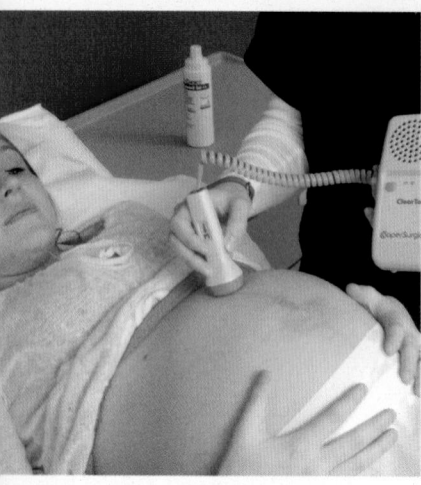 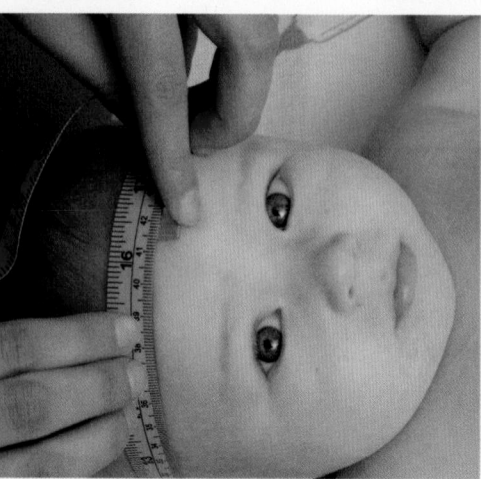 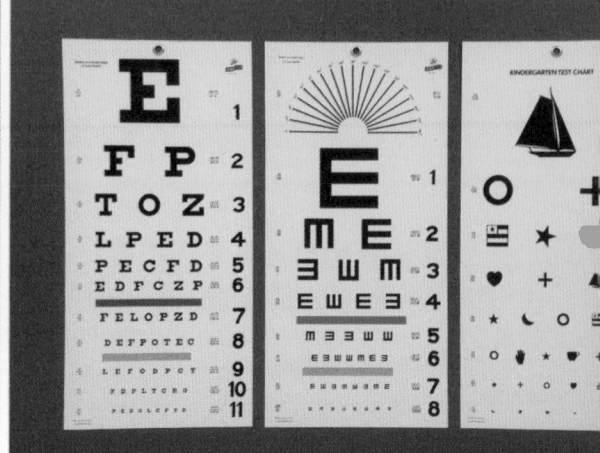

ATTRIBUTES OF PROFESSIONALISM

As a man or woman's body matures and secondary sexual characteristics emerge, specialty examinations and procedures are implemented to address patient needs. For female patients, breast health education and screening for other female cancers are a part of the annual care that the medical assistant will be involved in when employed in an OB/GYN setting. For male patients, these changes are usually managed by a family practitioner or internal medicine provider. Health issues specific to men include prostate cancer screening, treatment of erectile dysfunction, and disorders of the penis and testicles. Evaluation and treatment of sexually related systems can be a source of embarrassment for a patient. There are also social and religious diversity guidelines that must be known and followed in order to fully respect patients and their values when dealing with these specialized examinations.

Pediatric patients have their own set of normal values that apply to physical growth, developmental stages, and vital signs. An added consideration when working with the pediatric patient is the opinions, attitudes, and expectations of the child's parent or guardian. This adds an extra element when establishing a trusting rapport with the patient and his or her family, and it is one that cannot be overlooked when providing care.

When caring for older adults, you must understand that changes in sight, hearing, and psychologic

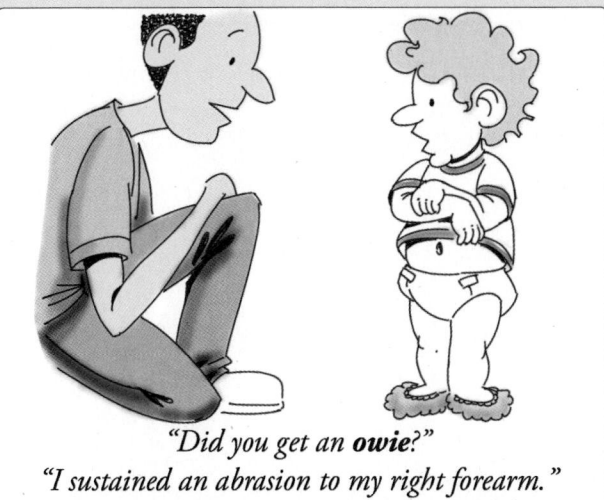

*"Did you get an **owie**?"*
"I sustained an abrasion to my right forearm."

outlook all have an impact on how the health care team interacts with the patient and his or her support system. Observing for elder abuse and reporting to the appropriate authorities is a responsibility of the medical assistant, so you must be alert and attune to both the verbal and nonverbal communication of each patient.

Listed below are a series of questions for you to ask yourself, to serve as a professionalism checklist. As you interact with patients and colleagues, these questions will help to guide you in the professional behavior and therapeutic communication that is expected every day from medical assistants.

Ask Yourself

COMMUNICATION
- [ ] Do I apply active listening skills?
- [ ] Do I demonstrate appropriate nonverbal communication?
- [ ] Do I explain to patients the rationale for performance of a procedure?
- [ ] Do I speak at each patient's level of understanding?
- [ ] Do I display appropriate body language?
- [ ] Do I respond honestly and diplomatically to my patients' concerns?
- [ ] Do I refrain from sharing my personal experiences?
- [ ] Do I include the patient's support system as indicated?
- [ ] Does my knowledge allow me to speak easily with all members of the health care team?
- [ ] Do I accurately and concisely update the provider on any aspect of a patient's care?

PRESENTATION
- [ ] Am I dressed and groomed appropriately?
- [ ] Do my actions attend to both the psychologic and the physiologic aspects of a patient's illness or condition?
- [ ] Am I courteous, patient, and respectful to patients?
- [ ] Do I display a positive attitude?
- [ ] Do I display a calm, professional, and caring manner?
- [ ] Do I demonstrate empathy to the patient?
- [ ] Do I show awareness of patients' concerns related to the procedure being performed?

COMPETENCY
- [ ] Do I pay attention to detail?
- [ ] Do I ask questions if I am out of my comfort zone or do not have the experience to carry out tasks?
- [ ] Do I display sound judgment?
- [ ] Am I knowledgeable and accountable?
- [ ] Do I incorporate critical thinking skills in performing patient assessment and care?

INITIATIVE
- [ ] Do I show initiative?
- [ ] Do I direct the patient to other resources when necessary or helpful, with the approval of the provider?
- [ ] Do I assist co-workers when appropriate?
- [ ] Do I make adaptations for patients with special needs?

INTEGRITY
- [ ] Do I demonstrate the principles of self-boundaries?
- [ ] Do I work within my scope of practice?
- [ ] Do I demonstrate respect for individual diversity?
- [ ] Do I demonstrate sensitivity to patient rights?
- [ ] Do I protect the integrity of the medical record?
- [ ] Do I protect and maintain confidentiality?
- [ ] Do I report situations that are harmful or illegal?

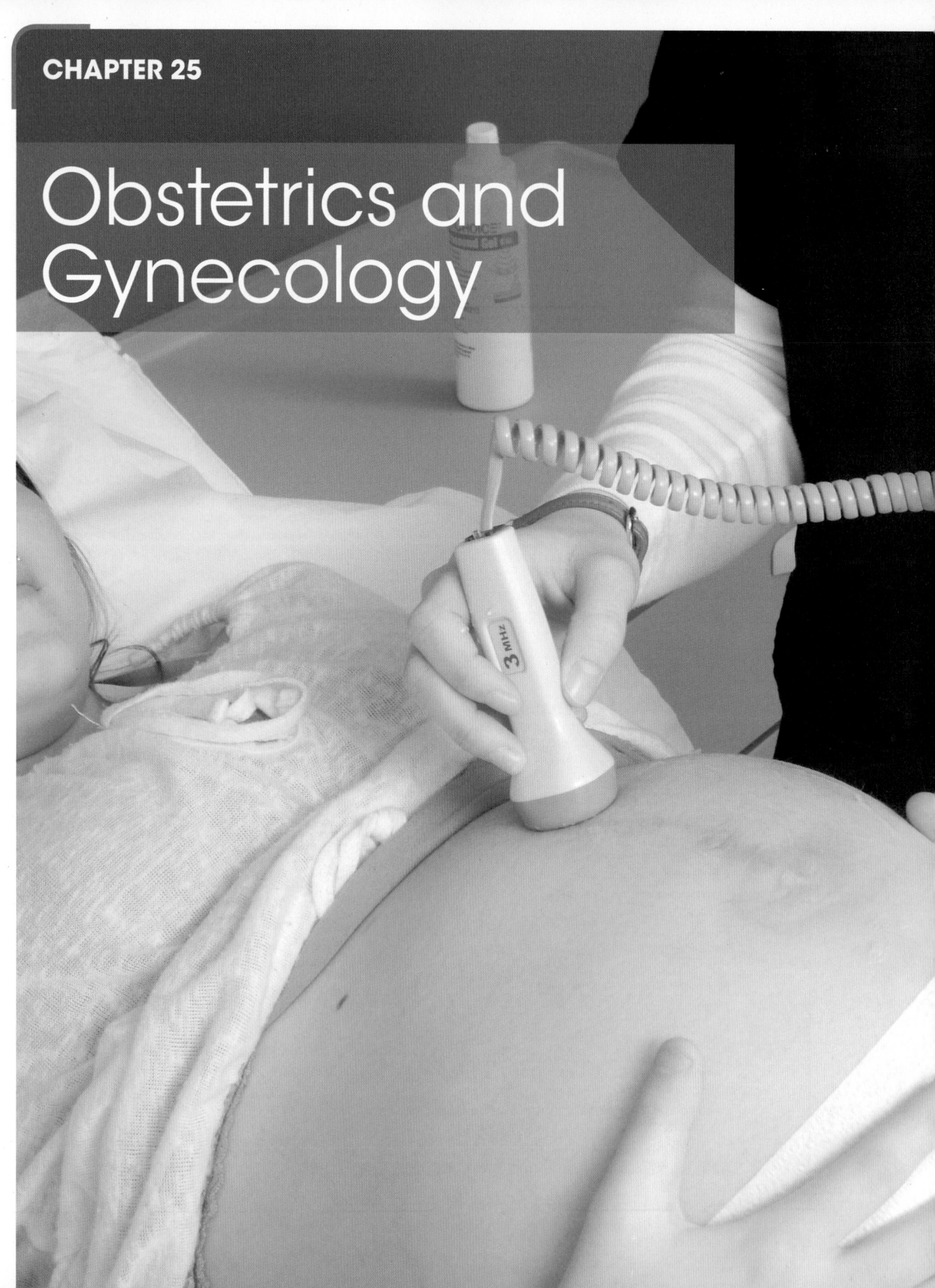

Obstetrics and Gynecology

1. Define and spell the key terms as presented in the glossary.

2. Summarize the importance of prenatal care, and discuss what examinations will be performed as part of the initial visit.

3. Identify the importance of the initial prenatal visit.

4. Outline 12 conditions or diseases that can cause a pregnant woman and her fetus to be at greater risk for problems during the pregnancy.

5. List signs and symptoms and their possible corresponding conditions that the provider searches for during the prenatal history and physical examination.

6. Calculate an expected date of confinement (EDC) or expected date of birth (EDB) using Nägele's rule.

7. Calculate an EDC (EDB) using a gestation wheel.

8. Define the purpose of ultrasonography and amniocentesis.

9. List and describe six types of abortion.

10. Describe what occurs in each of the three stages of labor.

11. Discuss what takes place during the postpartum examination.

12. List and describe the diseases and disorders that can affect the female patient.

13. Recognize the laboratory tests and procedures that can help diagnose the diseases and disorders that can affect the female patient.

14. Identify common sexually transmitted diseases.

15. Explain the medical assistant's responsibilities with a gynecologic examination.

16. Describe breast self-examination and the method of teaching a patient breast self-examination.

17. Discuss menopause.

18. Outline the findings and concerns surrounding hormone replacement therapy.

19. Describe 10 methods of contraception.

20. Explain reasons for impaired fertility.

21. Describe three therapies that assist in reproduction.

KEY TERMS

abortion	colposcopy	effacement
alpha-fetoprotein	condylomata	endometriosis
amniocentesis	congenital anomalies	erosion
amniotomy	contraception	formalin
bacterial vaginosis	coupling agent	fulgurated
Bartholin glands	cryosurgery	genitalia
bimanual examination	diethylstilbestrol (DES)	gestation
Braxton–Hicks	dilation	gestational diabetes
breast self-exam (BSE)	Down syndrome	gravidity
candidiasis	dysmenorrhea	human chorionic gonadotropin
carcinoma in situ	dyspareunia	hyperemesis gravidarum
cervical punch biopsy	dysplasia	hypoxia
Cesarean section(s)	eclampsia	hysterosalpingogram
chlamydia	ectopic pregnancy	intraepithelial

continues

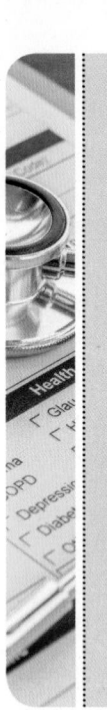

Key Terms, *continued*

involutes	Pap (Papanicolaou) test	prostaglandins
Lamaze	parity	puerperium
laparoscopy	parturition	sickle cell anemia
lochia	patency	supine hypotension
meconium	pelvic inflammatory	Tay–Sachs
menopausal hormone therapy (MHT)	disease (PID)	thalassemia
	placenta abruptio	titer
metrorrhagia	placenta previa	trichomoniasis
multigravida	polycystic	trimester
Nägele's rule	postcoital	ultrasonography
neonatal	preeclampsia	vesicles
nullipara	prenatal	viability
oxytocin	primigravidas	wet mount

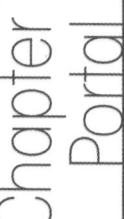

SCENARIO

Dr. Amy Cox is an OB/GYN in the obstetrics department of Inner City Health Care who has a fully packed schedule today. The morning hours are designated for prenatal visits and the afternoon for in-office GYN procedures.

It is important to understand the kind of prenatal visit that a patient requires. There are varied time requirements based on the patient's progress through her pregnancy. At predetermined gestational stages, there is screening scheduled to detect the risk of birth defects and genetic abnormalities, and to monitor the health of the mother during pregnancy. Other testing, such as ultrasound, monitors the progress of the baby or babies. First prenatal visits require more of the provider's time than the routine, regularly scheduled visits that occur throughout the pregnancy.

As a professional medical assistant, Gwen Carr, CMA (AAMA), must be aware of the needs related to each patient visit. She may be required to schedule the visit in an appropriate time slot on Dr. Cox's appointment calendar. She might be assisting Dr. Cox with a screening test or an exam. Gwen is the source for all patient teaching materials and handles the scheduling of outside testing for all of Dr. Cox's patients. She is a vital and indispensable part of the health care team.

Chapter Portal

Obstetrics is the medical specialty in which the provider treats the female patient from the prenatal period through labor and delivery, and during the 6-week postpartum period. Gynecology is the specialty that treats the medical and surgical disorders and diseases of the female reproductive tract. Both specialties are usually combined, and the provider who practices them is known as an obstetrician/gynecologist, or simply, an OB/GYN provider. Knowledge of female anatomy, laboratory tests and procedures for both specialties, diseases and disorders that affect the female patient during her nonpregnant and pregnant states, and patient education are essential for the medical assistant who will care for these patients. The goal of the OB/GYN specialty is to promote the health and well-being of the woman and her baby.

Integrity

HIPAA is important, especially when dealing with the cultural differences related to pregnancy. Some cultures demand modesty, and protecting these patients' privacy is critical. Infertility is a stigma in some cultures. Maintaining confidentiality is a requirement for all patients.

continues

OBSTETRICS

Obstetrics is the branch of medicine that provides care to the mother and fetus during pregnancy, labor, delivery, and the postpartum period known as the **puerperium**. Pregnancy is a period of approximately 40 weeks from the day conception takes place (Figure 25-1). The puerperium is the period of 6 weeks after delivery when the mother's body is returning to its prepregnant state. Visits to the provider for prenatal and postnatal care include the initial **prenatal** visit, return visits, and the 6-week postpartum checkup.

Initial Prenatal Visit

Procedure

The initial prenatal visit is of utmost importance and usually occurs after a woman has missed a second menstrual period or after an at-home pregnancy test result is positive (see Procedure 25-1). Some obstetricians recommend prepregnancy or preconception physical examinations. The information gained at this appointment can be used as a baseline on which to compare future tests and procedures. Any abnormalities can indicate a problem or complication necessitating further testing and assessment. Early detection and management of conditions such as **gestational diabetes**, urinary tract infections, anemia, and **preeclampsia** can prevent serious complications.

For more information on the tests and procedures conducted during the initial prenatal visit, see Table 25-1. Data are entered into the electronic medical record with each visit. This is reviewed with each subsequent visit to track and compare progress with expected milestones of pregnancy.

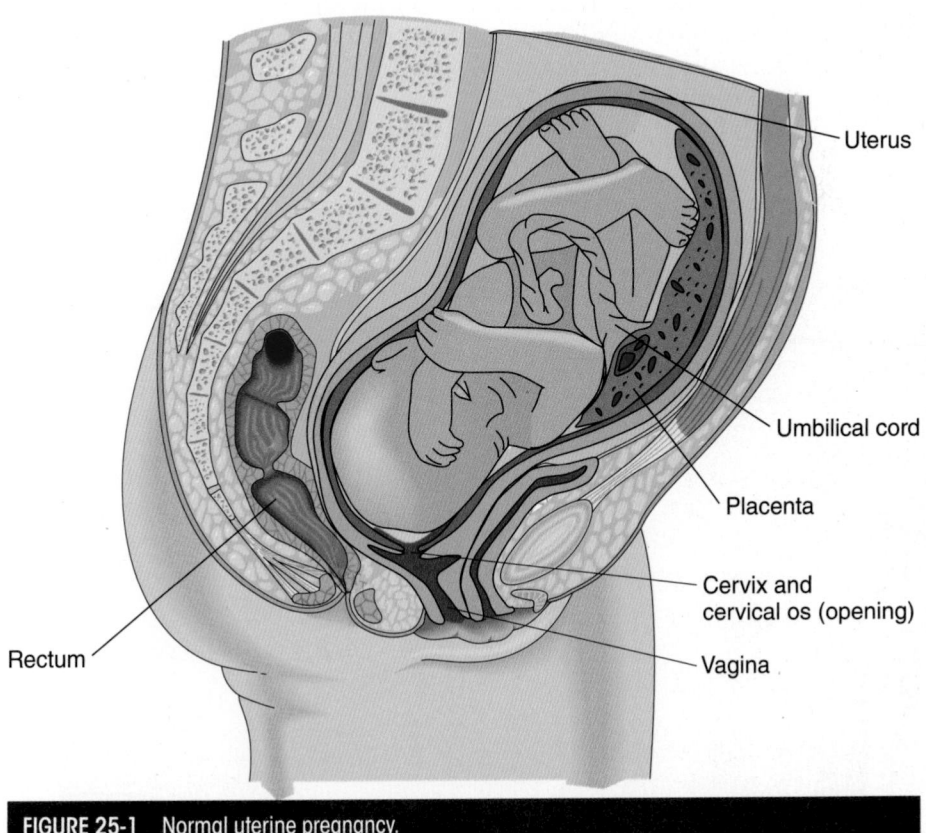

Uterus

Umbilical cord

Placenta

Cervix and cervical os (opening)

Vagina

Rectum

FIGURE 25-1 Normal uterine pregnancy.

Many formulas have been used for calculating the EDB (expected date of birth) or EDC (expected date of confinement). Although none is foolproof, **Nägele's rule** is the usual method used because it is reasonably accurate. Nägele's rule is to add 7 days to the first day of the last menstrual period (LMP), subtract 3 months, and add 1 year. An example is:

The first day of LMP = July 10, 2017

Add 7 days = July 17

Subtract 3 months = April 17

Add 1 year = April 17, 2018

Another method to calculate EDB or EDC is to add 7 days to LMP and count forward 9 months. Most women give birth within 7 days before or after the EDB or EDC.

Pregnancy wheels help determine the EDC. Line up the arrow of the first day of the LMP, then read off the date that corresponds to the 40-week designation (Figure 25-2).

Patient Education. Patient education includes such topics as nutrition, dental care, rest, and exercise, as well as discussion about over-the-counter (OTC) remedies, prescription medications, and herbal products. Alcohol and tobacco and their dangers and potential harm to fetus and mother should also be discussed. Medications, alcohol, cigarettes, and mind-altering substances taken by the mother have harmful effects on the fetus and should not be used.

Before the birth, the expectant mother is encouraged to choose a method of feeding the infant. During the initial prenatal visit, benefits of breast-feeding the newborn are discussed. If the mother is HIV negative, breast-feeding is encouraged because it offers many nutritional, psychologic, and immunologic benefits. Because the immune system of newborns is not fully developed, the high level of immunoglobulins in breast milk gives them protection against some pathogenic diseases of the respiratory and gastrointestinal tracts. Close contact between mother and newborn is certain with breast-feeding, and bonding can readily take place. Breast-fed infants seem to have fewer allergic reactions. For the mother, one benefit of breast-feeding is that the uterus **involutes**, or returns, more quickly to the nonpregnant state. Breast-feeding is the optimal way to feed a newborn. The services of a lactation consultant (available in most women's hospitals and some pediatric clinics) can be helpful especially during the initial phase of breast-feeding. The consultant can provide hands-on instructions to the patient to optimize the experience for the mother and baby.

Formal childbirth education classes given in various languages teach the fundamentals of labor, delivery, and newborn care and feeding. Other considerations include visiting the hospital where the delivery is planned to take a tour of the Labor and Delivery Department. This is a good time to complete any preadmission paperwork to make the admission process as seamless as possible.

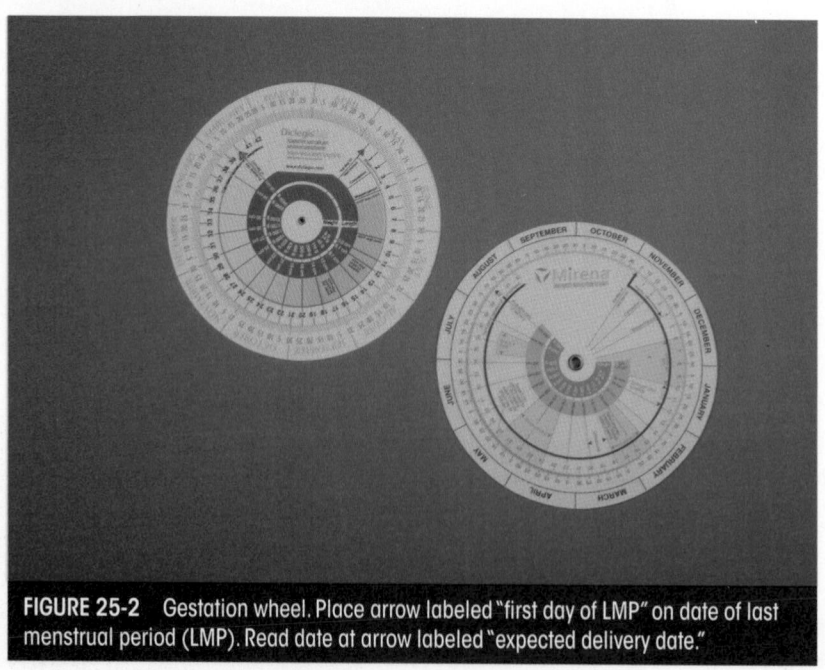

FIGURE 25-2 Gestation wheel. Place arrow labeled "first day of LMP" on date of last menstrual period (LMP). Read date at arrow labeled "expected delivery date."

TABLE 25-1

INITIAL PRENATAL VISIT (6 TO 10 WEEKS AFTER LMP)

COMPONENTS OF THE VISIT	DESCRIPTION

Patient history	Obtain the following information:
	• Date of last menstrual period (LMP)
	• Previous birth control
	• Past pregnancies (**gravidity**) (a woman who has been pregnant more than once is referred to as **multigravida**)
	• Number of pregnancies carried to the point of **viability** regardless of life or death at birth (**parity**) (a woman that has not carried a pregnancy to viability is considered **nullipara**)
	• FPAL:
	  ° **F** Number of full term deliveries (37 to 40 weeks' gestation)
	  ° **P** Number of preterm or premature deliveries (20 to 36 weeks' gestation)
	  ° **A** Number of abortions (either induced or spontaneous prior to 20 weeks' gestation)
	  ° **L** Number of living children born to the patient who are still alive at the time the history is taken
	  ° Example: A woman that has had four full term pregnancies, with four live births, but lost a child to leukemia at age 7 is referred to as 4-0-0-3 using the FPAL recording format
	• Hospitalizations
	• Medications
	• Allergies
	• Family medical history

Risk factors (see Table 25-2)	Record the following risk factors: • Maternal age (increase risk with age 35) • Use of street drugs • Rh-negative blood • History of premature labor and birth, abortions, or stillbirth • Familial genetic disorders • Previous **Cesarean section(s)** • Diabetes • Thyroid disorders • Sexually transmitted diseases • Hypertension • Nutritional deficiencies/eating disorders • Cardiac or kidney disorders • Seizure disorders
Physical examination	Conduct the following examinations: • Breast exam • Pap screening • Cervical culture • Possible ultrasound • Pelvic measurement • Maternal weight • Vital signs
Laboratory tests	Blood and urine screening
Gestational age	Conduct an early and accurate estimation of gestational age

TABLE 25-2

SIGNS AND SYMPTOMS OF POTENTIALLY SERIOUS CONDITIONS

SIGNS AND SYMPTOMS	POSSIBLE CONDITION
Rapid weight gain	Preeclampsia
Headaches	Preeclampsia
Hypertension	Preeclampsia
Vision changes	Preeclampsia
Severe nausea and vomiting	Hyperemesis gravidarum/dehydration
Bleeding, discharge, abdominal pain/cramping	Threatened abortion, placenta previa, placenta abruptio, ectopic pregnancy
Edema	Preeclampsia
One-sided pelvic or abdominal pain	Ectopic pregnancy (Figure 25-3)
Chills, fever	Vaginal infection, sexually transmitted disease, other infections

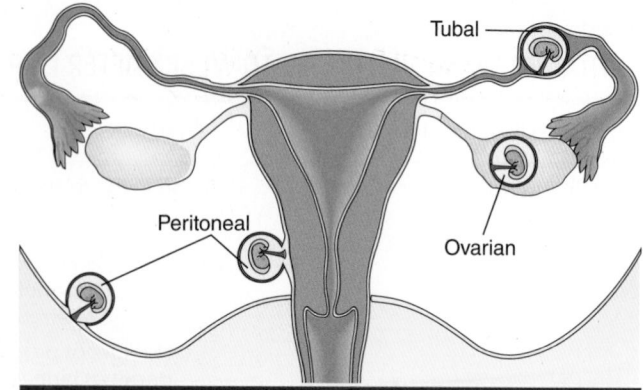

FIGURE 25-3 Sites of ectopic pregnancy.

- Are you comfortable with either a male or female provider?
- Are there any cultural practices that we need to be aware of during your pregnancy, childbirth, or postdelivery?

See Table 25-3 for more information on various cultural expectations and practices during pregnancy.

 Integrity
Respect for all cultures is of great importance, and judgments should not be made that some women are ignorant or lazy. Incorporating the patient's customs and beliefs demonstrates that you value cultural diversity and women's self-esteem.

All women should be fully involved in their care. Women with physical or emotional disabilities must have their particular needs addressed. When necessary, make adaptations whenever possible for women who are mentally challenged, blind, deaf, or physically incapacitated.

Laboratory Tests. The laboratory tests and procedures that may be part of the initial prenatal visit are described in Table 25-4.

 **Diversity**
Cultural Considerations during Pregnancy. Certain cultures expect women to observe practices believed to ensure a favorable pregnancy. It is helpful during the initial prenatal visit to include the following questions:

- Where were you born?
- What is your ethnic background?
- How long have you lived in the United States?
- What is your preferred language?
- Do you need an interpreter?

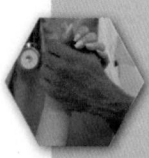

Patient Education

Whatever the pregnant woman ingests or inhales affects the fetus. Smoking during pregnancy poses serious risks to mother and fetus. Low birth weight, placenta abruptio, and deliveries before term are some of the possible effects to the fetus. Lung cancer, emphysema, and cardiovascular disease can affect the mother. Other kinds of substance abuse such as alcohol, cocaine, and other recreational drugs are commonly seen in pregnant women who are abused, such as in a domestic abuse situation; however, women do not have to be in an abusive situation to abuse drugs or alcohol. Ask the patient if she is in immediate danger. If so, a referral can be made to a community resource (e.g., women's shelter, hotline phone number, district attorney's office) or the provider can help devise a safety plan until the community resource steps in to help. (Chapters 6 and 34 provide more information about domestic violence and drug abuse.)

TABLE 25-3

CULTURAL CONSIDERATIONS DURING PREGNANCY

CULTURE	KEY ASPECTS
Spanish	Women wear a braided cord around their midsection to ward off nausea and ensure a safe birth.
Indian	Believe that "hot" foods are harmful and "cold" foods are beneficial during pregnancy. Believe in warding off the evil eye by burning red chillies and camphor. Believe that during an eclipse, pregnant women should remain inside the house or their babies will be born with a cleft lip or other deformity.
Mexican or Mesoamerican	Women should avoid strenuous physical activity during pregnancy. Prenatal care is sought later in pregnancy. Female caregivers are preferred. Believe that observing a lunar eclipse will cause the developing baby to have a cleft lip/palate. Prefer to labor at home. Forty days of rest after delivery with home remedies to aid in cleansing the impurities of birth.
Dutch	Prefer to treat pregnancy as a natural state. Prenatal screening not done unless familial indication. Prefer to give birth at home. Delivery is usually done by midwives. No pain medication given during labor or birth. Mother receives help with self-care, childcare, and housework from a nurse for several weeks after delivery.
Chinese	Women steer away from funerals, sex, and "evil spirits." Believe that the personality and spirit of the baby are strongly influenced by the state of the mother's mind and body during pregnancy. Drink strong herbal tea to assist with the pain of labor. New mothers take an entire month off from duties to stay in bed, heal, and connect with their newborns. Believe that exposure to cell phones, computers, or microwaves can cause miscarriages or birth defects.
Ethiopian	Consider pregnancy to be a natural, healthy occurrence and little changes in their day-to-day life.
Moroccan	Women wear loose clothing and leave their hair down and heads uncovered, believing that doing so will ease the birth process.
German	Midwives must be present at birth; physicians are optional. Must name their babies from a list of "accepted" names unless there is a compelling reason.
Japanese	Believe that labor pains must be endured as preparation for the challenges of motherhood. After delivery, mother and baby stay at the maternal grandparents' home for up to a month. Women are to lay in with their baby for 21 days. Laying in is a period of bed rest required even if there were no medical complications with the birth of the child.

TABLE 25-4

LABORATORY TESTS AT THE INITIAL PRENATAL VISIT

LABORATORY TEST	DISEASE OR CONDITION
Complete blood count (CBC), hemoglobin, and hematocrit	To detect anemia or infection
Urinalysis with microscopic examination (pH, specific gravity, color, glucose, albumin, proteins, white and red blood cell counts, casts, acetone, **human chorionic gonadotropin** [HCG])	To screen for diabetes mellitus, renal disease, infection, hypertensive disease, pregnancy
Blood type, Rh factor	To detect Rh incompatibility
Rubella titer	To determine immunity to rubella
Renal function Alpha-fetoprotein (if initial visit is at 16 to 18 weeks' gestation)	To evaluate renal impairment in women with history of diabetes mellitus, hypertension, or kidney disease
Genetic trait screening—cystic fibrosis, Tay–Sachs, thalassemia	To determine potential risk of genetic disorders in offspring
Tuberculin skin test	To screen for tuberculosis
Venereal disease research laboratory (VDRL) and rapid plasma reagin (RPR)	To detect syphilis
Human immunodeficiency virus (HIV)	To screen for HIV antibodies
Hepatitis B and C viruses	To screen for hepatitis B and C viruses
Blood glucose	To screen for gestational diabetes
Cardiac evaluation electrocardiogram (ECG), chest radiograph, or echocardiogram	To evaluate cardiac function in women with history of heart disease or hypertension
Pap smear	To check for cervical dysplasia, herpes simplex virus 2
Vaginal, cervical, or rectal smear or culture for gonorrhea, chlamydia, and *Streptococcus* group B	To check for gonorrhea, chlamydia, human papilloma virus (HPV)

Subsequent or Return Prenatal Visits

Procedure

Subsequent visits include weight, blood pressure, urinalysis, complete blood count with hemoglobin and hematocrit, measurement of the height of the uterine fundus (a tape measure is used by placing it on the anterior symphysis pubis and the crest of the uterus) (Figure 25-4), and fetal heart measurements (Figure 25-5). See Table 25-5 for more information on the procedures and patient education conducted during subsequent prenatal visits (see Procedure 25-1).

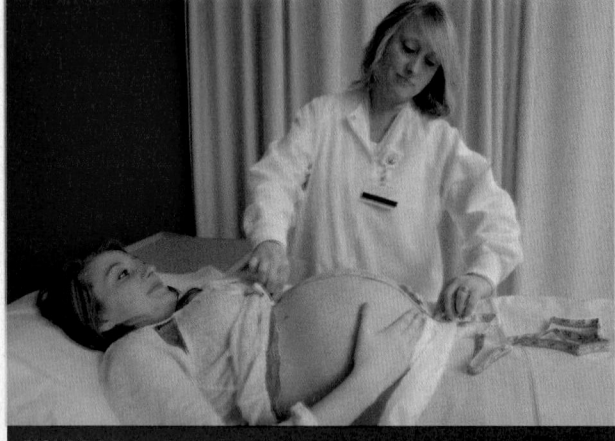

FIGURE 25-4 Fundal height is measured by placing the end of the tape at the symphysis pubis and extending it in either a curved or straight pattern to the fundus.

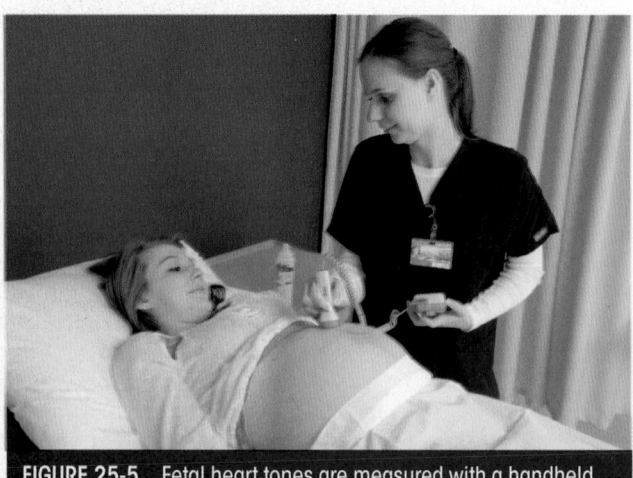

FIGURE 25-5 Fetal heart tones are measured with a handheld Doppler.

TABLE 25-5

SUBSEQUENT PRENATAL VISITS

TIMING	TEST OR PROCEDURE	PATIENT EDUCATION
Weeks 10 to 14	Update history Obtain vital signs, including maternal weight Review lab results Assess fetal heart tones (see Figure 25-5)	Provide patient education on the following topics: • Anemia and pregnancy, including dietary recommendations and prenatal vitamins • Bleeding in early pregnancy, including when to notify the provider
Weeks 15 to 18 (monthly visits)	Update history Obtain vital signs, including maternal weight Measure fundal height (see Figure 25-4) Assess fetal heart tones (see Figure 25-5)	Provide patient education on the following topics: • Breast- or bottle-feeding your baby, including benefits and preparation • Preeclampsia and its effect on pregnancy (see Table 25-2), including signs and symptoms and when to notify the provider
Weeks 19 to 24 (monthly visits)	Update history Obtain vital signs, including maternal weight Measure fundal height (see Figure 25-4) Assess fetal heart tones (see Figure 25-5) Fetal abnormality testing, including neural tube defects, Down syndrome, and trisomy 16 and 18 Possible ultrasound to screen for fetal anomalies, and secondarily to permit early detection of twins and other multiples	Provide patient education on the following topics: • Genetic disorders, including risk groups and how testing is performed • Pregnancy with multiples, including nutritional guidelines, risk factors, and exercise recommendations • Vaginal birth after C-section, including risks, benefits, and preparation • Chorionic villus sampling, including how procedure is performed and preparation • Amniocentesis, including purpose, how procedure is preformed, and preparation
Weeks 25 to 28 (monthly visits)	Update history Obtain vital signs, including maternal weight Measure fundal height (see Figure 25-4) Assess fetal heart tones (see Figure 25-5) Gestational diabetes screening Rhogam injection if mother is Rh negative	Provide patient education on the following topics: • Signs that labor has begun and timing, strength, and level of discomfort with contractions • Rh factor and how it can affect pregnancy, including diagnosis and intervention • Gestational diabetes, including diagnosis, management, and when to contact the provider • Vaginal birth, including expectations and preparation • Cesarean birth, including expectations and preparation
Weeks 29 to 34 (bi-weekly visits)	Update history Obtain vital signs, including maternal weight Measure fundal height (see Figure 25-4) Assess fetal heart tones (see Figure 25-5)	Provide patient education on the following topics: • Management of the discomforts of pregnancy, including heartburn, hemorrhoids, constipation, back aches, fatigue, and nasal stuffiness
Weeks 35 to delivery (weekly visits)	Update history Obtain vital signs, including maternal weight Measure fundal height (see Figure 25-4) Assess fetal heart tones (see Figure 25-5) Pelvic exam Group B strep screening	Provide patient education on the following topics: • Options for pain management during labor • Fetal heart monitoring during labor, including how to count and when to notify the provider • Group B strep and pregnancy, including the importance of obtaining a culture for diagnosis and the prescription of the appropriate antibiotic • Cord blood banking, including purpose and procedure • Counting fetal movements, including procedure and when to notify the provider

PROCEDURE 25-1

Procedure

Assisting with Routine Prenatal Visits

STANDARD PRECAUTIONS:

Handwashing

Gloves

Biohazard

PURPOSE:

To monitor the progress of the pregnancy.

EQUIPMENT/SUPPLIES:

- Scale
- Nonsterile gloves
- Patient gown
- Tape measure
- Sphygmomanometer
- Stethoscope
- Doppler fetoscope and coupling agent
- Urine specimen container
- Urinalysis testing supplies
- Biohazard waste container

PROCEDURE STEPS:

1. *Paying attention to detail*, assemble equipment.

2. Wash hands and follow Standard Precautions.

3. Introduce yourself to the patient. Identify patient using two patient identifiers.

4. *Explain the rationale for performance of the procedure*, *speaking at the patient's level of understanding*. Provide the patient with the opportunity to ask questions, *showing awareness of the patient's concerns related to the procedure*.

5. Provide the patient with the urine container and request that she empty her bladder. RATIONALE: An empty bladder will facilitate the examination of the uterus and will be more comfortable for the patient.

6. If a urine specimen is required, instruct the patient in the correct method of obtaining a clean catch urine specimen. RATIONALE: A clean catch urine specimen is utilized for several health screening tests.

7. *Considering any special needs of the patient*, instruct and then assist the patient to remove shoes, jacket, or sweater, and step on paper towels on the scale. Assist the patient to the center of the scale. Weigh patient. Accurately record findings. RATIONALE: Assesses gain or loss of weight to help determine fetal development and maternal nutrition.

8. Measure blood pressure and accurately record findings.

9. If this is a routine monthly visit without complications, a pelvic exam may not be required. Check with the provider.

10. *Being courteous and respectful*, provide patient with gown and drape.

11. *In a manner that protects the patient's personal boundaries*, have patient disrobe from waist down and put on a gown, open in the front. RATIONALE: An open gown facilitates access to the abdomen for examination and measurement of the fundal height.

12. Allowing the patient privacy, step out of the exam room and take this time to test the urine specimen while waiting for the provider. RATIONALE: Urinalysis is done to detect glucose and protein, which may indicate disease.

13. When finished with the testing procedures, return to the exam room and prepare the patient for the exam.

14. *Attending to any special needs*, assist patient onto examination table and drape her. RATIONALE: The patient may be off balance and unsteady on her feet because of the enlargement of the abdomen. Provide for her safety.

(continues)

15. Assist the provider as the examination is performed.
    - Hand the provider the tape measure to measure height of fundus.
    - Hand the provider the Doppler fetal pulse detector for measurement of fetal heart rate. The medical assistant may spread the coupling agent onto the patient's abdomen.

16. After the examination, assist patient to sit for a few moments. Assess her color and pulse and inquire about dizziness or faintness. RATIONALE: Orthostatic hypotension can occur when a patient rises from a recumbent position. Give the patient time for the blood pressure to go back to normal so she will not experience dizziness from decreased blood pressure.

17. Provide tissues so patient can wipe off coupling agent. Allow privacy for dressing after the exam.

18. When the patient is ready, provide any instructions or clarification of provider's orders, *speaking at the patient's level of understanding*.

19. After the patient has left the exam room, apply gloves. Discard disposable supplies per OSHA guidelines. Disinfect equipment used.

20. Remove gloves and discard them in the appropriate container.

21. Wash hands.

22. Set up for the next patient.

23. Accurately record all information in the patient's chart or electronic medical record.

DOCUMENTATION:

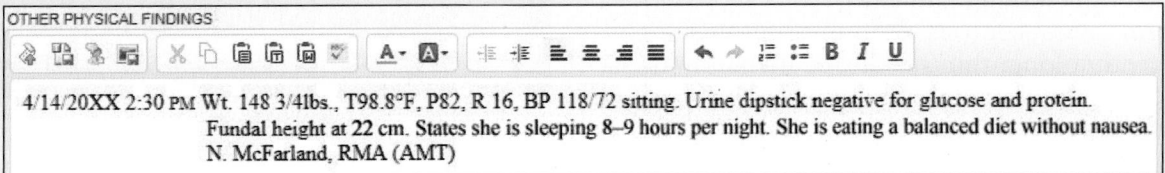

OTHER PHYSICAL FINDINGS

4/14/20XX 2:30 PM Wt. 148 3/4lbs., T98.8°F, P82, R 16, BP 118/72 sitting. Urine dipstick negative for glucose and protein. Fundal height at 22 cm. States she is sleeping 8–9 hours per night. She is eating a balanced diet without nausea. N. McFarland, RMA (AMT)

Courtesy of Harris CareTracker PM and EMR

Vaginal examinations are done only periodically up to 2 to 3 weeks before the EDB or EDC. Patients are encouraged to attend classes in the **Lamaze** method of childbirth, as well as classes in the care of the newborn.

Tests and Procedures **Alpha-fetoprotein**. Another test that may be done during a subsequent visit is the mother's serum alpha-fetoprotein (MSAFP) blood test. It is done about the 16th week of pregnancy. It is a screening test only, done to rule out neural tube defects, abdominal wall defects, and chromosomal problems such as Down syndrome. If the test is positive, additional testing such as an **amniocentesis** or an ultrasound will be used to help make a diagnosis.

Chorionic Villus Sampling (CVS). Chorionic villus sampling (CVS) is a test performed on women who are older than 35 years, have a history of chromosomal abnormalities, and/or are known carriers of a genetic disorder such as **thalassemia**, **sickle cell anemia**, **Down syndrome**, or **Tay–Sachs**. The test is done at about 8 to 10 weeks' **gestation** and has an advantage over amniocentesis because the latter cannot be done before the 14th week. In one method of the CVS test, a sample of tissue that surrounds the fetus is taken through a catheter by means of suction. The sample is analyzed in the laboratory for genetic abnormalities.

Ultrasonography/Amniocentesis. Two tests can be done that can supply vital information: **ultrasonography**, or ultrasound, and amniocentesis. An ultrasonogram is done simultaneously with an amniocentesis to avoid possible injury to the fetus or placenta.

Ultrasound can be performed in the first, second, or third **trimester**. It uses high-frequency sound waves to produce an image of the fetus. A **coupling agent** is spread onto the mother's abdomen to enhance penetration of sound waves through the tissue, and the scanning mechanism is moved over the abdomen. An image of the fetus can be viewed on a screen similar to a television screen. Photos are taken during the examination. The technique usually takes about a half hour. There are no known side effects to the fetus or mother, and ultrasound uses no X-rays. There is no pain involved, but slight discomfort can occur because the patient has a full bladder. (A quart of fluid should be consumed 1 hour before the test and finished within 15 or 20 minutes.) A full bladder is essential to a good-quality ultrasound because it supports the uterus in position for good imaging. This procedure may be used to identify the number of fetuses, check the age of the fetus (number of weeks' gestation), and detect some fetal abnormalities (e.g., Down syndrome; Figure 25-6).

A high-resolution three-dimensional ultrasonographic test is being used more and more frequently to check for Down syndrome. The test is useful because it can detect chromosomal abnormalities. It can be done sooner in a pregnancy than blood testing and could minimize the need for CVS or amniocentesis, both of which create risks for the mother and fetus.

An amniocentesis is the surgical puncturing, with a long, thin needle, of the amniotic sac through the woman's abdomen. The purpose of this test is to obtain, by aspiration, a sample of amniotic fluid that contains fetal cells. The procedure can be done as early as 14 weeks and helps to diagnose genetic problems, **congenital anomalies**

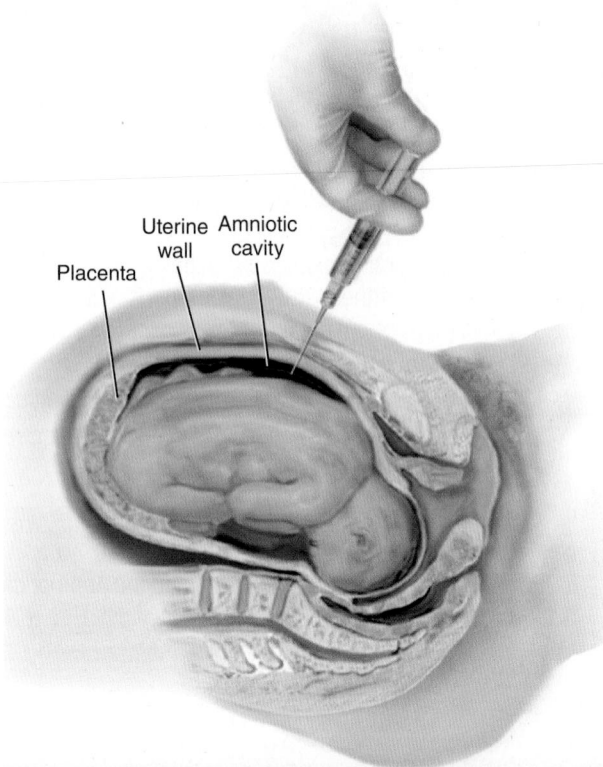

FIGURE 25-7 During amniocentesis, a sample of amniotic fluid is aspirated for evaluation. An ultrasonogram is done simultaneously with an amniocentesis to avoid possible injury to the fetus or placenta.

(present at birth), and chromosomal defects. It also can be used to determine the lung capacity of the fetus (Figure 25-7).

Ultrasonography is performed while the provider is doing the amniocentesis to identify the position of the fetus and placenta, thereby avoiding injury to either. There can be bleeding, leaking of amniotic fluid, and infection. Percutaneous umbilical blood sampling (PUBS) (also known as cordocentesis, fetal blood sampling, or umbilical vein sampling) is another procedure that can be done. It accesses fetal circulation by aspirating blood from the fetal umbilical cord vessels. Because the procedure is invasive, it is performed in conjunction with ultrasound. Many blood studies can be performed, and many conditions can be diagnosed using fetal cord blood, such as chromosomal abnormalities, infections within the uterus, and fetal hypoxia. Drug therapy and transfusions can be given through the umbilical vein in the fetal umbilical cord. With either of these procedures, there is a risk of miscarriage. Alerting patients to this potential risk is an important aspect of informed consent.

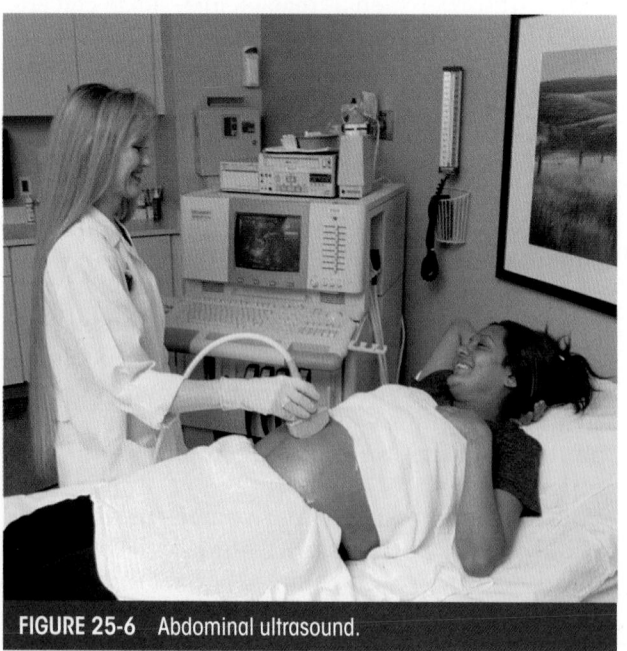

FIGURE 25-6 Abdominal ultrasound.

Fetal heart rate is another test. Monitoring can be done in one of two ways: a nonstress test monitors the fetus's heart rate while it is moving spontaneously, and a stress test monitors the fetal heart rate while the mother is stimulated with medication to have mild uterine contractions. Normally, the fetal heart rate will accelerate to a higher but safe limit while it is being stressed.

Entering data electronically during each visit allows immediate access to the patient's medical record and comparisons of vital signs, laboratory values, ultrasounds, amniocenteses, and all other diagnostic tests and procedures in previous data entries. Baseline values are important, and the timing of certain laboratory tests is crucial for accurate evaluation. Providers can refer back to these values throughout the pregnancy. The electronic medical record (EMR) is a communication mechanism for organizing a patient's care. All data entry should be dated and include the time and your signature.

Disorders of Pregnancy

The following sections address some problems that may occur during pregnancy.

Abortion/Interruption of Pregnancy. The interruption of pregnancy before the fetus is viable is known as **abortion**. Six types of abortion are listed here:

1. *Spontaneous.* Unknown etiology (miscarriage).
2. *Complete.* Expulsion of all products of conception, fetus, and placenta with no surgical intervention.
3. *Missed.* Fetus dies in the uterus and must be removed; usually a dilation and curettage (D&C) is the surgical procedure performed.
4. *Incomplete.* Only parts of the fetus and placenta are expelled. Tissue remains in the uterus and a D&C usually must be performed.
5. *Threatened.* Bleeding from the uterus, but there are no contractions or dilation of cervix. Pregnancy continues.
6. *Induced.* Evacuation of the fetus and placenta from the uterus at the patient's request or because the patient's health is in jeopardy.

Ectopic Pregnancy. An **ectopic pregnancy** indicates the implantation of an embryo outside of the uterus (see Figure 25-3). This may occur anywhere in the pelvic region, but occurs most commonly in the fallopian tube. This is a life-threatening condition for the mother. When the fertilized egg implants in other structures that do not have the capacity for the growth of the embryo, the structure may rupture. This causes uncontrolled bleeding at the site of the rupture.

Symptoms include early pregnancy symptoms such as breast tenderness or nausea. More serious symptoms include pain in the lower belly or pelvic area, abnormal vaginal bleeding, lower back pain, or mild cramping on one side of the abdomen. Postrupture symptoms include syncope; intense rectal pressure; hypotension; referred pain to the shoulder; and severe, sharp, and sudden pain in the lower abdomen.

Eclampsia. **Eclampsia** syndrome, also known as pregnancy-induced hypertension, can occur in pregnancy and result in convulsions unrelated to epilepsy or other brain conditions. Eclampsia occurs 1 in every 2,000 to 3,000 pregnancies. Risks for developing this condition include first or multiple gestation; pregnancy after age 35; being of African American heritage; and a history of diabetes, hypertension, or renal disease. Eclampsia is a potentially life-threatening disorder characterized by hypertension, generalized edema, and proteinuria. It can put the woman and her fetus in grave danger and can be fatal if not treated. Preeclampsia is less severe. The symptoms are the same, except there are no convulsions. This is why weight is measured, blood pressure is checked, and a urinalysis (including a check for protein) is routinely performed. Sudden significant weight gain, increase in blood pressure, and the presence of protein in the urine can indicate possible preeclampsia. The cause is unknown. Prophylaxis is of great importance. The problem is seen more often in women who have received inadequate prenatal care, especially poor nutrition; in **primigravidas** (pregnant for the first time) younger than 18 years; in women with preexisting cardiovascular and renal conditions; and in women who have diabetes.

Gestational Diabetes. Gestational diabetes first appears during the second or third trimester of the pregnancy and usually disappears after the woman has delivered her baby or when the pregnancy terminates for any other reason. Pregnancy hormones can block the action of insulin, resulting in elevated blood glucose. This type of diabetes is usually a milder form of the disease. Prompt detection (through blood and urine glucose testing) and therapy are essential to avoid fetal and **neonatal** (newborn) illness and death. Factors that increase the risk of developing gestational diabetes are a family history of diabetes, pregnancy after age 25, and being overweight before pregnancy.

A blood glucose sample is drawn 1 hour after the patient is given a high-glucose drink. If the test result is elevated, then a 3-hour glucose tolerance test is done. The patient with gestational diabetes requires more frequent prenatal visits to the provider. The fetus is evaluated at each visit. Ultrasound evaluation of fetal growth is performed more often. The patient must control her diet and monitor blood glucose levels at home several times daily. A nutritionist will help by teaching the patient about a diabetic diet. The appropriate number of calories and percentage of carbohydrates, proteins, and fats are calculated to keep the blood glucose as close to 100 mg/dL as possible. If the diabetic diet does not control blood glucose levels, insulin therapy is started. Usually the patient is admitted to the hospital if she has poorly controlled diabetes and the additional factor of hypertension.

Pregnant women with gestational diabetes have a strong possibility of developing diabetes within their lifetime. The provider will order a blood glucose (1-hour glucose tolerance) when the woman is 6 to 8 weeks' postpartum. The results will determine whether the patient's blood glucose level has dropped to the normal range.

Hyperemesis Gravidarum.
Hyperemesis gravidarum, or excessive vomiting during pregnancy, can be harmful and is more than simply morning sickness, which is a common complaint during the first trimester. The cause of the condition is not known, but it is thought to be related to the cells that become the placenta and to the production of pregnancy hormones. The symptoms include uncontrollable nausea and vomiting, inability to eat, and exhaustion from inability to sleep. Severe dehydration can result and starvation may ensue. This complication is usually not fatal, but it is a severe problem that warrants immediate treatment. Treatment includes intravenous fluids to replace those lost through vomiting and mild sedation to aid rest and sleep.

Placenta Previa.
Placenta previa occurs when the placenta implants low in the uterus and partially or completely covers the cervical os or opening of the uterus. It is an emergency. The cause is unknown. When labor ensues and the cervix begins to dilate, the placenta is pulled away from the wall of the uterus and causes bleeding. On occasion, the bleeding, which comes on suddenly and is painless, will stop spontaneously. If it continues, significant maternal blood is lost, and the fetus may suffer anoxia and die when the placenta separates from the blood supply (Figure 25-8A).

Ultrasonography can determine where the placenta is attached, at which time the diagnosis can be made and treatment begun. Treatment depends on the gestational age of the fetus and the percentage of placenta that covers the cervical os. A Cesarean section may be necessary to remove the placenta, control bleeding, and deliver the fetus safely.

Some of the factors associated with placenta previa are advanced maternal age, maternal smoking, and cocaine use. Maternal exposure to passive smoke and use of tobacco by the mother have been shown to be risky to the fetus, resulting in lower birth weight, premature birth, and infant death.

Placenta Abruptio.
Placenta abruptio occurs when the placenta prematurely and abruptly separates from the uterine lining (Figure 25-8B). It can result in fetal distress and death as well as maternal shock and death. It usually occurs late in pregnancy but can occur during labor.

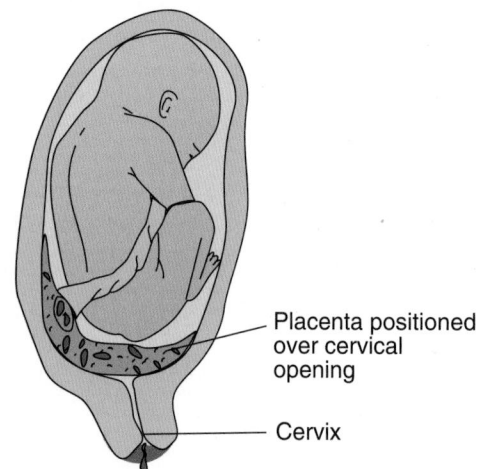

Placenta positioned over cervical opening

Cervix

Placenta previa

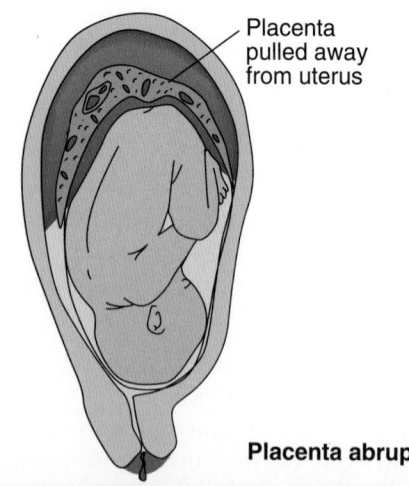

Placenta pulled away from uterus

Placenta abruptio

FIGURE 25-8 (A) Placenta previa. (B) Placenta abruptio.

Factors that contribute to this complication are multiple pregnancies, chronic hypertension, trauma to the uterus, and sudden release of amniotic fluid. Delivery as soon as possible either vaginally or by Cesarean section is indicated. The prognosis of the newborn depends on the extent of **hypoxia** suffered during labor and delivery.

The newborn infant should begin to cry and his or her color turn pink (hands and feet may remain blue for about a week). Abnormalities, if any, are documented. The Apgar score is an indication of the newborn's well-being. Assessments, in numbers from 1 to 10, are made at 1, 5, and 15 minutes. Five aspects of the newborn are evaluated: respiratory ease, heart rate, skin color, reflexes, and muscle tone. Each is assigned a number, which added together determine the newborn's Apgar score. The closer the score is to 10, the closer the newborn is to adapting to life outside the uterus. A lower score indicates a problem with the newborn's respirations, heart rate, color, and/or muscle tone. Oxygen and other measures may be necessary to stabilize a newborn with a low Apgar score (Table 25-6).

Impaired Fertility. The inability to conceive and bear a child after a period of unprotected sex is known as impaired fertility. One reason for this problem is that some couples delay pregnancy until later in life, when fertility is naturally lower. The increase in the incidence of **pelvic inflammatory disease (PID)**, endometriosis, substance abuse, and environmental factors such as pesticides and lead all can contribute to impaired fertility.

Diagnosis and treatment of impaired fertility require a physical, emotional, and financial investment over a long period. To diagnose impaired fertility in the female patient, a complete history and physical examination are performed. Endocrine system and anatomic and physiologic abnormalities are sought. Laboratory tests on urine and blood are performed. Proof of ovulation can be determined by retrieving an ovum from the uterine tube, performing an endometrial biopsy, assessing mucus characteristics, and taking the basal body temperature. Levels of estrogen, progesterone, follicle-stimulating hormone, and luteinizing hormone are also measured. A **hysterosalpingogram**, a radiograph of the uterus and tubes after the injection of dye, reveals defects in either the uterus or tubes. Laparoscopy can be performed to visualize the internal pelvic structures. Tubal patency, **endometriosis**, pelvic adhesions, or **polycystic** ovaries can be seen. Endometrial biopsy is done to examine the tissue and determine whether the endometrium is capable of accepting a fertilized ovum for implantation. Ultrasonography, either abdominal or transvaginal, can assess pelvic organs for abnormalities.

Tests that can be performed on a male to diagnose impaired fertility are semen analysis, hormone analysis, and biopsy of a testicle.

Once a diagnosis of impaired fertility has been made, a number of therapies are available to assist in reproduction. This is known as assisted reproductive technology (ART).

- *In vitro fertilization (IVF), indicated for fallopian tube blockage and endometriosis.* Eggs are retrieved from the woman's ovaries, fertilized with sperm from her partner in the laboratory, then transferred to her uterus.

- *Gamete intrafallopian transfer (GIFT).* Eggs are retrieved from the woman's ovaries. An egg

TABLE 25-6

APGAR SCORE FOR ASSESSING NEWBORNS

		APGAR SCORE*		
		0	**1**	**2**
A	**Activity**	Limp; no movement	Some flexion of arms and legs	Active motion
P	**Pulse**	No heart rate	Fewer than 100 beats per minute (bpm)	At least 100 bpm
G	**Grimace**	No response to airways being suctioned	Grimace during suctioning	Grimace, pull away, cough, or sneeze during suctioning
A	**Appearance**	Baby's entire body is bluish-gray or pale	Good body color; bluish hands or feet	Good color on body and extremities
R	**Respiration**	No respiration	Weak cry, whimpering, slow or irregular breathing	Strong cry and normal respiratory rate

*The APGAR score is obtained by assigning a number in each category based on the assessment of the newborn and then adding the numbers to determine the score

and a sperm from her partner are aspirated into a special catheter, then placed into the fallopian tube, where fertilization may occur naturally.

- *In vitro fertilization and gamete intrafallopian transfer (IVF + GIFT) with donor sperm.* Eggs are retrieved from the woman's ovaries, fertilized with donor sperm in the laboratory, aspirated into a special catheter, then placed into the fallopian tube, where fertilization may take place naturally.

Legal

New technology, testicular sperm extraction (TESE), allows sperm retrieval from the testicles if ejaculation is impossible. Sperm can be injected into the ovum, embryos can be frozen, and surrogate pregnancies are possible. With technology comes the ethical and legal questions of donor eggs and embryos, pregnancies in older women, how to define who the parents are, what to do with frozen embryos after the death or divorce of the adults involved, and other issues such as disposal of unused (extra) embryos.

Diversity

In some cultures, a woman is deemed the responsible party for impaired fertility, and the impairment is thought to be caused by her sins, evil spirits, or personal deficiencies. The virility of a male is questioned unless he is able to manifest his sexual potency by having a child.

Incompatibility.   The pregnant woman's blood type and Rh factor are determined at the first prenatal visit. If the woman has Rh-negative blood and the fetus has Rh-positive blood, which will happen if the father of the baby is Rh-positive, problems can occur. When the fetus's blood (red blood cells) leaks into the woman's body during birth, an Rh-negative woman may develop antibodies against the fetus's Rh-positive blood. As it takes time for these antibodies to develop, firstborn infants are not usually affected unless the mother has had previous pregnancies that ended in abortion or miscarriage. The antibodies can pass through the placenta and kill the RBCs in the fetus. The fetus becomes anemic and jaundiced. Death of the fetus is possible if too much fetal blood is destroyed. When an injection of Rh-immune globulin (RhoGAM) is given at around the 28th week of pregnancy and 72 hours postpartum, and after percutaneous umbilical blood sampling (PUBS), CVS, abortion, or amniocentesis, then sensitization is prevented. Rh incompatibility should not occur with any subsequent pregnancy. RhoGAM must be given after every birth, abortion, miscarriage, amniocentesis, CVS, and PUBS to prevent sensitization.

Parturition

Parturition, or labor, is the process during which the uterus, through contractions, expels the fetus and placenta. There are three stages of labor:

- *Stage I—dilation.* From onset of labor until complete **dilation** (expansion) and **effacement** (thinning and shortening) of the cervix
- *Stage II—expulsion.* From complete dilation and effacement through birth of the fetus (expulsion)
- *Stage III—placental.* From birth of the fetus through expulsion of the placenta

Labor is believed to be triggered by the release of **oxytocin** and **prostaglandins** after the level of other specific hormones decreases. When the oxytocin is released, it causes the muscles of the uterus to contract. **Braxton–Hicks** contractions, often referred to as false labor, can usually be differentiated from real labor because of their irregularity and tendency to disappear when the woman moves about and changes positions. When the woman is lying in

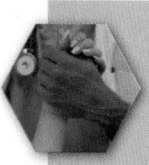

Patient Education

Alcohol Exposure

Alcohol along with tobacco exposure during pregnancy is common. Drinking during pregnancy is the leading cause of childhood intellectual developmental disorder. Two or more drinks a day while a woman is pregnant increases the risk of the newborn being born with fetal alcohol syndrome (FAS). Birth defects include small brain size; growth retardation; specific facial deformities (e.g., flat middle of the face, wide bridge of the nose, thin upper lip); and heart, kidney, and eye abnormalities. Behavioral problems (e.g., learning and attention difficulties, hyperactivity) occur. No safe amount of alcohol can be consumed during pregnancy, so abstention from all alcohol is necessary.

supine position, the heavy, large uterus can press on the inferior vena cava and aorta, reducing blood flow back to the heart. The patient becomes pale, sweaty, and dizzy, and blood pressure drops. The condition is known as **supine hypotension**. When the patient is turned onto her side, the pressure on the vena cava is removed and the hypotension resolves.

If fetal membranes do not spontaneously rupture during labor, an **amniotomy** (artificial rupture of the membranes) can be done. The procedure uses a sterile amniohook, and it may shorten the length of labor (Figure 25-9).

Signs and symptoms to watch for during labor that indicate complications are heavy vaginal bleeding, sudden increase or decrease in blood pressure, increased activity by the fetus, headache, extreme restlessness, and visual changes. **Meconium**, the first stool of the newborn, in the vaginal discharge can indicate fetal distress. Care must be taken to ensure that the newborn does not aspirate meconium-stained amniotic fluid at birth.

Postpartum Period

The postpartum period is the time known as the puerperium during which the body returns to its nonpregnant state. It usually lasts 4 to 6 weeks after delivery. The body undergoes changes during this time, as described in the "Postpartum Period" Quick Reference Guide.

An appointment in 6 weeks will evaluate the mother's general health, and the provider will discuss infant care, breast-feeding, the importance of

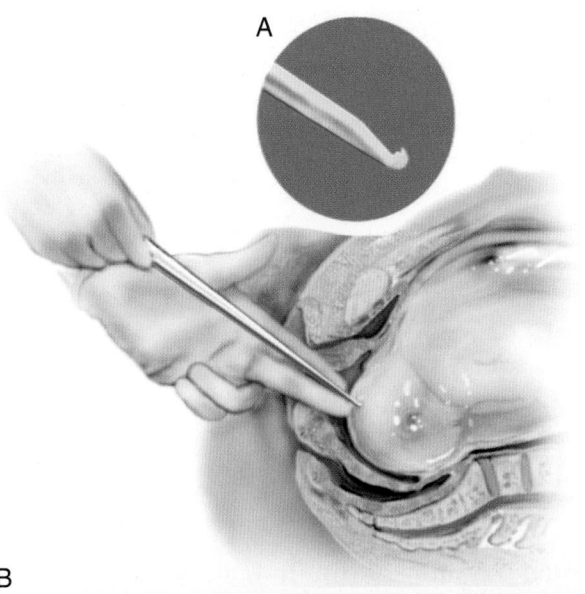

FIGURE 25-9 (A) Disposable amniohook used to rupture membranes. (B) Amniotomy technique.

exercise, good nutrition, and birth control. The medical assistant can stress the importance of yearly Pap smears and monthly breast self-examinations because these are important aspects of patient education.

Contraception

Voluntary prevention of pregnancy is known as **contraception**. The opportune time to discuss contraception with the mother is soon after delivery and before discharge from the hospital. She should know what method of contraception she and her partner will use before resuming sexual activity. Sexually transmitted disease (STD) protection should also be reviewed before discharge.

Written instructions about methods of contraception are important and help the patient understand options that are available.

Some nonprescription kinds of contraception are the various barrier methods: condoms, male (latex) and female (nonlatex); contraceptive foam; spermicide (nonoxynol-9) used with a condom to help prevent STDs; vaginal sponges that contain a spermicide; and abstinence.

Many types of prescription contraceptives are available (see Figures 25-10 through 25-14 and Table 25-7). They include hormonal contraception in the form of oral birth control pills; Implanon, a surgical implant of progestin in the upper arm, which provides up to 3 years of contraception; a diaphragm used with a spermicide; a cervical cap to fit over the cervix; an intrauterine device (a small device made of copper or progesterone-medicated plastic); and vaginal rings. Hormonal contraception methods work by changing the complex network of hormonal interactions that allow an ovum to leave the ovary and cause changes in the cervical mucus that allow sperm to enter the cervix. There are also changes that make the lining of the uterus unwelcoming toward implantation.

Sterilization is a surgical procedure that renders the individual infertile. The woman's uterine tubes are **fulgurated** (destroyed by means of an electric current), or bands and clips are placed around the tubes to block them (ligation). Both fulguration and ligation are considered to be permanent methods. Female sterilization can be performed immediately after giving birth or any time afterward during any phase of the menstrual cycle. Laparoscopic surgery is the usual approach. Tubal ligation and oral contraceptives are the top contraceptive choices in the United States (Figure 25-15).

The surgical procedure performed on a male to render him sterile is a vasectomy. It can be

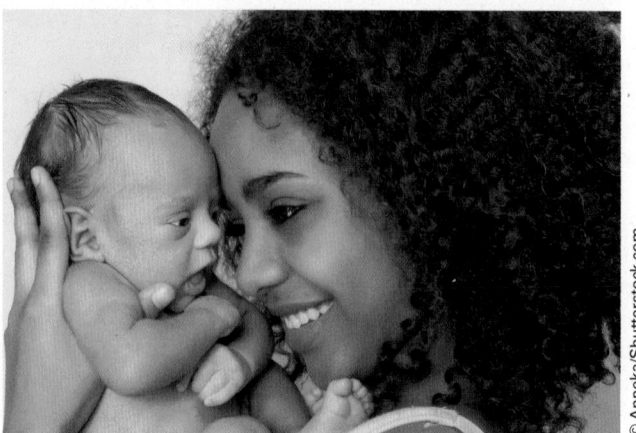

© Anneka/Shutterstock.com

Characteristics

- Uterus returns to normal size
- Need for good nutrition to restore homeostasis for the mother and to provide nutrition to the baby if breast feeding
- Emotional Adjustment due to hormonal shift

Patient Education

- Vaginal discharge (**lochia**) will appear, consisting of tissue, WBCs, mucous, and bacteria:
  - *Rubra.* Bright red, appears the first few days after delivery
  - *Serosa.* Pink or brown and indicates decreasing blood loss; occurs 3 to 10 days after delivery
  - *Alba.* Yellowish or white and may last from 2 to 6 weeks
- Expect return of menstruation in 2 months if not breast-feeding, 3 to 6 months if breast-feeding
- Eat a nutrient-rich, balanced diet
- Maintain adequate fluid intake of at least 8 glasses/day
- Continue prenatal vitamins
- Emphasize self-care
- Symptoms of postpartum depression include:
  - Loss of appetite
  - Difficulty sleeping
  - Lack of joy in life
  - Lack of interest in caring for the newborn
  - Thoughts of doing harm to oneself or the baby*

Seek medical treatment immediately if these symptoms are identified

performed on an outpatient basis under local anesthesia. Small incisions are made into the scrotum above and to the side of each testicle. Each vas deferens is identified, ligated twice, and then severed (Figure 25-16). It is important for the patient to realize that sterility is not immediate because some sperm remain in the sperm ducts after vasectomy. One week to several months may

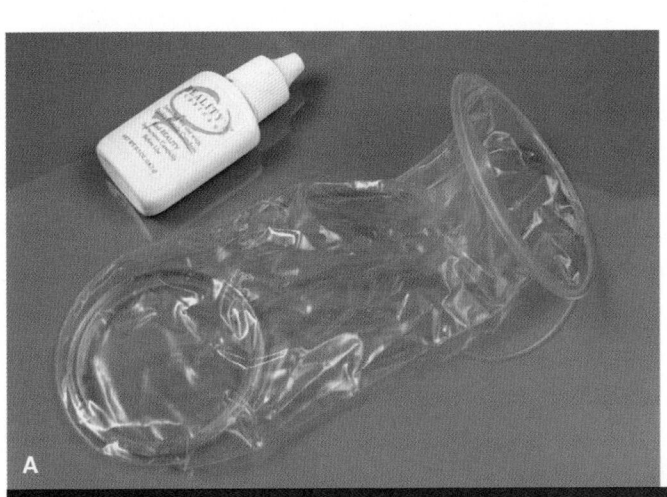

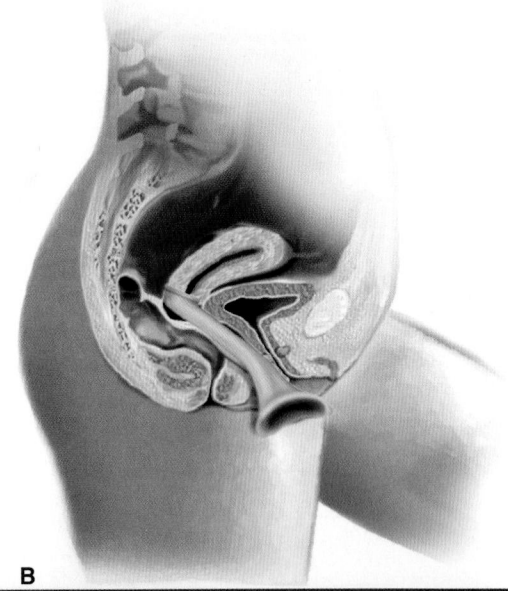

FIGURE 25-10 (A) Female condom. (B) Proper insertion of female condom.

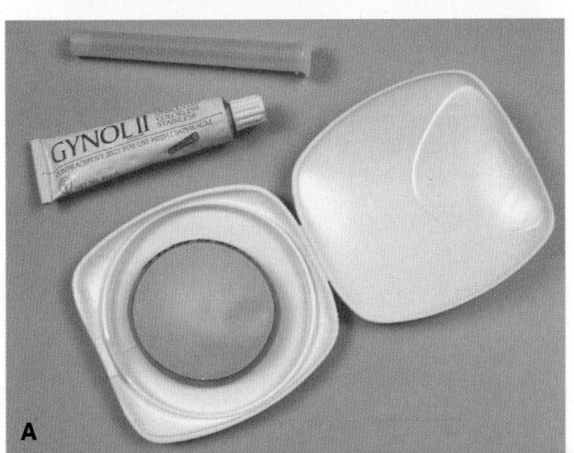

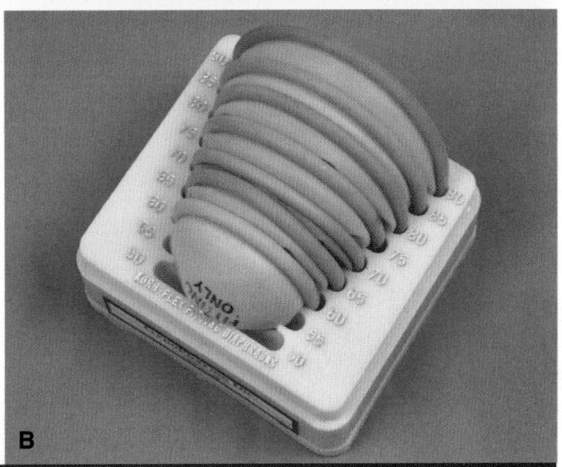

FIGURE 25-11 (A) Diaphragm with contraceptive jelly. (B) Various sizes of diaphragms. They must be fitted by the provider.

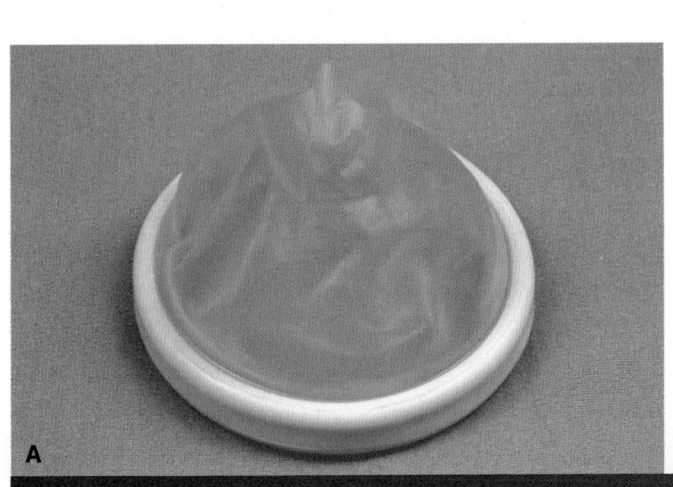

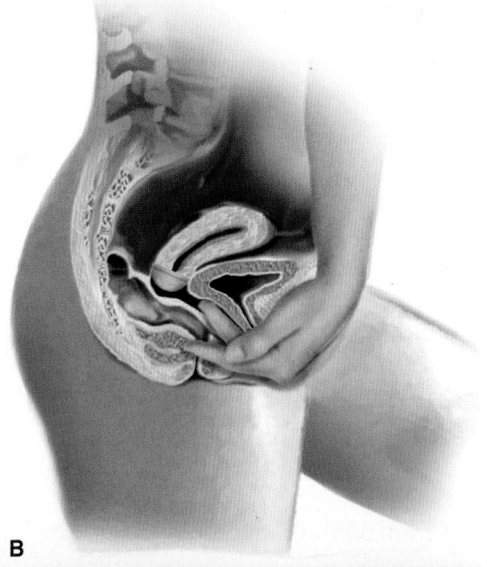

FIGURE 25-12 (A) Cervical cap. (B) Proper insertion of cervical cap.

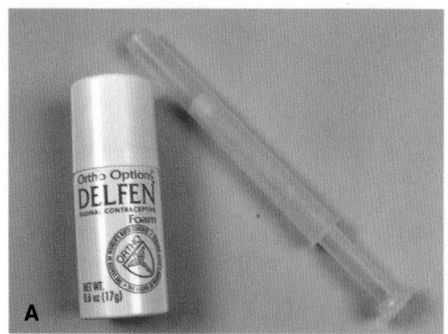

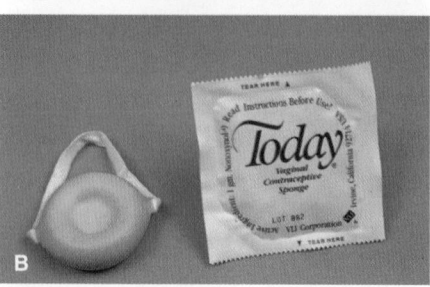

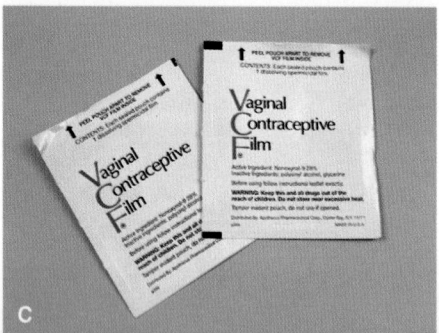

FIGURE 25-13 Spermicides. (A) Foam. (B) Sponge. (C) Film.

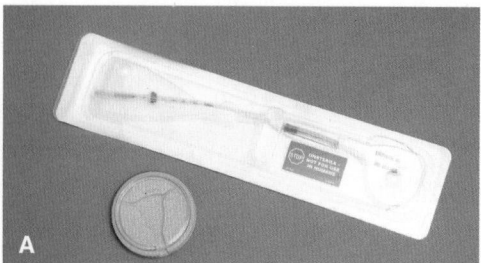

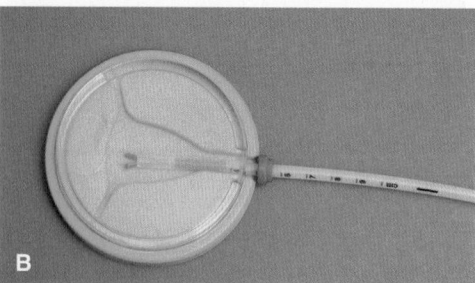

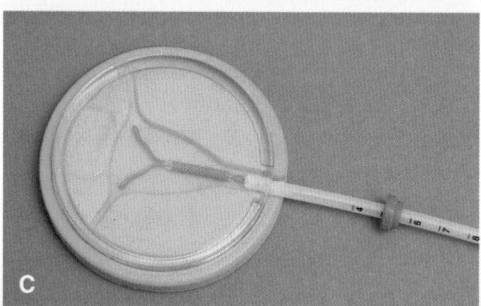

FIGURE 25-14 (A) Intrauterine device (IUD) and plastic uterus for patient education. (B, C) A plastic uterus can be used to demonstrate proper insertion and placement of an IUD during a patient education session.

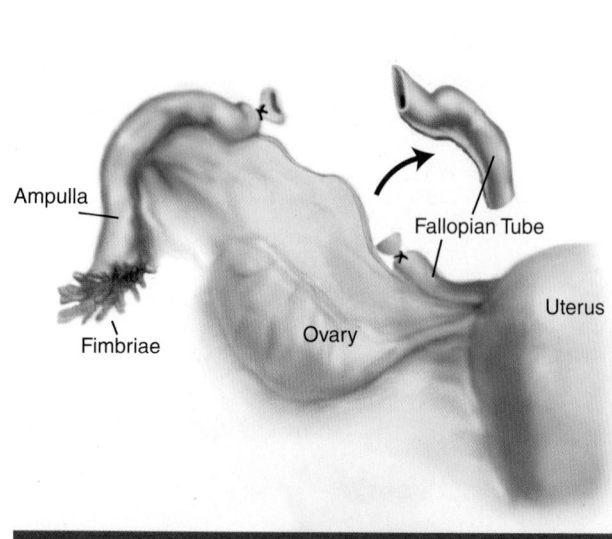

Ampulla

Fallopian Tube

Uterus

Ovary

Fimbriae

FIGURE 25-15 Tubal ligation.

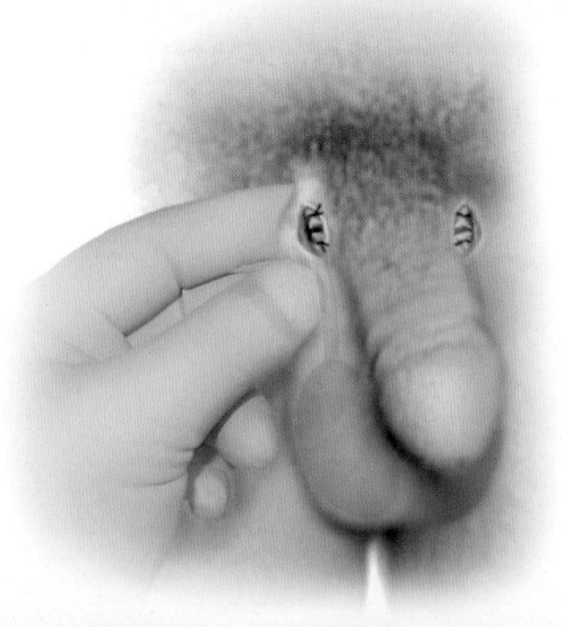

FIGURE 25-16 Vasectomy.

TABLE 25-7

VARIOUS CONTRACEPTION (BIRTH CONTROL) METHODS

METHOD	DESCRIPTION	EFFECTIVENESS	MECHANISM OF ACTION
Barrier (over-the-counter condom) (see Figure 25-10)	Male and female condoms available. Male condoms are latex; female condoms are nonlatex.	Less effective than hormonal methods or IUD. Use with spermicide. Use to protect from STDs.	Inhibits sperm from entering the vagina. Used only once. To prevent STDs and pregnancy, use a condom and another method of contraception.
Diaphragm (prescription needed) (see Figure 25-11)	Use with spermicide. Must be measured and fitted by provider. Fits up against the cervical opening so that cervix is within the cap.	Moderately effective if used correctly. Must fit perfectly. Spermicide is placed inside and around the diaphragm. Must remain in place for 6 hours after intercourse. Will last for years if cared for properly.	Provides barrier between sperm and opening to cervix.
Cervical cap (must be fitted by provider) (see Figure 25-12)	Made of rubber. Fitted to cover the cervix. Folded to insert into the vagina. Must be applied to cervix. Suction keeps the cap in place. Use with spermicide.	Moderately effective if used correctly, similar to diaphragm. Potential for infection because cap can be left in place up to 2 days. Must remain at least 6 hours after intercourse.	Provides rubber barrier between sperm and opening to cervix.
Spermicide sponge foam cream/gel (over the counter) (see Figure 25-13)	Chemical known as nonoxynol-9.	When used alone, failure rate is high compared to other methods. Used with condom, diaphragm, or cervical cap, it is more effective. No bathing or douching for 6 hours after intercourse. Must allow 15 minutes before engaging in intercourse. Reapply spermicide with repeated intercourse.	Destroys sperm cells.
Oral contraceptives (prescription needed for all hormonal contraceptives)	Various combinations of estrogen and progestin or progestin only. Newest oral contraceptives called extended hormonal contraceptives.	Highest effectiveness rate when taken correctly. Can help reduce dysmenorrheal and heavy menses. Pregnancy risk is highest when a woman misses more than 7 days of pills with extended hormonal contraceptives.	Prevents ovulation every month. Extended hormonal contraception delays menstruation. Continuous use eliminates menstruation.
Injection	Intramuscular injection (Depo-Provera) every 3 months. Lunelle, injected once per month.	Highly effective. One of the most effective contraceptives. Best given within first 5 days of normal menstrual cycle to be sure patient is not pregnant.	Stops ovulation for 1 month (Lunelle). Prevents ovulation for 3 months (Depo-Provera).
Patch	Applied to body and contraceptive is absorbed through the skin.	Highly effective. Worn for 1 week and then replaced same day of week for 3 consecutive weeks. Fourth week patch free.	Prevents ovulation for 1 month.
Vaginal ring	Small flexible ring inserted into the vagina. Releases steady flow of hormones. Left in for 3 weeks. Removed for 1 week.	Highly effective.	Prevents ovulation.

continues

Table 25-7, continued

METHOD	DESCRIPTION	EFFECTIVENESS	MECHANISM OF ACTION
Continuous contraception	No menstrual cycles for indefinite time period. Breakthrough bleeding possible. Continuous contraception for 3 months.	Effective. Highly effective.	Prevent ovulation. Reduce mood swings, migraines, and premenstrual syndrome (PMS). Prevent ovulation for 3 months.
Intrauterine device (IUD) (must be inserted by provider) (see Figure 25-14)	T-shaped device made of copper or drug-emitting plastic. The copper device is considered reliable for pregnancy prevention for up to 10 years (ParaGard) is Mirena, an IUD that releases hormones. Remains in place for 5 years. To prevent STDs, IUDs should be used in conjunction with a condom.	Both highly effective. One of the most effective contraceptives.	Copper slowly released into uterus and kills sperm. Hormones in Mirena cause thickening of the mucus in the cervix so sperm cannot reach the ovum.
Implantable (must be implanted by provider)	Device that is composed of one rod that is implanted in the upper arm. Lasts up to 3 years. Minor surgical procedure is required to implant and remove. Essure is a spring-like device implanted in the fallopian tubes via the cervix.	Highly effective. One of the most effective contraceptives. Becomes more effective as scar tissue grows thicker. Use another form of contraceptive for at least 3 months after implantation.	Inhibits ovulation and changes the cervical and endometrial mucus. Implanted device causes scar tissue to build up within the fallopian tubes, eventually blocking them. When blocked, neither sperm nor ovum can pass through. Provides permanent contraception.
Tubal ligation or hysterectomy (permanent method) (performed when the woman has a gynecologic problem that requires surgery and she wants permanent sterilization)	Sterilization procedure performed in which the fallopian tubes are tied or bands and/or clips are placed around the tubes to block them (ligation). The tubes can also be burned with electrocautery. Hysterectomy is the surgical removal of the uterus.	Considered permanent, but there is a small failure rate. Permanent sterilization.	Fallopian tubes are severed and/or burned, banded, and/or clipped. Because fallopian tubes now are incapable of transporting either sperm or ovum, fertilization is not possible. Uterus is surgically removed.
Family planning	Ovulation prediction (rhythm method). The woman charts her temperature and her changes in vaginal mucus and abstains from intercourse during the time she is ovulating (as predicted by temperature and mucus changes).	Can be effective if done correctly. However, method must be used consistently and the woman must realize that she may ovulate on a different day each month.	Prevents conception by avoidance intercourse during the period of ovulation.
Emergency contraception (**postcoital** contraception) also called Preven or Plan B (over the counter for ages 18 and over, prescription if under 18)	Prevents unintended pregnancy when the woman has had unprotected sexual intercourse. Prevents unwanted pregnancy. Pills (known as "morning after pills") that contain birth control hormones can be taken as soon after unprotected sex as possible and up to 5 days after and still prevent pregnancy. Take a second dose 12 hours after the first dose. Will not interrupt an established pregnancy and will not harm the embryo. No prescription needed.	Very effective.	Not the same as RU-486, an abortion pill. Prevents ovulation or stops fertilization.

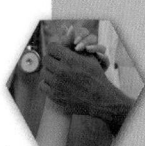

Patient Education

Post-IUD Insertion

1. Report any bleeding other than spotting that occurs in the first 2 days.

2. Report fever, vaginal discharge, or pain at once.

3. A small percentage of IUDs are expelled from the uterus into the vagina during the first year. If this occurs, another contraceptive should be used to prevent pregnancy.

4. There is a risk of perforation of the uterus, but this is most likely to occur during insertion.

5. An IUD does not protect against STDs.

6. Some women experience headaches, breast tenderness, and mood swings. These symptoms usually subside in a few months.

7. It is possible (but rare) to become pregnant with an IUD. It is recommended in this situation that the IUD be removed because it can cause miscarriage or premature birth.

8. The IUD can remain in place for as long as 10 years depending on the type.

9. An IUD must be removed by the provider.

10. An IUD is safe and highly effective.

---

elapse before the ducts are sperm free. Some form of contraception is necessary until two consecutive sperm counts are zero.

Another method of contraception approved by the Food and Drug Administration (FDA) is a medication called Mifepristone, known as RU-486, which is used to cause, or induce, an abortion. Its safety has been questioned by experts. Injectable contraceptives are available. Sayana Press and Depo-Provera are given intramuscularly every 3 months. Lunelle is given intramuscularly monthly. These injectables are best given within the first 5 days of the menstrual cycle to be certain the woman is not pregnant.

The majority of states mandate that health insurance cover the cost of contraception. The Affordable Care Act that was signed into law in March 2010 with the intent of making prevention affordable and accessible for all Americans requires health plans to cover preventative services and eliminate cost sharing. Contraceptive methods and counseling are covered under Health Resources and Services Administration Supported Women's Preventative Services: Required Health Plan Coverage Guidelines. All Food and Drug Administration–approved contraceptive methods, sterilization procedures, and patient education and counseling for all women with reproductive capacity are covered. There is an exception for group health plans sponsored by certain religious employers, and group health coverage in conjunction with such plans is exempt from the requirement to cover contraceptive services.

GYNECOLOGY

Gynecology is the specialty that studies diseases of the female reproductive tract and the breasts. The gynecologic examination is routinely performed in an office or clinic. It usually includes abdominal, pelvic, and breast examination and a Pap smear. It can be done as part of the female's complete physical examination, or it can be a separate examination performed in the gynecologist's office or gynecology clinic. Early diagnosis and treatment of problems associated with the female reproductive organs help the female to achieve optimum health of these organs and is the goal of the OB/GYN provider (Figure 25-17).

The Gynecologic Examination

Procedure

The American College of Obstetricians and Gynecologists recommends that women start seeing a gynecologist between the ages of 13 and 15. The goal of these visits is to assess the woman's health and to screen for cancer of the reproductive organs. They include a breast examination by the provider and instructions for the patient about how to perform her own **breast self-examination (BSE)**. They also include a pelvic examination and Pap smear (see Procedure 25-2). Pap tests are done to detect

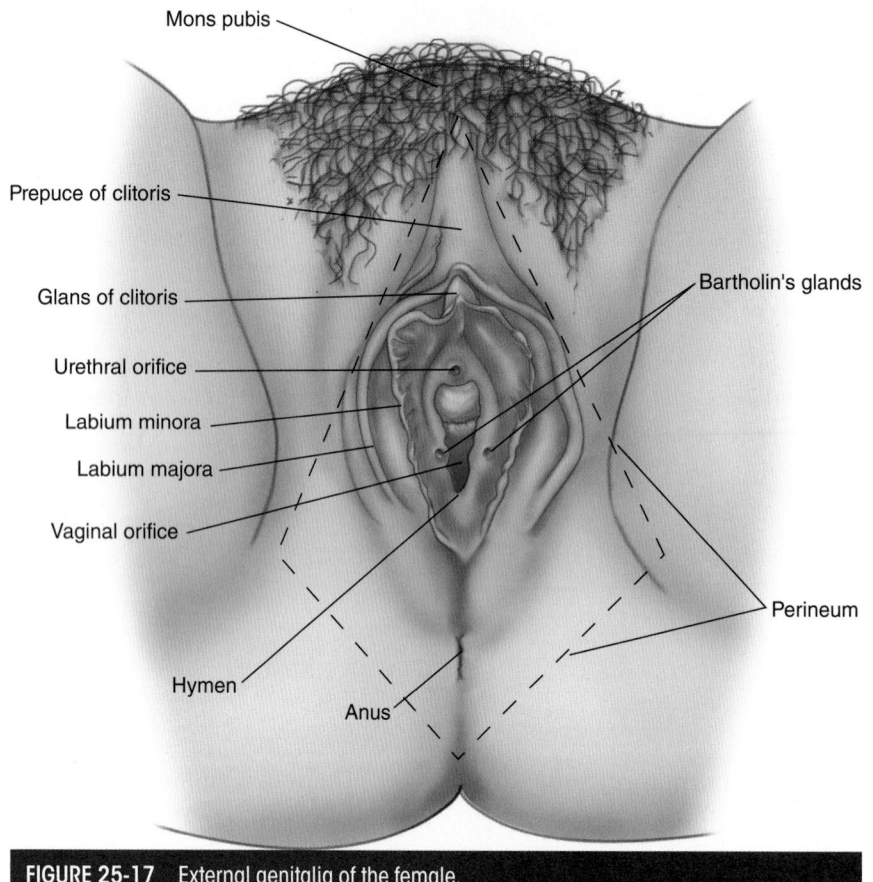

FIGURE 25-17 External genitalia of the female.

Labels: Mons pubis, Prepuce of clitoris, Glans of clitoris, Urethral orifice, Labium minora, Labium majora, Vaginal orifice, Hymen, Anus, Bartholin's glands, Perineum

cervical cancer. Women should be especially conscientious in scheduling annual Pap tests and mammograms if they have a family history of breast, uterine, ovarian, or cervical cancer. Early detection of cervical and breast cancers and appropriate treatment may cure the disease. Women who have had a hysterectomy because of cancer should continue to be tested for pelvic cancer annually by having a Pap smear. Because the cervix has been removed, the specimen cells are taken from the inner vaginal vault instead. Even after the hysterectomy, the woman still remains at risk for cancer cells to grow within the vagina and she should be encouraged to continue with her regular pelvic examinations and Pap tests. Others believe that in healthy women a Pap test done every 1 to 3 years is sufficient. The American Cancer Society (ACS) recommends that all women between the ages of 21 and 29 have a **Pap (Papanicolaou) test** every 3 years. HPV testing is not necessary in this age group unless it is needed after an abnormal Pap test result.

The recommendations change as a woman ages. Between 30 and 65, women should have a Pap test plus an HPV test (called co-testing) done every 5 years. This approach is preferred, but it is acceptable to have a Pap test alone every 3 years.

Women older than 65 who have had normal Pap results for the preceding 10 years do not need to be tested for cervical cancer. If there has been a diagnosis of precancer of the cervix, testing should continue for the next 20 years regardless of the woman's age. Screening schedules are based on the health history of the woman. HIV infection, organ transplant, diethylstilbestrol (DES) exposure, and so on are taken into consideration.

Pap testing is not needed by women who have had a complete hysterectomy for a noncancerous reason. If the procedure performed was only a partial hysterectomy, leaving the cervix intact, a Pap smear is still indicated. Also, if a partial or total hysterectomy has been performed for a cancerous or precancerous diagnosis, Pap tests are still indicated. It is best to discuss this with the provider prior to educating a patient regarding the need for continued Pap testing.

The American College of Obstetricians and Gynecologists established new guidelines for mammography in January 2016. These guidelines state that women should be offered a screening mammogram annually beginning at age 40. Younger women, aged 20 to 39, may have a mammogram every 1 to 3 years based on provider preferences

(Figure 25-18). Patients should be educated regarding the potential for false-positive and false-negative results and the follow up with additional imaging or biopsies that might be in order. Women who are estimated to have a lifetime risk of breast cancer of 20% or greater, based on risk models that rely largely on family history (such as BRCAPRO, BODACEA, or Claus), but who are either untested or test negative for BRCA gene mutations, can be offered enhanced screening. For women who test positive for BRCA1 and BRCA2 mutations, enhanced screening should be recommended and risk reduction methods discussed. Breast magnetic resonance imaging (MRI) is not recommended for screening women at average risk of developing breast cancer.

Human Papillomavirus (HPV) and Gardasil. There are more than 40 types of HPV that can infect sexually active males and females. The CDC reported in April 2016 that HIV infects about 79 million people. New infections will be diagnosed in almost 4 million people each year. HPV is so common that most sexually active men and women will get at least one type of HPV at some point in their lives. With these

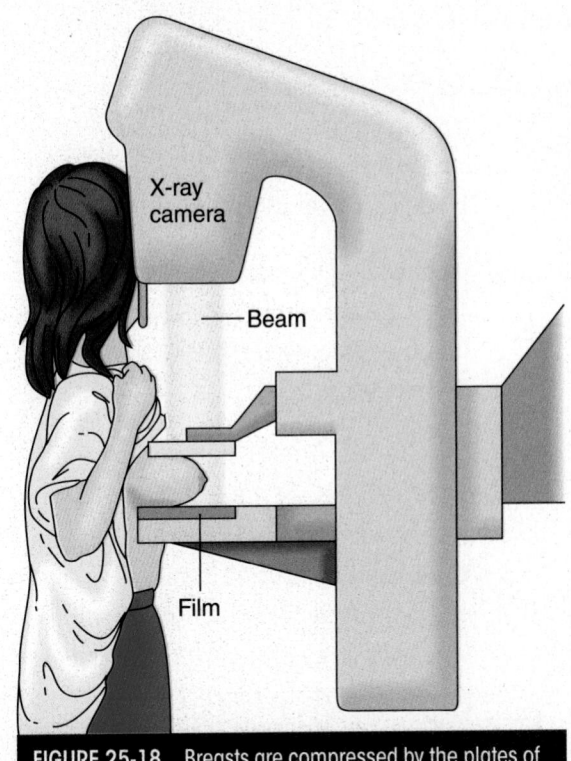

FIGURE 25-18 Breasts are compressed by the plates of mammographic X-ray unit.

PROCEDURE 25-2

Procedure

Assisting with Pelvic Examination and Pap Test (Conventional and ThinPrep Methods)

STANDARD PRECAUTIONS:

Handwashing

Gloves

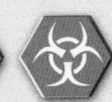
Biohazard

PURPOSE:

To assist the provider in collecting cervical cells for laboratory analysis for early detection of malignant cells of the cervix and to assess the health of the reproductive organs to detect diseases, leading to early diagnosis and treatment.

EQUIPMENT/SUPPLIES:

- Nonsterile gloves (2 to 3 pairs)
- Vaginal speculum, disposable or nondisposable
- Warm water or warming light
- Light source

- Drape sheet
- Patient gown
- Tissues
- Vaginal lubricant
- Lab requisition

- Urine specimen container
- Urine testing supplies
- Biohazard specimen bag
- Biohazard waste container
- Adjustable stool for provider

(continues)

Supplies for the Pap test according to the method used for ThinPrep Pap:
- Cervical spatula
- Brush and broom
- ThinPrep container with solution

For conventional Pap test:
- Microscope slides
- Fixative and/or specimen bottle
- Cervical spatula
- Cytology brush

PROCEDURE STEPS:

1. Wash hands and follow Standard Precautions.
2. ***Paying attention to detail***, assemble equipment.
3. ***Introduce yourself to the patient. Identify the patient.***
4. ***Explain the procedure, speaking at the patient's level of understanding.***
5. Request that patient empty her bladder. (If ordered by the provider, offer a specimen container and instruct patient to save a urine specimen.) RATIONALE: An empty bladder facilitates examination of the uterus and a urine specimen is frequently used for a urinalysis.
6. ***Being courteous and respectful***, provide patient with gown and request her to completely undress, ***being sure to protect the patient's personal boundaries***.
7. Instruct patient to sit at end of table when ready for pelvic examination. Drape patient for privacy. If performing conventional Pap test, label the frosted end of the slide with a marking pencil. Include patient's name on slide. Indicate site from where specimen is collected: c = cervix, v = vagina, e = endocervical.
8. Assist patient into lithotomy position. Patient's knees should be relaxed and thighs rotated out as far as comfortable. Drape for privacy and warmth.
9. Encourage patient to breathe slowly and deeply through the mouth during examination. RATIONALE: Allows for relaxation of pelvic muscles and easier insertion of vaginal speculum.
10. Warm vaginal speculum with either warm water or under heat lamp or place on a heating pad. *NOTE:* Do not lubricate speculum. Lubricant obscures exfoliated cervical cells when Pap test is being performed.
11. Hand speculum and spatula, cytology brush, and broom to the provider as needed.
12. Apply gloves.
13. For conventional Pap test, hold slides for provider to apply smear of exfoliated cells, one for vaginal (v), one for cervical (c), and one for endocervical (e), in that order. If spraying Pap fixative, spray it over the slide within 10 seconds at a distance of about 6 inches. Allow to dry for at least 10 minutes. If using Pap fixative in a bottle, place slide directly into bottle. If using ThinPrep, swish the cytology broom vigorously in the ThinPrep solution until all of the specimen has been deposited. Dispose of brush into biohazard container. RATIONALE: This maintains cell appearance and avoids contamination of cells. Avoid getting too close to slide with spray because this may destroy or damage cells. Slides must be fixed before they dry to protect the appearance of the cells.
14. For the ThinPrep Pap test, hand the speculum and cytology broom to the provider. Open the ThinPrep solution container. When the cells have been obtained, take the broom and vigorously swish it into the container of solution until all the cells have been deposited. RATIONALE: The ThinPrep procedure requires that all cells obtained from the cervix be presented in the solution for complete testing.
15. Replace the cap and label. Dispose of the broom into a biohazard waste container.
16. Place lubricant on provider's gloved fingers without touching gloves, for bimanual and rectal examinations. The provider will insert the index and middle fingers into the vagina. The other hand is placed on the lower abdomen. The size, shape, and position of the uterus and ovaries are palpated.

(continues)

17. The provider will insert one gloved finger into the rectum to check the ovaries and the tone of the rectal and pelvic muscles. Hemorrhoids, rectal fissures, or other lesions may be palpated.

18. Provide the patient tissues to wipe genitalia and rectum.

19. After the examination, assist the patient to a sitting position, allowing her to rest a while. Check her pulse and skin color. RATIONALE: Some patients, especially older adults, can experience orthostatic hypotension.

20. Apply disposable gloves. Discard disposable supplies per OSHA guidelines. If stainless steel speculum was used, soak in cool water. Sanitize and sterilize as soon as convenient.

21. Remove gloves and wash hands.

22. Assist patient down and off the table if necessary, *attending to any special needs of the patient*.

23. Assist the patient to dress if necessary; provide privacy.

24. Escort the patient to provider's office for discussion of examination results.

25. Prepare laboratory requisition (cytology request) form. Include provider name and address, date, source of specimen, patient's name and address, date of LMP, and hormone therapy, if any. Place slides in slide container or ThinPrep container into biohazard specimen bag. Place requisition into outer pocket of bag and send to laboratory.

26. Wash hands.

27. Accurately document procedure in patient's chart or electronic medical record.

DOCUMENTATION:

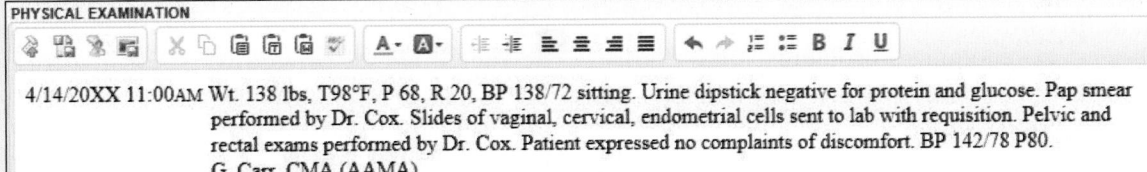

PHYSICAL EXAMINATION

4/14/20XX 11:00AM Wt. 138 lbs, T98°F, P 68, R 20, BP 138/72 sitting. Urine dipstick negative for protein and glucose. Pap smear performed by Dr. Cox. Slides of vaginal, cervical, endometrial cells sent to lab with requisition. Pelvic and rectal exams performed by Dr. Cox. Patient expressed no complaints of discomfort. BP 142/78 P80.
G. Carr, CMA (AAMA)

Courtesy of Harris CareTracker PM and EMR

alarming statistics, the FDA approved a vaccine in 2006 that targets the virus responsible for most cervical, vulvar, and vaginal cancers and condylomata (genital warts) for female administration. In 2009 this vaccine was approved by the FDA to prevent genital warts in men and boys. The vaccine, called Gardasil, protects against four types of HPV. Two of the four viruses are responsible for 70% of all cervical cancers. The other two viruses are responsible for 90% of condylomata.

HPV is spread through sexual contact. According to the CDC, by age 50 years, at least 80% of women will have had an HPV infection. However, most women with HPV do not get cervical cancer. Gardasil is 100% effective in protecting against two of the HPV strains if the individual has not been exposed to the virus previously. The vaccine will not protect people already exposed to the virus. The vaccine does not contain a live virus. It lasts for at least 5 years. The FDA approved Gardasil for girls and women aged 9 to 26 years. It is on the CDC's recommended vaccine schedule.

Screening for cervical cancer (Pap test) still is necessary because Gardasil does not protect against all HPV types. Pap tests also are essential for women who have not been vaccinated or who already are infected with HPV. The vaccine is not recommended during pregnancy.

The Advisory Committee on Immunization Practices (ACIP) recommends that preteen males and females 11 to 12 years of age be immunized with three doses of HPV vaccine, but the series can be started as early as age 9. The second and third doses should be given 2 and 6 months after the first dose. The immunization is most effective if administered prior to any sexual activity, thus the early administration recommendation.

HPV vaccines can be administered with other age-appropriate vaccines. Catch-up vaccinations are available for females 13 to 26 years of age who have not been vaccinated previously or who have not completed the full series. The vaccine is licensed for females and males 9 to 26 years of age. Each dose is 0.5 mL given intramuscularly.

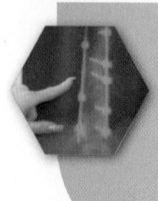

Critical Thinking

A 38-year-old woman has been diagnosed with HPV infection. What patient education materials are appropriate to provide to this patient?

Scheduling Pap Smear Tests. Encourage female patients to schedule their Pap smear and annual gynecologic examination on a date that will be easy to remember, such as April Fool's Day, Flag Day, tax day, or the first day of summer. Keep a tickler file to remind patients who "forget." Women may believe that because they have had a hysterectomy, they no longer need their annual examination and Pap smear. Every woman should have an annual (or at least regular) examination even if the Pap test is not included. A woman who has had a hysterectomy because of cancer should continue to have Pap smears on a regular basis. Many women are not aware of this and need to be educated.

Other gynecologic problems may arise between annual gynecologic examinations and require an appointment. They include symptoms and problems such as severe **dysmenorrhea** (painful menses), lower abdominal pain, **metrorrhagia** (bleeding between menstrual periods), **dyspareunia** (painful intercourse), sexual dysfunction, infertility, discomfort from menstrual symptoms, and infections or the development of STDs. Women experiencing these problems should have a gynecologic examination, and the provider will determine a diagnosis based on the examination, the patient's history, symptoms, signs, and laboratory data. The data from previous appointments are available to the provider via the computer. Comparisons can be made quickly with previous entries, saving time and possibly preventing errors.

Diversity

It is important to realize that patients' health practices related to culture, values, and belief systems are deeply ingrained and not easily changed. Being aware of some of these practices and beliefs will benefit both you and your patients. You will have a better understanding of their cultural heritage and beliefs that are different from yours, and this will help patients to be more comfortable. At times, it might be necessary to modify care according to the patient's cultural background and practice.

Female Circumcision. Female circumcision is an ancient cultural custom that has been practiced worldwide for more than 2,000 years. In 2016, it was estimated that more than 200 million girls and women currently alive have undergone female genital mutilation in the countries where the practice is concentrated. Each year, there are an estimated 3 million girls at risk of undergoing female genital mutilation. Central Africa is one of the main areas where various forms of the procedure are performed. These types of procedure may be performed on females at any time from birth until puberty, depending on the culture of the country of birth.

There are four different types of female circumcision: (1) removal of the prepuce of the clitoris; (2) clitoridectomy, which is removal of the prepuce and clitoris; (3) removal of the prepuce, clitoris, upper labia minora, and some labia majora; and (4) infibulation, which is removal of all external genitalia (prepuce, clitoris, labia majora, labia minora). Female circumcision is also known as female genital mutilation (FGM), and the World Health Organization defines it as "all procedures that involve partial or total removal of the external female genitalia, or other injury to female genital organs for non-medical reasons." Some reasons given for this practice are that it is a rite of passage, a sign of purity, an indication of marriage availability, an assurance of sexual faithfulness, protection from rape and abortion, and for socialization into the role of a woman. Surgery is usually performed by a lay midwife, and a razor or broken glass is used; infections and hemorrhages are common. If an infibulation is performed, the two sides of the vulva are sewn together. Scar tissue forms over the vagina. A small opening for urination and menstruation is made by insertion of a foreign object until the area heals. The most common reason given for this procedure is that it follows customs and tradition. During childbirth, the infibulation is cut to allow for delivery; it is then resutured after delivery.

Presentation   Integrity

There is opposition to this practice on the basis that it is a human rights violation. However, it is vital that a professional medical assistant always view patients as individuals whose cultural beliefs and practices may differ greatly from his/her own. Treat them as you would treat all patients, with respect and empathy (see

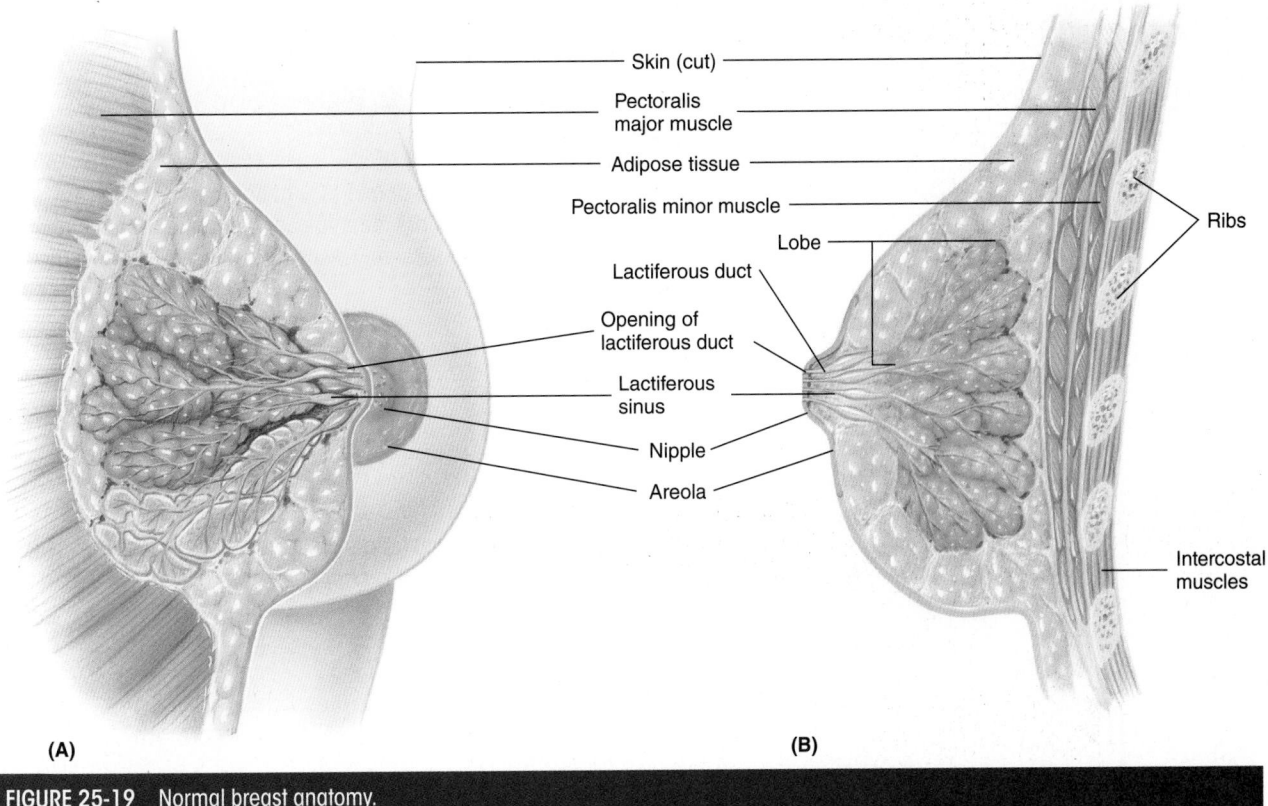

Skin (cut)

Pectoralis
major muscle

Adipose tissue

Pectoralis minor muscle

Ribs

Lobe

Lactiferous duct

Opening of
lactiferous duct

Lactiferous
sinus

Nipple

Areola

Intercostal
muscles

(A)

(B)

FIGURE 25-19 Normal breast anatomy.

Chapters 26 and 27 for information about male circumcision).

Breast Examination. The provider performs a breast examination on the patient as part of a gynecologic examination. (Normal breast anatomy is shown in Figure 25-19.) As the provider looks for redness, dimpling, and puckering, each breast is palpated and the axillae are felt for lumps or thickening. Part of the medical assistant's responsibility is to teach patients how to perform the breast self-examination (BSE). The provider may supply several pamphlets and a breast model with lumps and thickening to enhance patient education and awareness about the importance of the examination (Figure 25-20).

Breast Self-Examination (BSE). Breasts should be examined when they are not tender or swollen and at the same time each month, about one week after menses. It is important for women who are breast-feeding or pregnant or have breast implants to continue the routine BSE. Follow the steps described in the "Breast Self-Examination" Quick Reference Guide.

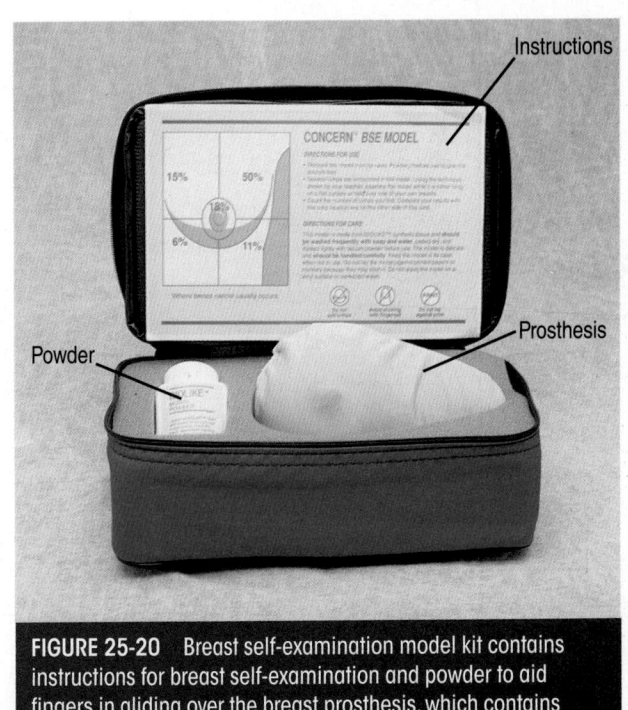

Instructions

Powder

Prosthesis

FIGURE 25-20 Breast self-examination model kit contains instructions for breast self-examination and powder to aid fingers in gliding over the breast prosthesis, which contains lumps and thickened areas for identification and location.

Illustration	BSE Steps
	1. Stand in front of a mirror and look at both breasts. Check your breasts for redness; dimpling; and change in shape, size, or contour. Look for any discharge. If any exists, note the color and location.
	2. Look in the mirror with hands pressing down on your hips, check your breasts for any change in normal shape.
	3. Raise your arms while still looking in the mirror and place your hands behind your head. This allows you to check the underside of your breasts.
	4. Place your left hand on your waist, roll your left shoulder forward, and check your left underarm area for enlarged lymph nodes. Also check the area above and below the collar bone. Repeat on the right side.

(continues)

Illustration	BSE Steps
	5. Place your left arm over your head. Gently use the pads of three or four fingers of your right hand, and glide the fingers over the entire left breast and axilla feeling for any lumps or thickening. Use an up-and-down pattern as you move around the breast, starting at your imaginary seam line (straight down from the underarm) and moving up and down to the middle of the breast bone. Be certain you have examined your entire breast, from the collarbone to the ribs. Repeat the procedure with the right breast.
	6. Lie flat on your back, place a small pillow under your left shoulder, and raise your left arm over your head. This spreads out the breast tissue, making it easier to examine. Use the same motion described in step 5 to examine your left breast. Body lotion, cream, or bath powder can be used during this step. Repeat the procedure with the right breast.

If any of the following are detected during the BSE, alert your provider immediately:

- Lump, hard knot, or thickening inside the breast or underarm area
- Swelling, warmth, redness, or darkening of the breast
- Change in the size or shape of the breast
- Dimpling or puckering of the skin
- Itchy, scaly sore or rash on the nipple
- Pulling in of the nipple or other parts of the breast
- Nipple discharge that starts suddenly
- New pain in one spot that does not go away

According to the American Cancer Society (ACS), breast cancer is among the top three causes of death in women along with lung cancer and colorectal cancer. Diagnosis of breast cancer is made by the provider using some or all of the following diagnostic tools: mammography, tissue biopsy, MRI, ultrasound, and MRI-guided breast biopsies.

Breast cancer risk factors include:

- A family history of breast cancer, especially in a first-degree relative (mother, sister, daughter)

- History of noncancerous breast lesions
- Being female (males can get breast cancer, but there is much less chance)
- Dense breast tissue
- A biopsy of a breast lesion that showed atypical hyperplasia
- Early menarche (younger than 12 years)
- Late menopause (after 55 years)
- No children, or first child after 30 years of age
- More than two to five alcoholic drinks per week
- BRCA1 and BRCA2 gene mutations
- Being Caucasian
- Obesity

The four standard treatment options for patients with breast cancer are surgery, radiation therapy, chemotherapy, and hormone therapy.

Hormone therapy prevents cancer recurrence by blocking receptor sites that encourage cell growth. Various therapies work in different manners. Tamoxifen acts against the effects of estrogen. In women who are at risk for breast cancer, tamoxifen reduces the chances of developing breast cancer. Tamoxifen for prevention of breast cancer continues to be studied. Hormone therapy is utilized for people with hormone receptor–positive cancer. The goal of this therapy is to lower the amount of estrogen present in the body and to block estrogen's effect on the cancer cells. Another type of hormone therapy with aromatase inhibitors, such as anastrozole, is particularly beneficial for postmenopausal women. This medication blocks the transformation of androgen into small amounts of estrogen.

Hormone therapy with a luteinizing hormone-releasing hormone (LHRH) agonist is given to some premenopausal women who have just been diagnosed with hormone receptor–positive breast cancer. LHRH agonists decrease the body's levels of estrogen and progesterone. Buserelin is an example of an LHRH agonist. Herceptin is a medication (nonhormone) that can be administered to women with breast cancer if a sample of breast cancer cells shows a particular abnormal protein. Herceptin targets the abnormal protein.

Assisting with a Gynecologic Examination. The gynecologic examination consists of four parts:

1. Breast examination
2. Inspection of external **genitalia** (labia minora, labia majora, urinary meatus, clitoris, **Bartholin glands**, and vagina) for swelling, lesions, or ulcerations
3. Pelvic examination of cervix, vagina, uterus, tubes, and ovaries, including a **bimanual examination**; may or may not include a Pap test
4. Rectal examination

The medical assistant should prepare the patient, equipment, and room before the examination.

Gynecologic Examination with Pap Equipment. In preparation for the annual examination, the patient is asked to avoid using tampons, foams, and gels; douching; and sexual intercourse for 2 days before the Pap test. Five days after menses is a good time to have a Pap test. Immediately before the pelvic examination, the patient is encouraged to empty her bladder. The urine may be collected for testing according to clinic policy or the provider's preference and depending on any urinary tract complaints or symptoms the patient may have.

It is the role of the professional medical assistant to set up the room, tray, and equipment necessary for the exam and Pap. Also, the provider may require your assistance during the examination in order to ensure that the patient is comfortable and that the laboratory specimens are managed correctly (see the "GYN Exam and Pap Smear" Quick Reference Guide).

Pap Smear. The federal government regulates laboratories that perform testing on Pap smears. Requirements are placed on the individuals who study the specimens for malignant cells, and they include specialized training. Limits are placed on the number of slides that can be read in one day. Proficiency testing, mandated by the Clinical Laboratory Improvement Act of 1988 (CLIA '88), ensures accuracy and precision of test results and is a requirement for Pap smear examination (Chapter 37 gives more information about CLIA '88).

One system for cytologic reporting of a Pap smear is a descriptive report that tells the provider exactly what cellular changes have taken place. The classification includes the grades of cervical **intraepithelial** neoplasia (CIN).

CIN 1 = mild **dysplasia** (abnormal tissue development)

CIN 2 = moderate dysplasia

CIN 3 = severe dysplasia or **carcinoma in situ**

Another system used to report Pap test results is the Bethesda system (TBS). The Bethesda system

Preprocedure

Activity	Rationale
Conduct a patient history to gather the following information: • LMP • Abnormal bleeding (breakthrough, postcoital) • Dysmenorrhea • Metrorrhagia • Perimenopausal irregularities • Hormone therapy (birth control, hormone replacement) • Exposure to **diethylstilbestrol (DES)** • Surgical history • Sexual history/habits • Symptoms of diseases/disorders	Documentation in the EHR assures continuity in care and easy reference to past laboratory results, medical and surgical history, and prescriptions. Obtaining a patient history for the provider will allow discussion of questions, concerns, or problems as a part of the exam. There is an increased risk for both cervical and vaginal cancer in daughters of women who were prescribed DES during pregnancy.
Perform exam setup to include the following equipment (see Figure 25-21): • Gooseneck lamp • Stool • Mayo stand • Gloves • Lubricating jelly • Speculum • Pap broom/brush or spatula **OR** • ThinPrep medium or slides and fixative • Hemoccult slides and developer	Having all supplies available for the provider will allow efficiency when exam is underway.
Conduct the following patient preparation: • Have patient undress and don gown, opening in the front • Seat patient on the exam table and explain the need for positioning during the examination • Provide comfort measures	It is important to protect the patient's modesty and provide a warm and comfortable environment to ease fears. Informing the patient regarding the process ahead of time sets expectations and decreases stress during the procedure. Keeping the patient warm and appropriately draped will reduce anxiety.

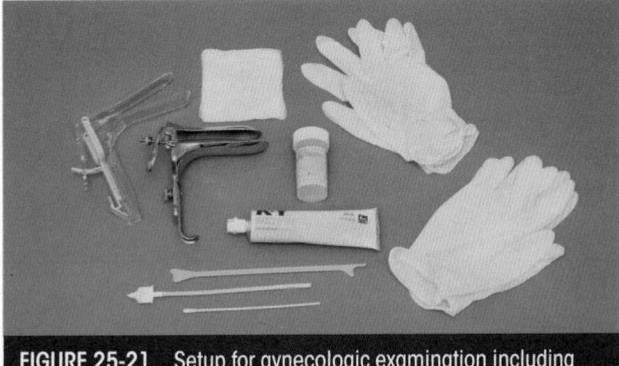

FIGURE 25-21 Setup for gynecologic examination including equipment for a ThinPrep Pap smear: transport medium container spatula, cytology brush and broom, specula (disposable and reusable), lubricant, gloves, tissues.

(continues)

During the Procedure

Activity	Rationale
Assist the patient into the supine position and provide a pillow for comfort.	Allows the provider access for breast exam.
Stand by to assist the patient into the lithotomy position.	Patient may need help with sliding down to the edge of the table and placing feet in stirrups.
After the provider is seated, assist in the adjustment of the lamp for optimal lighting.	Good visualization of the patient's anatomy is essential for obtaining the Pap specimens.
The provider will gently scrape the cervix with the spatula or the broom/brush to obtain cervical cells for evaluation (Figure 25-22).	Cervical cells obtained from the scraping are examined to diagnose precancerous and cancerous lesions of the cervix.
Stand by to assist the provider with the cervical specimen. • If using the spatula/slide method, appropriately label the slide and assist the provider with the application of cells to the slide followed by spraying with fixative. • If using the ThinPrep method, appropriately label the container and then vigorously swirl the brush/broom in the ThinPrep solution until the specimen is deposited. Also, ask the provider if other testing is required from the ThinPrep sample and indicate this on the Pap requisition.	Correct labeling of the specimen should contain: • Name • Date of birth • Patient number (if available) • Date and time of collection • If a Pap is indicated for posthysterectomy patients, the cells examined will be from the upper vaginal wall. Note "posthysterectomy" on the label of the container. With a ThinPrep Pap Test, multiple STDs may be identified—HPV, chlamydia, or gonorrhea.
Apply lubricant to provider's fingers for the bimanual exam (Figure 25-23).	Lubricant is needed as the provider will insert two fingers into the vagina to stabilize internal organs while the other hand is pressing against the outside of abdominal wall to determine the shape, mobility, consistency, and positioning of the uterus and ovaries.

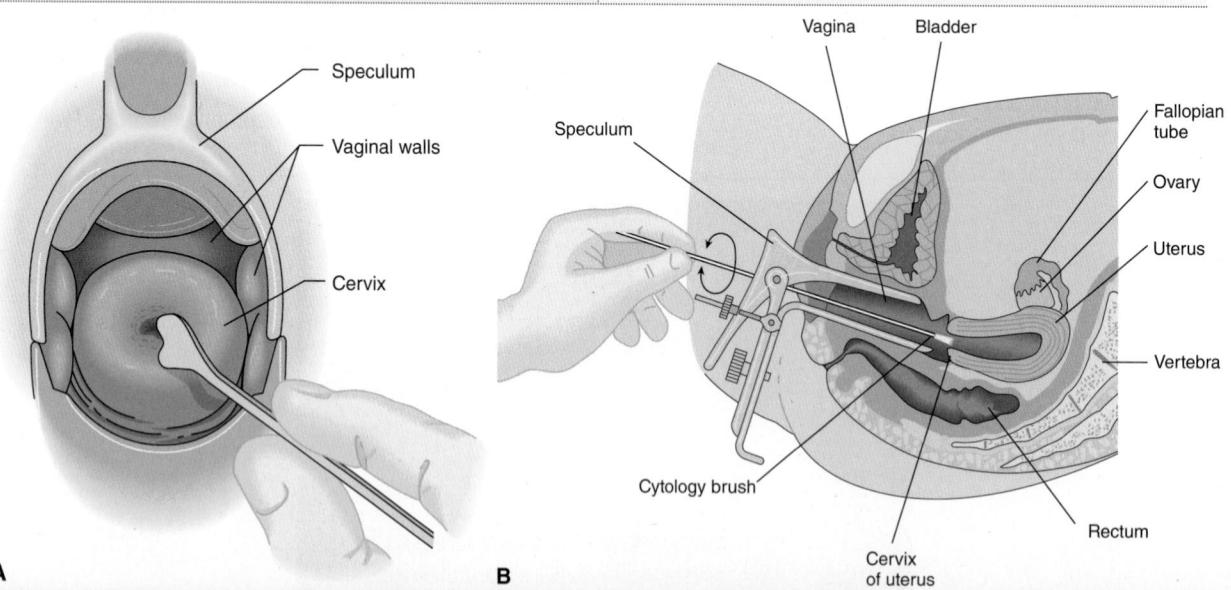

FIGURE 25-22 Use of speculum, cystology brush, and spatula to obtain material for a Pap smear. (A) The provider uses a spatula to obtain cells from the cervix. (B) The provider uses a cytology brush to obtain cells from the cervix.

(continues)

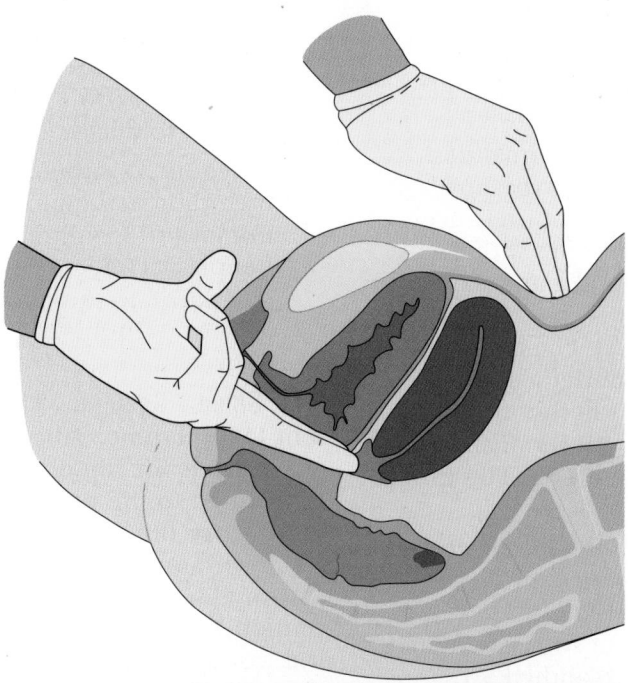

FIGURE 25-23 Bimanual pelvic examination.

Activity	Rationale
Apply additional lubricant for the rectal exam.	The rectal exam allows for evaluation of the posterior of the uterus and provides an opportunity to test for gastrointestinal (GI) bleeding.
Open Hemoccult slides for stool application.	Hemoccult is a screening tool for abnormal GI bleeding.

Postprocedure

Activity	Rationale
Assist the patient to a sitting position.	Patient may need support to return to a sitting position on the exam table.
Offer tissues.	Tissues may be needed to remove the lubricant after the exam.
Allow privacy.	The patient needs to dress and prepare for a discussion with the provider.
Provide patient education per provider's orders.	The history or exam may have initiated new orders. The medical assistant may be instructed by the provider to educate the patient on medications, procedures, lifestyle issues, or conditions.
Manage specimen(s): • Check labeling and requisition • Notify lab for pickup	Appropriate labeling and care of specimen ensures results will be accurately reported.

for reporting results of Pap tests has three main categories, some of which have subcategories:

Category 1 = negative for intraepithelial lesion or malignancy. This indicates that there is no sign of cancer or precancerous cells or other abnormalities found.

Category 2 = epithelial cell abnormalities. The cells of the lining of the cervix show changes that might be cancer or precancerous. There are several subgroups within this group for squamous cells and glandular cells.

1. *Atypical squamous cells (ASCs).* The name given to what the cells look like under a microscope. It is difficult to determine whether the abnormal cells are caused by an infection, an irritation, or a precancerous condition. This group is divided again:

   a. *Atypical squamous cells of uncertain significance (ASC-US) and atypical squamous cells where high-grade squamous intraepithelial lesions (SILs) cannot be excluded.* A repeat Pap test is done; biopsy and/or colposcopy and HPV DNA testing may be recommended.

   b. *Squamous interepithelial lesions (SILs).* There are low- and high-grade SILs. All patients in this category require a colposcopy. High-grade SILs can develop into cancer if not treated. Treatment can cure both high- and low-grade SILs and prevent cancer from developing. The Pap test does not identify which SIL the patient has; rather, it shows that the results fit into one of the abnormal categories.

   c. *Squamous cell carcinoma.* This test result shows that the woman likely has an invasive squamous cell carcinoma. Further testing, colposcopy, and biopsy are needed to be certain of the diagnosis. If the biopsy proves positive, the provider will recommend surgery, radiation, and/or chemotherapy.

   d. *Adenocarcinomas.* These carcinomas are abnormalities of glandular cells. If a clear decision cannot be made by the pathologist as to whether the cells are malignant, the term used is *atypical glandular cells (AGS).* Further testing is done to decide on a treatment plan.

Category 3 = other malignant neoplasms, including malignant melanoma, carcinoma, and lymphoma. These malignant neoplasms affect the cervix very rarely compared to squamous cell carcinoma and adenocarcinoma.

Pap Smear Results. The Pap smear usually is sent to a reference laboratory where a pathologist examines it for abnormal cells. The information is returned to the provider, and the report can be accessed in the EHR. Table 25-8 lists some of the terms used on the cytology report form.

An abnormal Pap smear result requires intervention by the provider. It is the professional medical assistant's role to assist the provider and the patient in follow-up.

Gynecologic Diseases and Conditions

The female reproductive system is affected by many diseases and conditions caused by hormonal imbalance, cysts, infection, and tumors. Some of the more common disorders and diseases are covered here.

Infertility. Most women, with unprotected intercourse, will be able to conceive within a year. The inability to conceive can be caused by a problem with either the male or the female individual. Some common causes of infertility in a female patient are:

- Endometriosis
- Certain medications
- Blocked fallopian tubes
- Problems ovulating

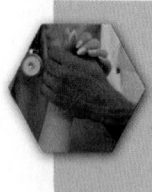

Patient Education

Many women think that if they have had a hysterectomy because of cancer they no longer need to have Pap smears performed. This is not true, and it is up to health care professionals to educate them. If the hysterectomy was performed because of cancer, the cancer cells can reappear in the vaginal vault after the surgery. During the pelvic examination, because the cervix has been removed, the provider will scrape the inner walls of the vaginal vault for cells to include in the Pap smear.

TABLE 25-8

TERMS AND ABBREVIATIONS USED IN CYTOLOGY PAP TEST REPORTS

TERM OR ABBREVIATION	MEANING
Atypical	not typical
CIN	cervical intraepithelial neoplasia
CIS	carcinoma in situ
condyloma	a lesion caused by human papillomavirus
dysplasia	precancerous lesion
epithelial	pertaining to epithelium
epithelium	cellular tissue that covers the surface of a body or that lines a body cavity
glandular	the cell making up the epithelium of a body cavity
HPV	human papillomavirus
lesion	a change in the tissue cells or a wound
malignant	a lesion that spreads out of the epithelium into underlying tissues
reactive changes	changes in cells caused by their reaction to infectious agents or a foreign body
reparative changes	changes in cells as they divide rapidly in an attempt to repair damaged tissue
SIL	squamous intraepithelial lesion (that lies within the squamous epithelium)
squamous	a type of cell that makes up the epithelium, the purpose of which is to protect underlying tissues

- Chronic stress
- Scar tissue from surgery, infection, or ectopic pregnancy
- Tumors

A woman who is having difficulty conceiving and has a history of any of the above will have a physical examination by a provider who specializes in infertility. The specialist will decide what tests and procedures are necessary. Hormone levels may be measured to look for hypothyroidism. Ovarian function can be determined through a surgical procedure, such as laparoscopy. A test for **patency** (openness) of the fallopian tubes can be performed by a hysterosalpingogram, a radiographic procedure done after injection of dye into the vagina, through the cervix, into the uterus, and out the fallopian tubes. The dye will pass through all of these organs if there is no blockage in any of them (see the "Impaired Fertility" section earlier in this chapter).

Menopause. The period of time that marks permanent cessation of menstrual activity is known as menopause. It usually occurs between the ages of 35 and 58 years. There may be a gradual decline in monthly menstrual flow, or a woman may suddenly cease to menstruate. Natural menopause occurs when the ovaries produce less and less estrogen. This causes the ovaries to cease ovulation and, therefore, menstruation stops. Surgical menopause is caused by the surgical removal of both ovaries (bilateral oophorectomy). Symptoms occur soon after ovulation ceases with both natural and surgical menopause. Symptoms may last for a few months to several years and may be mild to severe. Hot flashes, chills, nervousness, fatigue, apathy, mental depression, crying episodes, insomnia, palpitations, and headache are some common symptoms experienced. A long-term effect of lower estrogen levels is osteoporosis.

Menopausal hormone therapy (MHT) is prescribed to relieve the symptoms of menopause. An added benefit of this treatment is prevention of long-term biologic changes like bone loss related to decreasing levels of estrogen and progesterone that naturally occur in a woman's body during and after menopause.

MHT can be composed of singular hormones, such as estrogen alone, or in combination, like estrogen plus progesterone, or estrogen and progestin (a synthetic hormone with effects similar to those of progesterone). If a woman has had a hysterectomy, she is generally prescribed estrogen alone. Estrogen alone is dangerous to women who still have a uterus, as research has indicated that it should be prescribed with progestin to avoid an increased risk of endometrial cancer.

MHT risks and benefits have been explored in two research trials sponsored by the National Institutes of Health (NIH) as a part of the Women's Health Initiative (WHI). The trials studied more than 27,000 healthy women who were 50 to 79 years of age at the time of enrollment. Both trials were halted sooner than anticipated when it was determined that MHT was associated with specific health risks (see Figure 25-24).

Regardless of whether a woman chooses to use MHT (a decision based on discussions with her

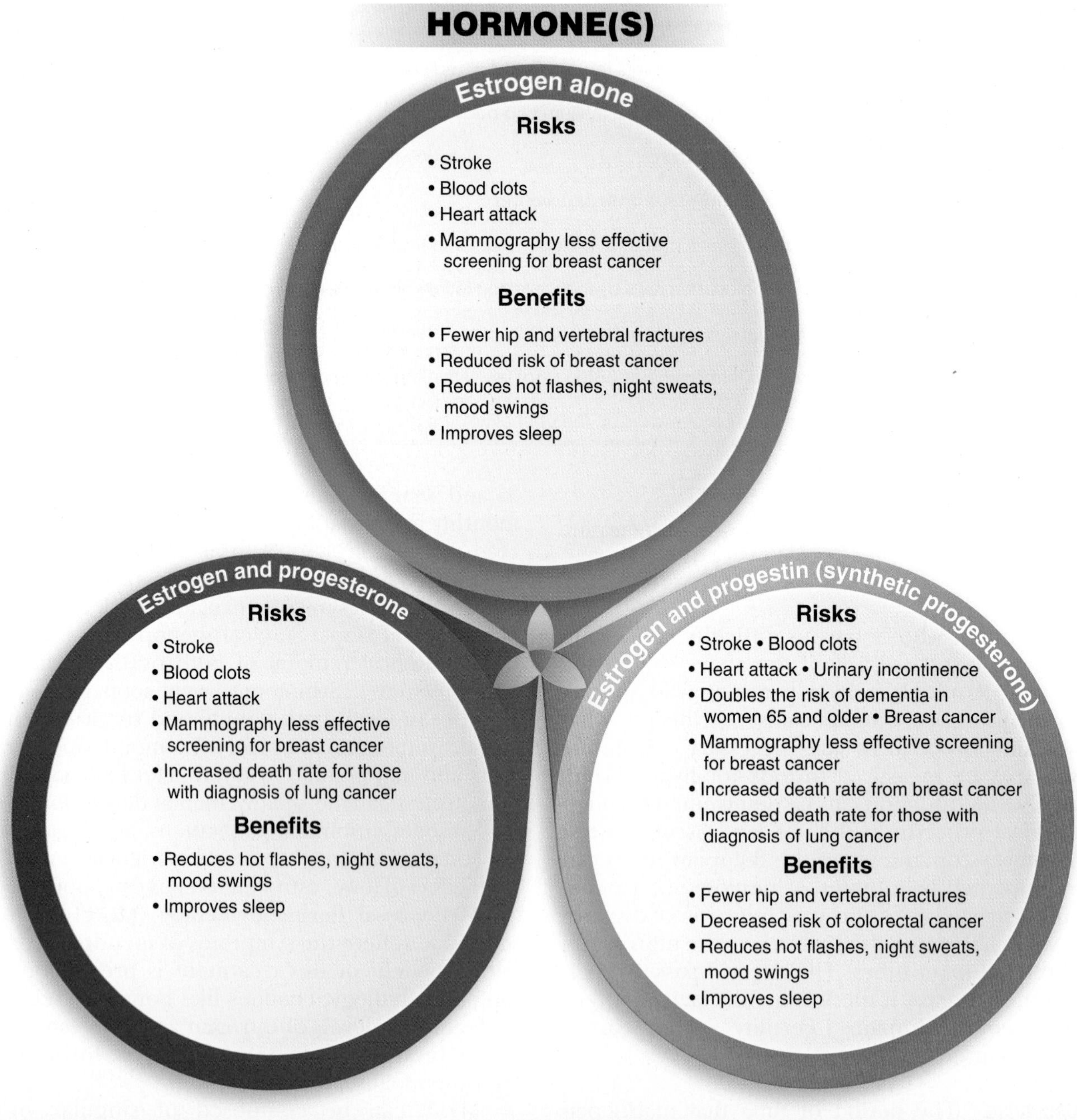

HORMONE(S)

Estrogen alone

Risks

- Stroke
- Blood clots
- Heart attack
- Mammography less effective screening for breast cancer

Benefits

- Fewer hip and vertebral fractures
- Reduced risk of breast cancer
- Reduces hot flashes, night sweats, mood swings
- Improves sleep

Estrogen and progesterone

Risks

- Stroke
- Blood clots
- Heart attack
- Mammography less effective screening for breast cancer
- Increased death rate for those with diagnosis of lung cancer

Benefits

- Reduces hot flashes, night sweats, mood swings
- Improves sleep

Estrogen and progestin (synthetic progesterone)

Risks

- Stroke • Blood clots
- Heart attack • Urinary incontinence
- Doubles the risk of dementia in women 65 and older • Breast cancer
- Mammography less effective screening for breast cancer
- Increased death rate from breast cancer
- Increased death rate for those with diagnosis of lung cancer

Benefits

- Fewer hip and vertebral fractures
- Decreased risk of colorectal cancer
- Reduces hot flashes, night sweats, mood swings
- Improves sleep

FIGURE 25-24 Risks and benefits of hormone replacement therapy.

provider) or decides against MHT, the following behaviors are beneficial to all women:

- Do not smoke.
- Keep blood pressure within normal limits.
- Keep cholesterol level within normal limits.
- Exercise regularly.
- Maintain a healthy weight.
- Get regular mammograms, with ultrasound if necessary, and Pap tests.
- Practice good nutrition (go to the USDA website at http://www.ChooseMyPlate.gov for information)
- Avoid regular alcohol use

Bioidentical hormone (hormones that are molecularly identical to those naturally occurring in the body) replacement therapy (BHRT) is gaining recognition as an alternative to traditional menopausal hormone therapy. While these hormones are derived from plant sources and not synthesized in a laboratory, they still must be manipulated to make them bioidentical. Most of these hormone combinations are specially formulated to the individual's needs. These compounded hormones are not subjected to the same rigid quality control as commercially available prescriptions. Though this therapy is gaining recognition, ACOG's position is that "there is no scientific evidence supporting the safety or efficacy of compounded bioidentical hormones."

Endometriosis. Endometriosis is a painful, common condition caused by endometrial tissue adhering to tissue and organs outside of the uterus. This endometrial tissue is primarily found in the pelvis, adhering to an ovary, a fallopian tube, or the pelvic peritoneum. It also can be found outside of the pelvis, even in the abdomen adhering to tissue and organs, such as the bowel. The cause is unknown. The abnormal and engorged endometrial tissue responds to hormonal stimulation (estrogen) and builds up along with the normal endometrium of the menstrual cycle. It sloughs off at time of menstruation and is painful. The blood has no way to leave the body and is discharged into the pelvic or abdominal cavities.

Because these pills suppress menstruation, endometriosis symptoms may respond to contraceptive medication and no further treatment may be necessary (Figure 25-25). However, long-term hormone treatment may help alleviate symptoms. Hysterectomy may be necessary if the woman does not respond to hormonal therapy.

Ovarian Cysts. Cysts that appear on the ovary are relatively common. As part of the menstrual cycle, the ovarian follicles enlarge and become graafian follicles. Only one graafian follicle ruptures at the time of ovulation. The follicles that do not rupture, but remain, are filled with fluid. They may enlarge and become cysts (Figure 25-26).

Ultrasonography will aid in viewing the ovaries. Most ovarian cysts resolve without treatment. Laparoscopy can be done to either drain or remove

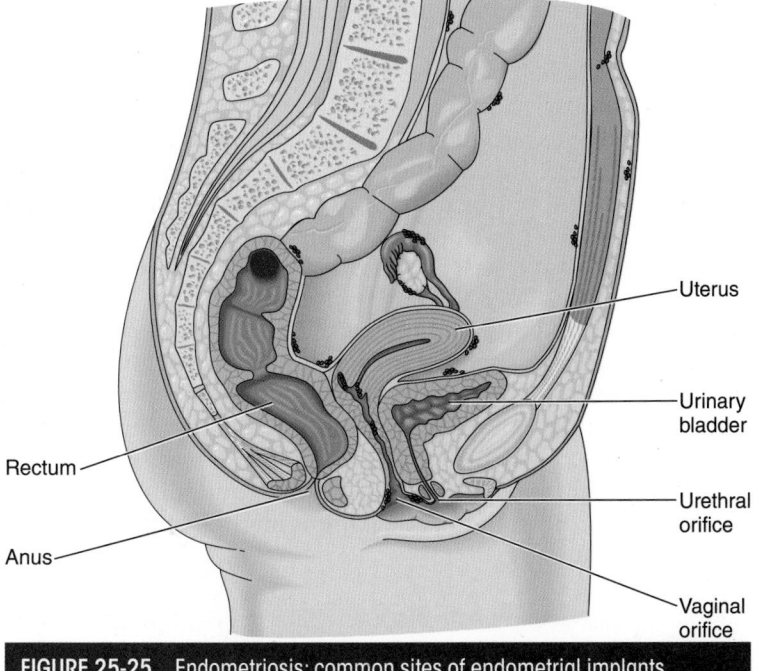

Uterus

Urinary bladder

Urethral orifice

Vaginal orifice

Rectum

Anus

FIGURE 25-25 Endometriosis; common sites of endometrial implants.

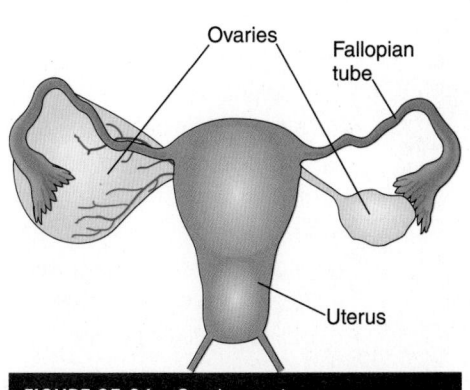

Ovaries

Fallopian tube

Uterus

FIGURE 25-26 Ovarian cyst.

the cyst. Contraceptive therapy is often helpful in resolving the cyst without surgery.

Direct viewing of the ovaries and surgery may be necessary because cancer of the ovary must be ruled out.

Ovarian Cancer. Ovarian cancer is the eighth most common cancer and the fifth leading cause of cancer death in women. It causes more deaths than any other kind of reproductive cancer. Because the symptoms of ovarian cancer are vague and usually do not appear until the disease has become established, it is difficult to make a diagnosis early in the disease process. Therefore, if a woman has any symptoms, the cancer usually has been present for some time. Symptoms may include pressure in the pelvis, lower abdominal discomfort, weight loss, bloating, and fluid in the abdomen. Diagnosis can be made by laparoscopic surgery and a biopsy. Hysterectomy and bilateral salpingo-oophorectomy are done, followed by radiation therapy or chemotherapy. The cause is not known.

Pelvic Inflammatory Disease (PID). PID involves some or all of the female reproductive tract and can be a serious infection. The causative microorganism is usually a sexually transmitted pathogen such as gonorrhea or chlamydia. The microorganism enters through the vagina and ascends through the cervix into the body of the uterus. It can spread out through the fallopian tubes into the pelvic cavity. Culture and sensitivity of the vaginal discharge are performed, and appropriate antibiotics are prescribed. Early treatment helps to lessen damage caused by scar tissue that forms in the pelvis and organs. Delayed treatment can cause septic shock, which can be life threatening. Infertility and ectopic pregnancy are long-range problems that also can occur.

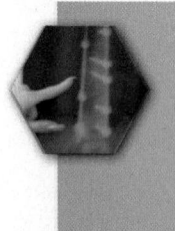

Critical Thinking

A 27-year-old woman wants to schedule an appointment because she has had some bright red bleeding after recent sexual intercourse. What conditions or diseases might this woman have? Discuss your reasons for choosing the conditions or diseases. What equipment and supplies might the provider require for her examination?

For more information on female reproductive system disorders and diagnostic tests, see Tables 25-9, 25-10, and 25-11.

Other Diagnostic Tests and Treatments for Reproductive System Diseases

Colposcopy. **Colposcopy** is examination of the vagina and cervix by means of a lighted instrument that has a three-dimensional magnifying lens called a colposcope. The examination is done to determine if areas in the vagina or the cervix contain precancerous cells or tissue. The procedure is performed after an abnormal Pap test. It can also be performed to evaluate a lesion noted during a pelvic examination and to follow up after treatment of cervical cancer. Because the instrument has the ability to magnify tissue, the cervix can be more readily examined and a biopsy taken.

The patient is placed in lithotomy position and is prepared as she would be for a gynecologic examination. A nonlubricated speculum is inserted into the vagina. The vagina is swabbed with a long cotton-tipped applicator that has been moistened with saline. (This provides better visualization of the cervical tissue.) The cervix is then swabbed with acetic acid to dissolve mucus and provide a good contrast between normal and abnormal tissue. A staining medium can be used as another means of identifying abnormal cells. If the provider finds an area of abnormal tissue, a biopsy can be performed using cervical punch biopsy forceps. The specimen is examined by a pathologist to determine whether malignant cells are present.

Endometrial Biopsy/Sampling. An endometrial biopsy/sampling is often performed when patients are experiencing abnormal periods, postmenopausal bleeding, or thickened uterine lining as diagnosed by ultrasound. It is a fairly simple procedure. The sampling device is housed in a long straw-like tube that slides through the cervical os quite easily. Once the end of the tube is inside the uterus, a plunger is pulled back. The action of pulling the plunger suctions a sampling of the endometrial tissue. This is a sterile procedure and requires application of a cleansing solution (such as Betadine) to the cervix before performing the biopsy. Endometrial biopsy/sampling is quick and almost painless for the patient. The patient might experience slight cramping.

Cervical Punch Biopsy. The **cervical punch biopsy** is usually done in conjunction with a colposcopy to obtain a sample of cervical tissue for pathologic

TABLE 25-9

FEMALE REPRODUCTIVE SYSTEM LABORATORY AND DIAGNOSTIC TESTS

DISEASE/DISORDER	MEDICAL TEST OR PROCEDURE	BLOOD TESTING	OTHER	RADIOGRAPHY	SURGERY
Bartholin gland infection	Pelvic examination		Exudate culture and sensitivity		Incision and drainage
Breast cancer	Monthly breast self-examination	Breast cancer gene detection BRCA1, BRCA2		Mammography Ultrasonography	Biopsy of breast lesion Lumpectomy
Cervical cancer	Pelvic examination Colposcopy		Pap smear		Cone biopsy Punch biopsy Dilation and curettage (D&C) Cryosurgery LEEP (loop electrosurgical excision procedure) Laser surgery Hysterectomy
Endometriosis	Pelvic examination		Urinalysis	Abdominal ultrasonography Chest radiograph	Laparoscopy Hysterectomy
Fibrocystic breasts	Monthly breast self-examination			Mammography Ultrasonography	Biopsy
Pelvic inflammatory disease	Pelvic examination	Complete blood count and differential (CBC)	Urinalysis Culture and sensitivity of vaginal discharge	Pelvic ultrasonography	Laparoscopy
TESTS FOR SEXUALLY TRANSMITTED DISEASES					
Chlamydia	Pelvic examination	Serology	Urinalysis Direct urethral or cervical smear using monoclonal antibodies ThinPrep Pap test		

continues

Table 25-9 continued

DISEASE/DISORDER	MEDICAL TEST OR PROCEDURE	BLOOD TESTING	OTHER	RADIOGRAPHY	SURGERY
Condylomata/HPV (genital warts)	Pelvic examination Pap smear		ThinPrep Pap test		Excisional biopsy
Neisseria gonorrhoeae Hepatitis B and C, and HIV	Pelvic examination	CBC Virology	Urinalysis Direct smear of vaginal discharge, anal canal, and oropharynx Thayer-Martin culture ThinPrep Pap test Liver function	Pelvic ultrasonography Abdominal ultrasonography	Liver biopsy
TESTS FOR VAGINITIS					
Candidiasis	Pelvic examination	Blood glucose	Urinalysis Wet mount: Direct vaginal smear with potassium hydroxide and/or saline (1 drop)		
Trichomoniasis	Pelvic examination		Urinalysis Wet mount: direct vaginal smear with isotonic saline (1 drop) and/or potassium hydroxide (KOH)		
Bacterial vaginosis	Pelvic examination	CBC	Culture and sensitivity of vaginal discharge		

TABLE 25-10

FEMALE REPRODUCTIVE SYSTEM DISORDERS AND CONDITIONS

Bartholin gland infection. Infection of the mucous glands that open near the vaginal opening.

Breast cancer. Most commonly diagnosed cancer in females. A genetic cause has been identified for some breast cancers. Some symptoms are lumps, thickening, swelling, dimpling, pain, and nipple discharge.

Cervical cancer. A carcinoma of the cervix of the uterus caused by a progressive cervical dysplasia. Most common in women ages 30 to 40 years. A significant risk factor is seen in women who become sexually active early in their lives and who have multiple sex partners. Presence of HPV poses greater risk.

Cystocele. Herniation of the urinary bladder into the vagina. May cause urgency and frequency. Injury to the bladder during delivery of a fetus is one cause.

Endometriosis. Presence of endometrium in sites other than inside the uterus. May be found on the ovaries, fallopian tubes, large bowel, lungs, and pleura. Causes pelvic pain, dysmenorrhea, and infertility.

Endometrial cancer. A cancer that originates in the endometrial tissue. It is most common in women over the age of 50 and in women who utilize estrogen-only hormone replacement therapy. Obesity and the use of the medication tamoxifen increase the risk.

Fibrocystic breasts. Benign cysts in breast tissue that increase or decrease in size during menses. Thought to be a normal variation in breast tissue due to monthly hormonal influence.

Pelvic inflammatory disease (PID). Pelvic reproductive organs become inflamed and infected by bacteria, viruses, or parasites. An ascending infection can ensue involving the vagina, cervix of uterus, body of uterus, fallopian tubes, and ovaries. Symptoms include vaginal discharge, pain, and fever. May cause infertility. Majority of cases caused by sexually transmitted disease *(Neisseria gonorrhoeae,* chlamydia).

Premenstrual syndrome (PMS). Cluster of symptoms that occur monthly before the onset of menses; thought to be caused by progesterone–estrogen imbalance. Symptoms include fluid retention, weight gain, irritability, and mood swings.

Rectocele. Herniation of the posterior wall of the vagina with the anterior wall of the rectum through the vagina.

Sexually transmitted diseases (STDs). Diseases caused by bacteria, viruses, and protozoa that are transmitted through sexual intercourse (vaginal, anal, oral) (see Table 25-11).

Vaginitis. Inflammation of the vagina that may be caused by bacteria, fungus, protozoa, chemical irritants, irritation from foreign bodies, vitamin deficiency, uncleanliness, and intestinal worms (see Table 25-9).

TABLE 25-11

COMMON SEXUALLY TRANSMITTED DISEASES

PATHOLOGY	SYMPTOMS	TEST	TREATMENT
AIDS	Flu-like, lymphadenopathy, infections, malignancies, pneumonia	HIV CBC	Medication: antiretroviral medications such as zidovudine, didanosine, ritonavir
Chlamydia	Usually asymptomatic	Vaginal culture ThinPrep Pap test Urinalysis	Doxycycline, azithromycin

continues

Table 25-11 continued

PATHOLOGY	SYMPTOMS	TEST	TREATMENT
Condylomata (HPV)	Warts on external and internal genitalia	Visual exam ThinPrep Pap test HPV	Cryocautery or chemocautery preferred but electrocautery can be used Keratolytic agents such as Podofilox, CO_2 laser
Gonorrhea	Usually asymptomatic; yellowish-green discharge with dysuria in advanced stages	Gram stain or Thayer-Martin culture ThinPrep Pap test	Ofloxacin, ceftriaxone, cefixine
Herpes simplex I and II	Itching and soreness followed by genital **vesicles**, which heal in 10 to 14 days	Visual exam Viral isolation by tissue culture	Acyclovir, Valtrex, Famvir
Syphilis	*Stage I.* Papule develops into ulcer, which develops into chancre on vulva *Stage II.* Fever, general malaise, dermal and mucosal lesions *Stage III.* Degeneration of central nervous system, lesions of internal structures	Venereal Disease Research Laboratory, fluorescent antibody test Dark-field exam Rapid plasma reagin (RPR) Culture and sensitivity of spinal fluid	Penicillin
Trichomonas	Milky white, frothy, malodorous discharge with genital burning and itching	Wet mount for microscopic examination	Oral Flagyl; partner(s) must also be treated

examination. The specimen is examined for malignant cells and the biopsy usually follows an abnormal Pap smear report.

The procedure is performed with the patient in lithotomy position and with a vaginal speculum in place. The provider may stain the cervix to aid in identifying abnormal tissue. If the colposcope is being used, it illuminates and magnifies the cervical tissue. The provider takes several tissue samples using the cervical punch biopsy forceps. If bleeding ensues, it can be controlled with a vaginal packing, or the area can be cauterized to stop the bleeding. The specimen is placed in a container with **formalin**, a completed requisition form is attached to the container, and it is sent to the pathology laboratory for examination. The patient may expect a small amount of bleeding and should notify the provider if bleeding ensues that is greater than a menstrual period. Discharge that has a strong, foul odor is to be expected and can last for up to a month after the procedure.

Cervical Cone Biopsy. Another type of biopsy, known as a cone biopsy, can be performed. An inverted cone of tissue is excised by scalpel or laser under general anesthesia. In this procedure, a larger sample of tissue is excised to rule out invasive cancer and to remove the lesion. It is the most comprehensive specimen to diagnose a premalignant or malignant lesion. This is also known as a cold knife biopsy.

Another type of cervical biopsy is the loop electrosurgical excision procedure (LEEP), also called large loop excision of the transformation zone (the border between ectocervix and exocervix). Precancers and cancers commonly develop in this area. Either type of cervical cone biopsy can be used as a treatment to completely remove many precancers and very early cancers.

Cryosurgery. **Cryosurgery** is used to treat tissue by freezing temperatures. Chronic cervicitis and cervical **erosion** are two common problems treated in this manner (see Chapter 30 for information about cryosurgery). The freezing temperature causes cells to die; they are then cast off from the cervix and eventually replaced with healthy cells about a month after the procedure.

The procedure is performed with the patient in lithotomy position. The cervix is swabbed to

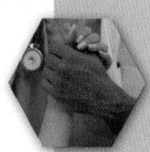

Patient Education

Post–Cervical Biopsy and Cervical Cone Biopsy

1. Rest for 24 hours after the procedure.
2. Do not lift heavy objects for 2 weeks.
3. Leave packing in place for 24 hours or as directed. Do not insert another tampon unless told to do so by the provider.
4. Report any bleeding greater than a normal menstrual period.

remove mucus. The cryo probe is placed against the affected area of the cervix and the machine is turned on. The liquid nitrogen flows over the area for about 3 minutes and freezes the tissue. The tissue is allowed to thaw, and the treatment is repeated for another 3 minutes. The patient may have some pain similar to dysmenorrhea that may last for about a half hour. There should be no strong, foul odor, but there can be discharge for up to a month. Patients should report any malodorous discharges because this may indicate an infection. Healing usually takes 4 to 6 weeks.

Wet Prep/Wet Mount for Yeast, Bacteria, and Trichomonas. The wet prep is a clinic procedure to determine the cause of vaginitis in women and urethritis in men. The provider takes a sample of the discharge on a cotton-tipped applicator. The medical assistant rinses it vigorously in a test tube containing a few drops (about 0.5 mL) of normal saline, pressing the swab against the inside of the test tube to express all the specimen, then places a drop of the solution onto a microscope slide and covers it with a coverslip. The provider then views it microscopically for the following:

- If a yeast infection is present, budding yeast will be seen.
- If a bacterial infection is present, clue cells will be seen. Clue cells are vaginal epithelial cells that appear fuzzy with no clear cell edge. They appear this way because the outside edge is covered with bacteria.
- If trichomonas are present, they appear as motile single-cell protozoa. Movement will be noted. The trichomonas are sometimes identified in a microscopic portion of the urinalysis as well (see Procedure 25-3).

Procedure

Potassium Hydroxide Prep for Fungus. After performing the previously mentioned test, a few drops of 10% potassium hydroxide (KOH) may be added to the remaining solution in the test tube and examined microscopically for fungi. The KOH destroys bacteria and vaginal epithelial cells, leaving only the cell walls of the fungus, which makes visualization easier. This slide is prepared in the same way as the wet prep: Place a drop of the solution onto a clean slide; cover with a coverslip. Dispose of all glass slides, coverslips, and test tubes in a sharps container (see Procedure 25-3).

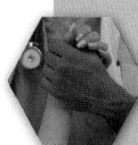

Patient Education

After Cryosurgery of Cervix

1. Expect a clear, watery, heavy discharge for several weeks, eventually tapering off.
2. Use only sanitary pads, not tampons. Change often, cleansing perineal area with each pad change.
3. Report signs of infection: fever, malodorous discharge, pain, nausea, or vomiting.
4. Do not engage in sexual intercourse, douche, or use tampons for 4 weeks (unless instructed otherwise by provider).
5. Expect a somewhat heavier than usual menstrual period the following month.
6. Report excessive bleeding.

PROCEDURE 25-3

Procedure

Wet Prep/Wet Mount and Potassium Hydroxide (KOH) Prep

STANDARD PRECAUTIONS:

Handwashing

Gloves

Biohazard

PURPOSE:

To test a vaginal specimen to determine the cause of vaginitis. The wet prep/wet mount tests for yeast, bacteria, and trichomonas; the KOH prep tests for yeast.

EQUIPMENT/SUPPLIES:

- Cotton-tipped applicator
- Small test tube
- Normal saline (0.5 mL, or a few drops)
- 10% potassium hydroxide (KOH; 0.5 mL, or a few drops)
- Two microscope slides and coverslips

- Microscope
- Vaginal speculum
- Patient drape
- Gloves
- Other equipment as necessary for a vaginal examination

PROCEDURE STEPS:

1. *Paying attention to detail*, assemble equipment for vaginal examination.
2. Wash hands and follow Standard Precautions.
3. Introduce yourself. Identify the patient.
4. *Explain the rationale for performance of the procedure, speaking at the patient's level of understanding. Show awareness of the patient's concerns. Help her to feel safe and comfortable.* Take time to answer any questions.
5. *Being courteous and respectful*, provide patient with a gown and request that the patient undress from the waist down.
6. *Considering any special needs of the patient*, once draped, assist the patient into the lithotomy position.
7. Don nonsterile gloves and place 0.5 mL normal saline into a small test tube preparation for the specimen.
8. *Working within your scope of practice*, assist the provider with vaginal exam and obtaining the specimen for evaluation.
9. Grasp the swab that contains vaginal discharge obtained by the provider and vigorously mix the swab in and out of the test tube containing saline, pressing the cotton tip against the inside of the test tube to express all of the specimen. RATIONALE: It is important to get as much of the sample as possible for a more accurate diagnosis.
10. Remove gloves and dispose of them in the appropriate container. Wash hands.
11. *Considering any special needs of the patient*, assist the patient back to a sitting position. Instruct her to dress and offer to assist if needed, *being sure to protect the patient's personal boundaries*. RATIONALE: While the provider is viewing the slide, your responsibility is the safety and comfort of the patient.
12. Place two slides prepared with the patient's name side by side on a flat surface. Apply a drop of the saline solution to each of the slides. Apply a drop of the KOH solution to one of the slides and cover both slides with a coverslip. The provider will view the slides under the microscope for yeast, bacteria, and trichomonas.

(continues)

13. Allow the slide with the KOH solutions to stand for 2 to 5 minutes before the provider examines it for the presence of yeast.

14. Dispose of the cotton-tipped applicator into a biohazard container. RATIONALE: All body fluid–contaminated supplies should be handled with care and disposed of according to Standard Precautions.

15. Dispose of any sharp items, including glass slides and cover slips in the appropriate biohazard container. RATIONALE: This prevents accidental injury and the spread of disease via microorganisms.

16. Disinfect the area and any equipment used for the procedure and slide exam. RATIONALE: As stated in Standard Precautions, all biohazard-contaminated surfaces must be disinfected after contamination.

17. Remove gloves and dispose of properly.

18. Wash hands.

19. Return to the patient and assist as needed, ***attending to any special needs of the patient***. RATIONALE: The patient may need assistance and direction.

20. Document the procedure in the patient's medical record.

DOCUMENTATION:

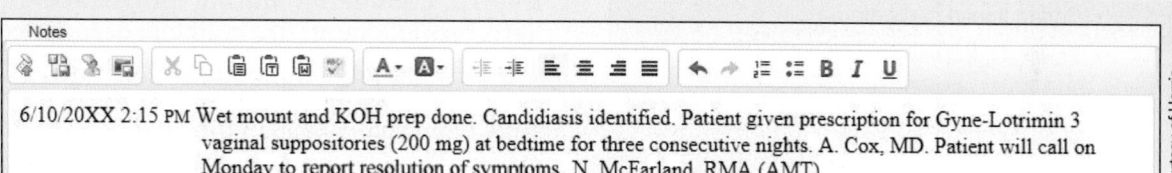

6/10/20XX 2:15 PM Wet mount and KOH prep done. Candidiasis identified. Patient given prescription for Gyne-Lotrimin 3 vaginal suppositories (200 mg) at bedtime for three consecutive nights. A. Cox, MD. Patient will call on Monday to report resolution of symptoms. N. McFarland, RMA (AMT)

Courtesy of Harris CareTracker PM and EMR

Amplified DNA Probe Test for Chlamydia and Gonorrhea. The amplified DNA probe test for chlamydia and gonorrhea is used as a screening tool for both men and women and on all pregnant women. It is not a culture. Two types of kits are available: the ProbeTec blue kit for urethral specimens from the male patient (see Chapter 27) and the ProbeTec pink kit for endocervical specimens from the female patient. The female kit contains preservative, swabs (one large swab and one small Mini-Tip Culturette Swab), and instructions. This test needs to be performed on the female patient before the digital/bimanual examination so that no lubricating jelly is present. Using the large swab, the provider will clean the cervix of any mucus, blood, or cellular debris and discard the swab. The Mini-Tip Culturette Swab is then inserted into the cervical canal and rotated for 15 to 30 seconds. It is then immediately placed into the transport tube. If the ProbeTec Wet Transport tube is used, the swab is broken off into the liquid before recapping. This test also may be used to look for chlamydia and gonorrhea in a urine specimen, following the manufacturer's instructions for collection and testing.

Laparoscopy. **Laparoscopy** is a procedure in which a lighted instrument is used to view the inside of the pelvic cavity. It can be helpful in diagnosing endometriosis and ovarian cysts or other abnormalities in the pelvic cavity. A tubal ligation, severing of the fallopian tubes, and an oophorectomy can be done laparoscopically. Laparoscopy can be done abdominally or vaginally (Figure 25-27).

Dilation and Curettage. Dilation and curettage (D&C) is a surgical procedure that involves dilating and scraping the cervix of endometrial tissue. It is commonly performed to remove any remaining tissue after an incomplete abortion or to examine the tissue if the patient has had abnormal uterine bleeding.

Diagnostic ultrasonography is used to help diagnose many gynecologic conditions, such as ovarian masses, fibroids, and endometriosis. The ultrasound can be performed transcervically or transvaginally.

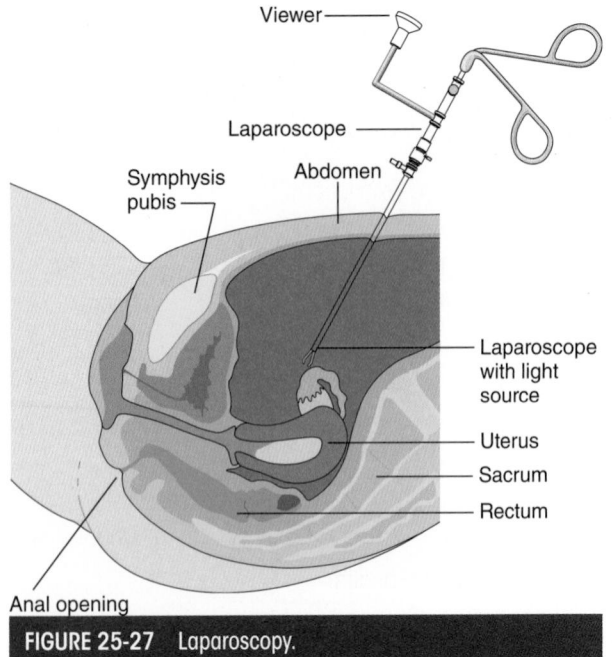

FIGURE 25-27 Laparoscopy.

Viewer

Laparoscope

Symphysis pubis

Abdomen

Laparoscope with light source

Uterus

Sacrum

Rectum

Anal opening

Complementary Therapy in Obstetrics and Gynecology

Most of the complementary therapy practiced today can be helpful to women in easing the discomforts of pregnancy and labor. In our stress-filled world, emotional calm can be provided through the use of some of these therapies.

Infants in neonatal intensive care unit benefit from a calm, warm touch and rocking, hugging, and singing softly.

Information should be obtained from the obstetrics patient at each visit about any form of complementary therapy (stress reduction, imagery, acupuncture, biofeedback, massage therapy, and music therapy, among others). Consultation with the provider concerning their safety during pregnancy is advisable.

Caution is advised when the use of herbal medicine is considered during pregnancy. Because herbal supplements are available over the counter and little is known about their effects on the fetus, women should be cautioned to avoid using any kind of herbal supplement during their first trimester. Women should ask their provider's advice about the use of such supplements after the first trimester.

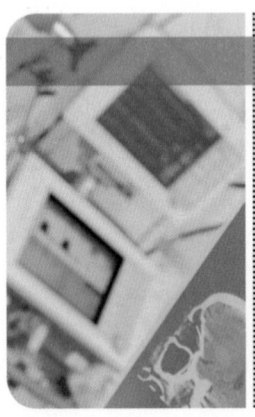

CASE STUDY 25-1

Refer to the scenario at the beginning of the chapter.

Mrs. Jennings has an appointment today in the obstetrics clinic at Inner City Health Care. Nancy McFarland, RMA (AMT), is responsible for preparing Mrs. Jennings for a repeat prenatal visit. Besides getting her patient ready, Nancy has other responsibilities to Mrs. Jennings. Vital signs and certain laboratory tests must be done.

CASE STUDY REVIEW

1. What are some potential problems with Mrs. Jennings's pregnancy that Nancy can discover and relay to Dr. Cox?

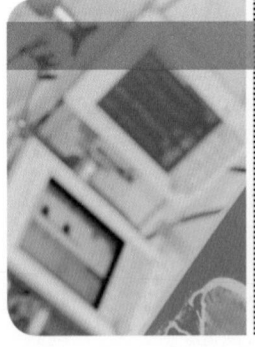

CASE STUDY 25-2

Maria Rodriguez has an appointment to see Dr. Cox today. It is her initial prenatal visit. She tells Nancy McFarland, the medical assistant, as she is escorted from the reception area that she has been feeling "pretty good."

CASE STUDY REVIEW

1. List three of the screening exams to be performed during the first prenatal visit.

2. What laboratory and other procedural tests may be performed at the initial visit?

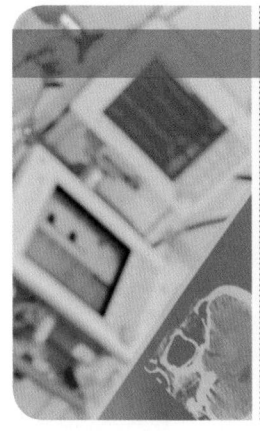

CASE STUDY 25-3

Renee Little has made an appointment with Dr. Cox because she has had symptoms of vaginitis. When she arrives at the clinic, you take her chief complaint and history. She tells you that she has milky-white, frothy vaginal discharge and that she itches in the genital area.

CASE STUDY REVIEW

1. How would you display your professional skills while taking the patient's chief complaint?
2. What tests/procedures will you prepare for Dr. Cox in consideration of Renee's symptoms?
3. What is the most likely causative microorganism for these symptoms?
4. Describe the treatment that Dr. Cox may prescribe.

Summary

- Obstetrics and gynecology are two specialties that are usually practiced by the same provider.
- The OB/GYN provider cares for the health and well-being of the female patient in her pregnant and nonpregnant states.
- Prenatal care begins with the detailed, initial, baseline assessment of maternal health.
- Prenatal care includes lab tests and extensive education.
- The prenatal history should be thorough and will alert the provider to indicators that might increase maternal and fetal risk factors.
- Return prenatal visits monitor the progress of the pregnancy in regard to both maternal and fetal health.
- During the pregnancy, several important tests may be performed. These screen for fetal developmental defects and genetic abnormalities. Other examinations monitor fetal growth and may be used to diagnose Down syndrome.
- Some problems occur during pregnancy that threaten the health and life of the mother and the fetus.
- These disorders include miscarriage, ectopic pregnancy, high blood pressure (eclampsia), gestational diabetes, disorders of the placenta, and hyperemesis gravidarum.
- OB/GYN providers often treat disorders that cause infertility.
- Knowledge of care standards for the mother during labor, delivery, and the postpartum period is necessary for the professional medical assistant.
- Birth control methods vary based on the preference of the patient. Methods include oral contraceptives; barrier methods such as the use of condoms, diaphragm, or cervical cap; use of spermicide alone; hormonal implantation; injection or cervical ring; IUD; and permanent solutions such as tubal ligation and vasectomy.
- Gynecology care includes an annual examination with a Pap test, breast exam, immunization for HPV, and patient education regarding monthly breast self-exams.
- It is the role of the professional medical assistant to assist with the Pap smear. This includes setting up the instrument tray, handing instruments, managing the specimen appropriately, and documenting the procedure.
- Women in middle age may be experiencing symptoms of menopause. This will be indicated by symptoms stated during the patient history.
- Some disorders of the GYN patient include endometriosis, ovarian cysts and ovarian cancer, and pelvic inflammatory disease.
- Diagnosis and treatment of these GYN disorders may include colposcopy, endometrial biopsy, cervical biopsies, and cryosurgery. The medical assistant will be expected to be knowledgeable and accountable as an assistant during these procedures.
- Performance of wet mount, potassium hydroxide prep, and testing for chlamydia and gonorrhea falls into the role of the MA.
- Assisting with invasive GYN procedures includes assisting the provider with a laparoscopy and D&C.

CERTIFICATION REVIEW

1. Which of the following conditions or diseases that an obstetrics patient experiences is considered to place her in the high-risk category?
   a. 19 years of age
   b. Both partners Rh negative
   c. Poor nutritional habits
   d. Poor hygiene

2. Using Nägele's rule, calculate the expected date of birth of the baby of a patient whose last menstrual period was August 20, 2017. Which of the following is the anticipated due date?
   a. November 27, 2018
   b. December 13, 2018
   c. May 27, 2018
   d. April 20, 2018
   e. June 9, 2018

3. The primary test performed at about the 16th week to check the fetus for neural tube defects is known as which of the following?
   a. Alpha-fetoprotein test
   b. Amniocentesis
   c. Chorionic villus sampling (CVS)
   d. Rubella titer

4. The release of which of the following hormones is thought to cause labor to begin?
   a. Progesterone
   b. Estrogen
   c. Oxytocin
   d. Thyroxine
   e. Follicle-stimulating hormone

5. After a cervical punch biopsy, it is normal for the patient to experience which of the following?
   a. Bleeding greater than a normal menstrual period
   b. No odor to vaginal discharge
   c. Malodorous vaginal discharge
   d. Severe abdominal cramps

6. Ultrasonography is done to check for which of the following?
   a. Gestational diabetes
   b. Preeclampsia
   c. Degree of effacement
   d. Number of weeks of gestation
   e. Group B strep infection

7. To diagnose pelvic inflammatory disease (PID), the provider may order which of the following?
   a. Culture and sensitivity
   b. Pap smear
   c. Urinalysis
   d. Ultrasonography

8. To make the diagnosis of trichomoniasis, the medical assistant will need to prepare for which of the following?
   a. Pap smear
   b. Ultrasonography
   c. Wet mount
   d. Culture and sensitivity
   e. Blood glucose

9. What is the primary purpose of colposcopy?
   a. To treat advanced cancer of the vagina and cervix
   b. To detect dysplastic cells of the cervix after an abnormal Pap test
   c. To treat PID in the fallopian tube
   d. To treat endometriosis of the pelvic cavity

10. Which of the following is/are primarily associated with abnormal Pap smears?
    a. Endometriosis
    b. Bartholin cysts
    c. Condylomata
    d. Ovarian cysts
    e. PID

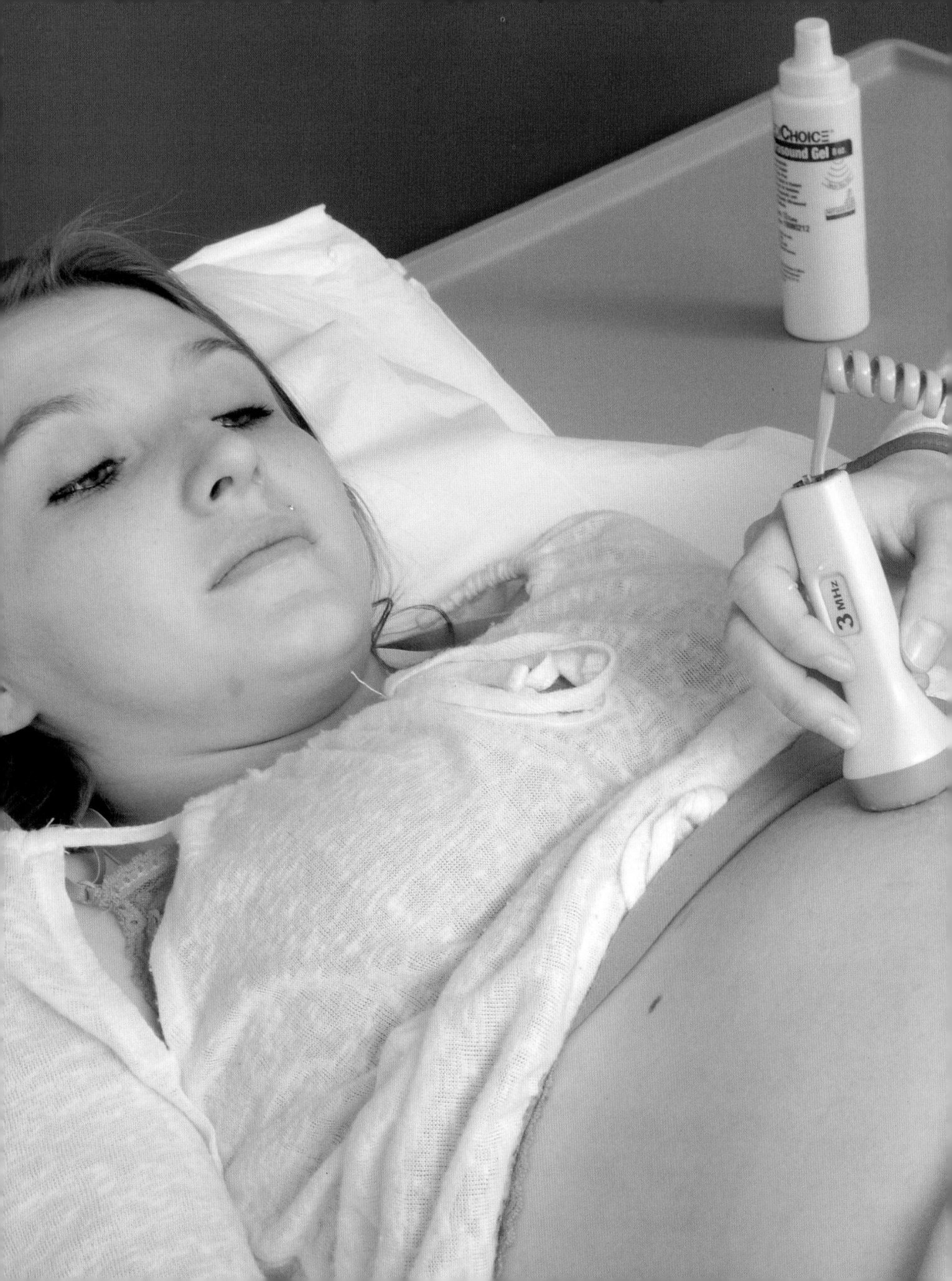

CHAPTER 26

Pediatrics

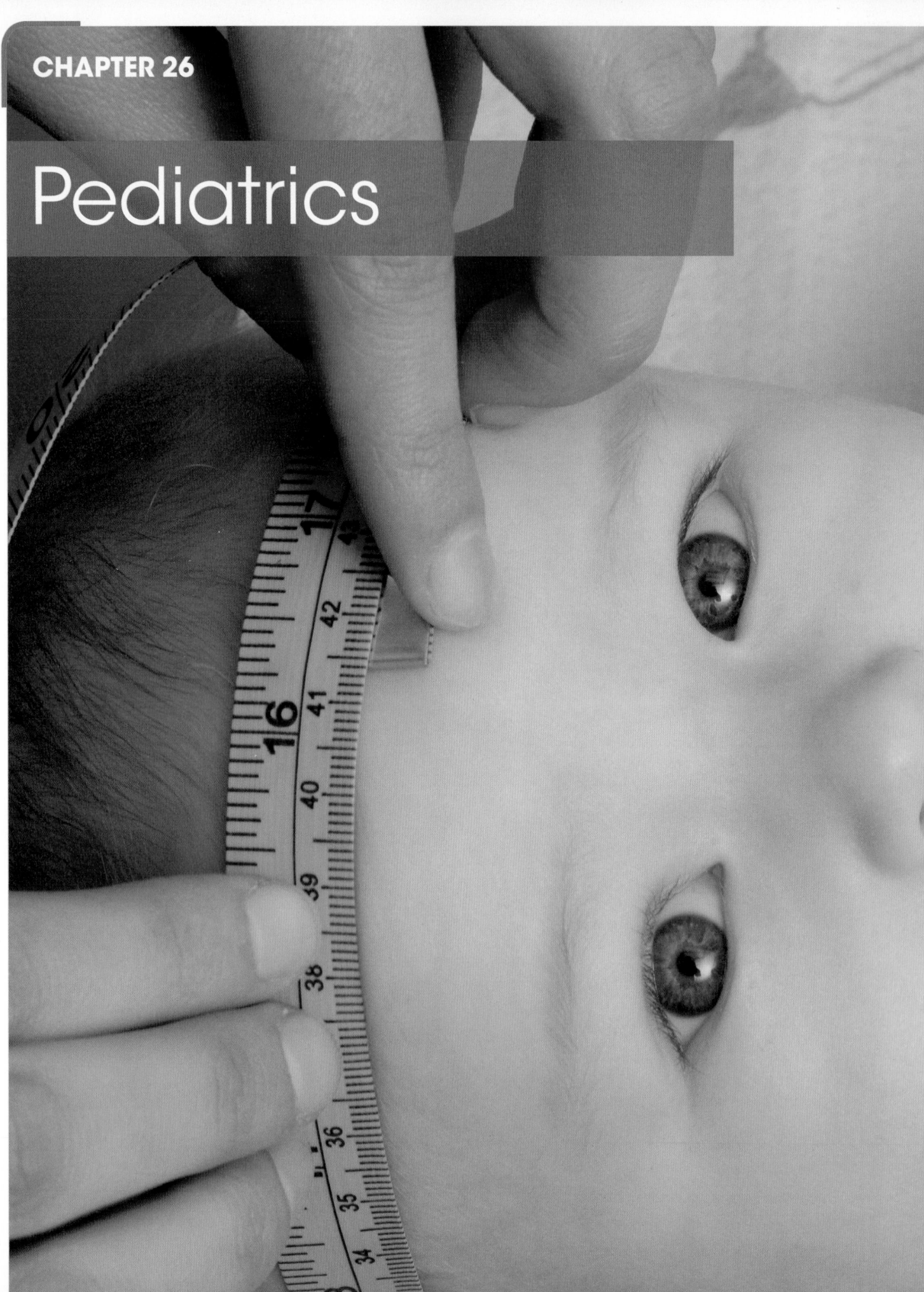

1. Define and spell the key terms as presented in the glossary.
2. Compare the various theories of human development.
3. Describe pediatric care, including measuring height, weight, head circumference, chest circumference, and vital signs.
4. Maintain growth charts.
5. Explain the process of collecting a urine specimen.
6. Discuss the process of screening for hearing and visual impairments.
7. Identify common pediatric diseases and disorders.
8. State the importance of immunizations and scheduling of them.
9. Describe infant holds for injections and procedures.

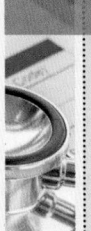

KEY TERMS

aerosolized	exudates	respiratory syncytial virus (RSV)
circumcision	fontanels	sensorineural
cochlear implantation	lyophilized	suppurative
conjunctivitis	myringotomy	syncope
DTaP (diphtheria, tetanus, pertussis)	neonate	tympanostomy
	phenylketonuria (PKU)	

SCENARIO

At Inner City Health Care, clinical assistant Joe Guerrero, CMA (AAMA), is responsible for encouraging parents to keep track of their children's immunization records. Joe teaches parents the importance of immunizations for long-term health protection and the importance of following recommended vaccination schedules for maximum benefit.

Chapter Portal

New techniques and developments occur frequently in medicine, and medical assistants must refine existing skills and learn new ones to be knowledgeable and proficient and to provide the most current, up-to-date quality care to patients. The medical assistant who works in a pediatrician's office or a pediatric ambulatory care setting that treats infants, children, and adolescents will need additional skills when providing pediatric care to patients.

Knowledge of the developmental stages, knowledge of diseases of infants and children, and the ability to gain the child's confidence and trust and the caregivers' cooperation are all skills required to provide for the physiologic, emotional, and psychologic needs of the pediatric patient. This chapter covers the specialty examination and the appropriate clinical procedures in pediatrics.

WHAT IS PEDIATRICS?

Pediatrics is the branch of medicine that cares for newborns, infants, children, and adolescents. Pediatricians are providers who diagnose and treat health problems and diseases specific to these age groups. This patient population has special needs, and medical assistants must be knowledgeable about the growth and developmental phases of life and diseases unique to pediatric patients. Children form judgments and have fears about health care providers. They need an atmosphere that is comfortable and one in which their physiologic, emotional, and psychologic needs are recognized and addressed.

Communication

Medical assistants must gain the confidence and trust of the child and parent(s), allay fear, and help to promote positive relationships between the child and the provider and must themselves develop a positive relationship with the child. Children are likely to be cooperative when being examined or during a procedure if good rapport has been established. It is important to be honest with young patients and approach them at their level of understanding. Allow children to touch and hold a "safe" instrument, such as a stethoscope, and explain its purpose to them. Doing so can reduce anxiety and fear (Figure 26-1). It is important also for the medical assistant to recognize pediatric patients by their names no matter what their ages.

Taking a history of the child; assessing the child; measuring vital signs, height, weight, vision, and hearing; laboratory work; administering injections; observing the parent–child interactions; and noting the child's development level are all responsibilities in which a medical assistant takes part.

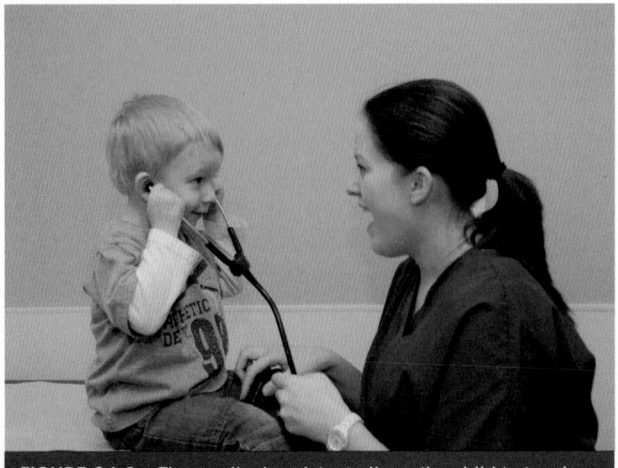

FIGURE 26-1 The medical assistant allows the child to touch the stethoscope and "listen" to her heartbeat to gain the child's cooperation.

The first physical examination of a newborn is performed immediately after delivery. The pediatrician assesses the **neonate's** ability to exist outside the mother's uterus. A scoring system is used to determine the neonate's physical condition at 1, 5, and 15 minutes after birth. It is known as the Apgar (appearance, pulse, grimace, activity, and respiration) score. Muscle tone, skin color, respiration, heart rate, and response to stimuli are each given a score of 0, 1, or 2, the highest total score being 10. Infants with low Apgar scores need immediate attention, such as stimulation, oxygen, medication, and so on. Their condition is monitored closely (see Chapter 25).

Tests are done to detect problems the neonate may have. **Phenylketonuria (PKU)**, iron deficiency anemia, lead poisoning, and hypothyroidism are problems for which neonates are screened shortly after delivery.

Many patients seen in the pediatric setting are babies or children who are not ill. They are considered "well-baby" or "well-child" patients and are having routine checkups. Ill babies or children are often called "sick-child" or "sick-baby" patients. Well-by appointments are regularly scheduled appointments during which time the provider examines the child and evaluates the growth and development of the child. Most clinics schedule well-baby appointments after birth according to the following time frame: 1, 2, 4, 6, 9, 12, 15, 18, 24, and 36 months, and yearly thereafter.

Well-baby checks include obtaining information regarding the child's sleep, appetite, and developmental progress. It is important to reinforce the importance of these regular provider appointments. These screening appointments allow the provider to identify potential problems early and plan interventions to maintain the health and development of the child.

IMMUNIZATIONS

Vaccines stimulate the immune system to produce antibodies against pathogens (see Chapter 21). Vaccines prevent dangerous and potentially deadly diseases. Vaccines help develop immunity by imitating an infection, but this "imitation" infection does not cause illness. It does, however, cause the immune system to develop the same response as it does to a real infection so the body can recognize and fight the vaccine-preventable disease in the future. Sometimes, after getting a vaccine, the imitation infection can cause minor symptoms, such as fever. Such minor symptoms are normal and should be expected as the body builds immunity.

Typically, immunizations are given during routinely scheduled appointments. The charts shown in Figures 26-2 and 26-3 include immunization schedules from the Centers for Disease Control Recommended Immunization Schedule for Persons Aged 0 through 18 Years. (To review the complete footnotes for these schedules, go to http://www.cdc.gov and search "Immunization Schedules.")

Immunizations are given by mouth, injection, and intranasal spray. The goal of the recommended immunization schedule is to protect infants and children early in life, when they are most vulnerable and before they are exposed to potentially life-threatening diseases. The initial doses of these vaccines need to be given before age 2 years, when children are most susceptible to infectious diseases. Vaccines protect children during these periods. HPV is the exception to this timeline. The Advisory Committee on Immunization Practices (ACIP) recommends routine vaccination with HPV4 or HPV2 for females ages 11 or 12 years and with HPV4 for males ages 11 or 12 years. Vaccination also is recommended for females ages 13 through 26 years and for males ages 13 through 21 years who were not vaccinated previously.

Preparation of Vaccines for Administration

Careful attention to both proper storage of vaccines and thorough patient preparation for immunization will promote effective vaccination results. Access to vaccination should be available to all patients, especially to families with young infants and children. Access involves cost

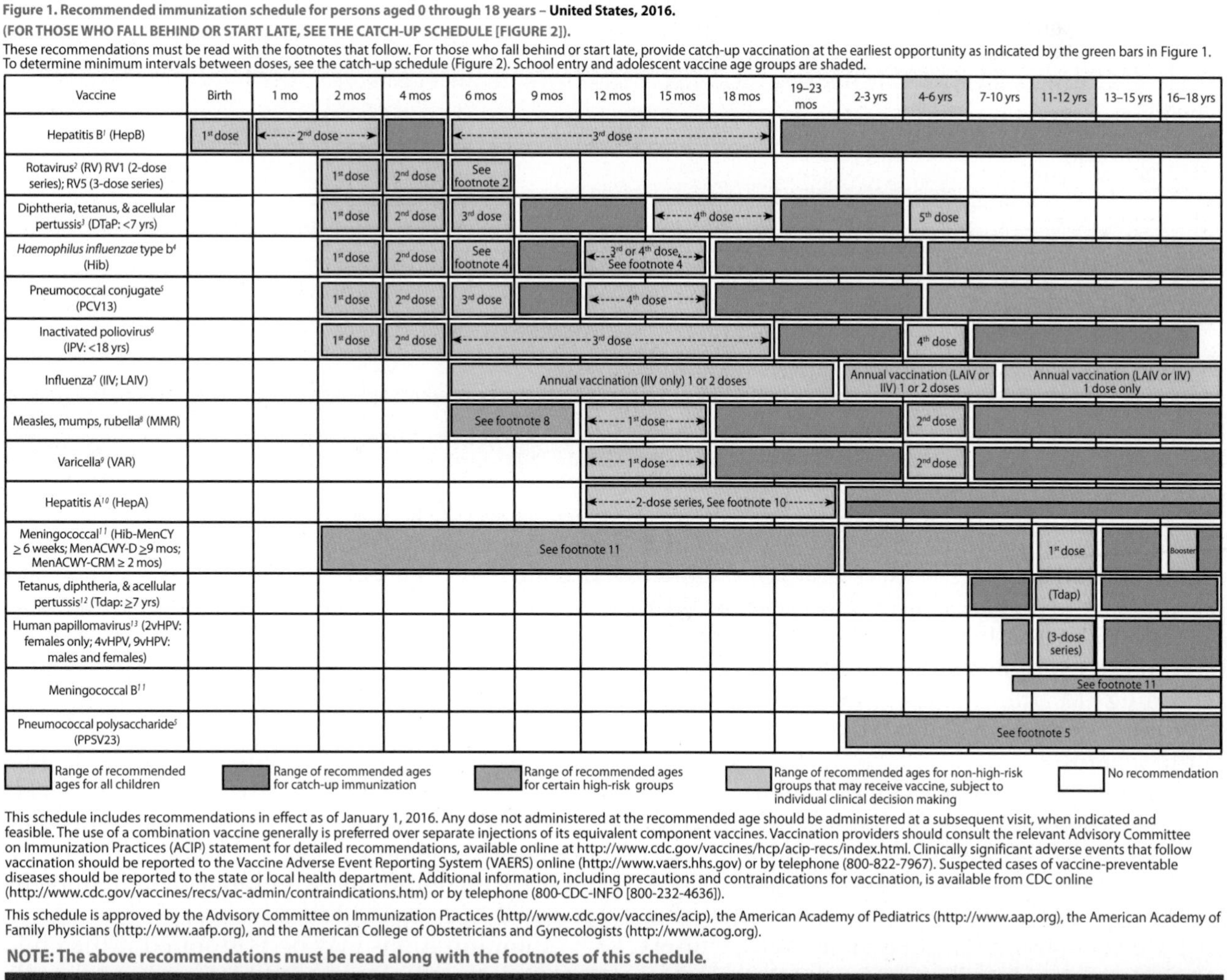

Figure 1. Recommended immunization schedule for persons aged 0 through 18 years – **United States, 2016.**
(FOR THOSE WHO FALL BEHIND OR START LATE, SEE THE CATCH-UP SCHEDULE [FIGURE 2]).

These recommendations must be read with the footnotes that follow. For those who fall behind or start late, provide catch-up vaccination at the earliest opportunity as indicated by the green bars in Figure 1. To determine minimum intervals between doses, see the catch-up schedule (Figure 2). School entry and adolescent vaccine age groups are shaded.

This schedule includes recommendations in effect as of January 1, 2016. Any dose not administered at the recommended age should be administered at a subsequent visit, when indicated and feasible. The use of a combination vaccine generally is preferred over separate injections of its equivalent component vaccines. Vaccination providers should consult the relevant Advisory Committee on Immunization Practices (ACIP) statement for detailed recommendations, available online at http://www.cdc.gov/vaccines/hcp/acip-recs/index.html. Clinically significant adverse events that follow vaccination should be reported to the Vaccine Adverse Event Reporting System (VAERS) online (http://www.vaers.hhs.gov) or by telephone (800-822-7967). Suspected cases of vaccine-preventable diseases should be reported to the state or local health department. Additional information, including precautions and contraindications for vaccination, is available from CDC online (http://www.cdc.gov/vaccines/recs/vac-admin/contraindications.htm) or by telephone (800-CDC-INFO [800-232-4636]).

This schedule is approved by the Advisory Committee on Immunization Practices (http://www.cdc.gov/vaccines/acip), the American Academy of Pediatrics (http://www.aap.org), the American Academy of Family Physicians (http://www.aafp.org), and the American College of Obstetricians and Gynecologists (http://www.acog.org).

NOTE: The above recommendations must be read along with the footnotes of this schedule.

FIGURE 26-2 The recommended schedule for persons ages 0 to 18 years is approved by the Advisory Committee on Immunization Practices (http://www.cdc.gov/vaccines/recs/acip), the American Academy of Pediatrics (http://www.aap.org), and the American Academy of Family Physicians (http://www.aafp.org).

Courtesy of the Centers for Disease Control and Prevention

The figure below provides catch-up schedules and minimum intervals between doses for children whose vaccinations have been delayed. A vaccine series does not need to be restarted, regardless of the time that has elapsed between doses. Use the section appropriate for the child's age. Always use this table in conjunction with Figure 1 and the footnotes that follow.

Vaccine	Minimum Age for Dose 1	Minimum Interval Between Doses			
		Dose 1 to Dose 2	Dose 2 to Dose 3	Dose 3 to Dose 4	Dose 4 to Dose 5
Children age 4 months through 6 years					
Hepatitis B[1]	Birth	4 weeks	8 weeks *and* at least 16 weeks after first dose. Minimum age for the final dose is 24 weeks.		
Rotavirus[2]	6 weeks	4 weeks	4 weeks[2]		
Diphtheria, tetanus, and acellular pertussis[3]	6 weeks	4 weeks	4 weeks	6 months	6 months[3]
Haemophilus influenzae type b[4]	6 weeks	4 weeks if first dose was administered before the 1st birthday. 8 weeks (as final dose) if first dose was administered at age 12 through 14 months. No further doses needed if first dose was administered at age 15 months or older.	4 weeks[4] if current age is younger than 12 months **and** first dose was administered at younger than age 7 months, **and** at least 1 previous dose was PRP-T (ActHib, Pentacel) or unknown. 8 weeks *and* age 12 through 59 months (as final dose)[4] • if current age is younger than 12 months **and** first dose was administered at age 7 through 11 months (wait until at least 12 months old); OR • if current age is 12 through 59 months **and** first dose was administered before the 1st birthday, **and** second dose administered at younger than 15 months; OR • if both doses were PRP-OMP (PedvaxHIB; Comvax) **and** were administered before the 1st birthday (wait until at least 12 months old). No further doses needed if previous dose was administered at age 15 months or older.	8 weeks (as final dose) This dose only necessary for children age 12 through 59 months who received 3 doses before the 1st birthday.	
Pneumococcal[5]	6 weeks	4 weeks if first dose administered before the 1st birthday. 8 weeks (as final dose for healthy children) if first dose was administered at the 1st birthday or after. No further doses needed for healthy children if first dose administered at age 24 months or older.	4 weeks if current age is younger than 12 months and previous dose given at <7months old. 8 weeks (as final dose for healthy children) if previous dose given between 7-11 months (wait until at least 12 months old); OR if current age is 12 months or older and at least 1 dose was given before age 12 months. No further doses needed for healthy children if previous dose administered at age 24 months or older.	8 weeks (as final dose) This dose only necessary for children aged 12 through 59 months who received 3 doses before age 12 months or for children at high risk who received 3 doses at any age.	
Inactivated poliovirus[6]	6 weeks	4 weeks[6]	4 weeks[6]	6 months[6] (minimum age 4 years for final dose).	
Measles, mumps, rubella[8]	12 months	4 weeks			
Varicella[9]	12 months	3 months			
Hepatitis A[10]	12 months	6 months			
Meningococcal[11] (Hib-MenCY ≥ 6 weeks; MenACWY-D ≥9 mos; MenACWY-CRM ≥ 2 mos)	6 weeks	8 weeks[11]	See footnote 11	See footnote 11	
Children and adolescents age 7 through 18 years					
Meningococcal[11] (Hib-MenCY ≥ 6 weeks; MenACWY-D ≥9 mos; MenACWY-CRM ≥ 2 mos)	Not Applicable (N/A)	8 weeks[11]			
Tetanus, diphtheria; tetanus, diphtheria, and acellular pertussis[12]	7 years[12]	4 weeks	4 weeks if first dose of DTaP/DT was administered before the 1st birthday. 6 months (as final dose) if first dose of DTaP/DT or Tdap/Td was administered at or after the 1st birthday.	6 months if first dose of DTaP/DT was administered before the 1st birthday.	
Human papillomavirus[13]	9 years	Routine dosing intervals are recommended.[13]			
Hepatitis A[10]	N/A	6 months			
Hepatitis B[1]	N/A	4 weeks	8 weeks **and** at least 16 weeks after first dose.		
Inactivated poliovirus[6]	N/A	4 weeks	4 weeks[6]	6 months[6]	
Measles, mumps, rubella[8]	N/A	4 weeks			
Varicella[9]	N/A	3 months if younger than age 13 years. 4 weeks if age 13 years or older.			

NOTE: The above recommendations must be read along with the footnotes of this schedule.

FIGURE 26-3 Catch-up immunization schedule for persons aged 4 months to 18 years who start late or who are more than a month behind.

Courtesy of the Centers for Disease Control and Prevention

of vaccines, appointment requirements, and time required to receive vaccines. Some clinics permit walk-in vaccination administration without cost or with a low co-payment fee. Routine well-infant examinations should be scheduled according to the recommended vaccination schedule to promote and facilitate maintenance of the schedule.

Specific manufacturer's guidelines for vaccine storage should be followed. Some vaccine preparations require refrigeration or protection from light.

Vaccines have trade names, and manufacturers have been tested for safety. The package insert of each vaccine describes the vaccine, including its route of administration, purpose, contraindications, and possible side effects (see Table 26-1). It is important to check with the parent prior to vaccine administration regarding any allergies. If a child has a known allergy to eggs, gelatin, any antibiotic, yeast, or latex, notify the provider. The presence of these allergies predicts an adverse reaction to many vaccines. A child with a damaged or suppressed immune system should not receive vaccines containing a live virus, such as MMR, varicella, or rotavirus. If the child's medical history includes diseases such as AIDS, leukemia, sickle cell disease, or cancer, or medical treatments such as steroids, chemotherapy, or radiation, this might indicate a compromised immune system and the provider must be made aware.

Immunizations may be postponed if the child has a moderate to severe cold, fever, or other illness. Be sure to inform the provider if your findings during the patient history or collection of vital signs indicate that this might be an issue.

Symptoms related to side effects, contraindications, and allergies must be known by the medical assistant, who will ensure that the parents are informed before the vaccines are given. After administration of vaccines, the medical assistant is responsible for documentation of the types of vaccines, site of administration, manufacturer's lot number, and side effects, if any have been reported by the parents (Figure 26-4). The provider will report any clinically significant adverse reactions to the Vaccine Adverse Event Reporting System (VAERS) and will file a VAERS events form for the National Immunization Program. VAERS is a national vaccine safety surveillance program co-sponsored by the Centers for Disease Control and Prevention (CDC) and the Food and Drug Administration (FDA).

Vaccine records can be kept electronically. Each child must have a personal immunization record as part of his or her permanent medical record. Parents must be provided with a Vaccine Information Statement (VIS). This contains useful information about the vaccine, including its risks and benefits. If parents have further questions, you may refer them to http://www.cdc.gov/vaccines.

It is mandated that the following information be included in the patient's electronic medical record with each immunization:

1. The vaccine manufacturer.

2. The lot number of the vaccine.

3. The date the vaccine is administered.

4. The name, office address, and title of the health care provider administering the vaccine.

5. The Vaccine Information Statement (VIS) edition date located in the lower right corner on the back of the VIS. When administering combination vaccines, all applicable VISs should be given and the individual VIS edition dates recorded.

6. The date the VIS is given to the patient, parent, or guardian.

The federally required information should be both permanent and accessible. Federal law does not require a parent, patient, or guardian to sign a consent form in order to receive a vaccination; providing them with the appropriate VIS(s) and answering their questions is sufficient under federal law.

Immunization record-keeping is mandated by both state and federal laws. An immunization information system (IIS) is a computerized database that records all immunization doses administered by participating providers to persons residing within a given geopolitical area. It is a lifetime registry that keeps track of immunizations for people of all ages. Immunization information systems now operate in all but one U.S. state. The IIS collects extensive amounts of information from the patient's EHR and serves several functions. For the provider, an IIS can provide consolidated immunization histories for use in determining appropriate client vaccinations. For organizations such as the CDC, an IIS provides aggregate data on vaccinations for use in surveillance and program operations, and in guiding public health action with the goals of improving vaccination rates and reducing vaccine-preventable disease.

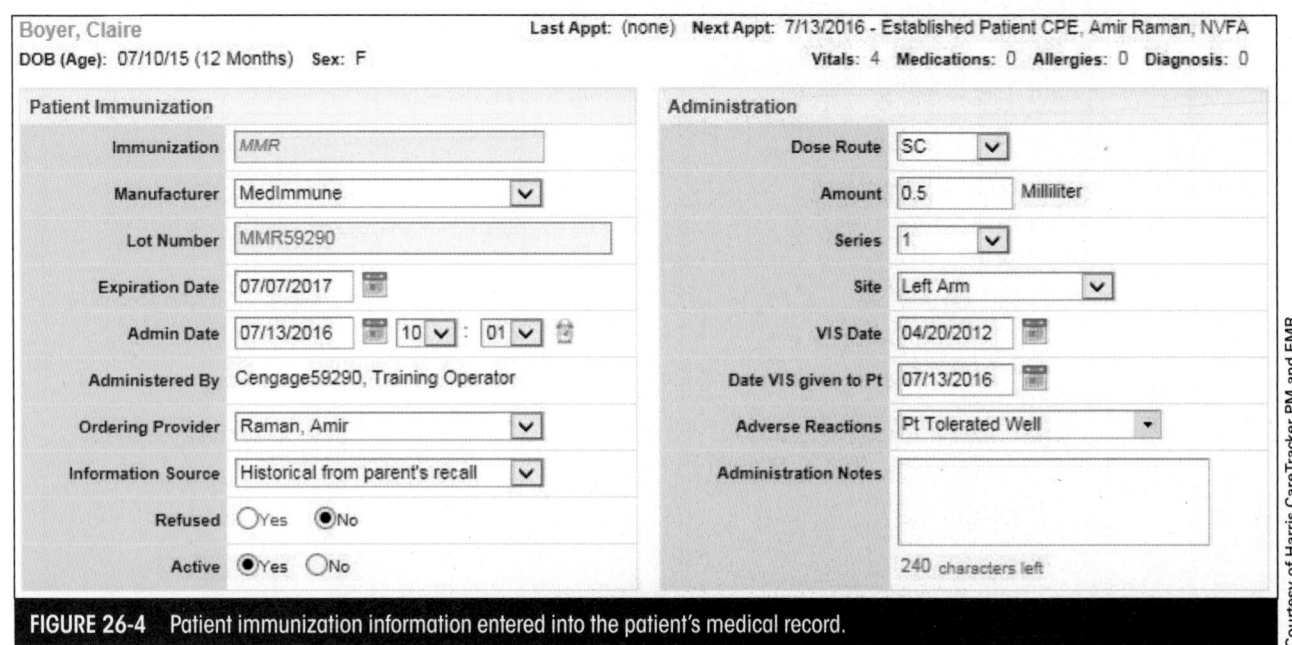

FIGURE 26-4 Patient immunization information entered into the patient's medical record.

Courtesy of Harris CareTracker PM and EMR

TABLE 26-1

VACCINE ADMINISTRATION GUIDELINES

VACCINE	DISEASE	ABOUT THE DISEASE	PRECAUTIONS AND CONTRAINDICATIONS	SIDE EFFECTS AND ADVERSE REACTIONS	VACCINE SCHEDULE	DOSE AND ROUTE OF ADMINISTRATION
DTaP, DT, Td	Diphtheria, tetanus, pertussis	Diphtheria can cause breathing problems, paralysis, heart failure, and death; tetanus causes paralysis of the jaw—cannot open mouth or swallow; pertussis (whooping cough) causes severe coughing so infants have difficulty eating, drinking, or breathing; can also cause brain damage/death	Moderate to severe acute illness, neurologic disorder, allergic reaction to prior dose	Local reactions, fussiness, seizures, fever, allergic reaction	2 months, 4 months, 6 months, 15 to 18 months, 4 to 6 years; not given at 7 years or older	0.5 mL IM
Inactive poliovirus (IPV)*	Poliomyelitis	Causes paralysis of skeletal muscles and diaphragm so that infants cannot breathe on their own	Allergic reaction to prior dose or to neomycin, streptomycin, or polymixin B; moderate to severe acute illness; pregnancy	Local reactions, allergic reaction	2 months, 4 months, 16 to 18 months, 4 to 6 years (booster)	0.5 mL IM or SQ
Haemophilus influenza type B (Hib)	Meningitis, pneumonia, epiglottitis, pericarditis	Causes bacterial meningitis, pneumonia, epiglottitis, septicemia, death	Moderate to severe acute illness, allergic reaction to prior dose	Fever, swelling, redness and/or pain; allergic reaction	2 months, 4 months, 6 months, 12 to 15 months (booster); children younger than 6 weeks old should not get vaccine	0.5 mL IM
Combination vaccines containing Hib • DTaP-Hib (TriHIBit) • Hepatitis B-Hib (Comvax)	Diphtheria, tetanus, pertussis, *Haemophilus influenzae*, hepatitis B and *Haemophilus influenzae*	See above information regarding diseases listed above	Moderate to severe acute illness	Local reaction, allergic reaction	Cannot be used at 2 months, 4 months, or 6 months; may be used as booster at 2 months, 4 months, 12 to 15 months; not given to infants younger than 6 weeks old	0.5 mL IM
Hepatitis A (HAV)	Hepatitis A	Anorexia, fatigue, itching, low-grade fever, nausea and vomiting, jaundice, death	Known allergies, pregnancy, decreased immune function	Redness, pain or swelling at the injection site, fever, loss of appetite, nausea and vomiting	Two doses given over a 6 to 18 month period beginning between the ages of 1 and 2 years	Less than or equal to 18 years old, 0.5 mL IM
Hepatitis B (HBV)	Hepatitis B	Anorexia, fatigue, diarrhea, vomiting, liver damage, cancer, death	Pregnancy, moderate to severe acute illness, allergic reaction to baker's yeast	Mild systemic effects, soreness, fever, allergic reaction	Within 12 hours of birth, 1 to 2 months, 6 months (3 doses needed)	Less than or equal to 19 years of age, 0.5 mL IM

continues

Table 26-1, continued

VACCINE	DISEASE	ABOUT THE DISEASE	PRECAUTIONS AND CONTRAINDICATIONS	SIDE EFFECTS AND ADVERSE REACTIONS	VACCINE SCHEDULE	DOSE AND ROUTE OF ADMINISTRATION
Pediatrix, DTap, HepV, IPV	Diphtheria, tetanus, pertussis, *Haemophilus influenzae*, hepatitis B, inactive poliovirus	See above information regarding diseases listed above	Moderate to severe acute illness	Mild systemic effects, local reaction, allergic reaction	2 months, 4 months, 6 months	0.5 mL IM
Td	Tetanus, diphtheria	See above information regarding diseases listed above	Moderate to severe acute illness, severe allergic reaction to prior dose	Soreness; swelling; severe allergic reaction; deep, aching pain in muscles of upper arm(s)	7 years or older then every 10 years for life	0.5 mL IM
MMR	Measles, mumps, rubella	Measles can cause otitis media, pneumonia, seizures, brain damage, death; mumps can cause fever, swollen glands, deafness, meningitis, swelling of testicles or ovaries, death; rubella can cause pregnant women to have miscarriages or babies born with severe anomalies	Do not give if allergic to gelatin or the antibiotic neomycin, moderate to severe acute illness, breast-feeding, pregnancy, immunosuppressed individuals	Fever, mild rash, swelling of glands in cheeks and neck, seizures, temporary pain in joints, severe allergic reaction	Two doses: 12 to 15 months and 4 to 6 years (or any age if longer than 28 days from first dose)	0.5 mL SQ
Varicella	Chickenpox	Severe skin infection, pneumonia, brain damage, death; shingles (herpes zoster) may occur years later	Do not give if allergic to gelatin or the antibiotic neomycin, moderate to severe acute illness	Soreness and swelling at site, fever, mild rash, seizures, pneumonia	12 to 18 months or any age if never had chickenpox	0.5 mL SQ
Influenza inactivated (IM) live, intranasal (IN) Ages 5 to 49	Influenza (flu)	Fever, cough, chills, aches, death	Do not give to pregnant women, egg allergy, history of Guillain-Barré syndrome	Soreness, redness, fever, aches, allergic reaction	All children 6 to 23 months	6 to 35 months, 0.25 mL; >3 years, 0.5 mL IM
Pneumococcal conjugate	Pneumonia, bacterial meningitis	Meningitis, septicemia, otitis media, pneumonia, deafness, brain damage	Moderate to severe illness, allergic reaction to prior dose	Redness, swelling at site, fever, drowsiness	2 months, 4 months, 6 months, 12 to 15 months	0.5 mL IM
Meningococcal conjugate	Meningitis	Infection of the brain and coverings of the spinal cord, septicemia, intellectual developmental disorder, seizures, stroke, death	Severe allergic reaction to prior dose	Allergic reaction, redness or pain at site, fever	Not for children younger than 2 years (two doses needed 3 months apart)	0.5 mL IM
Rotavirus (ROTA)	Kawasaki disease	Severe diarrhea, vomiting, fever, dehydration; cause unknown; serious in children; inflammation of small and medium-sized arteries, including coronary arteries; no test to diagnose disease (signs and symptoms used to help diagnose)	Serious allergic reaction from previous vaccine dose, serious allergic reaction to vaccine component	Allergic reaction	2 months, 4 months, 6 months	2.0 mL oral

Recommended Vaccination Schedule

The recommended vaccination schedule for infants and children is based on the premise that repeated doses of several vaccines are required and vaccine manufacturers recommend administering only compatible vaccines at any one visit to avoid drug interactions. If no contraindications are present at the various ages, vaccines should be administered according to the schedule to ensure complete vaccination by the age of 15 to 18 months, with booster vaccines on school entry and again every 10 years throughout adult life. Should any vaccine be missed for any reason, vaccine "catch-up" schedules are available to ensure adequate vaccine administration (see Figure 26-3).

Considerations for Vaccine Administration

- *Infection control.* Use Standard Precautions.
- *Handwashing.* Follow medical asepsis guidelines.
- *Gloving.* Wearing gloves may be prudent, but it is not required by OSHA.
- *Syringe selection.* A separate needle and syringe should be used for each injection. Selection of the syringe is determined by the volume of vaccine to be injected (see Table 26-2).
- *Needle selection.* Vaccine must reach the desired tissue site for optimal immune response (see Table 26-2).
- *Inspecting vaccine.* Each vaccine vial should be carefully inspected for damage or contamination and the expiration date prior to use.
- *Reconstitution.* Some vaccines are prepared in a **lyophilized** form that requires reconstitution, which should be done according to manufacturer guidelines. Read package instructions carefully. (See Chapter 35 for more information on reconstitution of medications.)
- *Prefilling syringes.* The CDC strongly discourages filling syringes in advance because of the

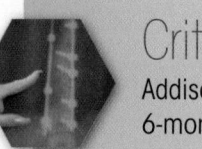
increased risk of administration errors. Under no circumstances should measles, mumps, and rubella (MMR); varicella; or zoster vaccines ever be reconstituted and drawn prior to the immediate need for them. These live virus vaccines are unstable and begin to deteriorate as soon as they are reconstituted with the diluent.

- *Labeling.* Once a vaccine is drawn into a syringe, the contents should be indicated on the syringe.
- *Multiple vaccinations.* When administering multiple vaccines, never mix vaccines in the same syringe unless approved for mixing by the Food and Drug Administration (FDA). It is recommended that separate limbs be utilized if multiple injections are required.

Vaccine doses range from 0.2 to 1 mL. The recommended maximum volume of medication for an intramuscular (IM) site varies among references and depends on the muscle mass of the individual. Simultaneous administration is sometimes required. Simultaneous administration of vaccines is defined as administering more than one vaccine on the same clinic day, at different anatomic sites, and not combined in the same syringe. If a vaccine and an immune globulin preparation are administered simultaneously (e.g., Td/Tdap and tetanus immune globulin [TIG] or hepatitis B vaccine and hepatitis B immune globulin [HBIG]), a separate anatomic site should be used for each injection. The location of each injection should be documented in the patient's chart or electronic

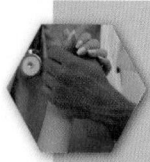

Patient Education

Encourage parents to be aware of different vaccines and to keep track of vaccination schedules. By posting recommended schedules in visible locations in the ambulatory care setting, parents can be reminded.

Figures 26-2 and 26-3 illustrate the recommended vaccination schedule for children and adolescents, which is supported by the American Academy of Pediatrics, the Advisory Committee on Immunization Practices (ACIP), the Committee on Infectious Diseases (COID), the Commission of Public Health and Scientific Affairs (COPHSA), and the American Academy of Family Physicians (AAFP).

medical record. Although the vastus lateralis is the preferred site for intramuscular injections, the deltoid is used for subcutaneous pediatric injections. Common injection sites for infants are noted in Figure 26-5 and for toddlers in Figure 26-6.

- *Nonstandard administration.* Deviation from the recommended route, site, and dosage of vaccine is strongly discouraged and can result in inadequate protection.
- *Needle gauge.* Use a 22- to 25-gauge needle.
- *Needle length.* Selection of the correct needle length is based on the tissue into which the vaccine solution is to be delivered. For a newborn or infant's intramuscular injection, a ⅝-inch needle is usually adequate. However, remember that for this age group, the needle should not be longer than 1 inch.

Children in the toddler age group require needle length from 1 to 1¼ inches if the anterolateral thigh is used. A needle that is ⅝ to 1 inch in length is the preferred choice if the deltoid muscle has adequate mass.

In the adolescent age group, both males and females weighing less than 130 pounds (60 kg), a ⅝- to 1-inch needle is sufficient to ensure IM injection. For females weighing 130 to 200 pounds (60 to 90 kg) and males weighting 130 to 260 pounds (60 to 118 kg), a 1- to 1½-inch needle is needed. If a female weighs more than 200 pounds (90 kg) or a male weighs more than 260 pounds (118 kg), a 1½-inch needle is required.

All subcutaneous injections for any age group require a needle that is no longer than ⅝ inch (see Table 26-2).

- *Injection site.* All subcutaneous injections are given in areas where there is adequate subcutaneous tissue. For all age groups, the anterolateral thigh is appropriate. For children and adolescents, the area above the triceps muscle on the posterior upper arm may also be used.

For the majority of infants (younger than 12 months), the anterolateral aspect of the thigh is the recommended site for intramuscular injection because it provides a large muscle mass. The muscles of the buttock are not used for administration of vaccines in infants and children because of concern about potential injury to the sciatic nerve, which has been well documented after injection of antimicrobial agents into the buttock. If there is a contraindication to use of the thigh, consult the provider.

For toddlers (1 to 3 years), the anterolateral thigh muscle is still the preferred injection site. At this age, the deltoid muscle may be developed adequately to be utilized for an intramuscular injection. No matter the site, care must be taken when selecting the needle length and administering the injection to avoid damage to underlying structures.

For adults and adolescents (11 years and older), the deltoid muscle is recommended for routine IM vaccinations. The anterolateral thigh can also be used.

- *Injection technique.* This is the most important factor to ensure efficient intramuscular vaccine delivery. Injectable pediatric vaccines are given either subcutaneously or intramuscularly.

All subcutaneous (SQ) injections, no matter the patient's age, are given in the same manner. The goal is to deliver the vaccine into the fatty tissues that just underlie the skin. For

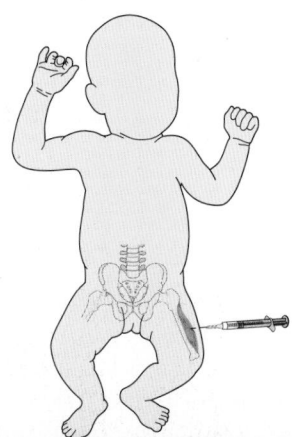

FIGURE 26-5 Injection site selection (vastus lateralis) for vaccine administration in the infant age group.

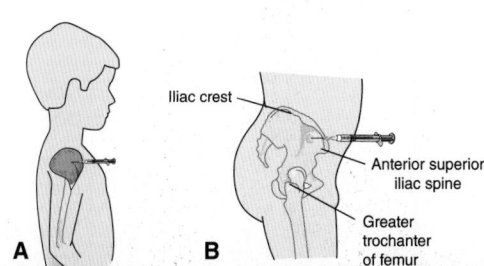

FIGURE 26-6 Injection site selection for vaccine administration in the toddler age group. (A) Deltoid. (B) Gluteal (ventrogluteal).

an SQ injection, a ⅝-inch, 23- or 25-gauge needle is inserted at a 45-degree angle to the skin. No aspiration is required for SQ injections prior to the delivery of the vaccine into the tissue.

Intramuscular (IM) injections are also delivered in the same manner no matter what the patient's age. Once the appropriate site, syringe, and needle have been selected, the 22- to 25-gauge, ⅝- to 1¼-inch needle is inserted into the tissue at a 90-degree angle. The depth of insertion is based on the patient's anatomic structure and should not exceed the depth required to deliver the vaccine into the muscle.

The maximum volume that can be delivered IM varies based on the age of the child. Consult with your provider to determine the limits set in your practice. Generally, a neonate or a very small infant should not have more than 0.5 mL injected IM. For a small child, a maximum of 1 mL is recommended. Larger children and adolescents may have up to 3 mL as the maximum volume injected. It is best to consult your provider if you are unsure, to avoid damage to the muscular tissue of your patient.

Table 26-2 gives information on administering vaccines.

Giving Injections to Pediatric Patients

Infants and toddlers who are receiving injections must be held in such a way that they cannot move. This is done for two reasons: to protect the child from injury and to provide access to an injection site. Parents must be informed of the procedure for administering injections. Their increased knowledge and understanding will allow the injection process to proceed with few complications.

Safety

Children who are 2 to about 4 years old are not emotionally developed enough to understand the need for cooperation. You will need help from the parent or another staff member to hold the child securely, thus avoiding injury. The deltoid is the preferred site for this age group. One method used to restrict the child's movement is to seat the child on the parent's lap. The parent wraps his or her legs around the child's legs to limit movement. The parent or staff member holds down the noninjection arm. The injection can be given once the child is securely immobilized (Figure 26-7).

Presentation   Communication

Once the child reaches toddlerhood, it is very likely that anticipation of the injection, or "shot," will cause high anxiety. It is important for the professional medical assistant to maintain a calm and deliberate manner when administering immunizations. Before beginning, explain the procedure to the parents and check for

---

TABLE 26-2

INJECTION GUIDE FOR INFANTS AND CHILDREN

TYPE OF INJECTION	ANGLE OF INJECTION (DEGREES)	AGE OF PATIENT	NEEDLE LENGTH (INCHES)	NEEDLE GAUGE	INJECTION SITE
Subcutaneous	45	Infant (newborn to 12 months)	⅝	23 to 25	Fatty subdermal tissue over anterolateral thigh muscle
	45	Children (12 months or older) adolescents and adults	⅝	23 to 25	Fatty tissue over the triceps, abdomen, or anterior thigh over the quadriceps muscle
Intramuscular injection	90	Newborn (0 to 28 days)	⅝	22 to 25	Vastus lateralis
	90	Infants (1 to 12 months)	1	22 to 25	Vastus lateralis
	90	Toddlers (1 to 2 years)	⅝ to 1 1 to 1¼	22 to 25 22 to 25	Deltoid muscle, vastus lateralis
	90	Children and teens (3 to 18 years)	⅝ to 1 1 to 1¼	22 to 25 22 to 25	Deltoid, vastus lateralis

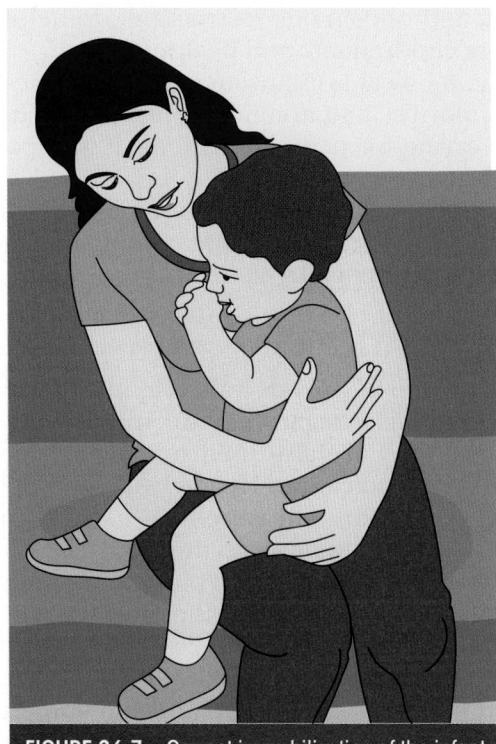

FIGURE 26-7 Correct immobilization of the infant or toddler prior to injection is a safety precaution.

understanding of their role during the injection. Examine the patient to determine the most appropriate injection site ahead of the actual injection. Prepare the syringes out of sight of the patient. When all medication checks have been performed (see Chapter 35), approach the patient in a calm and reassuring manner. Perform the skin prep and injection without unnecessary delay. This will reduce the stress on the child, the parent, and you, the medical assistant.

Adverse Reactions. Adverse reactions are defined as any undesirable aftereffect once a vaccine is given. These vaccine-related adverse effects are classified as local, systemic, or allergic. Localized reactions may include redness, irritation, and/or itching at the site of injection. Localized reactions are by far the most common. Systemic effects may include fever. Allergic reactions can be severe and life threatening. (Additional information is available at http://www.fda.gov).

Syncope, also known as fainting, can occur after vaccination and is most common among adolescents and young adults. It is important to protect this age group from secondary injuries, like head injury, with a syncopal episode. Patients should remain in the provider's office for at least 15 minutes for observation after vaccine administration. Your provider will indicate any interventions that need to be implemented if a reaction of any kind occurs.

Competency

Your role as the professional medical assistant may include education postimmunization. It is important to follow the provider's orders for postimmunization care. Parent education may include administering a nonaspirin pain reliever and encouraging increased fluid intake for fever and relief of discomfort. The application of a cool, moist cloth to an area of redness and swelling will increase feelings of comfort for the child.

Serious reactions are uncommon. However, it is important to educate parents that if their baby cries for 3 or more hours without stopping, seems limp or unresponsive, starts having seizures (convulsions), or is unresponsive, or if they are worried at all about how their baby looks or behaves, they should call the provider immediately.

Vaccine Safety. It is important for the medical assistant to know that parents may ask about vaccine safety and preservatives. The following information is helpful; however, the provider is the best individual to answer specific questions parents may have.

A 2013 CDC study added to the research showing that vaccines do not cause autism spectrum disorder (ASD). This study looked at the number of substances in vaccines that cause the body's immune system to produce disease-fighting antibodies during the first 2 years of life. The results showed little difference in the number of these substances in children with ASD and those without.

Thimerosal is one vaccine ingredient that has been studied specifically. Thimerosal is a mercury-based preservative used to prevent contamination of multidose vials of vaccines. Multiple research studies demonstrate that thimerosal does not cause ASD. In fact, a 2004 scientific review by the Institute of Medicine concluded that "the evidence favors rejection of a causal relationship between thimerosal-containing vaccines and autism."

Since 2003, there have been nine CDC-funded or -conducted studies that have found no link between thimerosal-containing vaccines and ASD, as well as no link between the measles, mumps, and rubella (MMR) vaccine and ASD in children.

Between 1999 and 2001, to reduce all types of mercury exposure in children, thimerosal was removed or reduced to trace amounts in all childhood vaccines except for some flu vaccines. This was done prior to studies that determined thimerosal was not harmful. It was done as a precaution. Currently, the only childhood vaccines that contain thimerosal are flu vaccines packaged in multidose vials. For patients or parents that are concerned, thimerosal-free alternatives are also available for flu vaccines.

Besides thimerosal, some people have had concerns about other vaccine ingredients in relation to ASD. However, no links have been found between any vaccine ingredients and ASD.

THEORIES OF GROWTH AND DEVELOPMENT

Before providing more in-depth information about the various stages of growth and development in children, it is important to review the major theorists who have contributed to understanding human growth and development.

There are at least eight or nine theories of human development put forth by Freud (psychosexual), Erickson (psychosocial), Sullivan (interpersonal), Piaget (cognitive), Kohlberg (moral), Bronfenbrenner (ecology), Pavlov and Skinner (behavioral), and Bandura (social learning). Each theory focuses on particular aspects of human development and its principles, strengths, and weaknesses.

No single theory can explain human development. It is important that the professional medical assistant understand these theories in order to assist in the assessment of a child or adolescent's appropriate maturation.

Table 26-3 provides more information about growth and development at the various stages of a child's life.

Professional   Legal

Communication with pediatric patients needs to be individualized and show acceptance, empathy, honesty, and openness. Confidentiality must be maintained regardless of age. Parents and caregivers are involved with the care of their youngsters; therefore, they have the legal right to know the medical matters relating to their minor children. Adolescents may share information with the medical assistant that they do not want their parents or other caregivers to know. It is important to stress that some matters may need to be shared with parents or caregivers, especially when adolescents are living at home (certain matters pertaining to birth control, abortion, pregnancy, and sexually transmitted diseases pose special problems). Some states allow minors to give their consent under these circumstances (see Chapter 6).

Medical assistants can teach parents and caregivers in various ways. Handouts, demonstrations, videos, and one-on-one instruction are helpful in keeping children safe and healthy.

The medical assistant must be caring, respectful, supportive, and nonjudgmental of all patients. When caring for pediatric patients it is important to reflect these values. Family beliefs and values also must be taken into account. This will foster care for pediatric patients that is compliant and in the best interest of all.

GROWTH PATTERNS

Growth patterns provide valuable information to the pediatrician regarding the infant's physical progress. They are also used to calculate pediatric doses of medication. Height, weight, and head circumference are measured at each regularly scheduled appointment at the pediatric facility. The measurements are then plotted on a physical growth percentile chart that is part of the patient's permanent record (Figure 26-8). Careful measuring of the infant or child and monitoring of growth patterns are essential and should be done in a consistent and accurate manner.

Length and Weight Measurements

Procedure

To record or plot length and weight measurements, you must first locate one growth value, either length or weight, in the vertical columns of the physical growth percentile chart shown in Figure 26-9. Find the child's age in months in the horizontal rows. Locate the area where the growth value lines intersect on the graph and plot the length and weight by marking with a dot. Connect dots from previous values with a ruler to provide a neat and accurate graphic recording. The date, age, measurements, and comments should also be indicated at the bottom of the chart (see Procedure 26-1).

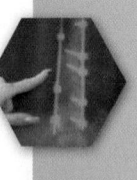

Critical Thinking

May Mobley has an appointment today for her 18-month checkup. She will be receiving her appropriate immunizations and the provider has asked that you perform a Denver Developmental Screening Test to assure that May is meeting her developmental benchmarks. After assessment, you see that May is delayed in several language activities. What is your best course of action? (*NOTE*: To review the Denver test form, go to http://denverii.com.)

TABLE 26-3

PEDIATRIC GROWTH AND DEVELOPMENT

AGE	VITAL SIGNS AND MEASUREMENTS	PHYSICAL ATTRIBUTES	GROWTH AND DEVELOPMENT THEORIES	PATIENT EDUCATION TO BE PROVIDED
Newborn (0 to 28 days) © Nadia Cruzova/Shutterstock.com	Respiratory rate, 50 to 63 breaths per minute Respiratory rhythm may be irregular in depth and rhythm, shallow, and abdominal Heart rate • 100 to 205 beats per minute when awake • 90 to 160 beats per minute when sleeping Blood pressure • Systolic, 67 to 84 mm Hg • Diastolic, 35 to 53 mm Hg • Not measured in newborns unless there is an indication Length, head circumference, weight (these vary by gestational age, genetics, and any underlying pathology)	Movements are mostly involuntary Visual acuity is increasing Sense of touch is most highly developed of the senses Reflexes • Moro (startle) • Rooting • Sucking and swallowing • Grasping Fontanels (both anterior and posterior are open)	Oral stage (Freud) Trust vs. mistrust (Erikson) Maslow • Physiological • Safety • Love and belonging Gratification of needs (Sullivan) Sensorimotor stage (Piaget)	Bottle-feeding guidelines Breast-feeding support Safe sleep guidelines Intake/output Stool types and frequency Diapering Cord care Hand washing Bathing/skin care Circumcision care Crying/sleep patterns Signs and symptoms of illness Safety

continues

continues

Table 26-3, continued

AGE	VITAL SIGNS AND MEASUREMENTS	PHYSICAL ATTRIBUTES	GROWTH AND DEVELOPMENT THEORIES	PATIENT EDUCATION TO BE PROVIDED
Infant (1 month to 1 year) 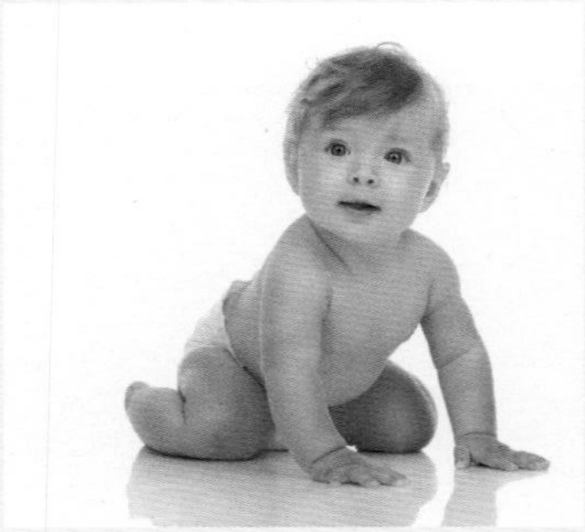	Respiratory rate, 30 to 53 breaths per minute Respiratory rhythm • Regular • Abdominal movement is normal Heart rate • 100 to 190 beats per minute while awake • 90 to 160 beats per minute while sleeping Blood pressure • Systolic, 72 to 104 mm Hg • Diastolic, 37 to 56 mm Hg • Not usually measured in infants unless there is an indication Length • Increases by about 1 inch per month • 50% increase from birth weight by 12 months Head circumference increases rapidly until age 6 months, then slows Weight • Double birth weight by 6 months • Triple birth weight by 12 months (vary by age, genetics, and any underlying pathology)	Increasing ability to control head • Head lag is measured by pulling the infant to a sitting position from supine by the arms • No head lag is expected by at 4 months Gross and fine motor skills develop (measured with an array of tools, e.g., the Denver Developmental Screening Tool) Verbalization • Babbles in what sounds like short sentences, complete with vocal inflections by age 1 year • Vocabulary is a few words (usually up to five) including *Mama* and *Dada* by age 1 year Crawling is expected between 6 and 10 months Walking is expected between 9 and 16 months Fontanels (posterior may close by 12 months)	Oral and anal stages (Freud) Trust vs. mistrust (Erikson) Maslow • Physiological • Safety • Love and belonging Gratification of needs (Sullivan) Sensorimotor stage (Piaget)	Adult–child interactions Safety Schedules and routines Developmental milestones Nutrition Signs and symptoms of illness Vaccines Frequency of well-child visits

© Dmitry Lobanov/Shutterstock.com

Table 26-3, continued

AGE	VITAL SIGNS AND MEASUREMENTS	PHYSICAL ATTRIBUTES	GROWTH AND DEVELOPMENT THEORIES	PATIENT EDUCATION TO BE PROVIDED
Toddler (1 to 3 years) © Samuel Borges Photography/Shutterstock.com	Respiratory rate, 22 to 37 breaths per minute Respiratory rhythm regular Heart rate • 98 to 140 beats per minute while awake • 80 to 120 beats per minute while sleeping Blood pressure • Systolic, 86 to 106 mm Hg • Diastolic, 42 to 63 mm Hg • Not usually measured in toddlers unless there is an indication Height increases by about 3 inches per year Weight gain of approximately 5 pounds per year (vary by age, genetics, and any underlying pathology)	Increasingly independent Gains bowel and bladder control Walks by age 12 to 15 months Climbs stairs by 18 months Gains verbal skills • By 2 years of age, 50% of words are intelligible • By 3 years of age, 75% of words are intelligible • Average vocabulary of 200 words at age 2 and up to 450 words by age 3 Able to follow commands and respond to simple questions by age 1, with ability increasing with age Eating habits change • Eats when hungry • Fewer calories needed related to slowing of growth	Anal stage (Freud) Autonomy vs. shame and doubt (Erikson) Maslow • Physiologic • Safety • Love and belonging • Esteem Delayed gratification (Sullivan) Piaget • Sensorimotor stage • Preoperational stage	Communicating with your child Safety, especially aspiration prevention Structure and rules Discipline and consequences Developmental milestones Nutrition Healthy eating habits Signs and symptoms of illness, especially otitis media, tonsillitis, and upper respiratory infection Vaccines Well-child visits Potty training
Preschool (4 to 5 years) © wong sze yuen/Shutterstock.com	Respiratory rate, 20 to 28 breaths per minute Respiratory rhythm regular Heart rate • 80 to 120 beats per minute while awake • 65 to 100 beats per minute while sleeping Blood pressure • Systolic, 89 to 112 mm Hg • Diastolic, 46 to 72 mm Hg Height increases by about 3 inches per year Weight gain of approximately 2 pounds per year (varies by age, genetics, and any underlying pathology)	Full control over bowel and bladder habits Able to • Run • Skip • Jump • Ride a bike • Jump rope • Feed self • Play with others • Share Interacts freely with others Vocabulary of 1,000 words by age 4 years Sexual curiosity begins Learning occurs through play and imitation of adults Creative and uses imagination Beginning of reading skills Participation in sports such as T-ball, karate, gymnastics	Phallic stage (Freud) Initiative vs. guilt (Erikson) Maslow • Physiologic • Safety • Love and belonging • Esteem Delayed gratification (Sullivan) Preoperational stage (Piaget)	Hand washing for children Frequency of well-child visits Laboratory testing Vision screening Physical activity needs Safety Vaccines Developmental milestones Nutrition Signs and symptoms of illness

continues

Table 26-3, continued

AGE	VITAL SIGNS AND MEASUREMENTS	PHYSICAL ATTRIBUTES	GROWTH AND DEVELOPMENT THEORIES	PATIENT EDUCATION TO BE PROVIDED
School-age (6 to 12 years) 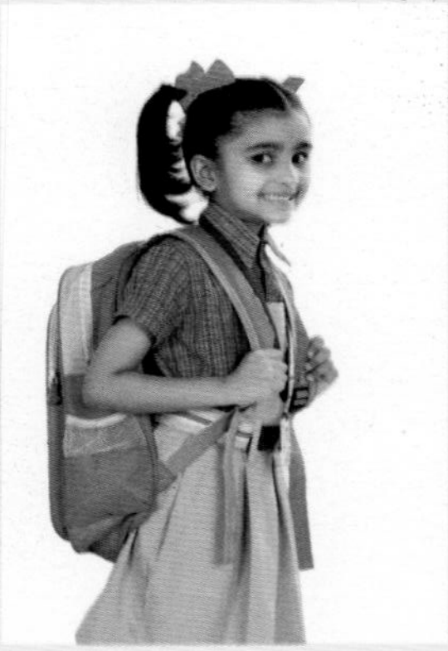	Respiratory rate, 18 to 25 breaths per minute Respiratory rhythm, regular Heart rate • 75 to 118 beats per minute while awake • 58 to 90 beats per minute while sleeping Blood pressure • Systolic, 97 to 115 mm Hg • Diastolic, 57 to 76 mm Hg Height increases by about 2 inches per year Weight gain of approximately 5 pounds per year (These vary by age, genetics, and any underlying pathology)	Improving mastery over motor skills Ages 6 to 8: • Participates in team sports • Develops ball skills with smaller ball • Enhanced game skills like hopscotch and jump rope • Rides a two-wheel bike • Runs up and down stairs Middle childhood: • Swims • Roller and ice skates • Jumps rope • Climbs fences • Uses a saw, hammer, and garden tools • Plays a variety of sports Immunity improved secondary to previous vaccines During the last years of the school-aged period, may begin to develop secondary sexual characteristics (breasts, body hair, etc.) Increasing importance of peer relationships Increasing independence from parents and family Language skills increase • Able to comprehend complex content • By age 6, vocabulary is 13,000 words • By age 12, understands 50,000 words	Latent period (Freud) Industry (competence) vs. inferiority (Erikson) Maslow • Physiologic • Safety • Love and belonging • Esteem Sullivan • Formation of peer group • Development of same-gender relationships Concrete operational stage (Piaget)	Need for physical exam every 2 years Need for booster immunizations Detection of use of recreational drugs, alcohol, or tobacco Nutritional counseling Detection of emotional issues (suicide, depression, eating disorders) Safety with a focus on accident prevention Bullying Stress reduction

© Rajesh Narayanan/Shutterstock.com

continues

Table 26-3, continued

AGE	VITAL SIGNS AND MEASUREMENTS	PHYSICAL ATTRIBUTES	GROWTH AND DEVELOPMENT THEORIES	PATIENT EDUCATION TO BE PROVIDED
Adolescent © Zurijeta/Shutterstock.com	Respiratory rate, 12 to 20 breaths per minute Respiratory rhythm, regular Heart rate • 60 to 100 beats per minute while awake • 60 to 90 beats per minute while sleeping Blood pressure • Systolic, 110 to 131 mm Hg • Diastolic, 64 to 83 mm Hg Height • Male: growth up to 6 inches or more • Female: growth up to 5 inches or more Weight • Male: gain up to 14 pounds • Female: gain up to 10 pounds (varies by age, genetics, and any underlying pathology)	Wide variety of physiologic changes Develops increased coordination and motor ability Greater physical strength and prolonged endurance Develops better distance judgment and hand-eye coordination Masters the skills necessary for adult sports, with practice Independence from parents and family Focuses on career goals	Genital stage (Freud) Identity vs. role confusion (Erikson) Maslow • Physiologic • Safety • Love and belonging • Esteem Sullivan • Identity • Forming lasting intimate relationships Formal operational stage (Piaget)	Recommended annual health screenings Detection of use of recreational drugs, alcohol, or tobacco Nutritional counseling Detection of emotional issues (suicide prevention, depression, eating disorders) Safety with a focus on accident prevention Bullying Stress reduction Sexually transmitted disease prevention and testing Tuberculosis testing Hepatitis B and C testing

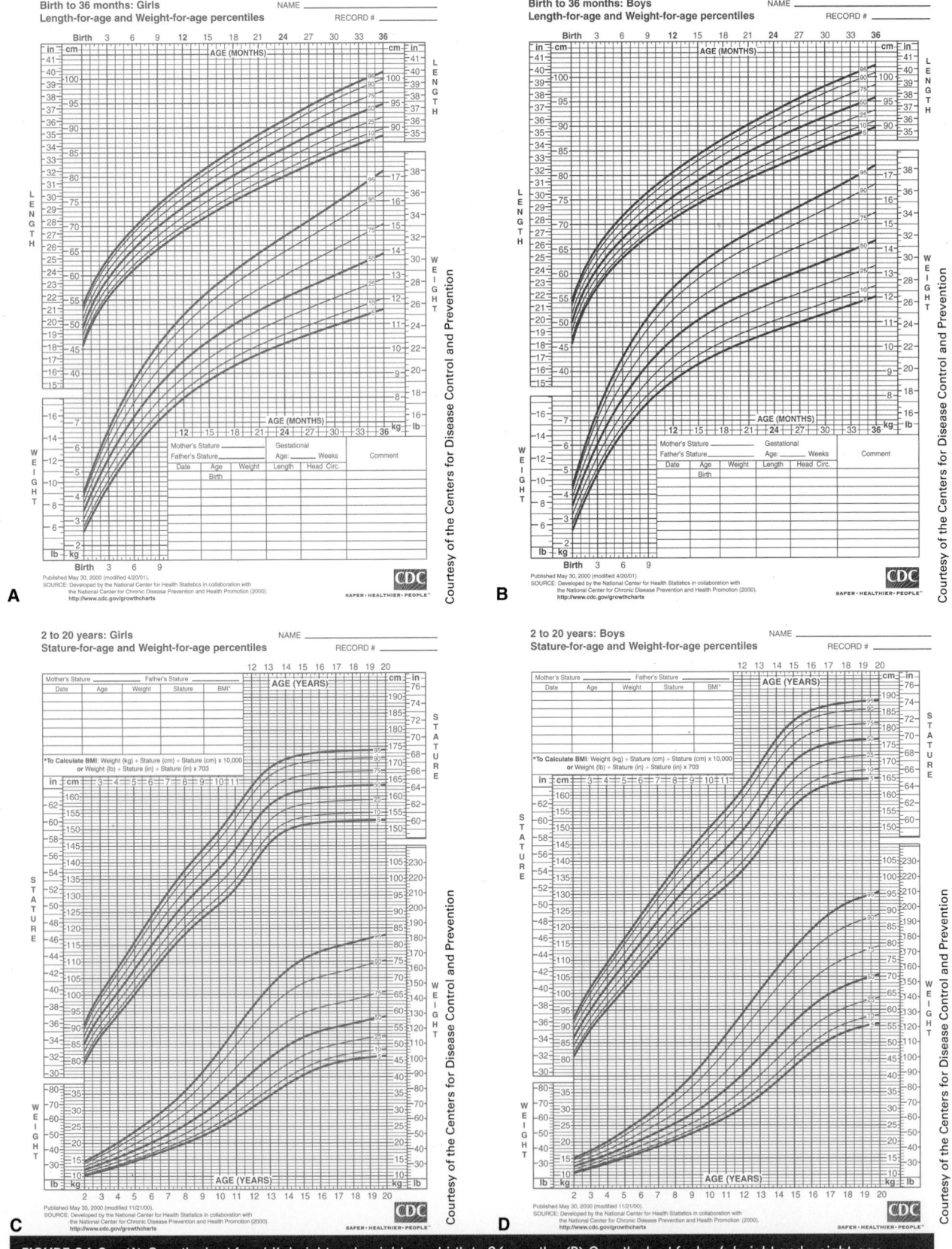

FIGURE 26-8 (A) Growth chart for girl's height and weight, age birth to 36 months. (B) Growth chart for boy's height and weight, age birth to 36 months. (C) Growth chart for girl's height and weight, age 2 to 20 years. (D) Growth chart for boy's height and weight, age 2 to 20 years. Note that the growth charts shown in (A) and (B) provide space at bottom right of chart for date, age, weight, length and head circumference.

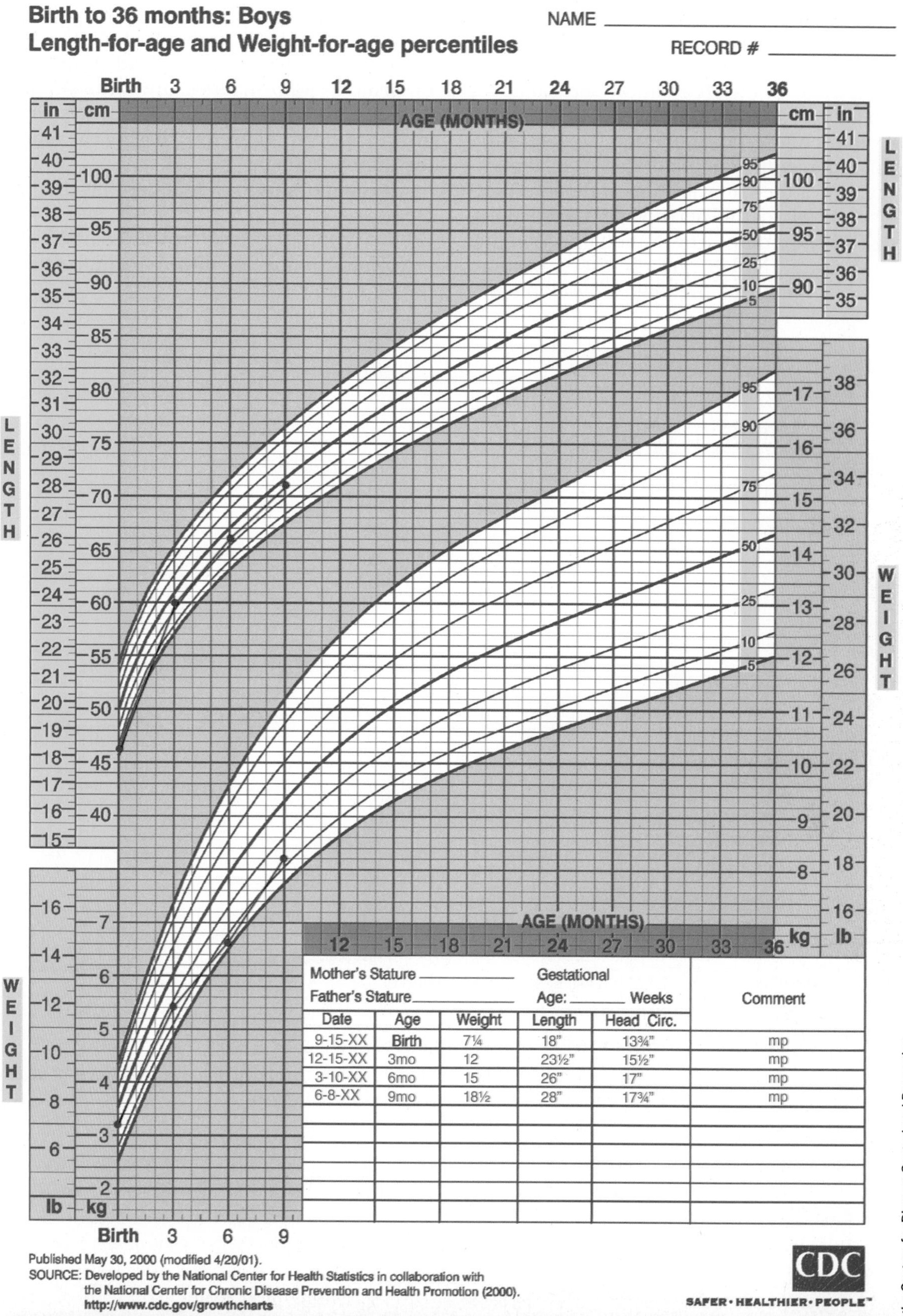

FIGURE 26-9 Sample growth chart information plotted at birth and 3, 6, and 9 months. Sections in this figure are highlighted to help you locate the values: length (yellow), weight (pink), age (green), and percentiles (white).

Published May 30, 2000 (modified 4/20/01).
SOURCE: Developed by the National Center for Health Statistics in collaboration with
the National Center for Chronic Disease Prevention and Health Promotion (2000).
http://www.cdc.gov/growthcharts

Date	Age	Weight	Length	Head Circ.	Comment
9-15-XX	Birth	7¼	18"	13¾"	mp
12-15-XX	3mo	12	23½"	15½"	mp
3-10-XX	6mo	15	26"	17"	mp
6-8-XX	9mo	18½	28"	17¾"	mp

Mother's Stature _____
Father's Stature _____
Gestational Age: _____ Weeks

Courtesy of the Centers for Disease Control and Prevention

The curved lines printed across the growth charts show the normal range of growth of infants and children in the United States. The numbers on the right side of the chart, in the vertical boxes between ages 34 and 35 months, show the percentiles of other children the same age. To determine into which percentile the infant falls in relation to other infants of the same age, follow the line (percentile) upward to the percentage values along the edge of the graph. The National Center for Health Statistics (NCHS) growth charts become a permanent record of the child's development.

These give the provider a quick way to check the child's growth in relation to that of other children the same age. Growth charts aid in the diagnosis of growth abnormalities and nutritional disorders and disease. Hereditary factors also influence growth patterns; therefore, having the family's history is important.

It is important to remember that children with Down syndrome, achondroplasia, and Turner syndrome require specific growth charts. These can be found online at http://pedinfo.org/growth.php.

PROCEDURE 26-1

Procedure

Maintain Pediatric Growth Charts

STANDARD PRECAUTIONS:

Handwashing

PURPOSE:

To record accurate measurements of a child's weight, length, and head circumference for medical records and to screen for growth abnormalities.

EQUIPMENT/SUPPLIES:

- Patient's medical record
- Pen
- Growth chart

PROCEDURE STEPS:

1. Assemble the equipment that you will need for the procedure.
2. Wash hands and follow Standard Precautions.
3. Introduce yourself to the child's parent or guardian. Identify patient using two identifiers.
4. *Explain the rationale for performance of the procedure to the parent, speaking at the parent's level of understanding. Show awareness of the parent's concerns related to the procedure*.
5. Select the appropriate growth chart based on the child's gender and age.
6. *Incorporating critical thinking skills when performing patient care*, obtain measurement data from the patient's chart and the appropriate growth chart depending on the infant or child's age. This includes patient's weight, height, and head circumference.
7. Using the length for age and weight for age percentiles chart, locate the patient's age on the growth chart.
8. Locate the patient's height on the growth chart. *Pay attention to detail* when plotting the child's length. RATIONALE: Depending on the child's length, you will find this in the left or right margin of the chart.

(continues)

9. Locate the patient's weight on the growth chart. ***Pay attention to detail*** when plotting the child's weight. RATIONALE: Depending on the child's weight, you will find this in the left or right margin of the chart.

10. Locate the spot on the graph where the age on the horizontal line and child's stature or length (height) on the vertical line intersect, and plot the measurement by making a dot on the chart.

11. Follow the curved line from the dot that was plotted up to the right to discover the percentile representing the child's growth compared to 100 normally growing children in the United States.

12. Repeat the process for the child's weight. RATIONALE: You can also determine the percentile in which the child falls by following the line on which the measurement is plotted to the side of the paper where the percentiles are indicated.

13. Using the head circumference for age and weight for length percentiles chart, locate the spot on the graph that represents the child's head circumference. Plot it the same way as you have done for the height and weight. RATONALE: The weight-to-length percentile is also determined on this graph by plotting them both and finding their intersection.

14. Complete the demographics box chart on the growth chart with the date, patient's age, weight, height, and head circumference. This will allow the provider to compare growth over time by comparing dates.

15. Your provider may request that you connect the dots of the measurements over time with a thin line as shown in Figure 26-9.

Height and Weight Measuring Devices

Various devices are available for measuring height and weight in children. Infants and small children are weighed on an infant platform scale, which provides a measurement in pounds and ounces as well as kilograms and grams (Figure 26-10). The scale has a platform with curved sides on which the child may sit or lie. Weigh the infant or child in as few clothes as possible, removing the diaper and shoes or slippers. A small sheet, cloth diaper, or paper towel should be placed on the scale before weighing the infant or child, to avoid the transfer of microorganisms from bare skin. (The scale is sanitized and disinfected between patients.)

Infant length can be measured using an infant measuring board, which consists of a rigid headboard and movable footboard. Place the measuring board on a table and position the infant on his or her back on the board, with the head touching the headboard. Move the footboard up until it touches the bottom of the infant's feet (Figure 26-11).

An infant can also be measured on a pad by placing a pin into the pad or making a pencil mark at the top of the head and a second pin or mark at the heel of the extended leg. The length is the distance between the two pins. A tape measure can also be used. (*NOTE:* 1 inch = 2.54 cm.)

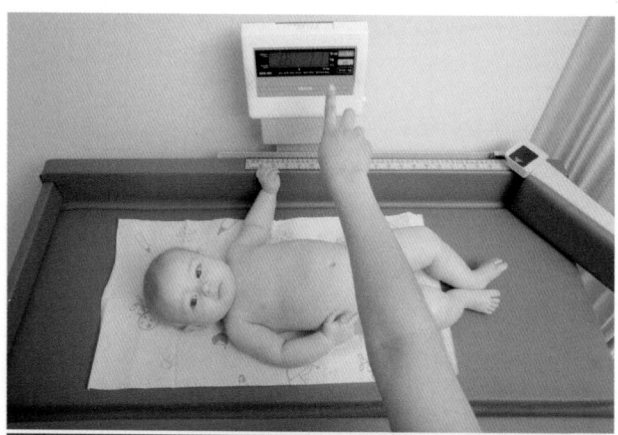

FIGURE 26-10 Infants who are able to sit and small children can be weighed on a platform scale.

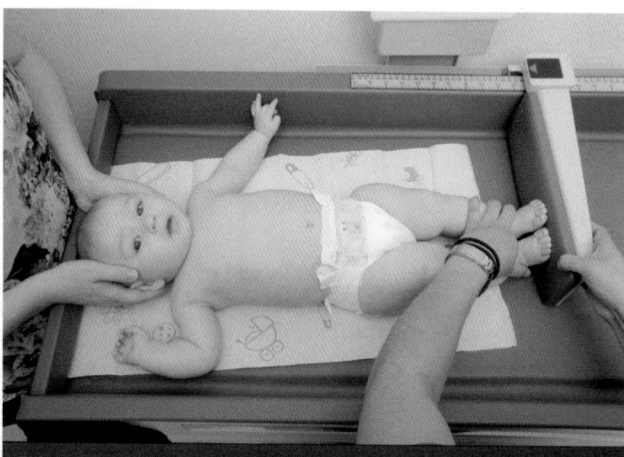

FIGURE 26-11 Measuring the recumbent length of an infant, from the vertex of the head to the heel.

A stature-measuring device can be used to measure height once the child is able to stand erect without support. The device consists of a movable headpiece attached to a rigid measuring bar and platform. A paper towel should be placed on the platform before use to avoid the potential transmission of microorganisms from bare feet.

Measuring Head Circumference

Head circumference measurement is routinely recorded on an infant's chart to alert the provider to any abnormal development. This procedure should be performed during routine visits until the child is 36 months old. Thereafter, it should be measured on a yearly basis until the age of 6 years. Head circumference measurement requires a flexible paper or metal measuring tape (Figure 26-12). A cloth tape may stretch and give a false measurement. Head circumference is plotted similarly to height and weight but on separate growth percentile charts for head measurements (Figure 26-13).

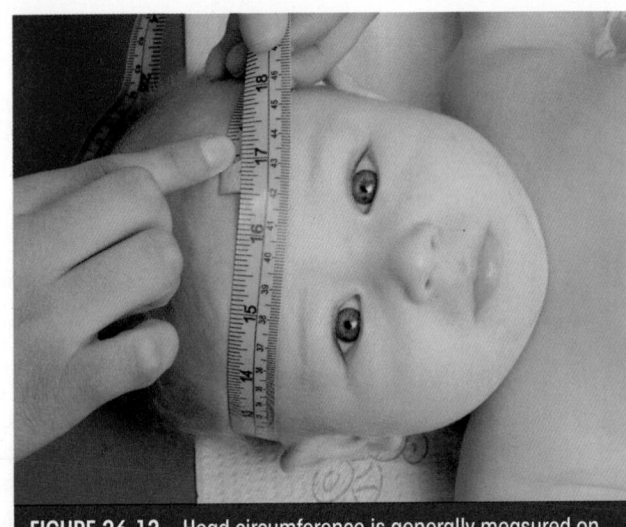

FIGURE 26-12 Head circumference is generally measured on infants and children until age three years.

Generally, head and chest circumference are equal at about 1 to 2 years of age. Rapid growth above the normal percentile may indicate hydrocephalus,

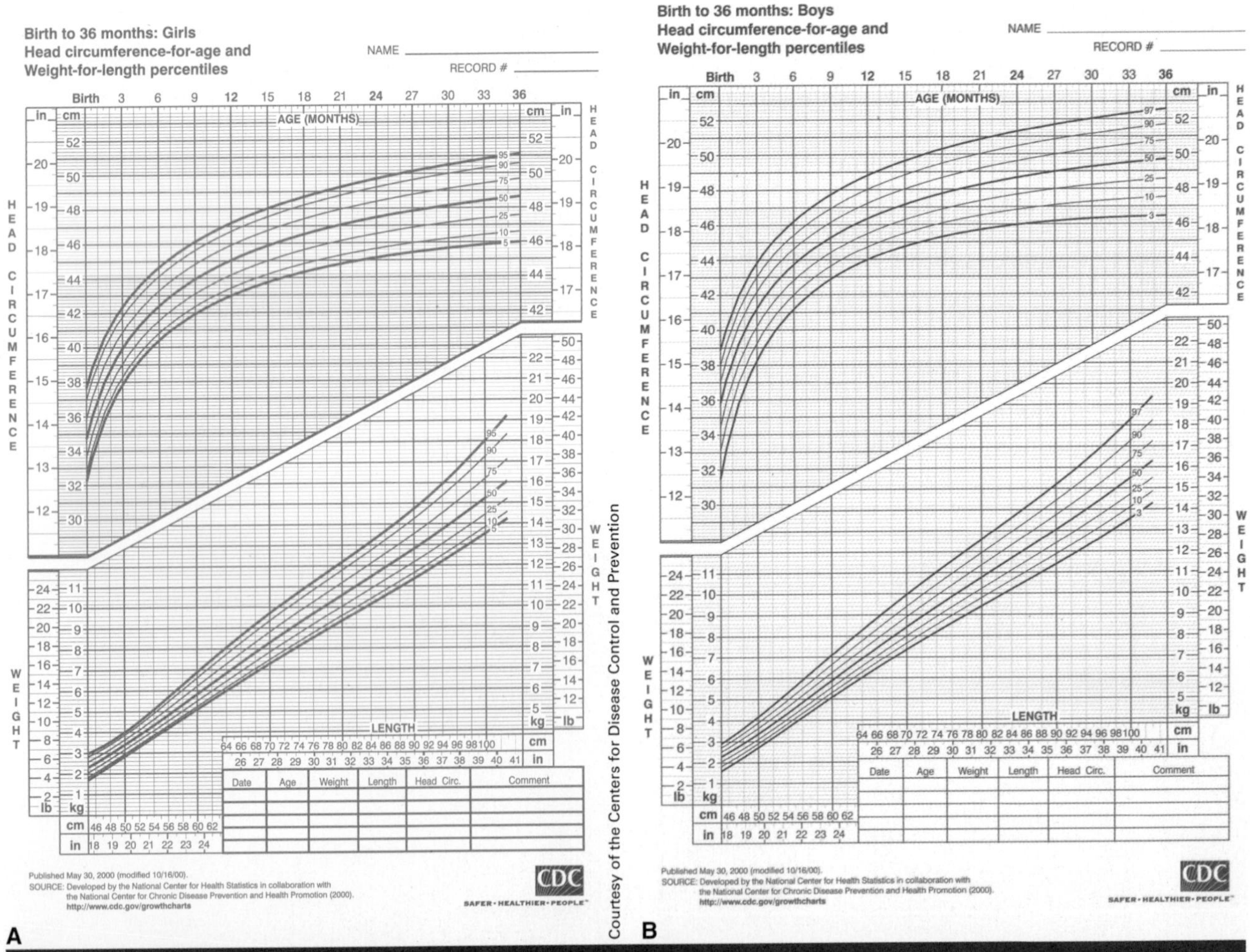

FIGURE 26-13 (A) Growth chart for girl's head circumference, birth to 36 months. (B) Growth chart for boy's head circumference, birth to 36 months.

a disorder in which excessive fluid accumulates around the brain causing an increase in intracranial pressure and possible brain damage. This could lead to mental and physical problems. Conversely, head growth that falls below the normal percentile may indicate microencephaly caused by a premature closure of the **fontanels**. In this instance, there is not enough room for the brain to develop, and intellectual developmental disorder can result. Head circumference for a newborn should be 12.5 to 14.5 inches (31.75 to 36.83 cm).

Measuring Chest Circumference

Measuring the chest circumference of an infant is not normally performed during routine examinations. It may be performed and monitored when there is a suspicion of overdevelopment or underdevelopment of the heart or lungs or calcification of rib cartilage. To measure the chest of an infant, snugly wrap the measuring tape around the chest at nipple level (Figure 26-14). It is preferable to read the measurement during the resting phase between respirations.

 Occasionally, it is necessary for the medical assistant to convert measurement results into inches or centimeters. To accomplish the task accurately, note that 1 inch equals 2.54 cm. (Procedure 26-2 gives steps for measuring infant chest and head circumference, weight, and height.)

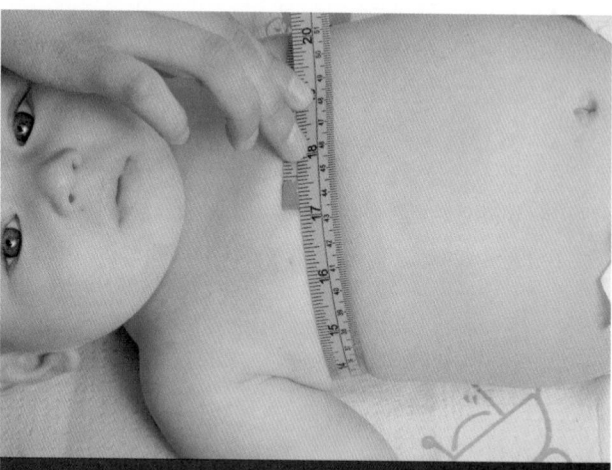

FIGURE 26-14 Chest circumference is measured at the level of the nipple using a flexible measuring tape.

Example:

To convert inches to centimeters, multiply the number of inches by 2.54:

10 inches × 2.54 = 25.4 centimeters

Example:

To convert centimeters to inches, divide the number of centimeters by 2.54:

10 centimeters ÷ 2.54 = 25.4 inches

PROCEDURE 26-2

Measuring the Infant: Weight, Length, and Head and Chest Circumference

Procedure

STANDARD PRECAUTIONS:

Handwashing   Biohazard

PURPOSE:

To obtain an accurate measurement of an infant's weight, length, and head and chest circumference for medical records and to screen for growth abnormalities.

EQUIPMENT/SUPPLIES:

- Infant scale
- Pen
- Paper protector
- Ruler

- Flexible measuring tape without elasticity
- Patient growth booklet/growth chart

- Biohazard waste container
- Disinfectant spray
- Disposable towels

(continues)

PROCEDURE STEPS:

1. Assemble the equipment that you will need for the procedure.
2. Wash hands and follow Standard Precautions.
3. Introduce yourself to the child's parent or guardian. Identify patient using two identifiers.
4. ***Explain rationale for performance of the procedure to parent, speaking at the parent's level of understanding. Show awareness of the parent's concerns related to the procedure.***
5. ***Being courteous and respectful,*** enlist the assistance of the parent to undress infant (including the diaper) while you prepare the scale.
6. ***Paying attention to detail,*** place a clean utility towel on scale and check balance scale for accuracy, being sure to compensate for the weight of the towel. RATIONALE: The protection that the paper utility towel affords helps to reduce transmission of microorganisms and provides warmth because the scale is cool.
7. If the infant is small, gently place him or her on his or her back on the scale. Larger infants can sit on the scale. Place your hand slightly above the infant's body to ensure safety (see Figure 26-10). Never leave the infant unattended on the scale at any time. RATIONALE: This will safeguard the infant from falling.
8. Read the scale when the infant is still to ensure accuracy of the weight obtained.
9. Record the patient weight on the table paper or on scratch paper, using pounds or kilograms as per the provider's preference.
10. Gently remove infant and apply diaper. (Parent can help with diapering and holding infant.)
11. Discard used protective paper towel per OSHA guidelines.
12. Proceed with the infant's height measurement by gently placing the infant on his or her back on the exam table. Ask the parent to gently hold the infant's feet while you place a mark on the table paper at the top of the patient's head. This will serve as the "zero" point for the measurement.
13. Gently straighten the infant's back and legs. It may be necessary to place a hand over the patient's knees to assist in keeping the legs in place.
14. Use a pen to place a mark on the table paper at the bottom of the patient's heel.
15. Measure the recumbent length from head to heel and record on scratch paper, using either inches or centimeters as directed by the provider.
16. The infant may remain on the examination table for measurement of the head circumference. Enlist the parent to assist in holding the child. An older toddler can sit for this measurement, but remember that for safety reasons, a child must not be left unattended on the table at any time.
17. Place the flexible nonelastic measuring tape around the infant's head from the occipital protuberance to the supraorbital prominence. RATIONALE: This is the largest part of the head.
18. Read the measurement and record this on scratch paper using inches or centimeters per the provider's preference.
19. Continue with the chest measurement. Use one thumb to hold the tape measure with the zero mark against the chest at the mid-sternal area.
20. With the other hand wrap the tape measure around the infant's back to meet the zero mark in the front. The tape should be positioned at the nipple line and below the axillary area. The measurement is taken during the resting phase of normal respiration.
21. Record the measurement to the nearest ⅛ inch or 0.1 cm per the provider's preferences.
22. Ask the parent to assist in dressing the child. Wash hands and record the findings in the medical record. Make a note of all information in the patient's growth chart or booklet as appropriate.
23. Sanitize the scale when the measurements are completed and wash your hands.

(continues)

DOCUMENTATION:

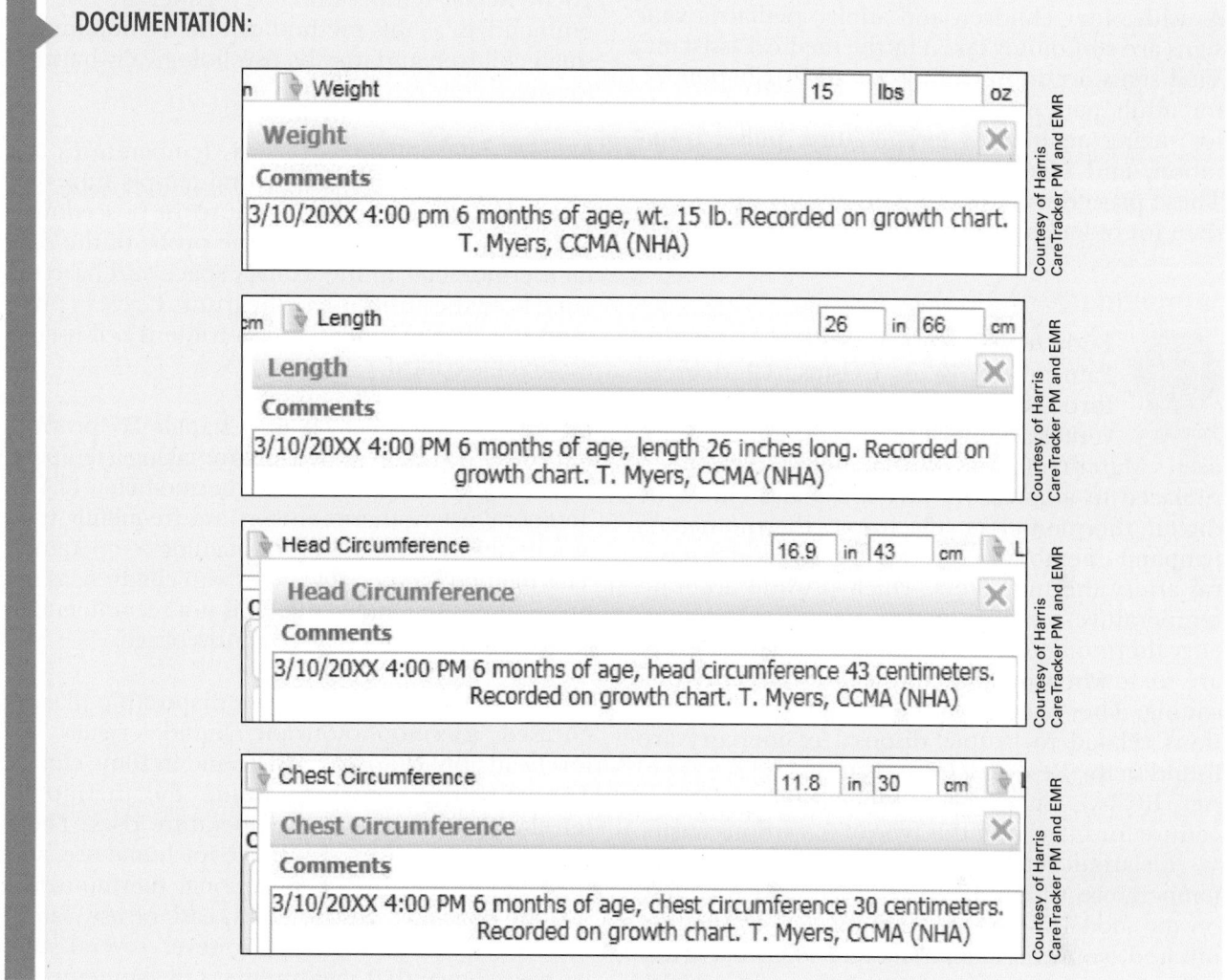

| Weight | 15 | lbs | | oz |

Weight   ✕

Comments

3/10/20XX 4:00 pm 6 months of age, wt. 15 lb. Recorded on growth chart.
T. Myers, CCMA (NHA)

Courtesy of Harris CareTracker PM and EMR

| Length | 26 | in | 66 | cm |

Length   ✕

Comments

3/10/20XX 4:00 PM 6 months of age, length 26 inches long. Recorded on
growth chart. T. Myers, CCMA (NHA)

Courtesy of Harris CareTracker PM and EMR

| Head Circumference | 16.9 | in | 43 | cm |

Head Circumference   ✕

Comments

3/10/20XX 4:00 PM 6 months of age, head circumference 43 centimeters.
Recorded on growth chart. T. Myers, CCMA (NHA)

Courtesy of Harris CareTracker PM and EMR

| Chest Circumference | 11.8 | in | 30 | cm |

Chest Circumference   ✕

Comments

3/10/20XX 4:00 PM 6 months of age, chest circumference 30 centimeters.
Recorded on growth chart. T. Myers, CCMA (NHA)

Courtesy of Harris CareTracker PM and EMR

Infant/Child Failure to Thrive

Sometimes an infant or child does not meet the expected standards of growth. A good definition of failure to thrive (FTT) is failure to maintain an established pattern of growth and development that responds to the provision of adequate nutritional and emotional needs to the child. Most cases of FTT are not related to neglectful caregiving, although FTT may be a sign of maltreatment, which should be considered during an evaluation for growth failure.

A thorough history must be taken in order to assist the provider in diagnosing FTT. The focus for this historical documentation includes maternal and neonatal medical histories, infant/child medical history, food intake and feeding, and psychosocial elements.

Many causes of an infant or a child failing to grow and thrive may be a manifestation of child neglect. Other reasons for an infant failing to thrive may be because the infant has a chronic disease; has a diet that is inadequate, especially in calories and proteins; has a disorder of the heart, brain, or kidneys; or has been improperly fed. Adequate nutrition is especially critical in the first few years of life to ensure physical growth and development.

Detecting FTT is important because the first 2 years of a child's life are a sensitive period of rapid brain growth when neurodevelopmental outcomes can be influenced. Motor, fine motor, speech, language, and cognitive delays have been documented in cases of FTT. Children with extreme failure to thrive in the first year may never catch up to their peers even if their physical growth improves. In about one third of these extreme cases, mental development remains below normal and roughly half will continue to have psychosocial and eating problems throughout life.

PEDIATRIC VITAL SIGNS

As with older children and adults, pediatric vital signs are commonly taken by the medical assistant. Vital signs are more fully covered in Chapter 23 for adult patients; however, specific procedures for taking an infant's temperature, pulse, respiration, and blood pressure are explained here. These procedures are done differently for infants than for older children and adults.

Temperature

Procedure

Body temperature may be measured in Fahrenheit (F) or Celsius (C) degrees through oral, rectal, axillary, or tympanic routes. Many types of thermometers are used. Mercury (glass) thermometers have been replaced in ambulatory care areas and clinics by digital thermometers; electronic thermometers; tympanic membrane sensors (aural); and temporal artery thermometers, which provide accurate temperature readings in less time. Broken mercury thermometers release vapors into the air that are toxic when inhaled and lead to mercury poisoning. They should not be used. Federal regulations related to proper disposal of mercury are found in the Resource Conservation and Recovery Act (RCRA). Check your facility's policy and procedure for managing this type of hazardous waste.

Electronic and digital thermometers can display temperature within 15 to 60 seconds, depending on the model used. A reading can be obtained on infrared tympanic membrane and temporal artery sensors in a matter of seconds (see Procedure 26-3).

Oral Temperature. The oral route is used for children older than 5 years. Caution the child against biting down on the thermometer. Do not take an oral temperature if the child has a history of seizures.

Aural Temperature. The aural route uses the tympanic membrane thermometer. It is used on children older than 2 years because it is considered less accurate for children younger than 2 years. Otitis media and impacted cerumen are two other reasons this route may not be selected. A reading can be obtained in a matter of seconds.

Rectal Temperature. Rectal temperatures are the most accurate from birth to 2 years, but care must be taken when utilizing this method. Place the child supine, with the knees flexed. An infant can also lie prone on a parent's lap. Do not force the thermometer. Rectal temperatures are not indicated for children who have had rectal surgery or for those who have diarrhea (see Procedure 26-3). Rectal temperatures are generally not recommended, as this method can be frightening for small children and may be psychologically harmful for older children.

Axillary Temperature. Axillary temperatures are often preferable to rectal or oral temperatures for toddlers and preschoolers because the procedure is safe and nonintrusive. Place the probe of the digital thermometer in the axillary space and have the child hold the arm close to the trunk. Leave in place until the "beep" is heard. This route is not used if accuracy is critical.

Temporal Artery Temperature. Chapter 23 provides information and the procedure for taking a temperature using a temporal artery thermometer (TAT). Temporal artery thermometers are frequently used as a noninvasive method for obtaining temperature. This method is especially useful with children, as the procedure is fast and gentle. It is not recommended for children younger than 3 months of age.

Skin Temperature. Single-use disposable plastic-encased thermophototropic liquid crystals for forehead application may be found in some clinics. The substance contained within the thermometer changes color as the temperature rises. These thermometers are most suitable for home use, and their advantages over conventional thermometers include convenient instruction, ease of use, safety, comfort, and rapid results. However, several studies have shown that measurement of skin temperature by these devices is inaccurate; they frequently record a normal temperature despite an elevated body temperature.

Pulse

Procedure

The apical pulse is heard at the apex of the heart, located at the fifth intercostal space left side, midclavicular line, that is, between the fifth and sixth ribs in the middle of the clavicle (usually below the nipple), left of the sternum. A stethoscope is required to obtain an apical pulse. The apical pulse is generally preferred over pulses from other locations for infants and small children (younger than 5 years). Each lub-dub sound is counted as one heartbeat. The pulse is counted for 1 full minute (see Procedure 26-4).

The normal pulse rate varies with age, decreasing as the child grows older (see Table 26-3). The heart rate may also vary considerably among children of the same age and size. The heart rate

PROCEDURE 26-3

Procedure

Taking an Infant's Rectal Temperature with a Digital Thermometer

STANDARD PRECAUTIONS:

Handwashing

Gloves

Biohazard

PURPOSE:

To obtain a rectal temperature using a digital thermometer.

EQUIPMENT/SUPPLIES:

- Digital thermometer (red probe) and probe cover
- Lubricating jelly
- 4 × 4 gauze sponges
- Gloves
- Biohazard waste container

PROCEDURE STEPS:

1. *Paying attention to detail*, assemble equipment.
2. Introduce yourself to the parent. Identify patient using two identifiers.
3. *Explain rationale for performance of the procedure to parent, speaking at the parent's level of understanding. Show awareness of the parent's concerns related to the procedure*. RATIONALE: Gain cooperation and assistance in disrobing infant and positioning properly.
4. Wash hands and follow Standard Precautions.
5. *Being courteous and respectful*, enlist the parent's assistance to undress the infant (including the diaper).
6. Position infant in a prone (Figure 26-15A) or supine (Figure 26-15B) position, having parent or another medical assistant safeguard infant.
7. Open the packet of lubricating jelly or squeeze a small amount onto a 4 × 4 gauze sponge.
8. Don nonsterile gloves.
9. Place a probe cover on thermometer. RATIONALE: Prevents microorganism cross-contamination.
10. Lubricate the thermometer with lubricating jelly. RATIONALE: Easier insertion of thermometer.
11. Spread buttocks, insert thermometer gently into the rectum past the sphincter; for an infant this is 0.5 inch (Figure 26-15B).

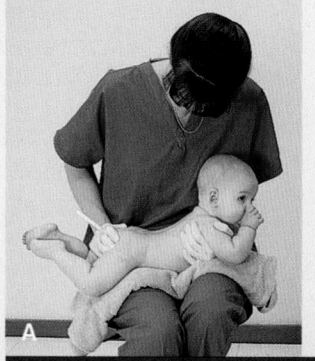
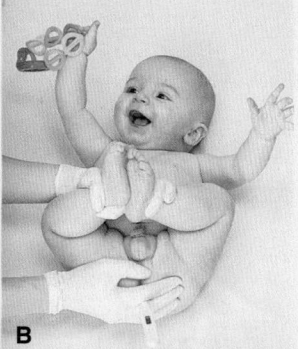

FIGURE 26-15   Taking the rectal temperature of an infant in (A) the prone position and (B) the supine position.

(continues)

12. Hold buttocks together while holding the thermometer. If necessary, restrain infant movement by placing your arm across infant's back. Parent can immobilize infant's legs. RATIONALE: Ensures infant's safety and comfort.

13. Hold thermometer in place until the "beep" is heard. Do not let go of the thermometer. RATIONALE: Movement by infant can cause thermometer to move and injure the infant.

14. Remove thermometer from rectum.

15. Enlist the parent's assistance in attending to the infant. Provide wipes to remove any leftover lubricating jelly. The diaper may be reapplied at this time.

16. Note temperature reading.

17. Remove probe cover by ejecting it into a biohazard container.

18. Wipe probe with antiseptic wipe. Replace thermometer on charger.

19. Remove gloves, discard in biohazard waste container.

20. Wash hands.

21. Accurately record all information in patient's medical record with the designation of (R) indicating rectal temperature.

DOCUMENTATION:

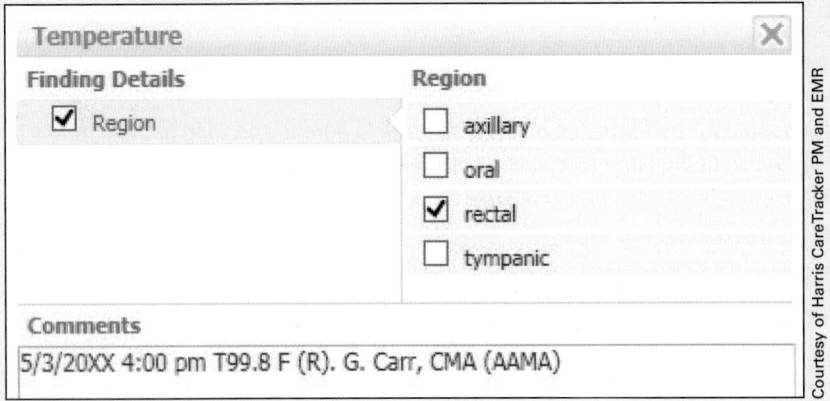

Courtesy of Harris CareTracker PM and EMR

PROCEDURE 26-4

Procedure

Taking an Apical Pulse on an Infant

STANDARD PRECAUTIONS:

Handwashing

PURPOSE:

To obtain an apical pulse rate.

EQUIPMENT/SUPPLIES:

- Stethoscope
- Watch with second hand
- Alcohol wipes

(continues)

PROCEDURE STEPS:

1. *Paying attention to detail*, assemble equipment.
2. Introduce yourself to the parent. Identify patient using two identifiers.
3. *Explain the rationale for performance of the procedure to the parent, speaking at the parent's level of understanding. Show awareness of the parent's concerns related to the procedure.* RATIONALE: Gains cooperation and assistance.
4. *Being courteous and respectful*, enlist the assistance of the parent to undress the infant (including the diaper).
5. Provide a drape for infant's warmth if necessary.
6. Wash hands and follow Standard Precautions.
7. Gently position the infant in a supine position or sitting on the parent's lap. RATIONALE: The supine position may offer easier access to apex of heart if the child is calm.
8. Locate the fifth intercostal space, midclavicular line, left of sternum. RATIONALE: Location of apex of heart.
9. Warm the stethoscope by rubbing the bell between hands, place on the site, and listen for the lub-dub sound of the heart.
10. Count the pulse for 1 minute while watching the second hand; each lub-dub equals one heartbeat or pulse.
11. Allow the parent to redress the infant.
12. Clean earpieces and diaphragm of stethoscope with alcohol wipes. RATIONALE: Prevents cross-contamination of microbes between patients.
13. Wash hands.
14. Accurately record the pulse in the patient's chart or electronic medical record. Designate (AP) to indicate apical pulse. Note any arrhythmias.

DOCUMENTATION:

Pulse Rate	X
Finding Details	**Region**
☐ Quality	☑ apical
☐ Location	☐ brachial
☐ Characterized BY	☐ corotid
☑ Region	☐ dorsalis pedis
	☐ femoral
	☐ popiteal
	☐ posterior tibial
	☐ radial
	☐ ulnar
Comments	
3/10/20XX 4:00 pm Pulse 140 (AP). Regular. J. Guerrero, CMA (AAMA)	

Courtesy of Harris CareTracker PM and EMR

increases in response to exercise, excitement, anxiety, and fever and decreases to a resting rate when the child is still.

Listen to the heart rate, noting whether the heart rhythm is regular or irregular. Children often have a normal cycle of irregular rhythm associated with respiration called sinus arrhythmia. In sinus arrhythmia, the child's heart rate is faster on inspiration and slower on expiration. Record whether the pulse is normal, bounding, or thready.

Respirations

Procedure

In older children and adolescents, the respiratory rate is counted in the same way as in an adult. In infants and children younger than 6 years, however, the respiratory rate is assessed by observing the rise and fall of the chest wall. Inspiration (when the chest or abdomen rises) and expiration (when the chest or abdomen falls) are counted as one respiration. Because these movements are often irregular, they should be counted for 1 full minute for accuracy. Normal respiratory rate varies with the child's age (see Table 26-3 and Procedure 26-5).

PROCEDURE 26-5

Procedure

Measuring Infant's Respiratory Rate

STANDARD PRECAUTIONS:

Handwashing

PURPOSE:

To measure respiratory effort by timing rate and observing rhythm and depth of respiration. The recording of this information assists the provider in the diagnosis of respiratory and cardiac diseases.

EQUIPMENT/SUPPLIES:

Watch with second hand

PROCEDURE STEPS:

1. Wash hands and follow Standard Precautions.
2. ***Identify the patient and explain the procedure to the parent, speaking at the parent's level of understanding. Show awareness of the parent's concerns related to the procedure.*** RATIONALE: Gains cooperation and assistance.
3. Position infant in a supine position.
4. Place hand on the chest to feel the rise and fall of the chest wall for 1 minute.
5. Note depth and rhythm while counting.
6. Wash hands.
7. Accurately record all information in patient's chart or electronic medical record. Note any irregularities in depth or rhythm.

DOCUMENTATION:

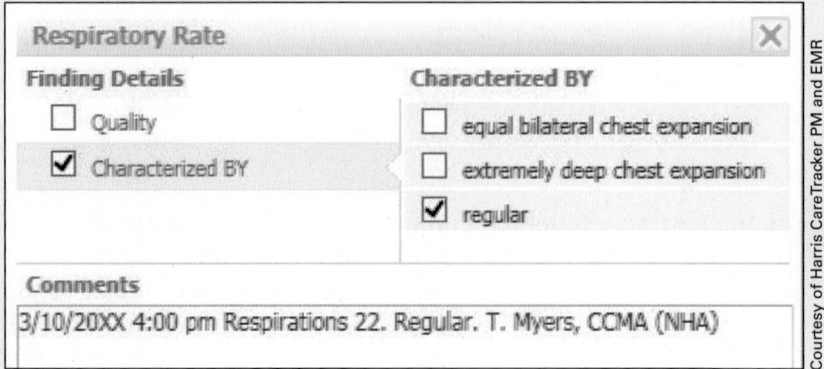

Blood Pressure

The blood pressure of an infant is not normally taken unless requested by the provider. In children 3 years of age and older, blood pressure should be measured annually as part of a routine vital sign assessment.

Blood pressure can be measured using electronic or aneroid equipment and a pediatric cuff. There are a variety of sizes available. Taking care to select the appropriate cuff will allow for the most accurate blood pressure reading. If the cuff is too small, pressure will be falsely high; if too large, falsely low. Sometimes it is difficult to hear the blood pressure in an infant or small child. Use a pediatric stethoscope over pulse sites if possible.

If the pulse still cannot be auscultated, the blood pressure can be measured by touch. Palpate for the pulse. Keeping your fingers on the pulse, pump up the cuff until the pulse is no longer felt. Slowly open the air valve as you watch the dial, and note the number where the pulse is again palpated. This is called the palpated systolic blood pressure.

COLLECTING A URINE SPECIMEN FROM AN INFANT

 Occasionally, the medical assistant is required to obtain a urine specimen from an infant for laboratory testing.
Procedure Special procedures and equipment are required for this procedure. The collection bag is clear plastic with adhesive tabs (clean catch bag) for application to the perineum of the infant (Figure 26-16; see Procedure 26-6).

The clean catch bag has been a popular way to obtain a clean catch specimen for urinalysis in pediatric patients. The urinalysis is essential to the provider's workup of the patient. Not only is it time consuming to wait for a child to void, but many times, the bag is empty. There are risks of contamination of the specimen by the bag method. According to the *Internet Journal of Emergency Medicine,* a procedure known as direct urethral bladder catheterization is the preferred method for obtaining a sterile urine specimen. A very small catheter (5 French) is used. Using sterile technique, the catheter is inserted through the urethra into the bladder of the pediatric patient. The procedures used on infants and children is the same as the procedures for performing urinary catheterization on male and female patients described in Chapter 29. Catheterization of a pediatric patient in order to obtain a sterile urine specimen is an invasive

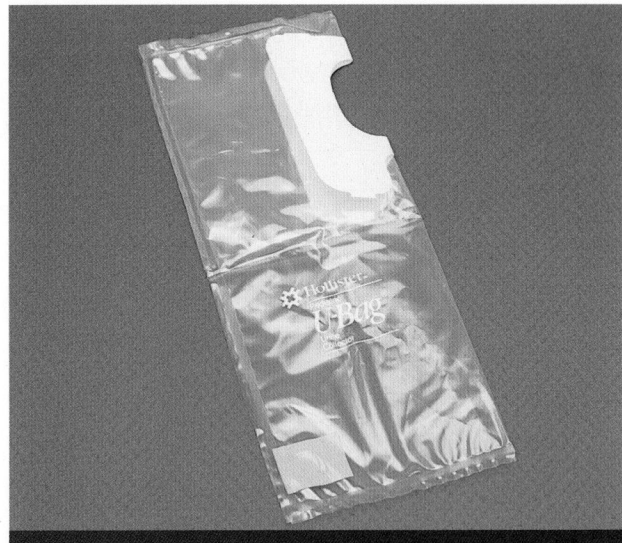

FIGURE 26-16 Pediatric urine collector. The collector is opened, and the paper backing is removed, exposing the adhesive surface. The collector is firmly attached over the child's cleansed genitalia to prevent leakage.

procedure performed by a licensed provider. A California study confirmed that catheterization is safe and effective, particularly in the emergency department, when a pediatric patient has a fever and symptoms of a urinary tract infection.

SCREENING INFANTS FOR HEARING IMPAIRMENT

In some hospitals, infants are screened for hearing impairment immediately after delivery. An automated system for checking hearing ability is used by some clinics. It is a more complex screening requiring the use of sensors. As the infant moves in response to sounds produced by the system, these responses are recorded by sensors attached to the infant. The procedure is a more definitive screening process. The medical assistant must maintain a quiet environment while these screening procedures are being performed because extraneous sounds may invalidate the results. For older children, a referral to an audiologist is indicated, especially if there is a delay in speech noted on developmental screening.

SCREENING INFANT AND CHILD VISUAL ACUITY

Measuring the visual acuity of an infant is difficult and is not usually performed unless visual impairment is suspected. Newborns will respond to light by tightly shutting their eyes and keeping them

Obtaining a Urine Specimen from an Infant or Young Child

Procedure

STANDARD PRECAUTIONS:

Handwashing   Gloves   Biohazard

PURPOSE:

To obtain a specimen of urine from an infant or young child.

EQUIPMENT/SUPPLIES:

- Pediatric urine collection bag
- Urine cup with label
- Marking pen
- Laboratory request form
- Biohazard transport bag

- Gloves
- Cleansing towelette
- Paper towel
- Biohazard waste container
- Nonsterile gloves

PROCEDURE STEPS:

1. ***Paying attention to detail***, assemble equipment.
2. Wash hands and follow Standard Precautions.
3. Introduce yourself to the parent or guardian. Identify patient using two identifiers.
4. ***Explain the rationale for performance of the procedure to the parent, speaking at the parent's level of understanding. Show awareness of the patient's concerns*** by allowing time for questions and answers. RATIONALE: Gains cooperation and assistance.
5. ***Being courteous and respectful***, enlist the assistance of the parent to disrobe patient and remove the diaper.
6. Don nonsterile gloves.
7. Place the infant on his or her back, spread legs to expose the genital area, and wash and dry the perineal area. RATIONALE: Cleaning the area reduces microorganism level and provides better quality urine specimen.
8. Apply collection bag by peeling away the coverings over the adhesive area. Apply the narrowest section of the exposed adhesive against the most posterior part of the perineum.
   a. Girls: spread perineum, place bag over labia
   b. Boys: place bag over penis and scrotum
9. Working outward from the point of first adherence, smooth the rest of the adhesive area against the skin. Press the adhesive firmly against the skin to secure. Avoid wrinkles, as they allow channels for leakage. Also, avoid taping across the leg area, as this will cause irritation when the leg is bent.
10. Replace diaper carefully so as not to disturb the properly positioned collection bag.
11. Wait for the infant to produce urine. Frequently check bag until the urine has been collected.
12. Remove bag carefully in order not to spill the collected urine.
13. Prepare specimen as required. Complete and print the appropriate requisition forms and carefully place both the prepared specimen and the forms in the appropriate compartments of the biohazard transport bag. Remove gloves and discard in biohazard waste container.

(continues)

14. Wash hands.

15. Accurately record collection in patient's medical record.

DOCUMENTATION:

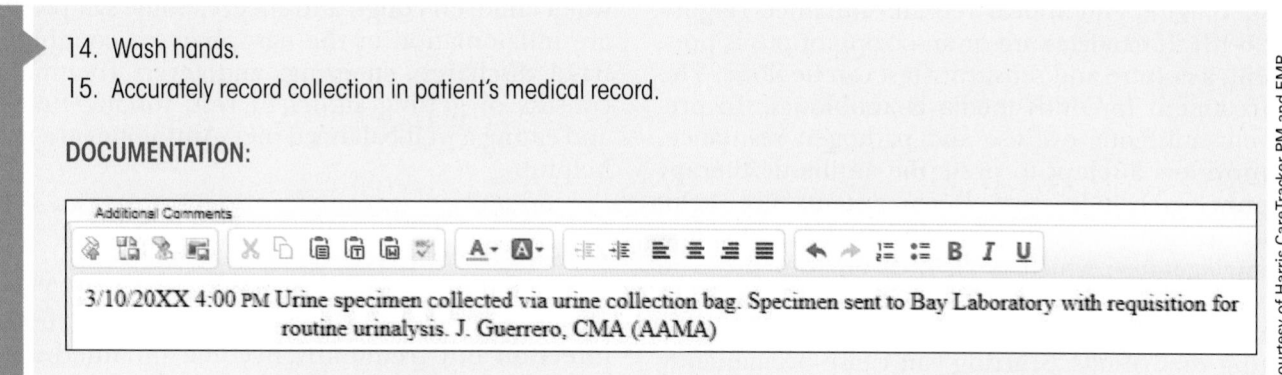

3/10/20XX 4:00 PM Urine specimen collected via urine collection bag. Specimen sent to Bay Laboratory with requisition for routine urinalysis. J. Guerrero, CMA (AAMA)

Courtesy of Harris CareTracker PM and EMR

closed until the light is removed. Older infants will follow an object up and down when it is placed directly in front of the eyes. It is estimated that a newborn has vision equivalent to 20/150, which will reach the adult level of 20/20 by the age of 6 months. The medical assistant will be required to maintain a nonstimulating environment while the provider is screening the infant, because any interference may invalidate results.

The kindergarten chart or Allen cards are used to test visual acuity in young children. The chart contains pictures in descending size, and the lines are labeled in the same manner as the Snellen chart. The child is asked to identify each picture as the medical assistant points to it. A standard Snellen chart is utilized for older children and adolescents.

The E chart is a series of E's pointing in different directions in descending size. The size and labeling are the same as the Snellen chart. This chart is used for older children. The child will be asked to point in the direction of each E as the medical assistant points to it (Figure 26-17).

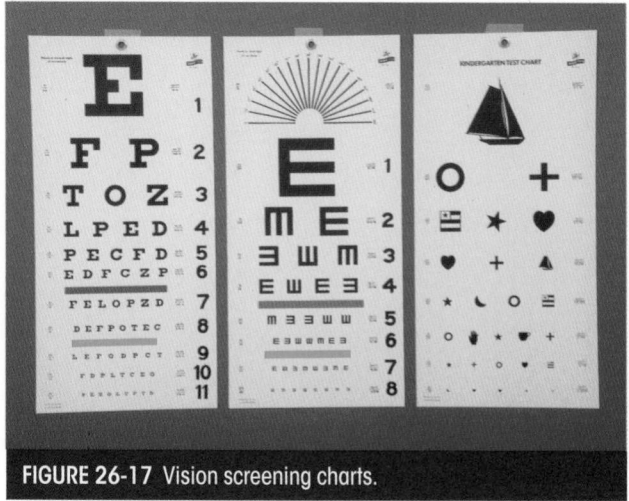

FIGURE 26-17 Vision screening charts.

Because their attention span is very limited, make a game out of measuring young children's visual acuity.

COMMON CHILDHOOD ILLNESSES

Young children grow and physically change very quickly. Their immune systems develop normally when they are healthy infants and children. Immunizations, together with their own developing immune system, give them protection from dangerous childhood diseases. Many life-threatening illnesses that were prevalent in the past have been controlled because of scheduled immunization, the child's own developing immune system, and the wise use of antibiotics for infections.

Otitis Media

Otitis media is a commonly occurring disorder in infants and young children. It is characterized by inflammation of the middle ear. Fluid accumulates behind the tympanic membrane, resulting in a degree of temporary hearing loss. It is commonly known as a middle ear infection. Because of the infant and young child's Eustachian tubes' connection to the nose and throat, bacteria that cause throat and respiratory infections can easily access the inner ear via a Eustachian tube. The fluid in the middle ear can become infected by the bacteria present in the nose and throat. The fluid turns to pus, and the resulting condition is known as **suppurative** otitis media. Pain and loss of hearing are common symptoms. Many young children have Eustachian tubes that are horizontal and narrow, which predisposes them to otitis media. As children develop physically, they can outgrow otitis media.

The provider can diagnosis otitis media by visually examining the tympanic membrane with an otoscope. In otitis media, the membrane will be bulging and appear red and inflamed (Figure 26-18). If **exudates** are or an oozing of pus is present, a culture and sensitivity test can be done. The treatment for otitis media is antibiotics. To prevent antibiotic overuse and pathogen resistance, providers attempt to prescribe antibiotic therapy only when necessary. Decongestants are helpful in some children. For chronic otitis media, a **myringotomy**, which is an incision into the tympanic membrane, may be necessary to prevent rupture of the tympanic membrane and the scarring that results. Scarring can cause permanently impaired hearing ability.

Tympanostomy is a surgical procedure in which pediatric ear tubes are placed through the tympanic membrane to promote ongoing drainage. Chronic otitis media that is left untreated can result in permanent hearing loss.

Hearing loss causes serious major problems in a child's development. Treatment of hearing loss depends on its cause. Hearing aids may be helpful to amplify sounds if the loss is caused by sounds not being conducted to the inner ear. Sensorineural hearing loss does not improve with hearing aids. **Cochlear implantation**, which has been approved by the FDA since 1990, is a procedure that can help children with bilateral **sensorineural** deafness.

The Common Cold

The common cold is aptly named because it is the most common and frequent disease that young children experience. Viruses are the usual microorganisms that cause a cold, and they are spread by direct contact and droplets through the air when children cough and sneeze. Some symptoms are inflammation of the nasopharynx, coughing, nasal discharge, sneezing, and fever. Treatment consists of getting sufficient rest, forcing fluids, and eating a well-balanced diet. Antibiotics are not helpful.

Tonsillitis

The tonsils are located in the back throat. They aid in protecting the respiratory tract from infection but frequently become inflamed and infected while doing their job. The cause most often is group A beta-hemolytic streptococcus or a virus. Fever; cough; sore throat; and red, swollen tonsils are common symptoms. Diagnosis can be made by doing a culture and sensitivity test of tonsillar exudate. Antibiotics will rid the child of infection if it is bacterial, and they must be taken as prescribed. Tonsillectomy is considered for older children who have chronic tonsillitis.

Pediculosis

Infestation with the head louse is known as pediculosis capitus and is common among school-aged children. The parasites suck blood from humans and are highly contagious. Diagnosis can be made by visual examination of the hair and scalp and observing the eggs (known as nits) on the hair. Special medications applied to the hair are an effective treatment.

Care must be taken to prevent reinfestation. Launder clothing, bed linens, and other items that

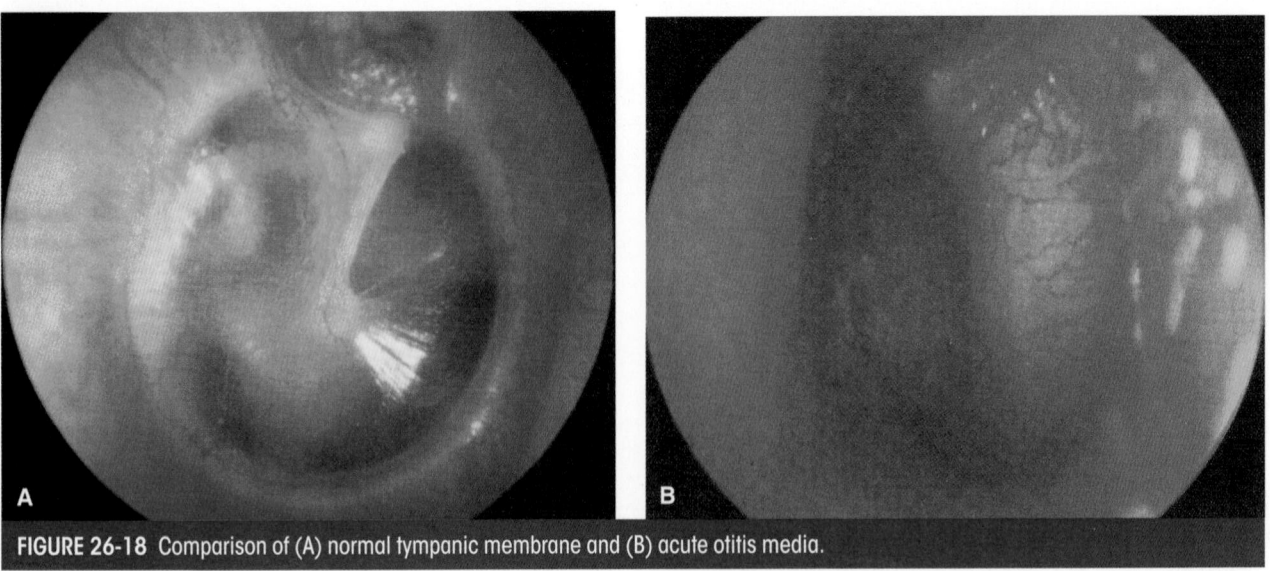

FIGURE 26-18 Comparison of (A) normal tympanic membrane and (B) acute otitis media.

the infested person wore or used during the 2 days before treatment. Ensure that the water used is at least 130°F in the laundry cycle and the heat high during the drying cycle. Clothing and items that are not washable can be dry-cleaned or stored in a sealed plastic bag. Soak combs and brushes in water that is at least 130°F for 5 to 10 minutes. Vacuum the floor and furniture, particularly where the infested person sat or lay. The risk of getting infested by a louse that has fallen onto a rug, carpet, or furniture is very low. Head lice can only survive a couple of days if they fall off a person and cannot feed. The nits (eggs or young form of the louse) cannot hatch and usually die within a week if they cannot remain at a temperature near that of the human body. The louse is not a vector for disease.

Asthma

Asthma has increased dramatically in the general population but especially in children. The cause of asthma is not known, but it can be brought on by environmental substances. Asthma triggers frequently include:

- Allergens such as pollen, dust mites, cockroaches, molds and animal dander
- Irritants in the air such as smoke, air pollution, chemical fumes, and strong odors
- Medications such as aspirin and acetaminophen
- Extreme weather conditions
- Exercise
- Stress

Spasms of the bronchi trap air and mucus in the lungs. The child will complain of a tight chest and will have shallow respirations and a nonproductive cough. The asthma attack may become an emergency situation.

The goal of asthma treatment is to keep symptoms under control all of the time. With this in mind, the provider may refer the child to an allergy specialist who will test the child for various allergies. Respiratory therapy is helpful for some children. There are many effective medicines to treat asthma. They include long-term control and quick relief medications. Immunotherapy (allergy shots) can also be helpful. Alternative therapies might also be useful such as breathing techniques, acupuncture, homeopathy, or herbal supplementation. It is important to emphasize consultation with the provider prior to beginning these therapies.

Croup

After having the common cold for several days, croup, which is a common viral condition, may begin as a "barking"-type cough, a high-pitched sound on inspiration (stridor), and respiratory distress. Symptoms begin as bedtime approaches and are worse at night. Croup most commonly occurs in children under the age of 5. The hallmark cough is due to inflammation of the larynx, trachea, and bronchi with swelling of the vocal cords. Respiratory obstruction can occur if severe, but children with croup generally are not seriously ill.

Parents should be instructed that comfort measures may include sitting in the bathroom with a hot shower running to create steam, or providing cool mist for inhalation. If the child has a fever, treatment with the appropriate dose of acetaminophen is indicated.

The provider should be notified if the child's respiratory effort includes a whistling sound that gets louder with each breath or if the child cannot speak or make verbal sounds for lack of breath, seems to be struggling to catch her breath, has bluish lips or fingernails, or has extreme difficulty swallowing saliva with resultant drooling. Be prepared to activate EMS upon the provider's order. These situations indicate a medical condition that must be treated for the safety of the child.

Pertussis (Whooping Cough)

Pertussis is a highly contagious respiratory tract infection caused by a bacterium. At the start, the disease appears to be a cold, but pertussis may become serious, especially in infants. Infected infants are at risk for pneumonia, seizures, brain diseases, and death. After about 2 weeks, the child has numerous rapid coughs that can last for months. Vaccines are available to prevent the disease. In recent years, there have been outbreaks of pertussis in college-age individuals and adults. The thinking by providers is that these people have lost their immunity to pertussis and need to be revaccinated with a booster vaccine.

Respiratory Syncytial Virus

Respiratory syncytial virus (RSV) affects the lungs. In most cases, the symptoms are relatively minor and mirror those of a cold. Death can occur in high-risk babies, such as premature infants, infants with a suppressed immune system, and infants with congestive heart failure. It is the most common cause of pneumonia in children under 1 year.

The virus spreads easily and rapidly through the air and can survive for an hour on hands and clothes and for several hours on toys, countertops, and other surfaces. There is no vaccine, but the infection can be treated with antiviral drugs such as ribavirin in **aerosolized** form. The drug inhibits the virus from replicating, so the sooner it is given, the better the results. This treatment is recommended only for severely ill and high-risk patients.

Instruct parents to call the provider or seek emergency medical treatment immediately if the child begins wheezing, breathing rapidly or struggling to breathe; refuses to drink anything; appears to be extremely lethargic; or starts to develop a bluish tinge on the lips and in the mouth.

Treatment includes hydration, bronchodilators, and—in rare cases—antiviral medications.

Fifth Disease

Erythemia infectiosum, or fifth disease, is a mildly to moderately contagious viral infection common among school-age children, particularly in the winter and spring. It manifests with an easily identifiable bright red rash on the cheeks that may occur on the arms and legs as well. It is commonly referred to as slapped cheek syndrome.

Fifth disease, so named because that was its location on a list of childhood illnesses in the 1960s, is a mild syndrome. It is spread by respiratory droplets and poses little risk to healthy children and adults. By the time the rash appears, the infected person is no longer contagious.

Fifth disease's rash may be accompanied by a low-grade fever and—less commonly—a sore throat, headache, and joint pain. There is little cause for concern unless the child has sickle-cell anemia, other anemias or a compromised immune system. There is no treatment required other than to treat the symptoms with an anti-inflammatory medication as needed for fever and joint pain. Prevention includes adhering to hand washing guidelines.

Hand, Foot, and Mouth Disease

Hand, foot, and mouth disease is a viral illness and most common in children under age 5 years due to the close proximity and behaviors of children of this age group. It is spread through saliva and the fluid from open blisters. Initial symptoms include fever, sore throat, and poor appetite. Later symptoms include painful sores that develop in the back of the throat and a skin rash, typically on the palms of the hands and soles of the feet. The rash may also occur on the trunk and diaper region.

This illness is self-limiting (usually 7 to 10 days) and requires no medical treatment.

Scarlet Fever

One group A streptococcal infection is commonly known as scarlet fever or scarlatina. It is characterized by a fever and a scarlet-colored rash on the neck, underarms, or groin. The illness is not usually severe but must be treated to avoid rare but serious long-term health problems. Appropriate antibiotic therapy must be initiated after a positive test for group A strep.

Scarlet fever most often occurs in children 5 to 15 years old. It is spread by droplet transmission to those in close contact with someone that has the illness or someone that harbors group A strep in their nose or throat. Prevention includes hand washing and education to include no sharing of utensils, glassware, towels, and other personal items.

Conjunctivitis

Conjunctivitis (pinkeye) is an inflammation or infection of the conjunctiva. When small blood vessels in the conjunctiva become inflamed, they are more visible, and that inflammation causes the eye to become pink or reddened. Conjunctivitis can be caused by viruses, bacteria, or any irritant. In childhood, conjunctivitis is commonly caused by bacteria; the infection is highly contagious and spreads quickly. Treatment includes antibiotic drops and comfort measures such as cool compresses to the eyes. Avoidance of contact with infected people, disinfection of household surfaces, and good hygienic practices can help prevent the spread of infectious pinkeye.

Child Abuse

Legal

Child abuse has increased significantly in recent years. By law, health care professionals, including medical assistants, as well as specified other people, must report suspected child abuse. The individual reporting the suspected abuse is protected against liability as a result of the reporting. If suspicion of abuse exists, the provider and other health care professionals should:

- Treat the child's injuries
- Send the child to the hospital if necessary
- Inform parents of the diagnosis
- Inform parents that the incident will be reported to the Department of Social Services, Children and Family Services, or Human Welfare. Depending on the laws of your state, notify the appropriate child welfare agency (see above). Find your local child welfare agency contact number at http://www.childwelfare.gov/. They will advise if local law enforcement must also be notified.
- Document all information
- Provide court testimony if requested

Child abuse is any physical or mental injury, sexual abuse, negligence, or mistreatment of a child under 18 years of age. Some signs of child abuse are:

- Bruises
- Broken bones
- Lacerations
- Burns (from cigarettes, rope, being immersed in scalding water, or being exposed to hot liquids such as coffee)
- Poor hygiene
- Failure to thrive
- Malnutrition
- Head injuries
- Neglected well-baby appointments

The AAP recommends that parents be taught to monitor television, videos, DVDs, and other types of media to limit viewing time and exposure to violence. Children 2 years and younger should not be exposed to any of these media. If a child's psychological and emotional needs are not being met due to extended "screen time," this may be considered neglect. However, this form of abuse is subtle and difficult to detect.

Diversity

The cultural background of the family should be taken into consideration, as should some folk medicine practices. Latin American and Russian cultures treat headaches and abdominal pain by placing a cup on the skin, creating a vacuum, and placing a small amount of burning material on the skin. These children may present with burns. To treat minor ailments, Southeast Asians rub a coin or spoon in hot oil and rub it onto the child's neck, spine, and ribs, and a burn may occur.

MALE CIRCUMCISION

Circumcision of the male involves the surgical removal of the foreskin (prepuce) of the penis. It is performed on a majority of males in the United States for hygienic reasons. Most circumcisions are performed in the hospital shortly after birth. Some people consider the procedure to be "cultural" surgery, as male circumcision is a religious rite in the Jewish and Muslim religions. The National Health and Nutrition Examination Survey collected data from 1999 to 2002 and found that the overall prevalence of male circumcision in the United States was 79%. According to the CDC, it is the neonatal surgical procedure most commonly performed in the United States. Female circumcision includes a variety of surgical procedures performed on a female's genitalia (see Chapter 25).

Those providing circumcision must be adequately trained, and both sterile techniques and effective pain management must be utilized. Significant acute complications are rare. In general, untrained providers who perform circumcisions have more complications than well-trained providers who perform the procedure, regardless of whether the former are physicians, nurses, or traditional religious providers.

In 2007, the American Academy of Pediatrics (AAP) convened a multidisciplinary workgroup of AAP members and other stakeholders to evaluate the evidence regarding male circumcision. Their evaluation of current evidence indicates that the health benefits of newborn male circumcision outweigh the risks. This group also determined that the benefits of newborn male circumcision justify access to this procedure for families who choose it. Identified benefits of male circumcision include preventing urinary tract infections, acquisition of HIV, transmission of some sexually transmitted infections, and penile cancer. Male circumcision does not appear to adversely affect penile sexual function/sensitivity or sexual satisfaction.

It is important that parents be provided factually correct, nonbiased information about circumcision, and they should receive this information from their provider before conception or early in pregnancy, which is when parents typically make circumcision decisions. Providers who counsel families about this decision should provide assistance by explaining the potential benefits and risks and ensuring that parents understand that circumcision is an elective procedure.

Those who advocate against circumcising male infants claim there is no medical reason to perform the procedure. Some believe that elective circumcision of males and females should not be performed by conscientious health care providers. Furthermore, some who are averse to the surgery say that a child is normal when born and that circumcision results in loss of a body part, is unnecessary, leaves a scar, and removes a functioning body part in the name of custom or tradition. It is viewed as a nonessential, pathologic procedure and a violation of basic human rights because infants are too young and helpless to consent or refuse.

How can parents decide what to do? Deeply rooted cultural and traditional customs can be difficult to sort through. With care, education, and research, parents can gain perspective about whether to circumcise their sons. The AAP has information regarding circumcision available on its Web site (http://www.aap.org).

Communication

Once a newborn male has been circumcised, it is important for the professional medical assistant to instruct the parents on care of the circumcised penis. Instruction should include:

- With every diaper change, the circumcision site should be gently cleansed with water and unscented soap (not a baby wipe) and allowed to dry.
- No tub baths until after the site is healed. A sponge bath is most appropriate.
- Apply petroleum jelly or antibiotic ointment, based on provider's preference, to the circumcision site with every diaper change until the site is healed.
- The provider must be notified if persistent bleeding, yellow discharge lasting more than a week, fever, swelling of the penis, or difficulty urinating are noted.

See Chapter 25 for information on female circumcision.

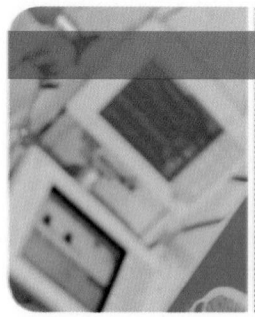

CASE STUDY 26-1

Refer to the scenario at the beginning of the chapter.

CASE STUDY REVIEW

1. In what ways can Joe learn about new vaccines that are required for pediatric patients?
2. Other than the provider giving information, describe two ways in which Joe can stay current with vaccines and immunizations.

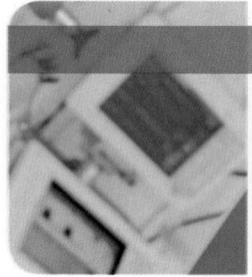

CASE STUDY 26-2

After examining Isaiah Little, Dr. King confirms the diagnosis of otitis media.

CASE STUDY REVIEW

1. Explain otitis media, the most common reason for its occurrence, and its treatment.
2. How can parents and caregivers be educated to help prevent otitis media?

Summary

- Caring for the health and well-being of infants and children throughout their various developmental stages and into adolescence is the responsibility of the pediatric practice.
- Careful observation of the parent or caregiver and the child is helpful to inform the treatment and care given to the child.
- The medical assistant is responsible for reporting to the provider any suspicion of child abuse.
- Opportunities abound for educating parents about topics that will keep their children healthy throughout life, including nutrition, sleep, immunizations, and exercise. Pamphlets, videos, and demonstrations are available to share with parents and caregivers.

Summary *continued*

- Children need respect and should be treated with empathy, love, and honesty; in doing so, a positive relationship can be developed with the child.

- Key aspects in the care of pediatric patients include a working knowledge of vaccine schedules and correct preparation and administration techniques.

- Growth and development expectations and theories are part of quality care of the pediatric patient. This requires proficiency in obtaining length, weight, and head and chest circumference.

- Pediatric vital signs vary based on the child's age. Variations from the normal ranges may indicate disease processes.

- Screening for vision and hearing, as well as specimens for laboratory testing, are part of the assessment of normal growth and development.

- There are common childhood illnesses that are seen frequently in the pediatric clinic. Knowledge of signs and symptoms of these illnesses will assist the medical assistant in obtaining a complete patient history.

- Education regarding postcircumcision care is needed in the clinical setting.

Study for Success

To reinforce your knowledge and skills of information presented in this chapter:

- Review the *Key Terms* and *Learning Outcomes*
- Consider the *Critical Thinking* features and *Case Studies* and discuss your conclusions
- Answer the questions in the *Certification Review*

- Perform the *Procedures* using the *Competency Assessment Checklists* on the *Student Companion Website*

Procedure

CERTIFICATION REVIEW

1. At what age should the first pneumococcal vaccine be given?
   a. Birth
   b. 1 month
   c. 2 months
   d. 3 months

2. Which of the following is a procedure to treat otitis media?
   a. Suppuration
   b. Tympanostomy
   c. Ear irrigation
   d. Otoscopy
   e. Myringectomy

3. Which of the following pathogens is usually responsible for causing tonsillitis?
   a. *Staphylococcus aureus*
   b. Meningococcus
   c. Beta-hemolytic streptococcus group A
   d. Beta-hemolytic streptococcus group B

4. Head circumference is measured on the child until what age?
   a. 12 months
   b. 24 months
   c. 36 months
   d. 48 months
   e. 52 months

5. An apical pulse is taken over which of the following sites?
   a. Second intercostal space on the left side
   b. Third intercostal space on the left side
   c. Fourth intercostal space on the left side
   d. Fifth intercostal space on the left side

6. What is the soft spot lying between the bones of the skull in a newborn and infant called?
   a. Frontal lobe
   b. Fontanel
   c. Foramen
   d. Cranium
   e. Sinus

7. Most childhood immunizations are administered within what time period?
   a. The first 6 months of life
   b. The first 12 months of life
   c. The first 16 months of life
   d. The first 24 months of life

8. The measurement of chest circumference is important to determine what?
   a. Underdevelopment of the infant's heart and lungs
   b. Overdevelopment of the infant's heart and lungs
   c. Calcification of rib cartilage
   d. Growth of the thymus
   e. All of these

9. When collecting a sterile urine specimen from an infant, it is important to use which method to ensure there is no contamination?
   a. Clean catch bag
   b. Direct catheterization
   c. Diaper extraction
   d. Voiding over the toilet

10. What is the most definitive method to test an infant's hearing?
    a. Automated system with the use of sensors
    b. Manual system with the use of sensors
    c. Observation and exposure to loud noises
    d. Extraneous sound monitoring
    e. Ambient sound system with sensors

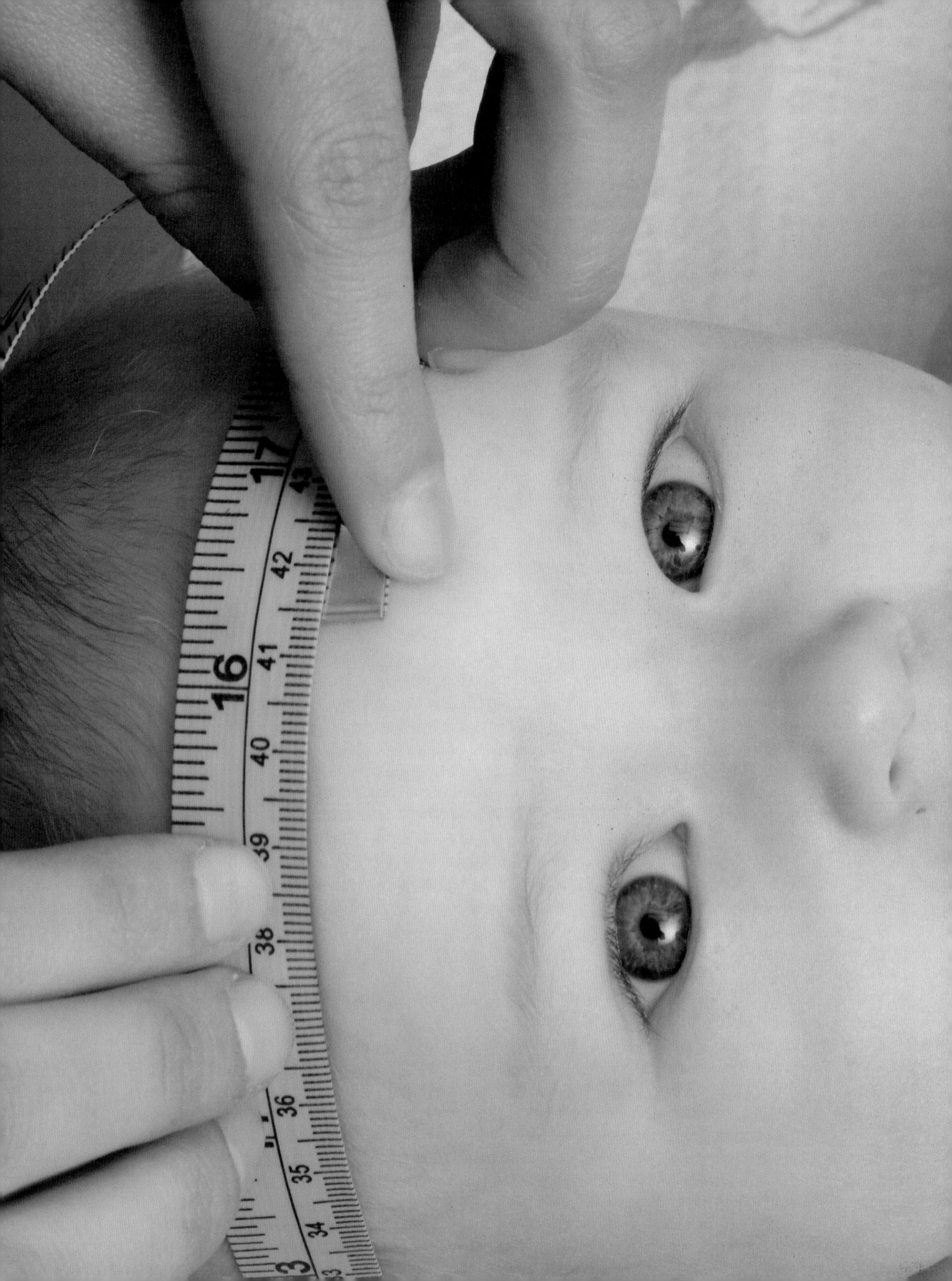

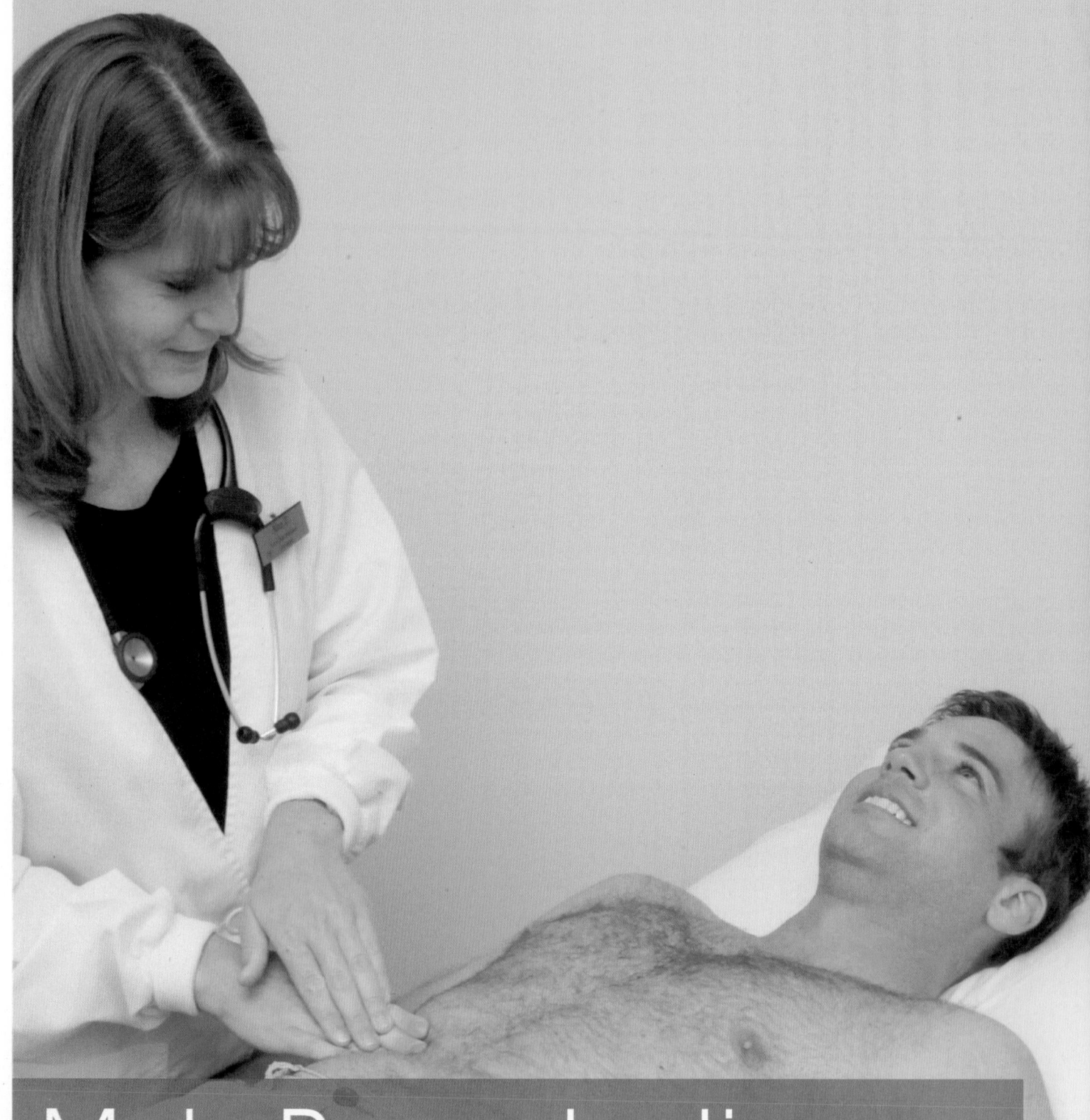

CHAPTER 27

Male Reproductive System

1. Define and spell the key terms as presented in the glossary.
2. Describe the structures and functions of the internal and external male organs.
3. Identify and label the anatomy of the male reproductive system.
4. Differentiate between diseases of the male reproductive system.
5. Analyze the pathology of the male reproductive organs.
6. Respond to known medical emergencies as they relate to certain male reproductive disorders.
7. Incorporate critical thinking skills when performing a health history related to the male reproductive system.
8. Use feedback techniques to obtain patient information regarding the history of male reproductive system functioning.
9. Explain male reproductive system diseases and disorders, their causes, and their treatments.
10. Describe the common diagnostic tests and procedures used for the male reproductive system.
11. Identify common treatments used for male reproductive disorders.
12. Teach testicular self-examination to a male patient.

KEY TERMS

balanitis

benign prostatic hyperplasia (BPH)

bulbourethral glands

circumcision

cryptorchidism

ejaculation

epididymitis

epispadias

erectile dysfunction (ED)

erection

highly active antiretroviral therapy (HAART)

hydrocele

hypogonadism

hypospadias

libido

male infertility

nocturia

orchiectomy

Peyronie disease

phimosis

prepuce

priapism

prostatectomy

prostate-specific antigen (PSA)

prostatitis

retention

scrotum

spermatic cord

spermatogenesis

spermatozoa

testes

testicular torsion

transurethral resection of the prostate (TURP)

varicocele

vas deferens

vasectomy

SCENARIO

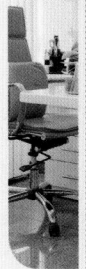

Mr. Greg Thomas, age 67, is a patient of Dr. Marita Carey at Inner City Health Care's Surgical Urology practice. Mr. Thomas is being seen today for a follow-up after his recent transurethral resection of the prostate (TURP). Wanda Slawson, CMA (AAMA), greets him in the waiting room and escorts him to the exam room in order to take his vital signs and his history since the surgical procedure. Mr. Thomas seems to be moving a little slower than usual and states, "I am having a little bit of trouble getting over this procedure." Wanda responds, "Having general anesthesia can take a week or so to get over. You look like you are doing pretty good as it has only been 4 days since your surgery!"

The male reproductive system consists of a number of specialized structures that serve the purpose of producing and delivering semen for sexual interaction and reproduction. It also has the important dual function of secreting male sex hormones that impact the growth and function of sexual organs and development of secondary sexual characteristics. This chapter will discuss the structure, function, and disease processes of this system.

Knowledge of the diseases, disorders, and conditions of the male reproductive system is essential for the medical assistant. There are specific diagnostic tests, procedures, and treatments that will be explored in this chapter. Included are quick reference guides and tables for ease of locating key information.

ANATOMY OF MALE REPRODUCTIVE SYSTEM

Males have a reproductive system that is both internal and external. The internal components are located near and interact closely with the urinary system and this must be kept in mind when considering the pathophysiology of this system.

External Anatomy

The male reproductive system has external and internal components. Unlike the female reproductive organs, most of the male reproductive organs are located outside of the abdomen or pelvis. The penis is the male sexual organ for intercourse. The scrotum is a sac-like structure that holds the testes. The testes generate sperm and male sex hormones.

⋙ QUICK REFERENCE GUIDE

⋙ ANATOMY OF THE PENIS

The penis (Figure 27-1) is the primary male sexual characteristic, and it is composed of the glans, corpus cavernosum, corpus spongiosum, and the urethra (all described in detail below). The penis has both a sexual and a reproductive function. The entire penis is sensitive, with an increased concentration of nerve endings in the glans. The reproductive function allows the delivery of semen deep into the female reproductive tract.

MEDICAL ANATOMY OF PENIS

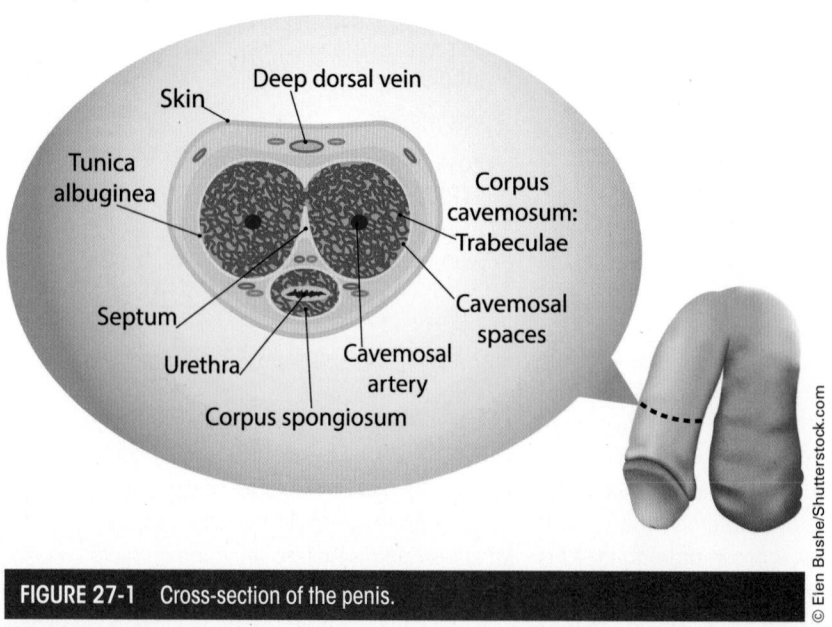

© Elen Bushe/Shutterstock.com

FIGURE 27-1 Cross-section of the penis.

(continues)

⟫ ANATOMIC PORTIONS OF THE PENIS

Portion	Description	Function
Glans (head)	Mucosa covered by the prepuce in uncircumcised males	Contains the urethral meatus for the exit of urine and semen from the body
	Circumcised males have epithelium covering	High concentration of nerve endings for erogenous stimulation
Shaft	Composed of the corpus carvernosum, corpus spongiosum, and urethra	Structures contained in the shaft fill with blood, and an erection occurs, enabling sexual activity
Corpus cavernosum	Cylinders made of erectile tissue located on each side of the penis that are rich in blood vessels	Tissues fill to form an erection
Corpus spongiosum	Spongy erectile tissue located on the posterior aspect of the penis	Enwraps the urethra to protect it from compression during ejaculation
Urethra	Fibromuscular tube connecting the bladder and ejaculatory ducts to the outside of the body	Provides an exit for urine and semen during ejaculation

⟫ KEYS TO PATIENT HISTORY

When conducting a patient history, the following questions related to penile function and possible diseases or disorders may be posed to the patient.

Questions Related to Penile Function:

- Have you had a **circumcision** (removal of the foreskin, also known as the **prepuce**)?
- Do you have a history of:
    ◦ Pain or burning when urinating?
    ◦ Discharge?
    ◦ Difficulties achieving or maintaining an **erection** (penile rigidity as a result of sexual or other types of stimulation)?
    ◦ Lack of external **ejaculation** (ejection of seminal fluid and sperm during male orgasm)?
- Have you had problems with pain, discharge, or lesions of:
    ◦ The penis?
    ◦ The glans?

Questions Related to Penile Diseases and Disorders:

- Have you ever suffered a penile injury?
- Do you have a history of:
    ◦ **Balanitis** (inflammation of the foreskin)?
    ◦ **Epispadias** (a condition at birth in which the opening of the urethra is not at the tip of the penis, but on the upper penile surface)?
    ◦ **Erectile dysfunction (ED)** (persistent inability to either achieve or maintain penile firmness sufficient for satisfactory sexual performance)?
    ◦ **Hypospadias** (a condition at birth in which the opening of the urethra is not at the tip of the penis, but on the underside)?
    ◦ Penile cancer?
    ◦ **Peyronie disease** (plaque causing the penis to bend or curve)?
    ◦ Tight foreskin (**phimosis**)?
    ◦ **Priapism** (persistent, frequently painful erection lasting more than 4 hours with or without sexual stimulation)?

⟫ ANATOMY OF THE SCROTUM

The scrotum (Figure 27-2) is composed of the testes, the epididymis, and a portion of the spermatic cord (all described in detail below). The muscles in the scrotal wall act to maintain the optimal temperature of the testes by contracting to draw the testes closer to the warmth of the body and relaxing to move them farther away from the body's warmth.

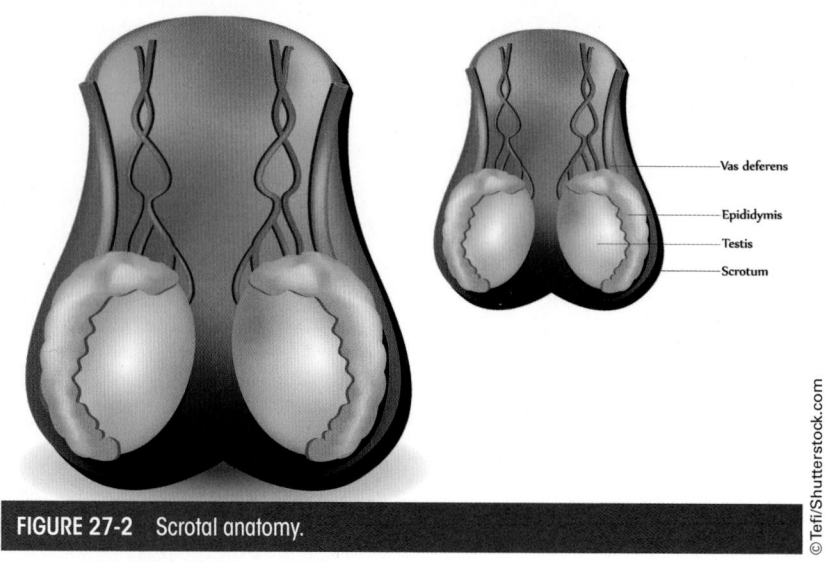

FIGURE 27-2 Scrotal anatomy.

© Tefi/Shutterstock.com

⟫ ANATOMIC PORTIONS OF THE SCROTUM

Anatomic Portion	Description	Function
Testes	Composed of two glandular organs with each testis measuring approximately 35 to 50 mm (1.5 to 2 in.) by 25 mm (1 in.) in diameter in the adult male (see Figure 27-2)	Secretion of the sex hormone testosterone follicle–stimulating hormone, and the production of **spermatozoa** or mature, mobile male sex cells (**spermatogenesis**)
Epididymis	Coiled tube-like structure that is more than 4.5 meters (15 ft) of convoluted tubules attached to the posterior of each testis that carries sperm from the testes to the ductus deferens	Spermatozoa produced in the testes enter the epididymis for storage and maturation until they develop the ability to swim and fertilize an ovum
Spermatic cord	Bundle of fibers, nerves, the vas deferens, testicular artery, and a network of veins that form a cord	Support the testes in the scrotum

⟫ KEYS TO PATIENT HISTORY

When conducting a patient history, the following questions related to scrotal function and possible diseases or disorders may be posed to the patient.

Questions Related to Scrotal Function:

- Have you had an **orchiectomy** (surgical removal of one or both testes)?
- Do you have a history of:
  - **Male infertility** (low sperm production, abnormal sperm function)?
  - Scrotal irritation?

(continues)

Questions Related to Scrotal Diseases and Disorders:

- Do you have a history of:
  - **Cryptorchidism** (failure of one or both of the testes to descend into the scrotum during infancy)?
  - **Epididymitis** (inflammation of the epididymis)?
  - **Hydrocele** (swelling of the scrotum due to painless buildup of watery fluid around one or both testes)?
  - **Hypogonadism** (failure to produce adequate amounts of testosterone)?
  - Orchitis (inflammation of one or both of the testes)?
  - Sexually transmitted parasites like scabies or public lice?
  - Testicular cancer?
  - Testicular trauma?
  - **Testicular torsion** (a twisting of the testes around the spermatic cord resulting in testicular ischemia)?
  - **Varicocele** (dilatation of veins found in the male spermatic cord)?

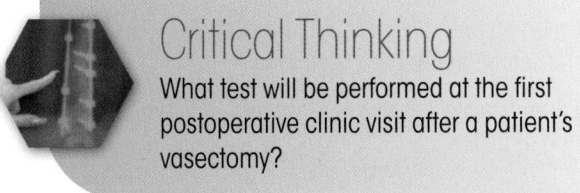

Critical Thinking

What test will be performed at the first postoperative clinic visit after a patient's vasectomy?

Internal Anatomy

The male reproductive system, though mostly external, does have internal components (see "Internal Anatomy" Quick Reference Guide). The main purpose of these structures is transporting the sperm from the testes to the outside of the body at the end of the penis. The prostate, seminal vesicles, and Cowper's gland manufacture fluid that, combined with the sperm, becomes ejaculate. The vas deferens is the structure that serves as the route from the testes to the urethra for ejaculation.

DISORDERS OF THE MALE REPRODUCTIVE SYSTEM

Balanitis

The swelling or inflammation of the glans penis is known as balanitis. If a male is uncircumcised, it is essential that the foreskin be retracted and the glans of the penis be cleansed as a part of daily hygiene. Also, care must be taken to remove any soap residue prior to returning the foreskin to its anatomic position. The exposure to soaps from inadequate rinsing and other potentially irritating substances is the major cause of balanitis. Infection, diabetes, and some autoimmune disorders might also be the basis for this disorder.

Treatment is based on the cause of the balanitis. Infection may be treated with oral or topical antibiotics. Patient education is important to limit balanitis due to errors in daily hygiene.

Benign Prostatic Hyperplasia

Enlargement of the prostate gland that is not due to infection or cancer is known as benign prostatic hyperplasia (BPH) (also known as benign prostatic hypertrophy). This condition is common in men over the age of 50 and is of concern because an enlarged prostate gland blocks the flow of urine and does not allow complete emptying of the bladder.

The most common symptoms involve not being able to sleep through the night because of **nocturia**. Your patient might also report a weak urine stream, dribbling at the end of the urine stream, or the feeling of being unable to completely empty the bladder.

Treatment is based on the severity of the symptoms. Treatment is indicated for complications such as sudden, painful inability to urinate; frequent urinary tract infections; or kidney damage caused by high pressure in the bladder due to urinary **retention**.

Evaluation will include a laboratory workup to assess prostate-specific antigen (PSA), rectal digital examination to palpate the prostate through the anterior wall of the rectum, and urinalysis. It is important to note that the PSA needs to be drawn prior to the digital examination as this manipulation

⋙ QUICK REFERENCE GUIDE

⋙ INTERNAL ANATOMY OF THE MALE REPRODUCTIVE SYSTEM

Anatomic Portion	Description	Function
Vas deferens	Muscular tube 30 to 35 cm (12 to 13 in.) long that contracts to propel sperm to the prostatic urethra. This structure is interrupted during the vasectomy procedure resulting in sterilization.	Connects the testes with the urethra inside the body of the prostate and conducts mature spermatozoa to the penis for ejaculation and potential fertilization of the female.
Prostate	Small, plum-sized, muscular gland located inferior to the urinary bladder in the pelvic body cavity; merges with the vas deferens at the ejaculatory duct	Produces milky-white, sugar-based secretions that make up a large portion of semen volume; function is to nourish sperm Produces alkaline secretions that serve to break down vaginal acidity to ensure sperm survival Contains the ejaculatory duct that releases sperm from the vas deferens into the urethra during ejaculation Smooth muscle contracts in the prostate to force the semen through the urethra Enhances pleasurable sensations during arousal and orgasm
Seminal vesicles	Positioned inferior to the urinary bladder and lateral to the vas deferens Unite with the vas deferens to form the two ejaculatory ducts prior to entering the prostate and then on to the prostatic urethra Approximately 5 to 10 cm in length (2 to 4 in.)	Secretes 70% to 85% of the fluid portion of semen Fluid is alkaline, assisting in neutralizing the acidity of the vaginal tract and prolonging the life span of sperm Produce a substance that contains proteins, enzymes, sugars, and vitamins to prolong spermatozoa life
Cowper's (or **bulbourethral**) glands	Two pea-sized glands located lateral and slightly posterior to the urethra	Excrete a mucous-like, salty, preejaculatory fluid that neutralizes acidity in the urethra to protect sperm as they exit

⋙ KEYS TO PATIENT HISTORY

When conducting a patient history, the following questions related to internal anatomy function and possible diseases or disorders may be posed to the patient.

Questions Related to Internal Anatomy Function:

- Have you undergone any of the following procedures?
  - **Prostatectomy** (surgical removal of all or a portion of the prostate)
  - **Transurethral resection of the prostate (TURP)** (surgical procedure to relieve urinary retention symptoms caused by benign prostatic hypertrophy (BPH) [see Figure 27-3])
  - **Vasectomy** (method of sterilization that includes cutting, tying, or cauterizing a portion of the vas deferens to interrupt the exit of sperm from the body)

(continues)

Questions Related to Internal Anatomy Diseases and Disorders:

- Do you have a history of:
  ◦ **Benign prostatic hyperplasia (BPH)** (enlarged prostate gland that is not cancerous in origin)?
  ◦ Bulbourethral gland infection?
  ◦ Bulbourethral gland stones?
  ◦ Cysts or abscesses?
  ◦ Elevated **prostate-specific antigen (PSA)** (protein produced by prostatic cells that when elevated may indicate prostatic cancer)?
  ◦ Prostate cancer?
  ◦ **Prostatitis** (inflammation of the prostate)?
  ◦ Seminal vesiculitis?

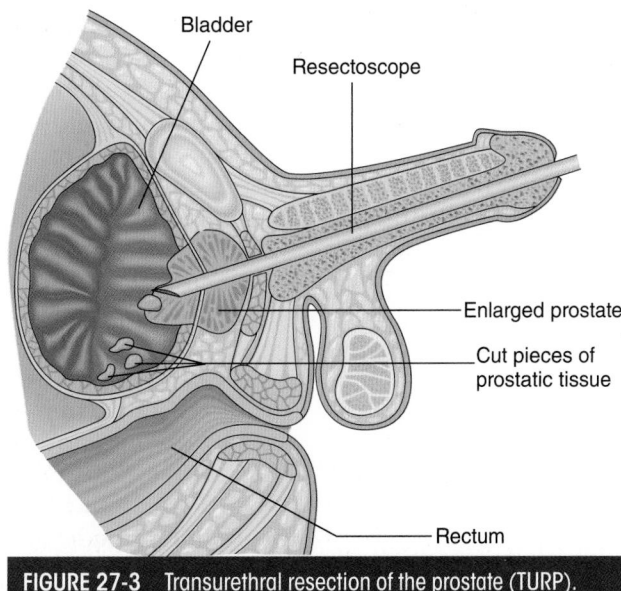

FIGURE 27-3 Transurethral resection of the prostate (TURP).

can cause a rise in the PSA. Diagnosis is also based on several procedures that measure the flow of urine from the bladder. These tests include:

- Urine flow studies to determine the strength and amount of urine flow

- Postvoiding residual urine studies to determine the amount of urine left in the bladder after voiding; this analysis can be conducted using an ultrasound or by accessing the bladder using a catheter to measure the amount of urine remaining

- Ultrasound of the prostate to measure its dimensions (performed transrectally)

More invasive methods include:

- Intravenous pyelogram (IVP) using venous access to inject a radiopaque medium that will allow the radiologist to observe the flow of urine through the urinary tract

- Prostate biopsy to rule out prostatic cancer

- Urodynamic studies to monitor pressures in the bladder, discover any urinary retention issues, and assess the function of the bladder muscles

If treatment is needed, medications that relax the bladder neck or shrink the prostate are utilized. If the symptoms are severe, surgery may be indicated. A transurethral resection of the prostate (TURP) is a common procedure (see Figure 27-3). As the name indicates, a scope is inserted in the urethra and small tools are utilized to access the prostate and carve away enough of the prostatic tissue that bulges into the urethra to allow adequate urine flow. A more invasive surgery is the open prostatectomy. This is indicated if the prostate is very large and there are other complicating factors. There are many associated risks with this procedure and the recovery time is much longer.

Recently, there have been strides in treatment modalities that allow the patient to recover more rapidly. One method is transurethral microwave thermotherapy (TUMT). This is one of several techniques that use heat provided by microwaves to destroy prostate tissue. Transurethral needle ablation (TUNA) is a newer approach that also uses heat. TUNA uses low-level radio waves delivered through twin needles to heat and kill obstructing prostate cells. A laser technique known as photoselective vaporization of the prostate (PVP), uses a high-energy GreenLight laser to vaporize tissue.

Other minimally invasive therapies for BPH access the prostate through the urethra using only a needle and suture to pull back the prostate tissue and relieve the pressure on the prostatic urethra. All of the above-mentioned therapies can be performed on an outpatient basis.

Cryptorchidism

Cryptorchidism is a condition that is present at birth in 3% to 5% of full-term male infants and usually resolves by one year of age. The lack of descent of one or both testicles is classified as cryptorchidism. The testes may be located in a number of anatomical areas: abdominal, inguinal, or prescrotal. Alternatively, the testes may be able to slide in and out of the scrotum but tend to reside below the inguinal ring.

Epididymitis

Inflammation of the epididymis can be caused by various factors. Most commonly, the causative factor is a bacterial infection. A sexually transmitted organism can cause an infection of the epididymis. Epididymitis can be a hallmark of sexual abuse in the pediatric setting, and reporting to a child protective agency is indicated. A patient of any age with epididymitis has symptoms that include pain in the groin, testicular area, flank, or abdomen; fever; discharge from the penis; and blood in the urine. There may be scrotal pain and swelling as well as pain upon urination.

The causative organism, *Chlamydia trachomatis*, is present in 50% to 60% of cases. Another common infectious organism is *Neisseria gonorrhoeae*. For men who participate in anal intercourse, *Escherichia coli* might be the infective agent. There are other conditions that lead to epididymitis. Retrograde urine flow can cause chemical epididymitis, as can some medications.

A diagnosis of epididymitis is based on physical examination, urinalysis, and urine culture. In addition, a urethral culture and the white blood cell count as part of a complete blood count might be included in the evaluation. In order to rule out other causes for this type of pain, your practitioner might prescribe a testicular ultrasound, computed tomography (CT) scan, or magnetic resonance imaging (MRI) of the affected area.

Treatment is based on the causative factor. If bacterial, this condition is treated with antibiotics. Once a diagnosis is made, an important aspect of care is counseling the patient to inform all sexual partners of the causative organism, because they must be treated as well.

Erectile Dysfunction (ED)

Also called impotence, erectile dysfunction (ED) occurs when a man is unable to achieve or to sustain an erection of the penis during sexual intercourse. This condition or dysfunction is not normal at any age and is different from other issues that impede sexual intercourse, such as lack of sexual drive, or libido.

Many men, at some point in their lives, can experience the inability to achieve an erection. This can happen on occasion from consuming too much alcohol or from extreme fatigue. This is not ED. The inability to achieve an erection more than 50% of the time is generally a reason for seeking treatment and is usually an indication of ED.

For an erection to occur, certain physiologic conditions must be present. There must be a stimulus from the brain and adequate circulation and nerve supply to the penis. If any of these conditions is impeded, an erection cannot be achieved. Some reasons why ED occurs include conditions or diseases that impair circulation (atherosclerosis) and nerve stimulation (nerve diseases) and psychological factors such as stress and depression. Medications such as those used to treat certain conditions such as hypertension can cause ED. Diabetes, multiple sclerosis, cerebral vascular accident (stroke), surgery on the prostate or bladder, and brain and spinal cord injuries are other causes of ED.

Treatment of the dysfunction is based on the cause. Referral to a urologist, psychologist, or both is made if appropriate. Blood and urine tests will be done after the provider examines the individual for medical problems. Medications the patient may be taking will be addressed. Some of the ways ED can be treated include oral medications (Viagra, Levitra, Cialis), penile injections (medication injected into the penis), sex therapy, surgery such as penile implants (device surgically implanted to overcome impotence), and vacuum pumps.

Professional

Because of the very nature of ED, many men are embarrassed if they have the disorder, feeling they are somehow less "manly" than other men. It is of extreme importance to be conscientious and sensitive when assisting the provider with the care of these patients. Confidentiality on the telephone and during in-person conversations must be maintained. Protect your patient's privacy at all times. It is not only the law, but it is also an important attribute of a professional medical assistant.

Some experts say ED should be considered a possible risk factor for heart disease if atherosclerosis is present.

Hypogonadism

The failure to produce adequate amounts of testosterone, sperm, or both is referred to as hypogonadism. Testosterone production tends to decline with age, as do healthy, mobile sperm populations. This is considered a normal part of aging. Hypogonadism is of concern when it impacts fertility.

Causes of hypogonadism may have a hormonal source or may be a result of genetic disorders, cryptorchidism, toxins, trauma, stress or chronic nutritional deficiencies. Other causative factors for hypogonadism include infection of the testicles from mumps, injury to the testicles, and cancer treatment. Some secondary causes are disorders of the hypothalamus or pituitary, inflammatory disease processes, HIV infection, and obesity.

The treatment for low levels of testosterone is simple and includes testosterone replacement therapy. The treatment for low sperm count is more complicated and includes medications, hormone supplementation, and assistive reproductive technologies.

Hypospadias and Epispadias

Hypospadias and epispadias are birth defects in boys in which the opening of the urethra is not located at the tip of the penis. Hypospadias is a more common defect than epispadias. In boys with hypospadias or epispadias, the urethra forms abnormally during weeks 8 to 14 of pregnancy.

With hypospadias, the abnormal opening can form anywhere from just below the end of the penis to the scrotum. There are different degrees of hypospadias; some can be minor and some more severe (Table 27-1).

There are associated difficulties sometimes for boys with hypospadias. There is an increased incidence of curvature of the penis (not Peyronie disease), cryptorchidism; sexual dysfunction; and, at a minimum, abnormal spraying of urine.

Male Infertility

A provider who is treating couples for infertility might order a semen analysis as an early test to determine if the source of nonconception is related to an insufficiency in the sperm count. Sperm present in semen may not be of a sufficient number or quality to allow fertilization. A semen analysis includes a measure of the volume of the ejaculate; the time it takes for the semen to become liquid; and the number of mature, mobile sperm in the semen. The semen is tested to reveal the pH, presence of fructose, and white blood cells. All of these components ensure the health of the sperm contained in the semen. If there is a determination of a low sperm count, treatment is based on the underlying cause.

TABLE 27-1

TYPES OF HYPOSPADIAS

NAME	DESCRIPTION	EXAMPLE
Subcoronal	Urethral opening near the glans of the penis	
Midshaft	Urethral opening along the shaft of the penis	
Penoscrotal	Urethral opening at the penis–scrotum junction	

Multiple causes of infertility are unrelated to a low sperm count. These causes include an infection in the genitourinary tract or the presence of an STD, either of which can block the tract and prohibit sperm from being fully ejaculated. An injury to the blood or nerve supply in the area, radiation exposure, stress, and hormonal imbalances are other factors that can promote infertility.

Treatment of a male patient with infertility depends on the cause. Treatments include surgery to remove a blockage, antibiotics to treat an infection, use of artificial insemination, or use of pharmaceuticals to treat the infertility.

Orchitis

Inflammation of one or both testicles is referred to as orchitis. The two most common causes of orchitis are bacterial infection or a viral infection called the mumps.

Sexually transmitted infections, especially gonorrhea or chlamydia, are common causes as well. Bacterial orchitis may result from epididymitis.

Orchitis causes pain and can cause male infertility. Treatment includes antibiotics and antiviral medications, which can cure or relieve the symptoms of orchitis.

Penile Cancer

The incidence of penile cancer is greater in uncircumcised men. There is also an increased rate in men who smoke, have been infected with human papillomavirus or HIV, or have accumulations of smegma (the oily substance secreted by the skin of the penis and foreskin). The most common symptoms include lesions that do not heal on the penis as well as penile pain and bleeding.

Although penile cancer is fairly uncommon, it is a psychologically devastating disease. Men commonly delay seeking medical treatment and physicians (especially men) delay intervention in preference for much less invasive treatment modalities such as topical steroids and antibiotics.

Usually a referral to a urologist is indicated, and the first step in treatment is a biopsy of the tissues. Treatment then depends on the severity of the lesions. Chemotherapy, radiation, and surgery are all components of the treatment regimen. A worst case scenario would be total removal of the penis, called a penectomy.

Peyronie Disease

Curvature of the penis during erection is known as Peyronie disease (Figure 27-4). It occurs due

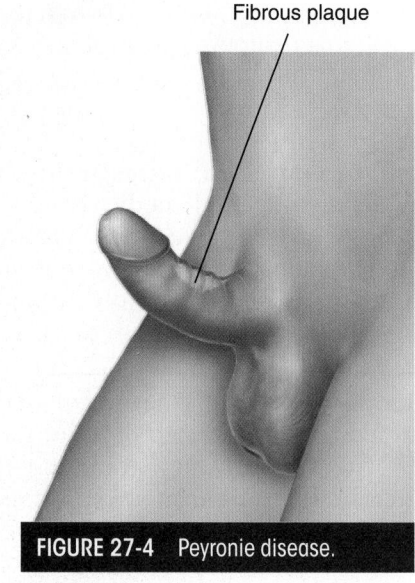

FIGURE 27-4   Peyronie disease.

to fibrous tissue that is present subcutaneously on the shaft of the penis. This tissue can be scarring from penile trauma, or it may be associated with other diseases that involve the formation of thickening and contracture of soft tissues.

Treatment includes medical interventions such as direct injections into the affected tissue, radiation therapy, and vitamin supplementation. For severe cases that interfere with sexual function, surgery may be suggested.

Phimosis

This condition is most common in children. Phimosis is the tightening of the foreskin so as not to allow retraction. By the age of 3 years, an uncircumcised male should be able to retract the foreskin from the tip of the penis.

The diagnosis of phimosis is usually made by a pediatrician, and the treatment involves steroid application, manual manipulation with lubrication, or a small incision to relieve the tension.

Priapism

Priapism is the result of filling of the erectile tissue in the penis that persists and interferes with the normal blood flow to the penile tissues. This interference can result in tissue death and permanent erectile dysfunction. Predisposing factors are sickle cell disease and the use of pharmacologic agents to enhance sexual function.

The treatment for priapism includes the application of ice packs to the groin area and increased physical activity. If these measures do not relieve the symptoms, emergency medical treatment is indicated.

Prostate Cancer

Prostate cancer is the leading cause of cancer-related death in men 75 and older. With the availability of better screening tools, like the PSA test, early diagnosis is enabling earlier treatment for men with this form of cancer. Many times, this blood test indicates prostate cancer before there are symptoms. If symptoms are present, they are very similar to those associated with BPH (see above).

A prostate cancer screen also includes a digital rectal examination by the health practitioner. If the transrectal examination shows irregularities in the surface of the prostate, further investigation is warranted. Transrectal ultrasonography and guided core needle biopsy are useful tools for diagnosis.

Prostate cancer is staged using a Gleason score. Treatment most often includes a prostatectomy and can be followed by chemotherapy and radiation. There is often an added component of hormone therapy. The surgical prostatectomy can lead to many complications with the urinary system and with sexual function. This can be psychologically stressful to the affected man. As a professional medical assistant, a referral to a support group as well as extensive patient teaching under the direction of your provider is indicated.

Prostatitis

Prostatitis is an inflammation of the prostate gland. This can be caused by a bacterial infection, an immune or nervous system disorder, irritation of the gland itself by the insertion of a Foley catheter, anal intercourse, and some types of athletic activities such as cycling. This condition can be acute or chronic.

Patients will present complaining of painful or difficult urination, nocturia, pain in the groin or lower back, pain in the testicular area, painful orgasms, or flu-like symptoms. In order to obtain an accurate diagnosis, your practitioner will do a thorough physical examination, order a blood culture, and might suggest a cystoscopy or urodynamic testing.

Treatments include antibiotics, alpha blockers to assist in the relaxation of the bladder and aid in the flow of urine, pain relievers, and prostate massage.

Testicular Cancer

This cancer most commonly affects young men between the ages of 15 and 40. At a higher risk are men who have a family history of testicular cancer or other risk factors including abnormal testicular development such as cryptorchidism and genetic abnormalities. Exposure to industrial or farming chemicals and human immunodeficiency virus (HIV) also increases risk.

There are many types of cancers that affect the testes. The most common is seminoma. Keys to successful treatment of any type of testicular cancer are early detection; rapid, appropriate treatment; and consistent follow-up to monitor for recurrence.

Diagnosis is made by ultrasound and other radiologic testing, biopsy, and blood testing for tumor markers. The procedure of choice for treatment is a radical orchiectomy with biopsy of surrounding tissues for staging purposes. Postsurgical treatment may include radiation, chemotherapy, or a combination thereof.

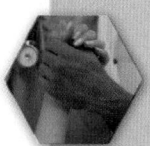

Patient Education

1. Other than skin cancer, prostate cancer is the most common cancer in American men.

2. The American Cancer Society's estimates for prostate cancer in the United States for 2016 are:
   - About 180,890 new cases of prostate cancer
   - About 26,120 deaths from prostate cancer

3. Approximately 1 man in 7 will be diagnosed with prostate cancer during his lifetime.

4. Prostate cancer is the second leading cause of cancer death in American men, behind only lung cancer. Approximately 1 man in 39 will die of prostate cancer.

5. A Gleason score indicates the risk of metastasis. This score ranges from 1 to 10.

6. Survival depends on the staging.

7. The treatment for prostate cancer can impact sexual performance and urinary control.

Procedure

The medical assistant may be directed by the provider to play a significant role in patient education. Primarily, it is essential to educate all males on the procedure for monthly testicular self-examination. Figure 27-5 illustrates the testicular self-examination procedure. Procedure 27-1 outlines instructions usually given to the patient by the medical assistant.

Testicular Torsion

As indicated in the "Anatomy of the Scrotum" Quick Reference Guide found on page 732, each testicle is suspended in the scrotum by the spermatic cord. A small percentage of males have a predisposition for a twisting of this cord, which is known as testicular torsion (see Figure 27-6). This creates an emergency situation if it is not resolved, with or without medical intervention. Testicular torsion is most common in males between the ages of 12 to 18 years. It can occur posttraumatically, after intense physical exercise, or without any evident reason.

A patient may see the practitioner complaining of sudden, severe pain in the scrotum with or without swelling. He might be nauseated, vomiting, and feel faint. To make the diagnosis, the

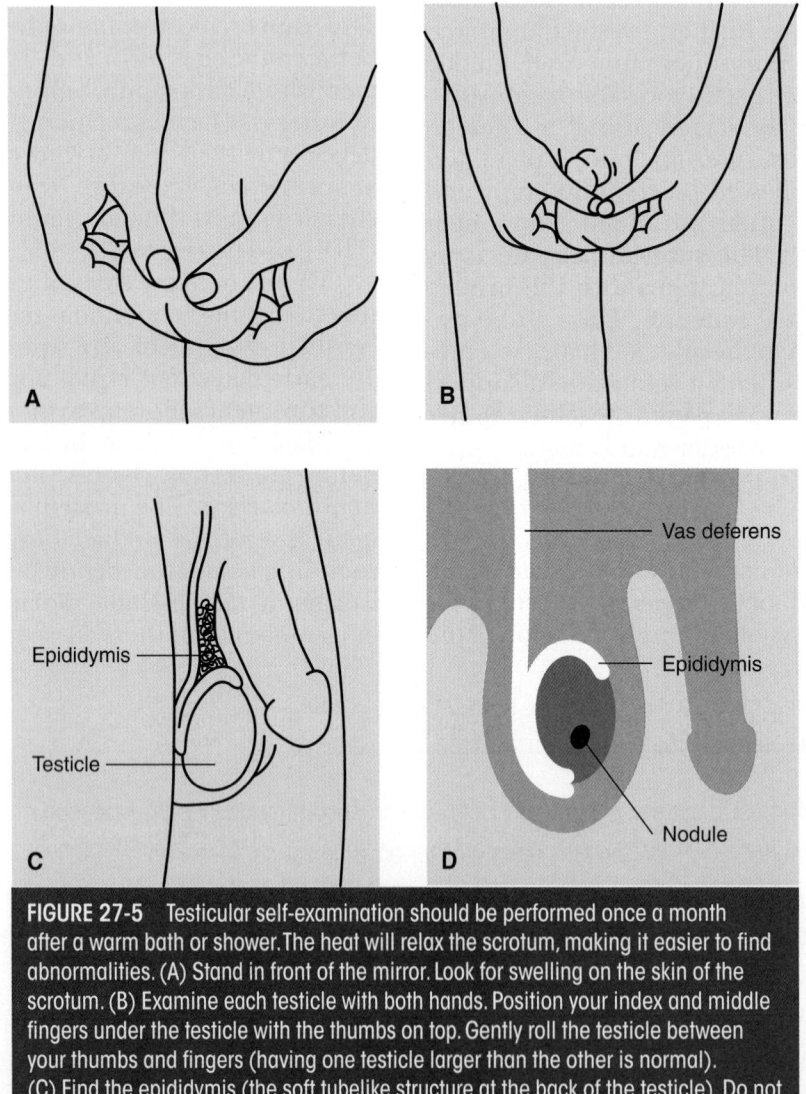

FIGURE 27-5 Testicular self-examination should be performed once a month after a warm bath or shower. The heat will relax the scrotum, making it easier to find abnormalities. (A) Stand in front of the mirror. Look for swelling on the skin of the scrotum. (B) Examine each testicle with both hands. Position your index and middle fingers under the testicle with the thumbs on top. Gently roll the testicle between your thumbs and fingers (having one testicle larger than the other is normal). (C) Find the epididymis (the soft tubelike structure at the back of the testicle). Do not mistake the epididymis for an abnormal lump. (D) If you find a lump, notify your provider immediately. Most lumps are found on the sides of the testicle, but some are located on the front. Testicular cancer is highly curable when detected early and treated promptly.

PROCEDURE 27-1

Procedure

Instructing Patients in Testicular Self-Examination

PURPOSE:

To provide a patient with information concerning testicular screening for the presence of a painless mass in the scrotum.

EQUIPMENT/SUPPLIES:

- Testicular self-examination card
- Anatomy illustration

PROCEDURE STEPS:

1. Introduce yourself and identify the patient using two identifiers. *Explain to the patient the rationale for performance of the procedure, showing awareness of the patient's concerns related to the procedure being performed.*

2. *Demonstrating empathy,* instruct the patient to examine his testicles monthly in a warm shower. Explain that this allows the skin to soften and the scrotal muscles to relax, making it easier to find abnormalities. RATIONALE: The warmth causes the scrotum to relax.

3. *Demonstrating respect for individual diversity,* explain the next steps of the procedure.

4. Instruct the patient that standing in front of a mirror and looking for swelling on the skin of the scrotum may reveal abnormalities.

5. The penis must be held out of the way and each testicle checked separately using both hands.

6. Placing the index and middle fingers underneath the testicle and the thumbs on top, roll the testicle gently between the fingers.

7. Look and feel for any hard lumps; smooth rounded bumps; or change in the size, shape, or consistency of the testes. It is normal to have one testis that is larger than the other.

8. Locate the epididymis.

9. It may be of assistance to provide a chart to the patient that illustrates the testes and epididymis. RATIONALE: A lump can be similar in size to the epididymis and needs to be distinguished from the epididymis.

10. Look for swelling or changes in the scrotal area.

11. Encourage the patient to report anything unusual to the provider.

12. Accurately record this patient education in patient's chart or electronic medical record.

DOCUMENTATION:

PROCEDURE NOTE

11/4/20XX 1:15 PM Patient provided an illustrated card outlining monthly testicular self-exam. Instructions for performing a
testicular self-examination reviewed. Understanding demonstrated by return demonstration on testicular self-exam.
J. Guerrero, CMA (AAMA)

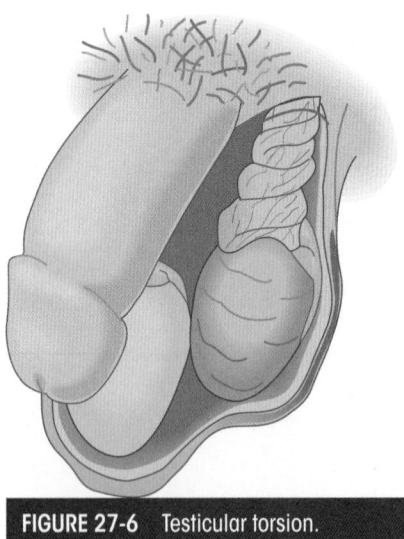

FIGURE 27-6 Testicular torsion.

practitioner will physically examine the testicles, looking for a palpable lump and visually evaluate whether one testicle is significantly higher than the other. Diagnosis might also include Doppler ultrasound to assess blood flow.

Treatment can include manual distortion, but the most common intervention is emergency surgery to release the torsion and secure the testicle to the inner layers of the scrotum to prevent future events.

Testicular Trauma

Even though the testicles are located on the exterior of the body, testicular trauma is less common than one might expect. Owing to the mobility of the scrotum, the testes are protected from most impacts.

Testicular trauma is usually caused by a direct blow to the area, an object that penetrates the scrotum, or an injury that involves the removal of the protective integument. If the scrotum is intact and the testes have been spared, the treatment is scrotal support, methods to decrease inflammation (i.e., anti-inflammatory drugs and ice), and bed rest. If there has been interruption in the integrity of the skin or damage to the internal structures, emergency medical treatment must include surgical intervention.

TREATMENT AND DIAGNOSIS OF DISEASES AND DISORDERS OF THE MALE REPRODUCTIVE SYSTEM

As discussed previously, most of the male reproductive system is externally located. Therefore, symptoms of disorders in these structures are usually evident soon after onset. Such symptoms should not be ignored out of embarrassment since most genital disorders can be cured by prompt treatment. Disorders of the internal structures such as testicular torsion can require emergency treatment. Table 27-2 outlines the diseases common to the internal and external structures of the male reproductive system.

Sexually Transmitted Diseases

Sexually transmitted diseases (STDs) affect both men and women; they can damage health and become life threatening (Table 27-3). (See Chapter 25 for additional information regarding STDs.)

ASSISTING WITH THE MALE REPRODUCTIVE EXAMINATION

Professional

A female medical assistant usually is not required to assist the provider with the examination of the male reproductive system. However, it is within your professional responsibility to assist your provider as requested. Remember to conduct yourself in a respectful, appropriate manner, including nonverbal communication.

Diversity

The provider examines the penis and the foreskin of the penis in an uncircumcised patient. In the United States, it is common for males to be circumcised shortly after birth. However, that is not the cultural expectation in many other countries. Remember that cultural norms vary from country to country. There are many men who require health care that are from other nations and cultures. It is important to understand that diversity is acceptable. The penis and testes are examined for swelling, masses, or discomfort. The provider performs a digital rectal examination to check the size of the prostate and also checks for an inguinal hernia.

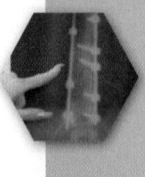

Critical Thinking

Mr. and Mrs. Jared Parris are being seen by the provider for a first visit to discuss their infertility issues. As these patients have never been seen by Dr. Carey before, what considerations should be taken when obtaining a patient history?

TABLE 27-2

DISEASES AND DISORDERS OF THE MALE REPRODUCTIVE SYSTEM

DISEASE/DISORDER	SYMPTOMS	LABORATORY DIAGNOSTICS	RADIOGRAPHY AND TECHNICAL DIAGNOSTICS	MEDICAL/SURGICAL DIAGNOSTICS	TREATMENTS
Balanitis	Redness, itching, pain and/or irritation of the head of the penis; tightened foreskin	Culture (rarely)	None	Physical examination, history	Localized soaks and frequent cleansing, antibiotics
Benign prostatic hyperplasia (BPH)	Dysuria, nocturia, frequency; weak urine stream; dribbling at the end of urination; inability to completely empty the bladder even with straining	Prostate-specific antigen (PSA), urinalysis	Intravenous pyelogram (IVP), pelvic ultrasound	Digital rectal examination, history, cystoscopy, ultrasound, and biopsy Symptoms: Frequent and/or urgent need to urinate Pain during ejaculation Pain during urination Dysuria (difficulty urinating) Urinary tract infections Difficulty emptying bladder Nocturia	Medications; surgical intervention (TURP); microwave, radio wave, or laser therapies
Cryptorchidism	Absence of one or both of the testes	None	Ultrasound	Physical examination, history	Hormonal therapy or surgical therapy, or a combination of both
Epididymitis	Discharge from the urethra; painful or urgent urination; a swollen, red or warm scrotum; testicle pain and tenderness, usually on one side; pain with ejaculation or with intercourse	Complete blood count, urinalysis (culture and sensitivity test), culture and sensitivity testing of urethral discharge	IVP; pelvic ultrasound	Physical examination, history	Antibiotics, scrotal support, surgery

continues

Table 27-2, continued

DISEASE/DISORDER	SYMPTOMS	LABORATORY DIAGNOSTICS	RADIOGRAPHY AND TECHNICAL DIAGNOSTICS	MEDICAL/SURGICAL DIAGNOSTICS	TREATMENTS
Erectile dysfunction (ED)	Inability to achieve or maintain an erection	Complete blood count, fasting blood sugar, lipid profile, testosterone level, urinalysis	Angiogram (rarely), magnetic resonance imaging (MRI) of the brain (rarely)	Physical examination, history; neurologic examination; psychological evaluation	Oral medications, localized injected medication, penile implant, penile pump, psychotherapy
Hypogonadism	Lack of male secondary sexual characteristics, ED, infertility, decreased libido	Testosterone level analysis, semen analysis, genetic studies, testicular biopsy	Pituitary imaging	Physical examination, history	Hormone replacement therapy, assistive reproductive technology
Hypospadias/Epispadias	Ureteral opening located other than at the tip of penis	None	Ultrasound	Physical examination, history	Surgical intervention
Male infertility	Inability to conceive	Testosterone level analysis, semen analysis	None	Physical examination, history	Hormone replacement therapy, assistive reproductive technology
Orchitis	Painful swelling in one or both testicles, elevated temperature, nausea and vomiting	Urinalysis, venereal disease research laboratory (VDRL) testing	None	Physical examination, history	Pain management, antibiotics or antiviral medication
Penile cancer	A growth or sore on the penis, color changes or thickening of the skin, rash or bumps under the foreskin, persistent drainage with a foul odor, bleeding, enlarged groin lymph nodes, irregular swelling of the head of the penis	None	Computerized tomography (CT) scan, (MRI)	Physical examination, history; biopsy	Surgical resection up to and including penectomy, laser therapy, radiation therapy, chemotherapy
Peyronie disease	Significant bend to the penis, erection difficulties, shortening of the penis, pain	None	Ultrasound or X-rays to reveal the presence of scar tissue	Physical examination	Medications, penile injections, surgical reconstruction

continues

Table 27-2, continued

DISEASE/DISORDER	SYMPTOMS	LABORATORY DIAGNOSTICS	RADIOGRAPHY AND TECHNICAL DIAGNOSTICS	MEDICAL/SURGICAL DIAGNOSTICS	TREATMENTS
Priapism	Unwanted erection lasting more than four hours, intermittent unwanted erection for several hours, rigid shaft but soft glans penis, painful or tender penis	None	None	Physical examination, history	Medication injection, pain management, therapeutic aspiration, surgical intervention, treatment of underlying conditions
Prostate cancer	Dysuria, nocturia, hematuria, frequency; pain or fullness in the pelvic area; bone pain with metastasis; erectile dysfunction	PSA, urinalysis, acid phosphatase (blood)	IVP; pelvic ultrasound	Digital rectal examination, history, cystoscopy, ultrasound, and biopsy	Prostatectomy: hormone manipulation; chemotherapy, radiation, or both
Prostatitis	Pain or burning sensation or difficult urination; nocturia; pain radiating to the low back, abdomen or groin	Complete blood count, urinalysis and culture, analysis of prostate secretion	Urodynamics (if not caused by a bacterium)	Digital rectal examination, history	Long-term treatment with antibiotics, prostate massage, increased fluid intake
Testicular cancer	A lump or enlargement in either testicle, pain in the testicle, feeling of heaviness in the scrotum, abdominal or groin aching, hydrocele	Blood for tumor markers	Testicular ultrasound	Physical examination (palpation of testis), history, biopsy	Excision of the testis, radiation therapy, chemotherapy
Testicular torsion	Acute onset of pain, nausea and vomiting, testicle retraction and/or transverse lie	None	Ultrasound, nuclear scan, Doppler sonogram	Physical examination, history; surgical exploration	Surgical intervention

TABLE 27-3

SEXUALLY TRANSMITTED DISEASES

DISEASE	KEY INFORMATION
Chlamydia	Common in male and female individuals. A prevalent sexually transmitted disease that often co-exists with gonorrhea. Can cause female infertility due to scarring from infection. Diagnosed by urinalysis; urethral smear. Treatment: Patient education, antibiotics, test/treat partner.
Condylomata acuminata or Genital warts	Result of an infection with the human papillomavirus (HPV). Most common sexually transmitted disease, surpassing even genital herpes. The most common anorectal infection affecting homosexual men. Treatment: Treated with topical chemical agents, immune therapy, and surgery. Due to the risk for communicability, as well as the risk for the development of squamous cell carcinoma, lesions must be treated.
Genital herpes (type II herpes simplex)	Painful viral disease that is dormant and recurs periodically. Characterized by blisters similar to chickenpox. Common in male and female individuals. Diagnosed by culture of lesion. Treatment: Symptoms are managed with oral antiviral medications.
Gonorrhea	Caused by a bacterium. Infection can spread, producing a stricture of the urethra or the vas deferens. Sterility can result if both vas deferentia become involved. Diagnosed by urethral smear. Treatment: Patient education, antibiotics, test/treat partner.
Hepatitis B and C virus and HIV infections	All are caused by a virus. Although there is no cure, symptoms of hepatitis B and C are managed with oral antiviral medications. The goal of treatment for HIV is support of the immune system with **highly active antiretroviral therapy (HAART)** medications.
Syphilis	Caused by a spirochete. Chancres develop and can subsequently heal. If untreated, the disease progresses to stages two and three. Severe damage to the cardiovascular system and brain; vision and hearing loss occur. General paralysis and death can result. Highly contagious. Diagnosed by urinalysis with culture, venereal disease research laboratory (VDRL) studies, culture of the lesion. Treatment: Patient education, antibiotics, test/treat partner.

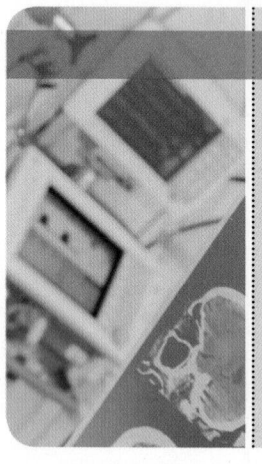

CASE STUDY 27-1

Refer to the scenario at the beginning of the chapter, the "Internal Anatomy" Quick Reference Guide, and the section regarding TURP to answer the following questions.

CASE STUDY REVIEW

1. What should Wanda do initially upon beginning the conversation with Mr. Thomas?
2. Understanding that speaking about matters of the male reproductive system might be sensitive, what is the most effective manner to ask the pertinent questions regarding his course since surgery to enter into patient history?
3. Using your critical thinking skills, list at least three questions that should be entered into Mr. Thomas's history.

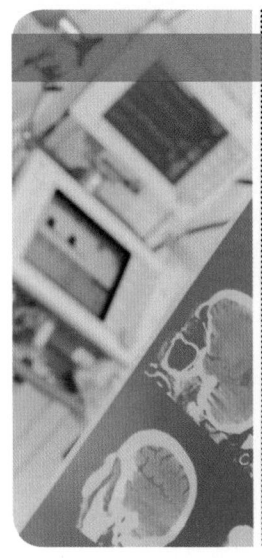

CASE STUDY 27-2

Mrs. Renee Southern and her little boy, Josh, are patients of Dr. Carey's. Mrs. Southern has brought 4-year-old Josh in today because she has a concern. Josh is uncircumcised. Wanda Slawson, CMA (AAMA), introduces herself and asks Mrs. Southern to state Josh's name and his birthdate as identifiers. Wanda greets Josh saying, "Hey, buddy! What's the name of your stuffed bear?" Wanda asks Mrs. Southern, "What brings Josh in to the office today?" Mrs. Southern responds, "I'm concerned because Josh's foreskin is so tight, it can't be pulled back during bath time."

CASE STUDY REVIEW

1. Reviewing your knowledge of common pediatric disorders of the reproductive system, what is this condition called?
2. Are there any special instruments that the provider might need to complete this child's exam?
3. How might you respond honestly and diplomatically to Mrs. Southern's concerns?

Summary

- A thorough knowledge of the diseases and disorders of the male reproductive system and the diagnostic tests and procedures that are performed for this specialty will enhance the quality of care given by the medical assistant.
- You should be familiar with both the internal and external anatomical structures of the male reproductive system, including descriptions of these structures and the functions of all structures.
- You should know the important elements to be documented in the patient's history related to the anatomy of the male reproductive system.
- You should be able to recognize male anatomical structures in a diagram.
- You should have knowledge of the common diseases and disorders of the male reproductive system, including symptoms, causes, and treatments.
- You should be able to provide appropriate patient education related to the male reproductive system.

Study for Success

To reinforce your knowledge and skills of information presented in this chapter:

- Review the *Key Terms* and *Learning Outcomes*
- Consider the *Critical Thinking* features and *Case Studies* and discuss your conclusions
- Answer the questions in the *Certification Review*

Procedure

- Perform the *Procedure* using the *Competency Assessment Checklist* on the *Student Companion Website*

CERTIFICATION REVIEW

1. Cancer of the prostate may be detected early by which of the following?
   a. Prostate-specific antigen
   b. Transurethral resection of the prostate
   c. Semen analysis
   d. Urine culture
2. The best preventive measure for testicular cancer is which of the following?
   a. Yearly physical examination
   b. Yearly intravenous pyelogram
   c. Monthly self-examination
   d. Monthly urinalysis with cultures
   e. Biannual testicular ultrasound
3. Benign prostatic hyperplasia (BPH) is thought to be caused by which of the following?
   a. Excessive consumption of alcohol
   b. Aging and hormonal changes
   c. Recurrent epididymitis
   d. Chronic chlamydia infections
4. Which of the following is a symptom of prostatitis?
   a. Painful urination
   b. Low sperm count
   c. Eruptions on the scrotum
   d. High testosterone level
   e. Elevated sexual drive
5. What is the most definitive way to diagnose cancer of the prostate?
   a. Ultrasonography
   b. Intravenous pyelogram
   c. Biopsy of the prostate
   d. Semen analysis
6. What is the definition of erectile dysfunction?
   a. The inability to achieve an erection
   b. The inability to sustain an erection
   c. Lack of libido
   d. Both a and b
   e. All of these
7. Which of the following is an important aspect of documentation of patient education regarding testicular examination?
   a. Patient questions
   b. Return demonstration
   c. Medical assistant name
   d. All of these
8. The vas deferens attaches to what structure?
   a. Bladder
   b. Penis
   c. Urethra
   d. Prostrate
   e. Scrotum
9. Prostate cancer is the leading cause of death in men from which age group?
   a. 45 to 55 years
   b. 55 to 65 years
   c. 65 to 75 years
   d. 75 years and older
10. The incidence of penile cancer is greater in what population?
    a. Men over 75 years
    b. Men with a history of STD
    c. Uncircumcised men
    d. Men who are infertile
    e. Men with greater exposure to UV light

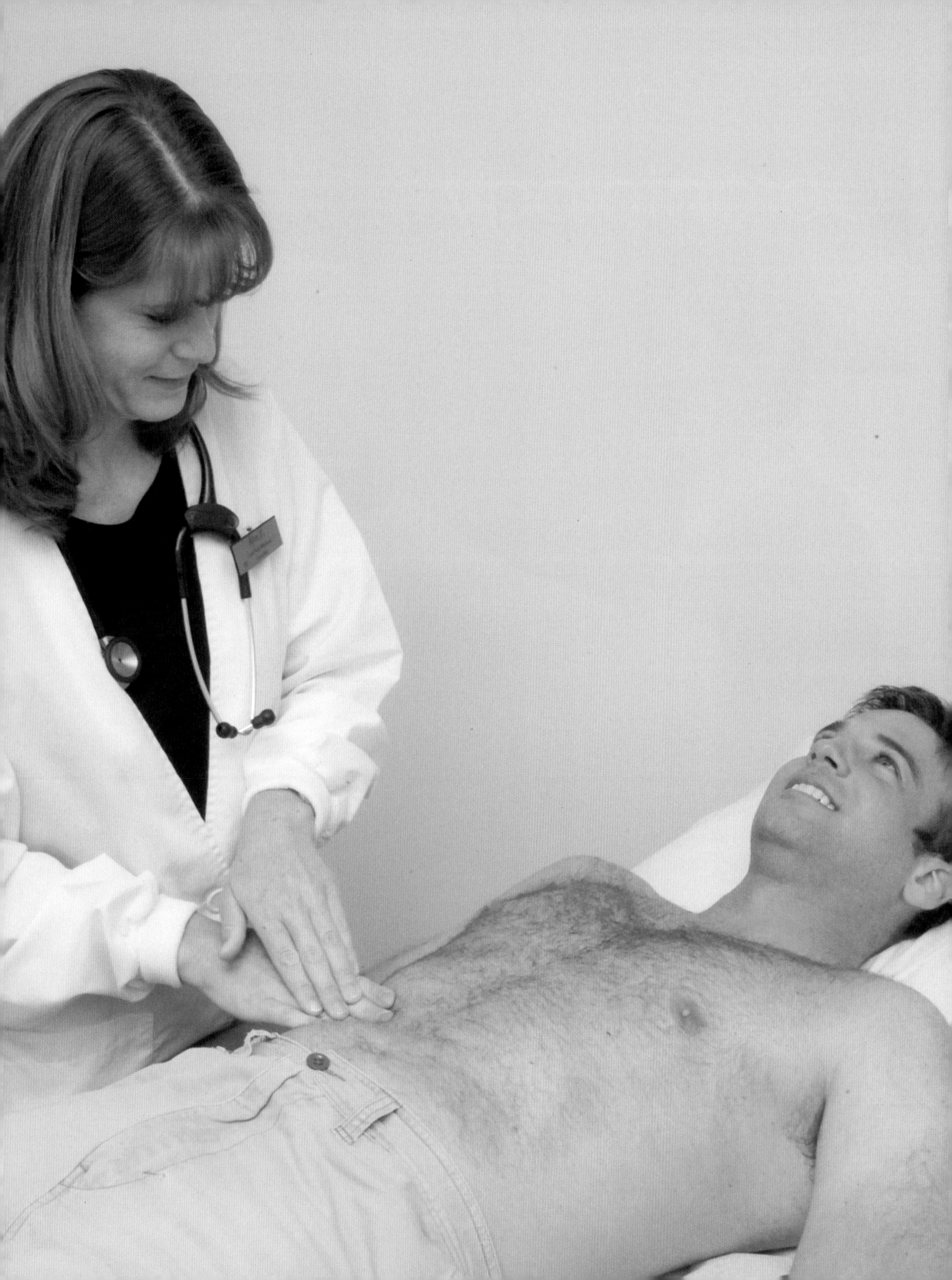

CHAPTER 28

Gerontology

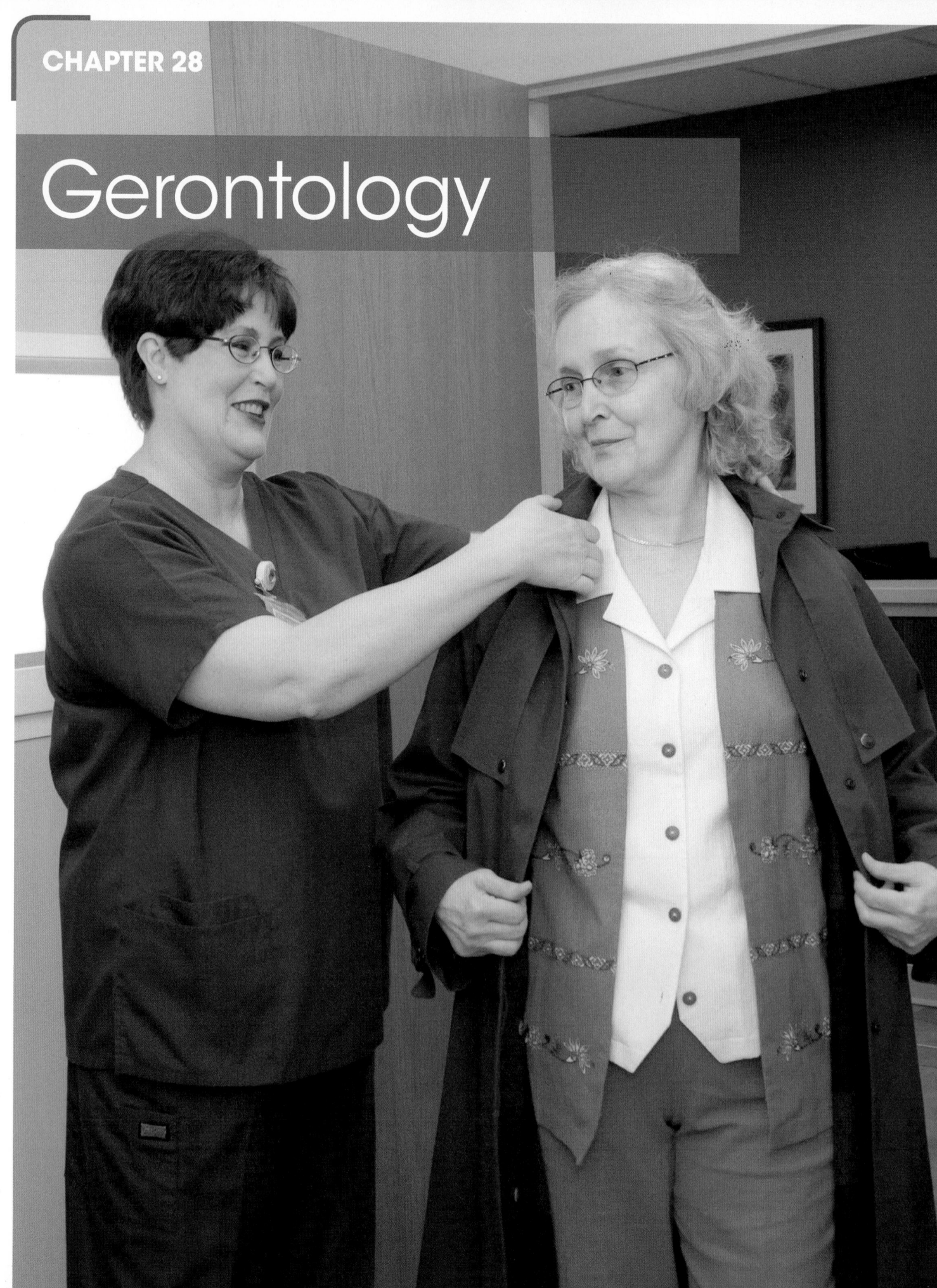

1. Define and spell the key terms as presented in the glossary.
2. Identify expected physiologic changes that occur as part of the aging process.
3. Recite five common functional changes that can occur as part of the aging process.
4. Describe prevention techniques for complications arising from age-related disorders.
5. Explain two myths about aging.
6. Summarize the importance of communication with older adults.
7. Identify several techniques or strategies to communicate with older adults who have visual and hearing impairments.
8. State strategies for healthy and successful aging.

KEY TERMS

ageism	glaucoma
andropause	hyperthermia
angina	hypothermia
arteriosclerosis	incontinence
cataracts	macular degeneration
cognitive functioning	menopause
cystitis	nevus
dementia	osteoporosis
dyspnea	pernicious anemia
esophagitis	presbycusis
geriatrician	presbyopia
geriatrics	residual urine
gerontology	transient ischemic attack (TIA)

SCENARIO

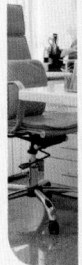

Mrs. Johnson is an 82-year-old patient of Dr. King, and she is scheduled for an appointment in the cardiac clinic. She is being evaluated for congestive heart failure and has had hypertension for many years. Her condition was difficult to control, but after patient education, she takes her medication according to her provider's orders. A part of her care plan is to walk at least one mile daily to enhance her overall wellness. Today she is volunteering in the gift shop at Inner City Hospital. She is an example of an older adult with chronic illnesses who has changed some longtime behaviors that were harmful to her health.

Gerontology is the scientific study of the problems associated with aging. Gerontology focuses on the resilience of the older adults in the areas of physiology, social science, psychology, public health, and policy. **Geriatrics** is the term indicating the medical care of older adults. A **geriatrician** is a doctor who is specially trained to evaluate and manage the unique health care needs and treatment preferences of older people.

Growing older should not be regarded as an affliction. It is a stage in life, like all others, that deserves to be celebrated and documented in all its natural grace and beauty. Increasingly, there is a need for greater attention to the population of elders as the numbers of older Americans increases. The most recent census data indicates that one in seven Americans is 65 years old or older. That percentage is anticipated to increase to one in five by 2040 (Figure 28-1).

Failing to integrate age into our efforts to understand and interpret human experience leads to a distorted view that risks reinforcing age discrimination and contributes to the widespread dread of getting older. Older adults have specialized needs just as do people in other stages of life. More than half of adults age 65 and older have three or more medical problems, such as heart disease, diabetes, arthritis, Alzheimer disease, or high blood pressure.

SOCIETAL BIAS

Diversity

In our culture, there is a deeply ingrained bias about aging. **Ageism** is discriminating against individuals or stereotyping groups on the basis of their age. Ageism is thought to be more even pervasive than racism or sexism. Myths and stereotypes are common regarding older adults, and the medical assistant can be an advocate for older adults and can be sensitive to these myths and stereotypes. Accurate information and useful concepts about aging must be communicated to the general public.

Older adults oftentimes are viewed as sick, frail, powerless, sexless, and burdensome. As a society, we are obsessed with the negative, rather than the positive, aspects of aging. The most popular myth is, "To be old is to be sick." Even in advanced old age, a majority of the older population has little functional disability. Because of better education about the practice of healthier lifestyles, to be old in the United States does not mean to be sick and frail. When it comes to health, there is no "typical" older person. Biological aging is only loosely associated with a person's age in years. Health in older age is not random. Such factors as genetics, good nutrition, regular exercise, stress reduction, yearly physical examinations, not smoking, and today's technology help forestall the aging process.

People from a disadvantaged environment are both more likely to experience poor health and less likely to have access to the services and the care that they may need.

The resilience of the elderly is well known and provides an opportunity for many to learn from this cohort of adults. As a society, our goal should be to lessen the struggles of such an amazing generation of adults. Aging is inevitable, but it is also something that should be revered. One might consider: What are we doing as a society to make sure that we adopt healthy lifestyles now to ensure a seamless transition into old age? This question is considered as we strive to meet the demands of a growing and diverse aging population.

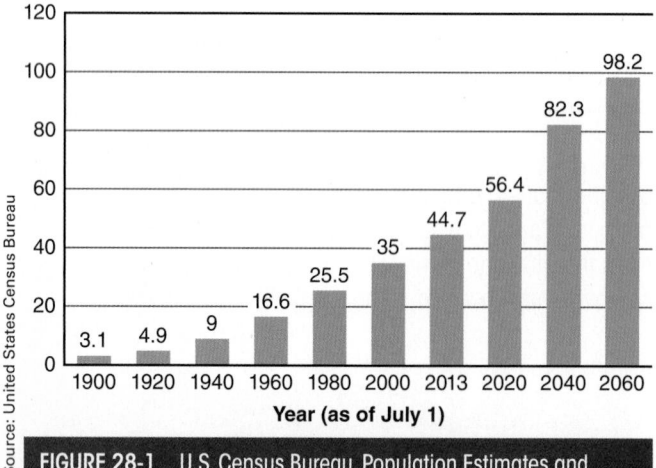

Number of Persons 65+, 1900 to 2060 (numbers in millions)

Data Source: United States Census Bureau

FIGURE 28-1 U.S. Census Bureau, Population Estimates and Projections.

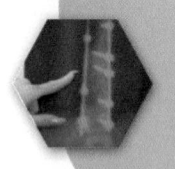

Critical Thinking

What do you consider common myths about older adults? What are your thoughts about these myths?

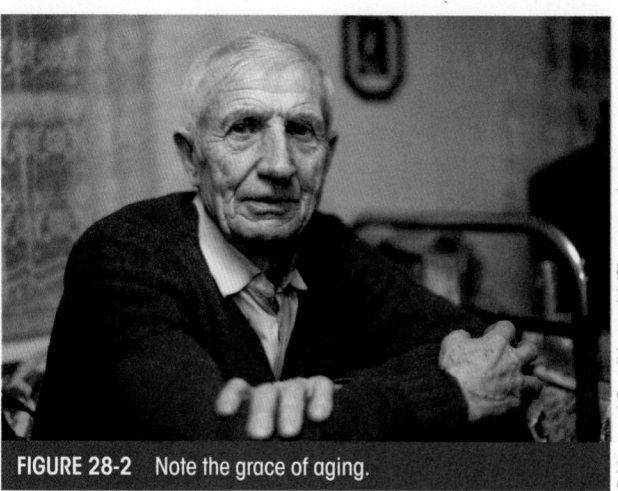

FIGURE 28-2 Note the grace of aging.

© Mostovyi Sergii Igorevich/Shutterstock.com

FACTS ABOUT AGING

Following are general facts about aging:

- Aging is a progressive, universal, and slow process.

- There are no diseases specific to aging.

- As people age, not all functional changes are related to disease. Interest, personal and financial resources, family structure, genetics, and attitude all play a part. The individual's lifestyle is a major factor. For example, smoking, misuse of chemicals such as alcohol or drugs, type of diet, and lack of exercise all play a part in how people age.

- Approximately 92% of older adults have at least one chronic disease, and 77% have at least two. Three chronic diseases—heart disease, cancer, stroke, and diabetes—cause almost two-thirds of all deaths of older adults in the United States each year.

- Every 15 seconds, an older adult is treated at the emergency department for a fall; every 29 minutes, an older adult dies following a fall.

- Among older adults, falls are the leading cause of fractures, hospital admissions for trauma, and injury deaths. Falls are also the most common cause of older adult traumatic brain injuries.

- One in four older adults (approximately 7.5 million) experiences some mental disorder including depression and anxiety disorders, and dementia. This number is expected to double to 15 million by 2030.

- Depression affects 7 million older Americans, and many do not receive treatment.

- The number of older adults with substance abuse problems is expected to rise to 5 million by 2020.

- There is a wider range of what is considered "normal" function among older adults than among younger people. There is a greater variability among older people in their physical abilities, sizes, and characteristics than among younger groups (Figure 28-2).

PHYSIOLOGIC CHANGES

Although aging is a normal process, not all individuals age in the same way or at the same rate, because no two people have exactly the same genetic inheritance, personal lifestyle, or experiences in life. All of these factors strongly influence the ways in which we grow older. Some believe that because of the wear and tear and stress the body endures during life, eventually the body loses its ability to function as well as it did. Others believe that one grows older, the body produces smaller and smaller amounts of various hormones and other chemicals that keep the body functioning. The fewer of these kinds of substances that are produced, the more susceptible an individual becomes to disease.

Every body system undergoes changes as we age. The changes are physiologic and psychological. As individuals move into their 60s and beyond, they will show physiologic changes that are part of the aging process.

Senses

See the "Sensory Changes in Older Adults" Quick Reference Guide for information on changes in vision, hearing, and taste and smell in older adults.

▶▶ SENSORY CHANGES IN OLDER ADULTS

Vision

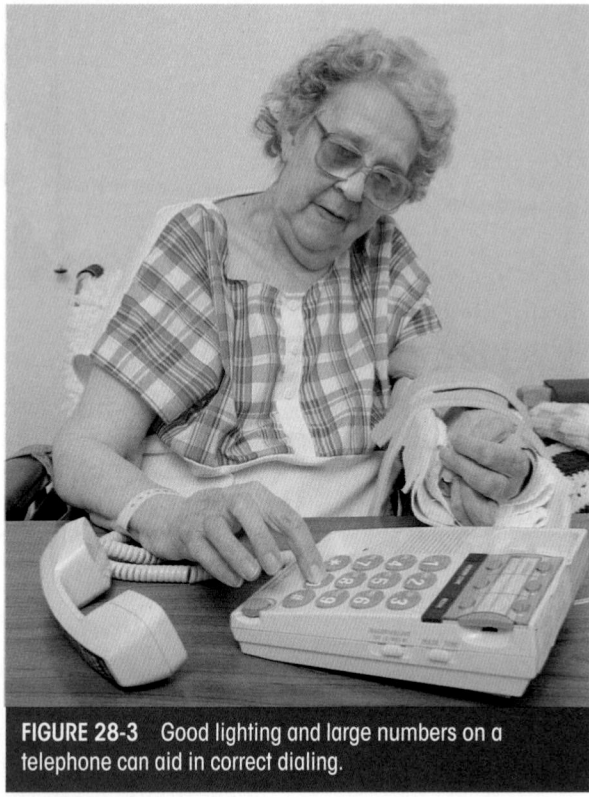

FIGURE 28-3 Good lighting and large numbers on a telephone can aid in correct dialing.

Disease/ Dysfunction	Description/Pathophysiology	Patient Education
Presbyopia	Blurred near vision caused by loss of elasticity of the lens of the eye	Signs and symptoms: • Eyestrain or headaches after reading or doing close work • Difficulty reading small print • Fatigue from doing close work • Requiring brighter lighting when reading (Figure 28-3) • Holding reading material at an arm's length to focus properly • Difficulty focusing • Squinting
Floaters	Tiny specks or "cobwebs" that seem to float across field of vision; most often noted in well-lit rooms or outdoors on a bright day	Signs of retinal detachment: • Many new floaters • Flashes of light See eye care professional immediately

(continues)

Disease/ Dysfunction	Description/Pathophysiology	Patient Education
Dry eyes	Lack of tears due to decreased production	Appropriate use of over-the-counter medications Need to contact the provider when eyes are burning and stinging, if eyes feel sticky and/or are often red, or if there are periods when eyes get so watery that tears spill over eyelids
Cataracts	Clouding of the structure called the lens; prevents light entering the eye and being interpreted by the retina	Signs and symptoms: • Clouded, blurred, or dim vision • Increasing difficulty with vision at night • Sensitivity to light and glare • Seeing "halos" around lights • Frequent changes in eyeglass or contact lens prescription • Fading or yellowing of colors • Double vision in a single eye Risk factors: • Diabetes • Excessive use of alcohol • High blood pressure • Excessive exposure to sunlight • Exposure to X-rays and radiation therapy • Family history • Obesity
Glaucoma	Group of related eye disorders that result in increased pressure in the eye causing damage to the optic nerve	Importance of regular eye exams to check for the development of glaucoma Use of prescribed eye drops Risk factors: • Increased intraocular pressure • Age >60 • Race: Increased incidence in African Americans and Hispanics/Latinos • Family history • History of diabetes, heart disease, high blood pressure, sickle cell anemia • Nearsightedness • History of eye trauma or surgery • Early estrogen deficiency • Corticosteroid use, especially eye drops

(continues)

Disease/ Dysfunction	Description/Pathophysiology	Patient Education
Age-related **macular degeneration**	Damage to the macula, which is responsible for sharp, central vision	Importance of routine eye exams Signs and symptoms: • Straight lines start to appear distorted, or the center of vision becomes distorted • Dark, blurry areas or whiteout appears in the center of vision • Diminished or changed color perception (very rarely) Risk factors: • Smoking doubles the risk • More common among Caucasians than among African Americans or Hispanics/Latinos • Family history To decrease risk: • Avoid smoking • Exercise regularly • Maintain normal blood pressure and cholesterol levels • Eat a healthy diet rich in green, leafy vegetables and fish

Hearing

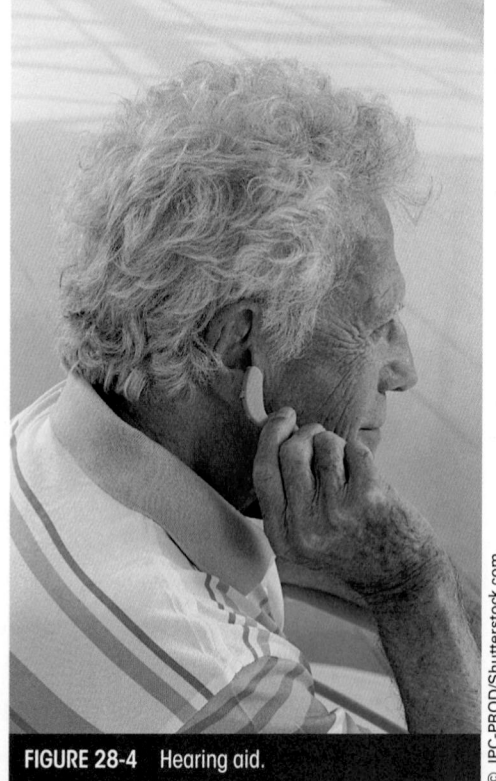

© JPC-PROD/Shutterstock.com

FIGURE 28-4 Hearing aid.

(continues)

Disease/ Dysfunction	Description/Pathophysiology	Patient Education
Presbycusis	Age-related hearing loss	Signs and symptoms: • Difficulty hearing people around you • Frequently asking people to repeat themselves • Feeling frustrated at not being able to hear • Some sounds being overly loud • Difficulty hearing in noisy areas • Difficulty differentiating certain sounds • Difficulty hearing/understanding higher-pitched voices • Ringing in the ears Risk factors: • Family history • Repeated exposure to loud noises • Smoking • Diabetes • Past history of chemotherapy Treatment-related teaching (Figure 28-4): • Hearing aid care • Hearing aid maintenance
Tinnitus	"Ringing in the ears"; it may also sound like blowing, roaring, buzzing, hissing, humming, whistling, or sizzling	Risk factors: • Exposure to loud noise • Hearing loss related to aging • High daily doses of aspirin • Eustachian tube dysfunction • Infections, such as otitis media or labyrinthitis • High blood pressure • Certain allergies • Diabetes
Vestibular Disorders	Damage to the vestibular system causes dizziness and/or balance problems; this system is involved in motion, equilibrium, and spatial orientation	Signs and symptoms: • Difficulty walking or standing Risk factors: • Decreased blood flow to the inner ear • Age (reduces nerve endings)

(continues)

Taste and Smell

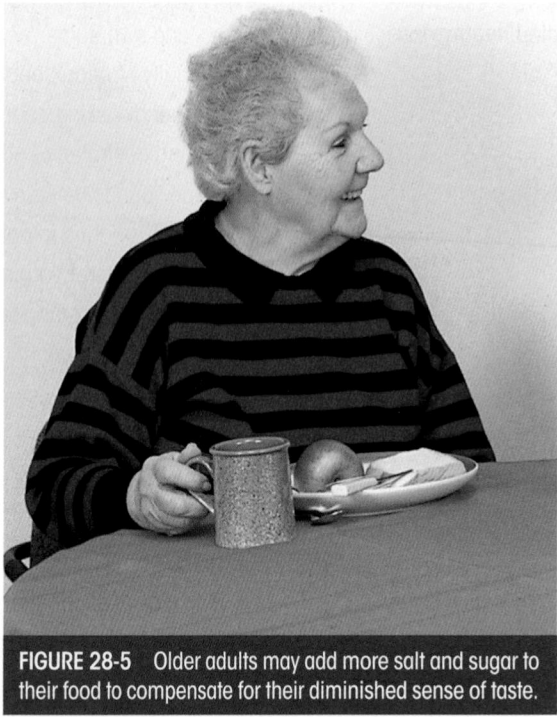

FIGURE 28-5 Older adults may add more salt and sugar to their food to compensate for their diminished sense of taste.

Disease/ Dysfunction	Description/Pathophysiology	Patient Education
Impaired taste	Lessening ability to distinguish flavors; sensitivity to taste declines after 60 years of age (Figure 28-5).	Risk factors: • Age (fewer taste buds with aging) • Loss of teeth leading to decreased chewing ability • Decrease in amount of saliva • Oral or pharyngeal diseases, such as candidiasis (thrush) • Smoking • Certain medications • Nutritional deficits
Impaired sense of smell*	Declining olfactory function results in loss of smell and a decreased ability to differentiate between smells	Risk factors: • Age (fewer olfactory cells with aging) • Neurologic disorders • Certain medications • Smoking Safety considerations: • Need for smoke alarm

A National Institutes of Health–supported study found that older adults that could no longer detect or distinguish smells were four times more likely to die in the next 5 years.

Integumentary System

Aging individuals' skin becomes more fragile with less subcutaneous and connective tissue. Exposure to sunlight is the major cause of wrinkled skin, liver spots, and leathery looking skin.

Sweat glands become smaller and the body becomes less sensitive to heat and cold. **Hyperthermia**, an unusually high fever, and **hypothermia**, an unusually low body temperature, are serious problems, and exposure to excessive hot or cold temperatures should be avoided (see Chapter 32).

Hair loses color and becomes thinner. The skin dries and is less elastic. Fingernails and toenails thicken.

The development of skin cancer on exposed skin surfaces is not uncommon in older adults. Basal and squamous cell carcinomas are the most common skin cancer types seen in this population. Both types of cancer can be serious if left untreated, but squamous cell cancer can metastasize. A complete skin assessment should be done on a yearly basis. Melanoma, a malignant tumor developing from a **nevus**, is the least common skin cancer, but it can be serious because it metastasizes readily. It is caused by exposure to the sun. Most skin cancers result from sun damage over the course of life. Due to their life span, seniors have had the most sun exposure and sustained the most damage from ultraviolet (UV) light. Many older adults live in the Sunbelt areas of the United States and should be particularly cautioned to wear sunscreen of SPF 15 or higher due to the higher UV radiation in these areas. However, people of all ages should protect their skin daily with a sunscreen of SPF 15 or higher, regardless of where they reside.

Nervous System

The brain shrinks in size as an individual ages because brain cells do not continue to divide throughout life as other cells do. Some loss of memory or delay in memory can be expected in many, but not all, aging people. Mental competence is the rule rather than the exception for older adults.

Problems with balance, temperature regulation, diminished pain sensation, and insomnia can occur as part of the physical changes of aging that affect the nervous system.

Chronic illnesses from which many older people suffer often require several different medications. Side effects of medication (over-the-counter, prescription, and herbals) can cause decreased mental capacity, as can malnutrition and substance abuse.

Loss of balance can be a problem for some older adults. Their coordination of muscles for movement may need more time for processing than it does with younger individuals. Older adults need to be reminded to be sure of their balance before starting to walk and to do so slowly. There is a general unsteadiness and lack of coordination not only because of the aging process, but also possibly because of medications the older adult takes. Older adults may need to use a cane to help steady their gait.

Table 28-1 lists diseases and disorders of the nervous system that may occur in older adults.

Musculoskeletal System

Musculoskeletal system changes are evident because older adults may have less muscle strength. This results in loss of mobility, and the activities of daily living become more difficult. Table 28-2 lists diseases and disorders of the musculoskeletal system that may occur in older adults. Poor nutrition, malnourishment, and lack of exercise all contribute to these conditions and prolong healing time as well (see Chapters 32 and 33).

Physical activity and a nutritious diet, including dairy products, can stall the development of bone and muscle loss; therefore, older adults should be encouraged to keep active by walking, gardening, swimming, bicycling, golfing, and so on. The pace of these activities should be suited to the individual's level of ability.

Respiratory System

Breathing capacity diminishes with age, and oxygen and carbon dioxide exchange is lessened. The rib and chest muscles become smaller and less efficient. Lungs lose their elasticity, and the older adult may experience **dyspnea** or possibly, shortness of breath (SOB), and become more prone to pneumonia.

As people age, there is a gradual decline in the muscle structure of the respiratory system, leading to a diminished ability to breathe deeply; thus, development of cough and pneumonia is not uncommon. Regular exercise can help to maintain the ability to breathe and cough effectively. People who have been active throughout their lives have greater lung capacity.

TABLE 28-1

DISEASES AND DISORDERS OF THE NERVOUS SYSTEM IN OLDER ADULTS

DISEASE/DYSFUNCTION	DESCRIPTION/PATHOPHYSIOLOGY	PATIENT EDUCATION
Dementia (e.g., related to Alzheimer disease)	Reduction in brain size and weight due primarily to a decrease in cerebral cortex volume Reduction in the number of neurons Decrease in blood flow	Signs and symptoms: • Significant impairment of core mental functions including memory, communication, ability to focus and pay attention, reasoning and judgement, and visual perception Risk factors: • Age • Family history • Heavy alcohol use • Depression • Diabetes • Smoking • Sleep apnea Safety considerations inside and outside of the home
Transient ischemic attack (TIA)	Known as a ministroke A temporary blockage of an artery in the brain	Risk factors: • Family history • Age—increased risk over age 55 • Sex—increased risk for males • Race—increased risk of death for African Americans • Diabetes • High blood pressure • Prior TIA • Sickle cell disease Signs, symptoms, and intervention (FAST): • Face drooping (F) • Arm weakness (A) • Speech (S) • Time to call 911 (T)
Stroke	Interruption of the blood supply in an area of the brain causing loss of neurologic function	Risk factors: • Age • High blood pressure • Previous TIA • Family history • Diabetes • Smoking • Elevated cholesterol • High blood pressure • Cardiovascular disease • Obesity Signs, symptoms, and intervention (FAST): • Face drooping (F) • Arm weakness (A) • Speech (S) • Time to call 911 (T)

TABLE 28-2

DISEASES AND DISORDERS OF THE MUSCULOSKELETAL SYSTEM IN OLDER ADULTS

DISEASE/DYSFUNCTION	DESCRIPTION/PATHOPHYSIOLOGY	PATIENT EDUCATION
Muscle loss	Decreased amount of muscle tissue and the number and size of muscle fibers Related to inactivity	Safety: • Careful transitions • Use of assistive devices
Osteoporosis (Figure 28-6)	Disease that results in demineralization of bones; an increased risk of fracture	Signs and symptoms: • Back pain caused by a fractured or collapsed vertebra • Loss of height over time • Stooped posture • Bone fracture that occurs much more easily than expected Risk factors: • Sex—increased in women • More common with increasing age • Race—increased in Caucasians and Asians • Small body frame in both men and women • Menopause • Abnormal thyroid function • Low dietary calcium • Alcohol use • Smoking • Certain medications such as steroids Maintain activity to increase bone mass

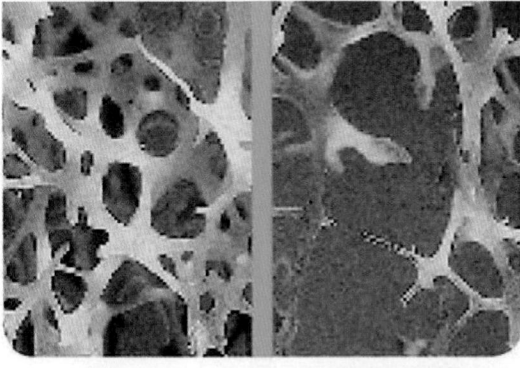

Normal Bone   Bone with Osteoporosis

Image courtesy of The 2004 Surgeon General's Report on Bone Health and Osteoporosis: What It Means to You. U.S. Department of Health and Human Services, Office of the Surgeon General, 2004.

FIGURE 28-6   Normal versus osteoporotic bone.

Cardiovascular System

Heart disease and blood vessel disorders are the major cause of death in the United States. Lifestyle has been implicated as the most significant cause of cardiovascular disease. Table 28-3 lists common diseases and disorders of the cardiovascular system that may occur in older adults. Regular exercise and a healthy diet are the most beneficial activities for older adults to help them maintain adequate cardiac output throughout their life spans.

Gastrointestinal System

Stomach secretions and motility slow as part of aging. Peristalsis slows, and food moves through the gastrointestinal tract more slowly. **Pernicious anemia** is a disorder that can occur when cells of the stomach lining fail to secrete intrinsic factor. Associated with the absence of hydrochloric acid, pernicious anemia affects the nervous system and red blood cell formation.

Fewer calories are needed during older adulthood because metabolism slows. Many older adults overeat if they are lonely and they may subsequently gain weight and become obese. Eating is a social as well as a physiologic event, and if they have no one to eat with, many older adults will not prepare a meal or eat properly to have good nutrition. Loss of vigor and vitality occur. Malnourishment is not uncommon.

TABLE 28-3

DISEASES AND DISORDERS OF THE CARDIOVASCULAR SYSTEM IN OLDER ADULTS

DISEASE/DYSFUNCTION	DESCRIPTION/PATHOPHYSIOLOGY	PATIENT EDUCATION
Atrial fibrillation	Abnormal heartbeat due to changes in the electrical system of the heart	Signs and symptoms: • Pulse that feels rapid, racing, pounding, fluttering, irregular, or too slow • Sensation of feeling the heart beat (palpitations) • Confusion • Dizziness, light-headedness
Arteriosclerosis	Loss of elasticity of the arteries due to a buildup of fatty deposits	Signs and symptoms: • **Angina** (chest pain caused by temporarily reduced blood flow to the heart muscle) • Dyspnea
Congestive heart failure (CHF)	Deceased ability of the heart muscle to pump blood to the body; may be related to elasticity of the heart muscle due to age or disease.	Signs and symptoms: • Cough • Fatigue, weakness, faintness • Loss of appetite • Need to urinate at night • Irregular pulse or palpitations • Dyspnea when active or upon lying down • Edema in feet and ankles • Weight gain

Poor eating habits, poor nutrition, overeating, or undereating can lead to dental problems. Poor dental hygiene leads to gum disease and loss of teeth, many times making the chewing of food difficult and discouraging. Sometimes cardiac problems, such as endocarditis and myocardial infarction, occur from gum disease due to the invasion of pathogens and inflammation. Other common diseases and disorders of the gastrointestinal system that may occur in older adults are listed in Table 28-4.

TABLE 28-4

DISEASES AND DISORDERS OF THE GASTROINTESTINAL SYSTEM IN OLDER ADULTS

DISEASE/DYSFUNCTION	DESCRIPTION/PATHOPHYSIOLOGY	PATIENT EDUCATION
Constipation	Due to infrequent bowel movements or the inability to completely evacuate the bowel, stool remains in the rectum longer and becomes more dense and dry due to continued fluid absorption from the feces; it may be related to decreased muscular contraction and medications that delay gastrointestinal motility	Managing constipation: • Increase fluid intake • Increase dietary fiber intake • Exercise
Esophagitis	Inflammation of the esophagus due to the intake of nonsteroidal anti-inflammatory (NSAID) medications	Reducing risk of esophagitis: • Take medications with a full glass of water • Take medications only in an upright sitting or standing position

Urinary System

With aging, the kidneys decrease in size, resulting in less urine production and output. With cardiovascular arteriosclerosis, blood flow to the kidney is less. Filtering of waste products from the blood is impaired. Medications are not excreted as quickly as they are in a young, healthy person. Levels of medication may increase to a dangerous level with impaired kidney filtration. The bladder walls become more inelastic, and the ability to empty the bladder completely becomes difficult.

Table 28-5 lists common diseases and disorders of the urinary system that may occur in older adults.

Reproductive System

Women experience **menopause** at about age 55 years. Estrogen produced by the ovaries ceases, and changes in the female are noticeable with shrinking of the genitalia. Hot flashes are not uncommon because of blood vessel dilation and contraction. Vaginal secretions diminish, the vagina becomes smaller, and infections are more likely. Estrogen replacement

TABLE 28-5

DISEASES AND DISORDERS OF THE URINARY SYSTEM IN OLDER ADULTS

DISEASE/DYSFUNCTION	DESCRIPTION/PATHOPHYSIOLOGY	PATIENT EDUCATION
Acute or chronic renal failure	The functional units of the kidney (nephrons) decrease in number with age; combined with the changes in the cardiovascular system, that lead to decreased blood flow to the kidney, the kidney is not able to function normally	Signs and symptoms: • Changes in urination • Swelling of the feet, ankles, hands, or face • Fatigue • Shortness of breath • Ammonia breath or an ammonia or metal taste in the mouth • Flank pain • Itching • Loss of appetite • Nausea and vomiting
Urinary retention	The inability to empty the bladder (**residual urine**) due to decreased function of the bladder wall muscle in the older adult	Signs and symptoms: • Urinary frequency—urinating eight or more times a day • Trouble beginning a urine stream • A weak or interrupted urine stream • An urgent need to urinate with little success when trying to urinate • Feeling the need to urinate after finishing urination
Cystitis	Infection and inflammation of the bladder, often related to urinary retention	Signs and symptoms: • Strong and frequent urge to urinate • Cloudy, bloody, or strong smelling urine • Pain or burning sensation when urinating • Nausea and vomiting • Muscle aches and abdominal pains
Incontinence	The inability to control the flow of urine from the bladder	Importance of skin care Collection/management devices Complications: • Skin breakdown • Depression/isolation Risk of urinary infection

therapy helps to lessen symptoms but is used only for short-term therapy in women who experience severe menopausal symptoms. Long-term use of estrogen and progesterone has been proved to increase the risk for heart disease and breast cancer (see Chapter 25 for more information regarding menopause and hormone therapy).

Men continue to produce sperm well after 50 years of age; however, testosterone levels diminish and midlife changes occur in men. This is known as **andropause**. It is about this time that many men older than 50 years experience benign hypertrophy of the prostate (see Chapter 27). Medication may help in some cases; otherwise, surgery (a prostatectomy) may be performed.

Aging men and women maintain their sexual desires, and many enjoy sexual intercourse more when children are no longer in the home. They have more privacy and time to relax.

SAFETY

Safety

As noted in the previous section, with age, our body systems change. These changes in normal functioning increase the risk of injury, specifically from falls. Changes in neurologic status, decreased visual acuity, and loss of muscle and bone strength predispose older adults to falling. Changes in circulatory function, gait, and certain medications also increase the risk of falling.

Falls can be serious and lead to a sequence of events that may limit a person's ability to care for himself or herself and even end in death. The statistics related to falls are alarming. More than 70% of all injury-related admissions to hospitals for people over 65 years of age are attributed to falls. This number increases dramatically in adults 80 years of age and older. Falls and their resulting complications are the ninth most common cause of death in the 65 and older population. Older Americans that are hospitalized after a fall have a nearly doubled length of stay compared to admissions for all other reasons. Among people ages 65 to 69, one out of every 200 falls results in a hip fracture. That number increases to one out of every 10 for those 85 and older. One-fourth of seniors who fracture a hip from a fall will die within 6 months of the injury. The most profound effect of falling is the loss of function necessary for independent living.

Falling is not a normal part of aging. Strength and balance exercises, managing medications, having vision checked, and a safe living environment are all steps that can be taken to prevent a fall.

Area of Home	Yes	No
Floors		
The traffic pattern is obstructed by furniture.		
Throw rugs are present.	○	○
There are objects on the floor (magazines, articles of clothing, shoes, etc.).	○	○
Cords are present in the walk areas (telephone, cable, electrical, etc.).	○	○
Stairs		
There are objects on the steps (magazines, articles of clothing, shoes, etc.).	○	○
The steps are in ill repair or are uneven.	○	○
Steps are poorly lit.	○	○
There is access to the light switch at only one end of the steps or stairs.	○	○
The carpet is torn or loose covering the stairs.	○	○
The handrails are loose or broken.	○	○
There is only a handrail on one side of the stairs.	○	○
Kitchen		
Items commonly used are placed on high shelves.	○	○
Step stool for common use is unsteady.	○	○
Bathroom:	○	○
Tub or shower floor is slippery.	○	○
Supportive handrails are missing for entering and exiting the bath.	○	○
Bedroom		
The light is far from the bed and difficult to reach.	○	○
The path to the bathroom is not well lit and is cluttered.	○	○

FIGURE 28-7 Home fall prevention checklist.

A safety checklist (Figure 28-7) is an effective tool to identify risk of falling and is *also* an essential teaching tool for all who provide care to older adults.

PSYCHOLOGICAL CHANGES

There is a great deal of variation in the psychological functioning of older adults. Among the factors that contribute are the person's health; psychosocial history; race; sex; and environmental aspects such as education, support system, and social class.

The level of decline in an older adult's intelligence can be affected by social factors. People who maintain their intelligence tend to be in better health, have had more education, be in a higher socioeconomic group, and be involved with others and in their community.

Dementia affects memory, personality, and **cognitive functioning** (awareness, reasoning, judgment, intuition) and is permanent. Alzheimer disease is a common form of dementia. Some research has shown that there may be a genetic, as well as environmental, link to Alzheimer disease.

Presentation

People who have had a stroke, which interferes with blood circulation to brain cells, may suffer from impaired brain functioning. Other forms of dementia include Parkinson disease, caused by a deficiency of dopamine, a chemical in the brain; syphilis, caused by a spirochete bacterium that causes brain damage (which manifests about 20 years after initial infection); and Huntington disease, a genetic disease. When caring for patients with dementia, protect them from injury, allow them to be as independent as possible, and do not be critical or judgmental of their behaviors (they are unintentional) or what they say. Scientists have not determined what is in the minds of patients with dementia. There is an ongoing study with the goal of understanding the mental processes of those with dementia and discovering appropriate interventions.

Depression in older adults can occur due to loss of a spouse, chronic illness, or financial problems. When caring for older adults, look for signs and symptoms of depression such as poor hygiene, insomnia or excessive sleep, crying, depressed mood (sad every day, most of the day), inability to concentrate, and increased alcohol consumption. Personality seems to help determine how individuals adapt to changes that they experience as they grow older.

THE MEDICAL ASSISTANT AND THE GERIATRIC PATIENT

Presentation   Communication

Many older adults experience dementia, mental illness, depression, stress, boredom, fear of the unknown, loss of independence, feelings of rejection and worthlessness, low self-esteem, loneliness, dependence, failed expectations, and disappointments. All of these factors coupled with the physiologic changes that can occur offer a special challenge to the medical assistant caring for the health and other needs of this group of patients. Allow patients time to ventilate and express their concerns, allow for private and confidential discussion, and empathize with their situation by showing awareness of their feelings, emotions, and behavior. Good communication is essential for quality care of older adults. Do not talk to older adults as if they were children. Speak slowly and clearly. Face the individual while talking. Write instructions in addition to verbalizing them.

Older Adults with Memory Impairments

Communication

Geriatric care poses challenges when attempting to communicate with older adults who have memory impairments. The inability to communicate on a meaningful

level can be frustrating and challenging, especially for the older person who is struggling to communicate but cannot find the right words. Following are some techniques that can be effective in improving verbal communication with older people experiencing memory impairment:

1. Talk to the person in a nondistracting place. It can be difficult for an older adult to concentrate or to sort things out when there are environmental distractions such as other conversations, equipment noises, or people walking by.

2. Begin conversations with orientating information. Identify yourself, and call older adults by their preferred names. Explain the purpose of your visit.

3. Use short words and short, simple sentences with specific descriptive nouns rather than vague pronouns. For example, "Do you have difficulty using your walker?" instead of, "Do you have difficulty using it?"

4. Speak slowly and say individual words clearly.

5. Never "talk down" or be condescending. This is demeaning. Speak in an adult manner as you would to a co-worker or friend. Provide the dignity and respect you wish to receive yourself.

6. Lower the tone (pitch) of your voice. A raised pitch is a signal that one is upset. A lower pitch is also easier for people with hearing impairments to understand.

7. Talk to the person in a warm and pleasant manner. Use nonverbal cues, such as facial expression, tone of voice, or touch, to show your feelings of affection and concern. Smiling, taking the older person's hand, or touching the person on the arm can vividly communicate that you are interested and really care.

8. When giving instructions, allow plenty of time for the information to be absorbed.

9. Give clear and simple instructions.

10. Ask the person to do one task at a time.

11. Listen actively. If you do not understand, apologize to the person by saying that you did not understand exactly what was said. It is extremely important to phrase responses in a way that does not damage the self-esteem of the older adult.

12. Avoid asking direct questions that require the person to remember a fact.

13. Focus on well behavior or things that you know the patient can still do.

14. Use humor when appropriate. If expressed naturally, humor brings much needed laughter, a dimension that is often lost in the health care setting.

15. Let the person know when you leave and if you will be returning.

16. When discussing a case with another staff member, do so in private to protect patient confidentiality.

Older Adults with Visual Impairments

Older adults with visual impairments need to know you are present, but do not approach the individual until you make your presence known. Help by explaining his or her location, and identify others who may also be present. See the "Sighted Guide Techniques" Quick Reference Guide for more information.

Older Adults with Hearing Impairments

Communication

For older adults who have hearing impairments to communicate and understand instructions, there are some techniques the medical assistant should keep in mind. These strategies will be beneficial and will facilitate communication and understanding. These techniques include:

1. Face the older adult who has a hearing impairment directly and on the same level when possible (if he or she is standing, the medical assistant should stand; if the patient is seated, the medical assistant should be seated).

2. Keep your hands away from your face while talking.

3. Reduce background noises when talking. Move to a quieter room away from extraneous sounds and activities.

4. Individuals who with hearing impairments hear and understand less when they are tired or sick.

5. Get the person's attention before beginning to speak and do not talk from another room.

6. Speak in a normal tone; do not shout.

7. Be sure that light is not shining in the eyes of the older adult who has a hearing impairment.

8. If the older adult who has a hearing impairment has trouble understanding, reword what you have said. Do not repeat the same words again and again.

9. Written instructions are useful, but the medical assistant must be certain that what is written is understood.

Elder Abuse

What is elder abuse? It is any form of mistreatment that results in harm or loss to an older person. The mistreatment can be divided generally into several categories. Physical abuse that results in pain, injury and/or impairment is only one type of abuse. Sexual abuse is the forcing a nonconsensual sexual contact of any kind. Psychological abuse is the willful infliction of mental or emotional anguish by threat, humiliation, or other verbal or nonverbal conduct. Abuse can be any of the aforementioned types of abuse if it is an escalating pattern of behavior and is used to exercise power and control. Another type of elder abuse is the illegal or improper use of an older person's funds, property, or resources. This is termed financial abuse. Neglect is also a type of abuse. This is the failure of a caregiver to fulfill his or her caregiving responsibilities.

Legal

Estimates indicate that 4% to 6% of all persons over the age of 65 are victims of abuse. This makes elder abuse a pervasive part of our culture. The laws in most states require helping professionals to report suspected abuse or neglect. These professionals are called mandated reporters. To report elder abuse, contact the Adult Protective Services (APS) agency in the state where the elder resides. You can find the APS reporting number for each state by visiting:

- The State Resources section of the National Center on Elder Abuse Web site
- The Eldercare Locator Web site or by calling 1-800-677-1116

Once reports are received by the elder protective services program, if appropriate, a caseworker will assess the situation to determine the nature and extent of the abuse. If abuse is confirmed, services will be provided to eliminate or alleviate abuse. Many social services are usually available. Mental health, legal, home caregiver services, and alternative living arrangements may be provided (see Chapter 6).

>> SIGHTED GUIDE TECHNIQUES

MAKING CONTACT

Introduce yourself. Ask the patient with the visual impairment if he or she would like assistance in order to navigate in unfamiliar surroundings. If he or she does, offer your arm by saying that you are offering your arm and by touching your hand or forearm against his or hers.

GRIP

The patient grips your arm just above the elbow. The grip must be firm but not so tight that it becomes uncomfortable.

STANCE

The patient stands next to you, slightly behind. His or her arm is bent and held close to his or her side. Relax your arm and let it hang naturally at your side (see Figure 28-8).

PACE

The pace should be comfortable for both of you. If the patient tightens his or her grip or pulls on your arm, slow down; your pace may be too fast or he or she may be anxious. You should alert the patient to obstacles such as curbs, stairs, doors, and thresholds. Be specific, but do not confuse him or her with too much information.

STAIRS

When approaching stairs, tell the patient. Let him or her know whether you are going to go up or down. Be sure you approach the stairs directly, not at an angle. Have the patient stand next to the handrail if there is one.

Before proceeding on the stairs, pause at the top (or bottom) of the stairs and describe anything unusual about them. The patient will find the handrail and reach forward with his or her foot to locate the edge of the first step. Start down (or up) the stairs, keeping yourself one step ahead. Keep a steady pace (see Figure 28-9).

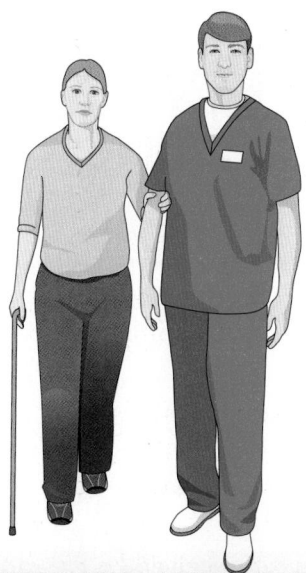

FIGURE 28-8 Notice how the medical assistant walks about a half step in front of the patient who is visually impaired toward the inside of the patient so that the patient can feel the medical assistant's body movements.

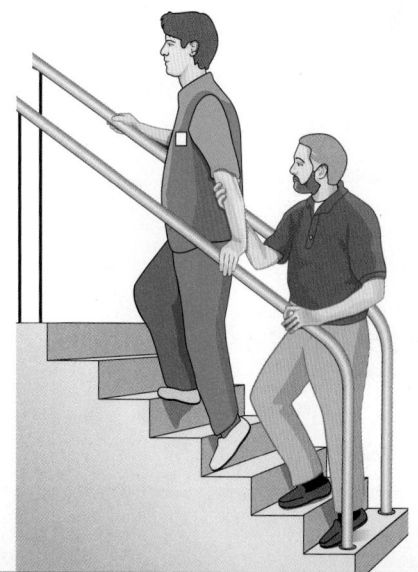

FIGURE 28-9 An example of the proper way to lead a patient who is visually impaired when ascending stairs.

(continues)

When you reach the top of a stair run, stop immediately. (Do not take an extra step.) Doing so lets the patient know that there are no more steps, and he or can then match his stride with yours.

The same procedure should be used when approaching curbs. Point out any changes in the terrain, even small ones.

SITTING

When guiding someone to a chair, assist the patient to walk up to the seat of the chair and then place your hand on the back of the chair. Let the patient trail your arm down to its back. Tell him or her which way the chair is facing, and he or she can then seat himself (see Figure 28-10).

If the chair lacks a back or is very large, bring the patient up to the chair so that his or her legs are against the front of it. He or she can then reach down to locate the arms and seat of the chair before he sits.

If the chair is at a table, describe the relationship of the chair, the table, and the patient. Place one of the patient's hands on the chair and the other hand on the table.

DOORS

When approaching a closed door, tell the patient its position when open. For example, "The door opens away and to the left." Or say, "Take the door with your left hand." After you open the door and begin to walk through, the patient will have his or her hand ready to help hold it open as you walk through together. The patient will move his or her arm across the front of his or her body to find the door with the palm of his or her hand (see Figure 28-11). He or she should close it behind you if it is not a self-closing door. Use the narrow passage technique (see below) in addition to this technique if the doorway is narrow.

NARROW PASSAGE TECHNIQUE

When coming to a narrow passage, tell the patient. Move your guiding arm to the center of your back. Slow your pace. He or she will move behind you and extend his or her arm, placing you in a single-file position. Once you pass through the narrow passage, bring your arm forward and return to the normal stance.

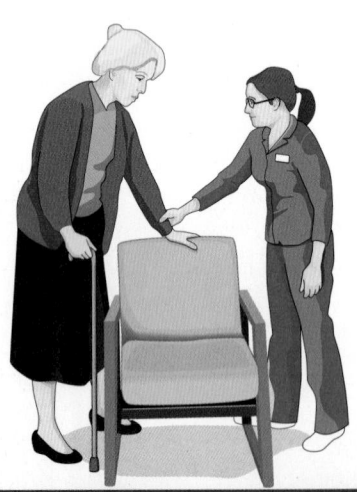

FIGURE 28-10   An example of the proper way to seat a patient who is visually impaired.

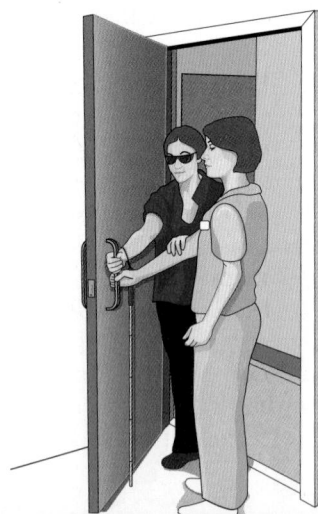

FIGURE 28-11   An example of the proper way to lead a patient who is visually impaired through a doorway.

The National Center for Elder Abuse (NCEA) is directed by the U.S. Administration on Aging. Their mission is to ensure that the elderly in America will live with dignity, integrity, and independence without abuse, neglect, or exploitation. This agency serves as a resource to local, state, and federal agencies for research, policy, and law as it affects the elderly. It is an excellent source for information on the latest policies relating to elder care in the United States.

Some signs and symptoms of mistreatment or abuse include:

PSYCHOLOGICAL SIGNS AND SYMPTOMS	PHYSICAL SIGNS AND SYMPTOMS
• Increasing depression	• Lack of personal care
• Anxiety	• Lack of supervision
• Withdrawn/timid	• Bruises
• Hostile	• Welts
• Unresponsive	• Lack of food
• Confused	• Beatings
• New poverty	• Neglect
• Longing for death	• Unsatisfactory living conditions
• Vague health complaints	
• Anxious to please	

There are other signs and symptoms, and not all of those listed by themselves indicate mistreatment, neglect, or abuse. If any seem to increase in number or severity, it may indicate a problem. By observing closely, you may be able to initiate corrective action to reduce or prevent the situation from deteriorating. Careful documentation in the patient's chart or electronic medical record over time can show continuous signs and symptoms of abuse. Usually the victim is frail (weak), physically or emotionally, and dependent on the abuser for basic survival needs. The victim may be afraid to speak out for fear of retaliation. Many times, the abuser is the caregiver or a member of the patient's family.

HEALTHY AND SUCCESSFUL AGING

Older adults are enjoying longer, healthier lives. Some reasons for healthy aging are the increase in the number of gerontologists (specialists who provide medical care only to older adult patients), greater awareness and involvement of older adults with their health care, improved nutrition, regular

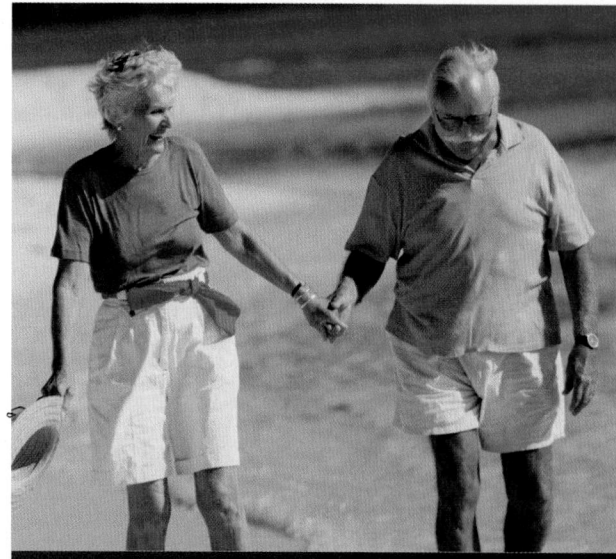

FIGURE 28-12 With improved geriatric care, older adults can look forward to longer, healthier lives.

exercise, new medications, and advancing medical technology (Figure 28-12).

Some tips for healthy aging according to the National Institute on Aging of the National Institutes of Health are:

1. Eat a balanced diet.
2. Exercise regularly.
3. Get regular checkups.
4. Don't smoke.
5. Wear a seatbelt when in the car.
6. Practice safety to avoid falls and fractures.
7. Keep in contact with family and friends and stay active through work, community, and recreation.
8. Avoid overexposure to the sun and cold.
9. Drink alcohol in moderation. Don't drink and drive.
10. Keep personal and financial records in order to simplify budgeting and investing. Plan for long-term financial needs, including housing.
11. Keep a positive attitude toward life and engage in activities that make you happy.
12. Get vaccines. The CDC recommends vaccines for pneumonia, influenza, herpes zoster, tetanus, diphtheria and pertussis, and chicken pox based on age and by health condition.

Successful aging requires that healthy living and daily activities be combined. To age successfully, individuals need to be continually involved in engaging activities, must pursue what makes them happy, and should make an effort to maintain a positive attitude. These healthy habits should begin in childhood when they can be established and encouraged. They become the responsibilities of each individual. Some activities that are important to successful aging are socialization with friends and family, intimacy, education, and

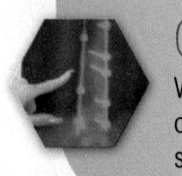

Critical Thinking

What are some strategies that older adults can employ to keep mentally and physically stimulated?

employment (for income and social satisfaction). For successful aging to happen, the older person must make a commitment to work at it.

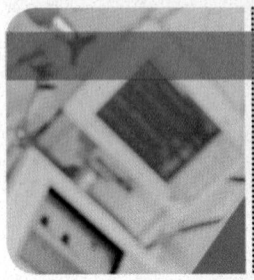

CASE STUDY 28-1

Refer to the scenario at the beginning of the chapter.

CASE STUDY REVIEW

1. Describe five strategies older adults such as Mrs. Johnson can use to help slow the aging process.

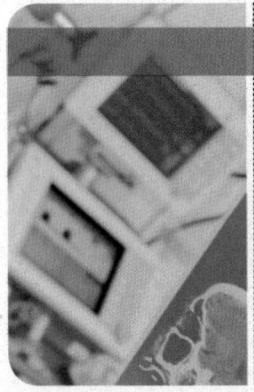

CASE STUDY 28-2

Adelaide Robinson, 83 years old, has an appointment Thursday morning for a recheck of her most recent complaint. She tells you that she is moving slower than she did just 6 months ago, and she has noticed less flexibility as well.

CASE STUDY REVIEW

1. What are the possible causes of Mrs. Robinson's complaints?
2. What effect will these problems have on Mrs. Robinson's daily routine?
3. What might Dr. King suggest Mrs. Robinson do to help alleviate symptoms?

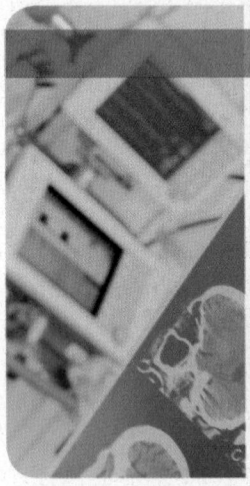

CASE STUDY 28-3

Sally Donovan, 92 years old, is in the gerontology clinic today. She currently lives with her 65-year-old son. You notice that she has lost 30 pounds since her last visit 2 months ago. Her demeanor is submissive and she looks to her son to answer any direct questions from the medical assistant and the provider. At checkout, her son opens her checkbook and writes the check for her co-payment, including signing her name on the signature line.

CASE STUDY REVIEW

1. What are the alarm signs for potential elder abuse with Ms. Donovan?
2. What are your next steps in reporting suspected elder abuse?
3. What might be some appropriate ways to include others in Ms. Donovan's support system in this situation?

Summary

- Many aging people live well into their 80s, 90s, and even to 100 years of age.

- Age impacts all of the body's systems.

- Some older adults, because of genetic inheritance, wear and tear, stress, and loss of chemicals and hormones, seem to age quickly and have little control over these factors.

- In order to maintain health, an active lifestyle, good nutrition, and proper medications are essential.

- Falls are a significant risk to the older adult as a means to end independent living. They can even result in death.

- Environmental safety is important to preserve function for as long as possible.

- The psychology of the older adult is commonly impacted by changes in his or her physiologic state and social changes. These changes may include dementia, depression, a decline in cognitive functioning, and personality changes.

- The medical assistant must be knowledgeable of the special care that must be provided to the older adult who has memory impairment, loss of sight or hearing, and/or decreased mobility.

- Patient education regarding nutrition, exercise, smoking cessation, limitation of alcohol intake, regular medical care, medication management, and social integration are important topics for the older adult to ensure healthy and successful aging.

Study for Success

To reinforce your knowledge and skills of information presented in this chapter:

- Review the *Key Terms* and *Learning Outcomes*
- Consider the *Critical Thinking* features and *Case Studies* and discuss your conclusions
- Answer the questions in the *Certification Review*

CERTIFICATION REVIEW

1. Which of the following is the most common chronic condition associated with older adults?
   a. Arteriosclerotic heart disease
   b. Cystitis
   c. Presbycusis
   d. Pernicious anemia

2. An eye disease common to older adults that is characterized by fluid pressure buildup is known as which of the following?
   a. Macular degeneration
   b. Presbyopia
   c. Cataract
   d. Glaucoma
   e. Conjunctivitis

3. Joint wear and tear in the older adult is characterized by which of the following?
   a. Cartilage covering the bone ends erodes
   b. Osteoporosis makes bones brittle
   c. Muscle fibers decrease
   d. Vertebrae become thinner

4. Inability to cough deeply and raise mucus makes older adults more susceptible to which of the following?
   a. Emphysema
   b. Asthma
   c. Pneumonia
   d. Bronchitis
   e. Pneumocystis

5. What does the term *residual urine* refer to?
   a. Catheterized urine for urinalysis
   b. First-voided specimen
   c. Amount of urine left in bladder after voiding
   d. Total amount of urine in the bladder when full

6. Age impacts which of the following body systems?
   a. Integumentary
   b. Musculoskeletal
   c. Cardiovascular
   d. Sensory
   e. All of these

7. With age, the damage to the retina that results in permanent loss of vision in the central visual field is known as which of the following?
   a. Cataracts
   b. Glaucoma
   c. Macular degeneration
   d. None of these
8. In order to prevent age-related disorders, which of the following behaviors are indicated?
   a. Eat a balanced diet
   b. Include at least five alcoholic drinks a day
   c. Increase exercise
   d. Take prescribed medications only if needed
   e. Both a and c
9. Patient education should be provided in a nondistracting environment, using short words and simple sentences, as well as speaking slowly and clearly. This demonstrates which of the following?
   a. Good communication techniques
   b. Professionalism
   c. Adhering to medicolegal guidelines
   d. Both a and b
10. Thinning of the long bones, pelvis, and vertebrae is a symptom of what condition?
   a. Osteomalacia
   b. Osteoarthritis
   c. Osteoporosis
   d. Osteochondroma
   e. Ochronosis

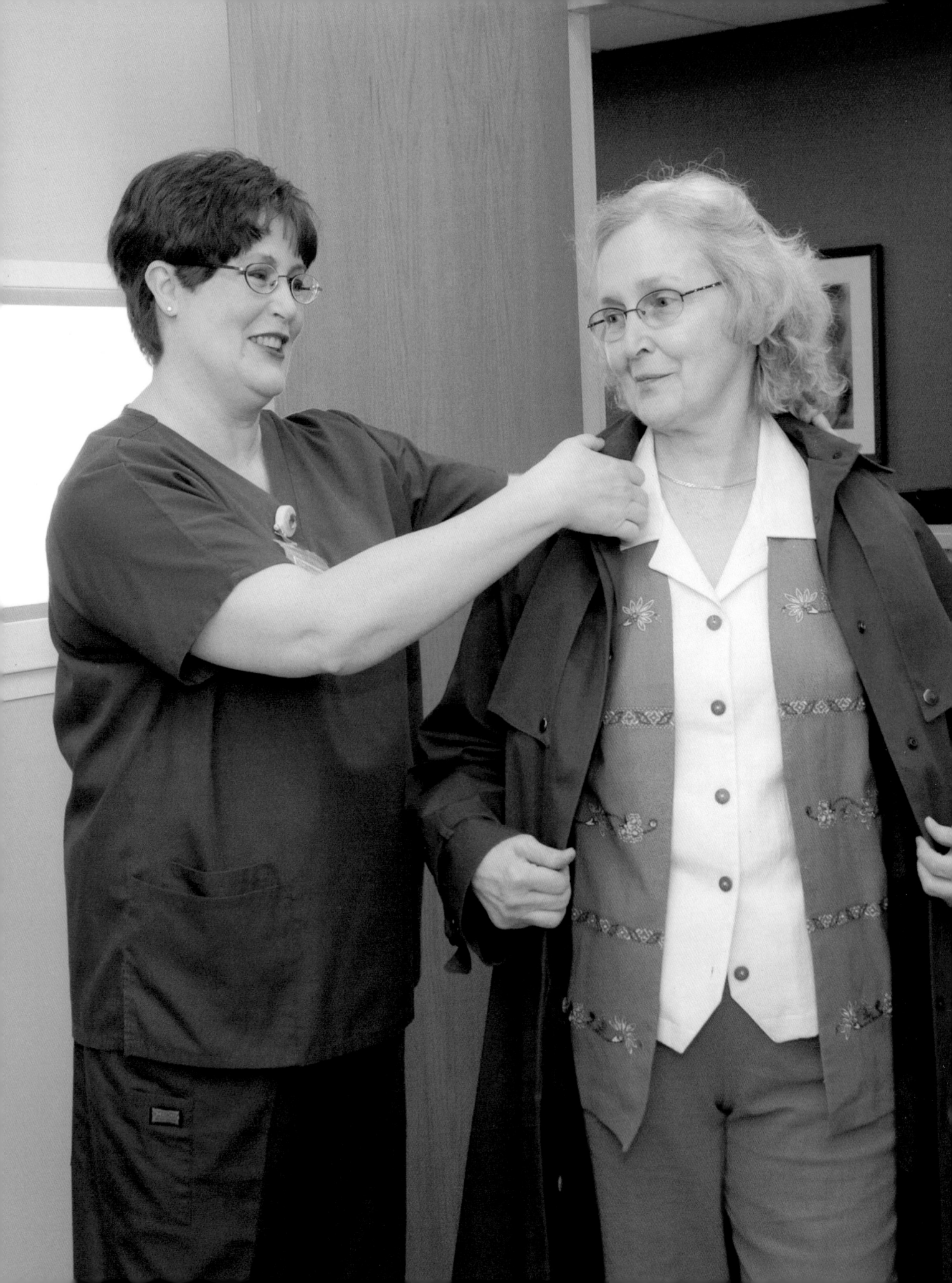

CHAPTER 29

Examinations and Procedures of Body Systems

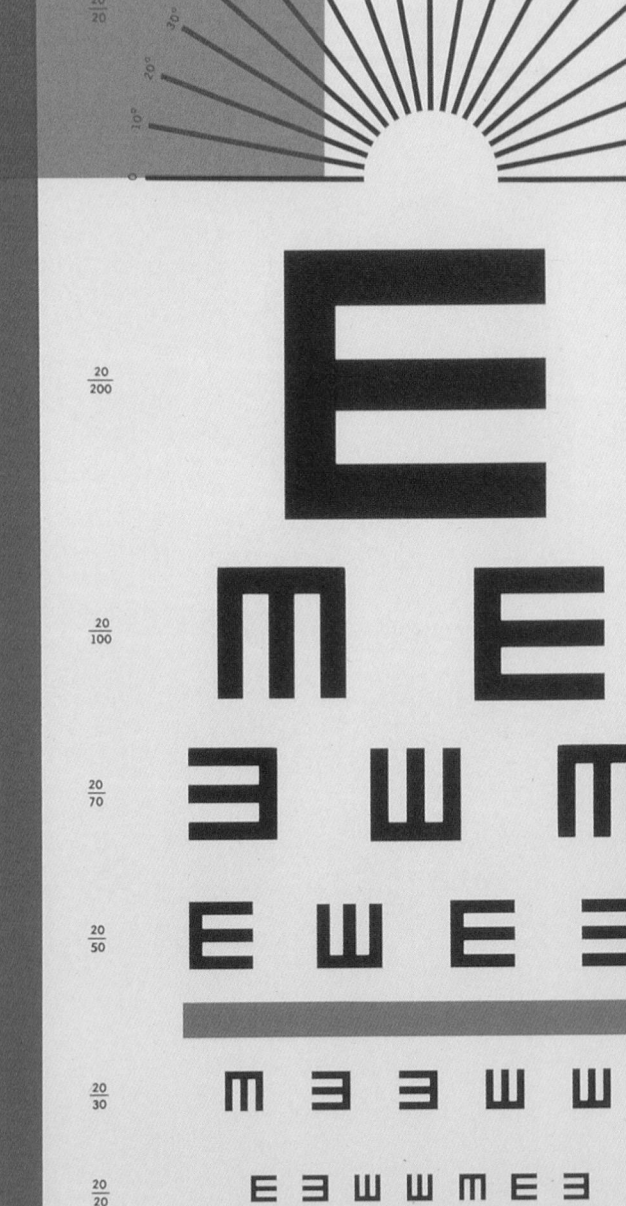

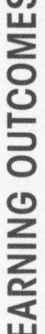

LEARNING OUTCOMES

1. Define and spell the key terms as presented in the glossary.
2. Identify major organs in each body system.
3. Recognize the normal function of each body system.
4. List basic integumentary assessment keys.
5. Discuss components of a neurologic examination.
6. Demonstrate essentials of a sensory system examination.
7. Clarify the value of each chart utilized in an eye exam.
8. Describe the proper use of a metered dose inhaler.
9. Summarize the role of the medical assistant during spirometry and pulse oximetry.
10. Explain oxygen administration using a nasal cannula.
11. Identify patient education information for sputum collections.
12. Cite patient preparation for occult blood testing.
13. Assemble items required by a provider for a neurologic examination and explain the medical assistant's role in the examination.
14. Differentiate the types of visual acuity charts and how to use them appropriately.
15. Compare the procedures of instillation and irrigation.
16. Describe how to perform a nasal irrigation.
17. Explain the medical assistant's role when assisting with audiometry.
18. Implement a urinary catheterization.

KEY TERMS

acute or adult respiratory distress syndrome (ARDS)

amblyopia

anaphylaxis

anorexia nervosa

aphasia

appendicular skeleton

auricle

axial skeleton

bariatrics

Bell's palsy

biopsy

bronchodilator

bulimia

carbuncle

cerebral vascular accident (CVA)

cerumen

chalazion

colonoscopy

comedones

conjunctivitis

deep tendon reflexes (DTRs)

demyelination

dermatophytosis

dislocation

dysuria

encephalitis

endoscope

epistaxis

erythema

external respiration

fibromyalgia

frequency

furuncle

gamma globulin

glaucoma

Key Terms, *continued*

gout	otoscope
hematochezia	oximetry
hematuria	polyps
hemoptysis	presbyopia
hordeolum	proteinuria
hyperopia	pruritus
inhalers	pyuria
internal respiration	rhizotomy
intravenous pyelogram (IVP)	rosacea
lesion	salicylates
malabsorption	sigmoidoscopy
malaise	Snellen chart
meningitis	spirometry
metered dose inhaler (MDI)	strabismus
morbid obesity	sudoriferous
myasthenia gravis	tic douloureux
myopia	tinea pedis
nebulizer	trabeculoplasty
nocturia	tympanostomy
nystagmus	urgency
oliguria	urticaria
otitis media	Wood's lamp examination

SCENARIO

At Inner City Health Care, a number of specialty examinations are scheduled for Tuesday the eighth. Administrative medical assistant Ellen Armstrong, CMAS (AMT), is careful to schedule patients requiring specialty procedures so that times do not overlap; before she schedules, Ellen makes certain examination rooms are available with an extra margin of time between patients. Clinical medical assistants Thomas Myers, CCMA (NHA), and Gwen Carr, CMA (AAMA), take responsibility to ensure that all supplies and equipment are assembled; that both provider and patient are comfortable with the physical environment; and that all safety precautions are followed before, during, and after the examination or procedure.

Chapter Portal

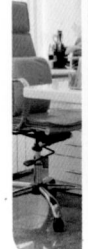

Initiative

New techniques and developments occur frequently in medicine, and medical assistants must refine existing skills and learn new ones to be knowledgeable and proficient and to provide the most appropriate quality care to patients. The medical assistant who works in a specialist's clinic or an ambulatory care setting that treats a variety of patient problems needs additional skills when providing specialty care to patients. Patients with conditions specific to a particular body system or body part need specialized care

continues

such as urinary catheterization or a lumbar puncture. The medical assistant aids the provider with a multitude of clinical procedures that are an integral part of each specialty examination.

This chapter covers specialty and body system examinations and the appropriate clinical procedures in urology; endoscopy; and the sensory, respiratory, musculoskeletal, neurologic, circulatory, blood and lymph, and integumentary systems.

Each specialty description includes tables that contain information on diseases, disorders, and diagnostic tests and procedures used to confirm diagnoses.

In a specialty practice, the uncommon may become commonplace in your practice as a professional medical assistant. It is important that you not lose sight of the importance of sterile technique and following procedures to protect the patient under your care.

INTEGUMENTARY SYSTEM

The integumentary system consists of the skin and its associated structures, such as hair, nails, nerve endings, and the sebaceous (oil) and **sudoriferous** (sweat) glands. This system provides protection for the body against invasion of microorganisms and trauma and helps regulate body temperature. Nerve endings sense pressure, touch, and pain. Structurally, the skin consists of two layers (Figure 29-1), which function differently from one another to perform specific activities.

- Epidermis is the outer layer of the skin that is composed of squamous epithelium and produces keratin and the pigment melanin.
- Dermis is the inner layer of the skin made up of connective tissue and contains blood vessels, nerve endings, and glands. This layer provides strength and elasticity.
- Subcutaneous connective tissue is the layer on which the skin and muscles lie and consists of elastic and fibrous connective tissue and adipose tissue. This layer guards against heat loss and provides insulation.

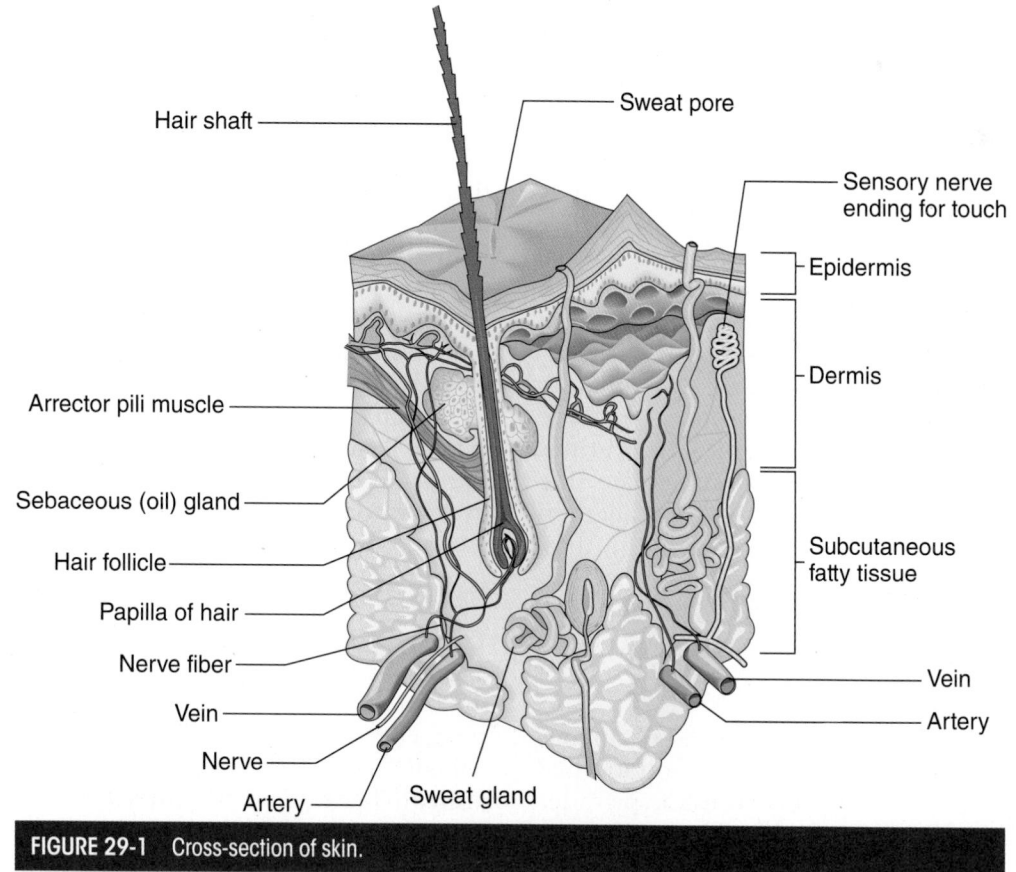

FIGURE 29-1 Cross-section of skin.

Skin disorders frequently produce a **lesion** unique to a specific skin disease, thus allowing for the diagnosis to be based on the appearance of the lesion, the patient's history, allergies, emotional well-being, drug use, and inherited diseases. If the lesion appears suspicious, the provider may perform a **biopsy** for tissue analysis. This procedure aids in the diagnosis and treatment of specific skin disorders. Table 29-1 lists integumentary system diseases and diagnostic procedures. Table 29-2 describes skin disorders of the integumentary system.

Diagnostic procedures involving the skin range from the simple to the complex. Simple observations such as skin color, texture, size and shape of a lesion, and patient history can lead to a quick diagnosis. Confirmatory procedures such as clinical studies of urine and blood, culture of a purulent lesion, radiographs, and biopsies of the affected tissues can further delineate the disease.

The clinical procedures for the skin most commonly performed by the medical assistant are obtaining wound cultures, applying sterile dressings to wound sites, and allergy skin testing.

Allergy Skin Testing

Medical assistants often perform allergy skin testing. When performing allergy skin tests, severe allergic reaction is a distinct possibility. As allergy testing elicits may elicit a serious reaction, known as **anaphylaxis**, the emergency cart (or crash cart) must be in easy reach (see Chapter 8). Emergency treatment must be available immediately and consists of the following: (1) notify provider immediately; (2) have patient lie down; (3) have epinephrine, Benadryl (diphenhydramine), and corticosteroid injections ready to be administered; and (4) check the patient's vital signs.

There can be a broad range of inflammatory responses to allergens. Some responses include **urticaria**, swelling at the injection site, **pruritus**, and redness. A reaction can be immediate, life threatening, and systemic in nature. The allergen reaches the circulatory system, triggering a massive release of substances (histamines) that can produce severe airway obstruction, vasodilation, hypotension, laryngeal edema, and anaphylactic shock (see Chapter 8).

Three Kinds of Skin Tests. The percutaneous (scratch) test, the patch test, and the intradermal test are the three skin test procedures the provider can perform on patients to evaluate for allergies.

Together with the patient's medical history, laboratory values, physical exam, and the skin test results, the provider compiles the data to determine the substances to which the patient is allergic.

Percutaneous Test. This type of testing is also known as a prick or scratch test. The back and arms are used for this type of testing. The skin surface is numbered in rows approximately 2 inches apart so that they can be identified. A small scratch is made on the surface of the skin and the allergen is placed on the scratch. As many as 50 allergens can be tested in one session. A reaction to the allergen usually occurs within 30 minutes. If the patient is allergic to a substance, a wheal will develop at the scratch site. The site is compared with a scratch test with no allergens (just an allergy-free fluid) introduced into it. The provider reads the results. Guidelines suggest that skin test records report the diameter of the wheal and the surrounding "flare" (measured in millimeters). The allergen extract should be wiped away from any scratch area that is exhibiting a number 4 reaction.

Patch Test. Patch testing does not require the use of needles. Instead, allergens are applied to patches, which are then placed on the patient's skin. Between 20 and 29 extracts of substances that can cause contact dermatitis are applied to the skin and left in place for a period of time determined by the provider. Instruct the patient to avoid bathing and activities that cause heavy sweating. The patient returns to the clinic to have the areas evaluated for skin irritation. This type of testing is utilized most often to detect the causes of contact dermatitis (see Figure 29-2).

Intradermal Test. A dose of 0.1 mL of an allergen is injected intradermally into the forearm, creating a bleb. The patient will be observed for up to 30 minutes to evaluate the reaction to the allergens. Intradermal testing is more sensitive than either the patch test or percutaneous testing. False positives are common.

NEUROLOGIC SYSTEM

The neurologic or nervous system functions to coordinate the activities of body systems and helps the body to adapt to its internal and external environments. Diagnosis and treatment of brain, spinal cord, and peripheral nerve disorders are often difficult because of the interdependence of one part of the system and another.

TABLE 29-1

INTEGUMENTARY SYSTEM DISORDERS

| DISEASE/DISORDER | LABORATORY/DIAGNOSTIC TESTS | | | SURGERY | MEDICAL TESTS OR PROCEDURES | TREATMENT |
	BLOOD TESTING	OTHER TESTING	RADIOGRAPHY			
Abscess (furuncle, carbuncle)	Complete blood count Blood glucose	Culture and sensitivity of wound exudate		Incision and drainage	Patient history Physical exam Sterile dressing application	Antibiotics (both oral and topical)
Acne		Culture of skin lesions			Patient history Physical exam	Topical cortico-steroids: Retin-A (tretinoin) Topical products containing benzoyl peroxide or salicylic acid Oral contraceptives for women
Athlete's foot		Skin scrapings Fungal culture			Patient history Physical exam **Wood's lamp examination**	Over-the-counter or prescription antifungal medications
Corn, callus, wart (verruca), mole (nevus)				Excisional biopsy Electrocautery	Patient history Physical exam Freezing with liquid nitrogen Laser therapy	Surgical excision Topical salicylic acid
Decubitus ulcers (treatment depends on staging)	Blood cultures	Wound cultures	Radiographs of adjoining bony structures	Rotational skin flap Debridement	Patient history Physical exam Application of protective dressings Application of pressure-reducing devices	Relieve pressure Antibiotics Nutritional supplementation Pain management Hyperbaric oxygen therapy

(continues)

Table 29-1 continued

DISEASE/DISORDER	LABORATORY/DIAGNOSTIC TESTS				MEDICAL TESTS OR PROCEDURES	TREATMENT
	BLOOD TESTING	OTHER TESTING	RADIOGRAPHY	SURGERY		
Dermatitis	**Gamma globulin** assay			Biopsy of lesion	Patient history Physical exam Skin scrapings Patch test for allergens	Depends on cause Topical corticosteroids Oral antihistamines
Dermatophytosis (ringworm)		Culture of lesion		Skin biopsy	Patient history Physical exam Wood's lamp examination Skin scrapings	Antifungal medication
Impetigo	Complete blood count	Gram stain of discharge from lesion			Patient history Physical exam	Antibiotics (topical or oral)
Melanoma			Chest radiograph	Biopsy of lesion Excision of lesion	Patient history Physical exam	Surgical excision Chemotherapy
Psoriasis				Skin biopsy	Patient history Physical exam	Medication Light therapy
Scleroderma	Sedimentation rate Rheumatoid arthritis factor Antinuclear antibodies	Urinalysis Kidney function tests	Gastrointestinal radiograph Chest radiograph	Tissue biopsy	Patient history Physical exam	Medication
Skin cancer				Biopsy of lesion Excision of lesion	Patient history Physical exam	Surgical excision Laser therapy Radiation therapy

TABLE 29-2

DESCRIPTION OF SKIN DISORDERS

Abscess. **Furuncle** ("boil"): Acute circumscribed infection of the subcutaneous tissues and surrounding tissues caused by *Staphylococci*. **Carbuncle**: A circumscribed inflammation and infection of the skin and deeper tissues accompanied by fever, leukocytosis, and sometimes prostration. Caused by *Staphylococcus* and common in patients with diabetes.

Acne. Chronic inflammatory disease caused by blocked sebaceous glands, characterized by **comedones** (blackheads), papules, and pustules.

Athlete's foot. Infection of the feet caused by fungus. It is also known as **tinea pedis**.

Corn and callus. Thickening and hyperplasia of the stratum corneum (outermost skin layer) caused by pressure or friction to the affected area.

Decubitus ulcers. Ulceration of skin layers due to pressure. The stage depends on the depth of tissue injury.

Dermatitis. Caused by a specific irritant characterized by **erythema** (redness), as in inflammation.

Dermatophytosis. A highly contagious fungal infection of the skin. Also known as ringworm. Common on hands and feet. When feet are infected, it is known as athlete's foot or tinea pedis.

Herpes zoster. An acute infectious disease caused by varicella-zoster virus. Characterized by inflammation of the ganglia of the spinal or cranial nerves. Painful vesicular eruptions occur along the course of the nerves.

Impetigo. Contagious small pustules caused by *Staphylococci, Streptococci,* or a combination of both and spread by direct contact.

Melanoma. A malignant pigmented skin lesion. Virulent and invasive. Can be caused by ultraviolet light exposure.

Nevus. A mole. Usually congenital.

Psoriasis. Chronic, genetically determined dermatitis, characterized by flat, reddened areas with silvery scales.

Scleroderma. Progressive thickening of the skin that involves collagen tissue. Systemic involvement occurs. Cause is unknown.

Skin cancer. Malignant lesions on the skin surface caused by exposure to ultraviolet rays.

Verruca. A wart caused by a virus.

The provider screens the patient during a physical examination for neurologic signs and symptoms. The medical assistant's role in a neurologic screening is to observe and evaluate the patient's mental status, assist or perform other tests as directed by the provider, and document findings. Most of the examination is performed in conjunction with the complete physical examination, but it can also be done when a patient is exhibiting specific signs and symptoms of a neurologic problem such as lack of sensation, seizures, confusion, paralysis, or **aphasia**, also known as the inability to speak.

The equipment and supplies used in a neurologic screening test the patient's reflexes, sense of touch, sense of smell, and degree of coordination, to name a few (Figure 29-3). The provider pays particular attention to symmetric strength and notes unequal weakness when comparing both sides of the body. A patient's sex and body build are considered when examining muscle mass and tone. Table 29-3 lists neurologic diagnostic procedures that are related to specific neurologic diseases. Table 29-4 describes common neurologic disorders.

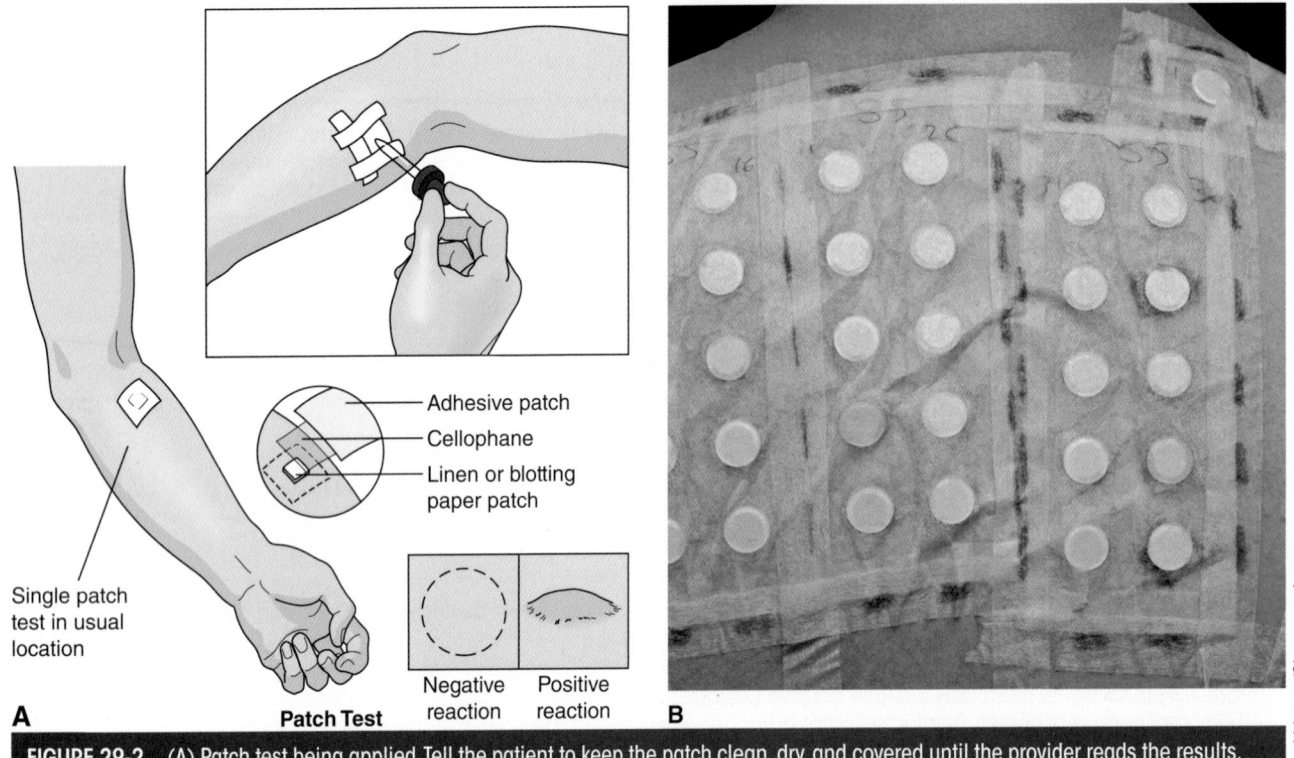

Single patch
test in usual
location

A   **Patch Test**

Adhesive patch
Cellophane
Linen or blotting
paper patch

Negative
reaction

Positive
reaction

B

© Andy Lidstone/Shutterstock.com

FIGURE 29-2 (A) Patch test being applied. Tell the patient to keep the patch clean, dry, and covered until the provider reads the results. (B) Skin allergy patch test on back.

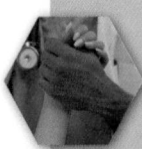

Patient Education

Early detection of skin changes can make a difference in the overall health and prognosis of patients who have risk factors associated with skin cancer. The Cancer Research Institute recommends a simple ABCDE method for identifying lesions that might be malignant.

A *Asymmetry.* Melanoma usually has an irregular shape; benign skin lesions usually have a smooth, rounded shape.

B *Borders.* As with shape, melanoma usually has wavy irregular borders, unlike benign lesions, which have smooth borders.

C *Colors.* As with asymmetry and borders, the colors present in the melanoma lesion are irregular and contain shades of brown and black; benign lesions are usually one shade of brown.

D *Diameter.* Melanoma lesions are usually larger (greater than 0.25 inch or 6 mm in diameter); benign lesions are usually smaller than that.

E *Evolution.* This has become the major factor to consider when diagnosing melanoma. If a lesion has undergone recent changes in size and/or color, it should be evaluated immediately.

It is important to instruct your patients that pink or white colors might be present in melanoma. These lesions can grow slowly or quite rapidly. It is essential that a patient seek medical intervention to increase the chance of surviving this type of cancer. There are several types of treatment, including surgical excision, chemotherapy and radiation, or immune therapy. Patients need to be aware that time is of the essence with this type of integumentary disease.

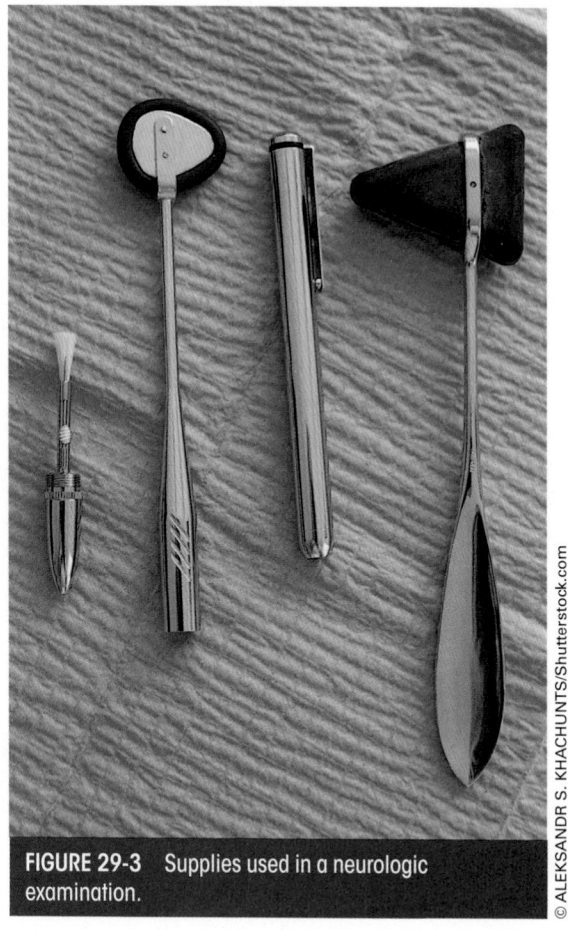

FIGURE 29-3 Supplies used in a neurologic examination.

© ALEKSANDR S. KHACHUNTS/Shutterstock.com

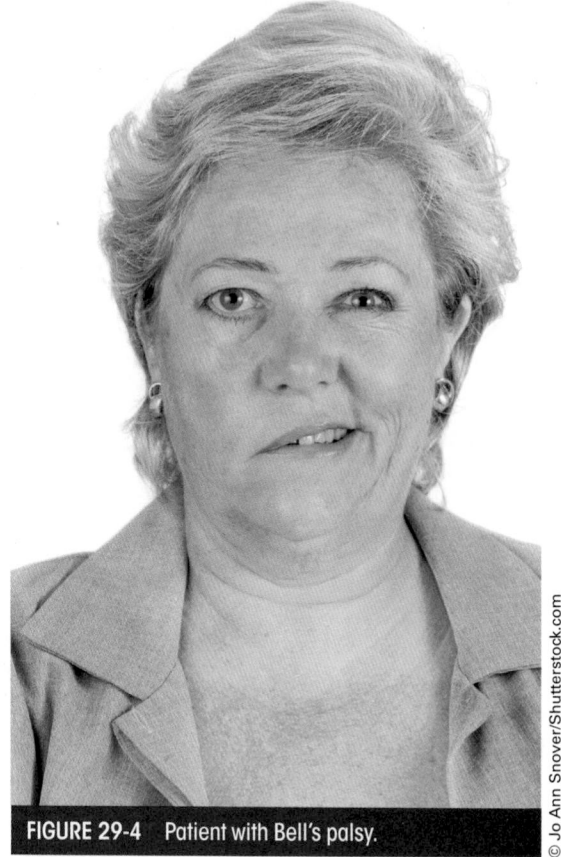

FIGURE 29-4 Patient with Bell's palsy.

© Jo Ann Snover/Shutterstock.com

Procedure

Procedures performed to confirm a diagnosis of a neurologic problem or disease are limited to the use of various diagnostic imaging and electrical impulse studies. The medical assistant's role is to aid the providers during certain procedures. Patient teaching by the medical assistant before a procedure and active reinforcement during a procedure will promote patient cooperation. Procedure 29-1 outlines steps involved in removing cerebrospinal fluid from the lumbar area.

Components of a Neurologic Screening

Procedure

During the neurologic screening examination, various functions are observed. Procedure 29-2 outlines the steps involved in a neurologic screening examination:

- History
  - Symptoms
  - Duration of symptoms

- Important factors to note
  - *Orientation.* Ability to state person, place, and time
  - *Changes in level of consciousness.* Periods of wakefulness, stupor, confusion, or lethargy; or history of coma
  - *Attention span.* Should be able to focus on examiner's questions and respond
  - *Judgement.* Ability to answer questions such as "What would you do if your house caught fire?" or "What are your plans for the future?"
  - *Changes in mental function or mood.* Verifying the patient's orientation to person, place, and time; history of depression and/or dementia; or the inability to express thoughts (aphasia)
  - *Headaches.* Frequency, location, severity, and duration; association with nausea or vomiting; aggravating and alleviating factors
  - *Visual changes.* Double vision, nystagmus

TABLE 29-3

NEUROLOGIC SYSTEM DISORDERS AND RELATED DIAGNOSTIC TESTING

| DISEASE/DISORDER | LABORATORY/DIAGNOSTIC TESTS | | | | MEDICAL TESTS OR PROCEDURES | TREATMENT |
	BLOOD TESTING	OTHER TESTING	RADIOGRAPHY	SURGERY		
Alzheimer	Vitamin deficiency testing Thyroid profile APOE-e4, the strongest risk gene for Alzheimer	Genetic: Autosomal dominant Alzheimer disease (ADAD)	Structural imaging with MRI or CT Positron emission tomography (PET) Amyloid imaging		Patient history Physical exam Mental status and neuropsychologic tests Mini-Mental State Examination (MMSE)	Cholinesterase inhibitor medications N-methyl-D-aspartate (NMDA) medications (memantine)
Amyotropic lateral sclerosis (ALS)	High-resolution serum protein electrophoresis, thyroid and parathyroid hormone levels Genetic testing	Pulmonary function tests 24-hour urine collection for heavy metals	Computed tomography (CT) of the cervical spine and head MRI of the head	Gastrostomy for swallowing difficulty Muscle or nerve biopsy	Patient history Physical exam Electromyography (EMG) Nerve conduction studies Nerve conduction velocity (NCV) Swallowing studies Lumbar puncture (spinal tap)	Treatment of the symptoms Medications to control spasms Physical therapy Caloric supplementation Assistive ventilation devices Riluzole (Rilutek): medication for slowing the progression of the disease
Bell's palsy (Paralysis of the VII cranial nerve) (see Figure 29-4)	Complete blood count		MRI or CT of brain		Patient history Physical exam	Warm moist heat Facial exercises Analgesics Eye care if unable to close eye Corticosteroids Antiviral drugs
Carpal tunnel syndrome			Wrist radiography		Patient history Physical exam Electromyography (EMG) Nerve conduction velocity study	Support of the extremity Anti-inflammatory medications Surgery to relieve pressure on the median nerve

Condition	Laboratory tests	Special tests	Diagnostic imaging	Procedures	Examinations	Treatments
Cerebral vascular accident (CVA) (stroke)			Cerebral angiography CT MRI	Angioplasty Carotid endarterectomy Coil or clip placement for hemorrhagic strokes	Patient history Physical exam Electroencephalography (EEG) Lumbar puncture	Anticoagulant therapy Physical therapy Speech therapy Tissue-plasminogen activator (tPA)
Epilepsy			CT MRI		Patient history Physical exam Electroencephalography	Antiepileptic medication
Herpes zoster	Varicella-zoster antibody Gamma globulins IgM and IgG response	Polymerase chain reaction (PCR) in skin scrapings			Patient history Physical exam Scrapings from lesion	Analgesics Corticosteroids Antiviral medication (Zovirax [acyclovir], Famvir [famciclovir]) Zostavax vaccine
Multiple sclerosis		Spinal fluid analysis	Bran scan CT MRI		Patient history Physical exam Lumbar puncture Evoked potentials (EP) testing	Corticosteroids Oral, injectable, and infusion disease-modifying medications Physical therapy Muscle relaxants Assistive devices Neuropsychology therapy
Parkinson disease	Complete blood count		Brain scans: PET MRI CT	Deep brain stimulator implant	Patient history Physical exam Neurologic exam	Dopamine-like medications Dopamine antagonist MAO-B inhibitors Catechol-O-methyltransferase inhibitors (COMT) Physical therapy

continues

Table 29-3 continued

	LABORATORY/DIAGNOSTIC TESTS					
DISEASE/DISORDER	BLOOD TESTING	OTHER TESTING	RADIOGRAPHY	SURGERY	MEDICAL TESTS OR PROCEDURES	TREATMENT
Rabies	Complete blood count Blood serum Reverse transcription polymerase chain reaction (RT-PCR)	Saliva Cerebrospinal fluid for antibodies to rabies virus			Patient history Physical exam Skin biopsies of hair follicles at the nape of the neck for rabies antigen in the cutaneous nerves at the base of hair follicles	Wash wound immediately with soap and water Antirabies injections Medication for convulsions
Reye syndrome	Complete blood count Serum ammonia	Liver function studies	Brain scan: CT MRI	Liver biopsy Skin biopsy	Patient history Physical exam Lumbar puncture Examination of cerebrospinal fluid	Supportive physical therapy Control of brain swelling
Sciatica			Myelogram CT MRI Spinal X-ray	Diskectomy (if caused by herniated disk) Spinal decompression surgery	Patient history Physical exam Electromyography (EMG) Steroid injections	Physical therapy Massage Exercise Analgesics Anti-inflammatory drugs Narcotics Antidepressants Antiseizure medications
Tic douloureux (trigeminal nerve neuralgia)			MRI	Surgery to dissect the trigeminal nerve **Rhizotomy**	Patient History Physical Exam	Analgesics Antiseizure medications Antidepressants
West Nile virus	Complete blood count	Cerebrospinal fluid	MRI		Patient history Physical exam Neurologic work-up	No specific treatment Supportive

TABLE 29-4

DESCRIPTION OF NEUROLOGIC DISORDERS

Amytropic lateral sclerosis (Lou Gehrig disease). Rapidly progressive, invariably fatal neurologic disease that attacks the nerve cells responsible for controlling voluntary muscles.

Bell's palsy. Paralysis of the seventh cranial nerve caused by acute inflammation. Usually characterized by unilateral facial paralysis and pain, but it can be bilateral (Figure 29-4).

Cerebral vascular accident (CVA). Loss of blood supply to the brain (anoxia). May be caused by a ruptured or clogged blood vessel or clot in the brain. Symptoms include sudden loss of consciousness and paralysis. Also referred to as a stroke.

Epilepsy. Episodes of seizures caused by changes in electrical brain potentials that result in disturbed brain impulses or function.

Encephalitis. Inflammation of the brain tissue. Usually due to a viral infection but may be caused by bacterial, fungal, parasitic, or rickettsial infections.

Headache. Pain in any part of the head. The pain may be unilateral or bilateral, located in one region or several. The type of pain varies from sharp and stabbing to a dull ache.

Herpes zoster. An acute infectious viral disease caused by the varicella-zoster virus (chicken pox). Painful vesicular eruptions. Also known as shingles.

Meningitis. Inflammation of the membranes of the spinal cord or brain. May be caused by bacterial, viral or fungal infection. Symptoms include a stiff neck, headache, anorexia, and irregular fever. Caused by either a bacterium or a virus.

Multiple sclerosis. Chronic progressive disease characterized by **demyelination** (destruction of nerve covering) of nerve fibers. The cause is unknown. First symptoms are visual disturbances and muscle weakness.

Parkinson disease. A slowly progressive disease, usually occurring in later life, caused by a degeneration of brain cells as a result of lack of dopamine in the brain. Muscle rigidity and akinesia are common symptoms.

Rabies. Caused by a virus and transmitted to humans by scratches or bites from animals infected with the virus. The disease infects the brain and spinal cord and causes acute encephalitis. It can be fatal.

Reye syndrome. A neurologic illness usually seen in young children after a viral infection such as influenza, varicella, or Epstein-Barr. There may be a connection between the viral infection and aspirin. The cause is unknown, but characteristic symptoms include vomiting, rash, lethargy and neurologic involvement, seizures, and coma.

Sciatica. Severe pain in the leg along the course of the sciatic nerve felt at the back of the thigh and running down the inside of the leg. Caused by compression of the nerve by a ruptured intervertebral disk or osteoarthritis. Characterized by sharp, shooting pain running down the back of the thigh. Leg movement aggravates the pain.

Tic douloureux. Degeneration of or pressure on the trigeminal (fifth cranial) nerve causing severe stabs of pain that radiate from the angle of the jaw along one of the branches. Pain may be felt in the eye, lip, nose, and/or tongue. Pain may come and go for hours.

West Nile virus infection. A potentially serious illness that affects the central nervous system. Symptoms may include headache, stupor, disorientation, tremors, convulsions, and coma. Spread by bite of infected mosquitoes.

Procedure

Assisting the Provider during a Lumbar Puncture or Cerebrospinal Fluid Aspiration

STANDARD PRECAUTIONS:

Handwashing

Gloves

PURPOSE:

To assemble supplies and position the patient for removal of cerebrospinal fluid from the lumbar area, which will be sent to the laboratory for analysis.

EQUIPMENT/SUPPLIES:

- Gown
- Sheet or blanket
- Waterproof drape
- Local anesthetic per provider's order (Xylocaine [lidocaine] 1% or 2%)
- Appropriately sized syringe and needle length and gauge for administration of anesthetic
- Sterile gloves for provider and medical assistant
- Gowns for provider and MA
- Sterile water
- Surgical prep kit that contains:
  - Antiseptic soap
  - Sponges
- Disposable sterile lumbar puncture tray that includes:
  - Skin antiseptic (providone-iodine) with applicator
  - Adhesive bandage
  - Spinal needle
  - Three to four vials for cerebrospinal fluid collection
  - Fenestrated drape
  - Manometer
  - Gauze sponges
- Laboratory requisition
- Examination light
- Biohazard container
- Sharps container

continues

PROCEDURE STEPS:

1. Introduce yourself and identify patient using two identifiers.
2. Assemble the required equipment.
3. Ask the patient about any allergies prior to starting the procedure.
4. Check to be sure that the consent for the procedure has been signed. If not, or if the patient has any further questions, notify the provider.
5. Encourage the patient to empty his or her bladder prior to positioning him or her on the table. Offer assistance as necessary. RATIONALE: The patient will be required to remain still during the procedure and for a period of time afterward.
6. This procedure can create anxiety in many patients, so **spend time attending to the patient's psychological and physiological needs** prior to the start of this procedure.
7. Position the patient in the lateral recumbent position. The patient's back should be at the edge of the exam table. Use a small pillow to support the patient's head. RATIONALE: This position achieves maximum alignment of the spine.
8. Drape the patient for warmth and privacy.
9. Instruct the patient to angle his or her chin toward the chest and to arch the back. He or she should also bring the knees toward the chest and hold them there if able (Figure 29-5). RATIONALE: This position widens the spaces between the lumbar vertebrae for ease of needle insertion.

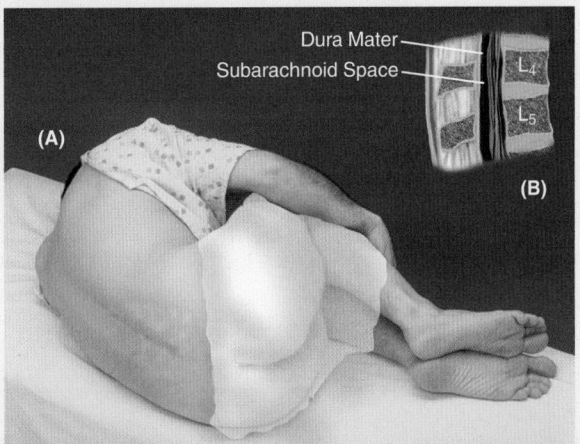

FIGURE 29-5 (A) Have the patient draw up the knees to the abdomen and grasp knees. Chin should flex on chest. (B) The site for the lumbar puncture.

10. Wash your hands and follow Standard Precautions.
11. Use a mayo stand as your base and open the sterile lumbar puncture tray in a manner that maintains sterility of all contents, as well as establishes a sterile field for the provider.
12. Being careful not to splash, pour sterile water into the provided area.
13. Don sterile gloves and prep the puncture site with the antiseptic soap solution. Begin at the puncture site location and cleanse in a circular manner to a diameter of at least 6 inches. Repeat this action three times using a new swab for each pass. If indicated by the provider's order, rinse the area and dry with a sterile towel.
14. Remove gloves and dispose of them properly. Wash hands.

continues

15. If needed, assist the provider to drape the puncture site with the sterile fenestrated drape. Be sure that the intended puncture site is centered in the opening.

16. Assist the provider to draw up the local anesthetic by inverting the vial and holding it steady while the provider withdraws the medication.

17. Encourage the patient to remain as still and calm as possible during the procedure, breathing slowly and evenly.

18. The patient must maintain the curved spinal position until the spinal needle is inserted and a free flow of cerebrospinal fluid (CSF) is obtained. If needed, assist the patient to stay in the correct position. RATIONALE: Movement by the patient could produce trauma to the spinal cord area.

19. When the manometer is applied, remind the patient to breathe slowly and remain quiet to ensure an accurate pressure reading.

20. The provider may request that the patient straighten his or her legs to obtain a more accurate reading. Assist the patient as necessary per the provider's instructions.

21. Assist the provider as needed by holding the specimen vials under the dripping CSF. Take care to maintain the sterility of the vial and the needle hub.

22. Once the procedure is complete, assist the provider to apply a sterile dressing to the puncture site by holding the sterile gauze in place while the provider applies an adhesive bandage.

23. Assist the patient to assume a supine position. Instruct the patient to remain in this position for 30 to 60 minutes, as instructed by the provider. RATIONALE: This will minimize the possibility of cerebrospinal fluid leaking from the puncture site and help to avoid a spinal headache.

24. Continue to monitor the patient's vital signs and to provide comfort measures, such as medication, if ordered.

25. Label the CSF vials with the date, patient name, and the order of collection (e.g. #1, #2, #3).

26. Place the specimens in the biohazard transport bag.

27. Dispose of all used supplies or equipment following Occupational Safety and Health Administration (OSHA) guidelines.

28. Remove gloves and wash your hands.

29. Complete the laboratory requisition form(s) and place them in the appropriate section of the biohazard transport bag.

30. Arrange for the bag to be transported to the appropriate laboratory for testing.

31. Using your knowledge of office policy, as well as the provider's particular orders, provide the patient with written instructions for aftercare.

32. Record the procedure, postprocedural vital signs, and the patient's tolerance of the procedure in the patient's medical record.

DOCUMENTATION:

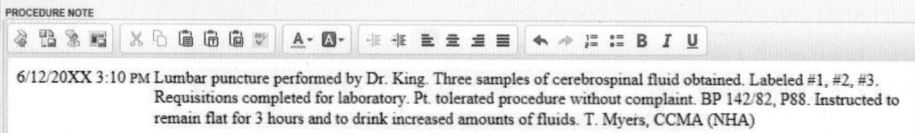

PROCEDURE NOTE

6/12/20XX 3:10 PM Lumbar puncture performed by Dr. King. Three samples of cerebrospinal fluid obtained. Labeled #1, #2, #3. Requisitions completed for laboratory. Pt. tolerated procedure without complaint. BP 142/82, P88. Instructed to remain flat for 3 hours and to drink increased amounts of fluids. T. Myers, CCMA (NHA)

Courtesy of Harris CareTracker PM and EMR

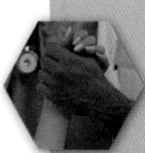

Patient Education

Post-Lumbar Puncture Instructions

1. You will be asked to remain in a supine position for at 30 to 60 minutes immediately after the procedure. You should recline on your ride home as much as possible, especially if you have the beginnings of a headache.

2. It is suggested that you find a comfortable reclining position and remain there for 6 to 8 hours after you arrive home. You may have bathroom privileges and sit up to eat.

3. Drink water and other liquids, at least eight to ten 8 oz glasses per day for several days.

4. Resume your regular activities the day after your procedure or as instructed by your provider. Avoid rigorous recreational exercise for the next 3 to 4 days. Expect to be able to return to work and mild exercise the following day if no headache is present.

5. Notify your provider if you develop a headache after the procedure; headache is the most common complication of a lumbar puncture.

○ *Changes in hearing or tinnitus*

○ *Dizziness/vertigo.* Related to position or movement, intermittent or constant, aggravating or alleviating factors

○ *Abnormal sensation.* Numbness, tingling, burning, absence of sensation

○ *Weakness.* Location, duration, paralysis, localized or generalized

○ *Pain.* Quality, quantity, description, continuous or intermittent

○ *Gait.* Balanced, staggering, shuffling

• Level of consciousness

○ *Awake.* Eyes open wide spontaneously and immediately to minimal stimuli

○ *Alert.* Responds quickly and appropriately

○ *Drowsy.* Has the appearance of sleepiness, but responds to stimuli

○ *Lethargic.* Sleeps intermittently, awakens to stimuli, but may drift off to sleep again once stimuli are removed

○ *Stuporous.* Can be awakened with more intense stimuli, can be disoriented when aroused, and returns to sleep once stimuli are removed

○ *Comatose.* No purposeful response even to painful stimuli, reflexes may be intact

• Memory (recall of past and present)

○ *Immediate.* Commonly a patient is given a verbal list of three objects and then asked to recite them correctly after 5 minutes

○ *Recent.* To check recent memory, the patient is asked about noteworthy current events

○ *Remote.* This test is recall of a patient's history such as birth date, name of children, first job, or hometown

• Cranial nerve function (see the "Cranial Nerve Assessment" Quick Reference Guide)

The provider continues with the neurologic examination by checking the patient for the following:

• *Motor function.* Aspects of the motor function exam are focused on evaluation of the muscles of the body. Muscle groups are examined to determine muscle mass, tone, and strength. Any abnormalities such as tenderness and involuntary or abnormal muscle movement should be noted. The exam also evaluates the symmetry of the muscles of the body, comparing right to left. Muscle strength is evaluated by applying resistance to the extremities during flexion and extension. This strength is usually rated on a scale of 0 to 5.

• *Sensory function.* It is important to evaluate the sensory as well as the motor function of the body to obtain a complete examination reflecting the status of the neurologic system. A number of tests can be used to test for appropriate sensory function. The aspects of sensation that are evaluated are pain, touch, joint position sense, and thermal perception. Pain is tested using a pin to gently prick the skin. Light touch is evaluated by touching the patient with a cotton ball. Vibration is tested with the use of a tuning fork.

CRANIAL NERVE ASSESSMENT

Cranial Nerve Number/ Name	Function	Assessment
I—Olfactory	Sense of smell	Ask patient to identify essence of coffee, peppermint, or vanilla using each nostril
II—Optic	Vision	Evaluate using Snellen chart and Ishihara test chart books
III—Oculomotor*	Control of pupil size and certain movements of the eye	Assess pupil size and light reflex and the ability to follow the light using a penlight
IV—Trochlear V—Abducens	Work in concert to control eye movement	Have patient turn eyes downward, temporally, and nasally Observe eye movement and pupillary constriction
VI—Trigeminal	Responsible for corneal reflexes, facial sensation, and the opening and closing of the mouth	*Motor.* Palpate jaws and temples while patient clenches teeth *Sensory.* Have patient close eyes, touch cotton ball to all areas of face and monitor the patient's response for appropriate report of sensation
VII—Facial	Controls the muscles of the face	*Motor.* Check symmetry and mobility of face by having patient frown, close eyes, lift eyebrows, and puff cheeks *Sensory.* Asses the patient's ability to identify taste (sugar, salt, lemon juice)
VIII—Acoustic (Vestibulocochlear)	Hearing	Can test with a variety of hearing examinations including air versus bone conduction using a tuning fork
IX—Glossopharyngeal X—Vagus**	Coordination of swallowing and movement of the uvula and soft palate	The practitioner evaluates the quality of the voice, the ability to cough and swallow, and the gag reflex
XI—Accessory	Controls the shoulders and the muscles of the neck	Evaluate by instructing the patient to shrug the shoulders and turn the face to each side against resistance
XII—Hypoglossal	Controls the movement of the tongue	Evaluate by asking the patient to open the mouth and move the tongue to commands; articulation of speech is also assessed

* Cranial nerves III, IV, and VI are examined together because they control eyelid elevation.

** The glossopharyngeal and vagus nerves are evaluated together because they work together in coordination.

- *Cerebellar function.* The cerebellum is a smaller brain structure than the cerebrum. However, it contains 50% of the total number of neurons in the brain. To evaluate the functionality of the cerebellum, a patient is asked to perform several tests. They are described as follows:
  - *Finger-to-nose (FTN) testing.* The patient is asked to alternately point from his or her nose to the examiner's finger. The examiner moves his finger to different locations to assess the patient's ability to adapt.
  - *Romberg test.* The patient is asked to stand still with his or her feet together and the arms straight at the sides. It is a normal result if the patient does not lose his or her balance.
  - *Heel-to-shin (HTS) test.* The patient is asked to run the heel of one foot along the shin of the opposite leg and to then alternate and repeat the procedure on the other side. There is an abnormal result if the patient cannot maintain coordination with rapid repeat of the exercise.
- *Reflex function.* The evaluation of **deep tendon reflexes (DTR)** examines the arc that sensation travels from the source to the spinal cord and back to the muscle tissue. The usual manner for testing DTR is to utilize a reflex hammer to tap on tendons in the upper and lower extremities. When the tendon is tapped, it activates the stretch fibers in the muscle and causes contraction of the muscle. If there is damage or injury, the impulse is delayed and the reaction is slowed. One of the aspects of assessment is symmetry. Reflexes should be bilaterally equal. Babinski's sign is an assessment of upper motor neurons. With this test, the handle of the reflex hammer strokes from the toes to the heel on the plantar aspect of the foot. If the great toe extends downward, the upper neurons are intact. Reflexes are rated on a 0 to 4+ scale, with 0 indicating no response and 4+ indicating a hyperactive response. Normal is midscale at 2+.
-  Competency *Gait and stance.* Specific neurologic disorders are identified by the rate, rhythm, and coordination of movement that represents gait. Gait characteristics can indicate a lack of integration of the peripheral and central nervous systems. It is the role of the medical assistant to be familiar with the components of a neurologic examination and to be able to accurately record the results of this exam at the direction of the provider (Procedure 29-2).

Additional tests:

- Angiography provides visualization of the circulation of the blood throughout the brain.
- Computed tomography (CT) uses a combination of X-rays and computer technology to produce horizontal or axial views of the brain and other structures to diagnose hemorrhage and tumors (see Chapter 31).
- Electroencephalography (EEG) records the electrical activity of the brain and helps to diagnose seizures and tumors.
- Magnetic resonance imaging (MRI) uses a magnetic field and pulses of radio wave energy to diagnose tumors and hemorrhage (see Chapter 31).
- Lumbar puncture (LP), also known as a spinal tap, and the examination of cerebrospinal fluid (CSF) are used in many diagnoses related to the brain and spinal cord. These diagnoses include:
  - Brain or spinal cord tumor
  - Cerebral hemorrhage
  - Meningitis
  - Encephalitis
  - Degenerative brain diseases (e.g., amyotrophic lateral sclerosis; Parkinson, Alzheimer, and Huntington diseases)
  - Autoimmune diseases (e.g., multiple sclerosis)
  - Inhalation anthrax
  - Guillain-Barré syndrome
  - Reye syndrome
- Positron emission tomography (PET) scans test brain function as they assess chemical activity and metabolic rates within the brain. These scans are used to diagnose movement disorders, cerebral vascular disorders, epilepsy, tumors, dementia, and other disorders.
- Electromyography (EMG) assesses nerve–muscle interaction. EMG measures the electrical potential of muscles at rest and during contraction. The test diagnoses diseases that interrupt the electrical signal from the muscle to the spinal cord and back via the nerve–muscle junctions. Diseases of the peripheral nervous system are easily diagnosed using EMG.

PROCEDURE 29-2

Procedure

Assisting the Provider with a Neurologic Screening Examination

STANDARD PRECAUTIONS:

Handwashing

PURPOSE:

To determine a patient's neurologic status.

EQUIPMENT/SUPPLIES:

- Percussion hammer
- Safety pin or sensory wheel
- Peppermint or alcohol prep for odor identification
- Cotton ball
- Solid objects such as keys, coins, paper clips
- Tuning fork
- Flashlight or penlight
- Tongue blade
- Nonsterile gloves

PROCEDURE STEPS:

1. Assemble the needed equipment.
2. Wash your hands and follow Standard Precautions where applicable.
3. Introduce yourself to the patient and confirm the patient's identity, using two identifiers.
4. ***Explain the rationale for the procedure to be performed, showing awareness of the patient's concerns.***
5. While interacting with the patient and taking down a health history, ***pay attention to detail*** and observe the patient's ability to manage cognitive functioning. Some things to look for include the patient's orientation to person, place, and time; the patient's memory, mood, and cognition; and the presence of appropriate behaviors.
6. Throughout the procedure, you may be asked to assist the provider with the various components of the neurologic exam, such as those that assess the patient's mental status, cranial nerve functioning, motor functioning, reflexes, coordination, and sensory functioning. In what manner and to what extent you will assist will often be determined by the needs and preference of the provider. RATIONALE: Knowing the components of the exam and the order in which they are administered will help you to assist the provider by ensuring that you are ready to provide equipment and materials as requested.
7. When the assessment is complete, record the procedure and its findings in the patient's medical record.

DOCUMENTATION:

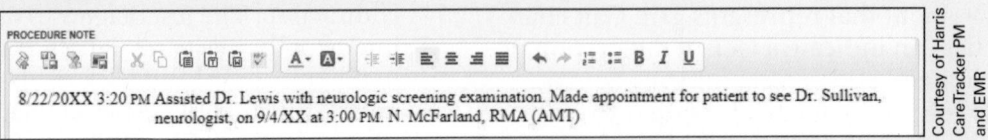

8/22/20XX 3:20 PM Assisted Dr. Lewis with neurologic screening examination. Made appointment for patient to see Dr. Sullivan, neurologist, on 9/4/XX at 3:00 PM. N. McFarland, RMA (AMT)

Courtesy of Harris CareTracker PM and EMR

SENSORY SYSTEM

The senses of vision, hearing, equilibrium (balance), smell, touch, and taste permit the body to detect information about the environment. The eyes, ears, nose, taste buds, and skin are all sense organs that contain specialized receptor organs. Table 29-5 lists diseases and disorders of the sensory system and diagnostic tests and procedures for eyes and ears.

The Eye

The eye is the primary organ for sight and is one of the few organs of the body that is externally exposed. Its accessory structures—the eyelids, eyelashes, lacrimal ducts, and extrinsic muscles—provide protection for the eye (Figure 29-6). The anterior portion of the eyeball protrudes outward and the remainder is protected by the orbit.

The intraocular structures consist of some parts of the eye visible externally and parts visible only through an ophthalmoscope. The intraocular structures include the following:

- *Sclera.* White area covering the outside of the eye except over the pupil and iris
- *Cornea.* Clear tissue covering the pupil and iris

- *Iris.* Round disk of smooth and radial muscles giving the eye its color
- *Pupil.* Round opening in the iris that changes size as the iris reacts to light and dark
- *Anterior chamber.* Space between cornea and iris/pupil filled with clear fluid called aqueous humor
- *Posterior chamber.* Space between the iris and lens that is filled with aqueous humor
- *Lens.* Clear fibers enclosed in a membrane; refract and focus light to the retina
- *Posterior cavity.* Space in the posterior part of the eyeball filled with thick, gelatinous material called vitreous humor
- *Posterior sclera.* White opaque layer covering the posterior part of the eyeball
- *Choroid layer.* Layer between the sclera and retina containing blood vessels
- *Retina.* Inside layer of the posterior part of the eye that receives the light rays (visual stimuli)

The mechanism of vision occurs after impulses leave the retina and travel through the optic nerves to the brain. At the optic chiasm, the nerve fibers cross and continue to the thalamus. These fibers synapse with other neurons that send the impulses to the right and left visual area of the occipital lobe of the brain. Because the

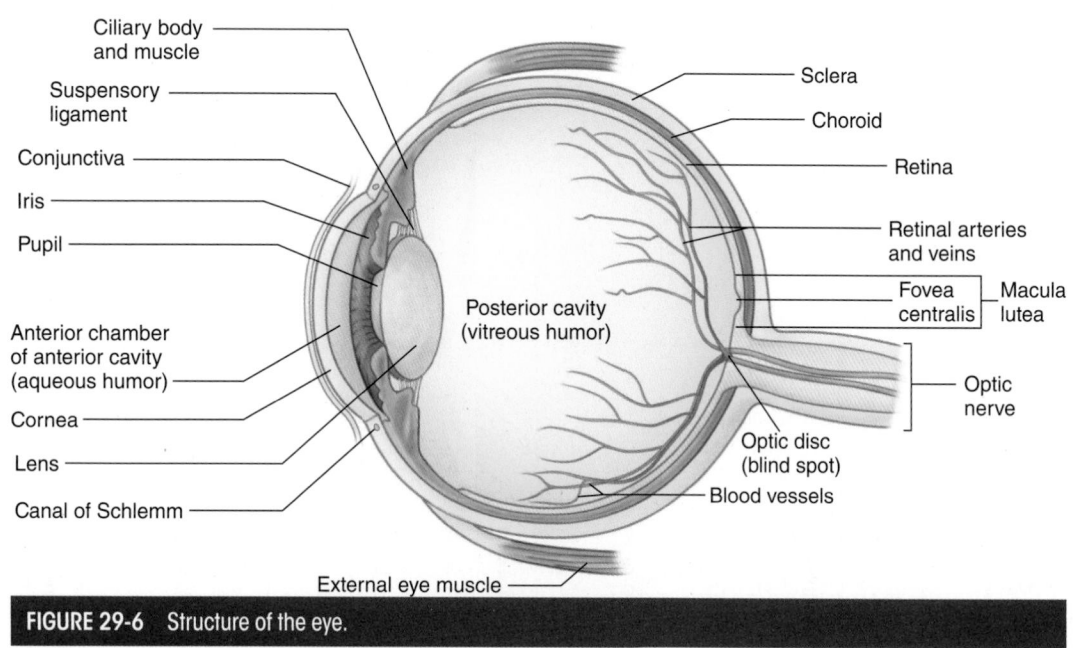

FIGURE 29-6 Structure of the eye.

TABLE 29-5

SENSORY SYSTEM DISORDERS

DISEASE/ DISORDER	LABORATORY/DIAGNOSTIC TESTS				MEDICAL TESTS OR PROCEDURES	TREATMENT
	BLOOD TESTING	OTHER TESTING	RADIOGRAPHY	SURGERY		
Amblyopia					Patient history Ophthalmologic examination	Cover the normal eye to force weaker eye to function
Astigmatism					Patient history Ophthalmic exam	Corrective lenses
Cataracts				Cataract surgery with intraocular lens replacement	Patient history Ophthalmologic examination Slit lamp	Phacoemulsification Surgical extraction
Chalazion				Preventative cleansing regimes Excision	Patient history Physical exam	Topical and oral antibiotics
Color blindness (achromatopia)					Patient history Examination using Ishihara color plates or Cambridge Color Test	Corrective lenses for green–red color blindness iPhone and iPad apps that help people with color blindness discriminate among colors
Conjunctivitis		Culture and sensitivity tests of eye discharge		Stained smears of conjunctival scrapings	Patient history Physical exam	Antibiotic drops or antibiotic ointment
Corneal abrasion		Fluorescein eye stain			Patient history Physical exam	Antibiotic ointment, dressing over affected eye

Diabetic retinopathy		Optical coherence tomography (OCT) exam	Focal laser treatment Scatter laser treatment Vitrectomy	Patient history Dilated eye exam Fluorescein angiography	Diabetic management with antiglycemic agents to prevent progression
Diplopia (double vision)				Patient history Ophthalmologic examination	Corrective lenses Treatment of underlying medical conditions
Epistaxis	Complete blood count			Patient history Blood pressure Application of pressure externally Nasal packing with or without anesthetic-vasoconstrictor solution Nasal tampon or balloon Packing with absorbable materials (Gelfoam, Surgicel) Chemical cauterization with silver nitrate	Evaluation and treatment of cause: Environmental irritants Foreign body Hypertension Hemophilia Drug use
External otitis (infection of the ear canal)	Complete blood count	Culture and sensitivity tests of exudate	Debridement	Patient history Otologic examination	Antibiotic therapy Topical acetic acid and corticosteroids
Glaucoma			Argon laser **trabeculoplasty** (ALT) Selective laser trabeculoplasty (SLT) Laser iridotomy (creating a small hole in the iris to increase fluid flow) Peripheral iridectomy (removal of a small piece of the iris)	Vision field testing Ophthalmologic examination including intraocular pressure Tonometry (measurement of the pressure in the eye) Gonioscopy (inspection of the eye's drainage angle)	Medicated eye drops Oral medication Laser

continues

Table 29-5 continued

DISEASE/DISORDER	LABORATORY/DIAGNOSTIC TESTS			SURGERY	MEDICAL TESTS OR PROCEDURES	TREATMENT
	BLOOD TESTING	OTHER TESTING	RADIOGRAPHY			
Impacted cerumen					Patient history Otologic examination Removal with curette irrigation with mineral oil, baby oil, glycerin, peroxide-based ear drops (such as Debrox), hydrogen peroxide, and saline solution	Patient education regarding the use of cotton-tipped applicators
Macular degeneration			Fluorescein angiography Optical coherence tomography	Laser surgery	Ophthalmologic examination Amsler grid Photodynamic therapy	Laser Intraocular injections Intravenous medication High-dose vitamins and minerals
Ménière's disease			MRI	Surgery to decrease fluid production or increase fluid reabsorption Surgery to interrupt vestibular nerve function Labyrinthectomy	Patient history Audiometry Middle ear injections with antibiotics or steroids	Motion sickness medications Antinausea medications Diuretics Meniett device Hearing aid for hearing loss in affected ear
Myopia				Radial keratotomy	Patient history Ophthalmologic examination	Corrective lenses
Nystagmus				Surgery to correct the position of the muscles controlling eye movement	Patient history Opticokinetic drum test Neurologic examination	Directed at cause (inner ear or central nervous system) Corrective lenses
Hyperopia				LASIK (laser-assisted in situ keratomileusis) surgery	Patient history Ophthalmic examination Astigmatoscopy	Corrective lenses

continues

Condition	Complete blood count	Culture and sensitivity	Imaging / Diagnostic	Procedure	Examination	Treatment
Presbyopia				Surgical placement of a KAMRA Inlay Conductive keratoplasty (CK)	Patient history Opthalmic examination Snellen chart	Corrective lenses
Nasal polyps			Nasal polypectomy	Biopsy of polyp (lesion) Nasal endoscopy	Patient history Nasal examination	Steroids Antihistamines Antibiotics
Otitis media	Complete blood count	Culture and sensitivity tests of exudate		Myringotomy Tympanostomy Tympanocentesis	Tympanography Pneumatic otoscopy Acoustic reflectometry	Antibiotics Comfort measures
Otosclerosis			CT	Stapedectomy	Patient history Audiometry Rinne test Tympanogram	Hearing aid
Retinal detachment			Ultrasound imaging	Laser surgery Cryosurgery to reattach retina Injection of air or gas into the eye Scleral buckling Vitrectomy	Patient history Ophthalmologic examination	
Retinoblastoma			CT of head MRI of head Ultrasound of the eye	Laser surgery Cryosurgery Removal of the eye (enucleation)	Patient history Ophthalmologic examination Bone marrow biopsy CSF exam	Radiation therapy Chemotherapy

Table 29-5 continued

DISEASE/DISORDER	LABORATORY/DIAGNOSTIC TESTS			SURGERY	MEDICAL TESTS OR PROCEDURES	TREATMENT
	BLOOD TESTING	OTHER TESTING	RADIOGRAPHY			
Sinusitis Functional endoscopic sinus surgery Balloon sinuplasty Caldwell Luc procedure	Complete blood count	Culture and sensitivity tests of exudate	Sinus radiographs		Patient history Physical exam Nasal endoscopy Allergy testing Nasal irrigation	Antibiotics for bacterial infection Antihistamines Saline lavage Nasal corticosteroids Decongestants
Strabismus				Eye muscle repair	Ophthalmologic examination Neurologic examination Corneal light reflex Cover/uncover test Visual acuity	Cover the normal eye to force weaker eye to function Corrective lenses
Stye (hordeolum)		Culture and sensitivity tests if exudate present		Incision and drainage		Antibiotic ointment
Vestibular neuritis (labyrinthitis)			CT of head MRI of head		EEG Electrostagmography Audiology/audiometry	Antihistamines Medications for nausea and vomiting Sedatives Environmental management to reduce vertigo

TABLE 29-6

DESCRIPTION OF EYE DISORDERS

REFRACTION AND OTHER DISORDERS

Astigmatism. Irregular lens curvature or cornea shape causing improper focusing of objects.

Cataract. Lens loses its transparent nature caused by changes in its proteins. Usually brought on by aging or exposure to sunlight.

Color blindness. Inability to distinguish among colors. Caused by an absence of a cone photopigment; a genetic disorder.

Conjunctivitis. Caused by a bacterial infection or irritant resulting in irritated and reddened conjunctiva. If caused by bacteria, conjunctivitis is treated with the appropriate antibiotic ophthalmic ointment or drops.

Corneal abrasion. Caused by an injury to the cornea by a foreign body resulting in pain, tearing, redness, and possible infection.

Diabetic retinopathy. Diabetes mellitus causes damage to the retina because the disease causes vascular changes. This is the leading cause of blindness in the United States.

Glaucoma. Condition caused by increased intraocular pressure due to a buildup of aqueous humor. This results in mild visual disturbances with little or no pain but can lead to severe visual impairment if untreated.

Nearsightedness (myopia). Caused by an elongated (irregularly shaped) eyeball; the image is focused in the front of the retina, resulting in the inability to focus on objects at a distance.

Farsightedness (hyperopia). Caused when the eyeball is irregularly shaped (shortened); the image is focused behind the retina, causing distance vision to be unclear.

Presbyopia. Attributed to the aging process when the lens loses its elasticity and the ability to accommodate. Vision is hampered when items are close.

Retinal detachment. Complete or partial separation of the retina from the choroid layer of the eye, leading to possible blindness.

Stye (hordeolum). Inflamed sebaceous gland of the eyelid caused by bacterial infection. Erythema and tenderness at site are common symptoms.

tracts cross at the optic chasm, the stimuli coming from the right visual fields are translated in the visual area of the left occipital area, and the stimuli coming from the left visual fields are translated in the visual area of the right occipital lobe. Table 29-6 describes common eye disorders. Figure 29-7 illustrates the visual pathways of the eye.

Signs and symptoms that are common to eye diseases and disorders are conjunctivitis; **hordeolum** (stye); decreased visual acuity; and any visual changes, such as seeing sudden flashes of light, that may indicate retinal detachment (see Figures 29-8 and 29-9).

Measuring Visual Acuity. A procedure commonly performed by the medical assistant is the measuring of a patient's visual acuity. This is a screening process used only when errors in refraction are suspected. The procedure must be performed in a well-lit, quiet area. While performing the procedure, the medical assistant must observe the patient for any action that may indicate difficulty with vision. These actions include squinting, wiping of the eyes, or leaning toward the chart. In near-vision acuity, these actions include holding the card nearer or farther than the stated position. The commonly used chart for distance visual acuity is the Snellen chart for the adult.

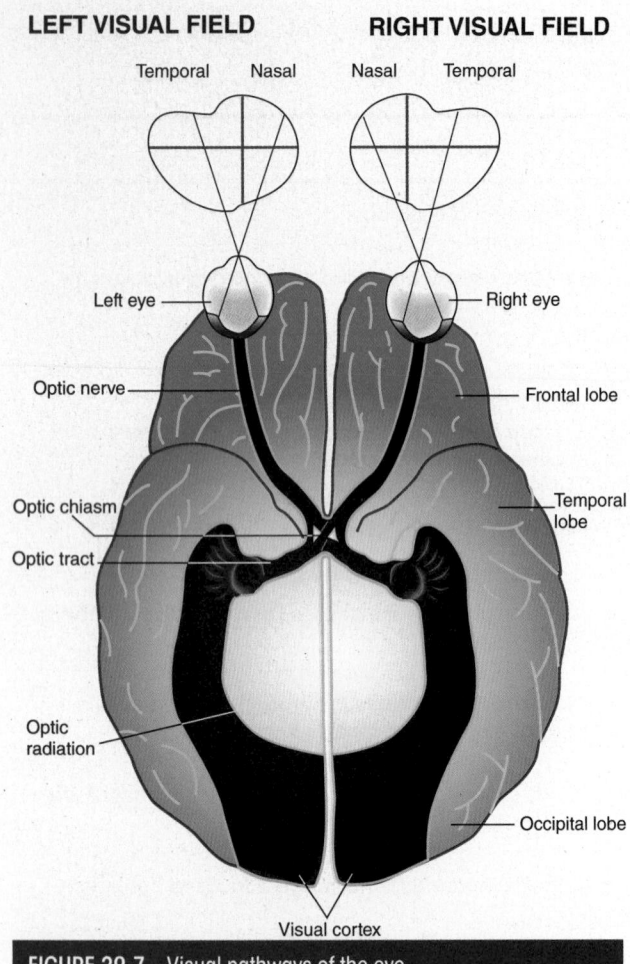

LEFT VISUAL FIELD   **RIGHT VISUAL FIELD**

Temporal   Nasal   Nasal   Temporal

Left eye —

Right eye

Optic nerve —

Frontal lobe

Optic chiasm —

Temporal lobe

Optic tract —

Optic radiation —

Occipital lobe

Visual cortex

FIGURE 29-7 Visual pathways of the eye.

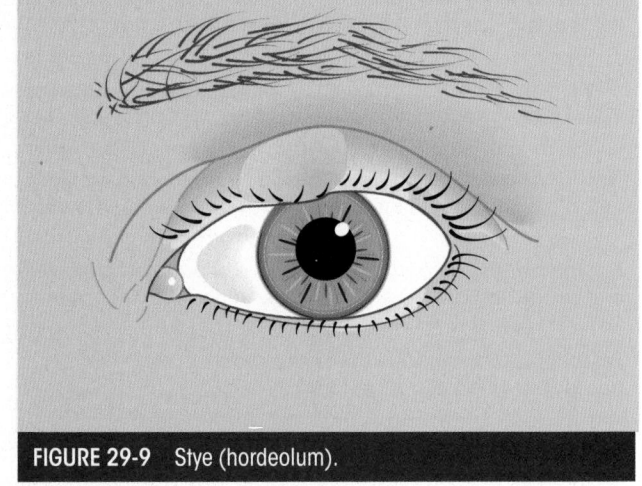

FIGURE 29-8 Conjunctivitis.

FIGURE 29-9 Stye (hordeolum).

Near vision is commonly checked by using the Jaeger chart.

The Jaeger chart used for checking clear vision is a small card that the patient holds between 14 and 16 inches from the eye. The medical assistant measures the distance for accuracy. This is the distance from which a person with normal vision is able to read printed material such as a newspaper. The Jaeger test consists of a series of reading material, the letters of which gradually become smaller. Record the last line number that the patient can easily read. The patient is checked with and without corrective lenses, and each eye is checked separately.

Errors in refraction is the term used to designate visual acuity abnormalities. The common visual abnormalities include myopia, or nearsightedness (the ability to see only near objects clearly); **hyperopia**, or farsightedness (the ability to see only distant objects clearly);

and astigmatism, which is uneven curvature of the cornea, resulting in a scattering of light rays producing blurry vision. **Presbyopia** is associated with the aging process and is an increase in farsightedness and a loss of lens elasticity that is necessary to accommodate for near vision (Figure 29-10).

The **Snellen chart** consists of the alphabet letters in various combinations starting at the top with a large E, and in lines of descending size toward the bottom. Each line is labeled with the visual acuity measurement. The Snellen chart for children has pictures. Patients who do not speak English may use a directional chart.

Recording Visual Acuity. Visual acuity, both near and far, is recorded in a fraction format.

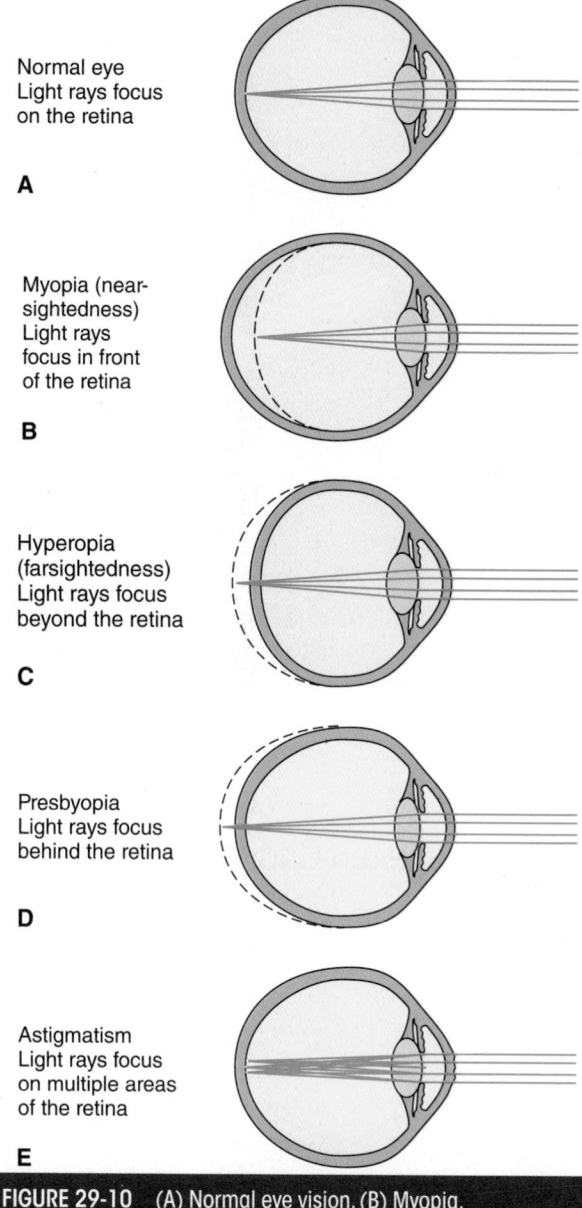

Normal eye
Light rays focus
on the retina

A

Myopia (near-
sightedness)
Light rays
focus in front
of the retina

B

Hyperopia
(farsightedness)
Light rays focus
beyond the retina

C

Presbyopia
Light rays focus
behind the retina

D

Astigmatism
Light rays focus
on multiple areas
of the retina

E

FIGURE 29-10 (A) Normal eye vision. (B) Myopia. (C) Hyperopia. (D) Presbyopia. (E) Astigmatism.

The numerator indicates the 20-foot distance between the patient and the chart. The denominator indicates the visual acuity of the patient in relationship to the normal seeing eye. Normal vision is 20/20. This means that at 20 feet the eye is seeing what the normal eye would see at 20 feet. Should the vision be 20/30, this indicates that the eye is seeing at 20 feet what the normal eye would see at 30 feet away. A visual acuity of 20/15 indicates that the eye is seeing at 20 feet what the person with normal visual acuity would be able to see at 15 feet. Vision is recorded

on the patient chart as right eye, left eye, and both eyes.

Example: Right 20/20   Left 20/20
Both 20/20

Patients should be screened with and without their corrective lenses and the results recorded in patients' charts or electronic medical records.

Color Vision. Checking color vision is not part of a routine examination. This procedure is usually performed on people who must distinguish color as part of their occupation (e.g., truck drivers, pilots, and salespeople). A commonly used color vision test is the Ishihara color graph. The Ishihara test chart book (Figure 29-11) contains pages composed of circles of varying sizes and colors. Inside the circles are numbers or lines that can be traced. The patient is seated for the procedure with the book held 14 to 16 inches away and is instructed to identify the numbers as the page is turned or is instructed to trace the line from the indicated starting point to the end. Inability to see the number or to follow the line may indicate color blindness. Should this occur, the medical assistant must inform the provider as to what number(s) could not be seen. The patient is then referred to an ophthalmologist.

The Cambridge Color Test is another method to assess color vision deficiencies. This testing allows for more detail in the changes in color discrimination over time. The test was developed by Professor John Mollon and colleagues at the University of Cambridge in England. The test is a refined tool for

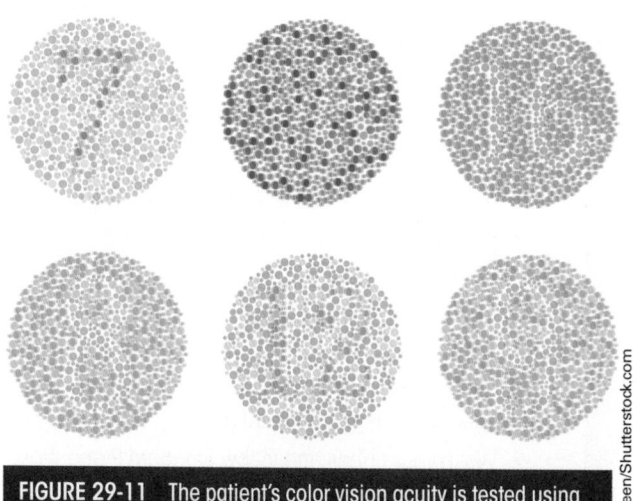

FIGURE 29-11 The patient's color vision acuity is tested using Ishihara plates.

© eveleen/Shutterstock.com

monitoring quantitatively over time the progression or remission of disease. Many drugs affect color vision, and pharmacologists will find the test well suited to monitoring the short- or long-term course of such side effects. There is also computer-controlled color vision testing that is available based on the Cambridge Color Test. (For more information on this testing method, go to http://www.crsltd.com and search for "Cambridge Color Test.")

The medical assistant will be responsible for assisting the provider in ophthalmologic examinations and performing the tests for visual acuity. Diagnostic procedures for the special senses involve the use of specialized instruments. The use of the ophthalmoscope (lighted instrument used to view inside the patient's eye; Figure 29-12) assists in identifying disease-related problems. The interior of the eye can be examined.

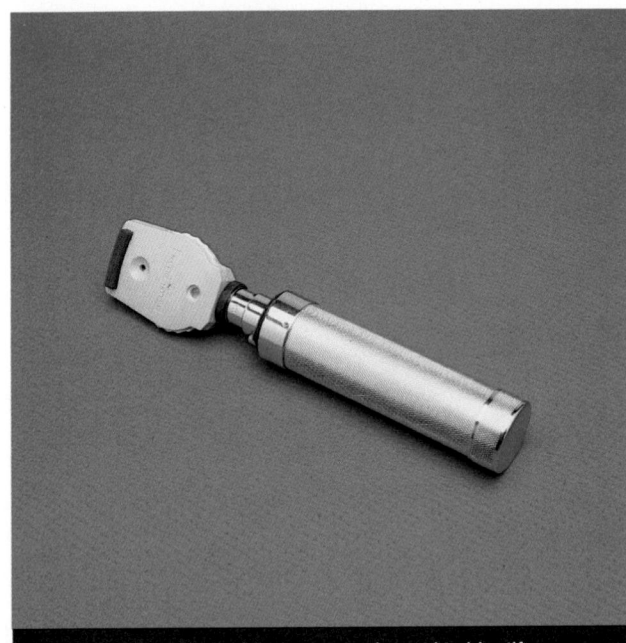

FIGURE 29-12 The ophthalmoscope is used to identify eye disorders.

 Procedures 29-3 through 29-8 list the steps for specialty procedures for the eye.

Procedure

PROCEDURE 29-3

Procedure

Performing Visual Acuity Testing Using a Snellen Chart

STANDARD PRECAUTIONS:

Handwashing

PURPOSE:
To perform a visual screening test to determine a patient's distance visual acuity.

EQUIPMENT/SUPPLIES:

- Snellen eye chart placed at eye level (appropriate for age and reading ability of the patient)
- Pointer
- Occluder
- Alcohol wipes

PROCEDURE STEPS:

1. Assemble the needed equipment.
2. Wash your hands and follow Standard Precautions where applicable.
3. Patients who already wear glasses or contacts should use these corrective devices for the test unless otherwise directed by the provider. Note this in the medical record.

continues

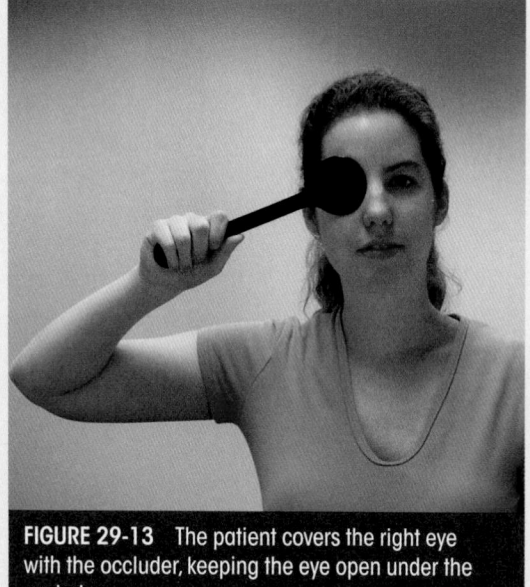

FIGURE 29-13 The patient covers the right eye with the occluder, keeping the eye open under the occluder.

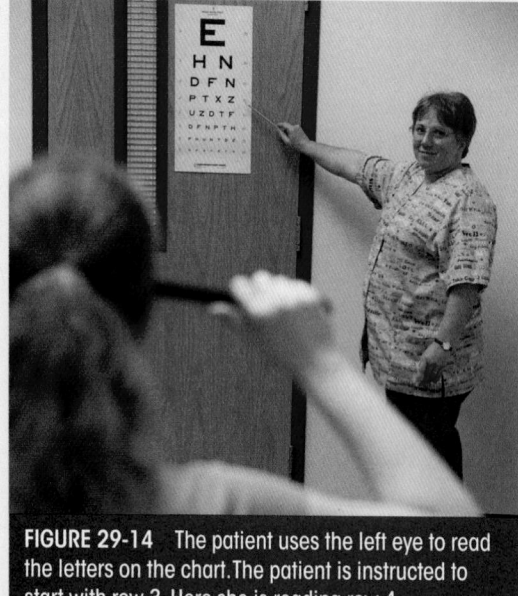

FIGURE 29-14 The patient uses the left eye to read the letters on the chart. The patient is instructed to start with row 3. Here she is reading row 4.

4. ***Explain the rationale for the performance of the procedure to the patient, showing awareness of the patient's concerns.***

5. To perform the distance visual acuity test, the patient will stand at a mark that has been measured 20 feet from the Snellen eye chart mounted on the far wall at eye level. **NOTE:** Depending on the age and cognitive ability of the patient, other eye charts, such as a Kindergarten or Sloan Letter chart, may be used for this test. Record the type of chart used in the patient's medical record.

6. Ask the patient to use the occluder to cover the right eye (Figure 29-13). Remind the patient to keep the covered eye open during the procedure and not to apply any pressure to the eyeball. RATIONALE: Closing of the eye not being tested may cause the person to squint when reading the chart.

7. Standing next to the chart, point to row 3 and instruct the patient to use the left eye to read and verbally identify each letter. If the patient is unable to read row 3, proceed to row 2 or 1 (Figure 29-14). RATIONALE: Pointing to each row helps the patient to focus on one row of letters at a time. Beginning at row 3 saves time.

8. Accurately record the results at the smallest line the patient can read with a maximum of two errors. RATIONALE: Distance visual acuity is generally recorded as a fraction, with the top number indicating the distance the patient is standing from the chart, in this case 20 feet, and the bottom line indicating the distance that a person with normal vision can read the same line. If the top line that can be read is noted as 20/60, it means that a person with normal vision could read this line at a distance of 60 feet. As the patient is taking the test, be aware of any behaviors that could indicate eye problems, such as leaning forward, squinting, or tearing from the eyes.

9. Repeat the procedure having the patient cover the left eye with the occluder and testing acuity of the right eye. Record the results when complete.

10. Repeat the procedure for a third time, this time with the patient using both eyes to read the chart. Record the results in the patient's medical record when finished.

11. Use an alcohol wipe to clean the occluder and then wash your hands.

DOCUMENTATION:

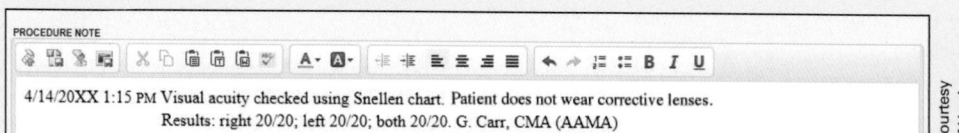

PROCEDURE NOTE

A· A· B I U

4/14/20XX 1:15 PM Visual acuity checked using Snellen chart. Patient does not wear corrective lenses.
Results: right 20/20; left 20/20; both 20/20. G. Carr, CMA (AAMA)

Courtesy of Harris CareTracker PM and EMR

PROCEDURE 29-4

Procedure

Measuring Near Visual Acuity

STANDARD PRECAUTIONS:

Handwashing

PURPOSE:

To measure the near vision of the patient.

EQUIPMENT/SUPPLIES:

- Appropriate near vision chart (Jaegar)
- Occluder
- Measuring tape
- Alcohol wipes

PROCEDURE STEPS:

1. Assemble the needed equipment.
2. To perform the near visual acuity test, you will need special test cards printed with a chart, known as the Jaeger chart, written in a language and reading level appropriate for that particular patient.
3. Wash your hands and follow Standard Precautions where applicable.
4. ***Explain the rationale for the performance of the procedure to the patient, showing awareness of the patient's concerns.***
5. Have the patient hold the card at a distance of 14 inches and instruct him or her to read aloud various paragraphs of the card with both eyes open. Use the measuring tape to ensure the appropriate distance.
6. Ask the patient to read until a line is reached where more than two mistakes are made. Ask the patient to repeat the line to ensure accuracy before recording the result. Normal vision for this test is 14/14.
7. If the patient wears corrective lenses, repeat the process again, this time with the lenses in place. Note the results in the patient's medical record.
8. Pay attention to the patient's behavior as the test is being performed. Note squinting or attempting to adjust distance for better visualization.
9. When the test is completed, return the test cards to proper storage.
10. Wash your hands and note any additional findings in the patient record.

DOCUMENTATION:

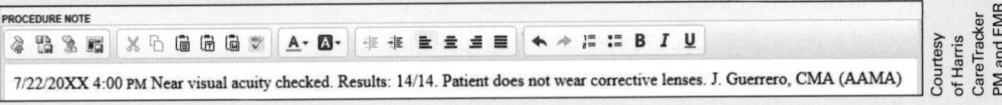

PROCEDURE NOTE

7/22/20XX 4:00 PM Near visual acuity checked. Results: 14/14. Patient does not wear corrective lenses. J. Guerrero, CMA (AAMA)

Courtesy of Harris CareTracker PM and EMR

PROCEDURE 29-5

Procedure

Testing Color Vision Using the Ishihara Plates

STANDARD PRECAUTIONS:

Handwashing

PURPOSE:

To assess a patient's ability to distinguish between the colors red and green.

Patient education:

1. Explain that the purpose of the test is to determine if the patient has a color vision deficiency.
2. Show the patient plate number 12 as an example of the test process.

EQUIPMENT/SUPPLIES:

- Ishihara Plates (1-2) (Figure 29-15)
- Measuring tape

PROCEDURE STEPS:

1. *Paying attention to detail*, assemble equipment and supplies.
2. Wash hands and follow Standard Precautions where applicable.
3. *Explain the rationale for the performance of the procedure to the patient, showing awareness of the patient's concerns*.

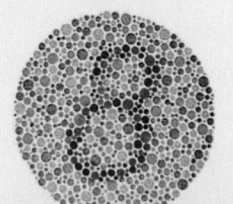 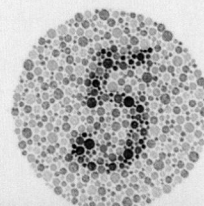

FIGURE 29-15 Ishihara plates are used to assess the patient's ability to distinguish between the colors red and green.

4. Using the measuring tape, set the plate or picture 30 inches from the patient. Ensure that there is adequate lighting as this is essential for appropriate interpretation.
5. Ask the patient to identify the number displayed on the plate or picture, and record the patient's answer. A result of 10 or more correct plates or pictures indicates normal color vision.
6. Wash your hands.
7. Return the plates to the storage area, covered and protected from sunlight. RATIONALE: Source for error: Test plates should be kept covered when not in use. Undue exposure to sunlight causes a fading of the color plates, thus leading to inaccurate test interpretation.
8. Update the provider with the test results and document the procedure in the patient's record.

DOCUMENTATION:

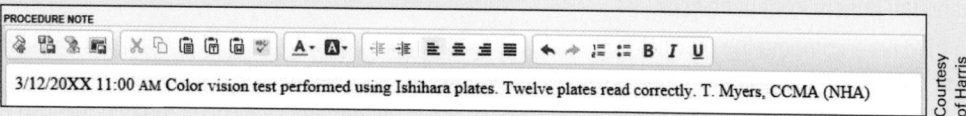

PROCEDURE NOTE

3/12/20XX 11:00 AM Color vision test performed using Ishihara plates. Twelve plates read correctly. T. Myers, CCMA (NHA)

Courtesy of Harris CareTracker PM and EMR

PROCEDURE 29-6

Procedure

Performing Eye Instillation

STANDARD PRECAUTIONS:

Handwashing

Gloves

PURPOSE:

To treat eye infections, soothe irritation, anesthetize, and dilate pupils. Ophthalmic medication is supplied in liquid or ointment form. Medication is sterile. In order to maintain sterility, take care not to touch any of the eye surface with the tip of the dispenser.

EQUIPMENT/SUPPLIES:

- Sterile eye dropper for single use
- Medication as ordered by provider
- Nonsterile disposable gloves
- Tissues

PROCEDURE STEPS:

1. ***Paying attention to detail***, assemble supplies needed for the procedure.

2. Wash your hands and follow Standard Precautions.

3. Verify the provider's orders, keeping in mind the "rights" of medication administration. If you are unfamiliar with a medication, refer to the *Physician's Desk Reference* (PDR) located within the electronic health records in order to educate yourself about the medication's name, mechanism of action, route of administration, and common side effects.

4. Check that the medication label is the same as that indicated on the physician's orders. Check for any special instructions related to the administration of the medication. Confirm that the expiration date is still within the allowable time period.

5. Introduce yourself to the patient and confirm his or her identity using two types of identifiers, such as name and date of birth. Confirm the procedure to be performed.

6. ***Speak to the level of the patient's understanding and explain the rationale for performance of the procedure***, making sure to provide the patient with the opportunity to ask questions.

7. Ask the patient about any allergies before administering any medication. Compare the medication to the provider's order for a second time.

8. Position the patient to sit or lie back.

9. For a third time, compare the provider's orders to the medication. Don gloves and open the bottle, being especially careful not to let the dropper tip touch anything when you remove the cap.

10. Instruct the patient to look up at the ceiling and expose the lower conjunctival sac of the affected eye by pulling gently downward on the lower lid (Figure 29-16).

continues

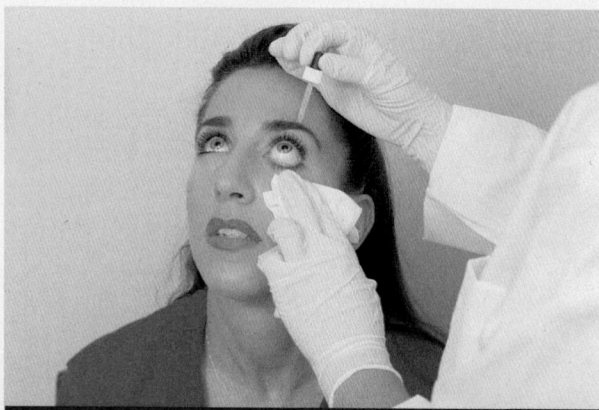

FIGURE 29-16 When medication is being instilled into the patient's eye, the patient should look up to the ceiling and the medical assistant should pull down on the lower lid. Contact with the eyeball should be avoided.

11. Placing the dropper tip as close to the eye as possible without touching it, brace the fingers not holding the dropper on the nose.

12. Gently squeeze the dropper and administer the appropriate amount of medication into the pouch formed by the lower lid as indicated by the provider's orders.

13. Instruct the patient to gently close the eye and keep it closed for at least 30 to 60 seconds in order to allow the medication to bathe the eye. RATIONALE: Movement distributes the medication evenly.

14. While the patient's eye is closed, gently place your finger in the medial corner of the patient's eye, near the lower tear duct, to inhibit the medication and any additional tearing caused by the drops from flowing into the tear drainage system.

15. Blot any excess medication or tears, using a tissue to wipe away from the infected eye. RATIONALE: Wipe from cleaner to dirtier.

16. Take a moment to instruct the patient on care of the eye, including any directions regarding the continued use of medication.

17. When finished, discard any waste into the appropriate container. Remove and discard gloves and wash your hands before recording the procedure in the patient's medical record. Make sure to include any instructions or patient education that you provided.

DOCUMENTATION:

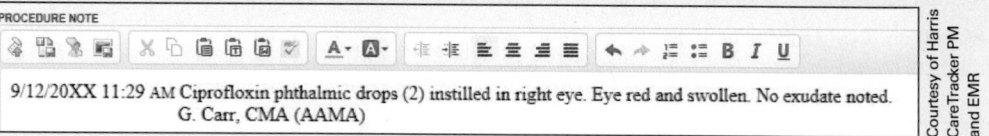

PROCEDURE NOTE

9/12/20XX 11:29 AM Ciprofloxin phthalmic drops (2) instilled in right eye. Eye red and swollen. No exudate noted. G. Carr, CMA (AAMA)

Courtesy of Harris CareTracker PM and EMR

PROCEDURE 29-7

Procedure

Performing Eye Patch Dressing Application

STANDARD PRECAUTIONS:

Handwashing

Gloves

PURPOSE:

To apply a sterile eye patch.

EQUIPMENT/SUPPLIES:

- Tape
- Sterile eye patch
- Sterile gloves

PROCEDURE STEPS:

1. ***Paying attention to detail,*** assemble supplies needed for the procedure.

2. Wash your hands and follow Standard Precautions.

3. Introduce yourself to the patient and confirm his or her identity using two types of identifiers, such as name and date of birth. Confirm the procedure to be performed.

4. ***Speak to the level of the patient's understanding and explain the rationale for performance of the procedure,*** making sure to provide the patient with the opportunity to ask questions.

5. Position the patient to sit or lie back.

6. Ask the patient to close both eyes.

7. Open the eye patch packaging using sterile technique and place the patch over the eye.

8. Secure the patch with three or four strips of 1-inch paper tape applied diagonally from mid-forehead to just in front of the ear. The completed tape application should form the shape of an oval.

9. When finished, discard any waste into the appropriate container. Remove and discard gloves and wash your hands before recording the procedure in the patient's medical record.

10. Instruct the patient regarding the length of time to wear patch and any return visits to the provider.

11. Accurately record the application of the sterile eye patch and patient education in the patient's chart or electronic medical record.

DOCUMENTATION:

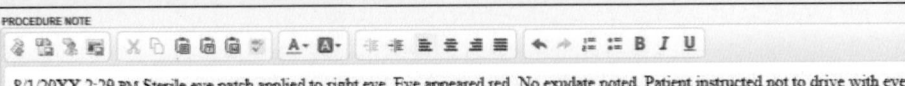

PROCEDURE NOTE

8/1/20XX 2:29 PM Sterile eye patch applied to right eye. Eye appeared red. No exudate noted. Patient instructed not to drive with eye patch on. Wife to drive patient home. Eye patch to remain in place for 3 days and will be removed at the next office visit 8/4/20XX. N. McFarland, RMA (AMT)

Courtesy of Harris CareTracker PM and EMR

PROCEDURE 29-8

Performing Eye Irrigation

Procedure

STANDARD PRECAUTIONS:

Handwashing   Gloves   Biohazard

PURPOSE:

To irrigate the patient's affected eye:

   a. To cleanse debris

   b. To cleanse discharge

   c. To remove chemicals

   d. To apply antiseptic

   e. To apply warmth for comfort

EQUIPMENT/SUPPLIES:

- Sterile irrigation solution as ordered by the provider
- Sterile bulb syringe
- Kidney-shaped basin
- Sterile basin
- 2-by-2 sterile gauze
- Sterile gloves in the appropriate size
- Towel
- Impervious pad (Chux)

PROCEDURE STEPS:

1. *Paying attention to detail*, assemble supplies needed for the procedure.

2. Wash your hands and follow Standard Precautions.

3. Refer to the provider's orders and select the correct solution and appropriate solution strength. The solution should be kept at body temperature.

4. Introduce yourself and confirm the patient's identity using two identifiers, such as name and date of birth.

5. *Speaking at the patient's level of understanding, explain the rationale for performance of the procedure.* Give the patient the opportunity to ask questions.

6. If the patient is wearing contact lenses, ask that they be removed for the procedure. Note this in the patient's medical record.

7. Position the patient in the supine position; check the eye solution against the medication indicated on the provider's orders to confirm that they are the same.

8. Check the expiration date to ensure it is within allowable limits.

9. On a flat surface near the patient, and *paying attention to detail*, create a sterile field by using a sterile impervious drape or the packaging for the sterile basin.

continues

10. Open the supplies, and without touching them, flip them one by one onto the sterile field, maintaining sterile technique at all times.

11. Make a third and final comparison of the solution and order before pouring the solution into the sterile basin. Be careful not to cause splashing.

12. Cover the shoulder with the waterproof pad and a towel to absorb any fluid that might splash.

13. Place a kidney shaped basin next to the affected side of the patient and instruct the patient to turn his or her head to the same side as the affected eye, nearest the basin. RATIONALE: The solution should flow away from the unaffected eye.

14. Don sterile gloves and fill the bulb syringe with the irrigating solution. Moisten the gauze sponges in the sterile saline. If indicated, and using one moistened gauze sponge at a time, clean the eyelid and eyelashes of the affected eye, moving from the nasal side to the outer aspect of the eyelid. Discard each sponge after one wipe. RATIONALE: Wipe from cleaner to dirtier.

15. Remove your gloves and dispose of them properly. Don a second set of sterile gloves.

16. Expose the lower conjunctiva by using the index finger and thumb of your nondominant hand to separate the eyelids. Instruct the patient to stare at a fixed spot during the procedure. RATIONALE: Facilitates flowing of solution.

17. Irrigate the affected eye by holding the syringe above the eye and gently squeezing the bulb to allow the solution to flow from the inner corner to the outer corner of the patient's eye (Figure 29-17). It is important that you do not touch either the eye or the conjunctival sac with the tip of the syringe at any time during the procedure. RATIONALE: Prevents a flow of solution into the unaffected eye causing cross-contamination.

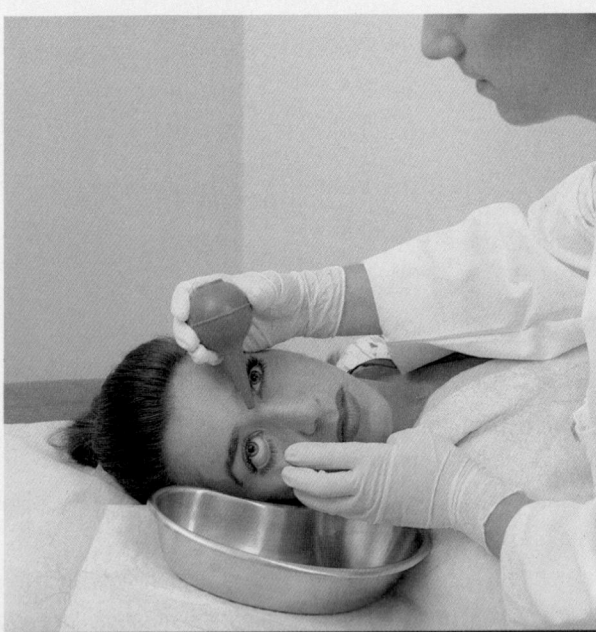

FIGURE 29-17 The medical assistant irrigates the patient's eye. Note that the solution will go from inner to outer canthus. The patient is turned toward the affected eye.

18. Repeat this procedure several times or until the debris is dislodged or until the ordered amount of irrigant is used.

19. Once done, dry the eyelid and eyelashes with a sterile gauze sponge.

20. If both eyes require irrigation, repeat the process as before, but use a new sterile kit for the second eye. RATIONALE: This will help to prevent cross-contamination.

continues

21. When finished with the irrigation process, consult with the provider before disposing of the setup as the patient may require stain to be added to check for corneal abrasions.

22. When the patient is ready to be released from your care, discard all supplies in the appropriate container.

23. Remove and discard gloves and wash your hands before documenting the irrigation procedure in the patient's medical record. Include the appearance of the eye, any drainage or debris, and the patient's response to the procedure.

DOCUMENTATION:

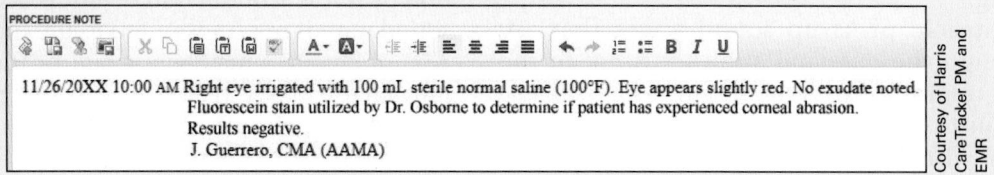

PROCEDURE NOTE

11/26/20XX 10:00 AM Right eye irrigated with 100 mL sterile normal saline (100°F). Eye appears slightly red. No exudate noted. Fluorescein stain utilized by Dr. Osborne to determine if patient has experienced corneal abrasion. Results negative.
J. Guerrero, CMA (AAMA)

Courtesy of Harris CareTracker PM and EMR

The Ear

The structures of hearing and equilibrium are divided into the external ear, the middle ear, and the inner ear (Figure 29-18). The external ear includes the pinna, or **auricle**, and the external auditory canal. The pinna is mostly cartilaginous tissue with a small amount of adipose tissue in the earlobe. The external auditory canal is about 1 inch in length and contains hair and wax-producing glands. *Cerumen* is the medical term for the wax that protects the ear canal. The external ear and middle ear are separated by the tympanic membrane, or eardrum.

The middle ear, also called the tympanic cavity, is a small space containing three bones—the malleus, incus, and stapes. Lay terms for these three smallest bones in the human body are the hammer, anvil, and stirrup. Next to the stapes is the oval window that leads to the inner ear. The Eustachian tube connects the middle ear to the throat.

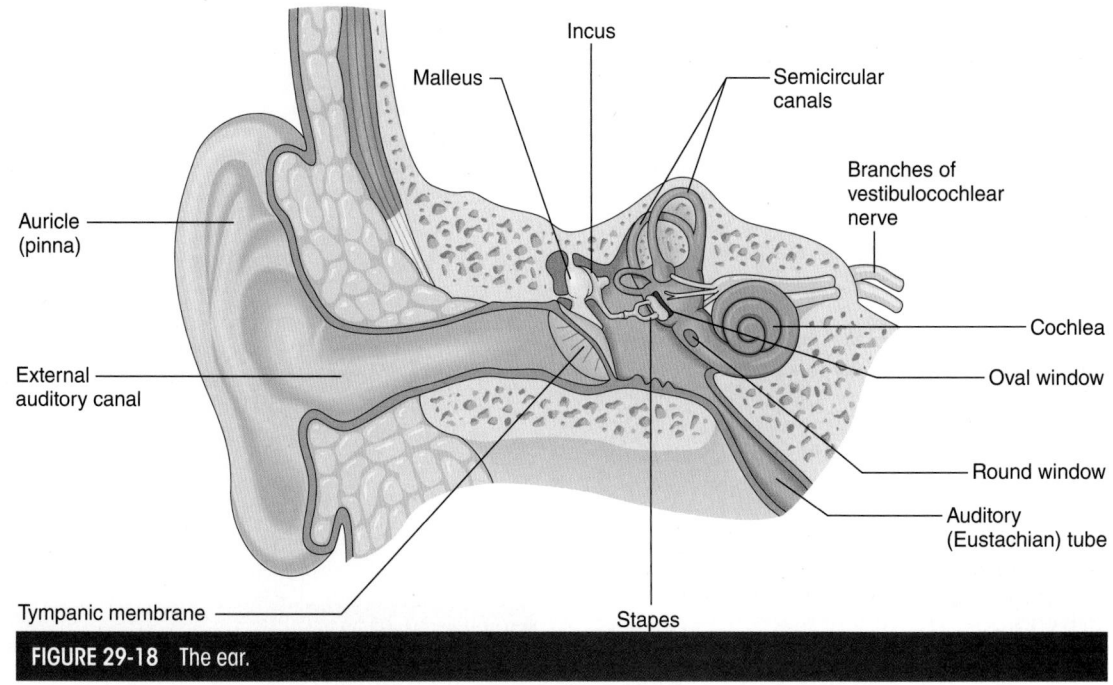

FIGURE 29-18 The ear.

The inner ear is the most sophisticated part of the ear. It is responsible for both hearing and equilibrium. The inner ear consists of a fluid-filled sterile space housing the vestibule, semicircular canals, round window, and cochlea. The structures in the vestibule are responsible for maintaining equilibrium during movement of the head. The semicircular canals assist the body to adjust to changes in direction. The movement of fluid in this area can cause symptoms of dizziness. The cochlea is the organ of hearing.

The auricle picks up sound waves that are sent through the external auditory canal to the tympanic membrane. The membrane vibrates in reaction to the sound striking it. These vibrations pass through the three tiny middle ear bones through the oval window and into the fluid in the cochlea. Receptor cells respond and transfer the sounds into electrical impulses that travel to the brain via the acoustic nerve. The receiving area of the brain for auditory impulses is in the temporal lobe. Diseases or conditions of the ear, if left untreated, can cause damage to nerves and tissues and can result in some degree of hearing impairment, from mild loss to deafness. Table 29-7 describes common diseases of the ear.

Measuring Auditory Ability. The simple methods of measuring gross hearing are usually performed by the provider. The patient may be instructed to place a finger in one ear while the provider whispers one or two words in the other. The patient is then asked to repeat the words. A ticking watch may be placed by the patient's ear to ascertain hearing. A vibrating tuning fork may be placed on the mastoid process behind the ear and then on top of the head. The patient is asked if the sound vibrations could be heard or felt. This procedure will identify nerve or conduction deafness. Conduction deafness occurs when the sound wave is not transmitted to the middle ear. This type of deafness may be a result of the presence of impacted ear wax (cerumen) in the ear canal or a scarred tympanic membrane. **Cerumen** is a substance secreted by glands at the outer third of the ear canal. In some individuals it can accumulate and block the canal and become impacted against the tympanic membrane (Figure 29-19). The sound waves cannot pass through the hardened cerumen to the middle ear, and conduction hearing loss results.

 To remove impacted cerumen, the provider may use a curette. The patient may have had ear drops prescribed before the physical removal of the impacted cerumen. The drops are instilled in an effort to

Procedure

TABLE 29-7

EAR DISORDERS

External otitis (swimmer's ear). Inflammation of ear canal. Symptoms are itchiness and crusting of ear canal.

Impacted cerumen. Caused by accumulation of hardened cerumen that has built up against the tympanic membrane. Impaired hearing and tinnitus can result.

Ménière's disease. Characterized by deafness, vertigo, nausea, and tinnitus. Probable cause is edema of the labyrinth.

Otitis media. Acute infection of the middle ear usually caused by bacteria. Symptoms are pain, fever, discharge, and decreased hearing acuity.

Otosclerosis. Conduction deafness caused by hardening of the stapes.

Tinnitis. Commonly known as ringing in the ears. However, the sound may be roaring, clicking, hissing, or buzzing. It may be soft or loud, high pitched or low pitched, in either one or both ears.

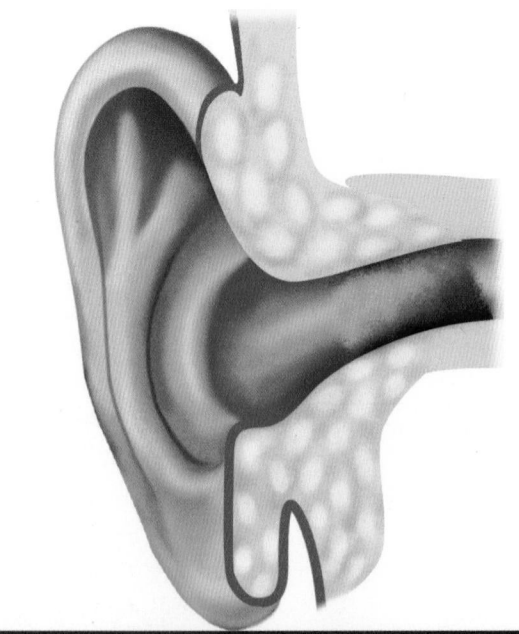

FIGURE 29-19 Impacted cerumen.

soften the cerumen to facilitate its removal. An ear irrigation may be performed by flushing the ear canal with warm water or a solution ordered by the provider. Commercial solutions are available for patients to use at home (see Procedure 29-9).

A tympanic membrane can become scarred from rupture or perforation. Scarring can occur from untreated acute otitis media or traumatic rupture. With acute otitis media, the tympanic membrane is red and bulges from accumulation of serous or purulent fluid behind it. The pressure of the fluid on the tympanic membrane may be so great that the membrane ruptures and drainage can be seen in the ear canal. The perforation or rupture will probably heal, but a small scar on the membrane will remain. Repeated ruptures from acute otitis media will cause repeated scarring and diminished hearing function, referred to as conduction hearing loss. A culture and sensitivity of any purulent or serous drainage will indicate the antibiotic to which the microorganism is sensitive.

A myringotomy is a surgical incision into the tympanic membrane made to remove accumulated fluid caused by infection. Because the procedure is surgical in nature, the tympanic membrane can be incised to allow the fluid to drain. Scarring is minimized because the incision is made with a scalpel in a controlled location and will heal with less scarring. Tubes may be placed in the opening made by the myringotomy, called a **tympanostomy**, to equalize pressure and prevent fluid from accumulating (see Chapter 26).

Nerve deafness is a result of injury or disease that affects the nerves leading from the inner ear to the auditory centers of the brain.

A more complex procedure for measuring hearing may be performed by the medical assistant but more often by an audiologist, using an audiometer (Figure 29-20). A quiet room with no distractions is required for the procedure to be accurate. The patient is seated facing away from the medical assistant and the audiometer, then ear phones are placed over the ears. The patient is instructed to raise a hand when a sound is heard. The audiometer has two dials, one for the various wavelengths and the other for wave intensity. Starting at the lowest pitch, the intensity is increased until the patient responds to the sound. The next pitch is then tested in the same manner. This process continues until the highest pitch sound is tested. The results are obtained

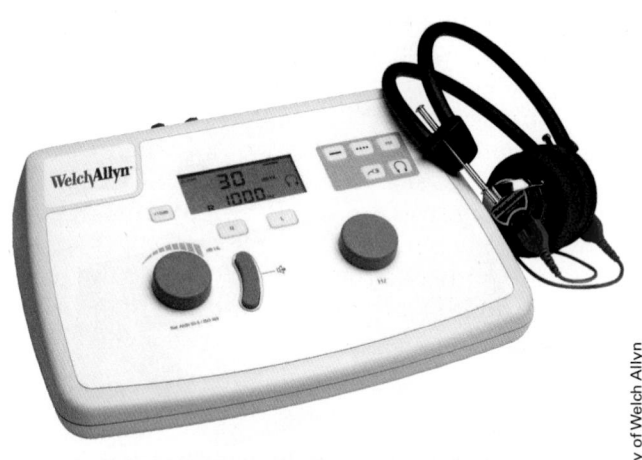

FIGURE 29-20 Audiometer.

by noting the number of intensity at which the sound was heard. When performing the procedure, the medical assistant must not develop a pattern that can be detected by the patient. The ears should be tested in an alternating fashion to ensure accuracy (see Procedure 29-10).

The medical assistant employed in an industrial medical facility may be required to monitor some employees' hearing. In this case, care must be taken to have the hearing test performed before the employee goes to work for the day. Hearing loss may result from the day's activities in some noisy facilities even when ear plugs are worn.

Tympanometry is a procedure used to ascertain the ability of the middle ear to transmit sound waves and is commonly performed on children to diagnose middle ear infections. A probe is inserted into the ear canal to measure the air pressure of the ear canal in relation to the air pressure found in the middle ear. Tympanogram is the recording produced by this procedure. The waves and peaks are measured, providing an indication of possible middle ear abnormalities (Figure 29-21).

The medical assistant or the provider may perform the audiometry test. Diagnostic procedures for the ear involve the use of specialized instruments, including the **otoscope** (lighted instrument to examine the tympanic membrane), which assists in identifying disease-related ear problems (Figure 29-22).

Procedures 29-9, 29-10, and 29-11 describe steps for ear irrigation, audiometry, and ear instillation.

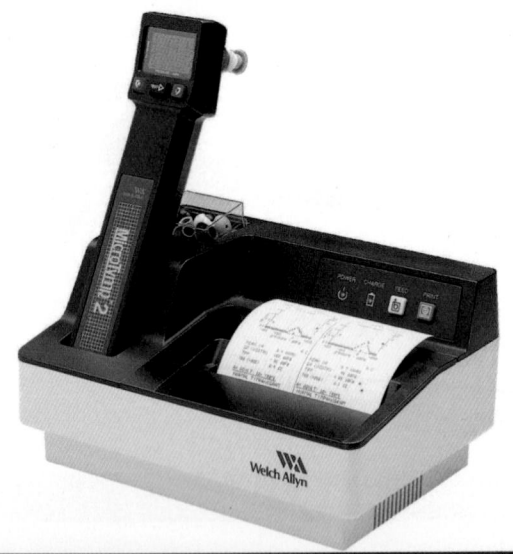

FIGURE 29-21 A portable tympanometric instrument with charger. A printout of the tympanogram can be seen. Testing is done in 1 second and is useful for diagnosing otitis media and other middle ear conditions, such as patency of tympanostomy tubes and otosclerosis.

Courtesy of Welch-Allyn

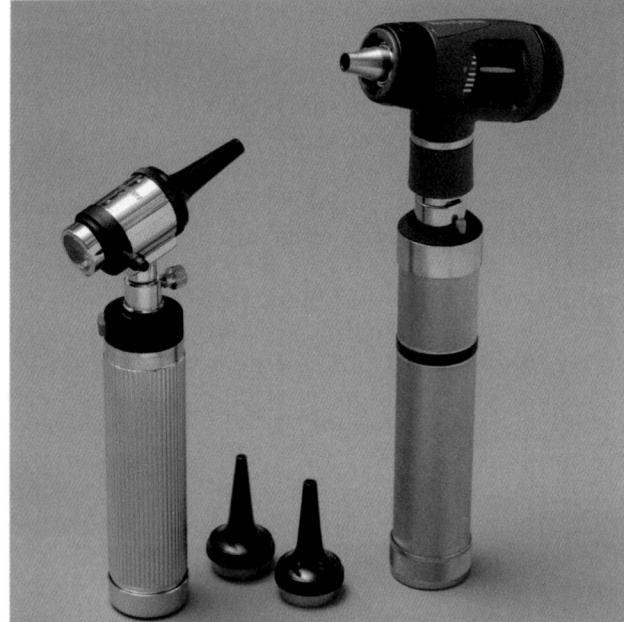

FIGURE 29-22 The otoscope is used to examine the patient's tympanic membrane.

PROCEDURE 29-9

Procedure

Performing Ear Irrigation

STANDARD PRECAUTIONS:

Handwashing

PURPOSE:

To remove impacted cerumen, discharge, or foreign materials from the ear canal as directed by the provider.

EQUIPMENT/SUPPLIES:

- Sterile irrigation solution as ordered by the provider, warmed to 98.6 to 103°F
- Nonsterile disposable gloves
- Kidney-shaped or emesis basin
- Sterile basin
- Impervious pad to protect the patient's clothing
- Bulb syringe

PROCEDURE STEPS:

1. *Paying attention to detail*, assemble supplies needed for the procedure.
2. Wash your hands and follow Standard Precautions.

continues

3. Refer to the provider's orders and select the correct solution and appropriate solution strength. The solution should be kept at approximately body temperature.

4. Introduce yourself and confirm the patient's identity using two identifiers, such as name and date of birth.

5. ***Speaking at the patient's level of understanding, explain the rationale for performance of the procedure.*** Give the patient the opportunity to ask questions. Explain to the patient that it is not uncommon to feel dizziness or some discomfort as the fluid comes in contact with the tympanic membrane.

6. Instruct the patient to take a comfortable position. Then compare the label on the sterile solution with the provider's order. Check the expiration date to ensure that the solution is within the allowable time limit.

7. Place the impervious drape over the patient's shoulder to protect clothing from any splashing solution.

8. Make a second check to compare the provider's orders with the label on the ear solution and pour the prewarmed solution into the sterile basin.

9. Instruct the patient to tilt his or her head in the direction of the affected side and make a third check to compare the solution to the provider's orders before donning gloves (Figure 29-23). RATIONALE: This position allows the solution to flow into the basin by gravity.

10. Place a kidney shaped basin under the affected ear and ask the patient to help you by holding it in place.

11. With the nondominant hand, gently pull the auricle upward and back to straighten the ear canal. RATIONALE: Allows better access to external ear canal.

12. Fill the bulb syringe with the warmed solution and squeeze it slightly to expel any air that might remain in the bulb's body or neck.

13. Carefully and gently insert the syringe tip into the affected ear. Do not occlude the external auditory canal. Instruct the patient to immediately inform you of any severe discomfort or pain. If reported, stop irrigating immediately and contact the provider for further instruction. RATIONALE: Avoids injury to the tympanic membrane and prevents occlusion of external auditory canal, allowing solution to drain out.

14. Very gently, squeeze the bulb syringe to deliver a slow, steady stream of warmed fluid into the ear canal in an upward direction.

15. Allow the fluid and any debris to drain out into the kidney basin. Repeat the irrigation as ordered by the provider.

16. Blot the outer ear dry and notify the provider to reexamine the ear to ensure that the procedure is complete.

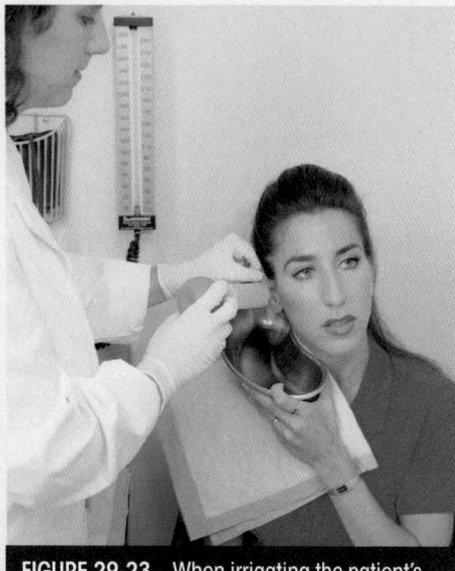

FIGURE 29-23 When irrigating the patient's ear, tip the affected ear to facilitate the flow of solution. The tip of the syringe does not occlude the opening to the external auditory canal.

continues

17. Once the provider confirms that the procedure is complete, ask the patient to lie on the affected side. Place a towel under the patient's ear to allow for complete drainage. Ask the patient to alert you to any dizziness or discomfort and advise the patient not to insert any foreign object into the ear, such as a finger or a cotton tipped applicator.

18. Empty the contents of the kidney basin following the guidelines set forth by OSHA.

19. Dispose of any remaining supplies appropriately.

20. Remove gloves and wash your hands.

21. Document the procedure in the patient's medical record, making sure to include the type and amount of irrigation utilized. Describe any cerumen, blood, or infectious drainage observed in the irrigation as well as any dizziness or discomfort reported by the patient.

DOCUMENTATION:

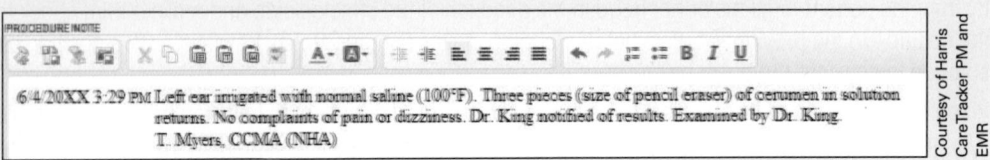

6/4/20XX 3:29 PM Left ear irrigated with normal saline (100°F). Three pieces (size of pencil eraser) of cerumen in solution returns. No complaints of pain or dizziness. Dr. King notified of results. Examined by Dr. King.
T. Myers, CCMA (NHA)

Courtesy of Harris CareTracker PM and EMR

PROCEDURE 29-10

Procedure

Assisting with Audiometry

STANDARD PRECAUTIONS:

Handwashing

PURPOSE:

To assist in testing patient for hearing loss.

Patient education:

1. Explain the use and purpose of the audiometer. Also explain that the test measures frequency of sound waves and ability of patient to hear various frequencies of sound waves (one frequency at a time).

2. When the patient hears a new frequency, he or she should signal the tester.

EQUIPMENT/SUPPLIES:

- Audiometer with headphones
- Quiet room

PROCEDURE STEPS:

1. ***Paying attention to detail***, assemble supplies needed for the procedure

2. Wash your hands and follow Standard Precautions.

3. ***Speaking at the patient's level of understanding***, explain to the patient that the test will measure the frequency of sound waves and the ability of the patient to hear various frequencies.

continues

4. Ensure that the room is free from extraneous noise and ask the patient to sit in a chair. RATIONALE: Outside interference may cause inaccurate test results, especially in the lower frequencies, which are more difficult to hear.

5. Before applying the headphones, instruct the patient to raise his or her hand when a new frequency is heard. Some audiometers also come with a handheld device to be given to the patient, who can depress the button when a sound is heard, rather than raising his or her hand. Adjust the headphones for fit and comfort. RATIONALE: Prepares to test each ear for hearing loss.

6. If you have been trained to perform the test, the provider may ask you to conduct the audiometry. Otherwise, you should be prepared to assist the provider while he or she conducts the procedure.

7. To begin the audiometry, the audiometer is set to a frequency of 1,000 at 20 decibels (dB) for basic screening. Test at 1,000; 2,000; and 4,000 frequencies. If the patient fails at 20 dB, retest at 30 dB beginning back at 1,000 frequency.

8. The patient will indicate when the first sound is heard. This information should then be plotted on the appropriate graph.

9. The frequency will be increased gradually and the patient's feedback will be plotted until the exam is complete. The procedure will then be repeated with the other ear.

10. If you have conducted the test, you must accurately relay the information you recorded to the provider for his or her interpretation.

11. Clean the equipment as indicated in the manufacturer's instructions.

12. Wash your hands and record the procedure in the patient's medical record.

DOCUMENTATION:

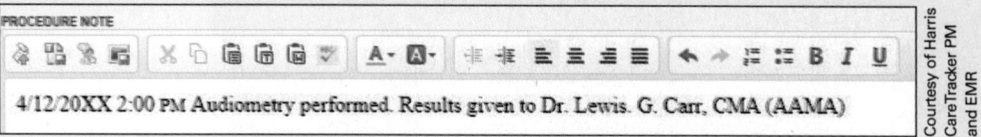

4/12/20XX 2:00 PM Audiometry performed. Results given to Dr. Lewis. G. Carr, CMA (AAMA)

Courtesy of Harris CareTracker PM and EMR

PROCEDURE 29-11

Performing Ear Instillation

Procedure

STANDARD PRECAUTIONS:

Handwashing   Gloves

PURPOSE:

To soften impacted cerumen, fight infection with antibiotics, or relieve pain.

EQUIPMENT/SUPPLIES:

- Otic medication as prescribed by the provider
- Sterile ear dropper
- Cotton balls
- Gloves

continues

PROCEDURE STEPS:

1. ***Paying attention to detail***, assemble supplies needed for the procedure.
2. Wash your hands and follow Standard Precautions.
3. Introduce yourself and confirm the identity of the patient using two identifiers, such as name and date of birth.
4. ***Confirm and explain the rationale for the procedure to be performed, speaking to the patient's level of understanding***.
5. Ask the patient to begin by either lying on the unaffected side or sitting with the head tilted so that the affected ear is facing upward. RATIONALE: Facilitates flow of medication.
6. Check the otic medication for accuracy against the provider's order. This should be done three times before the medication is administered in order to minimize the risk of medication error. RATIONALE: Only otic medication can be used in the ear. Checking the medication three times minimizes medication error.
7. Apply gloves.
8. Take an additional moment to check the expiration date to ensure that it is within allowable time limits.
9. Using the dropper, draw up the prescribed amount of medication.
10. If the patient is an adult, gently pull the top of the ear up and back (Figure 29-24). If the patient is a child, the earlobe should be gently pulled down and back.

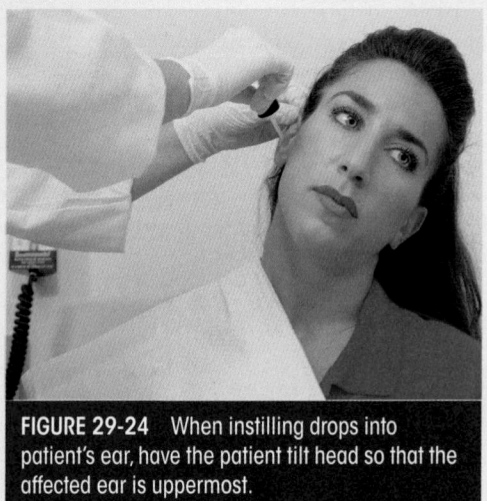

FIGURE 29-24 When instilling drops into patient's ear, have the patient tilt head so that the affected ear is uppermost.

11. Instill the prescribed dose of medication, usually specified by a number of drops, into the affected ear by squeezing the rubber bulb on the dropper.
12. Once the medication is administered, ask the patient to remain in position for about 5 minutes to keep the medication from dripping out.
13. When instructed by the provider, place a cotton ball into the external ear canal for about 15 minutes. RATIONALE: The cotton ball will help to contain the medicine in the ear.
14. Dispose of supplies into the appropriate container and then wash your hands thoroughly.
15. Document the procedure in the patient's medical record.

DOCUMENTATION:

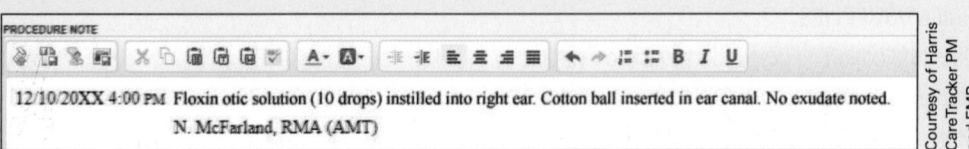

PROCEDURE NOTE

12/10/20XX 4:00 PM Floxin otic solution (10 drops) instilled into right ear. Cotton ball inserted in ear canal. No exudate noted.
　　　　　N. McFarland, RMA (AMT)

Courtesy of Harris CareTracker PM and EMR

The Nose

Procedure

The provider inspects the exterior surface of the patient's nose for skin lesions such as **rosacea**, squamous or basal cell carcinoma, and other dermatologic problems. The provider examines and palpates to determine if the nose is patent and the patient's ability to breathe in and out through each nostril.

The mucous membrane is checked for polyps, superficial blood vessels, and foreign bodies. The septum is noted for deviation. Epistaxis is a common problem and can be treated with nasal packing, nasal tampon, nasal balloon, or chemical cauterization. Procedures 29-12, 29-13, and 29-14 describe steps for specialized procedures and examinations for the nose.

PROCEDURE 29-12

Procedure

Assisting with Nasal Examination

STANDARD PRECAUTIONS:

Handwashing

Gloves

PURPOSE:

To assist the provider with the nasal examination when looking for polyps and engorged superficial blood vessels, and to assist in the possible removal of a foreign body.

Patient education:

When a foreign object is involved, instruct the patient not to blow the nose or to attempt to remove the object because this could cause tissue damage or push the object deeper into the nasal passage.

EQUIPMENT/SUPPLIES:

- Nasal speculum
- Light source
- Disposable, nonsterile gloves
- Bayonet forceps
- Kidney basin

PROCEDURE STEPS:

1. *Paying attention to detail*, assemble supplies needed for the procedure.
2. Wash your hands and follow Standard Precautions.
3. Introduce yourself and confirm the identity of the patient using two identifiers, such as name and date of birth.
4. *Confirm and explain the rationale for the procedure to be performed, speaking to the patient's level of understanding.* Take time to answer the patient's questions.
5. Assist the patient to assume a comfortably seated position and *allay any fears* the patient might have regarding the examination. If the patient has a foreign object in his or her nasal cavity, advise against blowing the nose or attempting to remove the object as this could cause further damage to the patient's nose.
6. As the provider performs the examination, be ready to assist by providing equipment and supplies as requested.

continues

7. When the examination is complete, discard any used supplies according to OSHA guidelines. Sanitize any reusable equipment following office procedure.

8. Remove and dispose of gloves and wash your hands before documenting the procedure in the patient's medical record.

DOCUMENTATION:

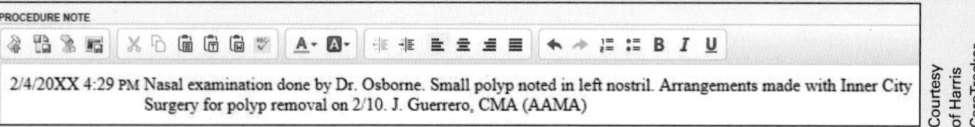

PROCEDURE NOTE

2/4/20XX 4:29 PM Nasal examination done by Dr. Osborne. Small polyp noted in left nostril. Arrangements made with Inner City Surgery for polyp removal on 2/10. J. Guerrero, CMA (AAMA)

Courtesy of Harris CareTracker PM and EMR

PROCEDURE 29-13

Procedure

Cautery Treatment of Epistaxis

STANDARD PRECAUTIONS:

Handwashing

Gloves

Biohazard

Goggles & Mask

PURPOSE:

Patient education:

Depending on the location and severity of the nosebleed, the provider will either pack the nasal canal or chemically cauterize the vessel. Generally, chemical cautery is attempted first; if that fails, nasal packing or a nasal balloon is inserted. If cauterization is performed, the patient should be instructed to not blow the nose or otherwise irritate/disturb the scab that will form. Cautery will sting, and the patient should be appropriately prepared.

EQUIPMENT/SUPPLIES:

- Patient gown and drapes
- Appropriate syringe and needles
- Kidney basin
- Tissues
- Vienna nasal speculum
- Hands-free light source
- Electrocautery
- Nonsterile, disposable gloves
- PPE as required based on severity of bleeding
- Sterile gloves for MA and provider
- Bayonet forceps
- Medications as ordered by provider (Xylocaine [lidocaine] with epinephrine or cocaine 4%)

continues

- Silver nitrate sticks
- Cotton balls or 2-by-2 gauze sponges
- Nasal packing or nasal tampons
- Absorbable packing (Gelfoam or Surigcel)
- Medicine cups
- Local anesthesia as ordered by provider
- Antibiotic/antiseptic ointment

PROCEDURE STEPS:

1. ***Paying attention to detail***, assemble supplies needed for the procedure.
2. Wash your hands and follow Standard Precautions.
3. Introduce yourself and confirm the identity of the patient using two identifiers, such as name and date of birth.
4. ***Confirm and explain the rationale for the procedure to be performed, speaking to the patient's level of understanding.*** Take time to answer the patient's questions.
5. Assist the patient to assume a comfortably seated position and ***allay any fears*** the patient might have regarding the procedure.
6. Monitor patient to ensure maintenance of airway and breathing.
7. Provide kidney basin and tissues to allow the patient to manage bleeding until the provider can intervene.
8. Instruct the patient to pinch all the soft structures of the nose between the thumb and index finger and press against the bones of the face. Have the patient lean forward with his or her head tilted forward until the provider can intervene.
9. If instructed by the provider, assist the provider in withdrawing the anesthetic ordered (Xylocaine or lidocaine with epinephrine, for example) by inverting the vial and holding it stable.
10. Remain with the patient as the anesthetic takes effect.
11. Assist the provider as requested. Don sterile gloves, if needed, to assist.
12. If the bleeding is controlled, skip to step 16.
13. If the bleeding continues, prepare the electrocautery unit or the silver nitrate sticks as ordered by the provider.
14. If the bleeding is controlled, skip to step 16.
15. If the bleeding continues, prepare nasal packing or tampons per provider's order.
16. ***Speaking at the level of the patient's understanding and including the patient's support system***, instruct the patient regarding postepistaxis care. For example:
    - Nasal packing should remain in place for 12 to 18 hours.
    - A follow-up appointment must be made with an otolaryngologist for further treatment.
    - Avoid aspirin or other anti-inflammatory medications.
17. When the procedure is complete, discard any used supplies according to OSHA guidelines. Sanitize any reusable equipment following office procedure.
18. Remove and dispose of gloves and wash your hands before documenting the procedure in the patient's medical record.

DOCUMENTATION:

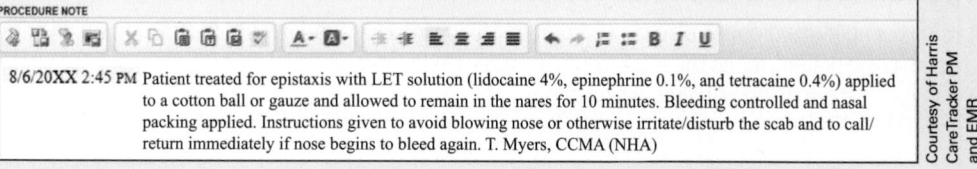

PROCEDURE NOTE

8/6/20XX 2:45 PM Patient treated for epistaxis with LET solution (lidocaine 4%, epinephrine 0.1%, and tetracaine 0.4%) applied to a cotton ball or gauze and allowed to remain in the nares for 10 minutes. Bleeding controlled and nasal packing applied. Instructions given to avoid blowing nose or otherwise irritate/disturb the scab and to call/ return immediately if nose begins to bleed again. T. Myers, CCMA (NHA)

Courtesy of Harris CareTracker PM and EMR

PROCEDURE 29-14

Procedure

Performing Nasal Instillation

STANDARD PRECAUTIONS:

Handwashing

PURPOSE:

To provide medication to the nasal membranes as ordered by the provider.

Patient education:

1. Instruct the patient to keep the head tilted back slightly during the procedure to allow the medication to cover the nasal tissues.
2. Instruct patient not to blow nose immediately after treatment. Medication could be forced out of nose.

EQUIPMENT/SUPPLIES:

- Nasal medication as prescribed by provider
- Sterile dropper (if required)
- Tissues
- Nonsterile disposable gloves

PROCEDURE STEPS:

1. ***Paying attention to detail***, assemble supplies needed for the procedure.
2. Wash your hands and follow Standard Precautions.
3. Introduce yourself and confirm the identity of the patient using two identifiers, such as name and date of birth.
4. ***Confirm and explain the rationale for the procedure to be performed***, *speaking to the patient's level of understanding.* Take time to answer the patient's questions.
5. Compare the medication to be used with that indicated on the provider's orders and check the expiration date.
6. Assist the patient to sit comfortably with their head tilted back slightly.
7. If the medication is not single use, you will have to calculate the amount of medication needed. Make a second check to ensure that the medication on hand is the same as ordered.
8. Don disposable gloves and make a third and final check to ensure proper medication administration.
9. Instruct the patient to keep the head tilted back and to inhale deeply during the instillation of the nasal drops.
10. Being careful not to touch the inside of the nasal passage with the dropper tip, instill the prescribed dose, or correct number of drops, into the center of the nostril. Repeat in the other nostril if indicated. RATIONALE: Touching the inside of the nostril will lead to contamination of the dropper.
11. Instruct the patient not to blow his or her nose, but do offer a tissue to help manage any drainage that occurs. RATIONALE: Allow time for medication to be absorbed by the nasal membranes.
12. If using a single-use dropper, dispose of it properly following OSHA guidelines. If using a multiuse dropper prescribed to the patient, recap the medication using sterile technique. Instruct the patient in home usage before giving the dropper to the patient to take home.

continues

13. Remove gloves and dispose of them before washing your hands thoroughly.

14. Document the administration in the patient's medical record, being sure to include the name of the medication, dose, route, date, time, and your initials.

DOCUMENTATION:

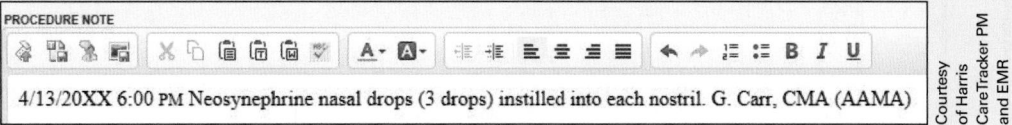

PROCEDURE NOTE

4/13/20XX 6:00 PM Neosynephrine nasal drops (3 drops) instilled into each nostril. G. Carr, CMA (AAMA)

Courtesy of Harris CareTracker PM and EMR

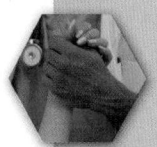

Patient Education

Nasal Irrigation

Advise the patient that commercial nasal irrigation kits are available at the pharmacy or department store, or the patient can make his or her own solution of salt and warm water (½ teaspoon salt to a pint of water). Use a bulb-type syringe for irrigation. Instruct patient not to blow nose for 5 minutes after the irrigation. This could force the solution into the sinuses or ears and possibly cause an infection in either or both.

RESPIRATORY SYSTEM

The respiratory process is all important to the life process. **External respiration** allows for the exchange of carbon dioxide and oxygen across the cell walls into the airspaces of the lungs. **Internal respiration** is the exchange of these two gases at the cellular levels of the organs.

The respiratory process begins with air entering the nose or mouth, where it passes through the pharynx, down into the trachea, and into the bronchi, and then enters the lungs. Gas exchange takes place when the blood filters through the alveoli (Figure 29-25). Table 29-8 lists diagnostic procedures for respiratory diseases and disorders. Table 29-9 describes respiratory disorders.

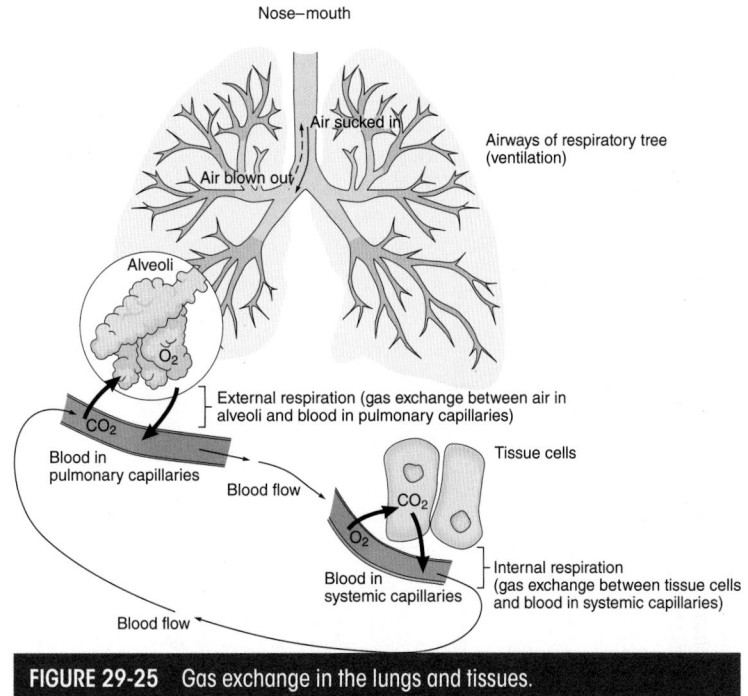

FIGURE 29-25 Gas exchange in the lungs and tissues.

TABLE 29-8

RESPIRATORY SYSTEM DISORDERS

DISEASE/DISORDER	LABORATORY/DIAGNOSTIC TESTS					MEDICAL TESTS OR PROCEDURES	TREATMENT
	BLOOD TESTING	OTHER TESTING	RADIOGRAPHY	SURGERY			
Acute or adult respiratory distress syndrome (ARDS)	Complete blood count Blood chemistry Prothrombin time Partial thromboplastin time Arterial blood gases Blood cultures	Electrocardiography Sputum cultures	Chest radiograph (CXR) CT of chest	Tracheotomy		Patient history Physical exam Thoracentesis	Antibiotics Ventilator Oxygen Nutritional Support
Asthma	Complete blood count Arterial blood gases	Sputum analysis Peak expiratory flow rate	Chest radiograph (CXR)			Patient history Physical exam Pulmonary function tests Skin testing for allergies Electrocardiogram	Medication (bronchodilators) Metered-dose inhaler Treatment of hypersensitivity Patient education on avoiding triggers and managing environmental allergens
Bronchitis	Complete blood count	Sputum culture and analysis	Chest radiograph (CXR)			Patient history Physical exam Bronchoscopy Pulmonary function testing	Antibiotics if secondary bacterial infection occurs Corticosteroids Oxygen Bronchodilators
Chronic obstructive pulmonary disease (COPD) Emphysema	Complete blood count Arterial blood gases		Chest radiograph (CXR) CT of chest	Lung volume reduction surgery Lung transplant		Patient history Physical exam Pulmonary function tests Pulse oximetry	Bronchodilators Phosphodiesterase-4 inhibitors Corticosteroids Antibiotics Careful administration of oxygen Patient teaching regarding smoking cessation

Condition	Blood Test	Other Lab Tests	Imaging	Surgical Procedures	Examinations/Procedures	Treatment
Cystic fibrosis	Immunoreactive trypsinogen (IRT)	Sweat chloride test, Fecal fat test, Genetic screening	Chest radiograph (CXR), CT scan	Lung transplant	Pulmonary function testing	Antibiotics, Bronchodilators, Enzyme therapy, Oxygen
Laryngitis	Complete blood count	Throat culture, Rapid strep test		Biopsy of vocal cords	Patient history, Physical exam, Laryngoscopy	Throat lozenges, Analgesics, Antibiotics, Steroids
Lung cancer	Complete blood count	Sputum cytology	Chest radiograph (CXR), CT scan	Biopsy of lung tissue, Wedge resection, Segmental resection, Pneumonectomy	Patient history, Physical exam, Bronchoscopy	Surgery, Chemotherapy, Radiation, Targeted drug therapy, Patient teaching regarding smoking cessation
Pharyngitis	Complete blood count	Throat culture, Rapid strep test			Patient history, Physical exam	Antibiotics if bacterial infection, Comfort measures such as lozenges or gargling with warm salty water
Pleurisy or Plural Effusion	Complete blood count	Culture and sensitivity of pleural fluid	Chest radiograph (CXR), CT of chest, Ultrasound	Pleural biopsy, Thoroscopy	Patient history, Physical exam, ECG, Thorocentesis	Taping of chest, Antibiotics if bacterial, Analgesics
Pneumonia	Complete blood count	Blood culture, Sputum culture, Pleural fluid culture	Chest radiograph (CXR), CT scan of chest	Pleurocentesis	Patient history, Physical exam, Pulse oximetry	Antibiotics if bacterial, Symptomatic treatment if viral

continues

Table 29-8 continued

DISEASE/DISORDER	BLOOD TESTING	OTHER TESTING	RADIOGRAPHY	SURGERY	MEDICAL TESTS OR PROCEDURES	TREATMENT
Pneumothorax	Arterial blood gases (ABGs)		Chest radiograph (CXR) CT of chest	Insertion of a chest tube Surgical repair of lung	Patient history Physical exam ECG	Oxygen Rest Chest tube insertion Pleurodesis
Pulmonary embolism (PE)	Arterial blood gases (ABG) Complete blood count (CBC) D-dimer	Electrocardiogram	Chest radiography (CXR) CT MRI Pulmonary angiography Ventilation/perfusion scan Ultrasound of chest	Placement of a vena caval filter Thrombectomy	Patient history Physical exam Venous Doppler studies	Oxygen Anticoagulants Thrombolytics
Severe acute respiratory syndrome (SARS)	Complete blood count Blood chemistry Serum antibodies of SARS	Throat or nasopharyngeal swab Viral culture	Chest radiography (CXR)			Antiviral drugs Corticosteroids Symptomatic treatment
Tonsillitis	Complete blood count Streptococcal antibody test	Throat culture		Tonsillectomy	Patient history Physical exam	Antibiotics Comfort measures such as rest; fluids; or gargling with warm salty water Analgesics Antipyretics
Tuberculosis	Complete blood count Interferon-gamma release assay (IGRA) tests for TB infection	Sputum culture Acid-fast smear of sputum	Chest radiograph (CXR) Bronchoscopy	Biopsy of lung tissue	Tuberculin skin test: Mantoux intradermal test	Multiple antituberculosis medications

TABLE 29-9

DESCRIPTION OF RESPIRATORY DISORDERS

Acute or adult respiratory distress syndrome (ARDS). A life-threatening condition that occurs when there is severe fluid buildup and hemorrhage in the lungs. ARDS is breathing failure that can occur in critically ill patients with underlying illnesses. There is a high mortality rate. Patients may be placed on isolation precautions (see Chapter 21).

Asthma. Inflammation and spasm of the smooth muscle of the bronchi brought on by an allergen or emotional upset. Characterized by dyspnea and wheezing.

Bronchitis. Inflammation of the bronchi, caused by viral or bacterial infection with a dry, painful cough, progressing to a productive cough of greenish yellow sputum. Symptoms include cough, slight fever, chills, malaise, and soreness under the sternum.

Cystic fibrosis. A genetic disease that causes an abnormal thickness and increased mucous secretions. These secretions build up in the respiratory, gastrointestinal, and other systems of the body. This buildup causes lung infections that can be life threatening, and intestinal digestive disorders.

Emphysema. Enlargement of the alveoli due to lost elasticity, usually brought on by a longtime irritant, such as cigarette smoking. Results in dyspnea, chronic cough, weight loss, and the appearance of a "barrel chest."

Epistaxis. A nosebleed. May be caused by trauma, chronic sinus irritation, drug abuse ("snorting" drugs), hypertension, blood disorders, and high altitude.

Influenza. A viral (various strains) infection of the upper respiratory tract. Sudden onset of chills, fever, cough, sore throat, and gastrointestinal disorders is common. Can range from mild to life threatening.

Laryngitis. Hoarseness, cough, and aphonia caused by infections from nose or throat.

Lung cancer. Cancer that may appear in trachea, air sacs, bronchi, and other lung tissues and cells.

Nasal polyp. A tumor of the nose that can bleed easily. Should be removed surgically.

Pharyngitis. Inflammation of the pharynx caused by bacteria, virus, or an irritant. Difficulty in swallowing, pain, redness, and inflammation of the pharynx are some of the signs and symptoms. *Streptococcus* is the most common bacterial infection; influenza virus and the common cold virus are the most common viral agents involved. May be accompanied by fever, malaise, and headache.

Pleurisy. Inflammation of the pleurae caused by bacteria or viruses. Symptoms include pain, fever, cough, chills, and dyspnea.

Pneumonia. Inflammation of the lungs caused by bacteria, fungi, viruses, and chemical irritants. Usually has sudden onset and is characterized by chills, fever, chest pain, cough, and purulent sputum. Symptoms include sore throat, fever, and lymphadenopathy.

Pneumothorax. The collapse of a lung due to disease or trauma. This results in a collection of air in the space around the lungs. This interferes with the lungs' ability to expand during inspiration.

Pulmonary embolism. A sudden blockage in a lung artery. Usually the blockage is caused by a blood clot that originated in a vessel in a lower extremity. The blockage causes damage to the lung tissue due to a lack of blood flow and oxygen.

Severe acute respiratory syndrome (SARS). An acute viral respiratory illness that begins with fever, headache, body aches, general malaise, and diarrhea. There may be mild respiratory symptoms at the onset. Most patients will develop pneumonia. The virus is spread by close person-to-person contact (i.e., kissing, hugging, sharing eating or drinking utensils, talking to someone within 3 feet [respiratory droplets], and touching someone directly). The patient will be placed on isolation precautions (see Chapter 21).

Sinusitis. Inflammation and infection of a sinus or sinuses. May be caused by allergies, bacteria, viruses, or polyps.

Tonsillitis. Inflammation of the tonsils usually caused by *Streptococcus*. Tonsils become red and enlarged causing severe pharyngitis and fever.

Tuberculosis. Inflammatory infiltrations, formation of tubercles, abscesses, fibrosis, and calcification. Can lead to infection of other body systems. Is highly infectious. Airborne precautions are necessary to prevent transmission of the disease.

SIGNS AND SYMPTOMS OF RESPIRATORY CONDITIONS AND DISORDERS

If a patient's chief complaint indicates a respiratory condition or disorder, medical attention is essential. Some signs and symptoms include:

- *Dyspnea.* Shortness of breath or air hunger
- *Chest pain.* Not only a symptom of cardiac disease
- *Fatigue.* Overall feeling of general tiredness or weakness due to decreased oxygen supply to the tissues
- *Hemoptysis.* Blood present in the sputum
- *Chills and fever.* Related to respiratory infection
- *Hoarseness.* Due to inflammation of the respiratory tract including the larynx
- *Wheezing.* A coarse whistling sound that arises from the lungs due to inflammatory or infectious narrowing of the respiratory passages
- *Cough, productive or nonproductive.* Productive cough results in bringing secretions up from the lower portions of the respiratory tract

Irrigating the nose, collecting sputum specimens, and assisting with pulmonary tests are the roles of the medical assistant.

Diagnostic Tests

A fundamental test, auscultation of the chest, is used to check for abnormalities in breathing rate and quality. Lung function tests can be done. Chest X-ray studies are useful in helping to diagnose tuberculosis (Figure 29-26), lung lesions, pneumonia, and other respiratory conditions.

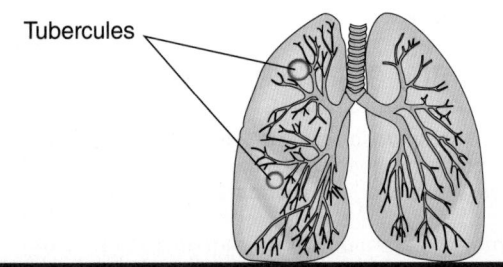

Tubercules

FIGURE 29-26 Tuberculosis.

Cultures of sputum can help diagnose infections in the respiratory tract. Bronchoscopy is used to take a sample of lung tissues (biopsy) for help in the determination of lung cancer and for culture of lung abscesses, washing, and irrigation. CT scanning allows very precise diagnosis of soft tissue disorders. This testing can be especially helpful in diagnosing diseases of the respiratory system.

Arterial blood gases (ABG) measure the amount of oxygen and carbon dioxide in the arterial blood. ABG also evaluate the mechanisms that help the body maintain a homeostatic pH. The quantities of oxygen and carbon dioxide found in the arterial blood indicate how well the process of internal respiration is functioning. This respiratory function requires that the lungs are functioning well to deliver oxygen to the alveoli and allow gas exchange across the capillary membrane, releasing carbon dioxide for exhalation. Higher amounts of carbon dioxide and lower amounts than normal of oxygen indicate poor lung function.

Multiple procedures and interventions relieve symptoms and treat various respiratory diseases. You will find the most common of these therapies in Procedures 29-15 through 29-17, which

---

PROCEDURE 29-15

Procedure

Administering Oxygen by Nasal Cannula for Minor Respiratory Distress

STANDARD PRECAUTIONS:

Handwashing

PURPOSE:

To provide a low dose of concentrated oxygen to a patient during periods of respiratory distress (e.g., chronic obstructive pulmonary disease).

continues

Patient education:

1. Demonstrate the position of the nasal prongs of the cannula into the nose. They face upward and the tab rests above the upper lip.

2. Describe how to clear the oxygen cylinder valve by turning it counterclockwise.

3. Oxygen supports combustion and a fire can start with oxygen in use. Friction, static electricity, a spark, or a lighted cigarette or cigar can cause ignition.

EQUIPMENT/SUPPLIES:

- Portable D cylinder oxygen tank with stand
- Disposable nasal cannula with 6-foot tubing
- Flowmeter with Christmas tree adapter
- Pressure regulator with gauge

PROCEDURE STEPS:

1. ***Paying attention to detail***, assemble supplies needed for the procedure.

2. Wash your hands and follow Standard Precautions.

3. Introduce yourself and confirm the identity of the patient using two identifiers, such as name and date of birth.

4. ***Confirm and explain the procedure to be performed, speaking to the patient's level of understanding.*** Take time to answer the patient's questions. It is important that the patient understand that oxygen is highly flammable and can be ignited by friction, static electricity, a spark, a lighted cigarette, or other smoking device.

5. Open the cylinder with one full turn in a counterclockwise direction.

6. Check the pressure gauge to ensure that oxygen is present in the tank. RATIONALE: This will determine the amount of pressure in the cylinder.

7. Attach the nasal cannula and tubing to the Christmas tree adapter on the flowmeter.

8. Adjust the flow rate according to the provider's order and check the cannula to ensure that oxygen is flowing.

9. Again, check the flow rate against the provider's order.

10. Carefully place the nasal cannula into the nares of the patient, taking the time to explain to the patient that the tips of the cannula should curve inward to follow the curve of the nasal passage (Figure 29-27). The tab should rest below the nose.

11. Check to make sure that the patient is comfortable, adjusting the tubing around the ears and at the chin (Figure 29-28). Make a third and final comparison between the flow rate and that ordered by the provider.

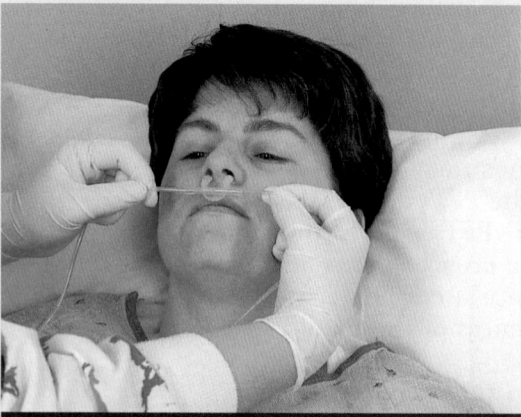

FIGURE 29-27 Insert cannula prongs into nostrils.

continues

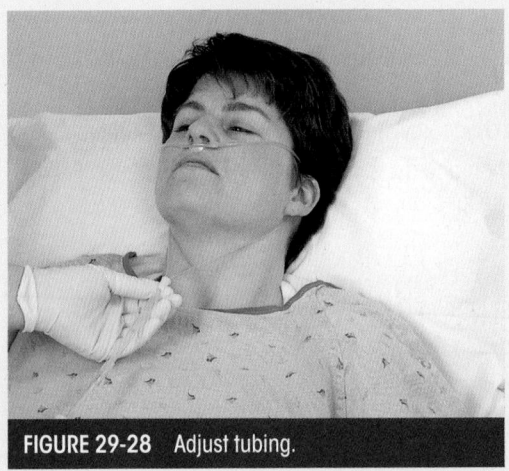

FIGURE 29-28   Adjust tubing.

12. Instruct the patient to continue to breathe deeply and slowly through the nose in order to achieve maximum benefit from the oxygen therapy. Remind the patient again about the dangerous flammability of oxygen.

13. Wash your hands and document the procedure in the patient's medical record, making sure to include the name of the medication (remember oxygen is a medication), the liter flow, route, date, time, and your initials.

DOCUMENTATION:

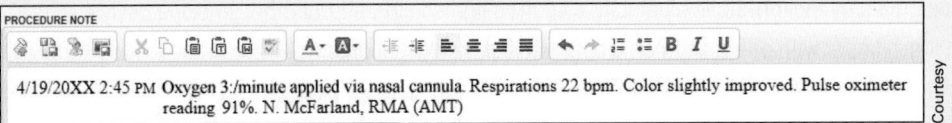

4/19/20XX 2:45 PM Oxygen 3:/minute applied via nasal cannula. Respirations 22 bpm. Color slightly improved. Pulse oximeter reading 91%. N. McFarland, RMA (AMT)

Courtesy of Harris CareTracker PM and EMR

provide detailed descriptions of the role of the medical assistant in common treatments and interventions.

Spirometry

Procedure

The measurements of airflow, lung volume, and lung capacity are known as pulmonary function tests (PFT). PFT measure how well air moves in and out of the lungs and how well the lungs utilize the oxygen delivered. The patient's height, age, and sex are used in interpreting the PFT values. Many times the provider requests the PFT be performed before the administration of a **bronchodilator** and again after the bronchodilator is used. This is useful in evaluating the effectiveness of the medication (see Procedure 29-16).

A commonly used tool in the medical office or clinic, **spirometry** (test to measure lung capacity) assists the provider in the evaluation of signs and symptoms of pulmonary disease by measuring the air capacity (airflow and volume) of the lungs

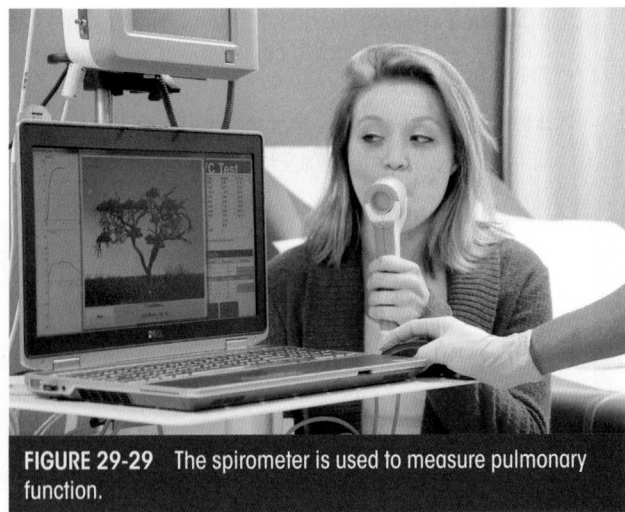

FIGURE 29-29   The spirometer is used to measure pulmonary function.

(Figure 29-29). Many components of lung function are measured, including the following:

1. Expiratory reserve volume (ERV) represents the maximum volume of air that can be exhaled from the lungs after normal expiration.

2. Forced vital capacity (FVC) represents the volume of air that can be forcibly exhaled from the lungs after taking the deepest breath possible.

3. Forced expiratory volume (FEV) is the volume of air that can be blown out in 1 second after full inspiration.

4. Forced expiratory flow (FEF) represents the speed of the air exiting the lungs in the middle of forced expiration.

5. Mean expiratory flow (MEF) is the measurement in liters per second of the peak of expiratory flow.

6. Tidal volume (VT) reflects the volume of air during either inspiration or exhalation during a single breath while resting.

7. Total lung capacity (TLC) is the maximum volume of air present in the lungs.

8. Maximum voluntary ventilation (MVV) is a good indicator of the health and strength of the respiratory muscles, the ability of the thorax to expand to allow lung movement, and airway resistance. This number is obtained by having the patient breathe in and out as fast as possible for 15 seconds. The result is reported in liters per second or per minute.

9. Residual volume (RV) measures the volume of air in the lungs after the patient has exhaled all the air possible.

10. Total lung capacity (TLC) is the amount of air that the lungs can hold. It is about 6 L in humans.

PROCEDURE 29-16

Procedure

Instructing Patient in the Use of a Metered Dose Inhaler with and without a Spacer

STANDARD PRECAUTIONS:

Handwashing

PURPOSE:

To instruct patient on the use of a handheld device known as a metered dose inhaler. The device delivers medication to the respiratory tract including the lungs. It is used to treat asthma, COPD, and other respiratory diseases and conditions.

Patient education:

1. Remind the patient to inhale slowly.
2. Tell him or her to place the mouth and lips around the mouthpiece.
3. The inhaler should be cleaned by rinsing the mouthpiece in warm water.
4. The prescribed dose should be adhered to.

EQUIPMENT/SUPPLIES:

- Handheld inhaler with mouthpiece
- Spacer
- Medication as ordered by practitioner

PROCEDURE STEPS:

1. *Paying attention to detail*, assemble supplies needed for the procedure (Figure 29-30).
2. Wash your hands and follow Standard Precautions.
3. Introduce yourself and confirm the identity of the patient using two identifiers, such as name and date of birth.

continues

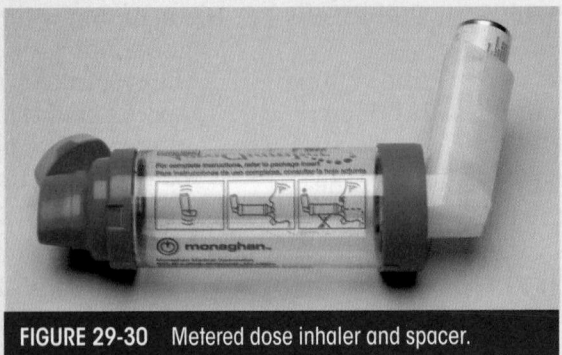

FIGURE 29-30 Metered dose inhaler and spacer.

4. Check the label on the medication against the medication indicated on the provider's order.

5. ***Confirm and explain the rationale for performance of the procedure, speaking to the patient's level of understanding.*** Take time to answer the patient's questions.

6. Again, check the medication against what the provider has ordered.

7. Take some time to educate the patient about the purpose of the medication and the purpose of the metered dose inhaler, otherwise known as an MDI. Explain to the patient in what manner this medication will help to manage his or her diagnosis, and explain the steps of the procedure. Make sure the patient is aware of the dose and frequency of the medication.

8. At this time, make a third check to ensure the medication and the provider's orders match.

9. If the patient is to use a spacer, show the patient how to remove the cap on the MDI and how to insert it into the appropriate end of the spacer.

10. Whether or not the patient is to use the spacer, the procedure will continue identically. Instruct the patient to shake the inhaler to mobilize the medication.

11. The patient should then exhale completely before inserting the mouthpiece between the teeth and closing the lips to create a tight seal.

12. Instruct the patient to inhale slowly while simultaneously pressing on the top of the inhaler to release the medication.

13. The patient should then remove the inhaler from the mouth, but should continue holding the breath for at least 10 seconds to allow the medication to enter the lungs.

14. If a second dose is required, the patient should wait at least 30 seconds before shaking the inhaler and repeating the procedure. The patient should be advised to never take more than the prescribed dose.

15. Advise the patient to rinse out his or her mouth, particularly if the medication is steroid based. Note any changes in condition or comments that the patient makes after the medication has been administered. RATIONALE: Rinsing prevents dry mouth, hoarseness, and microorganism growth.

16. Educate the patient that the medication canister should be stored at room temperature, and should not be exposed to water. The patient should also be made aware of the importance of removing the metal canister from the mouthpiece and, if applicable, the spacer. The mouthpiece and spacer should be washed with mild soap and water, and allowed to air dry nightly, or they should be washed in a dishwasher.

17. Before releasing the patient from your care, ensure that he or she knows how to reassemble the MDI and how to reload the medication into the MDI by spraying a puff into the air before using.

18. Document the procedure in the patient's chart along with any education that was provided.

DOCUMENTATION:

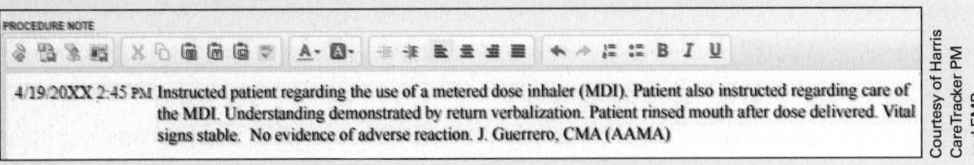

4/19/20XX 2:45 PM Instructed patient regarding the use of a metered dose inhaler (MDI). Patient also instructed regarding care of the MDI. Understanding demonstrated by return verbalization. Patient rinsed mouth after dose delivered. Vital signs stable. No evidence of adverse reaction. J. Guerrero, CMA (AAMA)

PROCEDURE 29-17

Procedure

Performing Spirometry Testing

STANDARD PRECAUTIONS:

Handwashing

Gloves

Biohazard

PURPOSE:

To prepare a patient for a spirometry to obtain optimum test results. To assist with diagnosis of asthma and chronic obstructive pulmonary disease (COPD).

Patient education:

1. Reinforce the importance of good posture during the process. RATIONALE: Good posture allows lungs to expand more fully.
2. Tell the patient that when blowing into the mouthpiece, the lips must seal tightly around it.
3. Explain the parameters needed for successful completion of the test.

Parameters:

1. Patient must refrain from the use of bronchodilators and tobacco for 24 hours before test.
2. Explain to the patient that maximum effort is required for accurate test results.
3. Patient must inhale deeply and quickly and exhale quickly and forcibly until no air can be expelled.

EQUIPMENT/SUPPLIES:

- Spirometer
- Disposable mouthpiece
- Biohazard container
- Sanitizing wipes

PROCEDURE STEPS:

1. ***Paying attention to detail***, assemble supplies needed for the procedure.
2. Wash your hands and follow Standard Precautions.
3. Introduce yourself and confirm the identity of the patient using two identifiers, such as name and date of birth.
4. ***Confirm and explain the rationale for the procedure to be performed***, *speaking to the patient's level of understanding.* Take time to answer the patient's questions.
5. The provider will have given the patient instructions for preparing for the spirometry test. Confirm that the patient has avoided the use of tobacco products and bronchodilators for 24 hours before the test. The patient should also not have eaten a large meal prior to arriving.
6. There are a variety of spirometers available for use, so be sure to follow manufacturer's guidelines for specifics regarding input of the patient's demographic data.
7. Place the disposable mouthpiece on the spirometer and place a nose clip on the patient's nose to ensure that all exhalation occurs through the oral airway.

continues

8. Inform the patient that several readings may be needed to achieve accurate test results and allow the patient to practice several times to become familiar with the machine. Remind the patient that it is important to maintain a tight seal around the mouthpiece and to use maximum effort to inhale completely and rapidly and then to exhale quickly and forcefully.

9. As the patient performs the test, coach him or her to inhale and exhale effectively to achieve maximum results for the provider's interpretation. Remind the patient to remain upright during the test and to continue exhaling until told to stop. Be encouraging. RATIONALE: Helps patient take as large an inhalation and exhalation as possible, which provides more accurate results.

10. The patient may become lightheaded, and if so, he or she should be instructed to sit down and rest between testing. At least three technically acceptable exhalations must be obtained.

11. At the conclusion of the procedure, remove the disposable mouthpiece and discard. Disinfect and sanitize the equipment per office policy, including removing the nose clip from the patient and cleansing appropriately.

12. Update the provider with the test results and document the procedure in the patient's medical record. Make sure to include the patient's response to the procedure as well as any education that you have provided.

DOCUMENTATION:

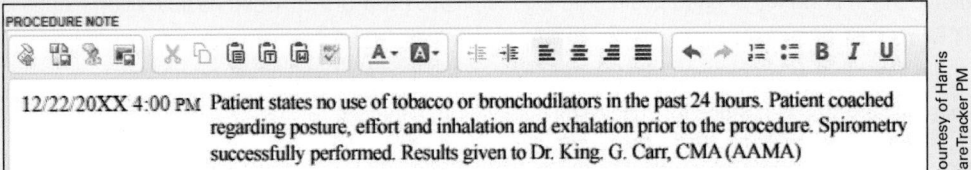

12/22/20XX 4:00 PM Patient states no use of tobacco or bronchodilators in the past 24 hours. Patient coached regarding posture, effort and inhalation and exhalation prior to the procedure. Spirometry successfully performed. Results given to Dr. King. G. Carr, CMA (AAMA)

Courtesy of Harris CareTracker PM and EMR

Most spirometers are computerized, and thus automatically calculate the lung functions. Results are stored in the electronic health record and are readily accessible for comparison. This information is vital to determining the health of a patient's respiratory system.

Peak Expiratory Flow Rates

Peak expiratory flow rates (PEFR) are measured using a peak flow meter (Figure 29-31). This is a fairly "low-tech" device as compared to a computerized spirometer that is utilized for PFT. A patient could utilize this tool at home to monitor asthma or other respiratory disorders. PEFR measures the amount of air that can be pushed from the lungs. Utilizing a peak flow meter can indicate a worsening of conditions, such as asthma, even before symptoms are noticeable. This allows early intervention to prevent serious episodes of illness.

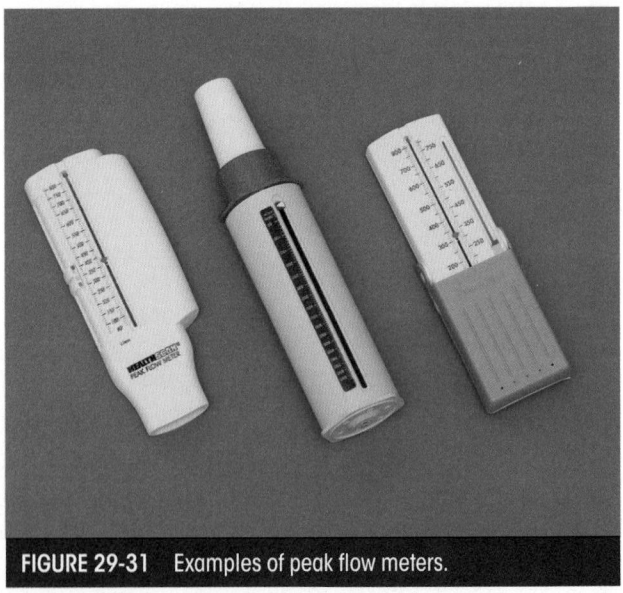

FIGURE 29-31 Examples of peak flow meters.

Pulse Oximetry

Pulse **oximetry** is a test that uses a small probe with an infrared light. The probe is placed on the earlobe, toe, finger, or bridge of the nose. It evaluates the amount of oxygen saturation in the blood. This test is helpful because cyanosis is not manifested until the saturation of oxygen is less than 85%. Pulse oximetry is useful in the diagnosis and evaluation of impaired respiratory and cardiac functions. A reading less than 95% indicates hypoxemia. It is not unusual for a patient being tested for sleep apnea to experience a pulse oximetry reading of under 75%.

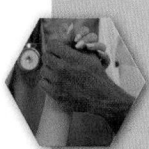

Patient Education

Instruct Patient on Use of Peak Flow Meter

1. Slide the indicator to the bottom of the scale (may be done by the medical assistant).

2. Sit up straight or stand.

3. Hold the peak flow meter upright.

4. Inhale as deeply as you possibly can.

5. Form a tight seal around the mouthpiece with your lips.

6. Blow out as quickly and as hard as you can to exhale all of the air out of your lungs.

7. The force of your exhalation will cause the indicator to rise in the meter.

8. The medical assistant will have you use the peak flow meter twice more and will record the highest number.

NOTE: For accurate results, it is very important to inhale and exhale as completely as possible.

Procedure

The pulse oximeter sensor is placed on the fingertip or earlobe most commonly. One side of the sensor is an infrared light, and the other side is a photo detector. The infrared light passes through the tissues and blood vessels, and the detector measures the amount of light absorbed by hemoglobulin. This noninvasive procedure measures the amount of hemoglobin and can be performed on any patient, but is especially useful in those with impaired heart and lung function. Postoperative patients are attached to an oxygen pulse oximeter in the recovery room. The patient is likely to have shallow, less effective respirations because of the anesthesia or narcotics. The patient must not be wearing nail polish (see Procedure 29-18 and Figure 29-32).

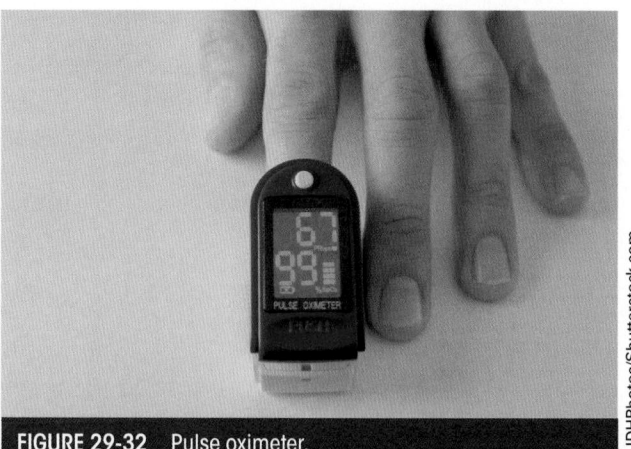

FIGURE 29-32 Pulse oximeter.

© JDHPhotos/Shutterstock.com

INHALERS

Inhalers are devices that are used to deliver medication into the lungs and are most often used to treat asthma. A number of different types of inhalers are available: **metered dose inhaler (MDI)**, metered dose inhaler with spacer (MDIS), dry powder inhaler (DPI), and nebulizer.

The MDIS is the preferred method. A tube that attaches to the inhaler and holds the medication until the patient can breathe it in is called the *spacer.* It makes the MDI easier to use and helps get the medication into the lungs better. A mask can be attached to the spacer for children or for an individual who has difficulty inhaling correctly with a conventional spacer. However, an MDI can be used without a spacer.

Some medications for asthma are in the form of a powder and can be taken with a handheld device known as a DPI. This device delivers medication to the lungs when the patient inhales through the device. However, some patients cannot inhale through the device with sufficient force to breathe in the medication well.

A **nebulizer** (see Figure 29-33) is an apparatus that changes the medication for asthma from a liquid form into a mist for ease of inhaling the medication into the lungs. Nebulizers work well for infants and young children and for any person who is unable to use an MDIS. The different types of nebulizers all work in essentially the same way. The nebulizer hose is connected to an air compressor. The medicine cup is filled with the appropriate dose of liquid along with saline. For a

PROCEDURE 29-18

Procedure

Pulse Oximetry

STANDARD PRECAUTIONS:

Handwashing

PURPOSE:

To measure arterial oxyhemoglobin saturation within seconds by using an external sensor.

EQUIPMENT/SUPPLIES:

- Pulse oximeter
- Sensor
- Soap and water or alcohol wipe
- Nail polish remover, if needed

PROCEDURE STEPS:

1. ***Paying attention to detail***, assemble supplies needed for the procedure.
2. Wash your hands and follow Standard Precautions.
3. Introduce yourself and confirm the identity of the patient using two identifiers, such as name and date of birth.
4. ***Confirm and explain the rationale for performance of the procedure, speaking to the patient's level of understanding.*** Take time to answer the patient's questions.
5. Select a site for the sensor. While the finger is the generally chosen site, other sensors are available for the forehead, the earlobe, or for infants, the toe. Alternate sites are particularly helpful if the fingers have decreased circulation.
6. To ensure that the site is clean, have the patient wash his or her hands with soap and warm water. The patient should also remove any fingernail polish if necessary. If a site other than a finger is to be used, clean the chosen area with an alcohol wipe before continuing. RATIONALE: Fingernail polish inhibits infrared light from passing through the oximeter.
7. There are many different brands of pulse oximeters. Refer to the manufacturer's instructions before operating. If required, secure the sensor to the cable and ensure that there is a tight connection between the cable and the pulse oximeter.
8. Insert the finger into the sensor. If an alternate site is to be used, apply the sensor in a manner appropriate for that site.
9. Turn the pulse oximeter on. You will see a pulse fluctuation on the digital readout.
10. Palpate the patient's pulse and compare it to the digital representation of the pulse to ensure an accurate reading. If trouble-shooting is required, refer to the manufacturer's information.
11. When the test is complete, update the provider with the results before documenting the procedure in the patient's medical record. Note the type of sensor used, the site of application, and the results.
12. Before putting the pulse oximeter away, check the battery life indicator. Change the batteries as needed or plug the oximeter in for recharging. Clean the unit when finished.

DOCUMENTATION:

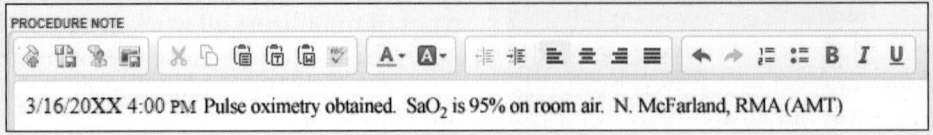

3/16/20XX 4:00 PM Pulse oximetry obtained. SaO_2 is 95% on room air. N. McFarland, RMA (AMT)

Courtesy of Harris CareTracker PM and EMR

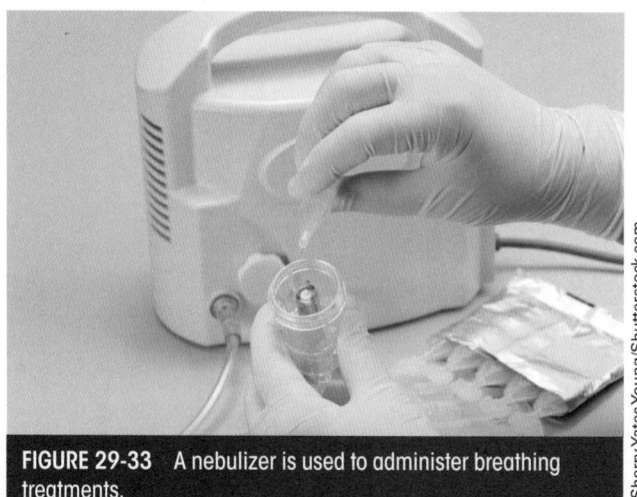

FIGURE 29-33 A nebulizer is used to administer breathing treatments.

© SherryYatesYoung/Shutterstock.com

single dose, the contents of the vial are squeezed into the medicine cup. The hose and mouthpiece are attached to the medicine cup. The patient puts the mouthpiece into the mouth and exhales, and then breathes through the mouth until all the medication is used, about 10 to 15 minutes. Alternatively, the nebulizer can be used with a mask. The mask must fit well to prevent medication from getting in the eyes. The medicine cup and mouthpiece are washed with water and allowed to air dry.

CIRCULATORY SYSTEM

The circulatory system is composed of the heart and a complex network of blood vessels. Their function is to pump and transport the blood to all parts of the body, thus supplying oxygen and removing waste products from body tissues. Table 29-10 lists circulatory system disorders and diagnostic procedures. Table 29-11 describes disorders of the circulatory system.

The variety of diagnostic procedures used to determine the patient's diagnosis is necessary because of the complexity of the cardiovascular system. The medical assistant assists with and performs some of the procedures used for clinical diagnosis. Electrocardiography (ECG) is explained in Chapter 36.

BLOOD AND LYMPH SYSTEM

The blood and lymph are excellent indicators of many underlying diseases. As blood circulates through body tissues and organs, it deposits nutrients and removes wastes. Failure to accomplish

this leaves the body in a disease state. Blood cells include erythrocytes, leukocytes, and platelets, and each has its own function. Studying the results of laboratory findings assists the provider in making a diagnosis.

Lymph is important because of its filtering properties. The body's immune system relies heavily on the fact that the lymph passes through the lymph glands and bacteria and other substances are filtered out. Table 29-12 describes diseases and disorders and the diagnostic procedures for the blood and lymphatic system; Table 29-13 describes certain blood and lymph system disorders.

Common laboratory and diagnostic procedures requested by the provider include some of the following:

- *Chemistry profile.* This test provides information on the functioning of several organ systems and can be an early diagnostic tool for many chronic illnesses such as diabetes, and kidney and liver disorders.

- *Coagulation studies.* Prothrombin time (PT), partial thromboplastin time (PTT), and international normalization ratio (INR) are all common lab tests that reflect the clotting time of blood.

- *Complete blood count (CBC).* This routine test includes a hemoglobin, hematocrit, and red and white blood cell count.

- *Differential.* The differential blood count distinguishes among the various types of white blood cells.

- *Erythrocyte sedimentation rate (ESR)* (sedimentation rate). This test is performed to time the speed of red blood cells settling to the bottom of a test tube.

- *Platelet count.* This test counts the number of platelets in a blood specimen.

- *Lipid profile.* High-density and low-density lipoproteins are measured as well as triglycerides to determine the risk for vascular disease. The lipid profile is a good measure of risk factors that are predictors of coronary heart disease.

- *Liver function studies.* These tests measure coagulation factors, prothrombin, and fibrinogen necessary for blood coagulation.

- *Thyroid profile.* This measure of thyroid hormones circulating in the bloodstream accurately reflects the function of the thyroid gland.

TABLE 29-10

CIRCULATORY SYSTEM DISORDERS

| DISEASE/DISORDER | LABORATORY/DIAGNOSTIC TESTS | | | SURGERY | MEDICAL TESTS OR PROCEDURES | TREATMENT |
	BLOOD TESTING	OTHER TESTING	RADIOGRAPHY			
Abdominal aortic aneurysm (Figure 29-34)			Abdominal radiography Abdominal ultrasound CT of abdomen Magnetic resonance angiography (MRA) MRI of abdomen	Abdominal Aortic Aneurysm repair Endovascular repair	Patient history Physical exam Abdominal ultrasound	This is an emergency, life-threatening condition
Angina pectoris	Cardiac enzymes		Chest radiograph (CXR) Cardiac CT scan Echocardiogram	Coronary artery bypass	Patient history Physical exam ECG Nuclear stress test Cardiac catheterization Balloon angioplasty Angiography with stent placement	Nitrate medications Aspirin Clot preventing medications (Plavix) Beta blocker medications Statins Antianginal medications (Ranexa [ranolazine]) Patient education on smoking cessation, weight reduction, diabetes management, stress management
Arteriosclerosis	Homocystine Fibrinogen Lipoproteina Lipid profile Creactive protein Glucose Lipid Profile		CT MRI Doppler ultrasound PET scan	Angiography	Patient history Physical exam ECG Stress test Cardiac catheterization Balloon angioplasty Stent placement	Cardiology management Lifestyle changes Risk factor management Percutaneous angioplasty

Condition	Laboratory tests	Diagnostic imaging	Procedures	Examinations	Medications / Treatment
Congestive heart failure	Chemistry panel Kidney function Liver function Thyroid function NT-proBNP	CXR Echocardiogram Cardiac computerized tomography (CT) scan Magnetic resonance imaging (MRI)	Myocardial biopsy Removal of part of myocardium Coronary bypass surgery Heart valve replacement Implantable cardioverter-defibrillators Pacemaker Heart transplant	Patient history Physical exam ECG Venous pressure Stress test Coronary angiography	ACE inhibitors Angiotensin II receptor blockers Beta blockers Diuretics Aldosterone antagonists Digoxin Heart transplant Lifestyle changes
Cardiomyopathy	B-type natriuretic peptide (BNP) Chemistry profile Complete blood count Thyroid panel	CXR Echocardiography MRI of heart CT scan	Pacemaker insertion Implantable cardioverter-defibrillator (ICD) insertion Heart transplant Septal myectomy Septal ablation Ventricular assist devices Heart transplant	Patient history Physical exam ECG Cardiac catheterization and biopsy	Beta blockers Digoxin Diuretics
Coronary artery disease	Electrolytes Blood chemistry panel: low-density, high-density lipoprotein, cholesterol, triglycerides High sensitivity C-reactive protein (hsCRP)	Thallium stress test CT of the heart	Coronary artery bypass	Patient history Physical exam ECG Balloon angioplasty Angioplasty with stent placement Cardiac catheterization	Statins Aspirin Beta blockers Nitrate medications ACE inhibitors Patient education on smoking cessation, weight reduction, increasing activity, stress reduction

continues

Table 29-10 continued

| DISEASE/DISORDER | LABORATORY/DIAGNOSTIC TESTS | | | MEDICAL TESTS OR PROCEDURES | TREATMENT |
	BLOOD TESTING	OTHER TESTING	RADIOGRAPHY	SURGERY	
Essential hypertension	Electrolytes Chemistry panel	Urinalysis Kidney function	Chest radiograph		Patient history Physical exam ECG Blood pressure measurement	Diuretics ACE inhibitors Angiotensin II receptor blockers Calcium channel blockers Renin inhibitors Vasodilators Diuretics Patient education on smoking cessation, weight reduction, increasing activity, stress reduction, limiting alcohol intake
Mitral valve stenosis			Transthoracic echocardiogram Ultrasonography Chest radiography Transesophageal echocardiogram	Valvotomy Valve replacement Balloon valvuloplasty	Patient history Physical exam ECG Cardiac catheterization	Diuretics Anticoagulants Beta blockers Calcium channel blockers Antibiotics
Myocardial infarction	Cardiac enzymes Complete blood count		Thallium stress test Echocardiogram CT MRI	Coronary artery bypass Balloon angioplasty Angioplast with stent placement	Patient History Physical Exam ECG Exercise Stress Test	Oxygen Aspirin Antiplatelet agents Thrombolytic Morphine Nitrite medications Beta blockers ACE inhibitors Patient education on smoking cessation, weight reduction, increasing activity, stress reduction, limiting alcohol intake

Pericarditis	Complete blood count Erythrocyte sedimentation rate Cardiac enzymes Bacterial antibodies	Urinalysis Blood culture	Chest radiograph Echocardiogram CT MRI	Pericardiocentesis Pericardiectomy	Patient history Physical exam ECG	Antibiotics Colchicine Steriods
Rheumatic fever	Complete blood count Streptococcalanti-bodies Erythrocyte sedimentation rate (ESR) Cardiac enzymes Kidney function Liver function	Throat culture	Echocardiography		Patient history Physical exam ECG	Antibiotic therapy Anti-inflammatories Anticonvulsants
Thrombophlebitis	Bleeding and clotting time Complete blood count D dimer	Urinalysis	Doppler ultrasonography Angiography Radioactive fibrinogen CT of affected area	Thrombectomy Placement of a vena caval filter Varicose vein stripping		Elevation of affected limb Anticoagulants Thrombolytic agents Support hose
Varicose veins			Venography Doppler ultrasonography	Ligation and stripping Laser surgery	Patient history Physical exam Sclerotherapy	Elastic stockings

TABLE 29-11

DESCRIPTION OF CIRCULATORY SYSTEM DISORDERS

Angina pectoris. Chest pain caused by lack of oxygen to the myocardium. Usual cause is coronary arteriosclerosis.

Aortic aneurysm. A bulge in a section of the wall of the aorta. It becomes weakened, bulging, and overstretched (Figure 29-34). The risk is rupture of this weakened area. The symptoms are abdominal, chest, or back pain. The provider may detect the aneurysm during an abdominal exam. This is an emergency condition that requires immediate intervention.

Congestive heart failure. A syndrome characterized by the heart's inability to pump blood adequately to the body tissues. Characterized by congestion in the lungs, or edema of lower extremities, dyspnea on exertion, cough, and related edema.

Coronary artery disease. Arteriosclerosis of the coronary arteries leading to impaired blood flow to the myocardium. Complete occlusion leads to myocardial infarction. May also be caused by thrombus in a coronary artery. Angina pectoris is the name of the chest pain caused by lack of oxygen to the myocardium.

Essential hypertension. Consistently high blood pressure of unknown cause.

Mitral valve stenosis. Narrowing of mitral valve obstructing flow from atrium to ventricle. Usual cause is a rheumatic heart disease as a result of a streptococcal infection (throat or scarlet fever). Thrombi can form. Atrial fibrillation is possible.

Myocardial infarction. Death of myocardial tissue caused by anoxia to the myocardium. Symptoms include dyspnea, chest pain, nausea, vomiting, and diaphoresis.

Pericarditis. Inflammation of the pericardium. Caused by tuberculosis, pyogenic organisms, uremia, and myocardial infarction. Characterized by fever, dry cough, dyspnea, and palpitations.

Rheumatic fever. A systemic disease affecting the heart, joints, and central nervous system after a group A beta-hemolytic streptococcal infection. May occur without symptoms. Symptoms include fever, migratory joint pain, pericarditis, and heart murmur.

Thrombophlebitis. An inflammation of a vein with thrombus formation, may be caused by trauma. Symptoms include pain and swelling in affected vein.

Varicose veins. Enlarged, twisted, and engorged veins, commonly occurring in the saphenous veins but may occur in any vein in the body. Caused by conditions that hamper venous return, such as pregnancy, standing for long periods of time, and obesity. Symptoms include pain in feet and ankles, swelling, and leg ulcers.

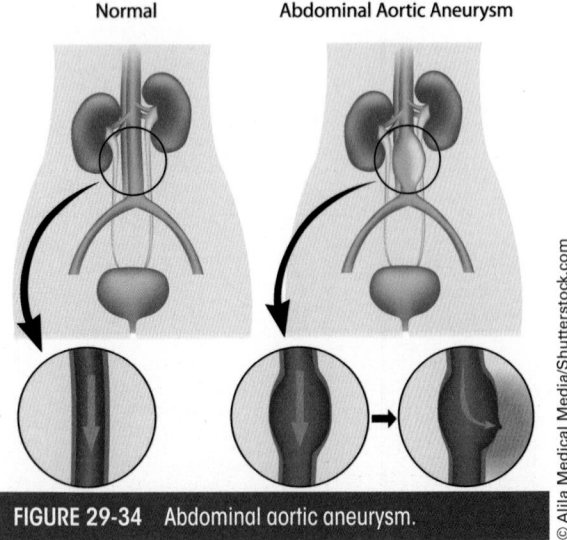

Normal   Abdominal Aortic Aneurysm

© Alila Medical Media/Shutterstock.com

FIGURE 29-34 Abdominal aortic aneurysm.

Procedures to collect blood specimens and venipuncture are explained in Chapter 39; hematology is discussed in Chapter 40.

MUSCULOSKELETAL SYSTEM

The muscular and skeletal systems interact to coordinate the supporting framework and movements of the body. The musculoskeletal system includes bones, joints, muscles, and surrounding tissue. The skeletal system provides support; protects vital organs; and allows for the attachment of ligaments, tendons, and muscles. The muscular system gives the body form and shape and is responsible for the coordination of movement.

Bones of the skeletal system store minerals for later use by the body. They are classified according

TABLE 29-12

BLOOD AND LYMPH SYSTEM DISORDERS

| DISEASE/DISORDER | LABORATORY/DIAGNOSTIC TESTS | | | MEDICAL TESTS OR PROCEDURES | TREATMENT |
	BLOOD TESTING	OTHER TESTING	RADIOGRAPHY	SURGERY	
Anemias	Ferritin Serum iron Complete blood count Red blood cell count Serum vitamin B$_{12}$	Gastric analysis	Ferrokinetic studies Radioactive vitamin B$_{12}$		Patient history Physical exam Bone marrow	Depends on cause Increase dietary intake of iron or folic acid Vitamin B$_{12}$ injections
Hemophilia	Complete blood count				Patient history Physical exam	Infusion of hormones or clotting factors based on the type of hemophilia Antifibrinolytics Fibrin sealants Physical therapy Patient education on avoidance of aspirin and ibuprofen, good dental hygiene, safety
Hodgkin disease	Complete blood count Liver function tests		Chest radiograph Lymphangiography Positron emission tomography (PET) scan	Lymph node biopsy Bone marrow biopsy	Patient history Physical exam Stem cell transplant	Radiation Chemotherapy
Infectious mononucleosis	Complete blood count Monoscreen Heterophile antibody Epstein-Barr virus Liver function tests				Patient history Physical exam	Analgesics Corticosteroids Comfort measures such as rest; increased fluids; and gargling with warm salty water

continues

Table 29-12 continued

DISEASE/DISORDER	LABORATORY/DIAGNOSTIC TESTS				SURGERY	MEDICAL TESTS OR PROCEDURES	TREATMENT
	BLOOD TESTING	OTHER TESTING	RADIOGRAPHY				
Leukemia	Complete blood count Liver function tests Platelet count Bleeding time				Bone marrow biopsy	Patient history Physical exam Bone marrow transplant Stem cell transplant	Chemotherapy Bone marrow transplant Targeted therapy Biological therapy Radiation therapy
Lymphedema			Lymphangiography MRI CT Doppler ultrasound			Patient history Physical exam	Antibiotics Surgery Lymphedema therapy Exercise Massage Complete decongestive therapy
Non-Hodgkin lymphoma	Complete blood count		CT MRI PET scan		Lymph node biopsy Bone marrow biopsy	Patient history Physical exam Bone marrow biopsy Lumbar puncture	Chemotherapy Radiation Radioimmunotherapy Stem cell therapy Biological therapy

TABLE 29-13

DESCRIPTION OF BLOOD AND LYMPH SYSTEM DISORDERS

Anemias. All anemias are manifested by a reduction in circulating red blood cells and the amount of hemoglobin, which is the volume of packed red blood cells per 100 mL blood. Symptoms include pallor of the skin, nailbeds, and mucous membranes; weakness; vertigo; headache; drowsiness; and general malaise.

- *Iron deficiency.* Lack of reserve iron in the body and in red blood cells that lack hemoglobin resulting from inadequate dietary intake of iron, iron **malabsorption** (poor absorption of nutrients), blood loss, or pregnancy.
- *Pernicious anemia.* Lack of intrinsic factor in the stomach secretions (hydrochloric acid). Vitamin B_{12} cannot be absorbed. Red blood cells cannot develop properly.
- *Sickle cell anemia.* A hereditary chronic anemia characterized by abnormal red blood cells causing lysis of the cells and the formation of clumps in the blood vessels, impairing circulation. Not curable.

Hodgkin disease. An idiopathic malignancy of the lymphatic system causing enlargement of lymphatic tissue, spleen, and liver. Symptoms include fever and night sweats. Often curable.

Leukemia. Overproduction of abnormal and immature white blood cells. Cause is unknown. Symptoms include anemia, fatigue, fever, and joint pain.

Lymphedema. Abnormal accumulation of lymph in the extremities caused by obstruction of the lymphatics. Symptoms include edema in arms or legs.

Non-Hodgkin lymphoma. A cancer of the immune system, specifically the lymphocytes.

to their shape. Bones provide for the attachment of muscles and joining of another bone, which allows for the passage of nerves and blood vessels. The skeletal system is divided into two parts: the **appendicular skeleton** (126 bones) and the **axial skeleton** (80 bones).

One of the top four reasons a patient visits a provider is back pain. During the visit, the provider evaluates the patient for contributory factors for the pain by assessing the patient for deformities, asymmetry, and signs of restricted motion. The provider performs a functional assessment by observing the patient's gait (manner of walking) for indications of decreased mobility and postural changes associated with aging or injury. Flexion tests with a goniometer (Figure 29-35) detect the degree of resistance applied to a given force, thus defining restricted motion and the amount of discomfort associated with movement. Supine straight-leg raising (SLR) tests detect the amount of hamstring flexibility and strength and can assess sciatic nerve damage.

There are more than 600 muscles in the body. Muscles are composed of bundles of muscle fibers, each with the ability to contract and relax. Any disease process that disrupts the balance between the muscular and skeletal systems severely hampers a

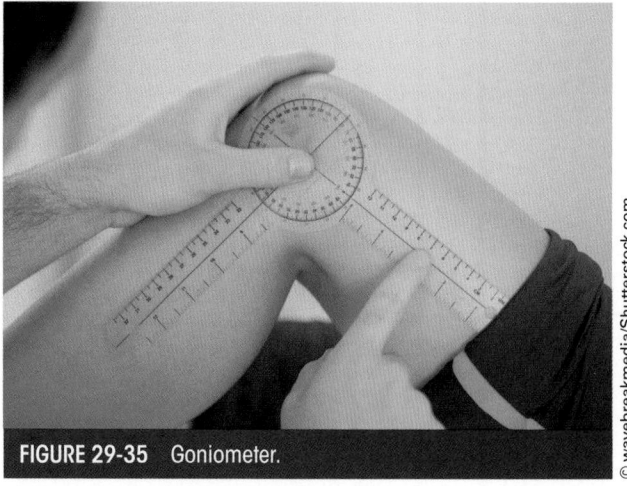

FIGURE 29-35 Goniometer.

© wavebreakmedia/Shutterstock.com

person's ability to move effectively and painlessly (Tables 29-14, 29-15, and 29-16).

Diagnostic procedures involving the skeletal system involve the extensive use of various forms of radiographs and visual examination techniques. A bone biopsy may be ordered when additional diagnostic data are required.

Muscular system diseases and disorders can be treated by electromyostimulation (EMS). Electrical

TABLE 29-14

MUSCULOSKELETAL SYSTEM DISORDERS

DISEASE/DISORDER	LABORATORY/DIAGNOSTIC TESTS					MEDICAL TESTS OR PROCEDURES	TREATMENT
	BLOOD TESTING	OTHER TESTING	RADIOGRAPHY	SURGERY			
Avascular necrosis			Magnetic resonance imaging (MRI) Radiograph Bone scan Computed tomography (CT)	Bone biopsy		Patient history Physical exam Measurement of intraosseous pressure	Analgesics Corticocorticosteroids Physical therapy Limited weight bearing Bone grafting Osteotomy Joint replacement Electrical stimulation
Bone cancer • Multiple myeloma • Osteosarcoma • Ewing sarcoma • Chondrosarcoma	Complete blood count		Radiograph CT MRI Bone scan PET scan	Needle biopsy Open biopsy		Patient history Physical exam	Surgical resection Amputation Radiation therapy Chemotherapy
Carpal tunnel syndrome	Erythrocyte sedimentation rate Uric acid Complete blood count		Wrist radiograph	Surgical repair		Patient history Physical exam EMG Nerve conduction study	Cortisone injection Physical therapy Anti-inflammatory drugs Splinting Surgery
Dislocation			Radiograph of affected joint MRI	Reduction		Patient history Physical exam	Reduction with anesthesia if necessary Surgical tightening of ligaments Immobilization Physical therapy

Condition	Laboratory Tests	Fluid Analysis / Other	Imaging	Surgical Procedures	Examination	Treatment
Gout	Uric acid Complete blood count Erythrocyte sedimentation rate	Synovial fluid analysis Urinalysis	Skeletal radiographs Ultrasound Dual energy CT scan		Patient history Physical exam	Bed rest when severe Ice to affected joint(s) Anti-inflammatory agents Analgesics Corticosteroids Antigout drugs
Herniated disk			Myelogram CT MRI	Surgical incision and release Surgical excision and spinal fusion	Patient history Physical exam EMG Epidural injection(s) of corticosteroids	Muscle relaxants Antinerve pain medications Analgesics Brace for affected disk area
Myasthenia gravis	Acetylcholine receptor antibodies	Detailed history and neurologic examination	CT MRI	Surgical excision of the thymus gland	Patient history Physical exam EMG Edrophonium test Repetitive nerve stimulation Ice pack test Pulmonary function test	Neostigmine Prednisone Immunosuppressants Plasmapheresis Intravenous immunoglobulin Monoclonal antibodies
Osteoarthritis	Complete blood count Sedimentation rate	Joint fluid analysis	Skeletal radiographs including vertebrae CT scan MRI	Surgery to replace knee, hip, or shoulder	Patient history Physical exam	Physical therapy Anti-inflammatory drugs Analgesics Muscle relaxants Corticosteroid injection into affected joint

continues

Table 29-14 continued

DISEASE/DISORDER	BLOOD TESTING	OTHER TESTING	RADIOGRAPHY	SURGERY	MEDICAL TESTS OR PROCEDURES	TREATMENT
Osteoporosis	Serum calcium Alkaline phosphatase Estrogen level Total protein Creatinine	Urine calcium Urine creatinine	Bone scan	Bone biopsy	Patient history Physical exam	Calcium supplements Vitamin D supplements and sunshine Osteoporosis medications (Boniva, Fosamax, Actonel) Hormonal therapy Weight-bearing exercises Patient education on smoking cessation, limiting alcohol intake, and fall prevention
Rheumatoid arthritis	Rheumatoid factor Antinuclear anti-body test Lupus erythematosus test Erythrocyte sedimentation rate Complete blood count C-reactive protein	Synovial fluid analysis	Skeletal radiographs MRI	Replacement of joint with artificial joint Synovectomy Joint fusion Tendon repair	Patient history Physical exam	Anti-inflammatory drugs Corticosteroids Immunosuppression drugs Disease-modifying anti-rheumatic drugs Biologic agents Splinting of affected joints Physical therapy
Rickets	Serum phosphorus Vitamin D Creatinine	Urine calcium Urine phosphorus Urine creatinine	Skeletal bone scan	Bone biopsy Surgery to correct deformities	Patient history Physical exam	Vitamin D and calcium supplements Sunlight exposure Bracing of affected extremities
Spinal curvatures • Scoliosis • Lordosis • Kyphosis			Radiographs of spine		Patient history Physical exam	Physical therapy Brace Spinal fusion Body cast

TABLE 29-15
MUSCULAR/CONNECTIVE TISSUE DISORDERS

| DISEASE/ DISORDER | LABORATORY/DIAGNOSTIC TESTS | | | | MEDICAL TESTS OR PROCEDURES | TREATMENT |
	BLOOD TESTING	OTHER TESTING	RADIOGRAPHY	SURGERY		
Back pain		Urinalysis	Radiograph of vertebrae CT MRI	Surgery may be necessary	Patient history Physical exam	Treatment depends on diagnosis Analgesics Anti-inflammatory medications Exercise Epidural corticosteroids Electronic stimulation device
Bursitis			MRI X-ray study of affected joint for calcium deposits	Excision of bursa	Patient history Physical exam	Moist heat immobilization Anti-inflammatory medications Local injection of corticosteroids
Fibromyalgia	Rheumatoid arthritis antibody Complete blood count Erythrocyte sedimentation rate Thyroid function tests		Skeletal radiographs		Patient history Physical exam Electromyography (EMG)	Anti-inflammatory medications may be useful Physical therapy Medication for sleep disturbances (antidepressants) Counseling Exercise
Strain, sprain			Radiographs of affected body part to rule out fracture	Surgery to tighten affected ligaments	Patient history Physical exam	Cold wet packs to area for 24 hours; follow with warm packs Anti-inflammatory medications Elevate and rest affected part Immobilization or movement of affected part (per provider's recommendation) Physical therapy*
Tendonitis			Arthrogram	Focused aspiration of scar tissue (FAST)	Patient history Physical exam	Moist heat Anti-inflammatory medications Local injection of corticosteroids Platelet-rich plasma therapy Physical therapy*

* Physical therapy should be encouraged from the onset. Patient can prevent further damage. Provide patient education.

TABLE 29-16

DESCRIPTION OF SKELETAL AND MUSCULAR DISORDERS

BONE

Carpal tunnel syndrome. Causes pain and weakness of hand and fingers. May cause paresthesia of hand and fingers. Caused by compression of the median nerve against the carpal bones. Usually results from repetitive tasks (such as using computer keyboard or mouse or rolling hair).

Cleft palate. Congenital disorder caused by nonunion of the maxillary bones. Surgical repair needed to close palate.

Fractures. Break in a bone classified according to angle, usually caused by trauma or disease.

Herniated disk. A rupture of the cushioning mass between two intervertebral disks of the spine most often caused by injury or osteoarthritis. Causes back pain that may radiate into buttock(s) and down leg.

Osteoporosis. Diminished bone mass caused by lack of calcium deposits in the bone, predisposing patients to fracture.

Paget disease. Chronic disease marked by a high rate of bone destruction and irregular bone repair. The new bone fractures easily. Cause unknown but may be hereditary.

Rickets. Abnormal bone softening caused by inadequate utilization of vitamin D, inadequate vitamin D intake, or loss of calcium. One symptom is night fever (known as osteomalacia in adults).

Spinal curvatures. Spinal defects with exaggerated curves caused by diseases of the spine, faulty posture, or congenital malformations.
- Scoliosis. Right or left sideway curvature of the spine
- Lordosis. Inward curvature of the lower spine (swayback)
- Kyphosis. Outward curvature of the upper spine (hunchback)

JOINTS

Dislocation. A bone forcibly displaced from its joint; usually caused by trauma.

Gout. Form of arthritis caused by metabolic disturbances in purine metabolism resulting in uric acid crystal deposits in the joints. Causes periodic attacks of arthritis pain and joint inflammation.

Osteoarthritis. Common, chronic inflammatory process of the joints, with overgrowth of bone and spur formation. Accompanies aging. Causes swollen joints and pain.

Rheumatoid arthritis. More serious and crippling form of arthritis caused by inflammation of the synovial tissues of several joints; may be caused by antigen–antibody reaction. Systemic symptoms include fatigue, body temperature elevation of affected joint, sensory disturbances, pain, and joint deformities.

MUSCLE DISORDERS

Back pain. Localized discomfort usually in the lumbar area caused by stretching or straining of muscles.

Bursitis. Inflammation of the cavity found in connective tissue of a joint that is lined with synovial fluid usually caused by trauma.

Fibromyalgia. Discomfort of muscles, tendons, ligaments, and soft tissues brought on by trauma, strain, and emotional stress.

Spasm. Sudden involuntary muscle contraction; can cause pain.

Sprains. Caused by trauma to a joint with torn ligament if severe.

Strain. Trauma to a muscle from violent contraction.

Tendonitis. Inflammation of tendons and attachments caused by trauma such as strain.

current directly stimulates motor nerves. A low-frequency charge of electricity is given to muscle(s) through electrodes placed on the skin to elicit muscle contraction. The therapy improves muscle strength and is used to help strengthen atrophied muscles caused by surgery or injuries. EMS therapy can reeducate muscles that have become paralyzed. It can be used in sports training to improve muscle strength.

Therapeutic treatment of muscular system injuries caused by trauma is clinically handled by the use of cold and hot therapy and physical therapy including ultrasound therapy. These procedures are discussed in Chapter 32.

Fractures, Casting, and Cast Removal

Closed fractures of the wrist, forearm, fingers, lower legs, or upper arm are often treated in the ambulatory care setting. Table 29-17 lists types of fractures (see Chapter 8).

Types of casting materials used are the plaster cast, synthetic or plastic cast, and air cast. Plaster casts are formed by wetting bandage rolls impregnated with calcium sulfate and molding them to the injured body part. Synthetic casts are formed by using tape embedded with a polyester/cotton combination, fiberglass, or plastic resin. Air casts are a type of inflatable immobilizer and are used for sprains and postcast support. The type of casting material used is dependent on provider preference and the body part to which a cast is being applied. Synthetic casts are lighter, stronger, and more water resistant, but they have less room for swelling.

- *Short arm cast (SAC)*. Extends from the fingers to just below the elbow (fracture or dislocation of wrist and forearm)
- *Long arm cast (LAC)*. Extends from the fingers to the axilla, with a bend at the elbow (fracture of the upper arm)
- *Long and short leg casts*. Extend from the thigh to the toes (LLC) or from below the knee to the toes (SLC) and usually include a walking heel

Procedure
The medical assistant's role in cast application and removal consists of setting up supplies and assisting the provider. Patient teaching of cast care is also a primary function of the medical assistant. Procedures 29-19 and 29-20 outline steps in applying a plaster cast and assisting in cast removal.

DIGESTIVE SYSTEM

The gastrointestinal (GI) system performs the following five functions:

1. Ingestion (taking in) of food and breaking it into smaller particles
2. Passage of food through the digestive system (peristalsis)
3. Digestion of food through secretions of digestive enzymes
4. Absorption of nutrients into the bloodstream
5. Elimination of the solid waste products of digestion (defecation)

TABLE 29-17

TYPES OF FRACTURES

Fractures can be simple, or closed, so called because the bone is broken with no penetration of the skin; or they can be compound, or open, so called because the broken bone has protruded through the skin and there is an open wound in addition to the fracture.

Two of the most common fractures are both simple fractures: Colles fracture and Pott fracture. Colles fracture is a fracture of the lower end of the radius. Pott fracture is a fracture of the lower part of the fibula and the malleolus of the tibia.

Fractures are described by their characteristics:

- *Greenstick.* The bone is bent on one side and fractured on the other.
- *Oblique.* The bone is fractured and runs obliquely to the axis of the bone.
- *Transverse.* The bone is fractured at a right angle to the axis of the bone.
- *Comminuted.* The bone is splintered into fragments.
- *Impacted.* The bone is fractured into fragments and the fragments have been driven into the interior of another bone. See Chapter 8.

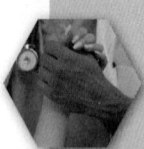

Patient Education

Cast Care Guidelines

The medical assistant should instruct the patient on managing and caring for a cast:

- Allow the casting material to dry by exposing it to the air and keeping it uncovered, even during the night. Applying pressure to the cast before drying can result in tissue damage under the pressure area.

- Elevate the casted extremity to aid in reducing swelling and pain. This allows for a better fitting cast, and thus less discomfort.

- Observe the fingers or toes for changes in color; temperature changes; and decreased sensation, pain, or tingling. This is called nerve and circulation assessment, and changes could indicate the cast is too tight.

- Do not place objects into the cast to scratch irritated skin. A break in the skin will provide a breeding ground for bacteria. Do not use powder or creams.

- Do not get the cast wet. This could lead to malformation of the cast, resulting in misalignment of the extremity and breakdown of the skin. Cover with waterproof covering when bathing. If the cast gets wet, dry it with a hair dryer.

- Cleaning a cast can be accomplished by using a damp cloth.

- When decorating a cast, use only water-soluble paints or marking pens. This allows the cast to breathe, thus preventing tissue damage.

- Do not cut or trim the cast. Use masking tape if there is a sharp edge, or use a nail file to smooth a rough edge.

Notify the provider if any of the following occurs:

1. Elevated temperature.
2. A bad odor coming from the cast may indicate an infection.
3. Numbness, tingling, severe pain, difficulty moving, severe swelling, or cold fingers or toes may indicate that the cast is too tight.
4. A burning sensation over a bony area may indicate that the cast is too tight.
5. If there is bleeding or pink to red discoloration on the cast, there may be bleeding from a wound under the cast.

PROCEDURE 29-19

Procedure

Assisting with Cast Application to Arm Fracture

STANDARD PRECAUTIONS:

Handwashing   Gloves

PURPOSE:

To assist provider in cast application.

continues

EQUIPMENT/SUPPLIES:

Cast material:

- Plaster or fiberglass casting material in the appropriate width
- Container of water with liner
- Stockinette (diameter based on limb to be immobilized)
- Synthetic rolled cast padding or Webril
- Bandage scissors
- Gloves
- Waterproof pad
- Medication per provider's orders

PROCEDURE STEPS:

1. ***Paying attention to detail***, assemble supplies needed for the procedure.
2. Wash your hands and follow Standard Precautions.
3. ***Introduce yourself and confirm the identity of the patient*** using two identifiers, such as name and date of birth.
4. ***Confirm and explain the rationale for the procedure to be performed***, *speaking to the patient's level of understanding.* Take time to answer the patient's questions.
5. If medication has been ordered, administer the medication as ordered by the provider.
6. Assist the patient to remove any clothing that might interfere or to put on a gown if necessary.
7. Use soap and water to cleanse the area to be casted as directed by the provider. If there is an open wound on the area to be casted then gloves should be worn. Follow the provider's orders regarding cleansing and dressing of the open wound.
8. Dry the area thoroughly.
9. Help the patient to assume a comfortable and accessible position.
10. Place a waterproof pad under the extremity to be casted and drape the area of cast application. Note and document neurovascular status, as well as any areas of skin lesions, or soft tissue injuries. RATIONALE: Appropriate documentation of skin conditions is needed to assist in evaluation of the extremity at a later time.
11. Don gloves.
12. Select the appropriate diameter of stockinette for the extremity to be casted. RATIONALE: Appropriate diameter is important as too tight can cause neurovascular impairment and too loose can wrinkle and contribute to skin breakdown.
13. Measure the stockinette to a length long enough to cover the area to be casted and add 2 or 3 inches to each end to allow for the stockinette to be folded back over the casting material. This will provide the patient with a padded edge. Assist the provider to apply stockinette, including creating an opening for the thumb. RATIONALE: A stockinette that is too large will form creases, thus allowing for injuries to tissues.
14. After the provider has determined the correct width of synthetic cast padding, assist by holding the extremities in alignment. RATIONALE: The stockinette and padding is applied to prohibit the development of pressure sores.
15. When directed, immerse the casting material (plaster or fiberglass) in water as instructed by the manufacturer. Gently squeeze the excess water from the material, but do not wring it.
16. Assist the provider as the casting material is applied, reassuring the patient as needed.
17. Once the cast has been applied, support the extremity in a manner that will not distort the molding of the casting material until it has set thoroughly.
18. Note any neurovascular changes that might indicate impairment of circulation.
19. A sling is usually applied, after the casting material has set, to further immobilize the arm and to provide comfort for the patient.

continues

20. Following clinic policy, provide the patient with any written instructions or cast care guidelines and make sure the patient understands what is expected prior to release. Arrange for a follow-up appointment to check the cast and the patient's progress. RATIONALE: Reviewing possible complications with the patient enhances the immediate reporting of circulatory impairment and infection.

21. Discard the liner, container, and other residue into the trash receptacle.

22. Discard the water bath in the sink or hopper being careful not to allow any casting material to enter the drain.

23. Remove and discard gloves and wash your hands.

24. Document the procedure in the patient's medical record. Make sure to include observations regarding the neuro-vascular status of the patient's affected limb both before and after the cast application, as well as the provision of patient education and the scheduled date of follow-up.

DOCUMENTATION:

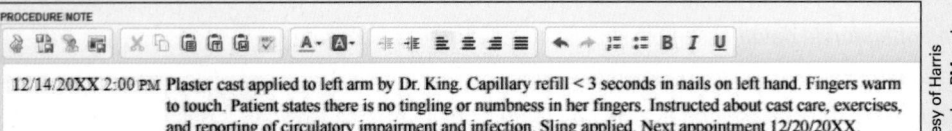

12/14/20XX 2:00 PM Plaster cast applied to left arm by Dr. King. Capillary refill < 3 seconds in nails on left hand. Fingers warm to touch. Patient states there is no tingling or numbness in her fingers. Instructed about cast care, exercises, and reporting of circulatory impairment and infection. Sling applied. Next appointment 12/20/20XX.
G. Carr, CMA (AAMA)

Courtesy of Harris CareTracker PM and EMR

PROCEDURE 29-20

Assisting with Cast Removal

Procedure

STANDARD PRECAUTIONS:

Handwashing

PURPOSE:

To assist the provider with removal of a cast.

EQUIPMENT/SUPPLIES:

- Cast cutter
- Cast spreader
- Bandage scissors
- Bag for disposing of cast materials
- Drape

PROCEDURE STEPS:

1. *Paying attention to detail*, assemble supplies needed for the procedure.

2. Wash your hands and follow Standard Precautions.

continues

3. Introduce yourself and confirm the identity of the patient using two identifiers, such as name and date of birth.

4. ***Confirm and explain the rationale for the procedure to be performed, speaking to the patient's level of understanding.*** Take time to answer the patient's questions. RATIONALE: Explaining the procedure reduces apprehension and fears about being cut with the blade.

5. Drape the area of cast removal, taking care to protect the patient's clothing.

6. ***Allay the patient's fears and help him or her feel safe and comfortable.*** Explain that the cast cutter will not damage soft tissue as it vibrates; it does not spin.

7. Explain that there might be a sensation of warmth and some pressure during the cutting of the cast.

8. Once the cast has been removed, cleanse the area under the cast of excess skin and dry completely. Apply lotion to moisturize the skin.

9. Reassure the patient that the muscle tone will return with physical activity.

10. Remove and discard gloves and wash your hands.

11. Document the procedure in the patient's medical record. Make sure to document patient education regarding post–cast removal care. Provide the patient with written instructions per office policy. Also, document the post–cast removal neurologic status, skin integrity, and bony assessment per the provider's preference. RATIONALE: Condition of the patient's extremity size, skin appearance, and color are important factors to note for further evaluation.

DOCUMENTATION:

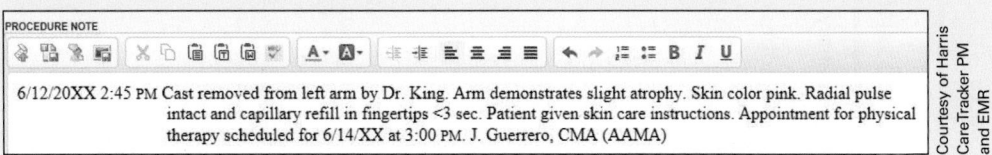

PROCEDURE NOTE

6/12/20XX 2:45 PM Cast removed from left arm by Dr. King. Arm demonstrates slight atrophy. Skin color pink. Radial pulse intact and capillary refill in fingertips <3 sec. Patient given skin care instructions. Appointment for physical therapy scheduled for 6/14/XX at 3:00 PM. J. Guerrero, CMA (AAMA)

Courtesy of Harris CareTracker PM and EMR

When any of these functions is hindered, the digestive system is considered to be malfunctioning.

The digestive process begins in the mouth and concludes at the anus. As food passes through the alimentary canal (also called the gastrointestinal tract or digestive tract), it is mixed with gastric juices and enzymes, allowing it to break down into smaller nutrients, which allows absorption through the walls of the small intestine. Peristalsis, or wave-like muscular contractions, moves the food and fluid mixture through the intestines. This movement creates gurgling, tinkling, or rumbling sounds that are referred to as bowel sounds. These should be present on auscultation in all four quadrants of the abdomen. Proper movement of intestinal contents creates a soft abdomen. If there are any abnormalities within the intestines, the consistency of the abdomen changes. It can be bloated, distended, or rigid. The provider will use palpation to assess the abdomen during a physical exam. Contents that have not been absorbed travel through the large intestine and are excreted through the anus. Tables 29-18 and 29-19 list common tests, procedures, disorders, and conditions of the digestive system. Figure 29-36 shows the major organs of the digestive system.

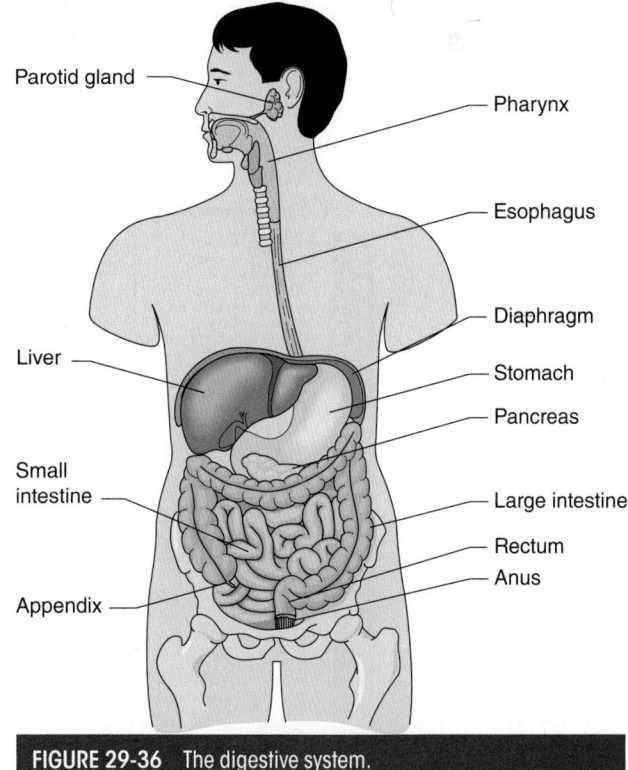

FIGURE 29-36 The digestive system.

TABLE 29-18

DIGESTIVE SYSTEMS DISORDERS

DISEASE/ DISORDER	LABORATORY/DIAGNOSTIC TESTS					MEDICAL TESTS OR PROCEDURES	TREATMENT
	BLOOD TESTING	URINE TESTING	OTHER	RADIOGRAPHY	SURGERY		
Anorexia nervosa	Complete blood count Electrolytes Blood glucose Liver function Kidney function Thyroid profile	Urinalysis	Psychological evaluation	Bone density scan Radiographs as needed		Patient history Physical exam Electrocardiography (ECG)	Replacement of fluids and electrolytes if needed Caloric supplementation Psychiatric care
Appendicitis	Complete blood count	Urinalysis Pregnancy test	Abdominal ultrasound Abdominal X-ray CT of abdomen		Appendectomy	Patient history Physical exam Rectal examination	Appendectomy Antibiotics
Bulimia	Complete blood count Electrolytes	Urinalysis	Psychological evaluation			Patient history Physical exam ECG	Replacement fluids and electrolytes if needed Caloric supplementation Care of esophagus and teeth erosion Psychiatric care
Celiac disease	Albumin Alkaline phosphatase Clotting factors abnormalities Cholesterol Complete blood count Liver enzymes Prothrombin time Genetic testing				Duodenal biopsy	Patient history Physical exam Endoscopy Capsule endoscopy	Gluten-free diet Vitamin and mineral supplementation Corticosteroids Patient education on gluten-free diet and reading food labels

Cholecystitis	Complete blood count Serum bilirubin	Urinalysis		Cholecystogram (oral or intravenous) Ultrasound of gallbladder CT Hepatobiliary iminodiacetic acid (HIDA) scan	Cholecystectomy	Patient history Physical exam	Fasting Antibiotics Pain medications Patient education on weight management, low-fat diet, and nutrition
Cholelithiasis	Complete blood count Serum bilirubin Metabolic profile			Radioisotope scan Ultrasound of gall bladder Intravenous cholangiogram CT scan Hepatobiliary iminodiacetic acid (HIDA) scan MRI of abdomen	Cholecystectomy	Patient history Physical exam Endoscopic retrograde cholangiopancreatography (ERCP)	Asymptomatic–no treatment other than diet modification (low-fat diet) Medications to dissolve gallstones
Colon cancer	Complete blood count Electrolytes Carcinoembryonic antigen (CEA)		Fecal occult blood testing	Barium enema Abdominal ultrasound CT scan of abdomen	Biopsy of colon Colectomy Endoscopic mucosal resection Resection of the colon Polypectomy Colostomy	Patient history Physical exam Sigmoidoscopy Colonoscopy	Chemotherapy Targeted drug therapy Radiation therapy

continues

Table 29-18 continued

DISEASE/DISORDER	LABORATORY/DIAGNOSTIC TESTS					MEDICAL TESTS OR PROCEDURES	TREATMENT
	BLOOD TESTING	URINE TESTING	OTHER	RADIOGRAPHY	SURGERY		
Crohn's disease	Complete blood count Electrolytes Sedimentation rate		Fecal occult blood testing	CT of abdomen Abdominal ultrasound Abdominal radiograph MRI of abdomen	Biopsy of colon Resection of the affected area of the colon Colostomy	Patient history Physical exam Upper GI series Lower GI series Barium enema Colonoscopy Sigmoidoscopy Stool culture Capsule endoscopy	Nutritional support Antibiotics Anti-inflammatories Oral 5-aminosalicylates Immune system suppressors Antidiarrheals Analgesics Vitamin and mineral Nutritional supplementation Patient education on low-fat diet, limiting dairy products, small meals, increasing fluid intake
Diverticulitis (Figure 29-28)	Complete blood count Erythrocyte sedimentation rate Liver function	Pregnancy test Urinalysis	Stool for culture and sensitivity	Abdominal radiography Barium enema	Colectomy in the case of perforation Colostomy	Patient history Physical exam Sigmoidoscopy Colonoscopy	Antibiotics Liquid diet Analgesics Patient education on high-fiber diet, increasing fluids, exercise
Drug-induced ulcer	Complete blood count Electrolytes		Fecal occult blood testing	Upper gastro-intestinal series	Biopsy of stomach	Patient history Physical exam Gastroscopy	Cessation of: Aspirin Anti-inflammatory drugs (ibuprofen, naproxen, etc.) Corticosteroids Iron Methotrexate treatments Histamine (H2) blocking agents (Pepcid (famotidine), Prilosec (omeprazole), Tagamet (cimetidine), Zantac (ranitidine))

Condition	Laboratory tests		Other tests	Radiology	Biopsy/Surgery	Examination	Treatment
Duodenal ulcer	Complete blood count H. pylori		Breath test H. pylori Occult blood test	Upper gastrointestinal series	Biopsy duodenum	Patient history Physical exam Upper endoscopy Esophagogastric duodenoscopy (EGD)	Medication: Gastric secretion-blocking agent Antibiotics Proton pump inhibitors Histamine (H2) blockers Antacids Patient education on small, frequent meals Gastrectomy if perforation
Enterobiasis (pinworm infection) (Figure 29-31)	Complete blood count		Stool sample for ova and parasites			Patient history Physical exam Perianal examination	Medications: Mebendazole Pyrantel Pamoate Albendazole Treat all members of the household
Gastric ulcer	Complete blood count Serum albumin Transferrin H. pylori		Guaiac test H. pylori (breath or stool) Culture stomach secretions Breath test	Upper gastrointestinal series Abdominal radiographs	Biopsy stomach lining Gastrectomy if perforation	Patient history Physical exam Upper endoscopy	Medication: Gastric secretion-blocking agent Histamine (H2) blockers Antacids Antibiotics Patient education on small, frequent meals; smoking cessation; limiting alcohol intake; stress reduction

continues

Table 29-18 continued

| DISEASE/ DISORDER | LABORATORY/DIAGNOSTIC TESTS | | | | RADIOGRAPHY | SURGERY | MEDICAL TESTS OR PROCEDURES | TREATMENT |
	BLOOD TESTING	URINE TESTING	OTHER					
Gastroenteritis	Complete blood count Electrolytes		Stool culture		Upper gastrointestinal series		Patient history Physical exam Upper endoscopy	Usually self-limiting Maintain electrolyte balance Antibiotics if indicated Infection control Patient education on comfort measures, rest
Gastritis	Complete blood count H. pylori		Samples of gastric content H. pylori (breath or stool)		Upper gastrointestinal series Abdominal X-ray	Biopsy of stomach	Patient history Physical exam Gastroscopy	Antacid Proton pump inhibitors Histamine (H2) blockers Antibiotics if needed Patient education on frequent small meals, limiting alcohol intake, stress reduction, irritating food avoidance
Gastro-esophageal reflux disease (GERD)					Esophageal ultrasonography Upper GI series	Surgery to reinforce the lower esophageal sphincter (Nissen fundoplication) Surgery to strengthen the lower esophageal sphincter (Linx)	Patient history Physical exam Esophageal manometry Ambulatory acid (pH) probe tests Gastroscopy Esophagoscopy	Medications: Antacid Proton pump inhibitors Histamine (H2) blockers Patient education on diet modification, weight loss, smoking cessation, remaining upright after meals, elevating head of bed

Hemorrhoids	Complete blood count				Hemorrhoidectomy Thrombectomy Hemorrhoidopexy Cryosurgery	Patient history Physical examination Anoscopy Proctoscopy Sigmoidoscopy Rubber band ligation	Topical creams Patient education on sitz baths, comfort measures, analgesia
Hepatitis	Protein Bilirubin Liver functions Alkaline phosphatase Gammaglobulin	Urinalysis		Ultrasonography of liver	Liver biopsy	Patient history Physical exam	Hepatitis A Immunoglobulin Hepatitis B No specific treatment Hepatitis C Medication (alpha-interferon; ribavirin) Patient education on rest, coping with nausea, limiting alcohol intake
Hiatal hernia (Figure 29-26)			pH studies of gastric secretions	Upper gastrointestinal series Chest radiograph Esophogram (barium swallow)	Biopsy	Patient history Physical exam Gastroscopy Esophageal manometry	Elevate head of bed for sleep Antacid medications (Prilosec, Tagamet, Zantac) Patient education on avoiding foods that irritate stomach and esophagus, avoiding overeating

continues

Table 29-18 continued

LABORATORY/DIAGNOSTIC TESTS

DISEASE/DISORDER	BLOOD TESTING	URINE TESTING	OTHER	RADIOGRAPHY	SURGERY	MEDICAL TESTS OR PROCEDURES	TREATMENT
Irritable bowel syndrome (IBS)	Testing to rule out celiac disease		Log of symptoms to include: Abdominal discomfort lasting more than 12 weeks; Change in frequency or consistency of stools; Feeling of being unable to empty your rectum; Mucus in stool; Abdominal bloating; Breath test for lactose intolerance; *H. pylori* testing (breath or stool); Stool for culture and ova and parasites	CT scan of abdomen; Abdominal radiographs; Lower GI series		Patient history; Physical exam; Sigmoidoscopy; Colonoscopy	Fiber supplements; Antidiarrheal medications; Anticholinergic drugs; Antidepressants; Antibiotics; IBS-specific medications: Lotronex, Amitiza; Patient education on stress reduction, high-fiber diet, avoiding problem foods, increasing fluids, avoiding dairy products, exercising
Pancreatic cancer	Complete blood count			Ultrasonography; CT scan; MRI; Endoscopic retrograde cholangiopancreatography (ERCP)	Whipple procedure (pancreatoduodenectomy)	Patient history; Physical exam; Percutaneous needle aspiration biopsy	Radiation therapy; Chemotherapy; Targeted therapy

Pancreatitis	Serum amylase Complete blood count Erythrocyte sedimentation rate	Stool for fats	CT scan Endoscopic retrograde cholangiopancreatography (ERCP) Endoscopic ultrasound MRI		Patient history Physical exam	Analgesics Fasting Fluid support Pancreatic enzyme supplementation Patient education on smoking cessation, limiting alcohol intake, low-fat diet, increased fluids
Rectal cancer	Complete blood count	Fecal occult blood testing	CT scan of the abdomen DNA stool testing	Surgical resection	Patient history Physical exam Colonoscopy Sigmoidoscopy	Chemotherapy Radiation therapy
Stomach cancer	Complete blood count Chemistry profile Liver function studies	Fecal occult blood testing	CT scan of the abdomen Magnetic resonance imaging (MRI) PET imaging Chest radiography	Laparoscopy Exploratory laparotomy Gastric biopsy Gastrectomy (subtotal or total)	Patient history Physical exam Upper endoscopy	Chemotherapy Radiation therapy Targeted therapy

TABLE 29-19

DESCRIPTION OF DIGESTIVE DISORDERS AND CONDITIONS

Anorexia nervosa. An eating disorder of psychological origin. Because of the need to avoid weight gain the individual does not eat and becomes emaciated (extremely thin) and malnourished.

Appendicitis. Acute inflammation of the appendix usually caused by infection or obstruction. Characterized by pain, nausea, vomiting, and fever.

Bulimia. A syndrome in which an individual binges on food and then purges by inducing vomiting. Laxative abuse is common. The reason individuals engage in this behavior is to avoid weight gain; it is of psychological origin.

Celiac disease. A genetic disease that damages the lining of the GI tract. This damage inhibits the ability to absorb nutrients in the small intestines. The ingestion of gluten causes an immune response that damages the villi in the small intestine that are important in the absorption of nutrients.

Cholecystitis. Inflammation of the gallbladder. Usual cause is gallstones, but other causes may be bacteria or chemical irritants.

Colon cancer. Common malignancy characterized by change in bowel habits, diarrhea or constipation, and abdominal discomfort as tumor grows.

Crohn disease. Chronic disease that exhibits inflammation of the ileum resulting in diarrhea, right lower quadrant pain, and attacks of diarrhea and frequent blood in the stools.

Diverticulitis. Inflammation of diverticula usually caused by impacted feces or bacteria in the sacs. Pain, cramplike, usually in left side of abdomen. Obstruction can develop.

Diverticulosis. Diverticula in colon without symptoms (see Figure 29-40).

Drug-induced ulcers. Ulcers of the stomach or duodenum caused by taking salicylates (aspirin), corticosteroids, anti-inflammatory medications (ibuprofen, naproxen), iron, and methotrexate.

Duodenal ulcer. Lesion in the mucous membrane of the small intestine usually caused by hyperacidity or *Helicobacter pylori*.

Enterobiasis (pinworms). Intestinal parasites causing intestinal and rectal infection. Pruritus of the anus is a symptom (Figure 29-37).

Gastric ulcer. Caused by *Helicobacter pylori*, a bacterium; salicylates; smoking; and alcohol.

Gastritis. Inflammation of the stomach lining usually caused by an undefined irritant that could be alcohol, bacteria, or viruses. It can result in stomach discomfort, nausea, or vomiting.

Gastroenteritis. Inflammation of the stomach and intestinal tract. Causes nausea, vomiting, and diarrhea. May be caused by ingestion of pathogen.

Gastroesophageal reflux disease (GERD). A small valve in the lower esophagus (between the stomach and esophagus) leaks, allowing stomach acid to back up from the stomach into the esophagus. It causes frequent heartburn and discomfort behind the sternum.

Hepatitis. Inflammation of the liver caused by infection from a virus resulting in hepatomegaly, anorexia, and jaundice.
- *Hepatitis A.* Spread by fecal contamination of food or water
- *Hepatitis B.* Spread by blood and body fluids contamination through sexual contact, contaminated needles, perinatal fluids, semen
- *Hepatitis C.* Spread by blood (e.g., transfusion), contaminated needles, and sexual contact

Refer to Chapter 21 for more information about hepatitis.

continues

Table 29-19 continued

Hiatal hernia. Congenital or traumatic protrusion of stomach through the diaphragm into the chest cavity (Figure 29-38).

Irritable bowel syndrome (IBS). A disorder whose symptoms include bloating, diarrhea, cramping, constipation, and abdominal pain. There is no permanent harm to the digestive tract and IBS can be managed by diet, stress management, and medications.

Rectal cancer. Cancer of the mucous membranes in the portion of the large intestine called the rectum. This malignancy can spread to the adjacent structures in the pelvis. The current survival rate is approximately 50% with treatment.

Stomach cancer. Uncommon in the United States, the worldwide diagnosis of stomach, or gastric, cancer is declining. Risk factors include salty or smoked food intake, diet low in fruits and vegetables, and a family history of stomach cancer.

Pancreatic cancer. Cancer of the pancreas (usually the head). One of the leading causes of cancer deaths in the United States. Most commonly seen in the 60- to 70-year age group.

Pancreatitis (acute and chronic). Inflammation of the pancreas. Acute: can be a life-threatening event; pancreatic enzymes begin to digest the pancreas, causing necrosis and hemorrhage. Chronic: a slow, progressive destruction of the pancreas thought to be from enzymes digesting the pancreas as seen in acute pancreatitis. May be idiopathic or related to alcoholism. Diabetes can be a complication of pancreatitis.

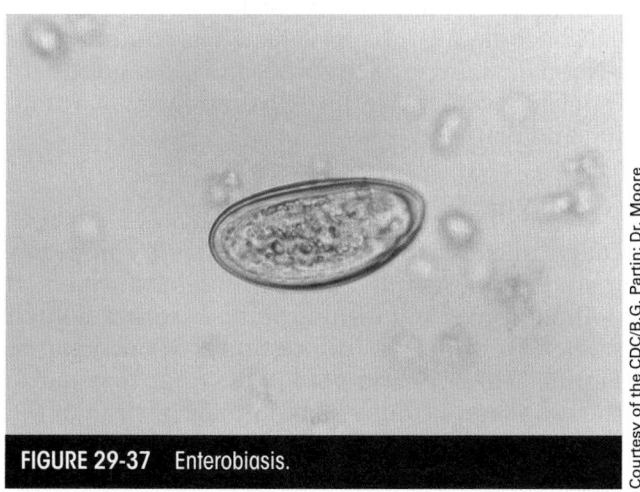

FIGURE 29-37 Enterobiasis.

Courtesy of the CDC/B.G. Partin; Dr. Moore

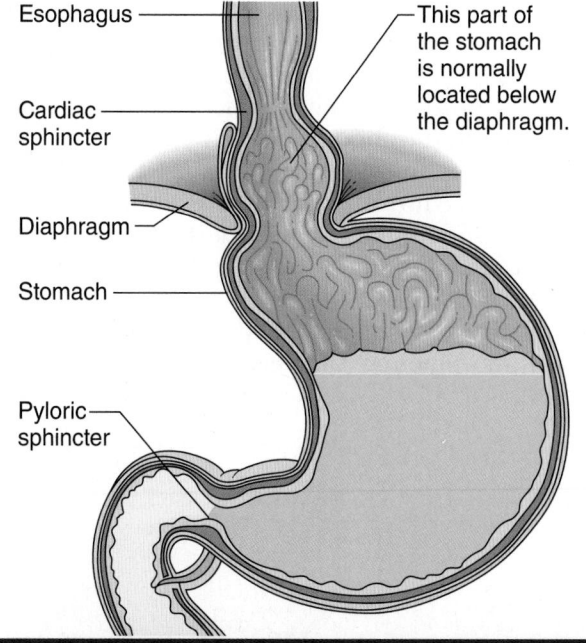

FIGURE 29-38 Hiatal hernia.

Signs and Symptoms of Digestive Conditions and Disorders

Common signs and symptoms of disorders and diseases of the digestive tract include nausea, vomiting, stomach cramping, diarrhea, heartburn, loss of appetite, weight loss, indigestion, fatigue, hematemesis (vomiting blood), melena (blood in feces), and **hematochezia** (bright red blood in feces).

Many disorders and diseases of the digestive tract can cause these signs and symptoms. Gastritis, a common ailment of the stomach, can be caused by caffeine, aspirin and other medications, spicy foods, and alcohol. It is characterized by epigastric pain, nausea, and vomiting of blood (hematemesis). Epigastric pain, chest pain, heartburn, and difficulty swallowing can also be caused by a pathologic condition known as a hiatal hernia (Figure 29-38). This pain occurs as a result of the upper portion of the stomach protruding through an enlarged opening in the diaphragm. This allows a backflow of gastric contents, including gastric acid, into the esophagus. The soft tissues of the esophagus cannot withstand this exposure to stomach contents and erosion occurs.

Gastroenteritis, described as inflammation of the stomach and small intestine, is a common ailment that can be caused by infection or ingesting foods that have been contaminated with pathogens. It can be caused by infections from contaminated food or water, drug reactions, and allergic reactions to particular foods. Peptic ulcers found in the stomach are called gastric ulcers and can be caused by the action of pepsin, an enzyme. These ulcers are an erosion (eating away of tissue) of the mucous lining of the stomach. **Salicylates** (such as aspirin), alcohol, smoking, oversecretion of hydrochloric acid, and stress seem to be implicated in this disease.

It has been discovered in recent years that some gastric ulcers may be caused by the bacterium *Helicobacter pylori* and require antibiotic treatment. Ulcers found in the duodenum are called duodenal ulcers and are similar to gastric ulcers. A duodenal ulcer is an erosion of the mucous lining of the duodenum, a part of the small intestine. If the ulcer is determined to be caused by the bacteria, antibiotics will be prescribed. Both types of ulcers seem to run a chronic course. If they are not controlled, the ulcerated area can perforate, creating a hole caused by ulceration, and hemorrhage ensues. Contents of the stomach or intestine can spill out into the abdominal cavity and cause a serious complication called peritonitis. Peritonitis is caused by the introduction of infectious organisms into the abdominal cavity that is covered by the mucous membrane called the peritoneum. See Figures 29-39 and 29-40.

Diarrhea is characterized by frequent liquid bowel movements. Diarrhea and vomiting may

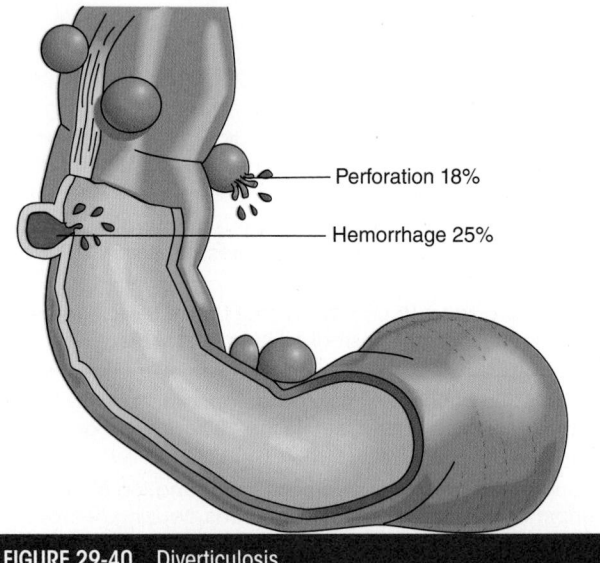

FIGURE 29-40 Diverticulosis.

Perforation 18%

Hemorrhage 25%

have many causes such as allergic reactions, infections from food or water, or stress. Dehydration can become a problem if diarrhea continues for several days. Infants, children, and older adults are especially vulnerable to dehydration from vomiting and diarrhea.

Diagnostic Tests

Diagnostic tests for the digestive system commonly include radiography and endoscopy, which is defined as viewing within the body with a lighted scope. An upper gastrointestinal (GI) series (see Figure 29-41) or barium swallow is done to visualize the esophagus, stomach, and upper portion of the small intestine. A lower GI series (see Figure 29-42) or barium enema visualizes the large intestine (see Chapter 31).

Endoscopic Procedures. An **endoscope** is an instrument or device that is used to observe the inside of a hollow organ or cavity. Using an endoscope, procedures can be done on many internal organs without surgical intervention. These are known as fiber optic endoscopic procedures or endoscopy, and they can be performed through a natural body opening or a small incision. A fiber optic endoscope permits the provider to observe within the body cavity for disorders such as polyps, tumors, cysts, stenoses, calculi, and malignancies. Biopsies and cultures can be taken during the procedure. Small lesions, such as polyps, can be totally removed during endoscopy. Photographs can be taken for documentation also.

An endoscopic procedure known as capsule video endoscopy (CVE), wireless capsule endoscopy

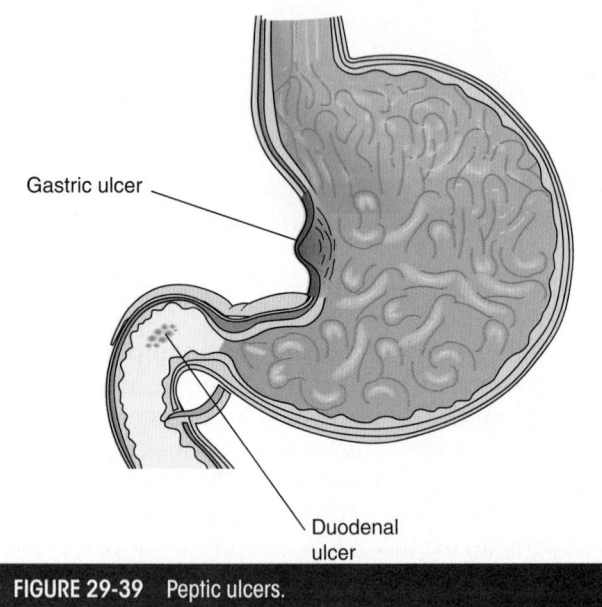

Gastric ulcer

Duodenal ulcer

FIGURE 29-39 Peptic ulcers.

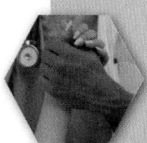

Patient Education

With the provider's direction, you may discuss with your patients the following topics about their digestive health:

1. Remind them that laxatives and enemas should be used only by direction of the provider.

2. Constipation may be avoided/relieved by including fresh fruits and vegetables, cereals, and grains in the diet; drinking plenty of liquids (water); and getting regular exercise.

3. Instruct them that if they have any of the following symptoms persistently it could mean that a disease or an abnormal condition is present and consulting the provider is strongly advised: heartburn or indigestion, nausea or vomiting (especially if coffee grounds consistency), constipation or diarrhea, excessive gas or bloating, or stool that is tarry (black) or other than a normal brown color.

4. Inform patients who are 40 years of age and older that they should routinely test their stool for occult blood every 2 years for screening of cancer of the colon, or more often if advised by the provider (if family history indicates). All patients older than 50 years should test annually for occult blood and have a colonoscopy.

5. Advise patients to include high-fiber foods in their diets, avoid fat (especially saturated fats) and cholesterol, and eat red meats sparingly.

6. Urge patients to eat a variety of foods (see ChooseMyPlate.gov) and to eat four to six small meals rather than one or two large meals daily to promote better utilization of nutrients and more energy.

7. Suggest to patients that they select snacks and beverages wisely such as fruits, vegetables, and juices over coffee/tea/soda and high-calorie sweets or salty chips.

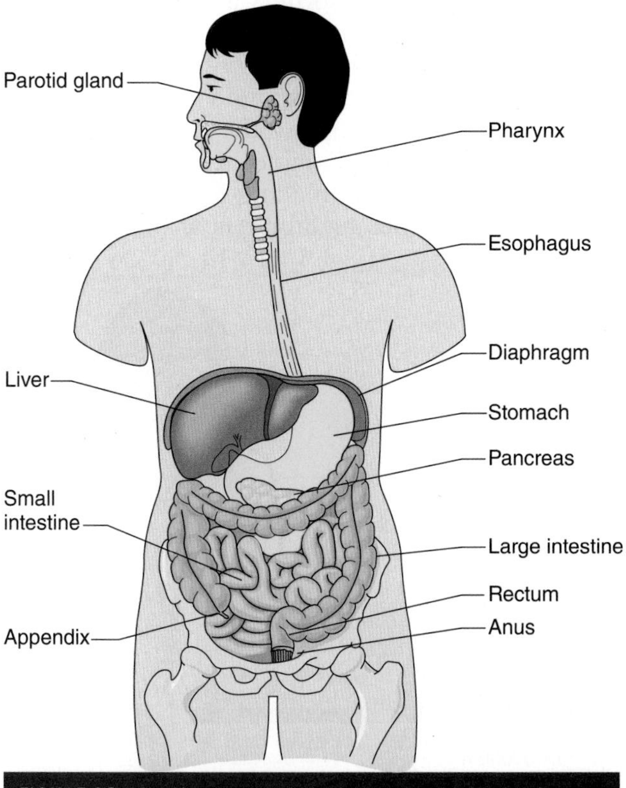

FIGURE 29-41 Upper gastrointestinal series; highlighted area is visualized.

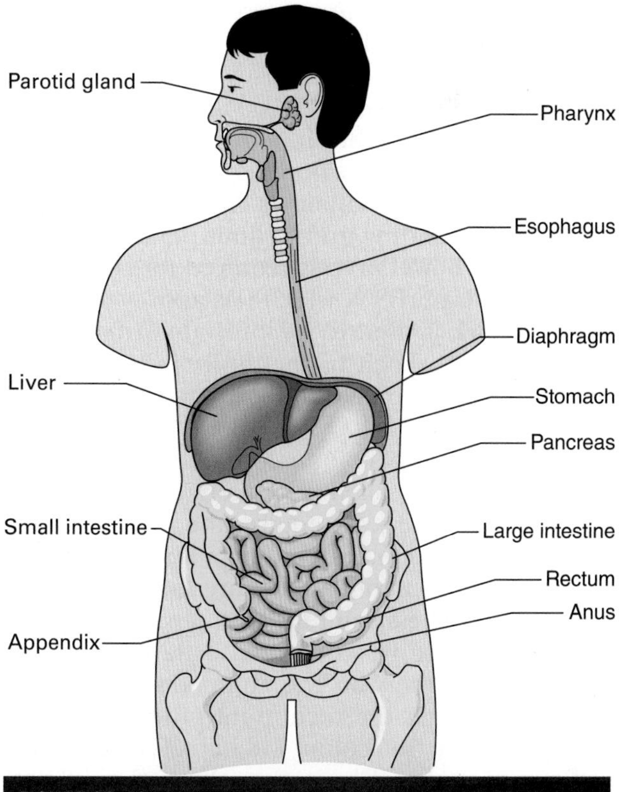

FIGURE 29-42 Lower gastrointestinal series; highlighted area is visualized.

(WCE), or PillCam (all three are the same type of endoscopy) can be performed. The patient must fast for 10 hours before the procedure and needs a bowel preparation similar to that used for a colonoscopy preparation. When the patient arrives at 7:30 AM at the gastroenterology clinic, sensor-like wires are attached to the abdominal wall (they look similar to electrocardiogram sensors) and an 8-hour battery-operated data recording device is attached to the patient's waist. The patient swallows a pill approximately the size of a vitamin that has a camera within it. The camera takes up to 57,000 color images (two photos per second) of the small intestine while the patient goes about normal activities. The camera "sees" areas overlooked by conventional endoscopy and small bowel X-ray studies. It photographs all 25 to 30 feet of the small intestine for evaluation of the patient's unexplained rectal bleeding, intermittent abdominal pain, and diarrhea. It can help diagnose polyps, cancer, Crohn disease, and other disorders and diseases. The patient returns after 8 hours and drops off the equipment and the data receiver.

The data from the recorder are downloaded onto a computer, and the photos are compressed into a video. The provider views the photographed images on a monitor.

The Food and Drug Administration (FDA) approved the capsule endoscopy (PillCam) in 2001. The FDA said the PillCam is safe and has few side effects. The patient excretes the camera in a bowel movement. The PillCam Colon was approved for use in the United States in 2014. This PillCam continues to take video for up to 10 hours, during which the patient is instructed to avoid stooping or bending and to limit physical activity. A thorough bowel prep is required for this procedure. A PillCam ESO, which was approved by the FDA in 2004, is used to look for abnormalities in the esophagus. Each of the devices is specifically programmed to image a designated part of the GI tract.

Another type of colonoscopy is known as virtual colonoscopy, also called computerized tomography (CT) colonography. It requires the same preparation as a conventional colonoscopy and can be used for patients who want a procedure they consider to be quicker and less painful.

The patient lies on the CT table, first on the back and then on the abdomen. A probe is inserted through the rectum into the colon. The probe inflates the colon with air. CT scan and radiography are used to create three-dimensional pictures of the colon, and software provides the radiographer with images on a monitor.

According to some gastroenterologists, virtual colonoscopy is not as good as a conventional colonoscopy because of the lower quality of images of the colon.

The medical assistant must be certain that the patient has signed a consent form before the procedure and that the patient has followed the preparatory instructions. Table 29-20 lists endoscopic procedures, their importance in diagnosis, and patient preparation.

Endoscopy allows the provider to look directly into the digestive organs with a lighted scope. Some examples of endoscopies used in the digestive tract are named by the organ being scoped:

Stomach: gastroscopy

Colon: colonoscopy

Sigmoid colon: sigmoidoscopy

Entire upper GI area: esophagogastroduodenoscopy (EGD); see Figure 29-43

Biopsies can be taken during an endoscopic procedure.

Sigmoidoscopy. **Sigmoidoscopy** is a diagnostic examination of the interior of the sigmoid colon. It is a useful aid in the diagnosis of cancer of the colon, ulcerations, polyps, tumors, bleeding, and other lower intestinal disorders. The sigmoidoscope is a flexible instrument with a light source and a magnifying lens, which permits visualization of the mucous membrane of the sigmoid colon.

Providers commonly use the flexible sigmoidoscope. Because it is flexible, it can be inserted farther into the colon, making it possible to view more of the mucous membranes of the intestines (Figure 29-44).

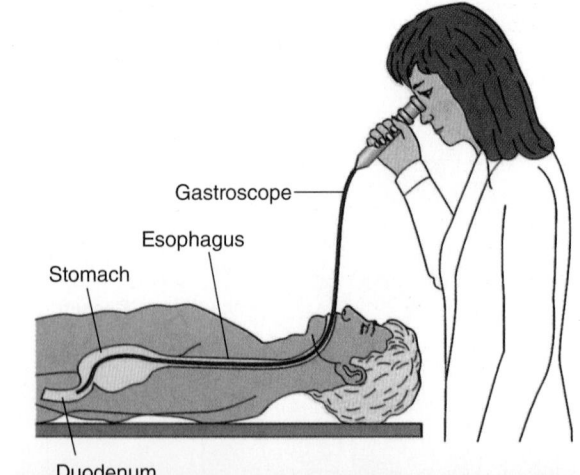

FIGURE 29-43 Esophagogastroduodenoscopy (EGD) procedure.

TABLE 29-20

ENDOSCOPIC PROCEDURES

ENDOSCOPIC PROCEDURE	IMPORTANCE IN DIAGNOSIS	PATIENT PREPARATION
Capsule video endoscopy (PillCam ESO)	Visualizes and detects abnormalities within the esophagus such as esophageal varices, Barrett esophagus, and esophageal cancers	Fasting for at least 2 hours before swallowing the PillCam ESO capsule with water
Capsule video endoscopy (PillCam SB)	Helps diagnose Crohn disease, polyps, and cancer of the small intestine	Laxative NPO (nothing by mouth) for 10 hours before procedure
Capsule video endoscopy (PillCam Colon)	Evaluates unexplained rectal bleeding, intermittent abdominal pain, and diarrhea	Laxative NPO for 10 hours before procedure
Colonoscopy (views entire colon)	Detects polyps, tumors, bleeding, and malignancies Can take biopsies, photos, and cultures, and remove polyps	Clear liquids for 2 days before NPO after 10:00 PM the night before Night before bowel preparation: laxatives and enemas
Endoscopic retrograde cholangiopancreatography (ERCP) (examines the liver, gallbladder, bile ducts, and pancreas)	Helps diagnose problems in the liver, gallbladder, bile ducts, and pancreas, such as cholelithiasis, stenoses, and malignancies of these organs and structures	NPO after 10:00 PM the night before
Esophagogastroduodenoscopy (EGD) (examines esophagus, stomach, and duodenum)	Detects abnormalities in the esophagus, stomach, and duodenum, such as hiatal hernia, stenoses, tumors, ulcers, erosion Performs biopsies, brushings, photos	NPO after 10:00 PM the night before
Gastroduodenoscopy	Examines stomach and duodenum for lesions, such as tumors, polyps, strictures, and ulcers	NPO after 10:00 PM the night before
Laparoscopy (examines the peritoneal cavity, abdomen, and pelvis)	A surgical procedure in which a fiber-optic instrument is inserted through the abdominal wall to view the organs in the abdomen and perform surgical procedures using a minimally invasive technique.	Laxative and enemas
Proctosigmoidoscopy (views sigmoid colon and rectum)	Detects polyps, rectal abscesses, tumors, fissures, and fistulas	Bowel preparation: 3-day special diet
Wireless capsule endoscopy	Evaluates unexplained rectal bleeding, intermittent abdominal pain, and diarrhea	NPO after midnight the night prior

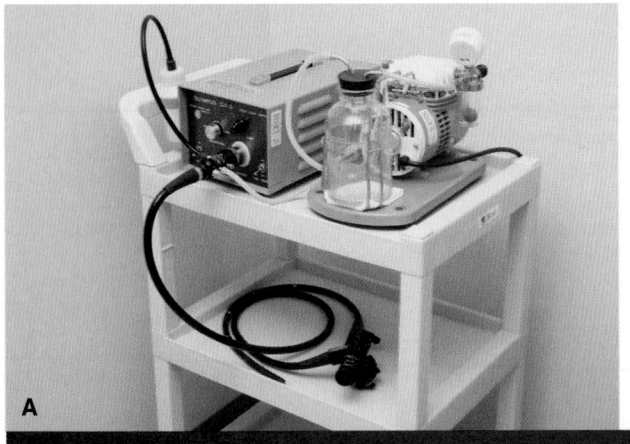
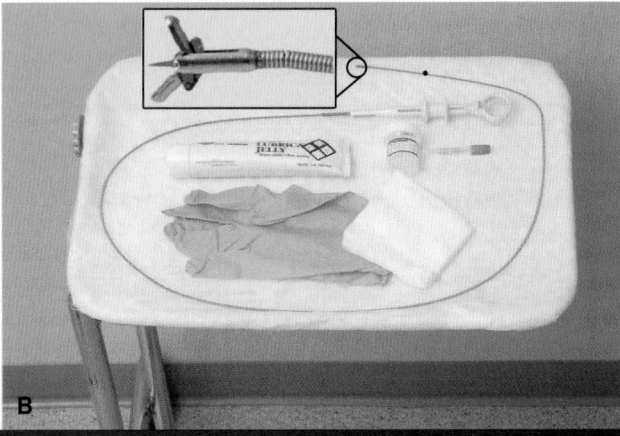

FIGURE 29-44 (A) Setup for a proctosigmoidoscopy with a flexible sigmoidoscope. (B) Control head of proctosigmoidoscopy.

As with any examination of the pelvic or abdominal cavity, you should advise the patient to empty the bladder and evacuate the bowel before the procedure begins. This will make the examination easier for both patient and examiner. During the procedure the patient should be instructed to breathe through the mouth deeply and slowly to relax abdominal muscles. Patients may feel the urge to defecate during a colon examination because of the stretching of the intestinal wall from the instrument passing through and air being introduced with it. If patients use the breathing technique mentioned, this discomfort can be relieved. Pain relievers and sedation are not usually necessary because of the short duration of the procedure. The procedure should last only a few minutes, especially if patients have followed preparation instructions.

Air is sometimes introduced into the sigmoid colon (by the examiner's use of the inflation bulb attached to the scope with tubing) to distend the wall of the colon for easier placement of the lumen of the endoscope. Patients find this to be uncomfortable and sometimes painful. The provider may need to use suction to remove mucus, blood, or fecal material that is obstructing the view of the sigmoid colon.

During these examinations, the medical assistant is responsible for having a working understanding of the instruments and equipment. It is often his or her role to assist the provider with positioning the patient for the procedure, handing instruments or equipment to the provider once the procedure begins, and offering comfort and support to the patient.

Most often it is the medical assistant who teaches the patient how to prepare for the sigmoidoscopy and explains how the test is performed. For successful examination, proper preparation is essential. Have patients restrict dairy products, raw fruits and vegetables, and grains and cereals from their diet, and encourage them to drink plenty of clear liquids and eat lightly the day before the scheduled appointment for the sigmoid colon examination. A plain commercial enema should be self-administered at home approximately 2 hours before the examination. The provider may vary the instructions according to the patient's condition. If patients are not completely informed about preparations and the examination is attempted with unsatisfactory results, the examination will have to be repeated, which is both costly and inconvenient. Satisfactory results are obtained by giving patients both oral and written instructions.

There are occasions when, during an appointment for which the patient was "worked in" to the schedules, the provider believes that the patient's condition warrants examination of the sigmoid colon. In this case, the provider will order an enema to be given to the patient in the clinic.

Administering an enema to a patient in the medical office or clinic is not a common procedure, but it is sometimes necessary for the successful completion of a sigmoidoscopy or other rectal examination. Even though a patient may have received proper instructions and carried them out before the scheduled appointment, there is no guarantee that the patient achieved success. In the event that the patient comes in for the appointment and the colon is not sufficiently evacuated of feces for a sigmoidoscopy, the provider may order a cleansing enema so that the examination can be completed. There are many considerations to be taken into account if the patient is not fully prepped. The provider will ultimately make the decision on how to proceed. Often the patient did follow the list of instructions but was not able to retain the enema solution long enough to get satisfactory results. You will more likely be able to encourage the patient to retain the contents of the enema longer. You may want to explain that the longer the contents are retained, the more successful the results will be. Otherwise, it may have to be repeated, or the examination rescheduled. Be certain that you use an examination room that is close to the rest room for the patient's convenience when you administer an enema. Your patience and understanding are needed, because many patients are embarrassed to have an enema administered to them.

Some examinations, such as diagnostic sigmoidoscopy and X-ray studies, require the use of laxatives by the patient the day before or the morning of the examination. This may present a problem in the patient's personal or employment schedule if instructions are not made clear before the appointment is made. Most patients are fearful of what the diagnostic examination will disclose. Helping them choose a convenient appointment time and explaining the reasons for the preparations they must undergo is usually appreciated.

Proper positioning of the patient during the sigmoidoscopy is important for both the provider's viewing of the rectum and sigmoid colon and the patient's comfort. Proctology tables are designed especially for this procedure. They provide support of the patient's chest and head with the arm resting against the headboard as the table is tilted to the knee-chest position. Patients who cannot tolerate this position are assisted into Sims' position for the examination. Many providers find this acceptable and it is more comfortable for the patient. You should ask about the provider's preference for patient position because there are many variations.

The provider may wish to view the intestinal mucosa after a normal bowel movement. More often, the patient is instructed to eat a light diet containing plenty of clear liquids and avoiding dairy products for 24 hours before the examination, and to have a plain cleansing enema the morning of, or 2 hours before, the examination. Still other providers may wish patients to use laxatives the day before and an enema the night before and also the morning of the examination.

When making a diagnosis of hemorrhoids, fissures, and ulcerations, the provider usually begins investigative procedures by examining the anus and the interior of the rectum with a proctoscope. During the sigmoidoscopy, the provider may want to take a biopsy of questionable tissue from the sigmoid colon to aid in confirming the diagnosis. It is a good rule to have all possible necessary items available. When the patient has been prepared and the provider is ready to begin the examination, the medical assistant hands the necessary instruments and supplies to the provider as needed. Remember to advise patients to report any problems, such as bleeding, discharge, swelling, or any other unusual discomfort, after the procedure. A biopsy laboratory request form must be completed and accompany the tissue to the laboratory. Containers for biopsy specimens have a formaldehyde solution to preserve the tissue until the analysis is done.

Whereas the proctosigmoidoscope examines the rectum and sigmoid colon with a flexible scope, a procedure known as a **colonoscopy** (viewing the colon with a lighted scope) can be scheduled in the outpatient department of the hospital or endoscopy center or performed in the office or clinic. A flexible fiber optic colonoscope is used, and the entire length of the large intestine (colon) can be examined for lesions such as tumors, polyps, fissures, and masses. Biopsies that consist of small tissue pieces can be removed with a snare-type instrument inserted through the colonoscope. The tissue is microscopically examined by a pathologist to determine whether a malignancy (cancer) is present in the colon (Figure 29-45). The patient may receive a muscle relaxant/tranquilizer to facilitate the examination.

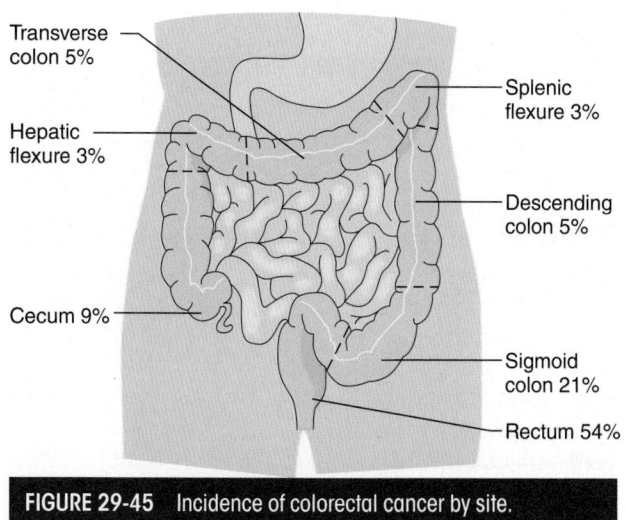

FIGURE 29-45 Incidence of colorectal cancer by site.

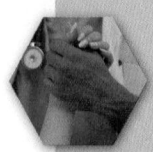

Patient Education

An important aspect of your role as a medical assistant is to provide patient education. Your provider may have created teaching materials specifically for patients or there might be preprinted educational materials in the clinic for this purpose. After a sigmoidoscopy, it is important that the patient follow instructions to avoid any complications after the procedure.

After sigmoidoscopy, patients should drink plenty of clear fluids to help relieve abdominal discomfort and flatulence. Prevention of constipation is essential. High-fiber foods and exercise will assist in reestablishing resumption of regular bowel habits. Patients may also find relief in lying in a prone position with a pillow across the mid-abdominal area to aid in the passage of gas.

Procedure

Fecal Occult Blood Test. Patients may be instructed to obtain three stool specimens at home for examination of a fecal sample for occult (hidden) blood. The patient will be given occult blood slides, applicators, and envelopes to take home (Figure 29-46). The patient will need to obtain two small stool samples from each of three separate bowel movements. Three separate samples are used to allow detection of blood from GI lesions that exhibit intermittent bleeding. The medical assistant's role is to instruct the patient about how to properly collect the stool specimens on the test slides, and then how to care for and store the slides until they are returned to the clinic by the patient (see Procedure 29-21). Biohazardous material (feces) cannot be sent through the U.S. Postal Service.

For patients who have daily bowel movements, this will not be a problem. For patients who have difficulty with daily elimination, collecting the samples may take several days. Patients should not use laxatives unless directed by the provider.

Positive tests for occult blood require further testing, because occult blood testing is a screening tool only. Sigmoidoscopy and colonoscopy help to identify the source of bleeding. If a lesion is found in either the rectum or colon, a biopsy can be performed and the sample sent to the laboratory for examination of cells for malignancy (see Procedure 29-21).

Radiographic Studies of the Digestive System. Endoscopic procedures are done routinely but have not replaced the need for radiographic studies of the gastrointestinal tract. Several diagnostic radiographic studies can be performed in order to study digestive structures and functions in the process of looking for disease. They include the upper GI series (barium swallow) (Figure 29-50), lower GI series (barium enema), and the cholecystogram. Table 29-21 lists the purpose, patient preparation, and procedures for each of these three studies.

READING AND INTERPRETING THE HEMOCCULT® TEST

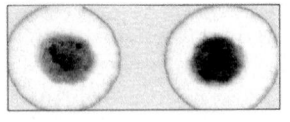

Negative Smears

Sample report: negative
No detectable blue on or at the edge of the smears indicates the test is negative for occult blood.

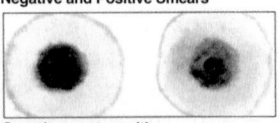

Negative and Positive Smears

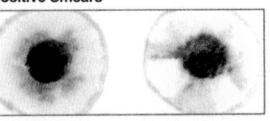

Positive Smears

Sample report: positive
Any trace of blue on or at the edge of one or more of the smears indicates the test is positive for occult blood.

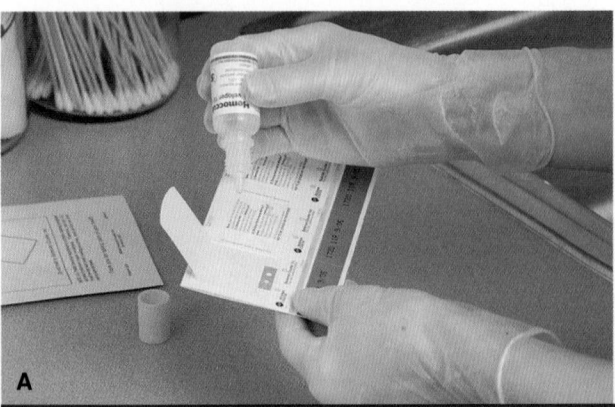

A   **B**

FIGURE 29-46 (A) Place the required number of drops of developing solution on the exposed guiac paper. (B) A change in color indicates the blood may be present in the stool.

PROCEDURE 29-21

Procedure

Performing Fecal Occult Blood Test

STANDARD PRECAUTIONS:

Handwashing

Gloves

Biohazard

PURPOSE:

To test feces for occult blood—collection and development of slides.

EQUIPMENT/SUPPLIES:

- Three occult slide test kits containing three slides, applicators, and envelope
- Prepared fecal slides from patient
- Occult blood developer
- Reference card that accompanies kit
- Nonsterile disposable gloves
- Clock or watch with a second hand

PROCEDURE STEPS:

1. *Paying attention to detail*, assemble supplies needed for the procedure. Be sure to check the expiration dates on the slides. RATIONALE: Outdated slides can give an inaccurate reading.
2. Wash your hands and follow Standard Precautions.
3. Introduce yourself and confirm the identity of the patient using two identifiers, such as name and date of birth.
4. *Confirm and explain the rationale for the procedure to be performed, speaking at the patient's level of understanding.* Take time to answer the patient's questions.
5. Complete the information on the front flap of all three slide packages (Figure 29-47). Be sure to include the patient's name, the date, and the specimen number. The prepared slide packets and an envelope should be given to the patient to take home.

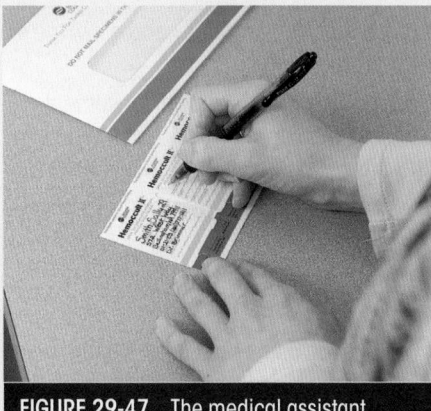

FIGURE 29-47 The medical assistant writes the patient's name, the date, and the specimen number on each occult slide.

continues

6. ***Speaking at the patient's level of understanding, explain the steps of the procedure***, most of which will be performed by the patient at home.

7. Instruct the patient to keep the slides at room temperature. The patient must follow specific dietary guidelines starting 2 days prior to testing, including not eating red meat, raw fruits, or vegetables. High doses of vitamin C greater than 250 mg a day, as well as aspirin and other nonsteroidal anti-inflammatory medications should be avoided for 7 days prior to and during the test period (Figure 29-48).

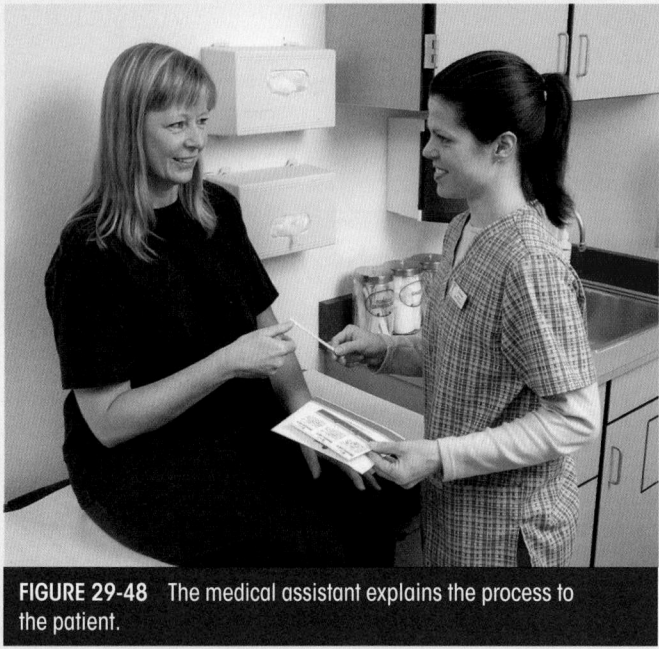

FIGURE 29-48   The medical assistant explains the process to the patient.

8. The stool sample should be collected in a clean dry container. In order for the test to be accurate, stool should not be collected during the menstrual cycle or if hemorrhoids are present.

9. The patient should write the date of collection on the front flap of the packet before opening it.

10. Instruct the patient to use one end of the wooden applicator to apply a thin smear of the stool sample from the container to box A on the slide.

11. The procedure should be repeated for box B using the other end of the applicator and a different area of the stool, as the presence of blood may be distributed unevenly.

12. Instruct the patient to dispose of the applicator properly and allow the stool samples to dry overnight. The covers should be closed after the samples have dried.

13. The patient will repeat this process for the next two bowel movements over subsequent days. Once completed, the patient will place the slides in the provided envelope and return them to the provider's office. The envelope should not be mailed. RATIONALE: Slides are considered biohazardous material.

14. When you are sure that the patient understands the procedure, record all information regarding instruction and the provision of the test kits in the patient's medical record.

15. When the completed kits are returned, you will need to develop the slides as soon as possible to ensure accuracy of the results.

16. After applying gloves, check the expiration dates on the developer and cover a flat dry work area with a protective barrier, such as paper towels.

continues

17. Open the window on the back of the slide packet and apply two drops of the developer directly over the smear in each box and one drop over each of the control windows (Figure 29-49). RATIONALE: Paper contains the chemical guaiac, which will help identify occult blood.

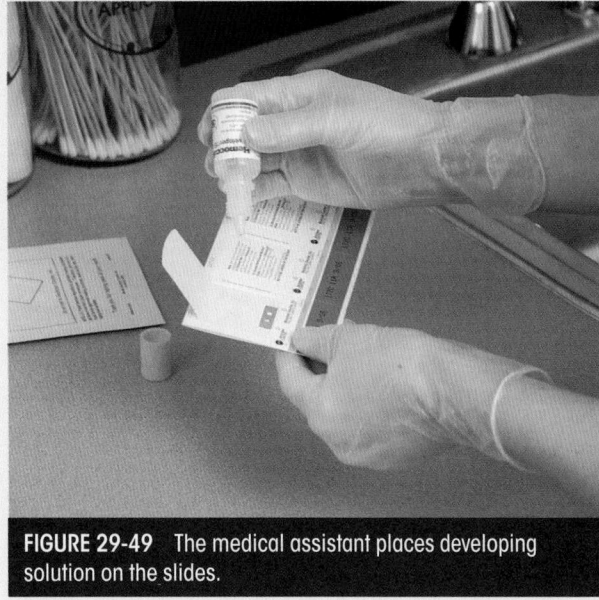

FIGURE 29-49 The medical assistant places developing solution on the slides.

18. It is important that the results be read within 30 to 60 seconds, unless otherwise specifically indicated by the test manufacturer.

19. A positive reaction will consist of a blue halo appearing around the perimeter of the specimen. Any blue color is considered positive.

20. Dispose of all supplies following OSHA guidelines and remove and discard gloves before washing your hands.

21. Record test results in the patient's medical record.

DOCUMENTATION:

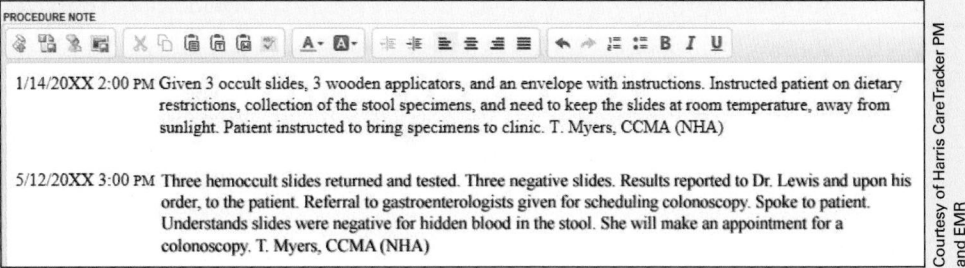

PROCEDURE NOTE

1/14/20XX 2:00 PM Given 3 occult slides, 3 wooden applicators, and an envelope with instructions. Instructed patient on dietary restrictions, collection of the stool specimens, and need to keep the slides at room temperature, away from sunlight. Patient instructed to bring specimens to clinic. T. Myers, CCMA (NHA)

5/12/20XX 3:00 PM Three hemoccult slides returned and tested. Three negative slides. Results reported to Dr. Lewis and upon his order, to the patient. Referral to gastroenterologists given for scheduling colonoscopy. Spoke to patient. Understands slides were negative for hidden blood in the stool. She will make an appointment for a colonoscopy. T. Myers, CCMA (NHA)

Courtesy of Harris CareTracker PM and EMR

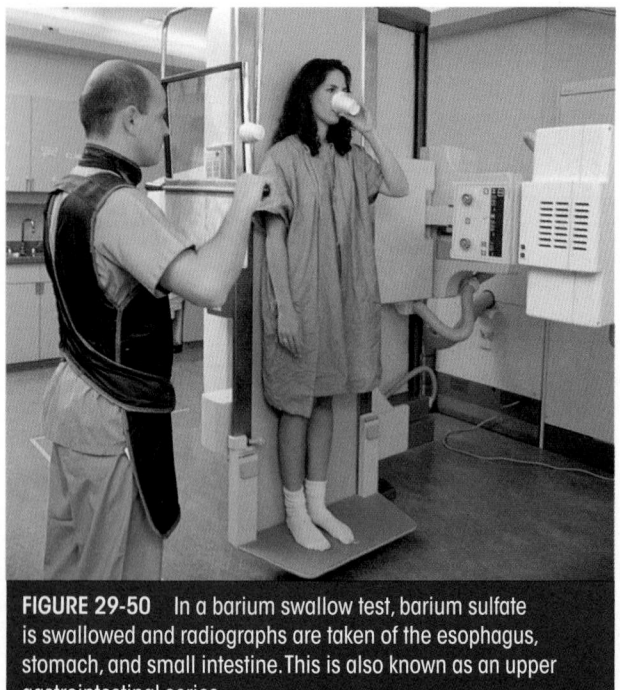

FIGURE 29-50 In a barium swallow test, barium sulfate is swallowed and radiographs are taken of the esophagus, stomach, and small intestine. This is also known as an upper gastrointestinal series.

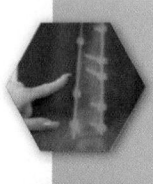

Critical Thinking

Phyllis Lomeli, a new patient of Dr. Reynolds, has been experiencing gastrointestinal problems. Dr. Reynolds has ordered fecal occult blood tests for the patient. What diet instructions does the medical assistant give to the patient? What directions and supplies does the medical assistant give to the patient? When the guaiac slides are returned by the patient, how does the medical assistant develop and interpret them?

TABLE 29-21

PATIENT PREPARATION AND PROCEDURE FOR RADIOGRAPHIC STUDIES OF THE DIGESTIVE SYSTEM

TEST	PURPOSE	PATIENT PREP	PROCEDURE	TIME
Barium swallow (upper gastrointestinal [GI] series)	To study the esophagus, stomach, and duodenum of the small intestine for disease (ulcers, tumors, hiatal hernia, esophageal varices)	Day before radiograph: • Light evening meal • NPO after midnight Day of test: • NPO Postprocedure: • Increase fluid intake • Take laxative as prescribed	• The patient is asked to drink a flavored barium mixture while standing in front of fluoroscope • The radiologist observes the passage down the digestive tract • The patient is turned to various positions to allow good visualization of the intestine • Radiographs are taken	1 hour
Barium enema (lower GI series)	To study the colon for disease (polyps, tumors, lesions)	Clear liquid 1 day prior (allowed: noncarbonated beverages, clear gelatin, clear broth, coffee and tea with sugar) No milk or milk products 8 oz water every hour until bedtime Prep kit: includes bottle of magnesium citrate, Dulcolax (bisacodyl) tab(s)	• The colon is filled with a barium sulfate mixture • The patient is turned in various positions to allow the barium to fill the colon; air is injected to move the barium along the colon • When the colon is full, radiographs are taken	1 to 2 hours

continues

Table 29-21 continued

TEST	PURPOSE	PATIENT PREP	PROCEDURE	TIME
		Day before radiograph: • Late afternoon drink bottle of magnesium citrate • Early evening take Dulcolax tab(s) as prescribed • Light evening meal; NPO except water, after dinner Morning of procedure: • NPO • Cleansing enema Postprocedure instructions: • Increase fluid intake and dietary fiber • Report to provider if no bowel movement within 24 hours of test		
Cholecystogram	To study the gall bladder for disease (stones, duct obstruction), inflammation	• Evening before test fat-free dinner • Take dye tablets with 8 oz water • Cathartic or cleansing enemas may be prescribed • NPO after dinner and tablets	• A series of radiographs is taken • A fatty meal may be given to stimulate the gall bladder to empty • Other radiographs can then be taken to check gall bladder function	1 hour

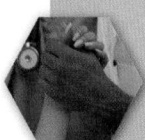

Patient Education

Your provider has ordered fecal occult blood testing to rule out colon cancer. It is important to instruct your patient on obtaining, handling, and storing the specimen until it can be returned to the clinic. The instructions for a successful and accurate test are provided here. First, always follow specific package instructions. These steps should be followed 2 days before the fecal occult blood test and continued until three slides have been prepared:

- Avoid red meats, processed meats, and liver. These foods release hemoglobin, which can produce a false-positive result.
- Avoid turnips, broccoli, cauliflower, and melons. These foods may contain a substance, peroxidase, that will cause a false-positive result.
- Avoid aspirin, iron supplements, and large doses of vitamin C for 7 days before the test. These substances may cause gastric bleeding that can mask bleeding from a lesion.
- Consume a high-fiber diet. Fiber provides roughage to promote bowel movement and encourage bleeding from any lesion that may be present.
- Do not begin the test during menses, for 3 days after menses, or if bleeding from hemorrhoids.
- Drink plenty of fluids to help prevent constipation.
- Store slides at room temperature and protect from heat, sun, and fluorescent lights.

Bariatrics

Millions of people in the United States are obese and are ill with or at serious risk for diabetes, heart disease, hypertension, certain cancers, stroke, sleep apnea, and many other conditions. Obesity affects every body system in a negative way. Emotional problems such as depression, rejection, low self-esteem, isolation, and chemical substance abuse are common. **Bariatrics** is the field of medicine that treats obesity and conditions associated with obesity.

Some obese patients decide, with their provider's recommendation, to undergo bariatric surgery because of the physical and emotional problems caused by their obesity. Prior to surgery, patients must participate with their provider to bring their existing medical problems, such as uncontrolled diabetes, severe hypertension, hyperlipidemia, and gallbladder disease, under control. Stabilization is important to prevent serious complications before, during, and after surgery.

Bariatric surgery is performed to treat obesity and to help the patient lose weight. It can be accomplished with a standard abdominal incision or laparoscope. Two procedures that can be performed are "banding," or "stapling," and gastric bypass surgery (Figure 29-51). With banding or stapling, the bottom of the esophagus (where it enters the stomach) is banded or stapled, thus shrinking the stomach. An adjustable port in the abdomen controls the tightness of the band or staples. In gastric bypass surgery, the surgeon creates a pouch out of a small portion of the stomach and attaches it directly to the small intestine, thereby bypassing the stomach and duodenum. As a result, absorption, which occurs in the small intestine, is reduced. Before surgery, patients are counseled about possible side effects, such as malabsorption, anemia, vomiting, diarrhea, hernias, and blood clots.

Bariatric surgery is considered for patients with **morbid obesity** who have tried numerous

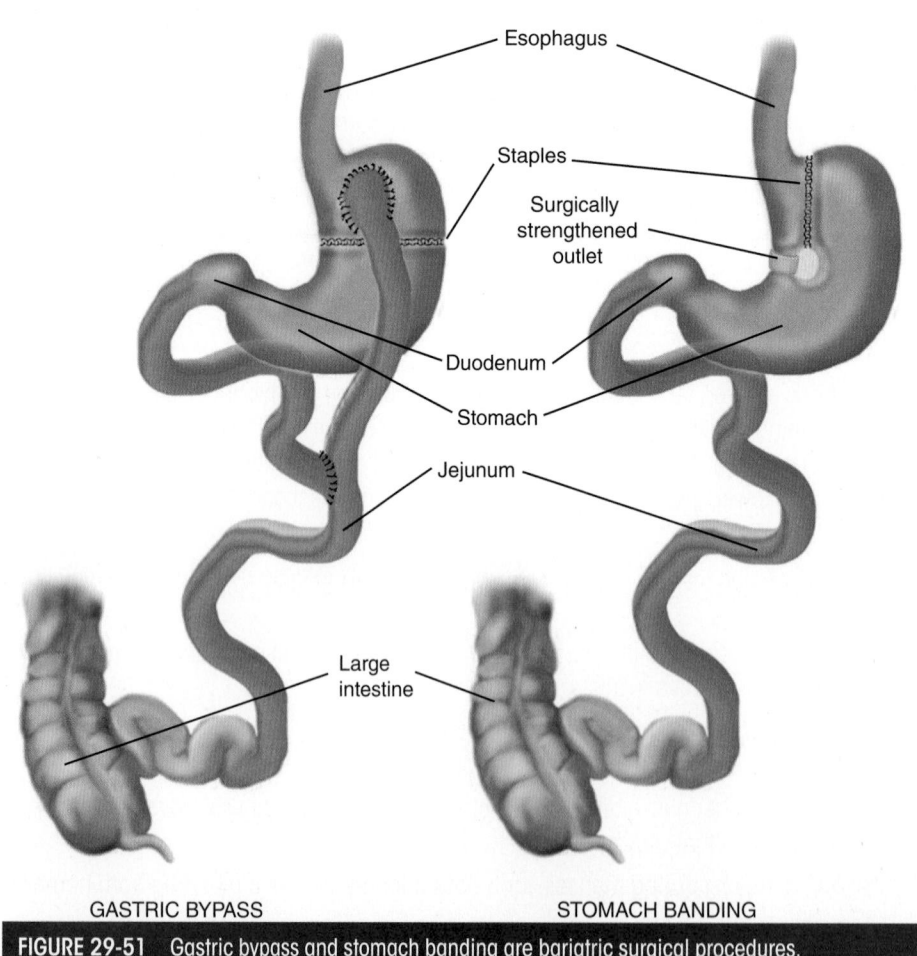

GASTRIC BYPASS   STOMACH BANDING

FIGURE 29-51 Gastric bypass and stomach banding are bariatric surgical procedures.

weight loss and exercise regimens without results and are at serious risk for heart disease, stroke, cancer, and other conditions. Body mass index (BMI) is another factor considered when providers evaluate patients for surgery. A BMI around 30 to 40 (a general guideline) is one of the criteria used to determine which patients are candidates for the surgery (normal BMI is 18.5 to 24.9). The presence of other diseases is also a factor in the evaluation.

Presentation Caring for bariatric patients is challenging. Their emotional health is important. Being nonjudgmental and showing empathy for these patients are very important. They often suffer from discrimination, prejudice, and isolation. Obesity is a chronic illness that requires patience and understanding.

URINARY SYSTEM

The urinary system includes the kidneys, ureters, and bladder. The main function of the kidneys is to form and excrete urine, which contains waste products harmful to body tissues. The kidneys also regulate water balance in the body and help maintain the acid–base balance of body fluids.

Collecting and processing urine for laboratory analysis is covered in Chapter 41. Several other clinical and diagnostic procedures of the urinary system are covered in this section, including urinary catheterization and an overview of performing a urine drug screen and a diagnostic X-ray study known as an intravenous pyelogram (IVP) or excretory urography used to diagnose disorders of the urinary tract.

Diagnostic tests, procedures, disorders, and conditions common to the urinary system are given in Tables 29-22 and 29-23.

Signs and Symptoms of Urinary Conditions and Disorders

Signs and symptoms of urinary tract diseases include any abnormality in urine or in the ability to urinate. Some common signs and symptoms are **dysuria** or painful urination, **proteinuria** or protein in the urine, **hematuria** or blood in the urine, **pyuria** or pus in the urine, **frequency, urgency, oliguria** or absence of urine production, and **nocturia** or excessive urination at night. Patients may report flank or low back pain or experience fever; nausea; vomiting; general **malaise**, known as general discomfort; and fatigue.

Urinary tract infection (UTI) is the most common disorder of the urinary system, and it manifests with many of the above signs and symptoms. UTI is a broad diagnosis covering any infection of the urinary tract including the urethra, ureters, bladder, and kidneys. UTI may be caused by virus or fungus, but by far the most common infection is caused by bacteria. The most common area is the bladder. The medical term for inflammation of the bladder is *cystitis*.

Bacteria may reach the urinary tract through the blood, called a hematogenous infection, or enter the tract through the urethra, known as an ascending infection. Hematogenous infection is less common and is usually the result of septicemia. In this case, the urinary tract is a site of secondary infection. Primary infection of septicemia may begin in the respiratory or gastrointestinal tract and is carried to the urinary tract through the blood.

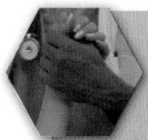

Patient Education

Several Web sites (e.g., CDC, Mayo Clinic, Weight Watchers) can automatically calculate BMI after inputting the patient's height and weight measurements. The following are formulas for determining BMI:

1. Multiply weight, in pounds, by 0.45 (130 pounds × 0.45 = 58.5).
2. Multiply height, in inches, by 0.025 (5 feet 6 inches or 66 inches × 0.025 = 1.65).
3. Multiply the answer from step 2 by itself (1.65 × 1.65 = 2.72).
4. Divide the answer from step 1 by the answer from step 3 (58.5 ÷ 2.72 = 21.48).
5. If the BMI is less than 18.5, the individual is underweight.
6. If the BMI is equal to or greater than 25, the individual is overweight.
7. A BMI equal to or greater than 30 indicates obesity.

TABLE 29-22

URINARY SYSTEM DISORDERS

| DISEASE/DISORDER | LABORATORY/DIAGNOSTIC TESTS | | | SURGERY | MEDICAL TESTS OR PROCEDURES | TREATMENT |
	BLOOD TESTING	URINE TESTING	RADIOGRAPHY			
Cancer of urinary bladder	Complete blood count	Urinalysis Culture and sensitivity of urine Urine cytology	Intravenous pyelogram Pelvic ultrasound CT scan of bladder	Cystoscopy with biopsy of the bladder Resection of cancer (transurethral resection of a bladder tumor [TURBT]) Cystectomy Urostomy	Patient history Physical exam	Radiation therapy Chemotherapy Biological therapy
Cystitis	Complete blood count	Urinalysis including microscopic examination Culture and sensitivity of urine	Intravenous pyelogram Ultrasound of bladder		Patient history Physical exam Cystoscopy	Appropriate antibiotic therapy Patient education on comfort measures (heating pad, sitz bath)
Glomerulonephritis	Blood urea nitrogen Creatinine Blood culture Sedimentation rate Electrolytes	Urinalysis Culture and sensitivity of urine	Intravenous pyelogram Ultrasound of kidneys X-ray of kidneys, ureters, and bladder	Kidney transplant	Patient history Physical exam Biopsy of kidney(s)	Diuretics Antihypertensives Dialysis (if necessary) Treatment for underlying cause (lupus, immune disease, or Goodpasture syndrome) Patient education on limiting salt intake, limiting protein and potassium intake, weight management, diabetes management, smoking cessation
Polycystic kidneys	Blood urea nitrogen Creatinine Electrolytes	Urinalysis	Intravenous pyelogram Ultrasound of kidneys CT scan	Kidney transplant	Patient history Physical exam	Dialysis Hypertension management Pain management Patient education on fluid management

Pyelonephritis	Blood urea nitrogen Creatinine Blood culture Electrolytes	Urinalysis Urine culture and sensitivity	Intravenous pyelogram Ultrasound of kidneys Voiding cystourethrogram		Patient history Physical exam	Appropriate antibiotics Patient education on increased fluids, heating pad application, pain management
Renal calculi	Complete blood count Uric acid Calcium	Urinalysis 24-hour urine collection	X-ray of kidneys, ureters, and bladder (KUB) Ultrasound of kidneys, ureters, and bladder Intravenous pyelogram	Cystoscopy Lithotripsy (crushing of a kidney stone) Surgery (nephrolithotomy) Uretoscope	Patient history Physical exam Examination of stones (composition)	Increase fluids Pain management Alpha blocker Patient education on increased fluid intake, limiting oxalate-rich foods, low-sodium diet, low-protein diet Diuretics Allopurinol
Urinary tract infection	Complete blood count	Urinalysis Culture and sensitivity of urine	CT scan of the urinary tract MRI	Cystoscopy	Patient history Physical exam	Appropriate antibiotics Patient education on alcohol avoidance, increased fluids, heating pad application for comfort

TABLE 29-23

DESCRIPTION OF URINARY DISORDERS AND CONDITIONS

Cancer of urinary bladder. Linked to cigarette smoking, industrial chemicals, and ingested toxins. Microscopic hematuria is one of the first signs.

Cystitis. Inflammation of the urinary bladder. More common in female patients due to the short length of the urethra. *Escherichia coli* may travel from the rectum to the bladder. Infectious organisms can invade the bladder during sexual intercourse. Frequency, burning, dysuria, and urgency are common symptoms.

Glomerulonephritis. Seen in children and young adults after streptococcal infection, strep throat, scarlet fever. Causes degenerative inflammation of glomeruli. Chills, fever, weakness are common symptoms. Edema and albumin in urine are common. Hypertension occurs.

Polycystic kidneys. A congenital anomaly. Kidneys contain multiple cysts and greatly dilated tubules do not open into renal pelvis. Hypertension, kidney failure, and death can result.

Pyelonephritis. Caused by pyogenic bacteria such as *E. coli, Streptococci, Staphylococci,* pregnancy, or calculi. May originate in the bladder and ascend to the kidneys. Pyuria, chills, fever, and sudden back pain are symptoms. Dysuria is common. Tenderness in suprapubic area.

Renal calculi. May be present with or without symptoms. Cause intense pain when they lodge in the ureter(s). Formed by certain salts (perhaps calcium). Urinary urgency, nausea and vomiting, fever.

Diagnostic Tests

The most commonly performed test to diagnose urinary system disorders is a urinalysis. Many different disorders of the urinary system can be identified, making this test extremely valuable. A specimen of urine can be analyzed for many components such as pH, specific gravity, protein, glucose, leukocytes, and blood. The specimen can be further analyzed by examination under the microscope to look for bacteria, white and red blood cells, crystals, and casts.

Procedure

Urine culture and sensitivity can be performed and will indicate if a UTI is present so the appropriate antibiotic can be prescribed by the provider. To obtain a urine specimen for culture, there are two ways to collect the specimen: clean catch or catheterization (insertion of sterile tube into urinary bladder) (see Procedures 29-22 and 29-23 and Chapter 41).

Blood tests can be done to determine whether waste products are being adequately filtered out of the circulatory system. A test for kidney function confirms the status of glomeruli function.

Two nitrogenous waste products normally filtered from the blood are urea and creatinine. A blood urea nitrogen (BUN) test checks the levels of these two wastes. High levels of waste products can result in uremia (waste products in the blood), a toxic condition of the blood that, if not reversed, leads to death (see Chapter 38).

IVP, kidney-ureter-bladder (KUB) radiograph, and cystogram are radiologic examinations of the urinary tract.

Intravenous Pyelogram. An **intravenous pyelogram (IVP)** is used to examine the urinary tract for blockage, narrowing, growths, and calculi. This urinary tract diagnostic radiograph is also used to diagnose disorders such as lesions; hydronephrosis, a collection of urine in the renal pelvis; and kidneys with many cysts, known as polycystic kidneys.

Patient Preparation for IVP. To study the urinary system, the IVP requires that the patient prepare with laxatives, enemas, and fasting (Table 29-24). The IVP consists of an intravenous injection of an iodine-based contrast medium that is used to define the structures of the urinary system. A retrograde pyelogram is a study of the urinary tract done by inserting a sterile catheter into the urinary meatus. Radiopaque contrast medium then flows upward into the kidneys. This diagnostic test is usually done in conjunction with cystoscopy. Patients should have iodine-sensitivity tests before the examination to determine the possibility of an allergic reaction. If there is an iodine and/or shellfish allergy, the patient will be required to be premedicated.

A voiding cystogram may be ordered in conjunction with an IVP. In this case, the contrast medium is instilled into the bladder by catheter and no special patient preparation is needed (see Chapter 31).

TABLE 29-24

INTRAVENOUS PYELOGRAM PROCEDURE AND PRECAUTIONS

PURPOSE	PATIENT EDUCATION	PRECAUTIONS
To examine the urinary tract—kidneys, ureters, bladder—for blockage, narrowing, growths, and calculi	1. Only clear liquids the day prior to the procedure 2. Laxatives as ordered 3. NPO after midnight the evening before the IVP 4. Cleansing enema(s) the morning of the procedure	Contrast medium of iodine used for visualization (check with patient regarding seafood or iodine allergies) Warn patients of a possible warm flushed sensation when dye is injected and that they may experience a metallic taste

Cystoscopy.   Cystoscopy is a sterile procedure that uses a lighted cystoscope to view the urethra and bladder. Inflammation, bladder calculi, **polyps**, and tumors can be seen using a cystoscope. A biopsy of the bladder can be done while performing a cystoscopy (Figure 29-52).

Biopsy of the Kidney.   Biopsies of the kidney will help confirm a diagnosis. Using radiology and ultrasonography, a fine-gauge needle is inserted through the flank to remove a piece of kidney tissue for analysis and determination of possible malignancy.

Urinary Catheterization

In some states, medical assistants can either perform or assist with urinary bladder catheterization, which is the introduction of a sterile catheter through the urethra into the bladder for withdrawal of urine. Figure 29-53 shows male

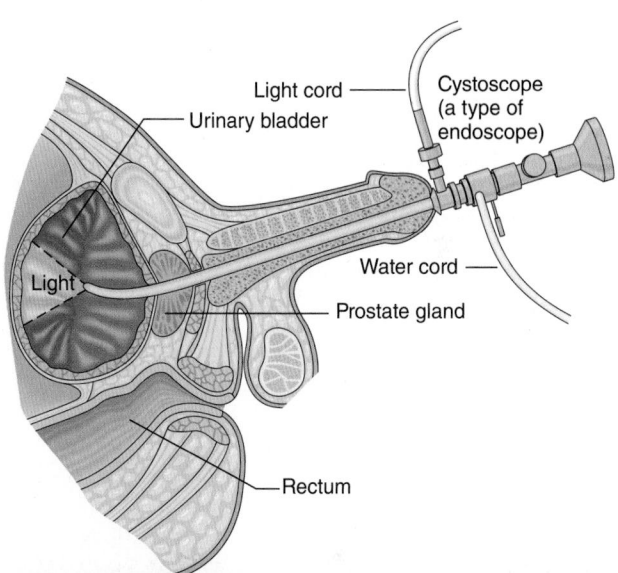

FIGURE 29-52   Cystoscopy.

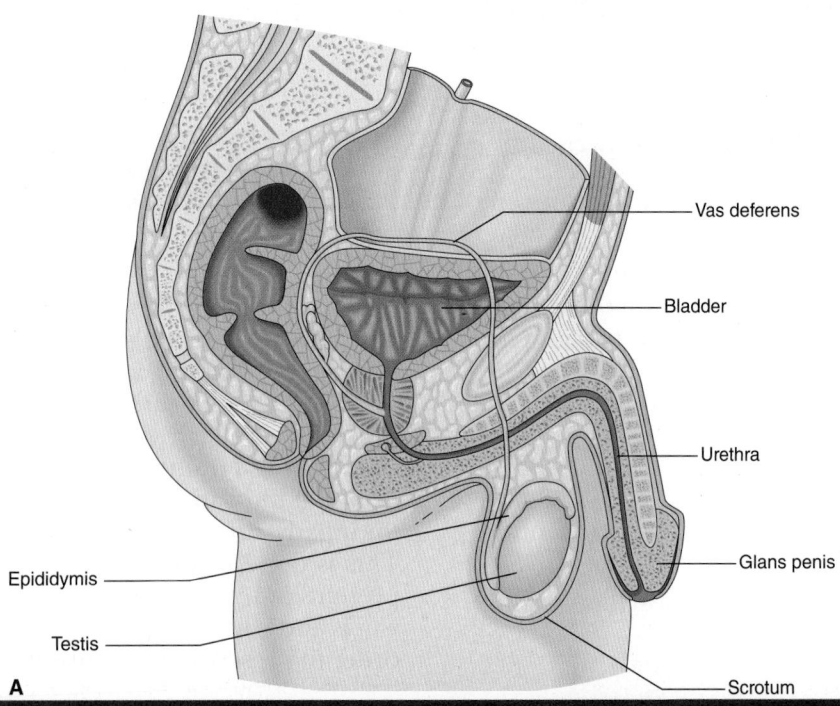

FIGURE 29-53   (A) Cross-sectional view of male anatomy showing urethra and bladder.

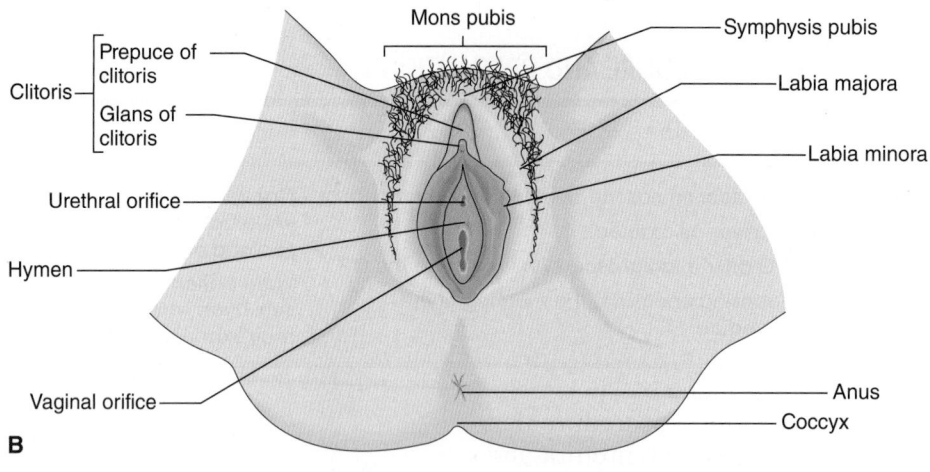

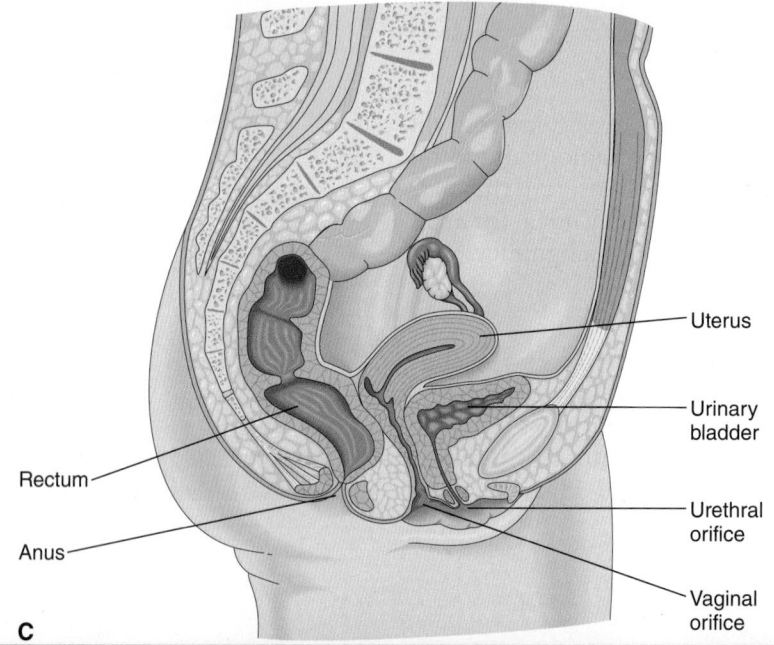

FIGURE 29-53 *(continued)* (B) External genitalia of the female. (C) Cross-sectional view of female anatomy showing urethra and bladder.

and female anatomy related to catheterization. There are basically four reasons to catheterize patients:

1. To obtain a sterile urine specimen for analysis
2. To relieve urinary retention
3. To instill medication into the bladder, after the bladder is emptied
4. To measure the amount of postvoid residual urine

In some cases, this procedure is done by a urologist; however, some providers in obstetrics/gynecology and general and family practice perform or have the medical assistant perform the catheterization. The provider may order a culture and sensitivity test of the urine obtained from catheterization if the patient is experiencing any of the following: dysuria, frequency, hematuria, or urgency. This is done to determine if microorganisms are present and, if so, what the causative microorganism is and which medication would eradicate it, in order to prescribe the appropriate antibiotics.

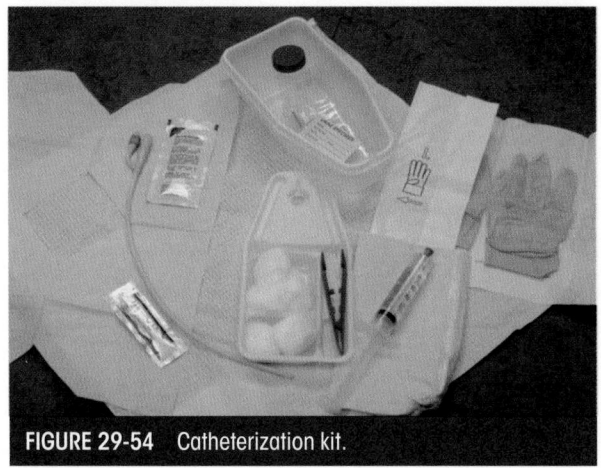
FIGURE 29-54 Catheterization kit.

Sterile technique must be maintained throughout the catheterization. Contamination of any items during the procedure requires discarding the items and obtaining new sterile equipment before continuing the procedure. Procedure 29-22 gives steps for performing a urinary catheterization of a male patient, and Procedure 29-23 gives these steps for a female patient.

Catheterization Equipment. Urinary catheters are sized according to a system of French (Fr) sizes. A common catheter size is Fr 12. The higher the number, the larger the diameter of the catheter. The provider specifies the catheter size when ordering the catheterization procedure. Urethral catheters, sometimes called straight catheters, are used when the catheter is to be removed after the procedure. The Foley catheter is used when the catheter will remain in the urinary bladder (indwelling catheter). A suprapubic catheter (indwelling) is placed in the bladder during a surgical procedure. An incision is made in the suprapubic area. The bladder empties through the catheter.

Sterile, disposable catheterization kits are available that contain all necessary items to perform the procedure (Figure 29-54). Figure 29-55 shows the types of urinary catheterizations.

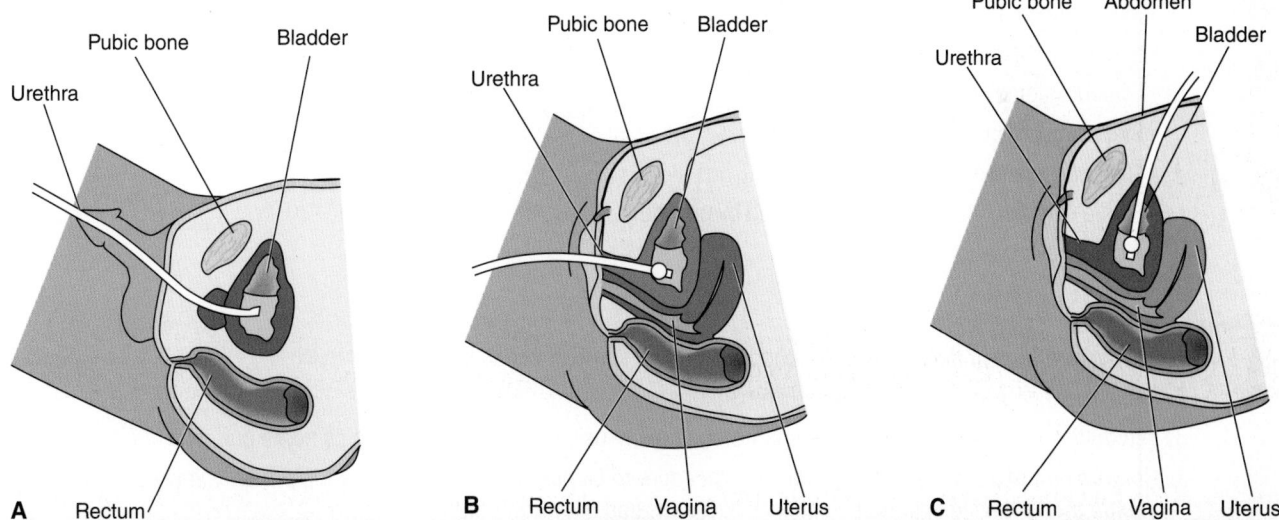
FIGURE 29-55 Types of urinary catheterizations: (A) Straight catheter. (B) Indwelling catheter. (C) Suprapubic catheter.

PROCEDURE 29-22

Procedure

Performing Urinary Catheterization of a Male Patient

STANDARD PRECAUTIONS:

Handwashing

Gloves

Biohazard

PURPOSE:

To obtain a sterile urine specimen for analysis or to relieve urinary retention.

EQUIPMENT/SUPPLIES:

- Catheterization kit (commercially available) containing:
  - Sterile gloves
  - Betadine solution or swabs
  - Lubricant
  - Sterile fenestrated drape
  - Sterile cotton balls
  - Sterile urine container with label
  - Sterile 2-by-2 gauze sponges
  - Forceps (sterile)
  - Sterile absorbent plastic pad
- Additional supplies needed:
  - Sterile catheter (size and type as ordered by provider)
  - Biohazard waste container

PROCEDURE STEPS:

1. ***Paying attention to detail***, assemble supplies needed for the procedure.
2. Wash your hands and follow Standard Precautions.
3. Introduce yourself and confirm the identity of the patient using two identifiers, such as name and date of birth.
4. ***Confirm and explain the rationale for the procedure to be performed***, *speaking at the patient's level of under-standing*. Take time to answer the patient's questions and allay any fears.
5. Make sure that the lighting is sufficient for the procedure.
6. ***Be courteous and respectful*** and ask the patient to disrobe below the waist. Provide a drape for the patient's lower body to help the patient to maintain personal boundaries for comfort.
7. ***Attend to any special needs the patient might have*** and help the patient onto the examination table and into the semi-Fowler's position.
8. Wash your hands again and open the outer wrapping of the sterile kit. This will serve as the sterile field. Using sterile technique, open the second kit containing the catheter.
9. Don the sterile gloves contained in the sterile kit.

continues

10. Take a few moments to set up the tray by opening the Betadine swabs. Open and dispense the lubricating jelly into one of the reservoirs in the plastic tray. Place the tip of the catheter into the lubricant and, using sterile technique, drop the sterile catheter in the field.

11. Utilizing sterile principles, place the sterile absorbent plastic pad under the patient's buttocks.

12. Ask the patient to keep knees apart while you open the fenestrated drape and place it over the genitals utilizing sterile technique (Figure 29-56). RATIONALE: This allows for access to the urinary meatus.

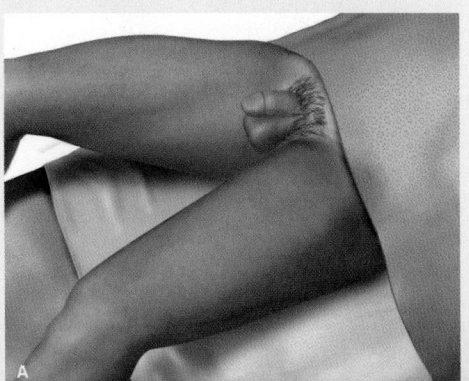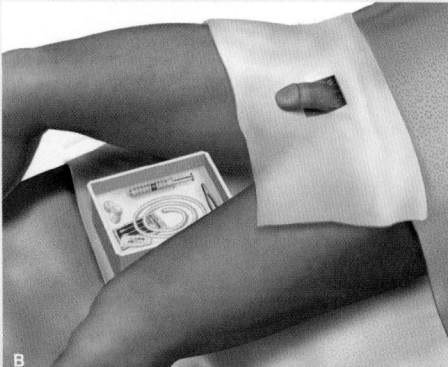

FIGURE 29-56 (A) First, have patient bend knees and separate legs. Then place sterile underpad between patient's legs. (B) Open fenestrated drape. Be careful not to contaminate sterile underpad or drape. Place over penis.

13. Instruct the patient to breathe slowly and deeply during the procedure to help relax the abdominal and pelvic muscles, making insertion of the catheter easier.

14. Use the nondominant hand to hold the penis just below the glans. If the patient is uncircumcised, the foreskin must be pulled back to expose the meatus by gently grasping the penis at the level of the glans and sliding the hand down the shaft, retracting the foreskin. RATIONALE: In order to maintain the sterility of the dominant hand, this must all be done with the nondominant hand.

15. With the dominant hand, cleanse the meatus in a circular motion using the Betadine swabs. Do this three times, using each of the swabs (Figure 29-57). RATIONALE: Ensures that as many microorganisms as possible will be removed from the meatus and surrounding area before insertion of the sterile catheter.

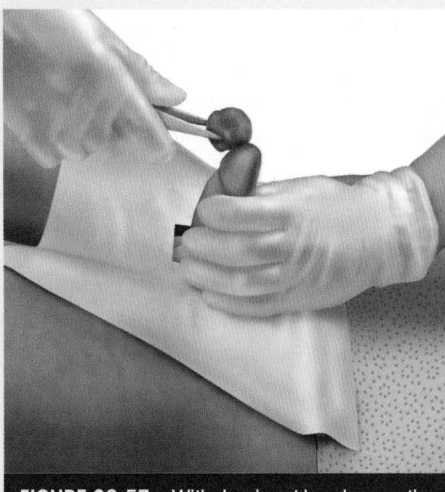

FIGURE 29-57 With dominant hand, grasp the Betadine swab and cleanse around the urinary meatus moving from the center toward the outside. Use all three cotton balls and Betadine.

continues

16. Continue using the dominant hand and pick up the catheter. While holding the penis upright and straight with the nondominant hand, insert the catheter slowly until urine begins to flow (Figure 29-58).

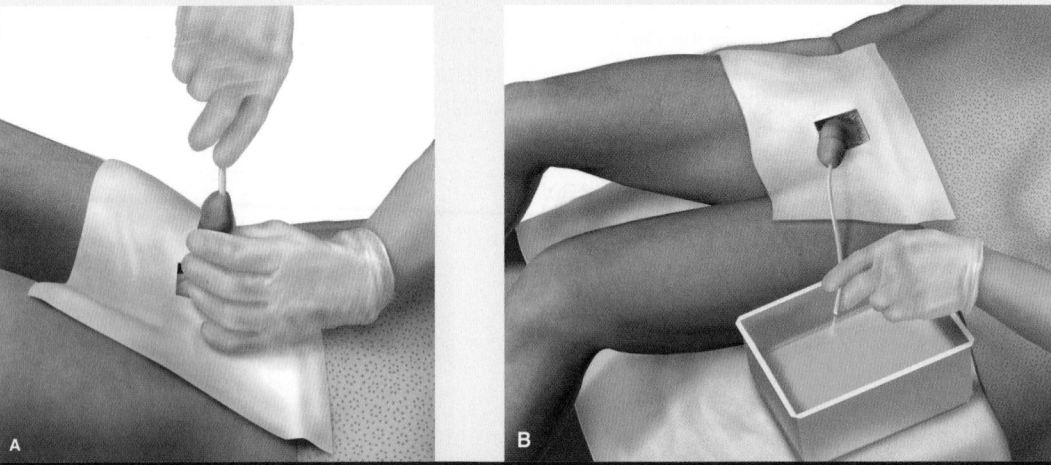

FIGURE 29-58 (A) With the dominant hand, take catheter out of lubricant. With the nondominant hand, hold the head of the penis so that the penis is an upright, straight position. Insert the catheter about 6 inches until urine flows into the sterile specimen cup. (B) Obtain a specimen if ordered.

17. You should not have to force the catheter. If any problems arise, stop the procedure and notify the provider.

18. Pinch or clamp off the catheter to interrupt the flow of urine and position the end of the catheter into the urine specimen container.

19. Collect the specimen by releasing the clamp and filling the collection container. If a urinalysis is required, you will use this collection after the catheterization is complete.

20. Allow the remaining urine to flow into the tray of the sterile catheterization kit until it ceases and then pinch the catheter closed.

21. Remove the catheter gently and slowly and clean off any Betadine from the perineum with 2-by-2 gauze squares.

22. Remove procedural items and dispose of them appropriately. Then remove and discard gloves and wash your hands thoroughly.

23. Help the patient to be comfortable, by either sitting up on the edge of the table, or allowing him to remain horizontal. Once the patient is ready to assume a seated position, assess his color and pulse.

24. If a urine specimen is required for urinalysis, don gloves and label and prepare a specimen container. Attach any laboratory requisition forms and prepare a biohazard transportation bag.

25. Remove gloves and wash your hands. Offer the patient tissues to clean up any lubricant. Provide the patient privacy to get dressed.

26. Clean the room and table.

27. Document the procedure in the patient's medical record, making sure to include the amount of urine collected, any specimens sent to the laboratory for testing, and any observations regarding the patient's tolerance for the procedure.

DOCUMENTATION:

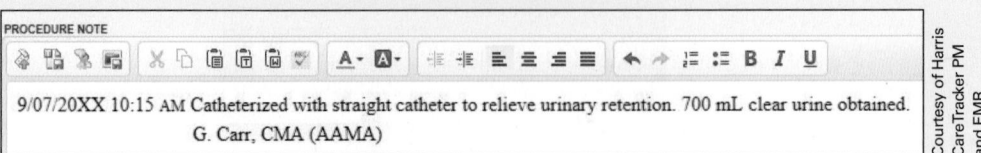

9/07/20XX 10:15 AM Catheterized with straight catheter to relieve urinary retention. 700 mL clear urine obtained. G. Carr, CMA (AAMA)

PROCEDURE 29-23

Procedure

Performing Urinary Catheterization of a Female Patient

STANDARD PRECAUTIONS:

Handwashing

Gloves

Biohazard

PURPOSE:

To obtain a sterile urine specimen for analysis or to relieve urinary retention.

EQUIPMENT/SUPPLIES:

- Catheterization kit (commercially available) containing:
  - Sterile gloves
  - Betadine solution or swabs
  - Lubricant
  - Sterile fenestrated drape
  - Sterile cotton balls
  - Sterile urine container with label
  - Sterile 2 × 2 gauze sponges
  - Forceps (sterile)
  - Sterile absorbent plastic pad
- Additional supplies needed:
  - Sterile catheter (size and type as ordered by provider)
  - Biohazard waste container

PROCEDURE STEPS:

1. ***Paying attention to detail,*** assemble supplies needed for the procedure.
2. Wash your hands and follow Standard Precautions.
3. Introduce yourself and confirm the identity of the patient using two identifiers, such as name and date of birth.
4. ***Confirm and explain the rationale for the procedure to be performed, speaking at the patient's level of understanding.*** Take time to answer the patient's questions and allay any fears.
5. Make sure that the lighting is sufficient for the procedure.
6. Be courteous and respectful and ask the patient to disrobe below the waist. Provide a drape for the patient's lower body to help the patient to maintain personal boundaries for comfort.
7. Attend to any special needs the patient might have and help the patient onto the examination table and into the dorsal lithotomy position. RATIONALE: This allows for access to the urinary meatus.
8. Wash your hands again and open the outer wrapping of the sterile kit. This will serve as the sterile field. Open the second kit containing the catheter using sterile technique.
9. Don the sterile gloves contained in the sterile kit.

continues

10. Take a few moments to set up the tray: Open the Betadine swabs; open and dispense the lubricating jelly into one of the reservoirs in the plastic tray; and place the tip of the catheter into the lubricant and, using sterile technique, drop the sterile catheter in the field.

11. Utilizing sterile principles, place the sterile absorbent plastic pad under the patient's buttocks.

12. Ask the patient to keep knees apart while you utilize sterile technique and open the fenestrated drape and place it over the genitals. RATIONALE: This position provides access to the genital area and good visualization of the urinary meatus once the labia is separated.

13. Instruct the patient to breathe slowly and deeply during the procedure. RATIONALE: This helps relax the abdominal and pelvic muscles, making insertion of the catheter easier.

14. Spread the labia with the nondominant hand. With the dominant hand, use the Betadine swabs to cleanse the urethral meatus, swabbing form anterior to posterior.

15. With a front to back motion, use each of the three swabs to cleanse the meatus. Discard each swab in the biohazard container after using.

16. Do not release the labia with the nondominant hand. RATIONALE: Holding the labia open will keep the urinary meatus from being contaminated while inserting the catheter.

17. Using the sterile dominant hand, pick up the catheter and hold it 3 to 4 inches from the lubricated end, keeping the other end of the catheter in the sterile tray.

18. Gently insert the lubricated tip of the catheter into the urinary meatus and advance until urine begins to flow.

19. You should not have to force the catheter. If any problems arise, stop the procedure and notify the provider.

20. Pinch or clamp off the catheter to interrupt the flow of urine and position the end of the catheter into the urine specimen container.

21. Collect the specimen by releasing the clamp and filling the collection container. If a urinalysis is required, you will use this collection after the catheterization is complete.

22. Allow the remaining urine to flow into the tray of the sterile catheterization kit until it ceases and then pinch the catheter closed.

23. Remove the catheter gently and slowly and clean off any Betadine from the perineum with 2-by-2 gauze squares.

24. Remove procedural items and dispose of them appropriately. Then remove and discard gloves and wash your hands thoroughly.

25. Help the patient to be comfortable, by either sitting up on the edge of the table, or allowing her to remain horizontal. Once the patient is ready to assume a seated position, assess her color and pulse.

26. If a urine specimen is required for urinalysis, don gloves and label and prepare a specimen container. Attach any laboratory requisition forms and prepare a biohazard transportation bag.

27. Remove gloves and wash your hands. Offer the patient tissues to clean up any lubricant. Provide the patient privacy to get dressed.

28. Clean the room and table.

29. Document the procedure in the patient's medical record, making sure to include the amount of urine collected, any specimens sent to the laboratory for testing, and any observations regarding the patient's tolerance for the procedure.

DOCUMENTATION:

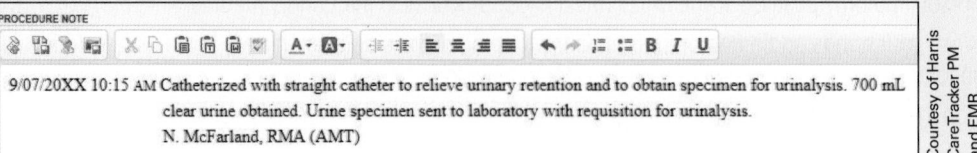

PROCEDURE NOTE

9/07/20XX 10:15 AM Catheterized with straight catheter to relieve urinary retention and to obtain specimen for urinalysis. 700 mL clear urine obtained. Urine specimen sent to laboratory with requisition for urinalysis.
N. McFarland, RMA (AMT)

Courtesy of Harris CareTracker PM and EMR

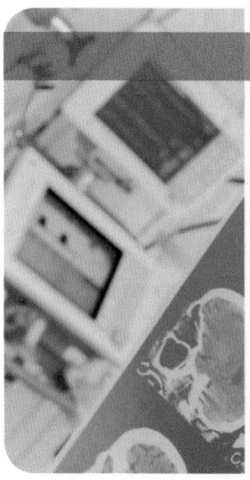

CASE STUDY 29-1

Refer to the scenario at the beginning of the chapter.

Both medical assistants are responsible for ensuring that the supplies and equipment needed for the specialty examinations are available and that safety precautions are followed before, during, and after the examination.

CASE STUDY REVIEW

1. Determine what supplies and equipment should be assembled for the following specialty examinations: fecal occult blood testing, performing an eye instillation, performing an ear irrigation, and performing color vision testing.
2. Explain four safety precautions that must be in place when allergy skin testing is being performed.

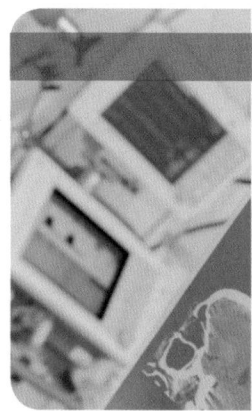

CASE STUDY 29-2

Corey Bayer is a 15-year-old patient at Inner City Health Care. He sustained an injury to his right wrist today during soccer practice. Dr. Osborne examined him and ordered a radiograph of the right forearm. The results show that Corey has sustained a Colles fracture of the right wrist. Dr. Osborne asks you to prepare the equipment to apply a cast.

CASE STUDY REVIEW

1. Describe cast application. What are the medical assistant's responsibilities?
2. After Corey's cast application, describe the cast care instructions that will be given to him and his mother.

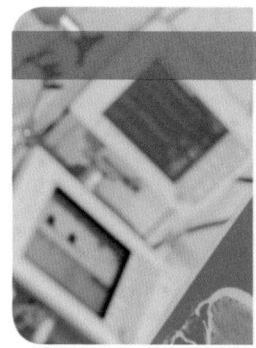

CASE STUDY 29-3

Dr. Osborne has scheduled Anita Blanchette for a spirometry test and wants you to telephone her the day before the test to prepare her so that optimal results are obtained.

CASE STUDY REVIEW

1. What information do you give to Anita before her spirometry so that the best test results can be obtained?
2. How would you explain the rationale for the performance of this procedure?

- A thorough knowledge and understanding of the various body system examinations and clinical procedures routinely performed as part of patient care will enhance the quality of care given.

- Some of the specialty procedures are performed on a routine basis in the ambulatory care setting; others are performed occasionally and perhaps only in larger settings that offer specialized and primary care.

- In order to feel comfortable assisting with the less common procedures, medical assistants may need to broaden their base of knowledge by conducting independent research.

- Medical assistants who are willing to constantly expand their clinical understanding will not only fine-tune their professional skills but will derive greater satisfaction from their job performance, and increase their career options.

- A grasp of the structures included in the integumentary system allows the medical assistant to assist the provider in testing patients for allergies.

- The neurologic exam screens for disorders of the nervous system. During this exam, sight, smell, hearing, touch, and taste are evaluated to reflect the health of the nervous system (including the cranial nerves).

- Coordination, gait, and reflexes are observed as a part of the neurologic examination.

- Evaluation of sight includes the use of a Snellen chart, Ishihara plates, and Jaeger charts. Familiarity with these tools allows the medical assistant to help with these exams.

- Hearing is evaluated using tools such as a tuning fork and an audiometer.

- Evaluation of the respiratory system includes auscultation of breath sounds, patient history, respiratory rate measurement, and spirometry.

- Proficiency in drawing venous blood samples allows for evaluation of the blood and lymph systems.

- Musculoskeletal evaluation includes assessment of bones, joints, muscles, and surrounding tissues. Treatment of musculoskeletal abnormalities includes splint and cast application.

- Gastrointestinal system health is demonstrated by active bowel sounds on auscultation, soft abdomen on palpation, negative occult blood testing, and endoscopic studies. The medical assistant is responsible for patient teaching to ensure that the patient is properly prepared for this type of testing.

- Often, the assessment of the urinary system includes catheterization of the patient to obtain sterile urine. Procedures such as an intravenous pyelogram, cystoscopy, or kidney biopsy require patient teaching so that the patient will be prepared for these invasive tests.

Study for Success

To reinforce your knowledge and skills of information presented in this chapter:

- Review the *Key Terms* and *Learning Outcomes*

- Consider the *Critical Thinking* features and *Case Studies* and discuss your conclusions

- Answer the questions in the *Certification Review*

- Perform the *Procedures* using the *Competency Assessment Checklists* on the *Student Companion Website*

Procedure

CERTIFICATION REVIEW

1. What is the name of the elevated skin lesions affecting the epidermis caused by the papillomaviruses?
   a. Scleroderma
   b. Moles
   c. Calluses
   d. Warts

2. What is the disorder that is characterized by discomfort of the muscles, tendons, ligaments, and soft tissues brought on by trauma, strain, and emotional stress?
   a. Carpal tunnel syndrome
   b. Bursitis
   c. Gout
   d. Fibromyalgia
   e. Tendonitis

3. What type of fracture has its bone fragments driven into each other?
   a. Greenstick
   b. Impacted
   c. Oblique
   d. Comminuted

4. What disease is caused by a degeneration of brain cells caused by lack of dopamine, bringing about muscle rigidity and akinesia?
   a. Multiple sclerosis
   b. Bell's palsy
   c. Parkinson disease
   d. Tic douloureux
   e. Lou Gehrig disease

5. Which of the following terms is the medical name for an acute circumscribed infection of the subcutaneous tissues caused by *Staphylococcus*?
   a. Comedone
   b. Carbuncle
   c. Verruca
   d. Psoriasis

6. A device that provides a specific amount of medication per puff of medication describes which of the following?
   a. A ventilator to increase lung volume
   b. A spacer that contains medication
   c. A metered dose inhaler
   d. A nebulizer
   e. A spirometer

7. A reflex hammer, alcohol swab, and cotton ball are supplies for which system assessment?
   a. Integumentary
   b. Musculoskeletal
   c. Neurologic
   d. Immune

8. Scratch, patch, and intradermal testing are part of which system testing?
   a. Integumentary
   b. Immune
   c. Respiratory
   d. Neurologic
   e. Gastrointestinal

9. Occult blood is a test that is commonly performed on which bodily substance?
   a. Feces
   b. Tears
   c. Saliva
   d. Wound exudate

10. Pulse oximetry, usually performed on a fingertip or earlobe, is a measure of which of the following?
    a. Pulse rate
    b. Respiratory rate
    c. Oxygen saturation
    d. Blood pressure
    e. Lung volume

UNIT VIII
ADVANCED TECHNIQUES AND PROCEDURES

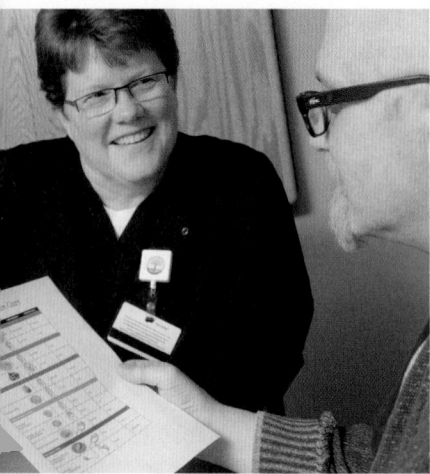
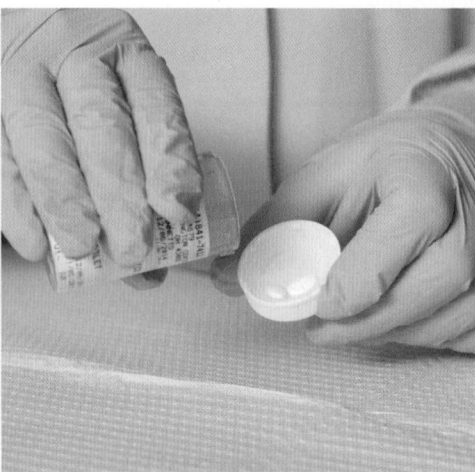
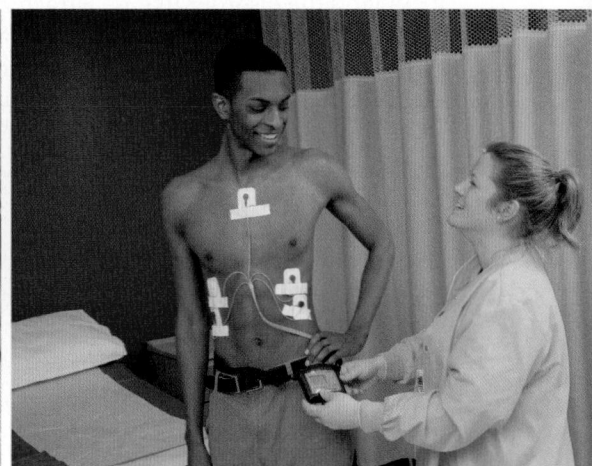

ATTRIBUTES OF PROFESSIONALISM

Providing clinical support to providers in an ambulatory care setting is the vital role of the professional medical assistant. The safety and quality of care provided to patients depends on the medical assistant's competence. In this unit, the focus shifts away from assisting with examinations and treatments that are less invasive to procedures that involve mandatory adherence to sterile technique and detailed attention to processes. There is great responsibility placed on the medical assistant in protecting the patient's health during these procedures.

Organization and the ability to multitask are characteristics that must be developed in order to successfully carry out this aspect of delivering patient care. Because of the demanding nature of the job, medical assistants must be able to handle stress and think clearly on the fly. Strong communication skills, the ability to listen well and share information clearly, and the ability to answer questions fully and succinctly are a part of the skill set that the medical assistant will utilize daily.

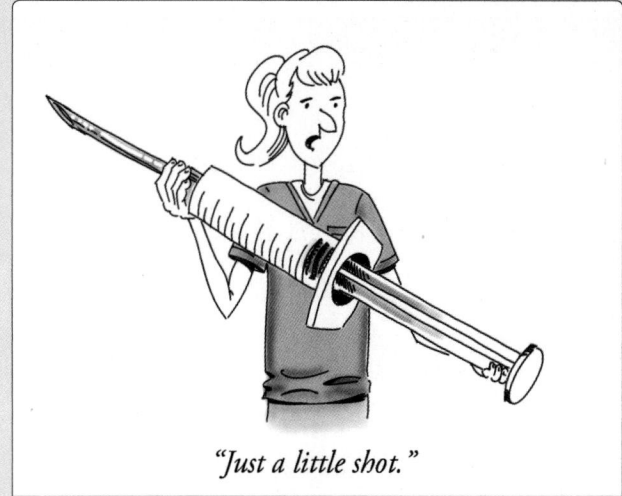

"Just a little shot."

Listed below are a series of questions for you to ask yourself, to serve as a professionalism checklist. As you interact with patients and colleagues, these questions will help to guide you in the professional behavior and therapeutic communication that is expected every day from medical assistants.

Ask Yourself

COMMUNICATION
- ☐ Do I apply active listening skills?
- ☐ Do I explain to patients the rationale for performance of a procedure?
- ☐ Do I speak at each patient's level of understanding?
- ☐ Do I respond honestly and diplomatically to my patients' concerns?
- ☐ Do I refrain from sharing my personal experiences?
- ☐ Do I include the patient's support system as indicated?
- ☐ Does my knowledge allow me to speak easily with all members of the health care team?
- ☐ Do I accurately and concisely update the provider on any aspect of a patient's care?

PRESENTATION
- ☐ Do my actions attend to both the psychological and the physiologic aspects of a patient's illness or condition?
- ☐ Am I courteous, patient, and respectful to patients?
- ☐ Do I display a calm, professional, and caring manner?
- ☐ Do I demonstrate empathy to the patient?
- ☐ Do I show awareness of patients' concerns related to the procedure being performed?

COMPETENCY
- ☐ Do I pay attention to detail?
- ☐ Do I ask questions if I am out of my comfort zone or do not have the experience to carry out tasks?
- ☐ Do I display sound judgment?
- ☐ Am I knowledgeable and accountable?
- ☐ Do I incorporate critical thinking skills in performing patient assessment and care?
- ☐ Do I recognize the implications for failure to comply with Centers for Disease Control and Prevention regulations in health care settings?

INITIATIVE
- ☐ Do I show initiative?
- ☐ Do I seek out opportunities to expand my knowledge base?
- ☐ Am I flexible and dependable?
- ☐ Do I direct the patient to other resources when necessary or helpful, with the approval of the provider?

INTEGRITY
- ☐ Do I demonstrate the principles of self-boundaries?
- ☐ Do I work within my scope of practice?
- ☐ Do I demonstrate sensitivity to patient rights?
- ☐ Do I protect the integrity of the medical record?
- ☐ Do I protect and maintain confidentiality?
- ☐ Do I immediately report any error I made?

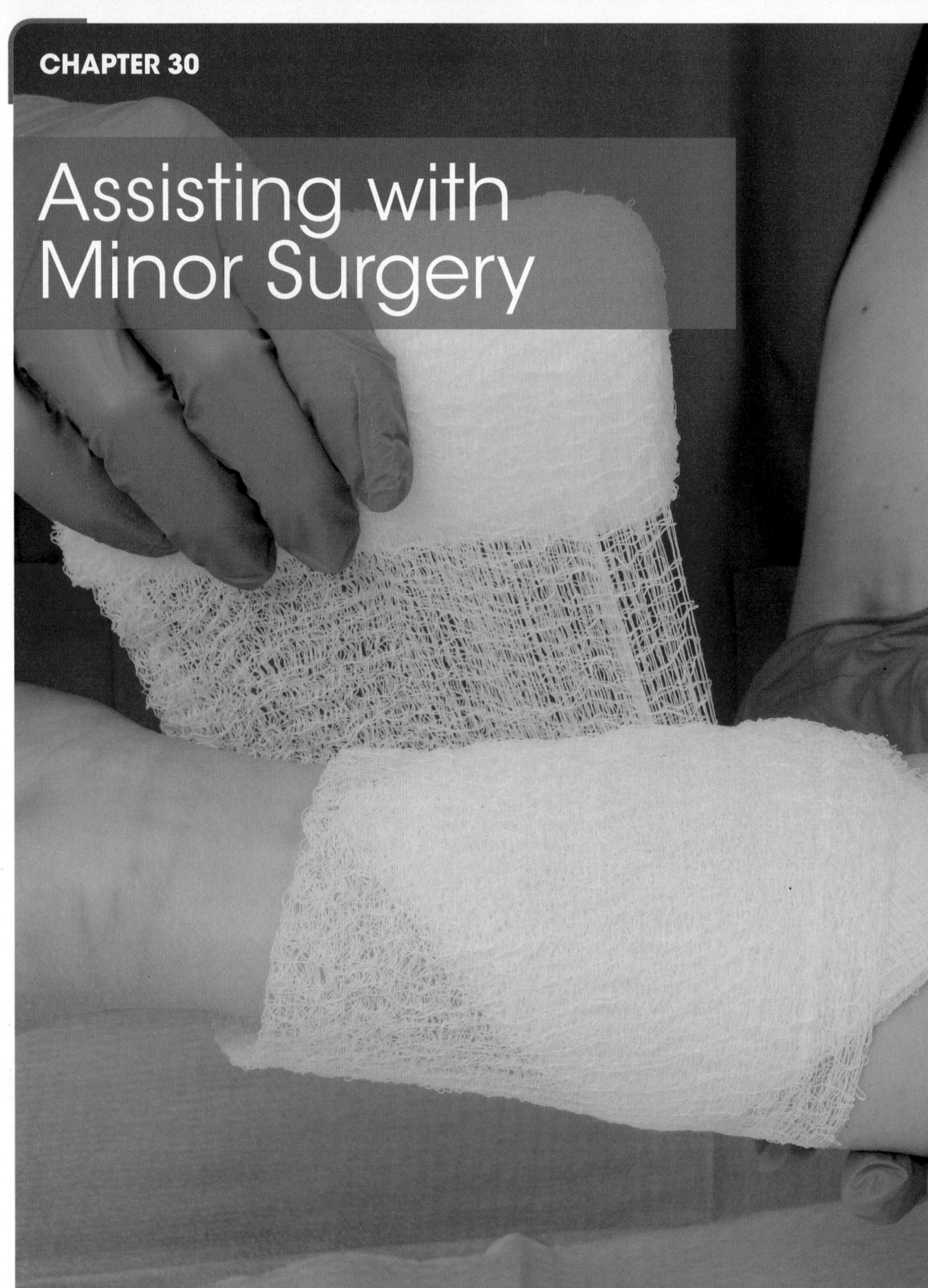

CHAPTER 30

Assisting with Minor Surgery

1. Define and spell the key terms as presented in the glossary.
2. Recognize surgical asepsis and differentiate between surgical asepsis and medical asepsis.
3. List eight basic rules to follow to protect sterile areas.
4. Cite four methods of sterilization.
5. Assemble supplies and equipment necessary to achieve surgical asepsis when using an autoclave.
6. Explain competent wrapping and operation of the autoclave.
7. Outline storage measures and expiration periods for autoclaved materials.
8. Explain the sizing standards of suture material and the criteria used to select the most appropriate type and size.
9. Given a variety of surgical instruments, be able to identify each and describe its intended use.
10. Demonstrate the ability to select the most appropriate type of dressings for a given situation.
11. Determine advantages and disadvantages of Betadine, Hibiclens, isopropyl alcohol, and hydrogen peroxide when each is used as a skin antiseptic.
12. Define anesthesia, and explain the advantages and disadvantages of epinephrine as an additive to injectable anesthetics.
13. Summarize five preoperative concerns to be addressed in patient preparation and education.
14. Summarize five postoperative concerns to be addressed with the patient and the caregiver.
15. Demonstrate applying sterile gloves.
16. Demonstrate setting up a surgical tray, including laying the field, applying supplies and instruments, pouring a sterile solution, using transfer forceps, and covering the sterile tray.
17. Explain what is meant by alternative surgical methods.

KEY TERMS

anesthesia	informed consent
approximate	isopropyl alcohol
autoclave	ligature
avascularized	Mayo stand/instrument trays
Betadine	nevi
caustic	preference cards
cautery	ratchets
contamination	sitz bath
electrosurgery	steam sterilization
epinephrine	sterile field
exudate	strictures
fenestrated	suppurant
friable	surgical asepsis
Hibiclens	suture
infection	swaged
inflammation	volatile

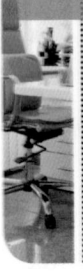

SCENARIO

Dr. Mark Beahm is a solo practitioner and runs a busy cosmetic surgery practice. He frequently performs smaller surgical procedures in his clinic. Today, Ms. Betty Jo Wells is in the clinic to have a suspicious skin lesion removed from her left forearm. This lesion is suspected basal cell carcinoma. Jessica Goodwin, RMA (AMT), is Dr. Beahm's lead medical assistant. It is her responsibility to prepare the room for the procedure, including the sterile tray. It is also her responsibility to care for the instruments and specimen after the procedure. Ms. Goodwin pulls Dr. Beahm's preference card and begins to collect the supplies needed for this procedure.

Clinic/ambulatory surgery differs from hospital surgery not only in complexity, but in the supplies, equipment, instruments, and personnel needed. Some office/ambulatory surgery is performed by the provider alone; some surgeries require the assistance of the medical assistant. Most ambulatory care settings do not need a large variety of surgical instruments but often need more than one of the more frequently used instruments. As a personal preference, special instruments may be purchased and maintained for a specific provider to use during a particular surgical procedure. These particular instruments are generally not used by the other providers.

The equipment and supplies used in office/ambulatory surgery are usually portable and easily maintained. Larger practices that perform many office/ambulatory surgeries generally can afford the space and expense of maintaining a special room just for that purpose. Often patient examination rooms serve as small surgical suites with portable **Mayo stands/instrument trays**, supplies, and equipment brought into the room for the procedure.

Whether assisting with minor surgery is a routine or an infrequent event for the medical assistant, it is nonetheless important to be knowledgeable about sterile technique, the use and care of instruments and the room, as well as patient preparation for the surgery. Medical assistants should understand the preferences of each provider on staff to make the surgical procedure comfortable and effective for both patient and provider.

SURGICAL ASEPSIS AND STERILIZATION

Surgical asepsis means all microbial life (pathogens and nonpathogens) is destroyed before an invasive procedure is performed. Therefore, all equipment to be used is sterile. The terms *surgical asepsis* and *sterile technique* often are used interchangeably.

Regardless of the number and complexity of surgical procedures performed in the clinic or ambulatory care center, surgical asepsis must be strictly maintained. Surgical asepsis uses practices known as sterile techniques and these techniques are always used during an invasive procedure. Some examples of invasive procedures include creating an opening in the skin such as a surgical incision, suturing a laceration, giving an injection, or inserting a sterile catheter into a sterile body cavity such as the urinary bladder.

Because microorganisms are on virtually every surface, such as skin, instruments, surgical instrument trays, clothing, and even in the air, it is necessary to destroy as many as possible before performing any surgical procedure. Surgical asepsis or sterile technique prevents microorganism entry into the body during an invasive procedure and, therefore, helps to protect the patient from infection. Once the items and areas are sterilized, every precaution must be taken to prevent **contamination** of the sterile items or areas either by a nonsterile item or surface or from airborne contamination. In this context, to contaminate means to make impure; for example, by introducing microorganisms or infectious material into or onto sterile goods or areas. The cardinal rule for maintaining surgical asepsis is "If in doubt, throw it out." There is no room for error when protecting a patient from the introduction of pathogens into the body during an invasive procedure. It is the responsibility of the medical assistant to scrupulously maintain sterility of all instruments, sutures, and other items utilized during a procedure.

Procedure

Living tissue surfaces such as skin cannot be sterilized but can be made as free of pathogens as possible before the use of a sterile covering. One example of this concept is the use of the surgical hand cleansing technique before applying sterile gloves (see Procedure 30-1). Another example of surgical asepsis is preparing the patient's skin with a surgical scrub solution before applying sterile drapes around the intended surgical site.

PROCEDURE 30-1

Procedure

Applying Sterile Gloves

STANDARD PRECAUTIONS:

Handwashing

PURPOSE:

To apply sterile gloves without compromising sterility. Because hands cannot be sterilized, everyone performing sterile procedures must wear sterile gloves.

EQUIPMENT/SUPPLIES:

- Packaged pair of sterile gloves of appropriate size
- Flat, clean, dry surface

PROCEDURE STEPS:

1. Remove rings and watch or other wrist wear. RATIONALE: Rings and watches can snag and tear gloves, and therefore interfere with barrier protection.

2. Wash hands using surgical asepsis.

3. Inspect glove package for tears or stains (Figure 30-1A). RATIONALE: Tears and stains indicate that the gloves are no longer considered sterile and must be disposed of or used for a nonsterile purpose.

4. Place the glove package on a clean, dry, flat surface at or above waist level. RATIONALE: Using a contaminated surface could compromise the sterility of the sterile package.

5. *Paying attention to detail,* peel open the package taking care not to touch the sterile inner surface of the package. Do not allow the gloves to slide beyond the sterile inner border (Figure 30-1B). RATIONALE: Care must be taken to maintain the sterility of the gloves.

6. Carefully place the inner packaging on a flat, dry surface. Ensure that the illustration of the hand on the outside of the packaging is positioned with the fingers pointed away from you. RATIONALE: Sterile gloves are packaged in this position for ease of application.

7. Carefully, flip open the inner paper wrapper to expose the folded edges. Smooth the edges open. There will be one last fold visible. Grasp this fold and open the final covering of sterile gloves. Be careful not to allow the sterile gloves to come into contact with your hands.

8. With the index finger and thumb of the nondominant hand, grasp the inner cuffed edge of the opposite glove. Without dragging or dangling the fingers over any nonsterile area, pick the glove straight up off the package surface. RATIONALE: Picking up the glove by grasping the inner cuff prevents the outer glove from becoming contaminated. Strict adherence must be made to the sterile principles.

9. With the palm up on the dominant hand, stand away from the sterile package and carefully slide the hand into the glove. It is imperative that the outer, sterile surface of the glove does not come into contact with anything.

10. Always hold the hands above the waist and away from the body with the palms up (Figure 30-1C).

11. With the newly gloved hand, pick up the remaining glove by slipping gloved fingers under the cuff. Lift the second glove up, again keeping it above the waist and away from the body. As before, do not allow the glove

(continues)

to drag outside of the sterile area or to touch anything (Figure 30-1D). RATIONALE: The outside of the second glove is sterile and may be touched only by another sterile surface.

12. With the palm up, slip the second hand into the glove. Again, it is important that the outside of the glove not touch any of your skin. You should be particularly careful of your thumb in this regard (Figure 30-1E).

13. Adjust the gloves as needed, but avoid touching any of your skin, particularly the wrist area. Do not allow your gloved hands to touch any nonsterile surface and keep them above the waist and away from your body (Figures 30-1F and G).

14. If, at any time, any part of the sterile, gloved hand touches a nonsterile object, the gloves must be discarded, and the gloving procedure should begin again with a new set of sterile gloves. Remember, "If in doubt, throw it out."

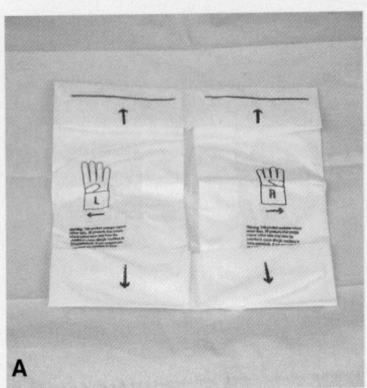

A

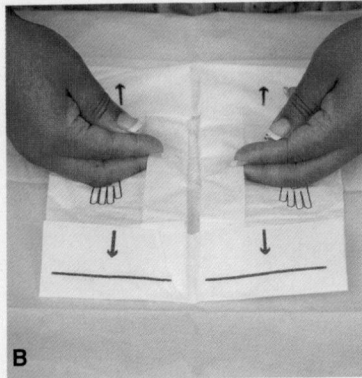

B

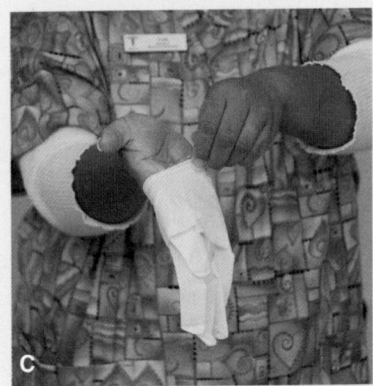

C

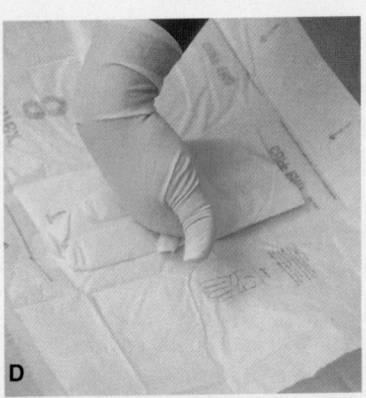

D

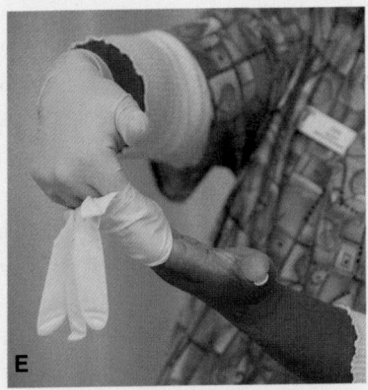

E

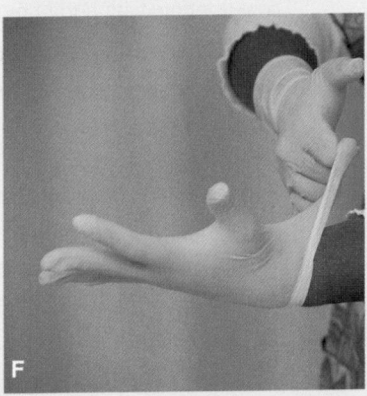

F

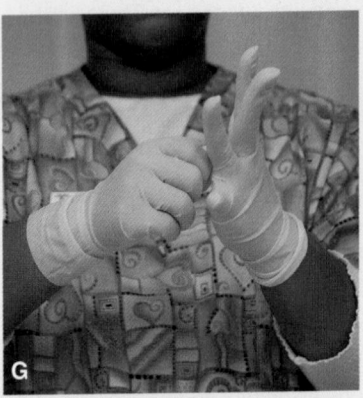

G

FIGURE 30-1 (A) Sterile gloves are packaged with right and left clearly marked. (B) Using only the fingertips, reach in from each side and grasp the edges of the paper. Pull out and lay paper flat without touching any area except the very edges. (C) With the nondominant hand, grasp the inner cuffed edge of the opposite glove. Pick the glove up and step away from the sterile area, keeping your hands above your waste and away from your body. With palm up on the dominant hand, slide the hand into the glove. (D) Step back to the sterile area. With the gloved hand, pick up the glove for the remaining hand by slipping four fingers under the outside of the cuff. (E) With palm up, slip the second hand into the glove. Keep the gloved thumb extended and away from the rest of the fingers. (F) Keeping hands above the waist and away from the body, pull on the second glove. (G) Adjust gloves if needed. Remember to avoid touching the wrist area. Keep gloved hands above the waist and away from the body at all times.

Refer to Chapter 21 for more complete information on the concepts of asepsis and aseptic techniques, including hand cleansing for medical asepsis.

The differences between hand cleansing for medical asepsis as discussed in Chapter 21 (see Procedure 21-1) and hand cleansing for surgical asepsis are addressed in the Table 30-1.

Hand Cleansing (Hand Hygiene) for Medical and Surgical Asepsis

Hand cleansing (hygiene) for medical asepsis is defined as removing pathogenic microorganisms from the hands after they become contaminated. Medical hand cleansing is used many times throughout the day to cleanse the skin after removing contaminated gloves, assisting with patient care, and touching surfaces that are used by and near to the patient.

Preparation for an invasive procedure requires a surgical hand scrub to achieve surgical asepsis for all health care personnel who will participate in any invasive procedure during an episode of patient care. This is a crucial step in preventing health care–associated infections (HAI). A major risk factor for HAI is the behavior of health care professionals regarding decontamination, hand hygiene/asepsis, and compliance with universal precautions.

The beginning steps of the surgical scrub involve antimicrobial soap; warm water; and vigorous scrubbing of hands, wrists, and forearms. This process begins with removing any jewelry. The scrub includes cleaning under the nails, applying the soap, and scrubbing the hands for at least 3 minutes. The first 2 minutes are focused on the fingers, palms, and the posterior aspect of the hands. Next, scrub the wrist area and the arms to at least a few inches above the elbows for an additional minute. Care should be taken to keep the hands above the elbows during the entire scrub process to avoid contamination from the bacteria-laden soap running across the already clean areas of skin. Always maintain the hands above the

TABLE 30-1

DIFFERENCES BETWEEN MEDICAL AND SURGICAL HAND CLEANSING (HYGIENE)

MEDICAL HAND CLEANSING (HYGIENE)	SURGICAL HAND CLEANSING (HYGIENE)
Liquid soap and water sufficient for most routine clinical activities	Performed before any invasive procedure
One-minute duration	Three- to 6-minute duration
Wash hands and wrists	Wash hands, wrists, and forearms to the elbows; brush may be used
Hands should be held down during rinsing	Hands should be held up during washing and rinsing
Scrub nails with brush and clean under each nail with cuticle stick	Scrub nails with brush and clean under each nail with cuticle stick
Alcohol-based preparations are practical alternatives to soap and water on visibly clean hands	Alcohol-based applications have no role in surgical asepsis
Apply lotion*	Do not apply lotion
Utilize Universal Precautions	Glove for sterility
	Higher level of decontamination

*The use of lotions is encouraged to help prevent chafing of the skin, especially with frequent hand cleansings. Nevertheless, studies have determined that lotions containing petroleum or mineral oil can break down latex and should be avoided if latex gloves are going to be worn within 1 hour after applying the lotion. If lotions are applied immediately before gloving, the use of water-based lotions is recommended. Of special interest to persons with latex sensitivities (see Chapter 21) is the fact that using lotions and creams containing petroleum products actually increases the amount of latex protein that is transferred from the gloves into the skin, thereby increasing the symptoms of latex sensitivity.

elbows while rinsing hands and arms, and avoid contact with any of the surfaces of the sink.

After a thorough drying of the hands and then the arms, taking care not to contaminate the areas of the hands that have been scrubbed, it is appropriate to don sterile gloves and prepare for the procedure.

Proper protocol when assisting with surgery requires the use of surgical hand cleansing at the beginning of each workday, as well as before every sterile technique, with the complementary use of medical hand cleansing before leaving the clinic and when returning and between patients and procedures. Any opening in the medical assistant's skin should be covered with a sterile adhesive dressing, and gloves are worn during any direct patient contact. See Chapter 21 for information on medical asepsis and Standard Precautions.

STERILE PRINCIPLES

Sterile principles are a set of guidelines designed to designate what items and areas are considered sterile and what actions cause contamination. Some areas are logical and clear, some are subtle and less clear. Some surfaces, such as skin, cannot be sterilized. Large items such as Mayo stands and their trays cannot fit into an autoclave for sterilization. To create sterile areas and surfaces where sterility is not possible, sterile barriers should be used; for example, sterile gloves can be worn over the hands. Sterile drapes can be applied to trays once they have been washed, rinsed, dried, and disinfected.

Guidelines to protect sterile items and areas include:

- A sterile object may not touch a nonsterile object.
- Sterile objects must not be wet. Moisture can draw microorganisms into or onto the sterile object.
- An acceptable border between a sterile area and a nonsterile area is 1 inch. The portion of a drape that hangs over the edge is considered nonsterile, no matter what its size. Sterile articles should be placed in the center of the **sterile field** and away from the edge as much as possible.
- Do not turn your back on a sterile field. If you cannot see the field, you cannot be aware of what touched it.
- Anything below the waist is considered contaminated. In support of this principle, all surgery trays should be positioned above waist level. All articles are to be held above the waist.

- All sterile objects (such as gloved hands) must be held in front and away from the body and above waist level.
- Do not cough, sneeze, or talk over a sterile field. Airborne particles may fall onto the sterile area and contaminate it.
- Do not reach over the sterile area. Contaminants may fall onto the area and clothing may touch, thereby contaminating the area. Spend as little time as possible reaching into the sterile area.
- Do not pass contaminated dressings or instruments over the sterile field.
- Arrange for the provider to place contaminated instruments into a separate container or area.
- Always be aware of your actions and the actions of others to determine whether the sterile field has been contaminated. When in doubt, err on the side of safety.
- When opening sterile packages, the outer wrapper is contaminated. It should be opened without touching the inner contents, and the contents are then dropped onto the sterile field. Double wrapping can be used (see Procedure 30-3).

Sterile solutions in bottles should be poured into sterile basins or cups on the sterile field without touching the rim of the bottle and without splashing solution onto the sterile field. If the sterile field is not polylined and becomes wet, it is considered contaminated because a field that is wet acts as a wick and draws microorganisms into the article. Using polylined drapes as sterile fields protects against contamination.

METHODS OF STERILIZATION

The goal of sterilization is to eradicate any living microorganisms from the materials being sterilized. This is done to prevent introduction of these organisms into a surgical field. There are four methods of sterilization:

1. Gas sterilization
2. Dry heat sterilization
3. Chemical ("cold") sterilization
4. Steam sterilization (autoclave)

Gas Sterilization

Gas sterilization is considered low-temperature chemical sterilization. Toxic gases permeate and destroy organisms on heat- or moisture-sensitive equipment. This method is best utilized in a hospital or large organizational setting. Ethylene oxide (EO) is toxic and must be properly vented to decrease the risk to health care workers. There is a long aeration time associated with this type of sterilization.

Dry Heat Sterilization

Dry heat sterilization requires higher temperatures than steam sterilization and requires longer exposure times as well. Procedures for wrapping are the same as when wrapping for steam sterilization (see Procedure 30-3). Dry heat is seldom used in today's medical office or clinic.

Chemical ("Cold") Sterilization

Procedure

Chemical sterilization, or cold sterilization, may use the same chemical agents used to chemically disinfect instruments or fomites. However, the exposure time for chemical sterilization is achieved through prolonged immersion. Items must be sanitized first.

The position of the Food and Drug Administration is that sterilization with liquid chemicals is different from sterilization with heat, moisture, or low-temperature gas. It is the position of the CDC that utilization of liquid sterilant is high-level disinfection and does not convey the same sterility assurances as the aforementioned methods.

Chemical sterilization is a method used in many medical clinics when the object being sterilized is too large or too heat sensitive for autoclaving (see following section for information on autoclaving). Fiber optic endoscopes are one of the most common items sterilized with the use of chemicals. These items are delicate and unable to withstand the high heat of an autoclave (Procedure 30-2).

PROCEDURE 30-2

Procedure

Using Chemical "Cold" Sterilization for Endoscopes

STANDARD PRECAUTIONS:

Handwashing   Goggles & Mask

PURPOSE:

To sterilize heat-sensitive items such as fiber optic endoscopes and delicate cutting instruments using appropriate chemical solutions.

EQUIPMENT/SUPPLIES:

- Chemical solution such as Cidex Steris System (peracetic acid)
- Airtight container
- Timer
- Sterile water
- Gloves (heavy-duty)
- Sterile towel
- Plastic-lined sterile drapes
- Sterile transfer forceps
- Sterile basin

(continues)

PROCEDURE STEPS:

1. Sanitize items that require chemical sterilization. Rinse and dry. RATIONALE: Recall that debris and body proteins must be scrubbed from items before sterilization. Ultrasonic cleaning is best.

2. *Paying attention to detail*, read manufacturer's instructions on original container of chemical sterilization solution. RATIONALE: Each brand of chemical sterilization solution has specific preparation instructions and germicidal properties; choose the solution that best fits the needs of the ambulatory care setting. Keep the solution in its original container to reduce chances of accidental poisoning.

3. Put on gloves. RATIONALE: Heavy-duty gloves help protect from sharp items puncturing the skin. Chemicals are harsh on the skin.

4. *Paying attention to detail*, prepare solution as indicated by manufacturer; place the date of opening or preparation on the container and initial it. RATIONALE: Following manufacturer's instructions ensures sterility. Note the expiration date of solution.

5. Pour solution carefully to avoid splashing into a container large enough to accommodate the instrument and allow complete immersion in the sterilizing solution. Be sure the container has an airtight lid (Figures 30-2A and B). RATIONALE: Chemicals should not be left exposed to open air to prevent evaporation and loss of potency, exposure to environmental contaminants, accidental inhalation, or poisoning. Splashing may cause skin or mucous membrane contact and result in injury.

6. Place sanitized and dried items into the solution, completely submerging items. Avoid splashing when placing items into airtight container. RATIONALE: Total immersion is necessary for sterility to be achieved.

7. Close lid of container, label with name of solution, date, and time required per manufacturer, and initial (Figure 30-2C). RATIONALE: Exposure time is the required time indicated by the manufacturer to achieve sterility. Initialing work ensures accountability and responsibility.

8. Do not open lid or add additional items during the processing time. RATIONALE: Adding to the container interrupts the sterilization process and limits the effectiveness of the chemical.

9. Following the recommended processing time, lift items from the container using sterile gloved hands or sterile transfer forceps. Carefully hold each item above sterile basin and pour copious amounts of sterile water over it and through it (endoscopes) until adequately rinsed of chemical solution. RATIONALE: Items once processed are sterile and must be handled appropriately. Using sterile gloved hands or sterile transfer forceps ensures sterile-to-sterile contact and no contamination of the items. Sterile water is poured through the inner channels of endoscopes to rinse chemicals from the inside, as well as the outside.

10. Hold items upright for a few seconds to allow excess sterile water to drip off.

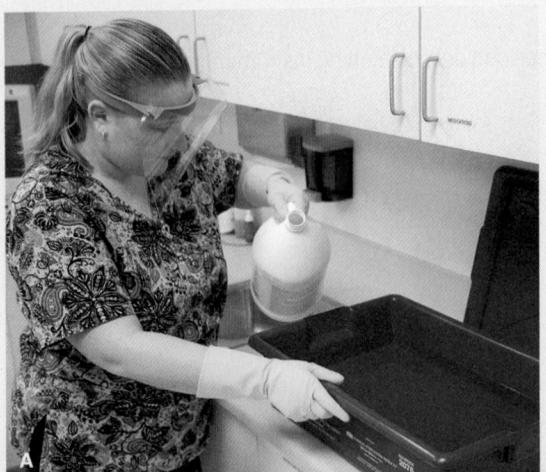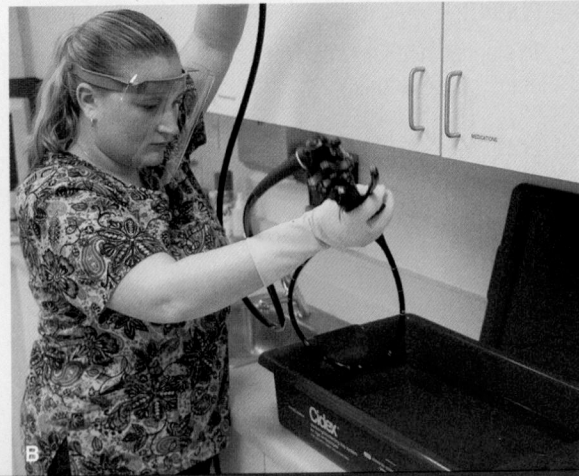

FIGURE 30-2　(A) Medical assistant pours chemical sterilization solution into a large soaking container. Note the use of heavy-duty gloves and face shield. (B) Medical assistant adds the endoscope to the chemical sterilization solution in the container.

(continues)

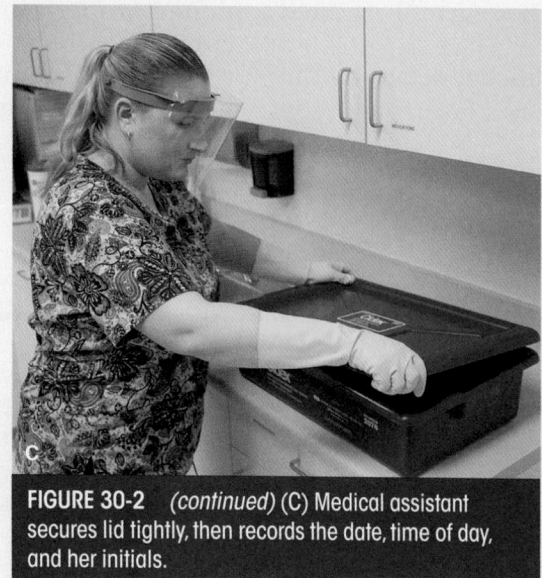

FIGURE 30-2 *(continued)* (C) Medical assistant secures lid tightly, then records the date, time of day, and her initials.

11. Place each sterile item on a sterile towel (which has been placed on a sterile field) and dry it with another sterile towel. The towel used for drying is removed from the sterile field. The use of sterile drapes that have a plastic polylined barrier layer between two layers of paper is recommended for the sterile field. RATIONALE: Plastic-lined sterile drapes create a barrier to prevent moisture from drawing contaminants from the metal surgical instrument tray or countertop up into the sterile area.

Steam Sterilization (Autoclave)

Procedure

Steam sterilization is the most widely used method of sterilization used in the medical clinic. An **autoclave**, basically a pressure cooker, is used to achieve sterilization. The autoclave uses steam under pressure to obtain higher temperatures than can be achieved with

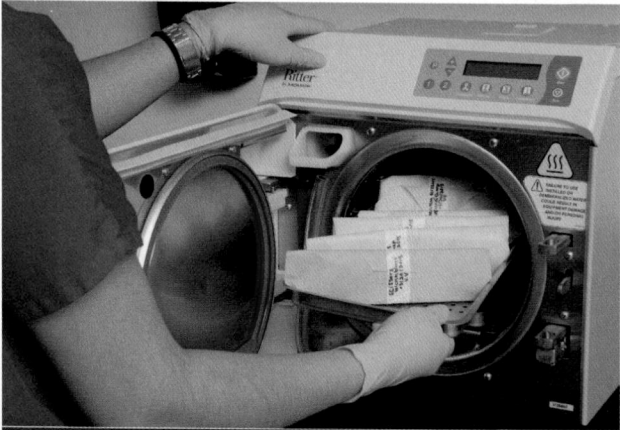

FIGURE 30-3 Commonly found in providers' offices, autoclaves are used for sterilization by steam pressure, usually at 270°F (118°C) for a specified length of time.

boiling (Figure 30-3). Water reaches a maximum temperature of 212°F through boiling. When under pressure, water is converted to steam and is then able to reach a temperature of 270°F and higher. Exposing items to this extremely high heat and at least 15 pounds of pressure for a specific amount of time ensures that all microorganisms and their spores are killed. The autoclave is an inner sterilizing chamber surrounded by a metal jacket. This creates a middle steam chamber between the inner sterilizing chamber and the jacket. Inside the jacket is a reservoir for water. When water is poured into the reservoir, the autoclave door closed and secured, and the autoclave turned on, several processes occur. The water in the reservoir heats until vapor is produced. The vapor enters the middle steam chamber inside the jacket. The air in the steam chamber is pushed out and replaced with steam. Because the air has been pushed out, the pressure increases. The increase of pressure causes the steam to then enter the inner sterilizing chamber (where the items and instruments for sterilization are placed), which pushes out the air. With the air being displaced with steam, the pressure increases in the inner chamber. The steam under pressure is able to reach a much higher temperature than boiling water. When the steam is able to reach all surfaces of the items placed in the autoclave and exposure is maintained for adequate amounts of time, sterility of those items is ensured (Procedure 30-4).

Table 30-2 lists some additional details on the various methods of sterilization.

How to Load Packages. It is of extreme importance that instruments and materials be positioned properly in the autoclave for the steam to circulate through and between packs and penetrate them. Do not overload the autoclave. Place items as loosely as possible inside the chamber.

TABLE 30-2

METHODS OF STERILIZATION

TYPE OF STERILIZATION	AGENTS USED	TIME REQUIRED	APPROPRIATE MATERIALS	SPECIAL CONSIDERATIONS
Gas	Ethylene oxide (EO) Temperature range 50 to 60°F	16 to 18 hours	Large loads of sensitive equipment	EO is a risk to health care workers EO is toxic and must not be inhaled Aeration times are prolonged for safety
Dry heat	Heat of 320 to 356°F	90 minutes to 3 hours	Instruments that corrode easily Powders Oils Ointments Rubber goods Plastic tubing	Instruments must be wrapped
Chemical or "cold"	Wavicide Cidex	Follow exposure time set by the manufacturer Cidex: 12 minutes Wavicide: 10 hours	Instruments that are too large or too heat sensitive for autoclaving (steam sterilization)	Instruments must be dry prior to placing them in the sterilant to avoid dilution of the chemical Instruments must be completely immersed in the sterilant Sterile gloves must be used to remove the instruments Sterile towels are used for drying and placing on a sterile surface A large container or basin with a well-fitting lid that is of a size to allow complete immersion of the instrument The lid must be securely placed on the container at all times (except when adding or removing instruments) in order to prevent evaporation A vent hood is required to avoid inhalation of fumes Use PPE to protect eyes and skin from contact with the sterilant Mix solution according to manufacturer's instructions to ensure effectiveness (FDA considers this high-level disinfection, not sterilization)
Steam or autoclave	Steam heat at 270°F and at least 15 pounds of pressure	20 to 40 minutes based on wrapping and number of items	Metal instruments Dressing materials	Unwrapped items need 20 minutes of sterilization Loosely wrapped items need 30 minutes of sterilization Tightly packed items need 40 minutes of sterilization If uncertain of sterilization time, refer to manufacturer's instructions Autoclaves must be cleaned with distilled water only

Leave a 1- to 3-inch space between packs and the walls of the autoclave. Correct positioning and spacing allows sterilization to take place provided the medical assistant adheres to proper temperature, pressure, and time requirements. For more information, see the "General Rules to Ensure Proper Sterilization Using an Autoclave" Quick Reference Guide.

Autoclave Maintenance and Cleaning. The autoclave, like any piece of equipment in the medical clinic, needs regular cleaning and maintenance. Frequency of cleaning the autoclave depends somewhat on its usage. If the autoclave is used every day, the inner chamber should be washed with a mild detergent and cloth, rinsed, and dried on a daily basis. The outer jacket should be wiped clean of dust

⯌ QUICK REFERENCE GUIDE

⯈ GENERAL RULES TO ENSURE PROPER STERILIZATION USING AN AUTOCLAVE

- Articles placed into the autoclave must have been sanitized, rinsed, and dried.
- The articles are wrapped and placed to allow adequate exposure of all surfaces (see Figure 30-4). Instruments inside packages should have hinges open and serrations exposed.
- To prevent formation of trapped air pockets, containers should be placed on their sides with lids loosely in place.
- Any wrapping material used must be approved for autoclave use.
- Timing should not start until the gauges read 15 pounds of pressure and 270°F.
- When the cycle is complete, the door must be opened slightly to allow steam to escape. The sterile wrapped articles will be hot and damp and should be left in the autoclave to cool and dry. Microorganisms can contaminate the sterile articles through the damp wrapping if the door is opened too wide or if articles are handled while damp.

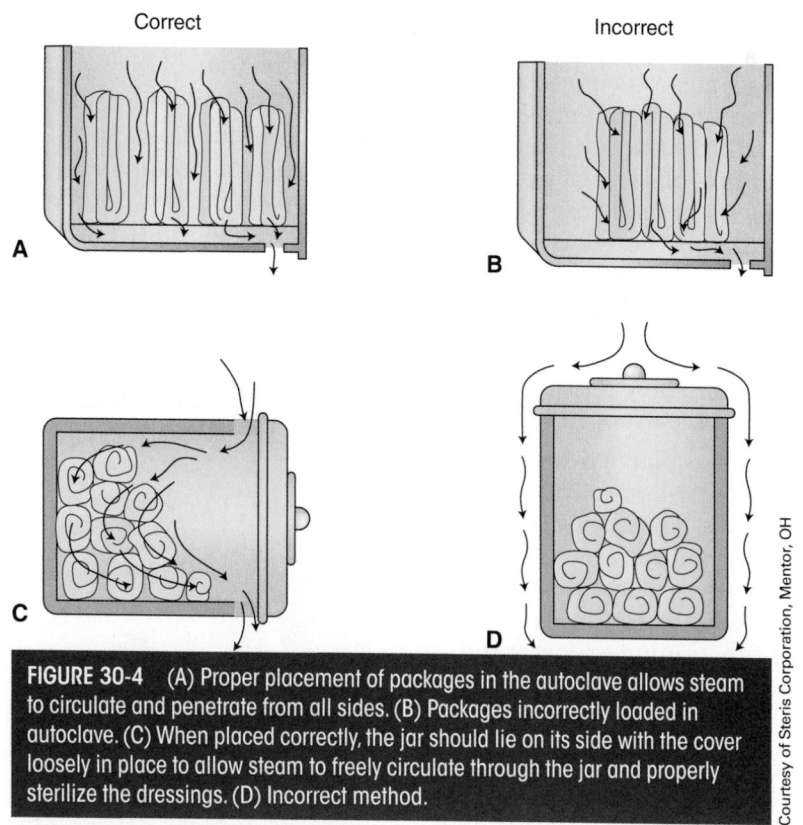

Correct   Incorrect

A   B

C   D

Courtesy of Steris Corporation, Mentor, OH

FIGURE 30-4 (A) Proper placement of packages in the autoclave allows steam to circulate and penetrate from all sides. (B) Packages incorrectly loaded in autoclave. (C) When placed correctly, the jar should lie on its side with the cover loosely in place to allow steam to freely circulate through the jar and properly sterilize the dressings. (D) Incorrect method.

and soil. Follow the manufacturer's instructions and recommendations for cleansers. Omni Cleaner XL is a well-known brand of autoclave cleanser.

At least once a week or following the manufacturer's instructions, the autoclave should be drained of water and cleaned thoroughly. Cleaning the autoclave requires that it be drained, filled with cleaning solution, run through a 20-minute heated cycle, drained of solution, filled with distilled rinse water, run through another 20-minute heated cycle, drained of rinse solution, and then filled with distilled water again. Then the inner shelves are removed and scrubbed, and the inner chamber is wiped clean. Because this process is fairly time consuming and puts the autoclave out of use for a while, consideration should be given to scheduling the weekly cleaning at a time when personnel can devote the time and when the autoclave is not in demand for sterilization processes.

During the cleaning process, attention should be given to inspecting the rubber seal for cracks or wear. An extra replacement rubber seal should always be kept on hand. The seals are available through medical supply sources. Refer to the manufacturer's instructions for regularly scheduled replacement of the rubber seal and other recommended maintenance procedures.

Quality Control and Assurance for Autoclave.
Quality control when using an autoclave consists of proper maintenance, proper operation, and observation of the temperature and pressure gauges. Equally important is the regular use of sterilization indicators and culture tests. Several types of sterilization indicators and culture methods are available:

- *Sterilization strips.* The strips contain a thermolabile dye that darkens when exposed to steam at the proper temperature and pressure for the proper amount of time. These indicators are placed in the center of the wrapped article.

- *Culture tests.* These are available as a culture strip containing heat-resistant spores. The strip is placed in the center of a wrapped article and placed in a fully loaded autoclave. After processing is complete, the article is unwrapped and the strip is placed into a culture medium. If the autoclave is functioning properly and the medical assistant has followed proper operating procedure, no growth should occur.

- *Biological indicators.* Also available through Becton-Dickinson Microbiology Systems is an ampule called the Kilit Ampule. These biological indicators are ampules that contain spores of the thermophile *Bacillus stearothermophilus*.

After being processed through the autoclave, the Kilit Ampule is sent to a cooperating laboratory for a week-long observation for survival of the bacilli spores. A written report of the results is generated by the laboratory and sent to the clinic for its records. The CDC recommends biological indicators.

Autoclave Wrapping Material and Packaging Supplies.
Wrapping or otherwise packaging surgical instruments and other surgical and medical articles before placing them in the autoclave will extend their shelf life. Before these articles are wrapped, they must first be sanitized, rinsed, and dried. Several materials are available for wrapping. Cost, convenience, visibility, time, space, and ease of use will help determine which to use. Many clinics use a combination of materials (Figure 30-5).

- Paper sterilization wrapping squares are available in many different sizes and types. This disposable type of material requires that a new paper be used each time items are sterilized, but it eliminates the need for laundering. Similar to cloth wrapping, paper wraps also lend themselves to larger sets of articles being wrapped together for surgery or procedural packs. As with muslin cloth, wrapping space and some personnel training are necessary. Paper wraps are opaque, making viewing of the contents impossible. Autoclave tape is required to seal the package.

- Sterilization pouches or bags may be plastic, paper, or a combination (Figure 30-6). They are fairly inexpensive and very easy to use. Because no wrapping is involved, additional work space is not required. Another advantage of bags is the visibility of the items inside. Some pouches are packaged on a continuous roll and are available

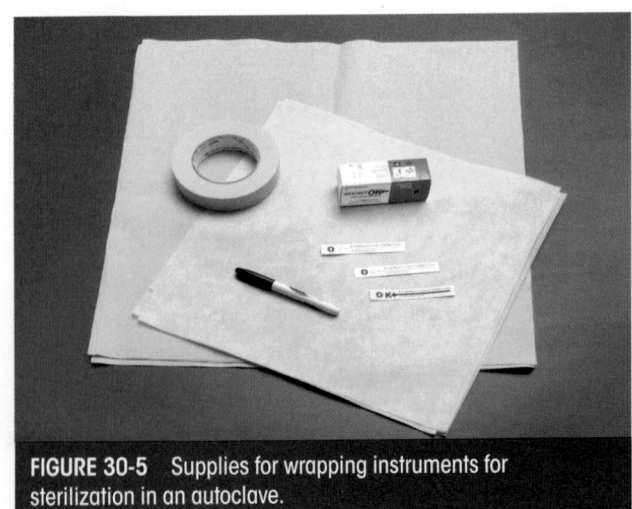

FIGURE 30-5 Supplies for wrapping instruments for sterilization in an autoclave.

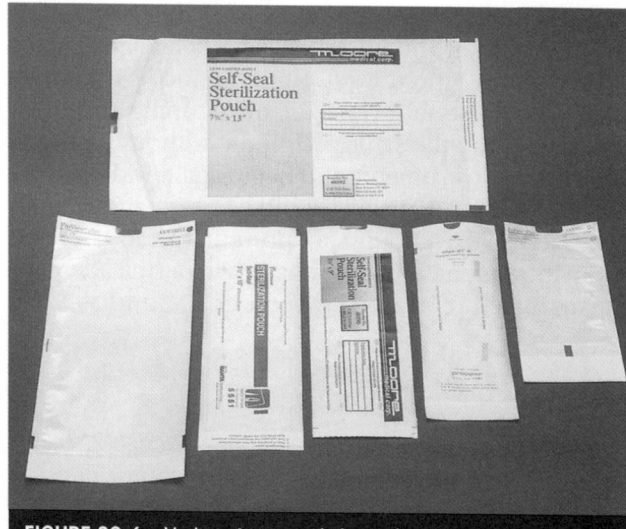

FIGURE 30-6 Various types and sizes of self-sealing bags for sterilization.

in a variety of widths. This allows the medical assistant to cut the bag to fit the article. Because both ends must be taped closed, it is difficult to remove the article while maintaining its sterility. Probably the best bag-type option is individual bags with the top end open for instrument placement and the bottom end factory closed with a peel-apart seal. The article is inserted into the top opening, the bag is taped closed, and the package is sterilized (Figure 30-7). When needed, the sterile article is removed through the factory-sealed bottom end in a peel-apart sterile fashion. These individual bags need to be purchased in several sizes and are expensive, but they have the advantages of ease of use and item visibility and are probably the preferred method for most medical clinics today.

Autoclave Tape. Autoclave tape is chemically treated to appear striped when exposed to heat. The striped pattern indicates exposure to high temperature but does not measure pounds of pressure or duration of exposure. Because of these limitations, autoclave tape does not ensure that the wrapped package is sterile, only that it has been in a heated autoclave. The tape is placed on the outside of the package, so it does not ensure that steam has penetrated to the inner article. It does help to determine if a package has been in the autoclave (Figure 30-8).

Labeling Packages for the Autoclave. Surgical packages should be labeled clearly. Clear bags usually have a designated place for labeling, and muslin- or paper-wrapped packages may be labeled across the autoclave tape. Proper labeling should include the name(s) of the articles in the pack, the date of sterilization, and the initials of the medical assistant responsible for the wrapping. The name of the instrument or article should be as specific as possible, especially when using the opaque cloth or paper wraps. If many instruments have been wrapped together for a specific surgery or for a specific provider, the label should clearly state which surgery or surgeon. For example, a "laceration repair set" could contain all the necessary instruments for repairing a laceration. "Dr. Peterson's vasectomy set" would contain all the instruments Dr. Peterson needs to perform a vasectomy, including, perhaps, personal preference instruments. The date of sterilization helps determine the expiration of sterility and a

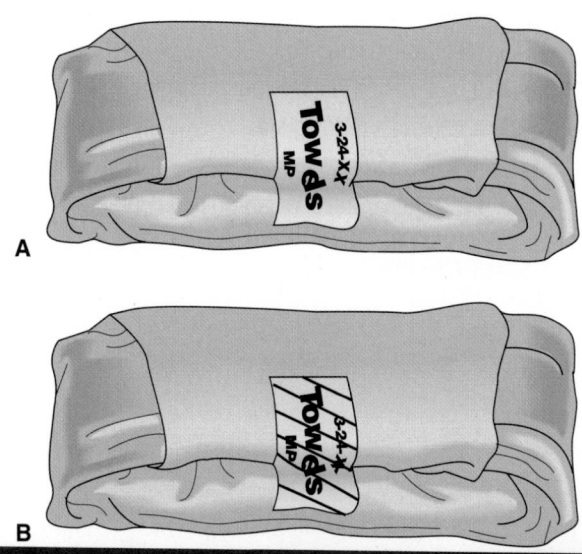

FIGURE 30-8 Package of towels (A) before and (B) after autoclaving. Note that the autoclave tape has a striped pattern indicating that the package was exposed to a high temperature. However, this does not assure sterility.

FIGURE 30-7 The medical assistant is placing a sanitized instrument into a sterilization bag for autoclaving by inserting the tips of the instrument in first.

"pull date" for resterilizing. Initialing the package allows for accountability, if necessary. Labels should always be written with a permanent marker. Ballpoint pen should never be used because the ink will smear when wet. Caution should be taken to avoid puncturing through the package during labeling.

Wrapping Techniques. Articles must be wrapped in a specific way to ensure they remain sterile when opened. Wrapped surgical instruments need to be double wrapped. Some methods include placing both layers of wrapping material together and double wrapping the pack in one process. A much more useful method is the "wrapping twice" technique (see Procedure 30-3). The wrapping twice technique allows for additional options at the time of opening. Wrapping twice allows for a completely wrapped inner sterile package to be placed on the surgical tray. This wrapping twice technique eliminates struggling to control multiple instruments during the unwrapping process; and, if the outer package becomes contaminated during the unwrapping, the medical assistant has the additional option of unwrapping the inner package using the same technique without having to discard the instruments and begin again with another sterile package. All packs should be neatly and securely wrapped—firm enough to prevent the instruments from movement, but loose enough to permit adequate steam penetration (see Procedures 30-2 and 30-3).

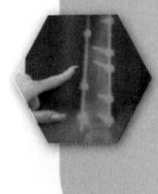

Critical Thinking

You have removed a double-wrapped instrument pack from the autoclave and notice a small tear in the outermost wrap. The innermost wrap appears to be intact. What would your action be? Why?

PROCEDURE 30-3

Preparing Instruments for Sterilization in an Autoclave

PURPOSE:

To properly wrap sanitized instruments for sterilization in an autoclave.

EQUIPMENT/SUPPLIES:

- Sanitized instruments
- Wrapping material
- Sterilization indicators
- 2-by-2 gauze (if instrument has hinges)
- Autoclave wrapping tape
- Autoclave tray
- Permanent marker or felt-tip pen (Figure 30-9A)

STANDARD PRECAUTIONS:

Handwashing

PROCEDURE STEPS:

1. Assemble the required equipment.
2. Wash hands and follow Standard Precautions.
3. Make sure you have a clean, dry surface of adequate space.

(continues)

4. Before wrapping an instrument for sterilization, make sure that it has been sanitized, rinsed, and dried.

5. Inspect all instruments for cleanliness and function. Set aside any that may need repair.

6. Select two wraps of adequate size in which to wrap the instruments.

7. Place the two squares of wrapping material at an angle in front of you on the dry surface so that one corner is pointed toward you.

8. Place the sanitized instrument or articles to be placed in the autoclave just below the center of the wrap. Open instruments with hinges as wide as possible and place a 2-by-2 gauze pad in the opening (Figure 30-9B). RATIONALE: Instruments with hinged parts that are not spread open before autoclaving may not be properly sterilized.

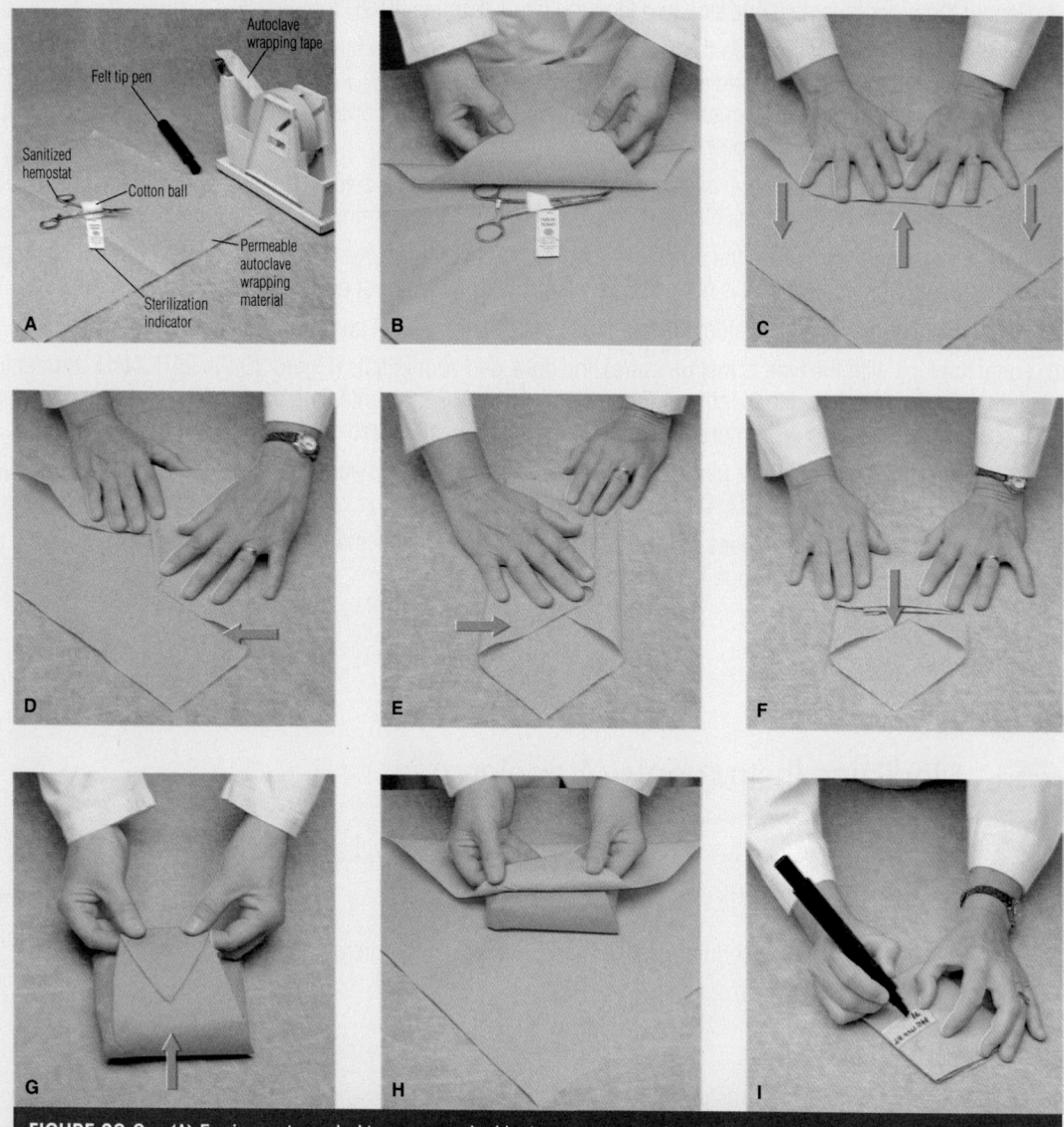

FIGURE 30-9 (A) Equipment needed to wrap surgical instruments or equipment for sterilization in an autoclave. (B) Place a cotton ball or folded gauze sponge between the hinge joints of instruments to keep them open. Do not ratchet instruments closed. Pad the tips of sharp instruments. Place a sterilization indicator in with the instruments to be wrapped. (C) The wrapping paper is folded toward center. A small corner is turned back on itself. (D) Fold one side toward center, leaving small corner turned back on itself. (E) Fold other side toward center, leaving small corner turned back on itself. (F) The package is folded up from the bottom and secured. (G) Fold corner back on itself. (H) Wrap first package in another wrap. Double wrapping allows more control of multiple instruments when setting up a surgical tray. (I) Wrapped package is secured with heat-sensitive autoclave tape and labeled with the date, contents, and medical assistant's initials.

(continues)

9. If the instrument is a sharps instrument you must cover the tips with some form of tip protector to ensure safety.

10. Place one sterilization indicator with the instruments. RATIONALE: This indicator will ascertain quality control of each individual package by changing color to confirm that the required temperature was reached during sterilization.

    NOTE: Quality control for autoclave operation can be evaluated with sterilization indicators.

11. Bring the corner of the wrap closest to you up and over the article and toward the center. Then fold it back toward you until it reaches the folded edge, creating a fan-fold effect.

12. Smooth the edges of the fold. At this point, the instrument should be completely covered (Figure 30-9C).

13. Repeat the process for first one side and then the other (Figures 30-9D thru 30-9F).

14. Finish by folding the package so that the top portion of the wrapping fully covers the package. If necessary, fold the corner back up over itself to create a flat bottom edge (Figure 30-9G). RATIONALE: Final edge should wrap entire package for assurance of adequate coverage and protection once contents are sterilized. If wrap does not cover adequately, unwrap and start over with larger wrapping material.

15. Double-wrap the now packaged instrument in the same manner as before using a second piece of wrapping (Figure 30-9H). RATIONALE: This allows for more control over the instruments when setting up a surgical tray.

16. Tape the exposed point using the autoclave tape. RATIONALE: Autoclave tape indicates whether the package has been through the autoclave; it is not a form of sterilization indicator or quality control.

17. Wrapped instruments are considered sterile until utilized or until the packaging is interrupted.

18. Label the tape with the type of instrument(s), the date, and your initials (Figure 30-9I). RATIONALE: Proper instrument labeling is required to identify wrapped sterilized instruments. Initialing packages ensures accountability and responsibility. Wrapped instruments are considered sterile until utilized or until the package is interrupted.

19. If the instruments are not to be placed in the autoclave immediately, wait to add the date to the package until you are ready to sterilize. RATIONALE: Dating is important to ensure "in first, out first" practices.

20. Alternatively, autoclave envelopes may be used. Include an indicator strip if the envelope does not have a built-in indicator strip. Label the package in the same way.

PROCEDURE 30-4

Procedure

Sterilizing Instruments (Autoclave)

PURPOSE:

To rid items for use in invasive procedures of all forms of microbial life (microorganisms).

EQUIPMENT/SUPPLIES:

- Steam sterilizer (autoclave)
- Autoclave manufacturer's instructions
- Wrapped sanitized instrument package(s) with sterilization indicators placed inside package (or unwrapped item if removed with sterile transfer forceps)

PROCEDURE STEPS:

1. *Paying attention to detail,* check water level in the autoclave reservoir and add distilled water to fill line if necessary. RATIONALE: Not enough or too much water will impair the efficiency of the autoclave. Distilled water will not leave deposits (tap water leaves deposits) inside the autoclave. Deposits can impair the efficiency of the autoclave.

(continues)

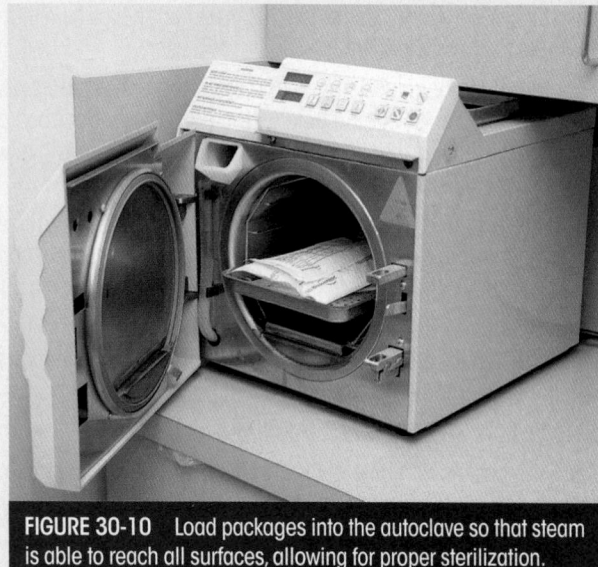

FIGURE 30-10 Load packages into the autoclave so that steam is able to reach all surfaces, allowing for proper sterilization.

2. Keep in mind that all autoclaves have manufacturer's instructions. If you are unsure of the proper method for cleaning and maintenance, refer to these instructions in order to ensure proper functioning of the autoclave.

3. Load the prepared packages into autoclave tray; allow room for steam to circulate (Figure 30-10). RATIONALE: Steam circulates in predictable patterns in an autoclave. When packages are loaded too closely or improperly, proper sterilization will not occur in individual packages.

4. If you are loading unwrapped instruments, make sure that they are lying flat on the tray with the handles in the open position to ensure that all surfaces are exposed for sterilization.

5. When you have finished loading the autoclave, close the door to seal it and then turn it on. RATIONALE: Pressure cannot be achieved without a proper seal.

6. Using the setting controls, select 270°F or 118°C at 15 psi for the number of minutes indicated by protocol. Note that the settings vary based on the materials to be autoclaved. RATIONALE: Proper heat, pressure levels, and exposure time must be achieved to kill all microorganisms within the autoclave. Careful note should be given to setting exposure time only after the proper temperature and pressure settings have been achieved.

Item	Required Exposure Time
Wrapped instrument packages or trays	40 minutes
Unwrapped items	20 minutes
Unwrapped items covered with cloth	30 minutes

7. When the autoclave has competed its full cycle, follow the manufacturer's instructions and vent the exhaust steam pressure. RATIONALE: Following the manufacturer's instructions carefully will ensure safe and proper use of the autoclave.

8. Once the pressure gauge on the autoclave indicates 0, and the temperature has decreased to at least 212°F, open the door approximately 1 inch. RATIONALE: You will not be able to open the door until the pressure is zero.

9. To avoid steam burns, use extreme caution when opening the door, keeping your face and hands clear of the opening.

10. Allow the contents to completely dry, approximately 30 to 45 minutes; do *not* touch contents until completely dry. RATIONALE: If packages are still wet or damp, microorganisms can enter a wrapped package, rendering it contaminated. Liquids travel along paper or cloth by capillary action and will be contaminated by microorganisms on countertops or from hands.

(continues)

11. If removing a tray that is still hot, be sure to utilize protective autoclave mitts. Set the tray aside on a clean, dry, flat surface to allow the contents to completely dry.

12. Remove the wrapped contents with dry, clean hands and store them in a clean, dry closed cupboard or drawer. RATIONALE: Sterilized wrapped packages can be held with clean hands, because only the interior contents require maintenance of sterility. If the outer wrapper is required to remain sterile, remove with sterile transfer forceps and place on a sterile field or in a sterile storage area.

13. Remove unwrapped contents with sterile transfer forceps; resanitize and resterilize the transfer forceps following use. RATIONALE: Sterile transfer forceps must have been sterilized immediately prior to or along with the unwrapped item if they are to be used immediately in a sterile procedure. Place onto sterile surface.

14. Perform quality control on a regular basis, based on usage. RATIONALE: Quality control and maintenance of an autoclave are critical to assurance of proper operation. Accountability and responsibility to monitor quality control should be the responsibility of the medical assistant(s) most often responsible for sterilization.

    a. Monitor sterilization indicators with each use of sterilized instruments.

    b. On a daily basis, clean the gasket with mild soap and distilled water. Never use bleach or abrasive cleaners.

    c. On a weekly basis, perform quality control by documenting sterilization indicator outcome on a log; date and initial quality-control log entries.

15. Weekly, the water should be drained and replaced with distilled water.

16. When necessary, service the autoclave according to the manufacturer's guidelines.

17. Maintain a log of cleaning, services, and quality-control measures performed.

COMMON SURGICAL PROCEDURES PERFORMED IN PROVIDERS' OFFICES AND CLINICS

Procedure

All surgery has commonalities as well as specifics. The following content on specific surgeries and surgical procedures includes lists of needed instruments, supplies, and equipment, as well as basic patient preparation and postoperative instructions for some of the more frequently performed surgeries. The following procedures are suggested protocol only because providers will have preferences and techniques unique to them and their practices.

Procedure 30-7, at the end of the chapter, outlines a medical assistant's role in assisting with minor surgery.

ADDITIONAL SURGICAL METHODS

Additional surgical methods are those methods not requiring the use of a surgical knife or scalpel but using other methods of cutting or destroying, such as electric current, heat, freezing, chemicals, or laser. The method used is determined by the provider's preference.

Electrosurgery

Electrosurgery uses an electric current in a concentrated area to either cut or destroy tissue whenever pathologic examination is not required. The equipment for electrosurgery consists of a power source, usually a small boxed unit, and a detachable, disposable handheld applicator.

Electrosurgery is useful in removing benign skin tags and warts. The main advantage of electrosurgery is that the bleeding is controlled through the cauterization of the blood vessels as the electric current is applied. The terms *electrocoagulation, electrofulguration, electrodessication, electroscission, electrosection,* and *eletrocautery* all refer to various uses of electric current to coagulate blood vessels, destroy tissue either with a spark or by drying, or cut tissue. Disposable battery-operated units designed for one-time use are available.

Cautery. The word *cautery* comes from the term *caustic* and means the application of a **caustic** chemical or destructive heat. Electrosurgery, cautery, and electrocautery are terms often used interchangeably. The burning of tissue, either chemically or electrically, is known as cauterization. Sometimes during surgical procedures unnecessary bleeding

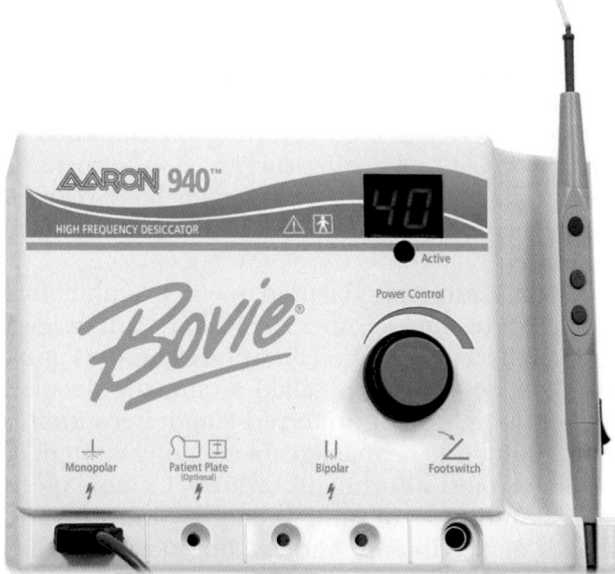

FIGURE 30-11 Electrosurgical equipment is used to destroy tissue, such as warts, or to coagulate blood vessels to decrease bleeding during surgery.

Courtesy of Bovie Medical Corporation

can be controlled by use of electrosurgical equipment (Figure 30-11). Tissues that do not need to be pathologically examined, such as benign skin tags, can be destroyed using cauterization. Some common chemicals used to destroy tissue and stop bleeding are silver nitrate, liquid nitrogen, and sodium hydroxide.

Chemical Tissue Destruction. Silver nitrate is available in a solid form, impregnated on the end of a wooden applicator stick (Figure 30-12). Silver nitrate is especially useful inside the nose to cauterize **friable**, easily broken blood vessels in the

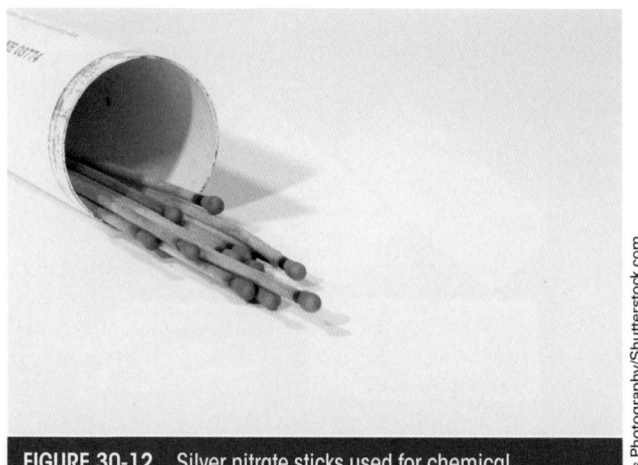

FIGURE 30-12 Silver nitrate sticks used for chemical cauterization.

© Rick's Photography/Shutterstock.com

treatment of epistaxis (nosebleed). Silver nitrate sticks are also known as caustic pencils.

Cryosurgery

Cryosurgery is the destruction of tissue by freezing. Some types of tissues react differently to heat than to cold in the rate of healing and level of scarring. The cryogenic substance most often used to destructively freeze tissue is liquid nitrogen. Liquid nitrogen, often incorrectly referred to as *dry ice*, is extremely **volatile** (easily evaporated) and must be kept in a covered insulated canister. Liquid nitrogen is obtained when nitrogen gas is compressed under cold temperatures into a liquid. It is most often used to destructively "freeze" warts. Liquid nitrogen can be applied to cervical erosions to facilitate healing and growth of normal tissue; to remove lesions on the anus; and for cataract extraction, retinal detachment, prostate gland destruction, and removal of superficial lesions in the nose and throat. Some units are single-purpose use. Cryosurgery offers less trauma, more control of bleeding, and less pain.

Many patients experience pain with liquid nitrogen because it is colder than other chemical cryosurgery options. Liquid nitrogen is usually kept in a large canister in a central location in the clinic and is carefully transferred to a small thermos for transport into the treatment room. The medical assistant must take care to keep the canister and thermos covered because of the volatile properties (evaporation rate) of the liquid nitrogen.

The cryogenic properties of solid liquid nitrogen make it useful for freezing warts and **nevi**. Nitrous oxide is another chemical used in cryosurgery. Nitrous oxide requires a gas cylinder, a regulator, a pressure gauge, and a cryogun with assorted tips. Nitrous oxide is applied in a more direct and controlled pattern because of the precision of the probes, and nitrous oxide does not evaporate as readily as liquid nitrogen. The tank, probes, and other supplies can be expensive. Nitrous oxide is not as cold as liquid nitrogen; therefore, although it is not so uncomfortable for the patient, it is not as destructive. It is not appropriate for use with cancerous lesions, which must be completely destroyed. Because nitrous oxide is a carcinogen, the Occupational Safety and Health Administration (OSHA) requires that all nitrous oxide systems have outside venting. It is not practical for most ambulatory clinics.

All volatile gases are dangerous to inhale, and appropriate ventilation must be used. Refer to the Material Safety Data Sheet (MSDS) information (available in printed form or on the manufacturers' Web sites) for specific cautions.

Laser Surgery

Laser is an acronym for light amplification by stimulated emission of radiation. The laser instrument converts light into an intense beam. By focusing the laser beam onto the target, the application can be extremely precise without damaging surrounding tissue. In recent years, laser surgery has become less expensive, more readily available, and consequently much more widespread as a treatment of choice for surgery in dermatology, ophthalmology, nerve surgery, vascular surgery, plastic surgery, and others. Most specialty surgery uses laser technology in various ways. Because many providers use laser technology in the ambulatory care setting, medical assistants must be familiar with the dangers involved with laser surgery, and safety precautions must be implemented. Attending a laser education and safety workshop is recommended for all personnel intending to work with lasers.

Safety

The following precautions are designed to heighten awareness and serve as a safety guide:

- When the laser beam is focused on the target tissue, the cells explode and vaporize. Care should be taken not to inhale the vapors.
- Whenever high levels of electricity are used, care should be taken to avoid burns and to ensure that the equipment is always in good working order.
- Safety glasses should be worn by the provider, the medical assistant, and the patient.
- If the patient's skin has been prepared with flammable products such as alcohol-based antiseptics, the skin must be dry with no pooling of liquid. Read the product label for alcohol and other flammable substances.
- Sterile water should be readily available to extinguish any fire if the laser beam accidently ignites cloth or paper in the area.

SUTURE MATERIALS AND SUPPLIES

Suture/Ligature

Procedure

The word *suture* can be used as a verb to describe the motion of sewing or as a noun to describe the material used to sew. Suturing, or sewing, a wound is a common procedure in provider's clinics. The purpose is to **approximate**, or bring together, the edges of a wound. Suturing hastens healing and lessens scarring. Whether the wound is an accidental laceration or a surgical incision, the suturing process is basically the same (see Procedure 30-10). When suture material is used for tying off the ends of tubular structures during surgery, it is termed **ligature**. The terms *suture* and *ligature* both refer to suture material, but they are named according to their uses.

Most suture material used in office/ambulatory surgical procedures comes already fused, or **swaged**, to a needle and packaged in various lengths (Figure 30-13). These are also called atraumatic needles. Eighteen inches is a preferred length because it is short enough to be manageable yet long enough to complete most suturing procedures. Combinations of sizes and types of suture materials and sizes and shapes of needles are endless, but most providers use a select few. Selection from among the many different suture materials and needles is based on the needs of the tissue and tissue healing. Sutures range in size on a scale from the smallest gauge below 0 (aught) to the largest gauge above 0. The scale from 6–0 to 4 includes all sizes from the smallest to the largest:

6–0, 5–0, 4–0, 3–0, 2–0, 0, 1, 2, 3, 4

Sometimes 2–0 is labeled 00, 3–0 labeled 000, 4–0 labeled 0000, and so on. Ambulatory care settings use sizes 6–0 to 3–0.

If the tissue being sutured is delicate, as on the face or neck, smaller suture material such as 6–0 is used; the finer the stitch, the less scarring. Some sutures are made from materials that dissolve when they come in contact with the tissue enzymes. These are referred to as absorbable

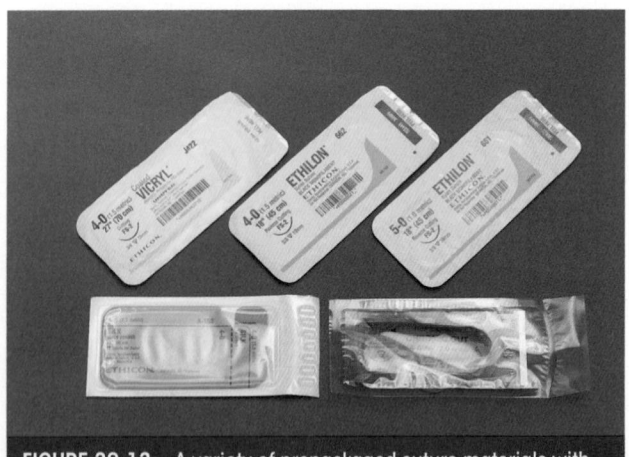

FIGURE 30-13 A variety of prepackaged suture materials with needles of various sizes and shapes.

sutures. The original absorbable suture was called surgical gut or "cat gut." It was made from sheep intestinal tissue. Left "natural" or uncoated, it is called plain gut suture. It dissolves or is absorbed in about 1 to 2 weeks. If more time is needed to heal, surgical gut may be coated with chromic salts and is called chromic gut. It allows for a longer period of healing before dissolution. Absorbable gut suture is used for underlying tissues where removal is not reasonable and areas where suture removal is inconvenient. Individual body chemistries influence the exact absorption rate of both plain and treated gut suture. Surgical gut is rarely used now, having been replaced by humanmade absorbable suture (such as Vicryl and PDS* II). Sutures are also made of nonabsorbable materials such as stainless steel, silk, cotton, nylon, and Dacron. Some are natural (cotton, silk) and some are synthetic/manmade (Dacron, Ethilon, Prolene). Each type of suture material comes in a variety of options such as different colors for ease of visualization, braiding for additional elasticity and strength, and coatings for lubrications and to lessen irritability to tissues.

Suture Needles

The atraumatic needles swaged to the suture material are also varied (see Figure 30-14). For office/ambulatory surgery, the needles are usually curved. They are categorized according to size, shape, radius of curve, and type of point. Needles may be termed *cutting needles*, *round taper point needles*, or *blunt point needles*.

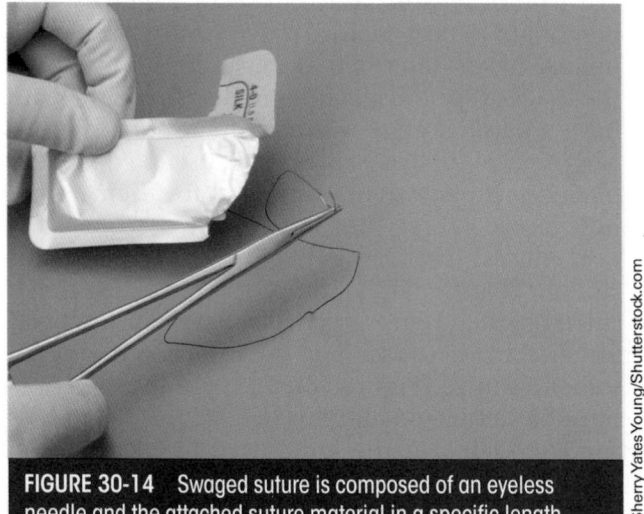

FIGURE 30-14 Swaged suture is composed of an eyeless needle and the attached suture material in a specific length.

© Sherry Yates Young/Shutterstock.com

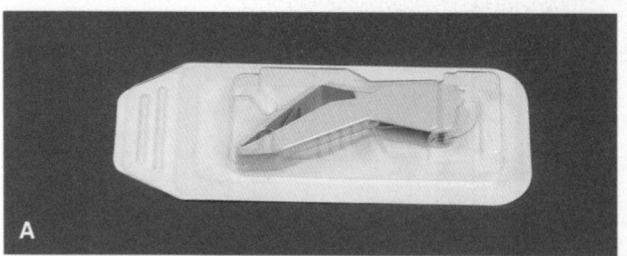

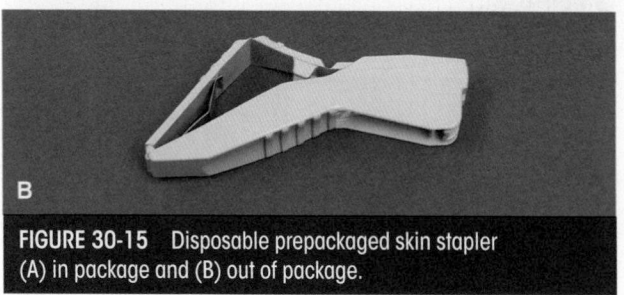

FIGURE 30-15 Disposable prepackaged skin stapler (A) in package and (B) out of package.

Staples

Many surgical incisions can be approximated using staples (made of stainless steel or titanium) and a stapler made for this purpose (Figure 30-15). The length, width, and number of staples depend on the tissue. They are safe to use, reduce blood loss, and reduce the length of time of the surgery. Wound healing is quicker, and there is less trauma. Staplers are made for specific types of tissues (e.g., blood vessels, skin, gastrointestinal tract). It is more difficult to remedy incorrectly placed staples than it is manually placed sutures.

Staple Removal. Staple removal (see Procedure 30-11) is done wearing sterile gloves and using sterile instruments. The staples are removed using a sterile prepackaged staple remover (Figure 30-16). The staple remover is carefully positioned under the staple and, when the handle is squeezed, the staple flattens out and it can be carefully lifted out. Cleanse with an antiseptic solution such as Betadine and pat dry. Be certain all staples have been removed by verifying that the number that were inserted matches the number you have removed.

INSTRUMENTS

Structural Features

Rarely does the phrase *form determines function* have as much meaning as when discussing surgical instruments. One can almost always correctly determine function simply by close examination of the instrument's design. Handles designed to be

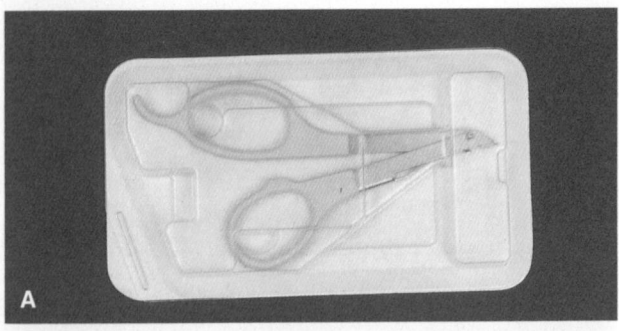

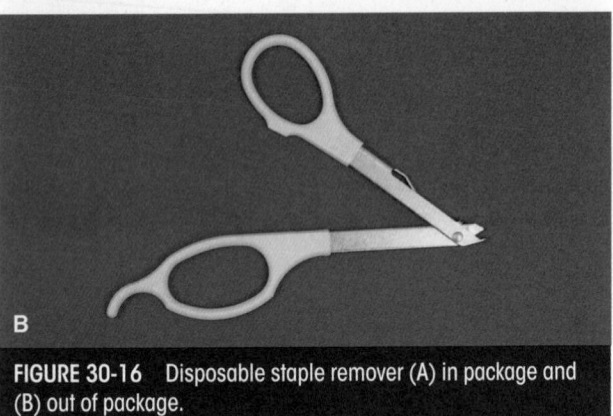

FIGURE 30-16 Disposable staple remover (A) in package and (B) out of package.

squeezed between the thumb and finger are called thumb handles. Ring handles are designed so that the thumb and finger can be inserted into rings. **Ratchets** are locking mechanisms located between the rings of the handles and are used for locking the instrument closed. Ratchets are designed to close in varying degrees of tightness. Serrations are the crevices etched into the surfaces of the jaws of hemostats, some forceps, and needle holders. The serrations provide a more secure grip during use with slippery tissues without actually puncturing the tissue. These serrated surfaces hold onto tissue and fluids and need added attention when preparing for sterilization by cleaning debris from this area.

For the purposes of grasping tissue, forceps with teeth are an option. Teeth may be numerous or few but are always sharp and should approximate tightly when the instrument is closed. This is a key assessment when sanitizing instruments. If the teeth do not approximate, the instrument should be set aside for repair. To help delicate tips match up properly, some thumb instruments have a guide pin built into the handle. The box-lock is a special type of hinge found on most ring-handled instruments, especially grasping instruments such as hemostats, forceps, and needle holders. This is also an area that requires special attention prior to sterilization. Because the box-lock provides strength

and aids in the prevention of warping, most instruments with ratchets also need the box-lock hinge. Other features include prongs, hooks, and loops (Figure 30-17).

Categories and Uses

Several companies publish and distribute large pictorial catalogs of well over 30,000 medical–surgical instruments. A glance through these references shows the many choices available. For ease of discussion, learning, and cataloging, most surgical instruments are placed according to their uses into three basic categories.

Instruments designed for specific purposes within medical specialties often do not readily fit into any one group and are called specialty instruments. This group includes long-handled gynecologic instruments, as well as other instruments designed to meet specific needs within specialty practices.

Scissors and Scalpels. Most of the cutting instruments are scissors. Scissors have ring handles and two blades and vary in size, shape, and function. Because scissors have two blades, the word *scissors* is always plural. Bandage scissors have one rounded tip to allow insertion under a bandage without causing injury to the patient. Bandage scissors do not have to be sterile to be used. The two most common styles are the Lister bandage scissors and the finer Knowles finger bandage scissors (Figure 30-18).

Operating scissors are used to cut tissues and generally have very sharp blades. The blades may be curved or straight, and the tips may be sharp, blunt, or a combination of each. They are described as sharp/sharp (s/s), blunt/blunt (b/b), or sharp/blunt (s/b) (Figure 30-19). A special type of scissors, Mayo dissecting scissors, may be straight or curved, with curved more often used, but are never described as sharp or blunt because the tips are specifically designed to be neither but have a beveled edge with slightly rounded points (Figure 30-20). Iris scissors are useful, delicately bladed scissors, originally named for their usefulness in eye surgery but now widely used in many procedures. Iris scissors may be either curved or straight (Figure 30-21). Suture scissors, also called stitch or stitch removal scissors, have a distinctively notched blade to facilitate the insertion of one tip under a suture (Figure 30-22). All of these scissors must be sterilized before use.

The scalpel is the knife used to cut the skin. The scalpel is actually a blade secured to a handle that, when combined, becomes a surgical knife or

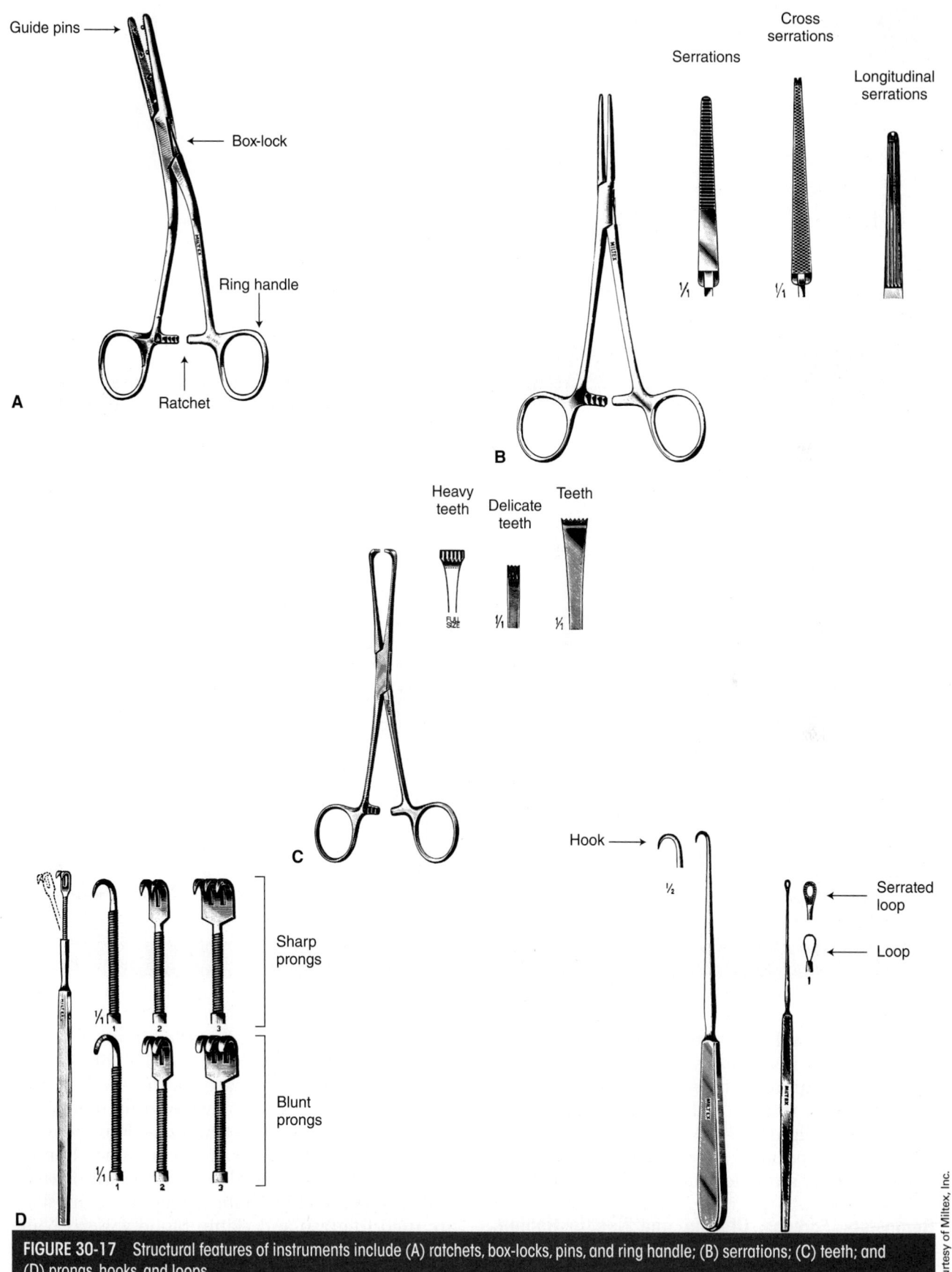

Guide pins

Box-lock

Ring handle

Ratchet

A

Serrations

Cross serrations

Longitudinal serrations

¹⁄₁ ¹⁄₁

B

Heavy teeth

Delicate teeth

Teeth

FULL SIZE

¹⁄₁ ¹⁄₁

C

Sharp prongs

Blunt prongs

¹⁄₁

¹⁄₁

Hook

¹⁄₂

Serrated loop

Loop

D

Courtesy of Miltex, Inc.

FIGURE 30-17 Structural features of instruments include (A) ratchets, box-locks, pins, and ring handle; (B) serrations; (C) teeth; and (D) prongs, hooks, and loops.

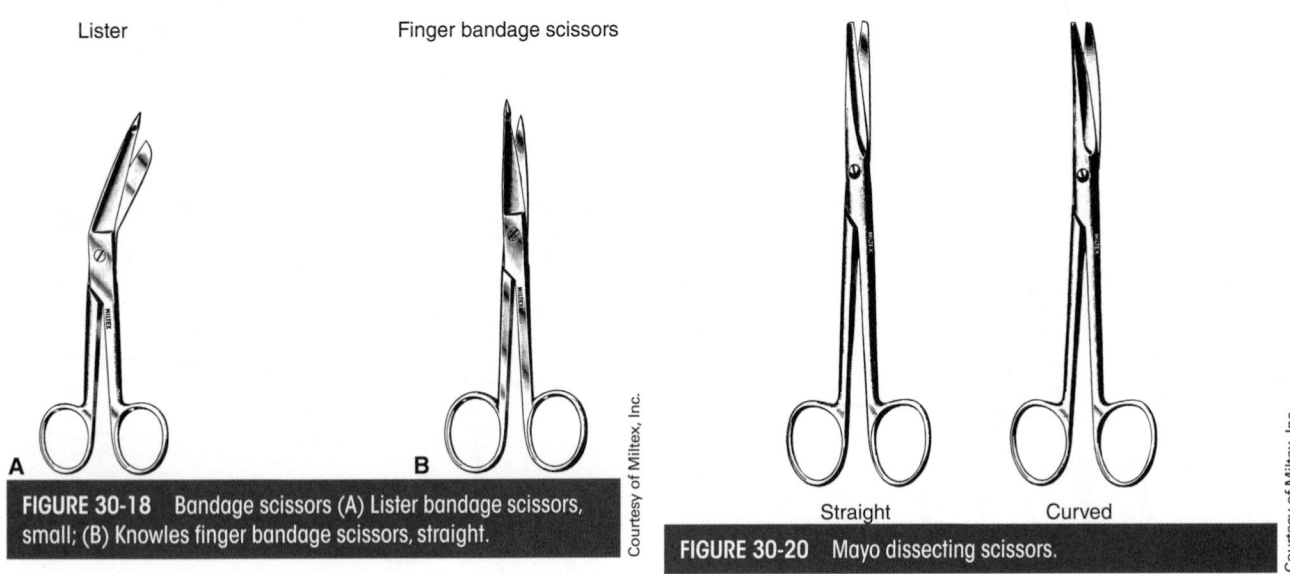

Lister   Finger bandage scissors

A   B

FIGURE 30-18 Bandage scissors (A) Lister bandage scissors, small; (B) Knowles finger bandage scissors, straight.

Courtesy of Miltex, Inc.

Straight   Curved

FIGURE 30-20 Mayo dissecting scissors.

Courtesy of Miltex, Inc.

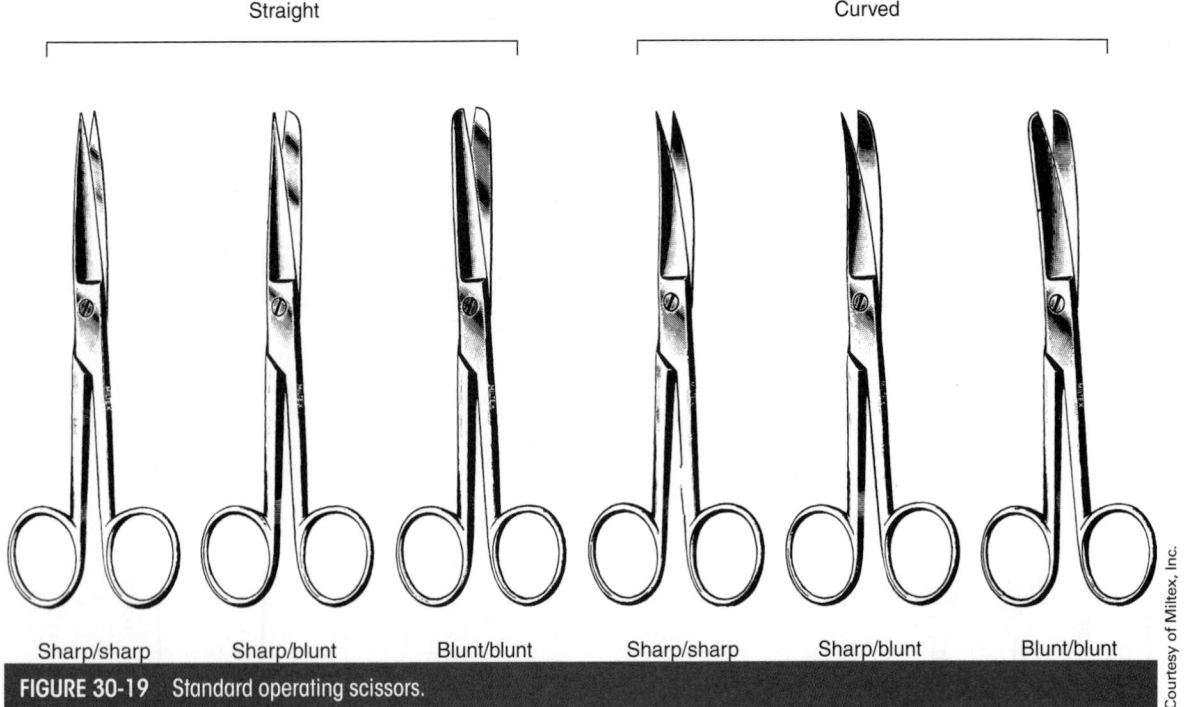

Straight   Curved

Sharp/sharp   Sharp/blunt   Blunt/blunt   Sharp/sharp   Sharp/blunt   Blunt/blunt

FIGURE 30-19 Standard operating scissors.

Courtesy of Miltex, Inc.

scalpel. Disposable one-piece units with a protective retractable blade are available. The most common blade sizes are #10, #11, and #15, with #11 often referred to as a "stab blade" because of its sharp point (Figure 30-23A). Handles vary in size, but the most popular are the sturdy #3 and #3L (long) and the more delicate #7 (Figure 30-23B).

Hemostats, Forceps, Clamps, and Needle Holders.
Grasping and clamping instruments are the largest of the instrument categories. They are used

for many different tasks. Included in this category are the towel clamps or clips, needle holders, and forceps. Many forceps have locking mechanisms called ratchets. Forceps may have ring handles or use a squeeze concept like tweezers. Forceps number in the hundreds, but most clinics need only a select few. Like the word *scissors*, the word *forceps* is always plural. Hemostatic forceps, or hemostats, are used to grasp and clamp blood vessels. Their name means literally to "stop blood." Because blood vessels are slippery, hemostatic forceps have

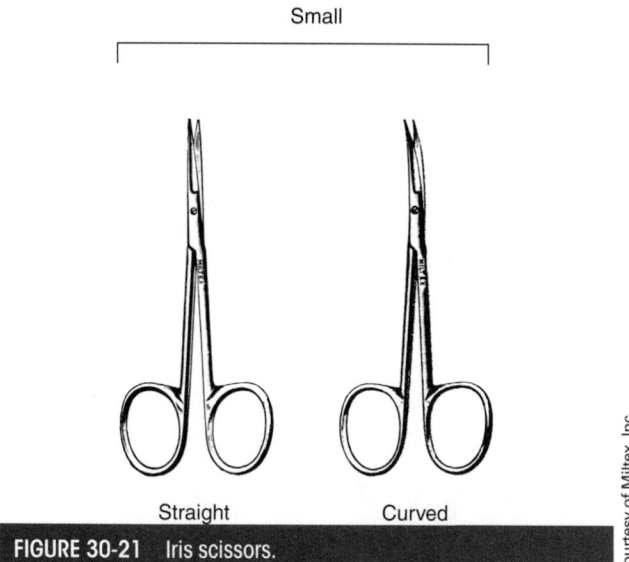

Small

Straight   Curved

FIGURE 30-21   Iris scissors.

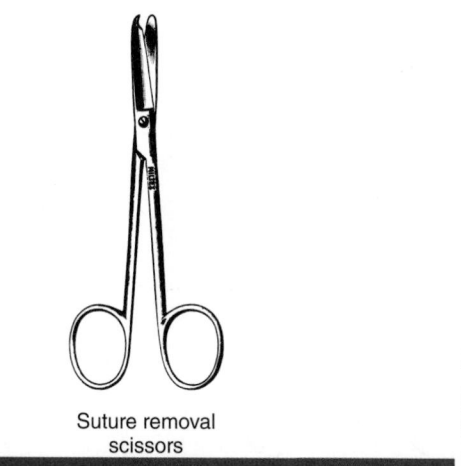

Suture removal
scissors

FIGURE 30-22   Suture or stitch removal scissors.

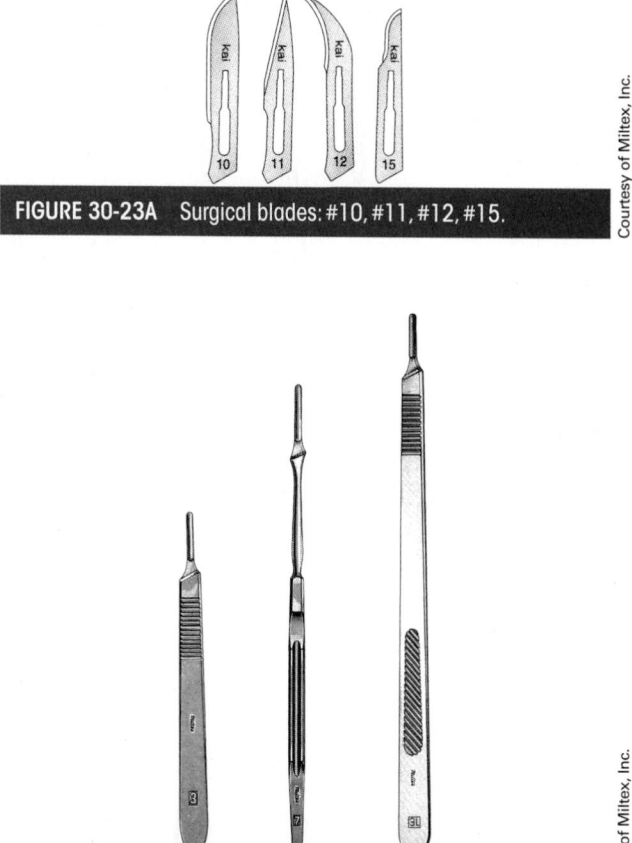

FIGURE 30-23A   Surgical blades: #10, #11, #12, #15.

FIGURE 30-23B   Scalpel handles: #3, #7, #3L.

serrations for grasping and ratchets for locking tightly. Mosquito hemostatic forceps have fine tips, with serrations along the entire length of the tips. The Kelly hemostats have serrations along only a partial length of the tips. The Kelly hemostatic forceps are sturdier, and some hemostatic forceps have teeth. All types may be straight or curved (Figure 30-24).

Allis tissue forceps are of a similar design to hemostatic forceps but have unique angular jaws with teeth. Thumb forceps are another type of grasping instrument, sometimes referred to as pickups. Thumb forceps do not have ring handles or ratchets but are more like common tweezers. Thumb forceps with teeth are called tissue forceps because of their ability to grasp tissue. Dressing forceps (plain) do not have teeth and are useful for dressing wounds and applying sterile skin closure strips. Dressing forceps are also used to insert sterile gauze packing strips into wounds to facilitate drainage. The Adson, a special type of thumb forceps, is easily differentiated by its shape. Adsons may have teeth or be plain and have a finer tip.

The Lucae bayonet-type forceps, used in nose and ear procedures, have a thumb handle and are curved to allow the simultaneous use of other instruments and scopes and to facilitate viewing. In contrast, the Hartman ear forceps, duckbill ear alligator–type forceps, and the Hartman nasal dressing forceps have ring handles but also are bent for ease of use in ear and nose procedures. Figure 30-25 shows examples of each.

Splinter forceps do not have teeth and are used for pulling splinters. Many splinter forceps such as the plain splinter forceps and the Walter splinter forceps are of the thumb-handled style, but the physician's splinter forceps have ring handles and the Virtus splinter forceps have a spring-type handle (Figure 30-26).

Sponge forceps such as the Foerster, or ring forceps, may have rings on the tips and, as the name implies, are used to hold surgical gauze

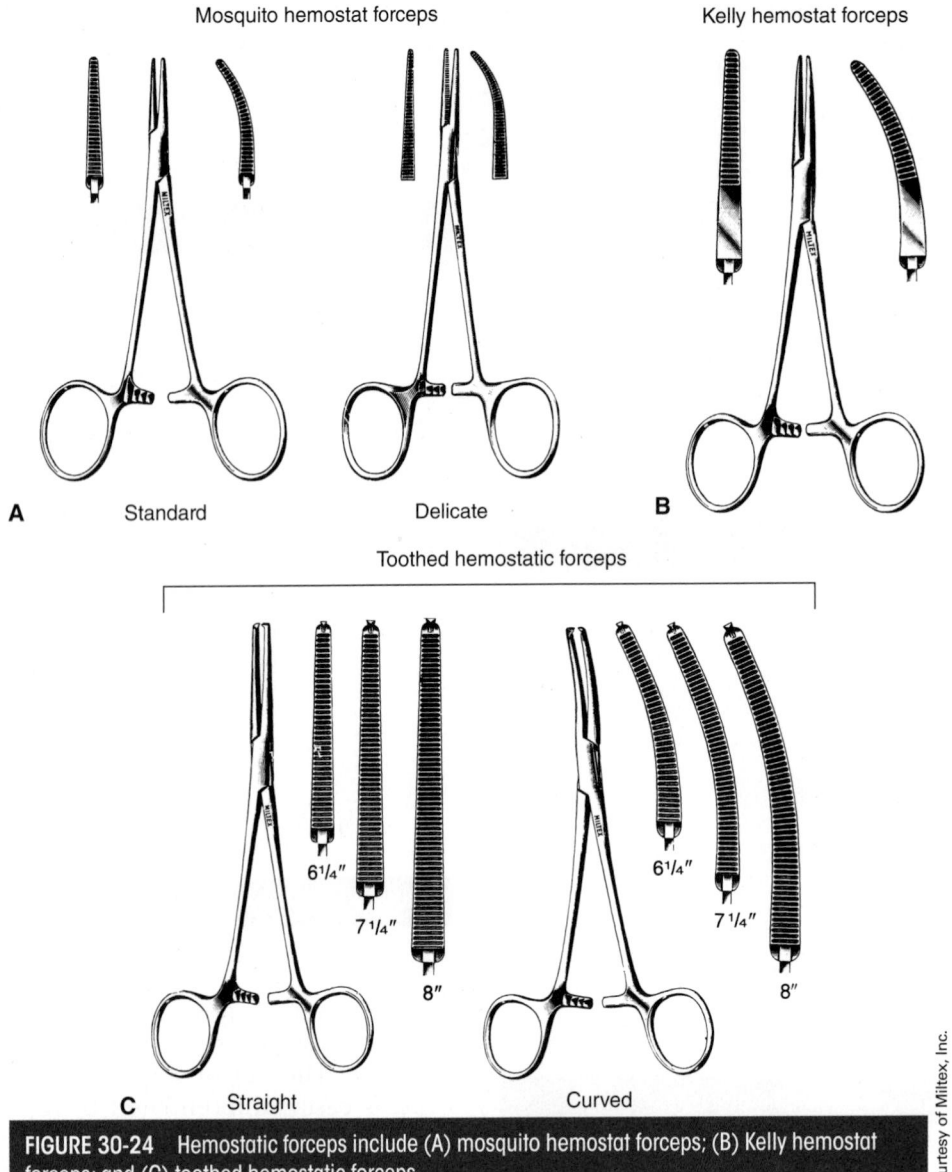

Mosquito hemostat forceps

Kelly hemostat forceps

A Standard   Delicate   B

Toothed hemostatic forceps

6¹/₄″
7¹/₄″
8″

6¹/₄″
7¹/₄″
8″

C Straight   Curved

Courtesy of Miltex, Inc.

FIGURE 30-24 Hemostatic forceps include (A) mosquito hemostat forceps; (B) Kelly hemostat forceps; and (C) toothed hemostatic forceps.

sponges. Sponge forceps may have long handles, making them useful for gynecologic procedures, and are called uterine sponge forceps. Many medical clinics use uterine sponge forceps as transfer forceps (Figure 30-27). (See the "Basic Surgery Setup" section later in this chapter.)

Towel clamps are used to attach surgical field drapes to each other and in some situations, such as when bisecting the vas deferens in a vasectomy, to clamp onto dissected tissue. In the case of a vasectomy, the Backhaus towel clamp is used to hold the dissected section of the vas deferens (Figure 30-28).

Needle holders are ratcheted instruments similar to hemostats but with a wider and more stout jaw. Often called needle drivers, they are designed to hold the needle firmly without crushing it while

suturing. Most needle holders have a vertical ditch in the center of the jaw to disperse tension and help prevent slipping of the needle. Needle holders such as the Crile-Wood may have a special groove in which to place the needle during suturing. Some needle holders come in various sizes and some are equipped with a cutting edge that eliminates the need for separate scissors to cut the suture material (Figure 30-29).

Specula, Scopes, Probes, Retractors, and Dilators.
The category of dilators and probes includes specula that are designed for enlarging and exploring body orifices (Figure 30-30). The vaginal speculum is available in various lengths and widths and may be made of metal or disposable plastic. The most

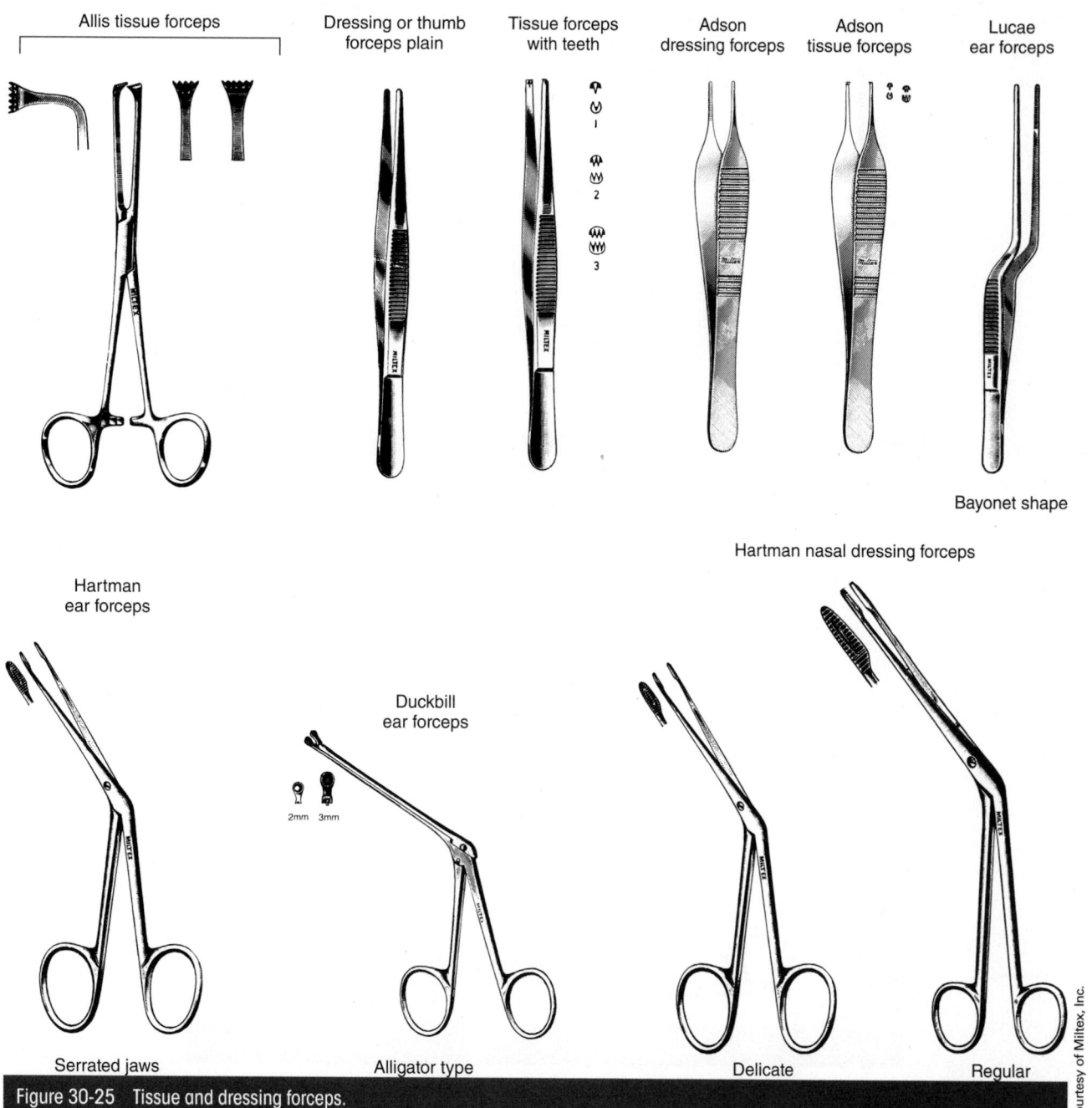

Allis tissue forceps

Dressing or thumb forceps plain

Tissue forceps with teeth

Adson dressing forceps

Adson tissue forceps

Lucae ear forceps

Bayonet shape

Hartman ear forceps

Hartman nasal dressing forceps

Duckbill ear forceps

2mm 3mm

Serrated jaws

Alligator type

Delicate

Regular

Courtesy of Miltex, Inc.

Figure 30-25 Tissue and dressing forceps.

common instrument for enlarging the nostril is the Vienna nasal speculum. This instrument is used with the Lucae bayonet forceps to perform procedures within the nose.

Scopes are lighted instruments used for viewing. The otoscope, used to visualize the ear canal and eardrum, has a small light aimed into an ear speculum. Ear specula may be disposable or reusable. If reused, they are sanitized, chemically disinfected, rinsed, and dried between uses. Proctoscopes, anoscopes (Figure 30-31), and rigid sigmoidoscopes are used for viewing the rectum, anus, and the sigmoid

portion of the large intestine and have guides called obturators to ease insertion. The light source for the proctoscopes and anoscopes is usually a separate lamp. Although the light sources cannot be sterilized, they can be meticulously disinfected. The speculum portion that is inserted into the rectum may be made of disposable plastic or metal. Both the metal speculum and its obturator can be sanitized and sterilized in the autoclave.

Another group of scopes are long, flexible, and much more complex and they use fiber optic light sources. Fiber optic scopes are considered

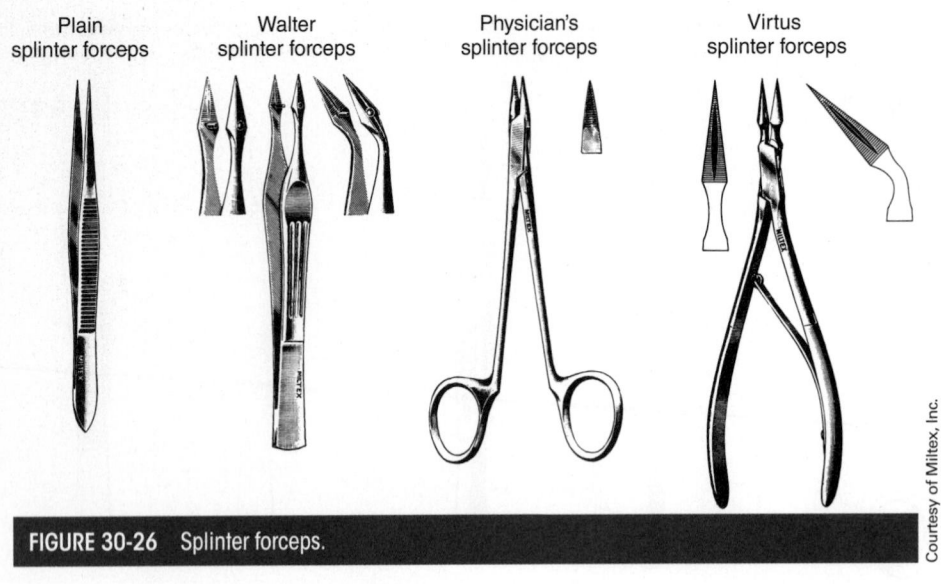

Plain splinter forceps Walter splinter forceps Physician's splinter forceps Virtus splinter forceps

FIGURE 30-26 Splinter forceps.

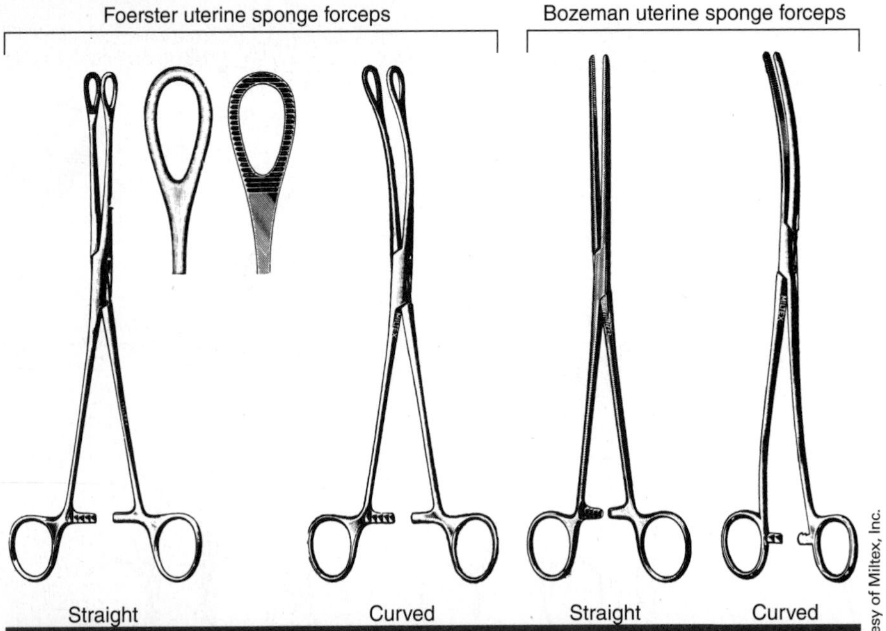

Courtesy of Miltex, Inc.

Foerster uterine sponge forceps   Bozeman uterine sponge forceps

Straight   Curved   Straight   Curved

FIGURE 30-27 Sponge forceps.

Courtesy of Miltex, Inc.

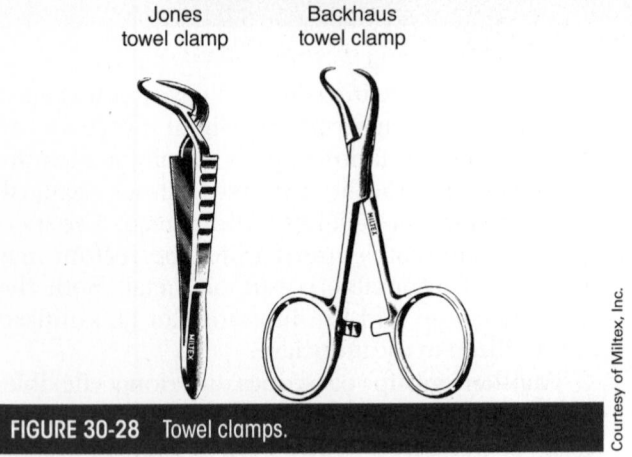

Jones towel clamp   Backhaus towel clamp

FIGURE 30-28 Towel clamps.

Courtesy of Miltex, Inc.

medical equipment rather than surgical instruments. Although considered to be medical equipment, these flexible scopes are inserted into body cavities and must be sanitized and sterilized between uses.

Probes are slender instruments used to probe into a hidden area, body cavity, or wound. Sounds are long, slender probing instruments used to determine the size and shape of the area being probed or to detect the presence of an unseen foreign body. Sounds may be calibrated in centimeters or inches (Figure 30-32).

Retractors used in office/ambulatory surgery are often called skin hooks and are used to hook onto and retract the edges of a wound to facilitate better

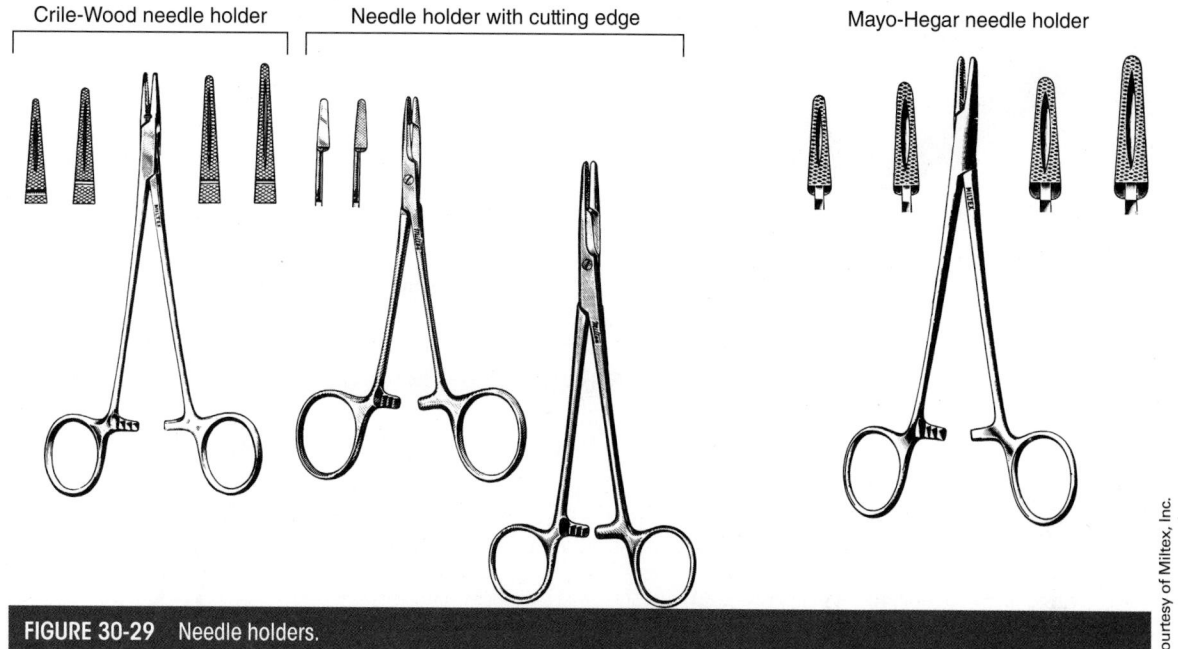

Crile-Wood needle holder   Needle holder with cutting edge   Mayo-Hegar needle holder

FIGURE 30-29   Needle holders.

Courtesy of Miltex, Inc.

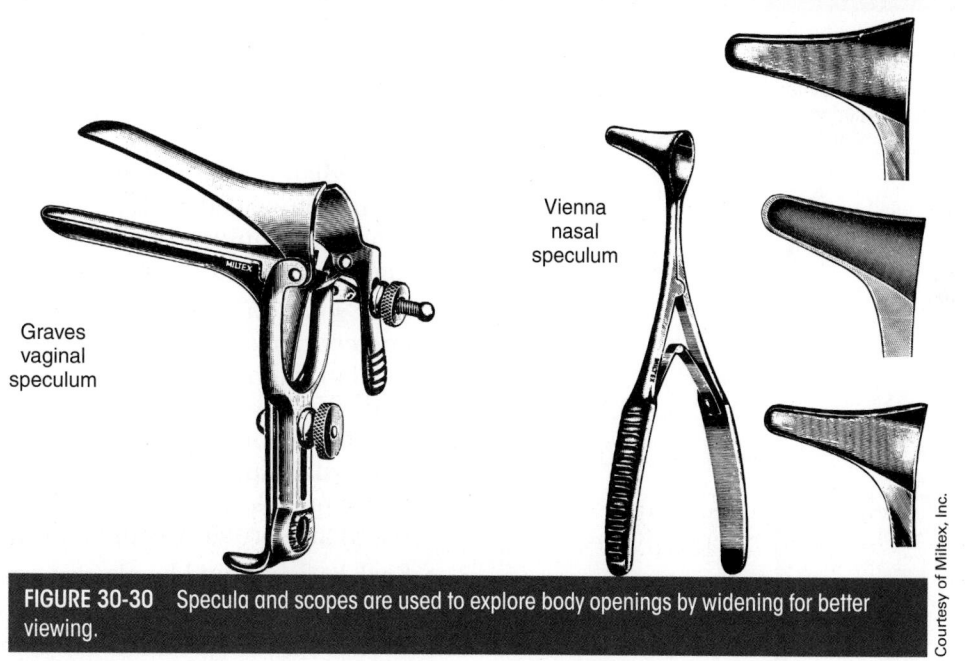

Graves
vaginal
speculum

Vienna
nasal
speculum

FIGURE 30-30   Specula and scopes are used to explore body openings by widening for better viewing.

Courtesy of Miltex, Inc.

viewing. Skin hooks are fine-tipped and delicate. As with all of the finer surgical instruments, special care should be taken to avoid damaging the delicate tips during the sanitization process (Figure 30-33).

Dilators are double-ended metal rods with smooth, rounded tips, ranging in calibrated sizes from small to large. Dilators are inserted into narrowed or constricted ducts and tubes for the purpose of gradually dilating or enlarging the opening. Hegar uterine dilators are used to dilate the cervix to gain access to the inside of the uterus. Esophageal dilators are used to relieve **strictures**, or narrowing, of the esophagus. Urethral dilators are used to relieve strictures of the urethra (Figure 30-34).

Care of Instruments

Medical–surgical instruments require special care to prevent excessive wear and tear and unnecessary damage. Careful and frequent inspections will

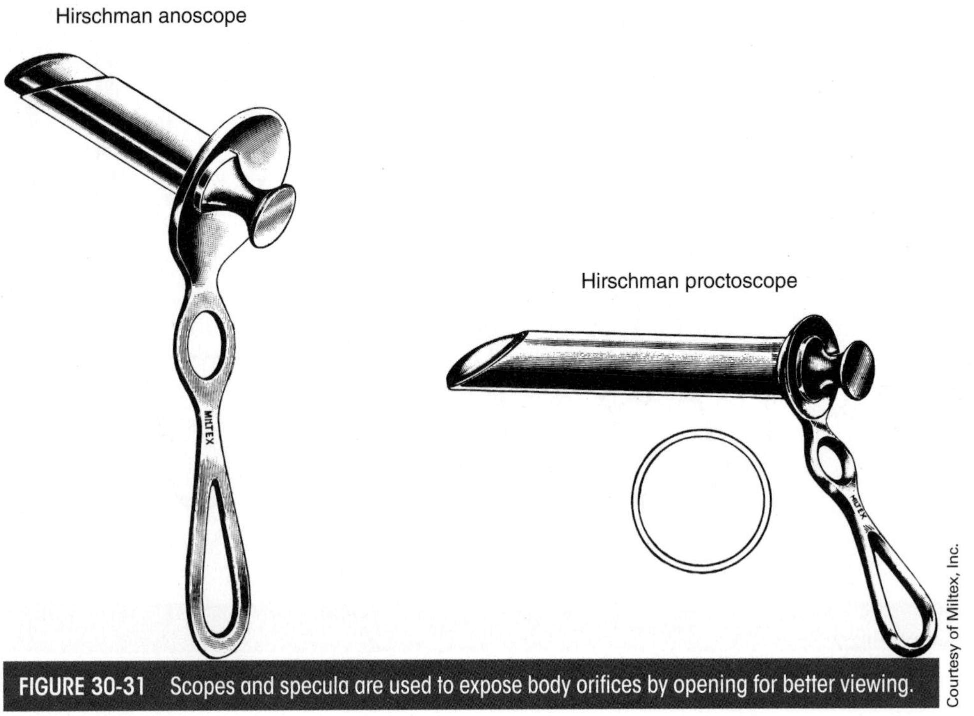

Hirschman anoscope

Hirschman proctoscope

Courtesy of Miltex, Inc.

FIGURE 30-31   Scopes and specula are used to expose body orifices by opening for better viewing.

Sims
uterine sound
(maleable)

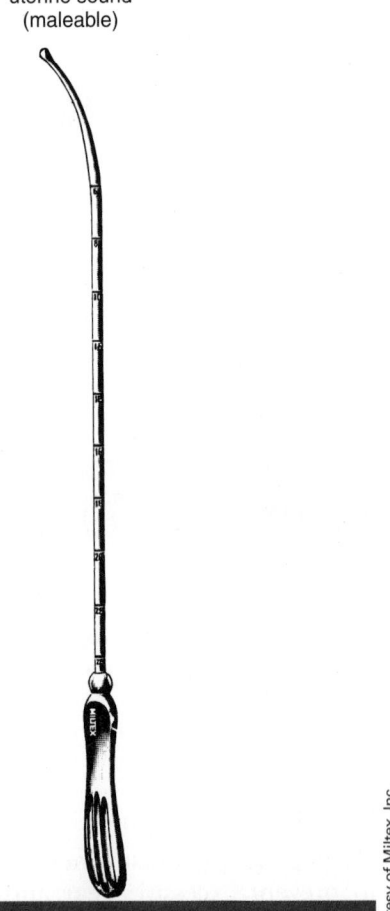

Courtesy of Miltex, Inc.

FIGURE 30-32   Uterine sound.

determine when instruments need to be replaced or repaired. Some basic rules and rationales include:

- Immediately after use, soiled instruments should be soaked. This prevents blood and other body fluids from drying onto the working surfaces of the instruments.

- Soak solutions should be at room temperature and contain a neutral pH detergent with a protein/blood solvent. The proteins in the body fluids will not coagulate on the instruments in cool water and the neutral pH detergent will help prevent spotting and corrosion of the metals. Solvents will help break up the blood and proteins in the body fluids.

- Soak basins should be plastic to prevent damaging points and edges. If a metal soak basin is used, placing a towel on the bottom as padding will help prevent damage to the instruments.

- Heavy-duty rubber gloves should be worn when cleaning instruments to lessen the likelihood of being stuck or cut with the sharp points and edges.

- Goggles should be worn to protect eyes from splashes.

- Delicate instruments should be separated from heavier instruments to prevent the delicate instruments from being bent or otherwise damaged.

- Sharp instruments should be carefully separated from the other instruments and washed

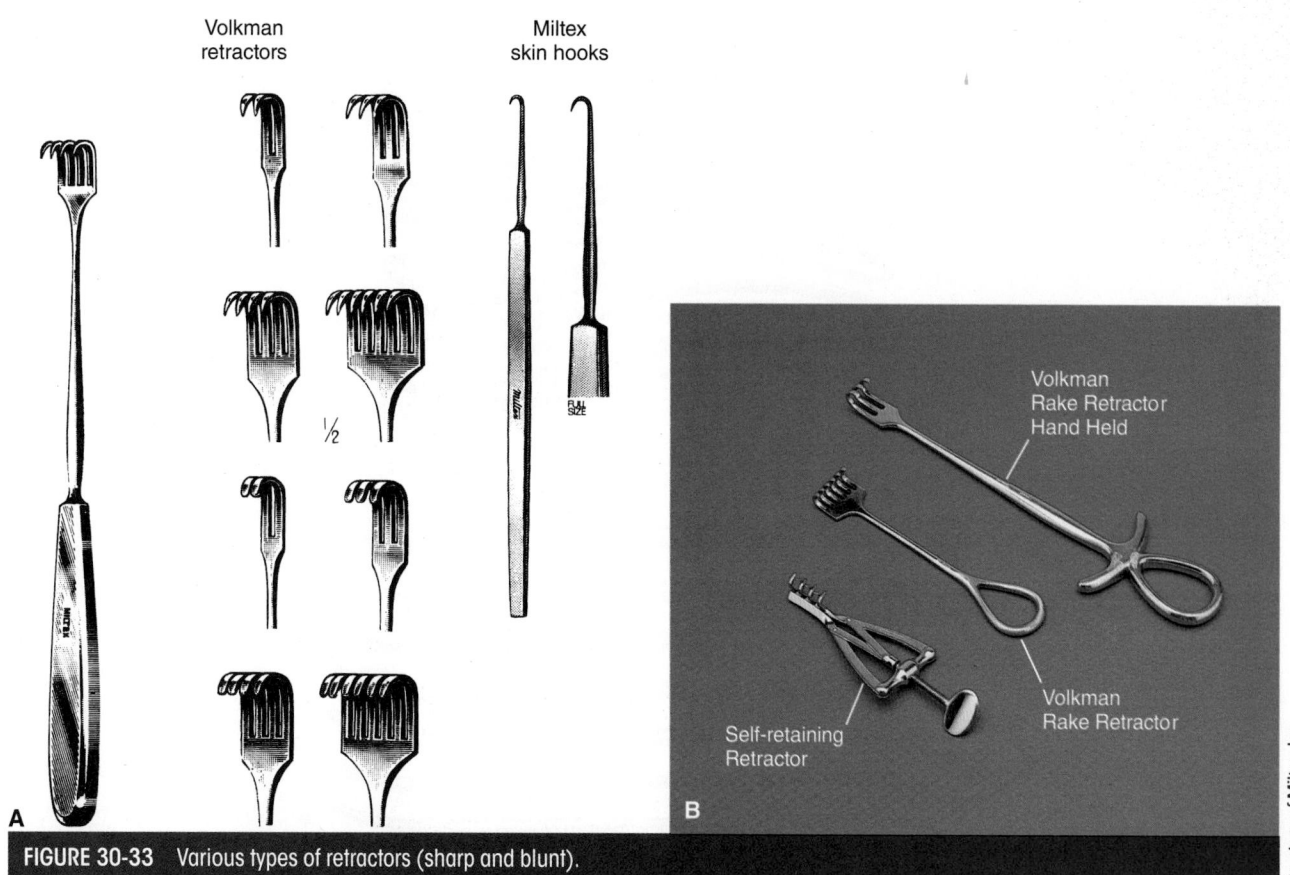

Volkman retractors

Miltex skin hooks

½

FULL SIZE

Volkman Rake Retractor Hand Held

Volkman Rake Retractor

Self-retaining Retractor

A

B

Courtesy of Miltex, Inc.

FIGURE 30-33 Various types of retractors (sharp and blunt).

with extreme caution. The danger of being cut or punctured by sharp instruments is greater when cleaning them than at most other times, and the sharp instruments are usually the most contaminated.

- A soft bristle brush should be used to scrub hinges, ratchets, and serrations. The brush should be firm enough to clean crevices thoroughly yet soft enough to prevent scratching instruments. Instruments with multiple parts must be taken completely apart.

- Immediately after sanitization, instruments should be thoroughly rinsed and dried to prevent spotting and water damage.

- Carefully inspect all surfaces, edges, and points. Check for nicks, dulling, and warping. Test blades for sharpness. Be sure the instrument is not bent or pitted. Handles should also be checked for nicks that may snag and tear surgical gloves, thus disrupting the protective barrier and causing contamination.

- Damaged or malfunctioning instruments should be repaired or replaced.

Ultrasonic Cleaning. Surgical instruments can be sanitized by using an ultrasonic cleaner. Instruments

are placed into an ultrasonic container with special cleaning solution. Sound waves vibrate to loosen debris and contaminants. Place instruments with ratchets or hinges into the cleaner in an open position. The articles, when finished, are rinsed well, dried, and wrapped for sterilization. The process of sanitizing contaminated instruments by ultrasound is safe for all instruments including delicate instruments. It is preferred for endoscopes. Follow manufacturer's directions for use and care of the ultrasonic cleaner (see Chapter 21).

Sanitization by use of an ultrasonic cleaner eliminates cleaning instruments by hand, thereby reducing the risk for contamination to the medical assistant.

- Instruments should be processed in the cleaner for the full recommended cycle time, usually 5 to 10 minutes.

- Place instruments in open position into the ultrasonic cleaner. Make sure that sharp blades and points do not touch other instruments.

- All instruments must be fully submerged.

- Do not place dissimilar metals (stainless steel, copper, chrome plated) in the same cleaning cycle.

Hegar dilators

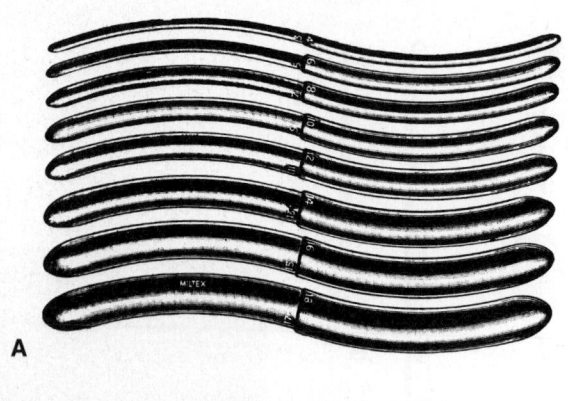

A

Pratt uterine dilators

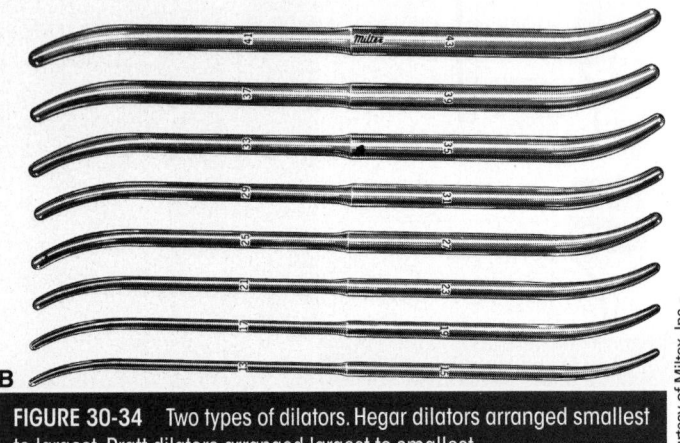

B

FIGURE 30-34 Two types of dilators. Hegar dilators arranged smallest to largest. Pratt dilators arranged largest to smallest.

- Change solution frequently—at least as often as the manufacturer recommends.
- Rinse instruments thoroughly with distilled water after ultrasonic cleaning to remove ultrasonic cleaning solution.

Chemical Sterilization. This type of sterilization is sometimes referred to as "cold" sterilization, which indicates that heat-sensitive items such as fiber optic endoscopes and delicate cutting instruments can be immersed in a chemical solution. The chemicals used are reliable and capable of destroying bacteria and their spores and, when used in strict accordance with the manufacturer's instructions regarding length of immersion time, can ensure sterility.

Procedure 30-2 gives steps for chemical ("cold") sterilization.

SUPPLIES AND EQUIPMENT

The supplies necessary for office/ambulatory surgery are often disposable and should be replenished as needed. Most medical–surgical supply companies have catalogs and Web sites available for ordering, and many companies have sales representatives who make regular stops or are available by telephone or email to assist in the ordering process. Sales representatives are familiar with the products marketed by their company and are extremely useful as resources. Samples of new products are often available for trial, and optional choices are always offered. Medical–surgical supply companies frequently offer special prices for larger quantity purchases. If a medical–surgical supply item is being used frequently and storage space is available, buying in larger quantities might be more cost effective. If a product currently being used is not meeting expectations, requesting optional trial products is usually the first step toward finding a better product. Following are some of the more commonly used supplies associated with office/ambulatory surgery.

Drapes

There are a variety of surgical drapes available for use in an ambulatory care setting. Drapes are used during surgery to create a sterile field over and around the surgical site. There are many types of drapes and the most appropriate should be selected to provide the best protection for the patient. Your provider will select the type of drape based on the type and complexity of the procedure. The drape may be impermeable, adherent, conformable, natural fiber, or antimicrobial. Natural fiber drapes are reusable after laundering and sterilization. Most adherent, conformable, and antimicrobial drapes are disposable. Care must be taken to appropriately manage these drapes after use. Disposable drape material must be placed in a biohazard container for disposal. Those drapes that are reusable must be managed utilizing Universal Precautions in the handling of materials contaminated with blood or body fluids.

Specialized drapes that are specific to a surgical site are referred to as **fenestrated** drapes. This specialized drape, being of either a reusable or disposable variety, has an opening large enough to accommodate the surgical field. This means that the area that needs to have the practitioner's attention, and no more, is exposed.

Sponges and Wicks

Surgical sponges are prepackaged squares of folded gauze used in surgery. In the provider's clinic, sponges are most often referred to by their size. A gauze square measuring 4 inches by 4 inches is called a 4-by-4 (Figure 30-35). The other most common size is 2-by-2. The gauze sponges are packaged in individual peel-apart packages of two or may be purchased in nonsterile bulk packages of 200. The individual packages are convenient, sterile, and useful for most purposes but cost more per sponge than the nonsterile bulk packages. For larger surgical needs, the medical assistant may wrap several bulk sponges together and autoclave them for later use. Most sponges are simply folded gauze, but some have cotton, rayon pads, or radiopaque fibers embedded in them to increase their absorption ability; to create a softer texture; and, in larger wounds, to be visible upon X-ray if left in the wound. The provider using the sponge may have a preference among the different types and uses. Gauze sponges are used in wound cleansing, in skin preparation, as absorbable sponges during surgery, as dressings and coverings, and for padding. The ambulatory care facility may prefer to have different sizes and types in stock to meet different needs.

Sterile surgical wicks or wound packing strips are used when an infected wound must remain open for drainage. The sterile wicking material is made of narrow strips of gauze packaged in long lengths in

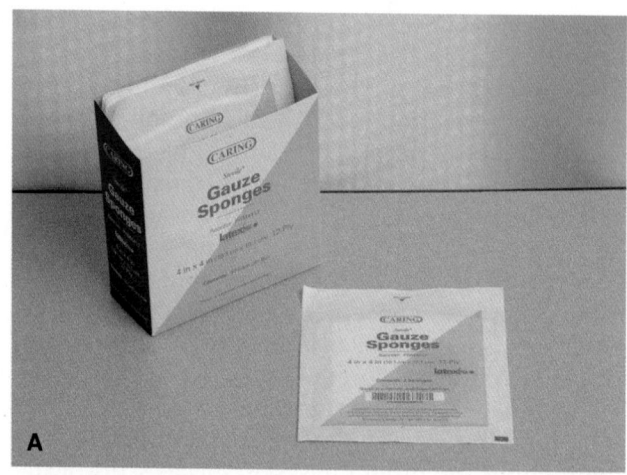

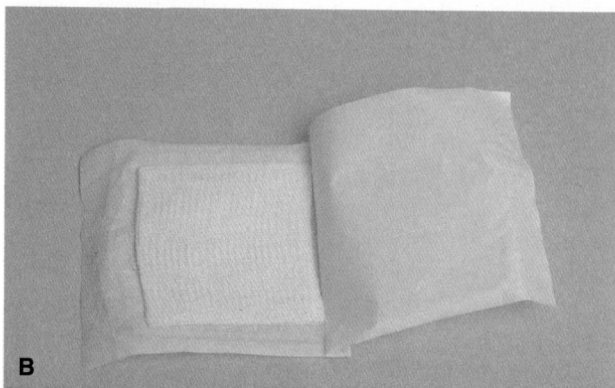

FIGURE 30-35 (A) Box of sterile gauze sponges. These are also referred to as 4-by-4s or, in surgery, as surgical sponges. (B) Peel-apart sterile open package of 4-by-4 gauze.

opaque glass bottles. The most recognizable product name is iodoform. Iodoform is sterile and packaged in multiple-use bottles. Extreme care should be taken to prevent contamination during removal of individual lengths. The bottle is opened using sterile technique, sterile dressing forceps or bayonet forceps are inserted into the bottle, the strip is cut to the desired length using sterile scissors, and the lid is applied without compromising the sterility of the remaining wicking material in the bottle.

Solutions/Creams/Ointments

Many different soaps and solutions are available and effective as skin cleansers, preoperative scrubs, paints, soaks, and antiseptics. **Betadine** (povidone-iodine) is a well-known antiseptic and is available as a surgical soap called a scrub and as a nonsoap solution for preoperative skin preparation/paint. Betadine comes in multiple-use bottles, in single use packaging, and in individually packaged swabs. **Hibiclens** is another effective antiseptic, and it does not have the staining tendencies of iodine. Medical–surgical supply companies can provide names and samples of other products. Cost, effectiveness, ease of use, shelf life, and personal preferences should all be considered. **Isopropyl alcohol**, a 70% alcohol solution, is of limited medical–surgical use, although because of its rapid volatility rate and its ability to dissolve oils, it is still preferred for skin preparation before injections and venipuncture. Isopropyl alcohol is available in bottles for use with cotton/rayon balls, but is most often found in convenient individually packaged pledgets. Isopropyl alcohol can be irritating and is not effective as a preoperative skin preparation. Hydrogen peroxide is a noncaustic mildly effective skin antiseptic. It bubbles on contact with mucous membranes and other moist skin surfaces, dissolving blood and proteins, and has a mechanical cleansing action. Hydrogen peroxide is ineffective as a skin prep before surgery but is useful for cleaning after surgery. Many providers do not recommend using hydrogen peroxide on surgical wounds because of its abrasive "scrubbing action," which can cause increased scarring and irritations. Do not use or recommend the use of hydrogen peroxide without consulting your provider.

Antibacterial creams and ointments are sometimes applied topically on wounds to aid healing. Antibacterial creams are usually white, water based, and nongreasy. Antibacterial ointments are usually clear and oil based. If a wound requires thorough cleaning between dressing changes, an antibacterial cream is preferred because of the ease of removal.

Some examples of sterile solutions are sterile saline, sterile distilled water, and Betadine.

Silvadene is the brand name of a sterile cream used on burns and other abrasion wounds. It is an excellent antibacterial cream but must be applied ⅛- to ¼-inch thick to help ensure that the dressing does not absorb all the cream, thus drying out the wound. Sterile tongue blades are handy to apply the Silvadene cream to large-area burns. Silvadene should be thoroughly removed and reapplied fresh with each dressing change. Silvadene is available by prescription only and comes in small tubes for individual use as well as larger jars for multiple uses. Silvadene is fairly expensive. When using a multiple-use jar, as with any multiple-use container, extreme caution must be taken to avoid contamination of the product.

Dressings and Bandages

Procedure

Dressings are sterile material applied directly onto the surface of a wound or surgical site. Bandages are supportive material applied over the top of dressings and are not sterile. A dressing, being sterile, should be handled with care to avoid contamination of the wound. Often a sterile nonstick pad or topical medication is applied to the wound to prevent the dressing from adhering to the wound.

Dressings are usually made of gauze and need to completely cover the wound. The dressings chosen should be adequately absorbent for any wound drainage. See Procedure 30-8 for directions on dressing changes.

Bandages are used to keep dressings in place, to provide padding and protection, and to immobilize. Bandaging may consist of rolled gauze wrapped around the wound area with an additional sturdier wrap applied overall. An elastic bandage may provide additional support, and a triangular bandage, sling, brace, or splint provides even more. A unique type of bandage is the tubular gauze bandage. Tubular gauze bandages are used to cover appendages such as fingers, arms, toes, and legs and come in various sizes according to the size of the body part being covered. Chapter 8 provides information about wounds and bandages. Figure 30-36 illustrates various bandage-wrapping techniques.

Anesthetics

The word *anesthesia* refers to the loss of feeling or sensation. An anesthetic is any mechanism that causes this loss of feeling. The application of extreme cold can be an anesthetic because it causes numbness to nerve endings and thus the loss of feeling. Anesthetics may be inhaled, topically applied, or sprayed, or injected directly into a vein (intravenously), the spinal column (intrathecally), or locally (subcutaneously) into the tissues at the site of the surgical procedure.

Injectable Anesthetics.   Most anesthetics used in office/ambulatory surgery are administered locally through injection into the subcutaneous tissues. The nerves exposed to the anesthetic become temporarily unable to conduct sensations and feelings to the brain, thereby causing a lack of pain sensation in the area during the surgery. All synthetic local anesthetics have names that end in *-caine*. Some of the most common are Xylocaine (lidocaine), Novocaine (procaine), Marcaine, and Carbocaine. Local anesthetics are available in single-dose vials or ampules of 10 mL, but most medical clinics prefer the cost-effectiveness of multiple-dose vials containing 30 to 50 mL. Local anesthetics are also available in varying strengths such as 0.5%, 1%, and 2%. Local anesthetic is chosen based on the mechanism of action. These decisions include the duration of

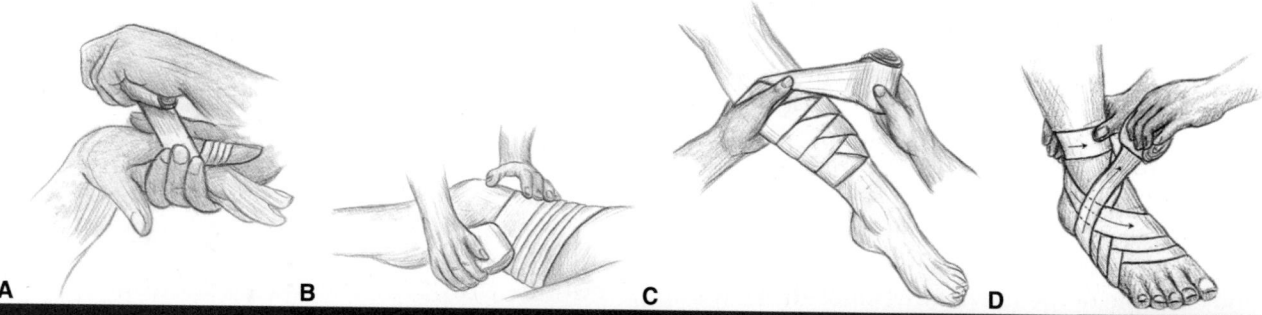

FIGURE 30-36 Bandage-wrapping techniques illustrating the circular, spiral, and figure-eight turns. (A) Circular turns are wrapped around a body part several times to anchor a bandage or to supply support. (B) Spiral turns begin with one or two circular turns, then proceed up the body part, with each turn covering two-thirds the width of the previous turn. (C) Reverse spiral turns begin with a circular turn. Then the bandage is reversed or twisted once each turn to accommodate a limb that gets larger as the bandaging progresses. (D) Figure-eight turns crisscross in the shape of a figure-eight and are used on a joint that requires movement.

anesthesia, and whether or not there are additives that constrict the local vasculature to reduce bleeding at the site.

Injectable anesthetics may contain an additive called **epinephrine**. Such an anesthetic will have a red label. Epinephrine causes vasoconstriction and is used when reduced blood flow to the area is desired. The medical assistant is often delegated the responsibility of filling the syringe with the prescribed amount and strength of the ordered anesthesia or may assist the provider in drawing up the medication. Be sure to identify the drug and dose for the provider. The professional medical assistant must make the practitioner aware that a patient has hypertension if an anesthetic with epinephrine is used. Epinephrine can increase blood pressure.

Competency Any time the medical assistant draws up a medication for the provider or pours a solution into a prep basin on the sterile tray, the original vial or bottle that the medication or solution comes from should be brought into the procedure room with the surgical/procedure tray and other supplies. It is the responsibility of the medical assistant to check the expiration date prior to providing the medication for the practitioner's use. The provider should check the vial and container before using the medication or solution to be sure it is exactly what has been ordered. A good practice is to set the vial or container on the counter within plain view for the provider to see. Often the provider verbally confirms what medication is in the syringe or what solution is in the prep basin before using them. An alternative is to use a sterile marker, while wearing sterile gloves, to label the syringe or container that the practitioner will utilize.

Anesthetics with epinephrine should not be used on fingers, toes, noses, or earlobes because of vasoconstriction. Patients with circulatory complications may have even more restrictions/cautions on the use of epinephrine. This is one reason why it is important to bring the vial into the procedure room with the patient.

Drawing Techniques. If the provider plans to inject the anesthesia before applying sterile gloves, either the medical assistant or the provider may draw up the medication. The filled syringe is then placed to the side, rather than directly on the sterile field. This allows the provider to anesthetize the patient before beginning the sterile procedure. After the anesthesia has taken effect, the provider performs a surgical hand cleansing, applies sterile gloves, and begins the surgery.

When the provider applies sterile gloves before injecting the anesthesia, the sterile syringe may be placed directly on the sterile field either empty or filled. One person wearing sterile gloves may handle the syringe and draw up the medication while another person not wearing sterile gloves holds the vial. The vial must be positioned so that the practitioner can easily read the label. The vial must also be held in a vertical position so that the practitioner can aspirate the fluid with a minimum of air and maintain the sterility of the syringe.

This method requires that the syringe and needle either be applied directly to the sterile tray or be handed directly to a "sterile" person. The medical assistant may draw up the anesthesia under sterile process when the sterile tray is set up. As stated previously, if the tray contains a filled syringe, the vial from which it was drawn should accompany the tray into the procedure room and be set on the counter for the provider to verify. Chapter 35 discusses the specific techniques for drawing up medications.

Topical Spray Anesthetics. Not all anesthesia is injectable. Topical (those that are applied to the surface) anesthetics are available in liquid and spray form. The most common topical anesthetic used in the medical clinic is ethyl chloride spray. Ethyl chloride freezes the skin to allow for simple piercing or lancing. The anesthetic action usually only lasts for a few seconds; therefore, the procedure must be performed quickly. It is highly flammable. One example of the use of ethyl chloride spray is to briefly numb an area before an injection. A lesion that is infected is extremely painful when injected with a local anesthetic; however, by using ethyl chloride spray before the injection, the patient is able to remain still. Ethyl chloride spray may also be used before installing intravenous lines.

The following Quick Reference Guide summarizes supplies and equipment commonly used in minor surgery.

PATIENT CARE AND PREPARATION
Patient Preparation and Education

For the patient who will undergo a planned surgical procedure, there is time for patient preparation. Patients may need to modify their diet, adjust

---

≫ QUICK REFERENCE GUIDE

≫ SUPPLIES AND EQUIPMENT COMMONLY USED IN MINOR SURGERY

Item	Use/Description
Anesthetics © EsHanPhot/Shutterstock.com	A product used to cause the loss of feeling. May be inhaled; topically applied; sprayed; or injected directly into a vein, the spinal column, or locally into the tissues at the site of the surgical procedure.
Bandages © xtrekx/Shutterstock.com	Nonsterile supportive materials applied over dressings to keep the dressings in place. May be rolled gauze, elastic bandage, or tubular gauze bandage.
Creams and ointments © felipe caparros/Shutterstock.com	Antibacterial. May be used topically on wounds to promote healing. Creams are water based; ointments are oil based.
Drapes © Keith A Frith/Shutterstock.com	Used to create a sterile field over and around the operation site. They are made in various sizes and of different materials. A fenestrated drape is commonly used in surgery.

(continues)

Item	Use/Description
Dressings © showcake/Shutterstock.com	Sterile material applied directly onto surface of a wound or surgical site. Usually made of natural or synthetic fibers. Must be adequately absorbent and must completely cover the wound.
Solutions © Denis Semenchenko/Shutterstock.com	Used as skin cleansers, preoperative scrubs, paints, soaks, and antiseptics. Most common are Betadine, an antiseptic often used in soap form as a scrub; Hibiclens, an effective antiseptic without iodine's staining properties; isopropyl alcohol, a 70% alcohol solution favored for skin preparation before injections and venipuncture but not effective as a preoperative skin preparation; and hydrogen peroxide, a mildly effective abrasive skin antiseptic.
Sponges © Sherry Yates Young/Shutterstock.com	Used in wound cleansing, in skin preparation, as absorbable sponges during surgery, as dressings and coverings, and for padding. Also called 4-by-4s. Typically made of folded gauze, though some have cotton or rayon pads embedded in them to increase absorption.
Wicks	Used when an infected wound needs to remain open for drainage. Wicking material is made of narrow strips of gauze packaged in long lengths in opaque glass bottles, which should be opened using sterile technique.

medication, acquire special supplies, adjust their personal home and work situations, obtain prior approval from their insurance, and prepare for the postoperative period. For the patient undergoing an unplanned procedure, such as a laceration repair, there is less time for preparation. In either case, the medical assistant needs to follow an established protocol related to wound care, patient education, patient health considerations, and consent. In the case of an accidental wound, the medical assistant needs to determine the cause of the wound and the date of the last tetanus injection. Chapter 26 provides specific information about tetanus and immunization schedules. The medical assistant must also check to determine whether the patient has allergies or sensitivities of any kind, particularly to medication and medically related substances.

Diet modifications include an absence of eating and drinking for several hours before the surgical procedure, as well as restricting the types and amounts of certain foods or liquids consumed before and directly after the procedure. When patients are aware of special dietary needs after surgery, they can shop early and be prepared. Examples of medication treatments are prescribing an antibiotic to be taken as a precaution against acquiring an infection after surgery and adjusting anticoagulant medications to prevent excessive bleeding during surgery. Each clinic, provider, procedure, and patient has individual requirements and preferences. The patient might be required to obtain special supplies for the convalescent period. For instance, immediately after a vasectomy a scrotal support is usually recommended. Crutches might be necessary after foot or leg surgery. Specific wound dressing and bandages might need to be purchased before the surgery in anticipation of postoperative needs. Having another person accompany the patient to the clinic for the surgery is required for the safe return home. Knowing the planned period for recovery allows the patient to make the necessary arrangements for work, childcare, and other personal situations.

Informed Consent

Legal

Before a surgical procedure, the patient's written consent must be obtained. For many medical and all surgical procedures, an **informed consent** form must be signed. An informed consent is a document that may be created specifically for a particular procedure or that may be an established document available for duplication. An informed consent document informs the patient of the medical or surgical procedure to be performed, describes the actual procedure in lay terms, cites alternative treatments, and lists possible undesirable outcomes and risks related to the procedure. Chapter 6 provides additional information about informed consent and a model consent farm.

The cost of the procedure is important information. Some insurances companies and Medicare require patients to sign an Advanced Beneficiary Notice (ABN) if their out-of-pocket expenses will exceed a certain amount. It is always a good idea to discuss financial arrangements with all patients before an elective procedure or surgery. In some clinics, the bookkeeper or office manager comes into the examination room, sits down with the patient, and goes over specific necessary forms and financial arrangements. Any questions the patient has about the surgery should be answered completely by the provider, and an assessment should be made that the patient understands the answers. Even in the best of circumstances, health care results cannot be guaranteed. Most of the difficult situations between providers' practices and patients come from misunderstandings about unexpected outcomes. If patients are informed completely, even unplanned results are better tolerated.

Medical Assisting Considerations

Initiative

The general health and condition of the patient before surgery is important when planning the recovery. A frail, weak person living alone may need home health care after even a simple surgical procedure. Some people may not be able to follow standard preoperative or postoperative instructions. The recovery may depend on the availability of supplies beyond what the patient can financially afford. If difficult circumstances can be identified before the surgery, arrangements can be made with home health care services, community assistance services, or friends and family. As a professional medical assistant, your role is to be a patient advocate. You must utilize the principles that you have learned in your training to provide holistic patient care. Understanding the health care benefits that your patient has access to beyond the care provided in the clinic could dictate the successful outcome of any intervention. It is the responsibility of the professional medical assistant to collaborate with the provider, the insurer, and the family to ensure the best interests and care of the patient.

This can help avoid complications. Prior medical history should also be established and questions should be asked about allergies and sensitivities to medications and medical substances. A pulse oximeter is applied to the patient to monitor blood oxygen percentage (see Chapter 29). Vital signs are watched carefully. The policy and procedure of the clinic or ambulatory surgery center will establish the guidelines for the safe discharge of the patient postprocedure.

Postoperative Instructions

Postoperative instructions should be written and clearly understood by the patient and his or her support system. The telephone number of the clinic and an after-hours number should be written on the postoperative instructions and brought to the attention of the patient and caregiver. It is good practice to plan to call patients within the first postoperative day to check on their condition.

Wounds, Wound Care, and the Healing Process

There are many different types of wounds based on the type of injury incurred. Wounds may be classified as open or closed, accidental, or intentional (surgical).

Lacerations, incisions, avulsions, and punctures are all examples of open wounds (Figure 30-37).

Ecchymosis, contusion, and hematoma are examples of closed wounds. They are caused by a blunt trauma that damages underlying tissues but leaves the skin intact (Figure 30-38).

Wounds are classified as superficial if the injury does not extend deeper than the subcutaneous tissues. Deep wounds extend beyond the subcutaneous layer. The size, location, and depth of the wound

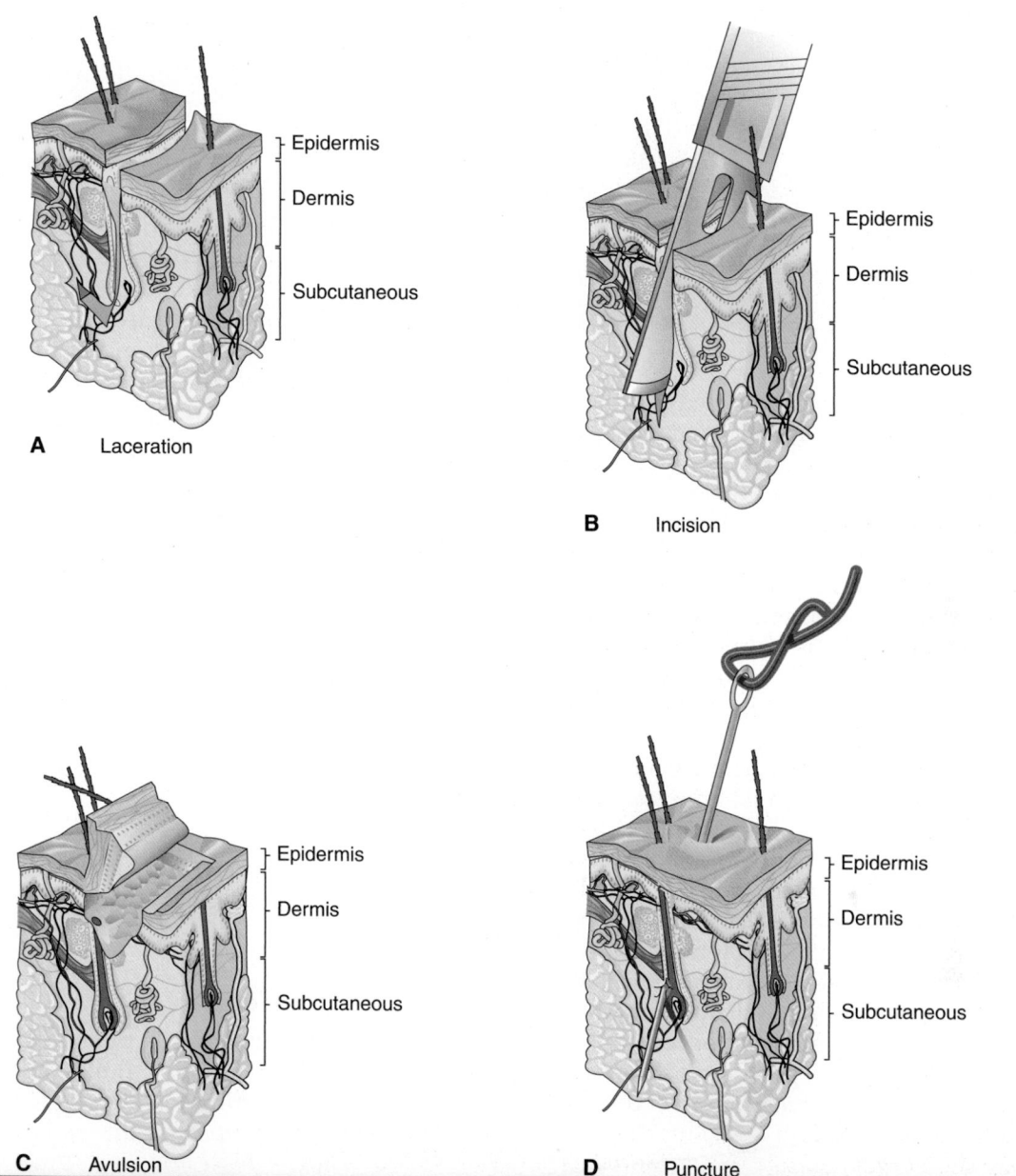

FIGURE 30-37 Open wounds. (A) Lacerations are accidental tearing of the body tissue usually made by sharp objects. The torn flesh may be smooth or jagged and often is difficult to clean and suture properly. There may be extensive bleeding. A cut from a sharp knife is an example of a laceration. (B) Incisions are intentional cuts typically made with a scalpel for surgical procedures. (C) Avulsions are accidental tearing away of a part or structures of the skin. (D) Punctures are holes or wounds made by a pointed object and can be either accidental or intentional. Puncture wounds have little bleeding because the point of entry is small. These wounds typically are not much larger than the instrument entering the skin. A puncture wound may also be the result of stepping on a nail.

are important descriptors both for the medical record and for proper insurance reimbursement. An appropriate description of a patient wound that is an intermediate laceration might be, "patient sustained a deep 3.5-cm laceration to the anterior surface of the right knee caused by a fall onto a rock." A puncture wound might be described as, "patient presents with a 2-cm deep puncture wound on the plantar surface of the left foot obtained from stepping on a rusty nail." Both statements describe not only the size, depth, location, and type of wound, but also the causative factor.

Inflammation is the body's natural reaction to trauma. Inflammation is also a normal process of wound healing. Occasionally, inflamed tissue will become infected if the trauma is caused by a

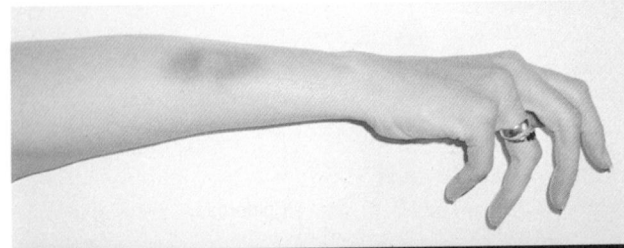

FIGURE 30-38 Closed wounds include contusions, ecchymoses, and hematomas. This photograph shows an ecchymosis.

pathogen. Although a certain degree of inflammation is expected, prevention of infection is a primary goal (see Chapter 21).

Chapter 8 describes wounds and emergency care of wounds.

Procedure

The best treatment of infection is prevention. Instructing the patient about proper wound care is extremely important. Encourage the patient to keep the wound clean and dry. In certain circumstances, the provider may prescribe a warm soak solution or the application of a topical antibacterial medication. If the wound becomes infected and a **suppurant** is present, the provider may order wound irrigation (see Procedure 30-9). Wound irrigation removes the accumulation of purulent **exudate** that delays healing. After the irrigation, a dry sterile dressing is applied (see Procedure 30-5). Protecting the wound from further trauma and contamination will aid in the healing process. Opinions will differ on whether a wound is best left open to the air or covered with a dressing. Most health care providers will agree that covering a wound is preferred whenever contamination is likely.

BASIC SURGERY SETUP

Preparing for surgery includes assembling supplies and equipment, setting up the surgery tray, getting the patient and room ready, and preparing to assist the provider during surgery. The specific instruments, supplies, and equipment needed for each surgery should be listed on individual **preference cards** or in a digital database that is easily accessible. The cards may be 3-by-5 or 5-by-7 and stored in a card file, they may be full sheets of procedures compiled in a manual or notebook, or procedures may be filed digitally. Each provider will have individual instrument sets for each surgical procedure performed. Information in the provider's preference listing should include provider glove size, standing preoperative and postoperative instructions, type of skin preparation, and any additional information specific to the provider's needs or to the surgical procedure. The card file, whether manual or digital, should be updated whenever changes are made, which is a task that may be the responsibility of the medical assistant.

Basic Rules and Concepts for Setup of Surgical Trays

In addition to basic sterile principles, the guidelines in Table 30-3 will help ensure the sterile field remains sterile.

SURGERY PROCESS

For ease in understanding the individual tasks involved in clinic surgery, Table 30-4 provides generic steps for setting up the surgical tray, preparing the room, preparing the patient, assisting

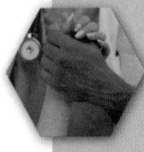

Patient Education

The basic signs of inflammation are redness, heat, swelling, pain, and loss of function. Any one or more of these may be present in varying intensities during the inflammatory process. Most wounds will have mild inflammation described as slightly red or pink, with mild warmth, slightly tender to the touch, and mildly swollen. The symptoms are caused by increased blood supply to the traumatized area and the infiltration of white blood cells in reaction to the trauma. Patients should be taught to watch for an increase in the intensity of redness, pain, swelling, and heat or any drainage, fever, or lymph gland swelling, which can indicate an **infection** from invading pathogens. Patients should be given instructions as to what actions to take if these symptoms of infection are noticed. They should also be instructed to take their temperature twice a day and phone the provider if their temperature reaches 101°F or higher.

The instructions should include a name and telephone numbers to call during the day or night. The medical assistant should reassure the patient not to hesitate to contact the center or provider if infection is suspected.

TABLE 30-3

GUIDELINES FOR STERILE TRAY SETUPS

Set up the sterile surgery tray just before the surgery to minimize the chance of accidental contamination.

If a tray is to be set up prior to a procedure or in another location, after the tray is set up, cover it with a sterile drape immediately.

Once the tray is prepared and covered, move it directly into the surgery area rather than leaving it in a common area.

Inform the patient and others in the surgery room that the tray is sterile and should not be touched. Patients are often curious about instruments and may attempt to look under the cover if not cautioned against it.

If you are interrupted while preparing the tray and it becomes necessary to leave the tray unattended, cover the tray and move it out of traffic paths to prevent it from being bumped.

with the surgery, and the terminal care process of the room and equipment. Table 30-4 is intended as a quick checklist only and does not include all the specific details necessary for each surgery. Refer to the individual surgical procedures that follow for more details.

TABLE 30-4

PREPARATIONS FOR MINOR SURGERY

TRAY SETUP

1. Wash hands.
2. Reference surgery card, manual, or computer.
3. Gather equipment and supplies.
4. Sanitize and disinfect Mayo instrument tray.
5. Wash hands.
6. Set up sterile field.
7. Place sterile instruments and supplies on the sterile field.
8. Apply sterile gloves or use sterile transfer forceps.
9. Arrange instruments and supplies in an organized and logical manner.
10. Medication may be drawn up with assistance (optional) (Figure 30-39).
11. Recheck tray for accuracy and completeness.
12. Remove gloves.
13. Cover tray using sterile technique.
14. Add sterile solution (skin antiseptic) to tray if required.

ROOM PREPARATION

In preparing a room for a surgical procedure, all equipment should be clean and in good working order. Be certain to have spare parts such as light bulbs and filters readily available. Turn on equipment before the procedure to make sure all is working properly.

1. Check room equipment (light, stool, equipment, examination table, waste receptacle).
2. Check room supplies (PPE, dressings, etc.).
3. Arrange accessory supplies on the side counter in a logical order (pathology specimen bottle containing preservative, laboratory requisition, sterile glove package, dressings/bandages, postoperative medications, and instructions).

PATIENT PREPARATION

1. Wash hands.
2. Greet patient and ensure identity.
3. Escort the patient to the procedure room and offer restroom facilities.
4. Discuss the patient's compliance to preoperative instructions.
5. Explain the procedure again and address any questions.
6. Review postoperative instructions.
7. Check for signed informed consent form and financial forms.
8. Have the patient remove appropriate clothing and position the patient on the examination table. Drape and then offer gown, pillow, and blanket for comfort.
9. Prepare the skin for the surgical procedure (see Procedure 30-6).

ASSISTING WITH THE SURGERY

1. Remove the sterile cover, using appropriate technique, from the surgical tray while the provider applies sterile gloves.
2. Assist the provider with stool and lamp adjustment as needed.
3. If you did not perform the skin preparation, assist the provider as needed during skin preparation and draping. The equipment and supplies for skin preparation are separate from the surgery tray and equipment.
4. Adjust the instrument tray and equipment around the provider.
5. Assist with drawing up local anesthetic or other medication as needed.
6. Apply clean gloves for protection or sterile gloves to assist.
7. Surgery begins.
8. The medical assistant either assists with sterile procedure or supports the patient as needed.
9. Assist the provider in placing the specimen, if one is obtained, in a sterile specimen container (Figure 30-40).
10. After surgery, assist with or perform dressing of wound.

(continues)

Table 30-4, continued

11. Clean any surrounding skin of blood or skin prep material

12. Remove gloves and dispose of properly.

13. Wash hands and don clean gloves.

14. Label any specimens obtained with the patient's name, date of birth, patient number (if available), date and time of procedure, and type of specimen.

15. Prepare lab requisition to accompany specimen.

16. Apply formalin or refrigerate as needed based on type of specimen and pathology testing to be performed.

17. Dispose of biohazardous waste materials.

18. Remove contaminated gloves; wash hands.

19. Assist the patient after surgery.

ASSISTING THE PATIENT AFTER SURGERY

1. Check patient vital signs.

2. Remain with patient to ensure patient safety. Allow patient to rest if necessary.

3. Assist patient off examination table and assist with clothing as necessary.

4. Review written postoperative instructions with patient and caregiver. Dressing should be kept clean and dry. Patient should report any signs of infection.

5. Clarify any medication orders with patient and support system.

6. If not previously arranged, schedule follow-up appointment.

7. Document postoperative instructions in patient chart or electronic medical record.

TERMINAL CARE OF THE ROOM AND EQUIPMENT

1. Apply barrier gloves, gown, and goggles (if appropriate).

2. Dispose of drapes, table cover, pillowcase, and so on. Use biohazardous waste receptacle whenever appropriate.

3. Transfer contaminated surgical tray to cleanup area.

4. Using forceps, isolate sharps from surgical tray and dispose of them into designated sharps container.

5. Place instruments into a soak solution.

6. Sanitize Mayo instrument tray and all surfaces (examination table, stool, counter, lamp, machinery, and equipment).

7. Dispose of contaminated barrier gloves and apply protective gloves.

8. Disinfect all surfaces (examination table, stool, counter, lamp, machinery, and equipment).

9. Allow to air dry.

10. Sanitize, dry, wrap, and sterilize instruments.

11. Ensure there are enough of each instrument and surgical set.

NOTE: During most surgical procedures, if tissue is excised, it is placed in a biopsy specimen jar containing formalin (a preservative) and sent to the pathology laboratory with an appropriately completed requisition (Figure 30-40).

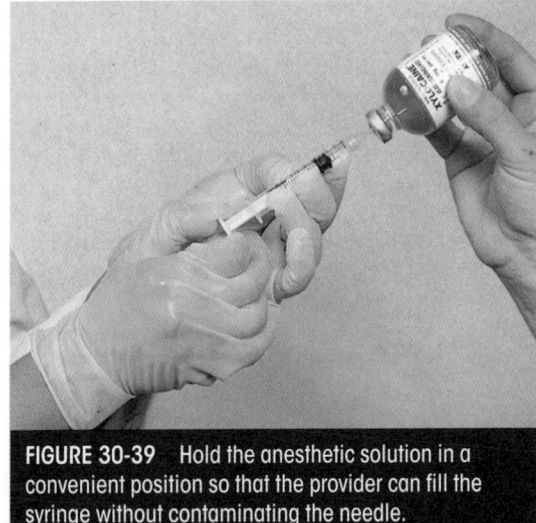

FIGURE 30-39 Hold the anesthetic solution in a convenient position so that the provider can fill the syringe without contaminating the needle.

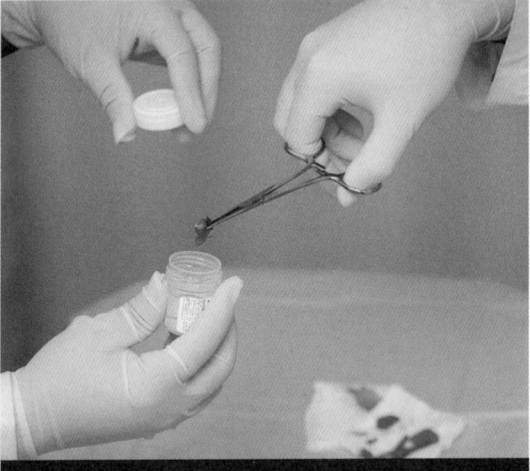

FIGURE 30-40 The provider places biopsy tissue into specimen jar. The specimen will be sent to the pathology laboratory for examination.

PREPARATION FOR SURGERY

Procedure

The following procedures are used in preparation for minor surgery:

- Applying sterile gloves (Procedure 30-1)
- Setting up a sterile field with instruments (Procedure 30-5)
- Preparing patient's skin before surgery (Procedure 30-6)

Setting up surgical trays for specific surgeries is addressed in the final procedures of this chapter:

- Excising sebaceous cyst (Procedure 30-13)
- Performing incision and drainage of localized infection (Procedure 30-14)

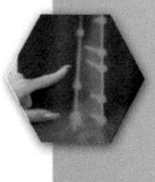

Critical Thinking

Dr. Woo asks you to assist him in repairing the laceration on Jaime Carrera's hand. Though you are unsure, you think you may have noticed a tiny hole in the palm of your left glove. What is your next step? Is this something that you should report to your provider?

- Aspirating joint fluid (Procedure 30-15)
- Performing hemorrhoid thrombectomy (Procedure 30-16)

Using Dry Sterile Transfer Forceps

Occasionally after a sterile tray has been set up and sterile gloves removed, an additional item needs to be applied to or removed from the tray. The use of dry sterile transfer forceps allows sterile items to be applied or sterile items on the tray to be rearranged without the application of another pair of sterile gloves (Figure 30-41). The practice of using wet sterile transfer forceps is no longer recommended. Instead, when the use of sterile transfer forceps is needed, dry sterile transfer forceps are unwrapped, used only once, and then reprocessed for sterilization and subsequent use.

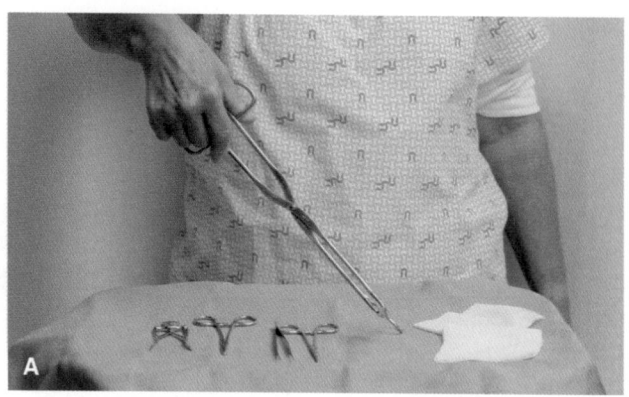

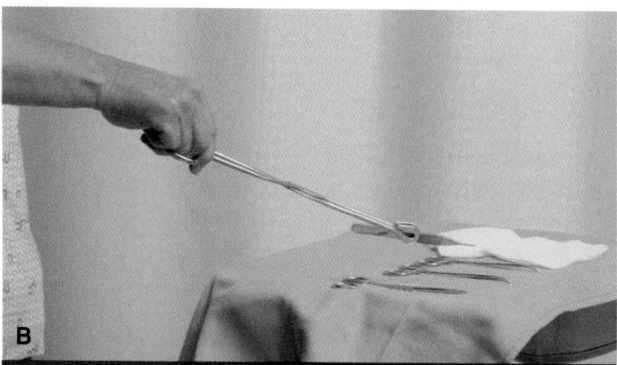

FIGURE 30-41 (A) If sterile gloves have been removed, use dry sterile transfer forceps to apply or rearrange sterile items on the Mayo stand. (B) Instruments and supplies can be moved around using dry sterile transfer forceps if necessary.

PROCEDURE 30-5

 Procedure

Setting Up a Sterile Field with Instruments

STANDARD PRECAUTIONS:

 Handwashing   Gloves 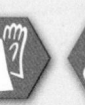 Goggles & Mask  Biohazard 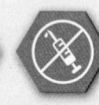 No Needle Recapping

PURPOSE:

To maintain sterility during surgical procedures that require surgical excision.

EQUIPMENT/SUPPLIES:

Mayo Stand:

- Needles and syringe for anesthesia
- Prep bowl/cup
- Gauze sponges

Side Table (Unsterile Field):

- Sterile gloves (in package)
- Labeled biopsy containers with formalin
- Appropriate laboratory requisition

(continues)

Mayo Stand:

- Scalpel and blade
- Operating scissors
- Fenestrated drape
- Hemostats (curved and straight)
- Thumb dressing forceps
- Thumb tissue forceps
- Needle holder
- Suture pack
- Transfer forceps
- Sterile disposable field drape

Side Table (Unsterile Field):

- Anesthesia vial
- Alcohol wipes
- Dressing, tape, bandages
- Biohazard container
- Betadine solution

PROCEDURE STEPS:

NOTE: The steps for preparing a sterile field require concentration and should never be hurried.

1. Wash your hands.
2. Don non-sterile gloves and sanitize and disinfect a Mayo instrument tray that has been adjusted to waist level with the stem to the right.
3. Check room and equipment for readiness and cleanliness.
4. Remove your gloves and wash your hands again before proceeding.
5. Select an appropriate disposable sterile field drape and place the drape package on a clean, dry, flat surface. Depending on the medical setting, the field drape may be either a disposable sterile polylined drape or reusable water-repellent sterile towels.
6. Open the package to expose the fan-folded surgical drape. RATIONALE: Sterile field drapes are fan-folded and positioned within the package to facilitate ease of use.
7. Using only the thumb and forefinger of one hand, carefully grasp the corner without touching the rest of the drape. Pick the drape up high enough to ensure that it touches nothing unsterile as it unfolds. RATIONALE: The drape or towel will naturally unfold as it is lifted, so care must be taken to ensure that it is lifted quickly and allowed to unfold without touching a nonsterile surface.
8. Keep the drape above waist level, away from your body, and grasp the opposing corner so that both corners along one edge of the drape are being held.
9. Reach over the Mayo tray with the drape, but do not allow the drape to drag across or otherwise touch the tray.
10. Gently pull the drape toward you as it is laid on the tray. It is extremely important that you do not reach over or touch the center of the drape. If any adjustments are needed, you must either reach under or walk around the draped tray. RATIONALE: Remember that all areas within one inch of the edges of the drape are considered unsterile. Items that are placed or that fall onto that area of the drape are considered contaminated and must be removed from the sterile field using sterile technique.
11. Grasping the taped end of the top flap, open the first flap away from you, taking care not to touch the inside of the flap (Figures 30-42A and B).
12. Now, grasping the tips of the side flaps that have just been folded back, pull the right-sided flap to the right. Follow with the left side. This will allow the inner portion of the package to be exposed without contamination. Do not reach over the package at any time (Figure 30-42C). RATIONALE: Pulling the tips of the flaps toward each side allows the inner portion of the package to be exposed without contamination.
13. Pull the last flap toward you by grasping the folded-back tip. It is very important that you do not touch the inner contents of the package (Figure 30-42D). RATIONALE: Pulling the last tip toward you allows you to avoid reaching over the inner contents of the package.
14. Gather all of the loose ends together to obtain a snug covering over the non-dominant hand. Then, close your covered hand over the inner package and gently drop the inner package on the sterile field (Figure 30-42E). RATIONALE: Gathering the loose edges prevents them from being dragged across the sterile field.

(continues)

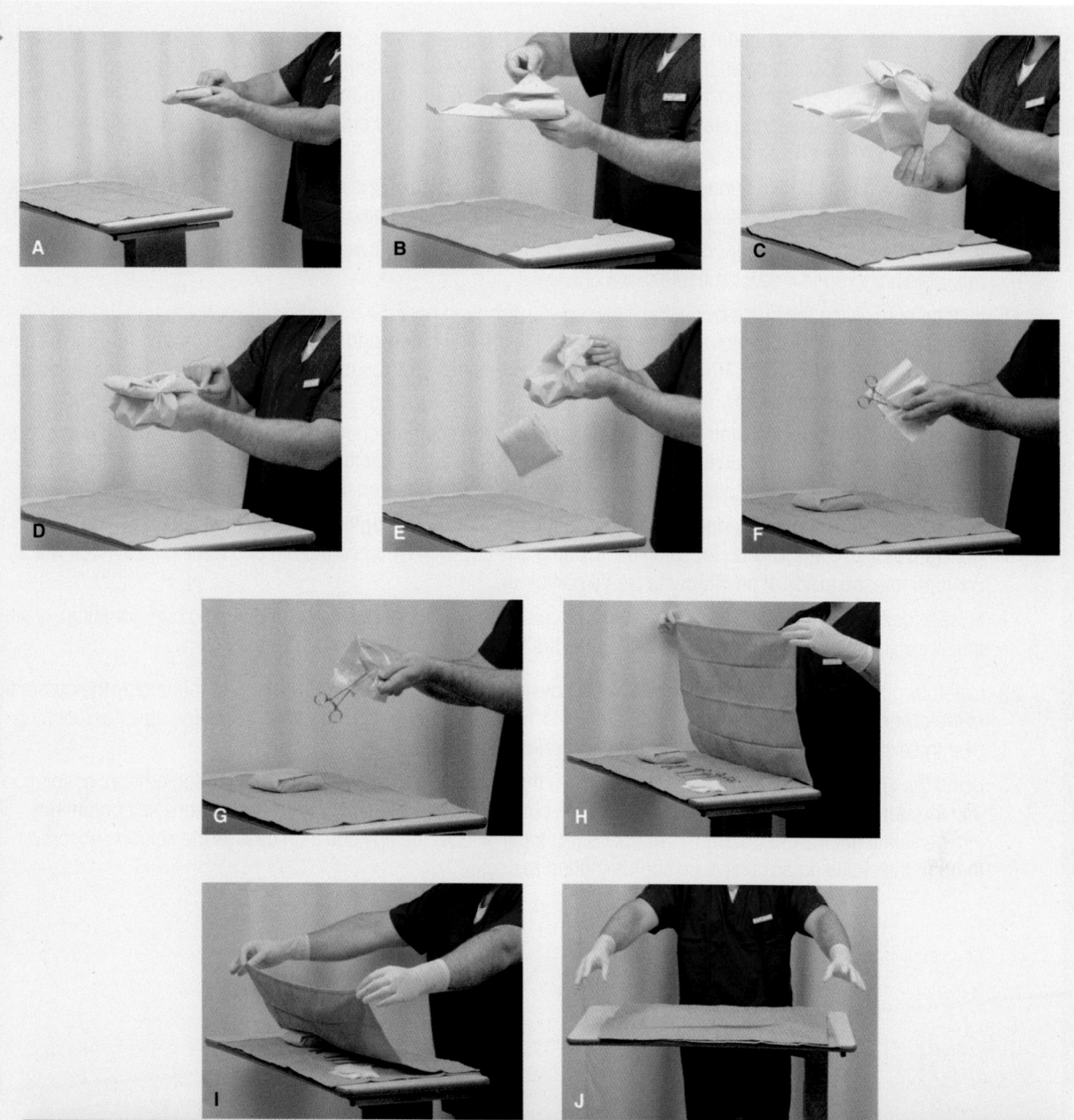

FIGURE 30-42 (A) To open a twice-wrapped pack, grasp the taped end of the top flap and open the first flap away from you. You should have the Mayo tray at or above waist height. Stand back from the sterile field. (B) Allow the pack to unroll on your hand. Do not touch the inside of the flap. Notice the medical assistant's thumb is under the flap, where he can securely grasp the inner pack. (C) Grasp just the folded back tips of the side flaps. First pull the right-sided tip to the right, then, reaching around or under, pull the left-sided tip to the left. Do not reach over the package. (D) Gather the loose edges together to form a snug covering over your nondominant hand. Securely grasping the wrapped inner pack, step toward your sterile field, and invert your hand. (E) Release (drop) the inner pack onto the center of the sterile field. Step back. (F) Open peel-apart packages using sterile technique, exposing sterile items slowly and gradually. Continue to peel back the sides of the package while securely holding onto the tip of the instrument. (G) Hold the sides of the package over your hand, step toward the Mayo tray, and apply the instrument, handle first, onto the sterile field. Apply other supplies as needed. Arrange instruments and supplies according to provider's preference using sterile gloves or sterile transfer forceps. (H) Apply the sterile drape cover to the surgical tray in a similar manner as the field was set up, except apply drape away from you. (I) Be sure the edges of the cover align with the edges of the field drape before letting go and applying the cover. (J) Do not adjust cover after it has been laid.

(continues)

15. Open the peel-apart instrument packages using sterile technique by grasping both edges of the flaps and pulling them apart with a rolling down motion, while keeping both hands together. As you peel, the sterile items should gradually be exposed between the two edges (Figure 30-42F). The instrument can then be offered either to the provider, who will be wearing sterile gloves, or it can be gently dropped onto the sterile field using a flipping motion (Figure 30-42G and H).

16. Apply sterile gloves before arranging the instruments and supplies on the sterile field. RATIONALE: All instruments and supplies should be organized in order of use with all handles pointed toward the user.

17. If the instruments and supplies are not to be used immediately, you will need to apply a sterile field cover. To do this, obtain and open a second sterile drape or towel.

18. Instead of applying the drape by pulling it toward you, this time hold the drape up between you and the field. Adjust the lower edge so that it is even with the lower edge of the first drape, and then with a forward motion, lay the cover over the sterile field (Figures 30-42I and J). RATIONALE: Ensures that you are never leaning your body over either the sterile field or instruments.

19. You will now add sterile solution to the field. Before using the solution, check the label of the container a minimum of three times to ensure that it matches that which has been ordered by the provider. Check the expiration date. RATIONALE: Eliminates the possibility of pouring the wrong solution or an outdated solution.

20. Without touching the inner surface, remove the cap from the solution bottle and place it upside down on a nonsterile surface. RATIONALE: Touching the inside of the cap with either your hand or a nonsterile surface will contaminate the inside of an otherwise sterile container.

21. Protect the label of the bottle with your palm, and pour a small amount of the solution into a cup, container, or sink that is outside the sterile field in order to cleanse the lip of the bottle.

22. Carefully pull back the upper right corner of the tray cover to expose the cup. Be careful to touch only the corner tip of the cover and not to reach over the exposed field. RATIONALE: Touching the underside of the cover or reaching over the exposed sterile field will contaminate the sterile surgical tray.

23. Using the cleansed lip of the bottle, approach from the corner of the tray and pour the needed amount of solution into the sterile cup (Figure 30-43). As you pour, be careful to avoid splashing, spilling, or otherwise contaminating the sterile field. RATIONALE: If this happens you must discard the tray and start over as the solution absorbed through the sterile drape can cause contamination to occur.

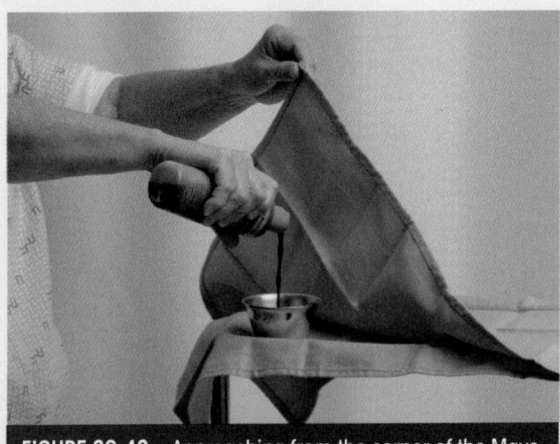

FIGURE 30-43 Approaching from the corner of the Mayo stand, pour the needed amount of solution into the sterile cup. Use the clean side of the container lip for pouring.

24. Replace the corner of the drape cover using sterile technique.

25. Replace the cap of the solution using sterile technique.

26. The sterile field is now ready for the provider's use. Remember that a sterile field is no longer sterile if left unattended, even if it was covered.

PROCEDURE 30-6

Procedure

Preparing Patient's Skin before Surgery

STANDARD PRECAUTIONS:

Handwashing

Gloves

NOTE: The skin and hair contain many microorganisms, and the patient's skin must be prepared before surgery to remove as many of the microorganisms as possible. Wound infection results when microorganisms enter the body. The patient may be told to scrub the site of the surgery using antimicrobial soap on the night before surgery. Because it is impossible to sterilize the skin, the operative site and an area surrounding it are scrubbed, shaved (hair harbors microorganisms), washed, and painted with an antiseptic such as Betadine solution. A skin prep self-contained unit is a sponge applicator with a cylinder of antiseptic solution inside. One brand is DuraPrep. It contains iodophor and isopropyl alcohol. The medical assistant can use the unit with nonsterile gloves. The unit is compressed, the seal to the inner cylinder is broken, and the sponge end becomes the applicator. The mixture is thick and should be allowed to dry; it should not be blotted. Because it contains alcohol, which can be a fire hazard, the site must be dry before draping. The chemical action decontaminates the patient's skin.

PURPOSE:

To remove as many microorganisms as possible from the patient's skin immediately before surgery.

EQUIPMENT/SUPPLIES:

- Absorbent pads
- Drape
- Disposable prep kit (includes antiseptic solution, several sponges, razor, and a container for water, or self-contained skin prep unit)
- Sterile water
- Betadine prep sticks
- Sterile gloves for medical assistant and provider (two pairs)

PROCEDURE STEPS:

1. *Paying attention to detail*, assemble your supplies.
2. Wash your hands following proper procedure.
3. Introduce yourself and identify the patient using two identifiers.
4. *Explain the rationale for performance of the procedure. Show awareness of the patient's concerns* and answer any questions.
5. Before draping or prepping the patient, take a moment to verify the location of the surgical site with the patient. Some facilities might even require that the site be indicated with an indelible ink pen to ensure that the correct site is identified.
6. Position the patient for comfort and for access to the site per provider's preference.
7. Wash your hands and place waterproof absorbent toweling under the area to be prepped. Check with the provider regarding the area to be shaved around the surgical site.
8. Don nonsterile gloves.

(continues)

9. Open the shave kit and place it in an area that is close to the incision site for ease of access. Pour sterile water into a well located in the kit. Add soap solution if needed, and soap the area to be shaved.

10. Begin to shave against the direction of hair growth. Shave at least 4 inches around the incision site or to the extent that the provider prefers.

11. Wipe away any hair that remains on the skin. Pat dry with absorbent material.

12. Discard razor in the sharps container and the other materials in the trash.

13. Dispose of gloves and wash your hands.

14. Open the disposable prep kit or assemble the items you will need. Don sterile gloves and pour the Betadine or other antiseptic solution onto the sponges or gauze.

15. Place the sterile towel under the operative site, taking care not to touch anything. Carefully, begin at the intended incision site and cleanse in an outward circular motion. It is important that you not return to the incision site with a used sponge, but instead begin each new cycle of cleansing with a new sterile sponge.

16. Blot the cleansed area dry with a sterile towel, being careful to maintain sterile technique.

17. Carefully, and without splashing, pour antiseptic solution into the sterile bowl and utilize Betadine paint sticks to paint the operative area with the solution three times. As before, take a fresh applicator after each pass and create a cleansed area that is much larger than the intended incisional area. Allow the solution to dry completely before proceeding.

18. Dispose of any used supplies in the proper containers. Remove gloves and wash your hands.

19. If directed, document the skin prep procedure in the patient's medical record.

PROCEDURE 30-7

Procedure

Assisting with Minor Surgery

STANDARD PRECAUTIONS:

Handwashing   Gloves   No Needle Recapping   Biohazard

PURPOSE:

To maintain sterility during surgical procedures that require surgical excision.

EQUIPMENT/SUPPLIES:

Mayo Stand

- Needles and syringe for anesthesia
- Prep bowl/cup
- Gauze sponges
- Scalpel and blade
- Operating scissors

Side Table (Unsterile Field)

- Sterile gloves (in package)
- Labeled biopsy containers with formalin
- Appropriate laboratory requisition
- Anesthesia vial
- Alcohol wipes

(continues)

Mayo Stand

- Fenestrated drape
- Hemostats (curved and straight)
- Thumb dressing forceps
- Thumb tissue forceps
- Needle holder
- Suture pack
- Transfer forceps

Side Table (Unsterile Field)

- Dressing, tape, bandages
- Biohazard container
- Betadine solution

PROCEDURE STEPS:

1. Check room and equipment for readiness and cleanliness.
2. Wash hands.
3. *Paying attention to detail,* set up side table of nonsterile items. RATIONALE: Nonsterile items cannot be placed onto a sterile field because they will contaminate it.
4. Perform surgical asepsis hand cleansing.
5. Set up sterile field on a sanitized and disinfected Mayo stand or on a clean, dry, flat surface (see Procedure 30-5).
6. *Paying attention to detail,* add sterile items to the sterile field.
7. Apply sterile gloves or use sterile transfer forceps (per Procedure 30-1).
8. Arrange instruments according to provider's instructions.
9. Remove sterile gloves and dispose of appropriately or remove forceps from area.
10. Wash hands.
11. Cover the sterile field with a sterile towel if not being used immediately.
12. Introduce yourself. *Identify the patient and explain the rationale for performance of the procedure at the patient's level of understanding. Show awareness of the patient's concerns by answering any questions.*
13. Prepare the patient based on the procedure to be performed and per provider's preference. Refer to Patient Preparation in Table 30-4.
14. Use appropriate skin prep.
15. *Paying attention to detail,* remove the sterile cover from the sterile setup as the provider applies sterile gloves. Lift the towel by grasping the tips of the corners farthest away from you and lifting toward you. Do not allow arms to pass over sterile field. RATIONALE: Avoids crossing over sterile field.
16. *Working within your scope of practice,* assist the provider as necessary, being certain to follow the principles of surgical asepsis.
    - Appropriately hold the vial of anesthetic agent while the provider withdraws the required dose.
    - The provider injects the local anesthetic, applies Betadine or other antiseptic to the surgical site, applies sterile drapes, and begins the surgery. Apply sterile gloves to assist as requested.
    - Adjust the instrument tray and equipment around the provider.
    - Ensure a good light source.
    - *Allay the patient's fears regarding the procedure being performed and help him or her to feel safe and comfortable.*
17. Hand instruments to the provider and receive used instruments from the provider and place in a basin or container out of the patient's line of sight.

(continues)

18. If necessary, hold biopsy container to receive specimen being excised. Do not contaminate the inside of the container. Assist with or apply sterile dressing to the operative site.

19. *Being courteous and respectful,* assist the patient as necessary. ***Attend to any special needs of the patient.***

20. The specimen container must be tightly covered; labeled with the patient's name, date, type, and source of specimen; and sent to the laboratory accompanied by the appropriate laboratory requisition.

21. Wearing appropriate personal protective equipment (PPE), clean surgical or examination room.

   • Dispose of used gauze sponges in biohazard container and knife blades and other disposable sharps in puncture-proof sharps container.

   • Rinse used surgical instruments; soak, sanitize, and sterilize for reuse (see Chapter 21).

   • Remove gloves and other PPE and dispose of per Occupational Safety and Health Administration (OSHA) guidelines.

22. Wash hands.

23. Accurately document in patient's chart or electronic medical record that the specimen was sent to the laboratory.

DOCUMENTATION:

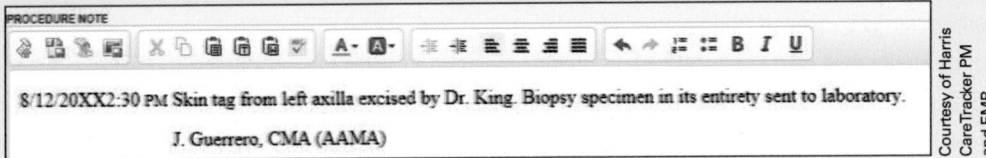

8/12/20XX 2:30 PM Skin tag from left axilla excised by Dr. King. Biopsy specimen in its entirety sent to laboratory.

J. Guerrero, CMA (AAMA)

Courtesy of Harris CareTracker PM and EMR

PROCEDURE 30-8

Procedure

Changing Dressings

STANDARD PRECAUTIONS:

Handwashing   Gloves   Biohazard

NOTE: After most surgical procedures have been completed, the wound is usually covered with a dry sterile dressing (DSD) that may need to be removed periodically so that the wound can be checked for healing or for suture removal. Another dry sterile dressing may then be applied. Burns require daily dressing changes.

PURPOSE:

To remove a wound dressing and apply a dry sterile dressing.

EQUIPMENT/SUPPLIES:

Sterile Field:

• Several sterile gauze sponges and other dressing material as needed or prepackaged sterile dressing kit

Unsterile Field:

• Nonsterile gloves
• Unopened sterile gloves

(continues)

Sterile Field:

- Sterile bowl with Betadine solution or prepared sterile Betadine swab sticks
- Sterile dressing forceps
- Sponge forceps

Unsterile Field:

- Hydrogen peroxide
- Unopened sterile water
- Cotton-tipped applicators
- Adhesive strips
- Antibacterial ointment/cream as ordered
- Tape
- Sponge forceps
- Bandage scissors
- Waterproof waste bag
- Biohazard waste container

PROCEDURE STEPS:

1. Check the provider's order and assemble the equipment you will need.

2. Wash your hands and follow Standard Precautions.

3. Check provider's order.

4. Introduce yourself to the patient and ***explain the rationale for the procedure to be performed. Speak at the patient's level of understanding,*** and answer any questions.

5. Prepare the sterile field and add sterile gauze sponges; a sterile bowl with a Betadine solution; and two sets of sterile forceps, one each for the dressing and the sponges.

6. Prepare a waterproof bag away from the sterile area, but still within reach.

7. Don gloves or use the forceps and loosen the tape on the bandage by pulling it toward the wound (Figure 30-44A).

8. Carefully remove the bandage and place it in a waterproof bag or directly into a pedal-operated biohazard container. Do not allow the contaminated dressing to pass over the sterile field. RATIONALE: Passing dirty (used) bandages or dressings over sterile field contaminates it.

9. Remove and dispose of gloves.

10. Don sterile gloves. Remove the dressing carefully, taking care not to cause any stress on the area when you do so. If the dressing is stuck to the wound, pour small amounts of sterile water or saline over the dressing and allow it to soak for a short time. Remove the dressing when you can do so without any resistance and discard it in the waterproof bag, being careful not to touch the outside of the bag with the dressing or the inside of the bag with your hands. Alternatively, utilize the pedal-operated biohazard container to dispose of the dressing. RATIONALE: Dirty (used) dressings can contaminate outside of bag.

11. Evaluate the wound for any drainage and note the amount and type in order to record accurately in the medical record.

12. Remove gloves and wash your hands.

13. Don a second pair of sterile gloves and clean the wound with antiseptic solution as ordered (Figure 30-44B). Discard the swabs or gauze into the biohazard container when finished.

14. Using sterile cotton– or Dacron-tipped applicators, apply cream or ointment to the wound as ordered, and follow by covering it with sterile gauze sponges (Figure 30-44C), using the roller bandages to secure the dressing (Figure 30-44D). Further secure the dressing with adhesive tape or elastic bandage as directed (Figure 30-44E).

15. Dispose of the waterproof bag in the biohazard waste container. Remove and dispose of the sterile gloves and wash your hands.

16. Document the procedure in the patient's medical record.

(continues)

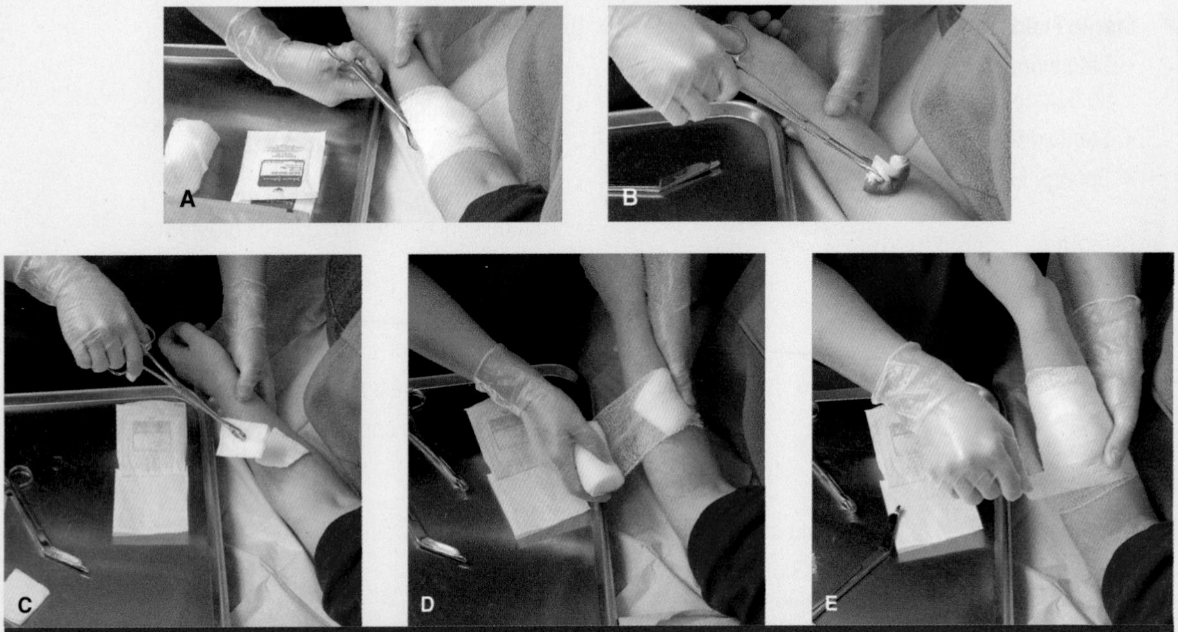

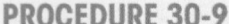

FIGURE 30-44 To change a dressing: (A) Gently remove dressing. Do not cause stress on wound. (B) Clean wound with Betadine solution using sponge forceps. (C) Using dressing forceps, new sterile sponge forceps, and a hemostat or sterile gloves, apply sterile gauze sponge(s) to wound. (D, E) Secure dressing with elastic bandage and adhesive tape or roller bandage.

DOCUMENTATION:

PROCEDURE NOTE

11/24/20XX 10:30AM Dressing change to laceration site left forearm. Small amount (dime-size) of serosanguinous discharge noted. No signs of redness or swelling in wound area. DSD applied. Patient states that she "feels fine and that my arm hurts very little" J. Guerrero, CMA (AAMA)

Courtesy of Harris CareTracker PM and EMR

PROCEDURE 30-9

Irrigating Wounds

Procedure

STANDARD PRECAUTIONS:

Handwashing

Gloves

Biohazard

PURPOSE:

To irrigate a wound to remove the accumulation of exudate that impairs and delays healing.

(continues)

EQUIPMENT/SUPPLIES:

On Mayo Tray:

- Sterile gloves in package
- Sterile irrigation kit (irrigating syringe, basin, and container for solution)
- Sterile dressing material in package

Side Area/Unsterile Field:

- Waterproof pad
- Sterile solution for irrigation (per provider's order)
- Nonsterile gloves
- Waterproof waste bag

PROCEDURE STEPS:

1. ***Paying attention to detail***, assemble any equipment or supplies you will need.
2. Wash your hands and follow Standard Precautions.
3. Refer to the provider's orders and select the correct solution and appropriate solution strength. The solution should be kept at body temperature.
4. Introduce yourself to the patient and ***explain the rationale for the procedure to be performed***. Take the time to answer questions, ***showing awareness of the patient's concerns***.
5. Place the waterproof pad under the body part that is to be irrigated, positioning the patient so that when the wound is irrigated, the solution will flow into the wound and then into a basin.
6. Don sterile gloves and remove and dispose of the dressing. Observe the wound and note its appearance, color, amount of discharge, and any odor present. RATIONALE: Allows ongoing assessment of the wound.
7. Remove gloves and wash your hands.
8. Maintaining sterile technique, open the sterile irrigation tray and the dressings. Use the inner kit wrapping as the foundation for your sterile field.
9. Being careful to avoid any splashing or spilling, pour the irrigation solution into a sterile solution bowl.
10. Don sterile gloves using proper procedure (see Procedure 30-1).
11. Fill the irrigating syringe with the sterile solution. Place the sterile basin against the edge of the wound to catch any irrigation solution.
12. Carefully wash out the wound with the flow of the solution (Figure 30-45A). Repeat this process until the solution runs clear and there is no drainage noted in or around the wound (Figure 30-45B).
13. Dry the area with sterile gauze and reassess the condition of the wound.
14. Apply a sterile dressing.
15. Remove and discard the sterile gloves in the appropriate biohazard container.
16. Wash your hands.
17. Document the procedure in the patient's medical record.

(continues)

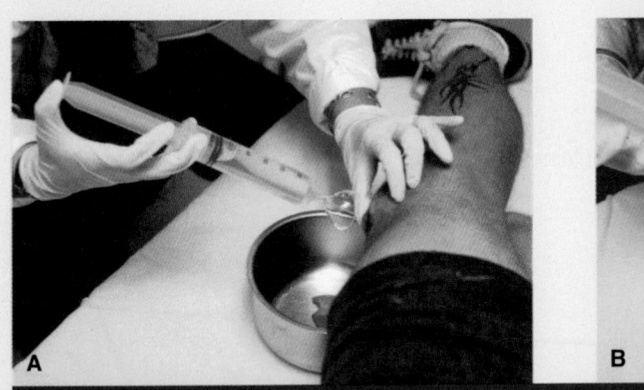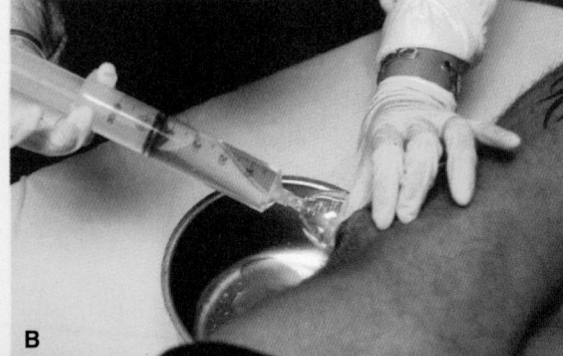

FIGURE 30-45 (A) Flush the wound gently. (B) Hold the syringe close to the wound, but do not touch the wound with the syringe.

DOCUMENTATION:

PROCEDURE NOTE

8/6/20XX 2:30 PM Dressing removed from abdominal wound. Wound red and filled with serosanguinous exudate. Irrigated with 900 mL sterile normal saline (fluid returns were clear). Wound slightly red and without exudate after irrigation. Wound slightly red and clean-appearing after irrigation. Wound dried with sterile 4 × 4s. Dry sterile dressing applied. Patient states, "I feel much better now that my wound has been cleaned out. It is throbbing a bit right now." Patient says she does not want anything for pain. G. Carr, CMA (AAMA)

Courtesy of Harris CareTracker PM and EMR

PROCEDURE 30-10

Suturing a Laceration or Repairing an Incision

Procedure

STANDARD PRECAUTIONS:

Handwashing Gloves No Needle Recapping Biohazard

PURPOSE:

Suturing is recommended if a laceration or incision is gaping; is bleeding uncontrollably; is located on the face, neck, or a bend of a body part; or extends deep into underlying tissue. Suturing facilitates healing by approximating the edges of the wound. Suturing decreases scarring, helps decrease the likelihood of infection, and promotes healing. The wound and the surrounding area must be meticulously cleaned of any dirt and debris. Many providers have standard orders for wound cleaning, such as a 10-minute soak in Hibiclens solution and sterile water, before suture repair of either a laceration or incision-type wound.

(continues)

EQUIPMENT/SUPPLIES:
Surgical Tray:

- Appropriate size syringe and gauge needle for administering anesthesia
- Hemostats (curved)
- Adson tissue forceps
- Iris scissors (curved)
- Suture material as ordered by provider
- Needle holder
- Gauze sponges
- Sterile water or saline

Side Table (Unsterile Field):

- Anesthetic as ordered by the provider
- Dressings, bandages, and tape
- Splint/brace/sling (optional)
- Sterile gloves in package
- Appropriate PPE

PROCEDURE STEPS:

1. If a wound is bleeding, the bleeding will need to be controlled before the wound can be sutured (see Procedure 8-3).
2. Introduce yourself. Identify the patient, using two identifiers, and ***explain the rationale for performance of the procedure, speaking at the patient's level of understanding.***
3. Before attending to the patient, make sure that your hands have been washed and you have donned the appropriate personal protective equipment. Once any bleeding has been controlled or has ceased, the patient can be prepped for suture repair.
4. After donning sterile gloves, assemble and set up the supplies and equipment that the provider will need to suture the laceration or incision. This will include a sterile surgical field as well as an anesthetic if ordered by the provider.
5. Wash your hands and follow Standard Precautions.
6. ***Speaking at the patient's level of understanding, confirm and explain the procedure to be done*** and take some time to answer questions.
7. Review the patient's health history in order to avoid possible complications. Make sure to gather information regarding any allergies, as well as the date of the last tetanus shot. Check with the provider to determine if a tetanus booster is indicated. Document this information in the patient's medical record.
8. Review the signed consent for the procedure. If the patient has questions, contact the provider.
9. Assess the cause of the wound and its severity, making sure to alert the provider to any update in information.
10. Assist the patient into a comfortable position. The provider may request that the wound prep include scrubbing with a Betadine soap solution. The provider may otherwise request that the wound be rinsed out with a Betadine solution (see Procedure 30-9).
11. As the provider sutures the wound, support the patient and be prepared to assist as requested.
12. Apply new gloves, and following the provider's preference, dress, bandage, or splint the wound (see Procedure 30-8).
13. Remove and discard gloves and wash your hands.
14. Obtain the patient's vital signs to assess the patient's stability postprocedure and document them in the patient's medical record.

(continues)

15. Take some time to educate the patient regarding the care of the wound and provide the patient with both written instructions for care as well as any signs or symptoms that might indicate infection. Be sure to include an after-hours contact number as well. Again, offer the patient the opportunity to ask questions.

16. Arrange for any necessary postoperative medication, as well as for a follow-up appointment. Make sure the patient's procedure is accurately documented in the medical record.

17. As needed, don personal protective equipment, commonly referred to as PPE, and dispose of used supplies as directed by the guidelines set forth by OSHA.

18. Sanitize instruments and sterilize for future use and clean the room. Finish by discarding all PPE and washing your hands.

DOCUMENTATION:

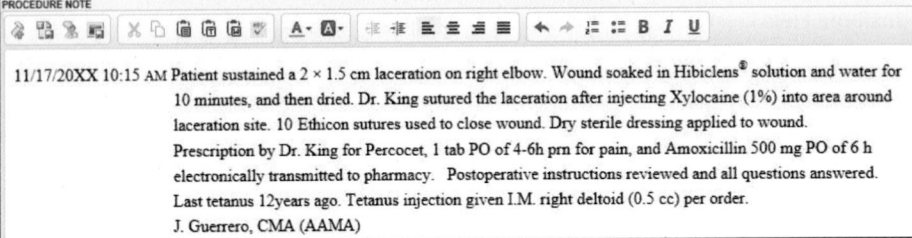

> **PROCEDURE NOTE**
>
> 11/17/20XX 10:15 AM Patient sustained a 2 × 1.5 cm laceration on right elbow. Wound soaked in Hibiclens® solution and water for 10 minutes, and then dried. Dr. King sutured the laceration after injecting Xylocaine (1%) into area around laceration site. 10 Ethicon sutures used to close wound. Dry sterile dressing applied to wound. Prescription by Dr. King for Percocet, 1 tab PO of 4-6h prn for pain, and Amoxicillin 500 mg PO of 6 h electronically transmitted to pharmacy. Postoperative instructions reviewed and all questions answered. Last tetanus 12years ago. Tetanus injection given I.M. right deltoid (0.5 cc) per order.
> J. Guerrero, CMA (AAMA)

Courtesy of Harris CareTracker PM and EMR

PROCEDURE 30-11

Removing Sutures/Staples

Procedure

STANDARD PRECAUTIONS:

Handwashing   Gloves   Biohazard

NOTE: Many minor surgical procedures require that suturing be done to approximate the skin edges to promote healing. Because these sutures or staples are nonabsorbable, they must be removed when the wound has healed. The patient returns to the office or clinic to have the sutures or staples removed. The medical assistant removes the dressing and checks the wound. The provider also checks the wound for degree of healing and determines that the sutures/staples can be removed.

PURPOSE:

To remove sutures or staples from a healed surgical wound (as per provider).

EQUIPMENT/SUPPLIES:

(See Figure 30-46)

- Gauze sponges
- Bandage scissors

(continues)

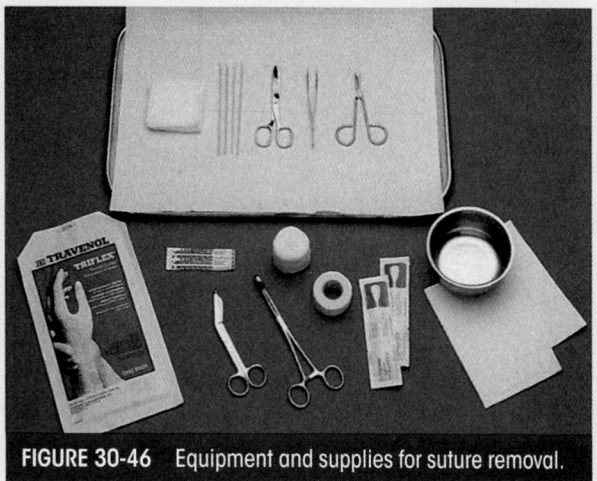

FIGURE 30-46   Equipment and supplies for suture removal.

- Biohazard waste container
- Tape
- Forceps
- Suture or stable removal kit (suture scissors or staple remover, thumb forceps, and 4-by-4 gauze)
- Sterile latex gloves
- Sterile saline or water, Betadine, Hibiclens, or hydrogen peroxide (per provider's order)
- Antibiotic cream if ordered

PROCEDURE STEPS:

1. Assemble the supplies you will need for the procedure.
2. Wash your hands and follow Standard Precautions.
3. Introduce yourself to the patient. Identify the patient using two patient identifiers. ***Speaking at the level of the patient's understanding, explain the rationale for performance of the procedure, showing awareness of the patient's concerns*** by taking the time to answer questions.
4. Apply nonsterile gloves and remove the bandage. Dispose of both the bandage and the gloves in a biohazard waste container.
5. Wash your hands again and open the suture or staple removal kit.
6. Examine the sutures. If they are covered with dried fluids, soak a sterile 4-by-4 gauze sponge with sterile water, sterile saline, Hibiclens, Betadine, or hydrogen peroxide as ordered by the provider.
7. Apply sterile gloves. Gently place the gauze sponge on the suture line to loosen the dried fluids so that they can be wiped away. This will allow an unobstructed view of the sutures.
8. Using the thumb forceps, gently pick up one knot of a suture and carefully pull it up toward the suture line. RATIONALE: Less pressure is exerted on suture line.
9. If the patient has staples to be removed, skip to step 13.
10. Using suture scissors, cut only one side of the suture as close to the knot as possible (Figure 30-47A). RATIONALE: Holding knot with forceps and cutting suture as close to skin as possible, the suture will be pulled out from under the skin, avoiding contamination of the wound.
11. Grasp the knot and pull slowly and continuously until the suture is free of the skin (Figure 30-47B).

(continues)

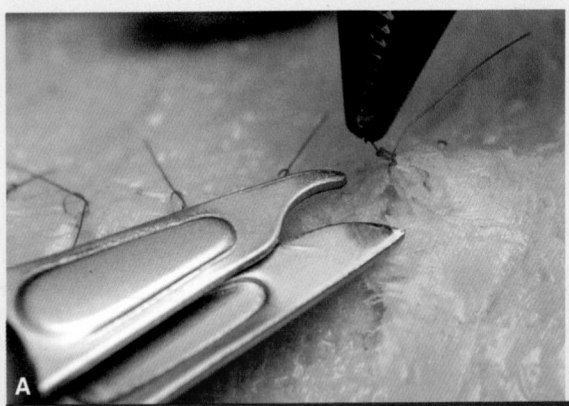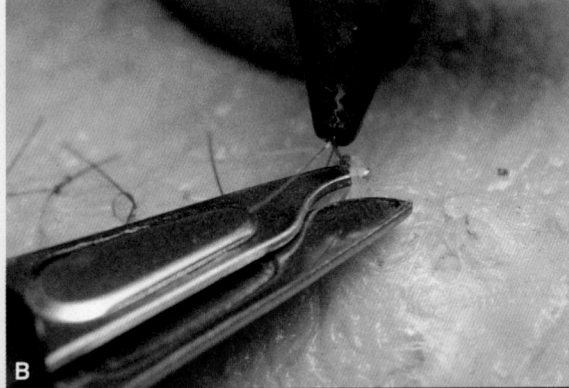

FIGURE 30-47 To remove sutures: (A) Grasp suture knot with thumb forceps. Place curved tip of suture removal scissors right next to the skin under the suture. Clip. (B) Gently pull the suture knot up and toward the incision with thumb forceps to remove.

12. Repeat this process until all of the sutures have been removed. Use caution as you proceed. If at any time the suture line appears to be opening as the sutures are removed, stop immediately and consult the provider. (Skip to step 16.)

13. If the patient needs to have staples removed, the process begins the same. After removing the bandage, observe the staples for any dried fluid, and remove as you would for sutures, using a 4-by-4 gauze soaked in sterile water and Hibiclens or Betadine.

14. Gently insert the staple remover under the first staple, positioning the two prongs beneath it and the single prong on top.

15. With slow continuous pressure, close the staple remover handles to extract the staple. Repeat until all of the staples have been removed, although as before, if the wound line begins to open at any time, stop and notify the provider.

16. The end of the procedure will be the same whether you are removing staples or sutures. Apply benzoin to both sides of the incision line and then apply Steri-Strips to support continued wound healing per provider's preference.

17. Apply an antibiotic ointment to the wound site, and cover it with sterile dressing as ordered by the provider.

18. Dispose of any used supplies according to the guidelines set forth by OSHA.

19. Remove your gloves and wash your hands before assessing the patient's post-procedural stability.

20. Document your assessment in the patient's medical record.

DOCUMENTATION:

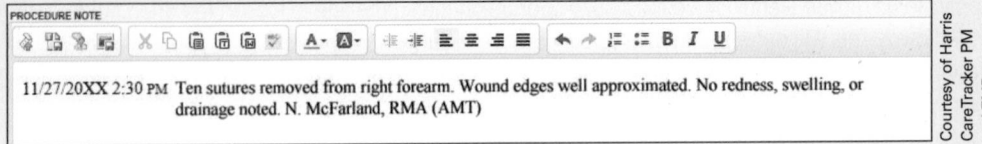

PROCEDURE NOTE

11/27/20XX 2:30 PM Ten sutures removed from right forearm. Wound edges well approximated. No redness, swelling, or drainage noted. N. McFarland, RMA (AMT)

Courtesy of Harris CareTracker PM and EMR

OR

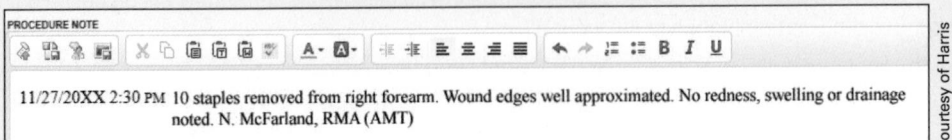

PROCEDURE NOTE

11/27/20XX 2:30 PM 10 staples removed from right forearm. Wound edges well approximated. No redness, swelling or drainage noted. N. McFarland, RMA (AMT)

Courtesy of Harris CareTracker PM and EMR

PROCEDURE 30-12

Procedure

Applying Sterile Adhesive Skin Closure Strips

STANDARD PRECAUTIONS:

Handwashing

Gloves

Biohazard

NOTE: On occasion, a superficial wound does not require sutures. However, the edges of the wound can be drawn together and sterile strips of adhesive can be used to hold the edges of the wound together to facilitate healing.

PURPOSE:
To approximate the edges of a wound after the removal of sutures. Sometimes used in lieu of sutures or to give additional support along with sutures.

EQUIPMENT/SUPPLIES:
Sterile Field:

- Suture removal instruments (if indicated)
- Sterile adhesive skin closure devices
- Iris scissors (straight)
- Adson dressing forceps
- Tincture of benzoin per provider's preference
- Sterile cup
- Sterile cotton-tipped applicators (for tincture of benzoin)

OR
- Sterile prepackaged benzoin swabs

Side Area (Unsterile Field):

- Prepackaged sterile gloves in the appropriate size
- Dressings
- Tape
- Waterproof bag

PROCEDURE STEPS:

1. Assemble the supplies you will need for the procedure.
2. Wash hands and follow Standard Precautions.
3. Introduce yourself to the patient. Identify patient using two patient identifiers.
4. Confirm the procedure to be performed. *Speaking at the level of the patient's understanding, explain the rationale for the performance of the procedure, and show awareness of the patient's concerns* by allowing for questions.

(continues)

5. Sterile adhesive skin closure strips can be used to both help support sutures at an incision line and continue to help support a wound line after the sutures or staples have been removed. If you are using the strips to support sutures or staples, open the strips and drop them onto the existing sterile field

6. Don sterile gloves before cleaning and drying the wound.

7. Apply tincture of benzoin up to the edges of the wound, using the cotton tipped applicator contained in the benzoin packaging. Allow it to dry. RATIONALE: This will help provide a better sticking surface for the strips. It is very important that the benzoin does not come into contact with the incision.

8. If needed, cut the strips to size before using the thumb forceps to carefully peel the strips from the backing.

9. Beginning at the center of the wound, place a strip across the wound, attaching it first to one side and then using slight tension to pull it gently toward the other side before attaching it there and pressing it in place. Continue to place strips to support the suture line in accordance with the provider's orders (Figure 30-48).

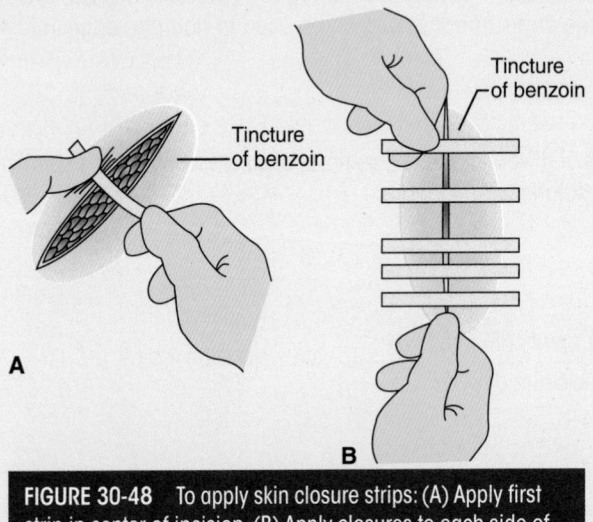

FIGURE 30-48 To apply skin closure strips: (A) Apply first strip in center of incision. (B) Apply closures to each side of center.

10. If you have applied strips to a wound postsuture or -staple removal, you will want to dress and bandage the wound as needed and will need to include home care instruction particular to the care of adhesive strips in addition to any postcare instructions provided for general postsuture wound care.

11. Document the appearance of the wound and use of skin closure strips in the patient record.

DOCUMENTATION:

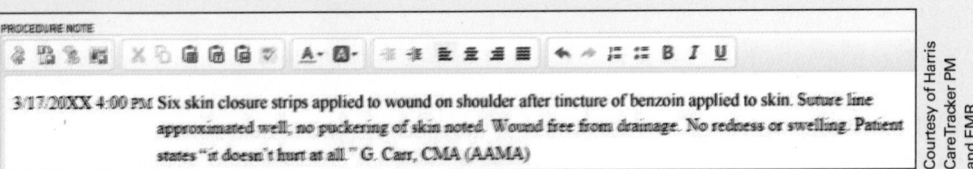

3/17/20XX 4:00 PM Six skin closure strips applied to wound on shoulder after tincture of benzoin applied to skin. Suture line approximated well; no puckering of skin noted. Wound free from drainage. No redness or swelling. Patient states "it doesn't hurt at all." G. Carr, CMA (AAMA)

PROCEDURE 30-13

Procedure

Excising a Sebaceous Cyst

STANDARD PRECAUTIONS:

Handwashing Gloves Goggles & Mask Gown Biohazard No Needle Recapping

NOTE: A sebaceous cyst is a benign retention cyst. Sebaceous cysts are caused by an oil duct becoming "plugged," which causes the sebum (oil) to accumulate in the gland. Eventually the oil gland becomes distended. Sebaceous cysts that become inflamed or infected need to be removed. The patient may also elect to have a noninflamed sebaceous cyst removed if it is unsightly or located in a bothersome area. Incision and drainage of sebaceous cysts is usually not the treatment of choice because they tend to recur if the entire cyst is not completely excised. Ideally, the entire cyst sac is removed intact, but occasionally the sac ruptures during removal and large amounts of malodorous biohazardous sebum can be expelled. In preparation for this occurrence, extra gauze sponges, gloves, and goggles should be available.

PURPOSE:

To remove an inflamed or infected sebaceous cyst. To remove a sebaceous cyst that is not inflamed or infected but is located on an area of the body where the cyst is unsightly or where it may become irritated from rubbing.

EQUIPMENT/SUPPLIES:

Sterile Field:

- Appropriate size syringe and gauge needle for administering anesthesia
- Iris scissors (curved)
- Mosquito hemostat (curved)
- Knife handle and blade
- Suture material as ordered by provider
- Needle holder
- Tissue forceps (two)
- Mayo scissors (curved)
- Sterile 4-by-4 gauze sponges
- Fenestrated drape
- Antiseptic solution as per provider preference

Side Area (Unsterile Field):

- Skin prep supplies
- Anesthetic as ordered by the provider
- Dressings, bandages, and tape
- Splint/brace/sling as indicated
- Prepackaged sterile gloves (appropriate sizes for medical assistant and provider)
- Nonsterile disposable gloves
- Appropriate PPE
- Alcohol pads
- Tube for culture
- Biohazard specimen transport bag
- Appropriate lab requisitions

PROCEDURE STEPS:

1. *Paying attention to detail* is important when preparing for surgical procedures. Begin by washing your hands and assembling the sterile tray following proper procedure.

2. Introduce yourself, identify the patient using two identifiers, and *explain the rationale for the procedure to be performed. Speak at the patient's level of understanding* and answer any questions.

(continues)

3. ***Show awareness of the patient's fears regarding the procedure being performed and help him or her to feel safe and comfortable.***

4. Don appropriate PPE, including goggles if indicated. RATIONALE: Purulent material may drain out of the wound and splash.

5. Don sterile gloves.

6. Prepare the patient's skin in a manner appropriate for the procedure to be performed.

7. Remove gloves and dispose of them in biohazard waste container.

8. As the provider prepares for the surgery, remove the sterile drape cover from the sterile field by grasping the tips of the corners farthest away from you and lifting the drape toward you. This method will protect the sterility of the field.

9. Be certain to follow the principles of surgical asepsis if holding the vial of anesthetic agent for the provider.

10. You may also be expected to provide supplies and equipment to the provider. If you are assisting the provider by handling sterile instruments, don sterile gloves. An important part of your role will be to help the patient to remain calm and provide support throughout the procedure.

11. Keep in mind that it is important that you work only within your scope of practice during the procedure.

12. As you receive used instruments from the provider, place them in a basin or container out of the patient's line of sight. If necessary, hold the biopsy container to receive the specimen being excised, being careful not to contaminate or touch the inside of the container in any way.

13. Once the procedure is complete, assist with the application of sterile dressing and any special needs the patient might have.

14. Make sure the specimen container is tightly covered and clearly labeled with the date, type and source of specimen, and patient's name. Arrange for the specimen to be sent to the lab accompanied by the appropriate laboratory requisition.

15. Wear appropriate personal protective equipment, or PPE, and thoroughly clean the procedure room by disposing of any used supplies in the appropriate containers.

16. Properly clean and sterilize any surgical instruments for reuse at a future time.

17. Remove gloves and other personal protective equipment and dispose of them properly.

18. After washing your hands, document the procedure in the patient's medical record, including any laboratory requisitions.

DOCUMENTATION:

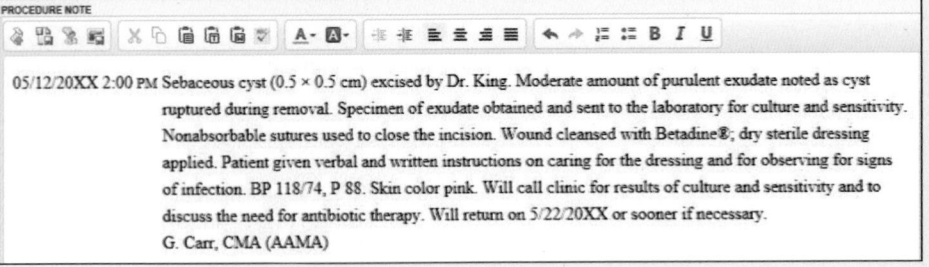

05/12/20XX 2:00 PM Sebaceous cyst (0.5 × 0.5 cm) excised by Dr. King. Moderate amount of purulent exudate noted as cyst ruptured during removal. Specimen of exudate obtained and sent to the laboratory for culture and sensitivity. Nonabsorbable sutures used to close the incision. Wound cleansed with Betadine®; dry sterile dressing applied. Patient given verbal and written instructions on caring for the dressing and for observing for signs of infection. BP 118/74, P 88. Skin color pink. Will call clinic for results of culture and sensitivity and to discuss the need for antibiotic therapy. Will return on 5/22/20XX or sooner if necessary.
G. Carr, CMA (AAMA)

Courtesy of Harris CareTracker PM and EMR

PROCEDURE 30-14

Procedure

Performing Incision and Drainage of Localized Infection

STANDARD PRECAUTIONS:

Handwashing

Gloves

Goggles & Mask

Gown

Biohazard

NOTE: An abscess is a localized accumulation of pus surrounded by inflamed tissue. The body attempts to isolate pus into a pocket, or abscess, as a means of protecting itself by walling off the pathogens and preventing them from spreading throughout the body. Incision and drainage is the procedure of cutting into an area (often an abscess) for the purposes of draining the fluid/material. A culture of the exudate can be done to identify microorganisms. Rather than suturing or otherwise closing the wound, the provider may place a gauze wick or a latex Penrose drain into the wound to facilitate continued drainage. The most commonly used type of wick is iodoform. Iodoform is available in 5-yard lengths and widths of ¼, ½, 1, and 2 inches. Iodoform is packaged sterile in glass bottles under, among others, the Johnson & Johnson brand name of Nu Gauze (see Figure 30-36). Care must be taken when removing the desired length from the bottle to avoid contaminating the remaining gauze. To accomplish this, the medical assistant might hold the bottle and remove the lid to allow the provider to reach into the bottle with a sterile thumb dressing forceps and pull out the desired length. Sterile scissors are then used to cut the strip without contaminating the remaining wick. The iodoform is packed into the wound with a short length exposed. After several hours or days of continued draining, the wick may be removed, and the wound allowed to heal without sutures. The patient may be prescribed an appropriate antibiotic.

The medical assistant should exercise caution by wearing appropriate PPE including goggles when assisting with this procedure because the exudate can be heavy and contains pathogenic microorganisms.

PURPOSE:

To incise and drain an abscess or other localized infection.

EQUIPMENT/SUPPLIES:

Surgical Tray:

- Appropriate size syringe and gauge needle for administering anesthesia
- Iris scissors (curved)
- Mosquito hemostat (curved)
- Knife handle and blade
- Suture material as ordered by provider
- Needle holder
- Tissue forceps (two)
- Mayo scissors (curved)
- Sterile 4-by-4 gauze sponges
- Fenestrated drape
- Antiseptic solution as per provider preference
- Sterile culture swabs
- Iodofom gauze or Penrose drain

Side Area (Unsterile Field):

- Skin prep supplies
- Anesthetic as ordered by the provider
- Dressings, bandages, and tape
- Splint/brace/sling as indicated
- Prepackaged sterile gloves (appropriate sizes for medical assistant and provider)
- Nonsterile disposable gloves
- PPE
- Alcohol pads
- Biohazard specimen transport bag
- Appropriate lab requisitions

(continues)

PROCEDURE STEPS:

1. Wash your hands and follow Standard Precautions.

2. Assemble and organize the equipment that the provider will need to incise and drain the infected site.

3. Introduce yourself to the patient, and use two identifiers to identify the patient.

4. ***Speaking at the patient's level of understanding, explain the rationale for performance of the procedure. Help to allay the patient's concerns by taking time to answer questions.***

5. Obtain a signed consent for the procedure from the patient before proceeding.

6. Take a patient health history, including any allergies and the date of the last tetanus shot. Check with the provider to determine if a tetanus booster is indicated. Be sure to document this information and to relay it to the provider as needed.

7. Don appropriate personal protective equipment including sterile gloves.

8. Prepare the skin as ordered by the provider. Then remove your gloves and discard them in a biohazard waste container.

9. ***Working within your scope of practice***, assist the provider as needed during the procedure. This might include holding the anesthesia vial as the provider aspirates the medication.

10. Once the abscess is incised, iodoform gauze or a latex Penrose drain will be inserted, but no sutures will be used. A specimen will most likely be taken for culture and sensitivity.

11. When the procedure is completed, don sterile gloves.

12. Using sterile water or saline and a 4-by-4 sterile sponge, clean the area around the wound. Dry it gently with a sterile sponge or sterile towels.

13. Dress or bandage the wound as directed. Have several thicknesses of dressing material standing by to absorb any exudate or accumulated fluid in the cavity.

14. Following the guidelines set forth by OSHA, dispose of any items used for the procedure.

15. Remove and discard gloves and wash your hands.

16. Obtain the patient's vital signs to assess postprocedure stability and document this information in the patient's medical record.

17. Take some time to educate the patient regarding the care of the wound and provide the patient with written instructions for care including the need to apply warm moist compresses to the wound. Stress the importance of using caution when handling contaminated items. Be sure to include an after-hours contact number with this information. Again, offer the patient the opportunity to ask questions.

18. Arrange for any necessary postoperative medication, as well as for a follow-up appointment.

19. Don nonsterile disposable gloves and clean the room.

20. Make sure the patient's procedure is accurately documented in the medical record along with the provision of patient education. Note if any culture specimen was obtained and whether it was sent to the laboratory.

DOCUMENTATION:

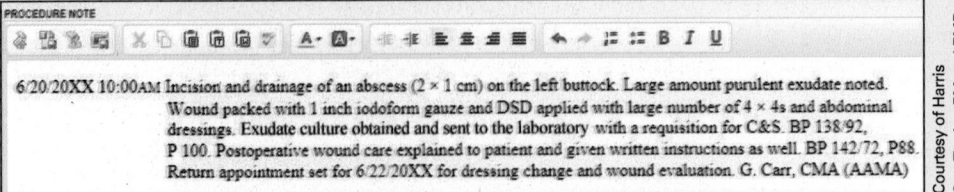

PROCEDURE NOTE

6/20/20XX 10:00AM Incision and drainage of an abscess (2 × 1 cm) on the left buttock. Large amount purulent exudate noted. Wound packed with 1 inch iodoform gauze and DSD applied with large number of 4 × 4s and abdominal dressings. Exudate culture obtained and sent to the laboratory with a requisition for C&S. BP 138/92, P 100. Postoperative wound care explained to patient and given written instructions as well. BP 142/72, P88. Return appointment set for 6/22/20XX for dressing change and wound evaluation. G. Carr, CMA (AAMA)

Courtesy of Harris CareTracker PM and EMR

PROCEDURE 30-15

Procedure

Aspirating Joint Fluid

STANDARD PRECAUTIONS:

Handwashing | Gloves | Goggles & Mask | Gown | Biohazard

NOTE: The most common reason for aspirating fluid is to remove excess fluid from a joint, often the knee. A long, sterile, sturdy needle is inserted into the joint capsule and fluid is removed. Often a long-acting anesthetic and cortisone are injected at the same time. The aspirated fluid can be diagnostically examined for blood, pus, and fatty substances and also cultured for pathogens. After surgery, the patient may be placed on anti-inflammatory medications to treat the inflammation and antibiotics if the culture is positive for pathogens.

PURPOSE:

To remove excess synovial fluid from a joint after injury.

EQUIPMENT/SUPPLIES:

Surgical Tray:

- Appropriate size syringe and gauge needle for administering anesthesia
- Sterile basin for aspirated fluid
- Appropriate size syringe and gauge needle for joint aspiration per provider preference
- Hemostat
- Sterile 4-by-4 gauze sponges
- Fenestrated drape
- Antiseptic solution as per provider preference

Side Area (Unsterile Field):

- Skin prep supplies
- Anesthetic as ordered by the provider
- Medication for joint injection per provider's orders
- Dressings, bandages, and tape
- Splint/brace/sling as indicated
- Prepackaged sterile gloves (appropriate sizes for medical assistant and provider)
- Nonsterile disposable gloves
- PPE
- Alcohol pads
- Culturettes
- Specimen container
- Biohazard specimen transport bag
- Supplies to obtain culture of joint fluid
- Specimen container
- Appropriate lab requisitions

PROCEDURE STEPS:

1. Assemble and organize the equipment that the provider will need to aspirate the joint.
2. Wash your hands and follow Standard Precautions.

(continues)

3. Introduce yourself and identify the patient using two identifiers. ***Speaking at the patient's level of understanding, explain the rationale for performance of the procedure. Help to allay the patient's concerns by taking time to answer questions.***

4. Obtain a signed consent for the procedure from the patient before proceeding.

5. Take a patient health history, including any allergies and the date of the last tetanus shot. Check with the provider to determine if a tetanus booster is indicated. Be sure to document this information and to relay it to the provider as needed.

6. Assist the patient to assume the position preferred by the provider.

7. Don appropriate personal protective equipment (PPE), including goggles and gloves.

8. Prepare the skin as ordered by the provider. Follow by removing your gloves and discarding them in the appropriate waste container.

9. ***Working within your scope of practice***, assist the provider as needed during the procedure. This might include cleaning and holding the anesthesia vial as the provider aspirates the medication.

10. After injecting the anesthesia, the provider will insert a long needle into the synovial sac to aspirate the fluid with a large syringe. Once the syringe is filled with fluid, it will be removed from the still-inserted needle using a hemostat and the aspirated fluid put into a sterile bowl. The syringe will then be reapplied to the needle and the process repeated until all excess joint fluid has been removed. Stand by to assist as needed.

11. When the procedure is completed, clean the area around the wound. Apply an adhesive bandage and dress with an elastic bandage to limit swelling.

12. Following the guidelines set forth by OSHA, dispose of any items used for the procedure.

13. Remove and discard gloves and wash your hands.

14. If sending the specimen to the laboratory, apply gloves and carefully insert culturette into the joint fluid. Close and set aside.

15. Remove and discard gloves and wash your hands.

16. Place the specimen and any lab requisition into a biohazard transport bag.

17. Obtain the patient's vital signs to assess postprocedure stability and document this information in the patient's medical record.

18. Take some time to educate the patient regarding the care of the wound and provide the patient with written instructions for care as well as any signs or symptoms that might indicate infection. Be sure to include an after-hours contact number with this information. Again, offer the patient the opportunity to ask questions.

19. Arrange for any necessary postoperative medication, as well as for a follow-up appointment. Make sure the patient's procedure is accurately documented in the medical record along with the provision of patient education.

20. Wearing appropriate personal protective equipment, set aside any instruments to be sanitized, and dispose of used supplies as directed by the guidelines set forth by OSHA.

21. Appropriately discard all PPE and wash your hands.

22. Document procedure, volume of joint aspirate, culture, and patient education in the medical record.

DOCUMENTATION:

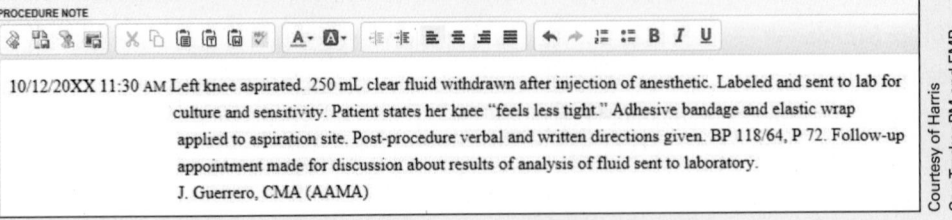

PROCEDURE NOTE

10/12/20XX 11:30 AM Left knee aspirated. 250 mL clear fluid withdrawn after injection of anesthetic. Labeled and sent to lab for culture and sensitivity. Patient states her knee "feels less tight." Adhesive bandage and elastic wrap applied to aspiration site. Post-procedure verbal and written directions given. BP 118/64, P 72. Follow-up appointment made for discussion about results of analysis of fluid sent to laboratory.
J. Guerrero, CMA (AAMA)

Courtesy of Harris
CareTracker PM and EMR

PROCEDURE 30-16

Procedure

Performing Hemorrhoid Thrombectomy

STANDARD PRECAUTIONS:

Handwashing

Gloves

Goggles & Mask

Gown

Biohazard

NOTE: Hemorrhoids are dilated or varicose veins in the rectum, either internal or external. Sometimes, a blood clot can form in a protruding portion of the hemorrhoid and the vessel can become inflamed. The hemorrhoid is incised with a scalpel blade and the clot removed with hemostat forceps. Suturing is not usually necessary. Soaking the area in a **sitz bath** aids in healing. Hemorrhoidectomy can be performed in much the same manner as a hemorrhoid thrombectomy, and the supplies and equipment are similar. The anal sphincter is dilated, the hemorrhoid pedicle is tied, and then each hemorrhoid is removed with either laser, electrosurgery, or cryosurgery. Another alternative is to ligate the internal hemorrhoids after visualizing the area with an anoscope. Two rubber bands are placed around the pedicle of each hemorrhoid. They will slough off after a week to 10 days because of the loss of blood supply to them (**avascularized** hemorrhoid).

PURPOSE:

To incise inflamed hemorrhoids and remove thrombus. To remove hemorrhoids with laser, electrosurgery, cryosurgery, or banding.

EQUIPMENT/SUPPLIES:

Surgical Tray:

- Appropriate size syringe and gauge needle for administering anesthesia
- Sterile basin
- Appropriate size syringe and gauge needle for joint aspiration per provider preference
- Mosquito hemostat (curved)
- Adson tissue forceps
- Knife handle and blade
- Disposable electrocautery handle
- Sterile 4-by-4 gauze sponges
- Fenestrated drape
- Antiseptic solution as per provider preference
- Sterile rubber band
- Medical tape

Side Area (Unsterile Field):

- Skin prep supplies
- Anesthetic as ordered by the provider
- Medication for joint injection per provider's orders
- 4-by-4 gauze sponges
- Prepackaged sterile gloves (appropriate sizes for medical assistant and provider)
- Nonsterile disposable gloves
- PPE
- Electrocautery unit
- Biohazard specimen transport bag
- Specimen container
- Appropriate lab requisitions

PROCEDURE STEPS:

1. Assemble and organize the equipment that the provider will need to perform the procedure.
2. Wash your hands and follow Standard Precautions.

(continues)

3. Introduce yourself and identify the patient using two identifiers. ***Speaking at the patient's level of understanding, explain the rationale for performance of the procedure. Show awareness of the patient's concerns*** by taking time to answer questions.

4. Obtain a signed consent for the procedure from the patient before proceeding.

5. Take a patient health history, including any allergies and the date of the last tetanus shot. Check with the provider to determine if a tetanus booster is indicated. Be sure to document this information and to relay it to the provider as needed.

6. Assist the patient to assume the position (usually Sims' position) as instructed by the provider. The buttocks may be taped open to provide better visualization of the area.

7. Don appropriate personal protective equipment (PPE), including goggles and gloves.

8. Prepare the skin as ordered by the provider. Follow by removing your gloves and discarding them in the appropriate waste container.

9. ***Working within your scope of practice***, assist the provider as needed during the procedure. This might include cleaning and holding the anesthesia vial as the provider aspirates the medication.

10. After injecting the anesthesia, the provider will grasp the exposed hemorrhoid with Adson tissue forceps or a curved hemostat. The hemorrhoid will then be lanced and the thrombus expressed. Or, the provider may grasp the hemorrhoid with the curved hemostat and apply a rubber band to interrupt the blood flow to the tissue. Alternately, the provider may use electrocautry to excise the hemorrhoid.

11. When the procedure is completed, clean the area around the wound. If the area is bleeding, use gloved hands to dress the wound with 4-by-4 gauze pads folded over once and taped into place in a transverse fashion.

12. Following the guidelines set forth by OSHA, dispose of any items used for the procedure.

13. Remove and discard gloves and wash your hands.

14. If sending the specimen to the laboratory, apply gloves and carefully add specimen to container. Close and set aside.

15. Remove and discard gloves and wash your hands.

16. Place the specimen and any lab requisition into a biohazard transport bag.

17. Obtain the patient's vital signs to assess postprocedure stability and document this information in the patient's medical record.

18. Take some time to educate the patient regarding the care of the wound and provide the patient with written instructions for care as well as any signs or symptoms that might indicate infection. Be sure to include an after-hours contact number with this information. Again, offer the patient the opportunity to ask questions.

19. Arrange for any necessary postoperative medication, as well as for a follow-up appointment.

20. Wearing appropriate personal protective equipment, set aside any instruments to be sanitized, and dispose of used supplies as directed by the guidelines set forth by OSHA.

21. Appropriately discard all PPE and washing your hands.

22. Make sure the patient's procedure and specimen sent is accurately documented in the medical record along with the provision of patient education.

DOCUMENTATION:

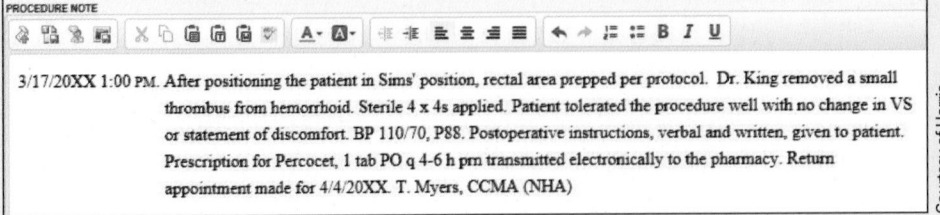

PROCEDURE NOTE

3/17/20XX 1:00 PM. After positioning the patient in Sims' position, rectal area prepped per protocol. Dr. King removed a small thrombus from hemorrhoid. Sterile 4 x 4s applied. Patient tolerated the procedure well with no change in VS or statement of discomfort. BP 110/70, P88. Postoperative instructions, verbal and written, given to patient. Prescription for Percocet, 1 tab PO q 4-6 h prn transmitted electronically to the pharmacy. Return appointment made for 4/4/20XX. T. Myers, CCMA (NHA)

Courtesy of Harris CareTracker PM and EMR

(continues)

OR

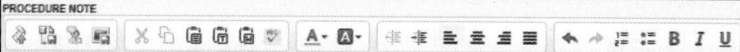

PROCEDURE NOTE

3/17/20XX 1:00 PM. After positioning in Sims' position, Dr. King treated internal hemorrhoids with electrosurgical equipment. Very little bleeding noted. Sterile 4x4s applied. Patient tolerated the procedure well with stable VS and no verbal complaints of discomfort. BP 110/68, P 72. Postoperative instructions given to patient (verbal and written). Prescription for Percocet 1 tab. PO q 4-6 h prn electronically transmitted to the pharmacy. Return appointment made for 4/4/20XX. T. Myers, CCMA (NHA)

Courtesy of Harris CareTracker PM and EMR

OR

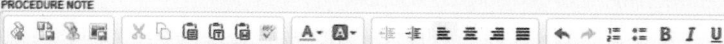

PROCEDURE NOTE

3/17/20XX 1:00 PM. After positioning in Sims' position, Dr. King treated external hemorrhoid by applying a sterile rubber band. Sterile 4x4s applied. Patient tolerated the procedure well with stable VS and no verbal complaints of discomfort. BP 110/68, P 72. Postoperative instructions given to patient (verbal and written). Prescription for Percocet 1 tab. PO q 4-6 h prn electronically transmitted to the pharmacy. Return appointment made for 4/4/20XX. T. Myers, CCMA (NHA)

Courtesy of Harris CareTracker PM and EMR

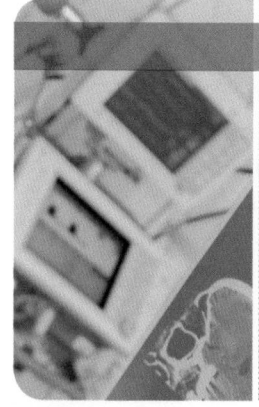

CASE STUDY 30-1

Refer to the scenario at the beginning of the chapter. Distinguish between the types of surgery that would be performed in a high-volume patient practice and surgery that would be performed in a smaller practice.

CASE STUDY REVIEW

1. Where would the medical assistant begin when preparing the equipment for Dr. Beahm and the procedure?
2. Describe the process for ensuring that the specimen obtained during the biopsy is delivered to the pathology lab in a condition to allow a diagnosis.

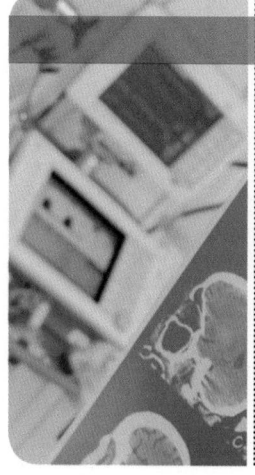

CASE STUDY 30-2

Cele Little, an 84-year-old patient at Dr. Beahm's clinic, is having office surgery performed on Thursday morning. Her sister, Dottie Tate, also a patient and also in her 80s, will come with Cele. A friend from the local senior citizen center has offered to drive them to the clinic and home again. Dottie is more nervous about the procedure, the removal of a bothersome cyst, than Cele. After talking with the sisters about the procedure, clinical assistant Jessica Goodwin, RMA (AMT), MLT, realizes this and wants to reassure Dottie but also wants her to be prepared to be a caregiver to Cele.

CASE STUDY REVIEW

1. Where should Jessica begin in her communication with the two sisters?
2. What specific advice should Jessica give Cele and Dottie before the procedure?
3. What instructions should Jessica give the sisters for after the procedure?

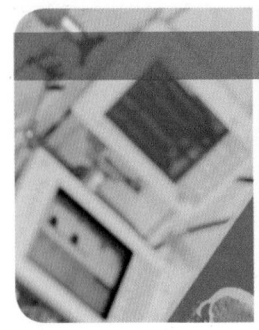

CASE STUDY 30-3

Letisha Brown has been scheduled to have a nevus excised from her upper back by Dr. Beahm.

CASE STUDY REVIEW

1. Explain how Jessica would prepare Ms. Brown for the surgery.
2. Explain how Jessica would care for her after the surgery.
3. What will become of the excised nevus? Explain Jessica's actions.

Summary

- In assisting with surgery in the ambulatory care setting, the medical assistant needs to know sterile principles and understand the difference between medical and surgical asepsis.

- Hand washing is a critical step in preventing the spread of infections. This is especially true when assisting with office surgery.

- Sterilization processes vary based on the type of instrument or material to be sterilized.

- Knowledge of suture materials, instruments, and other supplies such as dressings and bandages is also critical.

- In preparing for surgical procedures, the medical assistant's communication skills will allay patient apprehension

- Knowledge of common procedures performed in the clinic setting will aid the medical assistant in setting up the appropriate instruments and preparing the patient.

- There are alternate surgical methods such as electrosurgery, cryosurgery, and laser surgery.

- Suture materials and instruments vary based on the procedure to be performed. Knowledge of the variations and their use will assist the provider in preparing for the procedure.

- Dressings will be applied after any procedure that interrupts the skin integrity.

- Anesthesia is a part of the procedure that the medical assistant might be called upon to assist provider with. Assisting in drawing up anesthetic agents without breaking sterile technique is a role of the medical assistant.

- Patient education is the final step postprocedure regarding care of the incision site.

Study for Success

To reinforce your knowledge and skills of information presented in this chapter:

- Review the *Key Terms* and *Learning Outcomes*
- Consider the *Critical Thinking* features and *Case Studies* and discuss your conclusions
- Answer the questions in the *Certification Review*

Procedure

- Perform the *Procedures* using the *Competency Assessment Checklists* on the *Student Companion Website*

CERTIFICATION REVIEW

1. Which of the following describes the primary purpose of surgical asepsis?
   a. To prevent microorganisms from collecting on the Mayo stand
   b. To prevent microorganisms from causing inflammation
   c. To prevent microorganisms from entering the body during an invasive procedure
   d. To prevent microorganisms from multiplying

2. Which is true of the rule protecting sterile items?
   a. A sterile object can touch a nonsterile object under certain circumstances.
   b. It is safe to turn your back on the sterile field if you leave plenty of room between you and the field.
   c. Give the provider a separate container for contaminated instruments.
   d. An acceptable border between a sterile area and a nonsterile area is ½ inch.
   e. The portion of the drape that hangs over the edge of the Mayo stand is considered sterile.

3. Which of the following is the smallest size suture material?
   a. 0
   b. 2–0
   c. 4–0
   d. 1

4. Which of the following is an example of absorbable suture material?
   a. Vicryl
   b. Nylon
   c. Silk
   d. Cotton
   e. Nurolon

5. What is the purpose of adding epinephrine to the local anesthetic?
   a. To prevent an allergic reaction
   b. To reduce blood flow in the operative site through vasoconstriction
   c. To reduce patient discomfort during the procedure
   d. To maintain patient vital signs

6. Which of the following actions might the provider take if a sebaceous cyst were infected?
   a. Remove the cyst
   b. Do a biopsy of the cyst
   c. Perform cryosurgery on the cyst
   d. Incise and drain the cyst
   e. Cover the cyst with antibiotic ointment and a sterile dressing.

7. Which of the following are key methods to protect a sterile object?
   a. Sterile objects must not touch unsterile objects
   b. Never turn your back on a sterile field
   c. Anything below the waist is considered unsterile
   d. All of these

8. Which of the following is the gauge of the largest suture material?
   a. 0 silk
   b. 2–0 silk
   c. 3–0 silk
   d. 4–0 silk
   e. 5–0 silk

9. Which of the following is the definition of anesthesia?
   a. Loss of sensation
   b. Increased sensation
   c. Localized sensation
   d. General sensation

10. What is the purpose(s) of provider preference cards?
    a. Make setup for a procedure less difficult
    b. Make sure that the practitioner has the instruments needed
    c. Standardize procedures no matter which staff member sets up
    d. Both a and c
    e. All of these

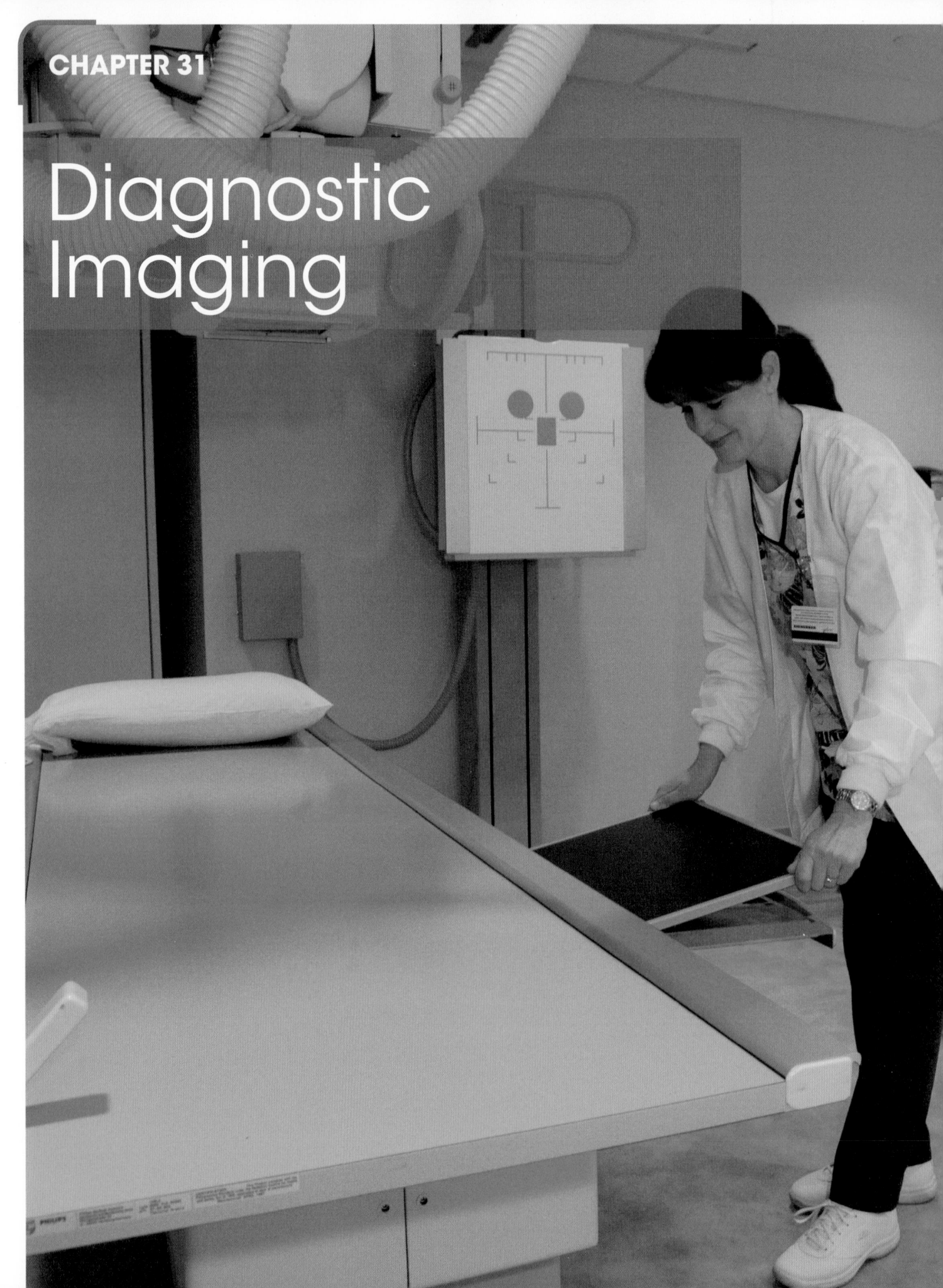

CHAPTER 31

Diagnostic Imaging

1. Define and spell the key terms as presented in the glossary.
2. Determine safety precautions for personnel and patients as they relate to ionizing radiation treatments.
3. Explain how fluoroscopy is used and explain its benefits.
4. Compare the various positions used during X-ray procedures.
5. Describe four X-ray procedures that require patient preparation.
6. Discuss the uses of ultrasonography, positron emission tomography, computerized tomography, magnetic resonance imaging, and flat plates.
7. Characterize how radiographs are stored.
8. Explain the differences among radiology, radiation therapy, and nuclear medicine.
9. Recall four possible side effects of radiation.

KEY TERMS

bone densitometry	oscilloscope
cathode	osteoporosis
claustrophobia	palliative
Doppler	positron emission tomography (PET)
dosimeter	radioactive
echocardiogram	radiographs
fluoroscope	radiolucent
implantable cardioverter-defibrillator (ICD)	radionuclides
ionizing radiation	radiopaque
isotopes	radiopharmaceuticals
magnetic resonance imaging (MRI)	stomatitis
mammogram	transducer
noninvasive	

SCENARIO

In the radiology department of Inner City Health Care, several patients are waiting to have their procedures performed. Gwen Carr, CMA (AAMA), brings Don Waite to the department for an excretory urogram known as an intravenous pyelogram. She is careful to make certain that Mr. Waite has been properly prepared for the procedure. She does not want the procedure to have to be repeated because of the inconvenience and anxiety it might cause Mr. Waite, nor does she want there to be additional expense and time spent repeating the procedure.

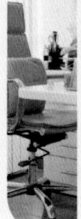

Chapter Portal

Radiology is a branch of medicine concerned with **radioactive** substances, including **radiographs**, radioactive **isotopes**, and **ionizing radiation**. There are three specialties into which radiology can be classified: diagnostic radiology, radiation therapy, and nuclear medicine. Radiology can further be classified as imaging, interventional, and therapeutic. All the specialties are extremely valuable tools that can be used to diagnose and treat diseases.

continues

X-rays were named when a German physicist, Wilhelm Roentgen, discovered them in 1895. He received the first Nobel Prize in physics for his discovery. Roentgen noticed while working with a **cathode** ray tube that the rays of energy emitted could pass through skin, paper, wood, and other solid materials. Because he didn't know what the rays were, he called them X-rays.

Radiologic procedures are not often performed in an office setting; rather, they are performed in the radiology department of a hospital, clinic, or a freestanding facility outside of the hospital or clinic.

Some radiographs, such as those used to look for a fractured bone, require no preparation, whereas others, such as an excretory urography (intravenous pyelogram [IVP]) or a computerized axial tomography (CAT) scan, require special preparation.

RADIATION SAFETY

Safety

X-rays, though invisible to the human eye, are extremely powerful, and they can be beneficial or they can be dangerous and harmful. Exposure to radiation can destroy tissue and permanently damage the eyes, bone marrow, and skin. X-rays are harmful to the developing embryo and fetus, causing severe anomalies and death.

One of the most important tasks of a medical assistant is to make sure that patients are adequately prepared for any radiologic procedure. Patient education is essential in preparing for many procedures. Without adequate patient education, the patient will not receive the desired outcome.

The benefit of X-rays is the ability to use the information obtained from them to diagnose and manage a patient's disease. The diagnostic benefits outweigh the risks that may result from X-ray exposure. Radiographers are educated to be certain that patients receive as low a dose of radiation as possible but still obtain a useful radiograph, and that they themselves and the patients are protected from exposure to radiation that is not necessary. Radiation is rarely used during pregnancy because of the danger it poses to the fetus and embryo. The first trimester is the most critical because severe congenital anomalies can be the result of the fetus's or embryo's exposure to radiation. Women are routinely asked if there is a possibility of their being pregnant. X-rays of fertile women should be taken only when necessary and with a minimal exposure to the fetus or embryo. If a radiologic examination is necessary, a radiologic physicist calculates the dosage of radiation to estimate how little radiation to which the fetus or embryo should be exposed. The past guideline stated that X-rays of fertile women should not be taken until 10 days after the onset on their last menstrual period. The thinking was that women

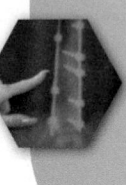
Critical Thinking
What are the effects of radiation on a fetus or an embryo? How might you respond honestly and diplomatically to a pregnant patient's concerns?

were unlikely to become pregnant during these 10 days. This guideline is now considered to be outdated because the ovum for the next menstrual cycle is most susceptible during this 10-day period.

Professional

In most states, medical assistants and other health care professionals who are not licensed to take radiographs are not allowed by law to take radiographs or assist with radiologic procedures. Licensure in those states is mandated because of the possibility of severe injury to an unlicensed individual and to patients. In some states, a limited license is required. The medical assistant must undergo additional training and is limited to "skeletal films" (arms, legs, and so forth). Education and training in radiologic techniques is of utmost importance for the safety of the patient and health care worker. Medical assistants must have a basic understanding of radiology and radiology safety to instruct patients in the correct preparation for procedures and to keep patients and themselves safe. They must protect themselves and their patients from radiation exposure by not participating in procedures for which they have not been adequately educated and trained.

Legal

The Consistency, Accuracy, Responsibility, and Excellence in Medical Imaging and Radiation Therapy Act of 2013 (CARE) was introduced before the

U.S. Congress in March of 2013. This Act would require health care personnel (excluding providers) who furnish the technical component of either medical imaging examinations or radiation therapy procedures for medical purposes to meet certain criteria. These criteria include:

1. Certification in each medical imaging or radiation therapy modality and service they furnish from a certification organization designated under this Act

2. State licensure or certification in the state where services and modalities are within the profession's scope of practice as defined by the state, and where requirements for licensure, certification, or registration meet or exceed standards established by the certification organization designated under this Act

If this Act passes, it would allow persons enrolled in a medical assisting program to participate in the radiologic care of a patient only if the medical assistant obtains further training and if it is allowed under state regulations. There are other stipulations that will be covered by this Act. The Secretary of Health and Human Services (HHS) must establish a program for designating certification organizations for the additional training. Also, a process must be outlined for individuals whose training or experience is determined to be greater than or equal to that of a graduate from a radiology program. The Secretary of HHS must publish a list of designated certification organizations. Presently, the law in some states requires only voluntary basic training standards. This situation allows individuals without formal education to perform imaging procedures.

The AAMA supports legislation that would require specific educational and certification standards for individuals performing medical imaging.

Personnel in the X-ray department and others who are exposed to X-rays must wear a **dosimeter**, a small badge-like device worn above the waist. The dosimeter contains a strip of film that measures the amount of X-rays to which a person is exposed. The dosimeter film is read on a regular basis, and radiation exposure is reported to a supervisor. Exposure can come from the X-ray beam itself or from scattered rays that are produced when going through the patient's body. Tracking of exposure to ionizing radiation is mandatory for health care professionals.

Patients must wear lead aprons over the reproductive organs, and technicians must shield

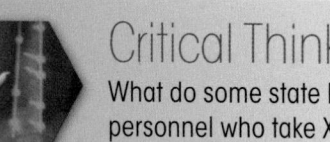

Critical Thinking

What do some state laws require of personnel who take X-rays? What does this indicate regarding scope of practice in your state?

themselves with lead aprons and gloves when they are assisting. However, shields are not necessary when technicians are standing behind the lead wall and working the control panel. In addition, walls in rooms where X-rays are taken are lead-lined to absorb scattering rays.

The World Health Organization held an international meeting in Geneva, Switzerland, on March 1 to 3, 2010, to discuss referral guidelines for appropriate use of radiation imaging. The meeting focused on standardizing an international evidence-based set of referral guidelines to limit unnecessary medical radiation exposure. As a result of this meeting, a guideline was developed in collaboration with experts and institutions to meet the goal of minimizing health risks while maximizing benefits to the patient. In the United States, the Food and Drug Administration (FDA) supports the efforts of the WHO and other organizations in the area of appropriate use of imaging exams through the development and adoption of appropriate-use guidelines. This is an important concept as it is estimated that 25% to 50% of high-tech imaging procedures fail to provide information that could improve patient welfare. There are many ramifications of this estimated overuse. Most importantly, the patient and health care staff are exposed to unnecessary radiation and it also drives up the cost of health care.

RADIOGRAPHY EQUIPMENT

There are three main parts to an X-ray machine: the table, the X-ray tube, and the control panel. The tube is where the X-rays are produced and then exit as a beam of electromagnetic radiation. Lead surrounds the tube except for the area where the beams of X-rays are sent out. The table on which the patient lies is movable in several directions, even upright or angled. The control panel is positioned behind a lead wall specially designed for shielding the radiographer from X-rays when an X-ray is being taken (Figure 31-1).

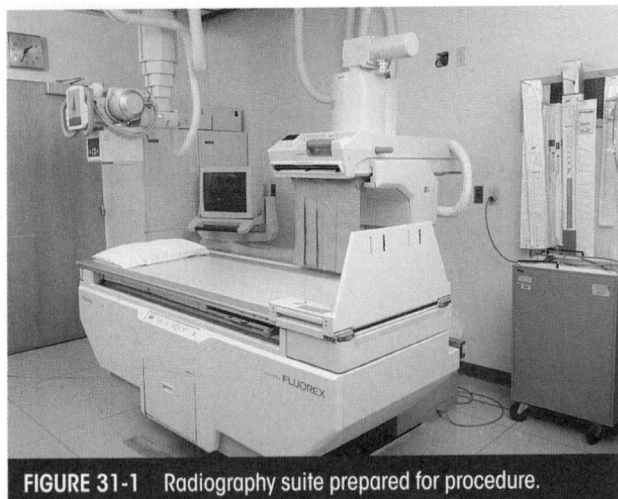

FIGURE 31-1 Radiography suite prepared for procedure.

Radiographic film is placed beneath or behind the patient's body and a radiograph, or X-ray film, is produced by sending X-rays from the tube of the machine through the body and onto the film. After the film is processed, an image is created (see Figures 31-2A and 31-2B).

Dense bone absorbs much of the radiation. Contrarily, soft tissue, like muscle, fat, and organs, allows more of the X-rays to pass freely through. Because of this absorption, bones appear white on the X-ray, soft tissue shows up in shades of gray, and air appears black.

Radiologic procedures can be done without using X-ray film. The technique is known as computed radiography (CR). CR uses very similar equipment to conventional X-rays. In place of radiographic film to create the image, an imaging plate is covered with a type of phosphor that is stimulated by the X-ray beam. When the X-rays fall on the cassette, a latent image is produced by exciting the electrons to a higher energy level. The imaging plate is processed through a special laser scanner, or CR reader, that reads and digitizes the image. This plate is housed in a special cassette and placed under the body part to be examined and the X-ray exposure is made. This type of imaging is useful when structures vary widely in their radiographic density. The technique provides clear images that assist the provider in making

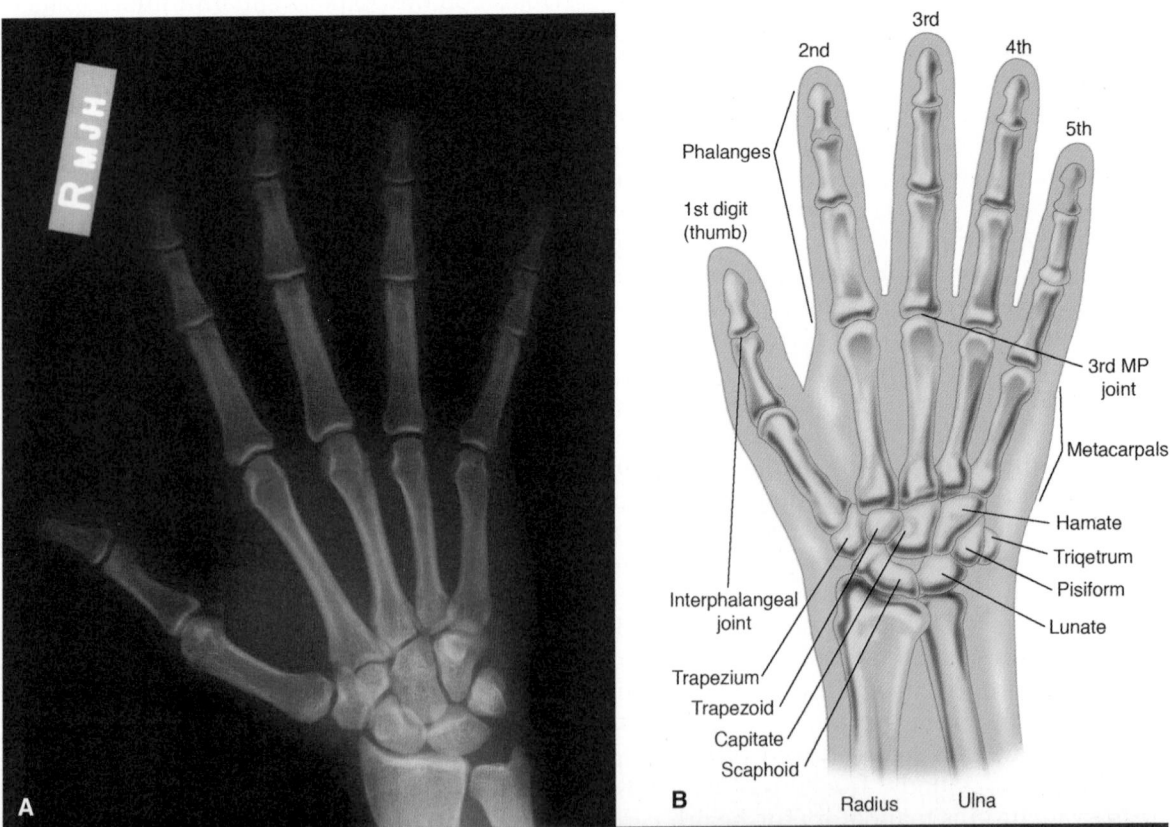

FIGURE 31-2 (A) Posteroanterior (PA) view of a hand. Note the dark spaces between the bones. This is because the bones (denser) pick up X-rays (absorb them) and appear white. The soft tissue (less dense) does not absorb X-rays and appears dark. (B) PA hand.

a diagnosis. The CR images can be sent to other providers digitally for consultation or referral. The process produces excellent images without film. It makes film storage unnecessary, thereby reducing costs. Transmission of patient data is quicker. Another benefit is that it limits the number of repeat X-rays required due to error in picking the correct exposure level.

CR equipment is costly, and technologists who use the equipment require training on its operation.

CONTRAST MEDIA

Various body structures are of different densities. Bone is denser than skin and, therefore, can absorb more X-rays, leaving fewer to be picked up by the X-ray film. Thus, an X-ray film of bone will appear white. Lung tissue is less dense, and the X-rays can penetrate with ease. Therefore, the lung appears black on the radiograph because the air does not slow the X-ray beams. If X-rays do not penetrate a structure easily, it is termed **radiopaque**; if they penetrate readily, it is termed **radiolucent**. Contrast media are radiopaque and help to obtain a radiographic image of an internal organ or structure that ordinarily would be difficult to see, because the contrast media cause the organs or structures of the body to absorb more radiation (Figures 31-3A and 31-3B). Some commonly used contrast media are barium sulfate, iodine compounds, air, and carbon dioxide. Barium is a chalky compound and, when mixed with water, can be swallowed by the patient or administered as an enema by a radiologic technician. It is not absorbed by the body. It is used for upper and lower gastrointestinal (GI) series of X-rays (Figures 31-4A and 31-4B). Iodine salts are radiopaque and are used for kidney, gall bladder, and thyroid examinations. Some individuals are allergic to the iodine salts used as contrast media. Patients are asked whether they have any allergies, particularly allergies to foods that contain iodine, such as fish.

Painful procedures utilizing air and carbon dioxide to visualize the spinal cord and joints have been replaced by use of **magnetic resonance imaging (MRI)** machines.

Although contrast media are widely used, they are not without risk. The effects can range all the way from minor changes in homeostasis to life-threatening situations. Informed consent may be required by the facility that is performing the study. Risk factors for adverse reactions include specific allergies (as mentioned above), asthma, and renal insufficiency.

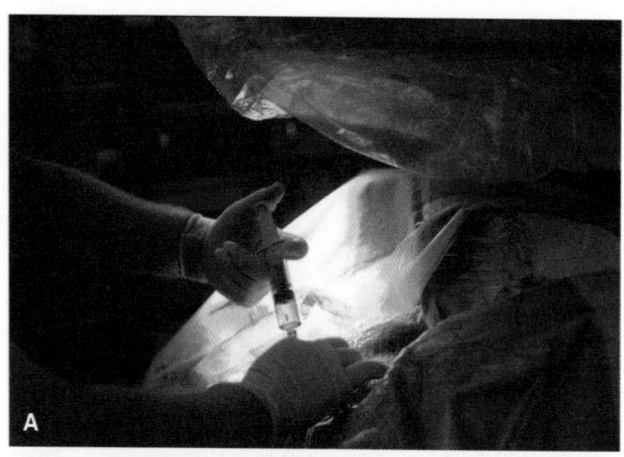

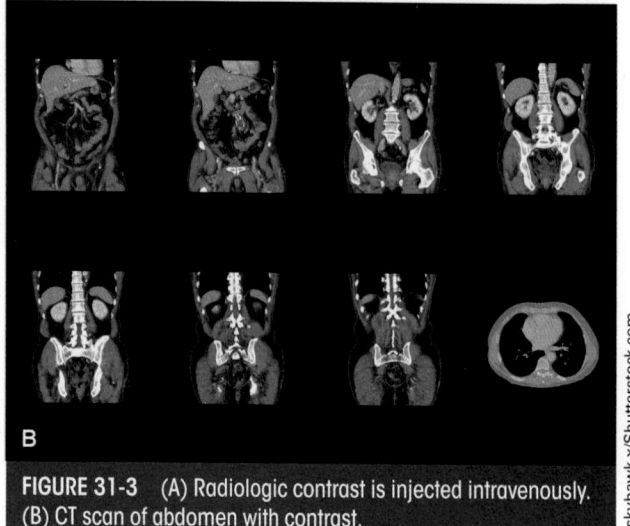

FIGURE 31-3 (A) Radiologic contrast is injected intravenously. (B) CT scan of abdomen with contrast.

© skyhawk x/Shutterstock.com

PATIENT PREPARATION

Legal   Communication

By law, without special education and training about X-rays, the medical assistant's role in X-ray procedures in most states is limited to giving patient preparation information and explanations about what the patient can anticipate.

A thorough knowledge of the procedure ordered by the provider is essential, and the medical assistant must be certain that patients understand the preparation they are about to undergo. Verbal explanations should be followed up with written instructions. Many patients, fearful of what the ordered X-ray will show, are anxious and frightened and can easily forget verbal instructions. Proper preparation is essential for the best radiographic results. Having to repeat a procedure because of inadequate preparation results in increased patient anxiety, time, expense, and inconvenience. See the "Radiologic Diagnostic Procedures" Quick Reference Guide for more information.

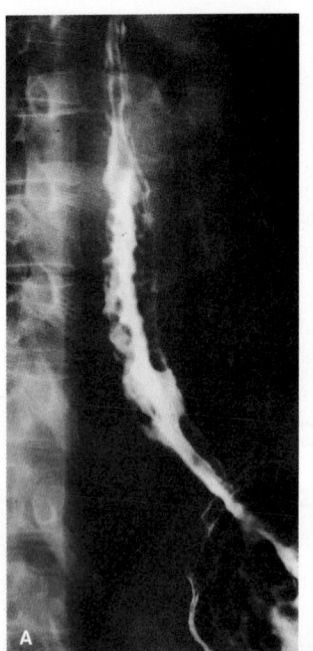
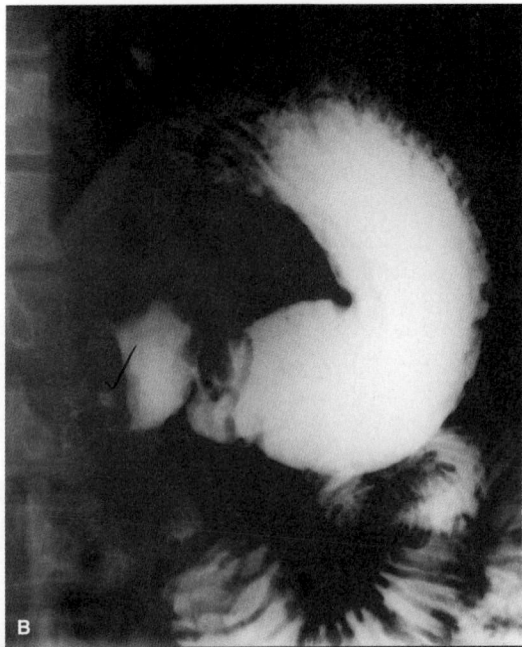

FIGURE 31-4 (A) Barium swallow showing esophageal varices. (B) Barium swallow showing duodenal ulcer.

QUICK REFERENCE GUIDE

RADIOLOGIC DIAGNOSTIC PROCEDURES

Test	Purpose	Patient Preparation	Procedure Information
Angiography	To visualize the inside of blood vessel walls. Helps to diagnose heart attacks, stroke, and aneurysm.	1. NPO 6 to 8 hours before examination. 2. If diabetic, ask provider for orders related to diabetic medications. 3. Inform provider if may be pregnant. 4. Inform provider of any allergies. 5. Inform patient that there might be a generalized feeling of warmness when the contrast is injected. Postprocedure: 1. Monitor arterial puncture site. 2. Do not lift heavy objects or participate in strenuous activity until cleared by provider.	1. Don patient gown. 2. Remove eyewear, jewelry, and dental devices. 3. Position supine on X-ray table. 4. Monitors applied for B/P, pulse, and pulse oximetry. 5. IV started. 6. May be given IV sedation. 7. Area of arterial catheter insertion shaved and prepped. 8. Catheter threaded to the appropriate site. 9. Contrast medium injected. 10. Images obtained over area of concern. 11. Digital angiography data can be stored on computer disk.

(continues)

Test	Purpose	Patient Preparation	Procedure Information
Barium swallow (upper gastrointestinal [GI] series) © Gam1983/Shutterstock.com	To study the esophagus, stomach, duodenum, and small intestine for disease (ulcers, tumors, hiatal hernia, esophageal varices).	1. 2 to 3 days prior: low-fiber diet. 2. Day prior: light evening meal. 3. NPO after midnight day of the procedure. 4. Remove all items that might be visible on X-ray (e.g., jewelry, dentures, clothing with zippers). 5. Inform provider if may be pregnant. 6. Inform the provider of any allergies. Postprocedure: 1. Increase fluid intake. 2. Take laxative as prescribed.	1. Don patient gown. 2. Remove eyewear, jewelry, and dental devices. 3. The patient is asked to drink about 1½ cups of flavored barium mixture while standing in front of the fluoroscope. 4. The radiologist observes the passage down the digestive tract. 5. The patient is turned to various positions to allow good visualization of the intestines. 6. Radiographs are taken over time as the barium moves through the digestive system.
Barium enema (lower GI series) © whitetherock photo/ Shutterstock.com	To study the colon for disease (polyps, tumors, lesions).	1. Prep kit (usually supplied by provider's clinic), which includes bottle of magnesium citrate and Dulcolax (bisacodyl) tablet(s). 2. Day prior: Clear liquids allowed: carbonated beverages, clear gelatin, clear broth, coffee and tea with sugar. No milk or milk products. 3. 8 oz of water every hour until bedtime. 4. Late afternoon: drink bottle of magnesium citrate. 5. Early evening: take Dulcolax tablet(s) as prescribed. 6. Liquid evening meal. NPO except water after dinner. 7. Morning of procedure: maintain NPO, to cleansing enema. 8. Inform provider if may be pregnant. 9. Inform provider of any allergies. Postprocedure: 1. Increase fluid intake and dietary fiber. 2. Report to provider if no bowel movement within 24 hours of test.	1. Don patient gown. 2. Remove eyewear, jewelry, and dental devices. 3. Lay in lateral position on specially designed table. 4. The colon is filled with a barium sulfate mixture by enema. 5. The patient is turned in various positions to allow the barium to fill the colon. Air is injected to move the barium along the colon. 6. When the colon is full, radiographs are taken.

(continues)

Test	Purpose	Patient Preparation	Procedure Information
Percutaneous transhepatic cholangiography	To view the bile ducts for possible calculi or lesions.	1. NPO after midnight day of procedure. 2. May have cleansing enema 1 hour before examination. 3. Inform provider if may be pregnant. 4. Inform provider of any allergies. 5. Inform patient that there might be a generalized feeling of warmness when the contrast is injected. Postprocedural: 1. Monitor insertion site for bleeding. 2. Avoid strenuous activity until cleared by provider.	1. Don patient gown. 2. Remove eyewear, jewelry, and dental devices. 3. Position supine on X-ray table. 4. Monitors applied for B/P, pulse, and pulse oximetry. 5. IV started. 6. May be given IV sedation. 7. Skin prep to upper right and center of abdomen. 8. Long, thin needle inserted through skin to liver. 9. Contrast medium injected and radiograph of bile ducts is taken.
Cholecystography © Santibhavank P/Shutterstock.com	To study the gall bladder for disease (stones, duct obstruction), inflammation.	1. Evening before test, fat-free dinner. 2. Take contrast agent tablets with 8 oz of water. 3. Cathartic or cleansing enemas may be prescribed. 4. NPO after dinner and tablets. 5. Inform provider if may be pregnant. 6. Inform provider of any allergies. 7. Inform patient that there might be a generalized feeling of warmness when the contrast is injected.	1. Don patient gown. 2. Remove eyewear, jewelry, and dental devices. 3. Position supine on X-ray table. 4. A series of radiographs is taken. 5. A high-fat beverage may be given to stimulate the gall bladder to empty. 6. Other radiographs can then be taken to check gall bladder function.
Cystography © Santibhavank P/Shutterstock.com	To view the urinary bladder for lesions, calculi.	1. Day prior: light evening meal. 2. Laxative in evening. 3. NPO after midnight day of test. 4. Empty bladder prior to exam. 5. Inform provider if may be pregnant. 6. Inform provider of any allergies. 7. Inform patient that there might be a generalized feeling of warmness when the contrast is injected.	1. Don patient gown. 2. Remove eyewear, jewelry, and dental devices. 3. Position supine on X-ray table. 4. Bladder will be catheterized. 5. Contrast instilled into bladder. 6. Radiographs of bladder and urethra will be taken.

(continues)

Test	Purpose	Patient Preparation	Procedure Information
		Postprocedure: 1. Increase fluid intake to flush contrast from bladder. 2. Normal postprocedure occurrences include bladder and/or urethral irritation and small amounts of blood noted in urine.	
Hysterosalpingography © whitetherock photo/Shutterstock.com	To view the uterus and fallopian tubes for blockage and lesions. To check for pelvic masses.	1. Laxative evening before. 2. Cleansing enema day of exam. 3. Meal prior to examination is withheld. 4. Prophylactic antibiotics may be ordered. 5. Prescription for oral sedation maybe given preprocedure. 6. Inform provider if may be pregnant. 7. Inform provider of allergies.	1. Don patient gown. 2. Remove eyewear, jewelry, and dental devices. 3. Position in lithotomy position on X-ray table. 4. Speculum will be placed in vagina. 5. A catheter is placed through the cervix into the uterus. 6. Contrast medium injected and radiographs taken of uterus and fallopian tubes. Carbon dioxide may also be used.
Excretory urography (intravenous pyelogram [IVP]) © Santibhavank P/Shutterstock.com	Visualization of kidneys, ureters, and bladder to detect kidney stones, lesions, strictures of urinary tract.	1. Eat a light evening meal. 2. NPO after midnight day of exam. 3. A laxative and enema are used to clean out the intestines to prevent a blocked view of the ureters behind the intestines. 4. Inform provider if the patient takes metformin for diabetes. This drug will interact with the contrast medium. 5. Inform provider if may be pregnant. 6. Inform provider if allergic to iodine. 7. Inform patient that there might be a generalized feeling of warmness when the contrast is injected. Postprocedure: 1. Force fluids to rid the body of the contrast medium.	1. Don patient gown. 2. Remove eyewear, jewelry, and dental devices. 3. Empty bladder. 4. Position supine on X-ray table. 5. IV started. 6. A contrast medium of iodine salts is given intravenously after it has been determined that the patient is not allergic to iodine. 7. Radiographs will be taken several minutes apart to observe the function of the urinary tract. 8. The patient is turned in various positions to allow the visualizations of the urinary structures.

(continues)

Test	Purpose	Patient Preparation	Procedure Information
Mammography © thailoei92/Shutterstock.com	To detect abnormalities in the breast, especially breast cancer.	1. Do not wear lotion, deodorant, or powders. 2. No contrast medium required. 3. Inform provider if may be pregnant.	1. Don patient gown. 2. Remove eyewear, jewelry, and dental devices. 3. Breast is positioned on the mammograph and compressed to flatten it. 4. Two radiographs are taken of each breast, from the side and from above.
Retrograde pyelography © Santibhavank P/Shutterstock.com	To view the kidneys and urinary tract for abnormalities.	1. Drink four to five glasses of water before examination unless sedated, then NPO. 2. Inform provider if allergic to iodine. 3. Inform provider if may be pregnant. 4. Inform patient that there might be a generalized feeling of warmness when the contrast is injected. Postprocedure: 1. Catheter may remain in place for a period of time. 2. May have painful urination with slight bleeding.	1. Don patient gown. 2. Remove eyewear, jewelry, and dental devices. 3. Position supine on X-ray table. 4. Monitors applied for B/P, pulse, and pulse oximetry. 5. IV started. 6. May be given IV sedation. 7. The provider will insert a scope into the bladder. 8. One or both ureters may be catheterized via the scope. 9. Contrast medium injected and radiographs taken of the kidneys, ureters, and urinary bladder.

POSITIONING THE PATIENT

The correct patient position is important for obtaining the best quality radiograph, and the type of examination that is necessary determines patient position. Some basic views are:

- *Anteroposterior view (AP).* The anterior surface of the body faces the X-ray tube and X-rays are directed from the front toward the back of the body.

- *Posteroanterior view (PA).* The posterior surface of the body faces the X-ray tube and X-rays are directed from back to front (see Figure 31-2).

- *Lateral view.* X-rays pass through the body from one side to the opposite side.

- *Right lateral view (RL).* X-rays are directed through the body from the left to the right side. The right side of the body is next to the film.

- *Left lateral view (LL).* X-rays are directed through the body from the right to the left side. The left side of the body is next to the film.

- *Oblique view.* The body is positioned at an angle.

- *Supine view.* The body is lying face up, on the back.

- *Prone view.* The body is lying face down, on the abdomen.

FLUOROSCOPY

Fluoroscopy is the process of using a **fluoroscope** to view internal organs and structures of the body so that they can be seen in motion immediately by the radiologist (Figure 31-5). The patient is usually given a contrast medium and placed between the X-ray tube and the fluoroscope. Fluoroscopy is used for procedures such as cardiac catheterization and for viewing the function of the stomach and intestinal structures to detect any abnormalities. A monitor and camera are available so that the radiographer can watch and take photos of the body system(s) in operation. In modern systems, the fluorescent screen is coupled to an electronic device that amplifies and transforms the glowing light into a video signal suitable for presentation on an electronic display. Electronic fluoroscopy systems create images that appear to be in real time by capturing and displaying images at a high frame rate, typically 25 or 30 frames per second. At these frame rates, the human visual system cannot distinguish frame-to-frame variation and motion

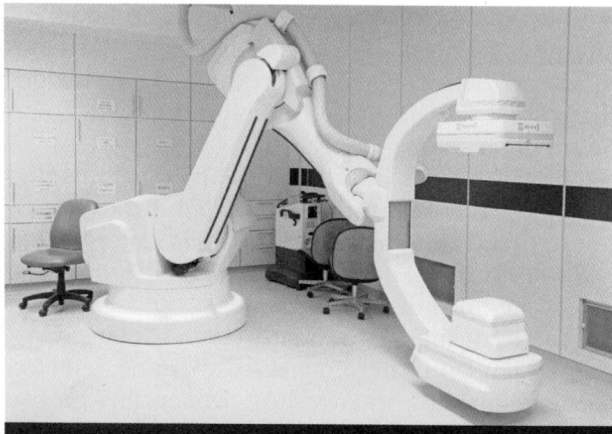

FIGURE 31-5 The fluoroscopic C-arm imaging intensifier (so named because of its shape) is utilized during procedures that require movement horizontally, vertically, and around the swivel axes, so that X-ray images of the patient can be produced from almost any angle.

© ChaNaWiT/Shutterstock.com

appears to be continuous, without visible flicker. Most fluoroscopes have radiographic properties and can be used for both fluoroscopy and still images. Still images can be taken and recorded during fluoroscopy.

BONE DENSITOMETRY

An enhanced form of X-ray technology that is used to measure bone loss is bone density scanning, also called dual-energy X-ray absorptiometry (DXA) or **bone densitometry**. X-rays check areas of the body (hip, hand, spine, foot) for signs of mineral loss and bone thinning. The DXA machine sends a beam of low-dose X-rays with two distinct energy peaks through the bones being examined. One peak is absorbed mainly by bone and the other by soft tissue. The soft tissue amount can be subtracted from the total and what remains is a patient's bone mineral density. The test is used to diagnose **osteoporosis**, which is often found in women after menopause. It can occur in men as well. Bone densitometry can assess an individual's risk for fractures. The lower the bone density, the greater the risk for fractures.

DIAGNOSTIC IMAGING
Positron Emission Tomography (PET)

Positron emission tomography (PET) is a radiographic procedure that uses a computer and a radioactive substance. The radioactive substance is injected into the patient's body and gives off charged particles. They combine with particles in the patient's body to produce color images that reveal the amount of metabolic activity in an organ or structure.

PET is primarily a diagnostic medical imaging modality. It makes use of specialized intravenously injected **radiopharmaceuticals**, called tracers, that emit positrons. These positrons can be detected out of the body due to high-energy releases. Using this method, changes in tissues can be detected at a cellular level and therefore disease can be detected sooner than with other testing. Depending on the type of imaging ordered, the tracer can be inhaled, taken orally, or injected. This type of study is considered a nuclear medicine imaging exam.

As the tracer, or radioactive material, accumulates in the organ or area of the body being examined, it gives off a small amount of energy in the form of gamma rays. Special cameras detect this energy, and with the help of a computer, create pictures offering details on both the structure and function of organs and tissues in the body. The PET scan can detect cancer and the effects of chemotherapy. Certain nuclear medicine treatment studies use specialized radiopharmaceuticals that isolate in the area to be treated. These agents emit their energy locally, irradiate tissue, and usually do not leave the body, unlike diagnostic radiopharmaceuticals. The properties and intent of diagnostic radiopharmaceuticals are different from therapeutic radiopharmaceuticals (Figures 31-6A and 31-6B).

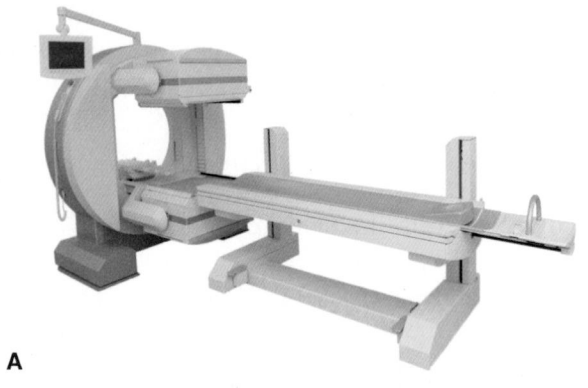

A

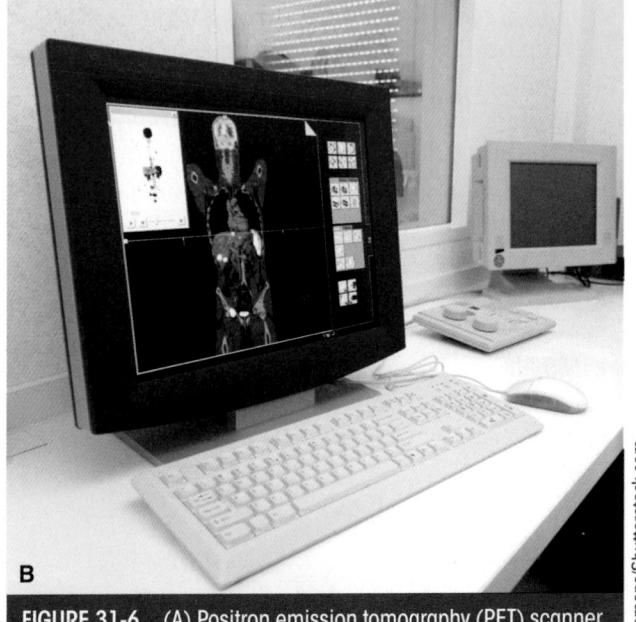

B

FIGURE 31-6 (A) Positron emission tomography (PET) scanner. (B) PET scan output images.

Computerized Tomography (CT)

CT uses a small amount of radiation. The beams penetrate body tissues to produce a series of cross-sectional images of the body part being examined. The procedure provides images of structures that cannot be seen with regular X-rays. It is a noninvasive test that usually requires no special preparation.

The CT machine has software and hardware for storing and managing information. The images can be examined on a computer monitor, and hard copies of the images can be made. It rotates 360 degrees around the patient to obtain cross-sectional images that are processed by a computer and can be viewed on a monitor and on film. It can also be used to guide biopsies, plan surgery, and identify internal organ injury due to trauma. It is ideal for early detection of tissue tumors such as childhood cancers and abdominal tumors, and it helps in directing radiation therapy for tumor masses. The cardiac CT is more useful

than cardiac stress testing for diagnosing coronary artery disease. On occasion, a contrast medium is injected for a better view of internal structures. If contrast medium is used, the patient must be NPO (have nothing by mouth) for 4 hours before being placed onto a motorized table that moves the body part to be examined into a scanner that surrounds that part of the patient. An entire body can be scanned in 15 to 20 minutes (Figures 31-7A and 31-7B). Newer multislice CT scanners produce thinner slices in a shorter time with greater detail.

Magnetic Resonance Imaging (MRI)

Images produced by MRI are of exceptionally high quality. No ionizing radiation is used, and it is a noninvasive, safe, and painless procedure that can

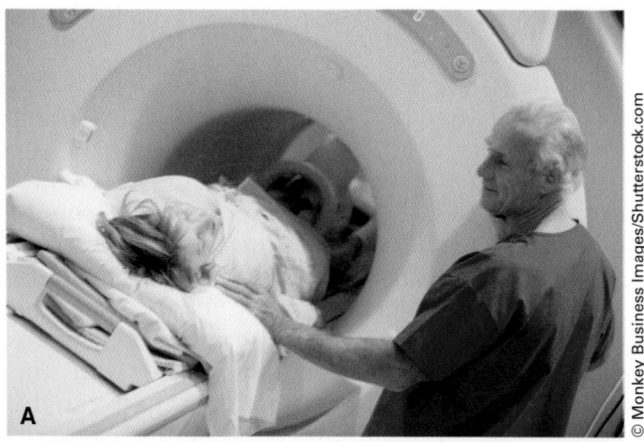

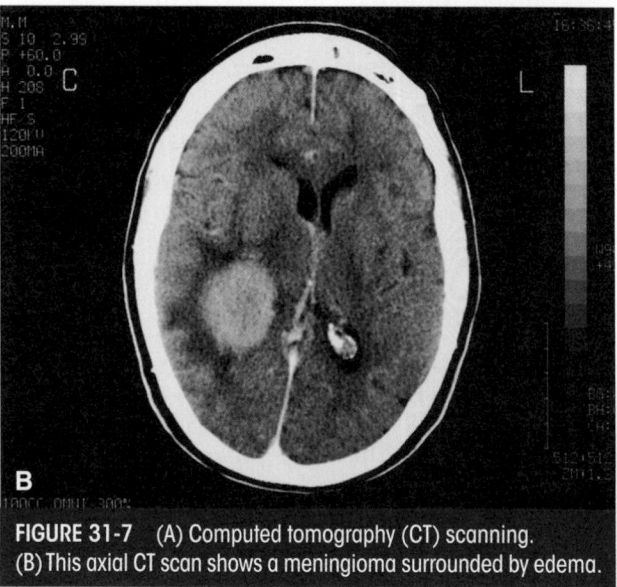

FIGURE 31-7 (A) Computed tomography (CT) scanning. (B) This axial CT scan shows a meningioma surrounded by edema.

produce computer-processed images. MRI uses radio waves and a large magnet to allow for examination of organs and structures inside the body. A strong magnetic field is created and this field aligns the protons inside the hydrogen atoms contained in the body tissues in a line parallel to the magnetic field. Then, short bursts of radio waves are emitted from the scanner and into the body. These waves bounce the protons back to their normal positions. When the radio wave burst stops, the protons line up again. When they do, they emit radio signals. Due to the varied composition of body tissues, the protons realign at different speeds. This results in varied signals. The signals are detected by a receiving device in the scanner. A software program creates an image based on the radio signals.

All body areas can be viewed by MRI, but it is especially helpful for soft tissues. It is good for the spine, pelvis, and joints and is superior for visualizing the brain and abdominal organs. It shows more detail than CT. The examiner can see through fluid-filled tissue with exceptional detail using an MRI machine.

Magnetic resonance angiography (MRA), a noninvasive test, evaluates arteries and veins throughout the body and is very useful for showing neck and brain blood flow. This technique uses a magnetic field and pulses of radio waves to image blood vessels inside the body. The computer converts the data into digital images of slices. No catheterization is needed, but a contrast medium may be given intravenously. The procedure helps diagnose blood vessel and heart disorders as well as strokes. Another imaging technique, functional MRI, measures split-second nerve cell activity of the brain.

Another application of the technology is breast imaging using an MRI. Hundreds of detailed pictures of the breast are taken from several angles. The patient lies on the table on her abdomen, and the breasts drop into a hollow in the table. Breast MRI is not used for routine breast cancer screening. Breast MRI is indicated for women known to be at higher than average risk for breast cancer, either because of a strong family history or a gene abnormality, gathering more information about an area of suspicion found on a mammogram or ultrasound, and monitoring for recurrence after treatment. Breast MRI does not take the place of conventional mammography and ultrasonography and is not routinely used to diagnose breast cancer.

Three types of MRI machines are available: closed MRI, open-air MRI, and open MRI. The conventional closed MRI has high magnetic strength. According to Lexington Medical Center, nine of ten MRI machines used in hospitals and clinics are closed MRI. This type of machine produces high-quality images.

The open-air MRI has open sides and ends (Figure 31-8). Most open machines have low-strength magnets and are not as powerful as the closed MRI. Images are of lesser quality.

The open MRI is an advanced MRI machine that is completely open on all sides. It eliminates patient **claustrophobia** and can accommodate obese patients. It has a powerful magnet that is much stronger than the magnet used in open air MRIs. Greater image detail results in information providers need to make a diagnosis (Figure 31-9).

A drawback to MRI and CT is that they cannot be used in patients with a pacemaker; an

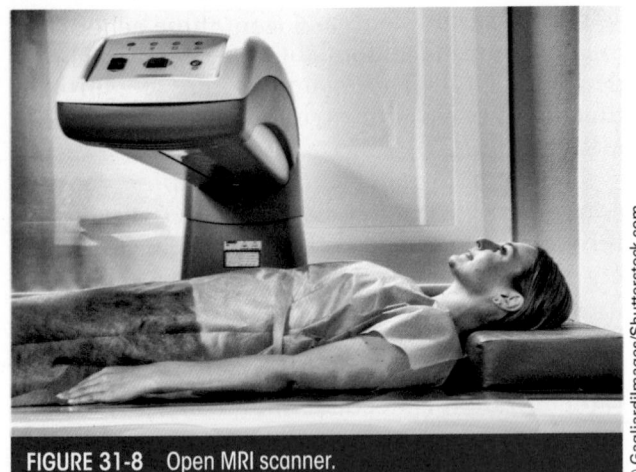

FIGURE 31-8 Open MRI scanner.

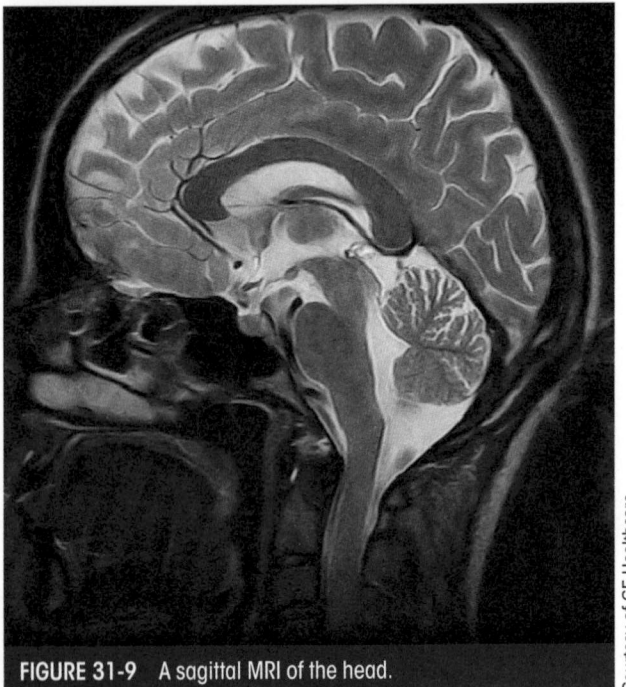

FIGURE 31-9 A sagittal MRI of the head.

radiographs or a CT scan for diagnosing fractured bones.

Patients are asked to remove all objects that have metal (watches, belts, hairpins, rings, other metal jewelry) and credit cards because of the strong magnet in the MRI machine. Loose, comfortable clothing without zippers or snaps should be worn. The procedure takes about 45 minutes to an hour, during which time the patient must remain still. The technician, although not in the room with the patient, has a camera and microphone with which to communicate with the patient. An intermittent tapping sound can be heard throughout the procedure, and earphones are available if the patient wants them.

X-Rays (Flat Plates)

Flat plates are also known as "plain" films because they require no special technique or use of contrast medium. This type of X-ray is used on various parts of the body and is helpful in diagnosing problems in the skull, abdomen, chest, sinuses, and bone.

Ultrasonography

Ultrasonography, CT, and MRI allow for greater imaging detail than conventional radiographs. Ultrasonography, or ultrasound, has been available longer than the other technologies. High-frequency sound waves (inaudible to the human ear) are used to image internal soft tissues. This procedure can be used to help diagnose problems in the abdominal organs, liver, gall bladder, uterus, ovaries, and spleen (Figure 31-10). It cannot be used for skeletal structures or the lungs.

implantable cardioverter-defibrillator (ICD); or metal clips, pins, or other permanent hardware left in place on an internal organ or structure as part of a surgical procedure. The metal may become damaged during testing. Controlled studies investigating whether patients with implantable devices such as a pacemaker and/or an ICD can undergo CT and/or MRI are inconclusive. The FDA has not approved either procedure for these patients. Some researchers found that compared with earlier models, which did cause minor difficulties in some patients, newer CTs and MRIs do not cause difficulties for patients with implantable devices. An MRI is not as useful as conventional

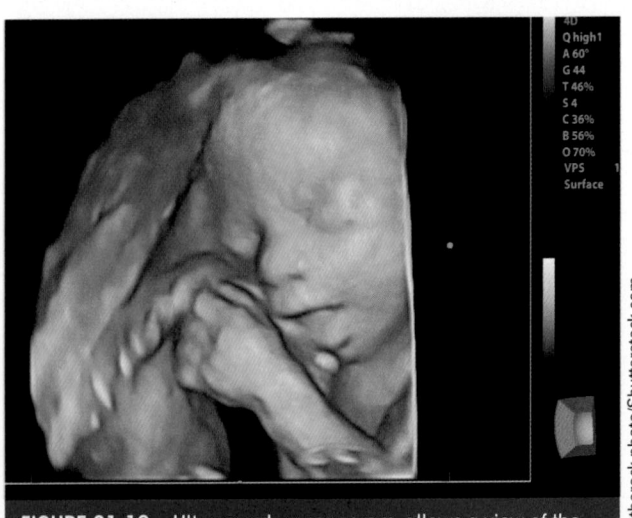

FIGURE 31-10 Ultrasound, or sonogram, allows a view of the baby in utero.

Doppler ultrasonography is a noninvasive technique used to evaluate blood flow through the major arteries and veins of the neck, arms, and legs. It can reveal blockages such as plaque or thrombi (blood clots). An **echocardiogram**, an ultrasound of the heart, can be used to view the heart and determine its size, shape, and position and the motion made by the valves opening and closing (Figures 31-11 and 31-12). Ultrasound has advantages over other methods of viewing internal organs and structures in that it uses no X-rays and allows for continuous viewing while organs and structures are in motion.

During ultrasound, a **transducer** is used with a coupling agent, and sound waves are emitted from the head of the transducer. The transducer is placed firmly on the patient's body over the organ to be examined. The sound waves pass through the skin, bounce off the body's tissues, and are reflected back to the transducer. These echoes are displayed on an **oscilloscope**, showing a visual pattern or picture. The image or record produced is known as a sonogram or echogram. Videotape and a permanent film for the patient's record can also be made. Integrating ultrasonography with a computer enables data storage and the production of three-dimensional images. Ultrasonography can be used to guide the provider while performing a biopsy.

Ultrasonography, because it is **noninvasive** (i.e., the procedure does not puncture skin or enter the body), is widely accepted for obstetrical use. Gestational age can be determined, congenital anomalies detected, multiple fetuses noted, ectopic pregnancy diagnosed, and fetal size and position determined (see Chapter 25).

Ultrasound takes 15 to 45 minutes, and the preparation depends on the body part being examined. An obstetrical ultrasound may require the patient to have a full bladder to push aside the intestines. An ultrasound of the gallbladder and liver requires the patient to have had nothing to eat or drink for 8 to 12 hours before the examination. The patient must remain still unless requested to change positions. Therapeutic ultrasonography is discussed in Chapter 32.

Mammography

More than any other X-ray, the **mammogram** must be of the highest resolution and contrast (Figure 31-13). High resolution and contrast call for an increase in exposure to radiation, but mammography currently is safer than ever because of strong regulations (it is the only radiography examination fully regulated by the federal government) and improved technology. The machines used for mammography must meet

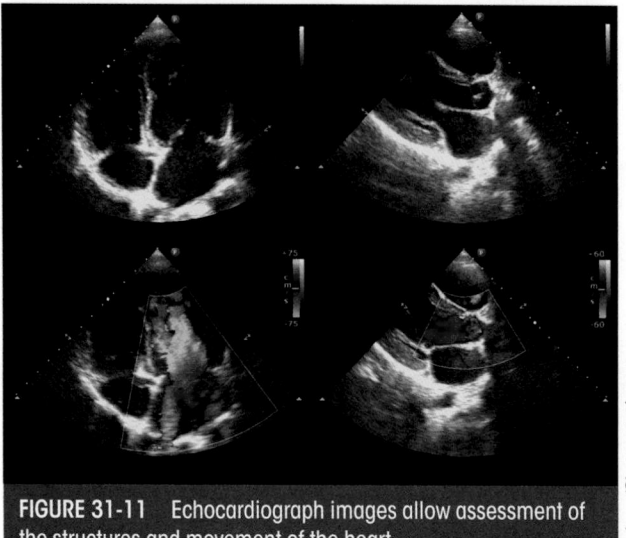

FIGURE 31-11 Echocardiograph images allow assessment of the structures and movement of the heart.

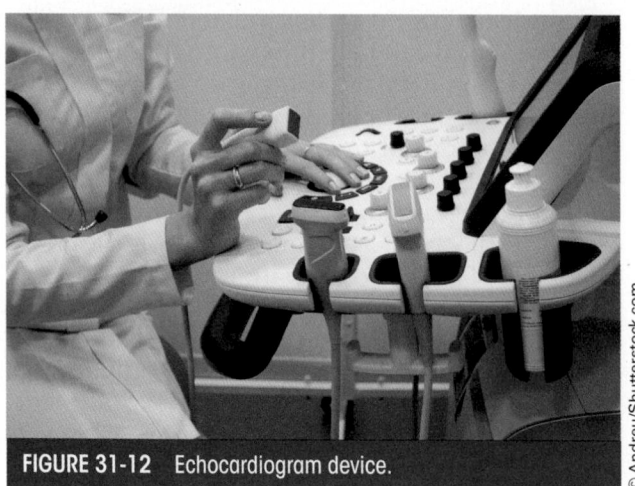

FIGURE 31-12 Echocardiogram device.

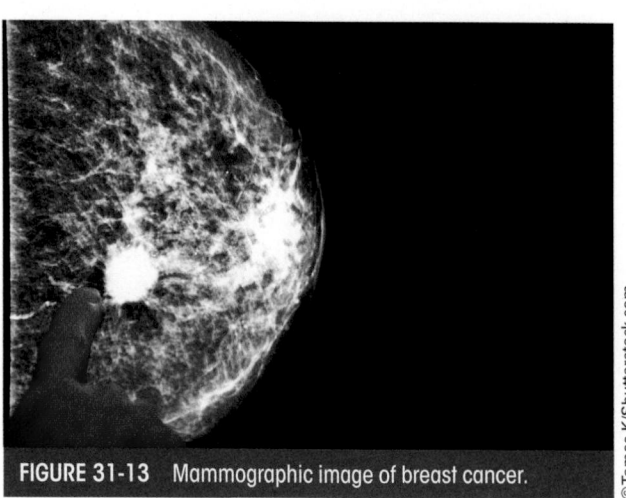

FIGURE 31-13 Mammographic image of breast cancer.

stringent requirements. They are used with special screens, film, and cassettes. Currently, the equipment can produce high-resolution and extremely high–contrast images with exposures that are lower than ever. Digitalization helps improve images. Although some newer mammography equipment is digitalized, according to some experts, it produces images that are only slightly better than those produced by non-digitalized equipment. Imaging techniques help providers perform biopsies of the breast, especially of abnormal areas that cannot be felt but are seen by conventional mammography or with ultrasound. A type of needle biopsy, stereotactic-guided biopsy, locates the exact location of the abnormal area in three dimensions using conventional mammography. (*Stereotactic* refers to use of a computer and scanning devices to create three-dimensional images.) A sterile needle is inserted into the precise location, and tissue or cell samples can be obtained. The samples are examined by a pathologist who looks for cancer cells.

Computer-Aided Detection (CAD).

Computer-aided detection uses the computer to bring suspicious areas on a mammogram to the radiologist's attention. The CAD scans the mammogram with a laser beam and converts it into a digital signal that is processed by the computer. The image is displayed on a video monitor, with the suspicious area highlighted. The radiologist can compare the digital image with the conventional mammogram to see if any of the highlighted areas were missed on the initial review and require further investigation. CAD technology may improve the accuracy of a screening mammogram. CAD provides a "second set of eyes" for the radiologist with the goal of increased analysis of suspicious areas. Researchers continue to seek ways to reduce patients' exposure to X-rays even further. Chapter 25 provides more information on mammography.

Filing Films and Reports

Because radiographs are part of the patient's permanent record, they must be safeguarded from the environment. Conditions such as heat, moisture, light, and radiation can damage them. Processed films are stored in special envelopes with the patient's name, date, and identification number marked on the outside. They are stored in a cool, dry place. The films are the property of the hospital or other facility where the films were taken and usually remain where they were taken. Storage on site makes them accessible for future use for comparison purposes and eliminates the possibility of their being lost as they could be if they were allowed to be taken away from the facility

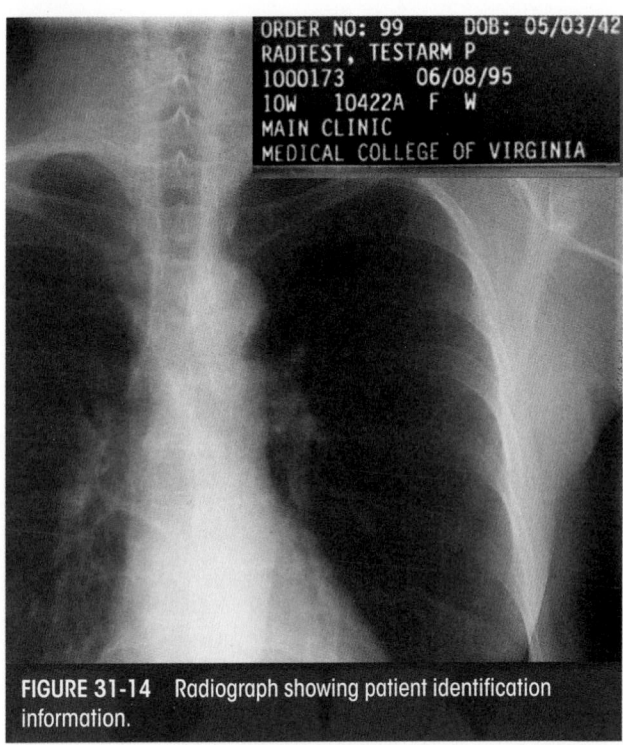

FIGURE 31-14 Radiograph showing patient identification information.

where they were processed. Written reports of the findings are prepared by the radiologist and sent to the patient's provider(s) (Figure 31-14). Computed radiography eliminates the need for hard copy film storage.

RADIATION THERAPY

Radiation therapy is generally used to treat tumors that cannot be surgically removed or that are inaccessible for surgical removal, and to treat a malignant tumor that was surgically excised but a portion of the tumor remains. It is a specialty within radiology. When used to treat inaccessible or inoperable tumors, the treatment is considered **palliative**. The treatment shrinks the tumor, thereby lessening symptoms related to the tumor. The treatments can be either external, with direct radiation aimed through the surface of the skin to an area within the body, or internal, using various applications of radioactivity such as seeds or beads that are planted inside the body and left there for a certain amount of time. The radiation therapy is the same as X-rays, with doses carefully calculated. The aim of radiation therapy is to target rapidly dividing malignant cell growth and to disrupt the DNA. The object is to destroy as many of the malignant cells as possible without harming healthy cells surrounding the tumor. Possible side effects are nausea, vomiting, hair loss, anorexia, bone marrow suppression, and **stomatitis**.

NUCLEAR MEDICINE

Nuclear medicine is the branch of medicine involved with the use of radioactive (i.e., emitting rays or particles from the nucleus) substances for diagnosis, therapy, and research. Specific training is necessary for this specialty.

Radioactive substances are administered to the patient either by mouth or by injection. The radioactive compounds, known as **radionuclides**, travel to an organ or area in the body that attracts them and creates an image of that area. The gamma rays omitted are detected by camera.

If the radionuclide is in an area that is abnormal, such as a tumor, the area is referred to as "hot." If the radionuclide does not concentrate in the abnormality, but surrounds it instead, the area is referred to as "cold." Both hot and cold areas are suggestive of abnormalities.

The provider may order a nuclear medicine scan for the following reasons: to analyze kidney function, image blood flow through the heart, scan the lungs, measure thyroid function, identify bleeding into the colon, determine the spread of cancer, bone scan, brain scan, and others. Nuclear imaging techniques use a camera and a nearby computer to detect emissions of the rays, measure the amount of radioactivity, and provide a digitalized image of the organ (e.g., the thyroid gland).

Data gathered from all of these diagnostic imaging devices are stored electronically in a hospital information system (HIS). Picture archiving and communication systems (PACS) store all radiologic exam results and are available online to providers on demand. The level of access to the data can be defined by each system. The benefits of these systems are that the examination reports and images will not become lost and no time is spent waiting for a report.

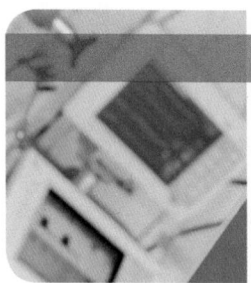

CASE STUDY 31-1

Refer to the scenario at the beginning of the chapter.

CASE STUDY REVIEW

1. What is the patient preparation for excretory urography (IVP)?
2. What should Gwen tell Mr. Waite about what to expect as he begins to have his procedure?

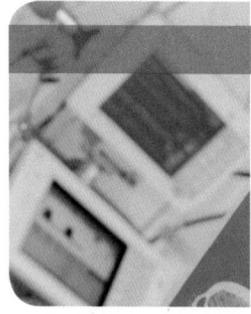

CASE STUDY 31-2

Gloria McDermott is scheduled to have a GI series of X-rays next week because of persistent episodes of stomach pain that is unrelieved by the medication Dr. King has prescribed for her.

CASE STUDY REVIEW

1. How will you explain to Ms. McDermott the purpose of the test?
2. What will you tell her about how to prepare for the test?

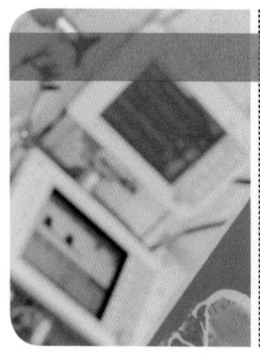

CASE STUDY 31-3

Ray Manard has had a series of X-rays, a GI series, a cholecystogram, and an MRI of his abdomen. He has scheduled an appointment with a gastroenterologist and asks you to get all of the films for him to take to the gastroenterologist.

CASE STUDY REVIEW

1. What is your response to his request?
2. Explain why the films should be kept on site.

- Radiology and diagnostic imaging are helpful in the diagnosis and treatment of diseases and conditions because procedures can be done to visualize internal structures and their functions.
- Radiation is not without its risks to personnel and patients, but by following specific safety precautions, the health and safety of all involved can be safeguarded.
- The three specialty areas are radiology, radiation therapy, and nuclear medicine.
- Principles of radiation safety should be followed to protect the patient and the health care staff from undue exposure to radiation.
- There are various types of equipment that function in different ways in order to visualize specific body parts.
- In order for some anatomic structures to be visualized, appropriate contrast media must be used.
- For many radiologic procedures, the medical assistant must educate the patient about the prep in order for the procedure to be successful.
- Patient positioning allows easy visualization of the structural areas being examined.
- Fluoroscopy is a radiologic technique that allows sequential, moving images to be obtained, as well as still films.
- As the patients age, osteoporosis is common. Bone densitometry allows measurement of bone strength.
- Positron emission tomography (PET) is a diagnostic imaging scan that requires an injection of radiopharmaceuticals.
- Computerized tomography (CT) utilizes low doses of radiation.
- Magnetic resonance imaging (MRI) allows detailed images of soft tissues.
- Flat plate films are also known a plain films. They are usually films of bony structures.
- Ultrasonography uses high frequency sound waves to image internal soft tissues.
- Mammograms are a part of screening for breast cancer.
- Radiation therapy is used to treat cancer that cannot be surgically removed.
- *Nuclear medicine* is the term used when referring to imaging that is completed after injection of radionuclides.

Study for Success

To reinforce your knowledge of and skills related to information presented in this chapter:

- Review the *Key Terms* and *Learning Outcomes*
- Consider the *Critical Thinking* features and *Case Studies* and discuss your conclusions
- Answer the questions in the *Certification Review*

CERTIFICATION REVIEW

1. Which of the following radiologic procedures does *not* require a contrast medium?
   a. Hysterosalpingogram
   b. Mammogram
   c. Cholecystogram
   d. Angiogram

2. A cholecystogram requires which type of contrast medium?
   a. Inhaled
   b. Oral
   c. Intravenous
   d. Topical
   e. Intramuscular

3. A cholangiogram will examine which of the following body structures?
   a. Upper GI tract
   b. Lower GI tract
   c. Bile ducts
   d. Kidneys and ureters
4. In which of the following positions does the posterior aspect of the body face the X-ray tube and the anterior face the film?
   a. Oblique
   b. Anteroposterior
   c. Posteroanterior
   d. Prone
   e. Supine
5. The radiologic procedure of choice for brain imaging is which of the following?
   a. Computerized tomography
   b. Positron emission tomography
   c. Magnetic resonance imaging
   d. Ultrasonography
6. Which of the following is a key way to limit your exposure to radiation as an allied health provider?
   a. Utilize a camera and microphone to communicate with patients during exams
   b. Allow the practitioner to perform all radiographic procedures
   c. Move quickly when in the room with patients
   d. Avoid holding patients manually during radiographic studies
   e. None of these

7. With a right lateral view, the beam of radiation travels in which direction?
   a. Through the body from the left to the right
   b. Through the body from front to the back
   c. Through the body from the right to the left
   d. Through the body from the back to the front
8. Which of the following statements is true regarding a CT scan?
   a. It uses a large amount of radiation.
   b. It produces cross-sectional images of the body.
   c. It allows imaging of structures that standard radiography cannot.
   d. It rotates 180 degrees around the patient to obtain cross-sectional images.
   e. Both b and c
9. What is the purpose of radiation therapy?
   a. To diagnose medical conditions
   b. To treat neoplasms that cannot be surgically removed
   c. To provide palliative therapy
   d. Both b and c
10. Which of the following is the best description of fluoroscopy?
    a. A form of X-ray that measures bone density
    b. Using a computer and contrast media
    c. X-rays that are viewed in motion
    d. The images cannot be seen in motion immediately by the provider
    e. None of these

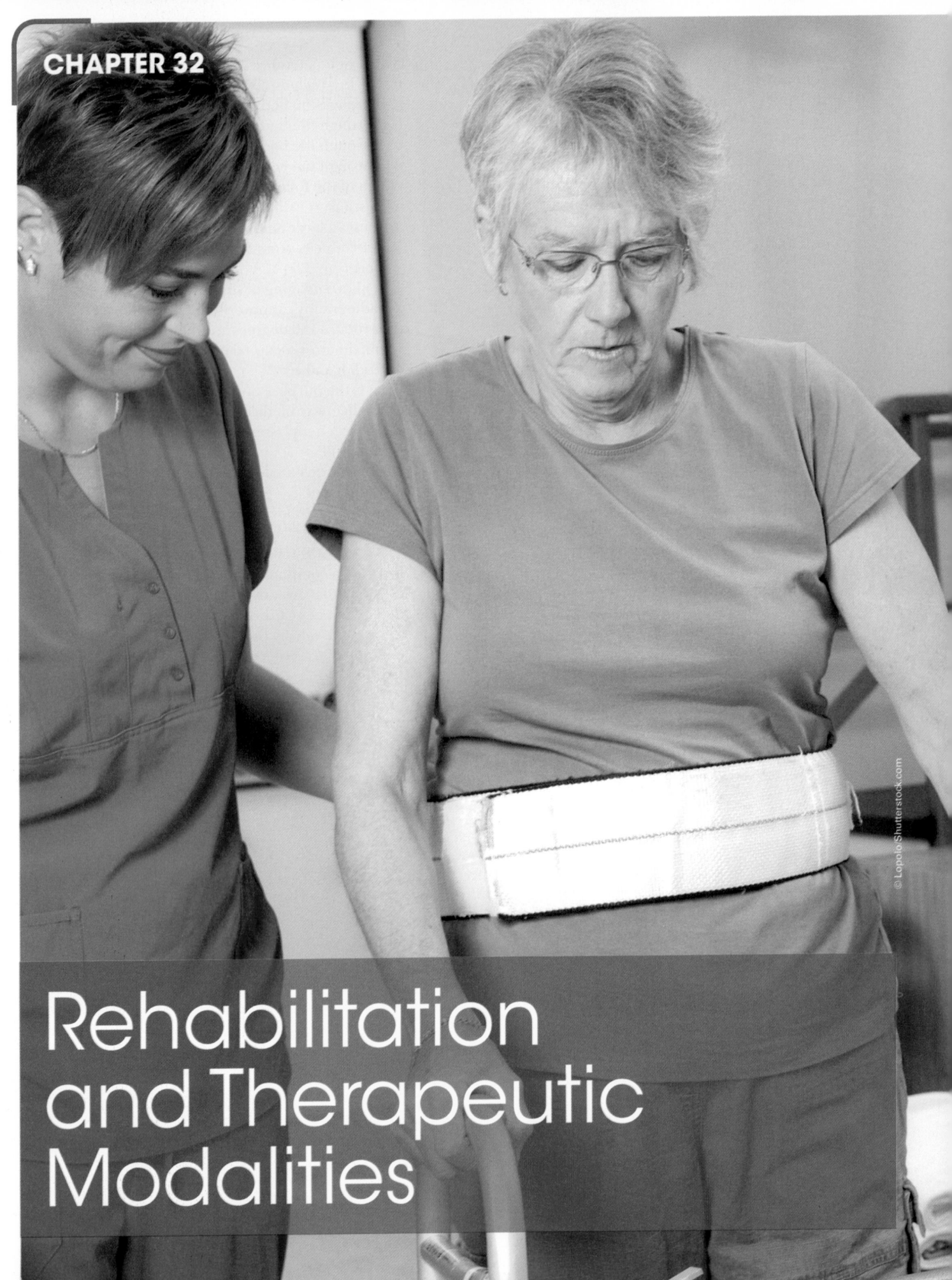

Rehabilitation and Therapeutic Modalities

LEARNING OUTCOMES

1. Define and spell the key terms as presented in the glossary.

2. Outline rehabilitation medicine and explain its importance in patient care.

3. Discuss the importance of correct posture and body mechanics, and demonstrate how to safely transfer patients and lift or move heavy objects using proper body mechanics.

4. Characterize safety precautions and techniques used when helping a patient to ambulate and demonstrate how to assist the patient to safely stand and walk.

5. Demonstrate how to safely care for the falling patient.

6. List assistive devices and the importance of each in helping patients to ambulate.

7. Demonstrate how to measure patients for a walker, crutches, and a cane, and help them ambulate safely with each device.

8. Simulate the ambulation gaits used with crutches.

9. Execute the safety precautions and techniques used when pushing a wheelchair.

10. Explain the importance of joint range of motion and the method used to measure joint movement.

11. Interpret the importance of therapeutic exercise and the types of therapeutic exercises used in patient rehabilitation.

12. Describe electromyography and its purpose.

13. Clarify the purpose of the electrostimulation of muscle.

14. Explain the body's physiologic reactions to heat and cold therapeutic modalities.

15. Be able to identify and describe the various types of hot and cold modalities, and describe how ultrasound works.

16. Describe various conditions for which massage therapy is used.

KEY TERMS

abduction	effleurage	modalities
activities of daily living (ADL)	electromyography (EMG)	petrissage
adduction	eversion	physiatry
ambulation	extension	plantar flexion
assistive device	flexion	pronation
axilla	gait	range of motion (ROM)
body mechanics	gait belt	rehabilitative medicine
circumduction	goniometer	rotation
contractures	goniometry	supination
cryotherapy	hemiplegia	thermotherapy
diathermy	hydrocollator	ultrasound
dorsiflexion	hyperextension	vasoconstriction
	inversion	

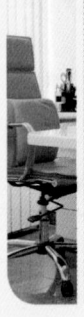

SCENARIO

In a large urgent care center such as Inner City Urgent Care, a team of therapists is responsible for providing patients with a high level of rehabilitative care. However, the clinical medical assistants at Inner City Urgent Care also are involved on a daily basis in the care of patients who have experienced injuries such as fractures or severe back pain. Clinical medical assistant Sam Tyler, CMA (AAMA), MLT, and clinical medical assistant Sarah Thomas, CMA (AAMA), are often responsible for transferring patients and getting them safely from the reception area to the examination room and from wheelchair to examination table. Although acutely aware of the needs and safety of the patient, Sam and Sarah also make sure they protect themselves by using proper body mechanics, by observing good posture, by using their arm and leg muscles and not their back muscles, and by always bending from the hips and knees, not the waist. Sam's and Sarah's observation of these important principles protects their health and ensures the safety of their patients.

Chapter Portal

Physical disability affects millions of people in the United States, regardless of age, race, or socio-economic status. Every year thousands of people survive strokes, head or spinal cord injury, or other debilitating illness or injury that leaves them unable to perform complete independent function. Some of these individuals recover completely. Others recover to their fullest ability, living the rest of their lives with some type of disability. Still other patients experience chronic conditions such as arthritis or severe back pain that incapacitate them to the extent they cannot work or completely care for themselves.

Rehabilitation medicine is a field of medical disciplines that uses physical and mechanical agents to aid in the diagnosis, treatment, and prevention of diseases and bodily injuries. Its goal is to aid in the restoration of those functions that have been affected by the patient's condition. For those who have experienced permanent loss of ability, it seeks to find practical substitutions for that loss, thereby assisting patients to make the most of their remaining abilities.

Physiatry is the term in the specialty that focuses on physical medicine and rehabilitation. Physiatrists treat a wide variety of medical conditions affecting the brain, spinal cord, nerves, bones, joints, ligaments, muscles, and tendons. Depending on the patient's condition, the rehabilitative services ordered can include a recommendation to one or several rehabilitation specialists. Most likely, that specialist will be a physical therapist, occupational therapist, speech therapist, or sports medicine specialist, although the field of rehabilitation medicine is certainly not limited to these four areas of specialty. Professional rehabilitation therapists, in whichever field they practice, are specifically trained and licensed in their field of expertise to assess, plan, and execute the patient's treatment in an overall effort to restore that patient to the highest level of physical and social independence possible. The medical assistant, as a member of an interdisciplinary health team, can use medical assisting skills to enable patients to regain normal or near-normal function after an illness or injury. Chapter 6 provides information on legal considerations and the Americans with Disabilities Act (ADA).

THE ROLE OF THE MEDICAL ASSISTANT IN REHABILITATION

Professional

As a medical assistant, you may find yourself working in one of the rehabilitation fields. Such opportunities might include an ambulatory care setting with a specialty in physical therapy or sports medicine, an orthopedic surgeon's practice, the occupational or speech therapy department of a large suburban hospital, or other outpatient clinic or medical clinic. For the more chronically ill, nursing homes and rehabilitation hospitals also focus on restoring patients to as much independence as possible.

Even if you do not work in the field of rehabilitation and therapeutic modalities, you may be referring patients for treatments and perhaps even performing insurance coding or rehabilitative and therapeutic modalities. Care of the total patient requires an understanding of rehabilitative medicine.

Whatever the rehabilitation setting, you will most likely find that you are a member of an interdisciplinary team of health care professionals who bring a broad knowledge base to patient care (see the "Specialized Fields of Rehabilitative Medicine" Quick Reference Guide). However, the provider is responsible for prescribing any type of **rehabilitative medicine**.

It is important to remember that patients seeking rehabilitation treatment may have sustained a tremendous loss of physical ability, leaving them vulnerable to feelings of helplessness and despair. They may be able to perform only limited **activities of daily living (ADL)** or normal daily self-care such as brushing their teeth, getting dressed, and eating. Perhaps they cannot even do the simple tasks we take for granted every day, leaving them completely dependent on another person for help. The goal of treatment is restoration of the highest level of function and health that is possible for each patient.

Understanding and encouragement are vital to the recovery process of these patients. While working with persons with disabilities, remember that certain tasks may be challenging for them. More than likely they are acutely aware of their impairment and feel frustrated at their loss of function and discouraged about the future. Some patients may suffer some speech impairment, making communication difficult or impossible. Respect for their dignity will build their self-esteem and have a positive effect on their treatment.

Patients' safety is essential. Many have a loss of ability to move and are vulnerable to falls. Patients and their support system can function at their highest level and in a safe manner if they are properly educated.

⯮ QUICK REFERENCE GUIDE

⯮ SPECIALIZED FIELDS OF REHABILITATIVE MEDICINE

Field	Description	Example
Physical therapy/ physiotherapy	The treatment of disorders with physical and mechanical agents and methods to restore normal function after injury or illness	© Tomislav Pinter/Shutterstock.com
Occupational therapy	The use of activities to help restore independent functioning after an injury or illness	© GBZero/Shutterstock.com

(continues)

Field	Description	Example
Speech therapy	The diagnosis and treatment of speech disorders	© Monkey Business Images/Shutterstock.com
Sports medicine	A branch of medicine that specializes in the treatment and prevention of injuries caused by athletic participation	© Aykut Erdogdu/Shutterstock.com

PRINCIPLES OF BODY MECHANICS

Safety

The medical assistant's work with persons with disabilities may require great physical effort, particularly if patients are incapable of lifting or moving themselves. Moving patients or heavy, awkward objects can be hazardous for the patient as well as the caregiver if not performed correctly.

Body mechanics is the practice of using certain key muscle groups together with good body alignment and proper body positioning to reduce the risk for injury to both patient and caregiver. Always be conscious of using proper body mechanics, not just on the job, but in everything that requires moving, lifting, pushing, or pulling heavy or awkward objects.

Posture

Practicing good body mechanics starts with good posture. Good posture protects the entire body, particularly the back, whether standing, sitting, or lying down. Following the principles of good posture allows all of the structural components of the body to work together to perform at a peak level and to avoid injury.

The central idea of good posture is body alignment. When standing, the body should be balanced. Keep your head in the midline and your earlobes equally distant from the shoulders. Hold your chest high while keeping your shoulders back and relaxed. Keep your abdominal muscles tight and pull in your buttocks. Balance your weight evenly on both feet and keep your knees relaxed.

Good posture when sitting includes keeping the spine in a neutral position. Sit with your buttocks against the back of the chair and rest your back on the chair back. Feet should be resting on the floor with knees level with hips. Keep your head and neck straight with your shoulders relaxed, not rounded, elevated, or pulled back.

Good posture when lying down includes maintaining your spine in a neutral position. A firm mattress for support is essential. When lying on your side, use a pillow between your knees to maintain proper alignment. If lying on your back, place the pillow under both knees to maintain proper positioning.

Refer to Figure 32-1 as a guide for proper posture when standing or sitting.

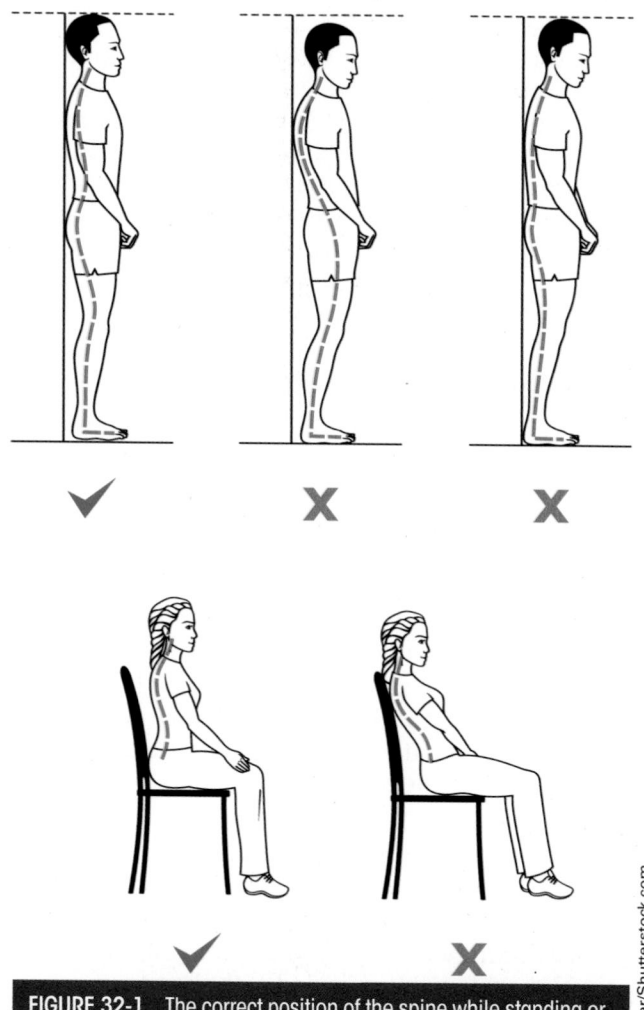

FIGURE 32-1   The correct position of the spine while standing or sitting.

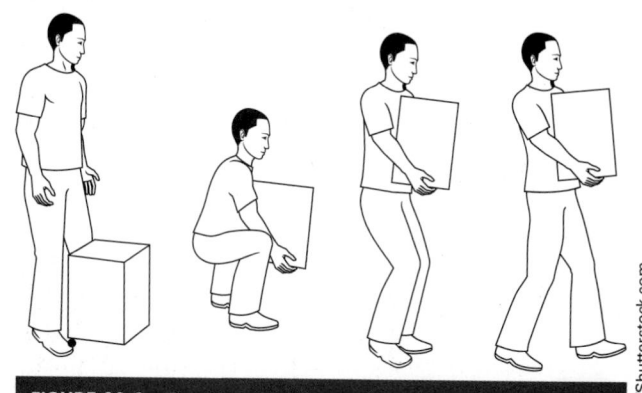

FIGURE 32-2   Provide a good base of support by keeping the back straight and feet apart.

USING THE BODY SAFELY AND EFFECTIVELY

Safety

The spine is a flexible rod, designed to bend in many directions and hold the back steady. However, the muscles of the back are small and not meant for lifting heavy loads. They can be easily damaged if called on to work beyond their natural ability. The muscles in the arms and legs, however, are large and were designed for heavy work. Rely on these muscles when lifting and carrying heavy objects, bending over or bending down, or moving patients.

It is important to keep several basic rules in mind whenever performing any task:

- Keep the back as straight as possible and feet shoulder-width apart to provide a good base of support (Figure 32-2).
- Always bend from the hips and knees, enabling the largest muscles of the legs to do the hard work, but *never* bend from the waist.

- Pivot the entire body instead of twisting it.
- Use the body's weight to push or pull any heavy object.
- Obtain help if unable to move a patient or object that is too heavy.
- Hold heavy objects close to the body.
- Make sure the path is clear and the area to receive the object is ready before lifting or moving it.
- Get into the habit of wearing a body support if a job includes much lifting.

Lifting Techniques

There is great risk for back injuries when dealing with patients who are immobile or partially immobile. The greatest risk occurs when attempting to assist a person to a sitting position from a reclining position, transferring a person from a bed to a chair, or when leaning over a person for a long period of time.

When lifting patients or moving or lifting heavy objects, certain techniques should be used to prevent back injury:

- Get as close as possible to the object or person being lifted, because this allows the center of gravity to be maintained over the base of support.
- Keep the feet apart, one slightly in front of the other, and knees slightly bent.
- Use the large muscles of the legs and arms to lift, not back muscles.
- Keep the back straight to transfer the workload to larger arm and leg muscles. Avoid twisting movements.
- Bend from the hips and knees, squat down, and push up with leg muscles.

TRANSFERRING PATIENTS

It may be necessary to transfer patients if they cannot walk or lift themselves. Such patients may have a wide variety of disabilities, ranging from severe back pain to **hemiplegia**, or paralysis of one side of the body resulting from a stroke, accident, or other condition. Frail older adults also require particular care when being transferred, because they are more prone to bruising and broken bones, and they may be unsteady on their feet.

Safety

As a safety precaution, it is important to remember good body mechanics when transferring patients. The act of lifting and moving someone can throw off one's center of gravity and therefore the base of support. Provide a wider base of support by moving the feet farther apart and bending slightly, using strong arm and leg muscles to lift.

Before beginning any transfer, observe certain precautions:

- Make sure the equipment is stable and firm. Lock the brakes of the wheelchair and make sure the examination table or other surface will not move during the transfer.
- Check that there are no obstructions to trip over when making the transfer.
- Take small shuffling steps, and avoid crossing the feet.
- It is best if the transfer surfaces being used are close to the same height. If possible, lower the examination table or bed to the height of the wheelchair.
- Position the equipment according to the patient's physical limitations or disability. If the patient is stronger on one side, make sure that is the side on which the transfer will take place. It not only makes the transfer easier, it gives the patient more confidence.

- Always use a **gait belt**, a safety belt worn around the patient's waist, when transferring a patient. Lift the patient by grasping the belt from underneath and lifting up. Utilization of a gait belt provides balance assistance during transfers and ambulation. This reduces the risk that either the patient or the staff will be injured. Never lift a patient by the arms, or under the armpits, because this could cause injury to you and the patient.
- Take advantage of any assistance the patient can provide in lifting and moving.
- Never have patients put their arms around your neck or on your shoulders, because it could cause you to be injured.
- Make sure both you and the patient are wearing footwear that will not slip or hinder the transfer process in any way. If a prosthesis or brace is involved, make sure it is secure and will not present a problem.
- Thoroughly explain to the patient what you intend to do, and make sure the patient understands what to expect during the transfer. Instructions need to be simple and repeated when necessary.
- Practice good body mechanics. Get close enough to the patient so you can lift with your legs. Always bend at the hips instead of the waist.
- Ascertain beforehand whether assistance from other staff will be needed with the transfer.
- Finally, take sufficient time when completing each step. Many patients will want to help themselves. Respect their courage and determination, but remember that safety is of the utmost importance.

Procedure

Procedure 32-1 gives the proper steps for transferring patients from a wheelchair to an examination table.

PROCEDURE 32-1

Procedure

Transferring Patient from Wheelchair to Examination Table

STANDARD PRECAUTIONS:

Handwashing

(continues)

PURPOSE:

To move a patient safely to and from a wheelchair to the examination table.

EQUIPMENT/SUPPLIES:

- Footstool with hand rail and nonskid rubber tips
- Gait belt

PROCEDURE STEPS:

1. Begin any transfer procedure by washing your hands.
2. Always take the time to **introduce yourself and to identify the patient**, using two identifiers. Before doing anything, **speak at the patient's level of understanding and explain what you will be doing** and the process to be followed. **Show awareness of the patient's concerns** by answering any questions.
3. Place the wheelchair next to the examination table, with the patient's strongest side facing the table so that he or she can use the stronger leg for balance during the transfer.
4. Check to ensure that the brake is locked.
5. Move the wheelchair footrests up and out of the way, or if possible, remove them completely.
6. Position the long-handled stool in front of the examination table and as close to the wheelchair as possible (Figure 32-3A)
7. Instruct the patient to place the feet flat on the floor, assisting as needed, and position the stool in front of the examination table, as close to the wheelchair as possible.
8. Place the gait belt snugly around the patient's waist and tuck the excess belting under the belt to avoid tripping or entanglement (Figure 32-3B)

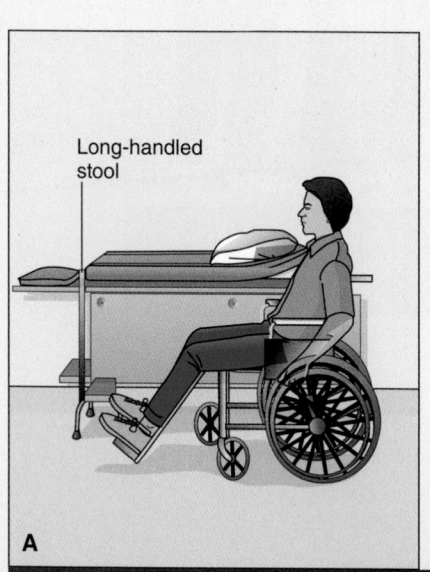

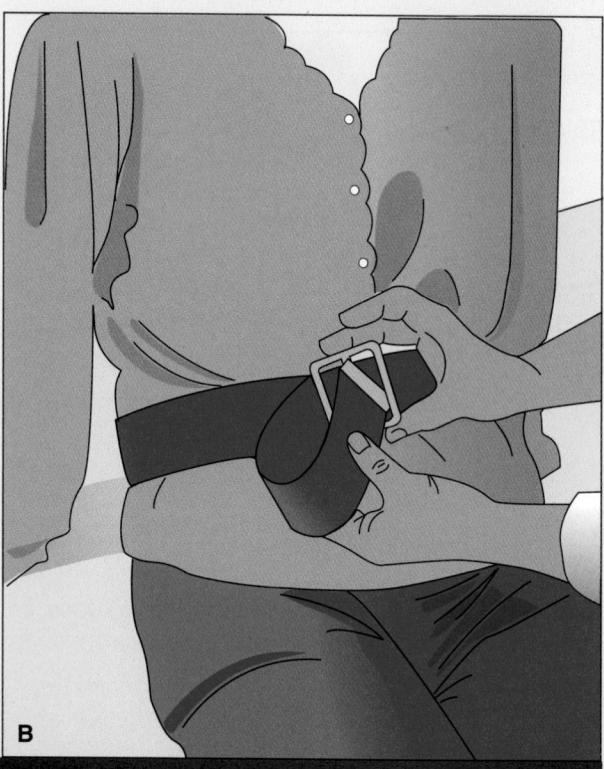

FIGURE 32-3 (A) Position the long-handled stool in front of the examination table and as close to the wheelchair as possible. (B) The gait belt is always applied snugly around the patient's waist before attempting to move or ambulate with the patient.

(continues)

9. Remind the patient to follow your instruction and signal, and stand directly in front of the patient with your feet slightly apart (Figure 32-3C).

10. Using good body mechanics, bend at the hips and knees and grasp the gait belt from underneath.

11. Have the patient place hands on the armrests and, on your signal, push up on the armrests as you assist the patient into a standing position.

12. Once standing, take a moment to assess the patient's strength, balance, and skin color. If there are any physical changes or if the patient implies or makes statements to indicate dizziness, carefully lower the patient back into the wheelchair and check vital signs.

13. However, if the patient appears steady, stable, and balanced, proceed by standing slightly behind and on the weaker side of the patient.

14. Grasp the gait belt with one hand, with your fingers under the belt, palm facing upward and elbow bent. Place the other hand on the patient's bent arm for support.

15. While continuing to hold onto the gait belt, have the patient grasp the handle of the footstool. Instruct the patient to carefully step up on the footstool.

16. Assist the patient to pivot so that the back is toward the examination table with the buttocks slightly above the table's edge (Figure 32-3D).

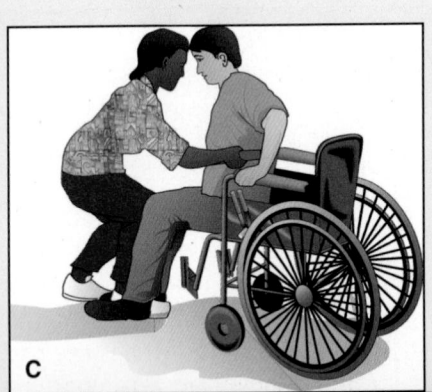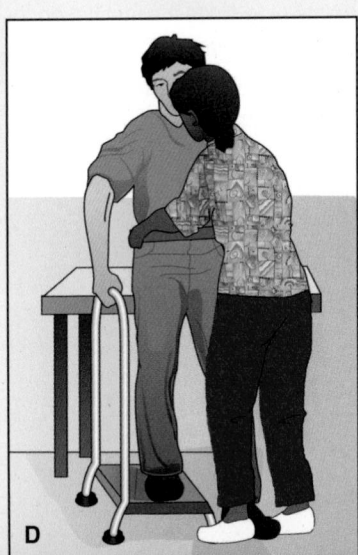

FIGURE 32-3   (C) Before lifting, observe proper body mechanics to avoid injuring yourself or the patient. (D) Check that the patient's foot is firmly placed on the stool before completing the transfer.

17. Steady the patient and instruct him or her to keep one hand on the safety handle of the footstool and one hand on the exam table. Ease the patient onto the table, making any adjustments as necessary.

18. Move the wheelchair and the footstool out of the way.

(continues)

> **Transfer Patient Back to Wheelchair**
>
> 19. When you are ready to transfer the patient back to the chair, position the wheelchair next to the table closest to the patient's strongest side. Lock the brakes.
>
> 20. Place the gait belt snugly around the patient's waist as before, tucking in any excess length.
>
> 21. Position your arms so that the one is under the patient's arm and around the shoulder and the other arm is under the patient's knees. Pivot the patient so that the legs dangle over the edge of the table.
>
> 22. Position the stool in front of the patient, near the foot of the table.
>
> 23. Instruct the patient that upon your signal, he or she should push off of the examination table. The patient should be aware that you will be pulling slightly forward so that the feet land squarely on the footstool.
>
> 24. Continue to hold onto the gait belt and instruct the patient to step onto the floor, leading with the strongest leg.
>
> 25. As soon as the patient steps down, he or she should pivot in one singular motion, so that the patient is facing away from the wheelchair.
>
> 26. Instruct the patient to swing the hands back and grasp the arms of the wheelchair, then bending from your hips and knees, gently lower the patient into the chair, controlling the rate of descent with the gait belt.
>
> 27. Help the patient to be comfortable and remove the gait belt.
>
> 28. Replace the footrests to their proper position to support the patient's feet and unlock the wheels.

ASSISTING PATIENTS TO AMBULATE

Despite great strides that have been made in providing access for persons with disabilities, **ambulation**, or walking, is a functional activity that still ensures the ultimate level of independence and freedom. For many patients, being able to ambulate again gives them tremendous satisfaction, because the act of walking more than anything else signifies their return to wellness. Some patients take months to walk again by undergoing exercises and treatment designed to strengthen specific muscles. They may still need help while in your clinic or in a clinic specializing in orthopedics or sports medicine.

Safety

Before assisting with any type of ambulation, there are several safety issues to remember:

- Make sure the patient is ready to walk. If a patient has trouble sitting well or cannot balance once standing up, walking should not be attempted.
- The patient should be wearing good shoes that are flat, are supportive, and have a rubber sole.
- Check to be certain there are plenty of handholds or railings within easy reach should the patient become unstable during walking.
- A gait belt provides a firm hold on the patient should the patient require assistance with stability at any time. For the patient just starting to walk, this device should be used and held by the caregiver throughout the session.
- Monitor the patient when standing and throughout the ambulation session for signs of fatigue and vertigo.
- Ambulate only as long as the patient has strength. Never push the patient beyond endurance.
- Never hurry a patient.
- Be ready should a patient start to fall. Generally, patients will fall toward their weaker side, but sometimes their legs lose stability and they go straight down.

Procedure

Procedures 32-2 and 32-3 detail the steps involved in assisting patients to stand and walk, and in caring for a falling patient.

PROCEDURE 32-2

Procedure

Assisting the Patient with Ambulation Using Assistive Devices

STANDARD PRECAUTIONS:

Handwashing

PURPOSE:

To help a patient ambulate safely.

EQUIPMENT/SUPPLIES:

Gait belt

PROCEDURE STEPS:

1. ***Introduce yourself to the patient. Identify the patient*** using two identifiers. ***Speaking at the patient's level of understanding***, explain what you are going to do and what is expected of the patient.

2. Before beginning any kind of assisted ambulation, the patient should be assessed by the provider. Make sure that the patient is wearing sturdy footwear with a flat nonslip sole.

3. Wash your hands before proceeding.

4. If the patient is to be using a walker, examine it to ensure that there are rubber tips secured on each leg. Check the handles for any rough or damaged edges that could injure the patient.

5. Place a gait belt snugly around the patient's waist, tucking in any excess length so that it is not a tripping hazard. Check to make sure that the walker is in the open and locked position and that it has been set at the appropriate height level, with the hand rests even with the patient's hip joint.

6. When the patient is standing with hands on the walker, the angle of the elbows should be approximately 30 degrees.

7. Once in a standing position, the patient should be instructed to step into the walker and hold onto the hand rests. Remind the patient to keep the walker out in front while ambulating.

8. Position yourself behind and slightly to the side of the patient, preferably on the patient's weaker side. Firmly grasp the gait belt (Figure 32-4).

9. Instruct the patient to lift the walker and place all four legs out in front, with the back legs even with the patient's toes. If the walker has wheels, the patient will simply roll the walker into position.

10. The patient should then lean forward with hands on the hand rests, thus transferring weight to the walker (Figure 32-5).

11. The patient should complete the movement by stepping into the walker, leading first with the stronger leg. Verbally coach the patient through the process as needed. Provide support by maintaining a grasp on the gait belt.

12. Assess the patient for strength, balance, and skin color before proceeding.

13. If the patient will be using crutches, check first to ensure that the crutches are in good working order, by examining the bar and hand rest to evaluate the padding. Check too to make sure the wing nuts are tightened appropriately.

(continues)

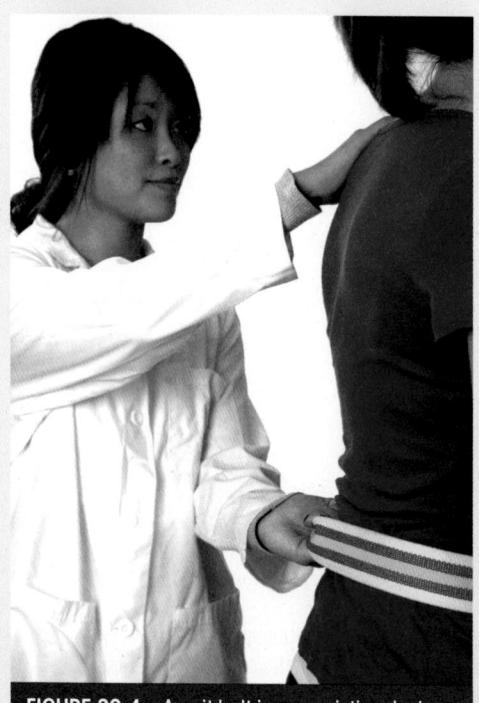

FIGURE 32-4 A gait belt is an assistive device which can be used to help safely transfer a person from a one area to another (e.g., wheelchair to bed), assist with sitting and standing, and aid in ambulation.

© aceshot1/Shutterstock.com

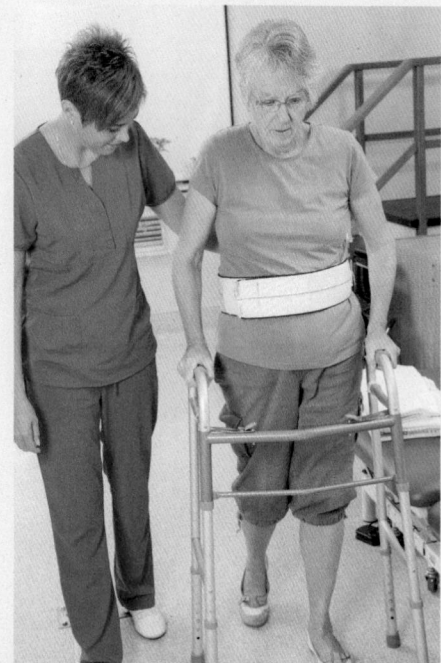

FIGURE 32-5 Walk slightly behind the person utilizing a walker, hold onto the gait belt from behind, and offer assistance only as needed.

© Lopolo/Shutterstock.com

14. Measure the appropriate height of the crutches by placing tape in the patient's axillary area. Measure the crutches to determine that the length of the crutch concludes at a spot that is 2 inches in front of and 6 inches to the side of the patient's foot. Adjust the crutches to meet this measurement.

15. Position the crutches and then instruct the patient to bear the weight of the body on the hands as he or she holds the hand rests. The patient should not bear weight using the axillary area (Figure 32-6).

16. Place both crutches at a comfortable distance in front of the patient's feet, and instruct the patient to stand tall, looking forward, not down.

17. The patient should then move the affected leg up until it is even with the crutches before transferring weight to the hands and moving the unaffected leg forward. This sequence should be repeated as the patient moves forward.

18. If the patient will be using a cane, you will again begin by assessing the equipment to ensure that the cane's rubber cover is not worn.

19. The cane should be placed close to the body at the side of the foot of the stronger leg. The handle should be level with the hip joint. This will allow the patient's elbow to remain at a flex of 20 to 30 degrees when weight bearing (Figure 32-7).

20. To move forward, instruct the patient to advance both the cane and the affected leg simultaneously, transferring the weight to the cane before bringing the unaffected leg up and past the cane.

21. The patient should repeat the sequence to continue forward. You should remain behind and slightly to the side of the patient with a tight grip on the gait belt as the patient ambulates.

22. When you are finished assisting the patient with ambulation, wash your hands and document the procedure in the patient's medical record. Include the date, time, duration, and method of ambulation, as well as the patient's response and any vital signs taken.

(continues)

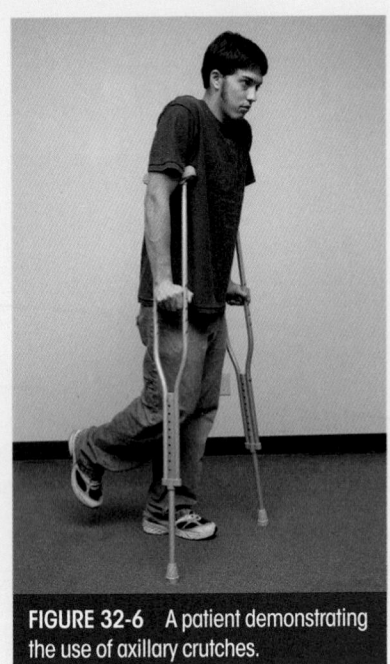

FIGURE 32-6 A patient demonstrating the use of axillary crutches.

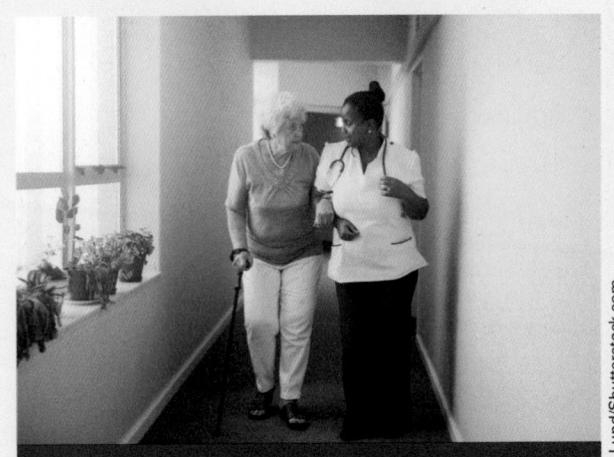

FIGURE 32-7 When using a cane as an assistive device, the patient holds it on the side of the strongest leg.

© Jacob Lund/Shutterstock.com

DOCUMENTATION:

> Assessment
>
> 7/14/20XX 2:30 PM Patient states she has been doing "fairly well" in physical therapy. She says she walks short distances, about 10 feet. Assisted with ambulation. Steady gait. Says she feels "very good." S. Tyler, CMA (AAMA)

Courtesy of Harris CareTracker PM and EMR

OR

> Assessment
>
> 7/14/20XX 2:30 PM Patient has been to physical therapy a total of 15 times. Dr. Woo wants patient to ambulate to see her progress. Assisted patient to ambulate with walker. Walked about 100 feet. Color pink. No c/o dizziness or lightheadedness. P 100, S. Thomas, CMA (AAMA)

Courtesy of Harris CareTracker PM and EMR

OR

> Assessment
>
> 7/14/20XX 2:30PM Patient fitted with crutches and instructed regarding crutch walking. Dr. Woo observed steady ambulation x 50 feet. Patient steady on feet. Manages coordinated crutch-walking. States, "I think I have the hang of this!" S. Tyler, CMA (AAMA)

Courtesy of Harris CareTracker PM and EMR

OR

> Assessment
>
> 7/14/20XX 2:30PM Patient doing well post-total knee replacement. Requires cane to ambulate steadily. Instructed regarding cane-walking. Ambulated steadily x 35 feet. Dr. Woo observed. No complaints of faintness or dizziness. Pulse regular at 88 bpm. S. Thomas, CMA (AAMA)

Courtesy of Harris CareTracker PM and EMR

PROCEDURE 32-3

Procedure

Caring for the Falling Patient

PURPOSE:

To help the patient fall safely to prevent injury.

EQUIPMENT/SUPPLIES:

Gait belt (should already be on patient)

PROCEDURE STEPS:

1. Firmly grip the gait belt. Never grab clothing as it can shift and become unstable.

2. As the patient falls backward, widen your stance to become a more stable base of support to accept the patient's weight (Figure 32-8). Provide support by utilizing a firm grip on the gait belt. Gently lower the patient to the floor.

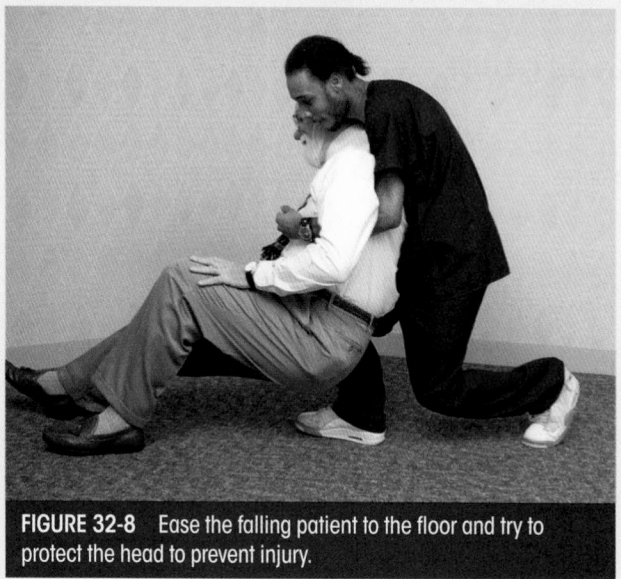

FIGURE 32-8 Ease the falling patient to the floor and try to protect the head to prevent injury.

3. Call for assistance.

4. Assess vital signs.

5. Notify the provider of the need for assessment prior to moving patient.

6. Accurately document in the patient's medical record indicating date, time, factual description of the event, response of patient, vital signs if taken, and any injuries noted by provider.

7. Complete occurrence report if required.

DOCUMENTATION:

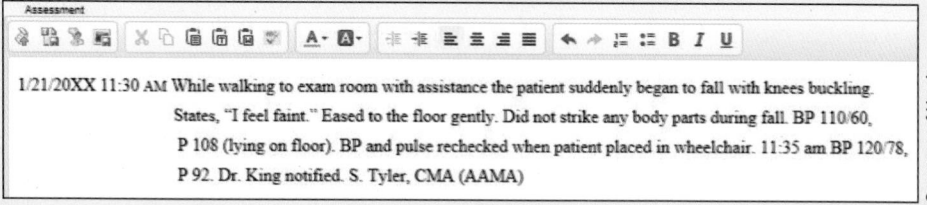

Assessment

1/21/20XX 11:30 AM While walking to exam room with assistance the patient suddenly began to fall with knees buckling. States, "I feel faint." Eased to the floor gently. Did not strike any body parts during fall. BP 110/60, P 108 (lying on floor). BP and pulse rechecked when patient placed in wheelchair. 11:35 am BP 120/78, P 92. Dr. King notified. S. Tyler, CMA (AAMA)

Courtesy of Harris CareTracker PM and EMR

ASSISTIVE DEVICES

For some patients, the extent of their physical disability may determine that ambulation is only possible with the help of an **assistive device**, or walking aid such as a walker, crutches, or cane. For others, their physical disability is such that mobility is not possible at all without the use of a wheelchair.

Some assistive devices provide stability and support, whereas others require more coordination. Depending on the patient's condition, one assistive device may be used until the patient has gained enough strength and coordination to move on to another type of assistive device, with the ultimate goal of walking unaided. The device a patient needs depends both on the disability and the patient's recuperation curve, and is prescribed after careful evaluation by the attending provider or other health professional (see the "Assistive Devices" Quick Reference Guide).

Whatever device a patient will be using, medical assistants may be called on to measure the patient for the correct size and to provide instruction in its proper use and care. Once the patient has become proficient on level surfaces, provide instruction on sitting; standing; turning around; and negotiating stairs, curbs, ramps, doors, and other obstacles. In addition, patients should be taught how to protect themselves should they fall while alone and how to get back up.

⬖ QUICK REFERENCE GUIDE

⟫ ASSISTIVE DEVICES

Assistive Device	Features	Considerations	Keys to Fitting
Walkers			
Standard	• Adjustable height • Rubber tips • Made of aluminum and is lightweight • Folds for storage or transport • Selection of hand grips based on need (foam grips or soft grip covers if hands tend to get sweaty; large grips for arthritic hands)	• Requires upper body strength • Provides maximum stability and support • Excellent for older adults • Cannot be used on uneven surfaces	• Height of the hand grip should be adjusted to just below the patient's waist, or at the top of the femur, • The elbow should be bent at a 15 to 20-degree angle when hands resting on hand grips
Rolling	• Legs have wheels • Otherwise same as regular walker • Made of aluminum and is lightweight • Folds for storage or transport	• Good for patients who need walker only for balance and not support • Can be easily pushed ahead while walking • Best for patients who primarily need a walker for balance • Two-wheeled models allow weight to be placed on the walker as movement occurs • Four-wheeled models allow faster walking speed with less stability • Cannot be used on uneven surfaces	• Height of the hand grip should be adjusted to just below the patient's waist, or at the top of the femur • The elbow should be bent at a 15 to 20-degree angle when hands resting on hand grips

© FamVeld/Shutterstock.com

(continues)

Assistive Device	Features	Considerations	Keys to Fitting
Crutches			
Axillary	• Made of aluminum or wood • Placed into **axilla** area	• Require good upper body strength and balance • Not recommended for older adults • Best for younger persons with lower extremity or hip fractures that will heal in a short time • Provide greatest range of ambulation • Can be utilized on stairs and in tight quarters • Easily transported	• Patient must stand tall • Measure with patient wearing good walking shoes • Adjust length so that axillary pad rests 2 to 3 finger breadths below the patient's axilla • Adjust hand grips so that elbows are bent at a 20-degree angle • Handgrips should be at level of crease of wrist when arms hang relaxed at side • Adjust overall length of each crutch until tip rests 2 inches lateral and 6 inches anteriorly to foot when positioned appropriately related to axilla
Forearm (Lofstrand or Canadian)	• Shorter than axillary crutches • Have metal cuff worn around forearm	• Less stable than axillary crutches • Best for long-term crutch use • Reduce stress on axillary vessels and nerves • Require upper body strength and more stability and coordination • Provide most maneuverability of all crutches • Can be utilized on stairs and in tight quarters • Easily transported	• Height is adjusted so that the elbow is flexed 15 to 30 degrees • Crutch should contact floor 2 inches lateral and 6 inches anterior to foot

(continues)

Assistive Device	Features	Considerations	Keys to Fitting
Platform	• Platform affixed to a crutch • Patient bears weight on forearm	• Best for patients with severe arthritis or poor use of hands • Do not require as much upper body strength • Can be adjusted to a height so that the arm can be bent at a 90-degree angle • Weight is borne on the forearm • Require good balance • Ideal for patients that require minimal weight transfer but cannot bear weight or grip with the hands • Can be utilized on stairs and in tight quarters • Easily transported	• Crutch should contact 2 inches below the skinfold of the armpit • Lower cuff should lie 0.5 to 1.5 inches below the back of the elbow to avoid bony contact on the arm
Canes			
Standard	• Single leg • Curved handle • Rubber tip	• Good for patients with only one good arm, lateral instability, or balance conditions	• Grip selection is a matter of personal preference • With cane in hand, elbow should be bent 15 degrees • With arm hanging relaxed at side, top of cane should be even with crease of wrist • Tip should be supple with good tread
Quad (four-point)	• Single cane resting on a platform with four legs • Rubber tips on legs	• Better for patients with more severe conditions • Does not require as much coordination, but still requires balance and upper body strength in one arm • More awkward to use • Appropriate for patients recovering from stroke	• Grip selection is a matter of personal preference • With cane in hand, elbow should be bent 15 degrees • With arm hanging relaxed at side, top of cane should be even with crease of wrist • Tip should be supple with good tread
Hemiwalker	• Has four legs that come all the way up to a handlebar • Rubber tips on all legs	• Provides most stability of all canes • Best for patients with hemiplegia who require extra support on one side • Folds for ease of storage or transport	• With arm hanging relaxed at side, top of cane should be even with crease of wrist

Walkers

Walkers are best used for patients who require maximum assistance with balance and coordination, because walkers provide stability and support when patients are standing or walking. They provide patients with the ability to ambulate independently with confidence. To use one, patients must be strong enough to be able to hold themselves upright while leaning on the walker.

Various styles of walkers are available. The two most widely used walkers are those that have rubber tips on the legs (stationary walkers), and those with wheels on the bottom of the legs (rolling walkers).

Procedure 32-2 provides steps for assisting a patient to ambulate with a walker.

Crutches

Crutches provide the ambulating patient with a great deal more mobility and flexibility. They provide good stability and support, therefore allowing for a broad range of gait patterns and ambulating speeds.

Axillary crutches are made of wood or aluminum and are used primarily for individuals who need crutches temporarily while a lower extremity heals. *Forearm crutches*, also known as Lofstrand or Canadian crutches, are shorter and provide less stability than axillary crutches. Forearm crutches are fixed with a metal or hard plastic cuff that fits around the patient's forearm. The weight is borne almost exclusively on the hand grip.

The *platform crutch* is a third type of crutch that is recommended for patients who cannot grip the handles of other types of crutches or bear weight through their wrists or hands. The crutch has a platform attached to the top that includes a hand grip. It is high enough for the patient to use with the elbow bent at a right angle.

Procedure 32-2 gives steps for teaching patients to ambulate with axillary crutches.

Crutch-Walking Gaits. The type of **gait**, or walk, a patient uses depends on the patient's injury and condition and is determined by the provider or licensed therapist. In crutch-walking gaits, each time the patient's foot or crutch touches the ground it is called a *point*. There are five gaits that are commonly used in crutch ambulation. The number of points in the gait relates to the number of feet and crutch tips that are on the ground at the same time.

Common crutch-walking gaits include two-point, three-point, four-point, swing-to, and swing-through gaits.

Two-Point Gait. There are two types of two-point gaits:

1. The first type is a non-weight-bearing gait. Patients place the crutch tips about 18 inches in front of them. They push off, taking the weight off their body and transferring it to their hands, and then bring their strong leg forward past the crutches.

2. The second gait, called the two-point alternating gait, is used when the patient can bear weight on both legs. The opposite foot and crutch are advanced forward at the same time (Figure 32-9). This gait is a more advanced gait and is used after the four-point gait has been mastered.

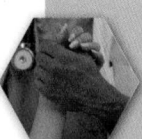

Patient Education

When instructing patients in the use of axillary crutches, impress on them the importance of putting all their weight on their hands, not on the axillae. Many patients using crutches for the first time mistakenly put the pressure on their axillae, which can damage the axillary nerve. Also reinforce the need for wearing flat nonskid shoes when using crutches.

Throw rugs and other obstacles in the home or work area are a danger to patients on crutches. Remind them to have such hazards removed. Teach patients to examine crutches daily for the following:

- Check that the wing nuts that adjust the crutches are tight.
- Check the crutch tips for wear and tear.
- Check the foam pads of the hand grips and axilla rests for tears.

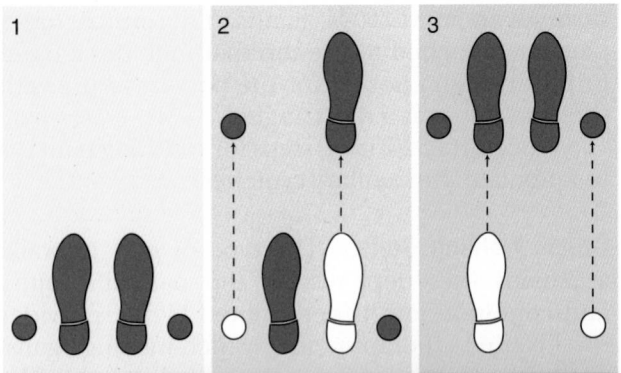

FIGURE 32-9 Two-point gait. The patient is bearing weight on both legs alternating weight distribution with opposing side crutch.

Three-Point Gait. This gait is used when the patient can only bear partial weight on one leg, or just touch that foot to the floor. Both the crutches and the weak leg are advanced at the same time. The body weight is then transferred forward to the crutches, and the stronger leg is advanced and placed slightly in front of the crutches (Figure 32-10).

FIGURE 32-10 Three-point gait. The left leg is the weaker leg and bears no weight.

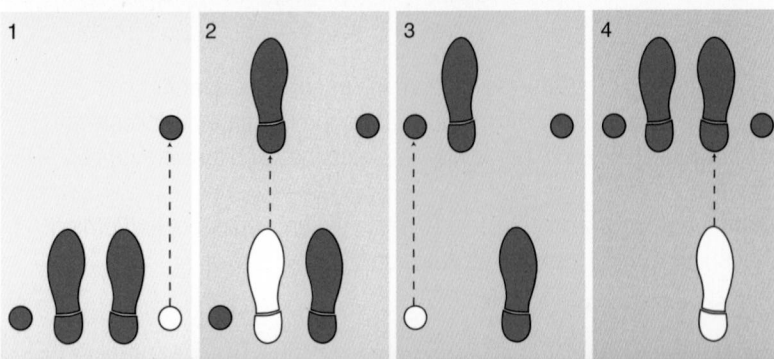

FIGURE 32-11 Four-point gait. The patient is bearing weight on both legs with consistent weight distribution with feet and both crutches.

Four-Point Alternating Gait. This is a slower gait that is used for patients who can bear weight on both legs and move each leg separately. The patient moves one crutch forward, then the opposite foot. The patient then moves the other crutch forward, then the opposite foot (Figure 32-11).

Swing-to Gait. Patients start with the crutches at their side. They move both crutches forward, transfer their weight forward, and swing both feet together up to the crutches.

Swing-through Gait. Patients start with the crutches at the side. They move both crutches forward. They then transfer the weight and swing both feet through the crutches, stopping slightly in front of the crutches.

Sitting. The patient backs into a straight chair with armrests until the seat of the chair touches the back of the legs. Crutches are held in the hand on the strong side and opposite the weak leg. With the other hand the patient can grasp the armrest of the chair and lower slowly into the chair.

Standing. The patient holds both crutches in the hand on the strong side, moves forward in the chair, grasps the armrest with the hand on the weaker side, then pushes up to a standing position.

Canes

A cane is used when the patient has one weak side and will need this assistive device for a longer period than crutches. It is also useful for patients who have a general but minor weakness on one side or those who have poor balance.

Canes come in three basic types. The first type of cane is called a *standard*, or single-tipped, cane. It has a curved handle for gripping, and the newer canes have a hand grip attached. The second type of cane is a four-legged, or *quad*, cane. It is a single cane that rests on a four-legged platform, provides stability and a wide base of support, and is for patients with more severe walking difficulties.

The third type of cane is a *hemi-walker*. It has four legs and a handle-bar for gripping and provides the best support of all canes. (See the "Assistive Devices" Quick Reference Guide for more information.)

Procedure 32-2 outlines the steps for teaching a patient how to walk safely with a cane.

Wheelchairs

Wheelchairs are mobile chairs that enable patients with severe ambulation conditions, or no ability to ambulate at all, to otherwise get around. Some must be moved manually, either by the patient or by someone else (Figure 32-12). Others are motorized and can be controlled completely by the patient (Figure 32-13).

With the many advancements in wheelchair design, patients with chronic conditions no longer are restricted to a home or hospital environment.

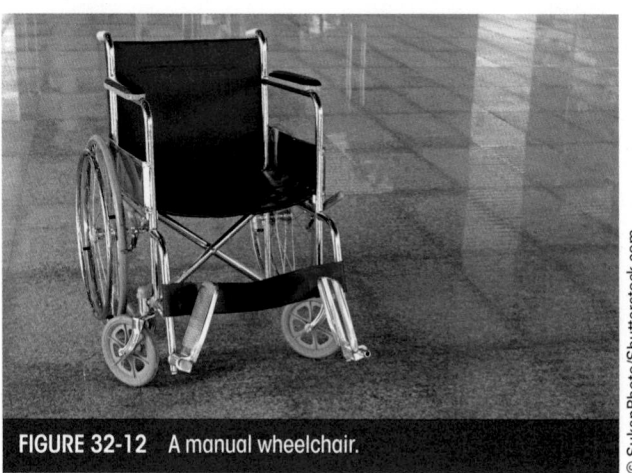

FIGURE 32-12 A manual wheelchair.

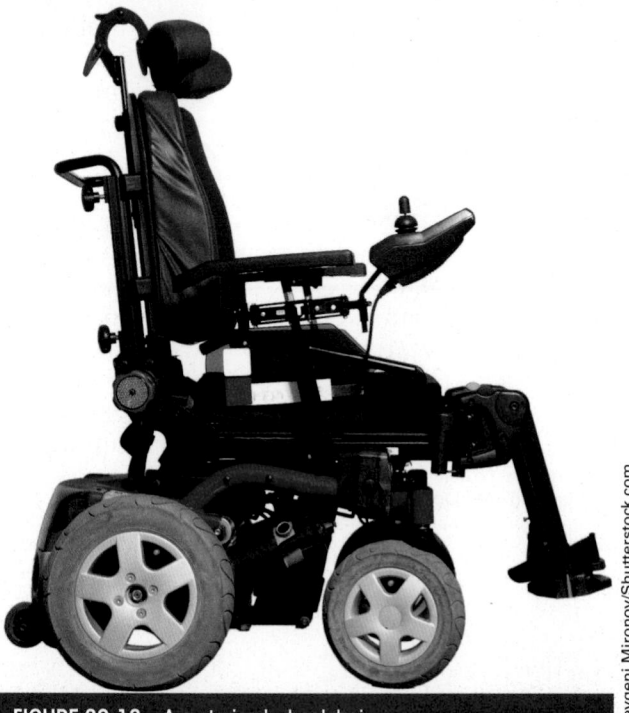

FIGURE 32-13 A motorized wheelchair.

Today, all public buildings and many private ones have handicapped access ramps as an alternative to stairs, remote-controlled doors, elevators that can accommodate a wheelchair, and other amenities that enable patients in wheelchairs to get around almost as well as if they were ambulating.

Many types of wheelchairs can be modified to suit a patient's particular disability and lifestyle. There are even wheelchairs that enable patients to participate in sports activities. Many car manufacturers can modify a van to accommodate a wheelchair, and some are equipped to allow patients with wheelchairs to drive.

Safety

Patients who will be using a wheelchair for a long time are taught how to maintain it. Depending on their abilities, they check it regularly to make sure all the parts are working correctly, and, if they are able, to make any necessary repairs. Patients are taught to use the wheelchair safely and how to maneuver into and out of difficult spaces.

If a patient is being pushed by someone else, that individual must learn basic safety rules for transporting a patient:

- Make sure that the brakes are locked when transferring a patient into and out of a wheelchair; if a patient must be left alone in the wheelchair for any length of time, lock the brakes (Figure 32-14).
- Make sure the patient's feet are placed on the footrests when the wheelchair is in use.
- Be certain the patient feels safe.
- Always back into and out of elevators.
- Stay to the right in corridors.
- Back down slanted ramps.

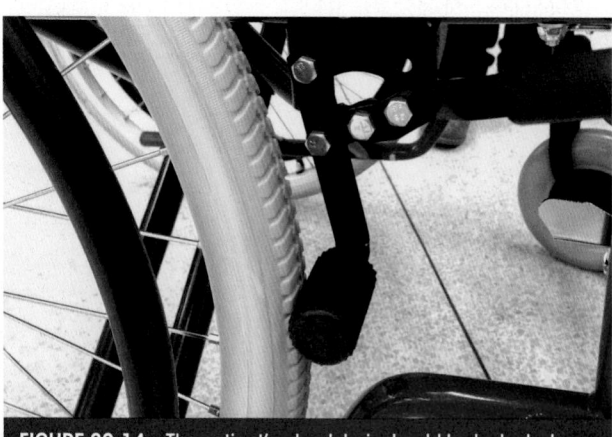

FIGURE 32-14 The patient's wheelchair should be locked when transferring a patient into and out of it, or when the patient is left alone in the wheelchair for any length of time.

THERAPEUTIC EXERCISES

Range of Motion

The musculoskeletal system is a complex joining of bones, joints, ligaments, and tendons. Not only does it give structure to the body and protect the body's vital organs but also it allows for movement so we can carry out a multitude of activities.

The bones of almost all the joints of the body are designed to move as well. Each joint has its own **range of motion (ROM)**, the amount of movement that is present in a joint.

Normal ROM varies among people and depends on several factors, such as age, sex, and whether the motion being performed is passive (assisted motion) or active (voluntary motion). There is a standard ROM for all movable joints, and it is this standard that is used when evaluating the joint movement of a particular patient.

The measurement of joint motion is called **goniometry**. Joint movement is measured with an instrument called a **goniometer** and is always expressed in degrees. For example, the average person lying flat with arms to the sides can move the elbows from a 20-degree hyperextension (extending the arm beyond its normal limits) to 0-degree extension, through to 150 degrees of flexion, or bending (Figure 32-15).

ROM evaluation is one of several tools used when developing a therapeutic program for a patient.

As a medical assistant, you need to be familiar with ROM exercises (Figure 32-16). ROM exercises are designed to maintain joint mobility and are performed either passively (someone else does the movement) or actively (the patient does the movement).

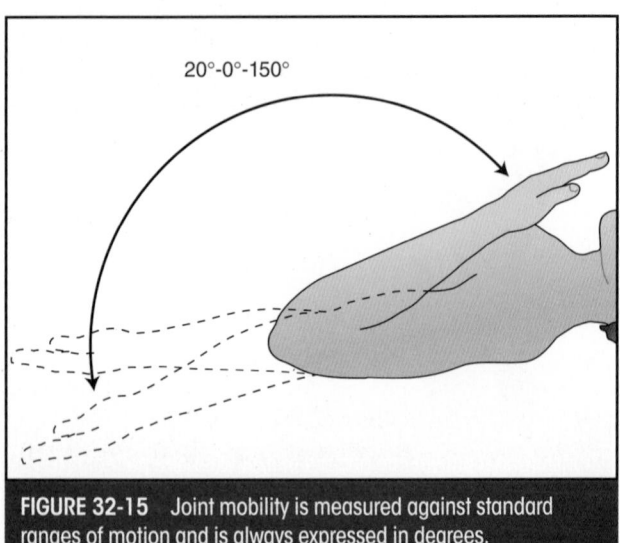

FIGURE 32-15 Joint mobility is measured against standard ranges of motion and is always expressed in degrees.

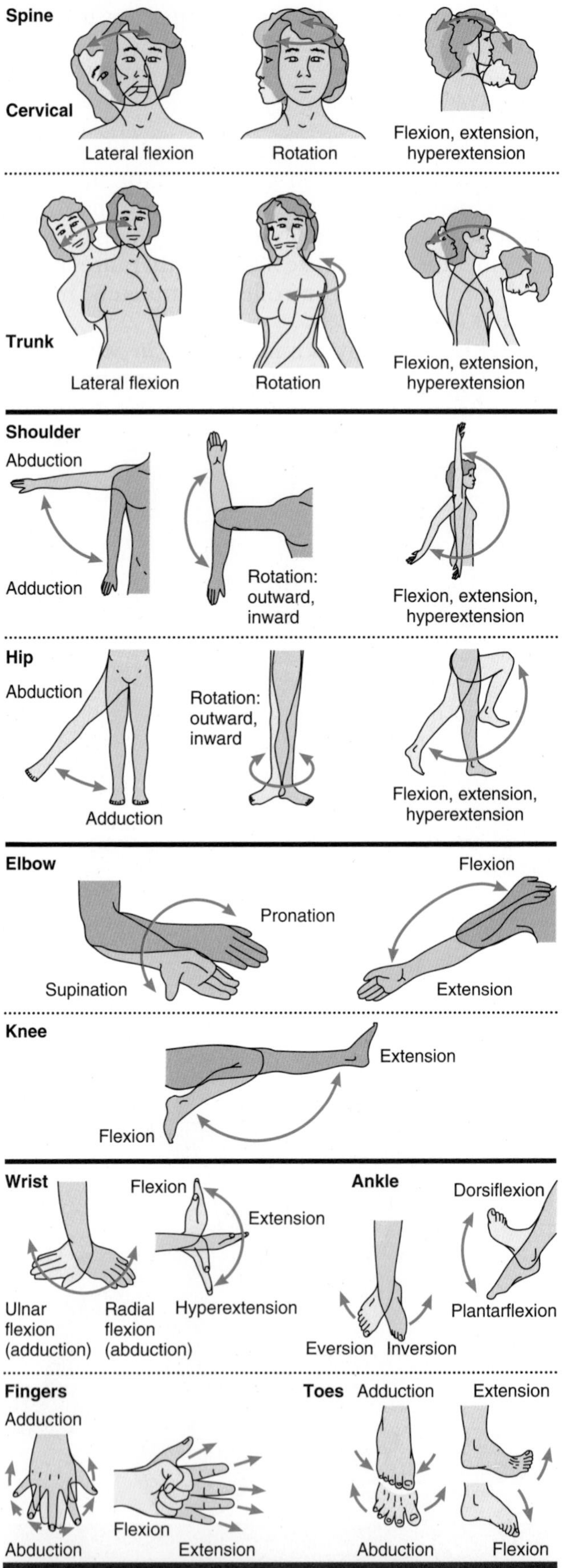

FIGURE 32-16 Range of motion (ROM) exercises for specific joints.

The importance of maintaining ROM is the prevention of contractures. **Contractures** occur when the body is in a nonmoving state. The usually flexible connective tissues become stiffened and are replaced with fiber-like tissues. This restricts movement and the immobility can become permanent. To avoid this complication of immobility, joints must be passively or actively in motion.

Joint movement has a special vocabulary, and it is helpful to learn the terms and their definitions (Table 32-1).

Before performing ROM exercises on a patient, the caregiver will need to observe general precautions:

- Always move the patient's limbs gently, within pain tolerance and within the flexibility of the limb.
- Use slow, careful movements that allow the muscles time to adjust to the movement.
- Always support the limb above and below the joint.
- It is best to perform passive ROM with the patient in the relaxed, supine position.
- ROM should never cause pain. If the patient reports pain at any time, the ROM exercises should be discontinued until the provider or other health care professional can determine the source of pain.
- Repeat each movement several times or as prescribed by the provider.
- Provide for patient privacy and drape if necessary for warmth and comfort.

Muscle Testing

The other tool used for evaluating the movement abilities of a patient is muscle testing. Whereas goniometry focuses on joint movement, muscle testing evaluates the motion, strength, and task potential of a given muscle. *ROM* testing for muscles determines how flexible and resilient a muscle may be. *Strength testing* shows how hard a muscle can work. As a medical assistant, you may assist with testing the patient for joint mobility, posture, and strength of muscles.

Types of Therapeutic Exercise

Without constant exercise, the musculoskeletal system would deteriorate. Joints would become stiff and contractures, or deformities, could develop. Muscles would atrophy, or shrink and lose strength. Bones would lose vital minerals such as calcium and phosphorus. The body's overall circulation would decrease, which in turn would create a separate set of unhealthy conditions. Like drugs, exercise has a powerful and systemic effect on the body. It involves the function of joints, bones, muscles, nerves, tendons, and ligaments, as well as the circulatory and respiratory systems. Therapeutic exercises are prescribed after careful evaluation by a trained specialist and are tailored to each patient depending on that patient's individual condition and rehabilitation goals. It is the role of the medical assistant to understand the goals and objectives of the therapeutic exercise program to better support and encourage patients to complete their program.

Whereas an athlete uses exercise to build strength and endurance to attain a certain level of performance, therapeutic exercises are prescribed for a variety of therapeutic and preventive effects. They are used most commonly to correct or prevent deformities, regain body movement after an accident or disease, restore joint motion after immobility, improve neuromuscular coordination, and improve or develop ADL.

Exercise is also used for another important reason: It can prevent many common problems brought on by inactivity, such as those associated with respiration and circulation.

TABLE 32-1

TERMINOLOGY OF JOINT MOVEMENT

Abduction	Motion away from the midline of the body
Adduction	Motion toward the midline of the body
Circumduction	Circular motion of a body part
Dorsiflexion	Moving the foot upward at the ankle joint
Eversion	Moving a body part outward
Extension	Straightening of a body part
Flexion	Bending of a body part
Hyperextension	A position of maximum extension, or extending a body part beyond its normal limits
Inversion	Moving a body part inward
Plantar flexion	Moving the foot downward at the ankle
Pronation	Moving the arm so the palm is down
Rotation	Turning a body part around its axis
Supination	Moving the arm so the palm is up

A variety of exercise programs are used for therapeutic or preventive purposes:

1. *Active exercises*, which are self-directed and performed by the patient without assistance
2. *Passive exercises*, which are performed by another person with no voluntary participation from the patient
3. *Assisted exercises*, which help the patient voluntarily move weakened muscles with the use of an assistive device, such as a therapy pool
4. *Active resistance exercises*, which provide voluntary movement against various types of manual or mechanical pressure to increase muscle strength

Electromyography

Electrical activity of muscles can be recorded on a graph or film to help determine how well muscles contract. **Electromyography (EMG)** is the instrument used to test the electrical activity of a muscle. An electrode (using a small-gauge needle) is inserted through skin into the muscle, and measurements of muscle strength are made.

Electrostimulation of Muscle

An electric current of low voltage can help stimulate muscles to exercise by stimulating the sensory and motor nerves for that muscle. It is helpful for a patient who has nerve damage to the muscle and cannot voluntarily move the muscle. The purpose is to prevent atrophy of the muscle and help restore muscle function.

The low current of electricity passing through the patient's muscle acts similarly to the patient's own nerves, causing the muscle to contract and relax. The stimulation is helpful to retrain a patient after experiencing an injury to a muscle or muscle group. Disposable gel electrodes are applied, and low-voltage current stimulates the muscles to prevent atrophy.

A method of using electric current to stimulate nerves is known as *transcutaneous electric nerve stimulation* (TENS). It is used for patients who have severe pain, for example, chronic lower back pain from an injury. In this method, electrodes are attached to the patient's skin over a painful area. This causes interference with the transmission of painful stimuli, thus reducing the patient's pain sensation. Many patients with chronic severe pain need narcotics to ease the pain. However, TENS can control the pain and lessen the need for addictive drugs. TENS can be used by patients at home.

THERAPEUTIC MODALITIES

Sometimes, therapeutic exercise is not the best or only way to restore injured or painful joints and tissues. A patient's condition may respond equally well to certain physical agents, called **modalities**, which take advantage of the properties of heat, cold, electricity, light, and water to improve circulation, minimize pain, and correct or alleviate muscular and joint malfunction.

Many modalities have been around for centuries, and some can easily be performed by the patient or caregiver at home. Modalities can be used locally to treat one small area at a time or systemically to alter a patient's temperature or soothe many groups of painful muscles or joints. The patient's condition and rehabilitation program both influence the modality or combination of modalities used.

A provider order is required for any therapeutic modality.

Heat and Cold

Heat, or **thermotherapy**, acts on the body by causing vasodilation (dilation of the blood vessels). The effect of heat increases circulation to an area and acts to speed up the repair process. Heat can be used to:

- Relax muscle spasms
- Relieve pain in a strained muscle or sprained joint
- Relieve localized congestion and swelling
- Increase drainage from an infected area
- Increase tissue metabolism and repair
- Combat local infection
- Increase circulation
- Improve mobility before exercise

However, because heat dilates the blood vessels and increases circulation, it also acts to speed up the inflammatory process, which can lead to more serious problems, such as increased bleeding and swelling. Heat should not be used longer than its prescribed length of time.

Cold applications, or **cryotherapy**, are used to constrict blood vessels and slow or stop the flow of blood to an area. This process, also called **vasoconstriction**, slows down the inflammatory process, which can reduce or prevent swelling of inflamed tissues, reduce bleeding, numb the pain sensation by acting as a topical anesthetic, and reduce drainage to an area.

By understanding how heat and cold affect the body, it is easier to observe whether they are having the desired therapeutic effect. Because heat and cold modalities can be extremely effective, they are widely used for treating certain physical conditions. However, the effects of heat and cold modalities depend on several conditions: the type of modality used, the length of time it is applied, the patient's condition, and the area or areas being treated.

Safety

Precautions for Heat and Cold Applications. When applying either heat or cold modalities, you need to take certain precautions to avoid injury. If misused, any therapeutic modality can actually cause more damage to the site it is trying to heal. Before starting any treatment, keep the following precautions in mind:

- Infants and patients who cannot report a burning sensation should be watched carefully. Infants and older adults are particularly susceptible to burns.

- Heat and cold sensitivity varies with patients; check patients frequently and never leave them alone.

- Never have a patient lie on a heating pad because severe burning can result. Place a rubber cover over the heating pad if using with moist dressings.

- Always wrap appliances, whether warm or cold, with cloth before applying them to the skin.

- Only soak or immerse patients in water between 104 and 113°F (40 to 45°C). Temperatures of 116°F (47°C) or greater can cause tissue damage.

- Never use heat within the first 48 hours of an acute inflammatory process and never apply heat to newly burned skin.

- Watch carefully persons with impaired circulation; cardiovascular, renal, sensorineural, or respiratory conditions; or osteoporosis. Tell the patient to report pain or numbness.

- Excessive cold can damage tissues.

- Lack of sensation to a therapy may indicate impaired circulation to an area, and the patient may be unable to report a burning sensation.

- Heat concentrates in metal materials, so have patients remove all jewelry and other metal objects, and administer the treatment on nonmetal tables and chairs.

- Document in the patient's chart or electronic medical record the type of modality, length of time applied, color of patient's skin, and any discomfort.

Moist and Dry Heat

Moist Heat Therapies. Moist heat refers to heat modalities that feel moist against the skin. Moist heat penetrates better than dry heat and aids in improving circulation, relaxation, and mobility.

Warm Soaks. Warm soaks are generally used for soaking the extremities and can be administered easily at home by the patient or caregiver. The patient's body part is gradually immersed in plain or medicated water no hotter than 110°F (44°C) for a short time, usually no more than about 15 minutes. The patient should be positioned to be comfortable. Observe the patient's skin for excessive redness and, if noticed, remove the limb at once. Always dry the skin carefully by patting, not rubbing, it.

Total body immersion in water 104 to 113°F can be achieved in a whirlpool bath or special Hubbard tank. This treatment is often prescribed to promote relaxation, circulation, and movement of limbs in preparation for exercise. The mechanical action of agitating water moving over the body in a whirlpool is called hydromassage and can both relax muscles and stimulate circulation. The Hubbard tank is a bit larger and provides room for limited body exercise without the effects of gravity.

Sitz Bath. A sitz bath is a bath of warm water in which only the hips and buttocks (perineum) are immersed for relief of pain and discomfort from conditions such as rectal surgery and episiotomy. It is therapeutic and cleansing and will help relieve discomfort by reducing swelling and will improve healing by stimulating blood flow.

Warm Wet Compresses and Packs. A warm wet compress is usually applied to a small area. It is prepared by soaking and wringing out either a square of gauze or other absorbent material (such as a clean washcloth) and applying it for a limited time to the affected area. Warm compresses can be administered easily at home. A warm pack is used

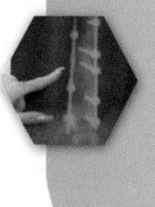

Critical Thinking

Dr. Cox orders 10 minutes of warm moist heat and a TENS unit application for 20 minutes to her patient Ray Maynard's lumbar area. How would these treatments ease Mr. Maynard's low back pain?

for a larger area and generally involves the use of a professional warm pack (**hydrocollator**) administered in the clinical setting. This type of warm pack is soaked in water 150 to 170°F, removed with tongs and drained, and placed over larger areas such as the back or shoulders. Check the color of the patient's skin frequently.

Paraffin Wax Bath. This type of treatment is most often used for chronic joint disease, such as rheumatoid arthritis. The bath mixture of seven parts paraffin to one part mineral oil is heated to melting (about 127°F) and the body part is dipped in the mixture several times until a thick coat of wax builds up. The body part is then wrapped in foil, cloth, or plastic wrap to help insulate the heat, then left on for 30 minutes or less. Once peeled off, the circulatory effects of this treatment can last up to several hours. It is an excellent modality for warming up joints before ROM or other exercises. This modality, ordered by the provider, will be carried out in the physical therapy department by a professional therapist (Figure 32-17).

Dry Heat Therapies. Dry heat applications feel dry against the skin and do not penetrate like moist heat. They are used more to improve circulation for the purposes of relieving swelling and healing wounds, as well as to relax muscles and reduce muscle spasms. Most dry heat modalities can be performed easily by the patient or caregiver at home.

Safety

Heating Pads and Packs. Heating pads and commercially prepared packs are used for smaller areas and should always be covered with a cloth before applying against the skin. Never let a patient lie directly on a heating pad because burns can result. Set the switch on the heating pad to a low or medium setting and observe the proper time of exposure.

An Aquamatic K-Pad is a commercial pad that is safer to use than a heating pad or commercially prepared pack because you can maintain a constant temperature and regulate that temperature more carefully. It is a pad with tubes that are filled with distilled water and heated by a control unit. The pad must be covered and left on the patient for no more than about 30 minutes. The temperature usually is set between 95 and 100°F.

Moist and Dry Cold

Moist Cold Therapies. Moist cold therapies are cold modalities that feel moist against the skin. Moist cold, as with moist heat, penetrates better than dry cold and is used to prevent swelling or edema, relieve pain or tenderness, and reduce body temperature. Most cold therapies can be performed easily at home by the patient or caregiver.

Cold Compresses and Packs. Cold compresses are used for smaller areas, and cold packs are used for larger areas. For a cold compress, immerse the cold cloth, gauze, or other clean material in a basin filled with ice and cold water or the prescribed solution. Wring out the cloth and apply it to the affected area. Keep the cloth cold by immersing it several times throughout the treatment or use a syringe to add cold water to the compress. Cold or ice packs are administered in the same manner. Check the patient's skin frequently.

Dry Cold Therapies. Dry cold treatments are used for the same reasons as moist cold treatments but

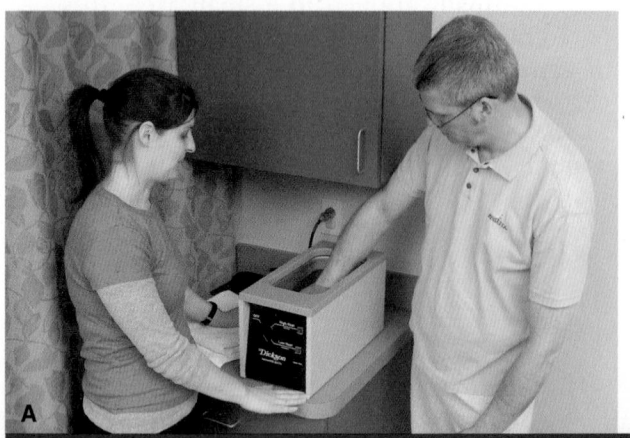
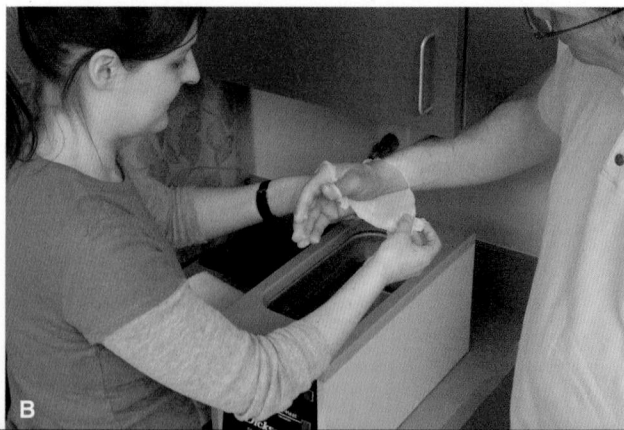

FIGURE 32-17 (A) A body part is dipped into the paraffin bath three or four times to create a layer of warm wax on the skin. (B) After the wax has been in place for 20 to 30 minutes, it is peeled off and discarded.

are better for bleeding and acute injuries. Dry cold is also an excellent therapy for sprains, strains, burns, or bruises.

The temperature used depends on the area being treated and the method used, as well as the patient's tolerance for cold temperatures. In general, the colder the temperature, the shorter the duration of exposure.

Ice Packs. Dry cold treatments include ice packs and commercially prepared chemical ice packs or cold packs. Always cover the pack with cloth before applying it to the skin. Generally, ice packs can be kept on the body longer than heat packs, about 30 minutes. Check color of patient's skin frequently (see Chapter 8). A commercial ice pack can be used for smaller areas and can usually be chilled in the freezer. Because they do not freeze and become solid, these ice packs are pliable, making them ideal for contouring to the body part being treated. The cold packs are usually single use. They must be activated by a blow to the pack before applying or by squeezing the pack.

Ultrasound

Ultrasound is a high-frequency acoustic vibration that is part of the electromagnetic spectrum, and its frequencies are beyond the perception of the human ear. This type of treatment uses high-frequency sound waves that are converted to heat in the deeper tissues. This type of heat therapy is referred to as **diathermy**.

Ultrasound is an effective form of treatment for chronic pain or acute injuries such as sprains or strains. It relaxes muscle spasms; increases the elasticity of tissue such as tendons and ligaments; and stimulates circulation, which, in turn, speeds up the healing process.

Safety

Ultrasound waves travel best in tissue that has a high concentration of water, such as muscles. They cannot penetrate and move through tissue such as bone that has a low water content. In fact, ultrasound treatment must be used carefully near bones, particularly those near the surface, because their waves are capable of concentrating in one area and causing damage.

Integrity

Because ultrasound waves cannot be conducted through air, a special gel is applied to the skin surface to act as a conduit. The sound waves are generated through an applicator that is rubbed over the gel. This applicator must be kept moving to prevent any internal damage caused by too high a concentration of sound waves. The duration of treatment lasts anywhere from 5 to 15 minutes, depending on the condition being treated and the recommendation of the physician or other health care provider. It is important to note that, because of its potential dangers, ultrasound treatment should only be administered if the medical assistant or other caregiver is specially trained in its safe and effective use.

Massage Therapy

Massage therapy has become recognized as a modality that is basic to physical therapy. The majority of states require a massage therapist to be licensed in order to practice the profession.

History shows massage therapy was one of the earliest practices for helping the body restore healthy functioning. It is used to relieve minor aches and pains, thus helping patients feel relaxed and refreshed. Massage therapy is safe and advantageous for most individuals, from infants to older adults.

Some physiologic benefits include increased metabolism, promotion of healing, soothing

Critical Thinking
How do heat and cold affect the body's physiology and for what conditions should each be used?

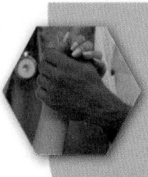
Patient Education
Neither heat nor cold applications should be left on the skin for prolonged periods, because both can have counterproductive effects if not monitored carefully. When applying heat or cold, periodically check the skin for signs of paleness or redness. If the patient experiences any numbness or tingling reaction, discontinue the application. Report the observations, and document.

of muscles, relief of discomfort and pain, and improvement of circulation. Massage therapy can be used to manage the pain associated with conditions such as whiplash injury, muscle spasm, sciatic nerve pain, arthritis, and many other health problems.

Therapists use their hands to handle or touch the soft tissues of the patients' body. The movements stimulate the patients' circulation, help relieve discomfort, improve range of motion, and relax muscles. Some of the movements include percussion (tapping), rubbing, pressing, **petrissage** (kneading), and **effleurage** (stroking) of the soft tissue (Figure 32-18).

Massage therapy is inappropriate for patients with open wounds, neuropathies, shock, severe

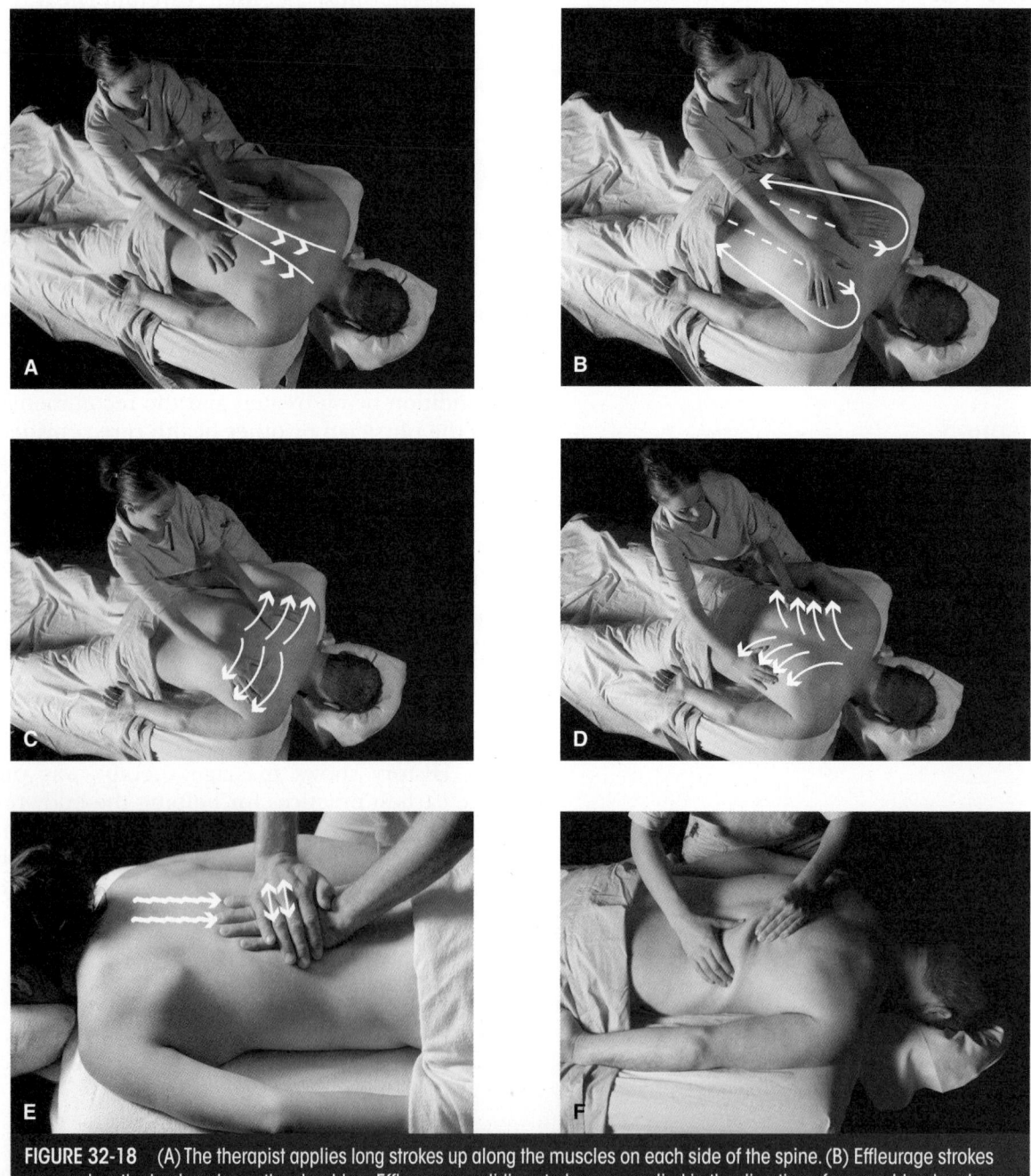

FIGURE 32-18   (A) The therapist applies long strokes up along the muscles on each side of the spine. (B) Effleurage strokes are used up the back and over the shoulders. Effleurage or gliding strokes are applied in the direction of venous blood and lymph flow. (C) The muscles of the back are stroked outward. (D) Fan stroking is applied to the back. (E) Vibration movements are applied to the vertebrae, and vibrations go back and forth as the therapist moves down along the spine. (F) Petrissage is applied to the entire side opposite the therapist.

upper respiratory illnesses, varicose veins, phlebitis, and high blood pressure. It is often inappropriate for patients with osteoporosis (bones can easily break).

There are psychological benefits as well. Massage therapy relieves stress and tension; refreshes the patient, thereby lessening fatigue; and regenerates energy.

Massage therapy has been accepted and recognized by the medical community and the community-at-large as a complementary or alternative form of medicine.

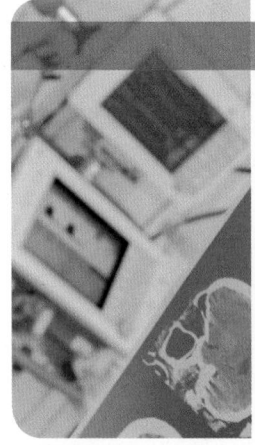

CASE STUDY 32-1

Refer to the scenario at the beginning of the chapter.

Mrs. Williams comes to Inner City Urgent Care because she fell when she tripped on a scatter rug at home. Her son helped her to the clinic. Her left ankle is swollen and painful.

CASE STUDY REVIEW

1. What action(s) should you take immediately to help Mrs. Williams?
2. After X-rays, Dr. Woo determined that Mrs. Williams has an ankle fracture, and he applied a cast to it. He wants you to fit Mrs. Williams to crutches and teach her how to use them. What gait will Dr. Woo have you teach the patient? Why?
3. In what way would you include Mrs. Williams's support system in education activities?

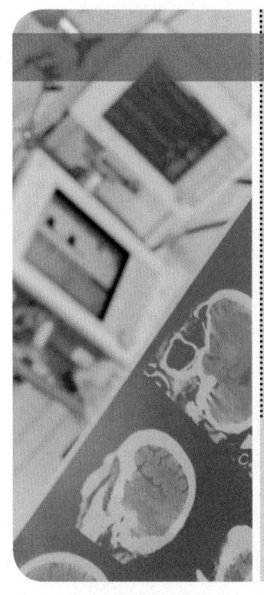

CASE STUDY 32-2

It is a mild summer afternoon in River City, where Inner City Urgent Care is located. The softball season is in full swing, and Inner City has treated its share of players and spectators who have had minor injuries. On this particular Tuesday, Bill Schwarz, a regular patient, comes in late in the day in obvious pain. Sam Tyler, CMA (AAMA), MLT, the clinical medical assistant on duty, quickly gets the patient into a wheelchair. From the patient's description of the situation and the pain, Sam suspects a sprained ankle. Dr. Woo is on call and is available to examine the patient immediately. Dr. Woo asks Sam to transfer Bill from the wheelchair to the examination table.

CASE STUDY REVIEW

1. What are some of the general principles the medical assistant should observe during any transfer?
2. Summarize the steps involved in transferring the patient from the wheelchair to the examination table.
3. What are possible treatment choices Dr. Woo may use?

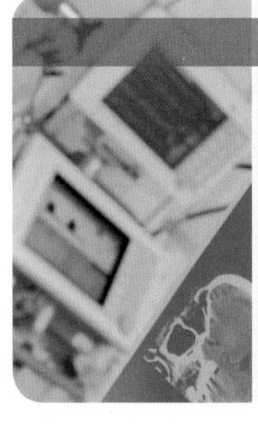

CASE STUDY 32-3

After diagnosing Mr. Schwarz with a sprained left ankle, Dr. Woo prescribed an Ace bandage to the ankle, crutches, and an ice pack to be applied to the ankle. He also gave Mr. Schwarz a prescription for pain relievers and has recommended that Mr. Schwarz stay off his feet as much as possible. He is to keep the leg elevated with an ice pack on it.

CASE STUDY REVIEW

1. Explain what you would tell Mr. Schwarz about applying the ice pack to his ankle at home.
2. What patient education can be used in this situation?
3. In what way could you demonstrate empathy to Mr. Schwarz?

- Rehabilitation medicine is a field of medical disciplines that specializes in both preventing disease or injury and restoring physical function. It uses a combination of physical and mechanical agents to aid in the diagnosis, treatment, and prevention of diseases or bodily injury, including exercise and a variety of treatment modalities.

- Much of what a medical assistant might do on the job in this field involves some form of lifting or moving of heavy objects.

- It is important to remember to use good body mechanics to prevent back or other injury. When transferring patients, good body mechanics ensures the safety of both caregiver and patient. If necessary, get someone to help with the transfer.

- Transferring patients from a wheelchair to the exam table is a common occurrence in some practices. There is risk of injury to the patient and the medical assistant if safe practices are not followed.

- Helping patients to ambulate safely after a period of sedentary recuperation is an important part of a rehabilitation program.

- Education is necessary for patients that require assistive devices to aid their mobility.

- Knowledge of the use of canes, crutches, walkers, and wheelchairs is essential for the medical assistant.

- Adjustments and fitting of assistive devices may be a part of a medical assistant's responsibilities.

- There are a number of types of therapeutic exercises.

- Joints and muscles must be exercised regularly to prevent muscle atrophy and joint contractures, as well as to improve circulation and maintain or improve overall health. A variety of therapeutic modalities might be used as part of the patient's rehabilitation program. These include using heat, cold, light, electricity, and water to act on the body to improve circulation, minimize pain, or correct or alleviate joint and muscle malfunction.

- Ultrasound and other electrical diathermies use an electrical current to create heat in the deeper tissues of the body.

Study for Success

To reinforce your knowledge and skills of information presented in this chapter:

- Review the *Key Terms* and *Learning Outcomes*

- Consider the *Critical Thinking* features and *Case Studies* and discuss your conclusions

- Answer the questions in the *Certification Review*

Procedure

- Perform the *Procedures* using the *Competency Assessment Checklists* on the *Student Companion Website*

CERTIFICATION REVIEW

1. What is the term that refers to brushing teeth, getting dressed, and eating?
   a. Rehabilitation medicine
   b. Activities of daily living
   c. Assistive behaviors
   d. Occupational therapy

2. What is the definition of hemiplegia?
   a. Inability of the patient to ambulate properly
   b. Severe back pain
   c. Paralysis of one side of the body
   d. Confinement to a wheelchair
   e. Paraplegia

3. Which of the following are considered ambulatory assistive devices?
   a. Gait belts
   b. Walkers, canes, and crutches
   c. Wheelchairs
   d. Stools with handholds
4. What is the medical term for movement away from the midline of the body?
   a. Adduction
   b. Pronation
   c. Extension
   d. Abduction
   e. Supination
5. What does supination involve?
   a. Placing the patient in the supine position
   b. Moving the arm so that the palm is up
   c. Bending a body part
   d. Straightening a body part
6. The use of a gait belt serves which function(s)?
   a. Assists in fall prevention
   b. Protects staff from accidental back injury
   c. Assists the patient with uncontrolled pain
   d. Teaches patients the proper gait
   e. Both a and b
7. What is the purpose of electrostimulation of a muscle?
   a. Stimulating the sensory and motor nerves in a muscle
   b. Preventing atrophy
   c. Restoring muscle function
   d. All of these

8. Massage therapy is sometimes utilized in combination with physical therapy. Which of the following is the purpose of this combination?
   a. Increased circulation
   b. Healing of bones
   c. Gait training
   d. Increased edema
   e. All of these
9. Which is the appropriate device to provide maximum assistance for a person with mobility problems?
   a. Cane
   b. Crutches
   c. Standard walker
   d. Splint
10. Which of the following is *not* an effect of ultrasound as a therapeutic modality?
    a. Provides heat to deeper tissues
    b. Decreases circulation
    c. Assists with management of chronic pain
    d. Decreases muscle spasms
    e. Treats acute injuries

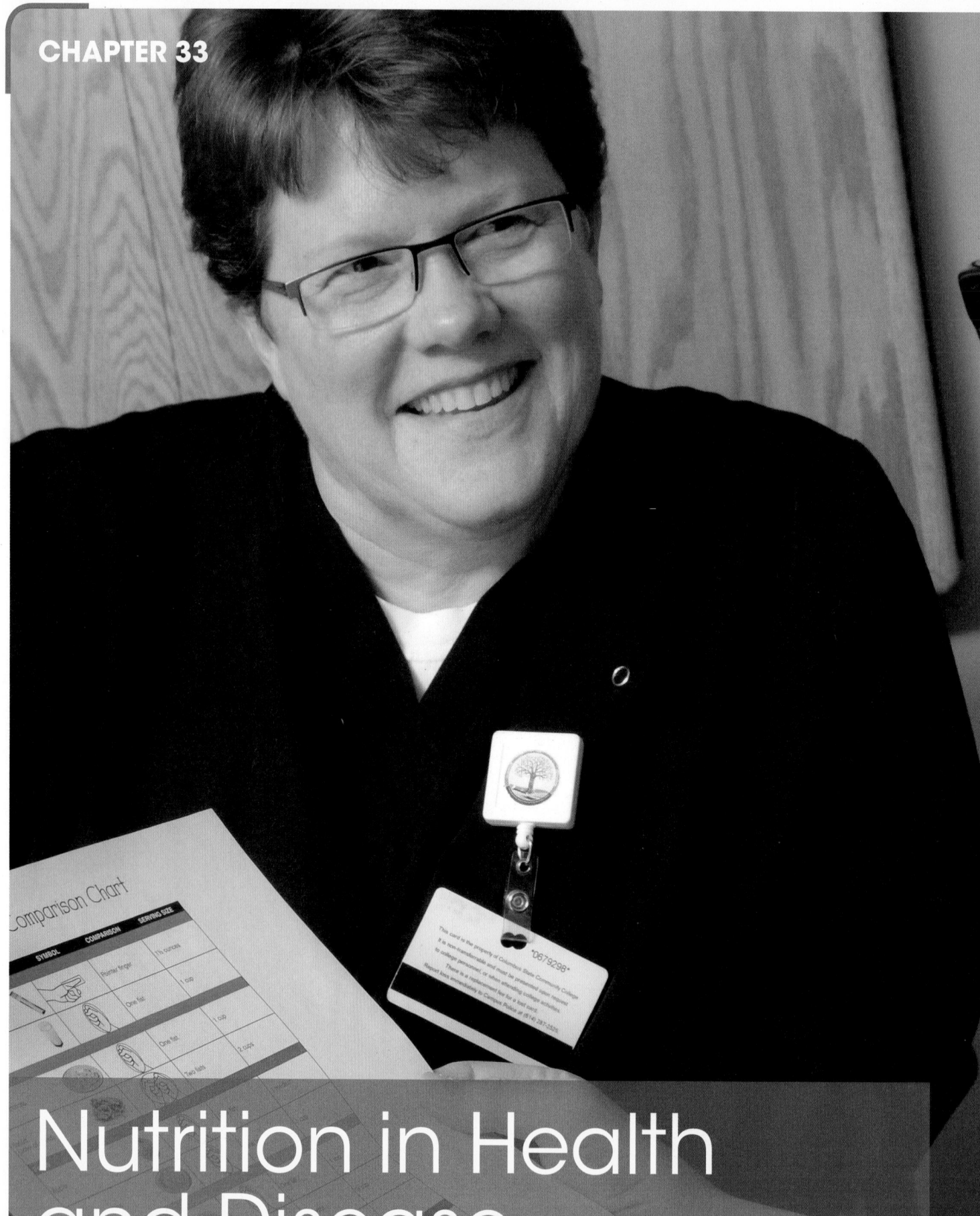

CHAPTER 33

Nutrition in Health and Disease

1. Define and spell the key terms as presented in the glossary.
2. Describe the relationship between nutrition and the functioning of the digestive system.
3. Identify the seven basic nutrient types.
4. Explain the relationship and balance among the three energy nutrients.
5. Distinguish between water-soluble and fat-soluble vitamins.
6. Discuss herbal supplements.
7. Explain the reason for nutrition labels on food packaging.
8. Read and interpret nutrition facts and ingredients on three food packages.
9. Discuss various therapeutic diets, and explain how each can help to control a particular disease state or accommodate a life cycle change.

KEY TERMS

amino acid	folic acid	nutrients
antioxidant	gingivitis	nutrition
ascorbic acid	glossitis	oxidation
basal metabolic rate (BMR)	glycogen	pellagra
beriberi	hemolysis	pernicious anemia
bulimia	homeostasis	photophobia
cachectic	hydrogenated	preservatives
calories	hypercalcemia	processed foods
carotene	hyperkalemia	pyridoxine
catalyst	hypermagnesemia	riboflavin
cellulose	hypernatremia	saturated fats
cheilosis	hyperphosphatemia	scurvy
cholecalciferol	hypocalcemia	thiamin
cobalamin	hypokalemia	tinnitus
coenzyme	hypomagnesemia	tocopherol
digestion	hyponatremia	trace minerals
diuretics	hypophosphatemia	vasoconstriction
electrochemical gradient	major minerals	vasodilation
electrolytes	megaloblastic anemia	water-soluble vitamin
extracellular	metabolism	Wernicke-Korsakoff syndrome
fat-soluble vitamin	niacin	xerophthalmia

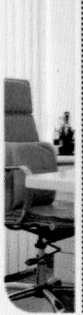

Becky Slack, RMA (AMT), works with Dr. Hannah, a pediatrician in a small town, rural setting. She initiated a discussion with Dr. Hannah about the recent increase in childhood obesity. The percentage of children ages 6 to 11 years in the United States who are obese increased from 7% in 1980 to current estimates at over 18%. The percentage of adolescents ages 12 to 19 years who were obese increased from 5% in 1980 to nearly 21% by 2012. Realizing the impact on their patient population, Ms. Slack wanted to know what solutions the practice might offer to these patients and their families. Dr. Hannah has agreed to collaborate with Ms. Slack to begin a nutritional education class that will be held at the clinic once a week. This class will include children and their parents who are concerned about weight. As treatment for obesity includes changes in diet and increased physical activity, this will be the focus of the education.

The human body is in a constant state of fluctuation. The outside environment is constantly changing, and the body requires **homeostasis**, or a stable internal environment, which, in turn, gives us a requirement for nutrients. Humans use nutrients for energy, repair, regulation, and essential biochemical processes essential to life. Some nutrients are manufactured by the body, but most are taken in via the digestive tract. Active regulation establishes a constant internal environment. **Nutrition** is the study of the interaction of the seven types of nutrients found in food and their relation to the function and sustainability of the body. The normal healthy individual will consume and use most of the building blocks that the body needs to stay healthy. However, some individuals either do not consume enough nutrients or consume too much of a particular type of nutrient. These are poor diets that can cause particular disease states, and these diets must be modified to return the patients to good health. In addition, specific disease states, such as diabetes mellitus, warrant a change from a normal diet to control the progression of the disease. The human body also goes through changes at different developmental stages in life. These changes come with new nutritional needs. Protecting health requires paying attention to strategies to prevent disease. The choices made regarding foods consumed and the quality of nutritional intake have a significant impact on quality of life and longevity. Healthy food choices contribute to living longer and preventing major health issues.

This chapter explores the balance of nutrients required for good health and examines therapeutic modifications to the diet that should take place at various life stages or in the presence of disease. The astute medical assistant will recognize the role of nutrition in maintaining health and will use a knowledge of nutritional principles to encourage patients to adopt a healthy lifestyle.

NUTRITION AND DIGESTION

Nutrition includes ingestion, digestion, absorption, and metabolism of food. Good nutrition results in longer life spans and healthier individuals through the control of preventable diseases. The food eaten by an individual is used to build and repair cells and tissues of the body. Therefore, it is important to have knowledge and information about nutrition and to make appropriate food choices for optimum health. A well-nourished individual is less susceptible to infection and disease.

Communication Competency

Patient education is important especially when the normal diet must be modified to treat the patient's illness. The medical assistant can answer patient questions only through a knowledge of both good nutrition and what constitutes the therapeutic diets prescribed by the provider.

Digestion involves the physical and chemical changes to food that the body makes to render it absorbable. Absorption is the transfer of the nutrients from the gastrointestinal tract into the

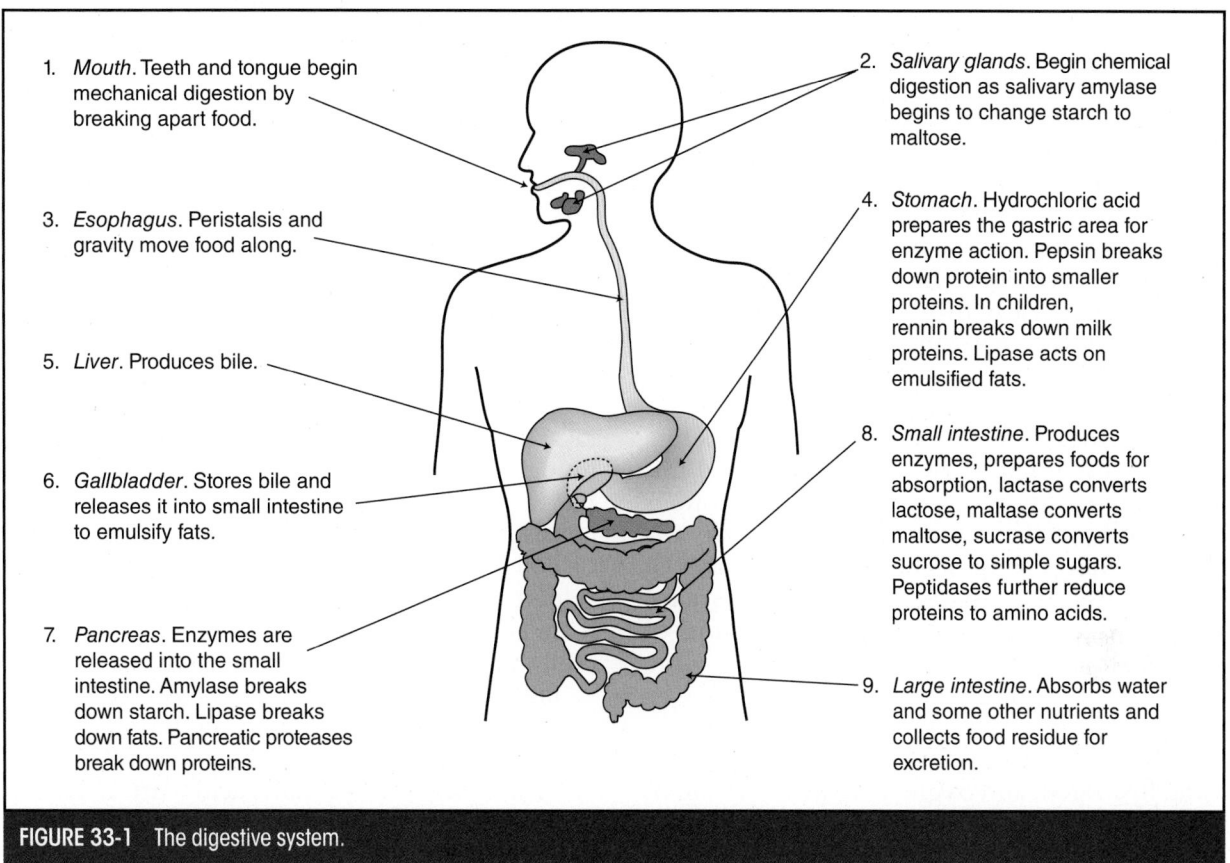

1. *Mouth*. Teeth and tongue begin mechanical digestion by breaking apart food.

2. *Salivary glands*. Begin chemical digestion as salivary amylase begins to change starch to maltose.

3. *Esophagus*. Peristalsis and gravity move food along.

4. *Stomach*. Hydrochloric acid prepares the gastric area for enzyme action. Pepsin breaks down protein into smaller proteins. In children, rennin breaks down milk proteins. Lipase acts on emulsified fats.

5. *Liver*. Produces bile.

6. *Gallbladder*. Stores bile and releases it into small intestine to emulsify fats.

7. *Pancreas*. Enzymes are released into the small intestine. Amylase breaks down starch. Lipase breaks down fats. Pancreatic proteases break down proteins.

8. *Small intestine*. Produces enzymes, prepares foods for absorption, lactase converts lactose, maltase converts maltose, sucrase converts sucrose to simple sugars. Peptidases further reduce proteins to amino acids.

9. *Large intestine*. Absorbs water and some other nutrients and collects food residue for excretion.

FIGURE 33-1 The digestive system.

bloodstream. Without absorption, the body would not receive the nutrients. Metabolism is the use of the nutrients that have been absorbed to maintain the living state of the cells and the entire body. Figure 33-1 shows the digestive system and its basic functions.

TYPES OF NUTRIENTS

Nutrients serve many purposes in the body. Some nutrients provide energy for the body to perform activities such as the pumping of the heart, the division of cells, or the contraction of muscles. Various nutrients also provide building blocks so that proteins or phospholipids can be made within the body, or they can act as catalysts to help processes such as the clotting mechanism proceed at a faster rate. Essentially, ingested substances that help the body stay in its homeostatic state can be called **nutrients**.

Nutrients can be divided into two groups: those that provide energy and those that do not. Both groups are necessary for good health. Those that provide energy are composed of three types: carbohydrates, fats (lipids), and proteins. Each of these three substances is used in ways other than

making energy, but it is important to remember that these are the only substances from which the body can derive energy. Nutrients that do not provide energy are also important and perform other vital functions as described previously. These nutrients include vitamins, minerals, water, and fiber.

Energy Nutrients (Organic)

The three energy nutrients—carbohydrates, fats, and proteins—have one thing in common: All can be converted into energy.

Carbohydrates. Carbohydrates provide the major source of energy and are made up of carbon, hydrogen, and oxygen. Although many compounds are made up of these three elements, it is the ratio of these elements that is important. Carbohydrates are made up of units called sugars. The scientific term for sugar is *saccharide*, and carbohydrates can exist as monosaccharides, disaccharides, or polysaccharides.

Glycogen is only ingested in small quantities, but is an important polysaccharide for storage of glucose within the body, specifically the liver. Fiber is a special polysaccharide because it cannot be digested. Fiber is important for slowing the rate of sugar absorption and in providing bulk for adequate elimination from the intestines.

Because the simple sugars are composed of only one or two units of sugar, their digestion takes little time, and absorption occurs soon after ingestion. The body initially experiences a large increase in sugar concentration in the blood, which is brought down to within a normal range by the release of insulin. The complex carbohydrates require more time to digest, and as a result there is a slower absorption of the single-carbohydrate units as the larger starch molecule is broken down. This is demonstrated in Figure 33-2. In this case, there would be a moderate increase in the sugar levels in the blood, and this would continue for a longer period. A continuous level of sugar in the bloodstream is necessary for a constant energy supply. The principle sources of carbohydrates are fruits, vegetables, cereal grains, and sugar. It is important to limit the amount of added sugar as a source of carbohydrates. One gram of carbohydrate contains 4 calories.

Fats. Fats, also called lipids, are also composed of carbon, hydrogen, and oxygen, but in a ratio different from carbohydrates. They exist as triglycerides in the body. A triglyceride has three fatty acids attached to a glycerol molecule (Figure 33-3). The fatty acid component of a triglyceride has several important characteristics. The first is whether it is essential to the diet. The only true essential fatty acid in the human diet is linoleic acid, and all other fatty acids the body requires can be derived from this. Another important characteristic of fatty acids is saturation. When a fatty acid is saturated, every carbon molecule on the fatty acid holds as many hydrogens as possible. If it does not hold all the hydrogens possible, it is called unsaturated. The more unsaturated the fatty acid, the more liquid the fat. For example, lard has saturated fatty acids and a thick consistency compared with olive oil, which has relatively unsaturated fatty acids and a thin consistency. If an unsaturated fat is **hydrogenated**, or combined with hydrogen, it becomes more saturated. **Saturated fats** are more common in foods from animal sources than from plant sources. Generally, saturated fatty acids tend to increase the level of fats and cholesterol in the blood. It is important to know that fats contain the most condensed caloric values. One gram of fat contains 9 calories.

Trans unsaturated fatty acids (trans fats) are unhealthy fats because they increase low-density lipoproteins (LDL), bad cholesterol, and decrease high-density lipoproteins (HDL), good cholesterol.

Trans fats are produced by a process known as hydrogenation. Vegetable oil (liquid) is heated and hydrogen is added to it. This makes the product solid at room temperature. It gives certain foods a longer shelf life and a better taste. The process, however, turns healthy fat into unhealthy fat, trans fat.

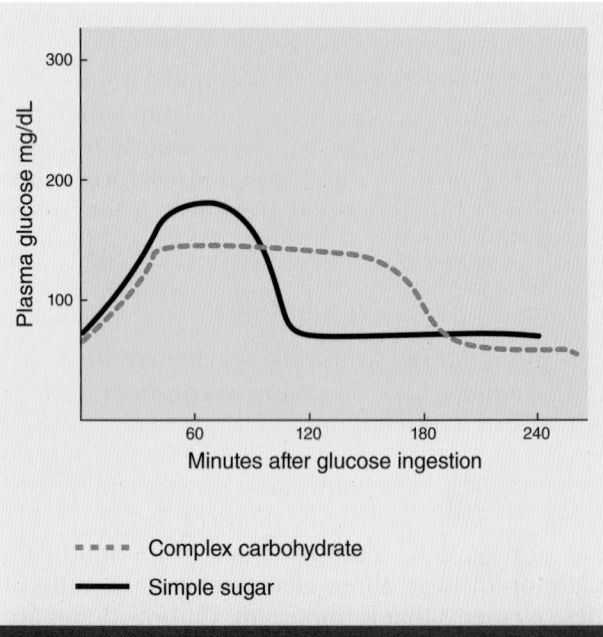

FIGURE 33-2 This graph shows how complex carbohydrates (red broken line) and simple sugar (black line) are used by the body (in minutes) after glucose ingestion. Simple sugar peaks to approximately 120 to 160 mg/dL in 60 minutes and returns to a normal level within 120 minutes. Complex carbohydrates never increase to more than approximately 130 to 140 mg/dL during a 60-minute period; that level is maintained for the next 180 minutes and then returns to normal.

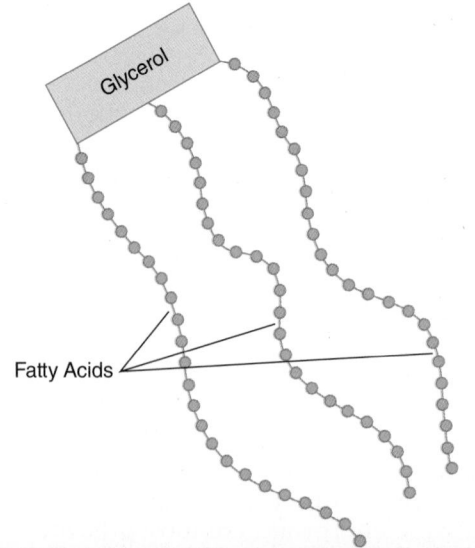

FIGURE 33-3 A triglyceride has three fatty acids attached to a glycerol molecule.

The FDA requires that all food packaging labels show the amount of trans fats per serving in the product. Every effort must be made to drastically limit or avoid these fats entirely. They are detrimental to human health. Table 33-1 lists some common foods and their grams of total fat and trans fat per serving.

An excellent tool for customized fat intake recommendations can be found at https://www.heart.org by searching for "My Fats Translator."

Proteins. Although protein is also composed of carbon, hydrogen, and oxygen, it contains one more important element: nitrogen. The basic structural unit of protein is the **amino acid**. There are 22 amino acids in proteins. Eight of these are needed in the diet for the body to function normally. One more, histidine, is essential only during childhood. The rest of the amino acids can be synthesized from the eight, provided that they are present in adequate quantities. A complete protein is so named because it has all eight of the essential amino acids. An incomplete protein does not contain all of these. The best sources for complete proteins are meats and animal products such as milk and eggs. Most plants provide only incomplete proteins and must be combined with complementary incomplete proteins to obtain all eight amino acids (Figure 33-4).

TABLE 33-1

GRAMS OF FAT PER SERVING OF SOME COMMON FOODS

PRODUCT	SERVING SIZE	TOTAL FAT	SATURATED FAT	TRANS FAT
Butter	1 tbsp	10.8	7.2	0.3
Cake (pound)	1 slice	16.4	3.4	4.3
Cookies (filled with cream)	3	6.1	1.2	1.9
Doughnut	1	18.2	4.7	5.0
French fries (fast food)	Medium	26.9	6.7	7.8
Granola bar	1 bar	7.1	4.4	0.4
Ground beef (95% lean)	4 oz.	6	3	0
Margarine (stick)	1 tbsp	11.0	2.1	2.8
Margarine (tub container)	1 tbsp	6.7	1.2	0.6
Mayonnaise	1 tbsp	10.8	1.6	0.0
Milk (whole)	1 cup	6.6	4.3	0.2
Peanut butter	1 oz.	14	3	0
Potato chips	Small bag	11.2	1.9	3.2
Ramen noodle soup	42 g	7.2	3.2	0.9
Shortening (solid)	1 tbsp	13.0	3.4	4.2
Wheat crackers	50 g	10.0	2.0	4.0
Yogurt (low fat)	1 cup	4	2	0

Source: Food and Drug Administration Center for Food Safety and Applied Nutrition; U.S. Department of Agriculture (USDA) National Nutritional Database.

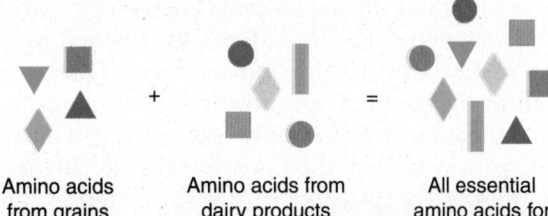

| Amino acids from grains | + | Amino acids from dairy products | = | All essential amino acids for complete protein |

FIGURE 33-4 Some foods, such as grains and dairy products, may not have all the essential amino acids when considered separately. Combined, however, these foods form a complete protein and therefore are considered complementary.

Although protein is described as an energy nutrient, its main function is not to provide energy but to provide amino acids to be used as building components of body proteins, which can be used as enzymes, hormones, and as the basic structural unit in all body tissues and cells. The body uses carbohydrates and fats as its primary energy sources; however, when these are in short supply, the body diverts its use of protein for structural purposes to use it as an energy source. This has detrimental effects on the body. Proteins are a component of every cell in the body. They provide the building blocks for growth and repair of bones, muscles, cartilage, skin, and blood.

Deficiencies in protein usually occur together with deficiencies in total calories. Foods high in protein are generally more expensive than those high in carbohydrates and fats. This leads to dietary choices that are based on economics for some families. Failure to thrive is caused by a lack of protein in infants and young children.

Energy Balance. Although all of the energy nutrients are capable of supplying energy to the body, they do so in different ways and in varying amounts. The amount of energy that a substance is able to supply can be measured in kilocalories. These are commonly referred to simply as **calories**.

Carbohydrates and proteins both give four calories for each respective gram. So, if 10 g of carbohydrate were ingested, it would yield 40 calories.

$$\frac{10 \text{ g}}{\text{carbohydrate}} \times \frac{4 \text{ calories}}{1 \text{ gram of carbohydrate}} = 40 \text{ calories}$$

Similarly, if 10 g protein were used for energy, it would yield 40 calories.

$$\frac{10 \text{ g}}{\text{protein}} \times \frac{4 \text{ calories}}{1 \text{ gram of protein}} = 40 \text{ calories}$$

Fats, in comparison, yield nine calories for every gram of fat. Fats, therefore, are a more energy-rich food source than carbohydrates or proteins. They give more calories for every gram used. If 10 g fat were used, it would yield 90 calories.

$$\frac{10 \text{ g}}{\text{fat}} \times \frac{9 \text{ calories}}{1 \text{ gram of fat}} = 90 \text{ calories}$$

The total of all changes, chemical and physical, that take place in the body is called **metabolism**. The metabolic rate is related to the changes in the body with respect to energy. It is the balance between the energy that is brought into the body and the energy used by the body. Energy is used during every action of the body, including voluntary activities such as walking or riding a bicycle and involuntary activities such as breathing and cellular repair.

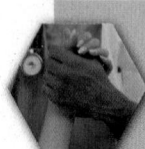

Patient Education

Trans Unsaturated Fatty Acids

Tips for Healthy Fat Consumption

- Use a margarine that is soft at room temperature; it is lower in trans fat. Some margarines are available that are entirely trans fat free.
- Olive oil is a wise choice for salads and for dipping bread, and butter is a better option than margarine.
- Olive oil and canola oil are best for sautéing and frying.
- Make foods from scratch to avoid trans fats. Foods such as breads, dips, salad dressings, cereals, and soups can be made without hydrogenated fats.

If a food label lists hydrogenated oil, partially hydrogenated oil, or shortening as one of its main ingredients (usually one of the first listed ingredients), it has a large amount of trans fats in it. Avoid the product altogether, or eat only small amounts.

The level of energy required for activities that occur when the body is at rest is called basal metabolism. The **basal metabolic rate (BMR)** varies according to several factors. For example, the BMR is higher in individuals with leaner body mass (muscle) because more energy is needed to fuel the muscles than to store fat. The BMR also is higher in individuals during periods of high growth rate, such as in children and pregnant women.

Ideally, an individual will take in as many calories as the body will use each day. When a person takes in more calories than will be used, the body will store the excess energy in the form of fat. When a person uses more energy than is brought into the body, the body breaks down these stores.

When the stores of fat are depleted, the body will start to break down its protein structures.

For an optimal energy balance in the body, the largest percentage of calories in the diet should come from carbohydrates. Ideally, the percentage should be 45% to 65% of total calories consumed, or 225 to 325 grams. The percentage of calories from fat should not be greater than 35%, with a percentage closer to 20% being preferred. This is approximately 40 to 80 grams of fat daily. The intake of saturated (animal) fat should not exceed 22 grams a day. Proteins should make up 10% to 35% of calories in the diet, or 46 grams of protein for women or 56 grams of protein for men (see the "Organic Nutrients" Quick Reference Guide).

⫸ QUICK REFERENCE GUIDE

⫸ ORGANIC NUTRIENTS

Nutrient	Daily Requirements	Sources	Calorie Calculation
Carbohydrates (sugars) © bitt24/Shutterstock.com	Children, 0 to 6 months: 60 grams Children, 7 to 12 months: 95 grams Children, 1 year through the teen years: 130 grams Adults: 225 to 325 grams based on overall recommended caloric intake	Monosaccharides: • Glucose and fructose—fruit and fruit juices, honey, sweet wine, syrup Disaccharides: • Sucrose—table sugar, syrup, cakes, cookies • Lactase—milk, ice cream, infant formula • Maltose—sweet potatoes, beer, high maltose corn syrup Sugar alcohols: • Erythritol and sorbitol—sugar alcohols used as sweetener • Glycerol—cane or corn syrup • Mannitol—mushrooms, strawberries, celery, onions Oligosaccharides: • Fruits and vegetables • Milk (human and cow) Polysaccharides: • Starch—cereal grains, potatoes, tapioca, yams • Cellulose—whole grains, green leafy vegetables, beans, peas, lentils • Glycogen—shellfish, animal liver	Carbohydrates contain 4 calories per gram

(continues)

Nutrient	Daily Requirements	Sources	Calorie Calculation
Fats (triglycerides) © Craevschii Family/Shutterstock.com	People of all ages: • 25% to 35% of total calorie intake • Limit saturated fat to 7%, which is 16 grams based on a 2,000 calorie diet • Limit trans fat to less than 1%, which is 2 grams based on a 2,000 calorie diet • Eat primarily monosaturated or polyunsaturated fats	Saturated fats: cheese, whole milk, butter Dietary cholesterol: eggs, liver, and organ meats Trans fatty acids: partially hydrogenated vegetable oils (e.g., margarine, shortening) Unsaturated fats: nuts, olives, vegetable oils, salmon, avocados	Fats contain 10 calories per gram
Proteins (amino acids) © nehopelon/Shutterstock.com	Children, 0 to 6 months: 9 grams Children, 7 to 12 months: 11 grams Children, 1 to 3 years: 13 grams Children, 4 to 8 years: 19 grams Children, 9 to 13 years: 34 grams Teenage boys: 52 grams Teenage girls: 46 grams Adult men: 56 grams Adult women: 46 grams If pregnant or breastfeeding: 71 grams	Seafood, white meat poultry, milk, cheese, yogurt, eggs, beans, soy, lean beef, lean pork	Proteins contain 4 calories per gram

Take note that these values are the percentage of the total calories derived from each energy nutrient—not the percentage of grams. This distinction is important because of the difference in calories derived from each energy nutrient. Figure 33-5 gives an example of these calculations. Note the percentages of fat, carbohydrate, and protein found in the "mystery" food. All fall outside of the recommended percentages for each.

Diversity

In many cultures outside of the United States, rice, bread, and noodles are the basis of the diet. In the United States, we have available great amounts of food from the dairy and meat groups. Unfortunately, dairy products and meats, although containing many good nutrients, also contain a great deal of fat. Studies have shown that many Americans are obese (defined as their weight being at least 20%

Label for Mystery Food:	Amount Per Serving
Calories	149
Total Fat	9g
Total Carbohydrate	14g
Total Protein	3g

The first calculation to make is one that converts grams to calories.

$$9 \text{ grams of fat} \times \frac{9 \text{ calories}}{\text{gram}} = 81 \text{ calories due to fat}$$

$$14 \text{ grams of carbohydrate} \times \frac{4 \text{ calories}}{\text{gram}} = 56 \text{ calories due to carbohydrate}$$

$$3 \text{ grams of protein} \times \frac{4 \text{ calories}}{\text{gram}} = 12 \text{ calories due to protein}$$

The next calculation is to find the percentage of total calories due to each of the energy nutrients.

$$\frac{81 \text{ calories due to fat}}{149 \text{ total calories}} = 54\%$$

$$\frac{56 \text{ calories due to carbohydrate}}{149 \text{ total calories}} = 38\%$$

$$\frac{12 \text{ calories due to protein}}{149 \text{ total calories}} = 8\%$$

FIGURE 33-5 Calculations of percentages of total calories from fat, carbohydrate, and protein.

greater than what their ideal weight should be). The U.S. diet is too high in fat, has too many calories, has too much salt and cholesterol, and has insufficient amounts of complex carbohydrates and fiber. As a result, many illnesses and diseases occur, such as heart disease, high blood pressure, diabetes, and cancer.

Because obesity in the United States has become such a serious problem, there was much interest in modifying the Food Guide Pyramid developed by the U.S. Department of Agriculture for maintaining ideal weight. Health experts believe that the emphasis on 6 to 11 daily servings from the bread, cereal, rice, and pasta groups (carbohydrates) is a contributing factor to obesity. Ongoing studies and research have led to a redesign of the pyramid with less emphasis on the carbohydrate group and more emphasis placed on fruits, vegetables, whole grains, legumes, and nuts.

This research was instrumental in developing the MyPlate Food Guidance System (Figure 33-6).

This food guide has specific information about portions and calories. It can help individuals get individualized nutrition and exercise advice.

Each color on the MyPlate guide represents a food group:

- *Orange* represents grains, which are divided into two groups: whole grains and refined grains. The recommendation is to eat 5 to 8 ounces of grain per day, at least half of which should be from whole grain breads, pasta, rice, cereal, or crackers.
- *Green* represents vegetables. For a low-calorie diet, 2½ cups of vegetables should come from all five vegetable groups several times a week.
- *Red* represents fruits. The recommended intake is 1½ to 2 cups daily.
- *Blue* represents dairy products. Three cups per day of fat-free or low-fat milk or milk products is recommended.
- *Purple* represents protein. The recommendation is to eat 5 to 6½ ounces of protein per day, choosing from lean meat, poultry, fish, eggs, processed soy products, beans, nuts, seeds, and peas.

The government ChooseMyPlate Web site allows individuals to input their age, gender, and activity level. After doing so, they get a recommendation about their personal daily calorie intake and physical activity level. Go to http://www.choosemyplate.gov and explore the interactive options. Download the ChooseMyPlate.gov brochure by searching for "Dietary Guidelines."

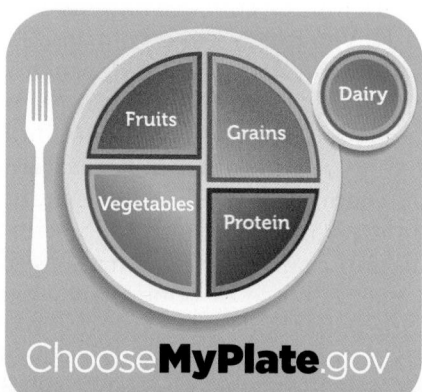

FIGURE 33-6 MyPlate is the "new generation" food icon to prompt consumers to think differently about their food choices.

Courtesy of the U.S. Department of Agriculture

Other Nutrients (Inorganic)

Many other nutrients are essential to maintaining good health. Although they do not provide the body with energy, they perform a variety of necessary functions. They include vitamins, antioxidants, herbal supplements, minerals, water, and fiber.

Vitamins. Vitamins are a class of nutrients in which each specific vitamin has a function entirely its own. They are complex molecules and are required by the body in minute quantities. Vitamins were first named as letters of the alphabet. These names have been supplemented with chemical names and both should be learned. Vitamins generally have one of two functions: to facilitate cellular metabolism by acting as a **coenzyme** with a catalyst, or to act as a component of tissue structure. A **catalyst** allows a chemical reaction to proceed at a much quicker rate and without as much energy input, and the coenzyme is the nonprotein part that acts with it. Neither a catalyst nor its coenzyme is used in the reaction; thus, each can be used again and again. Vitamins that work with catalysts are only needed in minute quantities.

Vitamins are divided into two classes based on solubility. The vitamins that are not soluble in water are said to be fat soluble. This is important because the **fat-soluble vitamins** are not carried into the bloodstream easily and are stored in fatty tissue, especially the liver. The **water-soluble vitamins** are not so easily stored, and blood levels must be maintained by constant dietary intake. Toxicity can occur with high doses of either type of vitamin, but is more likely to occur with the fat-soluble vitamins because they are stored in the body. The vitamins are listed in Table 33-2.

There are four fat-soluble vitamins: vitamins A, D, E, and K. Vitamin A has two forms. The form that is used by the body is retinol, which is found in animal foods. The form found in plants is carotene. **Carotene** is converted into retinol in the body. Vitamin D, also called **cholecalciferol**, is the fat-soluble vitamin involved in the metabolism of calcium in the body. It not only helps with absorption of this important mineral, but also with formation and maintenance of bone tissue. Vitamin D can be made in the body with exposure to sunlight. Another fat-soluble vitamin is vitamin E, or **tocopherol**. It too is an **antioxidant**, possibly reducing the likelihood of **oxidation** of substances. As the body breaks down nutrients, oxidation occurs. This process releases free radicals that can kill or change the cells of the body and create disease. This ability to reduce oxidation has recently led to suggestions that vitamin E may slow the aging process, but its true effectiveness is yet to be demonstrated. Vitamin K is a fat-soluble vitamin required for the production of prothrombin. Vitamin K is synthesized by intestinal bacteria, and bile is required for its absorption. About half of the body's requirement for vitamin K is fulfilled in this way. Supplementation of fat-soluble vitamins is rarely needed as there is a rich supply in the average diet. Care must be taken with supplementation because fat-soluble vitamins are stored for long periods of time and toxicity is a possibility.

Antioxidants. Antioxidants are an important topic in nutrition. Antioxidants are powerful and beneficial to us. The four primary antioxidants are vitamin A (beta carotene), vitamin C, vitamin E, and selenium.

When our bodies use oxygen to burn (oxidize) food for energy, the process results in the formation of free radicals. Most times our bodies take care of the free radicals by producing enzymes to fight them.

If free radicals are excessive, health can be seriously impaired. The radicals attack the cells' DNA and blood vessel cells, contributing to cardiovascular disease, strokes, arthritis, cataracts, and other diseases that may be degenerative in nature. Free radicals are not only a by-product of oxidation, they form with exposure to environmental influences such as water and air pollution, cigarette smoke, and certain foods, such as those that are fried.

Antioxidants fight free radicals through enzymes that are already in our bodies, those we ingest in food, and those we take as supplements. Vitamins A (as beta-carotene), C, and E along with selenium provide powerful benefits because they fight against oxidation that produces free radicals.

Vitamin C, or **ascorbic acid**, is a water-soluble vitamin. Vitamin C is a constituent of connective tissue and acts to hold cells together. The last group of water-soluble vitamins are the B-complex vitamins. It is important to remember that each vitamin in the B-complex is a separate vitamin with distinct functions. Vitamin B_1, or **thiamin**, helps in the conversion of glucose to energy. Vitamin B_2, or **riboflavin**, is also involved in energy production. A third B-complex vitamin, **niacin**, works with both thiamin and riboflavin in the production of energy. Lack of niacin results in gastrointestinal and central nervous system disturbances. All three of these vitamins are important throughout the body.

TABLE 33-2

VITAMIN SOURCES AND FUNCTIONS*

NAME	FOOD SOURCES	FUNCTIONS	DEFICIENCY/TOXICITY
FAT-SOLUBLE VITAMINS			
Vitamin A (carotene or retinol)	Animal: • Liver • Whole milk • Butter • Cream • Cod liver oil Plant: • Dark green leafy vegetables • Deep yellow or orange fruit • Fortified margarine Vitamin supplementation	As retinol from animal sources or carotene from plant sources converted to retinol: • Purplish-red light-sensitive pigment present in the retinas; responsible for night vision • Antioxidant • Maintenance of mucous membranes and skin • Growth and development of bones	Deficiency: • Night blindness • Preventable blindness in children • Increased risk of maternal mortality • **Xerophthalmia** • Respiratory infections • Bone growth ceases Toxicity: • Cessation of menstruation • Joint pain • Bone pain • Stunted growth • Enlargement of liver • Headache • Rough, dry skin
Vitamin D (cholecalciferol)	Animal: • Eggs • Liver • Fortified milk • The flesh of fatty fish: salmon, tuna, mackerel • Fish liver oil Plant: • Mushrooms Can be manufactured by the body with the skin's exposure to sunlight Vitamin supplementation	• Necessary for absorption of calcium and phosphorus to support bone health and growth • Essential to assist the immune system to fight infection • Muscle function • Supports respiratory system • Essential for brain development • Regulation of the neuromuscular system • Plays a major role in the life cycle of human cells • Anticancer properties	Deficiency: • Rickets • Osteomalacia • Osteoporosis • Skeletal deformities • Poorly developed teeth • Muscle spasms • Breast, colon, and prostate cancer • Depression • Autoimmune diseases • Over 200 diseases linked to vitamin D deficiency Toxicity: • Kidney stones • Kidney failure • Calcification of soft tissues • Hypertension • **Hypercalcemia** • **Tinnitus** • Cardiac arrhythmias

continues

Table 33-2 continued

NAME	FOOD SOURCES	FUNCTIONS	DEFICIENCY/TOXICITY
Vitamin E (alphatocopherol, beta-tocopherol, delta-tocopherol, gamma-tocopherol)	Animal: • Chicken • Pork • Egg yolks Plant: • Wheat germ • Spinach • Pumpkin • Asparagus • Collard greens • Avocado • Nuts and seeds (sunflower seeds, peanuts, almonds)	• Antioxidant • Supports the immune system • Assists in the formation of red blood cells • Assists in communication between cells • Cancer prevention	Deficiency: • Poor transmission of nerve impulses • Muscle weakness • Degeneration of the retina • Blindness • Cardiac arrhythmias • Dementia Toxicity: • Hypertension • Muscle weakness • Fatigue • Hemorrhagic stroke • Bleeding
Vitamin K (phytonadione)	Animal: • Animal liver • Milk Plant: • Green leafy vegetables (kale, spinach) • Cabbage • Fermented foods	• Bone formation • Blood clotting • Supports cartilage • Key in maintaining blood vessel walls • Associated with cell adhesion and migration • Anticancer properties	Deficiency: • Prolonged blood clotting • Excessive bleeding • Osteoporosis • Bone fractures • Heart disease • Kidney disease Toxicity • Hemolytic anemia • Jaundice • Liver damage

WATER-SOLUBLE VITAMINS

NAME	FOOD SOURCES	FUNCTIONS	DEFICIENCY/TOXICITY
Vitamin B$_1$ (thiamin)	Animal: • Liver • Eggs • Fish • Pork • Beef Plants: • Whole and enriched grains • Legumes • Brewer's yeast	• Assists in the conversion of carbohydrates into glucose • Metabolism of fats and proteins • Supports brain health • Maintenance of hair and skin • Maintenance of normal appetite and nervous system function	Deficiency: • **Beriberi** • Anorexia • Weight loss • Confusion • Short-term memory loss • Muscle weakness • Cardiac abnormalities • **Wernicke-Korsakoff syndrome** • Alzheimer disease Toxicity: • None (unused water-soluble vitamins are excreted by the kidneys)

continues

Table 33-2 continued

NAME	FOOD SOURCES	FUNCTIONS	DEFICIENCY/TOXICITY
Vitamin B₂ (riboflavin)	**Animal:** • Organ meats • Lamb • Milk • Natural yogurt • Salmon • Eggs **Plant:** • Green vegetables (broccoli, spinach, Brussels sprouts) • Enriched cereals and bread • Mushrooms • Sundried tomatoes • Almonds • Soybeans	• Assists in the conversion of carbohydrates into glucose • Metabolizes fats and protein • Supports liver, skin, hair, mucous membrane, and eye health • Assists in proper nervous system function	**Deficiency:** • **Cheilosis** • **Glossitis** • **Photophobia** • Slowed growth • Fatigue • Cataracts • Possible connection to autism **Toxicity** • None (unused water-soluble vitamins are excreted by the kidneys)
Vitamin B₃ (niacin, nicotinic acid)	**Animal:** • Milk • Eggs • Fish • Poultry **Intrinsic sources:** • Niacin synthesis from tryptophan	• Assists in the conversion of carbohydrates into glucose • Assists in the use of fats and protein • Supports the health of the liver, skin, hair, and eyes • Supports nervous system function • Assists in the building of various sex and stress-related hormones in the adrenal glands and other parts of the body • Improves circulation • Suppresses inflammation	**Deficiency:** • **Pellagra** • Depression • Fatigue • Canker sores • Alterations in circulation • Swollen, bright red tongue **Toxicity:** • Flushing of the skin • Headache • Dizziness • Blurred vision • Liver damage
Vitamin B₅ (pantothenic acid)	**Animal:** • Egg yolks • Beef (especially organ meats such as liver and kidney) • Poultry • Milk • Lobster • Salmon **Plant:** • Brewer's yeast • Corn • Cruciferous vegetables (cauliflower, broccoli) • Green vegetables (kale, broccoli) • Tomatoes • Avocado • Sunflower seeds • Peanuts	• Assists in the conversion of carbohydrates into glucose • Critical to the manufacture of red blood cells • Assists in production of sex and stress-related hormones produced in the adrenal glands • Maintains the health of the gastrointestinal tract • Needed to synthesize cholesterol • Assists the body to use other vitamins • Speeds wound healing	**Deficiency:** • Fatigue • Depression • Muscle cramps • Insomnia • Irritability **Toxicity:** • GI distress • Diarrhea

continues

Table 33-2 continued

NAME	FOOD SOURCES	FUNCTIONS	DEFICIENCY/TOXICITY
Vitamin B$_6$ (pyridoxine)	Animal: • Beef liver • Tuna • Salmon • Poultry • Milk • Eggs Plant: • Whole grain cereals • Legumes • Bananas • Squash • Spinach • Watermelon • Raisins	• Assists in the conversion of carbohydrates into glucose • Supports cardiovascular system • Vital component of neurotransmitters • Supports normal brain development and function • Plays a vital role in the function of approximately 100 enzymes that increase the speed of essential chemical reactions • Synthesis of nonessential amino acids • Conversion of tryptophan to niacin • Antibody production • Antioxidant to reduce homocysteine levels	Deficiency: • Increases risk of cardiovascular disease • Irritability • Depression • Dermatitis • Confusion • Decreases immune function • Abnormally acute hearing • Seizures • Painful, disfiguring dermatological lesions Toxicity: • Liver disease • Sensory neuropathy • Ataxia
Vitamin B$_7$, also known as Vitamin H (biotin)	Animal: • Cooked eggs, especially egg yolks • Sardines • Milk Plant: • Nuts (almonds, peanuts, pecans, walnuts) and nut butters • Soybeans • Legumes (beans, black eyed peas) • Whole grains • Cauliflower • Bananas • Mushrooms Biotin can be made by bacteria in the human intestine.	• Assists in the conversion of carbohydrates into glucose • Assists in the use of fats and protein • Strengthens hair and nails • Coenzyme in carbohydrate and amino acid metabolism	Deficiency: • Hair loss • Dry scaly skin • Cheilitis • Glossitis • Fatigue • Insomnia • Hallucinations • Numbness and tingling of the extremities Toxicity: • Unknown
Vitamin B$_9$ (folate or folic acid)	Animal: • Liver Plant: • Dark leafy greens (spinach, collard greens, romaine lettuce) • Asparagus • Citrus fruits (oranges, grapefruit) • Peas, beans, and lentils (kidney beans, green peas and beans, navy beans) • Avocado • Seeds and nuts (sunflower seeds, peanuts)	• Assists in the conversion of carbohydrates into glucose • Assists in the metabolism of fats and protein • Assists in the production of DNA and RNA • Required for the formation of RBCs • Supports brain function and health • Antioxidant to reduce homocysteine levels • Anticancer properties	Deficiency: • Anemia • Glossitis • Macrocytic anemia • Neural tube defects in the fetus • Poor growth • Gingivitis • Shortness of breath • Diarrhea • Forgetfulness and mental sluggishness Toxicity: • None

continues

Table 33-2 continued

NAME	FOOD SOURCES	FUNCTIONS	DEFICIENCY/TOXICITY
Vitamin B$_{12}$ (cobalamin)	**Animal:** • Shellfish • Organ meats • Beef • Pork • Poultry • Eggs • Milk • Cheese **Plant:** • Enriched cereals • Nutritional yeasts	• Assists in the conversion of carbohydrates into glucose • Assists in the use of fats and protein • Required for the formation of RBCs • Assists in the production of DNA and RNA • Important in protein metabolism • Maintenance of the central nervous system • Antioxidant to reduce homocysteine levels • Anticancer properties	Deficiency: • **Megaloblastic anemia** • **Pernicious anemia** • Fatigue • Weakness • Constipation • Loss of appetite and weight loss • Neurologic changes • Numbness and tingling in the hands and feet • Difficulty maintaining balance • Depression • Confusion, dementia, poor memory • Soreness of the mouth or tongue Toxicity: • None documented
Vitamin C (ascorbic acid)	**Fruit:** • Citrus (oranges, grapefruits, lemons) • Guava • Kiwi • Tomatoes **Vegetable:** • Dark green leafy vegetables (kale, collard greens, turnip greens) • Yellow bell peppers • Broccoli • Berries (strawberry, raspberries, blueberries)	• Prevention of scurvy • Formation of collagen for skin, cartilage, tendons, ligaments, and blood vessels • Healing of wounds • Release of stress hormones • Absorption of iron • Growth and repair of tissues in all parts of the body • Repair and maintenance of bones and teeth • Aids absorption of iron from the GI tract • Plays a role in prevention of heart disease, hypertension, common cold, osteoporosis, and age-related macular degeneration • Anticancer properties	Deficiency: • **Scurvy** • Dry and splitting hair • **Gingivitis** • Rough, dry, scaly skin • Poor wound healing • Bruising • Nosebleeds • High blood pressure • Gallbladder disease • Stroke Toxicity: • Abdominal cramps • Headache • Heartburn • Vomiting • Kidney stones

* Vitamins are divided into two classes based on water solubility: fat-soluble and water-soluble vitamins.

Vitamin B$_6$, or **pyridoxine**, has an important role in protein metabolism, especially the synthesis of proteins. It is also important in the metabolism of fats and carbohydrates. Another B-complex vitamin, **folic acid**, is involved in the formation of DNA and the formation of red blood cells. Vitamin B$_{12}$, or **cobalamin**, is another vitamin important to the functioning of red blood cells. Multivitamin supplements may help reduce the risk for certain diseases, especially in individuals who do not eat nutritionally sound diets. Individuals who may be more likely to suffer vitamin deficiencies because of poor nutrition include the elderly; individuals with mental challenges; young children without proper care; and patients with chronic diseases such as alcoholism, Crohn disease, cystic fibrosis, and celiac disease. Some studies show a reduced risk for coronary artery disease in patients who take a multivitamin coupled with antioxidants. Researchers believe that B vitamins and antioxidants may help keep plaque from forming in arteries.

Most patients who are healthy and eat a nutritious diet do not need a supplement in the form of a multivitamin. A balanced diet is the best overall source of nutrients as it provides the macronutrients and micronutrients that work together to repair and maintain the body and its functions. Some people may need a supplement because they are at risk for a disease such as cancer or heart disease. Examples of people at high risk are patients who have a chronic illness such as AIDS; patients who have gastrointestinal problems that impair digestion or absorption; patients who are dieting; patients who are vegans or vegetarians; pregnant and breastfeeding women; and patients older than 50 years (many adults older than 50 years have difficulty absorbing B vitamins from food, and their level of vitamin D may be low because of lack of sunshine and eating poorly).

Patients should check with their provider before beginning to take multivitamin supplements.

Herbal Supplements.
Herbs are medicinal plants and are also known as botanicals or phytomedicines. Many have been used as far back as Roman times and are considered to be herbal medicine.

Many patients use herbs for the treatment of illnesses and diseases and to maintain health. It is part of a movement toward alternative or complementary therapies. Herbal supplements can be found in health food stores, pharmacies, supermarkets, large outlet stores, through the mail, and on the Internet.

Herbal supplements are made from dried plants and plant juices. Herbal teas are made by placing the herb into boiling water. Many different compounds are found in herbs. For example, natural hormones can be found in soy products.

Some supplements are helpful; other supplements are harmful and are banned in several countries but may be available in the United States. The Food and Drug Administration (FDA) does not have authority over dietary supplements, although under the Dietary Supplement Health and Education Act of 1994, the FDA must prove a product is unsafe before it can order its removal from store shelves. An example of a potentially unsafe herbal supplement that the FDA removed from the shelves in 2004 is ephedra. It was used as an anorectic and as a bronchodilator, it acts as a stimulant, and it can increase blood pressure and pulse to dangerous levels. In 2005, a federal judge struck down the FDA's year-long ban on ephedra and supplements containing ephedra. A Utah supplement company had challenged the ban, which prompted the judge's ruling. In 2006, the ruling was appealed to the U.S. Court of Appeals for the Tenth Circuit in Denver, Colorado, and the court of appeals upheld the FDA's ban on ephedra. The sale of supplements containing ephedra alkaloids is illegal in the United States. Although ephedra is an illegal and banned substance, it is widely used by athletes. Ephedra extracts that do not contain ephedrine have not been banned by the FDA and are still sold legally today.

Be sure to ask patients about all substances or remedies they may be using, including herbs, vitamins, teas, and any others. Most patients do not consider supplements to be medicines and may not think to mention them when asked what medications they are taking. Herbs can interact unfavorably with certain prescription drugs, over-the-counter medications, and anesthetics.

Minerals.
Minerals differ from vitamins in two distinct ways. Vitamins are complex molecules. Minerals are singular elements. Another way that minerals differ from vitamins is that although vitamins are only required in minute quantities, some minerals are required in larger amounts. The foundation of the classification of minerals falls into two groups: major and trace minerals. No matter how small the quantity required of either a mineral or vitamin, all are vital to a healthy body. Some minerals are considered **electrolytes**, in that they become ionized and carry a positive or negative charge. The levels of these minerals in the bloodstream must be carefully balanced for the body to function in a healthy state.

There are seven **major minerals** (Table 33-3). They are calcium, phosphorus, sodium, potassium, magnesium, chloride, and iron.

Calcium (Ca) is the mineral present in the largest quantity in the body because of its involvement in the structure of bone and teeth. When there is a deficiency of calcium in the diet, calcium is taken from the bones to keep the blood calcium levels constant. The resulting deficient bone mass may put a person at risk for osteoporosis.

TABLE 33-3

MAJOR MINERAL SOURCES AND FUNCTIONS

NAME	FOOD SOURCES	FUNCTIONS	DEFICIENCY/TOXICITY
Calcium (Ca)	Animal: • Milk • Yogurt • Cottage cheese • Sardines • Salmon Plant: • Collard greens • Black eyed peas • White beans • Kale • Almonds • Oranges	• Development of bones and teeth • Maintenance of bones • Permeability of cell membranes • Mediates **vasoconstriction** and **vasodilation** • Transmission of nerve impulses • Blood clotting • Normal heart action • Stabilization of proteins	Deficiency (**hypocalcemia**): • Indicates abnormal parathyroid function • Osteoporosis • Osteomalacia • Rickets • Poor bone and teeth formation Toxicity (hypercalcemia): • Fatigue • Depression • Muscle weakness • Kidney stones • Gall stones
Phosphorus (P)	Animal: • Milk • Yogurt • Cheese • Eggs • Beef • Pork • Fish (salmon, halibut) • Poultry Plant: • Beans • Peas • Cereals • Nuts (almonds, peanuts) • Lentils Carbonated cola drinks contain high levels of phosphorus	• Essential for the structure of cell membranes • Regulation of acid–base balance • Supports cell signaling • Development of bones and teeth • Transfer of energy • Component of phospholipids • Buffer system • Structural component of bones • Essential for production and storage of energy in the cell (ATP)	Deficiency (**hypophosphatemia**): • Loss of appetite • Muscle weakness • Bone fragility • Numbness in the extremities • Rickets in children • Decreased immune function • Respiratory failure Toxicity (**hyperphosphatemia**): • Renal failure • Heart failure • Impairment of synthesis of the active form of vitamin D • Bone demineralization
Potassium (K)	Animal: • Milk • Yogurt • Cheese • Seafood (salmon, crab, cod) • Poultry • Ham Plant: • Tomatoes • Potatoes • Pumpkin • Mushrooms	• Works with sodium across cell membranes for regulation of membrane potential (**electrochemical gradient**) • Contraction of muscles • Maintaining water balance • Necessary for heart function • Transmission of nerve impulses • Carbohydrate and protein metabolism • Cofactor necessary for important enzyme in carbohydrate metabolism	Deficiency (**hypokalemia**): • Fatigue • Muscle weakness and cramps • Intestinal paralysis, which may lead to bloating, constipation, and abdominal pain • Muscular paralysis • Cardiac arrhythmias • Death Toxicity (**hyperkalemia**): • **Hemolysis** • Tingling of the hands and feet

continues

Table 33-3 continued

NAME	FOOD SOURCES	FUNCTIONS	DEFICIENCY/TOXICITY
	• Carrots • Green leafy vegetables (kale, spinach) • Beans (kidney, soy, pinto) • Plantains • Papayas • Pears • Dried fruits • Nuts (almonds, pistachios)		• Muscular weakness • Temporary paralysis • Cardiac arrhythmia • Cardiac arrest
Sodium (Na) Chloride (Cl) (listed together as they occur together in the body)	Animal: • Canned fish • Ham • Hot dogs • Processed meats Plant: • Cereals • Bread • Potato chips In sea salt, table salt, and other types of salt.	• Sodium with chloride as a major component of extracellular fluid • Maintenance of charge differences across cell membranes (membrane potential) • Transmission of nerve impulses • Muscle contraction • Cardiac function • Maintenance of blood volume and blood pressure	Deficiency (**hyponatremia**): • Headache • Nausea and vomiting • Muscle cramps • Fatigue • Disorientation • Fainting • Cerebral • Seizures • Coma • Brain damage • Death Toxicity (**hypernatremia**): • Nausea, vomiting, diarrhea, and abdominal cramps • Dizziness or fainting • Hypotension or hypertension • Diminished urine • Edema (swelling) • Congestive heart failure • Tachycardia • Shortness of breath • Convulsions • Coma • Death
Magnesium (Mg)	Animal: • Fish • Milk Plant: • Cereal • Brown rice • Spinach • Nuts (peanuts, hazelnuts) • Molasses • Bananas	• Magnesium-dependent metabolism of proteins and fats • Synthesis of DNA and RNA • Structural role in bone, cell membranes, and chromosomes • Active transport of ions like potassium and calcium across cell membranes • Formation of cell signaling molecules	Deficiency (**hypomagnesemia**): • Bone demineralization • Tremor • Muscle spasms • Tetany • Loss of appetite • Nausea and vomiting • Personality changes Toxicity (**hypermagnesemia**): • Hypotension • Nausea and vomiting

continues

Table 33-3 continued

NAME	FOOD SOURCES	FUNCTIONS	DEFICIENCY/TOXICITY
			• Urinary retention • Depression • Lethargy progressing to muscle weakness • Shortness of breath • Cardiac arrhythmias • Death
Iron (Fe)	Animal: • Beef • Chicken liver • Oysters • Tuna • Mussels Plant: • Raisins • Prunes • Swiss chard • Potatoes • Lentils • Nuts (hazelnuts, cashews)	• Maintaining protein structure • Oxygen transport and storage • Activities involved in energy production • Important role in cellular energy production • Antioxidant • DNA replication and repair • Critical role in immune functions—T lymphocytes	Deficiency: • Iron-deficiency anemia • Fatigue • Tachycardia • Palpitations • Tachypnea • Poor cognitive development in children • Abnormal behavior patterns • Altered brain function Toxicity: • Liver cancer • Neurodegenerative disease • Development of type II diabetes mellitus

Women older than 60 years are at greater risk for osteoporosis than are men. There are no symptoms of the disease, and the first indication for the patient is often when he or she sustains a fracture caused by weakened bones. Screening for osteoporosis includes bone density testing. This is important information as most adults in the United States older than 60 years do not consume enough calcium in their diets and risk development of osteoporosis. Supplemental estrogen for menopausal women was once a common preventative for bone loss. Since 2002, estrogen has not been given as a preventive measure because a large study by the Women's Health Initiative showed an increased risk for heart disease, stroke, cancer, and breast cancer in postmenopausal women who took estrogen. Now, the drugs of choice to treat osteoporosis are bisphosphonates. Bisphosphonates slow the breakdown and removal of bone. They are widely used for the prevention and treatment of osteoporosis in postmenopausal women.

Phosphorus (P) is another mineral important in bone formation. Phosphorus also is involved in numerous activities associated with energy metabolism, as well as maintaining a proper pH balance in the blood.

Sodium (Na) and potassium (K) are two minerals that act as electrolytes. Together they work to maintain proper water balance. They also help in maintenance of proper pH balance and are involved in nerve and muscular conduction and excitability. Magnesium (Mg) is another mineral that is involved with energy metabolism. It also functions in nerve and muscle excitability and is stored in bone. Magnesium is critical to more than 300 enzyme-driven biochemical reactions in the body. In particular, it is critical to glucose and fat breakdown, and creation of DNA and RNA.

Chloride (Cl) is important in pH balance and is the major **extracellular** (outside the cell) anion. It is also a major component of gastric secretions in the form of hydrochloric acid. Chloride is most often found in the body in combination with sodium. The last major mineral is iron (Fe). Iron is most important as a chemical component of heme. Heme is the oxygen-carrying molecule attached to a red blood cell.

The **trace minerals** are required in smaller quantities but are as important as the major minerals. Some of the more important trace minerals are copper, chromium, molybdenum, selenium, manganese, iodine, zinc, cobalt, and fluorine.

Copper, chromium, molybdenum, selenium, and manganese are trace minerals important as factors in a number of metabolic reactions. Selenium acts as an antioxidant and has received much recent publicity. Iodine is also involved in metabolism but is unique in that the only place iodine is found is in the thyroid hormone produced by the thyroid gland. Without it, the thyroid gland would be unable to regulate the overall metabolism of the body.

Zinc is an important constituent of many parts of the body but most notable is its involvement with the immune system and growth of tissues. Deficiencies lead to decreased ability to heal and reduced immune resistance. Cobalt is part of vitamin B_{12} and is therefore important for the functioning of red blood cells. Fluorine is involved in calcified tissues. Its involvement in strengthening teeth has led to the fluoridation of most public water supplies. Its role in the prevention of osteoporosis has been suggested but is still under investigation.

Water. Water is an important nutrient. The human body can go far longer without food than it can without water. Water has a multitude of functions in the body. It is the major solvent of the body and is the medium in which most biochemical reactions of the body take place. As a solvent, water is essential for the removal of toxic waste from the body. In addition, it is an important component of many structures; the body is composed of 50% to 65% water. Being the major component of blood, water serves as a transporter. Another function of water is its lubricating role, especially in joints and in the digestive system. In addition, water helps control temperature within the body by eliminating excess heat through the evaporation of water secreted in the form of perspiration.

Because the body cannot efficiently store water, water that is lost daily must continually be replenished. Water is lost through perspiration, feces, urine, and respiration. Water can be replenished in part from foods that are ingested, but additional water should also be consumed. It is suggested that six to eight glasses of water be taken in per day. Although other beverages are important sources of water, it should be considered that caffeine and alcohol are **diuretics** and may cause the body to lose water through increased urinary output.

Fiber. Although most fiber is carbohydrate in composition, it is discussed in its own section of this text because of its special characteristics. Fiber comes only from plant sources. An adequate supply of fruits, vegetables, and grains is necessary to ensure enough fiber in the diet. Fiber cannot be digested and therefore is not absorbed into the body. Although fiber is not digested, it is important for the proper functioning of the gastrointestinal tract because it adds bulk to feces as it is passed through the intestines; therefore, it gives the muscles of the intestinal tract something against which to work. Lack of fiber in the diet has been implicated in such gastrointestinal disorders as diverticulitis, constipation, and colorectal cancer.

There are several types of fiber. Most are carbohydrates and include **cellulose**, gums, mucilages, algal polysaccharides, pectins, and hemicellulose. Another important fiber, lignin, is not a carbohydrate. It is recommended that the diet contain 20 to 35 grams of fiber per day. The U.S. diet tends to include far less than this recommendation (approximately 11 grams), in part because of the consumption of processed foods. During processing, fiber is often removed. Fiber levels should be increased gradually to prevent gastrointestinal distress, which can include diarrhea and flatulence.

READING FOOD LABELS

Competency

When assisting patients in changing or modifying their diets, the medical assistant must be knowledgeable not only about types of nutrients, but also about how these nutrients are expressed in the foods we eat. The nutritional analysis presented on a package's food label is a helpful guide to understanding levels of fat, cholesterol, sodium, carbohydrate, protein, and vitamins contained in a particular food.

Many of the foods we eat are **processed foods** which are cooked or packaged with parts removed or ingredients added. We rely on the labels on the cans, bottles, and boxes to tell us what nutrients are inside. The government wants to make it easier for people to understand the labels.

The government also wants to prevent food companies from fooling people into thinking something has good nutrition when it really does not. Food companies often put words on their labels to make people believe a product is healthy. Words such as *healthy*, *light*, and *lite* are not adequately descriptive. To discover what is in the package and whether it is healthy, it is important to read the nutrition label (Figure 33-7).

Items on the Nutrition Label

Serving Size. The nutrition information given is for one serving of the food. In Figure 33-7, one serving is one-half cup of the food. The package contains four servings.

Calories. The label lists the number of calories per serving, as well as the number of calories from fat per serving. The latter number should be less than 30% of the total calories. For example, if there are 100 total calories, the calories from fat should be 30 or less.

The Percentage (%) Daily Value. The percentage (%) daily value is the amount of a nutrient obtained by eating one serving of the product. The amount is given in a percentage based on a diet of 2,000 calories a day. For example, if the packaged food has 3 grams of fat, the total fat from eating one serving is 5% of the total fat that should be ingested in an entire day.

Fat and Cholesterol. Because it is important to eat a low-fat diet, nutrition labels list both the total amount of fat and the amount of saturated fat and trans fat per serving. Saturated fat comes from an animal source and contains more cholesterol than unsaturated fat, which comes from a vegetable source. The cholesterol content is also listed.

Sodium. The amount of sodium per serving is listed. This category is especially important for patients on a sodium-restricted diet, such as those with cardiac disease and hypertension.

Carbohydrates. The total amount of carbohydrates per serving is listed together with the amount of carbohydrates that come from simple sugar. These two types of carbohydrates are separated for individuals who are trying to eat more complex carbohydrates and less simple sugar.

Other Information. The amounts of fiber, protein, and some vitamins and minerals are listed.

Ingredients. The ingredients contained in a packaged food are listed on the label. The item that is in the largest quantity is listed first. For example, if a product lists flour first and water second, there is more flour than water in the product. **Preservatives**, or chemicals, are added to food to keep it fresh longer, and artificial flavors and colors are often added to processed foods.

Comparing Labels

Look at some labels from snack foods that people eat when they want something crunchy and salty. Figure 33-8 shows labels from potato chips, pretzels, and snack crackers. When comparing products, compare equal amounts. These products list the serving as 30 or 28 grams. That is close enough to compare the labels.

In reviewing these labels, note the amount of fat and saturated fat in each item. It might be assumed that potato chips, which are fried, would be high in fat. It may be surprising that the snack crackers have high fat content. Pretzels are the clear winner for a low-fat snack among these options.

Although the labels show total fat and saturated fat, the amount of trans-fatty acids (TFA) is not listed. Previously, food labels included trans fats within the total fat amount. The FDA now requires the amount of TFA be listed in the label.

Nutrition Facts

Serving Size ½ cup (130g)
Servings Per Container About 4

Amount Per Serving

Calories 110

Calories from Fat 0

	% Daily Value*
Total Fat 0g	**0%**
Sodium 340mg	**14%**
Total Carbohydrate 20g	**7%**
Dietary Fiber 6g	**25%**
Sugars 2g	
Protein 8g	

Calcium 6%	•	Iron 10%

Not a significant source of saturated fat, trans fat, cholesterol, vitamin A and vitamin C.

*Percent Daily Values are based on a 2,000 calorie diet.

FIGURE 33-7 Labels on food packages give facts about the ingredients and nutrition of the food in the package.

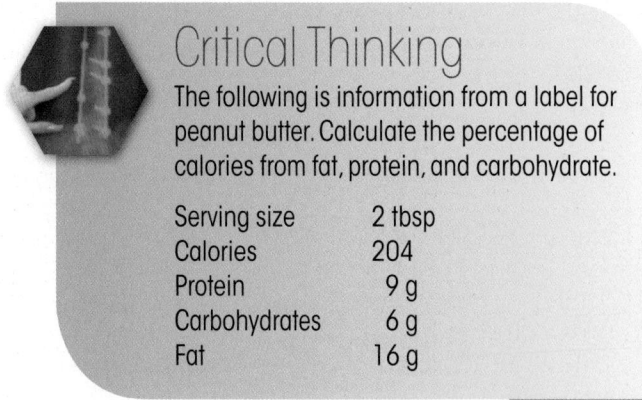

Critical Thinking

The following is information from a label for peanut butter. Calculate the percentage of calories from fat, protein, and carbohydrate.

Serving size	2 tbsp
Calories	204
Protein	9 g
Carbohydrates	6 g
Fat	16 g

Nutrition Facts (A) — Potato Chips

Serving Size 1 oz. (28g/About 15 chips)
Servings Per Container About 12

Amount Per Serving

Calories 140   Calories from Fat 60

	% Daily Value*
Total Fat 6g	**10%**
Saturated Fat 1g	**5%**
Polyunsaturated Fat 2g	
Monounsaturated Fat 3.5g	
Trans Fat 0g	
Cholesterol 0mg	**0%**
Sodium 130mg	**5%**
Potassium 75mg	**2%**
Total Carbohydrate 18g	**6%**
Dietary Fiber 2g	**9%**
Sugars 3g	
Protein 2g	

Vitamin A 0%	•	Vitamin C 0%
Calcium 0%	•	Iron 2%
Vitamin E 8%	•	Thiamin 2%
Niacin 2%	•	Vitamin B₆ 4%
Phosphorus 6%	•	Magnesium 4%
Zinc 2%		

*Percent Daily Values are based on a 2,000 calorie diet. Your Daily Values may be higher or lower depending on your calorie needs:

		Calories: 2,000	2,500
Total Fat	Less than	65g	80g
Sat Fat	Less than	20g	25g
Cholesterol	Less than	300mg	300mg
Sodium	Less than	2,400mg	2,400mg
Potassium		3,500mg	3,500mg
Total Carbohydrate		300g	375g
Dietary Fiber		25g	30g

Calories per gram:
Fat 9 • Carbohydrate 4 • Protein 4

Ingredients: Whole Corn, Sunflower Oil, Whole Wheat, Rice Flour, Whole Oat Flour, Sugar, Salt, Whey Protein Concentrate, Dry Buttermilk, Whey, Sour Cream (Cultured Cream, Nonfat Dry Milk), Onion Powder, Natural Flavors, Hydrolyzed Soy Protein, Cultured Whey, Corn Starch, Autolyzed Yeast Extract, Mozzarella Cheese (Pasteurized Part Skim Milk, Cheese Cultures, Salt, Enzymes), Citric Acid, Garlic Powder, Gum Arabic, Glycerol, Disodium Phosphate, Spice, and Artificial Color (Including Red 40, Blue 1).
CONTAINS WHEAT, MILK, AND SOY INGREDIENTS.

A

Nutrition Facts (B) — Wheat Crackers

Serving Size   6 Crackers (15g)
Servings Per Container   About 24

Amount Per Serving

Calories 60   Calories from Fat 15

	% Daily Value*
Total Fat 1.5g	**2%**
Saturated Fat 0.5g	**3%**
Trans Fat 0g	
Polyunsaturated Fat 0.5g	
Monounsaturated Fat 0.5g	
Cholesterol 0mg	**0%**
Sodium 160mg	**7%**
Total Carbohydrate 11g	**4%**
Dietary Fiber less than 1g	**1%**
Sugars 1g	
Protein 1g	

Vitamin A 0%	•	Vitamin C 0%
Calcium 0%	•	Iron 2%

*Percent Daily Values are based on a 2,000 calorie diet. Your Daily Values may be higher or lower depending on your calorie needs:

		Calories: 2,000	2,500
Total Fat	Less than	65g	80g
Sat. Fat	Less than	20g	25g
Cholesterol	Less than	300mg	300mg
Sodium	Less than	2,400mg	2,400mg
Total Carbohydrate		300g	375g
Dietary Fiber		25g	30g

Ingredients: Enriched flour (wheat flour, niacin, reduced iron, thiamin mononitrate [vitamin B₁], riboflavin [vitamin B₂], folic acid), partially hydrogenated soybean and/or cottonseed oil† with TBHQ for freshness, sugar, contains two percent or less of salt, leavening (baking soda, sodium acid pyrophosphate, monocalcium phosphate), corn syrup, high fructose corn syrup, sodium stearoyl lactylate, sodium sulfite, soy lecithin.
†Less than 0.5g *trans* fat per serving
CONTAINS WHEAT, AND SOY INGREDIENTS.

B

Nutrition Facts (C) — Pretzels

Serving Size 18 Pretzels (30g)
Servings Per Container about 8

Amount Per Serving

Calories 120   Calories from Fat 0

	% Daily Value*
Total Fat 0g	**0%**
Saturated Fat 0g	**0%**
Trans Fat 0g	
Cholesterol 0mg	**0%**
Sodium 320mg	**13%**
Total Carbohydrate 25g	**8%**
Dietary Fiber 2g	**8%**
Sugars 3g	
Protein 3g	

Vitamin A 0%	•	Vitamin C 0%
Calcium 0%	•	Iron 2%

*Percent Daily Values are based on a 2,000 calorie diet. Your Daily Values may be higher or lower depending on your calorie needs:

		Calories: 2,000	2,500
Total Fat	Less than	65g	80g
Sat Fat	Less than	20g	25g
Cholesterol	Less than	300mg	300mg
Sodium	Less than	2,400mg	2,400mg
Total Carbohydrate		300g	375g
Dietary Fiber		25g	30g

Calories per gram:
Fat 9 • Carbohydrate 4 • Protein 4

Ingredients: Organic wheat flour, water, organic oat flour and oat bran, organic evaporated cane juice, salt, yeast, sodium bicarbonate.
Allergy information: Produced in a facility that handles peanut butter.

C

FIGURE 33-8 Examples of food labels from (A) potato chips, (B) wheat crackers, and (C) pretzels.

All three snack items contain TFA. These snacks should be avoided or eaten sparingly.

In terms of sodium, calories, and sugar, pretzels have the most sodium, but all three are high in sodium.

All three are low in sugar. Their calories are nearly the same as are the amounts of fiber and protein. The pretzels have the most carbohydrates, and the crackers have the most artificial flavors, colors, and preservatives.

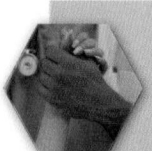

Patient Education

Encourage patients to read and evaluate food labels. Typically, they should look for:

- The lowest amount of total fat, saturated fat, and trans fat. Calories from fat should not be more than 30% of total calories.

- No cholesterol or low cholesterol. Total cholesterol should be less than 300 milligrams (mg) per day.

- Low sodium content. Total sodium should be less than 2,400 mg per day.

- High fiber. Fiber intake should be as high as possible.

- Vitamins and minerals. Some vitamins and minerals occur naturally and sometimes they are added to food during processing.

NUTRITION AT VARIOUS STAGES OF LIFE

For the nutrients discussed in the preceding sections, ranges of suggested normal requirements were given. These ranges should be used as a guide, remembering that each individual is unique, and requirements will vary.

Pregnancy and Lactation

Pregnancy and lactation both cause marked changes in a woman's body and both require an increase in various nutrients. During pregnancy, not only does the growth of the fetus require additional nutrients, but the growth of the placenta, the increase in adipose tissue in the mother, the increased volume of blood, and the growth of breast tissue also require additional nutrients.

The increased demand for nutrients is not just a demand for calories, but also for other specific nutrients to be increased, most notably protein. Protein requirements are nearly double during pregnancy. Because of the role vitamins play in metabolism and structure, they are needed in greater quantities than usual. In addition, calcium, phosphorus, and iron are needed in such high amounts that usually a vitamin supplement is prescribed. It is important that diet modifications are not simply an increase in calories but include quality foods high in minerals, vitamins, and protein.

Pregnancy is an important time for both fetus and mother. It is normal and healthy for the mother to gain weight. Her provider will determine the appropriate amount of weight gain based on the individual. A general rule of thumb is 25 to 35 pounds. During lactation, the requirement for higher levels of nutrients continues; however, overall, it is not as high as during pregnancy. A baby is more likely to be healthy and develop normally if the mother has good nutritional habits during pregnancy and breast-feeding. A baby born to a mother who is malnourished may suffer from intellectual disability and be of lower birth weight. Lower birth weight babies (less than 5.5 pounds) have a greater mortality rate than do babies of normal weight.

Breast-Feeding

There are several reasons why breast-feeding is encouraged. The nutrition the infant receives from breast milk is a perfect combination of water, lactose (sugar), fat, and protein. There are more than 100 ingredients in breast milk that are not found in formula milk. There are no allergic

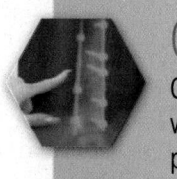

Critical Thinking

Consider your response to a teenage girl who refuses to gain weight during her pregnancy. Answer the following questions:

- How would you apply active listening skills to this situation?
- How do you respond honestly and diplomatically to your patient's concerns?

reactions to mother's milk. (On occasion, if the mother eats a particular food, the infant may react by being fussy.) Breast-feeding is nutritionally sound, economical, and sterile. Breast milk is easily digested and does not easily cause gastrointestinal upsets. Breast-fed babies receive temporary antibodies to many diseases from their mothers. Mother and infant bond during breast-feeding. Breast-feeding helps contract the uterus and bring it back to its nonpregnant state, thus helping to control postpartum bleeding.

While breast-feeding, the mother will continue to require nutritious foods taken from the MyPlate guidelines and will need to maintain the increased caloric intake that was required during pregnancy. If she consumes inadequate calories, the amount of milk produced will be decreased. When the mother terminates the period of breast-feeding (6 months is recommended for the greatest benefit to the infant), the mother's caloric intake should be reduced to avoid gaining weight.

Infancy

Infancy is a time of continuous growth. In the first year of life, the baby will triple birth weight. The infant will need two to three times more calories per kilogram (kg) of body weight than the normal adult. This is true for protein as well, and most of the vitamins and minerals are required at greater levels per kilogram. Most of these can be furnished with breast milk or formula; however, once iron stores have been used up, usually in 3 to 6 months, the infant will require an iron supplement, which is why pediatricians often prescribe an infant liquid iron supplement. Because of the high rate of growth, especially of the nervous system, infancy is an important time to be sure nutritional requirements are met. It is important to keep in mind that according to some pediatricians, overfeeding in infancy might lead to childhood obesity.

Childhood

Good eating habits develop during childhood. One way parents who have good eating habits can teach their children how to eat healthfully is by example. A family's healthy eating habits, physical activity, and an overall healthy lifestyle help children to adopt healthy habits. Poor habits can be established during childhood and are often difficult to alter. This can lead to lifelong health problems such as obesity, diabetes, and cardiovascular diseases. The effects of poor nutrition are not only physical but can be emotional as well. When an obese child is "picked on" in school, anxiety, low self-esteem, depression, and irritability can result.

Childhood obesity is a serious problem that can lead to type 2 diabetes mellitus because the disease is related to being overweight and having a poor diet. Children who are obese have a greatly increased chance of becoming obese as adults if they are obese before becoming a preteen (around age 11 years). Osteoporosis and cardiovascular diseases are other problems obesity can cause.

The availability of electronic devices such as computers, video games, and television, contribute greatly to a child's reluctance to be active. Bike riding, jumping rope, swimming, and running are activities that most children enjoy if encouraged to engage in them.

Fast foods and carbonated sodas contribute to obesity because of their high fat and sugar content. They are even banned from some schools because they are consumed readily and are poor choices at any age.

Clearly, parental education (and therefore education of their children) about exercise and good nutrition is an excellent way to stop childhood obesity and type 2 diabetes mellitus. By following MyPlate, as recommended by the USDA, parents and children can learn to be active every day and to make healthy food choices. The government Web site (http://www.ChooseMyPlate.gov) gives ideas on how everyone in the family can eat better and exercise more.

Adolescence

During adolescence, individuals experience the greatest levels of growth. The period of growth varies from person to person but generally begins sooner with girls. Except for times of pregnancy and lactation, the need for total nutrients is greatest at this stage of growth. At the end of the growth spurt, nutrient requirements decrease, and young adults must then also decrease the amount of food they consume and must exercise regularly.

Two particular nutrients that especially need to be altered during adolescence are iron and calcium. Iron requirements increase for the female individual as she begins menstruation. Calcium requirements increase for both male and female individuals because bone development is occurring at a rapid rate.

Bulimia and Anorexia Nervosa. Two eating disorders that may occur at any age are **bulimia** and anorexia nervosa, and they are serious in all affected individuals. Girls are more likely than boys to suffer from these problems, although eating disorders are on the rise among the male population. The diets of adolescent girls in general are deficient in calories, vitamins, protein, and, as previously mentioned, iron and calcium. Many girls have concerns about their weight coupled with poor eating habits; when taken to extremes, these can result in bulimia or anorexia nervosa. When a patient is diagnosed with bulimia or anorexia nervosa, the provider monitors the patient's weight gain or loss, orders laboratory tests at each clinic visit, and makes an appropriate treatment plan.

These tasks are facilitated by the patient's medical record, as the patient's weight pattern can be viewed graphically and test results can be easily accessed

Bulimia. Bulimia can be life threatening because it can result in an electrolyte imbalance. Dental caries, malnutrition, dehydration, and eroded mouth and esophagus are other problems related to the continuous exposure to stomach and digestive juices. Individuals with bulimia binge on food and then purge (vomit). Use of laxatives is common. Girls fear becoming overweight and usually binge on high-calorie dessert-type foods, then self-induce vomiting. Psychological therapy may help.

Anorexia Nervosa. Anorexia nervosa can be life threatening. It is characterized by an individual severely restricting caloric intake and exercising excessively. Problems that can occur are low blood pressure, alopecia, altered metabolism, amenorrhea, brain damage, and death.

Both bulimia and anorexia nervosa seem to have some basis in U.S. culture, with teenagers (mostly women) wanting to look like the slim supermodels and fashion models seen in movies and in magazines. Exposure to such media images may result in a teenager's body image becoming distorted.

These eating disorders are serious, and relapses are not unusual. Sometimes, they become a lifelong struggle, and repeated therapy sessions are needed.

Anorexia and bulimia are some of the most life-threatening disorders among the mental health disorders.

Older Adults

Aging is a natural process of the body. Although aging occurs in different stages and at different rates for each individual, some generalities can be made. As we age, our cellular metabolism tends to slow and, coupled with a general decline in physical activity, results in a decreased requirement for calories. At the same time, there may be an increase in nutrient requirement in special circumstances. There is always an increased requirement for nutrients, vitamins, and protein during illness, especially the prolonged illnesses that may occur in older adults. With aging, there may be increased breakdown of cells; as a result, there is an increased requirement for nutrients that repair and build cells and tissues. There is also a need to ingest more nutrients because of decreased absorption within the digestive tract. Thus, although there is less need for calories, there is more need for nutrient-rich foods. Less need for calories along with less physical activity may lead to weight gain if calorie intake is not reduced.

This may become difficult for older adults for several reasons. One reason may be an individual's psychological state. Loneliness and depression affect many older adults, especially after the loss of a spouse. Older adults may not like the idea of eating alone. The economic status of the individual also may present problems, as after retirement income generally decreases. Physiologically, taste tends to diminish with age and interest in food may decrease. In addition, problems with teeth and a decrease in salivary gland secretions may make eating painful. Many medications cause a decrease in saliva production. Also, decreased motility in the gastrointestinal tract may lead to constipation, making eating uncomfortable. All these factors, as well as a general unwillingness to break old habits, may make it difficult to change the diet to keep up with the body's aging process.

THERAPEUTIC DIETS

Presentation

Thus far, this chapter has examined the nutrient requirements of the body under normal conditions. There are times, however, when the body becomes diseased and nutrient requirements change. These changes may be necessitated by disease states such as diabetes mellitus or conditions resulting from a poor diet such as obesity. Therapeutic diets are designed to overcome or control these conditions.

Procedure

The diet can be modified in a number of ways. The number of overall calories can be adjusted, or one type of nutrient can be restricted or encouraged. The consistency, texture, and spiciness of food can be varied. The frequency of eating can be increased or decreased. When counseling patients, remember that habits are hard to change. The medical assistant should be supportive and encouraging (see Procedure 33-1).

Weight Control

Overweight and underweight are both weight disorders. The problem in defining overweight or underweight stems from the fact that there is no ideal weight for an entire population. There is only an ideal weight for the individual. Ideal weight can depend on many factors including age, sex, lean muscle mass, bone structure, and physical activity. Obesity is generally considered being more than 20% overweight. Underweight is weight 10% to 15% below average. Height–weight tables now generally give ranges that vary more than 20 pounds. The ratio of fat tissue to lean muscle mass is a better indicator than a specific weight of whether individuals are at their ideal weight.

Individuals will gain weight if they consume more calories than they need. Conversely, individuals will lose weight if they use more calories than they ingest. In either case, the individual must bring the amount of calories ingested into balance with the amount used. For the overweight individual, this means either decreasing calorie consumption or increasing calorie usage, or both. For the underweight individual, it usually means focusing entirely on increasing calorie consumption.

Weight loss has become a big business. However, individuals do not need to spend tremendous amounts of money to lose weight; patient education about low-calorie, low-salt foods and a moderate exercise program are basic starting points for weight loss. Because losing more than 1 to 2 pounds a week can put an individual into nutritional deficiency, goals should not be set higher than this. Modifications made to the diet should then be maintained even after the weight is lost and should be continued throughout life. Losing weight takes much effort, and the patient needs constant encouragement and support from medical personnel and family.

Obesity has become a serious health problem. It is defined as being severely overweight and having a body mass index (BMI) of 30 or above. BMI is calculated using height and weight to determine an individual's total amount of body fat. Go to https://www.nhlbi.nih.gov and search "BMI" to calculate your own BMI.

Genetics may play a role in obesity. Several genes affect the rate at which the body burns calories. Playing a major role in obesity are family eating habits, other lifestyle habits, physical activity levels, and psychological factors such as stress and depression. Major causes of obesity are lack of physical exercise, oversized portions of high-fat foods, and the accessibility of fast foods. Many people eat more food than their bodies need.

Obesity causes increased risk for hypertension, heart and lung disease, hip and knee problems, certain cancers, and diabetes, and it shortens the life span.

Parents can be role models and teach their children to eat nutritious foods and not to consume more calories than their bodies need. Parents should provide nourishing foods, limit inactivity such as television and computer time, engage the entire family in regular exercise, eat at regular mealtimes at the table, and encourage the family to drink plenty (six to eight glasses) of water daily. By parents setting good examples when their children are young, the children will learn that healthy eating habits and regular exercise will improve the quality of life (fewer illnesses) and prolong the length of life.

The American Heart Association and the American Cancer Society are community resources with information about reducing the risk for heart disease and cancer. Keeping weight under control and regular exercise help prevent heart attacks, hypertension, and certain cancers.

Because there has been a great deal of media attention given to the problem of obesity and the diseases it can cause, many people are looking for a quick fix to lose weight. There are many claims that people can lose weight without exercising or eating healthy foods. Most claims about weight loss products are deceptive or false.

Individuals who want to lose weight must strive to eat a healthful diet over time. A healthful diet together with regular exercise can reduce their risk for hypertension, coronary artery disease, and certain cancers (colon and breast).

Diabetes Mellitus

Diabetes mellitus is a disease in which there is either reduced or no production of insulin, or in which there is reduced or no response to insulin. Approximately 9% of the population has diabetes mellitus (type 1 or type 2) in some form. Most patients with type 2 diabetes are not dependent on insulin and can control their condition by monitoring diet, exercise, and weight.

Normally, after a meal, the body secretes the hormone insulin, which makes its way to all cells of the body. Insulin signals the cells that glucose is available and should be brought in so that it can be converted to energy. If the cells do not receive this signal, or do not respond to it, their ability to use glucose is markedly reduced. Because the body uses glucose as its main energy source, the ramifications of this affect almost every tissue of the body. In addition, the high level of glucose that remains in the bloodstream puts a tremendous strain on the kidneys and other major body organs, causing problems such as myocardial infarction, vascular diseases, neuropathy, and infections.

The effects of diabetes mellitus can be controlled with a general goal of maintaining a regular level of glucose in the bloodstream, avoiding large fluctuations between high and low levels. There are several ways suggested to accomplish this. Total calories need not be altered, unless the patient with diabetes is overweight. However, the ratio of carbohydrate, fat, and protein must be closely monitored. Total carbohydrates should be increased, but simple sugars should be avoided. Because of the slower rate of digestion and absorption of complex carbohydrates, these will be released over a longer period and will prevent a sudden high level of glucose in the bloodstream; thus, these are the type of carbohydrates people with diabetes need. Increasing fiber content also increases the time of absorption and decreases the likelihood of sudden increases in glucose levels in the bloodstream. Regular snacks may be added between meals to maintain levels of glucose. The trend is for patients to take charge of their own care. The medical assistant's role as educator will be an important one to facilitate patient self-management.

Type 2 Diabetes and Obesity. Obesity has become epidemic in the United States and is the most significant factor in the increase in diabetes. In 1990, obese adults made up approximately 15% of the population. Today, nationwide, roughly two out of three U.S. adults are overweight or obese. Children and young people who are obese are being diagnosed with type 2 diabetes at an extremely high rate. The longer individuals have diabetes, the greater their risk for development of the complications of the disease, including heart disease, stroke, kidney disease, blindness, and infections. Diabetes is a major cause of death.

Prevention of type 2 diabetes is of utmost importance. Changes in lifestyle such as weight loss, regular exercise, and a nutritious diet can prevent type 2 diabetes. If a patient has type 2 diabetes, it can be controlled by diet and exercise and by medication (see Chapter 35 for more information about diabetes and insulin).

Cardiovascular Disease

Cardiovascular disease is currently the leading cause of death in the United States. The unfortunate aspect of this situation is that much of it is preventable. Cardiovascular disease encompasses a variety of problems. Two of these problems, hypertension and atherosclerosis, often work hand in hand to perpetuate one another until a myocardial infarction occurs. It is important to remember that the conditions leading up to a myocardial infarction do not occur overnight. They develop slowly over many years, often asymptomatically. These conditions can be reduced or prevented with lifestyle modifications such as a healthy diet, moderate exercise, cessation of smoking, and weight management. This section focuses on a healthy diet to prevent cardiovascular disease.

Hypertension, or increased blood pressure, is often of unknown cause. Sometimes, it has a familial connection. When blood pressure is only moderately increased, certain diet modifications can be used to reduce it. If it is severe, drug therapy may be used in conjunction with diet therapy. One of the largest diet factors in controlling increased blood pressure is restricting sodium, because it can play such an important role in maintenance of water levels in the body. Salt sensitivity is a measure of how your blood pressure responds to salt and, therefore, sodium intake. With the increase of salt in the diet, the greater the concentration of sodium in the body. High sodium impacts water retention in the cells and tissues of the body. An increased volume of blood and water will increase the pressure on the blood vessel walls. Eliminating sodium includes more than simply eliminating use of table salt. Foods that are particularly high in sodium include smoked meats, luncheon meats, olives, pickles, chips, crackers, catsup, and cheese. In some cases, eliminating foods with only moderate salt levels may be indicated. These may include certain meats, breads containing baking powder or baking soda, shellfish, and some vegetables.

Atherosclerosis is another condition that can lead to a myocardial infarction. Atherosclerosis is narrowing of the arteries because of deposits of fatty substance. It should not be confused with arteriosclerosis, which is a narrowing of the arteries because of loss of the elasticity of the arterial wall. Atherosclerosis leads to arteriosclerosis, which generally occurs because of a lack of exercise and increased blood cholesterol levels. The elasticity can be regained by increasing activity, although it should be started slowly and under a provider's guidance. Atherosclerosis and arteriosclerosis often occur together. Smoking and hypertension will increase the likelihood of development of both of these conditions.

The conditions of atherosclerosis and arteriosclerosis facilitate each other. The fatty deposits associated with atherosclerosis tend to occur at points of damage to the inner walls of the artery. One of the causes of this damage is high pressure at points where there may be narrowing because of deposits that are already there, or because of the constriction of blood vessels due to nicotine. Carbon monoxide brought into the bloodstream during smoking also causes damage to the arterial walls. The deposits and hardening increase the blood pressure, which, in turn, causes more damage and more deposits. It is a cycle that is difficult to stop. The best solution is prevention.

Fats and cholesterol in the diet have been strongly implicated in atherosclerosis. It is not only total fat that is important, but also the types of fat ingested. The effect of high levels of fats and cholesterol in the diet will vary among individuals, and the key factor in atherosclerosis is the level of these substances in the bloodstream. Some individuals are able to ingest high amounts of fat and cholesterol without the body maintaining high levels in the blood. Unfortunately, this is not the case for everyone, and fat and cholesterol levels in the bloodstream must be closely monitored. Fat levels are measured by looking at triglycerides and lipoproteins. Lipoproteins are complex structures made of fatty acids and proteins and are used to carry fat and cholesterol in the bloodstream. LDL are used by the body to transport fats and cholesterol to the body tissues. These are the lipoproteins more likely to deposit cholesterol and fat onto the arterial wall. HDL carry fats and cholesterol to the liver to be broken down and used. These lipoproteins are more likely to remove fats and cholesterol from the deposits on the arterial walls. HDL levels can be increased by exercise.

The Nurses' Health Study, conducted by Harvard University, showed an association between the intake of hydrogenated fats (trans fats) and heart disease. The women who consumed high levels of foods that contained hydrogenated fats experienced a much greater risk for having a heart attack than did the women who consumed few hydrogenated fats. Harvard School of Public Health researchers have found that hydrogenated fats are in part responsible for the thousands of premature heart disease deaths in the United States every year. Trans fats have also been implicated in increasing the risk for type 2 diabetes.

If total serum cholesterol and LDL levels are found to be increased, the individual must modify the diet, and, if severe enough, drug therapy may be indicated. The percentage of calories from fat should be kept to less than 25% to 30% of total daily dietary intake, with less than a third of these coming from saturated fats. Cholesterol consumption should be less than 200 mg per day.

If a person experiences a myocardial infarction, it is important that the heart muscle be allowed to rest to facilitate proper healing. This includes bed rest initially, with a gradual progression to limited activity over about a 2-week period. Depending on the severity of damage from the MI and overall health, the recovery period is individualized. Rehabilitation consists of cessation of smoking; control of hypertension; weight reduction through a low-fat, low-calorie diet; and a program of exercise. All help to improve myocardial function.

Cancer

Some substances ingested or inhaled are thought to be carcinogenic. For example, nitrites that are found in foods such as smoked ham or bacon are thought to cause cancer of the stomach and esophagus. Smoking tobacco, although not a food, has been implicated in cancers of the mouth, larynx, esophagus, and lungs. High fat in the diet has been shown to be associated with cancer of the breast, uterus, and colon.

High fiber in the diet may protect from colon cancer. Foods with vitamins A and C protect from cancer of the stomach, lung, and bladder. Fruits and vegetables, legumes, and foods with soy may protect from certain cancers.

Wise choices of foods from MyPlate, avoiding foods with known carcinogens, keeping weight under control, and practicing a healthy lifestyle will improve the quality and length of life.

Cancer is a disease that comes in a variety of forms. It generally occurs when the normal regulatory mechanisms within a cell have broken down. The result is that cells continue to grow in an unrestrained manner, diverting energy and nutrients from the patient's body to the cells' uncontrolled growth. There are many stages through which these cells may go, and they will go through them at varying rates. The ramifications of this new growth will vary depending on what types of cells are affected.

For these reasons, each patient who has cancer will have varying nutritional requirements. However, there are some generalities that can be made. First, there is definitely a need for increased calories. Because the new cancerous growth has the ability to divert nutrients to itself, the result is that the body receives fewer nutrients. It will then break down its own tissue. In addition, there is an increased need for nutrient intake to supply the immune system with the energy and nutrients it needs in its attempt to destroy the cancerous cells.

The patient who is receiving chemotherapy or radiation treatment has an even greater need for increased nutrients. These therapies are directed at killing cells that are rapidly dividing. Affected cells include not only the cancerous cell but also healthy cells such as those of the lining of the gastrointestinal tract and hair follicles. Increased nutrients are needed for repair and replacement of the lost cells, and protein levels in particular should be increased. Because of the disturbance of the gastrointestinal lining, digestion and absorption may also be decreased. It is important that the patient maintain as healthy a nutritional status as is possible rather than have to make up for nutritional deficiencies.

The patient may experience loss of appetite, as well as nausea and vomiting. There are several ways to cope with this. First, food should be made as appealing as possible. If the patient has difficulty swallowing, food can be liquefied in a food processor or blender. Generally, food will be better tolerated if it is slightly chilled; extremes of temperature should be avoided. Several smaller meals may be easier to eat than three larger meals.

If patients lose large amounts of weight because of worry or concern or as a result of chemotherapy and/or radiation, they may become **cachectic**. In such cases, a tube is passed into the patient's stomach or duodenum through the nose, or directly into the jejunum, and liquid feedings are given through the tube. This is referred to a parenteral nutrition or tube feeding. Another method for providing nutrition to a patient who is unable to take in necessary amounts of food is through an intravenous catheter inserted into the subclavian vein to the superior vena cava, and this is known as total parenteral nutrition (TPN). Feedings via the catheter provide very good nutrition and can be given for prolonged periods.

Procedure

Providing Instruction for Health Maintenance and Disease Prevention

PURPOSE:

To instruct patients about how to exercise more responsibility for and take control of their health in order to extend their lives and enjoy healthy years.

With the provider's permission, medical assistants have many opportunities on a daily basis to educate patients about ways to stay healthy and reduce the risk of disease. Patient education boxes throughout this textbook relate specific behaviors patients can adopt to prevent diseases and measures they can take to preserve health.

EQUIPMENT/SUPPLIES:

- Discussion
- DVDs
- Print material
- Authenticated Web-based interactive information
- Community resources directories
- Seminars
- Classes (self-directed and self-paced)

PROCEDURE STEPS:

1. Gather materials to be utilized during the educational session for health maintenance and disease prevention.

2. Select a quiet and private area to begin the instruction.

3. *Introduce yourself and identify patient* using two patient identifiers.

4. Assess the patient's learning style and preference. *Involve the patient's support system.* RATIONALE: The patient's age, physical limitations, and learning preferences need to be taken into consideration by the medical assistant. The patient's family will learn along with the patient and provide instruction and encouragement to the patient at home.

5. *Speaking at the patient's level of understanding,* provide information to the patient regarding a specific illness, medical management, health maintenance, and/or disease prevention. Instruct patient, as appropriate, to:

   - Schedule regular screenings for illness as is age appropriate (e.g., yearly examinations, Pap smear, mammogram, occult blood testing, colonoscopy, urinalysis, ECG, CXR, anemia testing, chemistry profiles, hearing and vision testing)
   - Avoid tobacco
   - Exercise at least 30 minutes a day most days of the week
   - Maintain a balanced diet (http://www.choosemyplate.gov)
   - Practice safety to prevent injuries (make sure smoke detectors work, wear seat belts, do not drink and drive)
   - Control weight, blood pressure, and cholesterol
   - Watch sun exposure and use sun block factor of at least SPF 30 all year
   - Keep vaccine immunization current
   - Practice food safety by preparing food with clean hands and on clean surfaces

(continues)

6. Educate patients who do not have a home computer that they can access information at the public library. With the prevalence of smart phones and other widely available electronics, there are many ways to access the Internet for information on health maintenance.

7. Some examples of Web sites that could be useful are:
   - General health: http://www.healthfinder.gov
   - Cancer: http://www.cancer.org
   - Osteoporosis: http://www.nof.org
   - Nutrition: http://www.usda.gov or http://www.fda.gov/food
   - Alcohol and drug abuse: https://niaaa.nih.gov
   - Depression: http://www.nimh.nih.gov/health/topics/depression/index.shtml
   - Heart and lung health: http://www.nhlbi.nih.gov
   - Product safety: http://cpsc.gov
   - Heart health: http://heart.org
   - Lung health: http://lung.org

8. Accurately document in the patient's medical record indicating date, time, topic of education, demonstration of patient understanding and planned follow-up.

DOCUMENTATION:

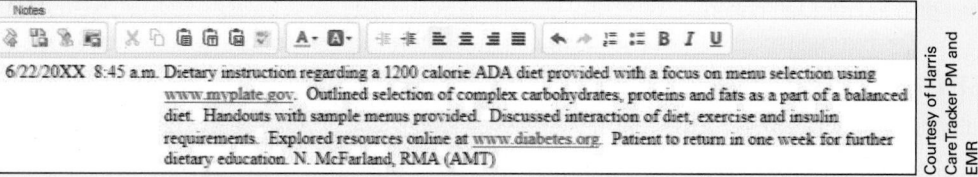

6/22/20XX 8:45 a.m. Dietary instruction regarding a 1200 calorie ADA diet provided with a focus on menu selection using www.myplate.gov. Outlined selection of complex carbohydrates, proteins and fats as a part of a balanced diet. Handouts with sample menus provided. Discussed interaction of diet, exercise and insulin requirements. Explored resources online at www.diabetes.org. Patient to return in one week for further dietary education. N. McFarland, RMA (AMT)

Courtesy of Harris CareTracker PM and EMR

SPECIAL DIETARY REQUIREMENTS

Allergies

More than 50 million Americans have allergies of some kind. An estimated one in 13 children and 3% to 4% percent of adults have food allergies, according to the Centers for Disease Control and Prevention (CDC). Food allergies can occur at any time, even to foods that have been consumed for years with no problems. Allergies to foods occur when the immune system reacts to a food or an ingredient in food as if it is a threat or a danger, much like it reacts to a pathogen. Allergies to foods tend to run in families. Allergies can be mild or as severe as anaphylaxis.

In order to manage food allergies, it is important to avoid those foods or additives that initiate the reaction. There are eight types of food that initiate the majority of allergic reactions. These foods are eggs, fish, shellfish, peanuts, milk, wheat, soy, and tree nuts.

Intake of these foods causes a variety of symptoms. Symptoms may be related to reactions in the integumentary, gastrointestinal, cardiovascular, and respiratory systems. It may take only moments or as long as several hours for the food allergy symptoms to present themselves. There is a severe type of food allergy, referred to as food protein–induced enterocolitis syndrome, or FPIES. FPIES produces dehydration due to profound vomiting and diarrhea. FPIES commonly occurs in infants and children and the diagnosis occurs when the infant or child is exposed to the new food. It is often confused with sepsis or other infectious process.

The first step for a patient to take when a food allergy is suspected is to see an allergist. The allergist will take a detailed history and order skin testing or blood tests to obtain a diagnosis. Food challenges may also be a part of the path to diagnosis. Once an allergy is confirmed, management includes avoiding the causative food.

It is important to read labels to discover ingredients that might cause a reaction, but also to avoid contact with food that might have contaminants during production with the allergy-related food.

If food allergies are severe, as in the case with peanut allergies, and anaphylaxis is a risk, the patient must carry an epinephrine (epi) pen for use if accidental exposure occurs. The epi pen should be used immediately upon the onset of symptoms and the dose may be repeated if instructed by the provider. Emergency medical service (EMS) must be called and upon arrival, the information that epinephrine has been utilized must be shared.

Several strides were made in 2013 related to food allergies. A study was published by the American Academy of Pediatrics indicating that introduction of solid foods earlier than 17 weeks may predispose children to food allergies. This study also encouraged breast-feeding for as long as possible. In the same year, President Obama signed into law the School Access to Emergency Epinephrine Act encouraging states to adopt laws requiring schools to have epinephrine auto-injectors on hand.

Lactose Intolerance

Although not considered a food allergy, other food intolerances exist. Lactose intolerance occurs when the body is unable to digest the natural sugar lactose, which is found in dairy products. The National Institute of Diabetes and Digestive and Kidney Diseases (NIDDK) estimates that 30 to 50 million Americans are lactose intolerant. The body produces an enzyme, lactase, which is responsible for breaking down this sugar. In the case of lactose intolerance, there is a shortage of this enzyme that is manufactured in the small intestine. While lactose intolerance is not life threatening, it can cause extreme discomfort.

If a person is lactose intolerant, symptoms begin within 30 minutes to 2 hours after ingesting dairy products. These symptoms include nausea, cramping, gas, bloating, and diarrhea and are brought on by lactose sugars reacting with bacteria found in the intestinal tract. Also, undigested lactose pulls fluids from the tissues into the intestine, leading to watery diarrhea. Diagnosis of lactose intolerance may include a lactose tolerance test, hydrogen breath test, and stool acidity test.

Treatment for lactose intolerance is aimed at reducing exposure to milk and other dairy products. Lactase can be added to dairy products in order to predigest lactose prior to ingestion. These over-the-counter additives such as Dairy Ease,

Lactaid, and others must be taken just before a meal or snack. Dairy products are important to the diet as sources of calcium, phosphorus, magnesium, and protein. Reduced lactose and lactose-free milk products are widely available in grocery stores. Patients should be cautioned to be label detectives—reading the fine print on labels to make sure that there are not "sneaky" sources of lactose such as caseinate in nondairy creamer.

Gluten Sensitivity

Another intolerance that has gained recognition in the past decade is gluten sensitivity. Around 1% of the population has celiac disease, an autoimmune disorder and a more serious form of gluten sensitivity. Another 18% of the population has a milder form of intolerance.

Gluten is found in grain products that come from wheat, oats, barley, and rye. The proteins in these grains are gut irritants and can cause an inflammatory response. This response results in a problem called intestinal permeability or "leaky gut" syndrome. Intestinal permeability allows substances other than the products of metabolism (protein, sugar, and fat) into the bloodstream. These other products include bacteria, viruses, and indigestible molecules (like gluten) that usually would travel through the intestine and be excreted in the stool. Gliadin, a component of gluten, in the bloodstream causes the immune system to react. This reaction is thought to be a causative factor in Crohn disease and ulcerative colitis, as gliadin is very similar to the cells lining the gut.

Diagnosis of gluten sensitivity can be done anecdotally by taking one of several online gluten sensitivity intolerance self-tests. A formal diagnosis requires a licensed provider to order medical diagnostic tests such as an immune assay, allergy skin testing, genetic testing, and/or an intestinal biopsy.

Treatment of gluten intolerance requires dietary modification to eliminate exposure to the proteins in grains that contain gluten. Antihistamines limit the symptoms by controlling the immune reactions that result in histamine release. If the allergy is severe enough, management of extreme reactions may include epinephrine administration and emergency care.

DIET AND CULTURE

Diversity   Professional

Medical assistants are likely to come into contact with patients from many different ethnic groups. Many of these patients will have diets based on traditional cultures, and some of the foods they eat, or the ways they combine foods, may be unfamiliar to the medical assistant. Often, diets in other cultures are sensible, with foods chosen or combined to make up a complete protein. The medical assistant who has some knowledge of ethnic food choices can help reassure patients that the dietary changes they need to make are within the parameters of their own cultures. Table 33-4 presents some highlights of the food choices of different ethnic groups.

TABLE 33-4

SAMPLE FOOD CHOICES OF VARIOUS CULTURAL, RELIGIOUS, AND ETHNIC GROUPS

CULTURE/REGION/GROUP	DIET AND FOOD CHOICES
Native American	It is thought that approximately half of the edible plants commonly eaten in the United States today originated with the Native Americans. Examples are corn, potatoes, squash, cranberries, pumpkins, peppers, beans, wild rice, and cocoa beans. In addition, they use wild fruits, game, and fish. Foods were commonly prepared as soups and stews, and also dried. The original Native American diets were probably more nutritionally adequate than their current diets, which frequently consist of too high a proportion of sweet and salty, snack-type, empty calorie foods. Native American diets today may be deficient in calcium, vitamins A and C, and riboflavin.
U.S. Southern	Hot breads such as corn bread and baking powder biscuits are common in the U.S. South because the wheat grown in the area does not make good quality yeast breads. Grits and rice are also popular carbohydrate foods. Favorite vegetables include sweet potatoes, squash, green beans, and lima beans. Green beans cooked with pork are commonly served. Watermelon, oranges, and peaches are popular fruits. Fried fish is served often, as are barbecued and stewed meats and poultry. There is a great deal of carbohydrate and fat in these diets and limited amounts of protein in some cases. Iron, calcium, and vitamins A and C may sometimes be deficient.
Mexican	Mexican food is a combination of Spanish and Native American foods. Beans, rice, chili peppers, tomatoes, and corn meal are favorites. Meat is often cooked with vegetables as in chili con carne. Cornmeal is used in a variety of ways to make tortillas and tamales, which serve as bread. The combination of beans and corn makes a complete protein. Although tortillas filled with cheese (called enchiladas) provide some calcium, the use of milk should be encouraged. Additional green and yellow vegetables and vitamin C–rich foods would also improve these diets.
Puerto Rican	Rice is the basic carbohydrate food in Puerto Rican diets. Vegetables and fruits commonly used include beans, plantains, tomatoes, and peppers. Bananas, pineapple, mangoes, and papayas are popular fruits. Favorite meats are chicken, beef, and pork. Milk is not used as much as would be desirable from the nutritional point of view.
Italian	Pastas with various tomato or fish sauces and cheese are popular Italian foods. Fish and highly seasoned foods are common to southern Italian cuisine, whereas meat and root vegetables are common to northern Italy. The eggs, cheese, tomatoes, green vegetables, and fruits common to Italian diets provide excellent sources of many nutrients, but additional milk and meat would improve the diet.
Northern and Western European	Northern and western European diets are similar to those of the U.S. Midwest, but with a greater use of dark breads, potatoes, and fish, and fewer green vegetable salads. Beef and pork are popular, as are various cooked vegetables, breads, cakes, and dairy products.
Central European	Citizens of central Europe obtain the greatest portion of their calories from potatoes and grain, especially rye and buckwheat. Pork is a popular meat. Cabbage cooked in many ways is a popular vegetable, as are carrots, onions, and turnips. Eggs and dairy products are used abundantly.
Middle Eastern	Grains, wheat, and rice provide energy in these diets. Chickpeas in the form of hummus are popular. Lamb and yogurt are commonly used, as are cabbage, grape leaves, eggplant, tomatoes, dates, olives, and figs. Black, very sweet (Turkish) coffee is a popular beverage.

continues

Table 33-4 continued

CULTURE/REGION/GROUP	DIET AND FOOD CHOICES
Chinese	The Chinese diet is varied. Rice is the primary energy food and is used in place of bread. Food is generally cut into small pieces. Vegetables are lightly cooked, and the cooking water is saved for future use. Soybeans are used in many ways, and eggs and pork are commonly served. Soy sauce is extensively used, but it is salty and could present a problem for patients on low-salt diets. Tea is a common beverage, but milk is not. This diet may be low in fat.
Japanese	Japanese diets include rice, soybean paste and curd, vegetables, fruits, and fish. Food is frequently served tempura style, which means fried. Soy sauce (shoyu) and tea are commonly used. Current Japanese diets have been greatly influenced by Western culture.
Southeast Asian	Many Indians are vegetarians who use eggs and dairy products. Rice, peas, and beans are frequently served. Spices, especially curry, are popular. Indian meals are not typically served in courses as Western meals are. They generally consist of one course with many dishes.
Thai, Vietnamese, Laotian, and Cambodian	Rice, curries, vegetables, and fruit are popular in Thailand, Vietnam, Laos, and Cambodia. Meat, chicken, and fish are used in small amounts. The wok (a deep, round fry pan) is used for sautéing many foods. A salty sauce made from fermented fish is commonly used.
Jewish	Interpretations of the Jewish dietary laws vary. Those who adhere to the Orthodox view consider tradition important and always observe the dietary laws. Foods prepared according to these laws are called kosher. Conservative Jews are inclined to observe the rules only at home. Reform Jews consider their dietary laws to be essentially ceremonial and thus minimize their significance. Essentially the laws require the following: • Slaughtering must be done by a qualified person, in a prescribed manner. The meat or poultry must be drained of blood, first by severing the jugular vein and carotid artery, then by soaking in brine before cooking. • Meat or meat products may not be prepared with milk or milk products. • The dishes used in the preparation and serving of meat dishes must be kept separate from those used for dairy foods. • A specified time, 6 hours, must elapse between consumption of meat and milk. • The mouth must be rinsed after eating fish and before eating meat. • There are prescribed fast days—Passover week, Yom Kippur, and Feast of Purim. • No cooking is done on the Sabbath—from sundown Friday to sundown Saturday. These laws forbid the eating of: • The flesh of animals without cloven (split) hooves or those that do not chew their cud • Hind quarters of any animal • Shellfish or fish without scales or fins • Fowl that are birds of prey • Creeping things and insects • Leavened (contains ingredients that cause it to rise) bread during the Passover Generally, the food served is rich. Fresh smoked and salted fish and chicken are popular, as are noodles, egg, and flour dishes. These diets can be deficient in fresh vegetables and milk.
Roman Catholic	Although the dietary restrictions of the Roman Catholic religion have been liberalized, meat is not allowed on Ash Wednesday and Fridays during Lent.
Eastern Orthodox	Followers of this religion include Christians from the Middle East, Russia, and Greece. Although interpretations of the dietary laws vary, meat, poultry, fish, and dairy products are restricted on Wednesdays and Fridays and during Lent and Advent.
Seventh Day Adventist	Generally, Seventh Day Adventists are ovo-lacto vegetarians, meaning they use milk products and eggs, but no meat, fish, or poultry. They may also use nuts, legumes, and meat analogues (substitutes) made from soybeans. They consider coffee, tea, and alcohol to be harmful.

continues

Table 33-4 continued

CULTURE/REGION/GROUP	DIET AND FOOD CHOICES
Mormon (Latter Day Saints)	The only dietary restriction observed by Mormons is the prohibition of coffee, tea, and alcoholic beverages.
Islamic	Adherents of Islam are called Muslims. Their dietary laws prohibit the use of pork and alcohol, and other meats must be slaughtered according to specific laws. During the month of Ramadan, Muslims do not eat or drink during daylight hours.
Hindu	To the Hindus, all life is sacred, and small animals contain the souls of ancestors. Consequently, Hindus are usually vegetarians. They do not use eggs because they represent life.
Vegetarians	There are several types of vegetarian diets. The common factor among them is that they do not include red meat. Some include eggs, some fish, some milk, and some even poultry. When carefully planned, these diets can be nutritious. They can contribute to a reduction of obesity, high blood pressure, heart disease, some cancers, and possibly diabetes. They must be carefully planned so they include all needed nutrients. Ovo-lacto vegetarians use dairy products and eggs but no meat, poultry, or fish. Lacto vegetarians use dairy products but no meat, poultry, or eggs.
Vegans	Vegans avoid all animal-based foods. They use soybeans, chickpeas, and meat analogues made from soybeans. It is important that their meals be carefully planned to include appropriate combinations of the nonessential amino acids to provide the needed amino acids. For example, beans served with corn or rice, or peanuts eaten with wheat, are better in such combinations than any of them would be if eaten alone. Vegans can show deficiencies of calcium; zinc; vitamins A, D, and B_{12}; and, of course, proteins.
Zen macrobiotic diets	The macrobiotic diet is a system of 10 diet plans developed from Zen Buddhism. Adherents progress from the lower number diets to the higher, gradually giving up foods in the following order: desserts, salads, fruits, animal foods, soups, and ultimately vegetables, until only cereals—usually brown rice—are consumed. Beverages are kept to a minimum, and only organic foods are used. Foods are grouped as Yang (male) or Yin (female). A ratio of 5:1 Yang to Yin is considered important. Most macrobiotic diets are nutritionally inadequate. As the adherents give up foods according to plans, their diets become increasingly inadequate. These diets can be especially dangerous because avid adherents promise medical cures from the diets that cannot be attained, and thus medical treatment may be delayed when needed.

Vegetarian diets are fairly common around the globe, including in the United States. With a good variety of grains, legumes, vegetables, fruits, and dairy products, a vegetarian diet can supply an individual with all the required nutrients. Pernicious anemia, a disease caused by lack of cobalamin (vitamin B_{12}), is sometimes associated with vegetarian diets that do not contain enough animal proteins (see the section on vitamins in this chapter). One type of vegetarian, the vegan, does not eat any product associated with animals, including milk or eggs. This type of diet is particularly susceptible to nutritional deficiencies. Patients who are vegan or vegetarian need additional dietary discussion to ensure that they are ingesting an adequate amount of amino acids and in the right combination to provide complete proteins. These complete proteins are necessary for cellular repair and maintenance of health.

In speaking with patients about diet and dietary changes, it is important to remember that patients choose their diets for a variety of reasons, including cultural, religious, or ethical beliefs. The medical assistant should respect the patient's reasons for following a certain diet while encouraging any necessary modifications.

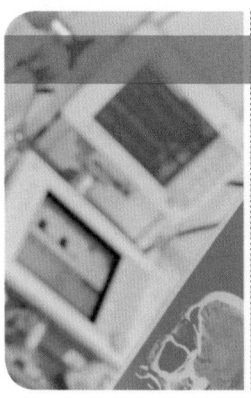

CASE STUDY 33-1

Refer to the scenario at the beginning of the chapter.

CASE STUDY REVIEW

1. What aspects of nutrition must be considered when Becky Slack, RMA (AMT), is considering the nutritional needs of an adolescent?
2. What are key ways that Becky can include parents in the educational process?
3. What guidelines should Becky follow when encouraging adolescents to incorporate exercise in their nutritional plans?

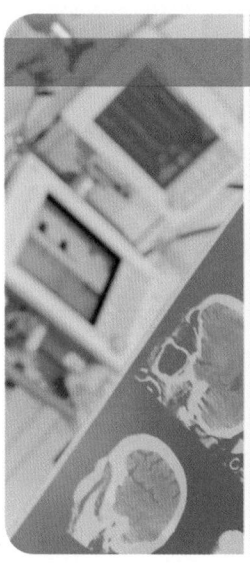

CASE STUDY 33-2

Anita Ferguson is a new patient at Inner City Health Care. She is a 16-year-old girl who is 4 months pregnant and came to the clinic only a couple of weeks ago. After Nancy McFarland, RMA (AMT), took Anita's medical history, and after Anita was examined by the provider, Nancy set aside time to answer any questions Anita might have about her pregnancy. Anita is obviously scared; she wants the baby, but she does not want her life to change. According to the history, Anita has lost a few pounds in the last 2 weeks.

CASE STUDY REVIEW

1. What patient education can Nancy provide to alert Anita to the importance of diet and weight gain during pregnancy?
2. What foods should Nancy encourage Anita to eat?
3. If Anita resists Nancy's suggestions and has not gained any weight by the next visit, how should Nancy proceed?

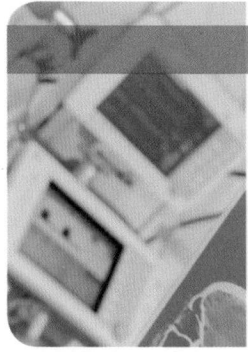

CASE STUDY 33-3

Dr. Lewis prescribed an 1,800-calorie American Diabetes Association (ADA) diet for Mrs. Johnson.

CASE STUDY REVIEW

1. Create a sample 1,800-calorie ADA diet with appropriate amounts of carbohydrates, protein, and fats.
2. Describe the patient education you would use to help Mrs. Johnson understand the diet and to help her reach her goal of improved health.

Summary

- The process of nourishing the body starts with the ingestion of food produced by plants and animals.

- The process of digestion starts in the mouth and continues through the gastrointestinal system until it ends in elimination of the waste products.

- Organic nutrients include carbohydrates, fats, and proteins that provide energy for the body.

- Inorganic nutrients do not contain carbon molecules. Examples of inorganic nutrients are vitamins, minerals, fiber, and water. These nutrients cannot provide energy but are responsible for many vital processes within the body.

- Energy balance occurs when the intake of calories equals the energy used by the body in order to maintain a stable weight.

- Herbal supplements may be medicinal in nature. They are used to treat medical conditions and can interact with pharmaceuticals.

- Learning how to read food labels is an important part of nutrition education.

- Nutritional needs change at various points in the life cycle. During pregnancy, lack of nutrients can be detrimental to the development of the fetus and the health of the expectant mother. The need for nutrients is great during infancy and childhood, with the greatest need for total nutrients occurring during adolescence. During adulthood, the requirement for calories decreases. With the decrease in basal metabolism that occurs with aging, the requirement for calories decreases even more.

- At times of disease, the diet of the individual must be modified to help relieve stress put on the body by the disease; to give energy to fight the disease; and, in cases where the disease is diet related, to decrease the severity of the disease.

- Nutritional status should be examined and adjustments made if necessary with the goal of helping patients maintain a healthy body.

Study for Success

To reinforce your knowledge and skills of information presented in this chapter:

- Review the *Key Terms* and *Learning Outcomes*

- Consider the *Critical Thinking* features and *Case Studies* and discuss your conclusions

- Answer the questions in the *Certification Review*

Procedure

- Perform the *Procedure* using the *Competency Assessment Checklists* on the *Student Companion Website*

CERTIFICATION REVIEW

1. The transfer of nutrients from the gastrointestinal tract into the bloodstream is which of the following processes?
   a. Ingestion
   b. Digestion
   c. Absorption
   d. Elimination

2. As a part of a healthy diet, fat is considered which of the following?
   a. A mineral
   b. A vitamin
   c. An energy nutrient
   d. Fiber
   e. An amino acid

3. The process that is the total of all chemical and physical changes that take place in the body is referred to by which of the following terms?
   a. Homeostasis
   b. Metabolism
   c. A catalyst
   d. An antioxidant
4. What is the significance for the provider in determining the patient's use of herbal supplements?
   a. The FDA has authority over these dietary supplements; therefore, they are safe.
   b. They are unsafe if bought in a supermarket.
   c. They may interact with over-the-counter and prescription medications.
   d. They are not considered medicines. It is not significant to inform the provider.
   e. Many providers prescribe holistic medications first when treating specific disorders.
5. What is another name for vitamin C?
   a. Tocopherol
   b. Carotene
   c. Biotin
   d. Ascorbic acid
6. What are the three energy nutrients?
   a. Vitamins, minerals, and herbal supplements
   b. Fat, carbohydrates, and protein
   c. Cholesterol, starch, and vitamins
   d. Sugar, starch, and fats
   e. Protein, vitamins, and fats

7. Fat-soluble vitamins include which of the following?
   a. A, D, E, and K
   b. C, B, and calcium
   c. A, C, and B
   d. None of these
8. Which of the following information can be found on a nutrition label?
   a. Vitamin content
   b. Protein content
   c. Fat content
   d. Calorie content
   e. All of these
9. What is the function of an antioxidant?
   a. Reduces the amount of fat in our diet
   b. Removes free radicals from our bodies
   c. Increases the amount of energy produced
   d. Impairs overall health
10. During which phase of life do humans triple their body weight?
    a. Infancy
    b. Childhood
    c. Adolescence
    d. Early adulthood
    e. Late adulthood

CHAPTER 34

Basic
Pharmacology

1. Define and spell the key terms as presented in the glossary.
2. Recall five medical uses for drugs.
3. Describe three types of drug names and give an example, for one drug, of all three names.
4. List five sources of drugs.
5. Outline the federal Food, Drug, and Cosmetic Act and the Controlled Substances Act of 1970.
6. Identify the five controlled substance schedules and describe appropriate storage of the substances.
7. Cite the law in terms of administering, prescribing, and dispensing drugs.
8. Describe how to use the four most commonly used sections of the *Physician's Desk Reference* (PDR).
9. Describe the principal actions of drugs and three undesirable reactions.
10. Identify the classifications of medications.
11. Rank the routes of drug administration and drug forms based on most rapid onset of action.
12. Employ correct procedure when handling and storing drugs.
13. Discuss emergency drugs and supplies.
14. Recall commonly abused drugs and describe their physical and emotional effects.
15. Critique the legal role and responsibilities of the medical assistant.

KEY TERMS

absorption	distribution
abuse	elimination
administer	pharmacogenomics
anaphylaxis	pharmacology
bioequivalent	pharmazooticals
biopharmaceuticals	prescribe
biotransformation	pruritus
contraindication	transdermal
controlled substances	urticaria
dispense	

SCENARIO

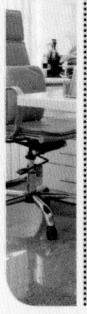

Claire Bloom, CMA (AAMA), is the lead medical assistant for Dr. Jim Hoback, a busy cardiologist. Due to the many look-alike and sound-alike drugs, Ms. Bloom knows that it is very important to have patients bring in their prescription bottles in order to obtain an accurate medication history. She has been assigned the responsibility of developing a policy and procedure to be approved by the provider outlining the appropriate steps for all staff members when taking a medication history. This need for a procedure was identified after a patient reported that he was taking the medication amiloride when in fact the medication that was prescribed was amlodipine. This is an example of one of the drugs on the Institute for Safe Medication Practices list of confused drug names.

Pharmacology is the study of drugs, the science that is concerned with the history, origin, sources, physical and chemical properties, uses, and effects of drugs on living organisms. Medical assistants in the ambulatory care setting need to understand basic pharmacology, including the uses, sources, forms, and delivery routes of drugs; they must know and be able to implement the intent of the law regarding controlled substances and other medications; and they must have a knowledge of drug classifications and actions to be able to caution patients who are taking prescription or nonprescription drugs. In addition, the medical assistant must be able to educate patients about a drug's intended purpose and the correct way to take the drug for maximum effectiveness.

This chapter provides an overview of pharmacology; it is considered a review for medical assistants who have had a formal course in the subject. Information on dosage, calculation, and medication administration can be found in Chapter 35.

USES OF MEDICATIONS

A drug is defined as a medicinal substance that may alter or modify the functions of a living organism. There are five medical uses for drugs:

- *Therapeutic.* Used in the treatment of a condition to relieve symptoms. An example is an antihistamine that may be used in the treatment of an allergy.
- *Diagnostic.* Used in conjunction with radiology and other diagnostic imaging procedures to allow the provider to pinpoint the location of a disease process. An example is dye tablets used in the X-ray study of the gallbladder.
- *Curative.* Used to kill or remove the causative agent of a disease. An example is an antibiotic.
- *Replacement.* Used to replace substances normally found in the body. Hormones and vitamins are examples.
- *Preventive or prophylactic.* Used to ward off or lessen the severity of a disease. Examples are immunizing agents such as vaccines.

RESEARCH AND DEVELOPMENT

It takes an average of 12 years for a drug to make it to market. Six to 7 of those years are spent in the clinical trial phase. The process begins with scientists researching an illness to begin to understand the mechanics of the disease. The goal is to understand the process of change from health to illness from the level of the cellular components. These identified areas are referred to as targets. From this information, the next step is to begin to design chemical compounds and **biopharmaceuticals** that will interrupt the disease process at the selected target.

According to the Tufts Center for the Study of Drug Development, the average cost to research and develop an effective drug is approximately $2.5 billion. Approximately half of that figure is true out-of-pocket funding and the other half is time costs (the time that investors are forgoing while the drug is in development). The estimated $2.5 billion is up dramatically from the last published study result of $800 million in 2003.

Many thousands and sometimes millions of compounds may enter the pipeline for only a few successful drugs to enter the market. For up to 20 years, the new drug is protected by a drug patent. This patent will not allow any other company to make or market the drug. Delaying the transition to generic production allows the originating pharmaceutical company to recoup the investment in research and development to develop the drug.

The Human Genome Project (HGP) was launched on October 1, 1990, and it was completed in 2003. In a joint effort, the U.S. Department of Energy and the National Institutes of Health identified 20,000 to 25,000 genes in human DNA. The sequences in the 3 billion base pairs were also determined. This information is stored in databases that could allow access to these technologies by the private sector, such as pharmaceutical companies. By discovering the pharmacogenomics, drug companies can focus on the creation of drugs specifically for genome targets. The process works in this manner: The structure of the genomes is understood, then the biology of the genomes is understood, leading to understanding the biology of the disease, and thus the science of medicine is advanced and eventually, delivery of health care is improved. This is especially true in the area of pharmaceuticals.

Pharmacogenomics is the study of the response of the body to various chemical compounds based on an individual's genetic inheritance. This knowledge could allow medications to be tailored to each individual and his or her disease process in the future. There is also potential for the creation of more effective medications. An added benefit is that the provider could prescribe the right drug the first time for a patient. Dosing could be customized more appropriately than current methods.

Utilizing **pharmacogenomics**, pharmaceutical companies could reduce the number of potential chemical compounds that are researched and get an effective drug to market more rapidly and at less cost. Genomic data can lead to specific target identification and scientifically informed drug design. Based on evidence from the genome data, scientists can tailor trial medications that have a higher efficacy with fewer side effects as well as guide gene therapies for illnesses such as cancer.

DRUG NAMES

Most drugs have three types of names: chemical, generic, and trade or brand name.

- The *chemical name* describes the drug's molecular structure and identifies its chemical structure. Chemical names begin with a lowercase letter.

- The *generic name* is the drug's official name and is assigned to the drug by the United States Adopted Names Council. A generic drug can be manufactured by more than one pharmaceutical company. When this is the case, each company markets the drug under its own unique trade or brand name. Generic names begin with a lowercase letter.

- A *trade* or *brand name* is registered by the U.S. Patent and Trademark Office and is approved by the U.S. Food and Drug Administration (FDA). The ® symbol following a drug's trade or brand name indicates that the name is registered and protected for 17 years. No other manufacturer can make or sell the drug during that time. Once the patent expires, any manufacturer can sell the drug under its generic name or a new trade name. The original trade name cannot be reused. The brand name begins with a capital letter.

Example:

Chemical name: 1, 4:3, 6-dian hydrosorbitol-2, 5 dinitrate

Generic name: isosorbide dinitrate

Trade/Brand name: Sorbitrate

When providers prescribe a drug, they may use either the generic or trade name. It is not uncommon for providers to prescribe the generic form of

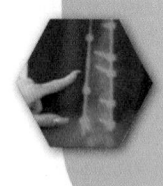

Critical Thinking

Describe how you can expand your knowledge base as it relates to the medications that are commonly used in your provider's practice.

a drug because it is usually less costly for the patient. To reduce costs, some insurance companies pay for only generic brands. Sometimes, providers specify drugs by their trade names. Some states allow patients to request that their pharmacist dispense the generic drug equivalent unless the provider has specified that the drug be dispensed by its trade name.

The U.S. Food and Drug Administration (FDA) maintains strict regulations regarding generic drugs. In order for a copy of a brand-name drug to be allowed to enter the market, generic drugs must have the same high quality, strength, purity, and stability as the innovator drug. Generics must be **bioequivalent** to the original. In some states, a pharmacist may select a generic form of a drug if not specifically directed otherwise by the provider. Generic and trade name drugs have the same chemical composition and must adhere to identical FDA standards; therefore, according to most state laws, they can be used interchangeably. The drug label reflects the drug products contained within.

HISTORY AND SOURCES OF DRUGS

Diversity

Drugs prepared from roots, herbs, bark, and other forms of plant life are among the earliest known pharmaceuticals. Their origin can be traced back to primitive cultures, where they were first used to evoke magical powers and to drive out evil spirits. Once it was discovered that certain plants were pharmacologically useful, a search was started for sources of drugs.

Today, this search continues. In addition to plants, drugs are derived from animals and minerals and are produced in laboratories using chemical, biochemical, and biotechnologic processes.

Plant Sources

The leaves, roots, stems, or fruit of certain plants may have medicinal properties. For example, the dried leaf of the foxglove plant (*Digitalis purpurea*) is a source of digitalis, a cardiac glycoside used in the treatment of certain heart conditions.

Herbals fit into this plant source category. The disadvantage of many natural herbals on the market today is that some drugs derived from plants may not be standardized. In any given crop, there may be plants that are more or less potent than their neighboring plants. This lack of consistency is related to the amount of sunshine and water a particular plant receives, as well as the nutrients in the soil. Another disadvantage of natural plant drugs is the pesticides that may be present. These may be humanmade pesticides applied to the plants or taken up by the plant through the environment (soil, water, and air); they may also be natural pesticides originating from the plant itself to defend itself from molds, insects, and other threats. These pesticides all pose biologic threats to our chemical and biologic functioning. These foreign chemicals can be interpreted by our bodies as irritants, free radicals, antigens, and/or antagonists. For these reasons, patients should be cautioned to purchase only reputable, standardized, natural herbal products.

Animal Sources

A few drugs are obtained from tissues such as the adrenal glands of animals. Drugs of this type are referred to as **pharmazooticals**. Specific examples of drugs obtained from animals are adrenaline and cortisone, extracted from the adrenal glands of animals. Adrenaline is used for allergic reactions and cortisone is an anti-inflammatory. Premarin is another example. It is derived from urine produced by pregnant mares. It is used for treating menopausal symptoms in some women.

Some drugs are derived from unusual animal sources. For example, Captopril, an ACE inhibitor that is widely utilized to treat hypertension, is derived from a chemical substance found in the Brazilian arrowhead viper.

Mineral Sources

Some naturally occurring mineral substances are used in medicine in a highly purified form. One such mineral is sulfur, which has been used as a key ingredient in certain bacteriostatic drugs. It is now prepared synthetically and used in the treatment of urinary and intestinal tract infections.

Lithium is used to treat episodes of mania associated with a diagnosis of bipolar disease. Lithium is a mineral that is present in some rocks and in the sea.

Herbal Supplements

With the increased interest in alternative or complementary medicine, many patients and some practitioners use herbal products for treatment, prophylaxis, and maintenance of health and care of disease. *Phytomedicine* is the term used to describe the use of plants to promote optimum health.

Diversity Native cultures since ancient times have had great respect for their medicine men and women because they knew about plants and herbs for medicinal purposes. Such diseases and conditions as cardiac arrhythmia, pain, blood thinning, digestive upsets, and increased urinary output (diuresis) have been successfully treated with herbal medicine.

Legal European providers use herbal medicines routinely in their practices and have had classes on the topic throughout medical school. In the United States, it was not until 1974 that the FDA passed an act known as the Dietary Supplement Health and Education Act (DSHEA). Pursuant to the Act, the FDA examines any dietary supplement, such as an herbal product, and may remove it from the market if it presents a significant or unreasonable risk for illness or injury when used according to its labeling or under ordinary conditions of use.

In accordance with DSHEA, the FDA gathers and thoroughly reviews evidence about the pharmacology of a product, uses peer-reviewed scientific literature on safety and effectiveness, examines adverse event reports, and includes public comments for information about associated health risks.

There is no efficacy, or proof of claim, oversight of herbal supplements by the FDA. Herbal supplements do not have to obtain the approval of the FDA prior to marketing. They are classified as dietary supplements. However, the FDA does monitor the quality of manufacturing to ensure that these compounds meet quality standards and do not include harmful substances such as pesticides.

Self-medication with herbal products is less common in the United States than it is worldwide, but sales in the United States have been increasing annually. There has been an abundance of interest by the public in herbal products because of media attention given to them and their benefits.

Some examples of herbs and their uses are as follows: cascara—laxative; feverfew—headaches; garlic—antibacterial; licorice—gastritis, cough, menopause; St. John's wort—depression and anxiety; and saw palmetto—prostate health.

Safety

There are risks associated with self-medicating with herbal products. Patients need to be informed that taking certain medications together with herbal products can produce dangerous interactions. It is important for you as the medical assistant to gather information about all medications, including prescription medications, over-the-counter medications, and herbals. Pregnant patients must take extra caution to inform their provider about what they are taking and should be cautioned about possible harm to the fetus (see Chapter 25). It is important to remember that any medication and any herb can cause an allergic reaction and have side effects.

The dietary supplement ephedra, also known as ma huang, has been prohibited from sale since April 2004 because, based on investigations in accordance with the DSHEA of 1994, ephedra was found to present an unreasonable risk for illness and injury. The herbal supplement had been promoted for use in weight loss and control and for enhancing performance in sports activities. Evidence showed modest effectiveness for weight loss with no clear health benefit. However, it was confirmed that, in many instances, the substance increased blood pressure and caused tachycardia, chest pain, myocardial infarction (MI), cerebral vascular accidents (CVA), seizures, psychosis, and death.

Once a dietary supplement is on the market and proves to be hazardous to the health of Americans, the FDA can file a claim against the manufacturer and issue a warning or have the supplement removed from the market.

Synthetic Drugs

Synthetic drugs are prepared in pharmaceutical laboratories. By combining various chemicals, scientists can produce compounds that are identical to a natural drug or create entirely new substances. An advantage of synthetic drugs over natural is the ability to standardize doses. Thousands of drugs are now produced synthetically. Examples are Motrin (ibuprofen), Feldene (piroxicam), and Prilosec (omeprazole).

Genetically Engineered Pharmaceuticals

Scientists are now capable of creating new strains of bacteria using a technique known as gene splicing. Through this process, hybrid forms of life have been created that benefit human beings by providing an alternative source of drugs, such as Humulin (insulin) for patients with diabetes and interferon for use in the treatment of cancer. These drugs can be manufactured in large quantities; thus, they are less expensive than natural substances.

DRUG REGULATIONS AND LEGAL CLASSIFICATIONS OF DRUGS

Safety   Legal

Qualified medical practitioners who prescribe, dispense, and/or administer drugs must comply with federal and state laws. These laws govern the manufacture, sale, possession, administration, dispensing, and prescribing of drugs. All drugs available for legal use are controlled by the federal Food, Drug, and Cosmetic Act. This law protects the public by ensuring the purity, strength, and composition of foods, drugs, and cosmetics. It also prohibits the movement in interstate commerce of altered and/or misbranded food, drugs, devices, and cosmetics. Enforcement of the act is the responsibility of the FDA, which is part of the Department of Health and Human Services (DHHS).

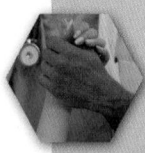

Patient Education

If you want to use herbal therapy, you should find a reputable herbalist and work with him or her and your practitioner. Herbal products are neither regulated nor standardized by any agency or organization (see previous section for information about DSHEA). Report at once any symptoms that seem unusual. Herbal products should be used for the shortest amount of time needed to obtain results. Keeping track of herbs taken, for what purpose they are being taken, and the effect on symptom control is important and provides information about those products that are helpful and those that are not. Journals, newsletters, and the Internet can provide information about herbal medicine. These publications can be explored for information and are a valuable resource. Relevant publications include *HerbalGram, Phytomedicine, Alternative Medicine Alert,* and the *Journal of Alternative and Complementary Medicine.*

Controlled Substances Act of 1970

Drugs with the potential for abuse or addiction are regulated by the Controlled Substances Act of 1970. It controls the manufacture, importation, compounding, selling, dealing in, and giving away of drugs that have the potential for abuse or addiction. These drugs are known as controlled substances and include heroin and cocaine and their derivatives, other narcotics, stimulants, and depressants. The Drug Enforcement Agency (DEA) of the U.S. Justice Department monitors and enforces the Act, which is also known as the Comprehensive Drug Abuse Prevention and Control Act. Under federal law, providers who prescribe, administer, or dispense controlled substances must register with the DEA and renew their registration as required by state law (Form DEA 224).

Applications for registration are available online (http://www.deadiversion.usdoj.gov). A licensed provider is issued a registration that must be renewed at regular intervals. The renewal form is sent approximately 2 months before the expiration date.

Controlled Substances Schedules. **Controlled substances** are classified according to five schedules:

- *Schedule I* is drugs that have a high potential for abuse and are not accepted for medical use within the United States. Examples are heroin, lysergic acid diethylamide (LSD), and marijuana.
- *Schedule II* drugs include those that also have a high abuse potential but also have an accepted medical use within the United States. Examples are amphetamines and cocaine. Because of their high potential for abuse, a special DEA form must be used to order these drugs for stock in an ambulatory setting. The form is not necessary for Schedules III and IV drugs. A written prescription is required for Schedule II drugs and the prescription cannot be renewed. According to the U.S. Department of Justice, Drug Enforcement Administration, Office of Diversion Control, "A prescription for a controlled substance must be written in ink or indelible pencil or typewritten and must be manually signed by the practitioner on the date when issued. An individual (secretary or nurse) may be designated by the practitioner to prepare prescriptions for the practitioner's signature." Examples of Schedule II drugs are morphine, codeine, Ritalin, and Percocet.

- *Schedule III* drugs have a low to moderate potential for physical dependency, yet have a high potential for psychological dependency. Some examples are barbiturates and various drug combinations containing codeine and paregoric. Prescriptions for Schedule III drugs can be either written or conveyed verbally. They can be refilled, but only five times within 6 months. Schedule III drugs are accepted for medical use in the United States.
- *Schedule IV* drugs have a lower potential for abuse and have an accepted medical use in the United States. Examples of these drugs are chloral hydrate and diazepam. Prescriptions for Schedule IV drugs may include refills, but refills are limited to five within 6 months.
- *Schedule V* drugs have the lowest abuse potential of controlled substances. Some examples from this schedule are Lomotil and Donnagel. Some drugs from Schedule V may include refills, but refills are limited to five within 6 months.

On occasion, the DEA will reclassify drugs and move them from one schedule to another.

So that they can be readily identified, the labels of controlled substance containers are marked with a large C with a Roman numeral to the right of it to indicate from which schedule the drug has come; for example, C_{II} indicates a Schedule II drug.

The provider's DEA number must appear on each prescription for controlled substances.

A copy of the federal law and a complete list of controlled substances and their schedules are available online at http://www.deadiversion.usdoj.gov by clicking on the "Resources" tab, selecting "Questions & Answers," and then "Prescriptions."

Storage of Controlled Substances. Federal law requires that all controlled substances be kept separate from other drugs. They must be stored in a well-constructed metal box or compartment that has a double lock. Controlled substances must be protected from possible misuse and abuse, and persons who administer controlled substances must record them both in the patient's record and in a narcotic count record. The record must be maintained on a daily basis and kept for a minimum of 2 to 3 years, depending on state laws. Patient name, address, date of administration of the controlled substance, drug name, dose, and route and method of administration must be included in the record.

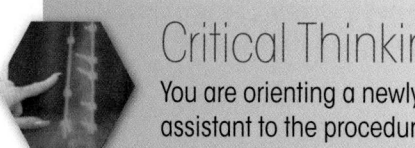

Critical Thinking

You are orienting a newly hired medical assistant to the procedure for monitoring controlled substances at your provider's practice. What might be some of the key aspects of controlled substance monitoring that need to be discussed?

Medical Assistant Role and Responsibilities. Medical assistants are required to know the legalities that surround controlled substances. Medical assistant responsibilities may include:

1. Monitor the provider's DEA registration renewal date

2. Maintain legally specified records and inventories of all drugs (Figure 34-1), including samples; this can be done electronically

3. Provide security for all drugs, in particular controlled substances

4. Provide security for prescription pads

5. Properly destroy expired drugs using the FDA guidelines and document such action

Controlled substances stored and used on the premises must be counted at the end of each workday, verified by two individuals for accuracy of count, and recorded on an audit sheet. An inventory record of Schedule II drugs must be submitted to the DEA every 2 years.

Because of the increase in clinic drug theft and substance abuse, as well as the stringent federal laws that apply to storing, dispensing, and administering controlled substances, many clinics do not keep controlled substances on the premises. However, agencies that have controlled substances on the premises for dispensing to patients in the ambulatory care setting must comply with the DEA's disposal policy.

Controlled Substance Disposal Policy (per DEA). The DEA Disposal Policy for Controlled Substances requires that controlled substances be accounted for when they are disposed of. More take-back programs are emerging to address drug abuse and diversion, environmental problems, and accidental poisoning by providing consumers with a safe and environmentally sound option for disposing of unused or expired drugs.

State- and community-driven take-back program initiatives focus on safely collecting and disposing of unwanted over-the-counter, prescription, and—in certain cases—veterinary medications.

Complete information regarding the disposal of expired controlled substances from the provider's perspective can be found at http://www.deadiversion.usdoj.gov by searching for "Drug Disposal." There are downloadable fact sheets and a copy of the Disposal of Controlled Substances; Final Rule (PDF) (September 4, 2014).

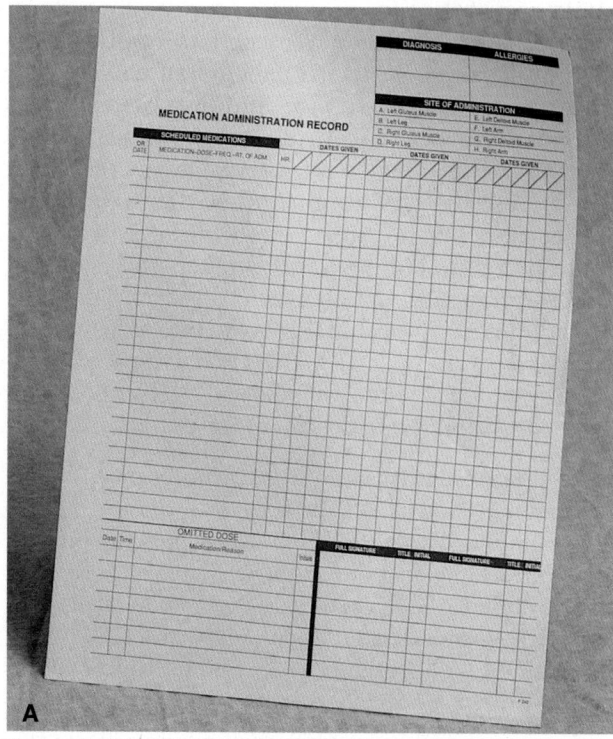

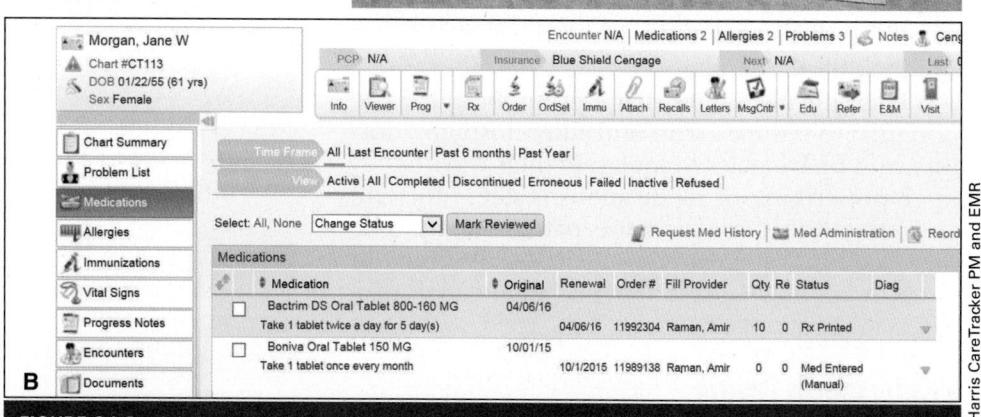

FIGURE 34-1 It is important to maintain patient medication records both for the safety of the patient and to protect the practice. (A) A paper-based patient medication record. (B) The patient medication record as part of the patient's electronic medical record.

Courtesy of Harris CareTracker PM and EMR

Competency

Integrity

6. Know and understand federal and state laws that regulate drugs, including all controlled substances and samples

7. In some states, medical assistants are allowed, under the supervision of the provider, to call in routine refills of medications that are exact and have no change in dosage

The electronic health record has the capability of storing information regarding the due date for the provider's DEA registration renewal, maintaining legal records and inventories on all drugs including samples, keeping track of expiration dates of drugs and when they are destroyed, accessing the latest information regarding new DEA laws, and e-prescribing.

The DEA has been reluctant to approve regulations covering e-prescribing of controlled substances. This reluctance and the lack of DEA policies have been a hurdle to widespread adoption of e-prescribing. Presently, some providers can e-prescribe medications other than controlled substances (which require handwritten and signed prescriptions). This requires two separate systems, e-prescribing and handwritten prescriptions, and providers object, viewing this as too time consuming.

On March 24, 2010, the DEA issued its 334-page *Interim Final Rule on Electronic Prescriptions for Controlled Substances.* In brief, it states:

> The regulations provide pharmacies, hospitals, and practitioners with the ability to use modern technology for controlled substance prescriptions while maintaining the closed system of controls on controlled substances dispensing…. Additionally, the regulations will reduce paperwork for DEA registrants who dispense controlled substances and have the potential to reduce prescription forgery.
>
> —*FCW* (http://www.deadiversion.usdoj.gov /ecomm/e_rx/)

This rule also states that e-prescribing has the potential to reduce errors and allow hospitals, doctors, and pharmacies to integrate their records.

E-prescribing of medications is safe, efficient, and effective. It can improve patient safety. The next section, on prescription drugs, discusses in more detail how e-prescribing is beneficial to providers and patients.

Prescription Drugs

State laws require that licensed practitioners who prescribe drugs must write and sign an order for the dispensing of drugs. This process is known as writing a prescription. In order for a prescription to be complete, it must contain the following:

- Date of issue
- Patient's name and address
- Practitioner's name, address, and DEA registration number
- Drug name
- Drug strength
- Dosage form
- Quantity prescribed
- Directions for use
- Number of refills (if any) authorized
- Manual signature of prescriber

Medical assistants may be instructed to provide patient education after the provider prescribes a new medication. A part of the education includes how to read warning labels on medication containers (Figure 34-2). Prescription drugs are also called legend drugs.

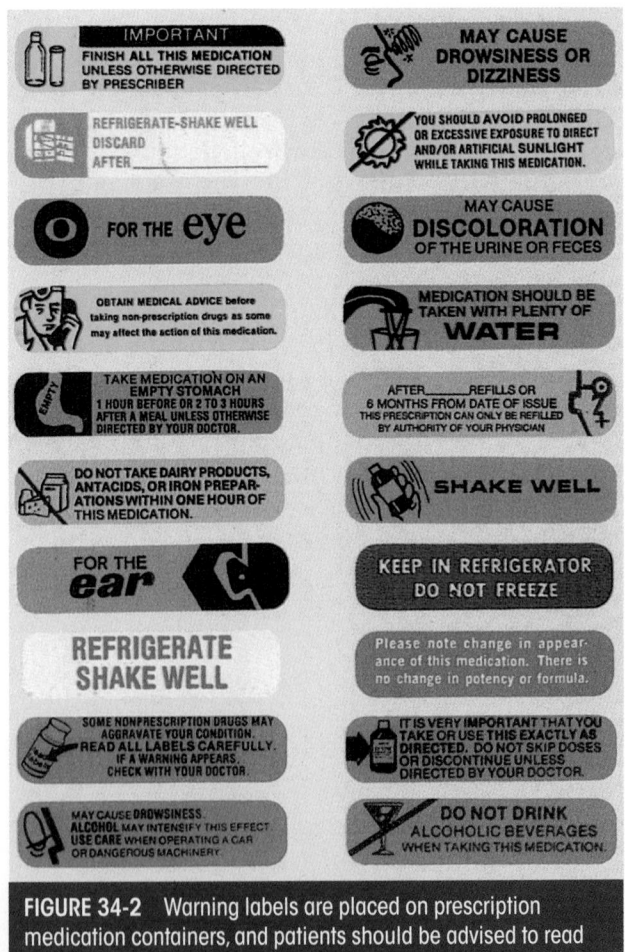

FIGURE 34-2 Warning labels are placed on prescription medication containers, and patients should be advised to read and adhere to the precautions or instructions.

Recent surveys of providers and other medical professionals reported that this group ranked computer systems high on timely access to records, better quality of care, and better documentation. E-prescribing is a feature many providers appreciate. With e-prescribing, providers have instantaneous and remote access to records in addition to many other features, including:

- Automatic alerts to allergies and drug interactions
- Automatic calculations of doses of medication according to the patient's age and weight
- Recommendations of brand and/or generic drug substitutions
- Printed prescriptions that are then faxed to the patient's pharmacy
- Integration with a drug reference such as the *Physician's Desk Reference* (PDR)
- Automatic processing of refills

Nonprescription Drugs

Drugs that are frequently referred to as over-the-counter (OTC) drugs fall into the category of nonprescription drugs. These drugs are readily accessible to the public. They do not require a prescription because the FDA considers them safe to use without a provider's advice. Examples of OTC drugs are aspirin, ibuprofen, and vitamins such as vitamin C. Although OTC drugs are considered safe, it is useful for the medical assistant to offer patients some guidelines (see "Patient Education" feature).

Prescription drugs can be reclassified to OTC if they meet the following criteria:

- The indication or indications of use for OTC must be similar to the prescription indication and must permit easy diagnosis and monitoring by the patient.
- There must be a low incidence of adverse reactions and drug interactions.
- The drug must not have properties that need additional monitoring or a very narrow margin for therapeutic effect.

The debate about the efficacy and safety of OTC medication continues. As far back as the early 1970s, this was a concern. At that point in time, the FDA launched the OTC Drug Review. As noted in the Federal Register on February 24, 2014, "The OTC Drug Review is one of the largest and most complex regulatory undertakings ever at FDA. It now consists of approximately 88 simultaneous rulemakings in 26 broad categories that encompass hundreds of thousands of OTC drug products marketed in the United States and some 800 active ingredients for over 1,400 different ingredient uses." The review continues to evaluate the way that the FDA ensures the safety and use of OTC medications by the American public, opening the door to the most expansive reform in the last 40 years.

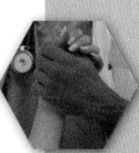

Patient Education

Guidelines for patients who take prescription medications include:

1. Take exactly as directed.
2. Inform the provider and/or the medical assistant of unusual or adverse reactions.
3. Continue to take the medication for the duration of the prescribed number of days, weeks, and so on.
4. If you want to discontinue the medication, inform your provider and/or the medical assistant.
5. Do not take other medications or herbs concurrently without checking with your provider or medical assistant.
6. Do not take someone else's prescribed medication.
7. Store all medications away from children.
8. Discard unused medication properly. Many states require that unused medications be turned in to a community's biohazard waste collection facility. Medication substances have been found in some water supplies.
9. Heed warning labels on medication containers.

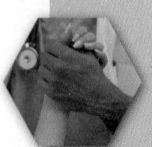

Patient Education

Because patients are more aware and better informed about their health care needs, they are becoming more involved in making choices and decisions about their health care. When they choose to take over-the-counter (OTC) drugs, they need information and guidance. Over the past few years, some drugs that had been available only with a prescription have been changed to OTC drugs. The safety of these drugs can be ensured only if patients take them as directed.

Patients need to realize that OTC medications:

1. Can interact with other drugs (either prescribed, herbal, or other OTCs) and cause undesirable or adverse reactions or complications

2. May be used in lieu of seeking professional help and thereby interfere with the need for medical care

3. Can mask symptoms and exacerbate an existing condition

4. May have several active ingredients, which may be found to be undesirable

5. Have a safe minimum dose, which may not have the desired therapeutic effect

Proper Disposal of Drugs

All drug labels contain an expiration date (Figure 34-3). When that date has been reached, the drug must be removed from the shelf and destroyed (see Procedure 34-1).

An expired drug cannot be dispensed or administered because it could be harmful.

If a medication is removed from its original container, and, for example, the patient refuses the medication, do not put it back in the container; it should not be used. Dispose of it as outlined earlier.

Expired controlled substances are handled differently. They must be returned to the pharmacy (as required by law). If a controlled substance (Schedule II) has been either dropped onto the floor or another surface (and is thus unfit to be given to a patient) or has spilled (if in liquid form), a witness should verify the incident and proper documentation must take place.

The local DEA office and local police must be notified and the appropriate paperwork completed if there has been a loss or theft of a controlled substance (Schedule II).

Administer, Prescribe, Dispense

There are three ways to handle drugs in the provider's clinic: prescribing, dispensing, or administering them. To **prescribe** a drug means that the licensed practitioner with prescriptive authority (provider, physician assistant, or nurse practitioner) gives a written order to be taken to the pharmacist to be filled. To **dispense** a drug means to provide the medication as ordered by the provider to the patient to be taken at another time. To **administer** a drug means to give it to the patient by mouth or injection or any other method of administration as ordered by the provider.

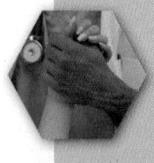

Patient Education

Many patients keep unused medications past their expiration date. This presents a potential health hazard, because some medications lose their potency after a period, whereas others become toxic. It is best to instruct patients to discard any unused portion of medications by the stated expiration date. Encourage patients to check their medicine cabinets at the same time every year so it becomes a routine practice. (See information on the National Take-Back Initiative.)

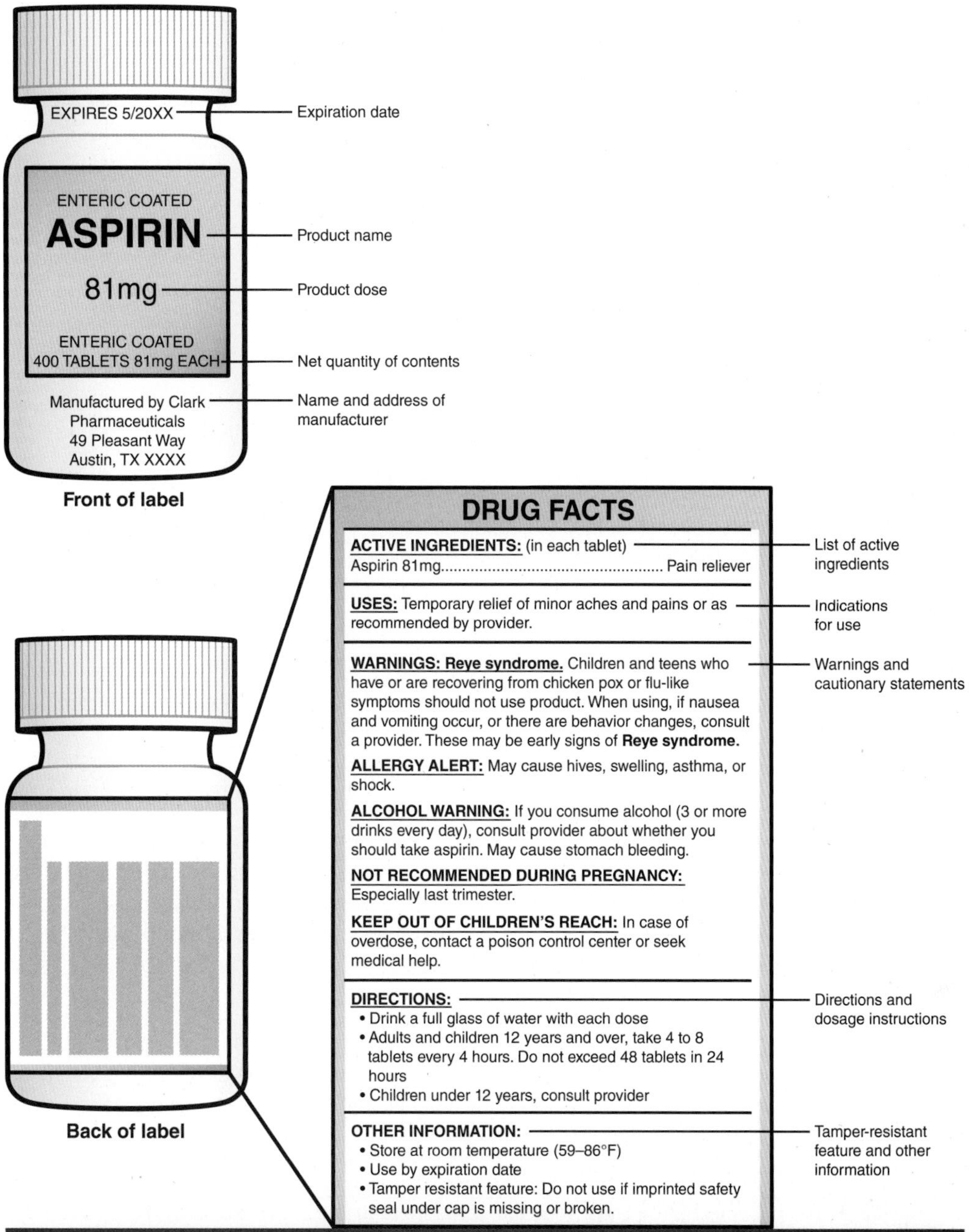

EXPIRES 5/20XX — Expiration date

ENTERIC COATED
ASPIRIN — Product name

81mg — Product dose

ENTERIC COATED
400 TABLETS 81mg EACH — Net quantity of contents

Manufactured by Clark — Name and address of
Pharmaceuticals   manufacturer
49 Pleasant Way
Austin, TX XXXX

Front of label

Back of label

DRUG FACTS

ACTIVE INGREDIENTS: (in each tablet) — List of active
Aspirin 81mg... Pain reliever   ingredients

USES: Temporary relief of minor aches and pains or as — Indications
recommended by provider.   for use

WARNINGS: Reye syndrome. Children and teens who — Warnings and
have or are recovering from chicken pox or flu-like   cautionary statements
symptoms should not use product. When using, if nausea
and vomiting occur, or there are behavior changes, consult
a provider. These may be early signs of **Reye syndrome.**

ALLERGY ALERT: May cause hives, swelling, asthma, or
shock.

ALCOHOL WARNING: If you consume alcohol (3 or more
drinks every day), consult provider about whether you
should take aspirin. May cause stomach bleeding.

NOT RECOMMENDED DURING PREGNANCY:
Especially last trimester.

KEEP OUT OF CHILDREN'S REACH: In case of
overdose, contact a poison control center or seek
medical help.

DIRECTIONS: — Directions and
• Drink a full glass of water with each dose   dosage instructions
• Adults and children 12 years and over, take 4 to 8
  tablets every 4 hours. Do not exceed 48 tablets in 24
  hours
• Children under 12 years, consult provider

OTHER INFORMATION: — Tamper-resistant
• Store at room temperature (59–86°F)   feature and other
• Use by expiration date   information
• Tamper resistant feature: Do not use if imprinted safety
  seal under cap is missing or broken.

FIGURE 34-3 Medication labels contain valuable information essential to the safe and effective use of the drug.

Competency

Integrity

Although state laws vary, some states allow certain professionals, including medical assistants, to prepare and administer medications under the licensed practitioner's supervision. Usually, it is the provider and pharmacist who dispense medications. However, medical assistants can also dispense samples of drugs under the provider's direction. Although medical assistants act as the provider's agent when they prepare and administer medications, they are ethically and legally responsible for their own actions and can be subject to legal action should harm come to a patient. The law requires that individuals who prepare and administer medications know the medications and their side effects.

PROCEDURE 34-1

Properly Disposing of Drugs

STANDARD PRECAUTIONS:

Handwashing

PURPOSE:

To properly dispose of drugs that have reached their expiration dates.

EQUIPMENT/SUPPLIES:

Drugs (oral and parenteral) that have reached their expiration dates

PROCEDURE STEPS:

1. Consult practice policy for disposal of expired medications.

2. Access the drug closet or narcotics cabinet and evaluate the expiration date on all medications.

3. Gather expired drugs, either prescription or OTC. RATIONALE: Expired drugs can be neither dispensed nor administered because they can be harmful to patients.

4. Medicine take-back programs for disposal are a good way to remove expired medications. Contact your city or county government's household trash and recycling service to learn about any special rules regarding which medicines can be taken back.

5. Consult the FDA Web site (http://www.fda.gov) for the most current recommendations for appropriate disposal of each medication. RATIONALE: Disposal of drugs into the sewage system, either by flushing down the toilet or down the sink, is discouraged everywhere and is prohibited in some states (medication substances have been found in some municipal water supplies).

6. Wash hands.

7. Accurately list medications selected for disposal, either in the medication log book or in a digital file. Document medication, dosage, expiration date and specifically the method of disposal. If medications are controlled substances, appropriately document their disposal using the required form and witness' signature.

DOCUMENTATION:

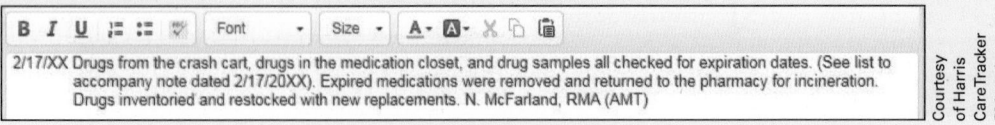

2/17/XX Drugs from the crash cart, drugs in the medication closet, and drug samples all checked for expiration dates. (See list to accompany note dated 2/17/20XX). Expired medications were removed and returned to the pharmacy for incineration. Drugs inventoried and restocked with new replacements. N. McFarland, RMA (AMT)

Courtesy of Harris CareTracker PM and EMR

It is imperative that any medication error be avoided and, if one does occur, that there is immediate notification of the practitioner to render aid, if needed, to the patient. Any medication error must be correctly documented according to the practice's policy and procedure on medication errors.

DRUG REFERENCES AND STANDARDS

The strength, purity, and quality of drugs differ depending on how they are manufactured. To control the differences, standards have been set. By law, the various drug products must meet standards that are set forth by the

FDA. A special reference book, *United States Pharmacopeia/National Formulary,* and Web site http://www.usp.org/usp-nf, list the drugs for which standards have been established. These resources are recognized by the U.S. government as the official list of drug standards, which are enforced by the FDA. Every 5 years, the information is updated in an attempt to include all drug products in the United States. Naturals and herbals are not regulated. Herbal medications and dietary supplements are not listed in the *Pharmocepeia.*

Other useful books used as references include the *Compendium of Drug Therapy,* the *Desk Reference for Nonprescription Drugs,* and the *Physician's Desk Reference* (PDR). When using the PDR, it is helpful to understand that each medication is described using the manufacturer's package insert. The format for each medication is similar, but not uniform, as is often found in other references. Also, there are color photographs of each medication included for easy recognition. The PDR is available online at http://www.pdr.net and is updated regularly. The printed version is still available if needed. The PDR is one of the most widely used reference books and is found in most offices and clinics. It is divided into sections of drug information, which are followed by other useful drug information such as a list of products, poison control's toll-free telephone numbers, conversion tables, and a guide to management of drug overdose.

Providers use electronic technology for assistance when they need references to drugs, their interactions, brand and generic names, and doses according to patients' needs. Some providers use tablets that give them the information they need.

How to Use the PDR

The four most commonly used sections of the PDR list drugs according to:

- Brand name and generic name index (Section 2)
- Classification or category (Section 3)
- Product identification guide (Section 4)
- Product information and alphabetical arrangement by manufacturer (Section 5)

Section 2 of the PDR is the alphabetized section used for finding the page numbers for generic and brand-name drugs. Each drug, whether generic or brand, has a page number listed to enable you to locate a specific drug. Each time a brand name appears, it is followed by the manufacturer's name and the page number to check for more information. When more than one page number appears, the first number refers to the photo section, in Section 4 (product identification guide); the last number refers to the prescribing category, in Section 3 (product category index). Generic drug names are underlined; brand names are not.

The PDR has many other sections within it, such as the Key to Controlled Substances category, the U.S. Food and Drug Administration telephone directory, telephone numbers for poison control centers, and herb and drug interactions.

The following guidelines will assist you as you learn to use the PDR.

If using the online version, type the brand name or generic name of the medication in the search box and follow the link. If using the printed version, turn to Section 2 and locate the drug in the alphabetical listing. The manufacturer's name will be in parentheses, followed by one or two page numbers. The first number is the product identification page number, in Section 4. The second number is the product information, in Section 5.

Example:

Look up Zithromax capsules in a current PDR.

Note all the information provided for a drug.

- *Description.* Gives the origin and chemical composition of the drug
- *Clinical pharmacology.* Indicates the effect of the drug on the body and the process by which the drug exerts this effect
- *Indications and uses.* States the various conditions, diseases, types of microorganisms, and so on for which the drug is used
- *Contraindications.* States when the drug should not be given based on other disease processes or medications
- *Warnings.* Gives the potential dangers of the drug
- *Precautions.* Explains how to use the medication safely, including physical impairments and drug interactions
- *Adverse reactions.* Lists the undesired side effects or toxicity of the drug

- *Dosage and administration.* States the amount (usual daily dose for adults and children) and time sequence of administration
- *How supplied.* Lists the various forms of the drug and their dosages

If you know the classification of the drug, turn to Section 3 and locate the category of the drug.

Example:

Antibiotics

Macrolide

Zithromax capsules (Pfizer)

NOTE: All controlled substances listed in the PDR are indicated with the symbol *C* with the Roman numeral II, III, IV, or V printed inside the *C* to designate the schedule in which the substance is classified.

Example:

Duramorph C$_{II}$, morphine sulfate USP

Other Reference Sources

On occasion, you may not find the drug that you are looking for listed in the PDR. When this happens:

- Refer to another drug reference book.
- Research medications online, making sure your source is reliable.
- Ask a pharmacist about the drug.
- Refer to the insert that comes in the drug package.

The package insert that most drug manufacturers provide with their products is an important source of information about a particular drug. It provides a brief description of the drug, including its clinical pharmacology, indications and usage, **contraindications** (any symptom or circumstance that indicates that the use of a particular drug is inappropriate when it would otherwise be advisable), warnings, precautions, drug interactions, adverse reactions, overdose, dosage, and administration. The package insert can be a valuable source of information about drugs that might not be listed elsewhere, or if a PDR is unavailable.

Information about some older medications, such as digoxin, can be found in the package insert because they may have been deleted from the current PDR.

CLASSIFICATION OF DRUGS

Drugs can be classified in a number of ways. Some examples are:

- Drugs used to treat or prevent disease (examples are hormones and vaccines) (see Chapter 21)
- Drugs that have a principal action on the body (examples are analgesics and anti-inflammatory drugs)
- Drugs that act on specific body systems or organs (examples are respiratory and cardiovascular drugs)
- Drug preparation (examples are suppository, liquid)
- Drugs that act on specific organisms
- Drugs that replace body chemicals

Table 34-1 lists common drug classifications.

PRINCIPAL ACTIONS OF DRUGS

Certain drugs have selective action, such as stimulants, which increase or speed up the functioning of the body's processes, and depressants, which decrease or slow down the functioning of the body's processes.

Other drugs may have what is known as:

- *Local action.* The drug primarily acts on the area to which it is administered.
- *Remote action.* A drug affects a part of the body that is distant from the site of administration.
- *Systemic action.* The drug is carried via the bloodstream throughout the body.
- *Synergistic action.* One drug increases or counteracts the action of another.

Factors That Affect Drug Action

The four principal factors that affect drug action are absorption, distribution, biotransformation, and elimination. These factors vary based on the individual patient, the form and chemical composition of the drug, and the method of administration.

1. **Absorption** is the process whereby the drug passes into the body fluids and tissues.
2. **Distribution** is the process whereby the drug is transported from the blood to the intended site of action, site of biotransformation, site of storage, and site of elimination.

TABLE 34-1

COMMON CLASSIFICATIONS OF DRUGS AND THEIR ACTIONS

CLASSIFICATION (WITH PHONETIC SPELLING)	ACTION	EXAMPLES OF DRUGS COMMONLY USED IN AMBULATORY CARE SETTING		SIDE EFFECTS
Analgesic (an″al-je′sik)	An agent that relieves pain without causing loss of consciousness	Tylenol (acetaminophen) Anacin, Bufferin, Bayer, Excedrin (acetylsalicylic acid or aspirin), Advil, Motrin (ibuprofen), Dilaudid (hydromorphone), Astormorph, Roxanol, MSIR (morphine), Lazanda, Actiq (fentanyl), Demerol (merperidine), Ultram (tramadol)		**Common:** GI changes, drowsiness, dry mouth, constipation, nausea, sedation **Severe:** Allergic reaction (rash, hives, tissue swelling, respiratory difficulty, chest tightness), respiratory depression, death, addiction
Anesthetic (an″es-thet′ik)	An agent that produces numbness May be local or general depending on the type and how administered	Xylocaine (lidocaine HCl) Novacaine (procaine HCl)	Both are local anesthetics	**Common:** Irritation, redness, changes in sensation, drowsiness, irregular heartbeat (based on route of administration) **Severe:** Allergic reaction (rash, hives, tissue swelling, respiratory difficulty, chest tightness)
Antacid (ant-as′id)	An agent that relieves heartburn or indigestion by neutralizing gastric acid	AlkaSeltzer, Bromoseltzer (sodium bicarbonate), Tums (calcium carbonate), aluminum-based Amphojel (aluminum hydroxide), Milk of Magnesia (magnesium hydroxide), Mylanta, Maalox, Riopan (magnesium hydroxide and aluminum hydroxide blend), Gaviscon (alginic acid) Acid reducers: H2 blockers: Zantac (ranitodine) Proton pump inhibitors: Prilosec (omeprazole)		**Common:** Constipation, loss of appetite, urinary changes, muscle weakness, increased thirst **Severe:** Aluminum intoxication, hypophosphatemia
Antianxiety (an″ti-ang-zi′e-te)	An agent that relieves anxiety by slowing down the nervous system, assisting with relaxation both physically and mentally	Benzodiazepines: Valium (diazepam), Librium (chlordiazepoxide HCl), Xanax (alprazolam) Nonbenzodiazepines: BuSpar (buspirone), alcohol		**Common:** Drowsiness, incoordination, muscle weakness, headache **Severe:** Allergic reaction (rash, hives, tissue swelling, respiratory difficulty, chest tightness), slurred speech, tremor, mood changes, mania
Antiarrhythmic (an″te-a-rith′mik)	An agent that controls cardiac arrhythmias such as tachycardia, atrial fibrillation, and premature beats	Calcium channel blockers: Norvasc (amlodipine), Vascor (bepridil), Cardizem (diltiazem), Cardene, Cardene SR (nicardipine), Adalat, Procardia (nifedipine) Beta-blockers: Tenormin (atenolol), Lopressor (metoprolol), Inderal (propranolol), Xylocaine (lidocaine HCl)		**Common:** Dizziness, nausea and vomiting, vision changes, decreased sexual ability **Severe:** Allergic reaction (rash, hives, tissue swelling, respiratory difficulty, chest tightness), slowed heart beat, heart failure

continues

Table 34-1 continued

CLASSIFICATION (WITH PHONETIC SPELLING)	ACTION	EXAMPLES OF DRUGS COMMONLY USED IN AMBULATORY CARE SETTING	SIDE EFFECTS
Antibiotic (an"ti-bi-ot'ik)	An agent that destroys or inhibits growth of microorganisms; used to treat bacterial infections	Penicillins: Penicillin G, Amoxil, Augmentin (penicillin) Cephalosporins: Ancef, Keflol (cefzalon), Rocephin (ceftriaxone), Fortaz (ceftazidime) Fluoroquinolones: Avelox (moxifloxacin) Sulfonamides: Bactrim DS, Septra DS (sulfamethoxazole and trimethoprim)	**Common:** Upset stomach, diarrhea, vomiting **Severe:** Allergic reaction (rash, hives, tissue swelling, respiratory difficulty, chest tightness)
Anticholesterol (an"ti-ko"less-ter-ol)	An agent that reduces cholesterol levels and fats (low-density lipids and triglycerides) in the bloodstream associated with vascular disease	Lipitor (atorvastatin), Zocor (simvastatin), Crestor (rosuvastation), Zetia	**Common:** Muscle pain or weakness, change in amount of urine produced **Severe:** Allergic reaction (rash, hives, tissue swelling, respiratory difficulty, chest tightness), renal changes / failure, liver damage, may cause or worsen diabetes
Anticholinergic (an"ti-ko"lin-er'jik)	An agent that blocks the action of the neurotransmitter acetylcholine in the parasympathetic nervous system; used to treat asthma, incontinence, gastrointestinal cramps, and muscular spasms	atropine, scopolamine, Artane (trihexyphenidyl HCl), Cogentin (benztropine mesylate)	**Common:** Dilated pupils, blurred vision, dizziness, constipation, dry mouth, drowsiness, sedation **Severe:** Allergic reaction (rash, hives, tissue swelling, respiratory difficulty, chest tightness), renal changes / failure, liver damage, tachycardia
Anticoagulant (an"ti-ko-ag'u-lant)	An agent that targets clotting factors to prevent or slow the formation of blood clots	Heparin (heparin sodium), Coumadin (warfarin), Pradaxa (dabigatran), Xarelto (rivaroxaban), Eliquis (apixaban), Lovenox (enoxaparin)	**Common:** Irritation at the site of injection **Severe:** Allergic reaction (rash, hives, tissue swelling, respiratory difficulty, chest tightness), bleeding gums, hematuria, gastric bleeding, shortness of breath, slurred speech
Anticonvulsant or antiepileptic (an"ti-kon-vul'sant)	An agent that prevents seizure activity in the brain	Tegretol (carbamazepine), Dilantin (phenytoin), Zarontin (ethosuximide), Depakene (valproate), Depakote (divalproex sodium)	**Common:** Constipation, dizziness, headache, nausea, vomiting, fatigue, blurred vision **Severe:** Allergic reaction (rash, hives, tissue swelling, respiratory difficulty, chest tightness), liver or pancreatic failure, decreased platelets, immune dysfunction

CLASSIFICATION (WITH PHONETIC SPELLING)	ACTION	EXAMPLES OF DRUGS COMMONLY USED IN AMBULATORY CARE SETTING	SIDE EFFECTS
Antidepressant (an"ti-dep-res'ant)	An agent that prevents or relieves the symptoms of depression	Monoamine oxidase (MAO) inhibitors: Marplan (isocarboxazid), Nardil (phenelzine sulfate), Tricyclic: Elavil (amitriptyline HCl), Tofranil (imipramine HCl) Selective serotonin reuptake inhibitors (SSRIs): Zoloft (sertraline HCl), Paxil (paroxetine HCl), Desyrel (trazodone), Prozac (fluoxetine)	**Common:** Anxiety, constipation, diarrhea, dizziness, drowsiness, GI symptoms **Severe:** Allergic reaction (rash, hives, tissue swelling, respiratory difficulty, chest tightness), bizarre behavior, severe mental status, and mood changes, fast or irregular heartbeat, suicidal thoughts or attempts
Antidiabetic (an"ti-di-a-bet'ik)	An agent that assists a person with diabetes control the level of glucose in the blood	Humulin and Novolin (regular insulin), NovoLog (insulin aspart), Humalog (insulin lispro), Humulin N, Novulin N (insulin isophane), Tresiba (insulin degludec), Lantus, Toujeo (insulin glargine), Precose (acarbose), Januvia (sitagliptin), Victoza (liraglutide)	**Common:** Bloating, gas, diarrhea, upset stomach, loss of appetite, skin rash, irritability **Severe:** Allergic reaction (rash, hives, tissue swelling, respiratory difficulty, chest tightness), low blood sugar, death, pancreatitis
Antidiarrheal (an"ti-di-a-re'al)	An agent that prevents or relieves diarrhea by slowing gastrointestinal motility but not treating the underlying condition	Pepto-Bismol (bismuth subsalicylate), Kaopectate (bismuth subsalicylate), Lomotil (atropine/ diphenoxylate), Immodium (loperamide)	**Common:** Darkening of stools or tongue, dizziness, drowsiness, fatigue **Severe:** Persistent vomiting or diarrhea, dizziness, abdominal pain, allergic reaction (rash, hives, tissue swelling, respiratory difficulty, chest tightness)
Antiemetic (an"ti-e-met'ik)	An agent that prevents or re-lieves nausea and vomiting	Dramamine (dimenhydrinate), Phenergan (promethazine), Reglan (metoclopramide), Marinol (dronabinol), Compazine (prochlorperazine), Droperidol (inapsine), Zofran (ondansetron)	**Common:** Dry mouth, vomiting, dizziness, drowsiness, weakness, headache, constipation **Severe:** Allergic reaction (rash, hives, tissue swelling, respiratory difficulty, chest tightness), blurred vision, irritation at injection site, hallucinations, loss of coordination, confusion, shortness of breath, twitching of face or tongue
Antifungal	An agent that treats fungal infections by killing or inactivating fungi	Mycelex (clotrimazole), Ecoza (econazole), Monistat (miconazole), Lamisil (terbinafine), Diflucan (fluconazole), Fungozone (amphotericin B), Mycostatin (nystatin)	**Common:** Nausea, abdominal pain, diarrhea, flatulence, headache, rash, indigestion **Severe:** Allergic reaction (rash, hives, tissue swelling, difficulty breathing, chest tightness), skin reaction (peeling or blistering), liver failure/damage
Antihistamine (an"ti-his'ta-min)	An agent that counteracts histamines that attach to the cells in the body and cause them to swell and leak fluid	Allegra (fexofenadine), Seldane (terfenadine), Zyrtec (cetirizine), Benadryl (diphenhydramine), Claritin (loratadine)	**Common:** Constipation, diarrhea, dizziness, dry mouth, excitability, loss of appetite, nausea and vomiting, blurred vision **Severe:** Allergic reaction (rash, hives, tissue swelling, respiratory difficulty, chest tightness), blurred vision, chest pain, loss of coordination, irregular heartbeat, urinary retention

continues

Table 34-1 continued

CLASSIFICATION (WITH PHONETIC SPELLING)	ACTION	EXAMPLES OF DRUGS COMMONLY USED IN AMBULATORY CARE SETTING	SIDE EFFECTS
Antihypertensive (an″ti-hi″per-ten′siv)	An agent that prevents hypertension by controlling or lowering systolic and diastolic blood pressure	Lopressor (metoprolol tartrate), Prinivil, Zestril (lisinopril), Tenormin (atenolol), Toprol XL (metoprolol succinate), Norvasc (amlodipine), Cardizem (diltiazem), Diovan (valsartan)	**Common:** Anxiety, confusion, constipation, dizziness, weakness, ringing in ears, sweating, thirst, dehydration, fatigue, syncope **Severe:** Allergic reaction (rash, hives, tissue swelling, respiratory difficulty, chest tightness), chest pain, fainting, cardiac arrhythmias, hallucination, shortness of breath, hypokalemia, reduced kidney function
Anti-inflammatory (an″ti-in-flam′a-to-re)	An agent that blocks or counteracts inflammatory reactions and pain at sites of injury or damage	Naprosyn (naproxen), Anacin, Bufferin, Bayer, Excedrin (acetylsalicylic acid or aspirin), Advil, Motrin (ibuprofen), Cataflam, Voltaren (diclofenac), Toradol (ketorolac), Mobic (meloxicam)	**Common:** Gastric irritation, abdominal pain, nausea, diarrhea, anemia, dizziness **Severe:** Allergic reaction (rash, hives, tissue swelling, respiratory difficulty, chest tightness), bleeding, kidney failure
Antineoplastic (an″ti-ne″o-plas′tik)	An agent that inhibits the maturation and proliferation of malignant cells	Otrezup (methotrexate), Cytoxin (cyclophosphamide), Efudex (fluorouracil), Platinol (cisplatin), Taxol (paclitaxel), Ellence (epirubicin), Nolvadex (tamoxifen), Iressa (gefitinib), Gleevec (imatinib)	**Common:** Loss of appetite, diarrhea, changes in skin color, hair loss, nausea, vomiting, weakness **Severe:** Allergic reaction (rash, hives, tissue swelling, respiratory difficulty, chest tightness), hematuria, tarry stools, fever, chills, hallucinations, infections, mouth sores, unusual bleeding or bruising, low blood counts
Antipsychotic or psychotropic	An agent that alters the effect of certain chemicals on the brain, as these chemicals have an effect on mood, emotions, and behavior	Haldol (haloperidol), Risperdal (risperidone), Zyprexa (olanzapine), Thorazine (chlorpromazine), Seroquel (quetiapine), Geodon (ziprasidone), Abilify (aripiprazole), Invega (paliperidone), Latuda (lurasidone)	**Common:** Constipation, diarrhea, drowsiness, dry mouth, headache, nausea, restlessness, weight gain, blurred vision **Severe:** Allergic reaction (rash, hives, tissue swelling, respiratory difficulty, chest tightness), chest pain, renal function changes, arrhythmias, seizures, rigidity, hypotension
Antipyretic (an″ti-pi-ret′ik)	An agent that reduces fever	Anacin, Bufferin, Bayer, Excedrin (acetylsalicylic acid or aspirin), Advil, Motrin (ibuprofen)	**Common:** GI changes **Severe:** Allergic reaction (rash, hives, tissue swelling, respiratory difficulty, chest tightness)
Antitussive (an″ti-tus′iv)	An agent that suppresses cough by acting on the center in the brain that controls the cough reflex	Pertussin, Romilar (dextromethorphan), Benlyn DM, Delsym (dextromethorphan), Zonatuss (benzonatate), Hycodan (codeine, oxycodone)	**Common:** Blurred vision, constipation, dizziness, drowsiness, nausea and vomiting **Severe:** Allergic reaction (rash, hives, tissue swelling, respiratory difficulty, chest tightness), breathing changes, especially slowed breathing, arrhythmias

CLASSIFICATION (WITH PHONETIC SPELLING)	ACTION	EXAMPLES OF DRUGS COMMONLY USED IN AMBULATORY CARE SETTING	SIDE EFFECTS
Antiulcer (an"ti-ul'ser) (H₂ blockers)	H2 antagonists: compete with histamine at H2 receptors, which results in a reduction in secretion of gastric acid Proton pump inhibitors: block the secretion of gastric acid by the gastric parietal cells	**H2 antagonists:** Tagamet (cimetidine), Zantac (ranitidine), Prilosec (omeprazole), Axid (nizatidine), Pepcid (famotidine) **Proton pump inhibitors:** Asiphex (rabeprazole), Protonix (pantoprazole), Nexium (esomeprazole), Prevacid (lansoprazole), Prolosec (omeprazole)	**H2 antagonists** **Common:** Drowsiness, dizziness, headache, dysuria, nausea and vomiting **Severe:** Allergic reaction (rash, hives, tissue swelling, respiratory difficulty, chest tightness), agitation, anxiety, confusion, hair loss, joint or muscle pain, inflammation of blood vessels **Proton pump inhibitors** **Common:** Headache, constipation, diarrhea, abdominal pain, nausea **Severe:** Allergic reaction (rash, hives, tissue swelling, respiratory difficulty, chest tightness), osteoporosis-related fractures, decreased vitamin B₁₂ absorption
Antiviral (an"ti-viral)	An agent that prevents and treats infections caused by viruses	Zovirax (acyclovir), Hepsera (adefovir), Symmetrel (amantadine), Vistide (cidofovir), Tivicay (dolutegravir), Prezista (darunavir), Videx (didanosine), Abreva (docosano)	**Common:** Nausea, diarrhea, fever, headache, pain, aggressive behavior, depression, fatigue, insomnia **Severe:** Allergic reaction (rash, hives, tissue swelling, respiratory difficulty, chest tightness), delirium, anemia, coma, psychosis, hepatitis, renal failure
Bronchodilator (brong"ko-dil-a'tor)	An agent that relaxes the smooth muscles in the lungs and allows widening of the bronchi to allow the flow of air into and out of the lungs	Proventil or Ventolin (salbutamol/albuterol), Asthmanefrin (racemic epinephrine), Brethine (terbutaline), Proventil (albuterol), Serevent (salmeterol), Arcapta Neohaler (indacaterol)	**Common:** Flushing, headache, dizziness, tremors, nausea, sweating, weakness, insomnia **Severe:** Allergic reaction (rash, hives, tissue swelling, respiratory difficulty, chest tightness), blurred vision, arrhythmias, worsening glaucoma
Contraceptive (kon"tra-sep'tiv)	Any device, method, or agent that prevents conception	Desogen, Ortho-Cept, Yasmin, Yaz (desogestrel/ethinyl estradiol), Amethyst, Lybrel, Nordette, Seasonique, Triphasil (levonorgestrel/ethinyl estradiol), Norinyl 1/50 (mestranol/norethindrone), Cyclafem 1/35, Loestrin, Microgestin, Nortrel (norethindrone/ethinyl estradiol), Ortho-Cyclen, TriNessa (norgestimate/ethinyl estradiol)	**Common:** Breast tenderness, bleeding between periods, headache, nervousness, nausea, vomiting, cramping, vaginal infection **Severe:** Allergic reaction (rash, hives, tissue swelling, respiratory difficulty, chest tightness), chest pain, depression, abnormal blood clotting, liver failure

continues

Table 34-1 continued

CLASSIFICATION (WITH PHONETIC SPELLING)	ACTION	EXAMPLES OF DRUGS COMMONLY USED IN AMBULATORY CARE SETTING	SIDE EFFECTS
Decongestant (de"con-gest'ant)	An agent that causes vasoconstriction in the small blood vessels of the nose, throat, and sinuses	Afrin (oxymetazoline), Neo-Synephrine (phenylephrine HCl), Sudafed (pseudoephedrine HCl)	**Common:** Increased nasal discharge, sneezing, stinging, burning, nasal dryness **Severe:** Allergic reaction (rash, hives, tissue swelling, respiratory difficulty, chest tightness), hypertension, arrhythmias, seizures
Diuretic (di"u-ret'ik)	An agent that increases the amount of water that is excreted from the body via the kidneys	Diuril (chlorothiazide), Lasix (furosemide), Osmitrol (mannitol), Diamox (acetazolamide), Bumex (bumetanide), Aldactone (spironolactone)	**Common:** Blurred vision, dizziness, headache, dry mouth, thirst, drowsiness, muscle pain, nausea and vomiting **Severe:** Allergic reaction (rash, hives, tissue swelling, respiratory difficulty, chest tightness), confusion, arrhythmia, oliguria, seizures, hypotension
Expectorant (ek-spek'to-rant)	An agent that increases the bronchial secretions to enhance the expulsion of mucus from the lungs	Musinex (galifenesin)	**Common:** Dizziness, excitability, headache, weakness **Severe:** Allergic reaction (rash, hives, tissue swelling, respiratory difficulty, chest tightness), severe drowsiness
Hypnotic (hip-not'ik)	An agent that slows the activity of the brain to allow for sleep	Nembutal (pentobarbital), secobarbital (Seconal), Xanax (alprazolam), Valium (diazepam), Librium (chlordiazepoxide), Ambien (zolpidem), Lunesta (eszopiclone)	**Common:** Clumsiness, dizziness, lightheadedness, confusion, fainting, impaired thinking and reactions **Severe:** Allergic reaction (rash, hives, tissue swelling, respiratory difficulty, chest tightness), confusion, hallucinations, fainting, depressed respirations, engaging in activities with no memory of these activities
Laxative (lak'sa-tiv)	An agent that increases stool motility, fluid content, bulk, and/or frequency	Colace (docusate sodium), Linzess (linaclotide), Enulose (lactulose), Miralax (polyethylene glycol), Metamucil (psyllium), Milk of Magnesia (magnesium hydroxide)	**Common:** Abdominal bloating or fullness, abdominal cramps, nausea, lightheadedness **Severe:** Allergic reaction (rash, hives, tissue swelling, respiratory difficulty, chest tightness), intestinal obstruction
Muscle relaxant (mus'el re-lak'sant)	An agent that works at the level of the brain or at the level of the muscle to decrease the tension in the muscle and improve mobility	Soma (carisoprodol), Flexeril (cyclobenzaprine), Dantrium (dantrolene), Lioresal (baclofen), Valium (diazepam), Robaxin (methocarbamol), Skelaxin (metaxalone)	**Common:** Blurred vision, confusion, dizziness, nasal stuffiness, nausea and vomiting, urinary retention **Severe:** Allergic reaction (rash, hives, tissue swelling, respiratory difficulty, chest tightness), memory loss, seizures, bradycardia, addiction

3. **Biotransformation** is the chemical alteration that a drug undergoes in the body, usually in the liver.

4. **Elimination** is the process whereby the drug is excreted from the body. Elimination occurs via the gastrointestinal tract, respiratory tract, skin, mucous membranes, and mammary glands.

Undesirable Actions of Drugs

Most drugs have the potential for causing an action other than their intended action. For example:

1. *Side effect.* An undesirable action of the drug that may limit the usefulness of the drug.

2. *Drug interaction.* Occurs when one drug potentiates, that is, increases or diminishes the action of another drug. These actions may be desirable or undesirable. Drugs may also interact with various foods, alcohol, tobacco, and other substances.

3. *Adverse reaction.* An unfavorable or harmful unintended action of a drug, such as an allergic reaction.

A patient may experience an allergic reaction to a drug after administration. It is often mild and may exhibit itself in the form of a rash, **urticaria**, or **pruritus**. On occasion, a severe allergic reaction or **anaphylaxis** can occur, which is hypersensitivity to a drug or other foreign protein. It is the least common allergic reaction but can become severe quickly and result in dyspnea and shock. Loss of consciousness and death can result. To help prevent an allergic reaction or minimize its risk, the medical assistant should make every effort to ensure that the patient has not had an allergic reaction to the medication she has been ordered to administer. The medical assistant should be aware of signs and symptoms of allergic reaction and notify the provider immediately so that appropriate emergency treatment can be given. The administration of epinephrine usually reverse the life-threatening symptoms of anaphylaxis, and they are followed by administration of an antihistamine and/or H1 and H2 blockers such as Benadryl (diphenhydramine), Tagamet (cimetidine), or Zantac (ranitidine). The patient needs to be immediately placed in the Trendelenburg position and supplemental oxygen applied. In severe cases that do not respond to this treatment, EMS is activated and the patient is transported to the nearest emergency department.

DRUG ROUTES

Drugs are manufactured in a variety of forms and for various purposes. The route of a drug is how it is administered to the patient, and thereby transported into the patient's body. Certain medications can be administered by more than one route, whereas others must be administered via a specific route.

The route of administration is determined by a number of factors. One factor is the action of the medication on the body, either local or systemic. Intravenous medication reaches the systemic circulation rapidly and quickly becomes effective. Injections of medications and medications absorbed through mucous membranes, such as suppositories and sublingual nitroglycerine, are absorbed quickly. Oral medications take longer to act because they first must be digested by the stomach and then must be absorbed into the bloodstream.

Another factor in route selection is the physical and emotional state of the patient. The patient's consciousness level, emotional status, and physical restrictions are considered when selecting a route to administer medication.

A third factor to consider is the drug's characteristics. An example is insulin. Insulin is destroyed by digestive enzymes; therefore, the route of administration must be by injection.

The most frequently used routes of administering medication to the patient are oral and parenteral; oral medications are taken by mouth, parenteral generally by injection. Other routes of administration include:

- Direct application to the skin, that is, topical (lotions, creams, liniments, ointments, transdermal [patch] systems)
- Sublingual (tablets, liquid, drops)
- Buccal (tablets)
- Rectal (suppositories, ointments)
- Vaginal (suppositories, creams, applications)
- Inhalation (sprays, aerosols)
- Instillation (liquid, drops)

FORMS OF DRUGS

Drugs are compounded in three basic types of preparations: liquids, solids, and semisolids. The ease with which a drug's ingredients can be dissolved largely determines the variety of forms manufactured. Some drug agents are soluble in water, others in alcohol, and others in a mixture of several solvents.

The method for administering a drug depends on its form, its properties, and the effects desired. When given orally, a drug may be in the form of a liquid, powder, tablet, capsule, or caplet. If it is to be injected, it must be in the form of a liquid. For topical use, the drug may be in the form of a liquid, powder, or semisolid. Oral and injectable medications are examples of preparations designed for internal use.

Liquid Preparations

Liquid preparations contain a drug that has been dissolved or suspended. Depending on the solvent used, the drug may be further classified as an aqueous (water) or alcohol preparation or as an aerosol or mist. When prescribed for internal use, liquid preparations other than emulsions are rapidly absorbed through the stomach, intestinal walls, or lungs.

Solid and Semisolid Preparations

Tablets, capsules, caplets, troches or lozenges, suppositories, and ointments are examples of solid and semisolid preparations. These products offer great flexibility as a means of dispensing different dosages of drugs. Figure 34-4 shows types of tablets and capsules.

Other Drug Delivery Systems

Technologic advances have introduced new ways by which drugs can be introduced into the patient. In addition to the conventional preparations, the following therapeutic systems offer special delivery of medication to targeted areas.

Transdermal System. The **transdermal** system of medication delivery consists of a small adhesive patch that may be applied to intact skin near the treatment site. For example, Transderm Scop, used for preventing motion sickness, may be applied behind the ear; Nitro-Dur (Figure 34-5), used for preventing angina pectoris, may be applied to the chest; Estraderm, used to treat menopausal symptoms, may be applied to the trunk; and Nicoderm, used to relieve the body's craving for nicotine, may be applied to any area above the waist. A transdermal system generally consists of four layers (Figure 34-6):

1. An impermeable backing that keeps the drug from leaking out of the system
2. A reservoir containing the drug

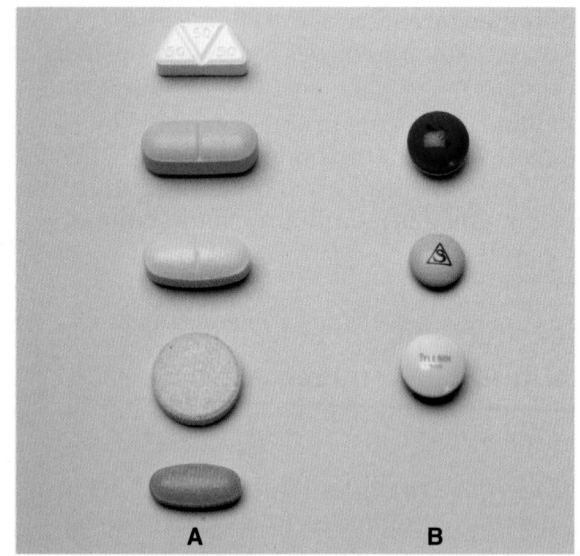

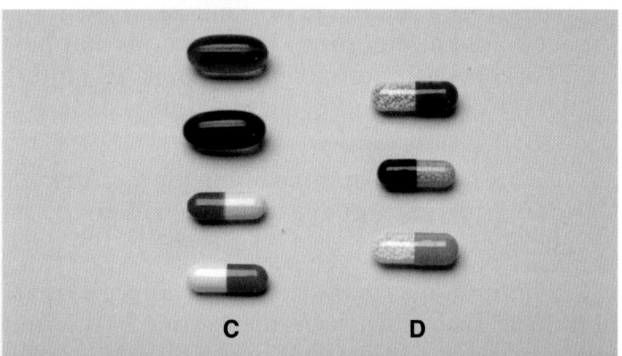

FIGURE 34-4 Drugs are manufactured in various forms, including solid preparations such as tablets and capsules. (A) Tablets, scored and unscored. (B) Enteric-coated tablets. (C) Capsules and gelatin-coated capsules. (D) Timed-release capsules.

3. A membrane with tiny holes that controls the rate of drug release
4. An adhesive layer or gel that keeps the device in place

Inhalation Medications. Respiratory diseases and conditions such as asthma, bronchiectasis (permanent dilation of one or more bronchi), bronchitis, and others may require treatment with inhalation medication from an aerosolized inhaler or a nebulizer. Some of the commonly prescribed medications are bronchodilators such as aminophylline, albuterol, Isuprel, epinephrine, and cortisone-type medications. Oxygen may be prescribed for hypoxia caused by respiratory diseases. Oxygen may also be prescribed for

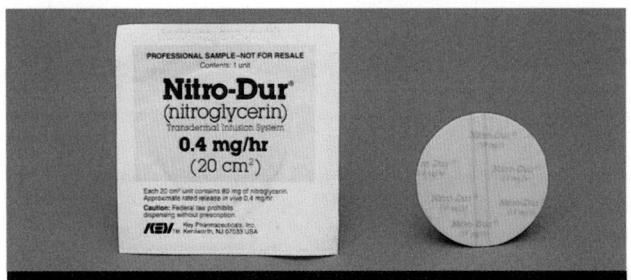

FIGURE 34-5 Nitro-Dur is a transdermal system of delivering medication used for prevention and for long-term management of angina pectoris. It can be applied to the chest.

cardiovascular collapse, congestive heart failure, and pneumonia, among other examples.

Implantable Devices. Implantable devices are available in several shapes and sizes and are positioned just beneath the skin near blood vessels

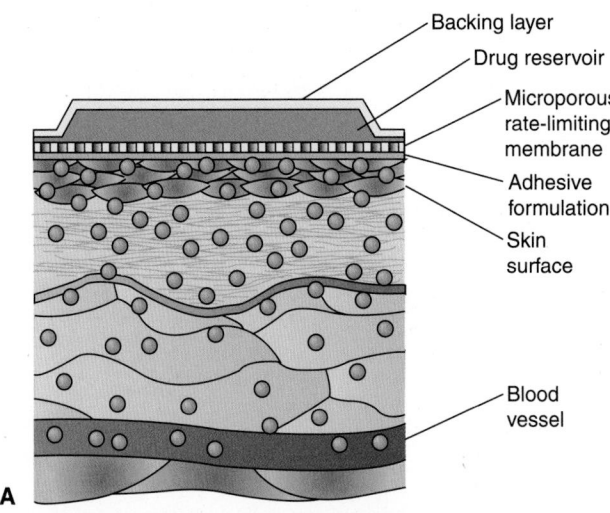

- Backing layer
- Drug reservoir
- Microporous rate-limiting membrane
- Adhesive formulation
- Skin surface
- Blood vessel

A

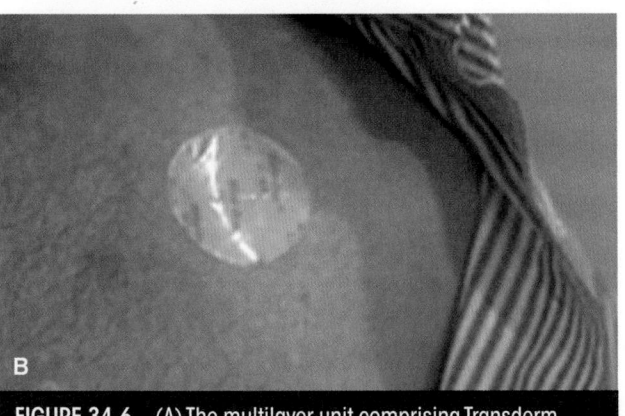

B

FIGURE 34-6 (A) The multilayer unit comprising Transderm Nitro delivers nitroglycerin into the bloodstream in a consistent, controlled manner for 24 hours. The thin unit contains a backing layer, a reservoir of nitroglycerin, a unique rate-limiting membrane, and an adhesive layer that has a priming dose of nitroglycerin. (B) The patch is applied to the skin.

Courtesy of Novartis

that lead directly to the area to be medicated. For example, an infusion pump that is about the size of a hockey puck can be implanted below the skin near the waist to provide continuous delivery of chemotherapy to patients with liver cancer, insulin to a diabetic, or narcotics to a chronic pain patient. This device, which has a refillable drug reservoir, is connected by an outlet catheter to the patient's blood vessel or directly into the spinal fluid. In addition to providing a continuous supply of medication, these devices have the advantage of delivering greater doses with fewer side effects than can be realized through the systemic route.

STORAGE AND HANDLING OF MEDICATIONS

Safety

Certain precautions should be followed if the ambulatory care setting keeps medications on the premises. The goal should be to store all medications in their original containers in a separate room in a locked cabinet. Many medications require storage in a certain manner, such as a dark area or a dark container (to keep light away from them) or in the refrigerator. Some must be kept in glass containers only because plastic may react with the medication's chemical composition. The drug label indicates proper storage and handling for each medication.

Keep medications that are for internal use separated from those intended for external use.

Access to medications is simplified if they are organized in the storage area either according to their classification (e.g., diuretic, hormones) or alphabetically. Always check expiration dates.

EMERGENCY MEDICATIONS AND SUPPLIES

The ambulatory care setting should maintain a tray, box, cabinet, or crash cart (see Chapter 8 for contents of crash cart) especially and solely for drugs and supplies needed in an emergency such as anaphylaxis or other form of shock. The drugs listed in Table 34-2 are a sample of some general drugs to keep readily available for emergencies.

Other supplies and equipment to keep together with the drugs on the emergency cart include:

- Intravenous (IV) materials such as IV fluids, needles, tubing, syringes, alcohol swabs, constriction band, and tape
- Sphygmomanometer

TABLE 34-2

EXAMPLES OF COMMON EMERGENCY DRUGS

DRUG	DESCRIPTION
Activated charcoal	A charcoal suspension; used to treat poisoning
Adrenaline (a-dren'a-lin) or epinephrine (ep-i-nef-rin)	A vasoconstrictor; relieves anaphylactic shock
Albuterol (al-bú-ter-ol)	A bronchodilator; relaxes smooth muscle of the respiratory tract
Atropine (a-trō-peen)	Helps restore heart rate
Benadryl (ben'a-dril)	An antihistamine that relieves allergic symptoms
Compazine (com-pa'zeen)	An antiemetic; relieves symptoms of nausea and vomiting
Dextrose (deks'trose) 50%	Used for hypoglycemia to counteract hyperinsulinism
Diazepam (di-i-az'-e-pam)	Helps control seizures; is used for anxiety
Digoxin (di-jox'in)	Cardiac drug; used for congestive heart failure, arrhythmias; slows and strengthens heartbeat
Diuril (di'ur-il)	Promotes excretion of urine
Hydrocortisone (hi"dro-cort'i-zon)	An anti-inflammatory; used to suppress swelling and shock
Insulin (in'sah-lin)	Regulation of blood sugar
Isuprel (licé-ū-prel)	Used for heart block
Lasix (lā-siks, -ziks)	Used for pulmonary edema
Lidocaine (li'-dō-kāne)	Used for local anesthesia
Morphine (mawr-feen)	A narcotic analgesic
Narcan (nar'can)	An antidote; used in narcotic overdose
Nitroglycerin (ni"tro-glis'er-in)	A vasodilator; dilates coronary arteries; used in treatment of angina pectoris
Valium (val'e-um)	Used for anxiety, as a muscle relaxant; used to calm anxious patients and to relax muscles; valium is a Schedule IV drug, and therefore must be kept in a locked cabinet
Verapamil (ver-ap'a-mil)	For cardiac arrhythmia, stable and unstable angina

NOTE: Ipecac syrup is no longer used to induce vomiting, because it has proven to be cardiotoxic, and several cases of aspiration have occurred.

- Stethoscope
- Oxygen and mask
- Airways
- Defibrillator
- Suction equipment (nasopharyngeal)
- Personal protective equipment

Check the tray on a regular basis (weekly or monthly, depending on use). Check the oxygen tank and gauge. Replace items that have been used as soon as possible, and discard drugs and supplies that have reached their expiration dates. Document that the tray has been checked and updated. (See Chapter 8 for more information about emergencies and emergency drugs used in the office and other ambulatory areas.)

Bioterrorism

Bioterrorism is the name given to the use of biologic weapons (pathogenic microorganisms) to create fear in people. There are many biologic agents that can be used in an attempt to cause serious diseases. Biological weapons do not cost a lot of money, yet the human casualties can be significant. Bioweapons are easy to transport; can be stockpiled; and when deployed, can cause more deaths than a tactical nuclear weapon. Terrorists have the opportunity to launch an attack and escape the area before the authorities even know that an attack has occurred.

In March 2015, the Blue Ribbon Study Panel on Biodefense arrived at the consensus that the government does not have a good answer to the question of who would be in charge if the United States were beset by a biological or chemical weapons attack. Therefore, it is logical that the response to these types of threats will originate at the local level. With this in mind, it is important for the medical assistant to be aware of these threats and be prepared to respond in the event of an emergency. At a minimum, PPE, including a respirator, and hand sanitizer must be kept on hand in preparation. A good place to begin to assist your provider or clinic to participate in preparedness is to access the Center for Disease Control and Prevention's "Bioterrorism Readiness Plan: A Template for Healthcare Facilities." This document can be accessed at http://emergency.cdc.gov by searching for the document by title.

The most dangerous such disease threats are anthrax, botulism, pneumonic/bubonic plague, smallpox, and tularemia. However, most bioterroristic diseases can be treated with pharmaceutical agents like antibiotics and antioxoids.

Anthrax, pneumonic/bubonic plague, and tularemia can all be treated with antibiotics. Botulism is treated with botulism antioxides supplied by public health authorities. Smallpox is treated by early vaccination (within 4 days). The Centers for Disease Control and Prevention has the vaccine.

Initiative Education plays a vital role in raising awareness and increasing the knowledge of health care professionals to aid them in being better prepared for threats to the public health. The World Health Organization,

the Centers for Disease Control and Prevention, and state and local public health departments are excellent resources for more information about bioterrorism. (See Chapter 8 for information about emergencies, Chapter 21 for infectious diseases.)

DRUG ABUSE

Safety

Legal

There has been an enormous increase in the **abuse**, or misuse, of legal and illegal drugs. Any drug can be abused, whether it is penicillin, alcohol, or a controlled substance such as cocaine. Medical assistants, while caring for patients, may unexpectedly come in contact with patients who abuse or misuse drugs.

Integrity

As a member of the health care team that commonly interacts on a face-to-face basis with patients, it is important to be able to recognize the symptoms of drug abuse in a patient or co-worker and report it to the provider. Health professionals, including providers, are among individuals who can have a problem with drug or alcohol abuse, and it must be reported to the proper professional association (see Chapter 6 for more information on drug abuse).

There are many programs available for treatment of drug abuse. Detoxification and rehabilitation are examples of treatment programs. The National Institute on Drug Abuse (NIDA), which is part of the National Institutes of Health of the U.S. Department of Health and Human Services, provides information, treatment options, and specific programs for drug abuse. The NIDA's mission is to advance science on the causes and consequences of drug use and addiction and to apply that knowledge to improve individual and public health. Information on drugs that are commonly abused, their effects on the body, treatment options, and much more can be found on their Web site, www.drugabuse.gov.

Table 34-3 gives examples of drug types most commonly abused.

The same social pressures that influence young people to try alcohol are responsible for introducing people of all ages to the previously mentioned drugs and other chemical substances. Because it is easier to prevent drug abuse than it is to break an established habit, most efforts to combat drug abuse are directed at the young. However, people of all ages, including older people, may be or become abusers.

TABLE 34-3

DRUGS OF ABUSE: USES AND EFFECTS

DRUG	CONTROLLED SUBSTANCE SCHEDULE	TRADE OR OTHER NAMES	MEDICAL USES	DEPENDENCE		TOLERANCE	DURATION (HOURS)	USUAL METHOD	POSSIBLE EFFECTS	EFFECTS OF OVERDOSE	WITHDRAWAL SYNDROME
				PHYSICAL	PSYCHOLOGICAL						
NARCOTICS											
Heroin	Substance I	Diamorphine, Horse, Smack, Black tar, *Chiva, Negra* (black tar)	None in United States, analgesic, antitussive	High	High	Yes	3 to 4	Injected, snorted, smoked	Euphoria, drowsiness, respiratory depression, constricted pupils, nausea	Slow and shallow breathing, clammy skin, convulsions, coma, possible death	Watery eyes, runny nose, yawning, loss of appetite, irritability, tremors, panic, cramps, nausea, chills, sweating
Morphine	Substance II	MS-Contin, Roxanol, Oramorph SR, MSIR	Analgesic	High	High	Yes	3 to 12	Oral, injected	Same as above	Same as above	Same as above
Hydrocodone	Substance II, Product III, V	Hydrocodone with acetaminophen, Vicodin, Vicoprofen, Tussionex, Lortab	Analgesic, antitussive	High	High	Yes	3 to 6	Oral	Same as above	Same as above	Same as above
Hydromorphone	Substance II	Dilaudid	Analgesic	High	High	Yes	3 to 4	Oral, injected	Same as above	Same as above	Same as above
Oxycodone	Substance II	Roxicet, Oxycodone with acetaminophen, OxyContin, Endocet, Percocet, Percodan	Analgesic	High	High	Yes	3 to 12	Oral	Same as above	Same as above	Same as above

DRUG	CONTROLLED SUBSTANCE SCHEDULE	TRADE OR OTHER NAMES	MEDICAL USES	PHYSICAL	PSYCHOLOGICAL	TOLERANCE	DURATION (HOURS)	USUAL METHOD	POSSIBLE EFFECTS	EFFECTS OF OVERDOSE	WITHDRAWAL SYNDROME
NARCOTICS											
Codeine	Substance II, Product III, V	Acetaminophen, Guaifenesin or Promethazine with Codeine, Fiorinal, Fioricet or Tylenol with Codeine	Analgesic, antitussive	Moderate	Moderate	Yes	3 to 4	Oral, injected	Same as above	Same as above	Same as above
Other Narcotics	Substance II, III, IV	Fentanyl, Demerol, Methadone, Darvon, Stadol, Talwin, Paregoric, Buprenex	Analgesic, antidiarrheal, antitussive	High-Low	High-Low	Yes	Variable	Oral, injected, snorted, smoked	Same as above	Same as above	Same as above
DEPRESSANTS											
Gamma Hydroxybutyric Acid	Substance I, Product III	GHB, Liquid Ecstasy, Liquid X, Sodium Oxybate, Xyrem	None in United States, anesthetic	Moderate	Moderate	Yes	3 to 6	Oral	Slurred speech, disorientation, drunken behavior without odor of alcohol, impaired memory of events, interacts with alcohol	Shallow respiration, clammy skin, dilated pupils, weak and rapid pulse, coma, possible death	Anxiety, insomnia, tremors, delirium, convulsions, possible death
Benzodiazepines	Substance IV	Valium, Xanax, Halcion, Ativan, Restoril, Rohypnol (Roofies, R-2), Klonopin	Antianxiety, sedative, anticonvulsant, hypnotic, muscle relaxant	Moderate	Moderate	Yes	1 to 8	Oral, injected	Same as above	Same as above	Same as above

continues

Table 34-3 continued

DRUG	CONTROLLED SUBSTANCE SCHEDULE	TRADE OR OTHER NAMES	MEDICAL USES	PHYSICAL	PSYCHOLOGICAL	TOLERANCE	DURATION (HOURS)	USUAL METHOD	POSSIBLE EFFECTS	EFFECTS OF OVERDOSE	WITHDRAWAL SYNDROME
DEPRESSANTS											
Other Depressants	Substance I, II, III, IV	Ambien, Sonata, Meprobamate, Chloral Hydrate, Barbiturates, Methaqualone (Quaalude)	Antianxiety, sedative, hypnotic	Moderate	Moderate	Yes	2 to 6	Oral	Slurred speech, disorientation, drunken behavior without odor of alcohol, impaired memory of events, interacts with alcohol	Shallow respiration, clammy skin, dilated pupils, weak and rapid pulse, coma, possible death	Anxiety, insomnia, tremors, delirium, convulsions, possible death
STIMULANTS											
Cocaine	Substance II	Coke, Flake, Snow, Crack, Coca, Blanca, Perico, Nieve, Soda	Local anesthetic	Possible	High	Yes	1 to 2	Snorted, smoked, injected	Increased alertness, excitation, euphoria, increased pulse rate and blood pressure, insomnia, loss of appetite	Agitation, increased body temperature, hallucinations, convulsions, possible death	Apathy, long periods of sleep, irritability, depression, disorientation
Amphetamine/Methamphetamine	Substance II	Crank, Ice, Cristal, Krystal Meth, Speed, Adderall, Dexedrine, Desoxyn	Attention deficit/hyperactivity disorder, narcolepsy, weight control	Possible	High	Yes	2 to 4	Oral, injected, smoked	Same as above	Same as above	Same as above
Methylphenidate	Substance II	Ritalin, Concerta, Focalin, Metadate	Attention deficit/hyperactivity disorder	Possible	High	Yes	2 to 4	Oral, injected, snorted, smoked	Same as above	Same as above	Same as above
Other Stimulants	Substance III, IV	Adipex P lontamin, Prelu-2, Didrex, Provigil	Vasoconstriction	Possible	Moderate	Yes	2 to 4	Oral	Same as above	Same as above	Same as above

HALLUCINOGENS

DRUG	CONTROLLED SUBSTANCE SCHEDULE	TRADE OR OTHER NAMES	MEDICAL USES	PHYSICAL	PSYCHOLOGICAL	TOLERANCE	DURATION (HOURS)	USUAL METHOD	POSSIBLE EFFECTS	EFFECTS OF OVERDOSE	WITHDRAWAL SYNDROME
MDMA and Analogs	Substance I	Ecstasy, XTC, Adam, MDA (Love Drug), MDEA (Eve), MBDB	None	None	Moderate	Yes	4 to 6	Oral, snorted, smoked	Heightened senses, teeth grinding, dehydration	Increased body temperature, electrolyte imbalance, cardiac arrest	Muscle aches, drowsiness, depression, acne
LSD	Substance I	Acid, Microdot, Sunshine, Boomers	None	None	Unknown	Yes	8 to 12	Oral	Illusions and hallucinations, altered perception of time and distance	Longer, more intense "trip" episodes	None
Phencyclidine and Analogs	Substance I, II, III	PCP, Angel Dust, Hog, Loveboat, Ketamine (Special K), PCE, PCPy, TCP	Anesthetic (ketamine)	Possible	High	Yes	1 to 12	Smoked, oral, injected, snorted	Illusions and hallucinations, altered perception of time and distance	Unable to direct movement, feel pain, remember	Drug-seeking behavior*
Other Hallucinogens	Substance I	Psilocybe mushrooms, Mescaline, Peyote Cactus, Ayahausca, DMT, Dextromethorphan (DXM)	None	None	None	Possible	4 to 8	Oral	Illusions and hallucinations, altered perception of time and distance	Unable to direct movement, feel pain, remember	Drug-seeking behavior*

CANNIBIS

DRUG	CONTROLLED SUBSTANCE SCHEDULE	TRADE OR OTHER NAMES	MEDICAL USES	PHYSICAL	PSYCHOLOGICAL	TOLERANCE	DURATION (HOURS)	USUAL METHOD	POSSIBLE EFFECTS	EFFECTS OF OVERDOSE	WITHDRAWAL SYNDROME
Marijuana	Substance I	Pot, Grass, Sinsemilla, Blunts, *Mota*, *Yerba*, *Grifa*	None	Unknown	Moderate	Yes	2 to 4	Smoked, oral	Euphoria, relaxed inhibitions, increased appetite, disorientation	Fatigue, paranoia, possible psychosis	Occasional reports of insomnia, hyperactivity, decreased appetite

continues

Table 34-3 continued

DRUG	CONTROLLED SUBSTANCE SCHEDULE	TRADE OR OTHER NAMES	MEDICAL USES	PHYSICAL	PSYCHOLOGICAL	TOLERANCE	DURATION (HOURS)	USUAL METHOD	POSSIBLE EFFECTS	EFFECTS OF OVERDOSE	WITHDRAWAL SYNDROME
CANNIBIS											
Tetrahydrocanna-binol	Substance I, Product III	THC, Marinol	Antinauseant, appetite stimulant	Yes	Moderate	Yes	2 to 4	Smoked, oral	Same as above	Same as above	Same as above
Hashish and Hashish Oil	Substance I	Hash, Hash oil	None	Unknown	Moderate	Yes	Same as above	inhalation or ingestion	Same as above	Same as above	Same as above
ANABOLIC STEROIDS											
Testosterone	Substance III	Depo Testosterone, Sustanon, Sten, Cypt	Hypogonad-ism	Unknown	Unknown	Unknown	14 to 28 days	Injected	Virilization, edema, testicular atrophy, gynecomastia, acne, aggressive behavior	Unknown	Possible depression
Other Anabolic Steroids	Substance III	Parabolan, Winstrol, Equipoise, Anadrol, Dianabol, Primabolin-Depo, D-Ball	Anemia, breast cancer	Unknown	Yes	Unknown	Variable	Oral, in-jected	Same as above	Same as above	Same as above
INHALANTS											
Amyl and Butyl Nitrite		Pearls, Poppers, Rush, Locker Room	Angina (amyl)	Unknown	Unknown	No	1	Inhaled	Flushing, hypotension, headache	Methemoglobin-emia	Agitation

DRUG	CONTROLLED SUBSTANCE SCHEDULE	TRADE OR OTHER NAMES	MEDICAL USES	PHYSICAL	PSYCHOLOGICAL	TOLERANCE	DURATION (HOURS)	USUAL METHOD	POSSIBLE EFFECTS	EFFECTS OF OVERDOSE	WITHDRAWAL SYNDROME
INHALANTS											
Nitrous Oxide		Laughing gas, balloons, Whippets	Anesthetic	Unknown	Low	No	0.5	Inhaled	Impaired memory, slurred speech, drunken behavior, slow-onset vitamin deficiency, organ damage	Vomiting, respiratory depression, loss of consciousness, possible death	Trembling, anxiety, insomnia, vitamin deficiency, confusion, hallucinations, convulsions
Other Inhalants		Adhesives, spray paint, hair spray, dry cleaning fluid, spot remover, lighter fluid	None	Unknown	High	No	0.5 to 2	Inhaled	Impaired memory, slurred speech, drunken behavior, slow-onset vitamin deficiency, organ damage	Vomiting, respiratory depression, loss of consciousness, possible death	Trembling, anxiety, insomnia, vitamin deficiency, confusion, hallucinations, convulsions
ALCOHOL											
Alcohol		Beer, wine, liquor	None	High	High	Yes	1 to 3	Oral	Impaired judgments, uncoordinated movements, slurred speech, blurred vision	Motor vehicle accidents, gastritis, liver damage, brain damage, domestic violence	Anxiety, shakiness, depression, hallucinations, sweats, increased blood pressure, seizures

*Not regulated

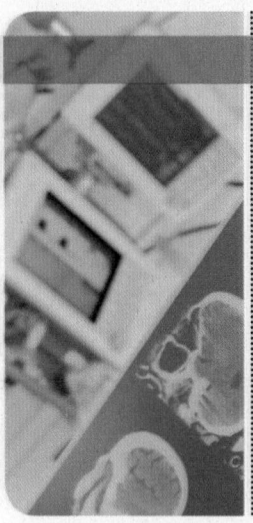

CASE STUDY 34-1

Refer to the scenario at the beginning of the chapter. Mrs. Maynard has an appointment to see Dr. Hoback this morning. She brings in her bag with all of her prescription medications. When Claire Bloom, CMA (AAMA), is updating Mrs. Maynard's electronic medical record, she becomes aware that there is a mistake in the record of Mrs. Maynard's medication history. The prescription bottle states "Zantac 150 mg by mouth twice a day." The electronic record reveals that the medication prescribed was "Zyrtec 10 mg by mouth once a day."

CASE STUDY REVIEW

1. What are the first steps that Ms. Bloom should take to clarify this issue?
2. What kind of questions would Ms. Bloom need to ask Mrs. Maynard about the medications?
3. What is the best method to communicate the recognition of this error to others on the health care team?

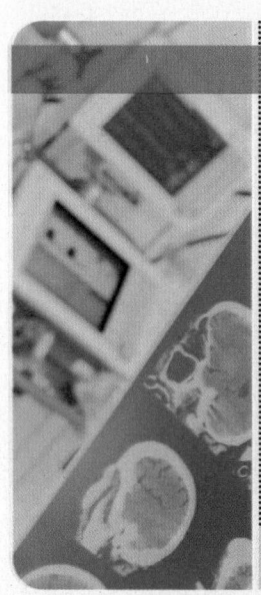

CASE STUDY 34-2

Maria Jover reports vaginal discharge and discomfort. Dr. King confirms the diagnosis of a yeast infection by performing a smear and identifying the microorganism. Dr. King prescribes over-the-counter vaginal suppositories. After asking Maria if she has any questions, clinical medical assistant Nancy McFarland, RMA (AMT), proceeds to help Maria understand the self-administration of this particular medication.

CASE STUDY REVIEW

1. The patient, Maria, asks Nancy McFarland whether she can use some vaginal suppositories she bought last year. How should Nancy respond?
2. Maria tells Nancy that the last time she had a vaginal yeast infection she used only some of the recommended number of suppositories because the infection cleared up. How should Nancy respond?
3. Maria does not really like using suppositories. Should Nancy ask Dr. King to prescribe another form of medication for the yeast infection? What other forms might be available?

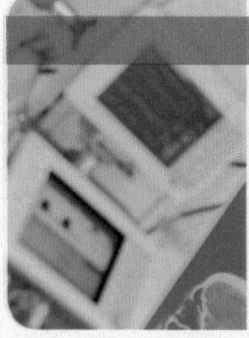

CASE STUDY 34-3

Dr. Lewis keeps a small quantity of various controlled substances on the premises for use in emergency situations.

CASE STUDY REVIEW

1. What are the legalities surrounding controlled substances that concern Joe Guerrero, CMA (AAMA), the clinical medical assistant?
2. What are his responsibilities?

- Medications fall into four specific categories: therapeutic, diagnostic, curative, and preventative.

- There is a long process that is followed during the research and development phase prior to a medication reaching the market.

- Drugs have several names that the medical assistant must be familiar with; the chemical name, the generic name, and the trade or brand name.

- Historically, drugs have come from natural sources. Drug companies use natural as well as chemical, biochemical, and biotechnical avenues to discover new medications.

- Medications that do not require a prescription are referred to as nonprescription or over-the-counter.

- Disposal of medications must be properly performed according to the type of medication, the governing laws, and with the protection of the environment in mind.

- Responsible medical assistants are familiar with medication classifications, principal actions, and routes of administration.

- Medical assistants must know state and federal laws that govern the storage, handling, and administration of medications and must understand their role and responsibilities in light of these laws.

- Knowledge of drug regulations; the legal classifications of drugs, including controlled substances; and prescribing, administering, and dispensing of drugs is essential to ensure compliance with the law.

- Available resources and reference books will provide valuable information about pharmaceutical products, their classifications, routes, forms, storage and handling, and side effects.

- Emergency drugs and supplies should be available on a crash cart or a tray or cabinet for the sole use in an office emergency.

- With the increase of drug abuse and misuse, it is important for medical assistants to recognize the signs of drug abuse in patients and coworkers and to report abuse to the provider or supervisor.

Study for Success

To reinforce your knowledge of and skills related to information presented in this chapter:

- Review the *Key Terms* and *Learning Outcomes*

- Consider the *Critical Thinking* features and *Case Studies* and discuss your conclusions

- Answer the questions in the *Certification Review*

Procedure

- Perform the *Procedure* using the *Competency Assessment Checklists* on the *Student Companion Website*

CERTIFICATION REVIEW

1. Which of the following drugs is commonly used in an emergency such as anaphylactic shock?
   a. Lomotil
   b. Interferon
   c. Cytoxan
   d. Epinephrine

2. Which of the following types of drugs do providers prescribe most frequently?
   a. Generic
   b. Official
   c. Chemical
   d. Brand
   e. Over-the-counter

3. Which of the following is an example of a drug that can be obtained from an animal source?
   a. Digitalis
   b. Cortisone
   c. Premarin
   d. Nexium
4. Which of the following is an example of a controlled substance?
   a. OxyContin
   b. Ventolin
   c. Inderal
   d. Aldomet
   e. Pristiq
5. After you have poured a medication and taken it to the patient, he refuses to take it. Which of the following actions is the next correct step?
   a. Give it to another patient who has the same medication prescribed
   b. Return the refused medication to its original container
   c. Save it for the next time the patient is due for another dose
   d. Notify the provider and await instructions
6. The substances that have the highest potential for abuse are designated as which schedule?
   a. Schedule I
   b. Schedule II
   c. Schedule III
   d. Schedule IV
   e. Schedule V

7. Which of the following are considered medical uses for drugs?
   a. Therapeutic, diagnostic, curative
   b. Diagnostic, curative, recreational
   c. Preventative, curative, holistic
   d. Replacement, prophylactic, research
8. Which of the following is a commonly abused drug in the United States?
   a. Aspirin
   b. Oxycodone
   c. Abilify
   d. Viagara
   e. Oxytocin
9. Which of the following is a category of drug names?
   a. Brand name
   b. Generic
   c. Chemical
   d. All of these
10. Which of the following routes of delivery results in the most rapid action of the medication given?
    a. Topical
    b. Oral
    c. Intradermal
    d. Intramuscular
    e. Intravenous

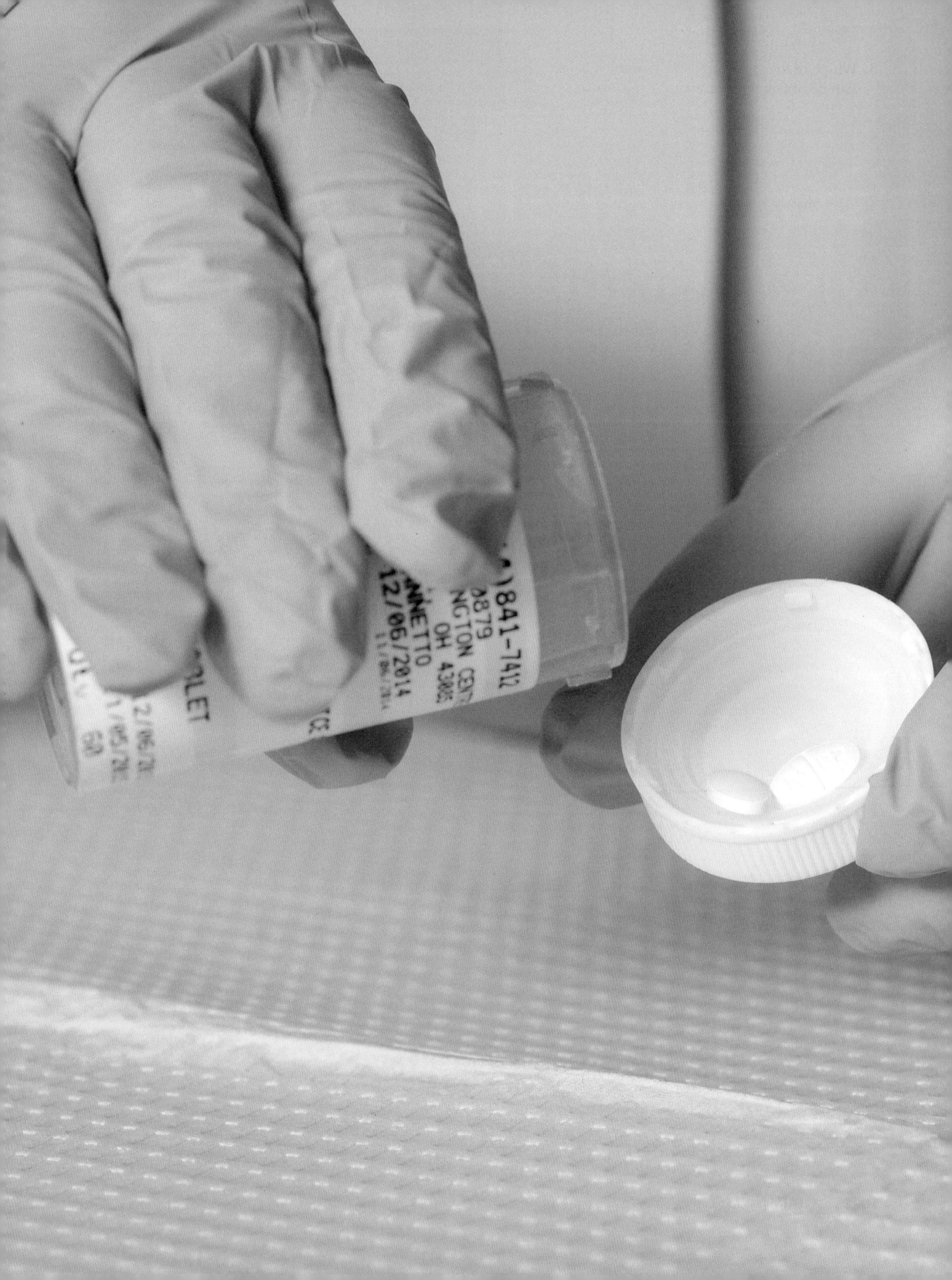

CHAPTER 35

Calculation of Medication Dosage and Medication Administration

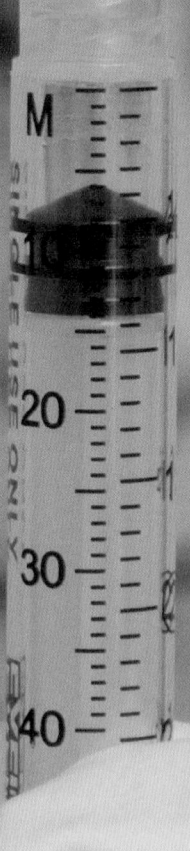

1. Define and spell the key terms as presented in the glossary.
2. Discuss the legal and ethical implications of medication administration.
3. Verify the medication order.
4. Identify abbreviations and symbols used in calculating medication dosage.
5. Describe the parts of a prescription.
6. Define drug dosage.
7. State what information is found on a medication label.
8. Understand ratio and proportion.
9. Use the metric, household, and apothecary systems of measurement and convert between the metric and apothecary systems.
10. Recognize units of medication dosage.
11. Correctly calculate dosages for adults and children.
12. List the guidelines to follow when preparing and administering medications.
13. Administer oral medications.
14. Select proper sites for administering parenteral medication.
15. Describe safe disposal of syringes, needles, and biohazard materials.
16. Explain intravenous therapy.
17. Choose site selection for administration of injections.
18. Characterize allergenic extracts.
19. Describe inhalation medication and its administration.

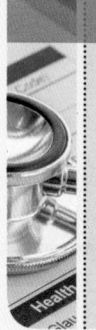

KEY TERMS

administering	meniscus	precipitate
apnea	nomogram	retrolental fibroplasias
body surface area (BSA)	parenteral	status asthmaticus
compounding	pharmacokinetics	unit dose
dispensing	phytomedicines	
hypoxemia	port	

SCENARIO

At Inner City Health Care, clinical medical assistant Joe Guerrero, CMA (AAMA), is careful to check the provider's order before preparing and administering medication. He checks the patient's medical record for the patient's name; the provider's order; and the date, time, and route the medication is to be administered. He then checks the medication and the order three times during the preparation of the medication before entering the patient's exam room. Once he enters the exam room, Joe identifies the patient and administers the medication. After giving the medication to the patient, Joe documents the fact in the patient's medical record.

Despite the fact that many ambulatory care centers use what is known as the unit dose type of medication preparation, there remains a responsibility for medical assistants to know and understand how to calculate dosages of medication and to safely administer them to patients.

This chapter addresses calculation of adult and pediatric dosages of medication using the metric and household systems. It also emphasizes the legal aspects of medication administration and discusses oral and parenteral medication administration.

LEGAL AND ETHICAL IMPLICATIONS OF MEDICATION ADMINISTRATION

Legal Competency

Members of the health care profession who prepare and administer medications are ethically and legally responsible for their own actions. Under law, these individuals are required to be licensed, registered, or otherwise authorized by a provider.

Each state has enacted laws governing the practice of medicine, nursing, and pharmacy. These laws vary from state to state; therefore, it is essential that medical assistants become familiar with the laws of the state in which they are employed before administering any medication. In some states, the only health professional authorized to give injections, other than a physician, is a registered nurse. In other states, legislation gives physicians broad authority to delegate responsibility for administering medication to other health care workers such as medical assistants. Laws have been passed in some states specifying which qualified and properly educated and trained persons may perform certain medical acts.

Regardless of the differences in state authorization laws, the courts will not permit the careless action of health care workers to go unpunished, especially when such actions result in harm or death to the patient. Under the law, those administering medications are expected to be knowledgeable about the drugs that they administer and the effects the drug(s) may or will have on the patient. Many states have uniform disciplinary acts. Never administer a medication without thorough knowledge of the drug. It is the medical assistant's responsibility to know the information listed in Table 35-1 about a medication before administering it to a patient. You are an agent of the provider and accountable for your actions.

Ethical Considerations

 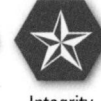

Legal Integrity

Anyone who has access to medications may be tempted to use them for personal benefit. To do so not only is unethical, but also is considered to be illegal. The conversion to personal use of medications intended for a patient, known as diversion, is unethical and illegal and may cause harm to the patient. This rule applies to any medication that belongs to your employer, even aspirin or drug samples, without proper authorization.

The Food and Drug Administration (FDA) defines a medication error as "any preventable event that may cause or lead to inappropriate medication use or patient harm while the medication is in the control of the health care professional,

TABLE 35-1

MEDICATION INFORMATION TO KNOW PRIOR TO ADMINISTERING TO PATIENT

1. Drug name (generic and brand)
2. Action
3. Uses
4. Contraindications
5. Warnings when indicated
6. Adverse reactions
7. Dosage and route
8. Implications for patient care
9. Patient teaching
10. Special considerations

patient, or consumer. Such events may be related to professional practice, health care products, procedures, and systems, including prescribing; order communication; product labeling, packaging, and nomenclature; compounding; dispensing; distribution; administration; education; monitoring; and use." It is essential that attention is focused on the administration of medications. However, mistakes are sometimes made. If there has been a medication error, it is the responsibility of the professional medical assistant to demonstrate integrity and report this error immediately. With more than 10,000 prescription medications available in the United States, it is impossible to be thoroughly familiar with each one. Therefore, a best practice is to reference the PDR or other source for medications that are commonly ordered by your provider. Use the method most convenient for quick access to create a reference that includes generic name, trade name, usual dosage and route, common side effects, and interactions.

The Medication Order

The medication order is given by the provider. It is for a specific patient and denotes the drug to be given, the dosage, the form of the drug, the time for or frequency of administration, and the route by which the drug is to be given.

The Prescription

Legal

The prescription is a written legal document that gives directions for **compounding**, **dispensing**, and **administering** a medication to a patient. There are eight parts to a prescription (Figure 35-1).

The purpose of a prescription is to control the sale and use of drugs that can be safely and effectively used only under the supervision of a licensed provider. Federal law divides medicines into two main classes: prescription or legend medicines and over-the-counter (OTC) medicines. The prescription is written by the provider and signed in ink or, more commonly, e-prescribed. The pharmacist fills the prescription according to the provider's order. Once the prescription has been filled, the assigned prescription number and all other information can be entered into a database. The hard copy of the prescription is filed and kept for a minimum of 7 years. There are state and federal laws, as well as Drug Enforcement Agency guidelines, that are applied to the prescribing provider and

Parts of a Prescription

1. The physician's name, address, telephone and fax numbers, and DEA registration number.
2. The patient's name, date of birth, address, and the date on which the prescription is written.
3. The superscription that includes the symbol Rx ("take thou").
4. The inscription that states the names and quantities of ingredients to be included in the medication.
5. The subscription that gives directions to the pharmacist for filling the prescription.
6. The signature (Sig) that gives the directions for the patient.
7. The physician's signature blanks. Where signed, indicates if a generic substitute is allowed or if the medication is to be dispensed as written.
8. REFILL 0 1 2 3 p.r.n. This is where the physician indicates whether or not the prescription can be refilled.

[1]
[2]
[3]
[4]
[5]
[6]
[7]
[8]

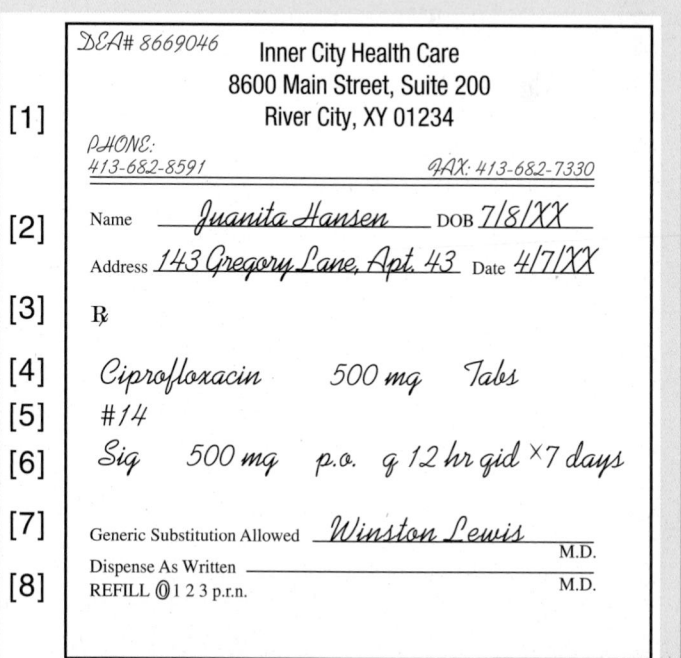

DEA# 8669046

Inner City Health Care
8600 Main Street, Suite 200
River City, XY 01234

PHONE:
413-682-8591   FAX: 413-682-7330

Name _Juanita Hansen_ DOB _7/8/XX_

Address _143 Gregory Lane, Apt. 43_ Date _4/7/XX_

Rx

Ciprofloxacin   500 mg   Tabs
#14
Sig   500 mg   p.o.   q 12 hr qid ×7 days

Generic Substitution Allowed _Winston Lewis_
_____ M.D.
Dispense As Written _____
REFILL ⓪ 1 2 3 p.r.n.   M.D.

FIGURE 35-1 Prescriptions are written legal documents that give directions for compounding, dispensing, and administering a medication. Prescriptions have eight distinct elements.

the pharmacy regarding controlled substances. Some examples are:

- There is a limit placed on the amount of time that a prescription is valid after the provider writes it and it is presented at the pharmacy to be filled.
- The number of days supply is limited.
- The refilling of a prescription for a controlled substance listed in Schedule II is prohibited.
- A prescription for controlled substances in Schedules III, IV, and V issued by a practitioner may be communicated orally, in writing, by facsimile, or digitally to the pharmacist, and may be refilled if so authorized on the prescription or by call-in.
- Schedules III and IV controlled substances may be refilled if authorized on the prescription. However, a specific number of refills must be stated.

HIPAA. E-prescribing is the process of electronically accessing the patient's medical history, prescribing a medication, and selecting a pharmacy.

The Medicare Prescription Drug, Improvement, and Modernization Act (MMA) of 2003 and the Health Insurance Portability and Accountability Act (HIPAA) of 1996 have recommended e-prescribing standards. Medicare incentivized providers to use electronic prescribing (eRx) until 2013 and currently some states require mandatory eRx. For example, as of 2016, providers in New York that are not prescribing electronically are subject to a 2% penalty on their Medicare Part B services.

Medication prescriptions handled electronically have reduced the problem of medication errors. Patients enjoy the ease of e-prescriptions because they do not have to drop off the prescription and then return to pick it up. There has been some question regarding the security and confidentiality of the use of electronic prescribing. However, there are few reports of breeches in security and this concern has lessened.

Prescriptions for Controlled Substances. Federal laws require that the provider follows specific procedures when prescribing controlled substances (Table 35-2).

All prescriptions for controlled substances must be dated and signed on the date issued, bearing the full name and address of the patient and the name, address, and Drug Enforcement Administration (DEA) number (see Chapter 34) of the provider. The prescription must be written in ink or typewritten and signed by the provider's own hand.

Prescription Abbreviations and Symbols. It is important to be knowledgeable of the most common abbreviations used by providers when an order for a prescription drug is given. The abbreviations are a clear and concise means of writing orders. This medical shorthand is an international language used by professional and nonprofessional people involved with patient care. Medical assistants should memorize all abbreviations in Table 35-3 so that they can prepare medications safely and accurately for administration.

The Joint Commission requires that facilities comply with its minimum requirement for the banning of certain abbreviations, acronyms, symbols listed in their "Do Not Use" list. This ban, as part of the Joint Commission's 2004 patient safety goals, has been applied to protect patients from errors during documentation. The ban was reaffirmed in 2005 by the Joint Commission. In 2010, the "Do Not Use" list was integrated into the Information Management standards to improve medication administration safety. This standard relates

TABLE 35-2

REQUIREMENTS FOR PRESCRIPTIONS FOR CONTROLLED SUBSTANCES

	VERBAL ORDER OR PRESCRIPTION	WRITTEN PRESCRIPTION	REFILLS
Schedule I	*Not for medicinal use*		
Schedule II	No	Yes	No
Schedule III	Yes	Yes	5 × within 6 months
Schedule IV	Yes	Yes	5 × within 6 months
Schedule V	Yes	Yes	5 × within 6 months

TABLE 35-3

COMMON PRESCRIPTION ABBREVIATIONS AND SYMBOLS

ABBREVIATION OR SYMBOL	ABBREVIATION MEANING	ABBREVIATION OR SYMBOL	ABBREVIATION MEANING
ac	before meals	pc	after meals
ad lib	as desired	per	by or with
aq	water	po	by mouth
bid	twice a day	prn	as needed
c̄	with	pt	patient
cap	capsule	q	every
dil	dilute	qh	every hour
elix	elixir	q (2, 3, 4) h	every (2, 3, 4) hours
G/gm	gram	qid	four times a day
gr	grain	qs	of sufficient quantity
gt	drop	Rx	take
h	hour	s̄	without
IM	intramuscular	sol	solution
IV	intravenous	ss	one-half
kg	kilogram	stat	at once
L	liter	tab	tablet
liq	liquid	Tbs	tablespoon
mg	milligram	tsp	teaspoon
mL	milliliter	tid	three times a day
mm	millimeter	tr	tincture
NPO	nothing by mouth	ung	ointment
p̄	after		

to documentation, both electronic and manual. The standard states that unapproved abbreviations cannot be used in any type of medication-related documentation. Table 35-4 lists abbreviations no longer allowed by the Joint Commission. Table 35-5 lists abbreviations and symbols that can be misinterpreted and are under consideration for possible inclusion in the "Do Not Use" list in the future.

TABLE 35-4

DANGEROUS ABBREVIATIONS NO LONGER ALLOWED

DO NOT USE	POSSIBLE MISINTERPRETATION	HOW TO AVOID PROBLEM
U (for unit)	Mistaken for 4, 0, or cc	Write out the word *unit*
IU (for international unit)	Mistaken for IV or 10	Write out *international unit*
Q.D., every day; Q.O.D., (every other day)	Mistaken for one another	Write *daily* Write *every other day*
Trailing zero (X.0 mg) Lack of preceding zero (.X mg)	Decimal point is missed and dose is either too much or not enough	Do not write a zero by itself after the decimal point (X mg) Always use zero before a decimal point (0.X mg)
ms mSO$_4$ MgSO$_4$	Can be interpreted to mean morphine sulfate or magnesium sulfate	Write out *morphine sulfate* Write out *magnesium sulfate*

TABLE 35-5

ADDITIONAL ABBREVIATIONS, ACRONYMS, AND SYMBOLS THAT MAY BE MISINTERPRETED (FOR POSSIBLE FUTURE INCLUSION IN THE OFFICIAL "DO NOT USE" LIST)

DO NOT USE	POSSIBLE MISINTERPRETATION	HOW TO AVOID PROBLEM
> (greater than) < (less than)	Can be misinterpreted as number 7 or the letter L Confused for one another	Write out *greater than* and *less than*
Apothecary units	Unfamiliar to many practitioners Confused with metric units	Use metric units
@	Mistaken for number 2	Write *at*
cc	Mistaken for U (units) when written poorly	Write out *mL* or *milliliters*
µg	Mistaken for mg (milligrams) causing 1,000 × overdose	Write out *mcg* or *micrograms*

Patients should be inquisitive when at the provider's office, clinic, pharmacy, or hospital and should ask questions about the medications they are prescribed or being given (see Patient Education box).

Many medications sound alike and look alike, which can cause confusion and errors. The Joint Commission recommends that pharmaceutical manufacturers examine their practices in naming their medications and make changes to alleviate confusion and errors. Table 35-6 lists a few sound-alike, look-alike medications. The Institute of Safe Medicine Practices (ISMP) publishes a list of "confused" drug names, the most recent of which was updated in 2015. This list can be found at https://www.ismp.org.

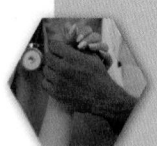

Patient Education

Patients should:

1. Question the provider, pharmacist, and staff administering the drug about the drug and its possible side effects.

2. Be sure the prescription has been written legibly. Many drugs sound alike (e.g., Ambien for insomnia and Amen for menstrual cycle control; Xanax for anxiety and Zantac for heartburn and ulcers; Fosamax for osteoporosis and Flomax for enlarged prostate).

3. Always check the label at the pharmacy to make sure it is clearly written.

4. Always check your medication at the pharmacy to be certain that the medication and directions are what you expect.

5. Have the provider or pharmacist explain the name and purpose of each new medication that is being prescribed. Be sure you understand.

6. Keep an updated list of all medications, prescriptions, OTC vitamins, minerals, and **phytomedicines**. Phytomedicines are medications that are plant based and used for prevention and treatment of various diseases.

7. Take medications as directed, and do not discontinue use until the appropriate date as indicated by the provider.

8. Store medicines away from heat and humidity in their original containers.

9. Ask the provider or pharmacist what you should do if you miss a dose.

TABLE 35-6

SOUND-ALIKE, LOOK-ALIKE MEDICATIONS

Accupril (hypertension)	Aciphex (heartburn, ulcers)
Rimantadine (flu)	Ranitidine (heartburn)
Oxycontin (pain)	Oxybutynin (urinary incontinence)
Paxil (depression)	Plavix (prevent heart attack and stroke)
Pravachol (high cholesterol)	Propranolol (hypertension)
Singulair (asthma)	Sinequan (depression, anxiety)
Clonazepam (anticonvulsant)	Chlorazepate (anxiety)
Darvon (analgesic)	Diovan (hypertension)
Clonazepam (anticonvulsant)	Lorazepam (anxiety)

DRUG DOSAGE

The dosage, or dose, is the amount of medicine that is prescribed for administration. It is determined by the provider or qualified practitioner, who considers the following important factors: age, weight, sex, and other factors as well.

Age

The usual adult dose is generally suitable for the 16- to 60-year age group. Infants, young children, adolescents, and older adults require an individualized dosage regimen.

Weight

The average adult dosage is based on 150 pounds (about 68 kilograms). Individuals who weigh less or more than this should have the dosage based on **body surface area (BSA)** or kilograms of body weight.

Sex

Many medications are contraindicated during pregnancy and breast-feeding. It is important that these two factors be known before any dose of medication is prescribed.

Other Factors

Other factors that determine the dosage of a medication include the following:

1. Physical and emotional condition of patient
2. Disease process, especially kidney disease because of impaired excretion
3. Presence of more than one disease process
4. Causative microorganism(s) and the severity of the infection
5. Patient's medical history, allergies, and idiosyncrasies
6. Safest method, route, time, and amount to effect the desired maximum result

Pediatric Considerations

The term **pharmacokinetics** refers to the way a drug moves into, through, and out of the body. For pediatric patients, pharmacokinetics dictate that drugs be administered in smaller but more frequent doses. Dosages are weight based in milligrams, micrograms, or milliequivalents per kilogram, which allows for much safer drug administration. Remember that children 16 years of age and younger are considered pediatric patients. At age 16, it is generally accepted that pharmacokinetics are similar to those of adults.

Only about one quarter of the drugs approved by the FDA are indicated for pediatric use. There is extensive testing required prior to approval to ensure safety in the less mature body systems of pediatric patients.

Medication errors occur with prescription as well as OTC medications. Reports to the FDA are considered to be voluntary, so the actual numbers are likely much higher. Medication errors lead to many thousands of deaths annually in the United States. There can be significant and life-altering results associated with these errors. Therefore, it is considered a best practice to always have a peer review the order, the calculation, and the medication prior to administering a drug to a pediatric patient.

THE MEDICATION LABEL

The medication label can be a source of valuable information to the medical assistant and the patient. Regardless of whether administering a prescription drug or a nonprescription product, an understanding of the information provided on the label is essential to the safe and effective use of any medicine. In addition to the name and address of the manufacturer, other important items of information on a medication label include:

- The trade, or brand, name for the medication
- The generic name (or listing of active and inactive ingredients)
- The National Drug Code (NDC) numbers that can be used to identify the manufacturer, the product, and the size of the container
- The dosage strength in a given amount of the medication
- The usual dosage and frequency of administration
- The route of administration
- Precautions and warnings
- The expiration date for the medication

Other information that may be on a medication label includes directions for storage and directions for mixing or reconstituting a powdered form of the drug. The ISMP has undertaken strategies to minimize the possibility of errors by encouraging drug labeling to be distinctive; bottle shape or label color should not be similar.

CALCULATION OF DRUG DOSAGES

Safety   Integrity

The preparation and administration of medications is one of the most critical tasks that medical assistants perform. Today, drugs are more potent and more likely to cause physiologic changes in the body; therefore, anyone who administers medications must do so with extreme care.

Incorrectly calculated or measured dosages are the leading cause of error in the administration of medications. A drug error is a violation of a patient's rights. It is important that medical assistants develop a working knowledge of mathematics to calculate a medication that is to be administered to a patient.

A recent study indicates the estimated number of deaths linked to preventable adverse events at 440,000—approximately one-sixth of all annual

U.S. deaths. This study looked at hospitalized patients and was not specifically studying medication errors. One can appreciate that a significant number of this almost half-million deaths are related to medication errors, as administering medications is the most frequent procedure performed on the hospitalized patient.

Barcoded medications are in wide use in acute care settings. For practices that administer a large number of medications on a routine basis, the use of barcoded medications is cost effective and increases the safety of medication administration for the patient. For smaller practices that do not frequently perform procedures or give specific injections, this option is not feasible. In either instance, administering barcoded medication or those without barcodes, the responsibility for safe medication administration rests with the medical assistant. You must follow the procedure for administering medications every time, no matter how familiar you are with the medication to be given or the receiving patient.

Digitally based practice management systems allow for entries of prescriptions and medication orders by the provider for easy reference by the medical assistant. This reduces errors that are caused by legibility and completeness problems. Patient records are also readily available and this improves patient safety and prevents medical errors and adverse drug events by checking allergies, previous medications, and dosages.

The Centers for Medicare and Medicaid Services (www.cms.gov) has initiated the EHR Incentive Program. As a part of this program, CMS has established 15 core measures to provide incentive payments to eligible providers, in- and outpatient clinics, urgent care facilities, surgery centers, and hospitals as they adopt, implement, upgrade, or demonstrate meaningful use of certified EHR technology. The fourth core measure addresses e-prescribing.

The objective of this core measure is the generation and transmission of permissible prescriptions electronically. Achievement of this objective is measured by proving that 40% of all permissible prescriptions written by the eligible professional are transmitted electronically using certified EHR technology. "Permissible prescriptions" refers to the current restrictions from the Department of Justice on the electronic prescribing of Schedules II through V controlled substances.

Understanding Ratio

Ratio is a method of expressing the relationship of a number, quantity, substance, or degree between two similar components. For example, the relationship of one to five is written 1:5. Note that numbers are side by side and separated by a colon.

In mathematics, a ratio may be expressed as a quotient, a fraction, or a decimal.

Ratio Expressed as a Quotient. A quotient is the number found when one number is divided by another number. The ratio one to five written as an equation to find the quotient is $1 \div 5 = x$.

Ratio Expressed as a Fraction. A fraction is part of the process of dividing or breaking a whole number into parts. The ratio one to five written as a fraction is $\frac{1}{5}$ or $\frac{1}{5}$.

Ratio Expressed as a Decimal. A decimal is a linear array of numbers based on 10 or any multiple of 10. To express the ratio one to five as a decimal, divide the denominator (5) into the numerator (1).

$$\text{(denominator)} \ 5\overline{)1.0}^{\ 0.2} \ \text{(numerator)}$$

The ratio may be expressed as:

A quotient	A fraction	A decimal
$1 \div 5$	$\frac{1}{5}$ ($\frac{1}{5}$)	0.2

Understanding Proportion

Proportion is comparing the relationship between a part, share, or portion with regard to size, amount, or number. In mathematics, a proportion expresses the relationship between two ratios. In setting up a proportion, the ratios are separated by a colon (:) or an equal sign (=) sign. In this text, the equal sign (=) is used to separate ratios.

Example:

$6 : 4 = 3 : 2$

Read as:

Six is to four equals as three is to two.

The four terms of a proportion are given special names. The *means* are the inner numbers, or the second and third terms of the proportion.

Example:

$$6 : 4 = 3 : 2 \quad (4) \quad (3)$$
$$means$$
$$4 \times 3 = 12 \ (means)$$

The *extremes* are the outer numbers, or the first and fourth terms, of the proportion.

Example:

$$6 : 4 = 3 : 2 \quad (6) \quad (2)$$
$$extremes$$

In a true proportion, the product of the means equals the product of the extremes.

Example:

means (16) (1)
$$8 : 16 = 1 : 2$$
extremes (8) (2)
$$16 \times 1 = 16 \ (means)$$
$$8 \times 2 = 16 \ (extremes)$$

Solving for X. The proportion is a useful mathematical tool. When a part, share, or portion of the problem is unknown, then x represents the unknown factor. You can determine the unknown by solving for x. The unknown factor x may appear anyplace in the proportion.

Now solve for x in the problem $3 : 4 = x : 12$.

1. Multiply the term that contains the x and place the product ($4x$) to the left of the equal sign.
2. Multiply the other terms and place the product (36) to the right of the equal sign.
3. To find x, divide the multiplier of x into the product of the other terms.

$$4x = 36$$
$$x = \frac{36}{4} \ or \ 36 \div 4$$
$$x = 9$$

After finding the unknown factor, check your mathematical skills by determining if you have a true proportion. This technique is called proof or proving your answer. To prove your answer:

1. Place the answer you found for x back into the formula where x was.

$$3 : 4 = 9 : 12$$

2. Now multiply the means by the means, and the extremes by the extremes.
3. The results will equal each other.

Formula: $3 : 4 = x : 12$

Proof: $3 : 4 = 9 : 12$

$$4 \times 9 = 36$$
$$3 \times 12 = 36$$

Weights and Measures

Two systems of measurement are used in pharmacology to calculate dosages: metric and household. The metric system is used throughout the world as the official language of communication in scientific and technical fields. It is based on the decimal system: the number 10 or multiples of 10.

Metric System Guidelines. The following guidelines are helpful when learning basic facts about the metric system:

1. Arabic numbers are used to designate whole numbers, for example, 1; 250; 500; 1,000.
2. Decimal fractions are used for quantities less than one, for example, 0.1, 0.01, 0.001, 0.0001.
3. To ensure accuracy, place a zero before the decimal point if there are no other numbers there, for example, 0.1, 0.001, 0.0001.
4. The Arabic number precedes the metric unit of measurement, for example, 10 grams, 2 millimeters, 5 liters.
5. The abbreviation for gram should be capitalized (Gm) or written as (g) to distinguish it from grain (gr).
6. The abbreviation for liter is capitalized (L).
7. Prefixes are written in lowercase letters, for example, milli, centi, deci, deka.
8. Capitalize the measurement and symbol when it is named after a person, for example, Celsius (C).
9. Periods are no longer used with most abbreviations or symbols.
10. Abbreviations for units are the same for singular and plural. An *s* is not added to an abbreviation to indicate a plural.

The Seven Common Metric Prefixes. It is important to know common metric prefixes to have a solid foundation for determining metric equivalents. When a metric prefix is combined with a root of physical quantity, you arrive at multiples or submultiples of the metric system.

Example:

- **milli** (prefix): one-thousandth of a unit
  meter (root): a measure of length
  millimeter: one-thousandth of a meter
- **kilo** (prefix): one thousand units
  liter (root): a measure of volume
  kiloliter: one thousand liters
- **micro** (prefix): one-millionth of a unit
  gram (root): a measure of mass and/or weight
  microgram: one-millionth of a gram

Prefixes

micro	=	one millionth of a unit, written as 0.000001
milli	=	one-thousandth of a unit, written as 0.001
centi	=	one-hundredth of a unit, written as 0.01
deci	=	one-tenth of a unit, written as 0.1
deka	=	10 units, written as 10 hecto
hecto	=	100 units, written as 100
kilo	=	1,000 units, written as 1,000

Fundamental Units

Following are the fundamental units of the metric system:

meter (m)	length
liter (L)	volume
gram (Gm, g)	mass and/or weight

The meter is the fundamental unit of length in the metric system and originally formed the foundation for the entire system. A meter is equal to 39.37 inches, which is slightly more than a yard, or 3.28 feet.

A millimeter is about the width of the head of a pin. It takes approximately 2.5 centimeters to make an inch; a decimeter is approximately 4 inches.

Length		Meter (m)
1 millimeter (mm)	=	0.001 meter
1 centimeter (cm)	=	0.01 meter
1 decimeter (dm)	=	0.1 meter
1 meter (m)	=	1 meter
1 dekameter (dam)	=	10 meters
1 hectometer (hm)	=	100 meters
1 kilometer (km)	=	1,000 meters

The liter is the metric unit of volume. A liter is equal to 1.056 quarts, which is 0.26 gallon or 2.1 pints.

A milliliter is equivalent to one cubic centimeter (cc), because the amount of space occupied by a milliliter is equal to one cubic centimeter. The weight of one milliliter of water equals approximately a gram. It takes approximately 15 milliliters to make 1 tablespoon.

Volume		Liter (L)
1 milliliter (mL)	=	0.001 liter
1 centiliter (cL)	=	0.01 liter
1 deciliter (dL)	=	0.1 liter
1 liter (L)	=	1 liter
1 dekaliter (daL)	=	10 liters
1 hectoliter (hL)	=	100 liters
1 kiloliter (kL)	=	1,000 liters

The gram is the metric unit of mass and weight. It equals approximately the weight of 1 cubic centimeter or 1 milliliter of water. A gram is equal to approximately 15 grains or 0.035 ounce.

Mass and Weight		Gram (Gm, g)
1 microgram (mcg)	=	0.000001 gram
1 milligram (mg)	=	0.001 gram
1 centigram (cg)	=	0.01 gram
1 decigram (dg)	=	0.1 gram
1 gram (Gm, g)	=	1 gram
1 dekagram (dag)	=	10 grams
1 hectogram (hg)	=	100 grams
1 kilogram (kg)	=	1,000 grams

The metric equivalents most frequently used in the medical field are:

Length

2.5 centimeters (cm)	= 1 inch

Volume

1,000 milliliters (mL)	= 1 liter (L)

Weight

1,000 micrograms (mcg)	= 1 milligram (mg)
1000 milligrams (mg)	= 1 gram (Gm, g)
1000 grams (g)	= 1 kilogram (kg)
1 kilogram	= 2.2 pounds (lb)

Household Measurements. Household measurements are approximate measurements. They are more frequently used in the home than in the medical field, but the medical assistant should be familiar with the common household measurements listed in Table 35-7.

TABLE 35-7

COMMON HOUSEHOLD MEASURES

60 drops (gtt)	is equal to:	1 teaspoon (t or tsp)
3 teaspoons (tsp)	is equal to:	1 tablespoon (T or Tbsp)
2 tablespoons (Tbsp)	is equal to:	1 ounce (oz)
8 ounces (oz)	is equal to:	1 measuring cup (c)
16 tablespoons or 8 ounces	is equal to:	1 measuring cup (c)
2 cups (c)	is equal to:	1 pint (pt)
2 pints (pt)	is equal to:	1 quart (qt)
4 quarts (qt)	is equal to:	1 gallon (gal)

Drop (gt) = approximate liquid measure depending on kind of liquid measured and the size of the opening from which it is dropped.

Because medications can be prescribed in either metric or household measurements, it is important to know equivalents between both to calculate the dose of prescribed medication (Table 35-8).

TABLE 35-8

APPROXIMATE EQUIVALENTS AMONG METRIC AND HOUSEHOLD SYSTEMS

METRIC	HOUSEHOLD
DRY	
1 Gm	¼ tsp
15 Gm	1 tbsp (3 tsp)
30 Gm	1 oz (2 tbsp)
1 kg	2.2 lb
LIQUID	
1 mL	15 gtt
5 mL	1 tsp
15 mL	1 tbsp (3 tsp)
30 mL	1 fl oz (2 tbs)
500 mL	1 pt or 2 cups
1,000 mL	4 cups (1 qt)
LENGTH	
2.5 cm	1 in
1 m	39.37 in

Metric System Conversion. The process of changing something into another form, state, substance, or product is known as *conversion*. In the metric system, changing from one unit to another involves multiplying or dividing by 10; 100; 1,000; and so forth. This can be done by the proportional method or by moving the decimal in the correct direction.

Proportional Method for Converting Metric Equivalents. There are six basic steps in the proportional method, plus an additional step to prove the answer. The following example will serve as a model for future applications of the proportional method of converting metric equivalents.

Example:

Convert 1,500 milligrams to grams.

$$1{,}500 \text{ mg} = \underline{\hspace{1cm}} \text{ g}$$

Step 1.

Because the unknown factor in the given formula is the number of grams contained in 1,500 milligrams, substitute the symbol x for grams in the equation.

Step 2.

Setting up the proportion requires that you know metric equivalents. For example, in this problem you have to know that 1,000 milligrams (mg) = 1 gram (g).

Step 3.

Since you know that 1,000 mg is equal to 1 g, you can create one-half of the equation. Write the equivalent and place it on the left of the equal sign.

$$1{,}000 \text{ mg} : 1 \text{ g} =$$

Step 4.

Now that you have the left side of the equation, set up the right side by using the designated metric value 1,500 mg : x g. Always write the smallest equivalent as to the largest equivalent, for example, mg : g. By being consistent, it is less likely errors will occur.

$$1{,}000 \text{ mg} : 1 \text{ g} = 1{,}500 \text{ mg} : x \text{ g}$$

Step 5.

Note that you have an equal equation:

$$mg : g = mg : g$$

The first values on either side of the equal sign are milligrams, and the second values on either side are grams.

Step 6.

Now solve for the unknown (x) by multiplication and division. Multiply the means by the means and the extremes by the extremes. *NOTE:* Once the proportion is correctly set up, simply use the numbers as you multiply and divide.

$$1{,}000 : 1 = 1{,}500 : x$$

$$
\begin{aligned}
1{,}000x &= 1{,}500 \\
x &= 1{,}500 \div 1{,}000 \\
x &= 1.5
\end{aligned}
$$

$$
\begin{array}{r}
1.5 \\
1{,}000\overline{)1{,}500.0} \\
\underline{1{,}000} \\
500.0 \\
\underline{500}
\end{array}
$$

Step 7.

To make sure the answer is correct, prove the work: Place the answer 1.5 g into the formula where *x* once was. Now multiply the means by the means and the extremes by the extremes.

$$
\begin{aligned}
1{,}000 \text{ mg} : 1 \text{ g} &= 1{,}500 \text{ mg} : 1.5 \text{ g} \\
1{,}500 &= 1{,}500
\end{aligned}
$$

MEDICATIONS MEASURED IN UNITS

Medications such as insulin, heparin, some antibiotics, hormones, vitamins, and vaccines are measured in units. These medications are standardized in units based on strength. The strength varies from one medicine to another, depending on the source, condition, and method by which it is obtained.

How to Calculate Unit Dosages

When calculating medications that are ordered in units, use either the proportional method or the formula method.

The Proportional Method.

Example:

The provider orders 4,000 USP units of heparin given deep subcutaneously. On hand is heparin 5,000 USP units per milliliter.

Step 1.

Use the following proportion to calculate the dose:

Known unit on hand	:	Known dosage form	=	Dose ordered	:	Unknown amount to be given
5,000 Units:		1 mL	=	4,000 Units:		*x* mL
		5,000*x*	=	4,000		
		x	=	$\frac{4}{5}$ = $\frac{4}{5}$ mL or 0.8 mL		

Use a tuberculin syringe to draw up 0.8 mL.

Step 2.

Convert $\frac{4}{5}$ mL to minims. *NOTE:* There are 15 or 16 minims per milliliter.

Multiply:

$$\frac{4}{\cancel{8}_{1}} \times \frac{\cancel{15}^{\,3}}{1} = \frac{4}{1} \times \frac{3}{1} = 12 \text{ minims}$$

Administer 12 minims (of 5,000 Units/mL for correct dose of 4,000 Units) to the patient.

The Formula Method.

Example:

The provider orders 450,000 units of Bicillin 1M. On hand is Bicillin 600,000 units per milliliter.

Step 1.

Use the following formula to calculate the dose:

$$\frac{\text{Dose ordered (desired)}}{\text{Dose on hand}} \times \frac{\text{Quantity}}{\text{(per mL)}} = \text{Amount to give}$$

$$\frac{450{,}000 \text{ units}}{600{,}000 \text{ units}} \times 1 \text{ mL} = \frac{4\cancel{50{,}000} \text{ units}}{6\cancel{00{,}000} \text{ units}} = \frac{45}{60} = \frac{3}{4}$$

$$\frac{3}{4} \times 1 \text{ mL} = \frac{3}{4} \text{ mL}$$

Step 2.

Convert the fraction ¾ mL to a decimal

Divide 3mL by 4mL or 3 ÷ 4 = 0.75 mL

The patient will receive 0.75 mL Bicillin 600,000 units for the ordered dose of 450,000 units.

Insulin

Insulin is a chemical substance (hormone) secreted by the beta cells of the islets of Langerhans in the pancreas. Insulin is necessary for the proper metabolism of blood glucose and maintenance of the correct blood sugar level. Inadequate secretion or no secretion of insulin, as in the disease diabetes mellitus, results in hyperglycemia and subsequent excessive production of ketone bodies. Eventual coma can occur.

Patients' needs are individualized according to the severity of their disease; treatment includes taking insulin, controlling diet, and exercise. The diet is well balanced and consists of the correct number of calories distributed among carbohydrates, fats, and proteins. Patients are taught to monitor blood and urine glucose levels at home throughout the day, because the dosage of insulin taken depends on the amounts of glucose detected. Uncontrolled diabetes mellitus can result in serious complications such as circulatory problems, especially in the feet and legs; kidney disease; loss of vision; bedsores; infection; and gangrene. Special care of the feet is essential. The mouth and teeth require excellent oral hygiene.

Diabetes

The National Institute of Diabetes and Digestive and Kidney Diseases, a department of the U.S. Department of Health and Human Services, identifies three main types of diabetes:

- *Type 1.* This type was previously known as juvenile diabetes as it most often has an onset prior to adulthood. However, type 1 diabetes can develop in adults. With this type of diabetes, the body no longer makes insulin or does not make enough insulin to support the body's metabolism. As a result, insulin must be injected based on blood glucose measurements.

- *Type 2.* This type was previously known as adult onset diabetes. It most commonly is diagnosed in the middle-aged population. First, there are symptoms of insulin resistance, or the inability of insulin to transport glucose into the cells to be used as energy. This advances to the need for oral hypoglycemic agents.

- *Gestational diabetes.* This type of diabetes develops when the hormones of pregnancy create insulin resistance. If the pancreas cannot secrete more insulin, the woman develops gestational diabetes. A woman that has gestational diabetes is at an increased risk of developing type 2 diabetes later in life.

Individuals with Insulin Dependent Diabetes Mellitus (IDDM) must take insulin on a regular basis to maintain life. Other insulin delivery devices besides the syringe and the needle can be used for injection. With an insulin pen, the patient can turn a dial on the top until the correct dose of insulin is displayed through a small window. Once the correct dose is chosen, the dial locks itself to prevent the pen from losing insulin or from the dial moving forward to give an unintended larger dose. The pen has a needle similar to the insulin syringe, and the patient presses the plunger and the dose of insulin is delivered under the skin.

The insulin pump is a small device outside of the body that pumps insulin through flexible tubing that is connected to a catheter that is under the skin of the abdomen, thigh, or buttocks. The pump is programmed to deliver a steady flow of the correct dose of insulin 24 hours a day. The pump can allow the patient to add insulin in a short time if needed. Although it is convenient and helps keep the patient's blood glucose under control, the pump can be damaged if the patient engages in certain physical activities. Patients still must regularly monitor their blood glucose levels.

The newest methods of delivering insulin include powdered insulin for inhalation and the insulin patch. Powered inhaled human insulin (Afrezza) is now available in 4-unit and 8-unit cartridges. An insulin patch is under development with some major advances in the process reported in 2016 from the University of North Carolina and North Carolina State University. Their "smart insulin patch" is filled with natural beta cells that can secrete doses of insulin to control blood glucose levels on demand with no risk of inducing hypoglycemia.

The dosage of insulin is expressed in units and is individualized by the provider for each patient. The amount of insulin that a person must take is based on blood and urine glucose levels, diet, exercise, and the individual's needs. See Table 35-9.

It is *extremely important that the exact dosage of insulin be given to the patient.* Too little or too much insulin can cause serious problems ranging from a blood sugar level too low or too high, to coma, and even death. It may be the medical assistant's responsibility to administer insulin and to teach patients and/or their families how to administer insulin.

When selecting an insulin syringe, an important factor is the number of units in one milliliter of insulin to be injected. Some insulins are U-100, or 100 units per 1 mL of insulin (the most common type), while other types of insulin may be U-500 for patients with a condition referred to as insulin resistance. It is important to select the correct syringe based on the type of insulin to be injected. Another factor to be considered is the total volume of insulin to be injected, as in the case of mixed dosing of insulin.

Insulin dosage should always be expressed in units rather than in milliliters. For example, if the provider orders 30 units of U-100 NPH insulin, use a U-100 syringe and draw up 30 units of U-100 NPH insulin. Markings on the syringe indicate the number of units. U-100 syringes are marked in 10-unit increments (Figure 35-2).

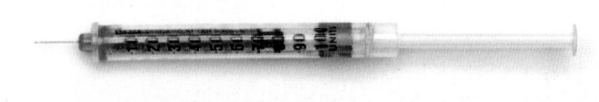

FIGURE 35-2 Standard U-100 insulin syringe. (*NOTE:* The red fluid shown is for ease of viewing, but true insulin is never red.)

TABLE 35-9

INSULIN PREPARATION UNITS 100

TYPE OF INSULIN	ONSET	PEAK	DURATION OF EFFECT	APPEARANCE
RAPID-ACTING				
Lispro (Humalog)	15 to 30 minutes	30 to 90 minutes	3 to 5 hours	Clear, colorless
Aspart (NovoLog)	10 to 20 minutes	40 to 50 minutes	3 to 5 hours	Clear, colorless
Glulisine (Apidra)	20 to 30 minutes	30 to 90 minutes	1 to 2½ hours	Clear, colorless
REGULAR OR SHORT-ACTING				
Regular (R) humulin or novolin	30 minutes to 1 hour	2-3 hours	30 minutes to 1 hour	Clear, colorless
Velosulin (for use in an insulin pump)	30 minutes to 1 hour	2 to 3 hours	2 to 3 hours	Clear, colorless
INTERMEDIATE-ACTING				
NPH(N)	1 to 2 hours	4 to 12 hours	18 to 24 hours	Cloudy, white
LONG-LASTING				
Insulin glargine (Basaglar, Lantus)	60 to 90 minutes	No peak time; this insulin is delivered steadily	20 to 24 hours	Cloudy, white
Insulin detemir (Levemir)	1 to 2 hours	6 to 8 hours	Up to 24 hours	Clear, colorless
PREMIXED				
Humulin 70/30	30 minutes	2 to 4 hours	14 to 24 hours	Cloudy, white
Novolin 70/30	30 minutes	2 to 13 hours	Up to 24 hours	Cloudy, white
Novolog 70/30	10 to 20 minutes	1 to 4 hours	Up to 24 hours	Clear
Humulin 50/50	30 minutes	2 to 5 hours	18 to 24 hours	Cloudy, white
Humalog mix 75/25	15 minutes	30 minutes to 2½ hours	16 to 20 hours	Clear

Precautions to Observe when Administering Insulin.
The following precautions must be observed when administering insulin:

- Be sure to use the proper insulin, the one ordered by the provider. Refer to Table 35-9 for various insulin preparations.
- Do not substitute one insulin for another.
- Use the correct syringe, matching the syringe type with the units per milliliter (e.g., U-100).
- Dosage of insulin is always measured in units and is individualized for each patient.
- Check the label for the name and type of insulin, strength, and expiration date.

- Make sure the insulin has the proper appearance. Refer to Table 35-9 for the proper appearance of various insulins.
- When insulin is not in use, store it in a cool place and avoid freezing.
- When mixing insulins in one syringe, be certain they are compatible. NPH and Regular are compatible. Regular and Lente are not compatible.
- Avoid shaking the insulin bottle. Roll gently in palms of hand to mix. This method prevents bubbles in the medication.
- Use a subcutaneous needle, but inject at a 90-degree angle (a 45-degree angle is appropriate for a thin person).
- Insulin pens are available prefilled with 300 units of insulin.
- Use a site rotation system and select an appropriate site. Insulin injection sites must be rotated to prevent tissue damage. Record the site used (Figure 35-3).
- Do not massage after injection.
- Always follow the provider's order and clinic policy when mixing insulins.

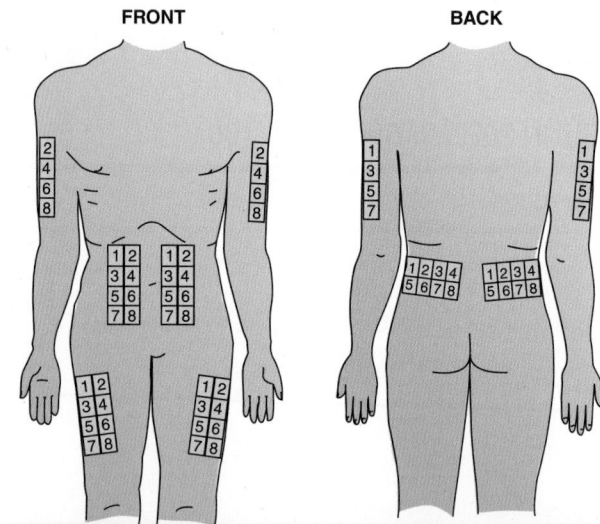

FRONT   **BACK**

FIGURE 35-3 Sites and rotation for insulin administration.

Oral Hypoglycemic Medication. Persons with type 2 diabetes mellitus are known to have non-insulin-dependent diabetes mellitus (NIDDM). Type 2 diabetes has a gradual onset and is usually seen in adults over 40 years of age. With the obesity epidemic in the United States, individuals are contracting type 2 diabetes at earlier ages (obesity contributes to and can cause type 2 diabetes). The pancreas in patients with type 1 diabetes secretes very little or no insulin; in type 2, the pancreas has some ability to secrete insulin. Most individuals with type 2 diabetes do not have to inject insulin, although a few do. Exercise and diet management may be sufficient for people with type 2 diabetes to lose enough weight and not require oral hypoglycemic medication. For the majority, however, exercise and diet are not enough to bring the blood sugar to an acceptable level. Medication works by stimulating the pancreas to secrete more insulin, by making cells more receptive to insulin, and by slowing the body's carbohydrate absorption. Some oral hypoglycemics are Prandin (repaglinide), Avandia (rosiglitazone maleate), Actose (pioglitazone hydrochloride), Precose (acarbose), Glyset (miglitol), DiaBeta (glyburide), Glucotrol (glipizide), Glucophage (metformin), and Starlix (nateglinide).

CALCULATING ADULT DOSAGES

Two measures, weight and volume, are used to determine the amount of medication that is to be administered. The weight of a medication may be expressed as any of the following:

- Milliequivalent (meq)
- Microgram (mcg)
- Milligram (mg)
- Gram (Gm, g)
- Unit

The volume of a medication may be expressed as a:

- Milliliter (mL)
- Minim (m)
- Dram (dr)
- Ounce (oz)
- Variety of household measures, such as the teaspoon (tsp)

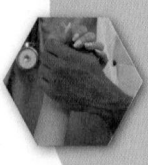

Patient Education

Encourage patients with diabetes to enroll in diabetic education classes, which are offered at most local hospitals. Patients also need to realize that treatment of diabetes is a lifelong commitment and that they must abide by everything that the hospital teaches.

Many different methods can be used when calculating the dosage to be administered. Two of the most useful methods—the proportional method and the formula method—are described next.

The Proportional Method Example.

Example:

The provider orders 0.2 g of Equanil tabs. The dose on hand is 400 mg tabs.

Step 1.

Determine whether the medication ordered and the medication on hand are available in the same unit of measure.

Step 2.

If the medication ordered and the medication on hand are not in the same unit of measure, convert so that both measures are expressed using the same unit of measure.

Conversion: To change 0.2 g to mg

$$1{,}000 \text{ mg} : 1 \text{ g} = x \text{ mg} : 0.2 \text{ g}$$

$$x = 200 \text{ mg}$$

or

multiply $0.2 \times 1{,}000 = 200$

Step 3.

Now use the following proportion to calculate the dosage. Remember that 0.2 g was converted to 200 mg.

Known unit on hand	:	Known dosage form	=	Dose ordered	:	Unknown amount to be given
400 mg	:	1 tab	=	200 mg	:	x tab

$$400 : 1 = 200 : x$$

$$400x = 200$$

$$x = \frac{\overset{1}{\cancel{200}}}{\underset{2}{\cancel{400}}} \quad \text{(Reduce fraction to lowest terms)}$$

$$x = \tfrac{1}{2} \text{ tab of 400 mg}$$

Step 4.

Prove your answer. Place your answer in the original formula in the x position.

$$400 \text{ mg} : 1 \text{ tab} = 200 \text{ mg} : \tfrac{1}{2} \text{ tab}$$
$$200 = \tfrac{1}{2} \text{ of } 400$$
$$200 = 200$$

Understanding the Formula Method

One of the simplest methods for calculating dosages is the formula method. One must know what is needed or ordered, what is available or the concentration, and the vehicle in which the medication will be delivered: tablet, mL, or capsule.

The formula looks like this:

$$\frac{\text{needed}}{\text{available}} \times \text{vehicle} = \text{dose}$$

Example:

Your provider orders 250 mg of Cephalexin po now to be given to Ms. Jones for her diagnosis of cystitis. The bottle of Cephalexin in the drug cabinet holds capsules that contain 250 mg.

Step 1.

Identify each part of the formula:

needed or ordered = 250 mg

available = 250 mg

vehicle = 1 capsule

Step 2.

The formula would be set up as follows: (needed 250 mg)

$$\frac{\text{(needed) 250 mg}}{\text{(available) 250 mg}} \times \text{(vehicle) 1 capsule} = \text{dose}$$

Step 3.

Determine whether the medication ordered and the medication on hand are in the same unit of measure.

As the needed dose is in mg and the available dose is in mg, there is no further need to address the concentration, and the mg aspect of the equation disappears. We will explore the management of differing concentrations a little later.

You equation now looks like this:

$$\frac{250}{250} \times 1 \text{ capsule} = \text{dose}$$

Step 4.

Do the math:

$$\frac{250}{250} \text{ is equal to 1}$$

Now multiple by the vehicle of 1 capsule:

$$1 \times 1 = 1 \text{ capsule}$$

The dose to be administered is 1 capsule.

Example:

The provider orders 5 mg of morphine to be given IM now. A check of the narcotics cabinet reveals that injectable morphine is available in 10 mg per 2 mL.

Step 1.

Identify each part of the formula.

needed or ordered: 5 mg; available: 10 mg

vehicle: 2 mL

Step 2.

The formula would be set up as follows:

$$\frac{\text{(needed) 5 mg}}{\text{(available) 10 mg}} \times \text{(vehicle) 2 mL} = \text{dose}$$

$$\frac{5\,mg}{10\,mg} \times 2\,mL = \text{dose}$$

Step 3.

Determine whether the medication ordered and the medication on hand are in the same unit of measure.

As the needed dose is in mg and the available dose is in mg, there is no further need to address the concentration, and the mg aspect of the equation disappears.

Step 4.

Do the math:

$$\frac{5}{10} = 0.5$$

Now multiply by the vehicle of 2 mL:

0.5 × 2 mL = dose

0.5 × 2 mL = 1 mL. 1 mL is the dose to be administered.

1 mL of morphine will be administered using the appropriate needle gauge and length in the appropriate volume syringe IM.

If the concentration of the needed medication differs from the concentration of the available medication, this must be resolved.

Example:

Your provider prescribes 500 mg cefadroxil po now. The medication available in the drug cabinet is 1 Gm cefadroxil in scored tablets.

Step 1.

Identify each part of the formula:

needed or ordered: 500 mg

available: 1 Gm

vehicle: 1 tablet

Step 2.

The equation would be set up as follows:

$$\frac{\text{(needed) 500 mg}}{\text{(available) 1 Gm}} \times 1\,\text{tablet} = \text{dose}$$

Step 3.

Determine whether the medication ordered and the medication on hand are in the same unit of measure. As the concentrations of the needed medication and the available medication differ, we must apply the principles discussed earlier in the chapter. The concentrations must be the same in order to determine the dose.

To accomplish this, multiply 1 Gm × 1,000 to convert Gms to mg. This results in 1000 mg. Insert this into the equation. It now looks like this:

$$\frac{500\,mg}{1000\,mg} \times 1\,\text{tablet} = \text{dose}$$

Step 4.

Do the math. As the needed and available doses are now in the same unit of measure, the mg portion of the equation disappears:

$$\frac{500}{1000} = 0.5$$

Now multiply by the vehicle:

0.5 × 1 tablet = 0.5 tablet. 0.5 tablet is the dose to be administered.

This formula can also be expanded to accommodate weight-based dosing.

Example:

Your provider orders amoxicillin suspension of 40 mg/kg/day BID for a pediatric patient. The amoxicillin that is available is in a concentration of 400 mg/5 mL. The child weighs 22 lbs.

Step 1.

The order is based on kilograms and the weight is noted in lbs; therefore, you must convert:

2.2 kg = 1 lb

lbs divided by 2.2 = weight in kgs

22 lbs divided by 2.2 = 10 kgs

Step 2.

Next we need to calculate the dose that we are to administer at this time.

40 mg/kg can be calculated for the child as 40 mg × 10 kg = 400 mg. Further, the dosage is to be divided into two times a day.

400 mg divided by 2 = 200 mg

The single dose that you are preparing right now is 200 mg.

Step 3.

Now that we have calculated the dose based on weight and taken the dosing interval into twice a day dosing, we can identify each part of the formula.

Needed or ordered: 200 mg

Available: 400 mg

Vehicle: 5mL

Step 4.

The equation would be set up as follows:

$$\frac{200 \text{ mg}}{400 \text{ mg}} \times 5 \text{ mL} = \text{dose}$$

Step 5.

Do the math. As the needed and available doses are now in the same unit of measure, the mg portion of the equation disappears:

$$\frac{200}{400} = 0.5$$

Now multiply by the vehicle:

$0.5 \times 5 \text{ mL} = \text{dose}$

$0.5 \times 5 \text{ mL} = 2.5 \text{ mL}.$ 2.5 mL is the dose to be administered.

CALCULATING CHILDREN'S DOSAGES

Each child is an individual differing from other children in age, size, and weight. In the past, formulas such as Young's, Clark's, and Fried's rules were used to calculate pediatric dosages. These formulas determined what fraction of an adult dose was appropriate for a child. Because each child does not develop in the same way during a given time span, these formulas have been replaced by more exact methods of determining the correct dosage of medication for a child.

Today, there are two basic methods used to calculate children's dosages:

- According to kilograms of body weight
- According to body surface area (BSA)

The body weight method is generally the method of choice, because most medications are ordered in this way and it is easier to calculate. The BSA is an exact method, but one must use a formula and a **nomogram** (a device-graph that shows a relation among numeric values) to determine a correct dosage (Figure 35-4).

Body Surface Area

The BSA is considered to be one of the most accurate methods of calculating medication dosages for infants and children up to 12 years of age. This method requires the use of a nomogram that estimates the BSA of the patient according to height and weight.

The body surface area is determined by drawing a straight line on a graph from the patient's height to the patient's weight. Intersection of the line with the surface area column is the estimated BSA. This figure is then placed in the following formula:

$$\frac{\text{BSA of child (m}^2)}{1.7 \text{ (m}^2)} \times \text{adult dose} = \text{child dose}$$

This formula is based on the average adult who weighs 140 pounds and has a body surface area of 1.7 square meters (1.7 m^2). There are also online resources for easily calculating BSA. See such tools at http://www.manuelsweb.com/bsa.htm.

Example:

Marion Carrera is a 4-year-old who is 40 inches tall and weighs 38 pounds (BSA 0.7). The provider has ordered Demerol for pain. The average adult dose of Demerol is 50 milligrams per milliliter. What dosage will be given to Marion according to the BSA method?

$$\frac{0.7 \text{ (m}^2)}{1.7 \text{ (m}^2)} \times \frac{50 \text{ mg}}{1} = \text{child's dose}$$

$$\frac{0.7 \text{ (m}^2)}{1.7 \text{ (m}^2)} \times \frac{50}{1} = \frac{35}{1.7} = 20.5 \text{ mg} = 20.5 \text{ or } 21 \text{ mg}$$

Now use the formula $\frac{\text{needed}}{\text{available}} \times \text{vehicle}$.

$$\frac{21 \text{ mg}}{50 \text{ mg}} \times 1 \text{ mL} = x \text{ mL}$$

$$\frac{21}{50} = 0.42 \text{ mL administered in a tuberculin syringe}$$

Kilograms of Body Weight

It may be the responsibility of the medical assistant to calculate the amount of dosage ordered by the provider according to the patient's body weight. There are a number of medications that are ordered in this manner; therefore, it is essential that you learn how to calculate dosage according to this method. The following example will guide you step by step through the mathematical process of calculating dosage according to kilograms of body weight.

There are 2.2 pounds in 1 kilogram.

Example:

The provider ordered the antiepileptic agent Depakene (valproic acid) 15 mg/kg/day capsules for Clark Kipperley, who weighs 110 pounds. The medication is to be given in three divided doses.

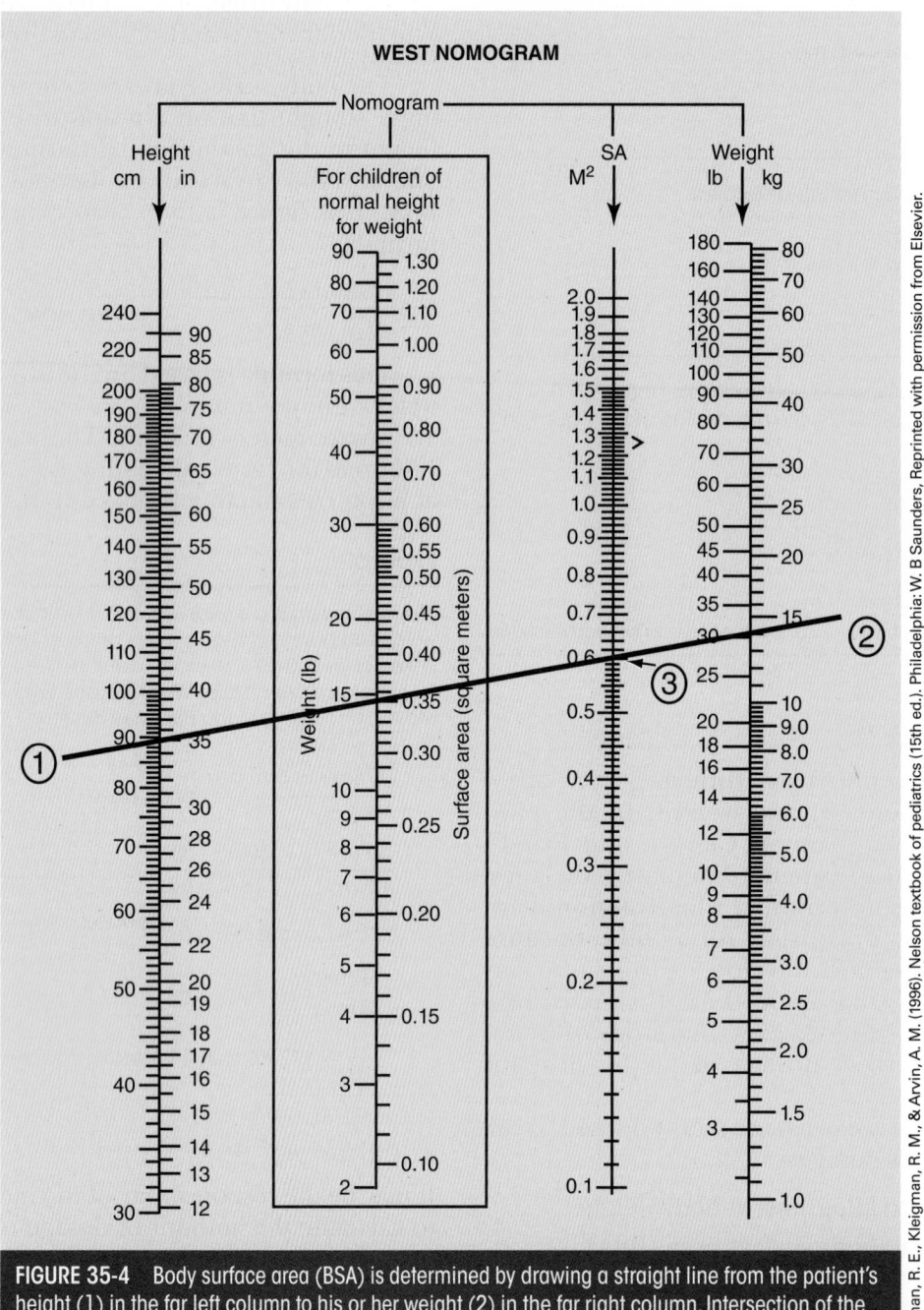

FIGURE 35-4 Body surface area (BSA) is determined by drawing a straight line from the patient's height (1) in the far left column to his or her weight (2) in the far right column. Intersection of the line with BSA column (3) is the estimated BSA (m²). For infants and children of normal height and weight, BSA may be estimated from weight alone by referring to the enclosed area.

From Behrman, R. E., Kleigman, R. M., & Arvin, A. M. (1996). Nelson textbook of pediatrics (15th ed.). Philadelphia: W. B Saunders, Reprinted with permission from Elsevier.

Step 1.

Convert the patient's weight to kilograms. To express pounds in kilograms, divide the weight in pounds by 2.2:

$$110 \text{ lb} \div 2.2 = 50 \text{ kg}$$

Step 2.

Now, calculate the prescribed dosage by placing 50 in the appropriate place:

$$15 \text{ mg/50 kg/day}$$

$$15 \text{ mg} \times 50 \text{ kg} = 750 \text{ mg/day}$$

Step 3.

To determine the amount of each dose, divide 750 mg by 3 (divided doses).

$$750 \text{ mg} \div 3 = 250 \text{ mg}$$

Depakene is available in 250 mg capsules and 250 mg/5 mL syrup. The provider ordered the medication in capsules, so Clark will receive a 250 mg capsule every 8 hours for a total of three doses a day.

In the same example, use the proportional method to calculate the dose using kilograms of body weight.

Step 1.

To convert 110 pounds to kilograms, set up the proportion as follows:

$$2.2 \text{ lb} : 1 \text{ kg} = 110 \text{ lb} : x \text{ kg}$$

Step 2.

Now, solve for *x*.

$$2.2 \text{ lb} : 1 = 110 \text{ lb} : x$$
$$2.2x = 110 \text{ lb}$$
$$x = 50 \text{ mg}$$

Step 3.

Now, calculate the prescribed dosage by placing 50 mg in the appropriate place: mg/50 kg/day.

$$15 \text{ mg} \times 50 \text{ kg} = 750 \text{ mg/day}$$

Step 4.

To determine the amount of each dose, divide 750 mg by 3 (divided doses).

$$750 \text{ mg} \div 3 = 250 \text{ mg per dose}$$

ADMINISTRATION OF MEDICATIONS

Regardless of a medication's form or the route by which it is administered, certain basic guidelines must be followed. These guidelines are:

1. 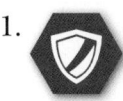 Practice medical asepsis (see Chapter 21 for specific medical asepsis rules). Wash your hands before and after administering a medication. Remember Occupational Safety and Health Administration (OSHA) guidelines and Standard Precautions (see Chapter 21 for Standard Precautions).

2. Work in a well-lighted area that is free from distractions.

3. Follow the Six Rights of proper drug administration (see following section).

4. Always check for allergies before administering any medication.

5. Give only drugs ordered by a licensed practitioner who is authorized to prescribe medications.

6. Never give a medication if there is any question about the order.

7. Be completely familiar with the drug that you are administering before giving it to the patient. Look it up in the PDR online, or in the electronic practice management software.

8. Always check the expiration date on the medication label.

9. Never give a drug if its normal appearance has been altered in any way (color, structure, consistency, or odor); it may be outdated, contaminated, or stored incorrectly.

10. Double check the provider's order that has been entered in the patient's medical record. Be sure to bring your tablet into the medication preparation area to allow verification of the order.

11. Give only those medications that you yourself have actually prepared for administration. Trust only your own actions.

12. Do not allow someone else to give a medication that you have prepared. Depend on yourself to give the correct medication.

13. Once you have prepared a medication for administration, do not leave it unattended; it could be misplaced or spilled.

14. Be careful in transporting the medication to the patient. Do not spill or drop. If it is spilled or dropped, follow the guidelines for disposal outlined in the practice's policy and procedure manual or consult with your provider.

15. When administering oral medications, stay with the patient until you are certain that the patient has swallowed the medication.

16. Shake (to mix) all liquid medications that contain a **precipitate** before pouring. A precipitate is a substance that separates from a solution if allowed to stand. Shaking ensures the even distribution of the active ingredients throughout the solution.

17. When pouring a liquid medication, hold the measuring device at eye level or place it on a flat surface and squat down so you can observe it at eye level. Read the correct amount at the lowest level of the **meniscus**, the curve seen at the top of a liquid in response to its container.

18. Do not contaminate the cap of a bottle while pouring a medication. Place the cap with the rim pointed upward to prevent contamination of that portion of the cap that comes into contact with the medication.

19. Keep all drugs not being administered in a safe storage place.

20. Carefully follow the procedural steps for the type of medication that you are administering.

21. ⬡ **Safety** Always keep safety precautions in mind. The United States Department of Health and Human Services, Public Health Service, and Centers for Disease Control and Prevention recommend following Standard Precautions for prevention of hepatitis B and C viruses, human immunodeficiency virus, and other bloodborne diseases (see Chapter 21 for specifics about Standard Precautions).

The "Six Rights" of Proper Drug Administration

The "Six Rights" have been developed as a checklist of activities to be followed by those who give medications. This easy-to-remember list should always be followed to ensure the proper administration of any drug:

1. *Right drug.* To be sure that the correct drug has been selected, compare the medication order with the label on the medication container. A frequent check of the medication label is a good way to avoid a medication error. One should make a practice of reading the label on each of the following three occasions:

   First: When the medication is taken from the storage area.

   Second: Just before removing it from its container.

   Third: On returning the medication container to storage or before discarding the empty container.

2. *Right dose.* It is essential that the patient receive the right dose. If the dose ordered and the dose on hand are *not the same,* carefully determine the correct dose through mathematical calculation. When calculating dosage, it is advisable to have another qualified person verify the accuracy of your calculations before the medication is administered.

3. *Right route.* Check the medication order to be sure that you have the right route of administration (Figure 35-5A).

4. *Right time.* You are responsible for medicating the patient at the proper time. Check the medication order to ensure that the drug is administered according to the time interval prescribed. For a drug to be maintained at the proper blood level, care must be taken to administer it at the right time.

5. *Right patient.* Before administering any medication, always be sure that you have the right patient. A good safety practice is to correctly identify the patient, using two identifiers, on each occasion when you administer a medication. In a hospital, the patient's identification bracelet is always checked. In the ambulatory care facility, ask the patient to state his or her name and date of birth, or the last four numbers of his or her Social Security number.

6. *Right documentation.* The recording process is the vital link between provider, patient, and medical assistant. It is an account of the essential data that are collected and preserved. The patient's chart is a legal document; therefore, all data should be recorded in ink or entered into the patient's electronic medical record. The data should be accurate and clearly stated. It is important that certain data about drug administration be entered into the patient's chart (Figure 35-5B):

   - Patient's name
   - Date and time of administration
   - Name of the medication and the dose administered

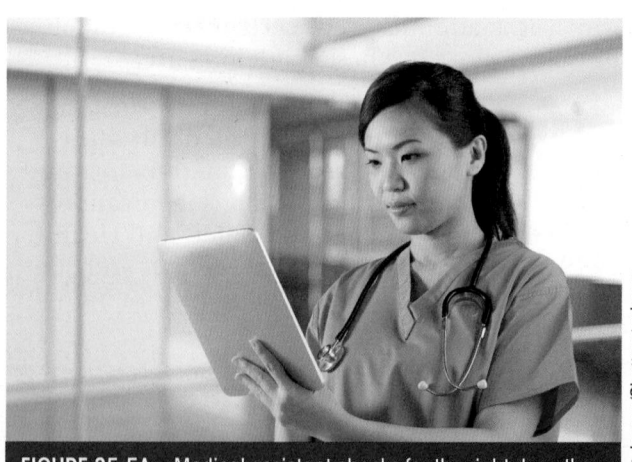

FIGURE 35-5A *Medical assistant checks for the right drug, the right route, and the right dose of medication to administer.*

© Stuart Jenner/Shutterstock.com

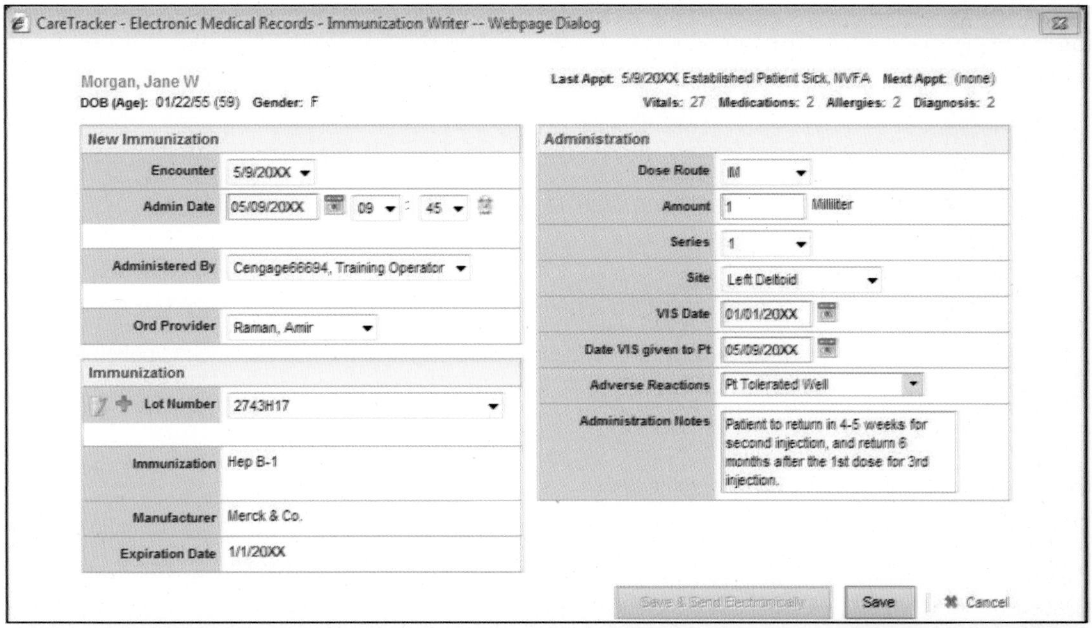

FIGURE 35-5B Medical assistant documents administration of medication in patient's chart.

- Route by which the medication was administered
- Any unusual reactions experienced by the patient
- Any complications in administering the drug (e.g., patient refusing to take the medication, difficulty in swallowing)
- **Safety** If the medication was *not* given, state why and dispose of the medication according to agency policy and federal and state laws
- Patient data, such as blood pressure, pulse, respirations, when appropriate
- Your name or initials and title

Medication Errors

Medication errors should not happen when personnel follow the "Six Rights" of proper drug administration and the essential medication guidelines; however, honest mistakes will be made periodically. A medication error is said to occur when any of the following happen:

1. A drug is given to the wrong patient
2. The incorrect drug is given
3. The drug is given via an incorrect route
4. The drug is given at the incorrect time
5. The incorrect dose is administered
6. Incorrect data are entered on the patient's chart or electronic medical record

Patient Assessment

Before administering any medication, carefully assess the patient's condition. An assessment should include, but is not limited to, the following conditions:

1. *Age.* Is the medication and route suitable for the patient at his or her particular stage in life? The stages of life include infancy, childhood, adolescence, adulthood, and old age. During infancy, early childhood, and the period of older adulthood, a lower dose of medication may be required than would be appropriate for the other stages in life. Also, very young children and some older adults are not able to swallow tablets or effectively chew chewables.

2. *Physical conditions.* Potential problems associated with the patient's physical condition must be considered. Female patients should not be given certain medications during pregnancy or while breast-feeding because they may be contraindicated.

When a Medication Error Occurs, Follow Standard Procedure:

1. Recognize that an error has been made.

2.  Stay calm. Assess the patient's condition and reactions to the medication.

   Competency

3. 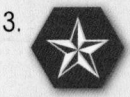 Report the error immediately to the provider. Give the details of the mistake and the patient's reactions.

   Integrity

4. Follow the provider's orders for correcting the error.

5. Prepare an incident or occurrence report following your clinic's policy. Include the following information and any other information required by your clinic's policy:

   • Patient identification

   • Location and time of the incident

   • Description of what happened including the type of error and the patient's reaction

   • Description of the steps taken to correct the error

   • Date, time, and your name

   • The incident report does not become a part of the medical record—it is not referenced in the documentation in the patient's chart; the intent is not to hide the error but to protect the medical assistant and the facility

3. *Body size.* The amount of medication given and size of the needle used are directly related to the size of the patient. Pediatric and geriatric patients usually have less subcutaneous and muscular tissue per BSA than the average adult. Small, thin patients usually require less medication, and a shorter needle may be used to reach the appropriate tissue level. On the other hand, the large or obese patient may or may not require more medication than the average adult and a longer needle to reach the appropriate tissue level.

4. *Sex.* Consider differences that are related to the sex of the patient. For example, pharmacokinetics in women are affected by lower body weight, slower gastrointestinal motility, less intestinal enzymatic activity, and slower filtration rate in the kidneys.

5. *Build.* Muscular patients have a greater density of muscle tissue. Obese patients have more adipose tissue. Older adults or those with chronic illness may have decreased amounts of both muscular and adipose tissue. Always inspect and palpate muscle tissue with this in mind when determining the appropriate needle length to reach muscle tissue.

6. *Skin texture.* Some patients have tougher skin than others. A young person's skin might have more tone than that of an older adult. Slightly more force is required to penetrate skin that is tough or lacking in tone.

7. *Injection site.* Always inspect and palpate the skin before administering an injection. The following body areas should be avoided when choosing the site for an injection:

• Any type of skin lesion

• Burned areas

• Inflamed areas

• Previous injection sites

• Traumatized areas

• Scar tissue (e.g., vaccination, keloid)

• Moles, warts, birthmarks, tumors, lumps, hard nodules

- Nerves, large blood vessels, bones
- Cyanotic areas
- Edematous areas
- Paralyzed areas
- Arm on same side as mastectomy, or other lymphatic compromise

Correct injection sites are illustrated later in this chapter.

ADMINISTRATION OF ORAL MEDICATIONS

Oral medications are easily and economically administered. There are, however, several disadvantages associated with the oral route. For instance, the drug may:

- Have an objectionable odor/taste
- Cause discoloration of the teeth, mouth, and tongue
- Irritate the gastric mucosa
- Be altered by digestive enzymes
- Be poorly absorbed from the digestive system because of illness or the nature of the medication
- Be refused by the patient
- Have less predictable effects on the body when given orally than when given by injection
- Not be able to be swallowed if in tablet, capsule, or caplet form

Equipment and Supplies for Oral Medications

Three measuring devices commonly used in the administration of oral medications are the medicine cup, the water cup, and the medicine dropper. The medicine cup (Figure 35-6) comes in various sizes and shapes, depending on its manufacturer and its intended use. Cups may be calibrated in fluid ounces, fluidrams, milliliters (mL), and/or tablespoons.

The water cup is a small plastic or paper cup that is disposable. The average water cup holds 3 ounces of liquid.

The medicine dropper (Figure 35-7) may be calibrated in milliliters, or drops. Medicine droppers are often included with the bottle of medication. Uncalibrated droppers may be provided

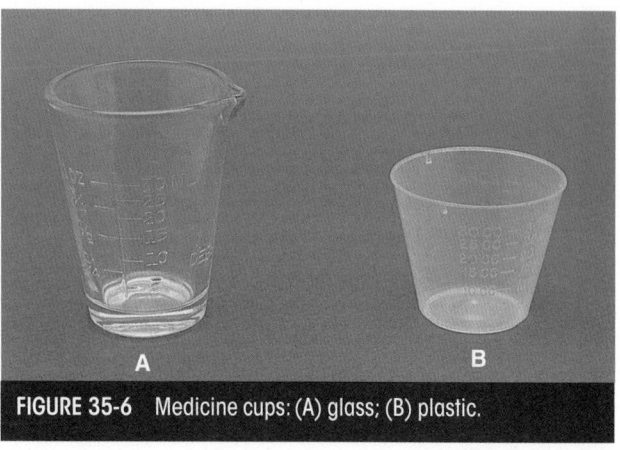

FIGURE 35-6 Medicine cups: (A) glass; (B) plastic.

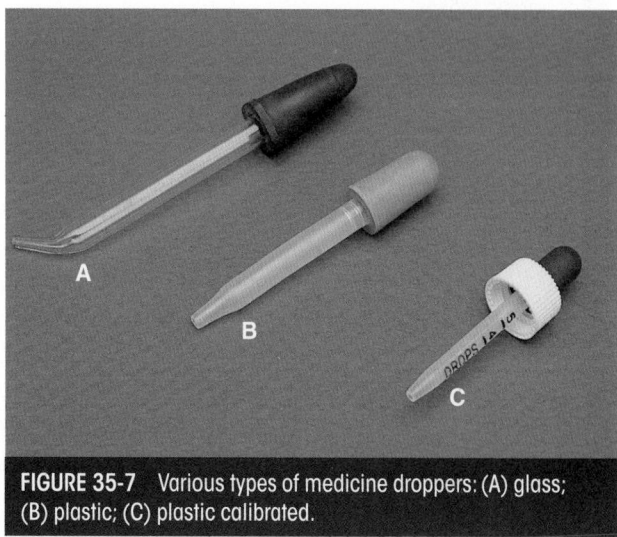

FIGURE 35-7 Various types of medicine droppers: (A) glass; (B) plastic; (C) plastic calibrated.

when the medicine is administered only in drops. The size of the drop varies with the size of the dropper opening, the angle at which it is held, the force exerted on the rubber bulb, and the viscosity of the medication.

It is important that the appropriate measuring device is selected for a particular medication and that the prescribed dosage is accurately measured. The selection of the measuring device depends on the physical structure of the medication (solid or liquid), the amount of medication prescribed, the size of the measuring device, and the calibrations on the container.

Procedure

Procedure 35-1 gives steps for administration of oral medications.

PROCEDURE 35-1

Procedure

Administering Oral Medications

STANDARD PRECAUTIONS:

Handwashing

PURPOSE:
To correctly administer an oral medication after receiving the provider's order and assembling the necessary equipment and supplies.

EQUIPMENT/SUPPLIES:
- Medication order per provider
- Tablet with patient's medical record open
- Correct medication
- Medicine cup
- Fluid for swallowing the medication (water, juice, or milk)

PROCEDURE STEPS:
1. **Paying attention to detail**, gather the supplies necessary to complete the procedure using the information in the provider's order as a guide. RATIONALE: A well-lighted area for preparing medications is important because you must be able to see well to accurately pour medications. A quiet area is free from distractions.

2. When you have assembled your supplies, perform medical asepsis hand washing procedure following the guidelines set forth by OSHA. RATIONALE: Medical asepsis helps fight transmission of microorganisms.

3. Review the "Six Rights" of medication administration and follow them when giving a patient any type of medication.

4. Review the provider's order and select the correct medication from the designated area. Take a moment to compare the medication label with the order. RATIONALE: This will help you prevent errors.

5. Check to make sure that the drug has not expired by locating and confirming the expiration date. RATIONALE: Outdated medication may have deteriorated or been altered in some way and may be harmful to the patient.

6. If you are unfamiliar with any particular drug, take a moment to consult the PDR, located in the electronic health record, or other comparable reference. You should be familiar with the drug's name, mechanism of action, route or routes of administration, and any common side effects.

7. Carefully calculate the dosage based on the order and the medication available. Correctly prepare the medication as multiple-dose solid, unit dose, or liquid medication.

8. If the medication is:
   a. In pill or capsule form, pour the desired amount in the cap (Figure 35-8A). Then pour the medication into a medicine cup.
   b. In liquid form, pour it directly into a measuring device to the calibrated line of the ordered amount (Figure 35-8B).
   c. In syrup or liquid form, it may also be given in disposable plastic measuring spoons or droppers.

(continues)

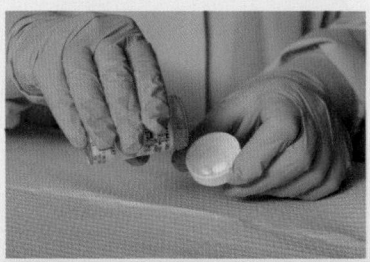 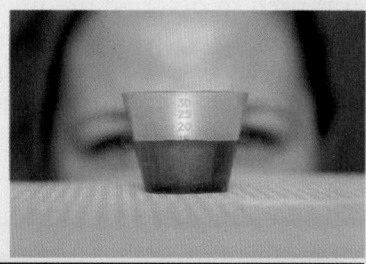

FIGURE 35-8 (A) Medical assistant pours capsules from the cover of the medicine container into a medicine cup before administering medicine to patient. The medication is poured into cover to avoid contamination of medicine. (B) Liquid medications should be read at eye level.

9. Make a second check of the provider's order and compare it to the medication label. RATIONALE: Though this might seem unnecessary, taking the time to perform a double-check can prevent careless mistakes that might endanger a patient.

10. If indicated, the patient may use water to assist with taking medication; however, some liquid medications, such as cough suppressant, should not be taken with water as it can wash away the desired coating.

11. Carefully transport the prepared medication to the patient exam room, bringing with you the original medication container and the provider's order.

12. *Introduce yourself* using your name and credentials and *verify the identity of the patient using two indicators* of identification, such as the patient's name and date of birth.

13. *Speaking at the level of the patient's understanding, explain the rationale for performance of the procedure to the patient.* State the name of the medication and why it is being given. Make sure the patient is comfortable and relaxed.

14. Review with the patient any known allergies to medications. Follow up by taking a moment to assess the patient visually for body size, physical condition, age, and gender. If necessary, take any vital signs as determined by the medication to be given.

15. For a third time, check the provider's order against the medication to be given.

16. Administer the medication, providing an adequate amount of fluid (as appropriate) to ensure ease of swallowing.

17. Have the patient open his mouth and move his tongue around to ensure that the patient has swallowed the medication.

18. If this is the first time a patient has taken a particular medication, *being courteous, patient, and respectful*, have the patient remain in the room and assess for signs of reaction every five minutes until it is determined that a reaction is unlikely.

19. *Paying attention to detail*, return the medication to the appropriate storage area and in the proper place.

20. Check on the patient.

21. Accurately document the medication type, dosage, route of administration, and any patient reaction. Sign and provide the date and time.

DOCUMENTATION:

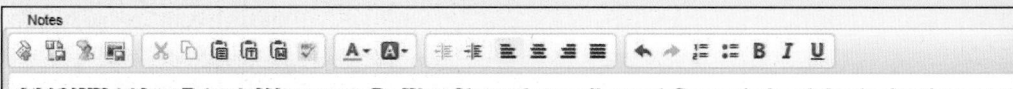

Notes

9/26/20XX 4:15 PM Tylenol, 500 mg po per Dr. King. Observed pt. swallow med. Gave pt. both verbal and written home care instructions for taking medication. T. Myers, CCMA (NHA)

Courtesy of Harris CareTracker PM and EMR

ADMINISTRATION OF PARENTERAL MEDICATIONS

The term **parenteral** is used to describe the injection of a substance into the body via a route other than the alimentary canal/digestive system. The most frequently used parenteral routes are subcutaneous, intramuscular, intradermal, and intravenous (see Quick Reference Guide):

- *Subcutaneous.* Just below the surface of the skin.
- *Intramuscular.* Within the muscle.
- *Intradermal.* Within the dermal layer of the skin.
- *Intravenous.* Within or into a vein.

 Medications that have been prepared for use by injection are available in multiple-dose form (vials) and in unit dose form (ampules and cartridge–needle units) (Figure 35-9) (see Procedure 35-2). **Unit dose** forms are premeasured amounts, packaged on a per-dose basis.

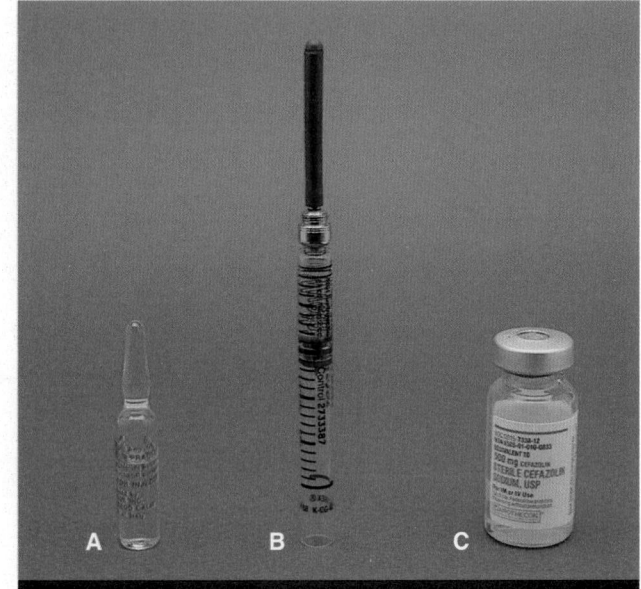

FIGURE 35-9 Medications given parenterally: (A) Ampule. (B) Sterile cartridge with premeasured medication. (C) Vial of powder for reconstitution.

▶▶ QUICK REFERENCE GUIDE

▶▶ INTRADERMAL, INTRAVENOUS, AND SUBCUTANEOUS MEDICATIONS

	Intradermal	Intravenous	Subcutaneous
	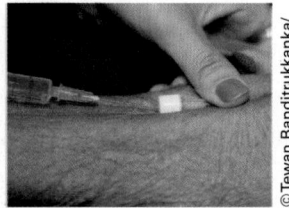	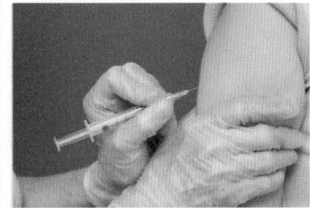 © Tewan Banditrukkanka/ www.Shutterstock.com	
Anatomic Site	Anterior forearm halfway between the wrist and elbow Back below the scapula	Hand Forearm Antecubital fossa in the metacarpal veins Dorsal venous arch Basilic, cephalic, or median cubital veins	Abdomen at least 2 inches away from the naval Posterior aspect of the upper arms anywhere between one hand's breadth below the shoulder and one hand's breadth above the elbow Upper, outer thighs between one hand's breadth below the uppermost aspect of the thigh and one hand's breadth above the knee

(continues)

Advantages of the Site	Hair is sparse Not over a bony prominence Veins and arteries are not as close to the surface Very slow absorption of the very small amount of the medication Excellent for allergy testing and testing for exposure to TB	Ease of access to superficial vessels with limited risk of damage to nerves and easy differentiation for arteries Rapid action due to distribution by the bloodstream	Thicker fat layers Ease of access Versatile—can be used for short- or long-term therapies Slower absorption of medication, up to 24 hours
Angle of Injection	10 to 15 degrees	25 to 30 degrees	45 degrees
Maximum Volume to Be Injected	0.1 mL	No limit; however, the rate of infusion is based on the medication and purpose of infusion	1.0 to 2.0 mL
Needle Size	25 to 27 G ⅜ to ⅝ inch	20 to 24 G 1 to 1½ inch Gauge and length selected based on age of patient and purpose of IV	25 to 27 G ⅜ to 1 inch
Syringe Size	1 mL	As large as is needed to dilute the medication to be administered	1 mL with unit or 0.1 mL marking 3 mL
Patient Position	Seated with arm support	Seated or reclining based on the medication's anticipated effects	Seated or prone depending on injection site chosen
Example Medications Given with This Route	Tuberculin purified protein derivative (PPD) Allergens for sensitivity testing	Antibiotics Morphine Benadryl Ativan	Heparin Insulin

Types of Packaging

- *Ampule.* A small, sterile, prefilled glass container that usually holds a single dose of a hypodermic solution.
- *Cartridge–needle unit.* A disposable sterile cartridge containing a premeasured amount of medication. This unit is designed for use in a nondisposable cartridge-holder syringe such as the Carpuject.
- *Vial.* A small, sterile, prefilled glass bottle with rubber stopper containing a hypodermic solution.

PROCEDURE 35-2

Withdrawing Medication from a Vial or Ampule

Procedure

STANDARD PRECAUTIONS:

Handwashing

Gloves

Biohazard

PURPOSE:

To effectively draw medication from a vial for parenteral injection.

EQUIPMENT/SUPPLIES:

- Medication order per provider
- Alcohol wipes
- Disposable nonsterile gloves
- Sharps container
- Correct medication
- Appropriately sized syringe and needle of the correct gauge and length

PROCEDURE STEPS:

1. Based on the information indicated in the provider's order, gather the correct supplies and equipment you will need.

2. Before withdrawing any medication from either a vial or ampule, perform medical asepsis handwashing procedure following the guidelines set forth by OSHA.

3. Review the "Rights" of medication administration and follow them when preparing to give a patient any type of medication.

4. Using the provider's order as a reference, select the correct medication from the medication area.

5. Take a moment to compare the medication label with the order. Also, check to make sure that the drug has not expired by locating and confirming the expiration date. RATIONALE: Labels can look very similar.

6. If you are unfamiliar with any particular drug, take a moment to consult the PDR, located within the electronic health record, or other comparable reference. You should be familiar with the drug's name (both generic and commercial), the mechanism of action, route or routes of administration, and any common side effects.

Withdrawing Medication from a Vial:

7. If the medication is contained in a multi-dose vial, label the vial with the name of the medication, the post-dilution strength, the date, time, your initials, and the expiration date. If the vial is single-use, it will be discarded appropriately in the sharps container when you have finished using it.

8. Select the appropriately sized needle and syringe. Carefully calculate the dosage based on the provider's order and the medication available.

9. Make a second check of the provider's order and compare it to the medication label. Though this might seem unnecessary, taking the time to perform a double-check can prevent careless mistakes that might endanger a patient.

10. When measuring from a vial, begin by removing the metal or plastic cap from the top of the vial.

11. Using a circular motion, clean the top of the vial with an alcohol wipe (Figure 35-10A).

12. Open the syringe and packaging and carefully remove the needle cover.

(continues)

13. Prepare to withdraw the medication from the vial by holding the syringe pointed upward at eye-level and pulling the syringe plunger back to the level of the expected amount of medication to be withdrawn. The syringe will be filled with air at this point.

14. Leaving the vial on the table or countertop, insert the needle through the center of the vial's diaphragm, making sure that the needle shaft does not come into contact with any other portion of the vial surface to avoid contamination (Figure 35-10B).

15. Push the plunger slowly to inject the air into the vial.

16. Holding the vial and needle steady, invert the vial with the needle still inside.

17. Keeping the syringe at eye level, carefully and slowly pull back the plunger to withdraw the correct amount of medication. Make sure that the tip of the needle remains below the surface of the liquid so that air doesn't enter the syringe (Figure 35-10C).

18. If air bubbles do enter the syringe, tap sharply on the syringe to remove them, and push them back into the vial (Figure 35-10D). If removing the air bubbles has reduced the dosage below the prescribed level, add the correct amount of medication before proceeding.

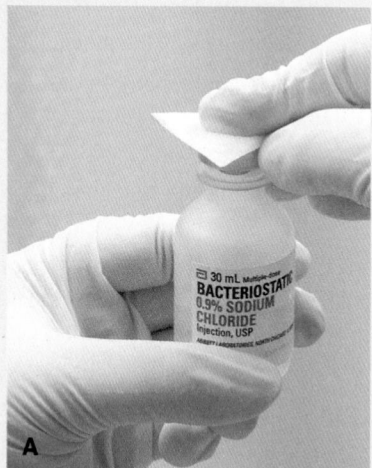
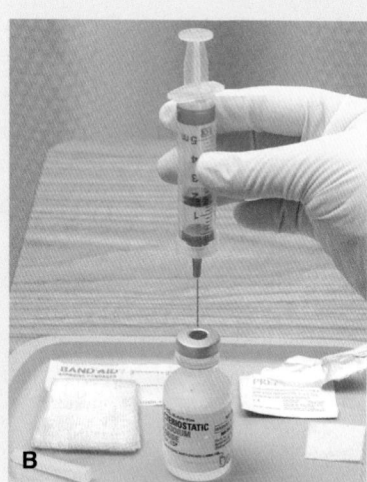
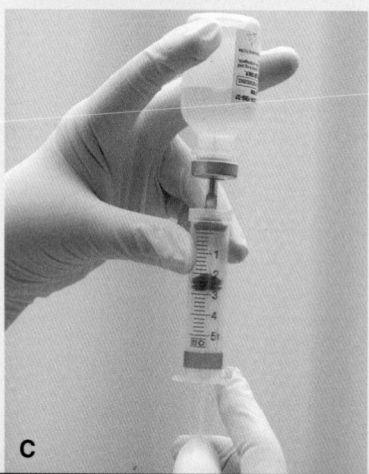
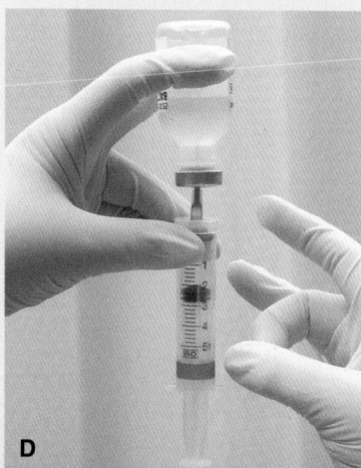

FIGURE 35-10 (A) Disinfect the rubber stopper on the medication vial with an alcohol wipe. (B) Keeping the bevel of the needle above the fluid level, inject an amount of air equal to medication quantity to be withdrawn. (C) Hold syringe pointed upward at eye level and with the bevel of the needle in the medication. Pull back plunger and aspirate the quantity to be withdrawn. (D) Tap syringe to eliminate air bubbles. Hand should hold syringe while tapping it.

(continues)

19. Check the measurement for accuracy before removing the needle from the vial and activating the safety device on the needle.

Withdrawing Medication from an Ampule:

20. When measuring from an ampule, the process for obtaining the medication will vary slightly. As with the vial, carefully compare the provider's order against the medication in the ampule.

21. Using the information on the ampule and in the order, calculate the amount of medication that you will need to withdraw.

22. Before withdrawing the medication, you need to ensure that none of the medication has become trapped in the neck of the ampule by tapping or flicking the top of the ampule (Figure 35-11A).

23. Thoroughly disinfect the neck of the ampule by wiping it with an alcohol wipe. Dry it with sterile gauze.

24. Apply gloves and remove the top of the ampule. You may use a safety device to help you with this process, or surround the neck completely with gauze and forcefully pull it toward you to snap it off (Figure 35-11B).

25. Discard the broken-off top into the sharps container.

26. Using a sterile syringe and filter needle, aspirate the required dose into the syringe (Figure 35-11C). RATIONALE: The filtered needle will prevent any glass particles from being aspirated with the medication.

27. You can also invert the ampule after you insert the needle and withdraw the medication. Do not inject air into the ampule before withdrawing the medication. RATIONALE: Surface tension will keep the medication from flowing out of the open end of the ampule.

28. Upon removal from the ampule, discard the ampule in the sharps container, and immediately cover the filter needle with the cap.

29. Replace the filter needle, using sterile technique, with one that is of an appropriate gauge and length for the injection. Discard the original filter needle into the sharps container. RATIONALE: Replacing the needle is indicated for two reasons: the filter needle is not appropriate for use during an injection and also, it is considered best practice to replace the needle after drawing up any medication that might be irritating to tissues.

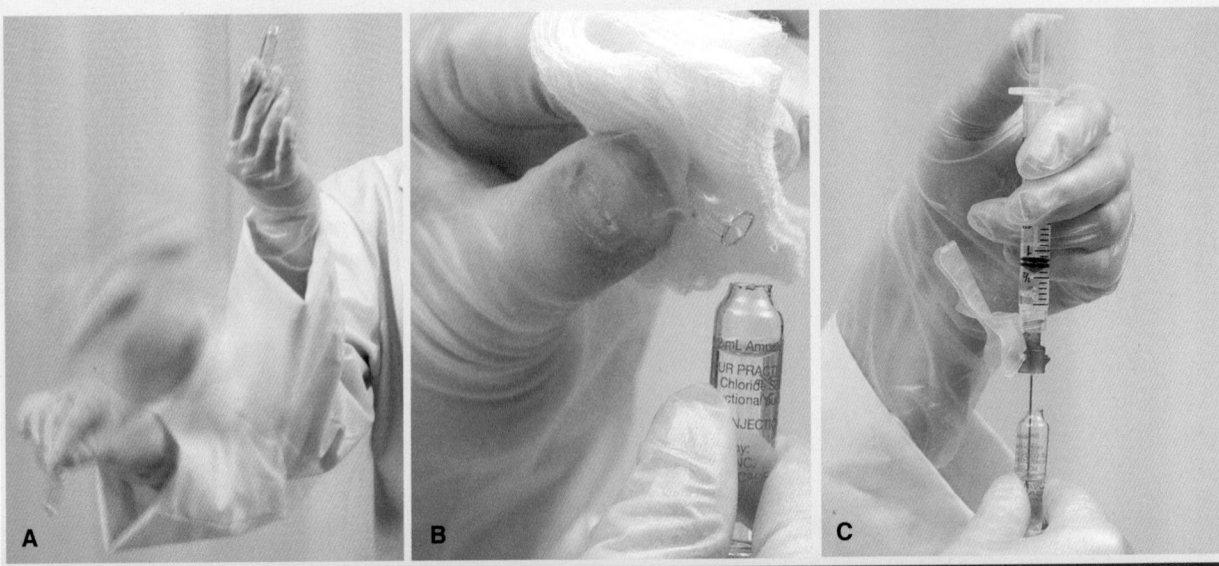

FIGURE 35-11 (A) Hold ampule by the top and force all the medication into the bottom of the ampule by a snap of the arm and wrist. (B) Remove top from ampule. Snap away from you by pulling top toward you. (C) Draw the required dose into syringe.

Hazards Associated with Parenteral Medications

Safety

Injecting medications must be done with extreme care. Sterile technique must be used because the needle and medication are being introduced into the patient's body and microorganisms must not be transmitted. Appropriate site selection and proper technique ensure effectiveness of the medication.

Additional dangers to be aware of when injecting medications parenterally include:

- Allergic reaction will be swift
- Injury to bone, nerve, or blood vessel
- Injecting into a blood vessel instead of tissue

Reasons for Parenteral Route Selection

The parenteral route is selected because of:

- Rapid response time to medication
- Accuracy of dosage
- Need for a concentration of medication injected into a joint or for local anesthetic

- Inability to administer orally because the medication is destroyed by gastric juices, or the patient is incapable of taking medication orally

Procedure

Because parenteral medications are intended for use by injection, they must be injected as liquids. Some medications are supplied in powder form and must be reconstituted to a liquid form for injection (see Procedure 35-3).

Because they must be in liquid form, the amount of a parenteral medication is expressed in terms of volume (milliliters or ounces). The strength of the drug contained in the liquid is usually expressed in terms of its weight (milliequivalents, micrograms, milligrams, grams, or units). Therefore, medications ordered for parenteral use are often ordered by both weight and volume.

The parenteral route of drug administration offers an effective mode of delivering medication to a patient when a rapid and direct result is desired. The effect of a parenteral medication is faster than one given by the oral route; however, the accuracy of dosage calculation for both is important.

PROCEDURE 35-3

Procedure

Reconstituting a Powder Medication for Administration

STANDARD PRECAUTIONS:

Handwashing

Gloves

Biohazard

PURPOSE:

To reconstitute a powdered medication for injection.

EQUIPMENT/SUPPLIES:

- Medication order per provider
- Powdered medication
- Diluent
- Appropriate syringe and needle gauge and length

- Alcohol wipes
- Nonsterile disposable gloves
- Sharps container

(continues)

PROCEDURE STEPS:

1. Based on the information indicated on the provider's order, gather the correct supplies and equipment you will need.

2. Before handling any medication, perform asepsis hand washing procedure following the guidelines set forth by OSHA. Put on gloves.

3. Review the "Rights" of medication administration and follow them when preparing to give a patient any type of medication.

4. Using the provider's order as a reference, select the correct medication from the medication area. It is important to take a moment to compare the medication label with the provider's order, as labels can look very similar. Check to make sure that the drug has not expired by locating and confirming the expiration date.

5. If you are unfamiliar with any particular drug, take a moment to consult the PDR, or other comparable reference, located in the electronic health record. You should be familiar with the drug's name (both generic and commercial), mechanism of action, route or routes of administration, and any common side effects.

6. Remove the tops from the diluent and powder medications and cleanse the tops and diaphragm of each with an alcohol wipe (Figure 35-12A).

7. Take a moment to look at the medicine in the vial. Check for any changes in color, any small pieces floating in the liquid, cloudiness, or any other changes. If any changes are noted, appropriately discard the vial.

8. Prepare the needle-syringe unit you will be using for the reconstituting. Fill the syringe with air equal to the amount of the diluent that is to be added to the powdered medication.

9. Carefully insert the needle through the rubber stopper on the vial of diluent and inject the air into the vial (Figure 35-12B).

10. Withdraw the appropriate amount to be added to the powdered medication. (Figure 35-12C).

11. Inject the diluent slowly into the powder bottle (Figure 35-12D).

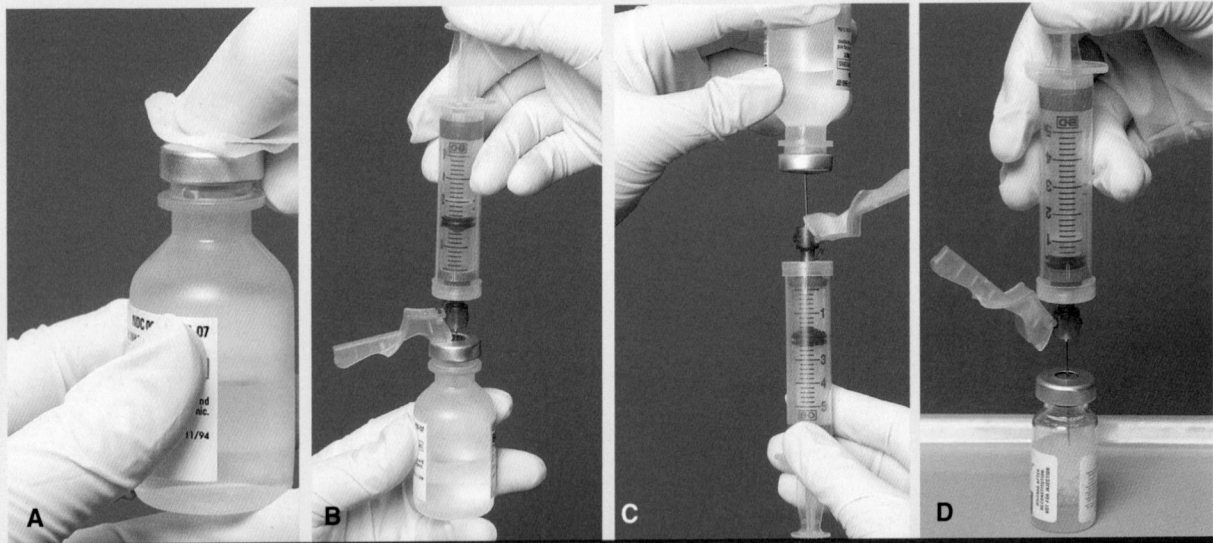

FIGURE 35-12   (A) Remove top from diluent and powdered medication. Wipe top of each with an alcohol wipe. (B) Inject air in an equal amount to diluent being removed from the vial. (C) Prepare to remove the needle from the vial after withdrawing diluent. (D) Inject diluent into vial containing powdered medication.

12. Withdraw the needle from the bottle and immediately activate the safety cap device to cover the needle. Discard the syringe and needle in a sharps container (Figure 35-12E).

13. Taking care not to shake the medication vial, roll it between the palm of your hands in order to mix the powder and diluent (Figure 35-12F).

(continues)

14. Cleanse the rubber stopper of the vial with an alcohol wipe and allow it to dry. Assemble a second sterile needle and syringe unit and withdraw the desired amount of medication (Figure 35-12G), tapping away any air bubbles that cling to the side of the syringe (Figure 35-12H).

15. Discard trash and the diluent vial in the sharps container.

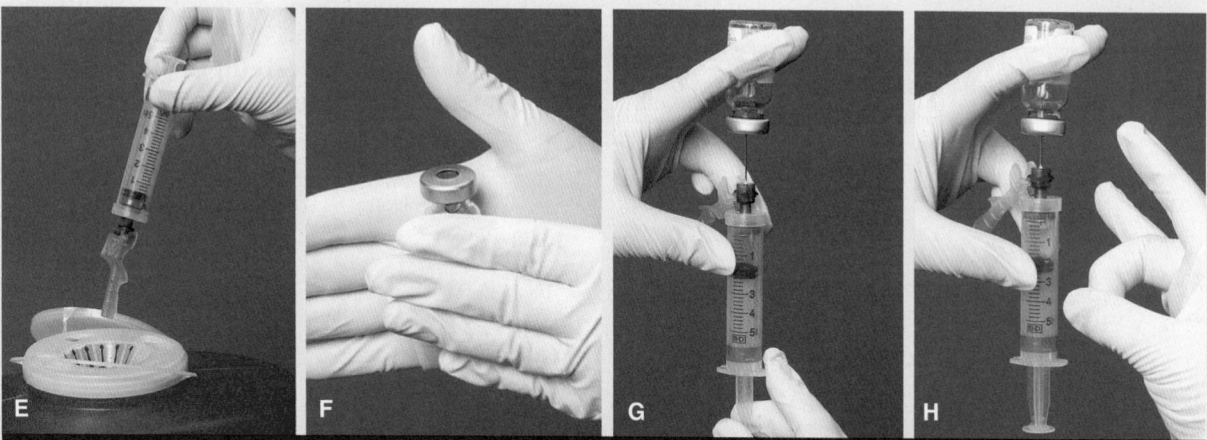

FIGURE 35-12 (E) Discard safety needle–syringe unit. (F) Roll vial of solution medication between palms of hands to mix well. Label vial with date, amount of diluent added, strength of dilution, time mixed, and your initials. (G) Use a second sterile needle–syringe unit to draw the prescribed dose of medication ordered by the provider. (H) Flick away any air bubbles that cling to the side of the syringe. Withdraw more medication if needed. Labeled, reconstituted medication will be taken to the room with the syringe and placed on the shelf or in the refrigerator according to the manufacturer's instructions after the injection is given.

Parenteral Equipment and Supplies

Syringes. Syringes are classified according to their intended use. In addition to the standard hypodermic syringes that are in general use, there are special-purpose syringes for irrigations or oral feedings, tuberculin syringes, and insulin syringes.

Disposable Syringes. Disposable syringes are those that are sterilize, prepackaged, nontoxic, nonpyrogenic, made of plastic, and ready for use. They are available as a syringe–needle unit or syringe only and are generally enclosed in individual peel-apart packages of durable paper or clear plastic. They are available in sizes from 1 to 60 milliliters. The 1-, 3-, and 5-mL syringes are the ones most often used when parenteral medications are administered.

A disposable syringe–needle unit consists of a syringe with an attached needle. The needle is covered by a hard plastic sheath to prevent it from accidentally penetrating

the package or sticking the user. The unit may be sealed within a peel-apart package or encased in a rigid plastic container that has been heat sealed to ensure sterility. Labeling usually includes the manufacturer's name, type and size of the syringe, gauge and length of the needle, and a reorder number. Packages are usually color-coded for ease of identification. Always read the label when choosing a syringe and needle combination. Disposable syringes are preferred for the administration of parenteral medications because they ensure sterility and sharp needles. Also, disposable syringes eliminate the need for resterilization, which is costly, time consuming, possibly unsafe if not done properly, and not generally accepted.

Combination Disposable/Nondisposable Cartridge-Injection Syringes. A cartridge-injection system, such as the plastic Carpuject (Figure 35-13), consists of a disposable cartridge–needle unit and a nondisposable cartridge-holder syringe. The cartridge–needle unit is factory sealed and sterile and con-

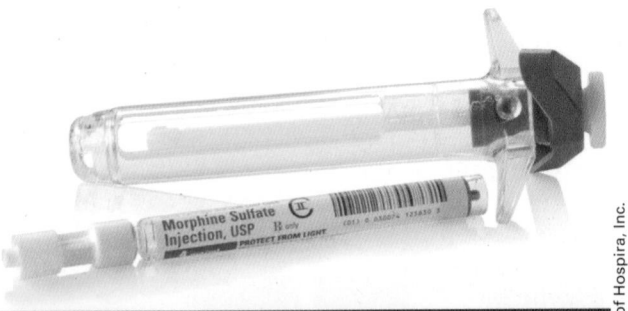

FIGURE 35-13 The Carpuject is a type of cartridge-injection system with a click-lock mechanism for safety.

Courtesy of Hospira, Inc.

tains a precisely measured unit dose of medicine. The cartridge-holder syringe may be made of durable chrome-plated brass or of plastic. These reusable syringes are designed for quick and safe loading and unloading of cartridge–needle units, which are manufactured in various sizes and dosage capacities and contain a wide range of medications (Figure 35-14).

The combination disposable/nondisposable syringe system is easy to use and convenient. When using this system, be careful to read the label and compare the medication order with the label. For

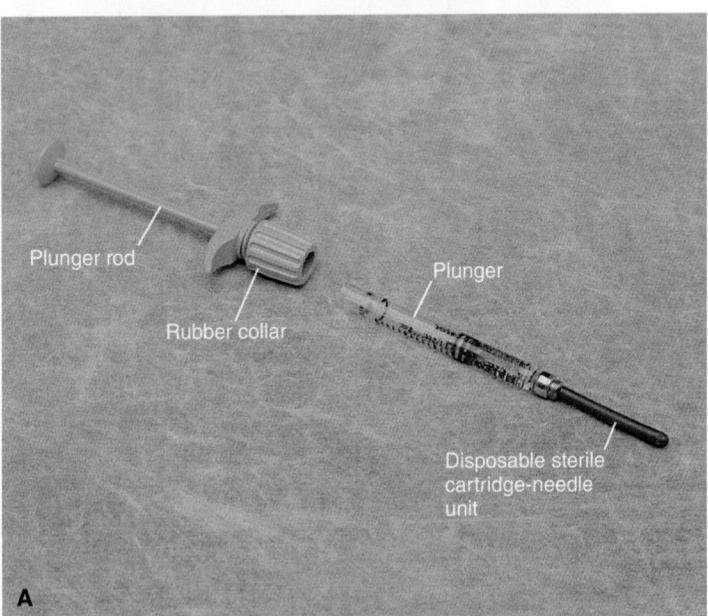

Plunger rod

Rubber collar

Plunger

Disposable sterile cartridge-needle unit

A

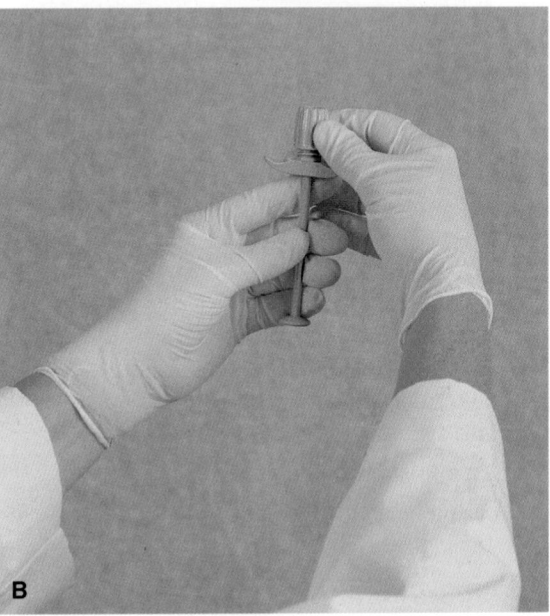

B

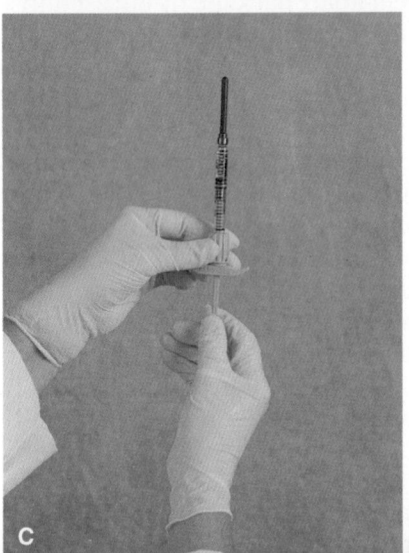

C

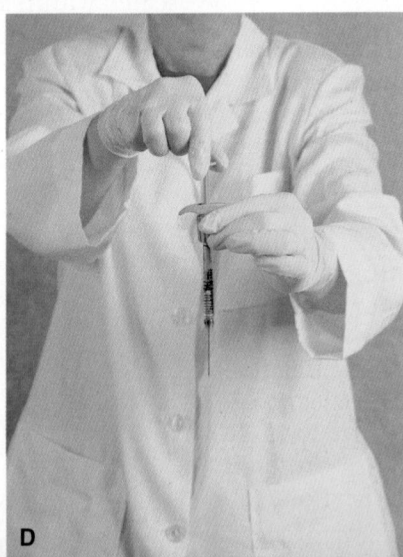

D

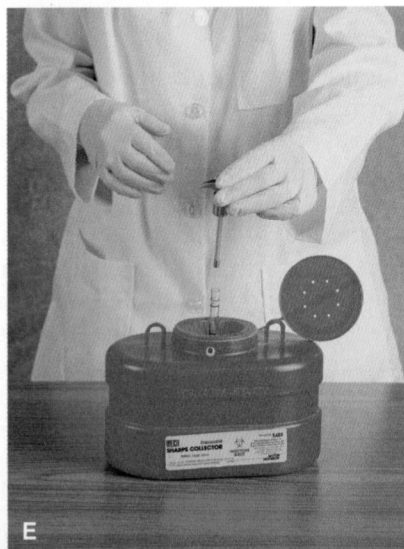

E

FIGURE 35-14 (A) Reusable cartridge holder with disposable sterile cartridge needle unit. (B) Turn ribbed collar to open position. (C) Insert the sterile cartridge-needle unit into the open end of the injector. The ribbed collar is firmly tightened. The plunger of the injector and the plunger of the cartridge-needle units are tightened and ready for use. (D) The medical assistant prepares to dispose of the cartridge-needle unit. The needle is not recapped. The plunger rod is disengaged by unscrewing. The ribbed collar is loosened. (E) The medical assistant holds the cartridge-needle unit over a sharps container, and the unit drops into the container.

example, the provider may order Morphine 5 mg and the cartridge is 10 mg/mL. Give 0.5 mL and properly discard the other 0.5 mL according to clinic policy. Another person must witness the disposal of the Morphone, which is a controlled substance.

Parts of a Syringe.   The component parts of a syringe are a barrel, plunger, flange, tip (Figure 35-15), and safety shield on a safety syringe.

- The *barrel* is the part that holds the medication and has graduated markings (calibrations) on its surface for use in measuring medications.
- The *plunger* is a movable cylinder designed for insertion within the barrel; it provides the mechanism by which a medication is drawn into or pushed out of the barrel.
- The *flange* is at the end of the barrel where the plunger is inserted. It forms a rim around the end of the barrel where the plunger is inserted and has appendages against which one places the index and middle fingers when drawing up solution for injection. The flange also prevents the syringe from rolling when laid on a flat surface.
- The *tip* is at the end of the barrel where the needle is attached.

- The *safety shield* is pulled over the needle while withdrawing it. Safety needles have a mechanism to sheath, retract, or blunt the needle.

The parts of a syringe that must remain sterile during the preparation and administration of a parenteral medication are the inside of the barrel, the section of the plunger that fits inside the barrel, and the syringe tip to which the needle is to be attached.

Types of Syringes and Uses.   Syringes are named according to their sizes and uses. Table 35-10 lists the types, sizes, calibrations, and uses of syringes for the administration of parenteral medications.

One should always choose a needle with sufficient length to reach the desired tissue level. A large person may require a longer needle to reach the correct body tissue than would be required for a smaller person. The delivery of medication to the proper tissue level is important. A concentrated or irritating medication that is intended for deep intramuscular injection could be delivered instead into the subcutaneous tissue of an obese patient if one selects a needle that is too short. Such an inappropriate injection may cause a sterile abscess and necrosis. This unnecessary complication can be avoided by considering the size of the patient when choosing the length of the needle.

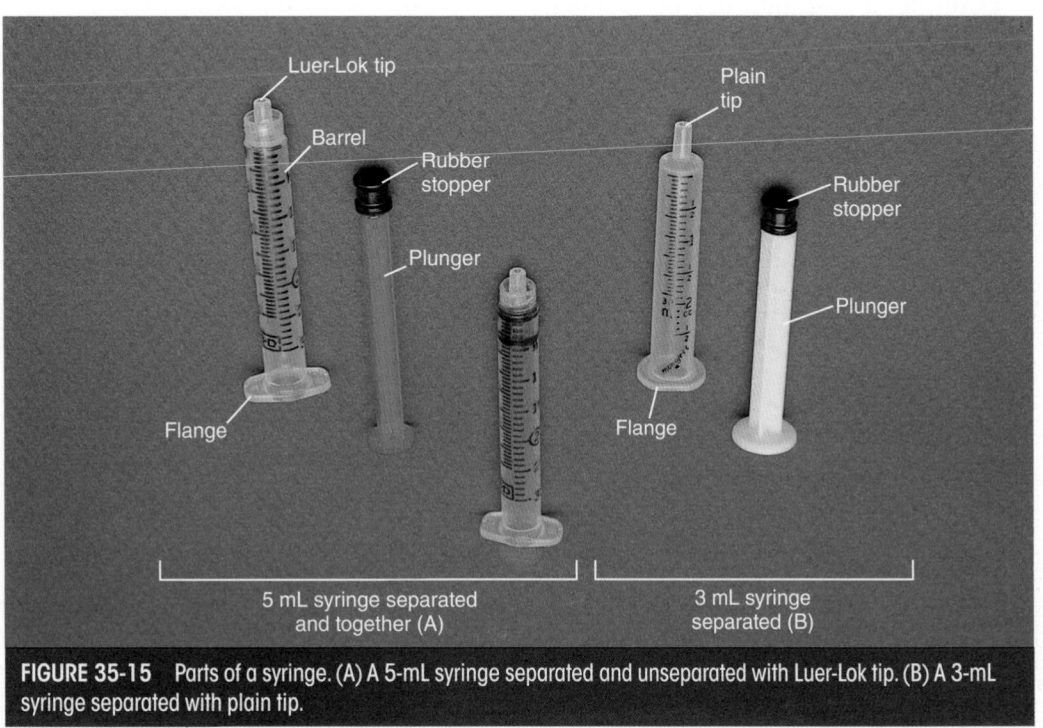

FIGURE 35-15   Parts of a syringe. (A) A 5-mL syringe separated and unseparated with Luer-Lok tip. (B) A 3-mL syringe separated with plain tip.

TABLE 35-10

THE MOST FREQUENTLY USED SYRINGES FOR PARENTERAL MEDICATIONS

TYPE OF SYRINGES	SIZE AND CALIBRATION	TYPICAL USES
Hypodermic	3 milliliter Calibrated 0.1 mL	Intramuscular and subcutaneous injections
Hypodermic	5 milliliter Calibrated 0.2 mL	Venipuncture and intramuscular injections
Hypodermic	Larger sizes (10, 30, and 60 milliliters) Calibrated 0.2 mL	Medical/surgical treatments, aspirations, irrigations, venipuncture, gavage (tube-to-stomach) feedings
Tuberculin	1 milliliter Calibrated 0.1 mL	Injection of minute amounts for intradermal injections, allergy testing, allergy injections
Insulin	U-100 (0.5 milliliter) U-100 (1 milliliter) Calibrated in units	Lo-Dose administration of insulin

Needles. Disposable needles are individually packaged in sterile paper or plastic containers. Disposable needles and syringe–needle units are available with a color-coded sheath. The sheath protects the needle and identifies its gauge and length. Common needle gauges (G) range from 16 to 32, and their lengths vary from ⅜ to 2 inches. The needle's gauge is determined by the diameter of the lumen or opening at its beveled tip. The larger the gauge, the smaller the diameter of its lumen. For example, a 25-gauge needle is much smaller than a 16-gauge needle.

See Figure 35-16 for various sizes and types of needles.

Parts of a Needle. Figure 35-17 shows the parts of a needle used to administer parenteral medications.

- The *point* is the sharpened end of the needle. The point is formed when the end of the shaft is ground away to form a flat, slanted surface called the *bevel*.

- The *lumen*, the hollow core of the needle, forms an oval-shaped opening when exposed at the beveled point.

- The hollow steel tube through which the medication passes is the *shaft*.

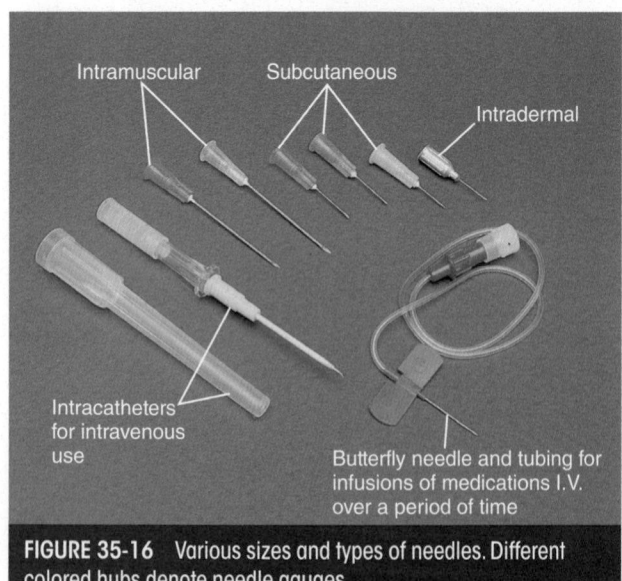

FIGURE 35-16 Various sizes and types of needles. Different colored hubs denote needle gauges.

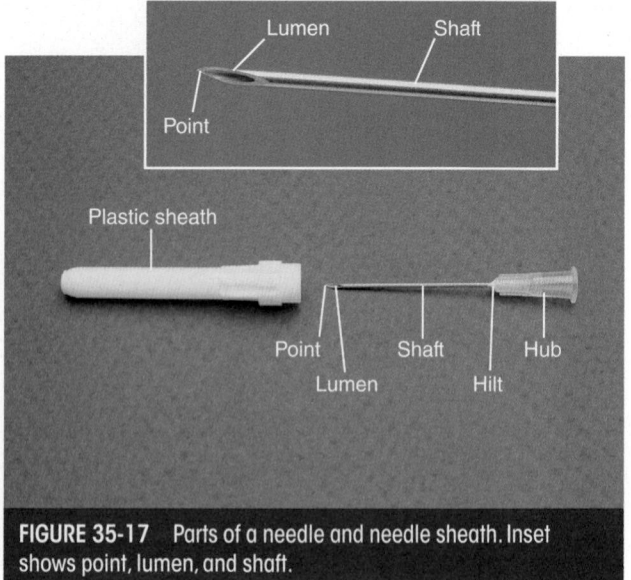

FIGURE 35-17 Parts of a needle and needle sheath. Inset shows point, lumen, and shaft.

- The other end of the shaft attaches to the *hub*, which is part of the needle unit that is designed to mount onto the syringe.
- The point at which the shaft attaches to the hub is called the *hilt*.

Safety Syringes. There are multiple manufacturers of safety syringes and multiple designs for the protection of the health care worker. Some safety syringes have covers that snap or slide over the used needle. There are other designs that have a needle that retracts into the plunger.

The Safe Disposal of Needles and Syringes

Safety

The careless disposal of used needles and syringes may present a health risk to any person coming into contact with the used equipment. An accidental stick by a contaminated needle could transmit diseases such as hepatitis B, hepatitis C, syphilis, Rocky Mountain spotted fever, tuberculosis, malaria, varicella zoster, and human immunodeficiency virus (HIV). Used needles and syringes should be discarded in a rigid, puncture-proof container (Figure 35-18). Never recap a needle after giving an injection. Do engage the safety feature. Most needlesticks occur while recapping. Refer to Chapter 21 for related OSHA regulations.

Most sharps-related injuries (needlesticks) occur in the hospital with inpatients. However, any health care worker who administers parenteral medications is at risk for an injury. Other sharps that can be involved in sharps-related injuries besides disposable needles include suture needles, butterfly needles, scalpel blades, phlebotomy needles, and IV catheter stylets.

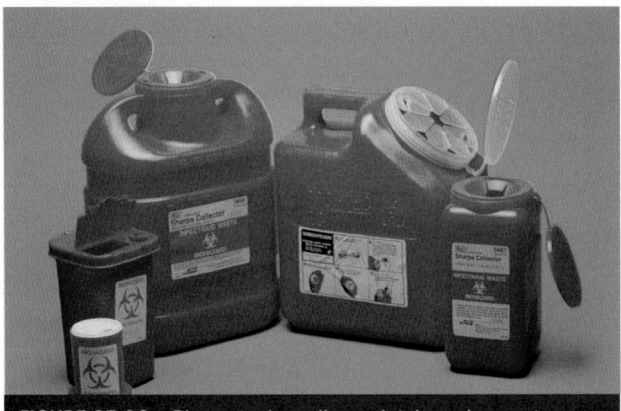

FIGURE 35-18 Place used needles, point down, in puncture-proof sharps containers.

A number of pathogens can enter the body during a sharps-related injury, but of greatest concern are hepatitis B and C viruses and HIV (see Chapter 21 for details about these and other bloodborne pathogens).

The National Alliance for the Primary Prevention of Sharps Injuries (NAPPSI) consists of medical device makers, health organizations, and health care providers whose goal is the prevention of sharps-related injuries. In addition to safety needles (see information in Chapter 21), laser scalpels, needleless drug delivery systems such as patches and inhaled medications, and needleless injection systems are available (fluid under pressure). There are glues and adhesives available to approximate surgical incisions. These alternative methods are helpful in reducing sharps-related injuries; however, phlebotomy and IV therapy still require a needle. Legal regulations (CDC and OSHA) require use of the safest needle available.

Proper use and disposal of sharps is of the utmost importance to health care workers and others. Avoid needles if there are other methods available, and never recap used needles. Engage the safety mechanism and dispose of needles and syringes immediately after use.

Sharps Collectors. Sharps collector systems eliminate the need to reshield the needle, thereby reducing the risk for an accidental needlestick.

Needles are placed into the container as a whole unit after safety mechanisms are engaged. Sharps containers need to be within reach any time injections are given.

PRINCIPLES OF INTRAVENOUS THERAPY

Patients who are unconscious, uncooperative, experiencing severe nausea and vomiting, have had severe burns, or have a significant amount of blood loss may need an intravenous infusion. All of these situations result in the patient losing body fluids, resulting in loss of homeostasis. The provider will order the fluids to be replaced by intravenous infusion according to the patient's condition or disease. The fluids will be specific for the needs of a particular patient. Some infusions maintain the patient's water (fluids) and electrolyte needs. For example, some elderly people who live alone and do not feel well, and perhaps have pneumonia, may not eat well or drink enough liquid to maintain the body's balance of fluids and electrolytes. If the situation goes on for a few days, during which time the patient becomes dehydrated, the patient will need IV fluids. Symptoms of dehydration are dry mouth, dark urine, and lightheadedness. It can lead to changes in the body's chemistry and become life threatening.

Severe nausea and vomiting can quickly dehydrate an individual and eventually can lead to kidney failure. The patient needs replacement of fluids and electrolytes through an intravenous infusion. (If a patient is vomiting, any attempt at taking in fluids orally is not likely to be successful.)

When a patient is prescribed intravenous fluids, the provider takes into consideration the patient's age, weight, height, and clinical laboratory results.

When patients are receiving an intravenous infusion, they must be watched carefully. The flow rate is ordered by the provider. Blood pressure should be monitored. Breathing and chest tightness should be reported. Excessive volume (too much fluid too quickly) can result in overhydration and possible serious adverse cardiac and pulmonary consequences.

Inserting a needle or cannula into a vein for purposes of an infusion is an invasive procedure, and the possibility exists for microorganisms to enter the patient's body. Everything must be sterile because microorganisms can enter the bloodstream and cause serious problems. Infection at the site of needle entry is possible. Phlebitis (inflammation of the vein) can occur from the patient moving about and causing the needle to irritate the vein. The IV fluid can infiltrate the tissues around the needle site, causing pain, swelling, and possibly tissue damage. The IV must be terminated and a new site used to restart it. Monitor the skin around the injection site for swelling and redness. Standard Precautions must be used to avoid exposure to the patient's blood and/or body fluids. The fluid is infused into the patient drop by drop. The flow of the solution is carefully monitored. The rate of the IV flow is crucial, and the number of drops per minute must be accurate. Other essential factors for IV infusion are that both the prescribed fluid amount and the amount of time required for the infusion to finish are correct, and that the drop factor is calculated using a mathematical formula.

Electronic devices for IV infusion are battery operated, electrically operated, or a combination of both. The devices are safe and accurate and can be programmed to a specific drop-per-minute rate. The devices have an alarm that signals if there is a problem and signals when the infusion is finished.

Equipment for an IV start comes in several pre-packaged sterile units. The IV catheter is selected based on the size and location of the vein as well as the type of fluid to be infused. In a separate IV start kit there is found a small quantity of tape, alcohol prep pads, and Tegaderm for application to the IV start site to secure the cannula. Also, the correct IV fluid to be infused and the tubing (Figure 35-19) for infusion must be collected prior to the IV start. The tubing has a roller-type clamp for adjusting the drop rate. Some tubing is made with a **port** that gives ready access for addition of

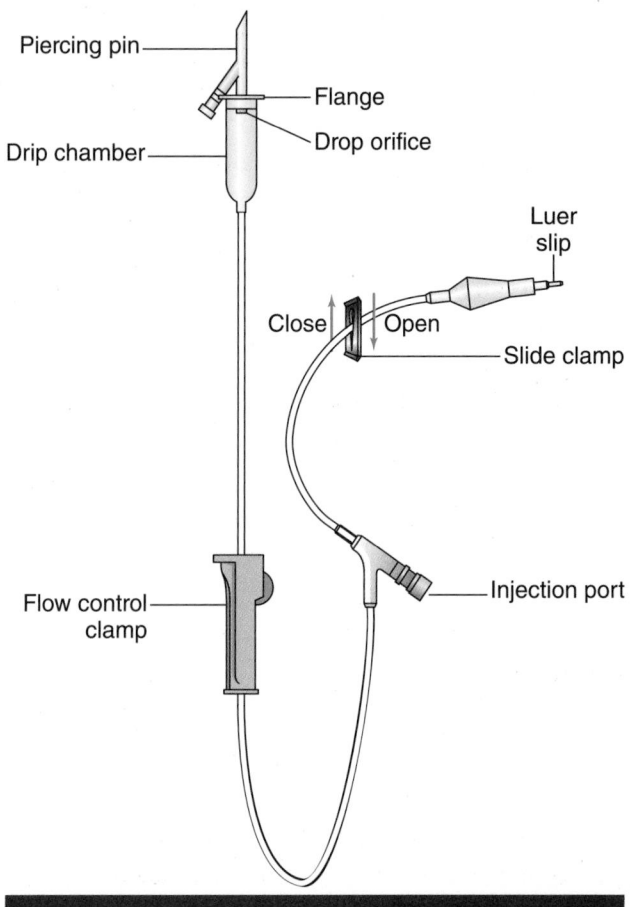

FIGURE 35-19A Basic IV administration set.

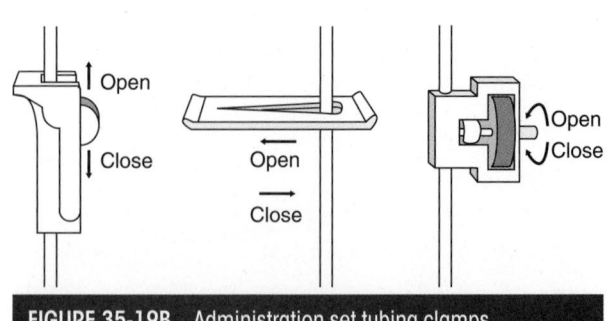

FIGURE 35-19B Administration set tubing clamps.

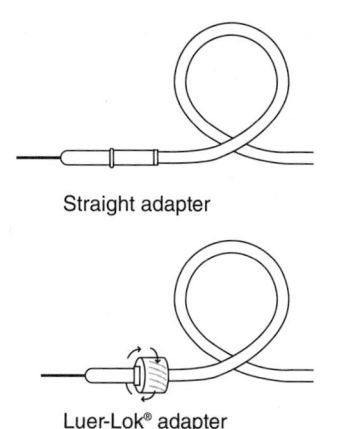

Straight adapter

Luer-Lok® adapter

FIGURE 35-19C Straight and Luer-Lok cannula hub adapters.

other fluids by using another infusion set simultaneously. The tubing can become kinked and slow down the flow of fluid. IV catheters are connected to the tubing using a straight connection or a Luer-Lock adaptor. The Luer-Lok connection is a more secure connection. This provides a lesser chance of loosening of the connection with leakage of fluid.

IV therapy or infusion is ordered by the provider for a variety of patient conditions. I.V. access allows medications to be administered when a rapid systemic response is needed, allows for rapid replacement of fluids to raise blood pressure when the patient is experiencing hypovolemic shock, and serves as a route for administering fluids and electrolytes, as well as nutritional supplementation. Access to a vein allows medications to be infused into the systemic circulation when a rapid onset is desired. The route provides a rapid route for countering poisonous substances or inappropriate medication response.

Veins may become very difficult to find as a result of a patient's condition (dehydration, hypotension, blood loss). The provider may order that for immediate accessibility, the vein should be kept opened (by continuous IV infusion). This is abbreviated KVO (keep vein open) or TKO (to be kept open).

Some IV solutions commonly used for infusions in ambulatory settings are:

- 5% dextrose in water
- Saline solutions
- Dextrose in normal saline
- Lactated Ringer's solution

Although IV therapy is not a procedure medical assistants perform, they must be knowledgeable about the procedure, understand the purpose for IV infusions, recognize the precautions concerning this invasive procedure, and realize that state laws vary regarding IV infusions. Monitoring the patient's condition and observing the IV site are roles that the medical assistant can perform in any state.

Legal

All persons providing health care to patients are legally responsible for their own actions. See Chapter 6 for legal considerations and Chapter 39 for information regarding phlebotomy.

It is important to realize that IV infusion is an invasive procedure much like the phlebotomy procedure. The veins for IV infusion are similar to those used for venipuncture in the hands and arms.

Integrity

The AAMA excludes the preparation and administration of intravenous medications from its list of clinical competencies for the medical assistant. It is important to understand the scope of practice for the medical assistant in the state in which you are employed. Questions regarding scope of practice can be directed to the American Association of Medical Assistants.

SITE SELECTION AND INJECTION ANGLE

The selection of a proper site for a subcutaneous, intramuscular, or intradermal injection and the correct angle of insertion for each will ensure that the medication is delivered to the correct tissue type (Figure 35-20).

A subcutaneous injection is given at an angle of 45 degrees just below the surface of the skin wherever there is subcutaneous tissue. The shaded areas shown in Figure 35-21A are the usual sites for subcutaneous injections because they are located away from bones, joints, nerves, and large blood vessels.

An intramuscular injection is given at a 90-degree angle, passing through the skin and subcutaneous tissue and penetrating deep into muscle tissue. Body areas used for intramuscular injections are the dorsogluteal area, ventrogluteal area, deltoid muscle, and vastus lateralis.

After locating an appropriate vein, an IV injection is given at a 25- to 30-degree angle penetrating the skin and introducing the needle into the vein. The antecubital, median cephalic, median basilic, and median cubital veins are common sites

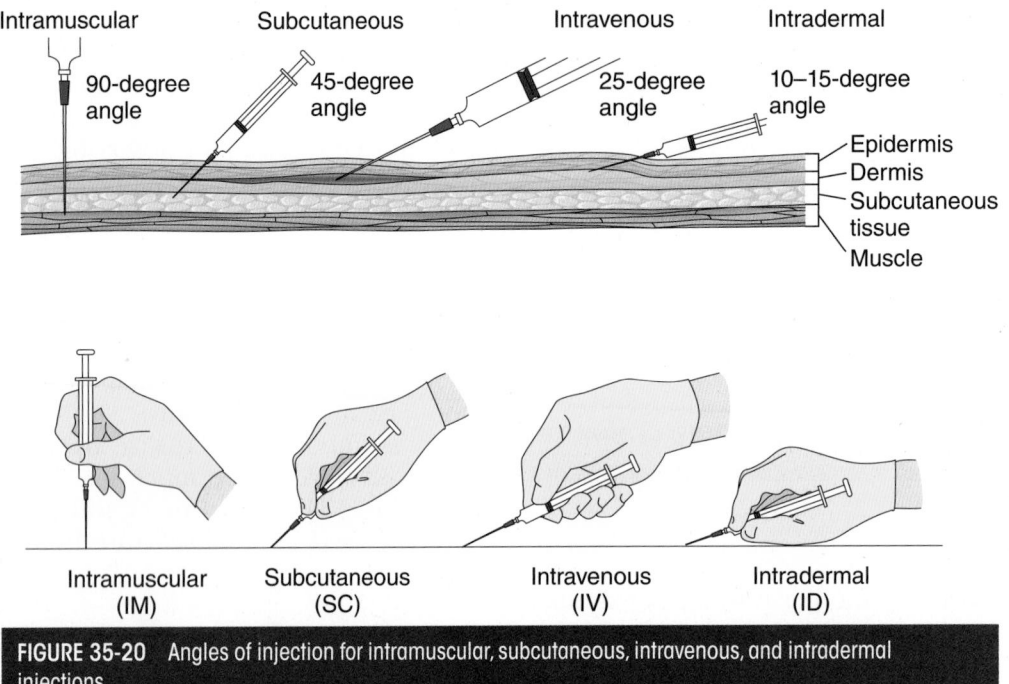

FIGURE 35-20 Angles of injection for intramuscular, subcutaneous, intravenous, and intradermal injections.

appropriate for IV injections (see Chapter 39 for more information about vein selection).

Intradermal injections are given at an angle between 10 and 15 degrees into the dermal layer of the skin. The body areas used for intradermal injections are the inner forearm and the middle of the back (Figure 35-21B). For further information, see the "Intramuscular Injections" Quick Reference Guide.

Marking the Correct Site for Intramuscular Injection

To give a safe injection, it is necessary to become familiar with the anatomic structures associated with the injection site. With knowledge of where such structures are located, it is easier to mark injection sites that avoid bones, nerves, and large blood vessels.

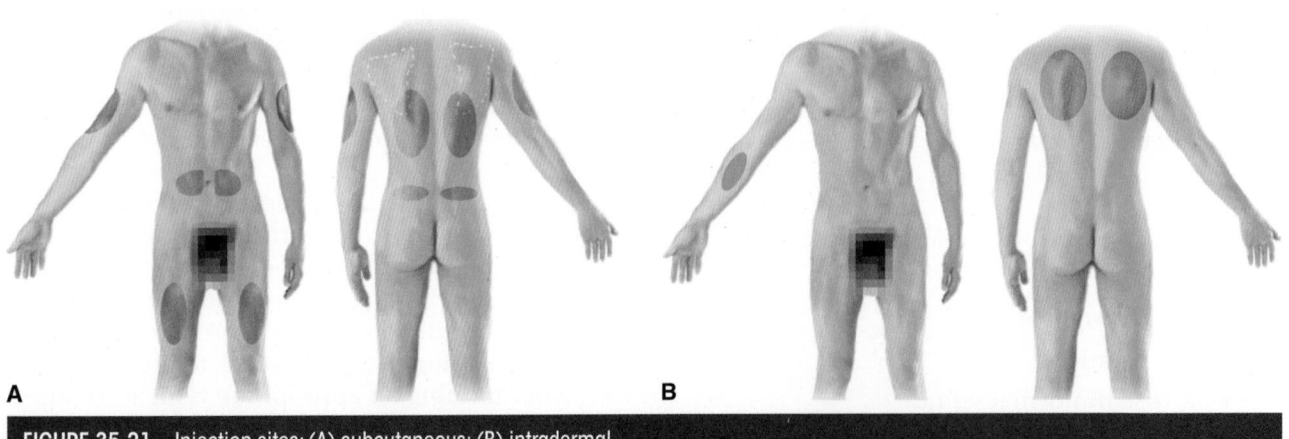

FIGURE 35-21 Injection sites: (A) subcutaneous; (B) intradermal.

INTRAMUSCULAR INJECTIONS

Site		Specifics	Advantages/ Disadvantages	Landmarks
Deltoid	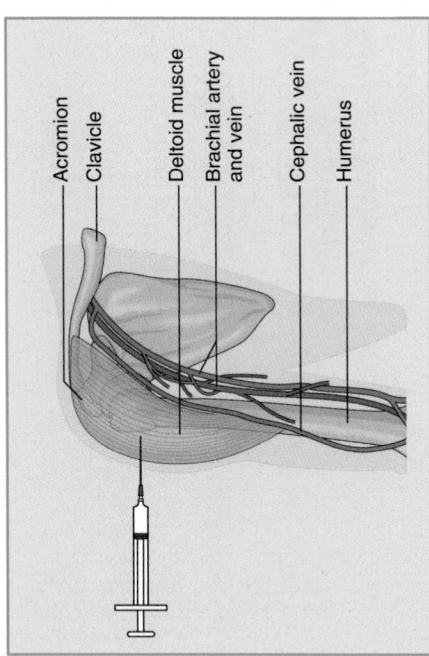	Volume of injection: 0.5 to 1.0 mL (based on muscle mass and age of patient) Needle sizes: 23 to 25 G ⅝ to 1½ inches Can be utilized for patients 15 months and older Patient positions: Sitting Prone Supine Lateral Angle of injection: 90 degrees The only site approved for hepatitis B vaccine injection	**Advantages:** Easily accessible General patient acceptance of site **Disadvantages:** Smaller muscle mass than other injection sites Increased risk of damage to brachial, axillary, and radial nerves and vascular structures Care must be taken to avoid bone injury to the acromion and humerus Irritating medications are contraindicated Not indicated for use in infants The upper and lower aspects of the deltoid are not suitable for injection	The deepest body of the deltoid muscle is located at the mid-axillary line, 1 to 3 finger breadths below the acromion process depending on the age and body size of the patient Inject just below the finger breadths

Image labels: Acromion, Clavicle, Deltoid muscle, Brachial artery and vein, Cephalic vein, Humerus

(continues)

Site	Specifics	Advantages/Disadvantages	Landmarks
Dorsogluteal	Volume of injection: 1.0 to 3.0 mL (based on muscle mass and age of patient) Needle size: 20 to 23 G 1 to 1½ inches Can be utilized in patients 2 years of age and older For patients with a higher BMI and therefore more subcutaneous tissue, a longer needle must be selected Patient position: Prone Angle of injection: 90 degrees	**Advantages:** Large muscle mass accommodates deep IM/Z-track injections Large muscle mass can tolerate relatively large quantities of medication Injections not visible to patient **Disadvantages:** Boundaries of the upper outer quadrant are often arbitrarily selected and may exceed margin of safety Danger of injury to major nerves and vascular structures if incorrect site or technique used Extreme caution should be utilized to avoid damage to the sciatic nerve or the superior gluteal artery or vein Subcutaneous fat is often very thick; therefore, an injection intended to be administered IM may be subcutaneous Contraindicated in infants and children Should not be utilized in emaciated or non-walking adults Slowest uptake of medication of the IM sites	Locate the greater trochanter at the top of the femur Locate the posterior iliac spine (many people have "dimples" over this bone) Draw an imaginary line between the two bones After locating the center of the imaginary line, find a point an inch superiorly; this is where to insert the needle Palpate the ileum and the trochanter in order to ensure proper anatomical site location and injection technique

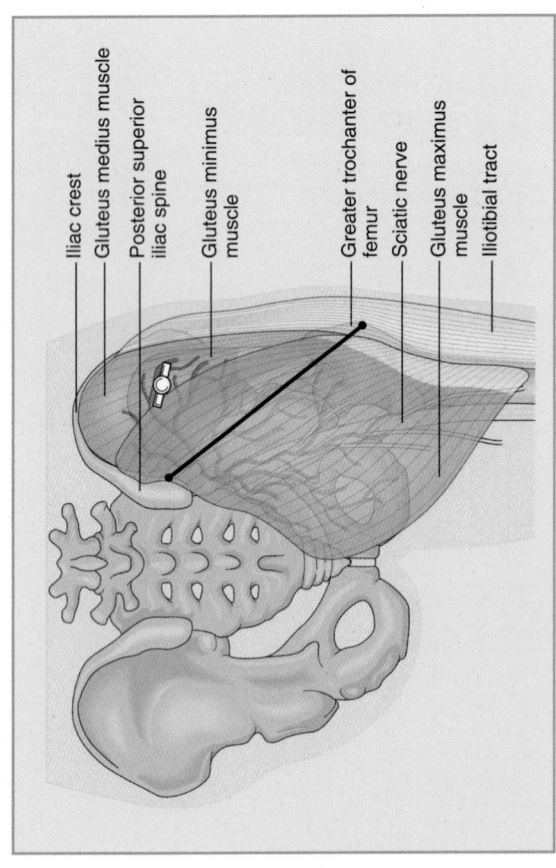

Iliac crest
Gluteus medius muscle
Posterior superior iliac spine
Gluteus minimus muscle
Greater trochanter of femur
Sciatic nerve
Gluteus maximus muscle
Iliotibial tract

(Referred to as the upper outer quadrant of the buttocks)

(continues)

Site	Specifics	Advantages/ Disadvantages	Landmarks
Ventrogluteal	Volume of injection: 1.0 to 3.0 mL (based on muscle mass and age of patient) Needle size: 20 to 23 G 1 to 1½ inches Can be utilized in patients 2 years of age and older Patient position: Supine Lateral Angle of injection: 90 degrees Serves as an alternative to dorsogluteal and vastus lateralis for deep IM/Z-track injections Preferred site for IM injections	**Advantages:** Area is relatively free of major nerves and vascular branches Well localized by anatomic landmarks Thin layer of subcutaneous fat Greatest thickness of gluteal mass for deep IM/Z-track injections Readily accessible from several patient positions **Disadvantages:** Health professional's unfamiliarity with the site	Locate the greater trochanter at the top of the femur Locate the anterior iliac crest Place the palm of your hand over the trochanter Point the index finger toward the anterior iliac crest Spread the second or middle finger toward the posterior of the body, making a *V;* the thumb should always be pointed toward the anterior of the body Form a V with the index and the long finger Inject in the exposed area between these fingers below the iliac crest

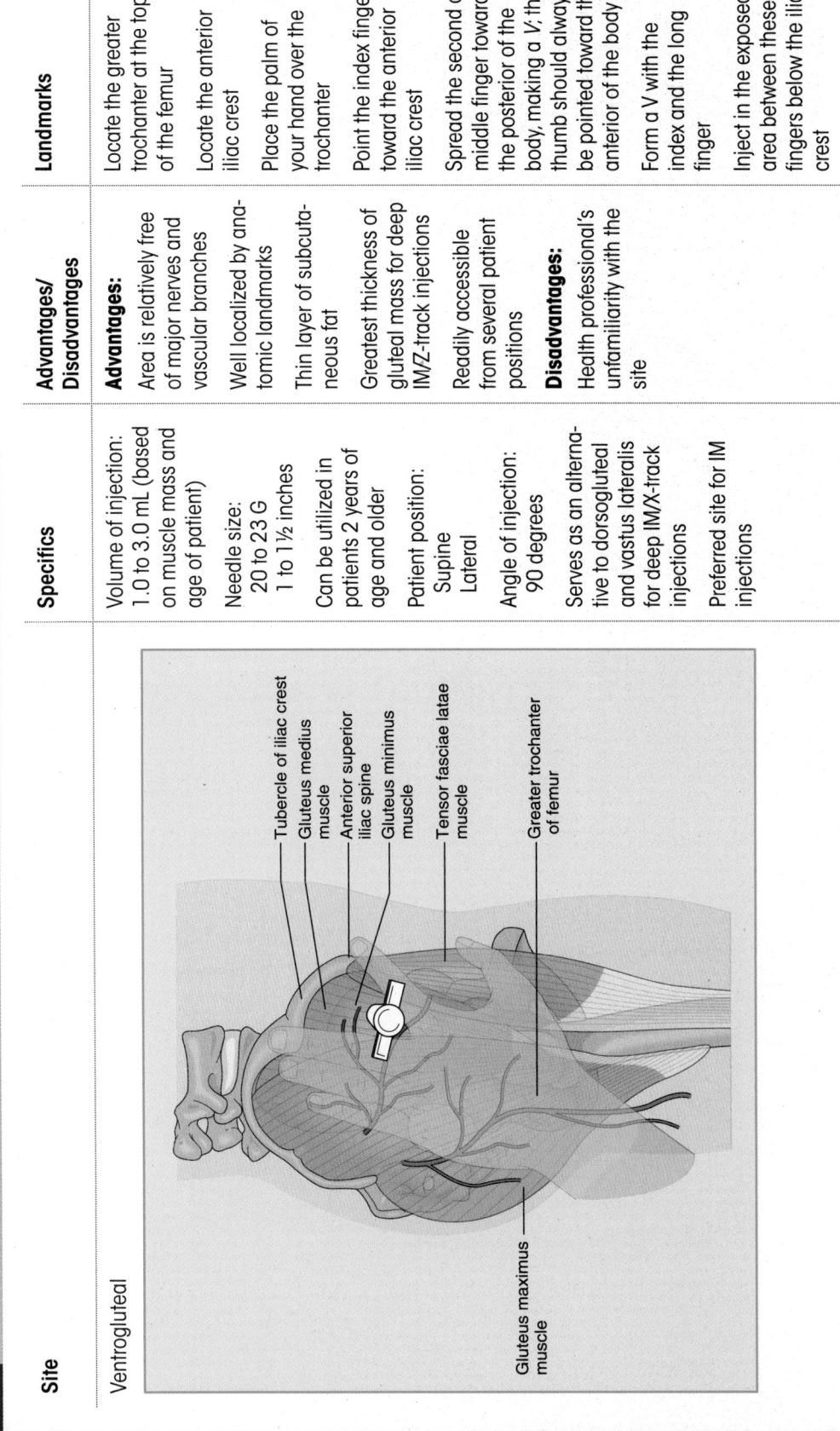

Tubercle of iliac crest
Gluteus medius muscle
Anterior superior iliac spine
Gluteus minimus muscle
Tensor fasciae latae muscle
Greater trochanter of femur
Gluteus maximus muscle

(continues)

Site	Specifics	Advantages/ Disadvantages	Landmarks
Vastus lateralis	Volume of injection (maximum): Infant—0.5 mL Pediatric—1.0 mL Adult— 2.0 mL	**Advantages:** Surface area provides sufficient space for several injections	Locate the greater trochanter
Adult	Needle sizes: Child—25 to 27 G, 1 inch Adult—21 to 23 G, 1½ inch	Free of major nerves and vascular branches	Find a location one hand's breadth be-low the level of the greater trochanter and one hand's breadth above the knee
	Appropriate for all ages	Suitable site for in-fants	

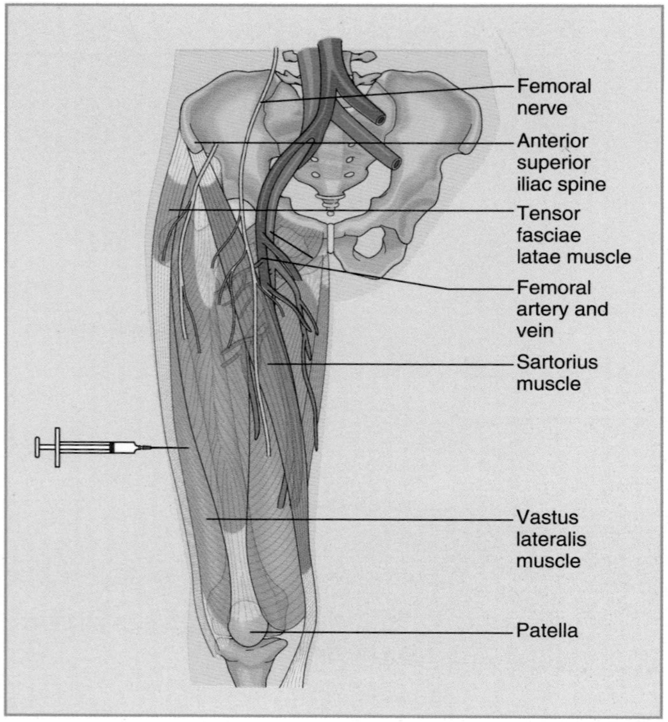

Femoral nerve
Anterior superior iliac spine
Tensor fasciae latae muscle
Femoral artery and vein
Sartorius muscle
Vastus lateralis muscle
Patella

(continues)

Site	Specifics	Advantages/Disadvantages	Landmarks
Pediatric	Patient positions: Sitting Supine Angle of injection: 45 degrees directed toward the knee for newborns to 2 years of age 90 degrees for ages 2 years to adults	**Disadvantages:** Uptake of medications injected in the thigh is slower than the deltoid, but more rapid than the dorsogluteal site	Inject in the area between the hand's breadth on the lateral aspect of the thigh

Anterior superior iliac spine

Greater trochanter of femur

Femoral artery and vein

Aponeurosis of vastus lateralis muscle

Femoral nerve

Vastus lateralis muscle

Patella

NOTE: Some sources list the maximum volume to be injected in the dorsogluteal site. Needle gauge selection is based on type of medication and location of injection. Consult with your provider or check your policy and procedure manual for guidance in these areas.

BASIC GUIDELINES FOR ADMINISTRATION OF INJECTIONS

Safety

Regardless of the type of injection, basic guidelines must be followed to safeguard the patient. These guidelines are presented according to the sequence of the events to which they relate:

1. Adhere to the "Six Rights" of proper drug administration.

2. Always evaluate each patient as an individual.

3. Select a needle–syringe unit that is the appropriate size for the proper administration of the specific parenteral medication.

4. Correctly prepare the appropriate parenteral equipment and supplies for use. Wash hands and put on gloves. Always use OSHA guidelines and follow Standard Precautions.

5. Select the correct site for the intended injection.

6. Prepare the patient properly for the injection.

7. For subcutaneous and intramuscular injections, use a smooth, quick, dart-like motion to insert the needle into the patient's skin. Use the correct angle of insertion, 45 or 90 degrees respectively, for the injection.

8. Once the needle is inserted, gently pull back on the plunger (aspirate) to ensure that the needle is not in a blood vessel.

   CAUTION: If blood appears in the syringe on aspiration, smoothly withdraw the needle, properly discard the used unit, and prepare another injection for administration. Repeat the preceding steps.

9. Slowly inject the medication.

10. With a quick, smooth motion, remove the needle from the injection site at the same angle as insertion. Immediately activate the safety mechanism and discard the syringe–needle unit in a puncture-proof container. Cover the injection site with a dry, sterile 2 × 2 gauze and gently massage the site.

    CAUTION: Do not massage the site when administering insulin, Imferon, heparin, or PPD.

11. Remove the gauze and check for bleeding. If bleeding occurs after applying pressure for 30 seconds, apply a sterile adhesive strip to the injection site (not for PPD injection site).

12. Remove gloves.

13. Observe the patient for any signs of hypersensitivity. Take precautions to ensure the patient's safety.

14. Properly and immediately discard the used equipment and supplies.

15. Wash hands.

16. Follow documentation procedures in the patient's chart or electronic medical record, noting administration of the medication.

17. Before releasing the patient, wait the appropriate amount of time and make sure the patient is given proper instructions and is not experiencing any unusual effects.

18. Return medications to shelf/storage.

Procedure

Procedures 35-4 through 35-6 provide steps as follows:

- Procedure 35-4: Administering an Intradermal Injection of Purified Protein Derivative (PPD)

- Procedure 35-5: Administering a Subcutaneous Injection

- Procedure 35-6: Administering an Intramuscular Injection

PROCEDURE 35-4

Procedure

Administering an Intradermal Injection of Purified Protein Derivative (PPD)

STANDARD PRECAUTIONS:

Handwashing

Gloves

Biohazard

(continues)

PURPOSE:
To correctly administer an intradermal injection of PPD.

EQUIPMENT/SUPPLIES:
- Medication order per provider
- Appropriate syringe and needle gauge and length
- Alcohol wipes
- Nonsterile disposable gloves
- Sharps container
- Adhesive bandage

PROCEDURE STEPS:

1. Using the information on the provider's order and ***paying attention to detail***, gather the appropriate supplies and equipment.

2. Before administering an injection to a patient, perform medical asepsis handwashing following the guidelines set forth by OSHA.

3. Review the "Rights" of medication administration and follow them when giving a patient any type of medication or injection.

4. Make sure you are working in a well-lit, quiet, clean area, and refer to the provider's order before selecting the correct medication from the designated area.

5. Take a moment to compare the medication label with the provider's order. This will help you prevent errors.

6. Check to make sure that the drug has not expired by locating and confirming the expiration date.

7. If you are unfamiliar with any particular drug, take a moment to consult the PDR, or other comparable reference, located in the electronic health record. You should be familiar with the drug's name, mechanism of action, route or routes of administration and any common side effects.

8. Carefully calculate the dosage based on the provider's order and the medication available.

9. If necessary prepare the parenteral medication as directed, taking care to be accurate and careful in your preparation. If you're using prepared medications, take a moment to roll the vial between your palms to ensure the medication is mixed thoroughly.

10. Make a second check of the provider's order and compare it to the medication label. RATIONALE: Though this might seem unnecessary, taking the time to perform a double-check can prevent careless mistakes that might endanger a patient.

11. Draw the proper amount of medication from the vial or ampule using proper technique.

12. Prepare for injection by changing the needle.

13. Properly discard any waste that might have been generated during preparation, including disposing of the needle in the sharps container.

14. Carefully transport the prepared syringe and order to the patient exam room along with the original medication container.

15. ***Introduce yourself and confirm the identity of the patient***, using two identifiers, such as name and date of birth.

16. ***Speaking to the level of the patient's understanding, explain the purpose of the medication and the procedure to be used for administration. Allay the patient's fears*** and allow time for questions. Make sure to ask about any allergies to medication at this time.

17. When the patient is ready, put on disposable gloves and prepare the area for injection by cleansing the site using an alcohol wipe. You should use a circular motion that begins at the site of injection and moves outward to a diameter of 2 inches. Allow the alcohol to air dry before proceeding.

(continues)

18. Perform a third and final check to ensure that the medication about to be given matches that indicated on the medication order. Carefully remove the needle cover and prepare to give the injection.

19. When administering an Intradermal Injection of Purified Protein Derivative, use your non-dominant hand to pull the skin taut. Have the patient take a breath and release it as you carefully insert the needle, bevel up, at an angle of 10 to 15 degrees and to a depth of 1/8 of an inch (Figure 35-22A).

20. Release the skin and steadily inject the PPD to form a "wheal" or "bleb" (Figure 35-22B).

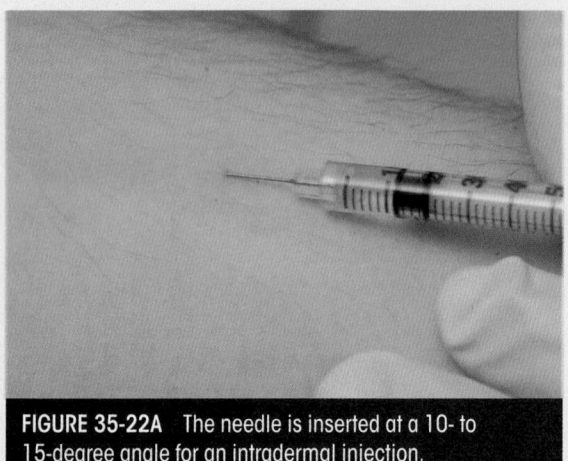

FIGURE 35-22A The needle is inserted at a 10- to 15-degree angle for an intradermal injection.

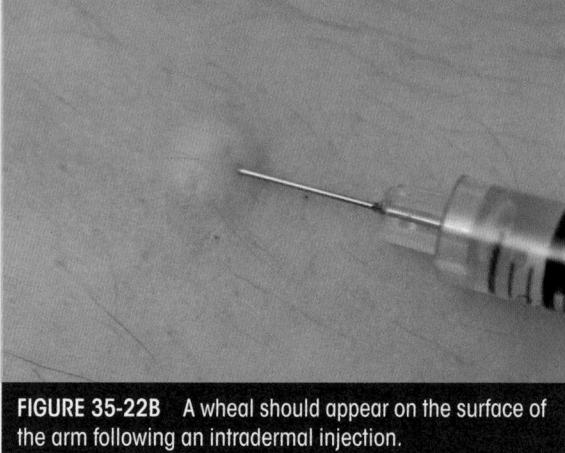

FIGURE 35-22B A wheal should appear on the surface of the arm following an intradermal injection.

21. When the medication has been administered in its entirety, remove the needle at the same angle it was inserted. RATIONALE: Minimizes leakage.

22. When the injection has been administered, immediately dispose of the needle and syringe in the sharps container.

23. You should never rub the injection site. Instruct the patient to not rub or massage the wheal.

24. Remove your gloves and discard them, and any other disposable items, into the appropriate waste container.

25. Wash your hands and return any supplies or medication to their proper place.

26. If this is the first time that the patient has received a PPD injection, the patient must be observed for 20 minutes to ensure no reaction. Assess the patient every 5 minutes during that time, taking into account color, pulse, respiratory rate, and self-report.

27. Advise the patient to return within 48–72 hours to have the injection site interpreted.

28. Accurately document the medication type, dosage, route of administration (including the site of injection if applicable) and any patient reaction. Sign and provide the date and time.

DOCUMENTATION:

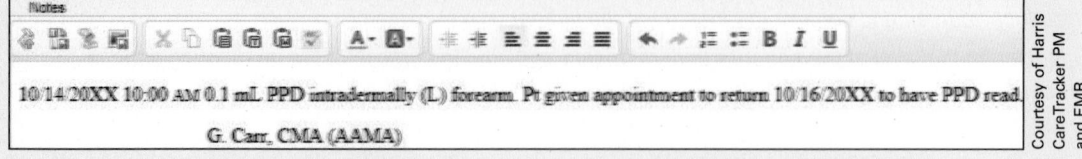

Notes:

10/14/20XX 10:00 AM 0.1 mL PPD intradermally (L) forearm. Pt given appointment to return 10/16/20XX to have PPD read.

G. Carr, CMA (AAMA)

Courtesy of Harris CareTracker PM and EMR

Procedure

Administering a Subcutaneous Injection

STANDARD PRECAUTIONS:

Handwashing

Gloves

Biohazard

PURPOSE:

To correctly administer a subcutaneous injection.

EQUIPMENT/SUPPLIES:

- Medication order per provider
- Appropriate syringe size and needle gauge and length
- Alcohol wipes
- Nonsterile disposable gloves
- Sharps container
- Adhesive bandage

PROCEDURE STEPS:

1. Using the information on the provider's order, and *paying attention to detail*, gather the appropriate supplies and equipment.

2. Before administering an injection to a patient, perform medical asepsis handwashing following the guidelines set forth by OSHA.

3. Review the "Rights" of medication administration and follow them when giving a patient any type of medication or injection.

4. Make sure you are working in a well-lit, quiet, clean area and refer to the provider's order before selecting the correct medication from the designated area.

5. Take a moment to compare the medication label with the provider's order.

6. Check to make sure that the drug has not expired by locating and confirming the expiration date.

7. If you are unfamiliar with any particular drug, take a moment to consult the PDR or other comparable reference, located in the electronic health record. You should be familiar with the drug's name, mechanism of action, route or routes of administration and any common side effects.

8. If needed, carefully calculate the dosage based on the order and the medication available. This order is insulin and the calculation is not needed.

9. If necessary, prepare the parenteral medication as directed, taking care to be accurate and careful in your preparation. If you're using a prepared medication, roll the vial between your palms to ensure the medication is mixed thoroughly.

10. Make a second check of the provider's order and compare it to the medication label. Though this might seem unnecessary, taking the time to perform a double-check can prevent careless mistakes that might endanger a patient.

11. Cleanse the diaphragm of the vial and withdraw the proper amount of medication from the vial using proper technique.

12. Properly discard any waste that might have been generated during preparation.

(continues)

13. Carefully transport the prepared syringe and order to the patient exam room along with the original medication container.

14. ***Introduce yourself and confirm the identity of the patient***, using two identifiers, such as name and date of birth.

15. ***Speaking to the patient's level of understanding, explain the purpose of the medication and the procedure to be used for administration. Allay the patient's fears*** and allow time for questions. Make sure to ask about any allergies to medication at this time.

16. Perform a third and final check to ensure that the medication about to be given matches that indicated on the order.

17. Position the patient and determine the most appropriate site to administer the injection.

18. When the patient is ready, put on disposable gloves and prepare the area for injection by cleansing the site using an alcohol wipe. You should use a circular motion beginning at the site of injection and moving outward to a diameter of two inches. Allow the alcohol to air dry before proceeding.

19. Carefully remove the needle cover and prepare to give the injection.

20. To administer a subcutaneous injection, grasp the skin around the targeted injection site using your non-dominant hand. Pinch upward to form a 1-inch fold.

21. Insert the needle quickly at an angle of 45-degrees (Figure 35-23). Slowly and steadily inject the medication. When all medication has been administered, remove the needle at the same angle it was inserted.

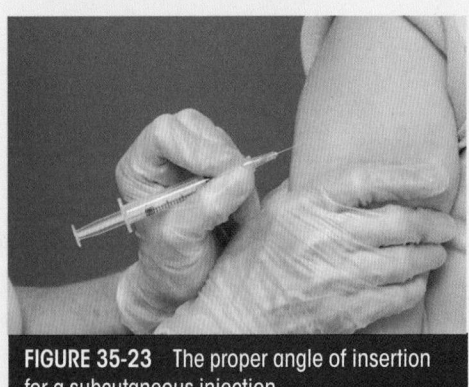

FIGURE 35-23 The proper angle of insertion for a subcutaneous injection.

22. When the injection has been administered, immediately activate the safety mechanism to cover the needle. Dispose of the needle and syringe in the sharps container.

23. If indicated, wipe the injection area with an alcohol wipe. Allow the area to dry and apply an adhesive bandage if needed.

24. Remove your gloves and discard them, and any other disposable items, into the appropriate waste container. Wash your hands and return any supplies or medication to their proper place.

25. If this is the first time the patient has received a particular medication, he or she should remain in the room for at least 20 minutes to ensure that there is no reaction. Assess the patient every 5 minutes during that time, taking into account color, pulse, respiratory rate, and self-report.

26. Accurately document the medication type, dosage, route of administration (including the site of injection if applicable) and any patient reaction. Sign and provide the date and time.

DOCUMENTATION:

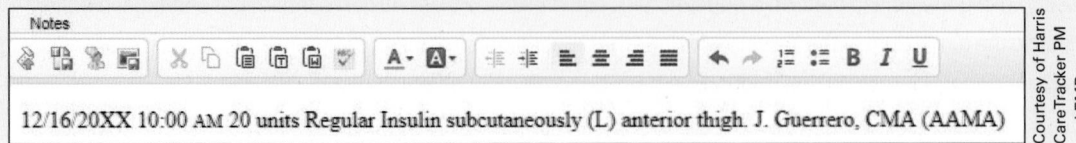

12/16/20XX 10:00 AM 20 units Regular Insulin subcutaneously (L) anterior thigh. J. Guerrero, CMA (AAMA)

Courtesy of Harris CareTracker PM and EMR

PROCEDURE 35-6

Procedure

Administering an Intramuscular Injection

STANDARD PRECAUTIONS:

Handwashing

Gloves

Biohazard

PURPOSE:
To correctly administer an intramuscular injection according to the provider's order.

EQUIPMENT/SUPPLIES:

- Medication order per provider
- Appropriate syringe size and needle gauge and length
- Alcohol wipes
- Nonsterile disposable gloves
- Sharps container
- Adhesive bandage

PROCEDURE STEPS:

1. Using the information on the provider's order and **paying attention to detail**, gather the appropriate supplies and equipment.

2. Before administering an injection to a patient, perform medical asepsis handwashing following the guidelines set forth by OSHA.

3. Review the "Rights" of medication administration and follow them when giving a patient any type of medication or injection.

4. Make sure you are working in a well-lit, quiet, clean area and review the order and select the correct medication from the designated area.

5. Take a moment to compare the medication label with the medication order.

6. Check to make sure that the drug has not expired by locating and confirming the expiration date.

7. If you are unfamiliar with any particular drug, take a moment to consult the PDR, or other comparable reference, located in the electronic health record. You should be familiar with the drug's name, mechanism of action, route or routes of administration, and any common side effects.

8. Carefully calculate the dosage based on the order and the medication available.

9. If necessary prepare the parenteral medication as directed, taking care to be accurate and careful in your preparation. If you're using an ampule, tap the ampule to release any medication into the main part of the ampule.

10. Don gloves and withdraw the proper amount of medication from the ampule using proper technique.

11. Properly discard any waste that might have been generated during preparation, including discarding the ampule in the sharps container.

12. Carefully transport the prepared syringe and order to the patient exam room along with the original medication container.

13. **Introduce yourself and confirm the identity of the patient**, using two identifiers, such as name and date of birth.

(continues)

14. ***Speaking to the level of the patient's understanding, explain the purpose of the medication and the procedure to be used for administration. Allay the patient's fears*** and allow time for questions. Make sure to ask about any allergies to medication at this time.

15. Perform a third and final check to ensure that the medication about to be given matches that indicated on the order.

16. When the patient is ready, put on disposable gloves and prepare the area for injection by cleansing the site using an alcohol wipe. Use a circular motion that begins at the site of injection and moves outward to a diameter of 2 inches. Allow the alcohol to air dry before proceeding.

17. To administer an intramuscular injection, carefully remove the needle cover and use your non-dominant hand to pull the area taut.

18. Using a "dart-like" motion, insert the needle to the hub at a 90-degree angle (Figure 35-24). Release the skin and aspirate the needle.

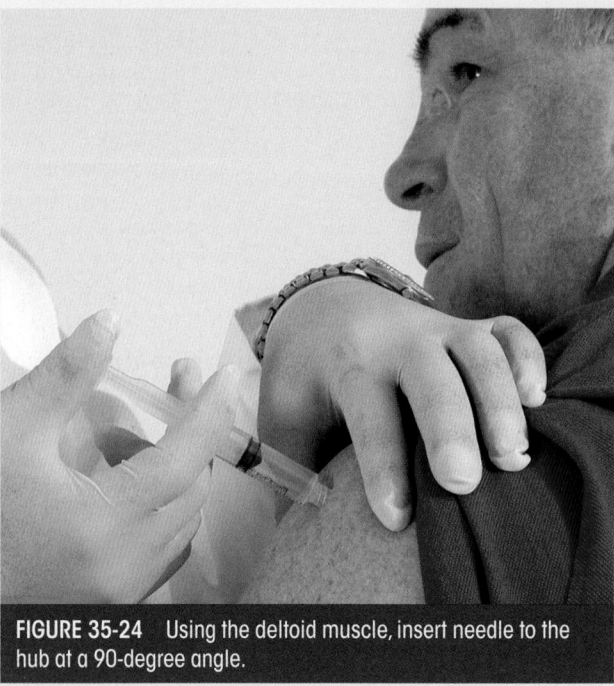

FIGURE 35-24 Using the deltoid muscle, insert needle to the hub at a 90-degree angle.

19. When performing an intramuscular injection, aspirate by holding the syringe steady and gently pulling back on the syringe plunger. If blood enters the syringe, remove the needle from the skin; discard both the needle and the syringe in the sharps container. Notify the provider.

20. If no blood is present upon aspiration, slowly and steadily inject the medication.

21. When all medication has been injected, remove the needle at the same angle of insertion.

22. When the injection has been administered, immediately activate the safety mechanism to cover the needle. Dispose the needle and syringe in the sharps container.

23. If indicated, wipe the injection area with an alcohol wipe and cover the site with an adhesive bandage. Remember not to use an adhesive bandage on a child under 3 years of age as this could constitute a choking hazard.

24. Remove your gloves and discard them, and any other disposable items, into the appropriate waste container. Wash your hands and return any supplies or medication to their proper place.

(continues)

25. If this is the first time the patient has received a particular medication, he or she should remain in the room for at least 20 minutes to ensure that there is no reaction. Assess the patient every 5 minutes during that time, taking into account color, pulse, respiratory rate, and self-report.

26. Accurately document the medication type, dosage, route of administration (including the site of injection if applicable) and any patient reaction. Sign and provide the date and time.

DOCUMENTATION:

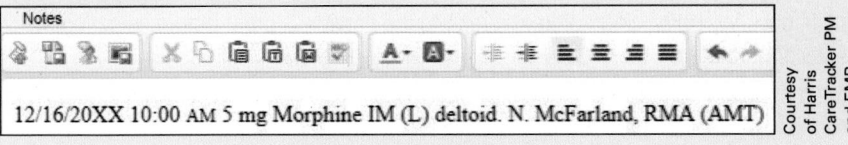

12/16/20XX 10:00 AM 5 mg Morphine IM (L) deltoid. N. McFarland, RMA (AMT)

Courtesy of Harris CareTracker PM and EMR

Z-TRACK METHOD OF INTRAMUSCULAR INJECTION

Procedure

Imferon is an example of a medication that is administered using the Z-track method. This medication and others that are irritating to the subcutaneous tissues and may discolor the skin are given in this manner. (The *Physician's Desk Reference* [PDR] is a good reference source for help in determining the correct route for specific injections.)

The Z-track technique is similar to an intramuscular injection, except that the skin is pulled to the side before needle insertion. This causes a displacement of the tissues and the medication enters in a manner that will not allow it to seep back into the subcutaneous tissues and up to the skin's surface. Because the medications are irritating, for the comfort of the patient, change the needle on the syringe after aspirating the medication from the ampule or vial and before injecting the patient with the medication (see Procedure 35-7).

PROCEDURE 35-7

Z-Track Intramuscular Injection Technique

Procedure

STANDARD PRECAUTIONS:

Handwashing

Gloves

Biohazard

PURPOSE:

To correctly administer a Z-track intramuscular injection.

EQUIPMENT/SUPPLIES:

- Medication order per provider
- Appropriately sized syringe and needle with correct gauge and length
- Alcohol wipes
- Disposable nonsterile gloves
- Adhesive bandage

(continues)

PROCEDURE STEPS:

1. Using the information on the provider's order and ***paying attention to detail***, gather the appropriate supplies and equipment.

2. Before administering an injection to a patient, perform medical asepsis handwashing following the guidelines set forth by OSHA.

3. Review the "Rights" of medication administration and follow them when giving a patient any type of medication or injection.

4. Make sure you are working in a well-lit, quiet, clean area and refer to the provider's order before selecting the correct medication from the designated area.

5. Take a moment to compare the medication label with the provider's order. Check to make sure the drug has not expired by locating and confirming the expiration date.

6. If you are unfamiliar with any particular drug, take a moment to consult the PDR, or other comparable reference, located in the electronic health record. You should be familiar with the drug's name, mechanism of action, route or routes of administration, and any common side effects.

7. Carefully calculate the dosage based on the order and the medication available.

8. If necessary, prepare the parenteral medication as directed, taking care to be accurate and careful in your preparation. If you're using prepared medications, take a moment to invert the vial several times, or roll it between your palms, to ensure the medication is mixed thoroughly.

9. Make a second check of the provider's order and compare it to the medication label. RATIONALE: Taking the time to perform a double-check can prevent careless mistakes that might endanger a patient.

10. Gather the appropriate needles and syringe. Withdraw the proper amount of medication from the vial using proper technique.

11. Change the needle after aspirating the medicine from the vial in order to avoid irritation of the patient's tissue.

12. Discard any waste generated during preparation before carefully transporting the medication and vial to the patient's room.

13. ***Introduce yourself to the patient*** using your full name and credentials and verify the identity of the patient, using two identifiers.

14. ***Speaking at the patient's level of understanding, explain the rationale for performance of the procedure***, answer questions, and otherwise ***allay the patient's fears.***

15. Review the provider's order and medication for a third and final time.

16. Assess the patient to determine the most appropriate site to administer the injection. Apply gloves. A Z-track intramuscular injection is often administered in the dorsogluteal muscle.

17. Cleanse the injection site using an alcohol wipe. Using a circular motion, work from the site of injection and circle outward to a diameter of 3 to 4 inches. Allow the skin to dry.

18. Remove the needle cover and using your non-dominant hand, place your fingers on the outside of the prepped area. Gently pull the skin laterally about 1 and a half inches from the chosen injection site. RATIONALE: This will keep the medication from leaking out.

19. Instruct the patient to take in a breath and release it. As the patient exhales, use a dart-like motion to insert the needle into the skin at an angle of 90-degrees (Figure 35-25).

20. Aspirate by holding the syringe steadily and gently pulling back on the syringe plunger. If blood enters the syringe, remove the needle and discard the syringe in the sharps container. Notify the provider immediately.

21. If no blood appears at aspiration, slowly and steadily inject the medication.

22. Remove the needle at the same angle of injection and immediately release the skin. RATIONALE: This will create a Z-Position and seal off the needle track.

(continues)

Procedure 35-7, continued

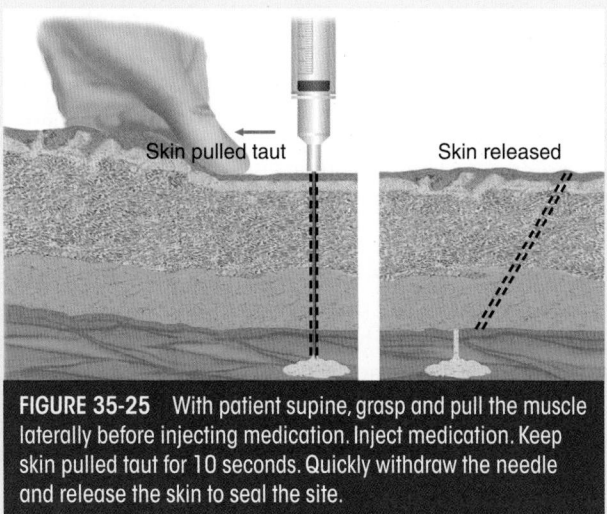

FIGURE 35-25 With patient supine, grasp and pull the muscle laterally before injecting medication. Inject medication. Keep skin pulled taut for 10 seconds. Quickly withdraw the needle and release the skin to seal the site.

23. Activate the safety mechanism to cover the needle and dispose of it immediately in the sharps container.

24. If the vial is single dose, it should also be disposed of in the sharps container. If it is not a single dose vial, the remaining medication will need to be returned to the medication cabinet or closet.

25. Cover the site with an adhesive bandage but do not massage.

26. Remove and discard gloves and wash your hands, while continuing to monitor the patient for possible side effects.

27. Accurately document the medication type, dosage, route of administration, the site of injection, and any patient reaction. Sign and provide the date and time.

DOCUMENTATION:

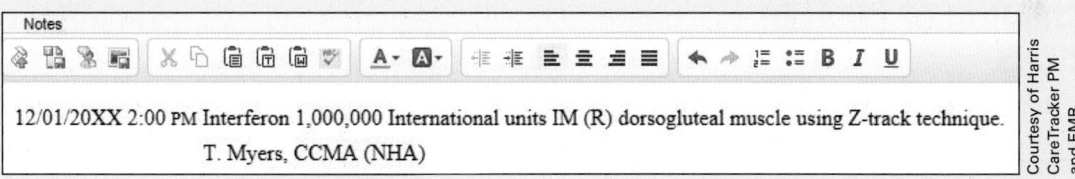

12/01/20XX 2:00 PM Interferon 1,000,000 International units IM (R) dorsogluteal muscle using Z-track technique.
T. Myers, CCMA (NHA)

Courtesy of Harris CareTracker PM and EMR

ADMINISTRATION OF ALLERGENIC EXTRACTS

It may be the responsibility of the medical assistant to administer allergenic extracts. It is important to observe the following:

- *Always* give allergic extracts in subcutaneous tissue, *never* in the muscle.
- Use a tuberculin syringe with a 25 G, ⅝-inch needle; 26 G, ⅜-inch needle; or 27 G, ½-inch needle or 1-mL allergist syringe (Figure 35-26).
- Use a site rotation system for each injected extract.

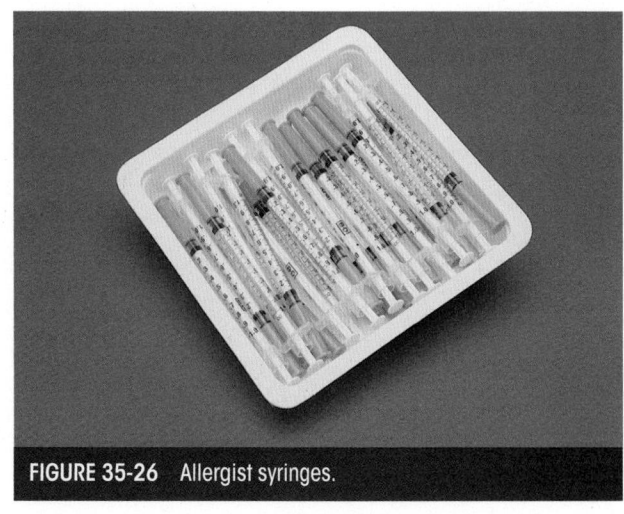

FIGURE 35-26 Allergist syringes.

- Allergen immunotherapy extract name and dilution from maintenance in volume per volume bottle letter (e.g., A, B), bottle color or number if used
- Expiration date of all dilutions
- Refrigerate allergenic extracts; they should retain potency for 10 to 12 weeks.
- Report adverse reactions such as itching, swelling, and redness immediately to the provider.
- Severe reactions such as anaphylactic shock have occurred; therefore, ensure emergency equipment and supplies are available for use. Epinephrine and Benadryl must be readily accessible. (See Chapters 8 and 34 for emergency supplies.)
- Perform allergy testing when the provider is present.
- Ensure the patient waits 20 to 30 minutes after injection to be certain there has been no reaction.

Susceptible individuals can experience development of allergic reactions to many foreign substances. Allergy testing can determine what particular pollens, molds, or other substances might be detrimental to a patient's health. Medication may be required to treat these allergies. Alternatively, knowing the cause of allergic reactions can assist in avoiding allergy triggers.

ADMINISTRATION OF INHALED MEDICATIONS

The act of drawing breath, vapor, or gas into the lungs is known as *inhalation*. Inhalation therapy may involve the administration of medicines; water vapor; and/or such gases as oxygen, carbon dioxide, and helium.

An inhaler may be used to deliver medications to the lungs. Medications that use an inhaler include bronchodilators, mucolytic agents, and steroids. Inhalers are useful in the delivery of treatment for chronic obstructive pulmonary disease (COPD) and reversible obstructive airway disease. An inhaler is a small, handheld apparatus, usually an aerosol unit, that contains a microcrystalline suspension of medication. When activated, it produces a fine mist or spray containing the medication. This suspension is then drawn into the respiratory tract, settling deep into the lungs and alveoli. See Chapter 29 for information about pulmonary diseases and procedures.

Implications for Patient Care

Patients should be instructed to follow the prescribed medication regimen. The prescribed medicine and the type of inhaler to be used will determine the method of administration. A handheld inhaler may be used for oral or nasal inhalation, depending on the type ordered by the provider.

Inhalation therapy may be contraindicated in patients with delicate fluid balance, cardiac arrhythmias, **status asthmaticus**, and hypersensitivity to the medication. As with any medication, the provider will determine the treatment regimen for each patient. See Chapter 29 for information about pulmonary diseases and procedures.

Administration of Oxygen

Oxygen is a colorless, odorless, tasteless gas that is essential for life. When the body does not have an adequate supply of oxygen, a state of **hypoxemia** (lack of oxygen in the blood) develops, and irreversible damage to vital organs is possible. When

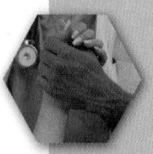

Patient Education

- Advise patients to avoid overuse of the inhaler. Tolerance, rebound bronchospasm, and adverse cardiac effects can occur from overuse. Instruct the patient to notify the provider should the prescribed dose of medication fail to produce the desired effect.
- Instruct the patient to perform good oral hygiene, including a thorough rinsing of the mouth and mouthpiece of equipment, after the inhalation treatment (to prevent the possible growth of fungi).
- Caution the patient against the continued use of a metered-dose canister after the prescribed number of actuations.
- If the medication contains adrenaline, fatalities can occur if heart rate and blood pressure increase significantly.

a lack of oxygen threatens a person's survival, supplemental oxygen must be prescribed and administered immediately, and arterial blood gas analysis will be necessary after oxygen administration has been started. If the situation is not an emergency or life threatening, pulse oximetry can be performed before the provider prescribes the dosage and method of administration. The normal range for SaO2 by pulse oximetry is between 90% and 100%. Oxygen is supplied in tanks (Figure 35-27) for use in the ambulatory care setting, but in a hospital setting, oxygen is piped in through a wall pipe system.

Dosage. When oxygen is to be administered, dosage is based on individual needs. Because supplemental oxygen is a considered a medication, the provider will prescribe the flow rate, concentration, method of delivery, and length of time for administration. Oxygen is ordered as liters per minute (LPM or L/min) and as percentage of oxygen concentration (%).

Communication

It is the medical assistant's responsibility to follow provider orders and adhere to the guidelines for proper drug administration. Always assess the patient as an individual, explain the procedure, and carefully observe the patient for signs of improvement or symptoms of oxygen toxicity.

A noninvasive technology that monitors the safety and efficacy of oxygen administration is the pulse oximeter. O_2 liter flow per minute can be titrated based on the results obtained from the pulse oximeter (see Chapter 29).

CAUTION: Oxygen toxicity may develop when 100% oxygen is breathed for a prolonged period. As with any other drug, toxicity depends on dose, time, and the patient's response. The higher the dose, the shorter the time required to develop toxicity. Symptoms of oxygen toxicity are substernal pain, nausea, vomiting, malaise, fatigue, numbness, and a tingling of the extremities.

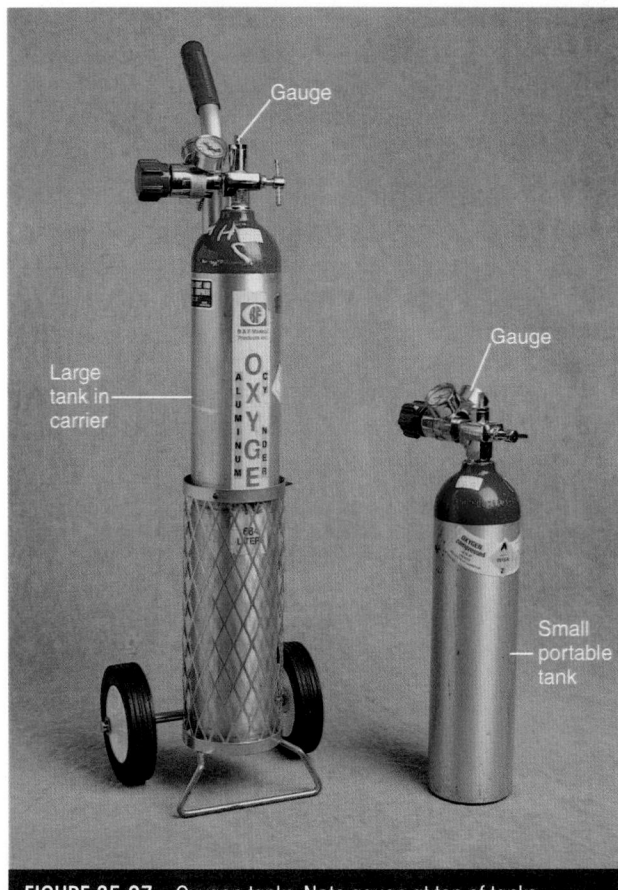

FIGURE 35-27 Oxygen tanks. Note gauge at top of tanks.

High concentrations of inhaled oxygen cause alveolar collapse, intraalveolar hemorrhage, hyaline membrane formation, disturbance of the central nervous system, and **retrolental fibroplasia** in newborns.

NOTE: **Apnea** (absence of breathing) can result when oxygen is given at a flow rate greater than 2 liters per minute to patients with COPD, especially those with emphysema.

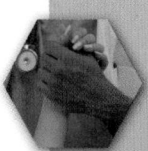

Patient Education

- Patients should be advised to avoid overuse of the inhaler. Tolerance, rebound bronchospasm, and adverse cardiac effects can occur from overuse. Instruct the patient to notify the provider should the prescribed dose of medication fail to produce the desired effect.

- Instruct the patient to perform good oral hygiene, including rinsing of the mouth and mouthpiece of equipment, after the inhalation treatment (to prevent the possible growth of fungi).

- Caution the patient against the continued use of a metered-dose canister after the prescribed number of actuations. If the medication contains adrenaline, fatalities can occur if heart rate and blood pressure increase significantly.

Methods of Oxygen Delivery. Many methods are available today for the delivery of oxygen. The more commonly prescribed methods include the use of nasal cannulas, nasal catheters, and masks. Other methods of delivery involve the use of isolettes, hoods, and tents.

Nasal Cannula. When a low concentration of oxygen is desired, the nasal cannula (Figure 35-28) is the simplest and most convenient method for the administration of oxygen. Made of plastic, the nasal cannula consists of two hollow prongs through which oxygen passes, and a strap or other device to secure it to the patient's head (Figure 35-29). Do not place the direct flow of oxygen against the patient's nasal mucosa, because this causes tissue dehydration. Flow rates greater than 2 to 4 L/min require humidification.

Mask. The common types of masks used for inhalation therapy include plastic disposable, partial rebreather, nonrebreather, and Venturi (Figure 35-30). These devices are used when the patient requires high humidity and a precise amount of oxygen. To be effective, the mask must be fitted snugly to the patient (Figure 35-31).

CAUTION: Oxygen must be humidified before delivery to the patient to prevent drying of the respiratory mucosa.

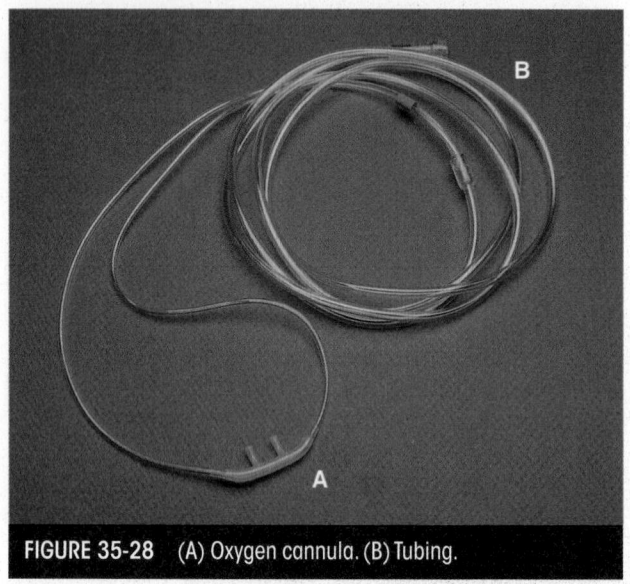

FIGURE 35-28 (A) Oxygen cannula. (B) Tubing.

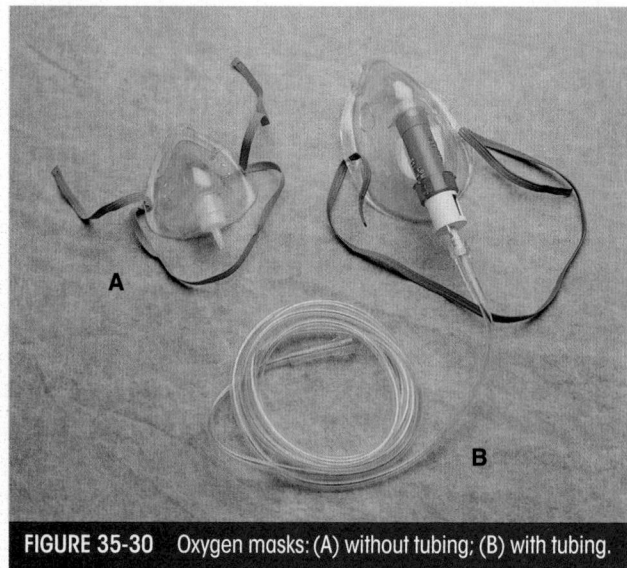

FIGURE 35-30 Oxygen masks: (A) without tubing; (B) with tubing.

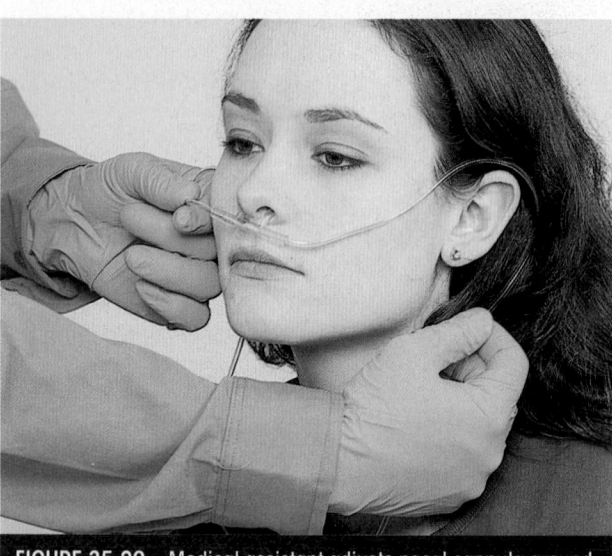

FIGURE 35-29 Medical assistant adjusts nasal cannula around patient's ears for oxygen administration.

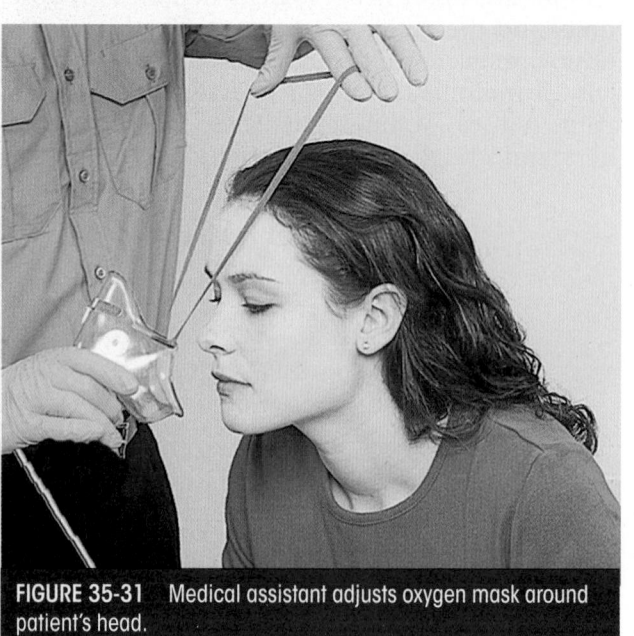

FIGURE 35-31 Medical assistant adjusts oxygen mask around patient's head.

Oxygen Safety Precautions. Oxygen supports combustion; thus, there is the danger of a fire being started when oxygen is in use. Extreme caution should be exercised when oxygen is being administered because ignition can be caused by friction, static electricity, or a lighted cigar or cigarette. In the provider's clinic, oxygen is generally stored in tanks. These tanks must be checked on a regular basis and replaced as necessary. See Chapter 29 for information about pulmonary diseases and procedures.

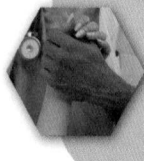

Patient Education

Explain safety measures to the patient who uses oxygen at home. Cigarettes, lighters, candles, and other smoking materials should not be used in the room where oxygen is used. Instruct the patient to wear non–static producing clothing, such as cotton.

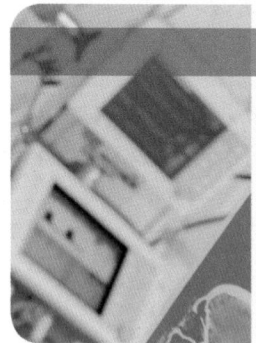

CASE STUDY 35-1

Refer to the scenario at the beginning of the chapter.

CASE STUDY REVIEW

1. Explain the consequences of preparing and administering a medication without referring to the provider's order in the patient's medical record.
2. Is it possible under normal circumstances to commit to memory the medication, dose, route, patient, and documentation?

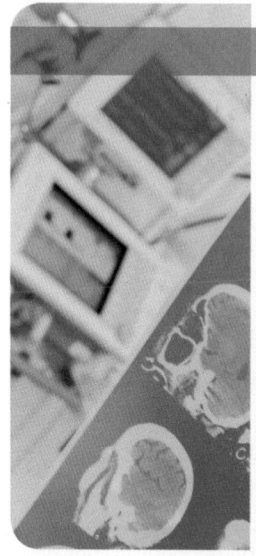

CASE STUDY 35-2

Abigail Johnson, a patient of Dr. Lewis, has been unable to keep her type 2 non–insulin dependent diabetes mellitus under control with oral hypoglycemics, and Dr. Lewis has decided that Abigail needs to begin to take insulin injections. Today in the clinic, her fasting blood glucose level is 190 mg/mL. Dr. Lewis prescribes Humulin insulin 10 units subcutaneously stat.

CASE STUDY REVIEW

1. What size insulin syringe should be used?
2. What does the medication label state are the number of units per milliliter? Show how to calculate the correct dosage.
3. Discuss the route of administration and the specifics regarding insulin administration that require it to be given slightly differently from other subcutaneous injections.
4. Describe several topics of discussion in which you would engage Abigail to help her learn how to better control her disease.

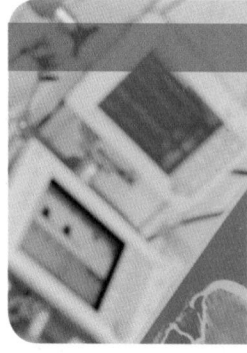

CASE STUDY 35-3

Alice Chambers weighs 28 pounds. Her pediatrician orders erythromycin 50 mg/kg/day po TID.

CASE STUDY REVIEW

1. Calculate Alice's weight in kilograms.
2. Calculate the daily dose of erythromycin Alice needs.
3. If the erythromycin is available as erythromycin 400mg per 5mL, calculate the dose to be given TID.

Summary

- Laws on both the federal and state level control the prescribing and administration of medications.

- Ethical and legal guidelines must be followed and anyone who has access to medications may not use them for personal benefit unless prescribed by a licensed provider.

- The prescription gives direction for compounding, dispensing, and administering a medication. Its purpose is to control the sale and use of drugs that can be safely and effectively administered under the supervision of a licensed provider.

- There are strict guidelines that pertain to the prescribing of controlled substances.

- Prescriptions often use abbreviations for dose, timing, and route.

- A medication's dosing is determined by age, weight, sex, physical condition, disease processes, causative factors, the patient's medical history, and safe and effective delivery to achieve the desired result.

- Pharmacokinetics is a term that refers to the way a drug is handled by the body. Pediatrics is a specialty that takes pharmacokinetics into consideration.

- Trade and generic name, the NDC, dosage strength, usual dosage and frequency, route, precautions, and expiration date information is found on the medication label.

- A working knowledge of the metric system is important for calculating medical dosages.

- There are several methods for calculating a medication's dose. These include ratio method and the formula method.

- Administering insulin subcutaneously is a part of the treatment plan for type 2 diabetes. There are many considerations when administering insulin. These include assuring that the proper insulin is given, using the correct syringe, the bottle should not be shaken, and rotating injection sites.

- Body surface area (BSA) is utilized when calculating pediatric medication dosages.

- The "Rights" of medication administration serve as a guide to limit the occurrence of medication errors.

- Prior to the administration of any medication, the patient's condition must be assessed.

- Oral medications are the most commonly prescribed. The administration of this type of medication requires few devices—a medicine cup, liquid for swallowing, and on some occasions a medicine dropper.

- Parenteral medication administration includes intradermal, subcutaneous, intramuscular, and intravenous routes.

- Parenteral routes provide rapid medication action.

- There are various sizes of syringes and various gauges and length of needles. Select the syringe and needle most appropriate to the medication being delivered, the injection type, the site of injection, and the patient's condition.

- Once used, needles and syringes must be disposed of in an OSHA-approved sharps container.

- The medical assistant may be tasked with the observation and management of intravenous infusions.

- The selection of intramuscular injection sites vary by the volume of medication to be injected and the age and condition of the patient.

- Intramuscular injection sites include deltoid, dorsogluteal, ventrogluteal, and vastus lateralis.

- Aseptic technique must be maintained during the administration of medications.

- The Z-track method of intramuscular injection is utilized when medication is irritating to the subcutaneous tissues and might discolor the skin.

- Allergy testing is administered using subcutaneous injection techniques.

- Oxygen is a medication that is administered via inhalation.

- Oxygen is delivered in liters/minute via nasal cannula.

CERTIFICATION REVIEW

1. What legal document gives directions for compounding, dispensing, and administering medication to a patient?
   a. Medication card
   b. Prescription
   c. Medication order
   d. Subscription

2. Which of the following abbreviation symbols represents "nothing by mouth"?
   a. Non rep
   b. NPO
   c. IM
   d. Mm
   e. NBM

3. Insulin-dependent diabetes mellitus is known as what?
   a. Type 1
   b. Type 2
   c. Type 3
   d. Type 4

4. The calculation of body surface area is utilized in which of the following circumstances?
   a. When calculating children's dosages
   b. When calculating adult dosages
   c. When determining an injection site
   d. When selecting an appropriately sized needle
   e. When calculating BMI

5. Which injection is given just below the surface of the skin at a 15-degree angle?
   a. Intramuscular injection
   b. Intradermal injection
   c. Subcutaneous injection
   d. Parenteral injection

6. Anatomic placement for deltoid injections is determined in what way?
   a. Measuring the circumference of the upper arm
   b. Locating a site 1 to 2 inches below the acromion
   c. Finding the largest muscle mass
   d. Finding the upper or lower aspect of the deltoid muscle
   e. Have the children flex their bicep to identify the deltoid

7. Pediatric dosages are carefully calculated based on which principle?
   a. Weight in kilograms
   b. Body surface area
   c. Divided dosing
   d. All of these

8. Which of the following is a part of the "Six Rights" of proper medication administration?
   a. Right patient
   b. Right medication
   c. Right time
   d. Right dose
   e. All of these

9. What action should be taken when a medication error occurs?
   a. Call poison control
   b. Inform the provider that an error has occurred
   c. Recognize that an error has occurred
   d. Assess the patient's condition

10. Which of the following is important when selecting a site for administering a prescribed medication?
    a. Anatomic structures
    b. Provider preference
    c. Treating each patient in exactly the same manner
    d. Knowledge of the Z-track method
    e. Equipment available

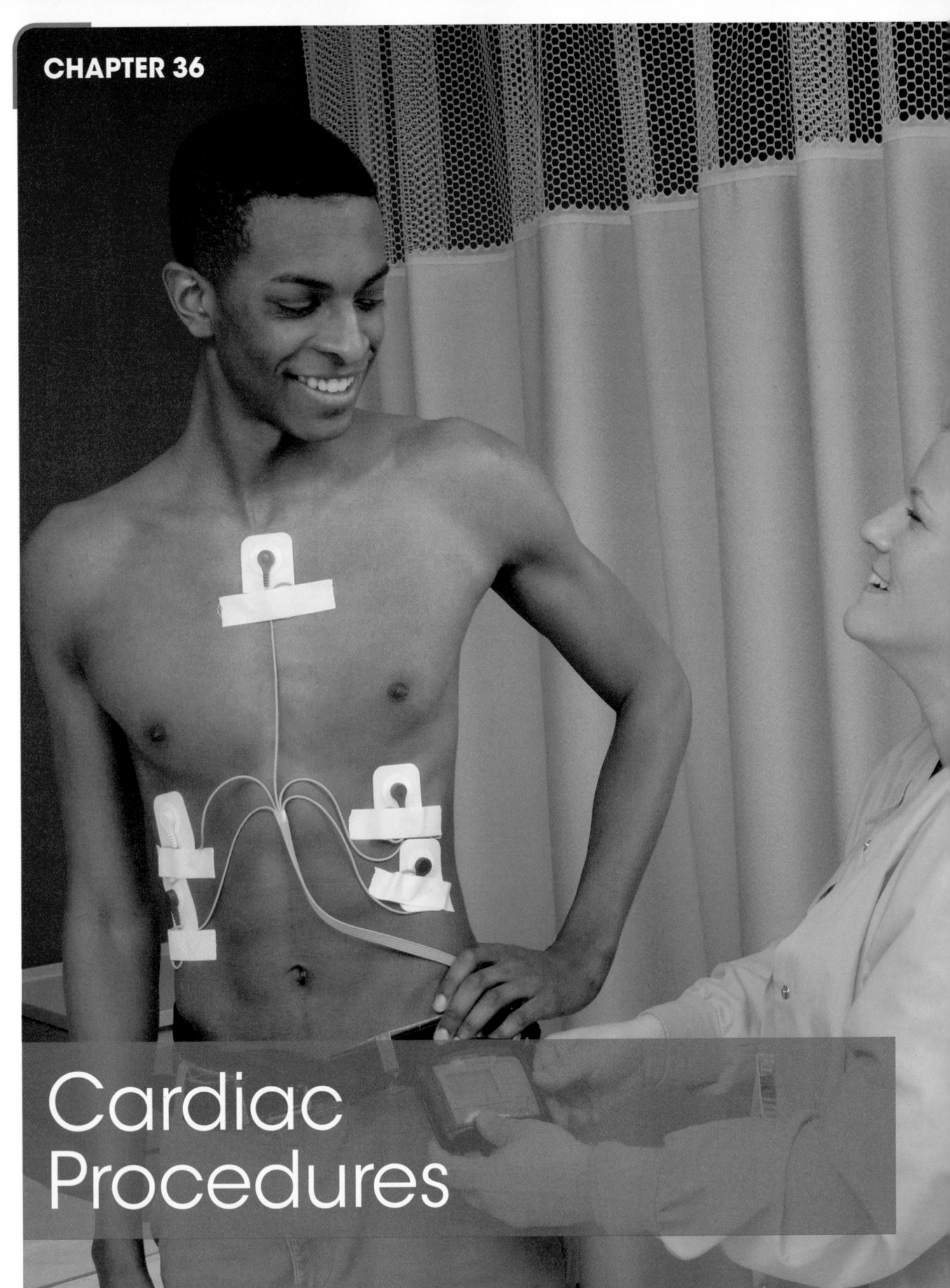

CHAPTER 36

Cardiac Procedures

1. Define and spell the key terms as presented in the glossary.
2. Follow the circulation of blood through the heart starting at the vena cavae.
3. Describe the electrical conduction system of the heart.
4. State three reasons why patients may need an electrocardiogram (ECG).
5. Identify the various positive and negative deflections and describe what each represents in the cardiac cycle.
6. Explain the purpose of standardization of the ECG.
7. Differentiate the 12 leads of an ECG and describe what area of the heart each lead represents.
8. Recite the function of ECG graph paper, electrodes (sensors), and electrolyte.
9. Describe various types of ECGs and their capabilities.
10. Compare and contrast each type of artifact and how each can be eliminated.
11. Name and describe the purposes of the various cardiac diagnostic tests and procedures as outlined in this chapter.
12. Identify the placement of Holter monitor electrodes.
13. Describe the reason for a patient activity diary during ambulatory electrocardiography.
14. Identify six arrhythmias and explain the cause of each.
15. Explain how to calculate heart rates from an ECG tracing.
16. Describe the procedure for mounting an ECG tracing.

KEY TERMS

amplified
amplitude
angina pectoris
angiogram
arrhythmias
artifacts
augmented
baseline
bipolar
calibration
cardiac catheterization
cardiac cycle
cardioversion
countershocks
defibrillation
defibrillator
deoxygenated
depolarization
diastole

electrocardiogram
electrocardiograph
electrocardiography
electrodes
electrolyte
galvanometer
Holter monitor
implantable cardioverter-
    defibrillator (ICD)
ischemia
isoelectric
lead wires
mounting
myocardial infarction
noninvasive
normal sinus rhythm
oscilloscope
percutaneous transluminal
    coronary angioplasty
    (PTCA)

precordial
radiopharmaceutical
repolarization
rhythm strip
sensors
sinus bradycardia
sinus tachycardia
sonographer
stylus
syncope
systole
test cable
thallium stress test
tracing
transducer
ultrasonography
unipolar

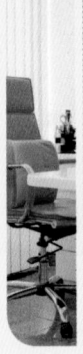

Chapter Portal

Many providers include an **electrocardiogram** (ECG or EKG) as part of a complete physical examination, especially for patients who are 40 years or older, for patients with a family history of cardiac disease, or for patients who have experienced chest pain. It is a noninvasive, safe, and painless procedure that can provide valuable information about the health of the patient's heart or suspected cardiac symptoms. A graphic representation of the heart's electrical activity, an ECG measures the amount of electrical activity produced by the heart and the time necessary for the electrical impulses to travel through the heart during each heartbeat.

Some reasons for **electrocardiography** are to (1) detect myocardial ischemia, (2) estimate damage to the myocardium caused by a myocardial infarction, (3) detect and evaluate cardiac arrhythmia, (4) assess effects of cardiac medication on the heart, and (5) determine if electrolyte imbalance is present. An ECG cannot always detect impending heart disorders or cardiovascular disease. The ECG is used in conjunction with other laboratory and diagnostic tests to assess total cardiac health. An ECG alone cannot diagnose disease. In a medical clinic or ambulatory care setting, it is often the medical assistant who records the ECG; therefore, special knowledge and skills are necessary and include these aspects of correct electrocardiography procedure: patient preparation, operation of the electrocardiograph, elimination of artifacts, mounting and labeling the ECG, and maintenance and care of the instrument.

ANATOMY OF THE HEART

The heart has four chambers: two upper chambers known as atria, and two lower chambers known as ventricles. **Deoxygenated** blood enters the right atrium from the superior and inferior vena cava and passes through the tricuspid valve into the right ventricle. In a healthy heart, the blood between right and left sides do not mix together. From the right ventricle, the blood then travels to the lungs via the pulmonary arteries. The deoxygenated blood releases carbon dioxide and picks up oxygen on the hemoglobin molecule in the capillary bed of the lungs. Oxygenated blood is pumped through the pulmonary vein into the left atrium, through the mitral valve, into the left ventricle. The oxygenated blood then passes through the aortic valve into the aorta and from the aorta to all cells, tissues, and organs of the body (Figure 36-1). The cycle begins again with each heartbeat.

On its external surface, the heart is surrounded by coronary arteries that supply the myocardium with its blood supply, from which oxygen and nutrients are obtained (see the section on the circulatory system in Chapter 29).

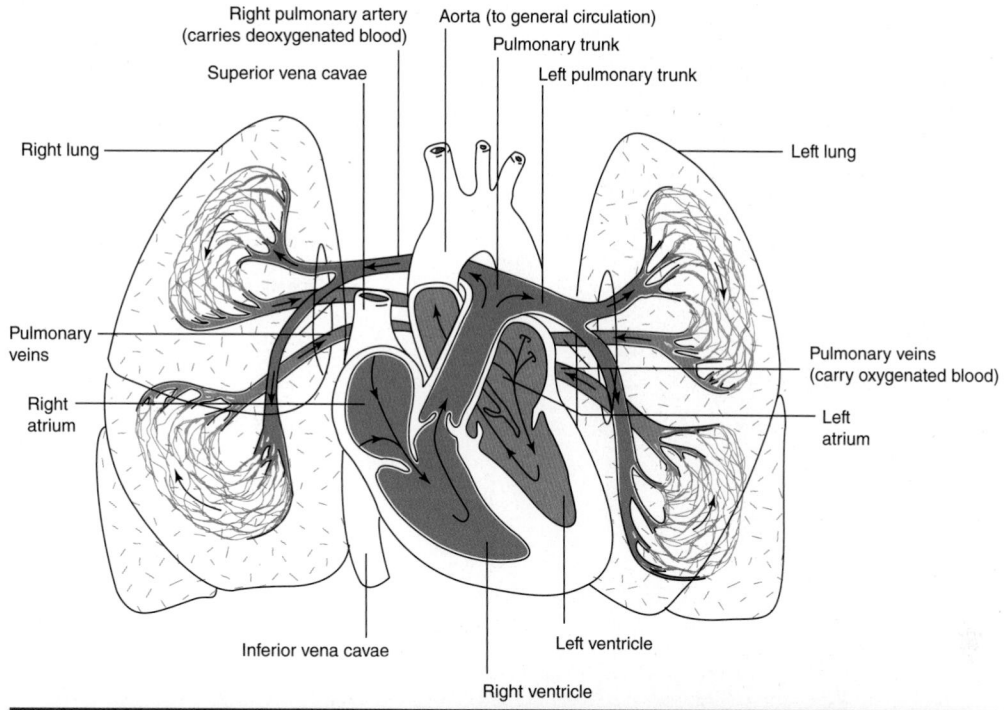

FIGURE 36-1 Flow of oxygenated and deoxygenated blood through the heart and lungs.

The labels in the figure:
Right pulmonary artery (carries deoxygenated blood)
Aorta (to general circulation)
Pulmonary trunk
Superior vena cavae
Left pulmonary trunk
Right lung
Left lung
Pulmonary veins
Pulmonary veins (carry oxygenated blood)
Right atrium
Left atrium
Inferior vena cavae
Left ventricle
Right ventricle

ELECTRICAL CONDUCTION SYSTEM OF THE HEART

There are basically two kinds of cardiac cells: electrical cardiac cells and myocardial cells. The electrical cells, which are located in distinct pathways around and through the heart, are sensitive to electrical impulses. Their pathways are referred to as the conduction system of the heart and have specific names.

The body's natural pacemaker, the sinoatrial (SA) node, is located in the upper part of the right atrium. The SA node is a bundle of specialized cardiac muscle cells that are self-excitatory or pacemaker cells. A healthy SA node "fires" at an intrinsic rate of 60 to 100 times a minute. It sends out an electrical impulse that begins and regulates the heartbeat. When the electrical impulses are sent along the pathways or conduction system of the heart (via the electrical cells), the myocardial cells contract, causing the heart muscle to pump the blood from chamber to chamber and through the lungs. The contraction of the cardiac cells is called **depolarization** (from the electrical discharge). The first chambers that contract under the influence of the electrical discharge from the SA node are the atria. From

the atria, the electrical impulses travel along the conduction system toward the ventricles, to the atrioventricular (AV) node, located at the base of the right atrium. The AV node responds to signals from the SA node. However, if there is suppression of the SA node, the AV node can fire intrinsically at a rate of 40 to 60 times per minute. With normal electrical conduction, the AV node picks up the signal sent by the SA node, regulates it, and sends the electrical impulse to the base of the heart via the bundle of His. This bundle of cardiac fibers travels down the septum between the ventricles and then divides into right and left bundle branches that conduct the electrical impulses on to the Purkinje fibers. These fibers disperse the electrical impulses to the right and left ventricles, causing them to contract. If there is an interruption in the electrical signals from the SA or the AV node, the Purkinje fibers can fire at a very slow and less effective rate of 15 to 40 times per minute.

Once the electrical conduction system completes the normal circuit to elicit a heartbeat, the heart recovers electrically (**repolarization**), then relaxes briefly (polarization). Then, a new impulse is begun by the SA node and the cycle begins again (Figure 36-2). This cycle is known as the **cardiac**

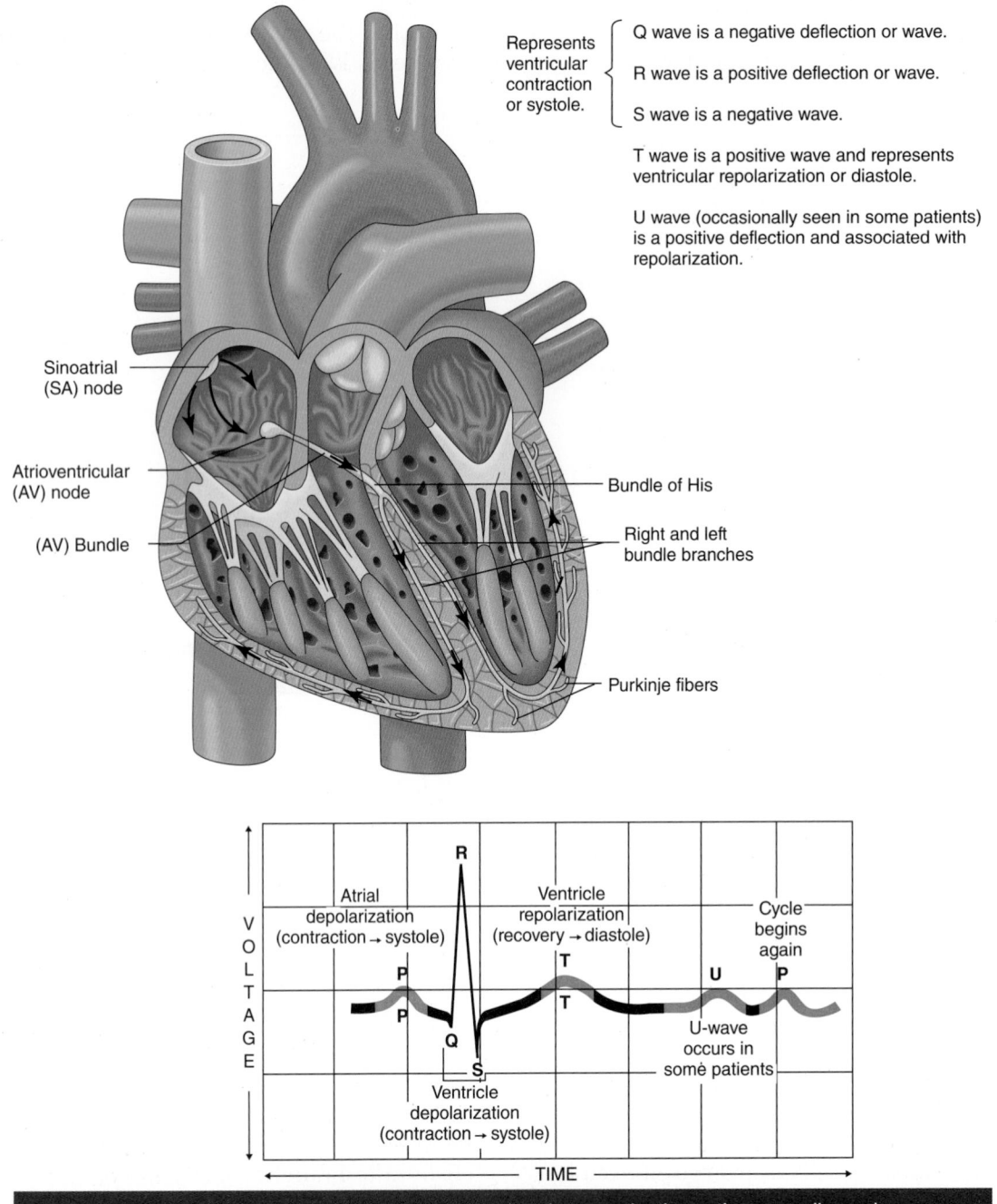

Q wave is a negative deflection or wave.

R wave is a positive deflection or wave.

S wave is a negative wave.

T wave is a positive wave and represents ventricular repolarization or diastole.

U wave (occasionally seen in some patients) is a positive deflection and associated with repolarization.

Represents ventricular contraction or systole.

Sinoatrial (SA) node

Atrioventricular (AV) node

(AV) Bundle

Bundle of His

Right and left bundle branches

Purkinje fibers

VOLTAGE

Atrial depolarization (contraction → systole)

Ventricle repolarization (recovery → diastole)

Cycle begins again

R

P

P

Q

S

Ventricle depolarization (contraction → systole)

T

T

U

P

U-wave occurs in some patients

TIME

FIGURE 36-2 The heartbeat is controlled by electrical impulses that comprise the continuous cardiac cycle.

cycle and it represents one heartbeat. The electrocardiograph records the electrical activity that causes the contraction (**systole**) and the relaxation (**diastole**) of the atria and ventricles. The ECG cycle is the recording and the graphic representation of the cardiac cycle. These electrical impulses can be recorded on special ECG paper or displayed on an **oscilloscope**.

THE CARDIAC CYCLE AND THE ECG CYCLE

The **baseline**, or **isoelectric**, line is the flat line that separates the various waves. It is present when there is no current flowing in the heart. The waves are either deflecting upward from the baseline, known as positive deflection, or deflecting downward from the baseline, known as negative deflection.

The P, QRS, and T waves, recorded during the ECG, represent the depolarization (contraction) and repolarization (recovery) of the myocardial cells. They are recorded on specialized graph paper. The electrocardiograph machine detects and amplifies the electrical impulses that occur as each heartbeat is conducted through the tissues and sends these data via the electrodes, the cables, and onto a computer-generated graph. This graph may contain a one-channel or single-lead recording or up to a 12-lead recording. The P wave is initiated when the SA node fires and represents atrial depolarization. It is recorded as a positive deflection. The QRS complex is initiated when the AV node fires and represents ventricular depolarization. It is measured from the end of the PR interval to the end of the S wave (see Figure 36-2). The T wave represents ventricular repolarization and is a positive deflection. The recovery of the atria is so slight that it is lost behind the QRS complex.

Each complete cardiac cycle takes about 0.8 second in a healthy heart. By observing and measuring the size, shape, and location of each wave on an ECG recording, the provider can analyze and interpret the conduction of electricity through the cardiac cells, the heart's rhythm and rate, and the health of the heart in general.

Calculation of Heart Rate on ECG Graph Paper

ECG graph paper is divided into 1-mm squares (small squares) and 5-mm squares (large squares). Each large square consists of 25 small squares and is 5 mm high and 5 mm wide. On the horizontal line, one small square represents 0.04 second. On the vertical line, one small square represents 1 mm of voltage. Because a large square is five small squares wide and five deep, each small square represents 0.2 second horizontal and 5 mm vertical. *NOTE:* Every fifth line, both horizontally and vertically, is darker than the other lines, making squares that are 5-by-5 mm (Figure 36-3). These measurements are accepted worldwide and enable

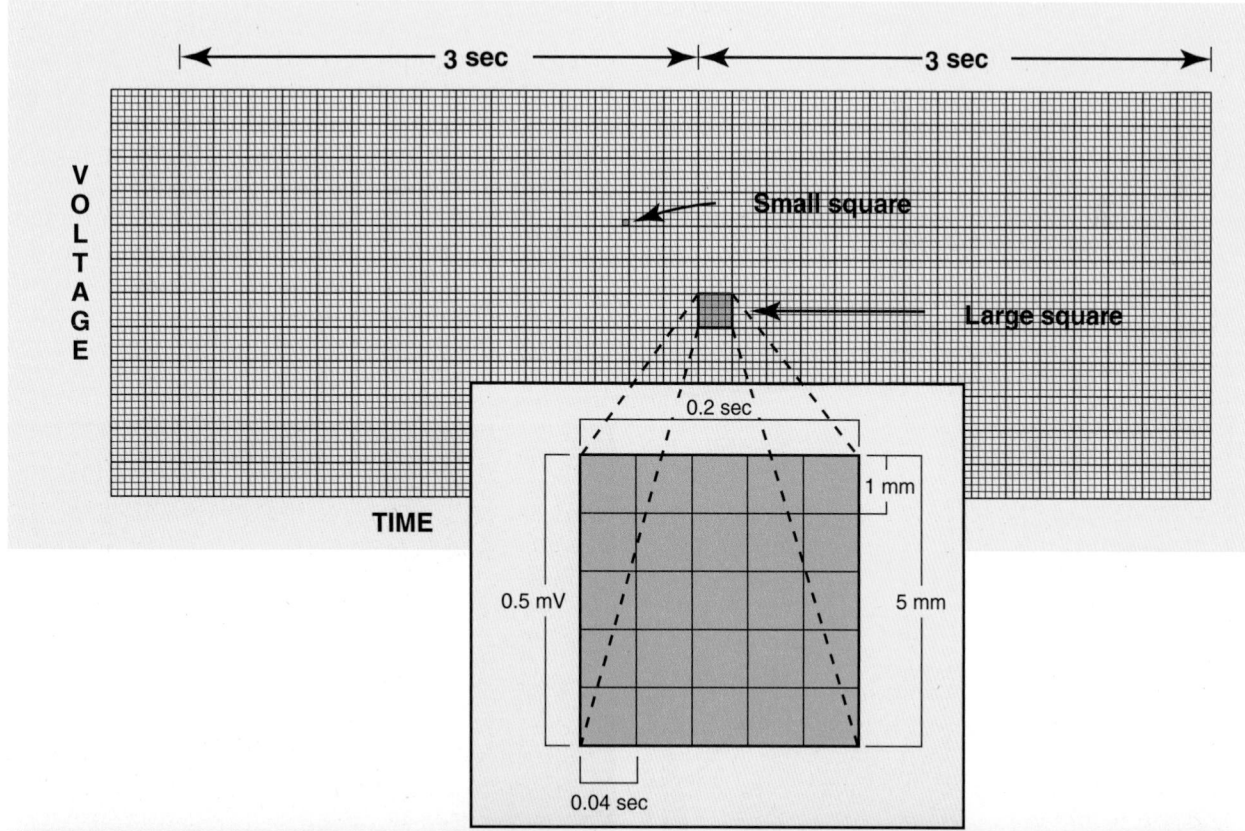

FIGURE 36-3 Electrocardiogram graph paper measurements allow medical professionals to determine the time and voltage of heartbeats. (A) The small square is 1 mm wide and 1 mm high. One small square = 0.04 second. (B) The large square consists of 25 small squares and measures 5 mm wide and 5 mm high. One large square = 0.04 second × 5, or 0.2 second.

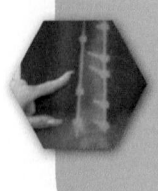

Critical Thinking

Explain the significance of the small and large boxes on ECG paper. For a particular patient, if there are 2.5 large boxes between each cardiac cycle, what is the heart rate in beats per minute?

the provider to interpret the time of each deflection on the horizontal line and cardiac electrical activity (voltage) on the vertical line to help determine cardiac health.

Because all cardiac complexes consist of P, QRS, and T waves, and the electrocardiograph paper measures time on the horizontal line, it is possible to calculate heart rate. Count the number of 5-mm boxes (number within the dark lines) between two R waves. Divide this number by 300. The result is the heart rate in beats per minute.

Example:

One small square (1 mm) = 0.04 second in time

One large square (5 mm) = 0.04 × 5 = 0.2 second

Divide 60 seconds (1 minute) by 0.2 second: 60 ÷ 0.2 = 300

Example:

There are three large squares between two R waves.

300 ÷ 3 = 100

The heart rate is 100 beats per minute.

TYPES OF ELECTROCARDIOGRAPHS

Single-Channel Electrocardiograph

A conventional 12-lead single-channel **electrocardiograph** can be used in either manual mode or automatic mode. When using automatic mode, the 12-lead ECG **tracing** is complete in less than 40 seconds. With a single-channel machine, only one lead can be recorded at a time. If not automatic, the single-channel ECG requires manually turning the lead selector on and off between each of the 12 leads. It may also require the leads to be coded so that they can be identified later and properly mounted. Lead coding and mounting are explained more fully later in this chapter. The ECG tracing from a single-channel machine will need to be cut and mounted onto special forms for filing into the patient record. Figure 36-4 shows a sample of a single-channel electrocardiograph machine and tracing.

Multichannel Electrocardiograph

An electrocardiograph that can simultaneously record several different leads is known as a multichannel electrocardiograph. The conventional electrocardiograph records one lead at a time. A three-channel machine, one type of multichannel electrocardiograph, records three channels at one time. It records leads I, II, and III; followed by aVR, aVL, and aVF; followed by V_1, V_2, and V_3; followed by V_4, V_5, and V_6. The advantage of the multichannel machine is its speed. The most common multichannel machine used in the provider's clinic is the three-channel machine. This type of machine requires three-channel recording paper that is

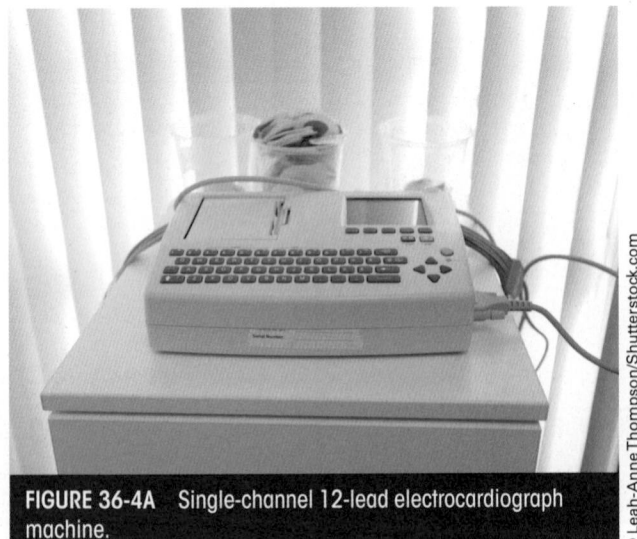

FIGURE 36-4A Single-channel 12-lead electrocardiograph machine.

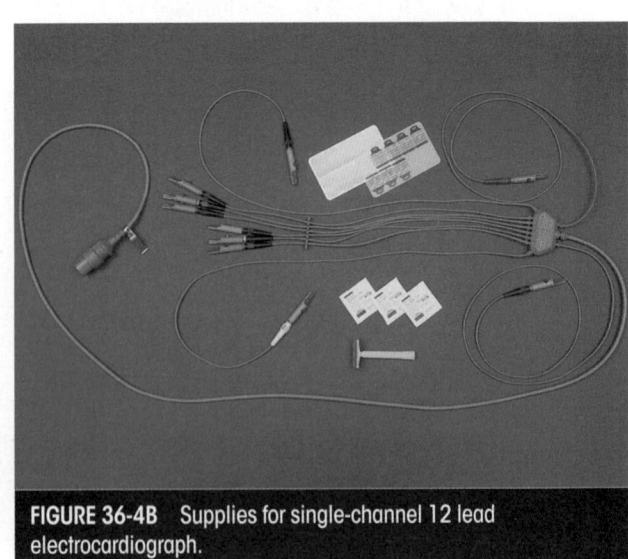

© Leah-Anne Thompson/Shutterstock.com

FIGURE 36-4B Supplies for single-channel 12 lead electrocardiograph.

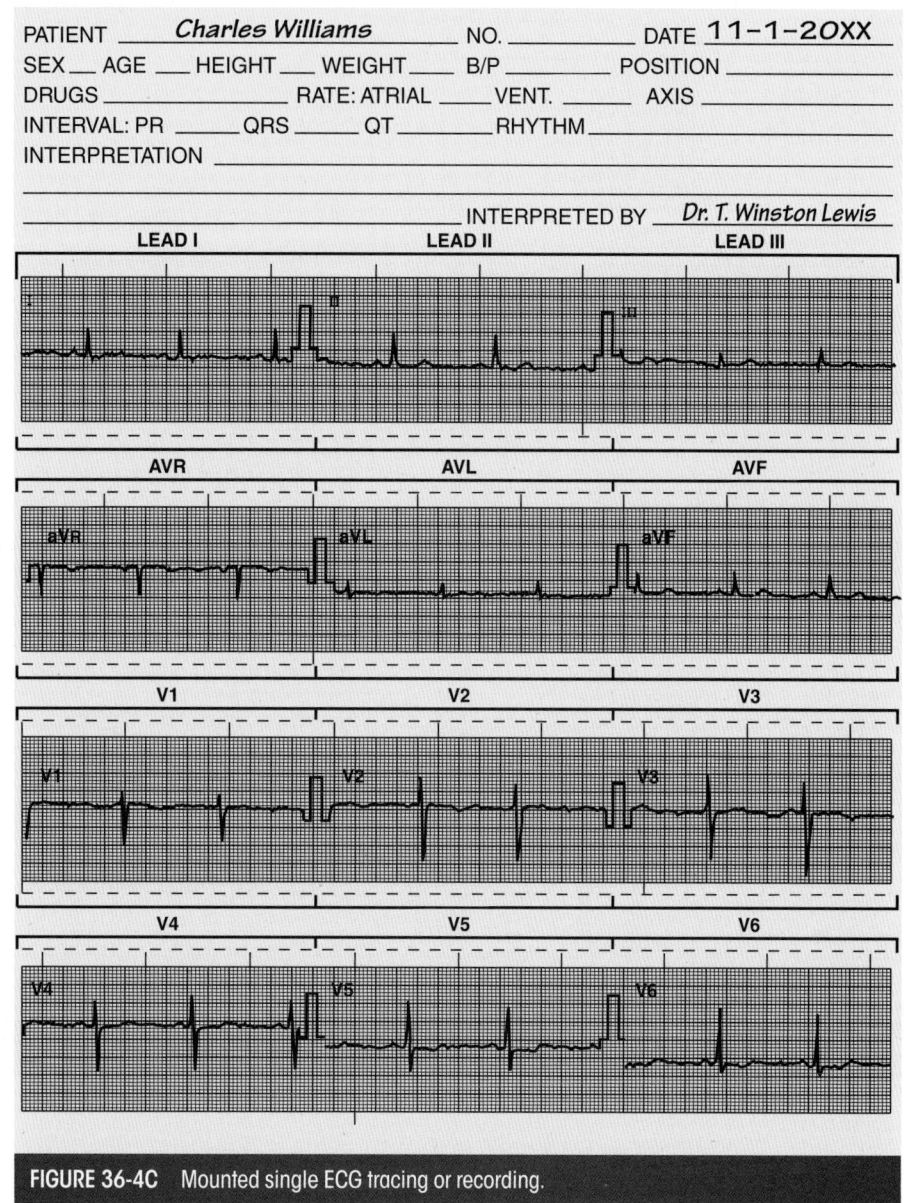

PATIENT _Charles Williams_ NO. _____ DATE 11–1–20XX
SEX ___ AGE ___ HEIGHT ___ WEIGHT ___ B/P _____ POSITION _____
DRUGS _____ RATE: ATRIAL ___ VENT. ___ AXIS _____
INTERVAL: PR ___ QRS ___ QT ___ RHYTHM _____
INTERPRETATION _____

_____ INTERPRETED BY _Dr. T. Winston Lewis_

LEAD I   LEAD II   LEAD III

AVR   AVL   AVF

V1   V2   V3

V4   V5   V6

FIGURE 36-4C Mounted single ECG tracing or recording.

8½-by-11 inches and fits into the patient record with no cutting or mounting. Figure 36-5 shows an example of a multichannel tracing. Other multichannel electrocardiograph machines are available, such as 6- and 12-channel machines. Some have a built-in rechargeable battery, an interpretation software program, a spirometery module, and transmission capability.

Automatic Electrocardiograph Machines

When using an automatic electrocardiograph, the lead length and switching of leads are done automatically by the electrocardiograph and there is no need to advance the control knob. For these reasons, both time and paper can be saved with the automatic machine. The automatic machine also comes equipped with a manual control that can be used if a longer tracing is necessary.

Electrocardiograph Telephone Transmissions

An electrocardiogram can be transmitted via a telephone line to an ECG interpretation site when using an electrocardiograph with such capabilities. A recording printout and interpretation (many times interpretation is done by a cardiologist or by a computer) are transmitted automatically on the electrocardiograph. Results of the ECG can be transmitted verbally as well.

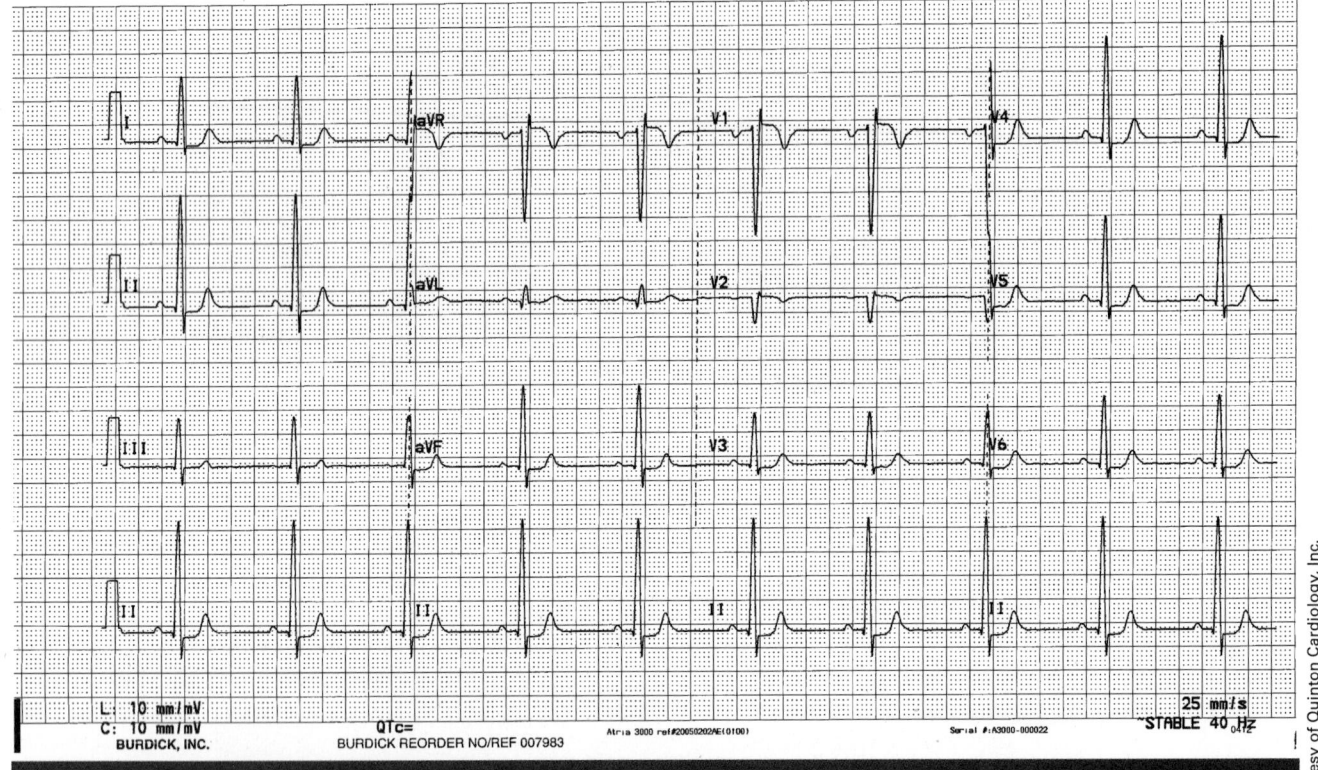

FIGURE 36-5 Example of three-channel electrocardiogram recording in which three leads are recorded simultaneously.

Facsimile Electrocardiograph

The provider may need a rapid, expert ECG interpretation from an off-site diagnostician. Direct ECG fax transmits from the electrocardiograph to a fax machine, and a high-quality facsimile is produced and sent to a diagnostician, who calls back with a reading. This saves time by eliminating the step of copying the report and sending it via a traditional fax machine.

Electrocardiograph via Smart Phone Application

As the availability of smart phone technology has become a part of everyday life, the frontier of health care applications is rapidly evolving. There are currently a number of apps that can be used to take a snapshot of various aspects of one's health

and transmit that information to the health care provider. One such app is Kardia by AlivCor. It is FDA approved and can capture a 30-second medical-grade ECG using either a smart phone or Apple watch. There is a required purchase of a sensor that communicates with the app. It is predicted that in the next 5 years this type of remote access to clinical consultations and uploads to a patient's electronic medical record will be the area of highest market potential.

Interpretive Electrocardiograph

The interpretive electrocardiograph has a built-in computer program that interprets the ECG tracing while it is being recorded, allowing for faster diagnosis and treatment. The provider in charge will review the tracing before a diagnosis is confirmed and treatment is begun.

ECG EQUIPMENT

Electrocardiograph Paper

ECG paper can be either black or dark blue and is wax- or plastic-coated with a white or pink background and colored lines. Older ECG systems that utilize a heated stylus need paper that is heat and pressure sensitive. The heat of the stylus can be adjusted to obtain a sharp, clear recording, or tracing. Newer models use a laser printer on ECG-specific computer paper. Medical assistants should learn how to adjust the proper control using the specific manual or instructions that accompany the electrocardiograph in their facility.

Electrolyte

Because the skin is a poor conductor of electricity, there are various types of conductive **electrolyte** substances applied with each electrode to pick up the electrical current. The impulses are transmitted to the electrocardiograph by metal tips on the patient lead wires or cables that are attached to the sensors. Because electrolyte substances must contain moisture to properly conduct impulses, they are manufactured in the forms of gels, lotions, pastes, presaturated pads or, more commonly, are contained within adhesive sensors. For our purposes in this text, we refer to the disposable self-adhesive sensors/electrodes.

Sensors or Electrodes

There are various types of **sensors** or **electrodes** made of metal or other conductive material. The sensors detect the electrical impulses on the body surface and relay them through cables, or lead wires, to the ECG machine.

Disposable Electrodes. Disposable sensors (electrodes) contain a layer of electrolyte gel on their adhesive surface and can be used on both the limbs and chest. They do not require additional electrolytes. These sensors are applied to the skin of the limbs and chest and held in place by the adhesive. The self-adhesive electrodes are discarded after use. They should be kept in an airtight bag because otherwise they dry out and then will not stick well or conduct the needed impulses for an accurate tracing. Skin preparation is essential for an accurate tracing. In order to provide the most conductive surface, it is recommended that the hair be cut or shaved from the area of electrode application. Then the dry, dead layer of the epidermis must be removed using soap and water, an alcohol prep pad, or a 4-by-4 gauze pad. Vigorously dry the skin to improve capillary circulation. Some providers encourage the use of an ECG prep pad that is similar to fine sand paper for the final step in preparation.

Lead Wires

Once the self-adhesive sensors are placed, a series of leads will connect the patient to the electrocardiograph. These leads will either snap onto the electrode pads (Figure 36-6A) or small clips, sometimes referred to as alligator clips, will grasp the tabs on a specific type of sensor (Figure 36-6B). This completes the circuit from the patient to the electrocardiograph.

Electrocardiograph Machine

Because the electrical activity that comes from the body is small, it is made larger, or **amplified**, by the

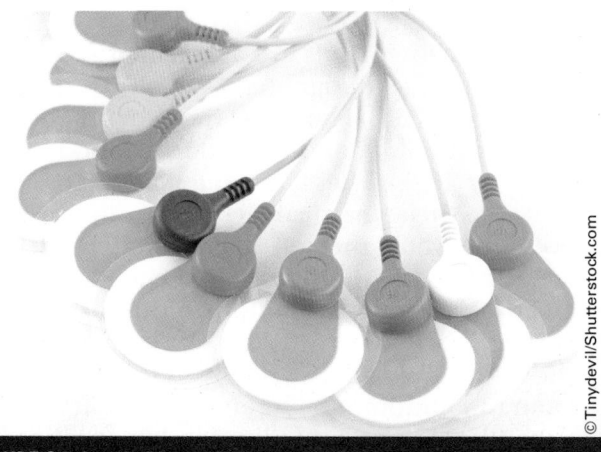
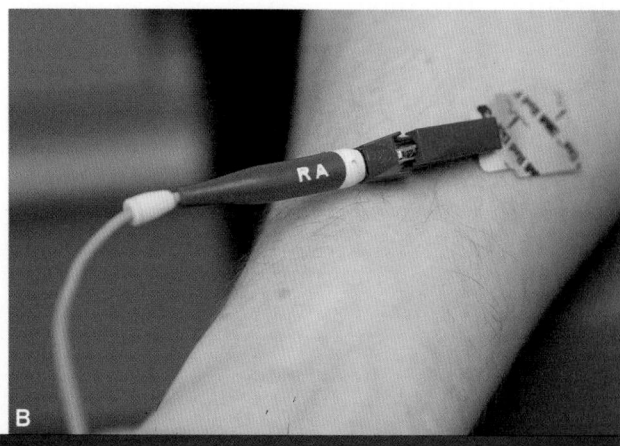

© Tinydevil/Shutterstock.com

FIGURE 36-6 (A) Disposable sensor with snap connections. (B) Alligator clip and disposable sensor.

amplifier of the electrocardiograph machine. The voltage is changed into a mechanical motion by the **galvanometer** and recorded on the paper by the heated stylus.

Care of Equipment

Once the ECG tracing is complete, remove the lead wires from the sensors, then remove the sensors from the patient. Dispose of the sensors. Check supplies on the machine so it is ready for the next use. Neatly and loosely place the lead wires on top of or beside the machine. Change the ECG paper when necessary according to the manufacturer's suggestions.

THE ELECTROCARDIOGRAPH AND SENSOR PLACEMENT

The standard ECG consists of 10 sensors that record 12 leads of the heart's electrical activity from different angles, allowing for a thorough three-dimensional interpretation of its activity. The electrical impulses given off by the heart are picked up by the electrodes and conducted into the machine through **lead wires**.

The electrodes are placed on the patient's four limbs and chest. The four limb leads are right arm (RA), left arm (LA), right leg (RL), and left leg (LL). The right leg electrode is not used as part of the recording. It is an electrical reference point only. The limb leads are placed on the fleshy, nonmuscular area of upper arms and lower legs. The chest leads are known as precordial leads, V leads, or C leads, and use an electrode for each of six areas on the chest wall or one electrode that is moved to six different positions on the chest wall. (This depends on the type of electrocardiograph being used.)

Older electrocardiographs may have plain lead wire tips for use with the older metal plates and suction cups. They can easily and inexpensively be converted to use the current self-adhesive sensor electrodes. The only conversion equipment necessary is a set of alligator clips that will fit over the end of the lead wire tips. Contact the manufacturer or a medical supplier for conversion sets.

Standard Limb or Bipolar Leads

The first three leads that are recorded on a standard ECG are called leads I, II, and III (Figure 36-7A). These are known as **bipolar** leads because each uses two limb electrodes that record simultaneously. Lead I records electrical activity between the right arm (RA) and left arm (LA), lead II records electrical activity between the right arm (RA) and left leg (LL), and lead III records activity between the left arm (LA) and left leg (LL). Lead II is used as a **rhythm strip** because it portrays the heart's rhythm better than the other leads. The rhythm strip is usually a separate longer recording of approximately 6 to 12 inches.

Augmented Leads

The next three leads are **augmented** (added to) leads and are designated aVR, aVL, and aVF (Figure 36-7B). The aV stands for augmented voltage; the R, L, and F stand for right, left, and foot (or leg). These are **unipolar** leads. Lead aVR records electrical activity from the midpoint between the left arm added to the left leg, directed to the right arm. Lead aVL records electrical activity from the midpoint between the right arm added to the left leg, directed to the left arm. Lead aVF records electrical activity from the midpoint between the right arm added to the left arm, directed to the left leg. Because these three leads produce such small electrical impulses, the electrocardiograph machine augments, or increases, their size to record them. Figure 36-7B will help you visualize the augmented process.

Chest Leads or Precordial Leads

The remaining six leads of the standard 12-lead ECG are the chest leads or **precordial** leads (Figure 36-7C). These are unipolar leads and are

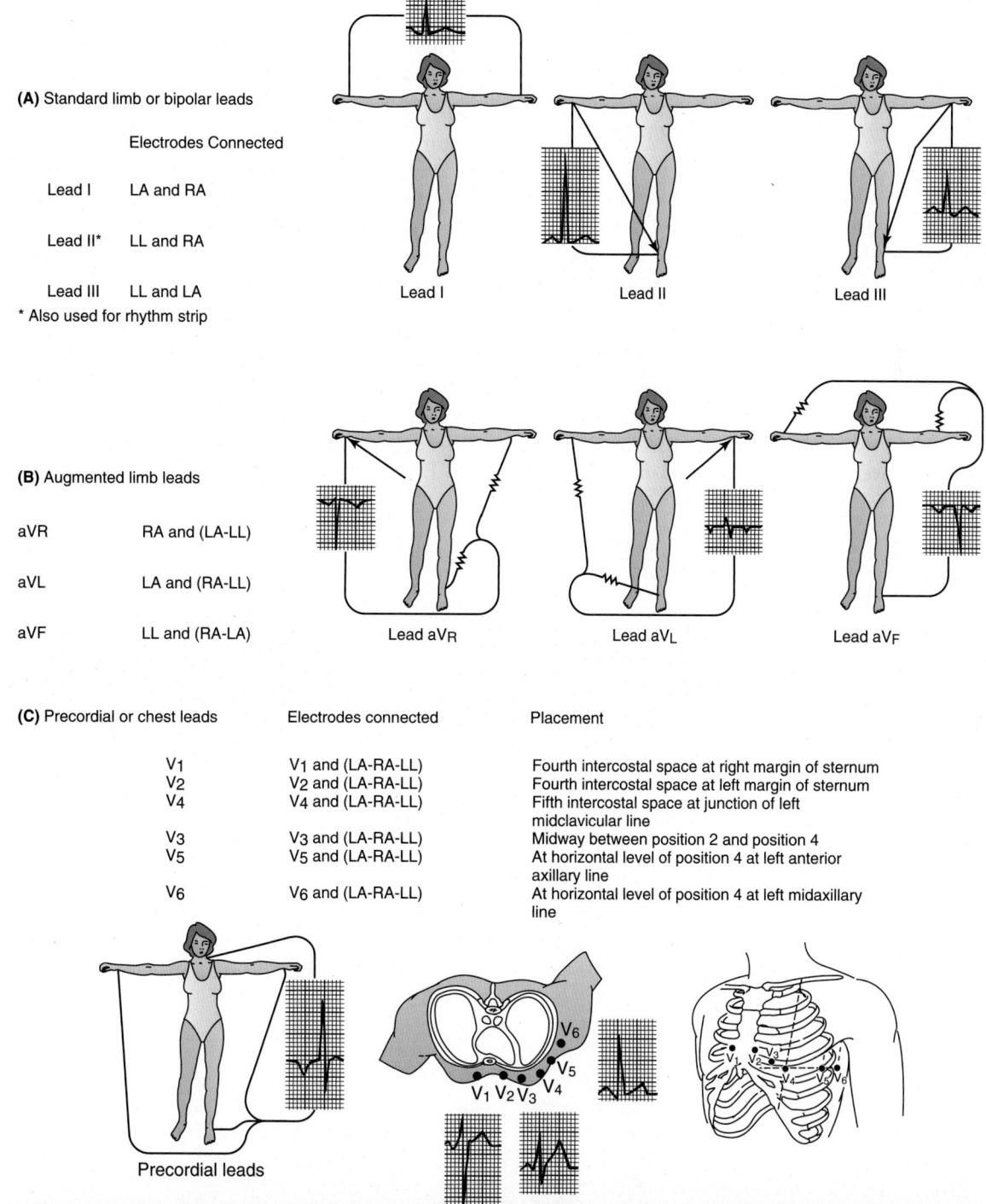

(A) Standard limb or bipolar leads

Electrodes Connected

Lead I   LA and RA

Lead II*   LL and RA

Lead III   LL and LA

* Also used for rhythm strip

Lead I   Lead II   Lead III

(B) Augmented limb leads

aVR   RA and (LA-LL)

aVL   LA and (RA-LL)

aVF   LL and (RA-LA)

Lead aV$_R$ Lead aV$_L$ Lead aV$_F$

(C) Precordial or chest leads

	Electrodes connected	Placement
V$_1$	V$_1$ and (LA-RA-LL)	Fourth intercostal space at right margin of sternum
V$_2$	V$_2$ and (LA-RA-LL)	Fourth intercostal space at left margin of sternum
V$_4$	V$_4$ and (LA-RA-LL)	Fifth intercostal space at junction of left midclavicular line
V$_3$	V$_3$ and (LA-RA-LL)	Midway between position 2 and position 4
V$_5$	V$_5$ and (LA-RA-LL)	At horizontal level of position 4 at left anterior axillary line
V$_6$	V$_6$ and (LA-RA-LL)	At horizontal level of position 4 at left midaxillary line

Precordial leads

FIGURE 36-7   Lead types, connections, and placement. (A) Standard limb or bipolar leads. (B) Augmented limb leads. (C) Precordial or chest leads.

designated V_1, V_2, V_3, V_4, V_5, and V_6. These leads record the heart's electrical impulse from a central point within the heart to one of six predesignated positions on the chest wall where an electrode is attached. The correct position *must* be used for each lead recording.

The anatomic positions for placement of the chest or precordial leads are:

V_1: fourth intercostal space at right margin of sternum

V_2: fourth intercostal space at left margin of sternum

V_4: fifth intercostal space on left midclavicular line

V_3: midway between V_2 and V_4 (*NOTE:* This is correct order, V_3 after V_4)

V_5: horizontal to V_4 at left anterior axillary line

V_6: horizontal to V_4 at left midaxillary line

When using an electrocardiograph with one chest wire, the chest electrode must be moved manually one by one to each of the six chest lead positions. This necessitates stopping the instrument between each chest lead to move the electrode to the next appropriate position on the chest wall. Some electrocardiographs have six lead wires, allowing all six chest leads to be applied at one time; therefore, there is no interruption between chest lead recordings (see Figure 36-10C in Procedure 36-1).

STANDARDIZATION AND ADJUSTMENT OF THE ELECTROCARDIOGRAPH

The value of an ECG recording depends on it being performed accurately. To ensure a precise and reliable recording, you must standardize the ECG instrument before every ECG performed. The standardization of the machine is a quality-assurance check to determine if the machine is set and working properly. Standardization measurements have been adopted internationally as a means of accurate **calibration** according to universal measurements. The universal standard is that 1 mV (millivolt) of cardiac electrical activity will deflect the stylus exactly 10 mm high. This is the equivalent of 10 small squares on the ECG paper. Figure 36-8 shows an example

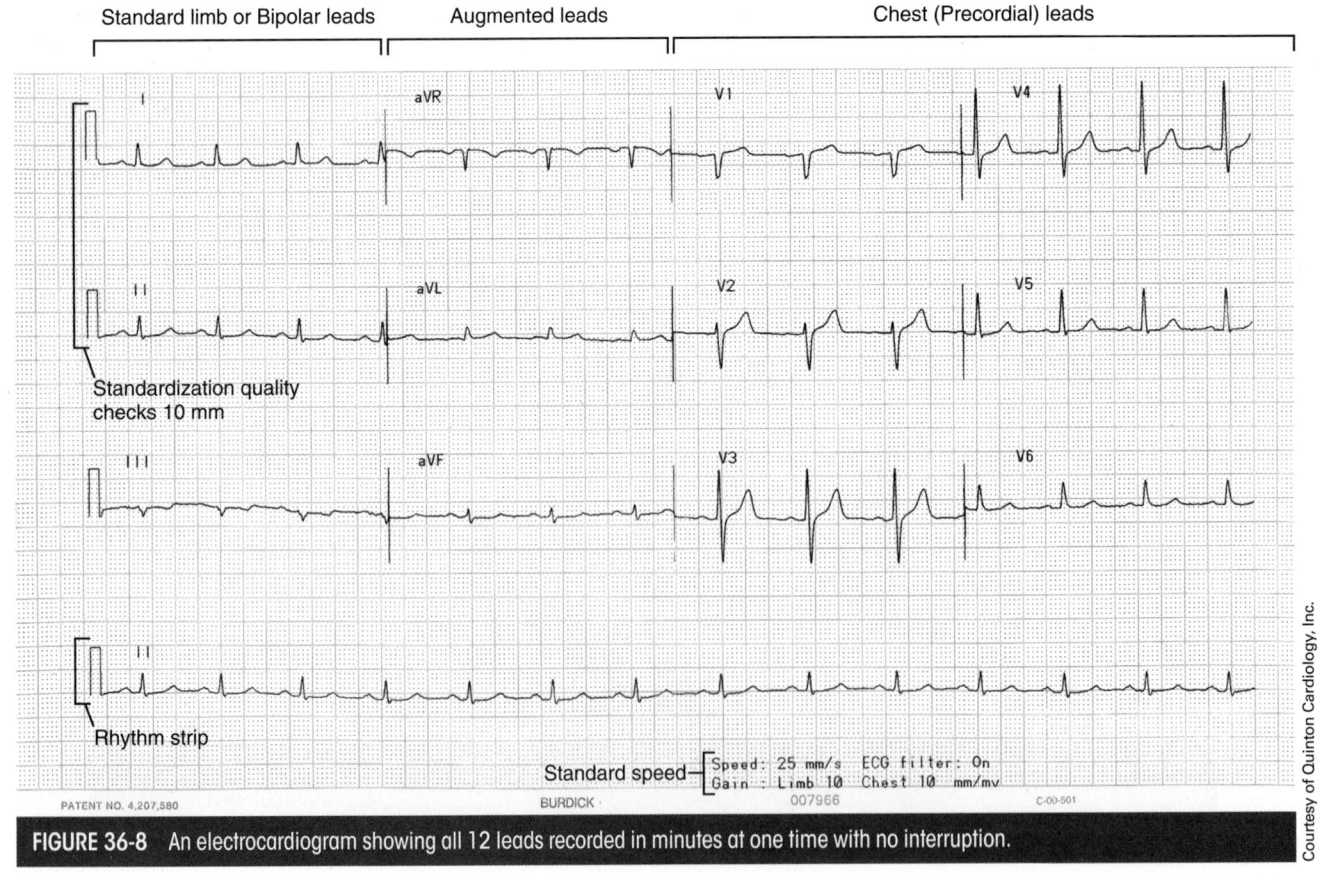

FIGURE 36-8 An electrocardiogram showing all 12 leads recorded in minutes at one time with no interruption.

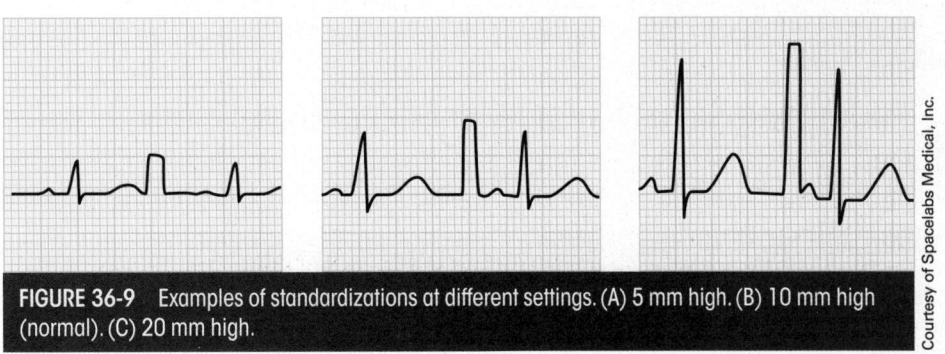

FIGURE 36-9 Examples of standardizations at different settings. (A) 5 mm high. (B) 10 mm high (normal). (C) 20 mm high.

Courtesy of Spacelabs Medical, Inc.

of the 10-mm standardization at the beginning of each row.

On occasion, a patient's R waves may be too large to be appropriately captured at standard sensitivity. In such instances, the medical assistant can record at one-half sensitivity the lead(s) in which the R wave is large. This action will record all ECG cycles at half their normal **amplitude**. See Figure 36-9 for examples of standardizations at different settings.

Safety

Conversely, the waves of the ECG cycles may be small, making it difficult to interpret. In this circumstance, the medical assistant can record the ECG cycles at twice the normal standard. This action will record ECG cycles at twice their normal amplitude. Whenever a change is made from a normal standardization (10 mm high) to either a one-half standardization (5 mm high) or a double standardization (20 mm high), the medical assistant must include the adjusted standardization mark with that particular lead to alert the provider to the change in standard. The standard must be returned to normal to prevent accidentally running the next lead at a standard other than normal. The paper is usually run at a speed of 25 mm/second. If cycles are too close together, the paper speed can be adjusted to 50 mm/second. Make a note on the ECG paper if paper speed or amplitude is changed.

STANDARD RESTING ELECTROCARDIOGRAPHY

Competency Procedure

Regardless of the type of electrocardiograph used, the basic components of the standard electrocardiography procedure remain the same. Patient preparation, placement

of limb and chest leads, attachment of lead wires, and elimination of artifacts vary little from one electrocardiograph to another. Procedure 36-1 explains a 12-lead ECG using a multiple-lead channel electrocardiograph. Before performing the procedure, medical assistants must be familiar with the electrocardiograph machine in their facility and should thoroughly review the manufacturer's instruction manual that accompanies the machine. Knowledge of the basic procedures included here can be adapted for all other electrocardiographs.

MOUNTING THE ECG TRACING

Commercially prepared **mounting** forms are available, and the medical assistant should mount the completed tracing after the provider has reviewed the entire recording. The mounting of the ECG recording depends on the machine. Some machines produce a strip already printed on a durable 8 ½ by 11 inch paper record. Some machines produce a long strip that will need to be cut apart and adhered to a mounting paper or card. There are many options within these two varieties. Included with any ECG recording should be the patient's name, date, address, age, sex, blood pressure, height and weight, and cardiac medications on the mounting form.

INTERFERENCE OR ARTIFACTS

The ECG is a valuable diagnostic aid to the provider and must be performed accurately. The medical assistant is responsible for obtaining a recording that can be easily read and interpreted by the provider.

There can be unusual and unwanted activity in the tracing not caused by the electrical activity of the heart. These defects in the ECG tracing are known as **artifacts**, and their appearance

Procedure

Performing Single-Channel or Multichannel Electrocardiogram

STANDARD PRECAUTIONS:

Handwashing

PURPOSE:

To obtain an accurate, graphic, artifact-free reading of the electrical activity of the patient's heart.

EQUIPMENT/SUPPLIES:

- Examination or ECG table with pillow and sheet or blanket
- Patient gown (open in front)
- Automated electrocardiograph with patient cable wires (Figure 36-10A)
- Alcohol wipes
- Disposable electrodes
- ECG paper
- 2-by-2 gauze squares
- Razor

PROCEDURE STEPS:

1. To begin the procedure, gather any needed equipment and wash your hands.

2. Introduce yourself and confirm the identity of the patient, using two types of identifiers. *Speaking at the patient's level of understanding, explain the rationale for performance of the procedure.*

3. Explain to the patient that the procedure will be painless and that the patient should remain quiet and still for the best quality tracing. RATIONALE: Patient cooperation ensures good quality tracing.

4. Provide a gown and ask the patient to remove any clothing from the waist up and to uncover the lower portion of the legs. While socks may be kept on during the procedure, nylon stockings may not. RATIONALE: Electropads must be placed on bare skin for optimum conductivity of electricity. All four limbs and chest must be uncovered for proper electrode placement.

5. Ask the patient to lay back on the exam table. If needed, you can make the patient comfortable with a sheet for warmth and modesty, or with pillows under the knees or head.

6. If the electrocardiograph is not battery powered, place the unit with the power cord facing away from the patient. Do not allow the cord to go under the table. RATIONALE: Helps reduce AC interference.

7. Adhesion can be improved by shaving the contact sites or by wiping them with alcohol to remove any natural oils. Allow the alcohol to dry thoroughly before applying the electrodes. RATIONALE: Skin oils can be removed by alcohol, thus improving the adherence of the sensor. By removing excess hair on the skin, the sensor will adhere better.

8. Apply the limb electrodes first on fleshy nonmuscular areas. Electrodes RA and LA should be placed between the shoulder and the elbow. RL and LL should be placed anywhere above the ankle and on the lower torso, at least 3 inches below the umbilical horizontal line. The hip area is often used. RATIONALE: Artifact can be reduced if sensors are placed on nonbony, nonmuscular areas of the limbs. Directing tabs properly reduces tension on the electrodes.

(continues)

9. Next, place the electrodes on the chest on the appropriate intercostal spaces, tabs facing downward. V1 should be placed on the fourth intercostal space to the right of the sternum. V2 should be placed at the fourth intercostal space to the left of the sternum. V3 is placed midway between V2 and V4. V4 is placed at the fifth intercostal space at the midclavicular line. V5 is placed at the anterior axillary line at the same level as V4. V6 is placed at the mid-axillary line at the same level as V4 and V5 (Figure 36-10B). RATIONALE: Following body contour prevents sensors from being pulled off.

10. Attach the appropriate cable from the ECG machine to each of the sensor tabs. Each lead will be color coded and labeled with an abbreviation to assist you in placing them on the appropriate electrode.

11. Supporting the patient cable on either the table or on the patient's abdomen, plug it into the electrocardiograph if it is not already connected. Turn the machine ON.

12. Enter the patient's information so it will appear on the patient's ECG printout. Remind the patient to stay quiet and still. Then press AUTO to signal to the machine to record and standardize the tracing. RATIONALE: The ECG machine automatically prints the information onto the ECG printout that has been entered.

13. A multichannel machine will print the tracing on a standard 8.5-by-11 inch sheet of paper (Figure 36-10C).

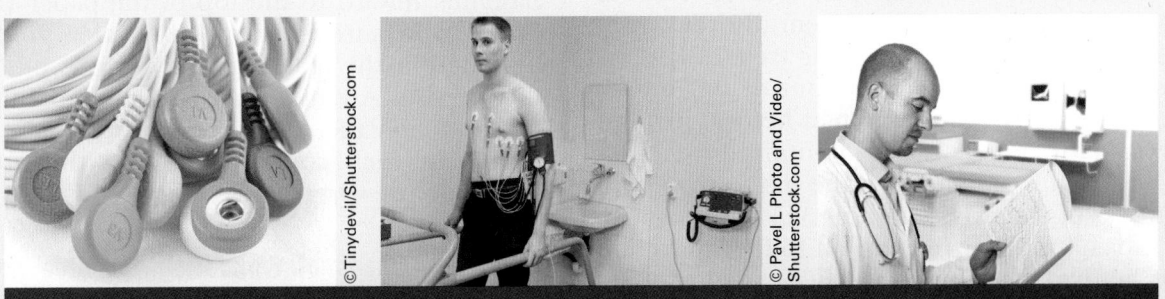

FIGURE 36-10   (A) Lead wires with nothing attached. (B) Lead wires attached to the patient's chest. (C) The machine prints each lead sequentially on a strip of ECG paper.

14. Check the quality of the tracing before disconnecting lead wires. Repeat the process if necessary after correcting the cause of the poor tracing. RATIONALE: Checking the tracing before removing the electrodes will save time if the ECG must be repeated.

15. If there are abnormal findings that put the patient at risk, consult the provider immediately.

16. Disconnect the lead cables and remove the electrodes from the patient.

17. Assist the patient to a sitting position. Verify that the patient's information is present and correct on the printout. Discard any used disposables and wash your hands. Direct the patient to dress.

18. Change the table paper and blanket. Wash your hands.

19. Document the procedure in the patient's medical record. Note the cause of a poor quality tracing, if applicable.

DOCUMENTATION:

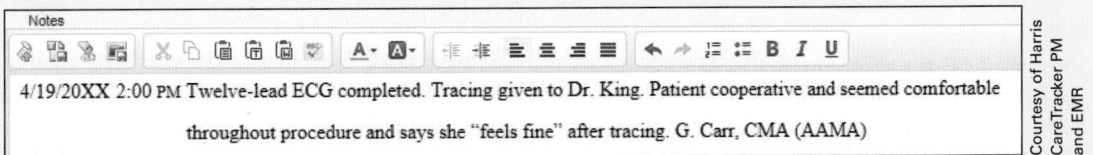

4/19/20XX 2:00 PM Twelve-lead ECG completed. Tracing given to Dr. King. Patient cooperative and seemed comfortable throughout procedure and says she "feels fine" after tracing. G. Carr, CMA (AAMA)

can make the ECG tracing difficult to read and interpret. Four of the more common artifacts are somatic tremor, alternating current (AC) interference, wandering baseline, and interrupted baseline. The medical assistant should understand the causes of each type of artifact and know how to eliminate them. The newer machines have filters, which will automatically filter out artifacts.

Somatic Tremor Artifacts

Somatic tremor artifact is also known as muscle tremor. It is characterized by unnatural baseline deflections such as jagged peaks or irregularity of spacing and height. The tracing appears fuzzy (Figure 36-11A). Somatic tremor occurs when the patient is apprehensive or uncomfortable, resulting in involuntary muscle movement. Voluntary muscle movement occurs when the patient moves, talks, coughs, and so on. Parkinson disease, a nervous system disorder, is an example of involuntary somatic tremor. It is not possible for the patient to control the muscle tremors. (Often, as mentioned before, involuntary somatic tremor can be minimized somewhat by having the patient slide the hands under the buttocks during the recording.)

It is natural for the patient to feel apprehensive before and during the ECG tracing. Reassurance and an explanation of the procedure will allay apprehension and relax muscles. Be certain the patient is comfortable. Use pillows for the head and under the knees; be sure the temperature of the room is comfortable. These simple techniques will help to minimize somatic tremor.

AC Interference

The AC interference artifact is caused by electrical interference and appears as a series of small regular peaks (Figure 36-11B). Electricity present in medical equipment or wires in the area can leak a small amount of energy into the room in which the ECG is being recorded. The current can be picked up by the patient's body and will be detected by the ECG tracing as an AC artifact.

Common Causes of AC Interference Artifacts. Some common causes of AC interferences are:

1. *Improper grounding of electrocardiograph.* The three-pronged plugs in the newer electrocardiographs should be inserted into a properly

grounded three-receptacle outlet. This reduces AC interference from improper grounding.
2. *Presence of other electrical equipment in the room.* Unplug other electrical equipment in the room (electrical examination tables, lamps, autoclaves, and so on).
3. *Electrical wiring in the floor, ceiling, or walls.* Move the ECG table away from walls.
4. *Crossed lead wires and lead wires not following body contour.* Straighten lead wires and be sure they are positioned to follow the patient's body contour.

Wandering Baseline Artifacts

A wandering baseline occurs when the isoelectric line changes position. This type of artifact appears as the complexes "wandering" across the ECG paper; for example, from the position of a normal baseline upward to the top of the paper (Figure 36-11C). Be sure to follow calibration guidelines provided by the manufacturer if this type of artifact persists. A wandering baseline makes it difficult to follow the complexes and to measure the timing of each component when the provider reads and interprets the tracing.

Common Causes of Wandering Baseline Artifacts. Wandering baseline artifacts can be caused by the following conditions:

1. *Electrodes applied too loosely or too tightly.* There should be equal tension on all four limb leads, metal tips should be firmly attached to the electrodes, and the cable attached to the patient should not have tension on it nor be dangling to cause pulling on the electrode.
2. *Corroded or dirty electrodes or metal tips of the lead wires.* Clean and rinse after each use.
3. *Inappropriate amount or poor-quality electrolyte gel or paste.* Each electrode should have the same amount of electrolyte gel or paste on it.
4. *Lotions, oils, or creams on the patient's skin that interfere with the adhesive sticking well.* Remove any of these substances before applying the electrode by cleansing the area with an alcohol wipe.

Wandering baseline artifacts are more often seen in older ECG machines that use metal electrodes and electrolyte. Newer machines use electrodes (sensors) that are disposable and self-adhesive, thereby eliminating several of the causes of wandering baseline artifacts.

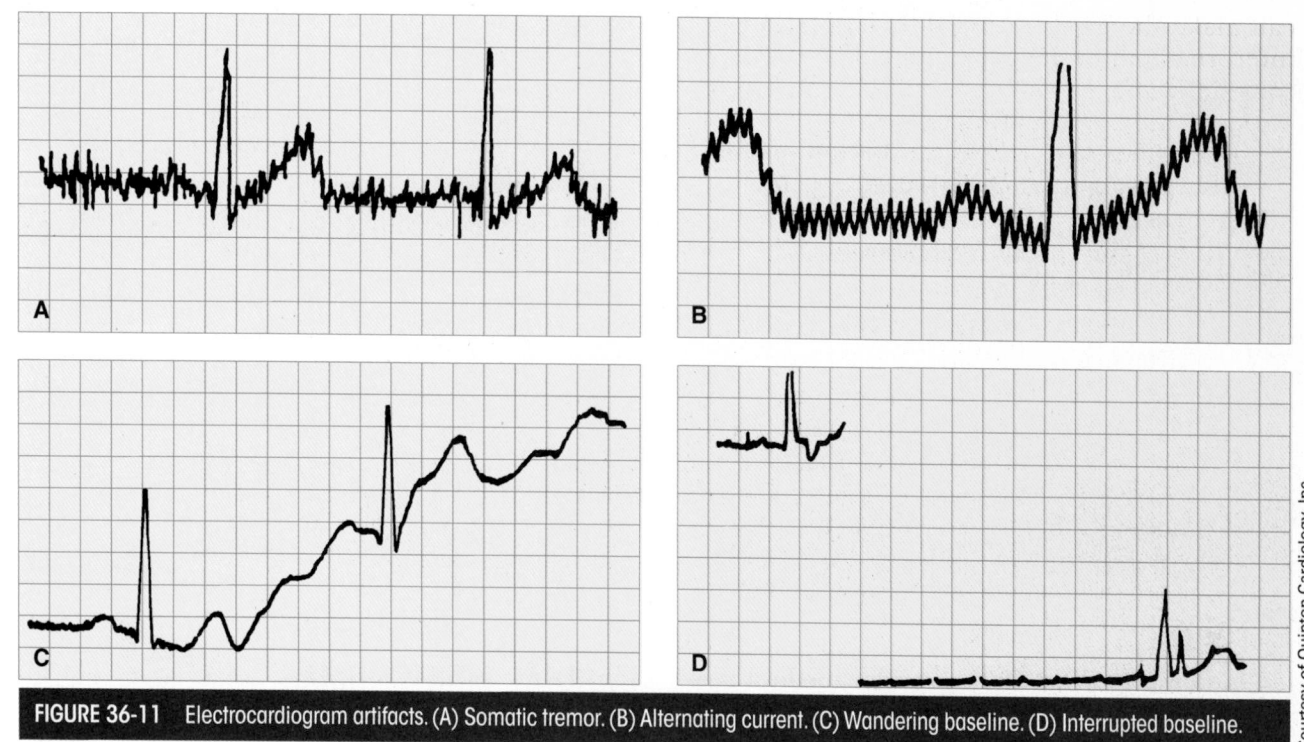

FIGURE 36-11 Electrocardiogram artifacts. (A) Somatic tremor. (B) Alternating current. (C) Wandering baseline. (D) Interrupted baseline.

Courtesy of Quinton Cardiology, Inc.

Interrupted Baseline Artifacts

On occasion, the baseline is interrupted and a break is seen between waves (Figure 36-11D). Possible causes are a broken cable, a lead wire that became detached from an electrode, or an electrode that came completely off.

Patients with Unique Problems

The medical assistant sometimes performs an ECG on a patient who has unique medical problems. With an obese patient, a woman with large breasts, or a patient with thick chest muscles, it is difficult to palpate the intercostal spaces. Place the chest leads on the chest as accurately as you can.

For a patient with a limb amputation or a cast, the medical assistant should apply the sensors as close to the preferred site as possible, higher on the limb. Place the sensor in a similar position on the other limb.

Do not place sensors on wounds, open areas, sutures, or staples. Try to situate the sensors as close as possible to the preferred site.

If the patient has dyspnea, the ECG can be taken with the patient in semi-Fowler's position (see Chapter 24 for descriptions of positions).

If you have difficulty performing an ECG on patients with certain medical problems or conditions, ask for assistance from your supervisor or clinic manager.

MYOCARDIAL INFARCTIONS (HEART ATTACKS)

Initiative

Coronary heart disease is the most common type of heart disease, killing nearly 380,000 people annually in the United States. **Myocardial infarctions** or, in lay terms, heart attacks, occur when the blood supply to the cardiac muscle is interrupted, causing tissue damage that interferes with the heart's ability to function. Heart disease historically has been considered to affect mostly men. However, these numbers are changing. Heart disease is now the primary cause of death in women. It is more deadly than all forms of cancer combined.

While 1 in 31 American women dies from breast cancer each year, 1 in 3 dies of heart disease.

Critical Thinking

You have just performed an annual ECG on your patient Ms. Cantrell. The tracing looks alarming. However, Ms. Cantrell is alert, oriented, and talking. What is your best course of action? Describe how critical thinking is a component of this decision.

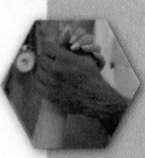

Patient Education

Atherosclerosis is the buildup of fatty deposits on the lining of coronary arteries causing narrowing and obstruction of the arteries. **Ischemia** or decreased blood flow to the heart muscle occurs when the heart is called on to work harder, for example, during increased physical activity, emotional stress, exposure to cold temperatures, and after a heavy meal. The heart's muscle tissue responds to these conditions and there are symptoms of pain or discomfort beneath the sternum, into the neck, jaw, left arm and shoulder, and throat. Rest usually relieves the pain. This condition is known as **angina pectoris** or simply angina.

Treatment of angina consists of rest and medication. Nitroglycerin may be prescribed in tablet or patch form. Change in lifestyle and other suggestions (Table 36-1) may be recommended. Tests that the provider may order include a 12-lead ECG, a stress ECG (stress test), blood tests, chest radiograph, and coronary **angiogram**.

Pain that does not subside after rest may indicate a more serious condition such as a complete obstruction of the coronary arteries and no blood flow to the heart muscle, a myocardial infarction, or heart attack. Seek immediate medical attention if pain persists.

With the approval of the provider, medical assistants are in an excellent position to offer healthy tips and suggestions from which patients can benefit. For instance, they can offer patient health tips regarding diet and exercise as a part of the clinic visit and provide handouts and informational Web sites for patients to research (Table 36-1). Patient education is an essential part of care for those patients in certain high-risk groups.

TABLE 36-1

BEHAVIORS TO ADOPT FOR A HEALTHY HEART

The provider may want the medical assistant to remind patients of the following healthy behaviors:

1. Avoid tobacco

2. Take medications as prescribed

3. Report any unusual symptoms or problems to the provider

4. Eat a low-fat, low-cholesterol, low-sodium diet

5. Exercise regularly with provider's permission

6. Get adequate rest

7. Keep weight under control and at an acceptable level

8. Practice stress reduction behaviors

CARDIAC ARRHYTHMIAS

The medical assistant should recognize cardiac **arrhythmias** (anything other than normal sinus rhythm) that occur during the ECG recording. Recognition and appropriate notification of the provider in a timely manner must be accomplished without alarming the patient. Knowledge of arrhythmias will allow the medical assistant to be prepared for the next steps in the care of the patient after notification of the provider (e.g., applying oxygen via nasal cannula). A word of caution: Always treat the patient, not the ECG tracing. Sometimes, the ECG tracing can look alarming due to artifacts or other disturbances. If the ECG demonstrates asystole, but the patient is alert and speaking with you, there is no need to initiate CPR and other lifesaving measures.

The normal, healthy ECG cycle represents the electrical activity of the heart muscle and consists of P, QRS, and T waves in a regularly appearing sequence or pattern. Every arrhythmia is an interruption in the rate or configuration of these waves.

The term *normal sinus rhythm* refers to an ECG tracing that has a P wave, a QRS complex, and a T wave for each cardiac cycle with a rate between 60 and 100 beats per minute (Figure 36-12A). A rate less than 60 beats/minute is known as **sinus bradycardia** (Figure 36-12B); a rate greater than 100 beats/minute is known as **sinus tachycardia** (Figure 36-12C). With both sinus bradycardia and sinus tachycardia, the elements of normal cardiac electrical conduction are present, but the rate is slower or faster than 60 to 100 beats per minute, respectively. These two heart rates, although regular in rhythm, are considered cardiac arrhythmias. See the "Cardiac Arrhythmias" Quick Reference Guide for more information on types of arrhythmias.

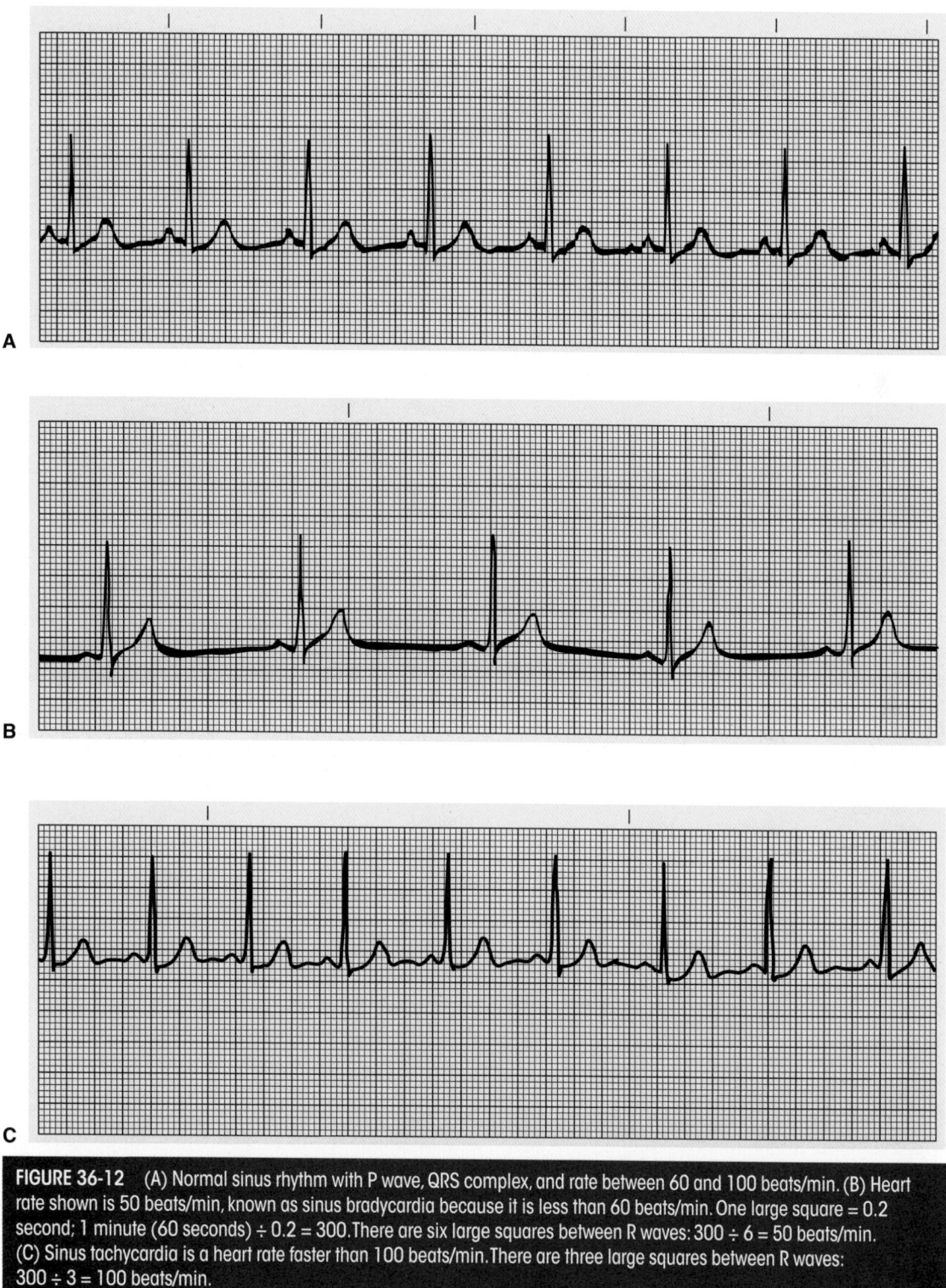

FIGURE 36-12 (A) Normal sinus rhythm with P wave, QRS complex, and rate between 60 and 100 beats/min. (B) Heart rate shown is 50 beats/min, known as sinus bradycardia because it is less than 60 beats/min. One large square = 0.2 second; 1 minute (60 seconds) ÷ 0.2 = 300. There are six large squares between R waves: 300 ÷ 6 = 50 beats/min. (C) Sinus tachycardia is a heart rate faster than 100 beats/min. There are three large squares between R waves: 300 ÷ 3 = 100 beats/min.

Atrial Arrhythmias

Type of Arrhythmia	Rate	Rhythm	Characteristics	Symptoms and Risk Factors
Premature atrial contractions (PAC) (Figure 36-13A)	Variable	Irregular	A cardiac cycle that occurs before the next cycle is due. P waves are present and vary in shape and are irregularly spaced. QRS complex is present and irregularly spaced	**Symptoms:** Heart palpitations **Risk Factors:** Tobacco and stimulant use, such as caffeine; can occur during exercise

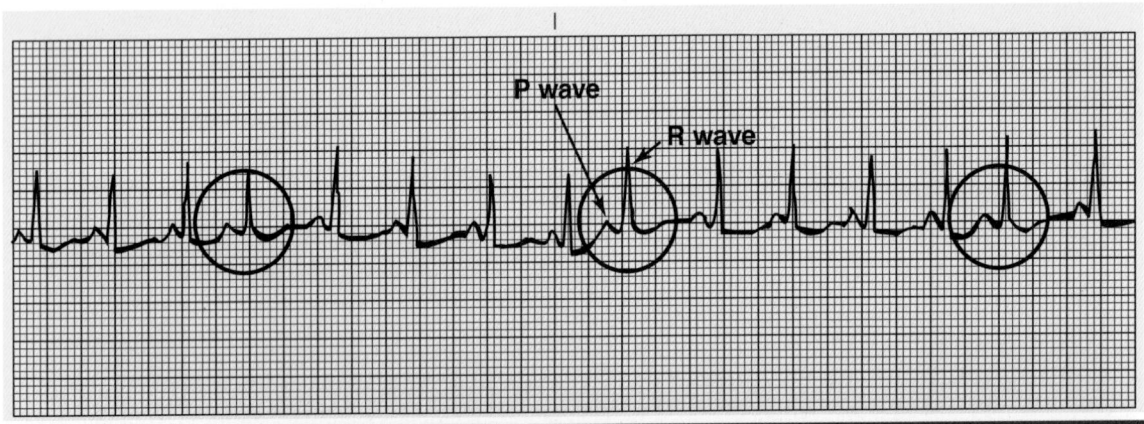

FIGURE 36-13A Premature atrial contractions.

Type of Arrhythmia	Rate	Rhythm	Characteristics	Symptoms and Risk Factors
Paroxysmal atrial tachycardia (PAT) (Figure 36-13B)	Between 160 and 250 beats/min	Regular	Unprovoked sudden onset and abrupt termination. P waves are abnormally shaped. QRS complex is present and regularly spaced	**Symptoms:** Fluttering in the chest, apprehension, shortness of breath, and, on occasion, dizziness **Risk Factors:** Cardiac disease

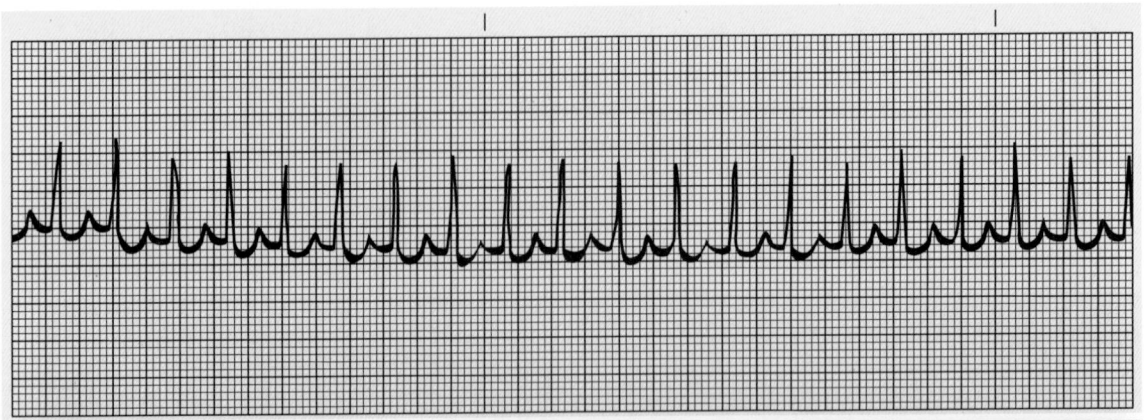

FIGURE 36-13B Paroxysmal atrial tachycardia.

(continues)

Type of Arrhythmia	Rate	Rhythm	Characteristics	Symptoms and Risk Factors
Atrial fibrillation (Figure 36-13C)	Artria can contract up to 500 beats/min but heart rate is usually < 120 beats/min	Irregularly irregular	Extremely rapid, incomplete contractions of the atria resulting in irregular and uncoordinated contractions of the ventricles at a much slower rate No distinct P waves QRS complexes are present but are irregularly spaced	**Symptoms:** Palpitations, weakness, fatigue, lightheadedness, dizziness, confusion, shortness of breath **Risk Factors:** Cardiac disease, congenital heart disease, mitral valve damage, hypertension, coronary artery disease, mitral valve prolapse

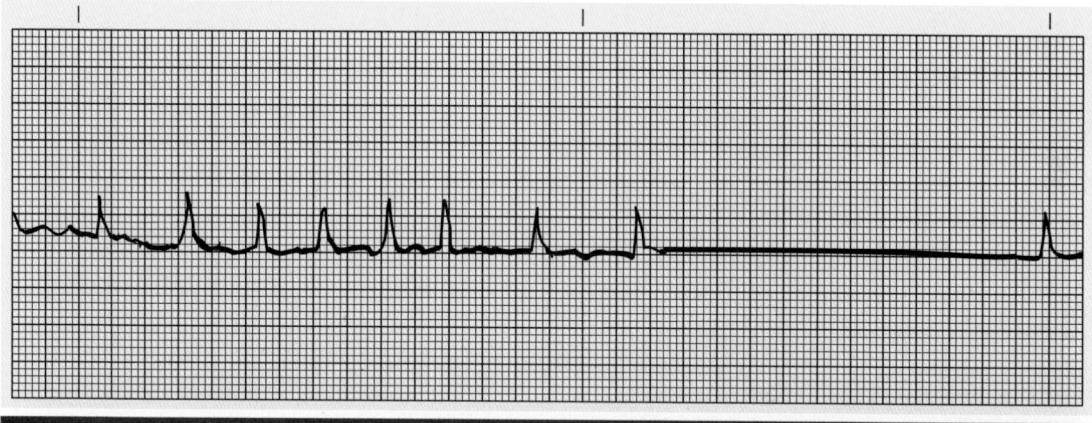

FIGURE 36-13C Atrial fibrillation.

Type of Arrhythmia	Rate	Rhythm	Characteristics	Symptoms and Risk Factors
Atrial flutter (Figure 36-13D)	Atria contract 250 to 300 beats/min but the heart rate is a maximum of approximately 150 beats/min	Regular	P waves have a picket fence pattern QRS complexes occur at a set ratio to P waves (e.g., 2:1, 3:1, or 4:1)	**Symptoms:** Increased heart rate, shortness of breath, lightheadedness, pressure in the chest **Risk Factors:** Smoking, heart disease, high blood pressure, heart valve conditions, lung disease, stress

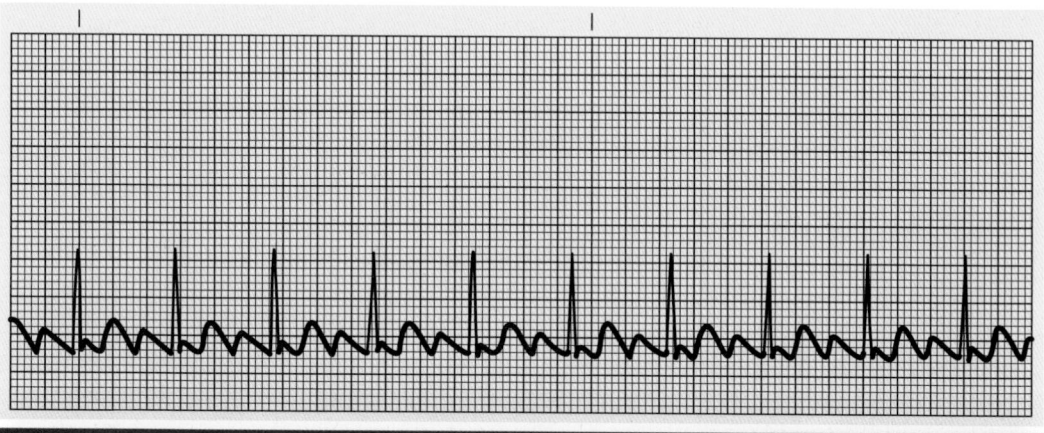

FIGURE 36-13D Atrial flutter.

(continues)

Ventricular Arrhythmias

Type of Arrhythmia	Rate	Rhythm	Characteristics	Symptoms and Risk Factors
Premature ventricular contractions (PVC) (Figure 36-14A)	Variable	Irregular	No P wave QRS complex that comes early in the cycle and is abnormally wide There will be a pause before the next normal cycle begins	**Symptoms:** Sensation of heart flutter, pounding, or skipping beats **Risk Factors:** Hypertension, coronary artery disease, lung disease, anxiety, tobacco and alcohol use, medications that contain epinephrine

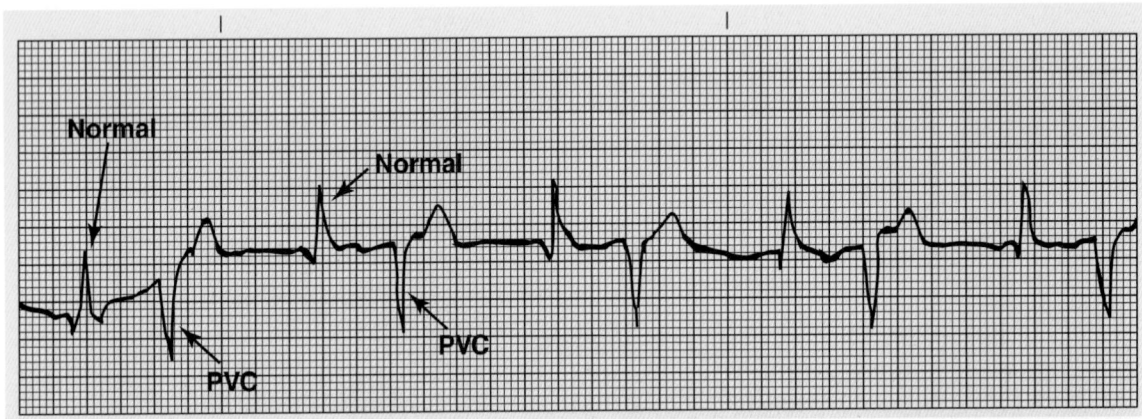

FIGURE 36-14A Premature ventricular contractions (PVCs).

Type of Arrhythmia	Rate	Rhythm	Characteristics	Symptoms and Risk Factors
Ventricular tachycardia (Figure 36-14B)	150 to 250 beats/min	Regular	No P waves QRS complexes are wide and distorted Life-threatening	**Symptoms:** Dizziness, fainting, fatigue, chest pain, shortness of breath **Risk Factors:** Cardiac disease (both acute and chronic), coronary artery disease, myocardial infarction

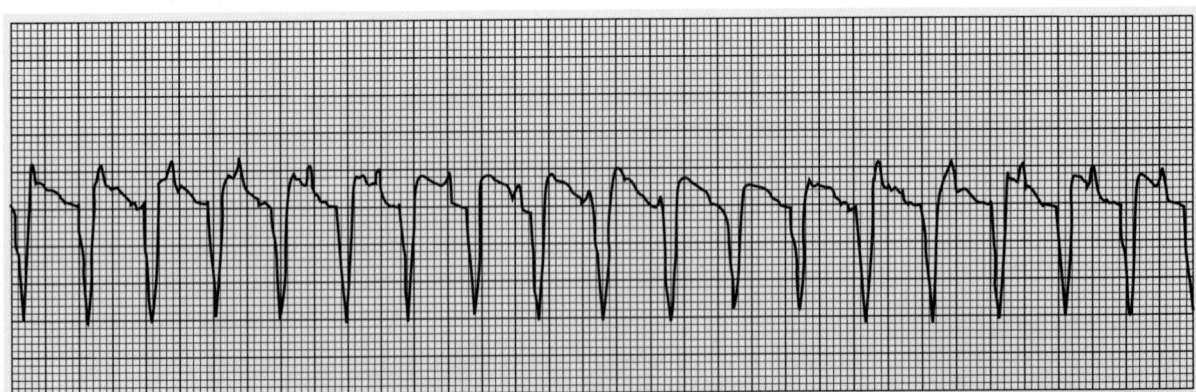

FIGURE 36-14B Ventricular tachycardia.

(continues)

Type of Arrhythmia	Rate	Rhythm	Characteristics	Symptoms and Risk Factors
Ventricular fibrillation (Figure 36-14C)	None	Disorganized	No P wave No QRS complexes, just chaotic wave-like lines with positive and negative deflection but no baseline Life-threatening	**Symptoms:** Chest pain, rapid heart rate, dizziness, nausea, shortness of breath, loss of consciousness **Risk Factors:** Myocardial infarction, existing cardiac disease

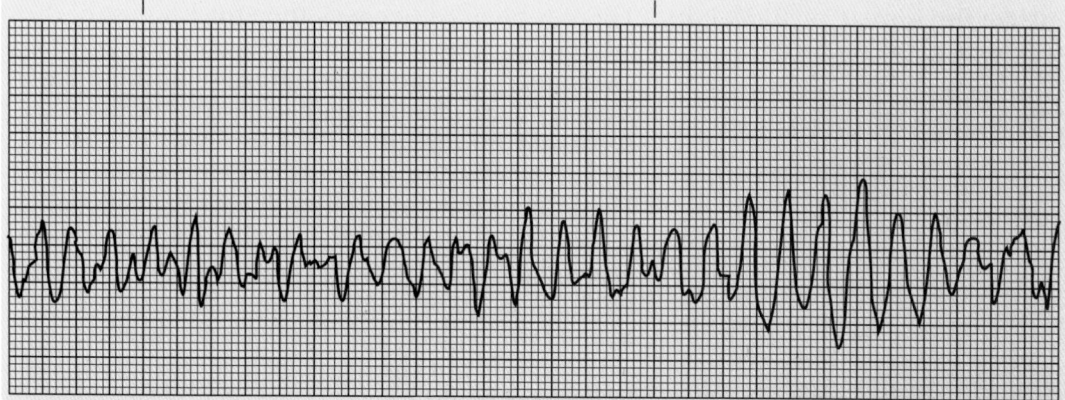

FIGURE 36-14C Ventricular fibrillation.

DEFIBRILLATION

Safety

A **defibrillator** is an electrical device that applies **countershocks** to the heart through electrodes or pads placed on the chest wall (Figure 36-15). The purpose is to convert cardiac arrhythmia into normal sinus rhythm. This is known as **defibrillation** or **cardioversion**. In most offices and clinics, a defibrillator is kept on a crash cart for quick access in emergency situations. The medical assistant should regularly check the equipment for proper operation and preparedness and assist the provider as needed.

Automated external defibrillators (AED) are widely used and are found in places where many people congregate, such as airports and the workplace, and in private homes of individuals at risk for cardiac arrest.

The devices are portable, small, and battery operated. In the past, emergency medical

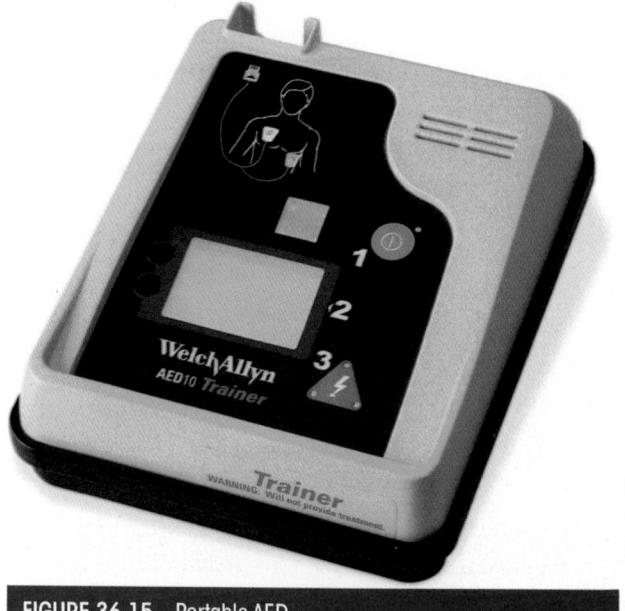

FIGURE 36-15 Portable AED.

Courtesy of Welch-Allyn

technicians, police officers, and firefighters trained in defibrillation techniques and who were the first to respond in an emergency were primarily the individuals who used these devices. Now, many citizens are certified to use AED (see Figure 36-15).

In an individual experiencing a myocardial infarction, ventricular fibrillation is not uncommon. If the fibrillation can be stopped within the first 5 minutes using a defibrillator, the life can be saved (see Chapter 8 for more about AED). AED are commonly found and come with very simple instructions about defibrillator pad placement. Once the unit is turned on, it uses a complex computer program to analyze the cardiac rhythm and provide audible instructions to the rescuer.

OTHER CARDIAC DIAGNOSTIC TESTS

Holter Monitor (Portable Ambulatory Electrocardiograph)

The Holter monitor is a portable continuous recording of cardiac activity for a 24-hour period (Figure 36-16). The patient is monitored while going about usual daily activities with no restrictions. This **noninvasive** test helps to diagnose cardiac arrhythmias by correlating them with the patient's symptoms. Some symptoms are **syncope**, fatigue, chest pain, and vertigo. This type of monitoring is useful for patients whose arrhythmias are sporadic and are not found on a 12-lead ECG tracing. Also, ambulatory monitoring helps assess the function of an artificial pacemaker and the effectiveness of antiarrhythmic medications.

Special electrodes attached to lead wires are placed in the appropriate areas of the patient's chest. Remember that skin preparation is an important aspect of ensuring accurate information. A special portable tape recorder, either digital or magnetic continually records the heart's electrical activity for a 24-hour period. The monitor is a battery-operated recorder that is placed in a leather pouch or bag and is worn by the patient either on a belt around the waist or by a strap over the patient's shoulder. Table 36-2 lists locations for placement of electrodes.

One kind of digital **Holter monitor** is a three-channel (five-lead) ECG that has Windows-based software technology. A keypad is used to enter the patient's information, such as date of recording and patient identification number. There is no need to check the effectiveness of the monitor by attaching it to a test cable and an ECG machine. Some monitors have a removable flash memory card and a flash card reader that can download information in 90 seconds. The monitor can hold up to 48 hours of ECG information. The tracing is interpreted and sent back digitally. It can be accessed and printed. The electrode placement is the same for a digital Holter monitor as it is for a magnetic tape Holter monitor, but electrode placement for both digital and magnetic tape is not the same as it is for a standard 12-lead resting ECG.

Other computerized continuous cardiac monitoring devices are available and are prescribed for patients according to the patient's symptoms and the practitioner's preference. The tracing can be read over the telephone or is computerized. Transtelephone monitor devices are frequently used by patients with a pacemaker and/or **implantable cardioverter-defibrillator (ICD)**. These patients have routine scheduled checks of their devices over the phone.

Some cardiac monitoring devices are sent directly to the patient from the supplier, complete with printed or telephone directions for the patient. When the specific time period has elapsed for the particular monitor being used, the patient is responsible for returning the device to the supplier.

 **Medical Assistant's Role.** The medical assistant is responsible for preparing the patient, instructing the patient, checking and replacing the battery, and applying and removing the monitor.

Communication   Competency

Holter Monitor Electrode Placement. Special disposable electrodes, which are round plastic and have a strong adhesive backing, are available for the Holter monitor. These disposable electrodes

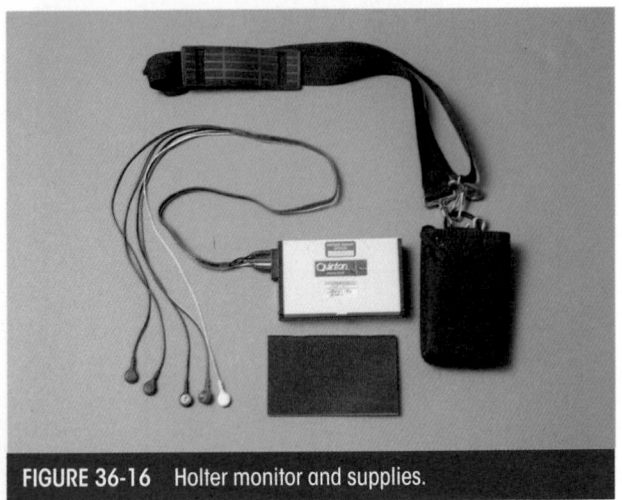

FIGURE 36-16 Holter monitor and supplies.

contain an electrolyte gel. There may be either four or five electrodes depending on whether the monitor has a built-in ground. Notice that the leads for the Holter monitor are applied to locations that are different from those of the electrodes of a resting ECG. Table 36-2 lists the locations for lead placement.

Procedure

Holter Monitor Attachment. Once the Holter monitor has been attached to the patient, the monitor should be checked for effectiveness by attaching the **test cable** to the monitor and the other end to an ECG instrument. A baseline strip can be recorded to verify the correct wave activity and lack of artifact. If there are inaccurate readings, the monitor may not have been applied properly. The medical assistant can reconnect the leads to the electrodes or reposition the electrodes and reconnect the leads (see Procedure 36-2). Prior to any lead placement, the skin should be cleansed with an alcohol wipe and rubbed with gauze to roughen it. Males should be shaved so that the electrodes adhere well. It is essential that the leads be applied appropriately and secured with waterproof tape to allow the collection of clean, interpretable data from the Holter monitor.

TABLE 36-2

HOLTER MONITOR ELECTRODE PLACEMENT

ELECTRODE	LEAD	LOCATION
A (black)	mV_1	Fourth intercostal space at right of the sternal edge
B (white)	mV_5	Right clavicle, just lateral to sternum
C (brown)	mV_1	Left clavicle, just lateral to the sternum
D (red)	mV_5	Fifth intercostal space at left axillary line
E (green)	Ground	Lower right chest wall

Patient Activity Diary. The patient activity diary is an important component of the monitoring procedures. As noted in the Patient Education box, all activities and emotional states, and the time of their occurrence, should be noted during the 24-hour monitoring time. Symptoms such as chest pain, shortness of breath, dizziness, and palpitations, and

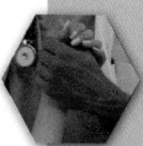

Patient Education

When preparing patients to wear a 24-hour Holter monitor, instruct them in the following:

1. Carry out the usual daily activities at the normal intensity level.

2. Keep a diary of daily activities, symptoms, and emotions, and note the time of occurrence.

3. Depress the event marker only briefly and only when experiencing a significant symptom. Overuse of the marker can mask the ECG tracing.

4. Add the details of the event in the diary including date, time, activities, and any other influencing factors. Symptoms that require documentation include:
   a. Chest pain or discomfort
   b. Dizziness or fainting
   c. Irregular heartbeats, such as a fluttery feeling in your chest
   d. Shortness of breath or trouble breathing
   e. Strong, pounding heartbeats

5. Do not shower, bathe, or swim while wearing the monitor because the recording could be interrupted or the monitor could be damaged.

6. Do not handle the electrodes. Doing so could cause artifacts.

7. Do not remove the recorder from its case.

8. Do not use an electric blanket. This can cause interference.

the time the event occurred, should also be noted. Patient symptoms recorded while being monitored can be compared with the patient's notations in the activity diary and correlated to the heart's activity. Symptoms can be further noted by the patient briefly depressing an event marker button located at one end of the monitor. This places an electronic "tag" on the tape. This signal can alert the person interpreting the ECG to look for a significant event or abnormality on the tape.

The following are examples of some of the daily activities that should be recorded by the patient in the patient activity diary:

- Eating meals
- Ascending and descending stairs
- Sexual activity
- Medications taken
- Times of sleep
- Smoking
- Bowel movements
- Physical exercise

Holter Monitor Removal. The patient is instructed to return to the clinic or ambulatory care center 24 hours after monitor application to have the monitor removed. Usually no appointment is necessary. The information is analyzed by a Holter monitor scanner or by a computer. This is usually done in the ECG department of a nearby hospital or the cardiologist's office. The provider can access the report from the electronic medical record with samples of any abnormalities that were picked up during the monitoring period. A follow-up appointment is scheduled with the provider to discuss the results.

PROCEDURE 36-2

Procedure

Applying a Holter Monitor

STANDARD PRECAUTIONS:

Handwashing

PURPOSE:
To record events that might indicate cardiac disease.

EQUIPMENT/SUPPLIES:

- Digital Holter monitor
- Carrying case with belt or shoulder strap
- SD memory card
- Disposable electrodes
- Disposable razor
- Alcohol wipes
- 4-by-4 gauze
- Patient activity diary
- Gloves

PROCEDURE STEPS:

1. Introduce yourself to the patient using your full name and credentials. Confirm the identity of the patient, using two identifiers, and *take a moment to make the patient at ease by explaining the rationale for the performance of the procedure at a level equal with his or her understanding.*

(continues)

2. Prepare the equipment by removing old (used) battery from the monitor and replacing it with a new battery. RATIONALE: Installing a new battery each 24-hour period will ensure the monitor will function because it will have sufficient power.

3. Ask the patient to remove his or her clothing from the waist up. Then wash your hands. Apply gloves. Have the patient sit up on the examination table for comfort and ease of access. Identify the correct electrode placement sites on the patient. Any sites with hair should be dry-shaved off.

4. Abrade areas where electrodes will be placed with dry 4-by-4 gauze until they are red or cleanse the areas with an alcohol wipe. RATIONALE: Shaved site and abraded skin help the electrodes to adhere better to the skin and facilitate easier removal.

5. Remove the electrodes from the package. Attach the lead wires to the electrodes.

6. Apply the adhesive-backed electrode to the appropriate site by applying firm pressure to the center of the electrode and moving outward toward the edges. Run your finger firmly around the outer rim. RATIONALE: Firmly attached electrodes help ensure a good quality tracing.

7. Continue to apply the remaining electrodes in the same manner (Figure 36-17).

8. Reinforce the electrode connection and ensure longevity by applying tape to the edges of the electrode pads.

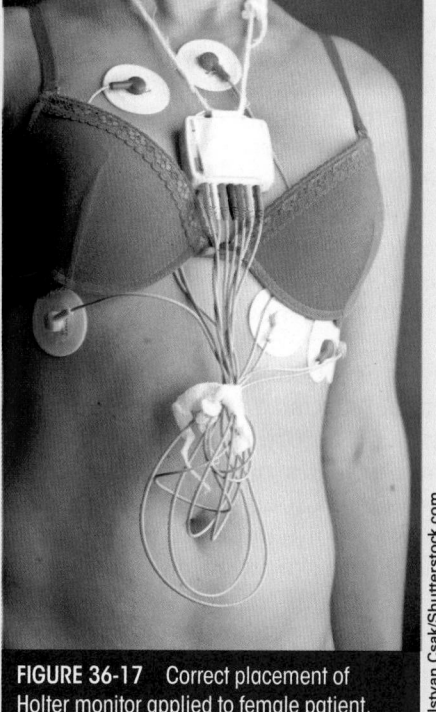

FIGURE 36-17 Correct placement of Holter monitor applied to female patient.

© Istvan Csak/Shutterstock.com

9. Place the electrode cable so that it extends from between the buttons of the patient's shirt, or from below the bottom of the shirt. Plug the wires into the recorder. When the recorder is placed in its carrying case and attached to the patient's belt or shoulder strap, there should be no pulling on the lead wires. RATIONALE: Pulling on electrodes could cause them to become detached.

10. Help the patient to dress. Remove gloves, then wash your hands.

11. Review care of the monitor with your patient.

12. Remind the patient that the Holter monitor must be kept dry, and that showers and baths should be avoided while it is in place. Instruct the patient to use the event diary to record activity and any adverse symptoms, such as palpitations or chest pain. Ask the patient to include time and duration when recording symptoms. Remind the patient what time the monitor will be removed on the following day.

13. Document the procedure and any patient education in the patient's medical record.

DOCUMENTATION:

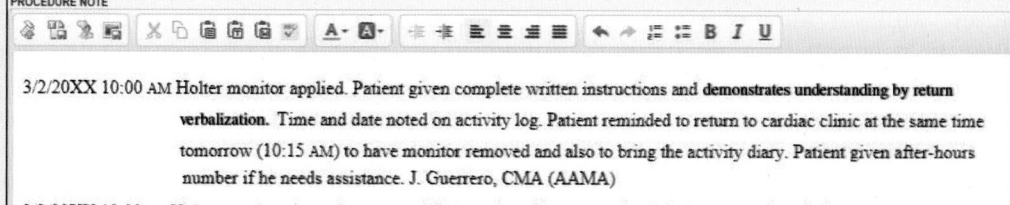

PROCEDURE NOTE

3/2/20XX 10:00 AM Holter monitor applied. Patient given complete written instructions and **demonstrates understanding by return verbalization.** Time and date noted on activity log. Patient reminded to return to cardiac clinic at the same time tomorrow (10:15 AM) to have monitor removed and also to bring the activity diary. Patient given after-hours number if he needs assistance. J. Guerrero, CMA (AAMA)

3/3/20XX 10:00AM Holter monitor electrodes removed from patient. Cassette and activity log returned or flash memory card removed for later analysis on the computer analysis system. J. Guerro, CMA (AAMA)

Courtesy of Harris CareTracker PM and EMR

Loop ECG

Another type of ambulatory electrocardiography is called *loop ECG*. It uses only two electrodes. It records a few minutes of the ECG at a time in the memory of the monitor. It constantly records new information and discards the oldest information. Thus, the memory contains only the last few minutes of the ECG recording. When a patient has an episode or event (symptoms), the patient pushes the record button and the recording remains in the device's memory. The recorded event is transmitted (played back) by telephone to the provider. The device then erases the event.

The recorder constantly refreshes its memory. It is suitable for capturing brief events and can be carried for long periods of time. Other types of recorders require a longer period of time, and if a patient is experiencing dizziness, it takes too long to apply a recorder. This may result in not being able to capture episodes associated with syncope.

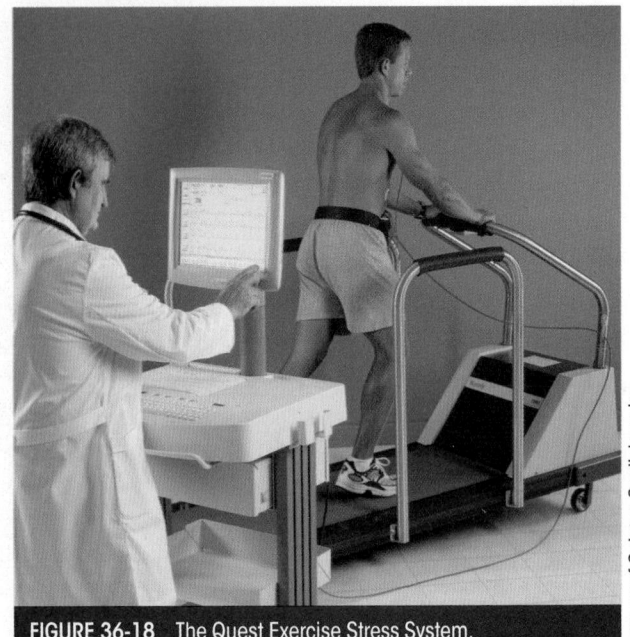

FIGURE 36-18 The Quest Exercise Stress System.

Courtesy of Quinton Cardiology, Inc.

Treadmill Stress Test or Exercise Tolerance ECG

On occasion patients have symptoms of cardiac problems that do not appear as abnormalities on a resting ECG. The provider may prescribe a treadmill stress test or exercise tolerance test to aid in the determination of the patient's diagnosis and prognosis. The test is done to diagnose heart disorders, to diagnose the probable cause of the patient's chest pain, and to assess the patient's cardiac ability after cardiac surgery. The treadmill stress test is a noninvasive ECG tracing taken under controlled conditions while the patient is closely monitored by the medical assistant and the provider. Frequent blood pressure readings are taken. The patient wears comfortable clothing and flat shoes such as sneakers with rubber soles and exercises on a treadmill at prescribed rates of speed (Figure 36-18). Electrodes are applied to the chest only.

As with the Holter monitor, the patient's skin should be cleansed with an alcohol wipe and rubbed with gauze to roughen it. Male patients should be shaved at the site of the electrodes to ensure electrode adherence.

The myocardium requires extra oxygen during exercise and in the presence of narrowed or obstructed coronary arteries; the additional workload on the myocardium will often be demonstrated as an abnormality on the ECG recording. The patient should have no pain, shortness of breath,

or excess fatigue. If any of these or other unusual symptoms occur, the provider may terminate the test because this could indicate cardiac disease.

At the conclusion of the test, the patient is allowed to rest. Monitoring continues until the vital signs and heart rate return to normal. Prior to the patient leaving the clinic, the patient should be instructed to rest, refrain from a hot bath or shower, avoid stimulants such as caffeine, and avoid extreme temperature changes for several hours.

Complications such as a myocardial infarction or a serious arrhythmia can occur during testing. Although these events are unusual, appropriate emergency equipment must be readily available (see crash cart information in Chapter 8), and the medical assistant should check them frequently for proper functioning. Some equipment to have available on a crash cart for cardiac emergencies includes oxygen, antiarrhythmic drugs, an Ambu bag, a defibrillator, an endotracheal tube, and a laryngoscope. One of the responsibilities of the medical assistant may be checking the supplies and plugging in the defibrillator.

Further diagnostic tests such as **cardiac catheterization** (angiogram) may be necessary to diagnose the extent of the atherosclerosis buildup and obstruction of the coronary arteries. A cardiac catheterization is an invasive procedure that is performed in an acute care setting. In order to visualize the coronary arteries and determine the extent of disease, if any, a large catheter is inserted into the femoral or brachial artery and threaded carefully to the origin of the coronary vessels via the inferior vena cava. Once the specially shaped tip of the catheter is engaged in the coronary artery, radiopaque contrast medium is injected into the vessel and visualized using radiographic techniques. The course of intervention is determined at this point if disease is noted.

Thallium Stress Test

Thallium stress test is similar to a treadmill stress test in that the patient has an ECG tracing done while exercising on the treadmill after having been given an injection of the radioactive substance thallium. The test shows how well blood flows to the heart muscle. It can help diagnose coronary artery blockage, the cause of a patient's chest pain, cardiac function, and status after myocardial infarction. It can also indicate the level of exercise a patient can safely engage in.

Thallium is a **radiopharmaceutical**. This means that thallium is a radioactive substance that serves as a radiotracer. The thallium is injected intravenously while the patient is being monitored on the treadmill and is exercising. After the stress test, the patient is scanned using a gamma camera in the diagnostic imaging department. The patient leaves the department for 3 or 4 hours (rests), then returns, and another scan is done. Therefore, the patient has been "scanned" during exercise and after a rest period of a few hours.

The thallium intravenous injection mixes with blood in the bloodstream and in the arteries and enters the heart muscle cells. If a portion of the heart does not receive a normal blood supply, then a smaller amount of thallium will be present in those heart muscle cells. To the cardiologist this finding indicates a degree of block in the heart's blood supply. The patient most likely has ischemia of the heart muscle or an infarct of the heart muscle.

Patients who cannot tolerate an exercise stress test because of serious heart disease or patients with special needs, such as patients who are confined to wheelchairs, can be given a vasodilator and undergo the ECG test seated in a chair or wheelchair. The medication will cause an increase in heart rate, thus simulating the stress of walking on a treadmill. The thallium stress test may be performed in a variety of settings—as an inpatient or outpatient in the hospital, the cardiology office, or clinic.

Echocardiography/Ultrasonography

Echocardiography is a noninvasive diagnostic test that uses ultrasound (ultrahigh-frequency sound waves) to image the internal structures of the heart. X-rays are not useful in such a situation. General anatomy, myocardial function, valve function, and heart chamber size can be evaluated. Echocardiography may be performed in a cardiologist's office.

During **ultrasonography**, a handheld **transducer** acts as a transmitter and receiver of the high-frequency sound waves as it is held against the chest wall and moved over the heart area. As the sound waves penetrate the skin and bounce off of internal structures, echoes are sent back to the transducer. A machine converts the images when the various structures provide different echoes. The images can then be examined by a computer and converted into photographs and films of structures and blood flow.

There is little patient preparation other than to have the patient lie on the examination table with the four-limb leads of a 12-lead electrocardiograph attached. The test is usually performed by a **sonographer**. The provider views the results later and informs the patient of the results.

Coronary MRI and CT Imaging

Magnetic resonance imaging (MRI) is useful in identifying the location and thickness of cardiac muscle scars due to damage. Although neither MRI nor computed tomography (CT) has replaced X-ray angiography (XRA) as the clinical standard for the diagnosis of coronary stenosis, their use in determining if a vessel is open is increasing. At the 64th Annual Scientific Session of the American College of Cardiology in 2015, three-dimensional heart imaging was presented as a tool to enhance traditional diagnosis of cardiac disease by improving diagnosis and outcomes. Using CT imaging in this manner results in guidance for further testing and intervention to prevent heart attack.

CARDIAC PROCEDURES

The following section discusses cardiac procedures performed in order to diagnose heart disease and arrhythmias. Some cardiac procedures for diagnosing diseases of the heart are computerized, and the results are stored in the patient's electronic medical record. The data are accessible on demand.

Procedures for Heart Disease

Percutaneous transluminal coronary angioplasty (PTCA) is a procedure that widens a narrowed or blocked coronary artery. One type of PTCA is balloon angioplasty. A catheter with a deflated balloon is inserted into the patient's femoral artery and gently advanced to the coronary arteries via the inferior vena cava. Once the tip of the catheter is engaged in the correct coronary artery, a very thin and flexible wire is advanced through the catheter and down the course of the coronary artery, past or through any lesion that has been identified during the coronary angioplasty. An additional, smaller catheter that holds a compressed balloon of a specified length is advanced over the flexible wire and positioned at the site of the blockage. Very precise inflation pressures and times are applied by the cardiologist with the hope of opening the occluded artery and establishing blood flow downstream to the heart muscle.

For complicated lesions, it is sometimes necessary to utilize a coronary stent. Stents are small mesh tubes that are compressed around a balloon that is much like the angioplasty balloon. Using radiographic visualization, the stent is positioned within the area of blockage. As the balloon is slowly and carefully inflated, the stent is deployed against the wall of the vessel. Once the stent is deployed, all of the interventional catheters and wires are removed. Over time, the stent becomes a part of the vessel wall after the inner layer of cells, or endothelium, regrows over the area that was stented. Thus, a stent is a permanent intervention and there is a standard regimen of care to ensure the best outcomes after insertion of a stent, including the use of anticoagulant medications.

Other cardiac procedures that can be performed to address heart disease are atherectomy and laser angioplasty. In atherectomy, the provider uses a very small device on the end of a catheter to cut away the blocked area inside the coronary artery. In laser angioplasty, the provider uses a laser beam to destroy the blockage in the artery.

Coronary artery bypass is a procedure in which a portion of a vein (typically the saphenous) is transplanted into one or more of the heart's coronary arteries. The transplanted vein circumvents or bypasses the blocked coronary artery, thus reestablishing blood supply to that portion of the heart. This is a major procedure and the recovery time is extended.

A balloon valvuloplasty is a less invasive procedure to address the narrowing of a heart valve. During this procedure, a large balloon loaded onto a catheter is threaded through the narrowed valve and is inflated in order to expand the opening. This procedure allows a more normal flow of blood through the valve. The aortic valve is the most common area where this type of treatment is appropriate. Balloon valvuloplasty might be used in some children, teens, and young adults in their 20s who have aortic valve stenosis.

A heart valve can be repaired or replaced. In a replacement procedure, a tissue or mechanical valve replaces the heart's damaged valve.

Procedures for Arrhythmias

A cardiac electrophysiologist is a specialist who provides care to patients with arrhythmias. After a study by the cardiac electrophysiologist determines the source of the patient's arrhythmia within the electrical conduction system of the heart, a catheter is inserted into the femoral artery and a special device with radio waves is aimed at the source of the abnormal heart rhythm. This is known as *cardiac ablation*. The tiny scar produced prevents the electrical conduction system from traveling through the scarred area, resulting in normal rhythm.

A permanent battery-operated pacemaker can be surgically implanted into the patient's chest wall for treatment of certain types of arrhythmias. Wires from the pacemaker are inserted into the heart to provide a steady, regular heartbeat.

An implantable cardioverter defibrillator (ICD) is a device surgically implanted into the patient's chest wall with wires leading into the heart. When the patient's heart rate is extremely low or the patient's heart stops beating, the defibrillator delivers a small electric shock to jar the heart back into a normal rhythm (works like AED; see the section on defibrillation earlier in this chapter and Chapter 8).

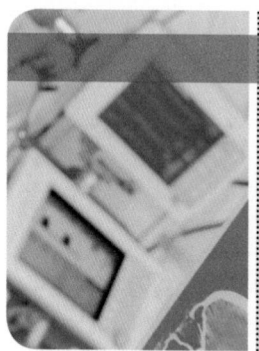

CASE STUDY 36-1

Refer to the scenario at the beginning of the chapter.

Gwen can empathize better with her patients now that she herself has had a baseline ECG.

CASE STUDY REVIEW

1. The feelings Gwen had while having her tracing are experienced by many patients. Explain what you can do for your patients to allay their fears when they are getting ready for an ECG and during the tracing.

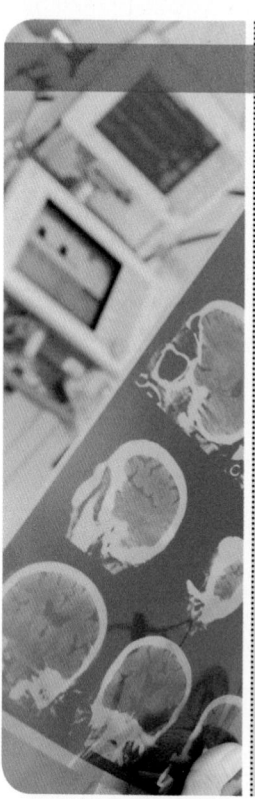

CASE STUDY 36-2

Abigail Johnson, who is in her mid-70s, arrives at Inner City Health Care reporting chest pain. She has been seen on two other occasions for similar pain and has a history of diabetes, hypertension, arteriosclerotic heart disease, and angina pectoris. Medical assistant Thomas Myers, CCMA (NHA), immediately alerts Dr. Rice of Mrs. Johnson's chest pain and then takes her into the cardiac examination and treatment room. Dr. Rice tells Thomas to have Mrs. Johnson take one of her nitroglycerin tablets and to perform an ECG on her. Mrs. Johnson is restless and anxious as Thomas prepares for the ECG and while the tracing is in progress. There is significant somatic tremor. Thomas attempts to allay Mrs. Johnson's apprehension to obtain a good quality ECG. The patient's pain subsides within a few minutes and she begins to feel better.

CASE STUDY REVIEW

1. What immediate action could Thomas have taken if Mrs. Johnson's pain had not subsided?

2. Mrs. Johnson tells Thomas that Dr. Rice explained arteriosclerotic heart disease and angina pectoris to her, but that she was nervous and understood little and that she is embarrassed to admit that to Dr. Rice. How can Thomas explain, in language that the patient can comprehend, what causes arteriosclerotic heart disease and angina, and what Mrs. Johnson experiences during an attack of angina? What strategies can Thomas teach Mrs. Johnson to promote healthier habits and prevent more serious heart problems?

3. Research what community resources are available for persons with Mrs. Johnson's heart condition. Explain how Mrs. Johnson can locate them and how she could benefit from them.

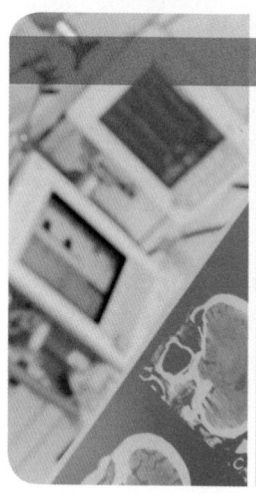

CASE STUDY 36-3

George Matthews, a 79-year-old patient of Dr. King, has a history of cardiovascular heart disease. He tells Dr. King that today he has been experiencing "palpitations and slow and fast heartbeats and sometimes dizziness." Dr. King orders a resting ECG that shows no evidence of arrhythmia and decides that a Holter monitor electrocardiograph for Mr. Matthews might be helpful in diagnosing a cardiac arrhythmia.

CASE STUDY REVIEW

1. Explain why Dr. King ordered Holter monitor electrocardiography for Mr. Matthews.

2. What instructions will you give to Mr. Matthews about wearing the monitor?

3. Mr. Matthews says he is not certain what activities should be recorded in the patient activity diary. Explain what activities he should record and why they are important.

Summary

- The heart has four chambers: two atria and two ventricles.

- Contraction of the heart and pumping oxygenated blood to the body is coordinated by an electrical conduction system that is represented by the electrocardiograph or ECG.

- Electrical stimulation of the heart starts in the aria in the sinoatrial (SA) node.

- The impulse originating in the SA node is conducted to the ventricles via the atrioventricular (AV) node.

- The Purkinje fibers carry the message of contraction to the base of the ventricles.

- The ECG is a representation of the SA node firing and the contraction of the atria in the P wave. The ventricular contraction is represented by the QRS complex.

- The electrocardiograph is a machine that is utilized in obtaining an ECG.

- ECG machines may be single or multichannel.

- Equipment needed to produce an ECG tracing includes electrocardiograph paper, the electrolyte conductor gel, sensors or electrode, and lead wires that connect the patient to the electrocardiograph machine.

- There are specific placement guidelines that must be followed for accurate ECG recording.

- Interference that can distort an ECG tracing is called an artifact.

- Abnormal cardiac rhythms are called arrhythmias. Some are life-threatening.

- Arrhythmias are named based on the part of the heart where they originate as well as their rate.

- Diagnostic testing assists the provider in accurate diagnosis of disease. Non-invasive testing includes Holter monitoring, loop ECG, treadmill, thallium stress testing, and cardiac ultrasonography.

- Invasive testing and treatment for cardiac disease includes coronary angiography, percutaneous transluminal coronary angioplasty, cardiac stenting and pacemaker/ICD placement.

Study for Success

To reinforce your knowledge of and skills related to information presented in this chapter:

- Review the *Key Terms* and *Learning Outcomes*

- Consider the *Critical Thinking* features and *Case Studies* and discuss your conclusions

- Answer the questions in the *Certification Review*

Procedure

- Perform the *Procedures* using the *Competency Assessment Checklists* on the *Student Companion Website*

CERTIFICATION REVIEW

1. Which of the following artifacts is caused by muscle tremors?
   a. Somatic tremor
   b. AC interference
   c. Wandering baseline
   d. Interrupted baseline

2. Which of the following arrhythmias occur in healthy individuals and can be caused by tobacco?
   a. Ventricular fibrillation
   b. Atrial fibrillation
   c. Asystole
   d. Premature atrial contractions
   e. Atrial flutter

3. One cardiac cycle (heartbeat) takes approximately how long?
   a. 0.2 second
   b. 0.4 second
   c. 0.6 second
   d. 0.8 second
4. Which of the following indicates ventricular depolarization?
   a. QRS complex
   b. P wave
   c. T wave
   d. ST segment
   e. U wave
5. What is another name for V leads?
   a. Precordial
   b. Augmented
   c. Standard
   d. Limb
6. An electrocardiograph is known as a 12-lead ECG. How many leads are placed on the patient?
   a. 4
   b. 6
   c. 10
   d. 12
   e. 14
7. Which of the following is a life-threatening arrhythmia?
   a. Atrial fibrillation
   b. Atrial flutter
   c. Premature ventricular contractions
   d. Ventricular fibrillation

8. The use of a defibrillator serves what purpose?
   a. To deliver a countershock to restore normal heart rhythm
   b. To deliver a countershock to keep respiratory rhythm
   c. To deliver a countershock and work as a pacemaker
   d. To deliver a countershock to synchronize pulse and respiration
   e. To deliver a countershock and summon emergency medical services
9. A treadmill or stress test is used to diagnose cardiac problems. What must be included in the preprocedure instructions?
   a. Rest the day before
   b. Avoid stimulants like coffee, caffeine, and tobacco
   c. Remain NPO
   d. All of these
10. When reading a patient's chart, the medical assistant sees a notation that the patient has had a PTCA. What medical phrase is this an abbreviation for?
   a. Partial transplant of coronary arteries
   b. Percutaneous transition of coronary arteries
   c. Percutaneous transluminal coronary angioplasty
   d. Primary tricuspid coronary appliance
   e. Post-traumatic cardiac arrhythmia

UNIT IX
LABORATORY PROCEDURES

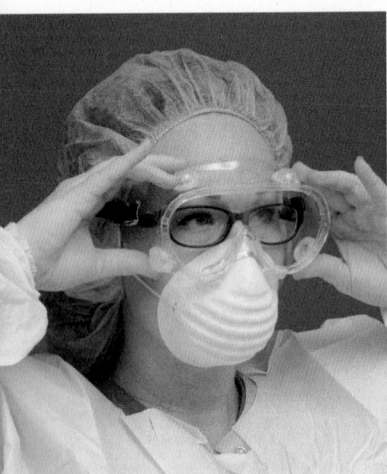
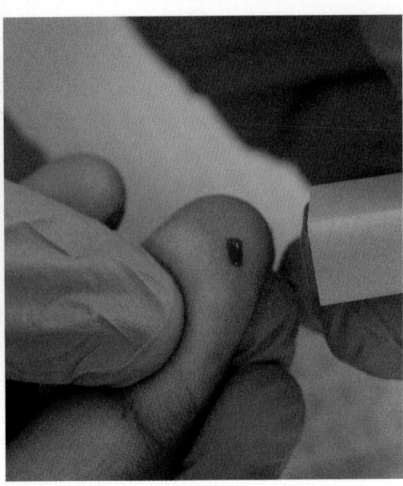
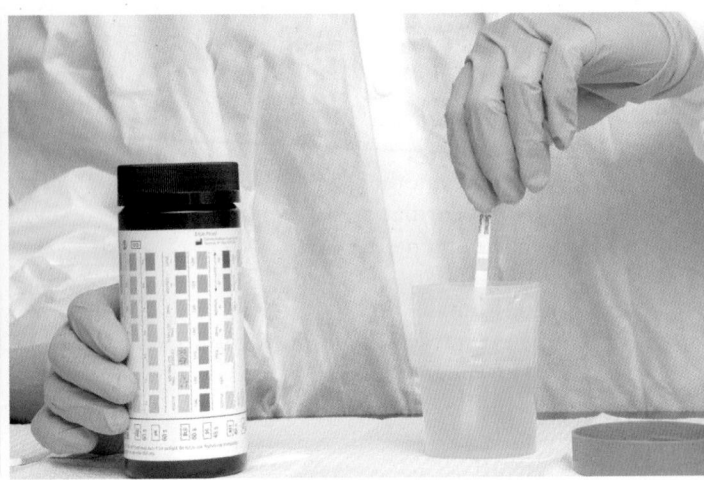

ATTRIBUTES OF PROFESSIONALISM

Many medical assistants will perform laboratory procedures as part of their clinical responsibilities. Administrative medical assistants will also utilize laboratory knowledge and training as well in working with patients, referrals, and medical health records. All medical assistants need to be well versed in legal guidelines, safety precautions, office protocols, scope of practice, and professional boundaries while assisting the providers and when helping patients with their laboratory procedures. Specimen collection in particular may cause patients to feel anxious and apprehensive. As a medical assistant you must exhibit appropriate concern for your patients, answering their questions honestly and helping to allay their fears.

Listed below are a series of questions for you to ask yourself, to serve as a professionalism checklist.

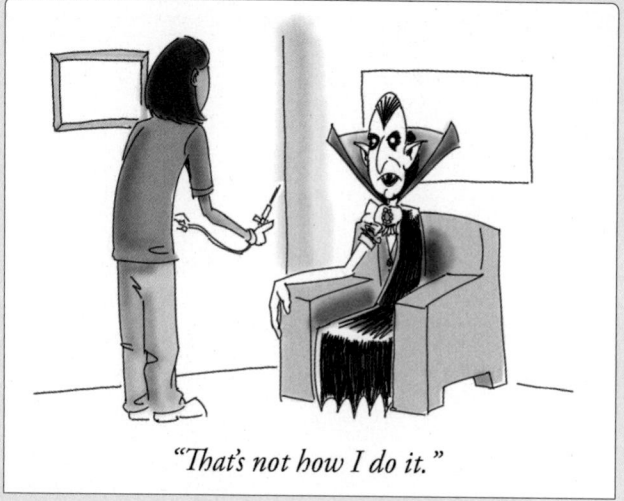

"That's not how I do it."

As you interact with patients and colleagues, these questions will help to guide you in the professional behavior that is expected every day from medical assistants.

Ask Yourself

COMMUNICATION
- ☐ Do I apply active listening skills?
- ☐ Do I demonstrate appropriate nonverbal communication?
- ☐ Do I explain to patients the rationale for performance of a procedure?
- ☐ Do I speak at each patient's level of understanding?
- ☐ Do I display appropriate body language?
- ☐ Do I respond honestly and diplomatically to my patients' concerns?
- ☐ Do I refrain from sharing my personal experiences?
- ☐ Do I include the patient's support system as indicated?
- ☐ Do I reassure patients of the accuracy of test results?
- ☐ Does my knowledge allow me to speak easily with all members of the health care team?

PRESENTATION
- ☐ Am I dressed and groomed appropriately?
- ☐ Do my actions attend to both the psychological and the physiologic aspects of a patient's illness or condition?
- ☐ Am I courteous, patient, and respectful to patients?
- ☐ Do I display a positive attitude?
- ☐ Do I display a calm, professional, and caring manner?

- ☐ Do I demonstrate empathy to the patient?
- ☐ Do I show awareness of patients' concerns related to the procedure being performed?

COMPETENCY
- ☐ Do I pay attention to detail?
- ☐ Do I incorporate critical thinking skills in performing patient assessment and care?
- ☐ Do I recognize the implications of failure to comply with CDC regulations in health care settings?

INITIATIVE
- ☐ Do I show initiative?
- ☐ Do I seek out opportunities to expand my knowledge base?
- ☐ Do I make adaptations for patients with special needs?

INTEGRITY
- ☐ Do I demonstrate the principles of self-boundaries?
- ☐ Do I work within my scope of practice?
- ☐ Do I demonstrate respect for individual diversity?
- ☐ Do I demonstrate sensitivity to patient rights?
- ☐ Do I protect and maintain confidentiality?
- ☐ Do I immediately report any error I made?

CHAPTER 37

Regulatory Guidelines for Safety and Quality in the Medical Laboratory

1. Define and spell the key terms as presented in the glossary.
2. Identify and discuss the contents of Clinical Laboratory Improvement Amendments (CLIA) and its importance to the medical assistant.
3. Describe how CLIA regulates the use of quality control in automated hematology instruments.
4. Recall the categories of testing and list several from the waived category.
5. Describe CMS form 116 and explain its purpose.
6. Identify personal safety precautions as established by the Occupational Safety and Health Administration (OSHA).
7. Describe the importance of Safety Data Sheets (SDS) in the health care setting.
8. Identify and comply with safety signs, symbols, and labels.
9. Evaluate the work environment to identify safe versus unsafe working conditions and safety techniques that can be used to prevent accidents and maintain a safe work environment.

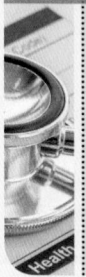

KEY TERMS

certificate of waiver (COW)
fume hoods
labile
proficiency testing
provider-performed microscopy procedures (PPMP)

quality assurance
quality control
Safety Data Sheet (SDS)
waived

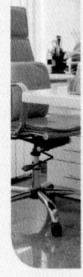

SCENARIO

At Inner City Health Care, clinical medical assistant Gwen Carr, CMA (AAMA), performs many laboratory tests, is always mindful of her legal scope of practice, and performs only those laboratory test that are within the CLIA-waived category. As Gwen interacts with patients to obtain laboratory specimens, she uses her best communication skills to make sure they understand her instructions, are comfortable with the laboratory tests, and always maintains professional boundaries. Gwen is also very careful when working with laboratory equipment and specimens, using precautions to assure her own safety and the safety of her patients, coworkers, and the public.

Chapter Portal

Laboratory safety is a concern for all—management, staff, and patients. An unsafe work environment and work practices can threaten the emotional and physical health of the health care worker as well as the patient. Injuries are also costly on many levels: personally to the injured individual, lost work days, workers' compensation, medical treatment, potential legal action, and potential fines from regulatory agencies. Appropriate orientation, annual reviews, periodic drills, and consistent enforcement of staff adherence to policy are all part of a successful laboratory safety program.

Also, in the course of performing your duties as a medical assistant, you will be in contact with blood and body fluids that may be highly infectious. It is of extreme importance that your health and safety, as well as the health and safety of your patients, be protected.

This chapter focuses on the federal regulations of the Clinical Laboratory Improvement Amendments (CLIA) and the Occupational Safety and Health Administration (OSHA) in relation to the providers' office laboratory (POL). CLIA and OSHA, together with the Centers of Disease Control and Prevention (CDC), regulate the safety of patients and health care workers. The purpose of CLIA is to safeguard the public by regulating all testing of specimens taken from the human body. The purpose of OSHA is to require employers to ensure employee safety in regard to occupational exposure to potentially harmful substances. Table 37-1 summarizes the guidelines and purposes of CDC, CLIA, and OSHA.

CLINICAL LABORATORY IMPROVEMENT AMENDMENTS (CLIA)

Safety

CLIA was designed to set safety policies and procedures that protect patients. In 1988, there was a public outcry as a result of articles published in the *Washington Post* and the *Wall Street Journal* and televised reports of deaths that were attributed to misread Pap smears. The public wanted action taken to ensure its safety, particularly in regard to laboratory testing. The outcry prompted the federal government to become more involved in regulating laboratories.

Legal

Although clinical laboratory controls were enacted into law in 1967, the issue of the misread Pap smears caused Congress to reexamine its regulations. Thus, CLIA'88 was passed that included amendments to the original law.

TABLE 37-1

FEDERAL HEALTH AND SAFETY GUIDELINES

GUIDELINES	ISSUING AGENCY	PURPOSE
Standard Precautions	Centers for Disease Control and Prevention (CDC)	To enhance Universal Precautions and techniques known as body substance isolation (BSI). Standard Precautions contain measures intended to protect all health care providers, patients, and visitors from infectious diseases.
Transmission-Based Precautions	CDC	Designed to reduce the risk for airborne, droplet, and contact transmission of pathogens. These are used in addition to Standard Precautions and are intended for specific categories of patients.
Universal Blood and Body Fluid Precautions (Universal Precautions)	CDC	To assist health care providers to greatly reduce the risk for contracting or transmitting infectious diseases, particularly AIDS and hepatitis B.
Clinical Laboratory Improvement Amendments of (CLIA)	Centers for Medicare & Medicaid Services (CMS), U.S. Department of Health and Human Services (DHHS)	Safeguards the public by regulating all testing of specimens taken from the body.
Occupational Safety and Health Administration (OSHA) Guidelines	OSHA, U.S. Department of Labor	Requires employers to ensure employee safety in regard to occupational exposure to potentially harmful substances.
Globally Harmonized System (GHS)	United Nations; also coincides with OSHA's SDS	Defines and classifies chemical hazards and communicates around the world for health and safety. Pictograms are an important part of the system to lessen language barriers.

States can seek exemptions from CLIA standards if they have regulations that are comparable to those imposed by CLIA. If the federal government grants the state an exemption, laboratories in that state are under the control of state standards and applicable fees, not federal standards and fees.

The Intention of CLIA

Legal

The intent of CLIA is to protect the public by regulating all laboratory tests performed on specimens taken from the human body, that is, tissue, blood, and body secretions and excretions, which are used in the diagnosis, treatment, and prevention of disease. The regulations require that all laboratories in the United States and its territories meet performance requirements that are based on how complex a test is and the risk factors associated with incorrect test results. Laboratories must comply with the requirements to be certified by the DHHS.

It is necessary to understand what CLIA regulations encompass and how they impact medical assistants and other health care workers who participate in testing human specimens because all laboratories, including POLs, must abide by the CLIA law. Data indicate that CLIA has helped to improve the quality of testing in the United States. The total number of quality deficiencies has decreased significantly from the first laboratory survey to the second.

General Program Description

Congress passed CLIA in 1988, establishing quality standards for all laboratory testing to ensure the accuracy, reliability, and timeliness of patient test results regardless of where the test was performed. A laboratory is defined as any facility that performs laboratory testing on specimens derived from humans for the purpose of providing information for the diagnosis, prevention, or treatment of disease, or impairment or assessment of health.

Regulations are based on the complexity of the test method; thus, the more complicated the test, the more stringent the requirements. Tests are categorized into waived tests, moderate complexity tests, **provider-performed microscopy procedures (PPMP)**, and high-complexity tests. CLIA specifies quality standards for proficiency testing, patient test management, **quality control**, personnel qualifications, and **quality assurance** as applicable. Because problems in cytology laboratories were the impetus for CLIA, there are also specific cytology requirements.

The Centers for Medicare & Medicaid Services (CMS) is charged with the implementation of CLIA, including laboratory registration, fee collection, surveys, surveyor guidelines and training, enforcement, approvals of providers, accrediting organizations, and exempt states.

To enroll in the CLIA program, laboratories must first register by completing an application, pay fees, be surveyed if applicable, and become certified. Waived and PPMP laboratories may apply directly for their certificate because they are not subject to routine inspections. Laboratories that must be surveyed routinely are those performing moderate- or high-complexity testing.

1. One of five certificates can be obtained:
   a. *Certificate of Waiver (COW)*. This certificate is issued to a laboratory to perform only waived tests.
   b. *Certificate for PPMP.* This certificate is issued to a laboratory in which a provider, mid-level practitioner, or dentist performs no moderate-complexity tests other than the PPMP procedures. This certificate permits the laboratory to also perform waived tests.
   c. *Certificate of Registration.* This certificate enables the entity to conduct moderate- and high-complexity laboratory testing until the entity is determined by survey to be in compliance with CLIA regulations.
   d. *Certificate of Compliance.* This certificate is issued to a laboratory after an inspection finds the laboratory to be in compliance with all applicable CLIA requirements.
   e. *Certificate of Accreditation.* This is a certificate that is issued to a laboratory on the basis of the laboratory's accreditation by an organization approved by CMS.

Table 37-2 shows the level of CLIA certifications.

Categories of Testing

CLIA has designated three main categories of testing and one subcategory, and each of these categories has different requirements for personnel and quality control.

1. **Waived** tests are simple, are unvarying, and require a minimum of judgment and interpretation. Test error carries minimal hazard to the patient. Waived tests represent the lowest percentage of the total number of tests performed and is the category for

TABLE 37-2

HOW TO TELL WHAT LEVEL OF CLIA IS REQUIRED

IF THESE TESTS ARE PERFORMED	THIS TYPE OF CERTIFICATE AND/OR SURVEY IS NEEDED
Waived tests only	Certificate of Waiver (COW)
Provider-performed microscopy procedure (PPMP)	Certificate of PPMP
Tests of moderate complexity	Certificate of Registration, CLIA survey, and Certificate of Compliance
Tests of high complexity	Certificate of Registration, survey by an accrediting agency, and Certificate of Accreditation

medical assistants performing laboratory test in the POL.

2. Moderate-complexity tests require a higher degree of training, personnel licensing, and more strict regulations. PPMP tests are moderate-complexity tests but represent a subcategory that was added at the request of providers (Table 37-3).

3. High-complexity tests include the most complex tests and have the highest level of qualification for personnel and regulations.

TABLE 37-3

EXAMPLES OF PROVIDER-PERFORMED MICROSCOPY PROCEDURES

All direct wet-mount preparations for the presence or absence of bacteria, fungi, parasites, and human cellular elements
All potassium hydroxide (KOH) preparations
Pinworm examinations
Fern tests
Postcoital direct, qualitative examinations of vaginal or cervical mucus
Urine sediment examinations
Nasal smears for granulocytes
Fecal leukocyte examinations
Qualitative semen analysis (limited to the presence or absence of sperm and detection of motility)

The following criteria are used to categorize moderate- and high-complexity tests:

- The degree of operator intervention needed
- The necessary knowledge and experience the operator possesses
- The degree of maintenance and troubleshooting needed to perform the tests

Even though most of the tests medical assistants perform fall into the waived category, POLs will often perform moderate-complexity tests, including the PPMP tests. POLs are not limited to any category as long as they have sufficiently trained and credentialed personnel, equipment, and approval.

Manufacturers of self-contained test kits apply for and receive Food and Drug Administration (FDA) approval for their particular test to be on the CLIA waived list. To find out if your particular brand of self-contained test kit is on the CLIA waived list, access an up-to-date listing at the FDA website (http://www.fda.gov) and use the key search term "Currently Waived Analytes" (be forewarned, though, that the list is very long).

Contents of the Law

Legal

The contents of CLIA are long and detailed and are available online at the CLIA website (www.cms.gov/clia). Most of the regulations are specific to nonwaived tests and laboratories that perform complex tests. See Table 37-4 for specific regulations of the waived testing categories that are applicable to medical assistants. CLIA requires that documentation be maintained for the categories listed in Table 37-5.

TABLE 37-4

SYNOPSIS OF CLIA CONTENTS RELATED TO THE WAIVED CATEGORY

All labs required to register regardless of size and category
A certificate (on CMS form 116) required to perform any tests
Waived category certification required, with renewal every 2 years
CMS must be notified within 6 months if changes occur in type of tests performed
Sanctions or penalties may be imposed for non-compliance
Requirements for correct collection, transport, storage, and reporting of results
CLIA maintains a list of laboratories that have had actions taken against them
Documentation must be maintained for all areas of sample processing (Table 37-5)

CMS Form 116. CMS form 116 for the clinical laboratory collects information regarding a laboratory's operation and is needed in order to evaluate fees, determine baseline data, update existing data, and fulfill legal requirements. The information obtained from the application will give the surveyor of the laboratory a perspective of the laboratory's operation and whether it will be subject to an on-site inspection.

Criteria for PPMP

To be categorized as a PPMP, the procedure must meet the following criteria:

1. The examination must be personally performed by the provider. Depending on state law, mid-level providers may require supervision.
2. The procedure must be categorized as moderately complex.
3. The primary instrument for performing the test is the microscope.
4. The specimen is **labile** (easily broken down), or a delay in performing the test could compromise the accuracy of the test result.
5. Control materials are not available to monitor the entire testing process.
6. Limited specimen handling or processing is required.

TABLE 37-5

CLIA DOCUMENTATION REQUIREMENTS

Specimen	Patient preparation
	Specimen collection procedure
	Proper labeling
	Preservation of specimen if applicable
Proficiency Testing	Corrective action taken
Quality Control and Quality Assurance	Any corrective action taken
Problem and Complaint Log	Patient name, birth date, identification or record number
	Name and address of laboratory
	Date and time of collection
	Name of test requested
	Working diagnosis
Results	Name and address of laboratory where test is performed
	Test name
	Test results, including normal ranges
	Disposition of unacceptable specimens
Log of Test Results	Printouts from instruments report
	Identification of person performing test
	Patient identification number
	Specimen identification
	Date and time specimen received and tested
	Specimen rejection log
	Results and dates of all tests done

Criteria for CLIA-Waived Tests

To be categorized as a laboratory performing waived tests, the procedures must meet the following criteria:

1. The tests must be simple laboratory examinations and procedures that are cleared by the FDA for home use, use methods that are simple and accurate so errors are negligible, or pose no reasonable risk for harm to the patient if performed incorrectly.
2. The tests performed must be on CLIA's waived test list.
3. The manufacturer's instructions for performing the tests must be followed.
4. Minimal scientific and technical knowledge is required to perform the test, or knowledge required to perform the test may be obtained through on-the-job instruction.
5. Minimal training is required for preanalytic, analytic, and postanalytic phases of the testing process, or limited experience is required to perform the test.
6. Reagents and materials are generally stable and reliable, or reagents and materials are prepackaged; premeasured; or require no special handling, precautions, or storage conditions.
7. Operational steps are either automatically executed (such as pipetting, temperature monitoring, or timing of steps) or easily controlled.
8. Calibration of quality-control materials are stable and readily available, and external proficiency testing materials, when available, are stable.
9. Test system troubleshooting is automatic or self-correcting, clearly described, or requires minimal judgment, and equipment maintenance is provided by the manufacturer, is seldom needed, or can be performed easily.
10. Minimal interpretation and judgment are required to perform preanalytic, analytic, and postanalytic processes, and resolution of problems requires limited independent interpretation and judgment.

CLIA Regulation for Quality Control in Automated Hematology

CLIA regulations require that three different procedures be performed in the quality-control protocol for automated hematology instruments. The procedures are regularly scheduled calibration, control sample testing each day prior to patient testing, and proficiency testing.

Impact of CLIA on Medical Assistants

Legal

CLIA requires every facility that tests human specimens for diagnosis, treatment, and prevention of disease to meet specific federal requirements. The law applies to any facility that performs tests for the preceding purposes. This includes any POLs and ambulatory care settings, two typical areas where medical assistants are employed. The law covers all facilities even if only one test or a few basic tests are done and even if there is no charge for the testing.

Medical assistants may be responsible not only for performing the tests but also for maintaining personnel records, including such information as education records and diplomas, state licenses, national certifications, continuing education, and recredentialing. Medical assistants may be involved with compiling a procedures manual on how to perform every test done; these must be reviewed every year. An instrument log must be available for each piece of equipment. Systems must be in place for calibration, quality control, quality assurance, and documentation.

Medical assistants are the only health care professionals trained specifically for the ambulatory setting, including the POL procedures. Lacking a medical laboratory technician or medical technologist in the POL, the burden of quality performance of the waived tests falls to the person specifically trained in that area, the medical assistant. Because laboratory training of the medical assistant focuses primarily on CLIA-waived tests, it is of major concern that medical assisting programs offer the best training possible in the areas of quality assurance, quality control, and following manufacturer's instructions. Keep in mind that the medical assistant may be the only health care professional in the POL who has formal training in the performance of the waived laboratory tests. Add that to the received findings of errors in processes at COW and PPMP laboratories, and medical assistants are definitely on the front lines of ensuring the best quality for test results performed in the POLs.

Where to Find More Information Regarding CLIA

You can obtain a list of categories and the complete CLIA guidelines from the CDC Web site (http://www.cdc.gov and use key search term "CLIA").

OSHA REGULATIONS

OSHA regulations are intended to ensure employers have a safe and healthy work environment for their employees. This applies to all workers, not just health care workers. Some of the regulations include hard hats and steel-toed shoes for construction workers, safety switches for machinery, fire prevention equipment in restaurants, and, of course, safety equipment and supplies for health care workers. Two OSHA standards have the greatest impact on medical personnel: *The Occupational Exposure to Hazardous Chemicals Standard* (expanded from *The Hazard Communication Standard* [*HCS*]) and *The Bloodborne Pathogen Standard*. *The Bloodborne Pathogen Standard* is reviewed in Chapter 21. This chapter discusses *The Occupational Exposure to Hazardous Chemicals Standard*. It is important to note that states have their own worker safety standards. Those state standards are required to be as strict or stricter than the federal OSHA standards.

The Standard for Occupational Exposure to Hazardous Chemicals in the Laboratory

In an effort to reduce the number of chemically related illnesses and injuries in the workplace, OSHA published its *Hazard Communications Standard* in 1983. This led many states to develop *right-to-know* laws. In 1992, OSHA expanded the *Hazard Communications Standard* and published *The Occupational Exposure to Hazardous Chemicals in the Laboratory Standard,* which specifically addresses clinical laboratories.

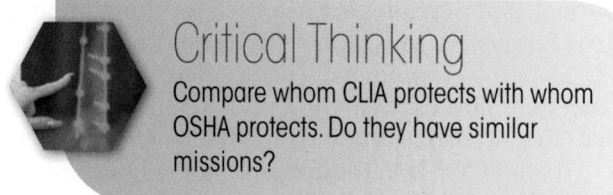

Critical Thinking

Compare whom CLIA protects with whom OSHA protects. Do they have similar missions?

The intention of this law is to heighten employee awareness of risks related to chemical exposure. It serves to improve work practices through employee training and identification of hazardous chemicals that exist in the workplace and the use of protective equipment to safeguard employees from harmful chemicals.

In 2012 the United States aligned HCS with the UN (United Nations) 2003 Globally Harmonized System of Classification and Labeling of Chemicals (GHS) (Figure 37-1) in order to improve the quality and consistency of handling chemicals in the workplace.

Chemical Hygiene Plan (CHP)

Legal

The Chemical Hygiene Plan (CHP) on hazardous chemicals is the core of the OSHA safety standard on hazardous chemicals. Certain specific control measures such as **fume hoods** and other safety features must be included in the plan. A designated employee is the chemical hygiene or safety officer. Provisions for housekeeping and maintenance of the facility are included. OSHA standards are not

---

STANDARDIZED CHEMICAL LABEL ELEMENTS

The standardized label elements included in the GHS are:

Symbols (hazard pictograms): Convey health, physical, and environmental hazard information, assigned to a GHS hazard class and category.

Signal Words: "Danger" or "Warning" are used to emphasize hazards and indicate the relative level of severity of the hazard, assigned to a GHS hazard class and category.

Hazard Statements: Standard phrases assigned to a hazard class and category that describe the nature of the hazard.

The symbols, signal words, and hazard statements have all been standardized and assigned to specific hazard categories and classes, as appropriate. This approach makes it easier for countries to implement the system and should make it easier for companies to comply with regulations based on the GHS.

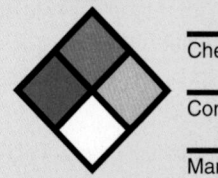

Chemical Name

Common Name

Manufacturer

FIGURE 37-1 Standardized label elements included in the Globally Harmonized System.

optional, and penalties are imposed for noncompliance. Employers must meet the requirements not only to be in compliance with the law but also to protect employees. (See the Quick Reference Guide titled "Requirements of a Chemical Hygiene Plan.")

To meet OSHA regulations, all laboratories and ambulatory care settings, including providers' offices, must be in compliance with a chemical hygiene plan. The primary component of the OSHA standard is that a written chemical hygiene plan and program must be operational if chemicals are stored in a facility and handled by employees. Some examples of chemicals include, but are not limited to, stains, ethyl alcohol, sodium hypochlorite (household bleach), formaldehyde, fixatives, preservatives, injectables such as chemotherapeutic agents, and acetone. Many laboratory accidents result in chemical-related illnesses ranging from eye irritation to pulmonary edema.

There are three primary goals that an employer must accomplish to be in compliance with the OSHA standard for chemical exposure. The first is that there must be an inventory taken and a list compiled of all chemicals considered hazardous. The following information must be documented on a Chemical Inventory Form (Figure 37-2): the quantity of chemicals stored per month or year; whether the substance is gas, liquid, or solid; the manufacturer's name and address; and the chemical hazard classification.

Second, a **Safety Data Sheet (SDS),** previously called a Material Safety Data Sheet (MSDS) (see Figure 37-3), manual must be assembled. The SDS are provided by the manufacturer when the chemicals are purchased and give detailed information about the chemicals. The SDS should be organized into a notebook for employee use and located in an area where employees can immediately access it. Every employee who is exposed to or works with chemicals must read the SDS about those chemicals and know where the manual is kept.

The various chemicals containers are labeled using the National Fire Protection Association's color and number method, while the SDS show the GHS numbering system. These two numbering systems are different, which can be confusing; however, the information on the labels is consistent

⬧ QUICK REFERENCE GUIDE

≫ REQUIREMENTS OF A CHEMICAL HYGIENE PLAN

Documentation

- Employers must have an operational written plan (a manual) relevant to the safety and health of employees.
- Written instructions on the use of PPE must be available.

Protocols

- Fume hoods or biohazard hoods must be checked regularly.

Training

- Training sessions must be held for employees regarding their right to know what hazardous chemicals are in their work environment.
- Instruction must be provided regarding disposal of hazardous waste produced in the workplace. (Usually a hazardous waste company is contracted by the employer.)

Employer Responsibility

- It is the employer's legal responsibility to provide medical attention for an employee should an accidental chemical spill and possible exposure occur.
- The responsibility for executing training sessions, keeping manuals current, and documenting is designated to an employee.
- Each employee's record must have a written statement, signed by the employer, stating the employer's responsibility to arrange for employee training and a safe work environment.

SAMPLE

CHEMICAL INVENTORY FORM

Office of _____

Date _____

Chemical Name	Catalog #	Quantity Stores L./gm. (monthly)	Physical State	Hazard Class				Manufacturer	Comments
				H	F	R	P		

(H) Health
0 - Minimal
1 - Slightly
2 - Moderate
3 - Serious
4 - Extreme

(F) Fire Hazard
0 - Will not burn
1 - Slight
2 - Moderate
3 - Serious
4 - Extreme

(R) Reactivity
0 - Stable is not reactive
　　with water
1 - Slight
2 - Moderate
3 - Serious
4 - Extreme

(P) Protection
A. - Goggles
B. - Goggles/Gloves
C. - Goggles/Gloves/Apron
D. - Face Shield/Gloves/Apron
E. - Goggles/Gloves/Mask
F. - Goggles/Gloves/Apron/Mask
X. - Gloves

FIGURE 37-2   Sample chemical inventory form for listing chemicals on the premises, including the quantity, physical state, hazard class, manufacturer, and comments.

Courtesy of POL Consultants, 2 Russ Farm Way, Delanco, NJ 08075, 856-824-0800

(see Figures 37-4 and 37-5). Each chemical label must contain the following:

1. Product name or identifier
2. Pictograms
3. Signal word (*Danger* or *Warning*)
4. Hazard statements
5. Precautionary statements
6. Name, address, and telephone number of the chemical manufacturer, importer, or other responsible party

Third, the employer is required to provide a hazard communication educational program to each employee within 30 days of employment and before the employee handles any hazardous chemicals. The training program should address locating and identifying hazardous chemicals, how to read and understand the labels on the chemicals, where the SDS manual is kept, how to interpret the GHS coloring and labeling system, when to use PPE, and procedures to follow for chemical spills. The training sessions must be documented, signed by the employer, and permanently retained in the employee's record (see Figure 37-6).

Importance of the Chemical Standard to Medical Assistants. Meeting the requirements set forth by OSHA is not optional. All must comply or face penalties. All employees,

Legal

HAZARD COMMUNICATION SAFETY DATA SHEETS

The Hazard Communication Standard (HCS) requires chemical manufacturers, distributors, or importers to provide Safety Data Sheets (SDSs) (formerly known as Material Safety Data Sheets or MSDSs) to communicate the hazards of hazardous chemical products. As of June 1, 2015, the HCS will require new SDSs to be in a uniform format, and include the section numbers, the headings, and associated information under the headings below:

Section 1, Identification includes product identifier; manufacturer or distributor name, address, phone number; emergency phone number; recommended use; restrictions on use.

Section 2, Hazard(s) identification includes all hazards regarding the chemical; required label elements.

Section 3, Composition/information on ingredients includes information on chemical ingredients; trade secret claims.

Section 4, First-aid measures includes important symptoms/ effects, acute, delayed; required treatment.

Section 5, Fire-fighting measures lists suitable extinguishing techniques, equipment, chemical hazards from fire.

Section 6, Accidental release measures lists emergency procedures; protective equipment; proper methods of containment and cleanup.

Section 7, Handling and storage lists precautions for safe handling and storage, including incompatibilities.

Section 8, Exposure controls/personal protection lists OSHA's Permissible Exposure Limits (PELs); ACGIH Threshold Limit Values (TLVs); and any other exposure limit used or recommended by the chemical manufacturer, importer, or employer preparing the SDS where available as well as appropriate engineering controls; personal protective equipment (PPE).

Section 9, Physical and chemical properties lists the chemical's characteristics.

Section 10, Stability and reactivity lists chemical stability and possibility of hazardous reactions.

Section 11, Toxicological information includes routes of exposure; related symptoms, acute and chronic effects; numerical measures of toxicity.

Section 12, Ecological information*

Section 13, Disposal considerations*

Section 14, Transport information*

Section 15, Regulatory information*

Section 16, Other information, includes the date of preparation or last revision.

*Note: Since other Agencies regulate this information, OSHA will not be enforcing Sections 12 through 15(29 CFR 1910.1200(g)(2)).

Employers must ensure that SDSs are readily accessible to employees. See Appendix D of 1910.1200 for a detailed description of SDS contents.

FIGURE 37-3 Example of a Safety Data Sheet (SDS) listing the required 16 categories.

Source: Occupational Safety and Health Administration, U.S. Department of Labor

1. Product identifier	**Sulfuric Acid**
2. Pictogram(s)	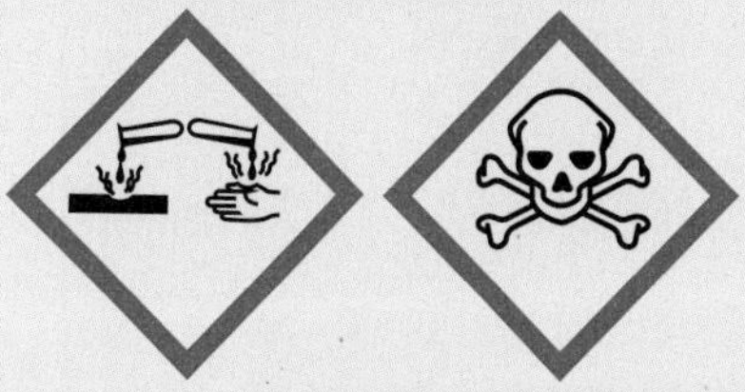
3. Signal Words	**Danger**
4. Hazard Statement	**Causes severe skin burns and eye damage.** **Fatal if inhaled, harmful to aquatic life**
5. Precautionary Statement	**Do Not breathe dust/fume/gas/vapors/sprays** **Wear protective gloves, cloths, eye, and face protection**
6. Supplier Information	**Supply Company, River City, XY, 12345** **Phone: 555-555-0123, Fax: 555-555-0234**

FIGURE 37-4 Safety Data Sheet information requirements for the Globally Harmonized System.

HCS Pictogram	Hazard	HCS Pictogram	Hazard	HCS Pictogram	Hazard
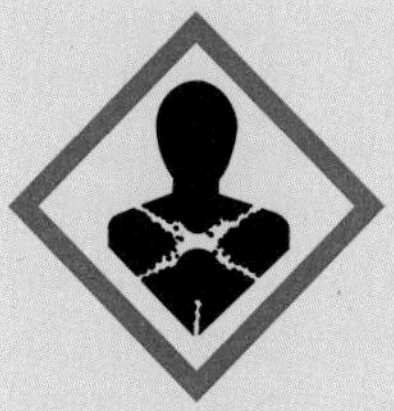	Health Hazard (long term)	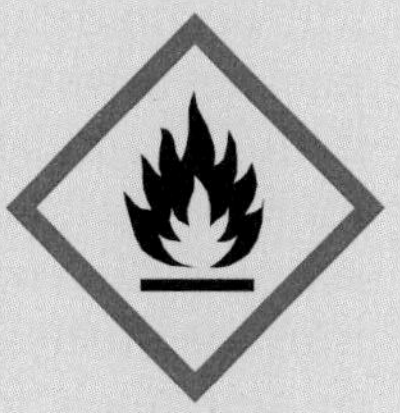	Flame	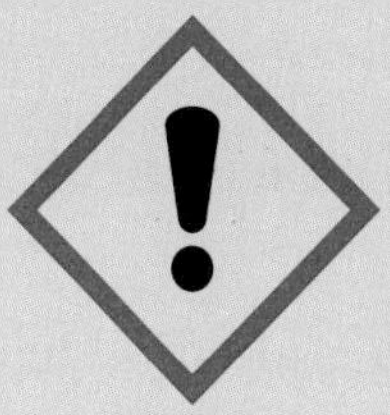	Exclamation Mark (immediate health hazard)
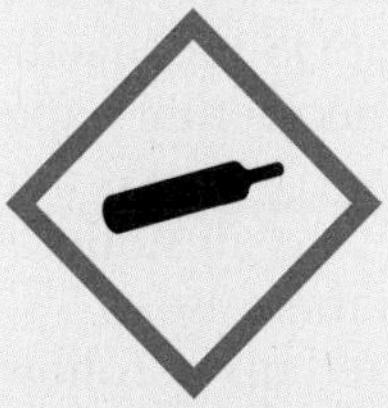	Gas Cylinder	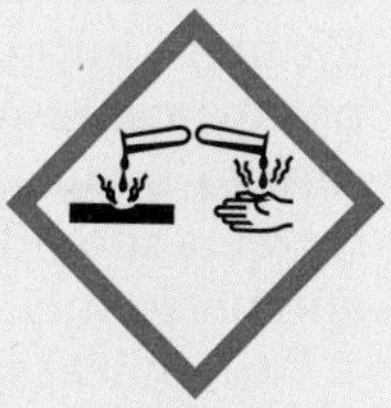	Corrosion	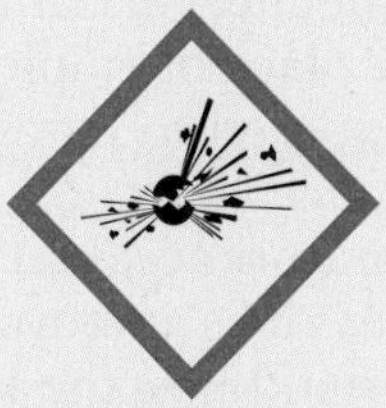	Exploding Bomb
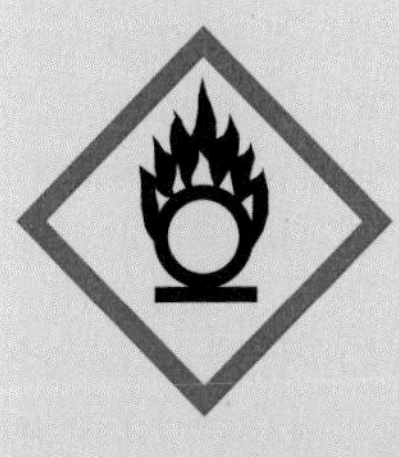	Flame over Circle (oxidizers)	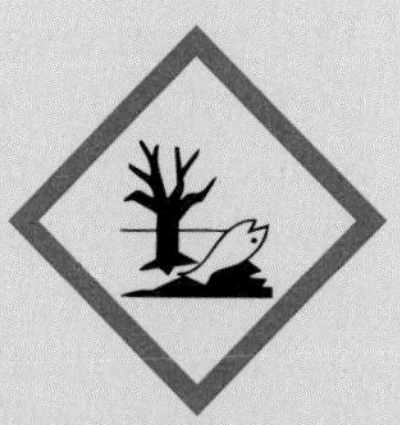	Environment (Non-mandatory)	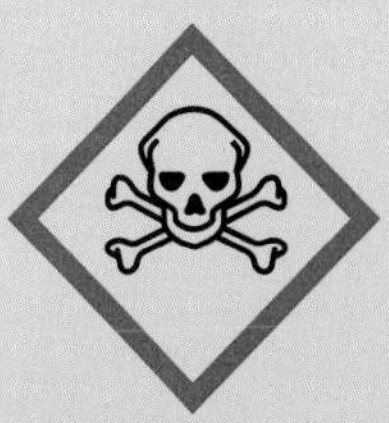	Skull and Crossbones (toxicity)

FIGURE 37-5 Pictograms of the *Hazard Communication Standard*.

Source: Occupational Safety and Health Administration, U.S. Department of Labor

SAMPLE

CERTIFICATE OF TRAINING

_____

First Name   Middle Initial   Last Name

has completed the

OSHA HAZARD COMMUNICATION
INFORMATION TRAINING PROGRAM

This certificate indicates your successful participation in a program instructing you of your rights as a worker and the proper handling of hazardous substances in the workplace.

_____   _____
Date   Employee Signature

_____
Instructor's Signature

_____
Employer's Signature

FIGURE 37-6 Sample certificate of training shows that the employee has completed an OSHA Hazard Communication Information Training Program.

including medical assistants, have the right to know about, be given information, and be educated regarding chemical hazards that they are exposed to in their place of employment. Medical assistants can be exposed to hazardous chemicals through skin contact, injection, or inhalation. Because many laboratory accidents result in chemical-related illnesses, it is important for medical assistants to understand how the law affects them, their place of employment, and their employer. Medical assistants and other health care providers should know what hazards they face, as well

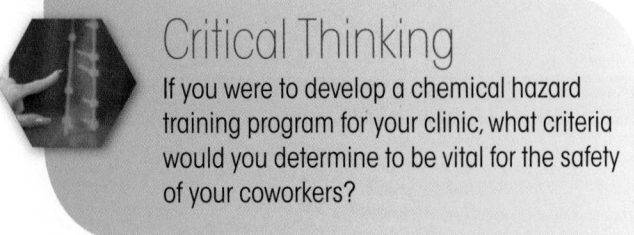

Critical Thinking

If you were to develop a chemical hazard training program for your clinic, what criteria would you determine to be vital for the safety of your coworkers?

as the proper technique for handling, storing, and disposing of hazardous chemicals. Medical assistants in administrative positions must use their knowledge and skills to provide a safe work environment for themselves and their staff.

OSHA REGULATIONS AND STUDENTS

All students with potential exposure to chemicals and bloodborne pathogens should follow all safety procedures as outlined by OSHA. Because students and unpaid volunteers in educational programs are not considered employees of a health care facility and are attending an educational institution, they do not fall under the OSHA guidelines. They should, however, take precautions to avoid contact with potentially infectious materials and toxic chemicals wherever learning is taking place. Instructors within medical assisting programs, as employees of the school, do fall under OSHA.

Avoiding Exposure to Chemicals

Students may come into contact with harmful chemicals when doing procedures that can cause such problems as burns to the skin and eyes. Students will be made aware of these through information packaged with kits and the SDS. As a general rule, if the chemical comes in contact with the skin, it must be flushed with water immediately and for five minutes afterward. Chemicals that get into the eye must be flushed for 15 minutes (unless contradicted on the label) followed by immediate medical care. See the "Eyewash Stations" Quick Reference Guide for more information. Refer to the SDS for specific postexposure procotol. In case of accidental exposure to hazardous chemicals, eyewash stations and showers should be readily available and all students and personnel should be trained in their use.

Chemical spills should be cleaned up by following the SDS procedure for the particular chemical. The same chemical biohazard spill cleanup kits used in POLs can be used in school laboratories. Students should be familiar with the contents of the kits and proficient in their use before an actual spill occurs.

Toxic fumes can occur with certain chemicals and certain tests can cause lung irritation and damage. This type of chemical should be handled under a fume hood that will exhaust the fumes by means of a ventilation system.

A student safety laboratory manual outlining an exposure control plan with emphasis on Standard Precautions, PPE, work practice controls, lists of

Eyewash Stations

- Eyewash stations must be readily available to employees wherever chemical exposure is possible
- Eyewash stations must be able to provide copious amounts of clean water at a low even pressure
- Eye flushing should begin immediately after exposure and continue for 20 minutes
- Eye wash stations must be regularly maintained
- Workers should receive training on the use of eyewash stations
- Medical attention should be obtained immediately after flushing

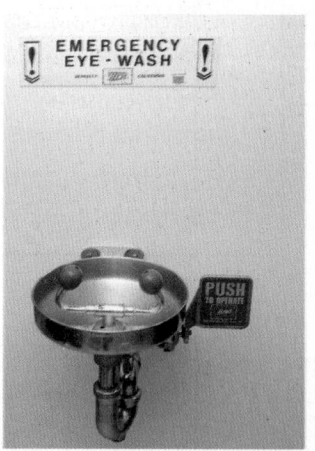

hazardous chemicals, and SDS should be compiled and accessible. Students should be thoroughly familiar with its contents. In addition, students should be educated as to the location and identification of hazardous chemicals just as employees are.

It is of utmost importance that students learn about and understand the OSHA standards and comply with them. In so doing, they will safeguard themselves from harmful chemicals and blood-borne pathogens.

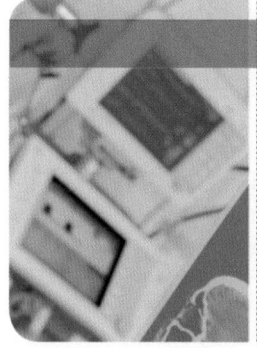

CASE STUDY 37-1

Refer to the scenario at the beginning of the chapter. Gwen examines the microscope slide even though the procedure is not a waived test. She compares her findings to Dr. Reynolds's assessment.

CASE STUDY REVIEW

1. Besides learning more about microscopic examinations and continuing her education, what benefit does Gwen obtain by putting forth this extra effort?
2. Do you think Dr. Reynolds will appreciate her extra effort?

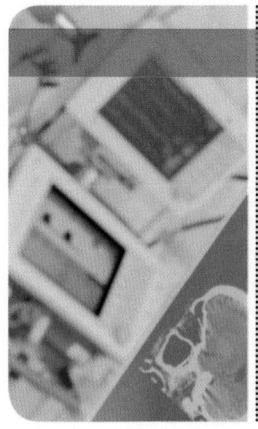

CASE STUDY 37-2

Marie Tyndall is a student in the Jackson Heights Community College Medical Assisting Program. She and two classmates have been assigned the project of creating a plan for cleaning up spills that might occur in the classroom laboratory and ensuring that all students using the laboratory have been trained in the proper procedure.

CASE STUDY REVIEW

1. What materials would her group need?
2. How would her group go about learning the proper steps in the cleanup process?
3. How would her group ensure that all other students in the laboratory also have the proper training?

- The spread of infectious diseases and accidents in the workplace can be prevented through education and safe practices.

- Medical assistants must understand the importance of the regulations and guidelines set forth by the federal government and follow through by helping employers implement them.

- Every medical office and ambulatory care setting must, by law, have clearly written and readily available manuals containing information about Standard Precautions, CLIA, and OSHA for the safe handling, storage, and disposal of blood, body fluids, and chemicals.

- Through consistent use of Standard Precautions and adherence to the CLIA and OSHA laws, health care providers can acquire the behaviors and techniques needed to safeguard themselves and their patients.

- Because of frequent changes in the laws, it is necessary for medical assistants and all other health care providers to keep abreast of the government mandates.

Study for Success

To reinforce your knowledge and skills of information presented in this chapter:

- Review the *Key Terms* and *Learning Outcomes*
- Consider the *Critical Thinking* features and *Case Studies* and discuss your conclusions
- Answer the questions in the *Certification Review*

CERTIFICATION REVIEW

1. What information do Safety Data Sheets contain?
   a. Flammability of the chemical
   b. Cost of the chemical per use
   c. Shelf life of the chemical
   d. Other chemical options available

2. Standard Precautions were issued by which agency?
   a. DHHS
   b. CDC
   c. CMS
   d. OSHA
   e. CLIA

3. Why was CLIA needed?
   a. To control the disposal of infectious waste
   b. For safety in the use of chemicals in the workplace
   c. To maintain quality of laboratory tests performed on specimens taken from the human body
   d. To prevent the transmission of the human immunodeficiency virus (HIV)

4. Which of the following is the core of the OSHA safety standard for chemical exposure?
   a. The employee safety manual
   b. The chemical hygiene plan
   c. The chemical control logs
   d. The SDS manual
   e. The chemical inventory form

5. Which is the agency that requires employers to ensure employee safety related to exposure to potentially harmful substances?
   a. CDC
   b. U.S. Public Health Service
   c. CMS
   d. OSHA

6. Which agency is charged with implementing CLIA?
   a. CDC
   b. U.S. Public Health Service
   c. CMS
   d. OSHA
   e. Clinical Laboratory Standards Institute (CLSI)

7. Which of the following does CLIA regulate?
   a. The chemicals used in the clinic
   b. The training of the personnel involved in testing
   c. The time allotted for the provider to respond to an abnormal test result
   d. The safety of the people within the laboratory
8. Medical assistants perform most of their tests in which CLIA category?
   a. Waived
   b. PPMP
   c. Noncomplex
   d. Moderately complex
   e. Highly complex
9. How many categories of testing are there in CLIA?
   a. 2
   b. 6
   c. More than 20
   d. 4
10. Which of the following does OSHA require?
    a. 15-minute breaks and at least a half hour for lunch for employees
    b. A COLA (cost of living) raise each year for employees
    c. Vacation time of at least one week a year for employees
    d. Personal protective equipment for employees
    e. Sufficient orientation period for employees

CHAPTER 38

Introduction to the Medical Laboratory

1. Define and spell the key terms as presented in the glossary.
2. Explain the reasons for performing laboratory testing.
3. Describe the main similarities and differences between an independent laboratory and a physicians' office laboratory (POL).
4. Explain the levels of laboratory personnel in relation to their education, skills, and duties, and where the medical assistant is placed in the hierarchy.
5. List eight different departments within the medical laboratory and determine the types of testing performed within each of those departments.
6. Name nine of the most common laboratory panels and explain the body system or function being surveyed.
7. Correlate the concepts of quality control and quality assurance in the medical laboratory.
8. Describe at least three methods of ensuring quality in the medical laboratory.
9. Demonstrate how to correctly complete a laboratory requisition.
10. Justify the rationale behind proper patient preparation before laboratory testing.
11. Explain where accurate and reliable information might be obtained about proper procurement, storage, and handling of laboratory specimens.
12. Demonstrate the proper use and care of a compound microscope.

KEY TERMS

baseline values	microbiology	quantitative tests
biopsy	mycology	reagents
clinical diagnosis	ova and parasite (O&P)	reference laboratories
control test	panel	reference ranges
cytology	parasitology	requisition
differential diagnosis	patient service centers	therapeutic drug monitoring (TDM)
DNA	peak	toxicology
hematology	physician's office laboratory (POL)	trough
histology	point-of-care testing (POCT)	virology
immunology	qualitative tests	

SCENARIO

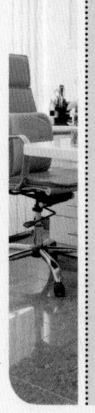

Dr. Winston Lewis's patient, Annette Samuels, has come into the Inner City Health Care clinic complaining of lower abdominal cramps and diarrhea. After discussion of her symptoms and a brief examination, Dr. Lewis's clinical diagnosis is an intestinal parasite infection. She asks Gwen Carr, CMA (AAMA), to obtain a stool sample from the patient. The sample will be sent to an outside independent lab to see if the parasite or its eggs can be visualized. This is called an **ova and parasite** test or O&P. Gwen is sensitive to Ms. Samuels's level of understanding as she gives her specific instructions on how to obtain the needed sample. She asks Ms. Samuels if she has questions and she has Annette repeat the instructions to be sure she understands them. When Ms. Samuels returns with the specimen, Gwen immediately labels it, and follows infection control protocol as she places it into a biohazard transport bag, then completes a lab requisition for the O&P test. Gwen reassures Ms. Samuels that the culture will take 24 to 48 hours, and responds honestly and diplomatically to Ms. Samuels's needs, assuring her that the test results will accurately determine her best treatment. Gwen tells Ms. Samuels that she will contact her the next day when the initial report is received.

f disease did not exist, we would have little need for clinical laboratories. If we were not susceptible to viral illnesses, if bacteria never infected our bodies, if our bodies always operated in their healthiest state regardless of what we did to them, and, perhaps most important of all, if we chose our parents wisely, there would be little that a clinical laboratory would be asked to do. But, since disease does exist and people do succumb to diseases and other conditions, clinics rely heavily on medical laboratories for patient care. Providers use laboratory tests to diagnose illnesses, assess patients' health, and manage chronic diseases such as diabetes and arthritis. Medical assistants working in clinics and laboratories may be responsible for patient preparation, obtaining specimens, and running the tests or sending specimens to outside independent laboratories. It is important for medical assistants to be aware of laboratory procedures to ensure accurate testing.

THE LABORATORY

The current health care environment offers numerous options in the methods used to process laboratory tests.

- The specimen may be obtained and the test performed within the physician's office laboratory (POL).
- The specimen may be procured and packaged for transport to a separate laboratory.
- The patient may be referred to a separate laboratory for collection and testing of the specimen.

Safety

Each laboratory setting has specific requirements for the training and qualifications of the health care personnel who work in that setting. The equipment, supplies, and paperwork, as well as the instructions given to the patient, are also determined by the type of laboratory. Whichever laboratory setting is selected, the focus should be on the safety of the public, the patient, and the health care personnel, while always maintaining quality testing to ensure accurate results.

Purposes of Laboratory Testing

Legal

Physicians depend on the ability of medical laboratories to help determine a patient's state of health or disease in some of the following ways.

To Record an Individual's State of Health. Blood tests may be performed periodically, usually during a routine physical examination, to be assured of healthy normal ranges, also known as **reference ranges.** Then in the future, if illness occurs, the patient's **baseline values** are available for comparison.

To Satisfy Employment, Insurance, or Legal Requirements. If an accident occurs, quite often blood is tested for the presence of drugs and alcohol. Such a determination can prove a person guilty or innocent of a crime. Sometimes, places of employment or life insurance companies request laboratory tests to be assured that their employees or clients are free of illegal or dangerous drugs. Employment-required drug and alcohol testing is a classic example of this reason for testing.

To Gain Statistics for Research and Clinical Trials. Laboratory tests are sometimes a part of the data gathered for research and for clinical trial information. When we read about the relationship between osteoporosis and hormone replacement therapy (HRT) that information has been gathered through research. Clinical trials might address the efficacy of certain medications, vitamins, and minerals on osteoporosis in women receiving HRT.

To Detect Asymptomatic Conditions or Diseases. Occasionally, a patient has no complaints of illness and is asymptomatic—that is, exhibits no symptoms that might be associated with a disease process—but during routine screening or testing in another, perhaps unrelated, area, a disorder may be discovered. An example is a young woman presenting at the office for an athletic physical. Routine urinalysis reveals she has a mild bladder infection, which is easily treated and of no concern to the sports physical requirements.

To Confirm a Clinical Diagnosis. When a patient reports specific symptoms and describes a particular condition (subjective information) and data are compiled through a clinical examination (objective information), the provider may be able to determine a diagnosis without the aid of laboratory tests. This is referred to as a **clinical diagnosis.** To confirm a clinical diagnosis, the provider orders laboratory tests. For example, a child has symptoms of a strep throat infection such as sudden onset of sore throat, fever, headache, and upset stomach. On visual examination, the provider discovers small abscesses on the child's tonsils. The provider is almost certain that the diagnosis will be strep throat, but a quick and simple strep test is performed to confirm the clinical diagnosis.

To Differentiate between Two or More Diseases.
Sometimes, a patient presents with a combination of symptoms that can be related to more than one condition. For the provider to diagnose accurately, a laboratory test is performed. In situations such as these, the provider chooses to perform the simplest and least invasive laboratory test to rule out a particular disease before requiring more extensive testing. This is known as a **differential diagnosis.** For example, if the child in the preceding case had a negative strep test but perhaps exhibited other more systemic symptoms, a blood test might confirm mononucleosis or another condition. The provider is then able to differentiate between the two diagnoses—strep throat and mononucleosis.

To Diagnose.
If symptoms are vague, thereby making a clinical diagnosis difficult for the provider, a series of laboratory tests may be required. Sometimes a **panel**, or group of related tests, is ordered. This helps narrow the field for diagnosis. For example, a patient presents with reports of severe fatigue, but preliminary testing does not indicate a diagnosis. Further testing will eventually either lead the provider in a specific direction or at least eliminate a wide variety of conditions.

To Determine the Effectiveness of Treatments.
After a patient has been diagnosed and has begun treatment, the provider monitors the patient's health to be sure that the treatment is therapeutic. For example, a patient diagnosed with epilepsy must take an effective amount of antiseizure medication. A blood test is used to check the level of medication in the patient's system. Sometimes, the provider wants to know the highest and lowest ranges of medication in the patient's blood to determine if the levels are within a therapeutic range, a process called **therapeutic drug monitoring (TDM)**, and to check for drug toxicity (if the drug level is too high). To measure the highest level of medication in the patient's blood serum (called the **peak**), the specimen is taken about a half hour after the patient has taken his or her regular dose of medicine. To measure the lowest level (called the **trough**), the specimen

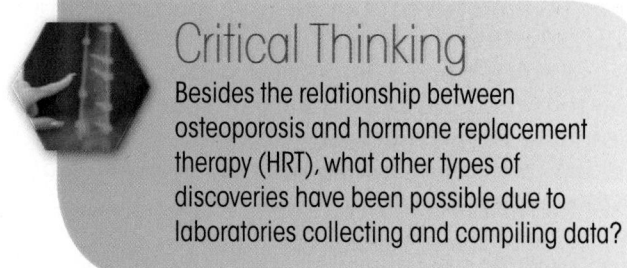

Critical Thinking
Besides the relationship between osteoporosis and hormone replacement therapy (HRT), what other types of discoveries have been possible due to laboratories collecting and compiling data?

is taken just before the patient takes his or her next scheduled dose of medicine. A periodic blood test can also be used to determine the effectiveness of dietary and lifestyle changes in reducing blood cholesterol levels.

To Prevent Diseases/Disorders.
Protection of the public, families, and co-workers can warrant laboratory tests. An example is protecting an unborn child from contracting genital herpes through the birthing process. A culture of the mother's cervical and vaginal mucosa helps to determine if the child is at risk. If the culture is positive, performing a caesarean (C-section) section is the treatment of choice to protect the newborn from contracting herpes. Because a newborn's immune system is not fully developed, herpes can cause serious illness and even death.

To Prevent the Exacerbation of Diseases.
Patients with chronic conditions require regular blood tests to prevent exacerbation of the disease. When the results of the blood test are obtained, the provider or patient determines whether it is necessary to adjust the diet or medication. For example, a patient with diabetes tests his or her blood regularly to measure the blood sugar, or glucose, level. If the blood sugar level is too high or too low, the patient may adjust the insulin dosage or have something to eat to return the blood sugar level to normal.

Types of Laboratories
There are many different types and locations of medical laboratories. They are identified by their size, capabilities, and affiliations. Independent laboratories may be located within medical centers or large clinics. They often have small satellite **patient service centers** located near more isolated medical facilities or in areas of convenience to patients. Satellite laboratories facilitate patients' specimens being obtained closer to their neighborhoods and ambulatory care settings. The specimens are

usually couriered back to the independent central laboratory for processing.

Hospital-based laboratories perform most of the tests required by that hospital, but even large hospitals use reference laboratories for specialized testing. **Reference laboratories** are independent, regionally located laboratories that service larger areas. Reference laboratories are used by hospitals and providers for complex, expensive, or specialized tests.

In a business sense, medical laboratories are quickly becoming more and more competitive. Growth and profitability depend on community relations and service, convenience, efficiency, cost, location, and even reputation. Competition often places the medical assistant and other medical personnel in a position of being asked to recommend a particular medical laboratory over another. Unless the provider has a valid reason for using a particular laboratory or not referring to a particular laboratory, the patient should choose the laboratory. The patient's insurance plan may also be a factor in determining which laboratory is used. Many insurance plans require the patient to use a particular laboratory or to choose a laboratory from those participating in the plan to guarantee payment for the tests. The medical assistant is then a resource for options rather than a referral service.

A laboratory physically set within the clinic is called a **physician's office laboratory (POL)**. Some of the more commonly performed medical laboratory tests can easily and inexpensively be performed in the office by the medical assistant. With a simple fingerstick and a few readily available medical supplies, a patient's blood glucose levels can be determined. Another commonly performed test in the ambulatory care setting is the urinalysis, in which urine is physically, chemically, and microscopically examined for irregularities. With the availability of the many varieties of self-contained kits, tests for strep throat, pregnancy, blood sugar (serum glucose) levels, and hidden (occult) blood in stool can be performed quickly. Other kits are being developed daily. Patients may use a kit at home that can be purchased without a prescription. Some of the home kits available to the general public are of the same quality as the kits used in medical offices. The major difference is that the person performing the test at home may not be trained, which may affect the accuracy of the test results. Consistent quality control measures might not be used by the

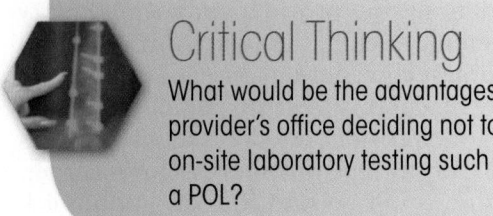

Critical Thinking

What would be the advantages of a provider's office deciding not to provide on-site laboratory testing such as in a POL?

nonmedical person (see Quality Control/Assurances in the Laboratory section). For example, a pregnancy test kit may be exposed to extreme temperatures while in the patient's care, on a grocer's shelf, or in the patient's home. These extreme temperatures may invalidate the chemical reaction in the test kit. More training, education, and credentialing are required as the complexity of the testing and equipment increases. (See CLIA in Chapter 37 for specific testing parameters.) If the results are not within normal limits, the provider needs to be consulted for confirmation and diagnosis/treatment.

Point-of-care testing (POCT) is sometimes referred to as near-patient testing or bedside testing, as it brings the laboratory services directly to the patient, wherever that may be. Medical conditions, location of the patient, and treatment methods often require laboratory results as quickly as possible so proper medical care can be administered without delay. POCT uses portable equipment and tests that provide rapid, accurate results when used correctly.

Laboratory Personnel

All independent medical laboratories must be managed by a pathologist, that is, a physician who specializes in disease processes. Additional staffing consists of clinical laboratory scientists, technicians, clinical laboratory assistants, phlebotomists, and medical assistants. Many agencies certify laboratory personnel. Table 38-1 gives specific information about laboratory personnel, their titles, training required, and duties performed within the clinical lab.

Professional

Laboratory Departments

Laboratories are usually divided into departments, which may then be further divided. There are many different options for laboratory organization, depending on the size and specialties

TABLE 38-1

LABORATORY PERSONNEL

CREDENTIAL/TITLE	EDUCATION REQUIRED	DUTIES PERFORMED
Physician Pathologist (MD) Scientist (PhD)	Board-certified medical doctor or PhD scientist (either must be CAP accredited)	Director of the lab Manages the laboratory Interprets biology results, Pap smears, and other cytology samples
Clinical Laboratory Scientist (CLS) Medical Technologist (MT) Registered Medical Technologist (RMT) Medical Laboratory Scientist (MLS)	Bachelor's degree in life sciences or medical technology, including 3 years of course work and 1 year of clinical experience Must be certified by ASCP, AMT, DHHS, ISCLT, NCA, or NRM	Qualified to perform analysis testing in all departments of the lab. Has leadership role; often trains, manages, and supervises other lab personnel; may perform routine lab tests as well as highly specialized lab tests. Troubleshoots problems with results, specimens, and/or instruments; works directly with the lab director/manager; performs quality control checks; evaluates new instruments implements new test procedures; often specializes in one area within the lab
Medical Laboratory Technician (MLT) Clinical Laboratory Technician (CLT)	Usually has associate's degree or certificate from an accredited MLT/CLT program May be certified by ASCP or NCA	Performs routine tests Performs microscopic exams and utilizes other lab equipment May specialize in one area in the lab
Phlebotomist/Phlebotomy Technician (PBT [ASCP]) Registered Phlebotomy Technician (RPT [AMT]) Certified Phlebotomy Technician (CPT [ASPT]) Clinical Laboratory Phlebotomist (CLP [AMT])	High school and additional phlebotomy training through a certificate program or on-the-job training; may be certified through ASCP AMT, ASPT, or NCA, and registered under state law	Performs venipuncture and skin puncture; may perform CLIA-waived testing; collects specimens Processes specimens for transport
Certified Medical Assistant (CMA [AAMA]) Registered Medical Assistant (RMA [AMT])	Generally, an associate's degree or certificate from an ABHES- or CAAHEP-accredited program in a community college, technical school, or proprietary school May be certified through AAMA or AMT May be registered under state law	May perform routine specimen procurement and waived testing as well as administrative duties, receptioning, computerized record-keeping, and billing Often works in POL

Credentialing associations: AAMA, American Association of Medical Assistants; ABHES, Accrediting Bureau of Health Education Schools; ASCP, American Society of Clinical Pathologists; ASPT, American Society for Phlebotomy Technicians; AMT, American Medical Technologists; CAAHEP, Commission on Accreditation of Allied Health Education Programs; CAP, College of American Pathologists; DHHS, Department of Health and Human Services; ISCLT, International Society of Clinical Laboratory Technology; NCA, National Credentialing Agency for Medical Laboratory Personnel; NRM, National Registry of Microbiologists

within the laboratory. See the "Departments of a Typical Medical Lab" Quick Reference Guide for descriptions of common departments. The various departments perform special tests categorized within their expertise. Table 38-2 shows some specific tests performed within each department. Knowing how the laboratory is organized is helpful to the medical assistant when test results are requested over the telephone or when there is a need to converse with laboratory personnel.

Department	Description
Hematology	Conducts quantitative and qualitative tests on the formed elements of the blood, such as: • Complete blood count and differential • Cellular analysis of other body fluids such as urine • Coagulation and clotting factors The **quantitative tests** involve actual number counts such as counting the number of white blood cells (WBC), red blood cells (RBC), or platelets, while the **qualitative tests** focus on the quality or characteristics of the item under study
Urinalysis	Physical, chemical, and microscopic analysis of urine (Figure 38-1)
Chemistry	Chemical composition of blood, cerebrospinal fluid, and joint fluid; some assay of enzymes, serum glucose, and electrolyte levels
Serology, **Immunology**/immunohematology	Evaluates the body's immune response and production of antibodies against viruses and bacteria, autoimmune responses (production of antibodies against one's own body)
Toxicology	Tests for toxic substances in blood and monitors drug usage, therapeutic levels of medication, or toxicity of drugs being used; determines levels of occupational exposure to metals and chemicals in the workplace; tests for drug use in preemployment physical exams
DNA	Tests to prove paternity and maternity of children; tests to prove guilt or innocence in criminal cases
Microbiology	**Mycology** (study of and identifying fungi), virology (the study of and identifying viruses, and bacteria
Parasitology	The study of parasites

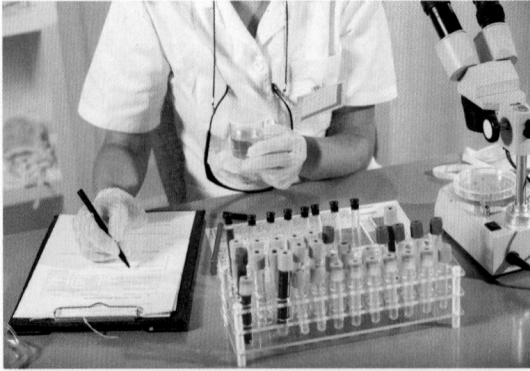

FIGURE 38-1 Clinical reference laboratories may have a separate urinalysis department where the laboratory professional tests urine for physical, chemical, and microbiologic properties.

© Jovanmandic/iStock.com

TABLE 38-2

CATEGORIES OF LABORATORY TESTS

HEMATOLOGY

White blood cell (WBC) count

Red blood cell (RBC) count

Differential white blood cell count (Diff)

RBC indices

Hemoglobin (Hgb)

Hematocrit (Hct)

Prothrombin time (PT)

Erythrocyte sedimentation rate (ESR)

Platelet count

CLINICAL CHEMISTRY

Glucose

Blood urea nitrogen (BUN)

Bicarbonate (CO_2)

Creatinine

Total protein

Albumin

Globulin

Calcium

Phosphorus

Chloride

Sodium

Potassium

Bilirubin

Cholesterol

Triglycerides

Uric acid

Lactate dehydrogenase (LD) (LDH)

Aspartate aminotransferase (AST) (SGOT)

Alanine aminotransferase (ALT) (SGPT)

Alkaline phosphatase (APT)

SEROLOGY (IMMUNOLOGY/IMMUNOHEMATOLOGY) AND BLOOD BANKING

Syphilis detection tests (VDRL, RPR)

C-reactive protein test (CRP)

ABO blood typing

Rh typing

Rh antibody titer test

Cross-match

Direct Coombs' test

Cold agglutinins

Rheumatoid arthritis factor (RA factor)

Mononucleosis test

Heterophil antibody titer test

Hepatitis tests

HIV tests: ELISA and Western blot

Antistreptolysin O (ASO) titer

Pregnancy tests

URINALYSIS

Physical analysis of urine:

Color

Clarity

Specific gravity

Chemical analysis of urine:

  pH

  Glucose

  Protein

  Ketones

  Blood

Bilirubin

Urobilinogen

Nitrite

Leukocyte esterase

Microscopic analysis of urine:

  Red blood cells

  White blood cells

  Epithelial cells

  Casts

  Crystals

continues

Table 38-2 continued

MICROBIOLOGY

Candidiasis	Pneumonia
Chlamydia	Streptococcal sore throat
Diphtheria	Tetanus
Gonorrhea	Tonsillitis
Meningitis	Tuberculosis
Pertussis	Bacteria (urinalysis)
Pharyngitis	

PARASITOLOGY (PARASITES)

Amebiasis	Scabies
Ascariasis (round worm)	Tapeworm disease
Hookworm disease	Toxoplasmosis
Malaria	Trichomoniasis
Pinworm disease (enterobiasis)	

CYTOLOGY (CELLS)

Chromosome studies
Pap test

HISTOLOGY (TISSUES)

Tissue analysis
Biopsy studies

DNA

DNA tests compare individuals according to their individual genotype

TOXICOLOGY

Tests for chemicals, specifically for drugs and other toxins in blood

There are two areas in medical laboratories that are experiencing the most growth. They are the toxicity and DNA departments. Besides drug testing in criminal cases and preemployment physicals, most states in the United States and its territories require toxicology tests in child protection cases. Drug testing is sometimes required for special assistance in low-income housing and other public financial assistance programs. The reasons for drug testing are wide and varied and are growing every year, making this department larger than in the past.

The second area within the medical laboratory growing larger each year is the DNA department. With the advent of DNA tests for proving paternity and maternity and the growing use of DNA testing for criminal cases, DNA testing is quickly becoming a major focus in many laboratories.

Panels of Laboratory Tests

Laboratory tests are often categorized into related groups to provide information about a particular body system or related body function. Blood serum (the part of blood that does not contain cells) tests are usually referred to as panels, formerly called profiles. Requisition forms are organized into panels for ease of ordering (Table 38-3). Please refer to Chapter 43 for additional information about each of the tests within the panels.

Medicare requires that providers order tests under their approved panels. Providers may not refer to panels by other names such as the previously named Chem Screen, SMAC, Chem 7, and so on. The panels listed in Table 38-3 are some more commonly ordered panels.

BILLING FOR LABORATORY SERVICES

Providers must justify which lab tests are ordered by using the correct diagnosis code. For example, if the clinical diagnosis is pneumonia, a urinalysis would not be justified and would not be covered. If a provider wants to order a test that probably will not be covered by insurance under CMS guidelines, the patient should sign a waiver. Medicare patients would sign an Advance Beneficiary Notice (ABN). The waiver/ABN notifies the patient that the test might not be covered and that the patient will have to pay for it.

QUALITY CONTROLS/ASSURANCES IN THE LABORATORY

Professional

The accuracy of any laboratory test result depends on all necessary safeguards being followed. These standards ensure the quality of the testing equipment, supplies, and personnel, and the accuracy of the test results. Many factors can compromise the accuracy of laboratory test results. Among these factors are collection of specimen, temperature, amount or age of specimen, time limits of test, and use of chemicals or reagents past their expiration dates. Even when laboratory guidelines are strictly followed, inaccurate results may be obtained if test kits have been exposed to extreme heat or cold, or if chemicals or reagents are used after their expiration date. It is important to follow all laboratory guidelines, and the medical assistant must also confirm that the specimen, chemicals, and test kits are handled and processed properly.

Control Tests

To further ensure accurate test results, **control test** samples are tested together with the patient's sample. The control samples have

TABLE 38-3

SOME OF THE MORE COMMONLY ORDERED BLOOD TEST PANELS

BASIC METABOLIC PANEL

BUN	Creatinine
Calcium, total	Glucose
CO_2 (bicarbonate)	Potassium
Chloride	Sodium

ELECTROLYTE PANEL

CO_2	Chloride
Potassium	Sodium

COMPREHENSIVE METABOLIC PANEL

Albumin	CO_2
Alkaline phosphatase	Chloride
ALT (SGPT)	Creatinine
AST (SGOT)	Glucose
Bilirubin, total	Potassium
BUN	Total protein
Calcium	Sodium

LIPID PANEL

Cholesterol	Triglyceride
HDL cholesterol and LDL cholesterol, calculated	

RENAL FUNCTION PANEL

Albumin	Creatinine
BUN	Glucose
Calcium, total	Phosphorus
CO_2	Potassium
Chloride	Sodium

HEPATIC FUNCTION PANEL

Albumin	Total protein
Alkaline phosphatase (ALP)	GGT
ALT (SGPT)	LDH
AST (SGOT)	PT
Bilirubin	

THYROID FUNCTION PANEL

TSH	T_4
T_3	

a known value, negative or positive result, or abnormal or normal result, which is compared with the results of the patient's test. One of the purposes of this control measure is to minimize human error. By being able to compare a sample of known value or positive or negative test result with the patient's test, the health care worker performing the test can accurately determine the result. An error in the testing method may be discovered if the control sample does not test accurately.

Another purpose of the control test is to check the **reagents,** or chemicals. If the control sample is not showing accurate results, it may be determined that the chemicals (reagents) are faulty or have expired. On receiving any test in the POL, the person responsible for quality assurance and quality control (probably the medical assistant performing the tests) should perform the calibration or control test provided by and as directed by the manufacturer. This ensures proper test function.

Proficiency Testing

CLIA requires laboratories to participate in an accredited proficiency program for certain identified tests (see Chapter 37 for CLIA requirements). Proficiency testing is similar to quality control in that "known" proficiency samples are tested the same as patient samples. The difference is an approved outside agency evaluates the accuracy of the testing and submits the performance records to CMS to ensure CLIA compliance.

Preventive Maintenance

Preventive maintenance helps identify potential problems before they actually occur. Procedures include manufacturer-recommended maintenance on equipment; daily temperature checks on refrigerators, freezers, and incubators; daily checks on expiration dates of reagents and supplies; and instrument log and centrifuge checks.

Instrument Validations

The quality of test results can be ensured by consistently checking the calibration and linear range of the instruments and machines. If the equipment is not maintained or is functioning improperly, accurate test results cannot be ensured.

The Medical Assistant's Role

Professional

Medical assistants are educated to perform administrative office duties, prepare patients, collect specimens, and perform waived tests in such a manner that patients and health care personnel are safe from contamination, patients are not harmed, samples are reliable, and tests are accurate. These four aspects of quality laboratory testing are critical for accuracy. When the patient is prepared properly, the specimen is obtained as expertly as possible, the reagents and equipment are in the best condition and calibration possible, and the test is performed by a trained professional, then the test results will be accurate. Professionals performing the lab tests should be able to explain the procedure to the patient; exactly follow the manufacturer's instructions; and follow proper protocol for labeling, handling, and processing the specimen. Labeling should always occur in the presence of the patient.

LABORATORY REQUISITIONS AND REPORTS

A printed **requisition** for laboratory work must be sent to the laboratory with the patient or with the specimen (Figure 38-2). These forms are preprinted with the most commonly requested tests separated into logical categories. Additional space is provided for entering special requests. The laboratories that patients use can provide your medical agency with these forms. Laboratory requisition forms are computer generated, and the provider's name, address, and other information necessary for proper reporting and record-keeping are often preprinted on the forms. If the requisitions are not preprinted, spaces are provided for the information to be written in. The information must be complete, accurate, and clearly legible. A properly completed requisition contains the following data (refer to numbered areas in Figure 38-2).

- *Section 1: Provider's name, account number, address, and telephone number.* This information is necessary if the office needs to be contacted for any clarification or further information and to report the results.
- *Section 2: Patient's name, address, and telephone number.* Be sure the name is complete and

Requested By

1

Courtesy Copy/Comments

Patient Information

Chart Number		Pre-Op? □Y □N	Surgery Date	Insurance Company (Name/Billing Address)
Social Security Number		Sex	Date of Birth (required)	
Patient Name	2			Guarantor (Responsible Party)
Mailing Address		City		Insurance Number
State	Zip	Patient Phone		Medicare Number

Insurance Information

3

REQUIRED REQUIRED REQUIRED

| ICD.9 Diagnosis Code(s) |

4

Physician Notice: For reimbursement, Medicare **requires ABN signature** review (see reverse side) be made for the following tests in **bold,** that may NOT be covered under "Medical Necessity".

☐ STAT	Phone Results ☐ # _____	Fasting ____ hrs	Last Dose Medication _____ Date/Time _____	Collected By ID _____	Date _____ Time _____
☐ ASAP					
☐ ROUTINE	FAX Report ☐ # _____				

Comments/Additional Tests

| SS = SST | L = LAV | B = BLUE | R = RED | G = GRAY | GN = GREEN | PK = PINK | U = URINE | C = CULTURE | S = SERUM | FROZEN | BIOPSY | SLIDES |

Alphabetical Test Listing	COLL CODE	Alphabetical Test Listing	COLL CODE	Alphabetical Test Listing	COLL CODE	Alphabetical Test Listing	COLL CODE	Microbiology
☐ ABO 50100 ☐ Rh 50200	R	☐ Creatinine 30570	S	☐ **Hepatitis Panel, Acute 40781**	S	☐ Prolactin 40450	S	Indicate Exact Specimen Source
☐ Albumin 30590	S	☐ Creatinine, Urine, 24hr 32100	U	• **Hep A Ab (IgM)** • **HBcAb (IgM)**		☐ Protein, Urine	U	
☐ Alkaline Phosphatase 30670	S	☐ Creatinine, Urine, Ran 32081	U	• **HBsAg** • **Hep C Ab**		☐ RAN 32180 ☐ 24hr 32200		☐ AFB Culture with Smear 64450
☐ **Alpha-fetoprotein 41150**	S	☐ Creatinine Clearance 32240	S,U	☐ **HIV-1 & -2 Antibody 42007**	S	☐ **PSA, Diagnostic 42158**	S	☐ C. difficile Toxin 68016
☐ ALT (SGPT) 30680	S	☐ C-Reactive Protein (CRP) 58200	S	☐ **HIV-1 RNA, PCR, Quant 42015**	L	☐ **PSA, Screen 41954**	S	☐ Chlamydia Only, Amplified 68361
☐ Amylase 31710	S	☐ CRP, Cardiac Risk 43575	S	☐ Homocysteine 43600	L	☐ **PSA Ratio, Free & Total 42147**	S	☐ Chlamydia/GC, Amplified 68395
☐ ANA (with Reflex) 69107	S	☐ **Digoxin 33060**	S	☐ Iron 30720	S	☐ **PT (Protime w/INR) 25000**	B	☐ Fungal Culture 64300
☐ Antibody Screen 50500	R	☐ Electrolytes 31310	S	☐ Iron, TRF Sat., (TIBC) 44210	S	☐ PTH (Whole Molecule) 40571	L	☐ Giardia Antigen 67031
☐ AST (SGOT) 30700	S	• Na • K • Cl • CO$_2$		☐ LDH 30710	S	☐ **PTT, Activated 25100**	B	☐ Gram Stain, Direct 60050
☐ **B$_{12}$ 41250**	S	☐ Electrophoresis, Serum 48010	S	☐ **LDL Direct 43571**	S	☐ **Reticulocyte Count 21150**	L	☐ Herpes simplex Virus Culture 68263
☐ B$_{12}$/Folate 41311	S	☐ Electrophoresis, Urine 48310	U	☐ LH 40500	S	☐ **Rheumatoid Factor 44480**	S	☐ Herpes/Varicella Virus Culture 68277
☐ Basic Metabolic Panel 31307	S	☐ **ESR (Sed Rate) 21050**	L	☐ **Lipase 31740**	S	☐ **RPR 58800**	S	☐ Influenza A & B, Direct Exam 65092
• Na • K • Cl • CO$_2$		☐ Estradiol 41600	S	☐ **Lipid Panel 1 43560**	S	☐ Rubella 58681	S	☐ KOH Prep 64200
• BUN • Creat • Gluc • Ca		☐ **Ferritin 41350**	S	• **Chol** • **HDL** • **Trig** • **LDL**		☐ Semen, Post Vasectomy 23540	Se	☐ Ova & Parasite 67002
☐ BNP 31379	L	☐ Folate 41300	S	• **Chol/HDL** • **LDL/HDL**		☐ T3, Free 40070	S	☐ Pinworm Prep 67200
☐ BUN 30550	S	☐ FSH 40400	S	☐ **Rflx Direct LDL, Trig> 400 43562**	S	☐ T3, Total 40200	S	☐ Polys (WBC's) 67455
☐ Bilirubin, Total 30640	S	☐ GGT 30690	S	☐ **Lithium 33320**	S	☐ **T4 (Thyroxine) 40000**	S	☐ Rapid Strep-A Antigen,
☐ Bilirubin, Direct 30650	S	☐ **Glucose 30550**	S	☐ Lymphocyte T-Cell Subsets 29100	LGN	☐ **T4, Free 40050**	S	Culture if Negative 65100
☐ **CA 125 41050**	S	☐ **Glucose Tolerance Test ___ hrs**	S	☐ Lymphocytes, T-Helper 29150	LGN	☐ **Free Thyroxine Index,**	S	☐ Rotavirus 68073
☐ **CA 19.9 42900**	S	☐ Glucose 2hr PP 31820	S	☐ **Magnesium 31280**	SS	**FTI (T4 + TU) 40025**		☐ Trichomonas Wet Mount 60103
☐ **CA 27.29 41061**	S	☐ **hCG-beta, Quantitative 41100**	S	☐ Microalbumin, Urine	U	☐ Thyroid Peroxidase Ab 34720	S	**Culture, Bacterial**
☐ Calcium 30610	S	☐ **hCG-beta, Tumor Marker 41110**	S	☐ Ran 43980 ☐ 24hr 42101		☐ **Theophylline 33430**	S	☐ Anaerobic 61653
☐ Carbamazepine (Tegretol) 33050	S	☐ **HCV RNA, PCR, Quant 40738**	L	☐ Timed ___hrs___min 42100		☐ Total Protein 30580	S	☐ Blood 60250
☐ Cardiolipin Abs, IgG, IgM 27500	S	☐ H. pylori, IgG 58322	S	☐ Microalbumin/Creat Ratio 43985	U	☐ **Triglycerides 30730**	S	☐ CSF 60450
☐ **CBC w/auto differential 20000**	S	☐ **Hemoglobin AIC (Glycol) 42550**	L	☐ Monotest 58550	S	☐ **Troponin I 31378**	S	☐ Catheter Tip 60420
☐ **Hemogram Only 20150**		☐ **Hepatic Function Panel 31306**	S	☐ **Occult Blood Screen 67100**	F	☐ **TSH 40250**	S	☐ E. coli – 0157, Only 61227
☐ CEA 41000	S	• **Alk Phos** • **Alb** • **DBil** • **TBil** • **TP**		☐ **Occult Blood Diagnostic 67105**	F	☐ **TSH with Reflex 40012**	S	☐ GC Only 60750
☐ **Cholesterol 30740**	S	• **ALT (SGPT)** • **AST (SGOT)**		☐ Phenytoin (Dilantin) 33360	S	☐ **Testosterone 40550**	S	☐ Genital, Full Culture 60800
☐ CK, Total 31350	S	☐ Hep A Ab, IgM 42114	S	☐ Phenytoin, Free & Total 87060	R	☐ Uric Acid 30630	S	☐ Group-B Strep Only, Genital 60217
☐ Comp Metabolic Panel 31305	S	☐ Hep B Core Ab, IgM 42141	S	☐ Phosphorus 30620	S	☐ **UA & Microscopic 24080**	U	☐ MRSA Screen, Nares 60867
• Na • K • Cl • CO$_2$ • Gluc		☐ Hep C Ab 40711	S	☐ **Potassium/NA 30510**	S	☐ **UA & Microscopic, Reflex**	U	☐ Sputum/Trach/Bronch 61100
• BUN • Creat • Ca • AST • ALT		☐ Hepatitis B Immunity Scrn 40770	S	☐ Prealbumin 44470	S	**with C&S if Indicated 11850**		☐ Stool, Full Culture 61150
• TP • Alb • A/G • Alk Phos • TBil		☐ HBsAg 42127	S	☐ Progesterone 41750	S			☐ Strep-A Screen, Throat 60207
								☐ Throat Culture 61350
								☐ **Urine Culture 61500**

5

| Lab Use Only |
| Veni ☐ A 95370 ☐ C 95372 |
| ☐ NH 99561 |
| Hfee ☐ 1 ☐ 2 ☐ 3 |

☐ Wound, 61657

source: _____

Many payors (including Medicare and Medicaid) have a necessity requirement for the diagnosis and treatment of the patient, therefore, only those tests which are medically necessary should be ordered.

FIGURE 38-2 Sample laboratory requisition form. 1. Physician information, 2. Patient information, 3. Billing information, 4. Specimen information, 5. Tests ordered.

spelled correctly. Avoid using alternate versions of the patient's name without also including the proper legal name. Make certain to include apartment numbers and ZIP codes. This information will be used for billing purposes, as well as medical records. Middle initials and date of birth are helpful when it is necessary to differentiate between patients.

- *Unique patient identifier.* This can be an identification number that is hospital or laboratory generated. In the outpatient setting, this can be the patient's date of birth.

- *Patient's age/date of birth and sex.* Age and sex both influence the results of some tests and should not be assumed.

- *Section 3: Patient's billing information, insurance, and identification number.* Because the patient is often not the person who is the subscriber to the insurance, the subscriber's name, address, telephone number, and insurance identification numbers are extremely important, especially if the patient does not live with the subscriber. Some patients have secondary insurance coverage. Be sure to include that information also. The laboratory would prefer to receive an additional sheet of information than to have incomplete insurance records in its business office.

- *Section 4: Source of specimen.* This information is especially important when dealing with tests such as cultures and biopsies. In the case of cultures, knowing the source of the specimen aids the laboratory in determining whether the specimen contains normal flora or is abnormal for that area of the body.

  - *Time and date of the specimen collection.* Some tests require that the specimen be tested fairly quickly after leaving the body; other tests must be performed after a certain amount of time has elapsed. The time and date of the specimen collection are important because accuracy can be compromised if the specimen is not sent to the laboratory in a reasonable amount of time.

  - *Medications the patient is taking.* Because medication can influence some test results, it is important that the laboratory be provided this information. Patients are often asked to refrain from taking certain medications before testing. Be sure to consult with the provider to verify orders. If a medication is not discontinued before testing, the type of medication, the dosage amount, and the time of the last dose must be included on the requisition.

- *Clinical diagnosis.* The provider's tentative diagnosis is useful to the laboratory in helping to differentiate between diagnoses or confirm a diagnosis. The clinical diagnosis may also alert the laboratory personnel to any possible special considerations of which to be aware. For example, if diabetes is suspected, the laboratory will give special consideration to the glucose value. The diagnosis, or preferably the ICD-9 code, is also necessary for billing.

- *Urgency of results.* Sometimes, the provider needs a test to be performed immediately (STAT) or would like a result as soon as possible (ASAP). The provider's orders need to be clearly stated on the requisition. Additional space is also provided for other special instructions if necessary.

- *Special collection/patient instructions.* Examples include fasting specimens, timed collections, and "do not collect from a specific area" instructions.

- *Section 5: Test requested.* This is usually a matter of putting a check mark in the appropriate box on the requisition, but it is surprising how often laboratories receive specimens with nicely completed requisitions and no indication of the test desired.

If copies of the results are to be sent to a second provider, the medical assistant must include the provider's full name, address, and fax number.

The laboratory will send back a printed report that will contain the following information:

- Name, address, and telephone number of the laboratory

- Referring provider's name, address, and identification numbers

- Patient's name, identification number, age, and sex

- Date the specimen was received by the laboratory

- Date and time the specimen was collected
- Date the laboratory reported the results
- Test name, results, and normal reference ranges if applicable

Lab requisitions may be electronically generated using an electronic health record (EHR) program and completed on screen and then either printed for the patient to take to the outside lab or sent electronically to the lab (Figure 38-3). Occasionally, a requisition will be faxed to a lab if the EHR is not available. Interestingly, today's medical clinic staff may perform a combination of electronic and manual communication with outside labs. Eventually, the electronic format will replace all manual methods.

Reports are sent to the provider by fax, manually delivered to the clinic, or—most often—sent electronically using EHR software

Interestingly, laboratory reference ranges can vary slightly from laboratory to laboratory.

An ongoing attempt to "harmonize" all laboratory test results to a "gold standard" is being discussed at the national level. A particular laboratory's normal range is always given on the report. Abnormal test results are always flagged in some way, either in a different color, a different column, or perhaps by a star or simply by *H* (for high) or *L* (for low). The provider is alerted to critical values (results that may indicate serious medical conditions) by a phone call from the laboratory. The provider should be alerted to any abnormal test results as soon as possible.

When the results are received as paper reports, before filing them, the medical assistant should attach them to the patient's chart for the provider to review and initial. Laboratories often electronically send computer-generated reports of test results directly to the provider and clinic (Figure 38-4).

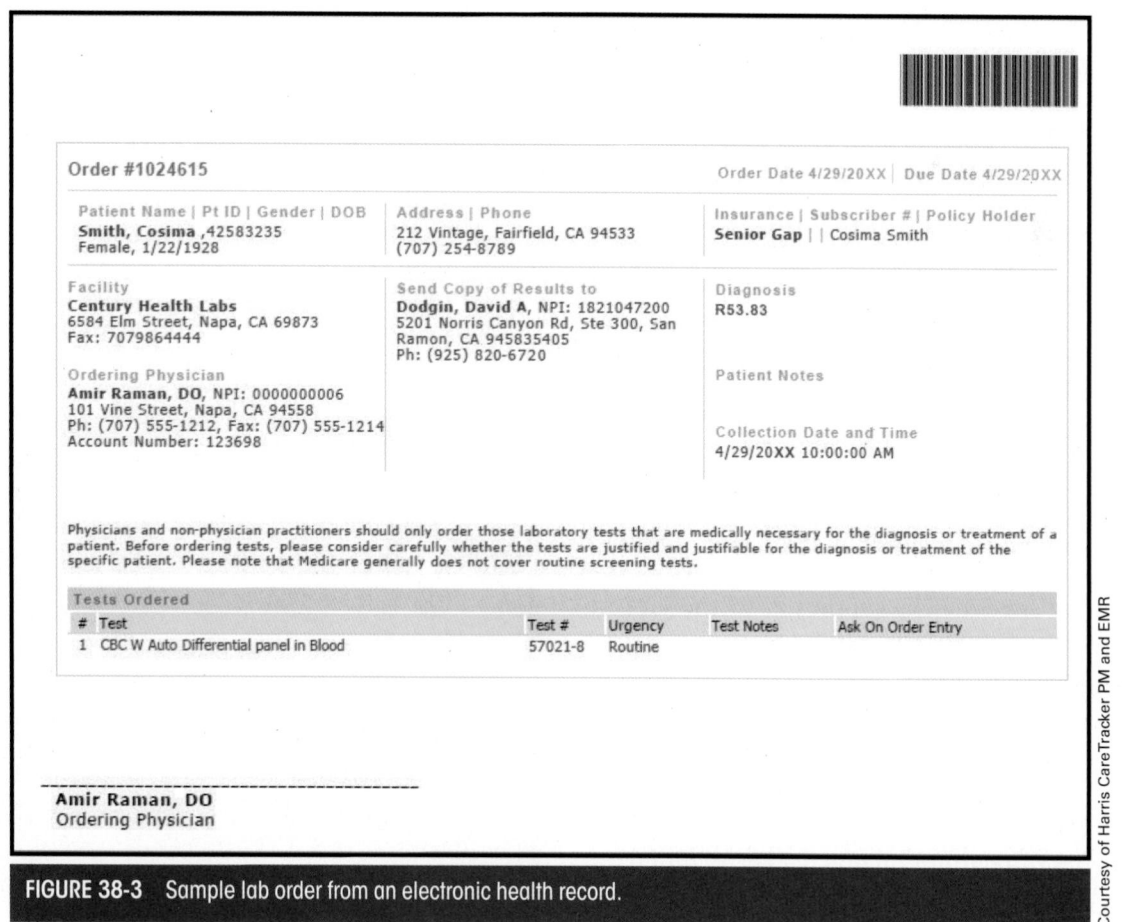

FIGURE 38-3 Sample lab order from an electronic health record.

Courtesy of Harris CareTracker PM and EMR

Patient: Black Doris L
ID: 161111
Birth Date: MAY 22 1924   Age: 90Y   Sex: F
Room: ED

Physician: Larkin, Alicia, FNP
Report To: ED

Sample ID: 70150072	Collected On:	03/11/XX @ 14:00	Received: 03/11/XX @ 14:17	
WHITE BLOOD CELL CT	7.7	X10^9		4.5 - 11.5
RED BLOOD CELLS H	5.5	x10^12		4.2 - 5.4
HEMOGLOBIN H	15.2	g/dl		12.0 - 15.0
HEMATOCRIT	48	%		35 - 49
MCV	88	f		80 - 100
MCH	32	X10^9		26.0 - 33.0
MCHC	35	%		32 - 36
PLATELET	327	X10^9		150 - 450
NEUT % - AUTO COUNT	68	%		50 - 70
MIXED CELL % - AUTOL	1	U/L		2 - 12
LYMPH% - AUTO COUNT	19	X10^9		18 - 42
NEUTROPHIL ABSOLUTE	6.5	x10^12		1.5 - 7.1
MIXED CELL ABSOLUTE	0.2	x10^12		0.2 - 1.0
LYMPHOCYTE ABSOLUTE	1.7	x10^12		0.8 - 2.8
RDW-CV	11.4	%		-
MEAN PLT VOLUME H	13.0			8.6 - 11.7

Original Print Date: 03/11/XX @ 14:47   Reviewed By:_____

FIGURE 38-4 Sample computerized laboratory report.

THE SPECIMEN

Proper Procurement, Storage, and Handling

Instructions for properly procuring, storing, and handling and transporting laboratory specimens can be obtained from each independent laboratory. Most laboratories will provide the office/clinic with a step-by-step instruction manual that is sometimes called a compendium, a laboratory manual, or a user manual and that is sometimes in electronic format. The laboratories will also be available to answer any additional questions by telephone.

Obtaining the specimen in the proper manner and using the right equipment will ensure that a high-quality specimen is submitted to the laboratory. Some guidelines are as follows:

- Check the provider's orders and identify the patient.
- Refer to the laboratory instruction manual or consult the laboratory for specific collection instructions.
- Instruct the patient on any necessary dietary restriction (see Patient Education box).
- Instruct the patient to ingest special food or take other substances if required.

- Select the appropriate container with the proper additives, if required (Figure 38-5).
- Label the specimen with the patient's name, identification number, date, type of specimen, time of collection, and provider's name. Label the container, not the lid, because the lid will be removed during testing. Label the container, not the packaging, because the packaging will be separated from the container

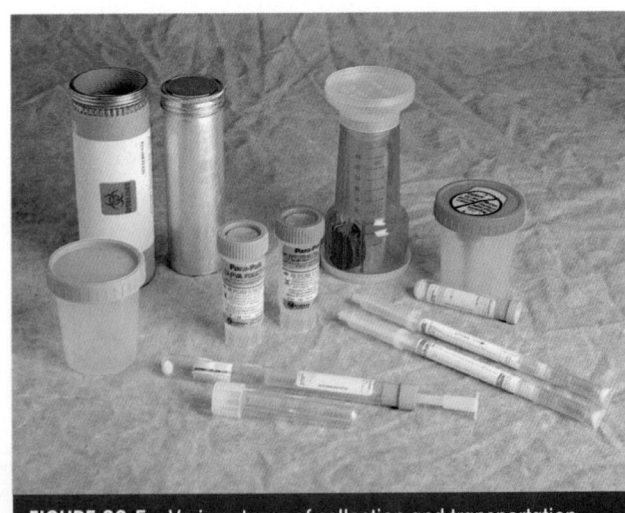

FIGURE 38-5 Various types of collection and transportation containers for laboratory specimens.

when testing is performed (e.g., throat swab packaging).

- Obtain the specimen or instruct the patient to provide the specimen according to the directions given by the laboratory.
- Follow applicable OSHA bloodborne pathogens guidelines (see Standard Precautions in Chapter 21) when packaging the specimen for transport so it will not leak or contaminate the courier or other office staff and so that it will safely arrive at the laboratory without being damaged or destroyed.
- Place any biologic specimen to be sent to an outside laboratory into an approved biologic transport bag (Figure 38-6 A–C). These bags, which have the universal symbol for biohazard caution stamped on them, contain two sections: one for the specimen and one for the requisition. The requisition and specimen are placed in the proper areas within the transport bag, and the bag is sealed. When the testing laboratory receives the bag, the opposite end is torn open so that the specimen and requisitions can be removed without contaminating the receiver.
- Document in the patient's chart or electronic medical record the type of specimen collected, the tests ordered, which laboratory the specimen is being sent to (even if it is being tested in your POL), how the patient tolerated the procedure (including any complications), and other pertinent information according to your office policy. Many offices also keep a copy of the laboratory requisition in the patient's chart for later reference. If the testing is performed in your POL, the results of the test should be recorded on a laboratory report form and, after the provider has initialed it, filed in the laboratory section of the chart.

If the clinic is using EHRs, lab requisitions often stay in a "pending" file until the results are reported from the laboratory. The medical assistant may be responsible for tracking pending lab tests until the reports are received.

Medical clinics and laboratories may share an interface software program that allows the report to be imported onto the provider's desktop as an "unsigned" document. Many clinics have policies in place that require the provider to electronically "sign" lab reports within 36 or 48 hours of receipt.

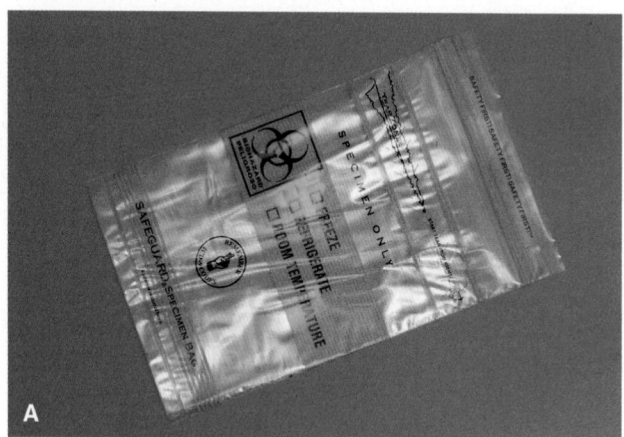

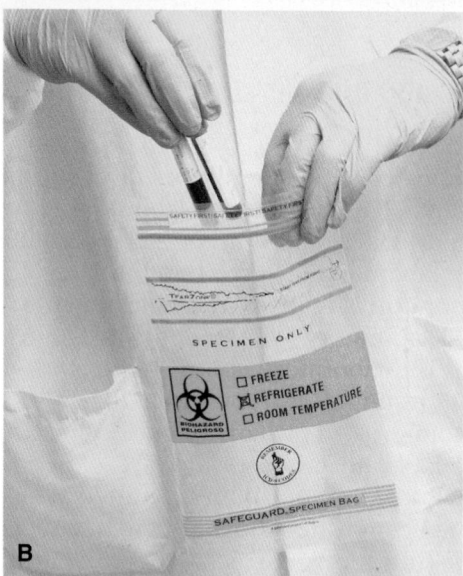

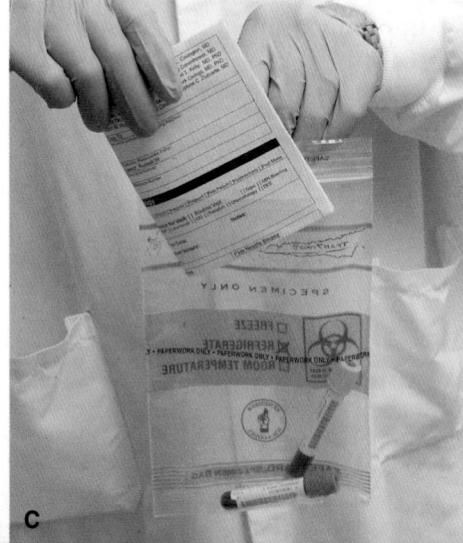

FIGURE 38-6 Preparing a biological specimen to be sent to an outside laboratory. (A) Laboratory specimen transport bag. (B) The medical assistant places the specimen into the transport bag and seals that part of the bag. (C) The medical assistant places the requisition into a separate compartment of the bag.

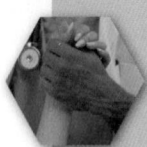
Processing and Sending Specimens to a Laboratory

Specimens collected by the medical assistant are often sent from the office to a laboratory many miles away or are picked up by a courier representing the outside laboratory. These are often large commercial laboratories that are not associated with a local hospital laboratory. The patient's insurance often dictates the laboratory contracted to perform the patient's testing. It is not unusual for several different laboratories to pick up at one location.

All laboratory test results are dependent on the quality of the specimen submitted. The quality of the specimen depends on patient preparation, proper collection, correct patient identification, and transportation of the specimen. If there is any doubt or question regarding the type of specimen to be collected, it is imperative that the appropriate laboratory be contacted to clarify the specimen needed. There are often differences between laboratories; the type of specimen acceptable for one laboratory is not necessarily the acceptable specimen for another laboratory.

MICROSCOPES

One of the most used pieces of equipment in the medical laboratory is the microscope. Consisting of light source, eyepieces, objectives, condenser, and diaphragm, the microscope enables us to see bacteria and other microorganisms that are much too small to be seen without magnification. For more information on the different kinds of microscopes, see the "Types of Microscopes" Quick Reference Guide.

 QUICK REFERENCE GUIDE

Types of Microscopes

≫ THE COMPOUND MICROSCOPE

The most commonly used microscope in the clinic is the compound microscope (Figure 38-7). As the name indicates, the image is compounded by the use of two different lenses. One lens compounds, or increases, the magnification produced by the other lens. The first lens system is located in the objectives, and the second lens system is in the eyepiece (ocular). The light source is a bulb in the base. The light is directed up through the specimen on the slide and into the objective lenses. The light, or image, is then reflected by the condenser onto the specimen to the ocular lenses for visualization.

The eyepiece may have a single (monocular) lens, or there may be two (binocular) lenses. This lens is not adjustable or changeable. The magnification in the eyepiece is usually 10 times (10×) the normal size of the object being viewed.

(continues)

The objective lenses are adjustable between low power (10 times magnification), high power (40 times magnification), and oil immersion. When viewing through the microscope under low power, more of the slide can be seen but with less detail than when using high power. When viewing under high power, a smaller portion of the field can be seen but with greater detail. The low-power objective lens magnification combined with the 10 times magnification of the ocular lens gives the ability to see microscopically 100 times the normal size (10× multiplied by 10× = 100×). Combining the 10× ocular lenses with the high-power (40×) objective lens increases magnification vision to 400 times the normal size (10× multiplied by 40× = 400×). This is enough magnification to see large microorganisms but is still not enough to see smaller organisms, such as bacteria, clearly. An oil-immersion lens is needed to view bacteria closely using a compound microscope.

The oil-immersion lens gives the ability to multiply the ocular lens magnification (10×) by a hundred (100×) to reach a possible total magnification of thousand times normal life size (10× multiplied by 100× = 1,000×). Because more light is needed to actually see this amount of magnification, the lens is immersed in oil. This prevents the scattering and loss of light rays, which naturally occur when light travels through air, consequently increasing the efficiency of the magnification.

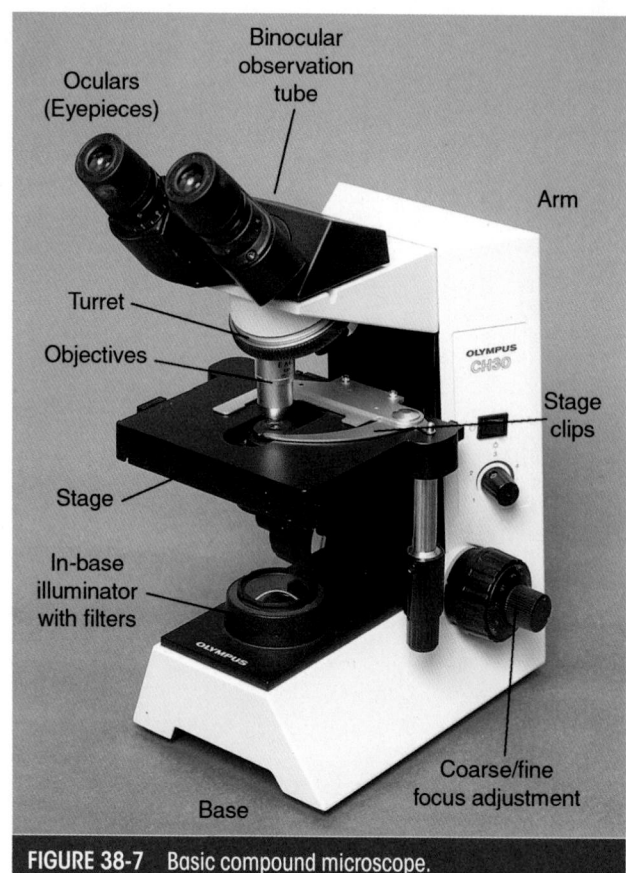

FIGURE 38-7 Basic compound microscope.

OTHER TYPES OF MICROSCOPES

Microscope	Description
Phase-contrast microscope	This microscope is specifically designed for viewing specimens that are transparent and unstained. Some microscopic specimens must be stained with a fluorescent dye to be examined in detail (e.g., when detecting specific bacteria).
Fluorescent microscope	This microscope is the instrument best suited for viewing luminescent specimens. In dark-field microscopy, the light is reflected from an angle, which causes the specimen to appear as a bright object on a dark field.
Electron microscope (Figure 38-8)	Special training is required to operate this sophisticated instrument. The electron microscope is large (several feet tall) and expensive; therefore, it is found only in larger regional and hospital laboratories. An electronic beam, rather than light, is passed through the specimen. The image is projected onto a fluorescent screen and may then be photographed and enlarged. The electron microscope provides views of extremely small organisms, such as viruses, in great detail and in three dimensions. Figure 38-9 shows blood cells visible using an electron microscope.

(continues)

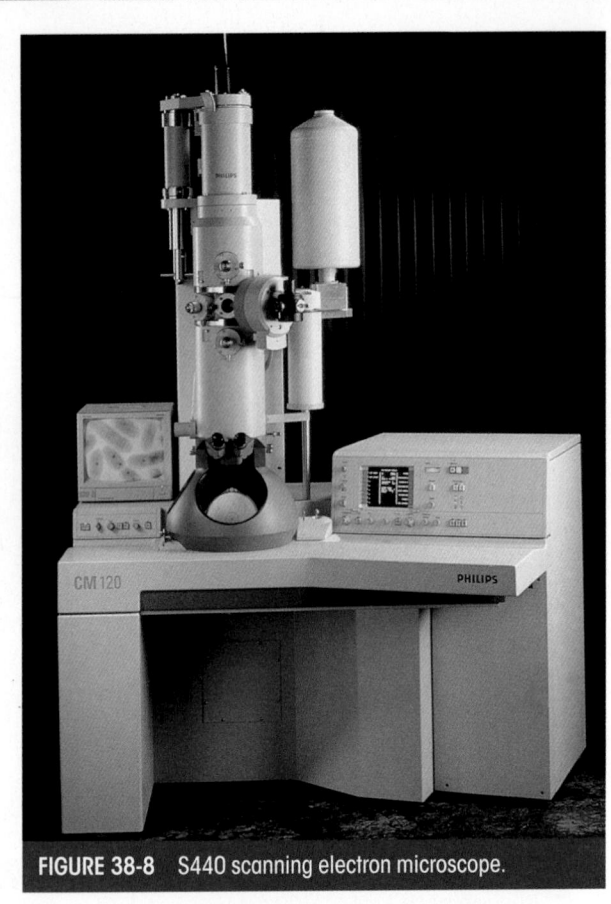

FIGURE 38-8 S440 scanning electron microscope.

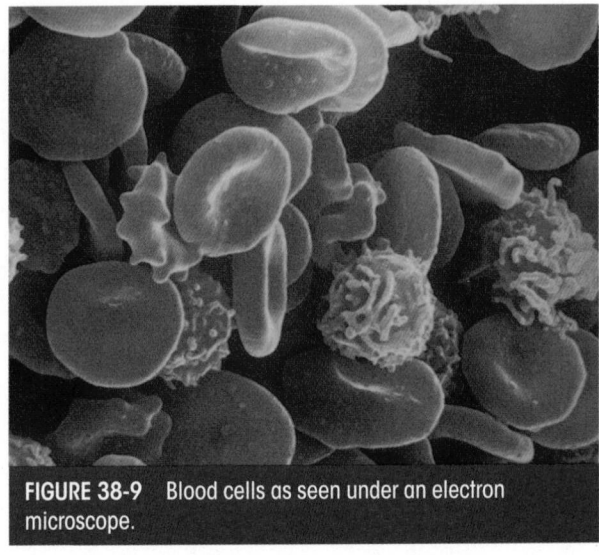

FIGURE 38-9 Blood cells as seen under an electron microscope.

How to Use a Compound Microscope

Professional

Microscopic exams are not within the medical assistant's scope of practice; however, it is beneficial to learn the basics in order to continue education and effectively assist the provider in microscopy procedures. Refer to Procedure 38-1 for step-by-step instructions in the use of a compound microscope. Besides needing to adjust a microscope's magnification, it may be necessary to adjust focus. The microscope contains a coarse adjustment and a fine adjustment. The coarse adjustment is to be used with the low-power (short) objective only. The coarse adjustment is used to bring the object into view. The fine adjustment may then be used to sharpen the image. Depending on the individual microscope, the coarse and fine adjustments may raise and lower the nosepiece, which houses the objectives, or they may raise and lower the stage, or platform, on which the slide rests.

It is important always to remember to raise the platform of the lower objectives using the coarse adjustment and the low-power objective *while viewing the slide from the side*. This allows the lens to come close to the slide without actually touching it. If the slide is not viewed from the side for the coarse adjustment, there is the possibility of running the objective through the slide and seriously damaging the lens and the microscope, or of breaking the slide. After bringing the slide and objective together, adjustments may be made through the ocular, always moving away from the slide. Once the item is in view, the fine adjustment may be used for clarity.

The bulb in the base directs light through the slide. The light first goes through a condenser and then through an iris diaphragm. The condenser is used to control the intensity of the light, and the iris diaphragm may be adjusted to control the amount of light.

Using the oil-immersion lens requires the use of a couple drops of transparent oil in order to magnify the view of the slide. Oil refracts light, which increases the resolution.

How to Care for a Microscope

Microscopes can be expensive and, like any precision instrument, should be treated with care. Some practices that will extend the life of a microscope and maintain the quality of its performance are:

- Always follow the manufacturer's and clinic's rules for the care and maintenance of the microscope.
- Carry the microscope with one hand securely supporting the base and the other hand holding the arm (Figure 38-10).
- Keep the microscope covered when it is not being used.
- Clean the lenses with special lens paper and lens cleaner after each use. Using standard tissue can scratch the lenses.
- When looking through the eyepiece and focusing, always move the platform away from, never toward, the eyepiece to prevent the

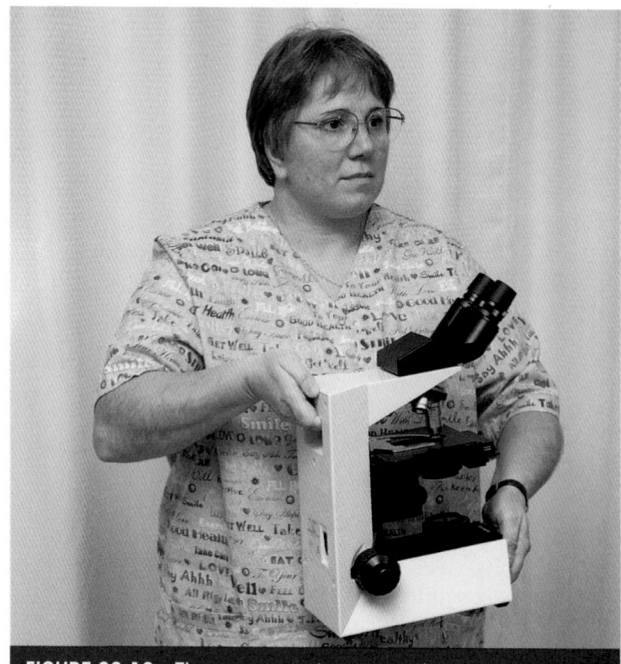

FIGURE 38-10 The proper way to carry a microscope.

objective from coming into contact with the slide. If you are actually looking at the platform, then you can move it closer to the eyepiece without allowing it to come into contact with the slide.

- Use oil only with the oil-immersion lens and clean the oil off after each use.

PROCEDURE 38-1

Using the Microscope

Procedure

STANDARD PRECAUTIONS:

Gloves

PURPOSE:

To properly use a microscope to view microscopic organisms using the coarse and fine adjustments, as well as the low- and high-power and oil-immersion objectives.

EQUIPMENT/SUPPLIES:

- Compound microscope
- Manufacturer's manual
- Lens paper
- Lens cleaner

- Alcohol or oil solvent
- Prepared slides (commercially available)
- Immersion oil

(continues)

PROCEDURE STEPS:

NOTE: The procedure will vary slightly according to microscope design. Consult the operating procedure in the microscope manual for specific instructions.

1. Wash hands.
2. Assemble equipment and materials.
3. Clean the ocular(s) and objectives with lens paper.
4. Use the coarse adjustment to raise the eyepiece or lens unit.
5. Rotate the 10×, or low-power, objective into position so that it is directly over the opening in the stage.
6. Turn on the microscope light.
7. Open the diaphragm until maximum light comes up through the condenser.
8. Place the slide on the stage (specimen side up).
9. Locate the coarse adjustment.
10. Look directly at the stage and 10× objective and turn the coarse adjustment until the objective is as close to the slide as it will go.

   NOTE: Do not lower any objective toward a slide while looking through the ocular(s).

11. Look into the ocular(s) and slowly turn the coarse adjustment in the opposite direction (as in step 10) to raise the objective (or lower the stage) until the object on the slide comes into view.
12. Locate the fine adjustment.
13. Turn the fine adjustment to sharpen the image.

   NOTE: If a binocular microscope is used, the oculars must be adjusted for each individual's visual acuity.

   a. Adjust the distance between the oculars so that one image is seen (as when using binoculars).

   b. Use the coarse and fine adjustments to bring the object into focus while looking through the right ocular with the right eye.

   c. Close the right eye, look into the left ocular with the left eye, and *use the knurled collar on the left ocular* to bring the object into sharp focus. (Do not turn the coarse or fine adjustment at this time.)

   d. Look into the oculars with both eyes to observe that the object is in clear focus. If it is not, repeat the procedure.

14. Scan the slide by either method:

   a. Use the stage knobs to move the slide left and right and backward and forward while looking through the ocular(s), or

   b. Move the slide with the fingers while looking through the ocular(s) (for microscope without movable stage).

15. Rotate the high-power (40×) objective into position while observing the objective and the slide to see that the objective does not strike the slide.
16. Look through the ocular(s) to view the object on the slide; it should be almost in focus.
17. Look through the ocular(s) and turn the fine adjustment until the object is in focus. Do not use the coarse adjustment.
18. Adjust the amount of light. This can be done by closing the diaphragm, lowering the condenser, or adjusting the light at the source.
19. Scan the slide as in step 14.
20. Rotate the oil-immersion objective to the side slightly (so that no objective is in position).
21. Place one drop of immersion oil on the portion of the slide that is directly over the condenser and a drop of oil onto the oil-immersion lens.
22. Rotate the oil-immersion objective into position.
23. Look through the ocular(s) and slowly turn the fine adjustment until the image is clear. Use only the fine adjustment to focus the oil-immersion objective.

(continues)

24. Adjust the amount of light using the procedure in step 18.
25. Scan the slide using the procedure in step 14.
26. Rotate the 10× objective into position (do not allow the 40× objective to touch the oil).
27. Remove the slide from the microscope stage and gently clean the oil from the slide with lens paper. Alcohol or a solvent cleaner, such as xylene, can be used to remove excess oil from the slide.
28. Clean the oculars, 10× objective, and 40× objective with clean lens paper and lens cleaner.
29. Clean the oil-immersion objective with lens paper and lens cleaner to remove all oil.
30. Clean any oil from the microscope stage and condenser.
31. Turn off the microscope light and disconnect.
32. Use the coarse adjustment to position the eyepiece in the lowest position.
33. Center the stage so that it does not project from either side of the microscope.
34. Cover the microscope and return it to storage.
35. Clean the work area; return slides to storage.
36. Wash hands.

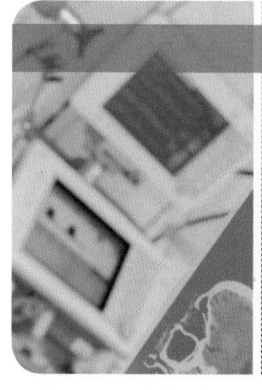

CASE STUDY 38-1

Refer to the scenario at the beginning of the chapter. Gwen sent Ms. Samuels to the lab for the O&P test rather than performing the test herself in the POL.

CASE STUDY REVIEW

1. Why didn't Gwen perform the microscopic examination of the stool sample for parasites and their eggs (O&P) herself in the POL rather than sending Ms. Samuels to an outside lab?
2. Why did Gwen give Ms. Samuels a biohazard transport bag along with the stool sample container?

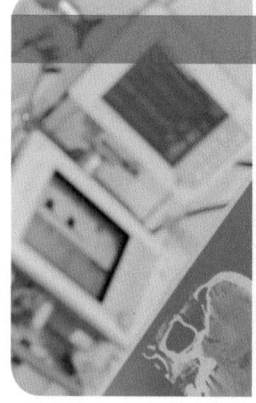

CASE STUDY 38-2

Refer to the scenario at the beginning of the chapter. Gwen noticed that Ms. Samuels appears to be apprehensive about giving a stool sample for the O&P test. Gwen wants to make sure Ms. Samuels is not embarrassed by the procedure so she shares a personal experience she had herself with intestinal parasites the previous year.

CASE STUDY REVIEW

1. How can Gwen assure Ms. Samuels that there is nothing to be embarrassed about?
2. Is it appropriate for Gwen to share her personal experiences in an attempt to reassure the patient?

Summary

- The fact that our bodies are susceptible to disease and abnormal conditions necessitates the existence and use of clinical laboratories.
- Laboratory personnel include doctors, scientists, technologists, technicians, as well as administrative and ancillary staff.
- Laboratories may be organized into departments that specialize in the types of tests performed.
- Quality controls and assurances are critical elements of laboratory testing.
- Requisitions and reports may be printed and faxed, hand carried, or sent electronically.
- Together with clinical laboratory personnel, medical assistants play an important role in laboratory testing by preparing patients for tests, obtaining specimens, and performing CLIA-waived tests or sending specimens to larger outside laboratories.
- Medical assistants are educated to perform these tasks in a manner that ensures the accuracy of the test and safeguards the health of patients and health care personnel.
- Medical assistants must be familiar with state and national laws pertaining to their scope of practice regarding laboratory testing.
- Various types of microscopes are used within medical laboratories, ranging from simple to complex.

Study for Success

To reinforce your knowledge and skills of information presented in this chapter:

- Review the *Key Terms* and *Learning Outcomes*
- Consider the *Critical Thinking* features and *Case Studies* and discuss your conclusions
- Answer the questions in the *Certification Review*

- Perform the *Procedure* using the *Competency Assessment Checklists* on the *Student Companion Website*

Procedure

CERTIFICATION REVIEW

1. Which of the following statements best describes POCT?
   a. It is performed in the exam room or at the patient's bedside.
   b. It must be performed by certified laboratory professionals.
   c. It provides for rapid, accurate results.
   d. The medical laboratory's role includes training and management of quality control.

2. Which of these professionals are qualified to manage an independent medical laboratory?
   a. Clinical laboratory technologist
   b. Pathologist
   c. Clinical laboratory technician
   d. Medical assistant
   e. Registered nurse

3. Which of the following describes the hematology department of a laboratory?
   a. It studies microorganisms and their activities.
   b. It studies blood and blood-forming tissues.
   c. It detects the presence of disease-producing human parasites or eggs present in specimens taken from the body.
   d. It detects the presence of abnormal tissues.

4. How is the quality of a patient's test results assured?
   a. Instrument calibration procedures
   b. Preventative maintenance procedures
   c. Quality control testing
   d. Confirming reagent expiration dates
   e. All of these

5. What document must accompany a patient or a specimen when sent to a medical laboratory?
   a. A printed requisition
   b. A report
   c. The patient's file
   d. An insurance form
6. What is the most commonly used microscope in the clinic?
   a. Fluorescent
   b. Electron
   c. Phase-contrast
   d. Compound
   e. Binocular
7. Testing a blood specimen for antibody–antigen reactions would be performed in which laboratory department?
   a. Hematology
   b. Chemistry
   c. Toxicology
   d. Immunohematology
8. When lab results indicate a serious medical condition, they are labeled with which of the following indicators?
   a. Provider attention
   b. High levels or low levels
   c. Critical values
   d. Dangerous levels
   e. Urgent results
9. Which of the following physicians specializes in the cause and development of diseases?
   a. Oncologist
   b. Pathologist
   c. Cytologist
   d. Medical technologist
10. Quantitative testing determines which of the following cellular factors?
   a. Size
   b. Shape
   c. Number
   d. Maturity
   e. Qualitative value

Phlebotomy: Venipuncture and Capillary Puncture

1. Define and spell the key terms as presented in the glossary.

2. Explain the medical assistant's responsibility to the patient in terms of quality of care and respect for the patient as a human being.

3. Explain why the medical assistant has a special responsibility to present a neat, pleasant, and competent demeanor.

4. Inventory a collection tray, explain the supplies and equipment used in blood collections, and demonstrate the ability to use them safely and comfortably.

5. Explain the importance of correct patient identification; complete specimen labeling; and proper handling, storage, and delivery.

6. Summarize the step-by-step procedure for drawing blood with a syringe, vacuum tube system, butterfly, or capillary puncture.

7. Choose appropriate blood collection tubes in proper order of draw.

8. Apply proper guidelines for handling specimens to eliminate rejection of specimens by the laboratory.

9. Explain how to handle the various reactions a patient might have to venipuncture.

KEY TERMS

additive	hematoma	serum
aliquot	hemoconcentration	thixotropic
anticoagulant	hemolysis	thrombocyte
buffy coat	hemolyzed	tourniquet
centrifuge	leukocyte	venipuncture
edematous	palpate	viscosity
erythrocyte	phlebotomy	
hematology	plasma	

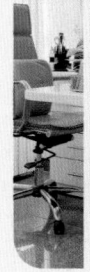

SCENARIO

At Inner City Health Care, medical assistant Thomas Myers, CCMA (NHA) often performs venipunctures. Thomas is personable and has an easygoing manner that makes patients feel comfortable with him. He takes time to talk to patients before performing a venipuncture to determine their feelings about the procedure and to learn about their previous experiences. Thomas is confident and professional in his interactions with patients. He is always well groomed, and he treats patients with respect. Using his social, technical, and administrative skills, Thomas is usually able to collect the necessary blood samples while providing a positive experience for patients.

Collecting blood samples from patients for diagnostic testing is known as **phlebotomy**. The health care professional who performs this duty varies at each health care setting and the task of phlebotomy may not be restricted to one individual. A variety of individuals are cross-trained to do phlebotomy and other related tasks. Many health care settings cannot justify having a dedicated phlebotomist available at all times, so medical assistants will often perform the phlebotomy procedure.

WHY COLLECT BLOOD?

Hematology is the study of blood and its components, fluids, and cells. Hematology also includes the study of blood-forming organs and blood diseases. Phlebotomy, also called **venipuncture**, is used to acquire the blood for testing. Blood is the fluid matrix for chemicals and blood cells to travel to and from our body cells, tissues, and organs. Testing the various components in the blood can determine disease processes, levels of chemicals and medications within our bodies, antibodies, and blood cell activities. The results of these various blood tests are critical for physicians and other health care providers in diagnosing and controlling diseases and conditions.

THE MEDICAL ASSISTANT'S ROLE IN PHLEBOTOMY

A phlebotomist is a person trained to obtain blood specimens by venipuncture and capillary puncture techniques. The phlebotomist's primary role is to collect blood as efficiently and safely as possible for accurate and reliable test results. How the medical assistant will be involved in phlebotomy will vary greatly from one health care facility to another. The medical assistant performing venipuncture will have direct contact with the patient and perform tasks that are critical to the patient's diagnosis and care. During the direct contact with the patient, the medical assistant will leave an impression with the patient. It can be positive or negative depending on the skill with which the medical assistant performs the venipuncture.

Professional

It is the medical assistant's responsibility to provide high-quality care to patients. The medical assistant must act professionally when working with patients. Professionalism is displayed by performing tasks in an efficient, competent manner; wearing clean, neat attire; and showing concern for patients and their feelings.

Patients will probably not tell family and friends that their blood was tested by qualified personnel on expensive state-of-the-art instruments but might share that the person drawing their blood sample was friendly and skilled. A smile and a kind word can reassure the patient and result in a more successful and professional encounter.

ANATOMY AND PHYSIOLOGY OF THE CIRCULATORY SYSTEM

To be prepared to collect blood, the medical assistant must understand the system that carries the blood and the composition of the blood. The system in which the blood is transported is the circulatory system. Blood forms in the organs of the body. The bone marrow is the primary factory for production of blood cells. The lymph nodes, thymus, and spleen are also sites for the production of blood cells. The function of blood is to carry oxygen to body tissues and to remove the waste product, carbon dioxide. The blood also carries nutrients to all parts of the body and moves waste products to the lungs, kidneys, liver, and skin for elimination (Figure 39-1).

The circulatory system consists of the heart and vessels. The heart pumps blood through the body by way of vessels—the arteries, veins, and capillaries. When blood flows away from the heart, it flows in arteries; blood flowing back to the heart flows through the veins. Tiny capillaries connect the arteries (and smaller arterioles) with the veins (and smaller venules) (Figure 39-2).

Arteries have a thick wall that helps them withstand the pressure of the pumping action of the heart. The arteries branch to form arterioles, which branch again to become capillaries. The capillaries then begin coming together to form venules, and the venules then become veins. As blood flows through the body, it follows this path of artery-arteriole-capillary-venule-vein. Oxygenated arterial

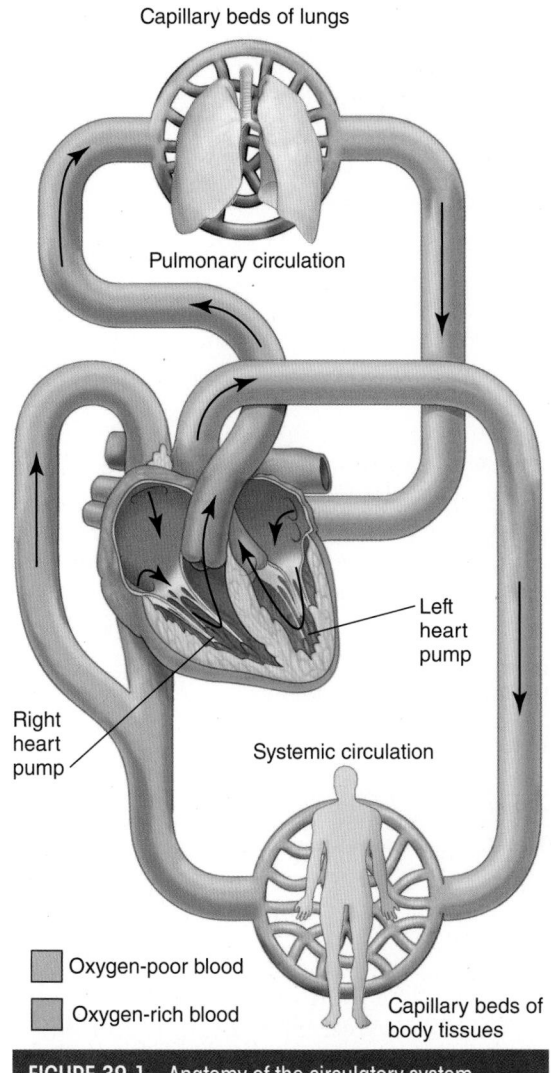

Capillary beds of lungs

Pulmonary circulation

Right heart pump

Left heart pump

Systemic circulation

☐ Oxygen-poor blood

☐ Oxygen-rich blood

Capillary beds of body tissues

FIGURE 39-1 Anatomy of the circulatory system.

ARTERIES TO VEINS	
Arteries	**Veins**
1. Carry blood from the heart, carry oxygenated blood (except pulmonary artery)	1. Carry blood to the heart, carry deoxygenated blood (except pulmonary vein)
2. The blood is normally bright red	2. The blood is normally dark red
3. Elastic walls that expand with surge of blood	3. Thin walls/less elastic
4. No valves	4. Valves
5. Can feel a pulse	5. No pulse

From Heart

To Heart

Artery   Arteriole   Capillaries   Venule   Vein

FIGURE 39-2 Blood flows from the heart through the larger arteries to arterioles to arterial capillary beds at the cellular level, then back to the heart through venous capillary beds into venules and finally larger veins.

blood, which contains a high level of oxygen, leaves the heart and carries the oxygen to the tissues by releasing the oxygen through the cell walls of the capillaries. At the same time, carbon dioxide is being absorbed by the blood, and then is transported to the lungs to be exhaled as a waste product. The flow of the blood also regulates body temperature. When the body gets warm, the capillaries in the extremities dilate and let off heat. This process cools the body. If the body becomes cold, the capillaries constrict and less blood flows through, thereby conserving heat for the rest of the body.

The body contains approximately 6 liters (L) of blood, 45% of which is formed elements. The formed cellular elements consist of **erythrocytes**, **leukocytes**, and **thrombocytes** (Figure 39-3). The remaining 55% of the blood is liquid. The liquid portion of uncoagulated blood is known as plasma. **Plasma** is the fluid that provides a matrix for blood cells, electrolytes, proteins, and chemicals to travel throughout the body via the blood vessels. Blood flowing through the body also contains a substance called fibrinogen. When blood cells are damaged or when blood is exposed to air (as in a wound), the clotting process converts the fibrinogen into fibrin. The fibrin is like a sticky spider web that traps the formed elements into the fibrin mass called a clot. The clear, straw-colored liquid that is left after the clot is formed is called **serum** and is used for many of the tests done in the laboratory. The main difference between serum and plasma is that plasma contains fibrinogen, and serum does not.

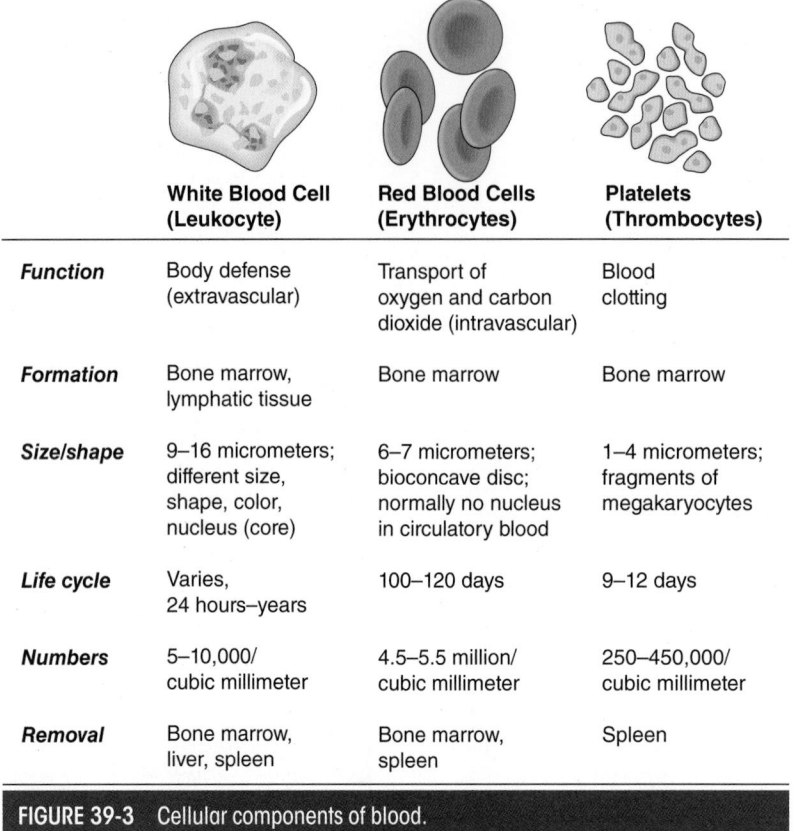

	White Blood Cell (Leukocyte)	Red Blood Cells (Erythrocytes)	Platelets (Thrombocytes)
Function	Body defense (extravascular)	Transport of oxygen and carbon dioxide (intravascular)	Blood clotting
Formation	Bone marrow, lymphatic tissue	Bone marrow	Bone marrow
Size/shape	9–16 micrometers; different size, shape, color, nucleus (core)	6–7 micrometers; bioconcave disc; normally no nucleus in circulatory blood	1–4 micrometers; fragments of megakaryocytes
Life cycle	Varies, 24 hours–years	100–120 days	9–12 days
Numbers	5–10,000/ cubic millimeter	4.5–5.5 million/ cubic millimeter	250–450,000/ cubic millimeter
Removal	Bone marrow, liver, spleen	Bone marrow, spleen	Spleen

FIGURE 39-3 Cellular components of blood.

BLOOD COLLECTION

Most laboratory tests are performed on serum, plasma, or whole blood. Collection tubes and methods will vary depending on the tests ordered. Always refer to your official laboratory manual for specific instructions.

Plasma, Serum, and Whole-Blood Collection

The formed elements (cells) and the liquid portion (serum or plasma) of the blood are usually separated for laboratory testing. To speed the removal of serum from a test tube of blood, the blood is allowed to clot naturally in the tube. A machine called a **centrifuge** spins the test tube of blood, causing the blood to separate according to weight. The centrifugal force pushes the blood clot to the bottom of the tube, leaving the clear serum on top.

To produce a plasma specimen, the blood must be prevented from clotting by the use of a chemical anticoagulant. Blood collected in a tube containing an **anticoagulant** can be centrifuged to separate the formed elements (cells) from the plasma. The bottom layer will contain the heavier erythrocytes. The thinner middle layer, called the **buffy coat**, will be a mixture of leukocytes and thrombocytes, On top of all these layers is the plasma layer. The plasma will contain fibrinogen and is therefore usually slightly hazy (Figure 39-4).

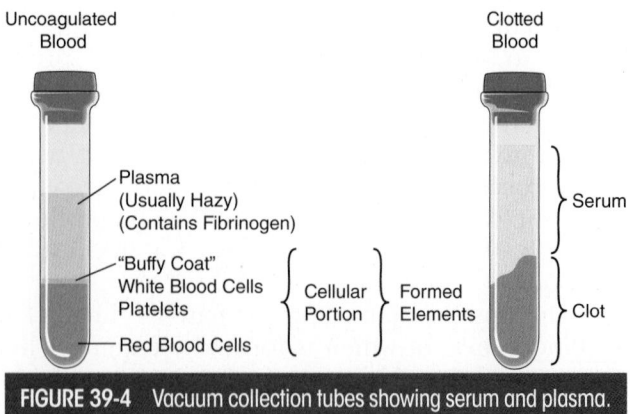

FIGURE 39-4 Vacuum collection tubes showing serum and plasma.

Whole-blood specimens are collected in anticoagulant tubes, mixed well, and maintained at room temperature.

Venipuncture Sites

The most commonly used method for blood collection is venipuncture. To obtain a blood sample, the medical assistant must locate a vein that is acceptable for blood collection. The preferred site for venipuncture is the antecubital space, which is located anterior to the elbow on the inside of the arm. The veins are near the surface and are large enough to give access to the blood (Figure 39-5). The median cubital vein is the vein that is used the majority of the time. When the median cubital vein is not available, palpate for other veins in the antecubital space. These veins include the basilic, cephalic, and median veins. When necessary, veins on the dorsal surface of the hand or wrist may be used for venipuncture, but they are more painful for the patient and will require a smaller needle and the use of a butterfly apparatus.

The veins of the feet are an alternative when the arms are not available. The provider's written permission is needed before drawing blood from the veins of the legs and feet. Due to the potential of harm to the patient, the person performing a foot draw must be specially trained and certified for that procedure.

The arteries in the arm consist of the brachial artery in the brachial region of the arm and the radial and ulnar arteries in the wrist (Figure 39-6). Arterial punctures and drawing blood from arteries are not generally done by a medical assistant. Refer to individual state laws for specific training and certification/registration requirements.

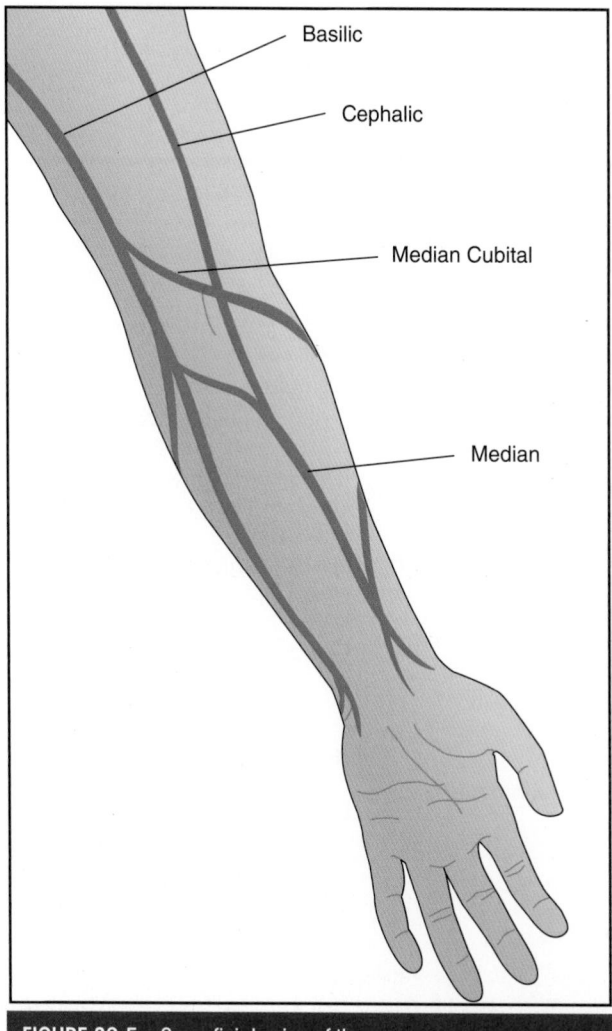

FIGURE 39-5 Superficial veins of the arm.

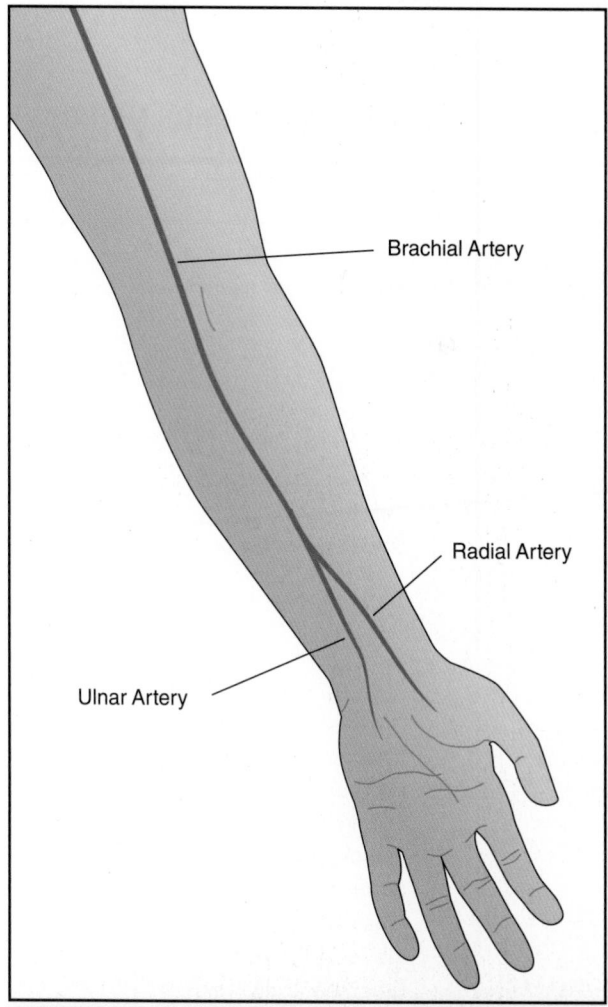

FIGURE 39-6 Arteries of the arm.

VENIPUNCTURE EQUIPMENT

All methods of venipuncture require the invasive procedure of puncturing a vein to obtain a blood sample. The three methods used to perform venipuncture are the syringe method, the vacuum tube method, and the butterfly method. Each method has advantages and disadvantages (Table 39-1). It is important that the well-trained medical assistant be comfortable with each method when drawing blood from a wide range of patients in a variety of situations. If the syringe and/or butterfly methods are used, the specimen will ultimately be transferred into a vacuum tube. This is because vacuum tubes contain the chemicals and substances necessary for the blood tests to be performed.

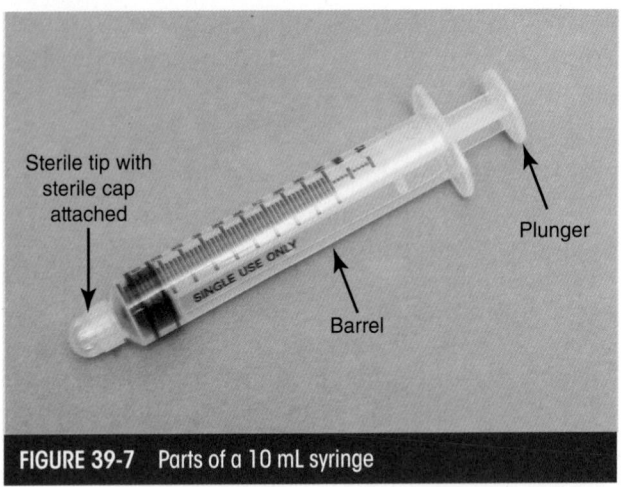

FIGURE 39-7 Parts of a 10 mL syringe

Syringes

Syringes used in venipuncture (Figure 39-7) come in a variety of sizes; the most commonly used are the 5 and 10 mL sizes. Each manufacturer has its own packaging and coloring; thus, there is really no significance related to the color and design of syringes. Some syringes are designed with a Luer-Lok tip that allows the needle to be securely

COMPARISON OF BLOOD COLLECTION METHODS

METHOD	INDICATIONS FOR USE	ADVANTAGES	DISADVANTAGES
Vacuum tube	Routine collection Multiple tubes are needed Whenever possible	Fast Relatively safe Best specimen quality Large collection amount possible	May not work well with: 　Small veins 　Fragile veins 　Difficult draws 　Small children 　Hand or feet draws
Butterfly assembly	Small or fragile veins Difficult draws Small children or older adults	Least likely to collapse vein Less painful to patient Can attach syringe Can attach vacuum tube adapter Least likely to pass through small veins Good specimen quality	Syringe attachment not as safe because tube transfer is necessary Specimen may become hemolyzed (rupture of RBCs) Not recommended for large amounts of blood
Syringe	Children Infants Older adults Oncology patients Severely burned patients Obese patients Inaccessible veins Extremely fragile veins When specimen requires a drop of blood	Easier to perform Allows for smaller amount of specimen	Not recommended for dehydrated patients Not recommended for patients with poor circulation Cannot be used for: 　Blood cultures 　Erythrocyte sedimentation rate

Source: Courtesy of Sheri R. Greimes, CMA (AAMA), PBT (ASCP).

twisted onto the syringe. The Luer-Lok tip may be preferred to the push-on tip for additional safety for the user.

Needles

Needles attached to syringes that are used for venipuncture do not differ in design from needles used for injections They come in a wide variety of lengths and gauges. The most common sizes for venipuncture needles are gauges 20, 21, and 22 and about 1 or 1.5 inches in length (Table 39-2). Sixteen-gauge needles are larger and are often used for blood-banking procedures. Remember the larger the number, the smaller the gauge.

Another type of needle used in venipuncture is the special needle, designed for use with the vacuum tube method. This needle has a double end—the longer needle to puncture the vein and the shorter needle to puncture into the vacuum tube. These needles also come in a variety of gauges and lengths; the most common is the same as the standard needle described previously: 20, 21, and 22 gauge, 1 to 1.5 inches in length. When selecting a double-ended needle for use with the vacuum tube, you will use a multidraw needle, which enables drawing of more than one tube of blood. Multidraw needles come with a rubber sheath over the shorter needle, which goes into the vacuum tube (Figure 39-8). This rubber sheath prevents blood from leaking out of the needle during tube changes. Multidraw needles are sometimes referred to as multiple sample needles.

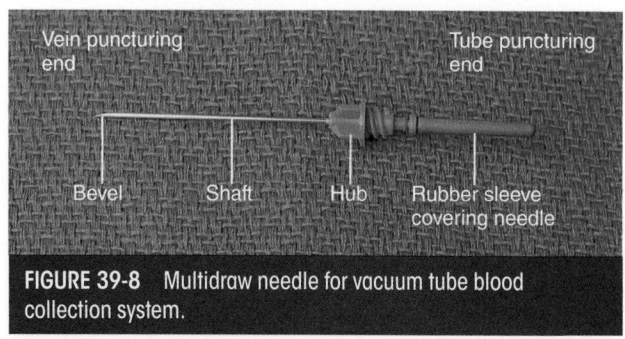

FIGURE 39-8 Multidraw needle for vacuum tube blood collection system.

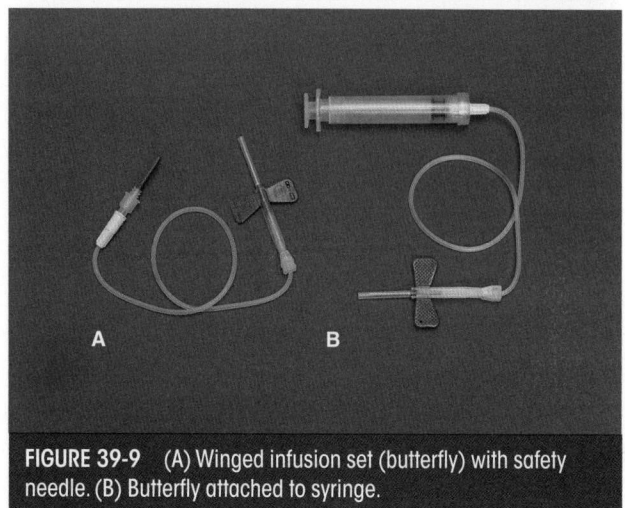

FIGURE 39-9 (A) Winged infusion set (butterfly) with safety needle. (B) Butterfly attached to syringe.

Another type of needle used in venipuncture is on an infusion set called the butterfly collection system (Figure 39-9). Because the butterfly system is used on small and/or fragile veins, the needles are smaller, usually 21 or 23 gauge. Patients who have fragile blood cells may benefit from an even a smaller (25-gauge) needle. Evidently the smaller gauge does not cause damage to fragile blood cells as previously thought.

More details about each collection method are discussed later in this chapter.

Safety Needles and Blood Collection Systems

The Occupational Safety and Health Administration (OSHA) requires that safety needles be made available to employees to prevent on-the-job needlestick injuries. There are a variety of safety needles and blood collection systems currently available to reduce the risk for accidental needlesticks. These systems are often referred to as needlestick prevention devices (NPDs). A common type of safety mechanism is a device in which a cover is snapped over the needle after it is removed from the vein (Figures 39-10 and 39-11).

TABLE 39-2

NEEDLE GAUGES USED IN PHLEBOTOMY

GAUGE SIZE	COMMENTS
23	Used sometimes with butterfly system
22	Preferred for pediatric phlebotomy or very small veins of the hands or feet
21	Most common size used with vacuum tubes
20	Appropriate, but large for common phlebotomy
18	Not used for phlebotomy, but sometimes used in blood banking/donations
16	Most commonly used in blood banking/donations

Vacuum Tubes and Adapters/Holders

Vacuum tubes are vacuum-packed test tubes with either twist-on caps or rubber stoppers. They are available in a variety of sizes for a variety of uses (Figure 39-12). Vacuum tubes come plain or with added chemicals or other substances necessary for the appropriate test to be run. The color of the rubber stopper designates the additive inside the tube. Although most colors are universal regardless of manufacturer, the shades may vary and can be confusing to beginners. It is always best to read the label to determine the additive if the shade is different.

Plastic holders or tube adapters (Figure 39-13) are used in conjunction with the vacuum tubes. Adapters that fit inside the holder to accommodate smaller pediatric vacuum tubes are available. Safety holders are equipped with clickable needle-release mechanisms to minimize the risk for accidental needlesticks. Some plastic holders are reusable, but there is much debate about the appropriateness of reusing them, even after disinfection. They are fairly inexpensive and the inner threads will eventually wear out; therefore, replacing them frequently is always good practice.

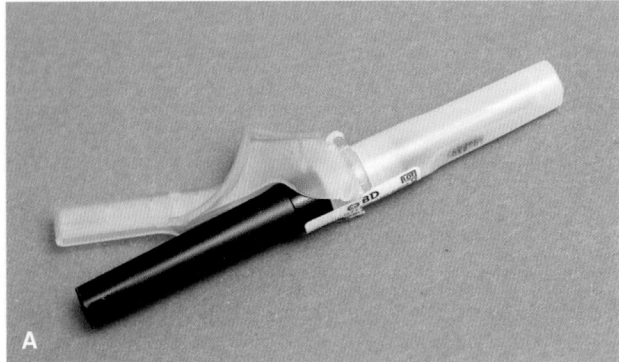

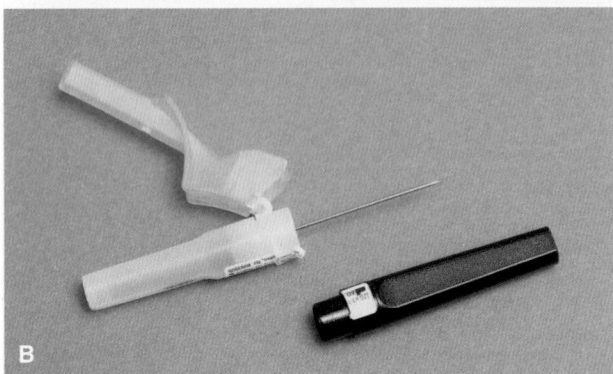

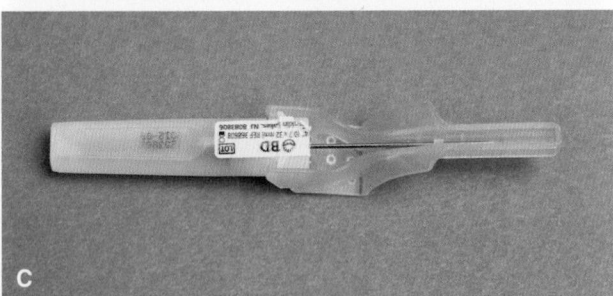

FIGURE 39-10 Eclipse safety needles for use with vacuum tubes. (A) Needle capped, safety mechanism not engaged. (B) Needle exposed, safety mechanism not engaged. (C) Safety mechanism engaged.

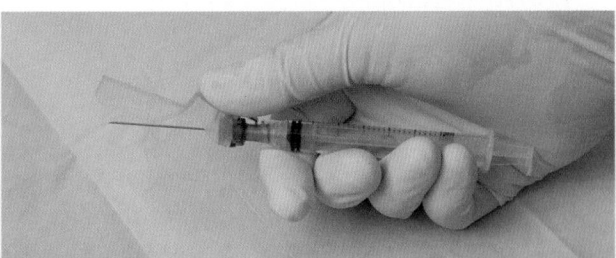

FIGURE 39-11 With the thumb and forefinger, press the safety mechanism over the needle; or an even safer technique is to press it against a hard surface such as the edge of the counter. Be sure to listen for the click. Once engaged, the safety mechanism should be firmly locked in place.

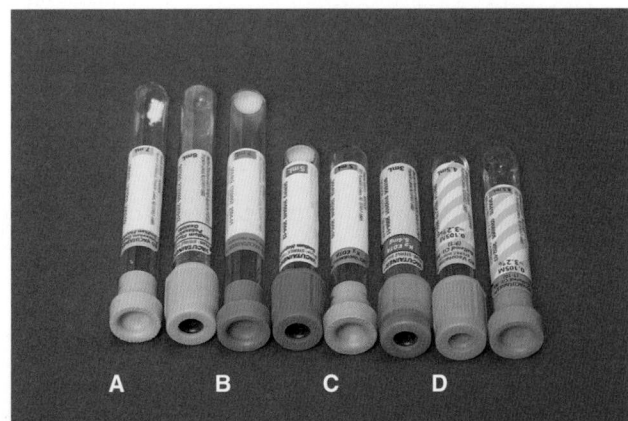

FIGURE 39-12 Standard anticoagulant tubes with conventional rubber stopper and Hemogard twist-off closures. (A) Gray-top tube contains antiglycolytic agent; left tube with rubber stopper, right tube with twist-off Hemogard top. (B) Green-top tube contains heparin anticoagulant; left tube with rubber stopper, right tube with twist-off Hemogard top. (C) Lavender-top tube contains EDTA anticoagulant; left tube with rubber stopper, right tube with twist-off Hemogard top. (D) Light blue–top tube contains sodium citrate; left tube with twist-off Hemogard top, right tube with rubber stopper.

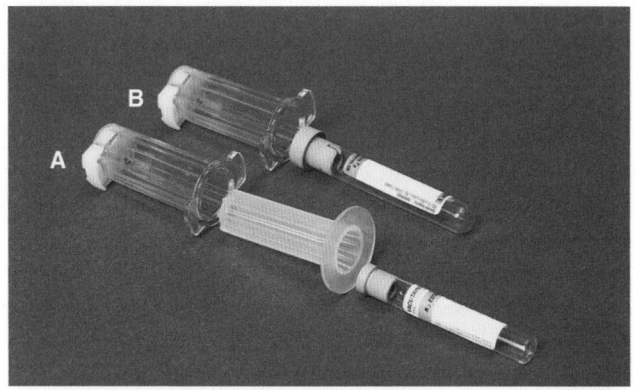

FIGURE 39-13 Holders for vacuum tube system. (A) Adult holder. (B) Pediatric tube using an adapter.

Critical Thinking

You are preparing to perform a venipuncture on a geriatric patient who has fragile veins. Which system would you use: a syringe or a vacuum tube system? What would make one technique more successful than the other in this case?

Anticoagulants, Additives, and Gels

Different tests require different types of blood specimens. Since coagulation/clotting occurs naturally (see the simplified process in Table 39-3), if a step is prevented, the blood does not clot. Some specimens require a serum sample and need to be drawn in a tube that allows the blood to clot. Others require a whole-blood or plasma specimen and need to be drawn in a tube that does not allow the blood to clot. **Additives** are put into the tubes during manufacturing (Figure 39-14). Some tubes

TABLE 39-3

STEPS TO BLOOD CLOTTING (SIMPLIFIED)

1. Uncoagulated blood

2. Calcium utilized

3. Prothrombin converts to thrombin

4. Fibrinogen converts to fibrin

5. Clot forms

Red Top		
Contains:	None	
Effects on Specimen:	Blood clots, and the serum is separated by centrifugation	
Uses:	Chemistries, immunology and serology, blood bank (cross-match)	

Red-Gray Mottled Top ("Tiger top")		
Contains:	Serum separating tube (SST) with clot activator	
Effects on Specimen:	Forms clot quickly and separates the serum with SST gel at the bottom of the tube	
Uses:	Blood type screening and chemistries	

Gold Top		
Contains:	Separating gel and clot activator	
Effects on Specimen:	Serum separator tube (SST) contains a gel at the bottom to separate the blood from serum on centrifugation	
Uses:	Serology, endocrine, immunology, including HIV testing	

Light Green Top		
Contains:	Plasma separating tube (Na heparin)	
Effects on Specimen:	Anticoagulants with lithium heparin: plasma is separated with PST gel at the bottom of the tube	
Uses:	Chemistries	

Lavender/Purple Top		
Contains:	EDTA (liquid form)	
Effects on Specimen:	Forms calcium salts to remove calcium	
Uses:	Hematology (CBC) and blood bank (cross-match); requires a full draw—invert 8 times to prevent clotting and platelet clumping	

Light Blue Top		
Contains:	Sodium citrate (Na citrate)	
Effects on Specimen:	Forms calcium salts to remove calcium	
Uses:	Coagulation tests (PT, PTT, TCT, CMV), tube must be filled 100%	

FIGURE 39-14 Collection tubes and their additives for phlebotomy.

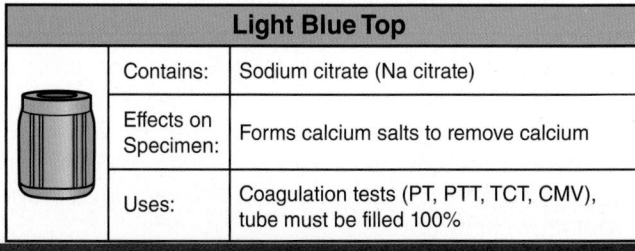

Figure 39-14, continued

Dark Green Top		
	Contains:	Sodium heparin or lithium heparin
	Effects on Specimen:	Inactivates thrombin and thromboplastin
	Uses:	Ammonia, lactate, HLA typing For lithium level, use sodium heparin For ammonia level, use sodium or lithium heparin

Dark Blue/Royal Blue Top		
	Contains:	Sodium heparin or Na$_2$ EDTA
	Effects on Specimen:	Forms calcium salts Tube is designed to contain no contaminating metals
	Uses:	Toxicology and trace element testing (zinc, copper, lead, mercury) and drug level testing

Light Gray Top		
	Contains:	Sodium fluoride and potassium oxalate
	Effects on Specimen:	Antiglycolytic agent preserves glucose up to 5 days
	Uses:	For lithium level, use sodium heparin Glucose requires a full draw (may cause hemolysis if short draw)

Yellow Top		
	Contains:	ACD (acid-citrate-dextrose)
	Effects on Specimen:	Complement inactivation
	Uses:	Paternity testing, DNA studies

Tan/Brown Top		
	Contains:	Sodium heparin
	Effects on Specimen:	Inactivates thrombin and thromboplastin
	Uses:	Serum lead determination

Black Top		
	Contains:	Sodium citrate (buffered)
	Effects on Specimen:	Forms calcium salts to remove calcium
	Uses:	Westergren sedimentation rate; requires a full draw

Orange Top		
	Contains:	Thrombin
	Effects on Specimen:	Quickly clots blood
	Uses:	STAT serum chemistries

FIGURE 39-14 *(continued)*

also contain **thixotropic** gel plugs, which act as separators between the blood cells/clot and the serum/plasma. A chemical additive may be a chemical to help preserve the blood or a substance to accelerate the clotting process (called a clot activator) (see Table 39-4). An anticoagulant is a chemical additive that prevents the clotting by removing calcium in the form of calcium salts or by inhibiting the conversion of prothrombin to thrombin.

The step removed depends on the anticoagulant used. The basic anticoagulants used consist of oxalates, citrates, ethylenediaminetetraacetic acid (EDTA), or heparin. It is important to use the correct anticoagulant for the test because the improper anticoagulant can alter test results. Refer to Figure 39-14, which shows the color-coded stoppers for each tube.

Clot activators consist of silica (small glass) particles on the sides of the tubes that initiate the clotting process. The silica particles work as a catalyst for the clotting process by promoting the clotting process.

Serum and plasma tubes are also available with a thixotropic separator gel (Figure 39-15). The gel is an inert material that undergoes a temporary change in **viscosity** during centrifugation. When centrifuged, the gel changes to a liquid and moves up the sides of the tube to create a barrier between the blood cells or clot and the liquid portion of the blood. The gel then forms a solid plug and separates the cells/clot from the plasma/serum, thus protecting the serum from contamination from any **hemolyzed** (ruptured) RBCs (Figure 39-16).

TABLE 39-4

ACTIONS OF ADDITIVES

ADDITIVE	ACTION
Potassium oxalate	Binds calcium
Sodium fluoride	Inhibits glycolysis
Sodium citrate	Binds calcium
EDTA	Binds calcium
Lithium heparin	Inhibits prothrombin to thrombin
No additive	Clot naturally forms
Sodium polyanethol sulfonate (SPS)	Binds calcium
Glass particles/silica	Promotes clotting
Ammonium heparin	Inhibits prothrombin to thrombin

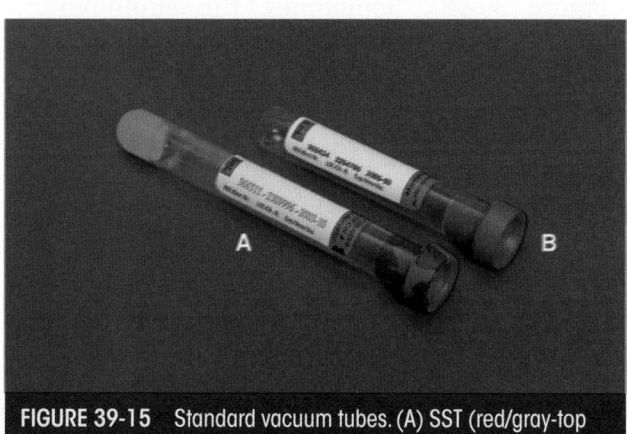

FIGURE 39-15 Standard vacuum tubes. (A) SST (red/gray-top or speckled-top) tube contains clot activators and thixotropic gel. (B) Standard red-top (glass) tube contains no anticoagulant but might contain glass particles/silica on the inside walls to irritate the thrombocytes to promote clotting.

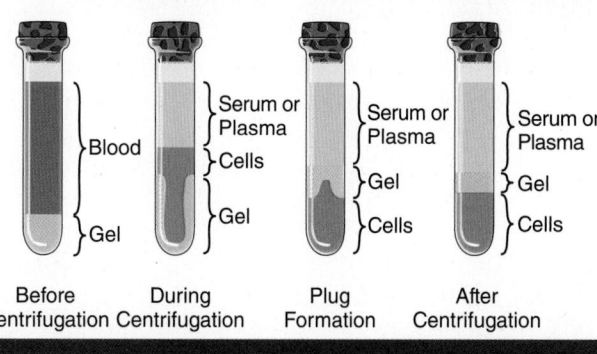

FIGURE 39-16 Separator thixotropic gel tube showing how stages of the centrifugation process works.

Order of Draw

The order in which blood is drawn or mixed with additives is important. The Clinical Laboratory Standards Institute (CLSI) establishes laboratory procedures, including specimen procurement. The order in which the vacuum tubes are to be used, designated in the CLSI's latest publication (2011), is listed in Table 39-5. The rationale behind a specific order of draw is to prevent cross-contamination. Sterile collection bottles (for blood cultures) need to be filled first to prevent cross-contamination. After the sterile culture tubes are drawn, the order for the other tubes is related to the additives in them. The clot activator in the red and speckled-top tubes is now considered an additive, even though it is not a chemical anticoagulant. It does not matter whether the blood is drawn directly into a vacuum tube or into a syringe, then transferred to the vacuum tube. The order of the tubes remains the same for either method.

Tourniquets

The **tourniquet**, when applied to the arm, constricts the flow of blood in the arm and makes the veins more prominent. The tourniquet is a soft, pliable, rubber or elastic strip (preferably latex free) approximately 1-inch wide by 15- to 18-inches long (Figure 39-17). The elastic strip is the best tourniquet for all conditions. The elastic strip can easily be released with one hand. Being about 1-inch wide, it does not cut into the patient's

TABLE 39-5

CLSI STANDARD ORDER OF DRAW

Blood culture tubes or vials	Yellow top or culture bottles
Sodium citrate	Light blue top
Serum tubes	Red top and red/gray and gold top (SST)
Heparin tubes	Green tops, light and dark
EDTA tubes	Lavender top, then pink, white, or royal blue
Glycolytic inhibitor	Gray top
Fibrin degradable products	Dark blue

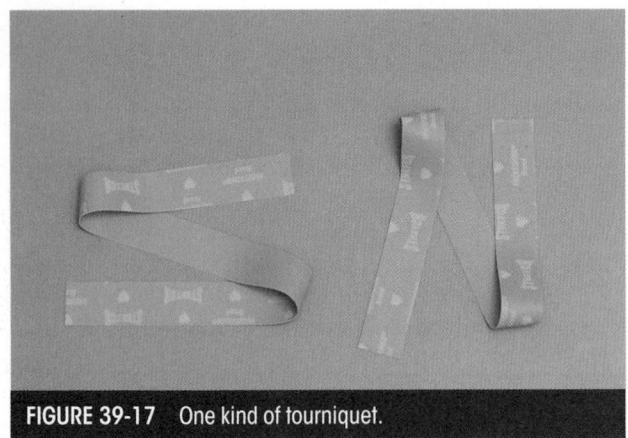

FIGURE 39-17 One kind of tourniquet.

arm; rather, distributes pressure. The tourniquet can easily be disinfected but is inexpensive enough that it should be replaced often. If the tourniquet is obviously contaminated, it should be discarded into biohazard waste. If a patient has been identified as having a latex hypersensitivity, you must use a nonlatex tourniquet. Latex-free tourniquets are readily available and inexpensive, so they can be used for all patients regardless of latex allergy or hypersensitivity.

A blood pressure cuff can also be used as a tourniquet. Its use is primarily for veins that are difficult to locate using a standard tourniquet. The blood pressure should be taken first, and then the cuff should be maintained slightly below the diastolic pressure (average: 40 mm Hg).

Specimen Collection Trays

Unless a designated drawing station is available, the medical assistant may need a portable specimen collection tray to hold all the equipment necessary for proper specimen collection. The tray can be taken to the patient in the examination room so that whatever procedure is performed, the phlebotomy procedure can be conducted without the medical assistant searching for the proper equipment. Trays vary depending on the type of collection being performed. Because trays are also used to transport blood specimens, OSHA's *Bloodborne Pathogen Standard* requires each tray to be all red or prominently labeled with an approved biohazard symbol. The tray is usually preferred because it is more portable and can easily be taken to the patient. Trays (without supplies) are available from medical supply manufacturers in a variety of sizes and shapes (Figure 39-18). Sometimes, the equipment is stored in a special drawer for venipuncture equipment in each examination room or in a central laboratory area. Whichever storage system is used, restocking is a continual responsibility that aims to keep supplies readily available for the next time they are needed.

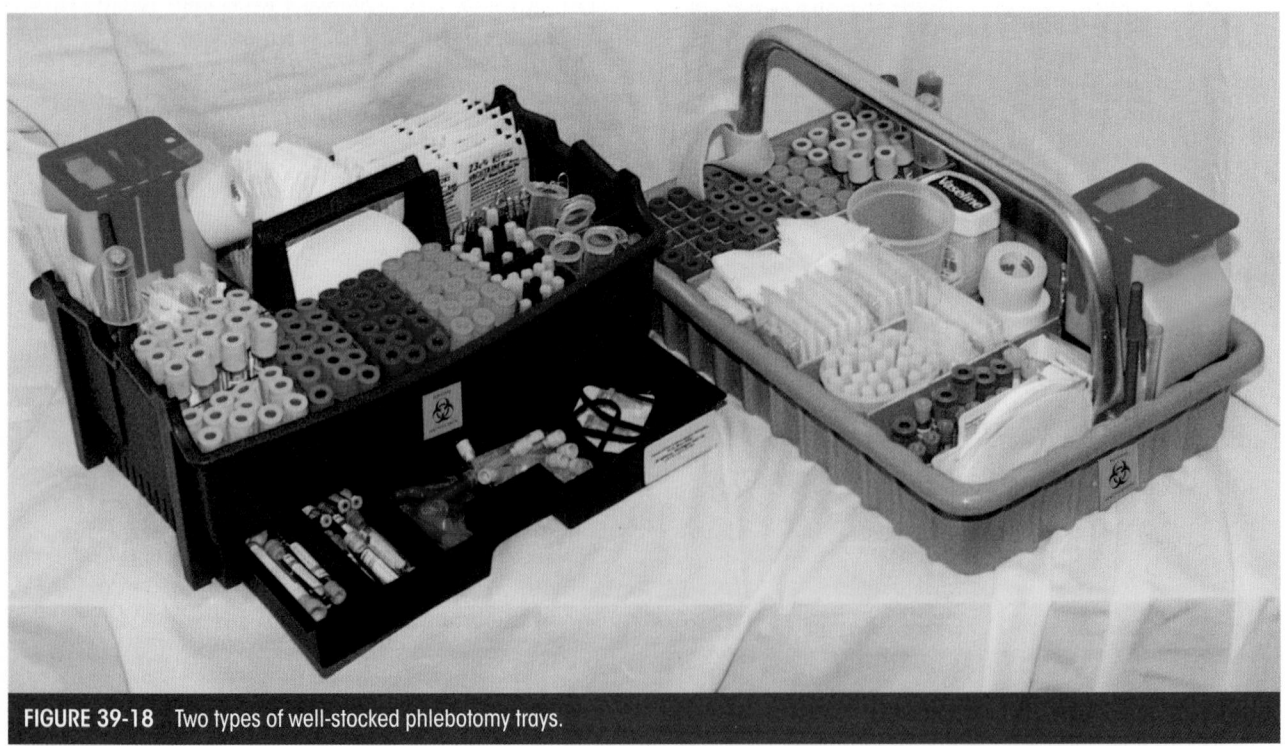

FIGURE 39-18 Two types of well-stocked phlebotomy trays.

VENIPUNCTURE PRINCIPLES

Professional

The first step to a successful venipuncture is putting the patient at ease. The medical assistant uses many skills when interacting with patients during phlebotomy. In addition to the technical skills related to performing the procedure safely and confidently, and the quality assurance skills of correct labeling and handling of the specimens, the skills that will affect the patient the most will be the medical assistant's interpersonal and therapeutic communication skills.

Therapeutic communication skills (see Chapter 4) are used by the medical assistant to obtain cooperation from the patient. Some patients will be calm, whereas others may be extremely frightened. The nicest individual may be irritable and may even become physically or emotionally abusive when placed in an unfamiliar health care setting. The medical assistant uses interpersonal and therapeutic communication skills and professional behavior to put each patient at ease, reassure patients, and encourage cooperation. When greeting the patient, adhere to the following guidelines:

1. Reassure the patient that the procedure is going to be simple and there will be only a slight inconvenience.

2. Be friendly and outgoing and talk to the patient conversationally as you explain the procedure. Polite conversation with all patients gives them the feeling someone cares about them.

3. Do not tell the patient that the procedure will not be painful. Explain that the procedure can be slightly uncomfortable but you will take care to cause the least discomfort possible. If the patient seems overly concerned about pain, check frequently with him or her to see how he or she is doing. If the patient seems extremely apprehensive, ask if he or she would prefer to lie down during the procedure. This may prevent further problems if the patient faints.

4. Exhibit professional concern for patients, because this will result in more satisfied patients who will return in the future for care from the same provider.

Procedure

After assessing the patient's level of concern and calming the patient if needed, the medical assistant will explain the procedure and then use technical skills to perform the phlebotomy procedure with minimal discomfort to the patient (see Procedure 39-1). As important as it is to obtain a good specimen, it is equally important to treat the patient with empathy. Using social and technical skills, the medical assistant can provide a positive experience for the patient. A patient who has had a positive experience will talk with friends and neighbors about that experience, which could result in a positive reputation in the community for the facility.

Preparing Supplies

Prepare all supplies and equipment before the venipuncture. Place all tubes within easy reach to avoid crossing over the patient and possibly moving the needle after it is in the patient. Remember that occasionally a tube will not fill completely; therefore, it is best to have a few spare tubes or to keep the phlebotomy tray within reach.

Patient and Specimen Identification

Proper patient and specimen identification is essential to accurate patient testing. The results of specimen testing will be incorrect if the specimen is not accurately identified. When entering the room, it is best not to say: "Mr. Jones, I'm here to draw your blood," assuming that if the patient says "Okay" he is Mr. Jones. The patient may not have been paying attention and may answer okay even if it is not his name. Instead, ask the patient to state his or her full name and date of birth. If the patient is unable to communicate with you, or if you are in an inpatient environment such as a hospital or extended care facility, always check the patient's identification wristband or check with the caretaker. In ambulatory settings, a good policy is to ask for picture identification from non-English-speaking patients.

Once the medical assistant has identified the patient and the blood is drawn, the specimen needs to be labeled for proper identification. Labeling should include the patient's first and last name, middle initial, date of birth, any assigned identification number, the date, the time, and the initials of the person collecting the specimen. Either apply a computer generated label or write the required information clearly and legibly, using a permanent marker, before leaving the patient's presence. By doing so, if the tubes are taken to the physician's office laboratory or an outside reference laboratory, the specimens will be properly identified. Any paperwork or forms accompanying the specimens must be checked with the blood tubes to verify that names and numbers match.

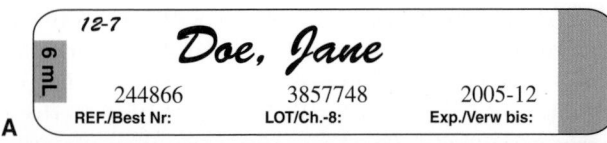

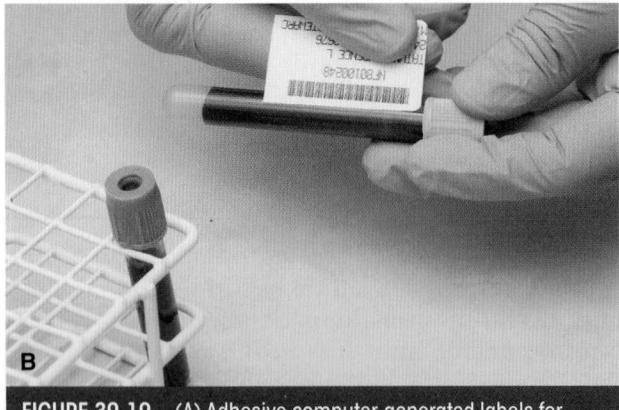

FIGURE 39-19 (A) Adhesive computer-generated labels for identifying specimen tubes from one patient. (B) The medical assistant applies a computer-generated label to the patient's specimen tube.

Many clinics use computerized systems for test requisitions, labeling, and result reporting. The computer label has several advantages in that it lists the specific tests that are ordered, the specimen needed, and specimen requirements. The label is also adhesive so it can be attached directly to the tube. Smaller labels can also be printed at the same time for smaller specimens. A portion of a specimen that has been taken for use or storage is called an **aliquot**. Labels may also contain bar codes to assist in electronic patient and specimen identification (Figure 39-19A and B) With computerized systems, the medical assistant will verify by entering information into the computer when the blood is drawn.

Positioning the Patient

The position of the patient is critical for proper patient blood collection. The best position is the position that is comfortable for the patient and the health care professional. The patient might tell you of a past unpleasant experience in which he fainted or felt dizzy during a phlebotomy procedure. In that case, lying down is the position of choice for the patient. Specially designed chairs assist the patient in staying fairly upright and safe if she or he becomes lightheaded or faints.

Selecting the Appropriate Vein

The appropriate venipuncture site can vary depending on the patient. The usual site that is first checked is the antecubital region of the arm.

The primary vein used in the antecubital region of the arm is the median cubital vein. This is usually the prominent vein in the middle of the bend of the arm (see Figure 39-5). The basilic or cephalic vein can be used as an alternative. However, these veins may not be accessible or may not be prominent enough to obtain a blood sample. Check both arms as one may be a better choice than the other. The next alternate site is the back of the hand. The veins in the back of the hand have the tendency to "roll" more than the arm veins because they are not supported by as much tissue and are closer to the surface. To avoid this, the vein will have to be held in place securely while a smaller-gauge needle or a butterfly is used. The hand veins are ideal for a 3- to 5-mL syringe with a 22-gauge needle. Careful, slow pulling on the syringe will obtain the blood sample without collapsing the vein or causing hemolysis of the specimen. The veins at the back of the wrist are also an alternative, but they are generally more painful than the other sites.

Applying the Tourniquet

A tourniquet must be used to assist the medical assistant in feeling a vein. The tourniquet is applied 3 to 4 inches above the intended puncture site. It is applied tightly enough to slow the flow of blood in the veins but not so tightly as to prevent the flow of blood in the arteries (Figures 39-20A–D). With the tourniquet applied, the venous blood is unable to return past the tourniquet so the veins swell a bit, making the veins more prominent. The veins can then be **palpated** (examined with the fingertips) to determine their direction, depth, and size. The tourniquet should be on the arm no longer than 1 minute. A tourniquet that is left on too long will cause **hemoconcentration** of the blood, that is, an increased concentration of constituents in the blood sample that may lead to inaccurate test results. If the tourniquet is removed, CLSI requires it not be reapplied to the same arm for 2 full minutes. If the patient has sensitive skin or a skin problem, the tourniquet can be applied over the patient's upper arm clothing or a piece of gauze pad. This will minimize the discomfort felt by the patient.

The tourniquet often causes greater discomfort for patients than the venipuncture itself. The tourniquet should ideally be removed as soon as blood flow is established. This is not practical for the novice medical assistant. The act of removing the tourniquet may move the needle or vein just enough so that no more blood can be obtained

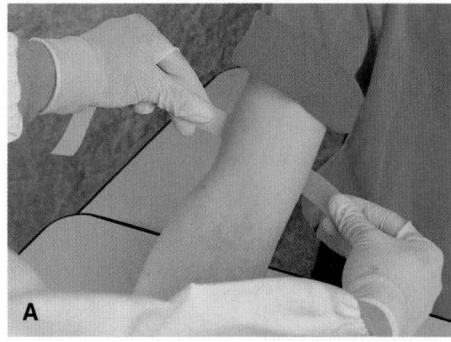

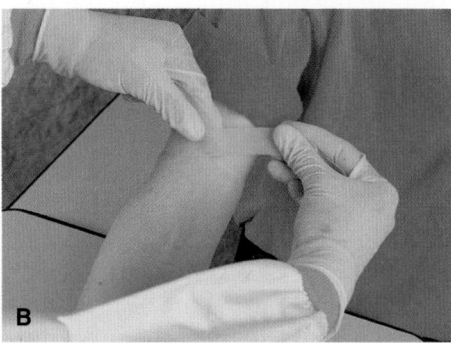

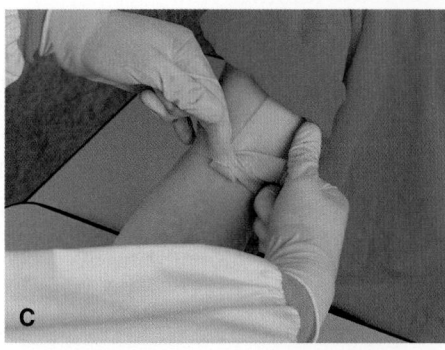

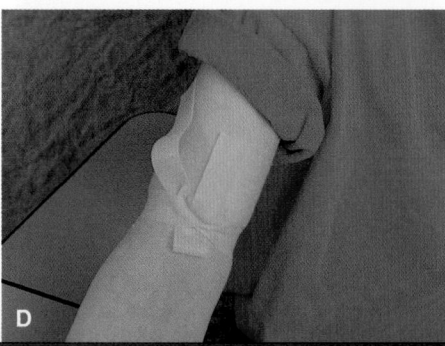

FIGURE 39-20 Applying a tourniquet. (A) Wrap the tourniquet around the arm 3 to 4 inches above the venipuncture site. Keeping the tourniquet flat to the skin will help minimize the discomfort felt by the patient. (B) Stretch the tourniquet tight and cross the ends. (C) While holding the ends tight, tuck one portion of the tourniquet under the other. (D) The tourniquet should not be loose and the ends should be secure. The ends of the tourniquet should be pointed upward and not hanging into the intended venipuncture site.

and a second venipuncture must be performed. It is recommended to wait until just before the needle is removed from the patient to remove the tourniquet. The tourniquet must be removed prior to removing the needle from the vein. If the needle is removed while the tourniquet is still in place, the vein will bleed heavily. Blood will be forced out of the needle hole and into the surrounding tissue, resulting in a **hematoma** (an accumulation of blood in the tissues) or bruising around the venipuncture site. As with any procedure, practice makes for a smoother and more skillful performance.

Performing a Safe and Successful Venipuncture

The first step in successful collection of a venous blood specimen is to find the site that will give the best blood return. Rather than relying on visualizing the vein, rely on touch. While you practice, close your eyes while palpating. The vein should be palpated with the tip of the middle or ring fingers, which tend to be more sensitive than the index finger. Feel for and trace the path of the vein several times. Avoid using the thumb because it has a pulse and is not as sensitive as the rest of the fingers. The vein will feel soft and bouncy to the touch. The roundness of the vein and the direction it follows may be determined. Feel for turns that veins take along their path. Palpate the path of the vein to determine the direction for needle insertion and feel the contour, across the vessel, to find the "bouncy" touch. Both actions will assure a better approach and site selection for the blood draw. All veins are not straight up and down the arm. If no veins become prominent, release the tourniquet and change arms. You might need to retie the tourniquet tighter (after waiting the requisite 2 full minutes). Be careful to not stop the flow of arterial blood into the arm. If the tourniquet is tied tightly enough to stop arterial blood flow, the patient will no longer have a pulse in the wrist. If this occurs, immediately remove the tourniquet because this indicates that blood has ceased flowing below the tourniquet.

If the "vein" that is felt has a pulsing action to it, it is an artery, not a vein, and the vessel should not be punctured. Tendons can be deceptive and give the appearance of veins. However, they do not have the soft, bouncy feel and will be hard to the touch. Puncturing a tendon will give no blood return and will be painful to the patient. Nerves also run the length of the arm. The nerves cannot be seen or felt. Avoid deep insertion or probing with the needle to diminish the chance of damaging nerves and other tissues. If the patient complains that the venipuncture is extremely painful, it is best to stop and try another site. Do not subject the patient to more than two attempts. If the venipuncture is that difficult, ask another health care professional to try. The medical assistant should not change the direction of the needle once inserted. Doing so can cause serious damage to the patient.

Arms that are **edematous** or swollen due to poor lymphatic action, such as after a mastectomy, should never be used for venipuncture, nor should a tourniquet be applied to a compromised arm. Using the tourniquet in this instance may cause tissue damage, and compromised circulation hinders healing. Areas of scarring or bruising should also be avoided because of possible injury, or excessive discomfort to the patient.

Safety

Puncturing an Artery. If you accidentally puncture an artery, you will see that the blood is a brighter color. This is due to the oxygenation of arterial blood versus venous blood. Go ahead and calmly fill the tubes.

Critical Thinking
You are having a difficult time getting the needle to cooperate when putting together a butterfly system and you accidentally contaminate it. The patient has the tourniquet already on his or her arm. What do you do? Why? Is there something else you could have done?

Often the laboratory can run the blood tests on arterial blood just as with venous blood. After the needle is removed, pressure needs to be held for a full 3 minutes (5 minutes or longer if the patient is taking a blood thinner such as aspirin or Coumadin (warfarin)). As with any phlebotomy procedure, make sure the bleeding has stopped before the patient leaves your care. While the patient is still there, check with the lab. If the test requires venous blood, you will need to repeat the procedure. To do so, you would use another site.

Procedure

PROCEDURE 39-1
Palpating a Vein and Preparing a Patient for Venipuncture

STANDARD PRECAUTIONS:

Handwashing   Gloves

PURPOSE:
To palpate a vein and assess patient preparation prior to performing venipuncture.

EQUIPMENT/SUPPLIES:
- Gloves
- Tourniquet

PROCEDURE STEPS:
1. Introduce yourself by name and credentials. Identify the patient *and explain the rationale for performance of the procedure, showing awareness of the patient's concerns related to the procedure being performed.* Ask the patient's name and verify it with the computer label or identification number. If a fasting specimen is required, verify that the patient has not had anything to eat or drink except water for 12 hours. RATIONALE: Proper identification of the patient and specimen and ensuring that the patient has properly prepared for the blood tests are quality-control and quality-assurance measures.

(continues)

2. Wash hands. Put on gloves.

3. Apply tourniquet 3 to 4 inches above the venipuncture site (see Figure 39-20). Apply tightly enough to slow venous blood flow but not so tight that blood flow in arteries is stopped. RATIONALE: Applying the tourniquet too tightly can lead to excessive engorgement of the veins, causing blood to enter the tissues during puncture, further causing a hematoma.

4. Have the patient close the hand. Then place the patient's arm in a downward position. Do not allow the patient to pump his or her hand. RATIONALE: Having the patient close his or her hand and positioning the arm below the heart causes enlargement of the vein, allowing for an easier, more successful puncture. Pumping of the hand can lead to excessive engorgement of the vein, causing blood to leak into surrounding tissue during the puncture, which will cause a hematoma to occur.

5. Palpate the antecubital space of the arm, feeling for the basilic or cephalic vein with the tip of your middle or ring finger. Feel for a soft bounce and a roundness to the vein. RATIONALE: The tip of the middle or ring finger is less callused and more sensitive than the tip of the index finger. Veins will have a soft round feel.

6. After locating an acceptable vein, mentally map the location, ***incorporating critical thinking skills when performing patient care.*** Visualize the puncture site. Follow the direction of the vein with your fingertip, making a mental note of any turns, dips, and twists. RATIONALE: Mentally mapping the location and visualizing the puncture site will help in planning a successful direction.

7. If a vein cannot be found in the antecubital space of either arm, then the hand veins may be checked following the same procedure. The butterfly technique is more successful for hand venipuncture. RATIONALE: Butterfly is more successful because the hand veins have a greater tendency to roll and are smaller than the veins in the arm.

SPECIMEN COLLECTION

The patient has been identified, requisition/orders and tubes have been verified, equipment has been assembled, and the patient is in a comfortable position. Hand washing is the most critical step to preventing the spread of infection. Before touching the patient, medical assistants should wash their hands. It is good practice to wash your hands in view of the patient to give the patient confidence in your technique. The next steps are to tie the tourniquet, apply gloves, and palpate for the best site. Some authorities suggest putting on gloves first and then palpating for the vein. This technique is required for the patient who is isolated because of a communicable disease and is good practice for all patients. After the best vein is selected, the site is cleansed with a gauze pad that has a 70% isopropyl alcohol solution on it. Commercially prepared alcohol pads are called alcohol pledgets. They remove any oil, sweat, perfume, lotions, and skin contaminations. This process is often referred to as "defatting" the skin. The site is allowed to air dry since puncturing the skin through wet alcohol can cause hemolysis of the specimen and give the patient a stinging sensation. Residual alcohol can also contaminate the specimen. After the site is dry, the venipuncture is performed by the appropriate method.

Standard Precautions require that personal protective equipment be worn when there is a chance of coming in contact with blood or body fluid. Safety glasses and a mask must be worn if there is a potential for blood splatter. Refer to your facility procedures and requirements for full PPE requirements.

The Syringe Technique

Procedure

The syringe technique is used less often than the vacuum tube method. The syringe is ideal for collecting small volumes of blood from fragile, thin, or "rolling" veins or veins on the back of the hand or from the foot. Pulling on the plunger of the syringe creates suction. Vein collapse can be avoided by pulling the plunger slowly and by resting between pulls to allow the vein to refill. Because pediatric and geriatric patients often have thin and fragile veins, the syringe is the preferred method of venipuncture for them. The use of a syringe larger than 15 mL is not recommended. If more than 12 mL is needed, the butterfly collection method should be considered. Syringe draws are also ideal in special procedures when the blood must be transferred to a different container (see Procedure 39-2). For more information on proper syringe technique, see the "Correct Hand and Needle Positions" Quick Reference Guide.

Correct Hand and Needle Positions

≫ CORRECT HAND POSITION TO HOLD A SYRINGE

1. The needle is attached to the syringe.

2. Hold the syringe and needle system in your dominant hand, cradling it on your four fingers. A right-handed person would hold the syringe in the right hand, leaving the left hand to pull on the plunger. A left-handed person would do the opposite.

3. Place the thumb on top of the syringe (Figure 39-21).

4. With the syringe held in this position, turn it slightly so the bevel of the needle is facing up.

5. Hold the hand in such a position that by tilting the point of the needle down slightly the needle will enter the skin at a 15-degree angle and about a half inch below the point where the vein was felt.

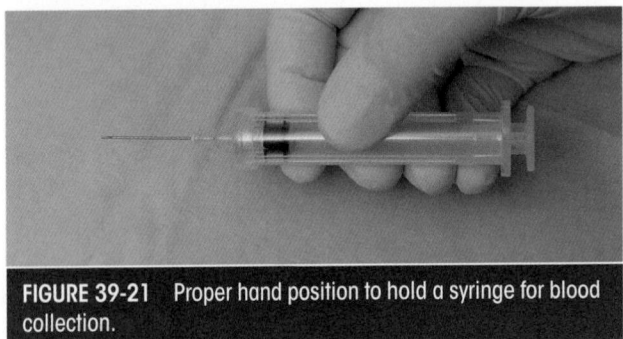

FIGURE 39-21 Proper hand position to hold a syringe for blood collection.

≫ CORRECT NEEDLE POSITION

The patient might experience the least amount of pain if the bevel of the needle is facing upward when the needle is inserted into the vein. The bevel of the needle is upward when the opening in the needle is visible when you look straight down on the needle as it is inserted. This position also helps prevent the suction from causing the inside wall of the vein to adhere to the needle bevel, thus occluding the needle.

The needle should be inserted at a 15-degree angle to the surface of the skin (Figure 39-22).

The skin should be held taut until the needle has been inserted. This technique allows the point of the needle to enter the skin with little drag or bunching of the skin, thereby reducing the discomfort of the puncture.

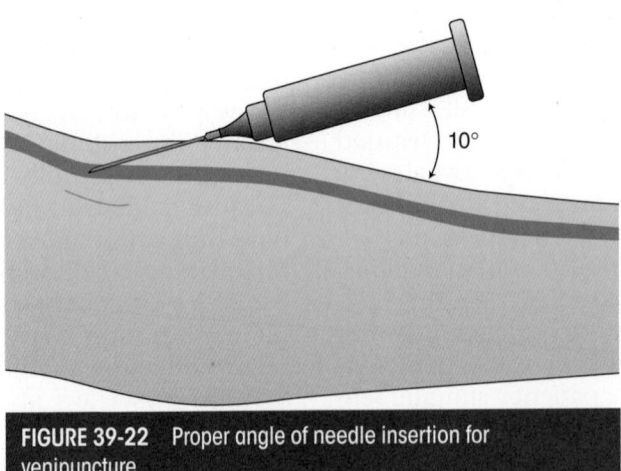

FIGURE 39-22 Proper angle of needle insertion for venipuncture.

When a syringe is used, the blood obtained must be placed in appropriate containers. The order of filling the tubes is important. Refer to Table 39-5.

The use of an unguarded needle to transfer blood from a syringe to a vacuum tube or culture bottle is unsafe and prohibited by OSHA. The use of a safety system such as the BD Vacutainer Blood Transfer Device is recommended (Figure 39-23). After drawing the blood into the syringe, activate the needle's safety mechanism, then remove the needle and dispose of it. Connect the needleless syringe to the transfer device. Insert a vacuum tube to the device and allow the blood to transfer from the syringe to the tube using the tube's vacuum. Never push on the syringe plunger or force the blood into the tube. This could cause the tube's stopper to pop off. When the appropriate tubes have been filled, dispose of the entire syringe and transfer assembly as one unit according to your clinic policies.

Immediately after filling, mix any tubes containing additives (Figure 39-24).

 Safety Techniques. When transferring blood from a syringe to a vacuum tube, keep these safety precautions in mind:

- Never transfer to a vacuum tube using a needle. When transferring from a syringe to a vacuum tube, use a safety transfer device.

- Never push the blood into the vacuum tube. It will fill on its own.

- Always wear gloves, goggles, and face guard when performing this procedure.

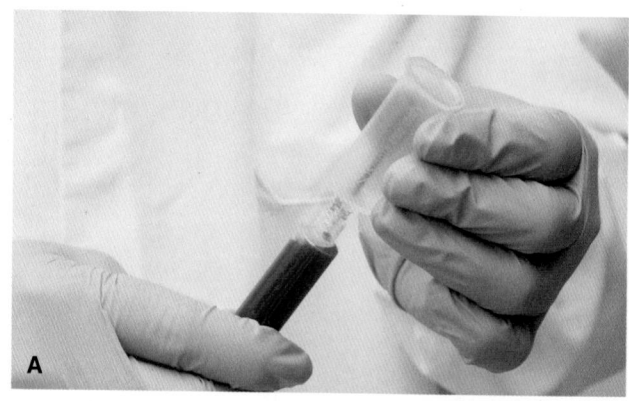

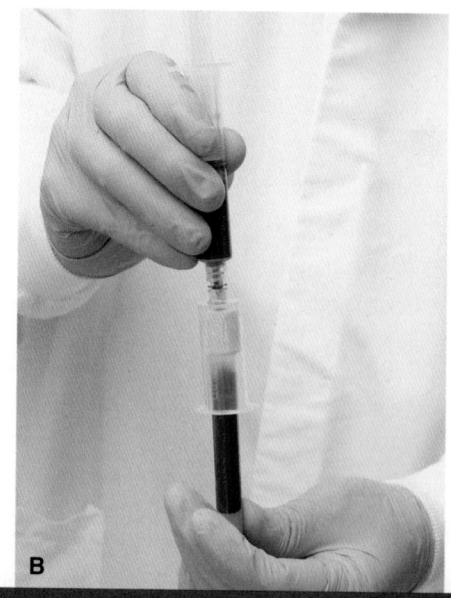

FIGURE 39-23 (A) The medical assistant attaches the BD Vacutainer Blood Transfer Device. (B) The device is used to safely transfer blood from a syringe to a vacuum tube.

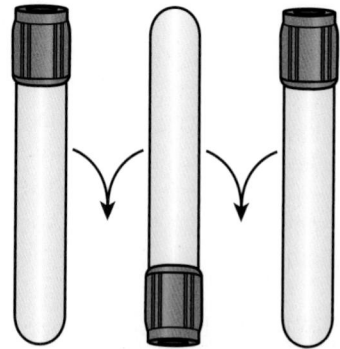

BD Vacutainer™ Tube Type	Closure Color	Number of Inversions
EDTA	Lavender	8–10
Sodium citrate	Light blue	3–4
SST with gel	Tiger (red gray) or gold	5
Serum	Red	5
Sodium fluoride	Gray	8–10
Heparin	Green	8–10

FIGURE 39-24 Vacuum tubes should be inverted several times (not shaken) to mix the additives well.

PROCEDURE 39-2

Venipuncture by Syringe

Procedure

STANDARD PRECAUTIONS:

Handwashing

Gloves

Goggles & Mask

No Needle Recapping

Biohazard

PURPOSE:

To obtain venous blood acceptable for laboratory testing as requested by the provider.

EQUIPMENT/SUPPLIES:

- Gloves
- Goggles and mask
- 10 mL syringe, 21-gauge needle
- Vacuum tube(s) or special collection tube(s)
- Tourniquet
- 70% isopropyl alcohol pledget
- Gauze pads

- Adhesive bandage or tape
- Sharps container and red biohazard bag
- Test tube rack
- Computer-generated label or thin-tipped permanent marker
- Biohazard transport bag (optional)
- Lab requisition (optional)

PROCEDURE STEPS:

1. Assemble the supplies. RATIONALE: Organizing supplies before the procedure ensures a more timely and professional process.

2. Introduce yourself by name and credentials. Position and identify the patient. Ask the patient's name and verify it with the tests ordered and the computer label or identification number. If a fasting specimen is required, verify that the patient has not had anything to eat or drink except water for 12 hours. RATIONALE: Properly identifying the patient and the tests ordered and ensuring that the patient is properly prepared for the blood tests are all quality-control and quality-assurance measures.

3. *Explain the rationale for performance of the procedure and expectations to the patient. Show awareness of the patient's concerns related to the procedure being performed.* RATIONALE: Explaining the procedure and allaying the patient's fears will assure the patient that you are concerned about any apprehension he or she may have and that you are open to discussing the concerns.

4. Wash hands and apply gloves and goggles/mask. RATIONALE: Clean hands further protect the patient. Gloves protect you. Goggles/mask should be worn if there is a possibility of blood splatter.

5. Open the sterile needle and sterile syringe packages and assemble if necessary. Pull the plunger halfway out and push it all the way in again. RATIONALE: Preparing the equipment ahead of time ensures a smoother process. Syringes can stick when new, so pulling once on the plunger prevents it from sticking during the venipuncture.

6. Select the proper vacuum tubes for later transfer of the specimen; tap all tubes containing anticoagulants and check the expiration dates. Arrange them in a holding rack in proper order. RATIONALE: Having the supplies ready and in the rack reduces confusion later. The rack is a safety item so you are not holding the tube while transferring the specimen. Tapping the tubes ensures that all the additive is dislodged from the stopper and wall of the tubes. Checking expiration dates is a quality-assurance measure.

7. Apply the tourniquet and palpate to select a site (Figure 39-25A). See Procedure 39-1. RATIONALE: Applying the tourniquet causes the vein to enlarge for easier venipuncture.

(continues)

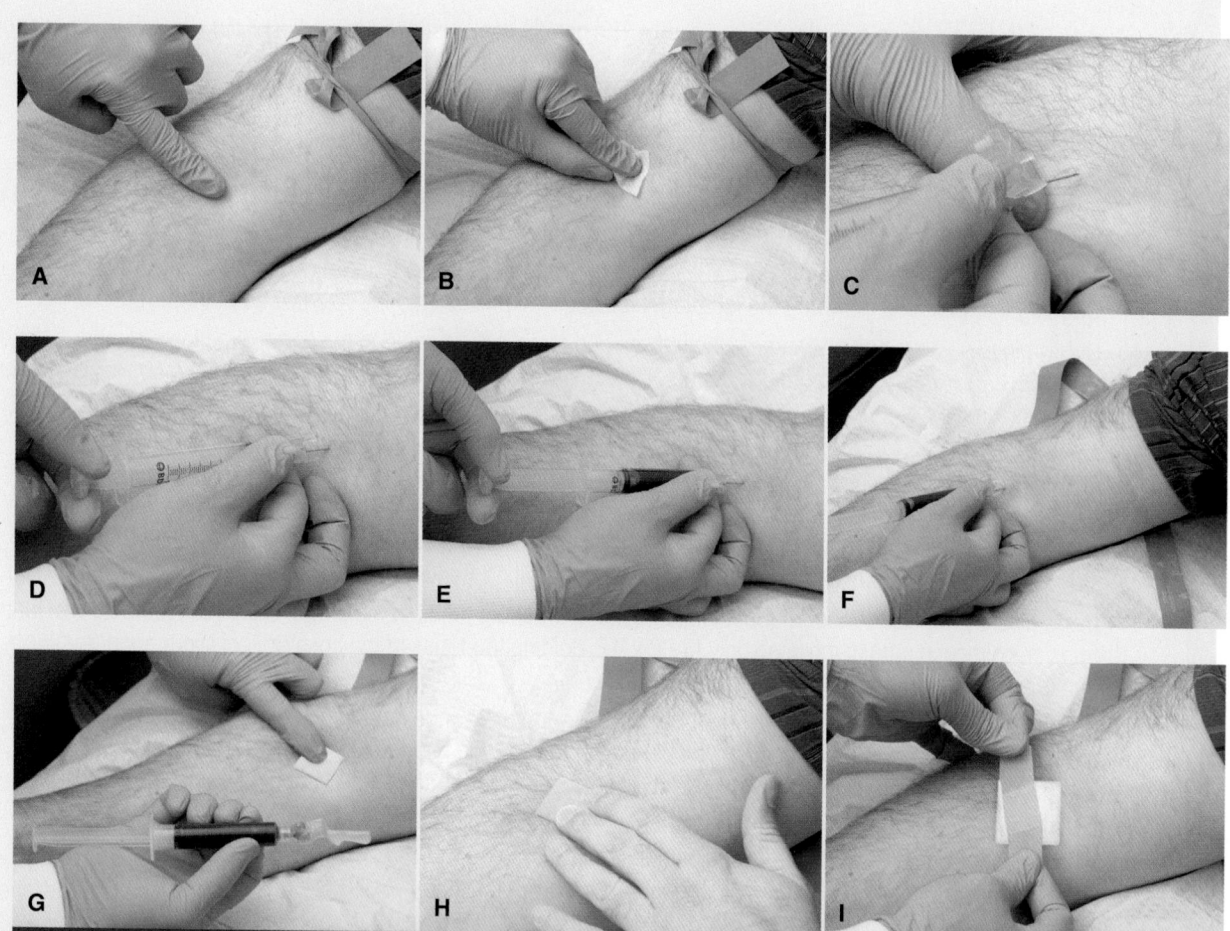

FIGURE 39-25 Performing a venipuncture with the syringe method. (A) Apply tourniquet and find vein. (B) Apply alcohol in one quick motion and allow to dry. Area can be wiped with a clean 2 × 2 gauze. (C) Draw skin taut below the puncture site and insert needle bevel up. (D) Let go of skin and use that hand to pull back on the plunger. (E) Withdraw blood slowly, until the syringe is full. (F) Release tourniquet. (G) Apply a clean gauze compress immediately after withdrawing needle. (H) Have the patient apply pressure to the site until a clot forms. (I) Apply a bandage over the site.

8. Ask the patient to close the hand. The patient must not pump the hand. Place the arm in a downward position. RATIONALE: Closing the hand and placing the arm in a downward position further enlarges the vein, allowing for easier venipuncture. Pumping the hand can lower the quality of the specimen collected.

9. Select a vein, noting the location and direction of the vein. ***Incorporate critical thinking skills when performing patient care.*** RATIONALE: This allows you to prepare mentally for the venipuncture.

10. Cleanse the site with an alcohol swab with one firm swipe (Figure 39-25B). Avoid touching the site after cleansing. RATIONALE: Alcohol removes body oils, sweat, and other contaminants. The site should stay as clean as possible.

11. Draw the skin taut with your thumb by placing it 1 to 2 inches below the puncture site. RATIONALE: This will anchor the vein.

12. With the bevel up, line up the needle with the direction of the vein and perform the puncture (Figure 39-25C). The point of the needle should enter the skin about ¼ inch below where the vein was palpated. With experience, a sensation of entering the vein can be felt. Once the vein has been entered, do not move the needle from side to

(continues)

side. Do not push down or pull up on the needle. The needle can be slightly moved in or out very gently if needed to access the vein. RATIONALE: Lining up the needle with the vein is a mental exercise to help the needle enter the vein in the proper direction. Entering the skin a fraction of an inch below the palpated site will aid in entering the vein at the correct site. This will align the needle so that it will enter the vein.

13. Let go of the skin and use that hand to pull back on the plunger (Figure 39-25D). Pull gently and only as fast as the syringe fills (Figure 39-25E). If the vein collapses, stop pulling on the plunger and let the vein refill. RATIONALE: Pulling too rapidly or too hard can cause the vein to collapse.

14. When the syringe is full, have the patient open the hand. Remove the tourniquet (Figure 39-25F). RATIONALE: Opening the hand and removing the tourniquet releases the pressure so the needle can be removed.

15. Lightly place a gauze pad above the puncture site and remove the needle in the same direction as inserted (Figure 39-25G). RATIONALE: Holding the gauze pad above the site allows for immediate pressure to be applied once the needle is removed.

16. Apply pressure to the site for 2 to 3 minutes, or a minimum of 5 minutes if the patient is taking prescribed anticoagulants (blood thinners) such as warfarin (Coumadin) or is taking aspirin or an herbal blood thinner such as ginkgo biloba. Let the patient assist by holding the pressure if desired (Figure 39-25H). The patient can elevate the arm but should be instructed not to bend the elbow. RATIONALE: Two to 3 minutes is usually enough time for the bleeding to stop. Elevating the arm while holding pressure aids in the clotting. Bending the elbow can cause a hematoma to form.

17. Using a safety transfer device, aliquot blood into the appropriate tubes in the proper order (see Table 39-5). During transfer, hold each tube at the base only. RATIONALE: Holding the tubes at the base protects your hand from accidental needlestick during the transfer process.

18. Puncture the vacuum tube through the rubber stopper with the syringe needle and allow the blood to enter the tube until the flow stops. Never push on the plunger or force blood into the tube. RATIONALE: Pushing on the plunger and forcing blood into the vacuum tube can cause the rubber stopper to pop off, splashing blood.

19. Implement safety mechanism or devices on the needle immediately. RATIONALE: Immediate implementation of safety mechanisms will protect from accidental needlesticks.

20. Mix any anticoagulant tubes immediately. RATIONALE: Mixing the anticoagulants right away minimizes the chance of microclots forming.

21. Discard the syringe and needle into a sharps container and the contaminated gauze pad and other contaminated waste into a red biohazard bag. RATIONALE: Proper disposal of sharps and biohazard waste protects all personnel.

22. Label all tubes before leaving the room. If any special treatment is required for the specimens, institute the handling protocol right away. RATIONALE: Labeling the tubes right away lessens the chances of a mix-up error. Proper handling of specimens ensures an accurate test result.

23. Check the patient. Observe him or her for signs of stress. RATIONALE: Venipuncture can be stressful for some patients.

24. When sufficient pressure has been applied to stop the bleeding, apply a small pressure bandage by applying a gauze pad to the puncture site, and placing an adhesive bandage or tape over it (Figure 39-25I). Instruct the patient to remove the bandage in 20 minutes. If the patient is sensitive or allergic to latex, be sure to use nonlatex paper tape. If the bleeding has not stopped after 2 to 3 minutes, have the patient continue to hold direct pressure on the site for another 5 minutes with his or her arm elevated above the heart. He or she can do this by lying down with his or her arm on a pillow. Recheck after 5 minutes. RATIONALE: The patient should not leave your care until the bleeding has stopped.

25. Disinfect tray and supplies and dispose of all contaminated items properly. Remove gloves using proper technique. RATIONALE: Proper disposal and disinfection of all contaminated supplies and equipment protects from exposure to biohazard substances.

26. Wash hands, record the procedure, and complete the laboratory requisition in the presence of the patient. RATIONALE: Washing hands after removing gloves offers further protection from biohazard substances and lessens the chance of cross-contamination to the patient's chart and the laboratory requisition. Completing the documentation and requisition as soon as possible after the procedure ensures the patient's sample is with the right requisition and improves accuracy.

(continues)

27. Place specimen and requisition into biohazard transport bag and notify the laboratory that the specimen is ready for pickup.

DOCUMENTATION:

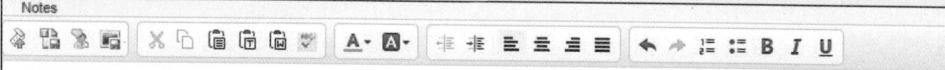

Notes

11/13/XX 2:54 PM Venipuncture performed right arm for CBC and sed rate. Specimens sent to Inner City Lab. Identification. #987654321. Patient tolerated the procedure well and will call back tomorrow for the test results.
  J. Guerrero, CMA (AAMA)

Courtesy of Harris CareTracker PM and EMR

Vacuum Tube Specimen Collection

The vacuum tube system has many advantages over the syringe method in that it tends to be quicker and allows for multiple tubes to be drawn. When the syringe method is used, a vacuum is created as the medical assistant pulls on the syringe plunger, but with the vacuum tube method, the vacuum is already in the tube.

The similarity between the vacuum tube system and the syringe system is that the holder and needle are held in the same manner (Figure 39-26). The syringe is held in a manner that allows the medical assistant access to pull on the plunger. The vacuum tube holder is held in a manner that allows tubes to be changed without switching hands.

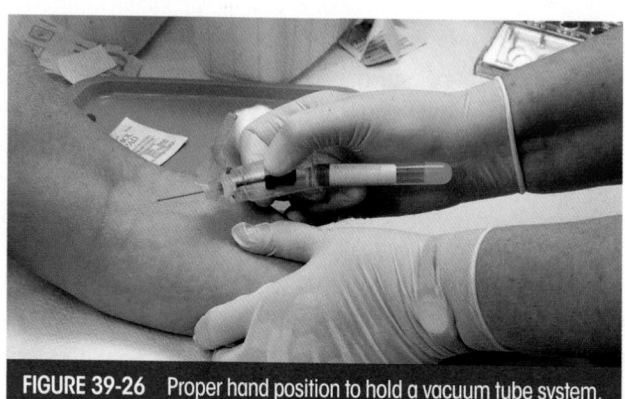

FIGURE 39-26 Proper hand position to hold a vacuum tube system.

Procedure

The procedure for venipuncture with the vacuum tube system follows the same steps as the syringe method with only slight variations (see Procedure 39-3).

Procedure

PROCEDURE 39-3

Venipuncture by Vacuum Tube System

STANDARD PRECAUTIONS:

Handwashing   Gloves   Goggles & Mask   No Needle Recapping   Biohazard

PURPOSE:

To obtain venous blood acceptable for laboratory testing as requested by a provider.

EQUIPMENT/SUPPLIES:

- Gloves
- Goggles and mask
- Vacuum tube adapter/holder

- Lab requisition (optional)
- Computer-generated label or thin-tipped permanent marker

(continues)

- 70% isopropyl alcohol pledget
- 2 × 2 gauze
- 21-gauge multidraw needle
- Vacuum tube(s) or special collection tube(s)

- Tourniquet
- Adhesive bandage or tape
- Sharps container and biohazard red bag
- Biohazard transport bag

PROCEDURE STEPS:

1. Introduce yourself by name and credentials. RATIONALE: The patient has a right to know who is performing a procedure on him or her and what your credentials are. You will also be exhibiting professionalism.

2. ***Explain the rationale for performance of the procedure and expectations to the patient. Show awareness of the patient's concerns related to the procedure being performed.*** RATIONALE: Explaining the procedure and allaying the patient's fears will assure the patient that you are concerned about any apprehension he or she may have and that you are open to discussing the concerns.

3. Position and identify the patient. Ask the patient's name and verify it with the tests ordered and the computer label or identification number. If a fasting specimen is required, verify that the patient has not had anything to eat or drink except water for 12 hours. RATIONALE: Properly identifying the patient and the tests ordered and ensuring that the patient is properly prepared for the blood tests are all quality-control and quality-assurance measures.

4. Wash hands and apply gloves and goggles/mask. RATIONALE: Clean hands further protect the patient. Gloves protect you. Goggles/mask should be worn if there is a possibility of blood splatter.

5. Break the seal on the shorter needle and then thread the shorter needle into the holder/adapter. Select the first tube and gently place it into the holder/adapter (do not puncture the tube yet). RATIONALE: Preparing the equipment ahead of time ensures a smoother process.

6. Tap all tubes containing anticoagulants and check the expiration dates. RATIONALE: Tapping the tubes ensures that all of the additive is dislodged from the stopper and wall of the tubes. Checking expiration dates is a quality-assurance measure.

7. Select a site and apply the tourniquet (see Procedure 39-1). RATIONALE: Applying the tourniquet causes the vein to enlarge for easier venipuncture.

8. Ask the patient to close the hand. The patient must not pump the hand. Place the arm in a downward position. RATIONALE: Closing the hand and placing the arm in a downward position further enlarges the vein, allowing for easier venipuncture. Pumping the hand can lower the quality of the specimen collected.

9. Select a vein, noting the location and direction of the vein. ***Incorporate critical thinking skills when performing patient care.*** RATIONALE: This allows you to prepare mentally for the venipuncture (Figure 39-27A).

10. Cleanse the site with an alcohol swab with one firm swipe. RATIONALE: Alcohol removes body oils and contamination (Figure 39-27B).

11. Avoid touching the site after cleansing. RATIONALE: The site should stay as clean as possible.

12. Draw the skin taut with your thumb by placing it 1 to 2 inches below the puncture site. RATIONALE: This will anchor the vein.

13. With the bevel up, line up the needle with the direction of the vein and perform the puncture. The point of the needle should enter the skin about ¼ inch below where the vein was palpated. With experience, a sensation of entering the vein can be felt. Once the vein has been entered, do not move the needle. RATIONALE: Lining up the needle with the vein is a mental exercise to help the needle enter the vein in the proper direction. Entering the skin a fraction of an inch below the palpated site will aid in entering the vein at the palpated site (Figure 39-27C).

14. Let go of the skin and use that hand to grasp the flange of the vacuum tube holder and push the tube forward until the needle has completely entered the tube (Figure 39-27D). Do not change hands while performing venipuncture. The hand performing the venipuncture is the hand that is holding the vacuum tube holder. The other hand is free for tube insertion and removal. RATIONALE: Using the flange of the adapter helps you hold the needle steady while changing tubes. Changing hands while performing venipuncture could cause the needle to move.

(continues)

15. Fill the tube until the vacuum is exhausted and the blood flow stops. Rotate tubes so the label is down. RATIONALE: Letting the tubes completely fill will ensure the right ratio of blood to additive. Positioning the label down enables you to see the tube filling.

16. When the blood flow ceases, gently remove the vacuum tube from the needle and holder. Do this by grasping the tube with the fingers and palm of your spare hand and using your thumb to push off from the flange of the holder (Figure 39-27E). RATIONALE: Using the flange will help steady the needle.

17. Immediately mix the blood in the anticoagulant tubes by gently inverting them several times. RATIONALE: Mixing the anticoagulant tubes right away minimizes the chance of microclots forming.

18. Insert the second tube onto the needle using the same motion as with the first tube (Figure 39-27F). Let it fill; then remove it with the same motion as with the first tube. Invert it several times if it contains anticoagulants. RATIONALE: Mixing the additives prevents the blood from coagulating.

19. When the last tube has filled, remove it from the needle (Figure 39-27G). Ask the patient to open his or her hand. Then release the tourniquet. RATIONALE: Removing the last tube from the needle prevents any residual suction from drawing blood through the tissues when the needle is removed from the vein. Opening the hand and removing the tourniquet relieves pressure so the needle can be removed without causing excessive blood loss through the puncture site.

20. Lightly place the gauze pad above the puncture site and smoothly remove the needle from the arm in the same direction of insertion. RATIONALE: Holding the gauze pad above the site allows for immediate pressure to be applied once the needle is removed.

21. Immediately activate the safety device. RATIONALE: Activating the safety device protects you from accidental needlesticks.

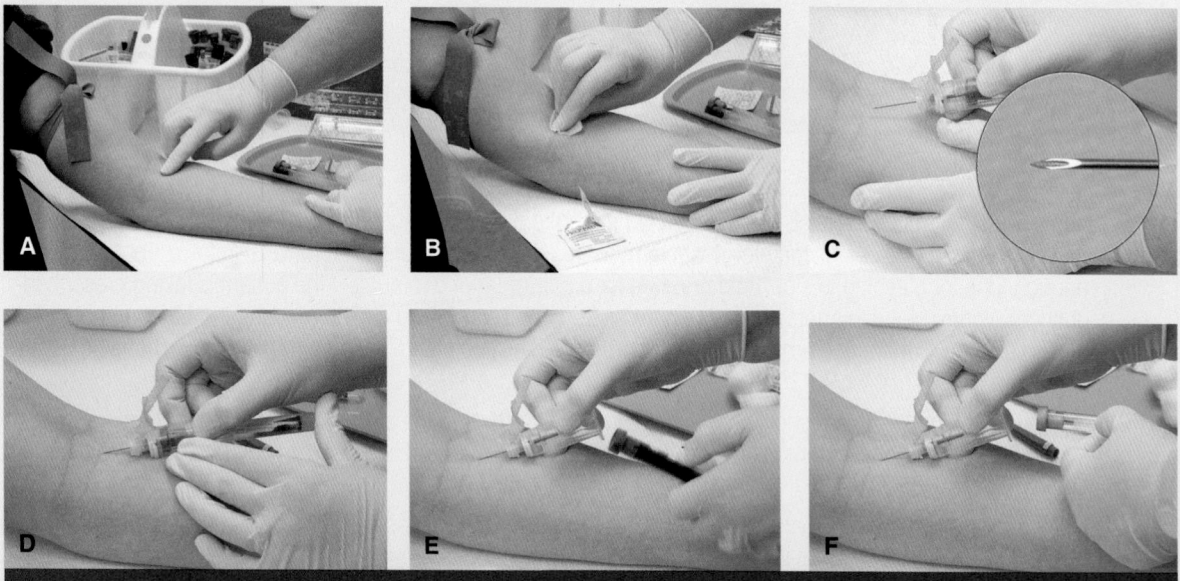

FIGURE 39-27 Performing a venipuncture with a vacuum tube assembly. (A) After tying the tourniquet, palpate the vein. (B) Cleanse the site with alcohol. Allow area to dry or wipe with a clean 2 × 2 gauze. (C) While holding the skin taut, hold needle with bevel up and penetrate the vein with a smooth rapid movement. (D) Grasp the flange of the vacuum tube holder to push the vacuum tube onto the needle. (E) When the tube has stopped filling, remove it gently from the needle and holder using the flange to push from. Invert it several times to mix the additives. (F) Place another tube onto the needle and let it fill.

(continues)

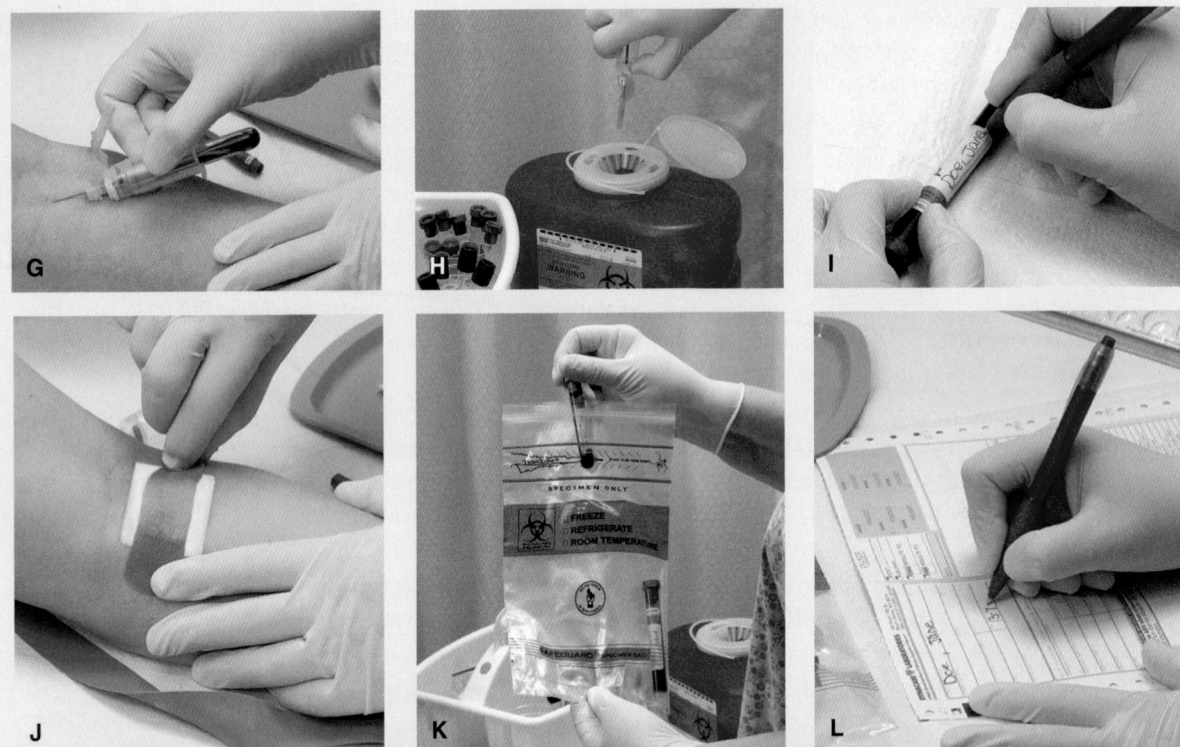

FIGURE 39-27 *(continued)* (G) When the last tube has filled, gently remove it from the holder. Release the tourniquet (not shown) and smoothly remove the needle from the vein, immediately applying pressure with the gauze compress. Mix well by inverting several times. (H) Dispose of the needle and holder into a nearby sharps container. (I) Properly label the tubes. (J) Check the patient and apply a bandage. (K) Package the specimens properly for transport (be aware of special storage or treatment needed, such as centrifugation or refrigeration). (L) Complete the laboratory requisition and document the procedure in the patient's chart or electronic medical record.

22. Apply pressure on the site for 2 to 3 minutes. Let the patient assist by holding the pressure. Ask him or her not to bend the arm, but he or she can elevate the arm while applying pressure. RATIONALE: Two to 3 minutes is usually enough time for bleeding to stop. Hold pressure for a minimum of 5 minutes if the patient is taking prescribed anticoagulants (blood thinners) such as warfarin (Coumadin) or taking aspirin or an herbal blood thinner such as ginkgo biloba. Elevating the arm while holding pressure aids in clotting. Bending the elbow can cause a hematoma to form.

23. Dispose of the needle into a sharps container (Figure 39-27H) and the contaminated gauze pad and other con-taminated waste into a red biohazard bag. RATIONALE: Proper disposal of sharps and biohazard waste protects all personnel.

24. Label all the tubes before leaving the patient (Figure 39-27I). If any special treatment is required for the specimens, institute the handling protocol right away. RATIONALE: Labeling the tubes right away lessens the chance of a mix-up error. Proper handling of the specimens ensures accurate test results.

25. Check the patient. Observe him or her for signs of stress. He or she should stop bleeding within 2 to 3 minutes. If the bleeding has stopped, apply a small pressure bandage by applying a gauze pad to the site, and placing an adhesive bandage or tape over it (Figure 39-27J). The patient should be instructed to remove the bandage in about 20 minutes. If the patient is sensitive to latex, be sure to use a nonlatex paper tape. If the bleeding has not stopped, have the patient continue to hold direct pressure for another 5 minutes with the arm elevated above

(continues)

heart level. This can be achieved by having him or her lie down with the arm up on a pillow. Recheck the site after 5 minutes of additional direct pressure. RATIONALE: Check the patient for signs of distress because venipuncture can be stressful for some people. The patient should not leave your care until the bleeding has stopped.

26. Disinfect all surfaces and supplies/equipment. Remove gloves using proper technique. Dispose of contaminated items appropriately. RATIONALE: Proper disposal and disinfection of all contaminated supplies and equipment offers protection from exposure to dangerous biohazard substances.

27. Wash hands, record the procedure, and complete the laboratory requisition in the presence of the patient. Place the specimen and requisition into the biohazard transport bag and notify the laboratory that the specimen is ready for pickup (Figure 39-27K and L). RATIONALE: Washing hands after removing gloves further protects you from biohazard substances and lessens the chance of cross-contamination to the patient's chart and the laboratory requisition. Completing the documentation and the requisition as soon as possible and in the presence of the patient improves accuracy and ensures that the patient's sample is with the right requisition.

DOCUMENTATION:

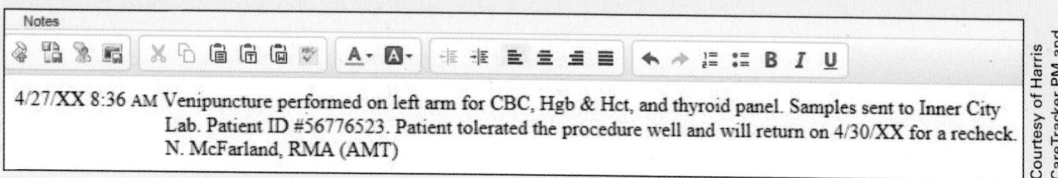

4/27/XX 8:36 AM Venipuncture performed on left arm for CBC, Hgb & Hct, and thyroid panel. Samples sent to Inner City Lab. Patient ID #56776523. Patient tolerated the procedure well and will return on 4/30/XX for a recheck.
N. McFarland, RMA (AMT)

Courtesy of Harris CareTracker PM and EMR

Butterfly Needle Collection System

Procedure

The butterfly collection system allows for either a syringe draw or a vacuum tube draw. (see Procedure 39-4). The butterfly collection system has on one end a 21- or 23-gauge needle with attached plastic wings. Several inches of tubing leads from the winged needle to a hub that can be attached to another needle that is covered with a rubber sheath. The sheath-covered needle can attach to either a syringe or a vacuum tube holder depending on which technique is desired (Figure 39-28). The sample may also be drawn into a syringe (if a slower draw is desired) and then transferred to vacuum tubes as needed.

The butterfly system is used for small, fragile veins that are difficult to puncture with the vacuum tube system and standard vacuum tube system needle. The butterfly collection system works well on children who have small veins and the tendency to move while blood is being collected. The butterfly system also facilitates drawing from veins that have a tendency to collapse and is especially useful for veins on the back of the patient's hand. Instead of entering the vein at the usual 15-degree angle, the needle is inserted at a 5- to 10-degree angle, and then threaded into the vein.

Although the butterfly collection system has many benefits, it is not used for all collections. It is a bit more expensive than the needle system and the additional expense is usually not cost effective for all blood draws.

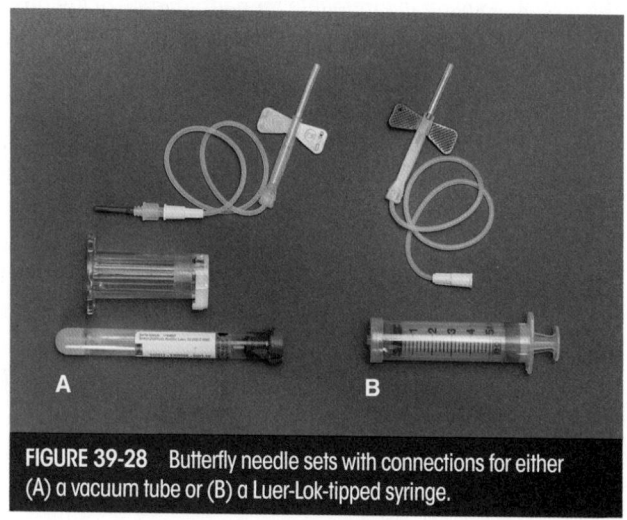

FIGURE 39-28 Butterfly needle sets with connections for either (A) a vacuum tube or (B) a Luer-Lok-tipped syringe.

PROCEDURE 39-4

Procedure

Venipuncture by Butterfly Needle System

STANDARD PRECAUTIONS:

   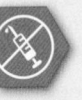 

Handwashing   Gloves   Goggles & Mask   No Needle Recapping   Biohazard

PURPOSE:

To obtain venous blood acceptable for laboratory testing as requested by a provider.

EQUIPMENT/SUPPLIES:

- Gloves
- Goggles and mask
- Vacuum tube holder if using a vacuum tube connection
- A 10 to 15 mL syringe if using a syringe connection
- Butterfly needle system with 21-gauge needle (use a multisample needle system with a vacuum tube holder or a hypodermic needle for syringe attachment)
- Vacuum tubes (for aliquot specimens)

- Tourniquet
- 70% isopropyl alcohol swab
- 2 × 2 gauze
- Adhesive bandage or tape
- Sharps container and red biohazard bag
- Computer-generated label or thin-tipped permanent marker
- Lab transport bag and requisition (optional)

PROCEDURE STEPS:

1. Assemble the supplies. RATIONALE: Organizing supplies before the procedure ensures a more timely and professional process.

2. Introduce yourself by name and credentials. RATIONALE: The patient has a right to know who is performing a procedure on him or her and what your credentials are. You will also be exhibiting professionalism.

3. Position and identify the patient. Ask the patient's name and verify it with the computer label or identification number. If a fasting specimen is required, verify that the patient has not had anything to eat or drink except water for 12 hours. RATIONALE: Properly identifying the patient and the tests ordered and verifying that the patient is properly prepared are quality-control and quality-assurance measures.

4. ***Explain the rationale for performance of the procedure and expectations to the patient. Show awareness of the patient's concerns related to the procedure being performed.*** RATIONALE: Explaining the procedure and allaying the patient's fears will assure the patient that you are concerned about any apprehension he or she may have and that you are open to discussing the concerns.

5. Wash hands. Put on gloves, as well as goggles and mask if there is a potential for blood splatter. RATIONALE: Clean hands further protect the patient. Gloves and goggles/face shield protect you from any potential splatters.

6. Open the package of butterfly needle system. If using the multisample needle, connect the needle to the vacuum tube holder/adapter. If using the hypodermic needle and syringe, connect the needle to the syringe (Figure 39-29A). If using a syringe, set the vacuum tubes in a rack for later use. RATIONALE: The more organized you are before the venipuncture, the smoother the procedure will go.

7. Tap the vacuum tubes to be sure any additive is dislodged from the stopper and sides of the tube. Check the expiration dates. RATIONALE: Dislodging the additive will ensure the proper ratio in the specimen. The tubes' expiration date should not have passed.

8. Apply the tourniquet. RATIONALE: Applying a tourniquet enlarges the vein, making it more accessible.

(continues)

9. Ask the patient to close his or her hand (Figure 39-29B). The patient should not pump the hand. If possible, place the arm in a downward position. RATIONALE: Pumping the hand can lead to excessive engorgement of the vein, which can cause blood to enter the tissues during the puncture, which will cause a hematoma.

10. Select the vein, noting the direction and location of the vein. ***Incorporate critical thinking skills when performing patient care***. RATIONALE: You will want to enter the vein in the same direction it is positioned.

11. Cleanse the site with an alcohol swab using one swift firm swipe and allow the site to dry (Figure 39-29C). RATIONALE: Alcohol removes body oils and other contaminants. Puncturing the skin through wet alcohol can cause stinging and hemolysis of the specimen and will contaminate the specimen.

12. Avoid touching the site after cleansing. RATIONALE: Touching the skin will contaminate it.

13. Draw the skin taut by placing your thumb 1 to 2 inches below the site and pulling down firmly. RATIONALE: This will anchor the vein.

14. Hold the wings of the butterfly together with the bevel of the needle up, line up the needle with the vein, and smoothly insert it into the vein at about a 5- to 10-degree angle (Figure 39-29D). RATIONALE: This process will cause the least amount of discomfort and provide the greatest success.

15. Remove your hand from holding the skin taut. RATIONALE: You will need one hand free to handle the other equipment.

16. If using a vacuum tube holder, grasp the flange of the vacuum tube holder and push the tube forward until the needle has completely entered the tube. RATIONALE: Using the flange when inserting and removing vacuum tubes will help the needle stay in position.

17. If using a syringe, pull gently on the syringe (Figure 39-29E). RATIONALE: Pulling too rapidly can cause the vein to collapse.

18. Do not change hands while performing venipuncture. The hand performing the venipuncture is the hand that is holding the vacuum tube holder. The other hand is for inserting and removing the vacuum tubes. RATIONALE: Changing hands can cause the needle to change position.

19. If you are collecting directly into vacuum tubes, remove and replace the vacuum tubes as explained in Procedure 39-3 until you have drawn the necessary amounts. If you are drawing into a syringe, you will be limited to the size of the syringe being used. RATIONALE: You do not have the option of removing and replacing the syringe during a draw.

20. When the syringe is filled, ask the patient to open his or her hand. Then release the tourniquet. RATIONALE: Opening of the hand and releasing the tourniquet takes the pressure off the vein and allows the blood to flow freely through the arm.

21. Lightly place a gauze pad above the puncture site and smoothly remove the needle from the arm in the same direction of insertion (Figure 39-29F). RATIONALE: You are getting the gauze pad ready so you can apply pressure on the puncture site immediately upon removing the needle.

22. Activate the safety device of the butterfly needle immediately (Figure 39-29G). RATIONALE: The safety devices offer better protection if activated immediately.

23. Apply pressure on the site. Let the patient assist by holding the pressure (Figure 39-29H). If blood was drawn from the arm, ask him or her to not bend the arm. He or she can elevate the arm while applying pressure, though. RATIONALE: Applying pressure and elevating the arm lessens the chance of bruising, whereas bending the elbow increases the chance of hematoma formation.

24. If using a syringe, aliquot blood into the appropriate tubes as outlined in Procedure 39-2. RATIONALE: Following proper procedure when transferring blood from the syringe into the vacuum tubes ensures the best specimens for testing.

25. Dispose of the needle into a sharps container (Figure 39-29I). RATIONALE: Immediate disposal of contaminated needles is the safest practice.

26. Label all the tubes. RATIONALE: Not labeling the tubes right away increases the likelihood of a mix-up error.

27. Check the patient. Observe him or her for signs of stress. RATIONALE: Patient safety is a primary concern. Venipuncture can be difficult for some patients.

28. The patient should stop bleeding within 2 to 3 minutes. If the bleeding has stopped, provide a small pressure bandage by applying a gauze pad to the site, and placing an adhesive bandage or tape over it (Figure 39-29J).

(continues)

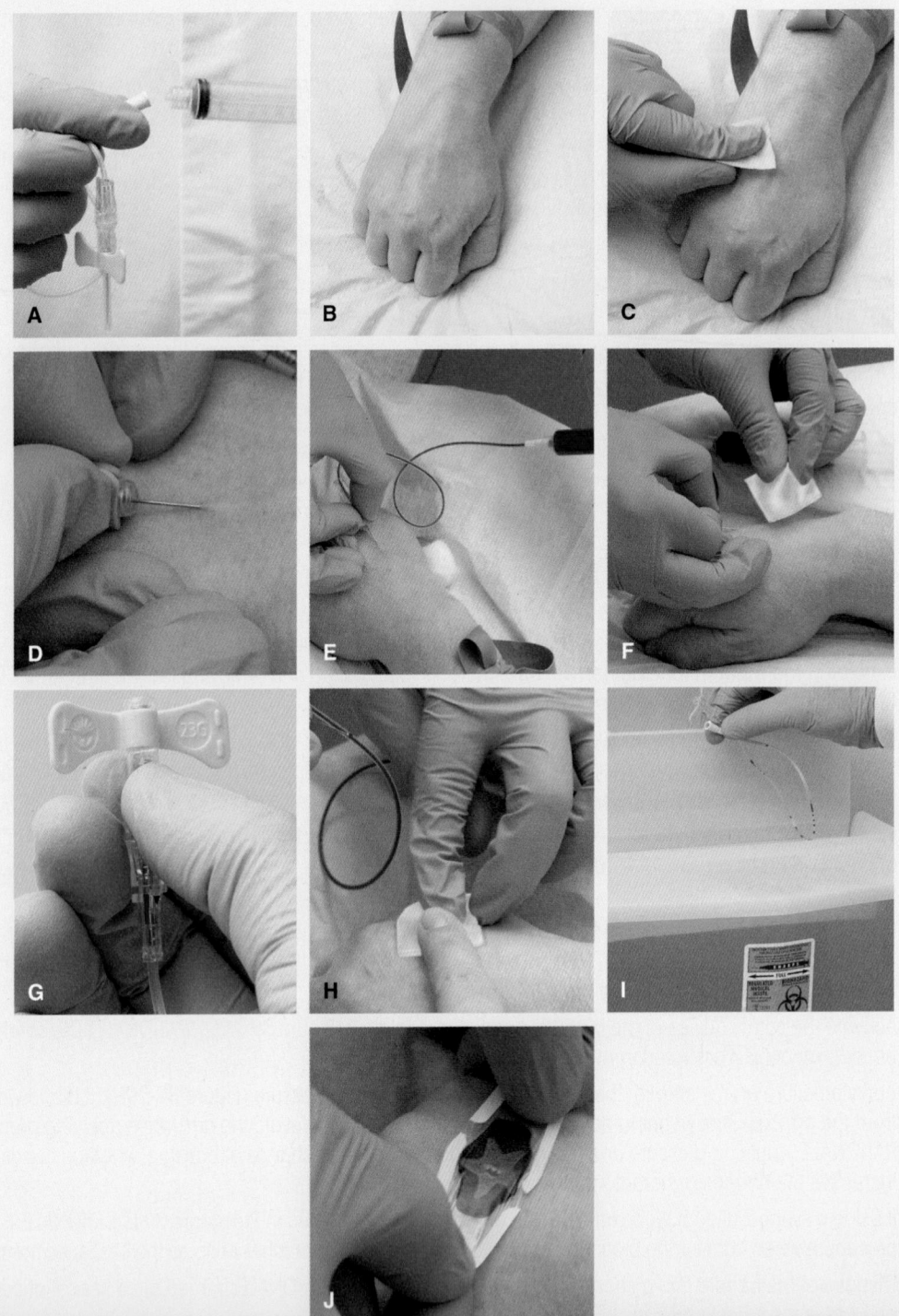

FIGURE 39-29 Performing a venipuncture with the butterfly needle system. (A) Open the package with the butterfly needle system and assemble the needle. In this case, the needle is connected to the syringe. (B) Apply the tourniquet and ask the patient to close his hand. (C) Cleanse the site using one swift wipe and allow to air dry. (D) Draw skin taut. While holding the wings of the butterfly together, line up the needle with the vein, and insert at a 5- to 10-degree angle. (E) Pull gently on the syringe, allowing it to fill. (F) When filled, have the patient relax his hand, and release the tourniquet. Place a 2 × 2 gauze above the puncture site and remove the needle. (G) Activate the safety device of the butterfly needle. (H) Apply pressure on the site, and ask the patient to continue holding the pressure. (I) Dispose of the entire butterfly system into a sharps container. (J) Apply a bandage to the site.

(continues)

The patient should be instructed to remove the bandage in about 20 minutes. If the patient is sensitive to latex, be sure to use a nonlatex paper tape. If the bleeding has not stopped, have the patient continue to hold pressure for another 5 minutes with the arm elevated above heart level, then recheck. RATIONALE: The patient should not be released from your care until the bleeding has stopped.

29. Clean up tray and supplies; dispose of contaminated gauze pad. Remove gloves using proper technique. Discard gloves into biohazard container and disinfect goggles. RATIONALE: Proper disposal and disinfection of contaminated supplies and equipment offers protection from exposure to biohazard substances.

30. Wash hands, record the procedure, and complete the laboratory requisition. Place the specimen and requisition into the biohazard transfer bag in the presence of the patient and notify the laboratory that the specimen is ready for pickup. RATIONALE: Washing hands after removing the gloves further protects from biohazard substances and lessens the chance of cross-contamination to the patient's chart and laboratory requisition. Completing the documentation and requisition as soon as possible after the procedure and in the presence of the patient improves accuracy and ensures the patient's sample is with the right requisition.

DOCUMENTATION:

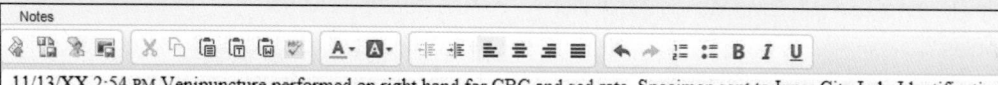

Notes

11/13/XX 2:54 PM Venipuncture performed on right hand for CBC and sed rate. Specimen sent to Inner City Lab. Identification #987654321. Patient tolerated the procedure well and will call back tomorrow for the test results.
J. Guerrero, CMA (AAMA)

Courtesy of Harris CareTracker PM and EMR

Blood Cultures

Procedure

Occasionally, a patient will need to have blood collected for culture (see Procedure 39-5). The culture will determine if the patient has pathogens in the blood. Normally, blood is sterile. When drawing blood for cultures, use a surgical solution, often povidone-iodine (brand named Betadine), rather than alcohol and sterile rather than clean procedure. This means using sterile gloves; do not wipe away the surgical solution, touch the puncture site, or in any way compromise the sterile process. The blood is collected into special transport bottles, which are like vacuum tubes but shaped differently (Figure 39-30). The blood culture bottle contains transport media to preserve any microorganisms present while they are transported to the laboratory for culture. Because it is unknown whether the pathogen is anaerobic (living without oxygen) or aerobic (living with oxygen), blood is collected to test for both. The aerobic bottle is filled first, then the anaerobic bottle is filled.

Patient Reactions to Blood Draws

Patients can have a variety of reactions to having their blood drawn. The medical assistant must anticipate these reactions and respond appropriately as quickly as possible. The most common patient reactions are fear and pain. To determine his or her possible reaction, ask the patient if he or she has had blood drawn in the past. Watch for sweating, shaking, and other indicators of potential untoward events. Other possible patient reactions and the medical assistant's appropriate responses are listed in Table 39-6.

The Unsuccessful Venipuncture

Methods of vein stimulation are shown in Table 39-7. When a blood sample cannot be obtained, it may be necessary to change the position of the needle. Rotate the needle half a turn. The bevel of the needle may be against the wall of the vein. If the needle has not penetrated the vein far enough, advance it further into the vein.

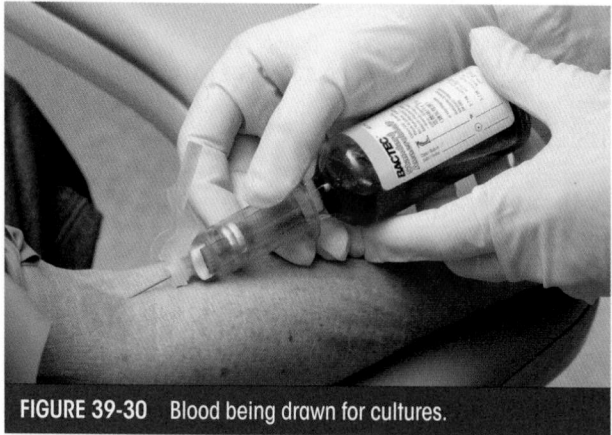

FIGURE 39-30 Blood being drawn for cultures.

Obtaining Blood for Blood Culture

STANDARD PRECAUTIONS:

   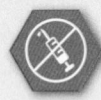 

Handwashing   Gloves   Goggles & Mask   No Needle Recapping   Biohazard

PURPOSE:

While performing venipuncture from two separate sites, prepare two culture bottles of blood from each site for culture (four total).

EQUIPMENT/SUPPLIES:

- Nonsterile gloves for use with povidone-iodine solution
- Sterile gloves
- Laboratory requisition and transport bag
- Computer-generated label or thin-tipped permanent marker
- Blood culture bottles, anaerobic and aerobic (usually four: two bottles each for two sets of cultures)

- 70% isopropyl alcohol
- Povidone-iodine solution swabs or towelettes
- Venipuncture supplies (according to method used) for two separate sites
- Red biohazard bag
- Sharps container
- Biohazard transport bag

PROCEDURE STEPS:

1. Identify the patient and introduce yourself by name and credentials. RATIONALE: Identifying the patient and rechecking the provider's orders will ensure the proper tests will be performed on the right patient. Introducing yourself and stating your credentials demonstrates professionalism and helps to reassure the patient.

2. *Explain the rationale for performance of the procedure and expectations to the patient. Show awareness of the patient's concerns related to the procedure being performed.* RATIONALE: Explaining the procedure and allaying the patient's fears will assure the patient that you are concerned about any apprehension he or she may have and that you are open to discussing the concerns.

3. Ensure that the patient has not initiated antimicrobial therapy. RATIONALE: Antibiotic therapy can interfere with the culture results. If the patient has started antibiotics, the name and strength of the antibiotic, dosage, duration, and last dose must be documented clearly on the laboratory report.

4. Wash hands and put on gloves. RATIONALE: Washing hands before any laboratory process prevents contamination of the specimen. Gloving provides personal protection.

5. Assemble equipment and supplies according to the venipuncture procedure being used and the laboratory requirements (Figure 39-31A). Check expiration dates on all collection and culture supplies. RATIONALE: Organizing your work area prevents confusion and error due to missing supplies. Usually two separate sites are used for collection, with two bottles (one aerobe and one anaerobe) from each site. Occasionally, three sites will be necessary. Expired supplies and culture bottles must not be used.

6. Place the culture bottles on a flat surface that will be within reach during the procedure. Mark the correct fill line on both bottles at 10 mL per bottle (1 to 3 mL per bottle for pediatric patients). RATIONALE: Marking the fill line helps in viewing the proper amount during the procedure.

7. Prepare the venipuncture site with isopropyl alcohol and allow to dry, then apply povidone-iodine in progressively larger concentric circles from the inside outward (Figure 39-31B). The iodine must remain on the skin for

(continues)

1 full minute and be allowed to dry naturally. The venipuncture site should not be touched after the skin is disinfected. RATIONALE: Alcohol removes oils and other debris, and the povidone-iodine is a more thorough antiseptic. One full minute is required to ensure antisepsis. Touching the site may recontaminate it.

8. Cleanse the bottle tops with alcohol and the povidone-iodine solution. RATIONALE: The bottle tops need to be disinfected to remove contamination. *NOTE:* Some laboratory guidelines state that iodine can disintegrate the rubber stopper and therefore should not be used. Follow your laboratory guidelines as stated in your laboratory manual.

9. Remove the preparation gloves and apply the sterile gloves using sterile procedure. RATIONALE: Sterile gloves will ensure the procedure will be as sterile as possible.

10. Perform venipuncture according to the method used. Insert the aerobic culture bottle onto the needle (Figure 39-31C). Fill to the appropriate line, usually 10 mL per bottle (1 to 3 mL for pediatric patients). Remove the first bottle, invert 8 to 10 times, and apply the second (anaerobic) bottle. Fill. Remove the second bottle and invert 8 to 10 times. RATIONALE: Follow your laboratory manual guidelines. The aerobic bottle should be filled first because there will be some residual air in the needle. The anaerobic bottle will then collect only blood. Inverting the bottles ensures the culture media will be well mixed with the blood.

11. Complete the venipuncture procedure as determined by the method used. ***Incorporate critical thinking skills when performing patient care***. Remove the remaining iodine from the skin with isopropyl alcohol. RATIONALE: The next two bottles will be filled from a different site. The iodine solution can irritate the skin and should be removed.

12. Perform venipuncture at the second site, repeating the process as stated above. The second and subsequent culture bottles must be collected within 30 minutes of the first. RATIONALE: The 30-minute time frame allows for an accurate assessment of the microorganisms present on that particular date and at that particular time.

13. The culture bottles should be stored at room temperature and not refrigerated. RATIONALE: Room temperature is ideal for the cultures so organisms are not destroyed.

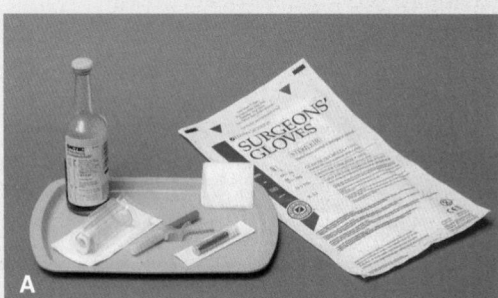
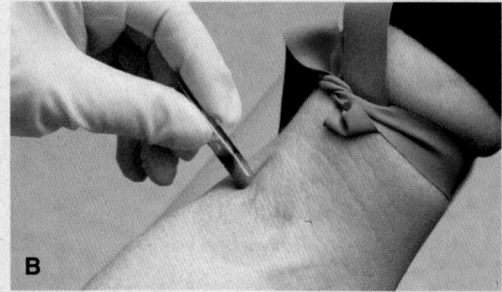
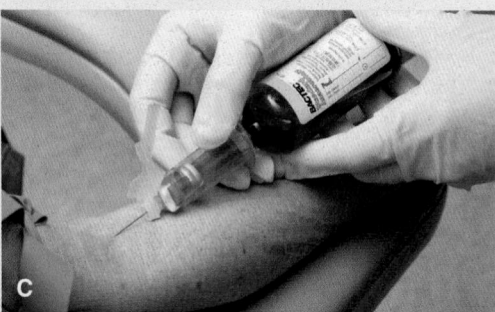

FIGURE 39-31 Obtaining blood for blood culture. (A) Assemble equipment and supplies (only one culture bottle shown). (B) Prepare the venipuncture site with alcohol and allow to dry, then apply povidone-iodine in concentric circles from the inside outward. Allow the iodine to dry naturally. (C) Perform venipuncture. Insert the aerobic culture bottle onto the needle and fill to the appropriate line.

(continues)

14. Label the bottles with the patient's name, date, time, and other required information. RATIONALE: Labeling with the required information prevents mix-ups of specimens and ensures a quality timeline. Specimens will be rejected if not labeled properly.

15. Dispose of all contaminated supplies, disinfect all surfaces, remove gloves, and wash hands. RATIONALE: Using appropriate disposal techniques and disinfecting all surfaces according to Standard Precautions safely controls biohazard substances.

16. Complete the laboratory requisition in the presence of the patient, including the date and time of each specimen collected, any antibiotic therapy the patient is on, the name and strength of the antibiotic, as well as the dosage, duration, and last dose taken. Include the clinical diagnosis and any special organisms suspected or to rule out. The laboratory requisition must indicate if the culture is for *brucella* or *francisella*. The information on the laboratory requisition should match exactly the information given on the bottles. RATIONALE: Labeling with the required information prevents mix-ups of specimens, ensures a quality timeline, and ensures the laboratory will have the necessary information. Specimens will be rejected if there is a discrepancy between the information on the bottle and the information on the laboratory requisition.

17. Place the specimen and the requisition in the biohazard transport bag in their separate compartments and notify the laboratory that the specimen is ready for pickup. RATIONALE: The biohazard transport bag separates the specimen from the requisition and protects laboratory personnel.

18. Document the procedure in the laboratory section of the patient's chart or electronic medical record. RATIONALE: Necessary information and the patient's chart or electronic medical record will be accurate and complete.

DOCUMENTATION:

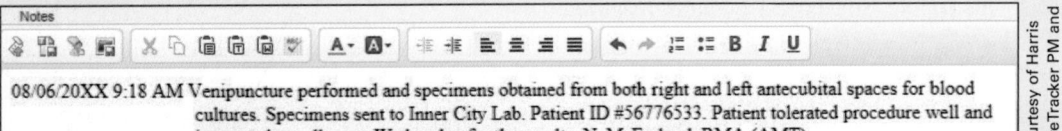

08/06/20XX 9:18 AM Venipuncture performed and specimens obtained from both right and left antecubital spaces for blood cultures. Specimens sent to Inner City Lab. Patient ID #56776533. Patient tolerated procedure well and instructed to call us on Wednesday for the results. N. McFarland, RMA (AMT)

Courtesy of Harris CareTracker PM and EMR

TABLE 39-6

PATIENT REACTIONS TO BLOOD DRAWS

PATIENT REACTION	MEDICAL ASSISTANT RESPONSE
Syncope (fainting)	Immediately remove the tourniquet, then the needle, and stop the patient from falling. Lower the patient's head and arms. Wipe the patient's forehead and back of the neck with a cold compress if necessary. If the patient does not respond, notify the provider, and place a pillow under the patient's legs.
Nausea	Apply cold compresses to the patient's forehead. Give the patient an emesis basin, and have facial tissues ready if the nausea does not diminish. Advise the patient that deep slow breathing through the mouth may help lessen the nausea.
Insulin shock or hypoglycemia	The first signs of insulin shock are a cold sweat and pallor similar to signs of syncope. The patient becomes weak and shaky, sudden mental confusion may follow, and it appears as though the patient's personality changes instantly. Call the provider if the patient loses consciousness. This can happen especially to patients having a fasting blood sugar test.
Convulsions	The patient loses consciousness and exhibits violent or mild convulsive motions. Do not try to restrain the patient. Move objects or furniture out of the way to prevent the patient from striking objects and being hurt. Help the patient to the floor and into a reclining position. The patient usually recovers within a few minutes. Notify the provider about the patient's reaction. The provider will determine when to release the patient.

TABLE 39-7

METHODS OF VEIN STIMULATION

1. Position the patient's arm lower than his or her heart.

2. Reapply the tourniquet; it may not be tight enough.

3. Massage the arm from the wrist to the elbow to encourage venous return.

4. Tap sharply at the specific vein with your fingertips. This can cause the vein to dilate. Do not slap the antecubital space. Doing so can cause the entire area to become red and reactive.

5. Use a blood pressure cuff in place of the tourniquet. Pump it to about 40 to 60 mm Hg.

6. Warm the venipuncture site with a warming device or a warm washcloth (not hotter than 100°F).

7. Have the patient make a fist. Do not have the patient pump the fist; that can cause a false high level of potassium in the specimen.

TABLE 39-8

QUALITY ASSURANCE FOR SPECIMEN COLLECTION AND PROCESSING

1. Each specimen must have its own label attached to the specimen's primary container.

2. Each specimen must have a laboratory requisition label.

3. Labels must have the patient's complete name and identification number, date of birth, date and time, and your signature.

4. Specimens in syringes with needles still attached are unacceptable.

5. Specimens must be in the appropriate anticoagulant.

6. Blood collection tubes with anticoagulant must be at least 75% full. All blood collection tubes for coagulation testing must be at least 90% full.

7. Anticoagulated blood specimens must be well mixed and free of clots.

8. The specimen may need to be recollected if the results do not agree with what the provider believes is the patient's diagnosis.

9. Do not combine partially filled tubes.

10. Do not mix tubes of different additives.

11. As soon as possible, invert tubes 8 to 10 times to prevent microclots from forming (see Figure 39-24).

12. Mix tubes gently to prevent hemolysis of the specimen.

13. Specimens must be processed properly between the draw and the laboratory. This may include refrigeration or as directed by the manual.

Advance it only slightly; a small change may mean the difference between a failed and a successful venipuncture. If the needle has penetrated too far into the vein, pull back a little. Always withdraw the needle slowly when the venipuncture has been unsuccessful. The blood often may start coming just as it seems the needle is ready to come out of the skin. The tube used may not have sufficient vacuum. Try another tube before withdrawing the needle. Probing the site is never appropriate.

Criteria for Rejection of a Specimen

The primary goal of a venipuncture procedure is to provide an acceptable specimen for laboratory testing as requested by the provider. Certain general criteria must be met for a specimen to be acceptable. If the criteria are not met, the laboratory will reject the specimen and another venipuncture of the patient must be performed.

Table 39-8 lists quality-assurance controls for specimen collection and processing. The list is not all-inclusive.

Factors Affecting Laboratory Values

Competency   Integrity

Numerous variables can affect laboratory test results. The specimens are tested by analytic instruments that give accurate and precise results, but these results will be accurate only if the specimen is collected correctly. The medical assistant is responsible for collecting and caring for the specimen properly. When in doubt of how to care for a specimen, refer to the manual supplied by the laboratory or contact the laboratory for specific instructions. It is always better to ask the question and perform the proper procedure than not to ask and have to repeat the venipuncture. In addition, if you ever do need to repeat a venipuncture because of improper collection or handling of the specimen, the patient should not be billed for the second collection. Patient physiologic factors may also contribute to inaccurate results. Other factors that can alter results are listed in Table 39-9.

TABLE 39-9

FACTORS AFFECTING LABORATORY RESULTS

FACTOR	EFFECT
Blood alcohol	When drawing a specimen for blood alcohol testing, a nonalcohol-based antiseptic should be used to clean the venipuncture site. The cleansing alcohol may falsely elevate the test result.
Diurnal rhythm	Some specimens must be drawn at timed intervals because of medication or diurnal (daily) rhythm. The exact time of collection must be noted on the specimen label.
Exercise	Strenuous short-term exercise can make the heart work harder and increase cardiac enzymes. Long-term exercise such as that performed by highly trained runners can cause erroneous results due to runner's anemia.
Fasting	If the patient is not in fasting state when fasting is required, test results may not be accurate.
Hemolysis	Destruction of red blood cell membrane and release of intercellular contents into serum/plasma can be caused by not allowing alcohol to air-dry at the venipuncture site, using a needle that is too small (less than 22 gauge), forcing the blood into a Vacutainer tube from a syringe, or shaking the Vacutainer tube instead of mixing by gentle inversion when mixing tubes with additives.
Heparin	Using the incorrect heparin additive can interfere with tests being run on the patient.
Stress	In children, violent crying before a specimen is collected can increase the white blood cell count.
Tourniquet on too long	Hemoconcentration can occur, causing a change in chemical concentration.
Volume	Not enough blood will cause a dilution factor, which can change the size of the cells and therefore produce a variation in test results.

Occasionally, a specimen requires protection from light, incubation, refrigeration, or chilling immediately after collection. Any delay in implementing these requirements will alter the results. The laboratory manual will direct you as to which specimens need to be chilled.

The medical assistant is not the only person who can adversely affect test results. The patient can knowingly or unknowingly alter the results by certain actions. For example, a patient has consumed a cup of coffee but claims not to have had anything to eat or drink. The patient is often under the misconception that a small cup of sweetened black coffee will not be a problem. Caffeine and sugar can both affect metabolism and thus can affect the test results.

CAPILLARY PUNCTURE

Venipuncture is the most frequently performed phlebotomy procedure, but it is not the procedure of choice in all circumstances. An alternative to venipuncture is capillary puncture, also known as dermal puncture or skin puncture.

Capillary puncture is a method of obtaining one to several drops of blood for a variety of tests. With proper instruments, tests such as a complete blood count, RBC count, white blood cell (WBC) count, hemoglobin, and hematocrit can be run. One drop of blood can be used to test glucose blood levels, a few drops of blood can fill capillary tubes, and several drops can complete a phenylketonuria (PKU) test card. Tests that cannot be run on capillary blood specimens are sedimentation rates, blood cultures, coagulation studies, and any other tests requiring large amounts of serum or plasma.

Capillary puncture is the method of choice with two types of patients: when patient blood volume is a concern, such as with infants, and when vein access is difficult, such as with burned or scarred patients. Capillary puncture should not be used when a patient is edematous, is dehydrated, or has poor peripheral circulation.

Composition of Capillary Blood

Blood obtained via capillary puncture is a mixture of blood from arterioles, venules, capillaries, and interstitial fluid. In most instances, a capillary puncture specimen most resembles arterial blood. There may be significant differences between specimens obtained by capillary puncture and those collected by venipuncture. For example, the glucose level may be increased in capillary blood, whereas the potassium, calcium, and total protein levels may be decreased. It is therefore important to always note on the specimen label when capillary blood has been obtained.

Capillary Puncture Sites

The usual site for capillary puncture in adults and children is the fingertip (Figure 39-32). In adults, the ring finger is often selected because it usually is not callused. In infants, the lateral or medial plantar surface of the heel pad is usually used, and the procedure is often called a heelstick. The heelstick is most often performed when testing for PKU, which is covered in detail in Chapter 43.

Preparing the Capillary Puncture Site

The area selected for a capillary puncture must be carefully prepared. The puncture site will be warm if blood circulation is adequate. Coolness of the skin indicates decreased circulation. To increase circulation, the site can be gently massaged, or a warm, moist towel, face cloth, or warm pack (at a temperature not higher than 100°F) can be placed on the site for 3 to 5 minutes.

Alcohol-soaked gauze should be used to cleanse and disinfect the puncture site. Since residual alcohol at the puncture site can cause hemolysis of the blood sample, as well as a stinging sensation to the patient, the site should then be allowed to air-dry, or dried with a gauze pad. A cotton ball is not recommended because the tiny cotton fibers can stay on the puncture site and promote clotting, which is not desirable at this point. Povidone-iodine should not be used to clean the puncture site because blood contaminated with iodine may falsely increase certain blood chemistries.

Performing the Puncture

Safety glasses, a mask, and gloves should be worn by the medical assistant while performing capillary puncture. Some patients bleed quite readily from the puncture, so be sure to have extra gauze on hand. The patient's hand and finger should be held so the puncture site is readily accessible. The puncture is made at the tip of the fleshy pad and slightly to the side (see Figure 39-32). The skin near the chosen site should be pulled taut. If the tips of the fingers are heavily callused or thickened, a lancet with a longer point may be used. Capillary punctures are performed using semi-automated devices such as the disposable Microtainer Safety Flow Lancet (Figure 39-33).

After cleansing the puncture site, twist off the indicator as directed on the tab. Press the safety lancet firmly against the puncture site. Hold the lancet between your fingers and press the white button with your thumb. The lancet should not bounce off the skin. The puncture should be performed in one quick, steady movement. Once you have depressed the plunger, the button will lock into the housing and the needle will be permanently encapsulated. Practice working the lancets until you are comfortable with the process.

Collecting the Capillary Blood Sample

The first drop of blood is wiped away with dry, sterile gauze because it contains tissue fluid, which dilutes the blood drop and can also activate clotting. The second and following drops of blood are used for test samples. Depending on the tests to be performed, the blood may be collected in capillary tubes or other capillary collecting devices. Capillary tubes are small-diameter glass or plastic tubes that are open at both ends. Capillary tubes are extremely fragile and care should be taken to

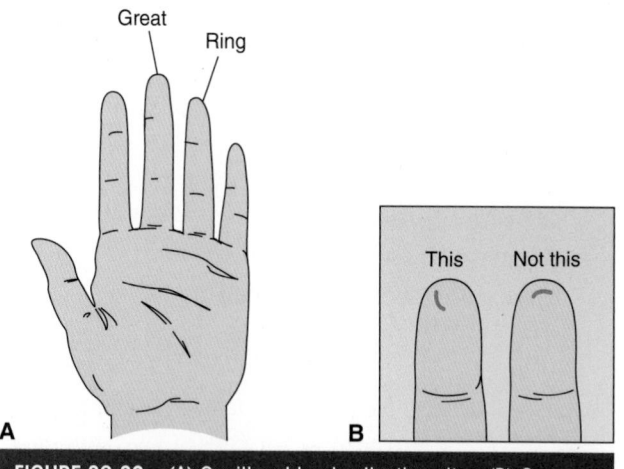

FIGURE 39-32 (A) Capillary blood collection sites. (B) Correct direction of capillary puncture.

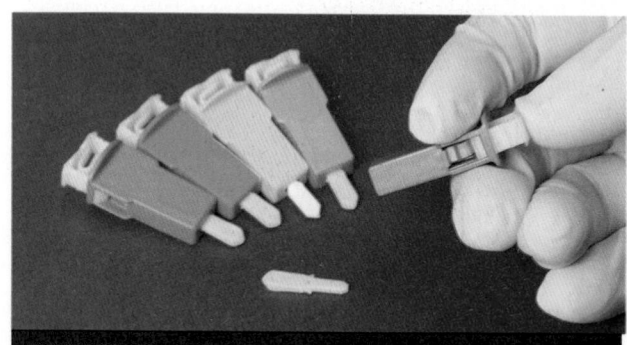

FIGURE 39-33 Microtainer brand lancets are available in different types for various purposes. They are color coded and have specific information on their packaging.

prevent breakage. The tubes have a colored line around one end. A red or black line indicates that the tube contains heparin, an anticoagulant, and will yield a nonclotted specimen. A blue line indicates that the tube contains no anticoagulant and will yield a clotted specimen. Capillary tubes are used for many tests, depending on the equipment available. Chapter 40 explains how to use capillary tubes to check hematocrit levels. When capillary tubes are used for hematocrit tests, they are called microhematocrit tubes.

It may be necessary to massage the finger to increase the blood flow. It is best to massage the whole hand, taking care not to apply direct pressure near the puncture site. Squeezing the fingertip should be avoided; this forces tissue fluid into the blood sample and dilutes it or may cause hemolysis. Do not use a scooping technique when collecting blood from the puncture site. Scooping can break the RBC membranes, leading to hemolysis.

Procedure 39-6 shows the basic steps to follow when filling a capillary tube. During the filling of the tubes, if the flow of blood begins to slow, wipe the puncture site firmly with dry gauze (not a cotton ball). This action will dislodge the platelet plug and allow the blood to flow freely. Be sure the patient is relaxed. Have the patient take a deep breath. After filling the required number of tubes, apply a gauze compress to the puncture site. The patient can usually help hold the compress. The compression should be held in place for 1 to 3 minutes, depending on the patient. If the patient is taking aspirin, Coumadin (warfarin), or other anticoagulants, compression should be for at least 5 minutes.

In many ways the procedure for capillary puncture is similar to the other collection procedures discussed in this chapter (e.g., patient identification, safety precautions, specimen labeling). Procedure 39-6 provides a detailed description of capillary puncture, and Procedure 39-7 provides instruction on how to obtain a capillary specimen for transport using a Microtainer transport unit.

PROCEDURE 39-6

Capillary Puncture

Procedure

STANDARD PRECAUTIONS:

   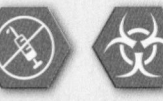

Handwashing   Gloves   Goggles & Mask   No Needle Recapping   Biohazard

PURPOSE:

To obtain capillary blood acceptable for laboratory testing as requested by a provider.

EQUIPMENT/SUPPLIES:

- Gloves
- 70% isopropyl alcohol swab
- Microcollection tubes or capillary tubes
- Safety lancet
- 2 × 2 gauze
- Adhesive bandage or tape

- Sharps container
- Red biohazard bag
- Computer-generated label or thin-tipped permanent marker
- Laboratory requisition (optional)
- Biohazard transport bag (optional)

PROCEDURE STEPS:

1. Assemble the supplies. RATIONALE: Organizing the supplies before the procedure ensures a more timely and professional process.

(continues)

2. Identify the patient, introduce yourself by name and credentials, and recheck the provider's orders. RATIONALE: Introducing yourself will establish a professional relationship with the patient and might help put him or her at ease. Identifying the patient and rechecking the provider's orders will ensure the proper tests will be performed on the right patient.

3. *Explain the rationale for performance of the procedure and expectations to the patient. Show awareness of the patient's concerns related to the procedure being performed*. RATIONALE: Explaining the procedure and allaying the patient's fears will assure the patient that you are concerned about any apprehension he or she may have and that you are open to discussing the concerns.

4. Wash hands and apply gloves. RATIONALE: Washing your hands protects the patient, and applying gloves protects you.

5. Select the puncture site on the fleshy part of the ring or middle finger, avoiding the very tip and the extreme sides (Figure 39-34A). *Incorporate critical thinking skills when performing patient care*. RATIONALE: The ring and middle fingers generally will have fewer calluses and less scarring. The tip and sides are more sensitive than the fleshy part.

6. Have the patient wash his or her hands in very warm water; if necessary, apply a warming pack to the fingertip; encourage the patient to relax; and provide a comfortable, professional atmosphere. RATIONALE: The patient washing his or her hands in very warm water provides two benefits: His or her hands will be cleaner and warmer, and the warmth encourages blood flow to the area. Applying a warming pack to the fingertips will further encourage blood flow. A relaxed patient in a comfortable, professional atmosphere is more likely to provide a better sample.

7. Clean the selected puncture site with the alcohol swab and allow it to air dry or dry it with a gauze pad (Figure 39-34B). RATIONALE: Alcohol will remove any residual soap or debris. Allowing the alcohol to dry will prevent irritation and stinging. If the site is wiped dry, the irritation of the gauze pad will further encourage blood to the area.

8. Holding the distal phalange firmly, perform the puncture across the lines of the fingerprint rather than along the lines (Figure 39-34C). RATIONALE: Holding the distal phalange firmly will add support to the finger and prevent the patient from pulling back on the finger during the puncture. Puncturing across the fingerprint will assist the blood to form a drop rather than flow across the fingertip.

9. Dispose of the lancet into the sharps container (Figure 39-34D). RATIONALE: Disposing of biohazard supplies appropriately lessens the chance of accidental needlesticks.

10. Using a gauze pad, wipe away the first drop. RATIONALE: The first drop usually contains contamination from the alcohol and tissue fluid and would not be a good representation of the blood sample needed. Using gauze rather than cotton to wipe it away lessens the likelihood of it clotting too quickly.

11. Let a fresh drop accumulate on the fingertip (Figure 39-34E). Collect the specimen according to the test being performed (Figure 39-34F). (See Chapter 40 for hemoglobin and hematocrit; see Chapter 43 for PKU, glucose, and other specialty tests performed on capillary blood.)

12. Wipe the blood from the microhematocrit tube (Figure 39-34G) and apply a plug.

13. Have the patient hold firm, direct pressure on the site with a gauze pad for at least 2 minutes. If the bleeding has stopped, an adhesive strip can be applied. If the bleeding has not stopped yet, hold firm, direct pressure on the site for another 5 minutes and then recheck. Adhesive strips are not recommended for patients younger than 2 years. RATIONALE: The bleeding should be stopped before the patient leaves your care. Adhesive strips for children younger than 2 years are not recommended because they are a choking hazard.

14. Disinfect the area and equipment, remove gloves, and dispose of them into a biohazard waste container/red bag. Wash hands. RATIONALE: Biohazard waste should be controlled for everyone's protection. Hand washing after removing gloves further protects you.

15. Record the procedure. If the test is being sent to an outside laboratory, complete the requisition in the presence of the patient, insert both into the biohazard transport bag, and alert the laboratory to pick up the specimen. If the test is to be performed in your POL, proceed with the completion of the test immediately, record the results, and notify the provider of the results. RATIONALE: Documentation is critical for good patient records. Completing the laboratory requisition in the presence of the patient provides accurate insurance and personal information if needed for the insurance forms and for your medical records.

(continues)

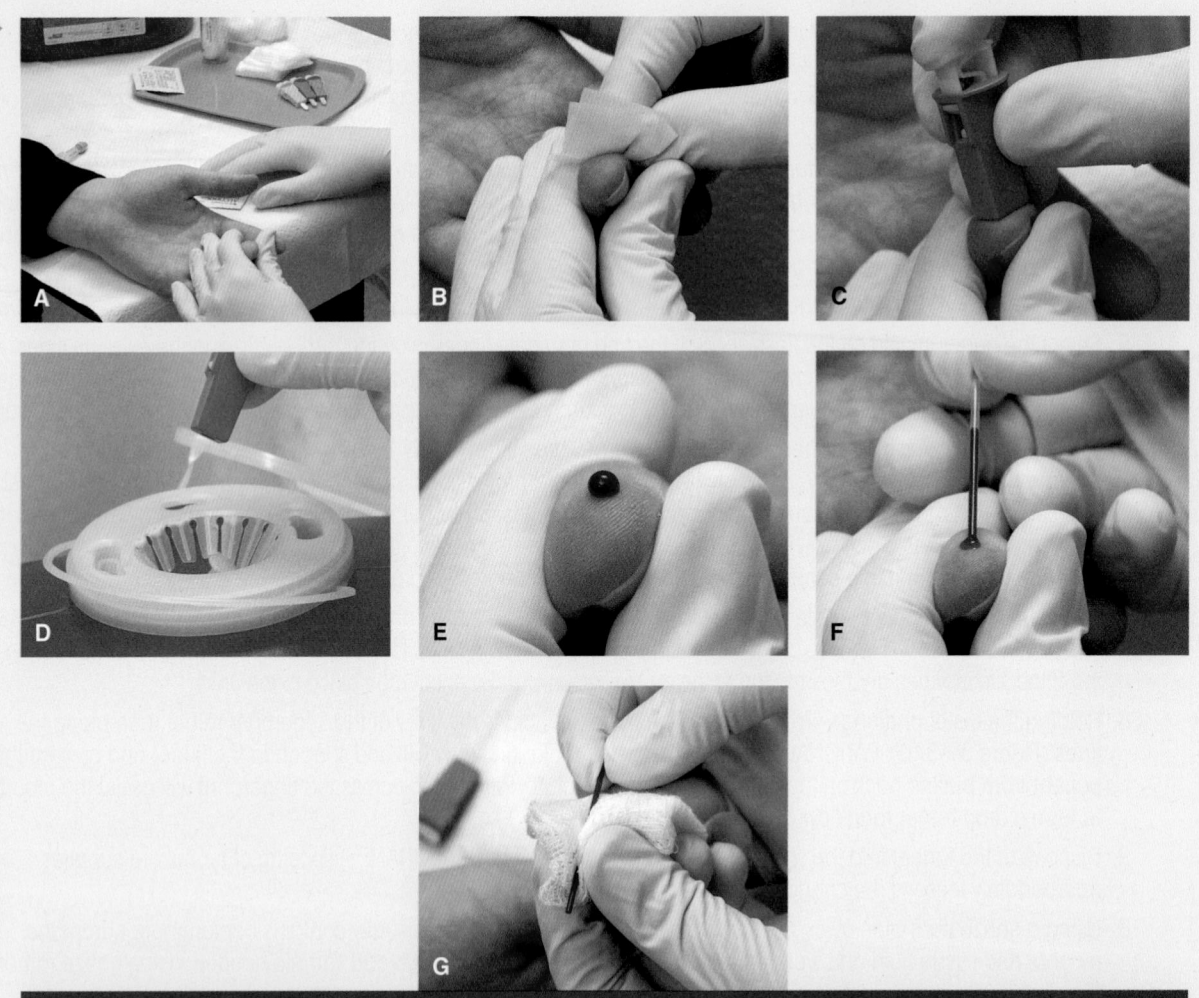

FIGURE 39-34 Collecting a specimen into a capillary tube through capillary puncture. (A) Assemble the necessary equipment and supplies and examine the finger for the best puncture site. (B) Clean the site with alcohol and allow the area to dry. (C) Perform the puncture. (D) Discard the lancet into a nearby sharps container. (E) Wipe off the first drop (not shown) and allow a well-rounded drop to form. (F) Holding the capillary tube horizontally, touch the end to the drop and allow the tube to fill. (G) Carefully wipe the residue blood off the tube.

DOCUMENTATION:

Notes

4/27/XX 8:15 AM Capillary puncture performed left ring finger for HgbA1c. Patient tolerated the procedure well. Dr. Lewis is scheduled to see the patient today to discuss progress. J. Guerrero, CMA (AAMA)

Courtesy of Harris CareTracker PM and EMR

Procedure

Obtaining a Capillary Specimen for Transport Using a Microtainer Transport Unit

STANDARD PRECAUTIONS:

Handwashing   Gloves   Goggles & Mask   No Needle Recapping   Biohazard

PURPOSE:

To obtain a specimen of capillary blood for transport to a laboratory for testing, using a Microtainer.

EQUIPMENT/SUPPLIES:

- Capillary puncture supplies as used in Procedure 39-6
- Gloves
- Gauze pads
- Adhesive bandage
- Sharps container and biohazard waste receptacle
- Microtainer tube transport unit

- Laboratory requisition
- Computer-generated label or thin-tipped permanent marker
- Small sturdy container with a tight-fitting lid (such as a urine specimen cup or red-top vacuum tube)
- Biohazard specimen transport bag

PROCEDURE STEPS:

1. Begin by completing steps 1 through 10 in Procedure 39-6. Then continue on with the procedure steps below.

2. Scoop the drop into the Microtainer tube (Figure 39-35A). RATIONALE: This is the method used to get the specimen into the tip of the Microtainer tube.

3. Tip the Microtainer tube, allowing the drop to slide into the tube (Figure 39-35B). RATIONALE: As soon as a drop is obtained on the scoop it should be moved into the tube, where it can mix with the additive.

4. Gently agitate the tube. RATIONALE: Agitating the tube allows the additive to mix with the blood.

5. Continue collection of blood until the tube is filled (Figure 39-35C). RATIONALE: The tube must be filled to the fill line to ensure the proper ratio of blood to additive.

6. Provide the patient with a gauze pad and ask him or her to hold pressure on the puncture site. RATIONALE: The pressure with a gauze pad will encourage the wound to clot.

7. Remove the scoop from the Microtainer unit and discard the scoop into the sharps container (Figure 39-35D). RATIONALE: The scoop is contaminated with blood and therefore is considered to be biohazard waste. Being hard plastic, it is capable of scratching someone, so the sharps container is safer than the red bag waste receptacle.

8. Remove the colored cap from the back of the Microtainer tube and place it securely onto the opening. RATIONALE: Placing the cap securely onto the Microtainer tube will ensure the specimen will stay in the Microtainer tube during handling and transport.

9. Place the capped Microtainer tube into a small sturdy container with a tight-fitting lid. RATIONALE: Placing the Microtainer tube in another container protects it from being uncapped and (because of its small size) lost in transport. The Microtainer tube is also not large enough for adequate labeling.

10. Label the container. RATIONALE: Proper labeling ensures the proper tests on the right specimen.

(continues)

11. Fill out the laboratory requisition while the patient is present. Place the specimen and the requisition into the bio-hazard transport bag in their separate compartments. RATIONALE: Any questions about the patient's address and insurance can be answered immediately if the patient is present while you complete the form.

12. Check the patient's puncture site. If bleeding has stopped, apply an adhesive strip, answer any questions the patient has, and release the patient. RATIONALE: Caring for the patient both physically and emotionally shows a professional dedication to your job.

13. Document the procedure in patient's chart or electronic medical record and notify the laboratory that the specimen is ready for pickup. RATIONALE: Documentation ensures that the proper information is recorded into the patient's chart or electronic medical record.

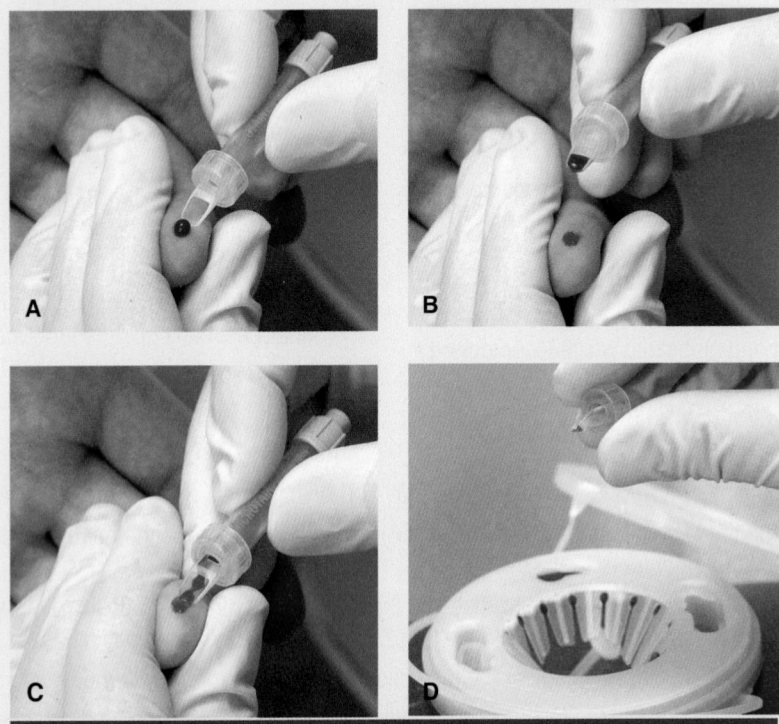

FIGURE 39-35 Collecting a capillary specimen for transport. (A) After wiping away the first drop (not shown), allow drop to form. Touch the scoop on the collection Microtainer tube to the blood droplet. (B) Tip the collection Microtainer tube up so that the blood flows into the tube. Agitate it gently to mix the anticoagulant with the blood. (C) Continue collecting the blood until the collection Microtainer tube is filled to the marked level. (D) Remove the scoop from the collection Microtainer tube and dispose of the scoop into a nearby sharps container.

DOCUMENTATION:

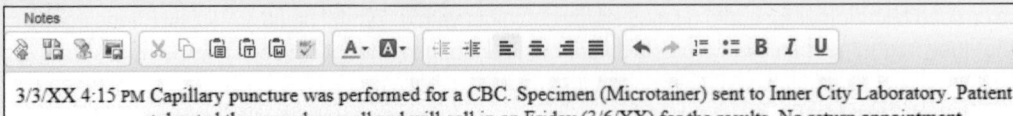

3/3/XX 4:15 PM Capillary puncture was performed for a CBC. Specimen (Microtainer) sent to Inner City Laboratory. Patient tolerated the procedure well and will call in on Friday (3/6/XX) for the results. No return appointment scheduled. N. McFarland, RMA (AMT)

Courtesy of Harris CareTracker PM and EMR

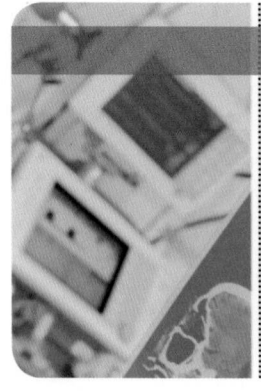

CASE STUDY 39-1

Refer to the scenario at the beginning of the chapter.

CASE STUDY REVIEW

1. What types of information will patients share with Thomas about their previous venipuncture experiences?
2. How can Thomas use that information to better serve the patients?
3. Do you think patients are a good source of information about their bodies and their reactions to past experiences?

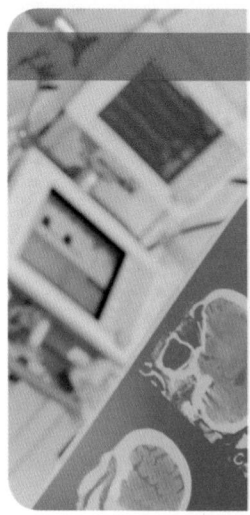

CASE STUDY 39-2

Inner City Health Care is short-staffed today, and medical assistant Nancy McFarland, RMA (AMT), is feeling pressed for time. She has many tasks to complete, but first she must perform a venipuncture. She greets the patient, Katy Friend, in a perfunctory manner to discourage time-wasting conversation. Although Katy appears apprehensive, she is not resistant, so Nancy quickly assembles the necessary supplies, applies the tourniquet, and inserts the needle. While she is drawing her blood, Katy faints.

CASE STUDY REVIEW

1. What should Nancy do now?
2. What could Nancy have done to prevent this situation from occurring?
3. In the future, what are some steps Nancy can take to provide a positive experience for venipuncture patients?

Summary

- Phlebotomy skills improve with hands-on practice.
- Safety is of the utmost consideration when performing phlebotomy procedures.
- Sharps must be deposited into official sharps containers.
- Contaminated supplies must be disposed of into a red bag or biohazard container.
- Frequent hand washing between patients as well as before and after each procedure will lessen chances of cross-contamination.
- Wearing gloves and appropriate PPE with each phlebotomy procedure will ensure safety for both the patient and the medical assistant.
- Accurate blood test results require that lab specimens be collected using the correct method of draw and order of draw, and that the specimens are processed and handled appropriately according to the laboratory manual.
- Good communication skills are critical in putting the patient at ease while drawing his or her blood.
- Medical assistants who always present a professional image show a greater level of concern for positive interaction with the patient, the families, and the public.
- Active listening skills and the ability to respond appropriately, honestly, and diplomatically while being cognizant of professional boundaries will all help provide for a more positive experience.
- Safe practice requires that medical assistants are aware of and abide by current laws and regulations regarding their scope of practice, credentials, and professional training requirements when performing clinical patient procedures.

Study For Success

To reinforce your knowledge and skills of information presented in this chapter:

- Review the *Key Terms* and *Learning Outcomes*
- Consider the *Critical Thinking* features and *Case Studies* and discuss your conclusions

Procedure

- Answer the questions in the *Certification Review*
- Perform the *Procedures* using the *Competency Assessment Checklists on the Student Companion Website*

CERTIFICATION REVIEW

1. What is the most common patient concern when having blood drawn?
   a. Nerve damage
   b. Hematomas
   c. Infection
   d. Pain

2. What is the purpose of an anticoagulant in a vacuum tube?
   a. To dilute the blood before testing
   b. To ensure the sterility of the tube
   c. To separate the blood cells into layers
   d. To make the blood clot faster
   e. To prevent the blood from clotting

3. When collecting a blood sample with a vacuum tube system, why is the last tube withdrawn from the holder before removing the needle from the patient?
   a. To avoid hematoma at the venipuncture site
   b. To avoid dripping blood out the end of the needle
   c. To prevent clotting of the blood
   d. To eliminate pain for the patient

4. Leaving the tourniquet on a patient's arm for an extended length of time before drawing blood may cause which of the following?
   a. Hemoconcentration
   b. Specimen hemolysis
   c. Stress
   d. Bruising
   e. Pain

5. When drawing multiple specimens in vacuum tubes, it is important to fill which of the following color-stoppered tubes first?
   a. Light blue
   b. Green
   c. Lavender
   d. Red

6. What organization determines proper lab procedures?
   a. OSHA
   b. L&I
   c. CLIA
   d. CSLI
   e. CMS

7. What is the single most important way to prevent the spread of infection from patient to patient?
   a. Gowning and gloving
   b. Hand washing
   c. Always wearing masks
   d. Avoiding breathing on clients

8. Which is the anticoagulant of choice when drawing coagulation studies such as PT?
   a. No anticoagulant (red top tube)
   b. Sodium citrate (light blue top tube)
   c. EDTA (lavender top tube)
   d. Heparin (green top tube
   e. SST (red mottled top tube)

9. When the medical assistant cannot perform a venipuncture successfully after two attempts, what is the best course?
   a. Try at least two more times
   b. Notify the provider
   c. Ask another health care professional to try
   d. Request the test for the next day

10. What might happen if the blood is drawn too quickly from a small vein?
    a. The vein might collapse.
    b. A bruise might form.
    c. The blood cells might disintegrate.
    d. The vein could roll.
    e. The patient will experience more discomfort.

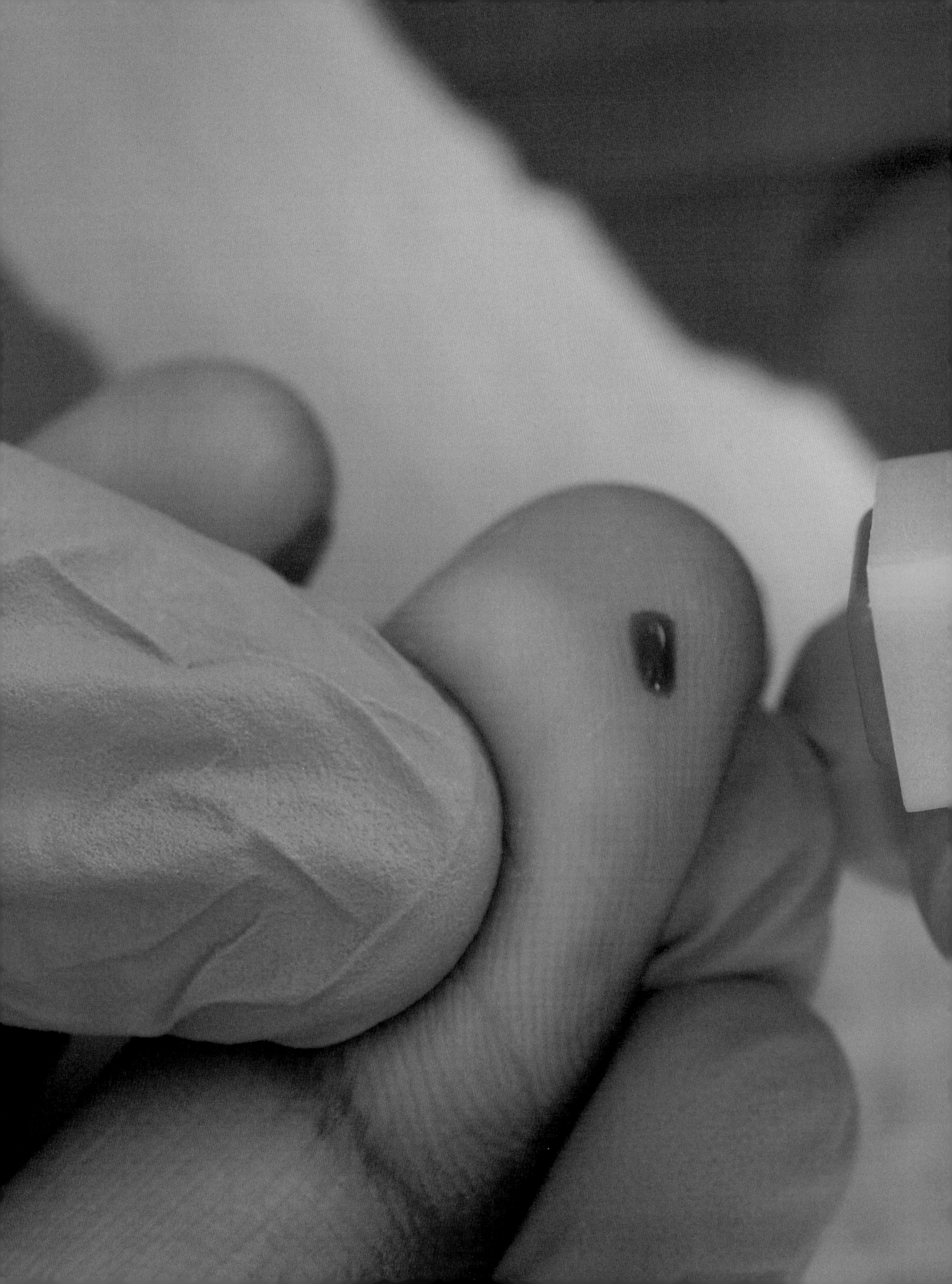

Hematology

1. Define and spell the key terms as presented in the glossary.

2. Describe the process of hematopoiesis.

3. List the five types of normal white blood cells and give the identifying characteristics and role of each.

4. Explain to a fellow student the role of the red blood cells and the platelets.

5. Distinguish between normal and abnormal blood test results.

6. Discuss how the clinical science of hematology and the complete blood count (CBC) are used in the diagnosis and treatment of disease.

7. Discuss how the hemoglobin, hematocrit, RBC indices, WBC differential, and ESR are used to diagnose patients.

8. Apply mathematical computations to solve the equation of erythrocyte indices (using RBC count, hemoglobin, and hematocrit).

9. Describe CRP and its uses as a screening test for general infection and inflammation.

KEY TERMS

anisocytosis

basophils

C-reactive protein (CRP)

complete blood count (CBC)

eosinophils

erythrocytes (red blood cells [RBCs])

erythrocyte indices

erythrocyte sedimentation rate (ESR)

erythropoietin

hematocrit (Hct or crit)

hematopoiesis

hemoglobin (Hgb)

hemoglobinopathies

hypochromic

leukocytes (white blood cells [WBCs])

lymphocyte

macrocytic

microcytic

monocytes

neutrophils

normochromic

normocytic

protime

reticulocyte (retic)

rouleaux

thrombocytes (platelets)

thrombocytopenia

thrombocytosis

SCENARIO

The providers at Inner City Health Care often order hematologic tests to assist them in diagnosing and treating patients. As she performs the tests in the providers' office laboratory, medical assistant Gwen Carr, CMA (AAMA), uses her knowledge of hematology every day. Gwen is comfortable performing waived lab tests because she understands the purposes and procedures of the tests. As a competent professional working within her scope of practice, she always follows all safety and quality-control guidelines to protect herself and others and to ensure the accuracy of test results.

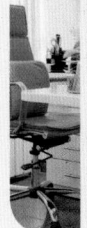

Chapter Portal

Hematology is the study of the blood cells and coagulation in both normal and diseased states. The two main components of the blood are plasma (the liquid portion) and cells. Cells of the blood are also known as the formed elements of the blood. The study of hematology is usually limited to the cellular components of the blood and does not include the chemistry of the blood. See Chapter 43 for the chemistry of blood and tests related to blood chemistry.

The cellular components of blood include **erythrocytes (red blood cells [RBCs]), leukocytes (white blood cells [WBCs]), and thrombocytes (platelets).** Blood has many different functions as discussed later in this chapter.

THE FORMATION OF BLOOD CELLS

Hematopoiesis is defined as the formation of blood cells (Figure 40-1). The blood-forming tissues of the body and hematopoiesis are included in the study of hematology. In the embryo, hematopoiesis occurs in the yolk sac, liver, and spleen. After we are born, the primary site for the production of erythrocytes, granulocytes, and platelets is the bone marrow. Lymphocytes are also produced in the bone marrow, as well as in the lymph nodes. At birth, most of the bone marrow in the body is capable of producing blood cells. This process is confined to the bone marrow of the ribs, vertebrae, sternum, and iliac crest by the age of 20 years. Bone marrow that is producing cells is known as red marrow. With aging, the area for hematopoiesis is reduced and the red bone marrow is replaced by yellow marrow, which is stored

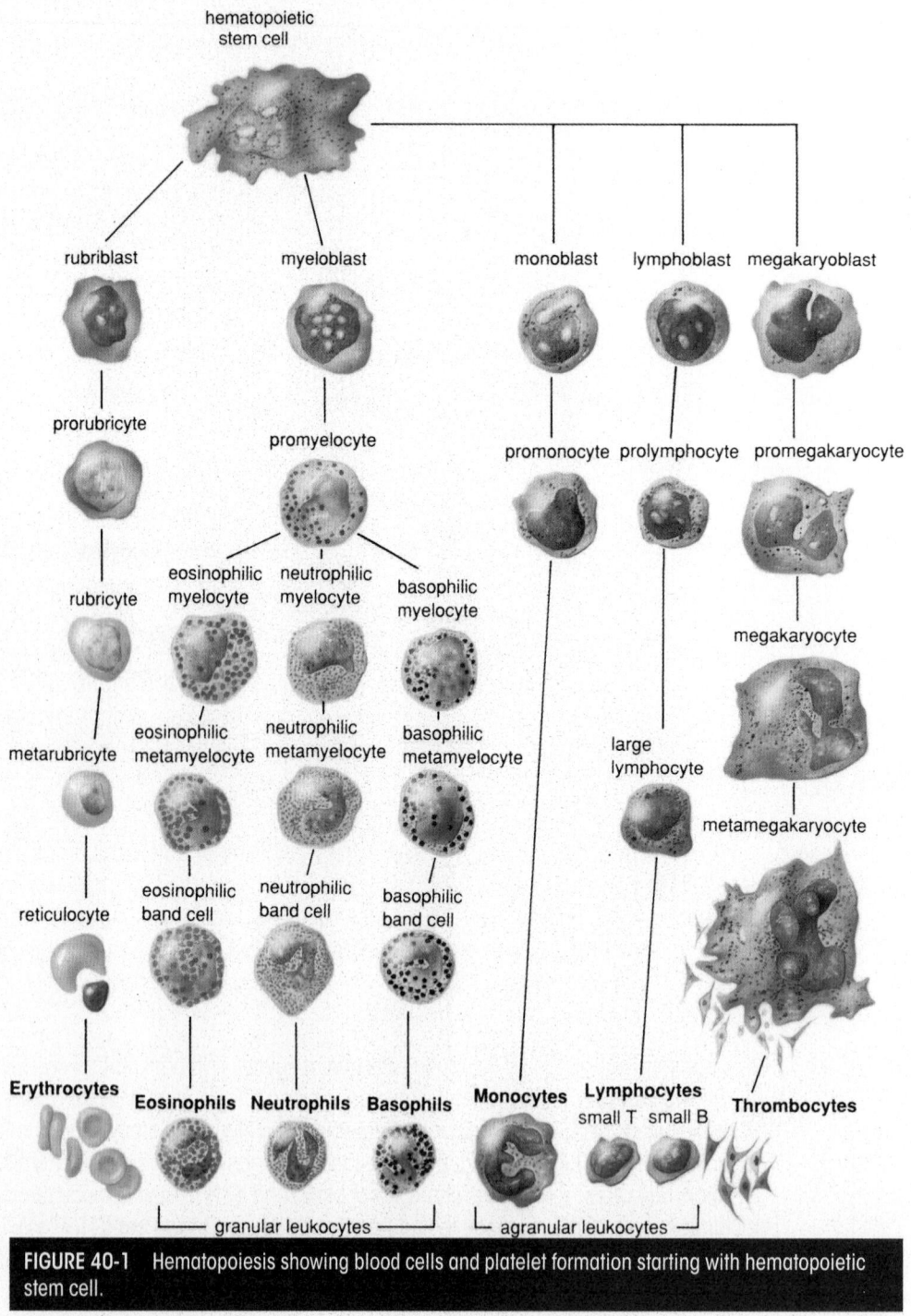

FIGURE 40-1 Hematopoiesis showing blood cells and platelet formation starting with hematopoietic stem cell.

fat. When a provider collects a bone marrow sample in an adult, the site chosen for sampling is the sternum or the iliac crest because this is where the blood cells are still being produced.

HEMATOLOGIC TESTS

Hematologic tests are the second most common tests performed in the physician's office laboratory (POL). The most common test is the urinalysis. The cellular components of the blood may be affected by changes in either the blood-forming organs or in other tissues of the body. The study of these changes forms the basis of hematologic tests performed in the POL.

Hematologic tests performed in the clinical laboratory include:

- Hemoglobin
- Hematocrit
- WBC count
- Differential WBC count
- RBC count
- RBC indices
- Platelet count
- Erythrocyte sedimentation rate (ESR)
- Prothrombin time (PT)

The results of these hematologic tests provide valuable information used by the provider in making a diagnosis, evaluating a patient's progress, and regulating further treatment.

The laboratory test ordered most frequently on blood in the ambulatory care setting is the **complete blood count (CBC)**. The exact number of parameters included in the CBC will vary from laboratory to laboratory (Figure 40-2). The CBC generally includes:

- Hemoglobin determination
- Hematocrit determination
- RBC count (and indices)
- WBC count (and differential)
- Platelet count

Competency   Integrity

All these tests can be performed by manual testing procedures or with an automated hematology analyzer. Manual blood cell counts are considered by the Clinical Laboratory Improvement Act (CLIA) to be of moderate to high complexity, whereas the automated tests are considered to be moderately complex; therefore, neither are within the medical assistant's scope of practice. The manual blood cell counts are performed only at reference laboratories by medical technicians. The automated cell count analyzers may be located in the POL, but the testing and interpretation of the tests, maintenance of the analyzers, as well as training and supervision of laboratory personnel is performed by the medical technician.

Laboratory tests ordered by the provider are recorded in the patient's medical record in the progress notes section and a lab report is completed. The lab report is filed in the lab section of the patient's record. All test results are noted by the provider before the patient is notified. Accurate and timely documentation are important in all medical laboratory procedures.

HEMOGLOBIN AND HEMATOCRIT TESTS

Hemoglobin (Hgb) and **hematocrit (Hct or crit)** tests are part of the CBC; however, they are frequently ordered separate from a CBC. They have a unique relationship with each other and are rarely ordered individually. Both the hemoglobin and the hematocrit tests are performed to obtain similar information about RBCs in relation to the rest of the blood sample, but they also give decidedly different information. In normal results, the hemoglobin often will be about one third the number of the hematocrit.

Hemoglobin

Hemoglobin is the major component of the RBC and serves to transport oxygen and carbon dioxide through the body. Hemoglobin, which is responsible for about 85% of the dry weight of the RBC, is a conjugated (combined) protein composed of heme and globin. A single hemoglobin molecule consists of four globin chains with a heme group attached to each globin (Figure 40-3). The central component of each heme group is an iron molecule. One oxygen molecule can be transported to each heme group; therefore, each RBC can carry four oxygen molecules.

Synthesis of the heme portion of the hemoglobin molecule requires iron, which is usually obtained through our diets. The daily iron requirement for an adult man is about 0.5 mg/day, whereas a menstruating woman requires about four times that much, or 2 mg/day.

Hemoglobin carries about 95% of the oxygen to the body cells and carries away about 27% of the carbon dioxide. The RBCs pick up the oxygen in the lungs from when we breathe in, and they drop

A	Test	Results	Abnormal Results	Units	Reference Range

Patient Name
Thompson, Adam
Ordering Provider
Anthony Brockton MD

DOB
1/1/1942

Age
71

Gender
M

Report Status: **Final**
Reported: **11/10/20XX 7:17:14 PM**
Accession:
Collected: **8/12/20XX**

A	Test	Results	Abnormal Results	Units	Reference Range
CBC	**W Auto Differential panel in Blood**				
N	Granulocytes %				
N	Erythrocyte distribution width				
N	Neutrophils.band form #				
N	Platelet distribution width				
N	Platelet mean volume				
N	Neutrophils.band form %				
N	Lymphocytes Variant %				
N	Lymphocytes Variant #				
N	Hematocrit %	41.2		%	39.0–50.0
N	Leukocytes other #				
N	Auto Differential panel in Blood				
N	Other cells %				
N	Complete blood count (hemogram) panel in Blood by Automated count				
N	Other cells #				
N	Monocytes %	12.9		%	0.0–13.0
N	Leukocytes #	5.2		Thous/cu. mm	3.9–11.1
N	Basophils #				
H	**Basophils %**		0.3	%	**0.0–2.0**
N	Eosinophils #				
N	Eosinophils %	0.6		%	0.0–8.0
N	Hemoglobin	14.5		g/dL	13.2–16.9
N	Lymphocytes #				
N	Lymphocytes %	46.1		%	15.0–48.0
N	Monocytes #				
N	Neutrophils #				
N	Neutrophils %	40.1		%	38.0–80.0
N	Platelets #	172		Thous/cu. mm	140–390
H	**Erythrocyte mean corpuscular hemoglobin**	41.4		pg	**27.0–34.0 pg**
N	Erythrocyte mean corpuscular hemoglobin concentration	35.3		%	32.0–35.5 g/dL
H	**Erythrocyte mean corpuscular volume**	117		fL	**78.0–100.0 fL**

FIGURE 40-2 Hematology report form.

off the carbon dioxide in the lungs to be expelled when we breathe out. The rest of the carbon dioxide is removed through other processes. Oxygenated hemoglobin is bright red, and hemoglobin unbound to oxygen is darker. This explains the bright red color of arterial blood (moving from the lungs and to the cells) and the darker color of venous blood (going back to the lungs).

A second function of hemoglobin is as a blood buffer; that is, hemoglobin helps maintain the proper pH balance of the blood as it picks up and drops off oxygen and carbon dioxide.

The production of new RBCs and consequently the formation of new hemoglobin is triggered by a hormone called **erythropoietin**, which is produced in the kidneys. The erythropoietin

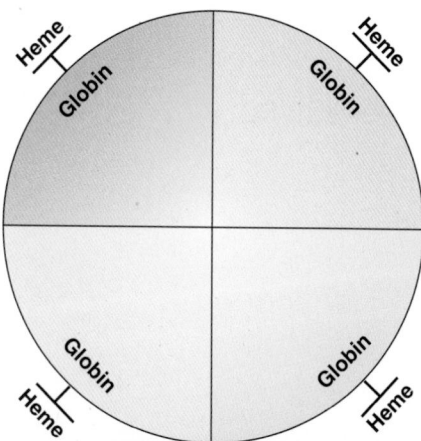

FIGURE 40-3 Representation of a normal hemoglobin molecule containing four globin chains with a heme group attached to each globin. One oxygen molecule can be transported by each heme group.

process is activated when the body cells sense a low oxygen level.

There are several forms of hemoglobin. Hemoglobin A (Hgb A) is the most common form found in adults. The other hemoglobin types are abnormal and are responsible for a group of diseases known as **hemoglobinopathies**. These abnormal forms of hemoglobin include hemoglobin S (Hgb S), hemoglobin C, and hemoglobin E. Hgb S is the most common abnormal form of hemoglobin observed in the laboratory. It is the form of hemoglobin that causes sickle cell anemia. When Hgb S molecules are subjected to certain conditions, they alter the physical structure of the RBCs. The RBCs assume a sickle shape, which makes it difficult, if not impossible, for the cell to pass through a capillary bed.

The most frequent hemoglobin disease seen in the ambulatory care setting is anemia, with iron deficiency anemia being the most common type. A decrease of available iron in the body is the most common cause of this type of anemia. Lack of available iron can be caused by insufficient intake through the diet (called nutritional anemia); losing iron because of a bleeding problem (called hemorrhagic anemia); or less commonly, congenital defects, industrial toxins, diseases of the bone marrow (aplastic anemia), and a variety of other disorders. In nutritional anemia, the laboratory finding usually shows a normal or near-normal hematocrit (because these patients have the right percentage of RBCs), but low hemoglobin. Their RBCs are hypochromic (pale) because they lack oxygen. The main symptom of anemia, fatigue, is also caused by lack of oxygen.

Procedure

Hemoglobin is measured in the POL using an automated CLIA-waived POCT (point-of-care testing) device (Figure 40-4). These devices are infrared analyzers that measure the density of the hemoglobin pigment by light refraction. The more hemoglobin present in the sample, the more light is refracted. POCT is a quick method, uses only a small drop of blood, and gives immediate results. Many such devices will also connect electronically to patient management systems, eliminating the need for manual documentation of the test results (Procedure 40-1).

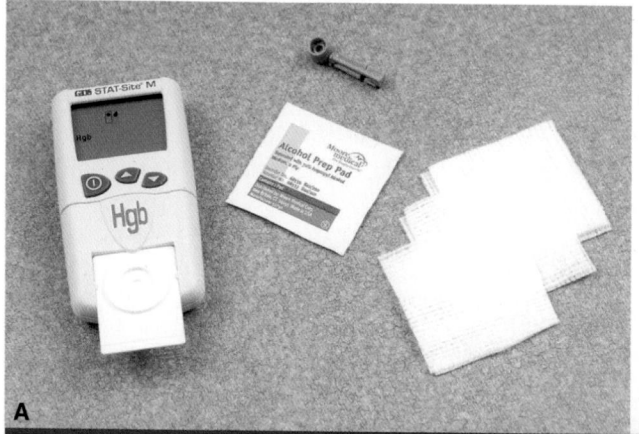
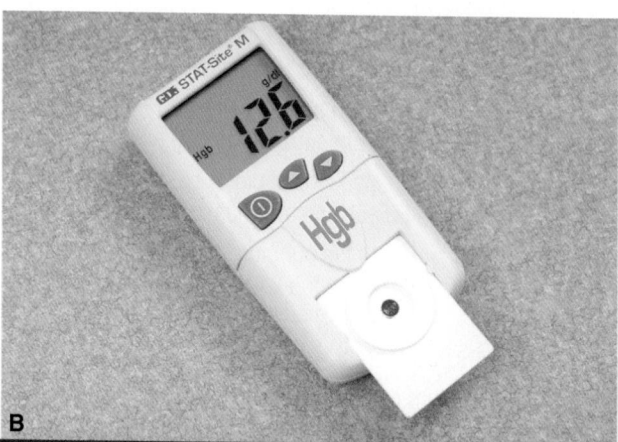

FIGURE 40-4 (A) A handheld hemoglobinometer that is commonly found in the physician's office laboratory. (B) Results after performing a hemoglobin test on capillary blood.

PROCEDURE 40-1

Procedure

Hemoglobin Determination Using a CLIA-Waived Hemoglobin Analyzer

STANDARD PRECAUTIONS:

Handwashing

Gloves

No Needle Recapping

Biohazard

PURPOSE:

To properly and safely perform an automated hemoglobin determination to evaluate the oxygen-carrying capacity of the blood.

EQUIPMENT/SUPPLIES:

- Gloves
- Biohazard container
- Sharps container
- Capillary puncture equipment
- 70% isopropyl alcohol pledget

- Safety lancet
- 2 × 2 gauze
- Adhesive bandage
- CLIA-waived hemoglobin analyzer with test strips or slides

PROCEDURE STEPS:

1. Assemble and organize equipment and supplies. RATIONALE: Being organized helps the process go more smoothly and professionally.

2. Wash hands and put on gloves. RATIONALE: Hand washing and gloving protects the patient and you.

3. Turn on the analyzer and calibrate or standardize according to the manufacturer's instructions (Figure 40-5A). RATIONALE: Turn on the analyzer to warm the machine up; calibrate to maintain quality controls.

4. Introduce yourself by name and credential, identify the patient, and recheck the provider's orders. RATIONALE: Introducing yourself and stating your credentials demonstrates professionalism and helps to reassure the patient. Identifying the patient and rechecking the provider's orders will ensure the proper tests will be performed on the right patient.

5. ***Explain the rationale for performance of the procedure to the patient, showing awareness of the patient's concerns.*** Allay the patient's fears regarding the procedure to help him or her feel safe and comfortable. RATIONALE: Explaining the procedure and allaying the patient's fears will assure the patient that you are concerned about any apprehension he or she may have and that you are open to discussing the patient's concerns.

6. Select the site, prepare the site, and perform the capillary puncture (see Chapter 39, Procedure 39-6). Wipe away the first drop with gauze. RATIONALE: The first drop may be contaminated with tissue fluid.

7. Apply the second drop of blood into the slide reservoir using the appropriate technique for the analyzer (Figure 40-5B). RATIONALE: Each machine has a slightly different applicator device and technique.

8. Apply gauze to the puncture site and ask the patient to hold pressure for 2 minutes. RATIONALE: The puncture should clot during the 2 minutes the pressure is held.

9. Place the slide into the analyzer and perform appropriate steps as required by the manufacturer's instructions. RATIONALE: Each manufacturer has specific processes for use with its analyzer.

10. Read and make a note of the test results (Figure 40-5C). RATIONALE: Making a note helps you retain the results until they can be charted in the patient's medical record.

(continues)

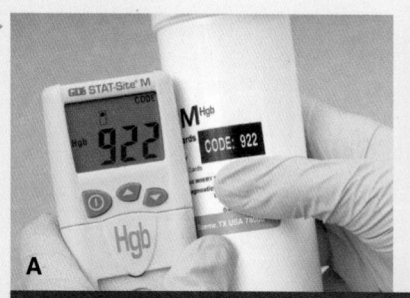
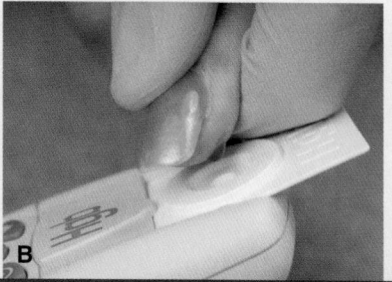
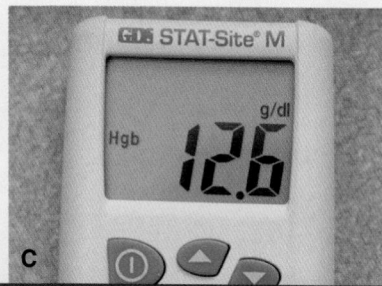

FIGURE 40-5 (A) Turn on the machine and perform control testing if necessary. Always follow the manufacturer's instructions. (B) Place the patient's drop of blood into the slide reservoir. (C) Read and record the hemoglobin value.

11. Assess the patient and apply a bandage strip to the puncture site. RATIONALE: The patient should not leave your care until the bleeding has stopped. Do not apply a fingertip bandage to an infant or young child because it could pose a choking hazard.

12. Disinfect the analyzer according to the manufacturer's instructions. Discard all contaminated equipment and supplies into appropriate biohazard waste receptacles. Disinfect counter space. RATIONALE: Using disinfectants not recommended by the manufacturer could harm the analyzer. Use sharps containers for sharp supplies and red bags for contaminated gauze and gloves.

13. Remove gloves and discard into biohazard container, and wash hands. RATIONALE: Washing hands removes residual contamination.

14. Document the procedure in the patient's medical record in the progress notes charting section and complete a lab report. File the lab report in the lab section of the patient's record. RATIONALE: Accurate and timely documentation are important in medical laboratory procedures.

DOCUMENTATION:

PROCEDURE NOTE

08/06/20XX Capillary puncture performed for hemoglobin determination. Specimen tested in our lab. Results: 14.5 gm/dL. Dr. Rice notified of results and report filed in patient records. Patient tolerated the procedure well and Dr. Rice discussed results with her. Joe Guerrero, CMA (AAMA)

Courtesy of Harris CareTracker PM and EMR

TABLE 40-1

NORMAL HEMOGLOBIN VALUES, OR REFERENCE RANGES, BY AGE AND SEX

Newborn	15 to 20 g/dL
Age 3 months	9 to 14 g/dL
Age 10 months	12 to 14.5 g/dL
Adult female	12 to 16 g/dL
Adult male	13 to 18 g/dL

The normal reference values for hemoglobin vary according to both the age and sex of the individual (Table 40-1).

Hematocrit

Procedure

Hematocrit (packed RBC volume) is the ratio of the volume of packed RBCs to that of the whole-blood specimen. Packed RBC volume is expressed as a percentage of the whole specimen. This is achieved manually or by automated methods. Most medical assistants working in ambulatory care settings use the manual microhematocrit method (see Procedure 40-2). It requires only a few drops of blood either directly into a microhematocrit tube obtained by capillary draw, or the sample can be taken from a vacuum tube containing ethylene-di-aminetetraacetic acid (EDTA) after a venipuncture. Chapter 39 explains both capillary draw and venipuncture.

The cellular components of the blood sample separate into layers when they are centrifuged

PROCEDURE 40-2

Procedure

Microhematocrit Determination

STANDARD PRECAUTIONS:

Handwashing

Gloves

Biohazard

PURPOSE:

To properly and safely perform a microhematocrit determination.

EQUIPMENT/SUPPLIES:

- Gloves
- Biohazard container
- Sharps container
- Capillary puncture equipment
  - 70% isopropyl alcohol pledget
  - Safety lancet
  - 2 × 2 gauze
  - Adhesive bandage
- Microhematocrit tubes: heparinized, plastic, self-sealing (Figure 40-6)
- Microhematocrit tube holder
- Microhematocrit centrifuge and reader

FIGURE 40-6 Self-sealing microhematocrit (capillary blood) tubes.

ClearCrit is a trademark of Separation Technology, Inc.

PROCEDURE STEPS:

1. Assemble and organize equipment and supplies. RATIONALE: Being organized helps the process go more smoothly and professionally.

2. Wash hands and put on gloves. RATIONALE: Hand washing and gloving protects the patient and you.

3. Introduce yourself by name and credential, identify the patient, and recheck the provider's orders. RATIONALE: Introducing yourself and stating your credentials demonstrates professionalism and helps to reassure the patient. Identifying the patient and rechecking the provider's orders will ensure the proper tests will be performed on the right patient.

4. ***Explain the rationale for performance of the procedure to the patient, showing awareness of the patient's concerns***. Allay the patient's fears regarding the procedure to help him or her feel safe and comfortable. RATIONALE: Explaining the procedure and allaying the patient's fears will assure the patient that you are concerned about any apprehension he or she may have and that you are open to discussing the patient's concerns.

5. Select the site, prepare the site, and perform the capillary puncture (see Chapter 39). Wipe away the first drop with gauze. RATIONALE: The first drop may be contaminated with tissue fluid. Using gauze rather than a cotton ball will discourage a clot from forming.

6. Allow the second drop of blood to form on the patient's finger. Holding the microhematocrit tube horizontally, touch the end onto the top of the blood drop and let the tube fill by capillary action until the self-sealing tube stops filling (Figures 40-7A and B).

7. With a 2 × 2 gauze pad, wipe off the end of the tube. Place the filled microhematocrit tube into the tube holder. RATIONALE: Wiping the end of the tube of blood lessens contamination of the centrifuge.

8. Repeat the procedure with one more tube. RATIONALE: The two tubes balance one another in the centrifuge and the amounts are averaged to get the hematocrit results.

(continues)

9. Apply a gauze compress to the puncture site and ask the patient to hold pressure for 2 minutes. RATIONALE: The puncture site should clot during the 2 minutes the pressure is held.

10. Place the tubes into the centrifuge with sealed ends outward against the gasket. Make certain the tubes balance each other across the centrifuge (see Figure 40-8). Fasten the lid securely, lock into place, and turn the centrifuge on. Set the timer and spin for the appropriate amount of time as specified in the manufacturer's instructions. RATIONALE: Centrifugal force requires that the plugged ends be to the outside to prevent the specimen from leaking out. Balancing the tubes and locking the lid ensures laboratory safety and prevents breakage.

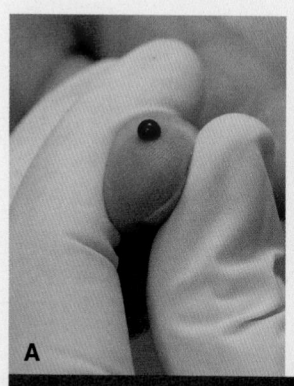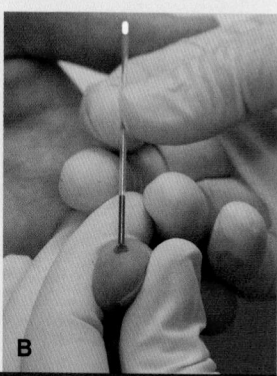

FIGURE 40-7 (A) Perform the capillary puncture, and wipe away the first drop with gauze (not shown). Allow the second drop of blood to form on the patient's finger. (B) Holding the microhematocrit tube horizontally, touch the end onto the top of the blood drop and let the tube fill by capillary action until it is approximately ¾ full.

11. ***Incorporating critical thinking skills when performing patient assessment and care***, assess the patient and apply a bandage strip to the puncture site. RATIONALE: The patient should not leave your care until the bleeding has stopped. Do not apply a fingertip bandage to an infant or young child because it could pose a choking hazard.

12. Allow the centrifuge to come to a complete stop before touching it. Remove the tubes. Using a reader or accompanying graph, determine the hematocrit level. Read and make a note of the test results as shown in Figure 40-10. RATIONALE: A spinning centrifuge is very dangerous and can cause a friction burn if touched. Making a note helps you retain the results until they can be charted in the patient's medical record.

13. Discard all contaminated equipment and supplies into appropriate biohazard waste receptacles. Disinfect the counter space and centrifuge according to manufacturer's instructions. RATIONALE: Using disinfectants not recommended by the manufacturer could harm the analyzer. Use sharps containers for sharp supplies and red biohazard bags for contaminated gauze and gloves.

14. Remove gloves and discard into biohazard container, and wash hands. RATIONALE: Washing hands removes residual contamination.

15. Document the procedure in the patient's medical record in the progress notes charting section and complete a lab report. Notify the provider of the results and file the lab report in the lab section of the patient's record. RATIONALE: Accurate and timely documentation are important in medical laboratory procedures.

DOCUMENTATION:

PROCEDURE NOTE

A ▾ A ▾ B *I* U

08/06/20XX Capillary puncture performed on patient's left middle finger for hematocrit determination. Specimen tested in our labs. Result: Hct reading is 38%. Dr. Rice notified of result and report filed. Patient tolerated the procedure well and Dr. Rice discussed results with her. Joe Guerrero, CMA (AAMA)

Courtesy of Harris CareTracker PM and EMR

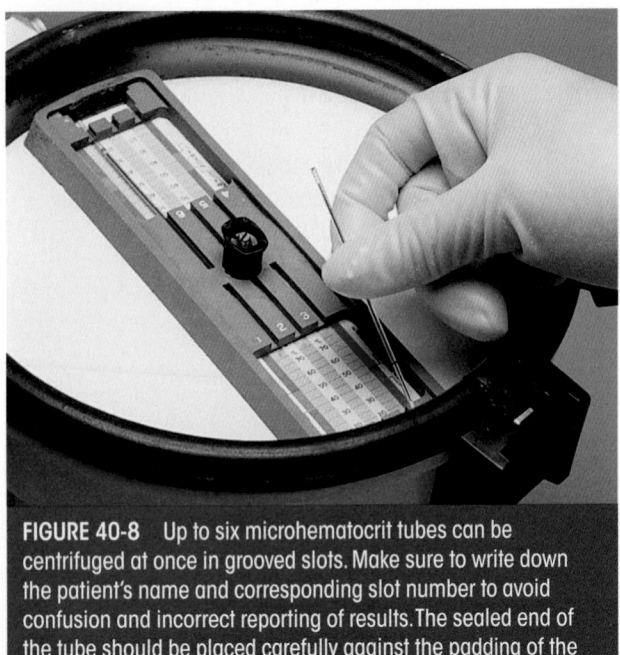

FIGURE 40-8 Up to six microhematocrit tubes can be centrifuged at once in grooved slots. Make sure to write down the patient's name and corresponding slot number to avoid confusion and incorrect reporting of results. The sealed end of the tube should be placed carefully against the padding of the centrifuge wall.

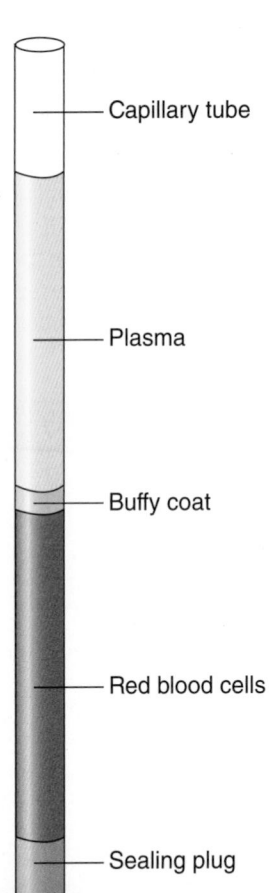

Capillary tube

Plasma

Buffy coat

Red blood cells

Sealing plug

FIGURE 40-9 Diagram of packed cell column in the hematocrit tube showing separation of cellular components after centrifugation.

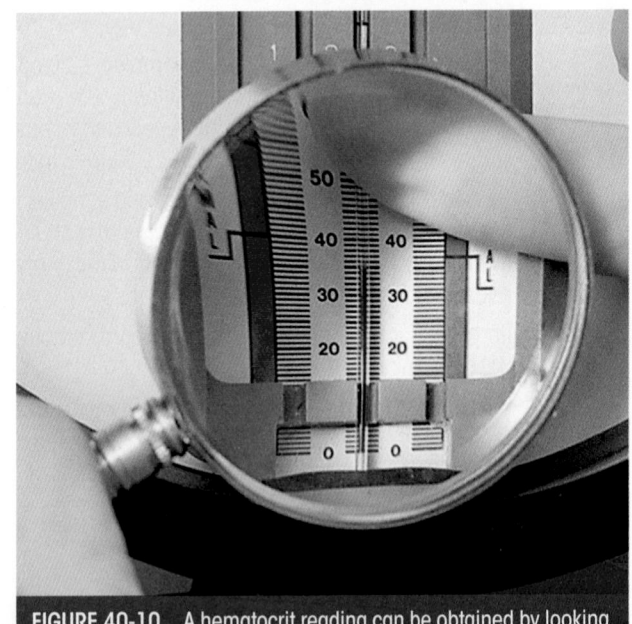

FIGURE 40-10 A hematocrit reading can be obtained by looking down onto the tube against the values chart within the centrifuge. The reading is obtained after centrifugation by placing the sealed end against the padding and reading the hematocrit at the bottom of the meniscus. The reading in the photo is 35 percent.

at high speeds in a microhematocrit centrifuge machine (Figure 40-8). The cellular layers arrange themselves with the RBCs at the bottom of the tube. RBCs are the most numerous and the heaviest of the cellular components. WBCs and platelets form a thin layer called the buffy coat on top of the erythrocytes. The buffy coat has a whitish tan appearance. The plasma often is so clear it is difficult to see (Figure 40-9).

The hematocrit is measured on a scale (Figure 40-10). Two tubes are measured and the amounts are then averaged. As an added benefit, the WBC count of the sample can be estimated by measuring the buffy coat thickness. Each 0.1 mm of the buffy coat equals approximately 1,000 WBC/mm^3. Therefore, a buffy coat of 1 mm would equal a leukocyte count of approximately 10,000 WBCs/mm^3, and a 0.5 mm reading would equal 5,000 WBCs/mm^3. The cell counts may be reported in units of microliters (mcL), which are equivalent to cubic millimeters. Keep in mind this WBC estimation is exactly that—an estimation. It is not considered reliably accurate, nor does it replace a WBC count.

The normal values of hematocrit vary according to the age and sex of the individual (Table 40-2).

Sources of error associated with the microhematocrit method include improper centrifugation, which results in increased trapped plasma,

TABLE 40-2

NORMAL HEMATOCRIT VALUES, OR REFERENCE RANGES, BY AGE AND/OR SEX

Newborn	45% to 60%
1-year-old child	27% to 44%
Adult female	36% to 46%
Adult male	40% to 55%

and improper reading of the packed RBC volume, such as including the buffy coat layer.

Procedure

Procedure 40-2 explains the microhematocrit method of determining blood hematocrit levels. Review the sections in Chapter 39 on capillary tubes and capillary draw, together with Procedure 39-6.

WHITE AND RED BLOOD CELL COUNTS

Professional

WBC and RBC counts can be performed using either a manual or an automated method. Because neither method is considered CLIA-waived, neither is within the scope of practice for the medical assistant. The Chapter Portal section discusses the functions of blood cells, and you will learn much more in your anatomy and physiology course. The formation of blood cells is shown in Figure 40-1. Because blood cell counts are not performed by medical assistants, this section does not discuss the test process itself but rather the diagnostic implications of the cell count with the differential and indices.

White Blood Cells and Differential

WBCs do not necessarily remain within the blood vessels like RBCs do. They leave the blood vessels and travel to the tissues of the body to find and destroy pathogens. When a "bacterial battle" is fought in an area and many WBCs have died,

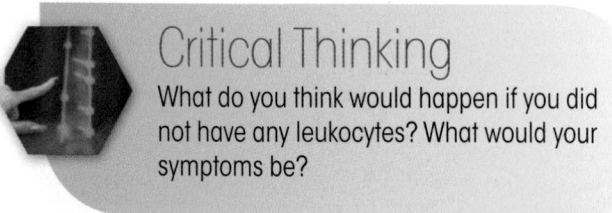

Critical Thinking
What do you think would happen if you did not have any leukocytes? What would your symptoms be?

the "battlefield" may be too large for the phagocytes to clean up. In these cases, pus can occur. A localized accumulation of pus is called an abscess and often must be incised (lanced) to aid in the removal of the pus. This procedure is called an incision and drainage. Antibiotics are useful in some cases to help the leukocytes fight off the bacteria and remove the infection. When leukocytes travel into the tissues, most of them do not return to the bloodstream. The **lymphocyte** is the only type that does; it travels to the lymphatic system, where it is specialized and matured (hence, the name lymphocyte), then returns to the bloodstream to await a mission. The normal values for WBCs vary with age. Babies need more, because they have not yet built up antibody protections (Table 40-3).

WBCs, or leukocytes, can be divided into two basic groups: granulocytes, which contain granules within their cytoplasm, and agranulocytes, which do not contain granules. The presence of granules can be visualized by the trained eye after a staining process during the manual WBC count. Even during the automated method, the leukocyte is identified by the contents of the cytoplasm and the shape of its nuclei. The granulocytes are the **neutrophils**, **basophils**, and **eosinophils** (notice they all end in *-phil,* which will help you remember their cytoplasm is "filled" with granules). The agranulocytes are the lymphocytes and the monocytes.

The nuclei of the different types of leukocytes differ from each other, as well as the cytoplasm. All three of the granulocytes contain nuclei that are multilobed or segmented (sometimes they are even called segs). They are described as being polymorphonuclear cells (*poly* means

TABLE 40-3

NORMAL LEUKOCYTE COUNTS

AGE	LEUKOCYTE COUNT (CELLS/MM³)	
	AVERAGE	REFERENCE RANGE
Newborn	18,000	9,000 to 30,000
1-year-old child	11,000	6,000 to 14,000
6-year-old child	8,000	4,500 to 12,000
Adult	7,000	4,500 to 11,000

"many," *morpho* means "shape," and *nuclear* means "nucleus"). The immature neutrophil has a nucleus that has not yet formed lobes and is called a band cell (or stab cell) because its nucleus looks sort of like a comma mark. The agranulocytes do not form lobed nuclei; their nuclei are rounded in a single mass. Because of their single nuclei, the agranulocytes are sometimes called mononuclear (meaning "one nucleus"). The "Leukocyte Function" Quick Reference Guide will help clarify the various leukocytes, their morphology, and their purposes.

Each of the five types of WBCs provides specialized protection. Some of their methods include phagocytosis, detoxification, inflammation, and immune response.

Phagocytosis is an engulfing process performed by all leukocytes, but especially the neutrophils and the monocytes. Once the bacteria or particles are engulfed, the material is destroyed by enzymes present in the leukocyte. Phagocytosis is vitally important as a means of protection; we would die if our leukocytes lost their ability to perform this process.

⋗ QUICK REFERENCE GUIDE

≫ LEUKOCYTE FUNCTION

Cell Type	Function
Granulocytes	
Neutrophils	Perform phagocytosis of bacteria and fungi
• Mature neutrophils are called segs	First responders in infections
• Immature neutrophils are called bands or stabs	
Eosinophils	Detoxify toxins and harmful substances
	Neutralize histamine
	Destroy parasitic worms

(continues)

Cell Type	Function
Granulocytes	
Basophils	Mediate inflammation, allergic/antigen response
	Release histamine to increase inflammation
Agranulocytes	
Monocytes	Perform phagocytosis to clean up
	Present pathogens to lymphocytes for antibody formation
Lymphocytes	Destroy viruses
B cells	Coordinate immune response
T cells	Make antibodies

Detoxification is a neutralizing process that is effective against poisons and other harmful substances. Eosinophils use detoxification to control allergic reactions and histamine production.

Inflammation is a general process that occurs as a sequence of events. Chapter 21 explains the inflammatory process in more detail. The leukocyte most actively involved in inflammation is the basophil, which releases histamine into injured tissue to increase inflammation (antihistamines work to reduce inflammation). Basophils also contain the anticoagulant heparin. The basophil synchronizes the entire inflammatory process; thus, the poison is rendered harmless, the offending agents are eliminated, and the area is cleaned up of all the necrotic tissue and is ready for repair.

Immune response is a series of complicated and involved specific antigen–antibody reactions. Simply stated, when a harmful substance enters the human body, the adaptive immune response provided by the lymphocyte destroys the harmful substance. A "memory" is created so that the next time the body is exposed, it recognizes the intruder and is better able to prevent the illness again. This is called immunity. Immunity can be permanent or temporary, passively acquired or actively acquired. Passively acquired immunity is gifted to us either in utero (congenital or natural) or through an injection (artificial). Actively acquired immunity requires us to actively fight off a disease, and because we actively take part in creating the immunity, it is usually permanent. Passively acquired immunities do not make us sick, but they usually do not last longer than 6 months.

Not only do the leukocytes fight off pathogens/toxins in a variety of ways, they also are fairly specific in the types of pathogens they do battle with (see Table 40-4). Neutrophils are the most numerous of all leukocytes and for good reason. They are there to destroy bacteria, which is our most common enemy. The second largest group is the lymphocytes, and they fight our second most common enemy: viruses. Lymphocytes are also involved in immune responses, which explains why we can have immunity to viruses and not to other substances or microbes. Basophils release histamine to increase inflammation in injured tissues. Inflammation usually is our friend, but sometimes the inflammation is too severe, which is what can happen in an allergic reaction. Eosinophils are especially well suited to battle the inflammation

accompanying allergic-type reactions because they neutralize the histamines. **Monocytes** can be likened to the "cleanup crew" because these "big eaters" come in later to clean up the battlefield of the cellular debris and other substances.

Red Blood Cells

RBCs (erythrocytes) are very different from WBCs in composition, function, and numbers (Table 40-5).

Remember that erythrocytes are responsible for carrying oxygen to the body's cells and bringing back the carbon dioxide. To have room to carry the oxygen and carbon dioxide molecules, the erythrocyte leaves its nucleus in the bone marrow where it is formed. The nucleus is used again and again to create other erythrocytes. Our bodies are efficient at recycling raw materials. If an erythrocyte is released from the bone marrow before it is mature, it may retain some of its nucleus material. It is then called a **reticulocyte (retic)** (see Figure 40-1). About 1% of the circulating erythrocytes are reticulocytes, and an increase in the number of circulating reticulocytes is an indication that the body needs more erythrocytes. This can occur in cases of hemorrhage and anemia. Erythrocytes can be of varying sizes. When erythrocytes are of normal size, they are called **normocytic**. Those that are larger are called **macrocytic**, and those that are smaller are called **microcytic**. When the erythrocytes show marked variation in size, the condition is called **anisocytosis**. The normal erythrocyte has a round or slightly oval shape. If the shape of the erythrocytes shows marked variation, the condition is known as poikilocytosis.

The RBC should contain hemoglobin that fills about half of the cell. The RBC is biconcave, so most of the hemoglobin is seen around the outer part of the cell. The central area of the RBC is

---

TABLE 40-4

NORMAL VALUES FOR A DIFFERENTIAL LEUKOCYTE COUNT IN ADULTS

Neutrophil bands: 3% to 5%
Neutrophil bands increase in appendicitis and many other diseases.

Neutrophil segs: 54% to 62%
Segmented neutrophils increase in appendicitis and many other diseases. An elevation in neutrophils usually is indicative of an infectious disease.

Lymphocytes: 25% to 33%
Lymphocytes increase with infectious mononucleosis, lymphocytic leukemia, and many diseases of viral origin.

Monocytes: 3% to 7%
Monocytes increase in tuberculosis and monocytic leukemia.

Eosinophils: 1% to 3%
Eosinophils increase with allergic reactions, hay fever, and parasitic infections.

Basophils: 0% to 1%
Basophils increase in polycythemia vera, chicken pox, and ulcerative colitis.

TABLE 40-5

NORMAL ERYTHROCYTE COUNTS

AGE	REFERENCE RANGE
Newborn	5.00 to 6.5 $\times$ 10^6/mm^3
1-year-old child	4.0 to 5.0 $\times$ 10^6/mm^3
Adult female	4.0 to 5.5 $\times$ 10^6/mm^3
Adult male	4.5 to 6.0 $\times$ 10^6/mm^3

pale. RBCs with the proper amount of hemoglobin are called **normochromic**. Those that do not have enough hemoglobin, that demonstrate too large of a pale central area, are called **hypochromic**.

Both WBCs and RBCs change in reaction to diseases. Table 40-6 lists a few examples of changes that might occur.

PLATELETS

The normal number of platelets (thrombocytes) is 150,000 to 450,000 per microliter of blood. If the platelet count is above 450,000, the patient is said to have **thrombocytosis**, and a count lower than 150,000 is known as **thrombocytopenia**. Low platelet counts are usually related to leukemia or certain drugs. High platelet counts can be from cancers, anemia, and many other conditions.

Thrombocytes are actually fragments of cells. Like mature erythrocytes, thrombocytes have no nuclei. Thrombocytes are involved in the clotting of blood, or coagulation. Coagulation is a complex series of events and contains 13 distinct steps. A brief overview is provided here. When the body is physically injured, chemicals are released. Included in these chemicals are thromboplastin from injured tissues and plasma proteins and factors released from platelets. These chemicals form prothrombin activator. Prothrombin activator (with calcium) converts (activates) a blood protein called prothrombin into thrombin. Thrombin converts another blood protein called fibrinogen into fibrin. Fibrin is stringy and traps the sticky blood cells in a web at the site of injury, forming a plug of sorts. Eventually, the plug starts drying up, shrinks (pulling the edges of a wound together), and forms a scab.

What is really fascinating about the clotting of blood is why blood does not normally clot inside the blood vessels. Two chemicals made in the human body prevent that from happening. One is heparin, which is released from basophils and endothelial cells, and the other is antithrombin, which is released by the liver. The body needs blood to clot to stop bleeding, but it is important that blood not clot inside the body, where it could cause problems and even death.

ERYTHROCYTE INDICES

The **erythrocyte indices** include the mean corpuscular (cell) volume (MCV), the mean corpuscular hemoglobin (MCH), and the mean corpuscular hemoglobin concentration (MCHC). These indices (plural for *index*) are calculations that provide information about the size of the RBCs and the hemoglobin content. The blood parameters needed to calculate all three indices are RBC count, hematocrit, and hemoglobin. The erythrocyte indices values are important in the diagnosis or classification and treatment of different types of anemia. Table 40-7 shows normal values for the erythrocyte indices.

Before the automated hematology instrument became commonly used in the ambulatory care setting, erythrocyte indices were not included as a part of the CBC because the RBC count was not an accurate measurement.

Understanding RBC Indices

If we think of the RBCs as water balloons filled with red-colored water, we might better understand the indices: The red-colored water signifies the hemoglobin inside the RBC. We have a basket of water balloons to signify our blood sample.

Because each water balloon is a different size (as are our RBCs), we would need to measure the size of all of them to get the average volume or mass. We would add together the size/mass of all the balloons in our basket, then divide that number by the number of balloons in the basket. This gives us the average (mean) mass (volume), or MCV.

TABLE 40-6

EXAMPLES OF BLOOD CELL CHANGES IN DISEASED STATES

DISEASED STATES	BLOOD CELL CHANGES
Acute appendicitis	WBC numbers increases rapidly Higher percentage of neutrophils Increase in bands (stabs)
Viral infections	Often reduction in WBCs Higher percentage of lymphocytes Infectious mononucleosis shows increased atypical lymphocytes
Iron deficiency anemia	RBCs with less hemoglobin content, hypochromic

TABLE 40-7

NORMAL VALUES FOR THE ERYTHROCYTE INDICES

MCV	80 to 100 femoliter
MCH	27 to 33 picograms/cell
MCHC	32 to 36 grams/deciliter

MCH is the average amount of water in the balloons. To measure this, we would pop each balloon, measure the total amount of water, and then divide by how many balloons there were. This would give us the average (mean) amount of red water (hemoglobin), or MCH.

Using the same water balloon comparison for explaining MCHC, it would be the intensity of the red water within all the balloons. Some of the balloons might contain light red water, some might contain dark red water. The average of the intensity would give us the average (mean) intensity (concentration), or MCHC.

All of these numbers together tell us about how many RBCs there are in the sample, their average size (volume), how much they contain (amount hemoglobin), and the average concentration/intensity of the hemoglobin within all of them.

Understanding the relationship between MCV, MCH, and MCHC helps us better understand what is happening when a patient is anemic due to low hemoglobin within each RBC versus a patient who is anemic due to low RBC count and so forth.

Using Erythrocyte Indices to Diagnose

MCH and MCV can be increased in various types of anemias, hypothyroidism, and liver disease. MCH and MCV can be decreased in some anemias and occasionally in hyperthyroidism.

MCHC is increased in hereditary spherocytosis. It is normal in macrocytosis. MCHC is decreased in iron deficiency anemia. The stained blood smear of a person with iron deficiency anemia demonstrates RBCs that are both hypochromic and microcytic.

ERYTHROCYTE SEDIMENTATION RATES (ESR OR SED RATE)

Procedure

The **erythrocyte sedimentation rate (ESR)**, as the name implies, is a measurement of the rate at which the RBCs in a well-mixed, anticoagulated blood sample will fall, or settle, toward the bottom when it is placed in a vertical tube. This test is commonly referred to in the laboratory as a sed rate (see Procedure 40-3). The ESR has been used for many years in the diagnosis and treatment of many disease states of the body, especially systemic inflammation. It is an inexpensive, accurate, and easy test to perform. Two factors that influence the sedimentation rate are the condition of the surface membrane of the RBC and changes in the level of fibrinogen in the plasma of the blood. During disease conditions in the body, the surface membrane of the RBC is altered, as are the levels of fibrinogen, and this affects the rate at which the RBCs fall in the tube. RBCs will demonstrate this change even after the disease has subsided because RBCs have an average life of 120 days. For this reason, the ESR is a more accurate tool in diagnosing the onset of a disease than in checking the progress of treatment.

There is a commercial rapid ESR test available that uses centrifugation with results in 4 minutes. Two traditional manual methods of performing the ESR test are the Wintrobe method and the Westergren method. All of these methods will provide the same information, but the manual methods take at least an hour after the tubes are set up.

The erythrocytes in normal, nondiseased blood tend to remain suspended in the plasma. They do not aggregate (clump) together to form rouleaux. **Rouleaux** are a phenomenon whereby RBCs form aggregates that look like rolls or stacks of coins (Figure 40-11).

This aggregate form causes the rate of sedimentation to increase. RBCs have membrane properties

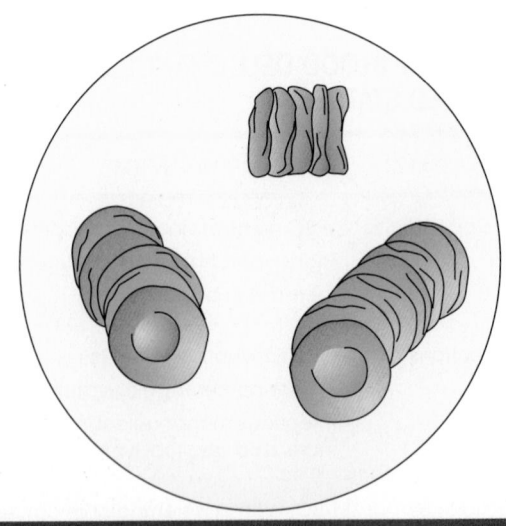

FIGURE 40-11 Erythrocytes forming rouleaux.

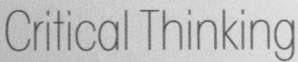

Critical Thinking

The stained blood smear of a person with iron deficiency anemia demonstrates RBCs that are both hypochromic and microcytic. Can you explain why?

PROCEDURE 40-3

Procedure

Erythrocyte Sedimentation Rate

STANDARD PRECAUTIONS:

Handwashing   Gloves   Goggles & Mask   Gown   No Needle Recapping   Biohazard

PURPOSE:

To properly and safely examine a blood sample by using either the Sediplast (Westergren) or Wintrobe method to determine the ESR.

EQUIPMENT/SUPPLIES:

- Gloves
- Sample of venous blood collected in EDTA
- Sediplast kit (or other ESR kit)
    - Sedivial containing 0.2 mL sodium citrate
    - Sediplast autozeroing pipette
    - Sediplast rack
- Wintrobe method:
    - Wintrobe sedimentation tube (disposable or reusable)
    - Wintrobe sedimentation rack
    - Long-stem Pasteur-type pipette with rubber bulb
- Timer
- Disinfectant
- Biohazard disposal container
- Acrylic face shield or goggles and mask
- Sharps container

NOTE: Consult the manufacturer's package insert for specific instructions for the ESR kit being used.

PROCEDURE STEPS:

1. Wash hands and put on gloves.
2. Assemble equipment and materials.
3. Gently mix the EDTA tube of blood for 2 minutes.
4. Perform either method a (Sediplast ESR) or method b (Wintrobe):
    a. Sediplast ESR (modified Westergren) method:
        (1) Remove stopper on sedivial and fill to the indicated one milliliter mark with 0.8 mL blood. Replace stopper and invert vial several times to mix (or mix using pipette).
        (2) Place sedivial in Sediplast rack on a level surface.
        (3) Gently insert the disposable Sediplast pipette through the pierceable stopper with a twisting motion and push down until the pipette rests on the bottom of the vial. The pipette will autozero the blood and any excess will flow into the sealed reservoir compartment.

(continues)

(4) Set timer for 1 hour.

(5) Return blood sample to proper storage. (If no laboratory work will be performed during the incubation, remove gloves, discard appropriately, and wash hands. Reapply gloves before handling test materials.)

(6) Let the pipette stand undisturbed for exactly 1 hour, and then read the results of the ESR: Use the scale on the tube to measure the distance from the top of the plasma to the top of the RBCs.

(7) Record the sedimentation rate: ESR 1 hr = ___ mm.

(8) Dispose of tube and vial in appropriate biohazard container.

   b. Wintrobe method:

(1) Place tube in Wintrobe sedimentation rack.

(2) Check the leveling bubble to ensure that the Wintrobe rack is level.

(3) Fill Wintrobe tube to the zero mark with well-mixed blood using the Pasteur pipette and being careful not to over fill. **NOTE:** Tube must be filled from the bottom to avoid getting air bubbles in the tube.

(4) Follow steps 4 through 8 as stated above in the Westergren method. Clean work area with surface disinfectant.

5. Remove gloves and discard in biohazard container.

6. Wash hands.

7. Document the procedure in the patient's medical record in the progress notes charting section and complete a lab report. Notify the provider of the results and then file the lab report in the lab section of the patient record. RATIONALE: Accurate and timely documentation are important in medical laboratory procedures.

DOCUMENTATION:

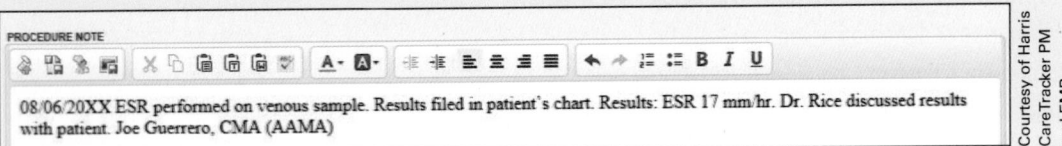

PROCEDURE NOTE

08/06/20XX ESR performed on venous sample. Results filed in patient's chart. Results: ESR 17 mm/hr. Dr. Rice discussed results with patient. Joe Guerrero, CMA (AAMA)

Courtesy of Harris CareTracker PM and EMR

---

that tend to make them remain separated in the plasma. During certain disease states, this repelling property is lost and the RBCs tend to aggregate.

Wintrobe and Westergren Methods

A well-mixed EDTA venous blood sample is transferred to a Wintrobe tube. The blood is added to the left zero mark at the top of the tube. After the tube stands for exactly an hour in an exact vertical position, the test is read by determining the number of millimeters (mm) the red cells have settled. The tube has a total capacity of 100 mm. The test is reported in millimeters per hour (Figure 40-12). Table 40-8 lists normal values for the Wintrobe method of ESR. Table 40-9 lists normal values for the Westergren method of ESR.

Using the ESR to Screen

ESRs are increased in infections, acute stress, inflammatory diseases, tissue destruction, and other conditions that lead to an increase in plasma fibrinogen. They are also increased with menstruation, pregnancy, lupus, malignant neoplasms, and multiple myeloma. With anemia, the ESR increases according to the severity of the condition.

The ESR may be normal in osteoarthritis and in some cases of cirrhosis and malaria. ESR values are decreased in polycythemia, spherocytosis, and sickle cell anemia.

C-REACTIVE PROTEINS

Another screening blood test for inflammation is **C-reactive protein (CRP)**. The CRP level will rise and drop more quickly than the ESR, giving the

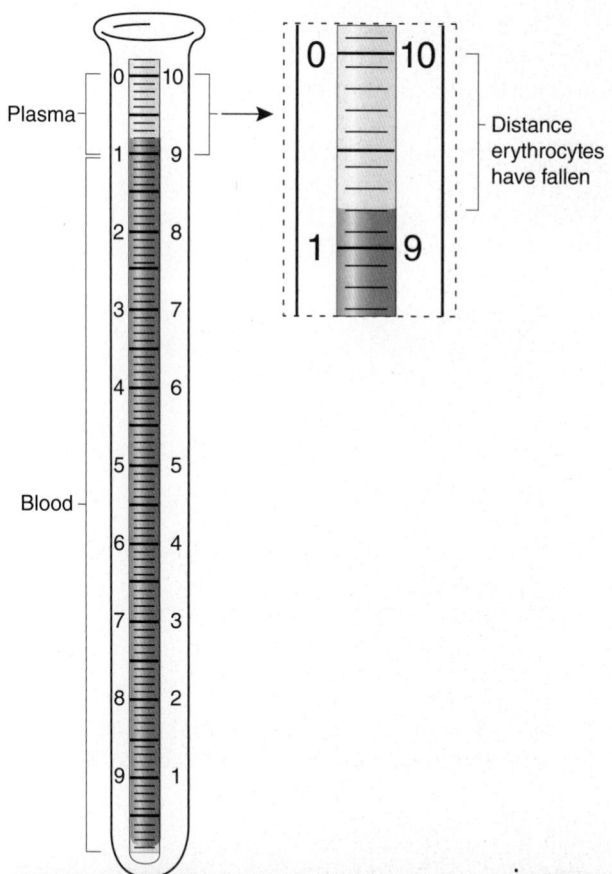

FIGURE 40-12 Wintrobe sedimentation tube showing settling of cells. The example shows a sedimentation of 8 mm.

provider more timely information about the effectiveness of treatment. The CRP is not affected by as many other factors as the ESR, making it a better inflammation indicator than the ESR.

Like the ESR, CRP is helpful in determining systemic inflammatory conditions such as autoimmune diseases, inflammatory bowel conditions, and some forms of arthritis. While it is not specifically diagnostic for any one disease, it can serve as a marker for general infection and inflammation, and, once the disease or condition is diagnosed, it can help determine the effectiveness of treatment.

CRP is made by the liver and released into the bloodstream. It increases when infection and

TABLE 40-8

NORMAL VALUES FOR THE WINTROBE METHOD OF ESR

Male patients	0 to 9 mm/hr
Female patients	0 to 20 mm/hr

TABLE 40-9

NORMAL VALUES FOR THE WESTERGREN METHOD OF ESR

Male patients younger than 50 years	0 to 15 mm/hr
Male patients older than 50 years	0 to 20 mm/hr
Female patients younger than 50 years	0 to 20 mm/hr
Female patients older than 50 years	0 to 30 mm/hr

inflammation are present. It has been used for many years as an indicator of serious bacterial infections.

Due to more recent studies showing the correlation between vascular inflammation and heart disease, a more sensitive CRP-related test called hsCRP (highly sensitive C-reactive protein) has gained popularity in detecting vascular inflammation that can indicate coronary artery disease and cardiovascular disease. hsCRP is used in conjunction with the traditional lipid profile and cardiac risk assessment.

COAGULATION STUDIES (INR AND PROTIME)

Persons prone to forming blood clots often are medicated with anticoagulants (blood thinners) such as Coumadin (warfarin), Pradaxa (diabigatran), Eliquis (apixaban), or Xarelto (rivaroxaban). Patients on Coumadin (warfarin) are monitored regularly to ensure that their blood can clot within a reasonable amount of time, which ensures that the patient is taking the correct dosage of the blood thinning medication. The method of monitoring coagulation time is called prothrombin time (PT) or, more commonly, **protime**. Protime is reported as the time (seconds) it takes for the patient's blood to clot and as the international normalized ratio (INR). We still refer to both tests as protime. Currently, the INR is more useful because it is standardized, that is, it can be universally applied, which is in contrast to the timing test, which can vary quite a bit from facility to facility. Normal blood will clot in about 11 to 13 seconds. The provider will want the patient taking anticoagulant medication to have a protime of approximately 16 to 18 seconds and INR of 2.0 to 2.6 (sometimes higher). If blood clots too soon, the anticoagulant medication is not at a therapeutic level.

If blood clotting takes too long (prolonged clotting), then the patient is taking too much medication. An INR of 1.0 is considered ineffective; 5.0 is considered dangerous.

Because activities of daily living, such as eating particular foods, drinking alcohol, fluctuations in body fluids (from diarrhea or vomiting or dehydration), and taking vitamins or supplements can interfere with clotting factors, protime usually is tested on a regular basis (weekly at the beginning of treatment, then monthly or less frequently as treatment progresses). If the patient experiences frequent abnormal or unexplained bruising or bleeding that might indicate an imbalance in clotting ability, then the protime test can be run "on demand." Some foods rich in vitamin K (e.g., dark leafy vegetables), alcohol, vitamins and supplements, aspirin, and many other medications can interfere with anticoagulant therapy. Health care professionals must interview the patient carefully about what is being ingested. Patient education and compliance are important components of effective treatment with anticoagulants.

The protime test is also used as a screening test for people who have liver disease, have clotting factor disease, or are vitamin K deficient.

Procedure

Protime is a simple CLIA-waived test that is performed on a drop of blood (Figure 40-13) using a POCT Protime analyzer. Procedure 40-4 describes the step-by-step process.

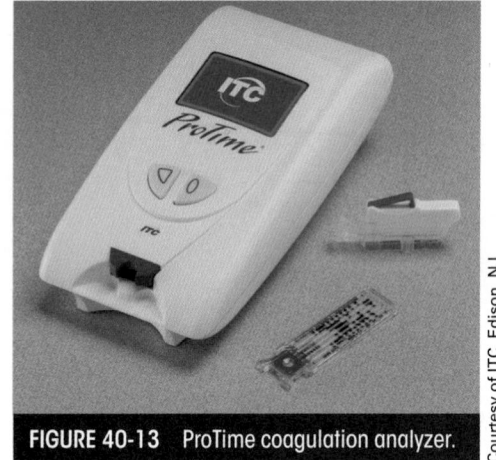

FIGURE 40-13 ProTime coagulation analyzer.

Courtesy of ITC, Edison, NJ

PROCEDURE 40-4

Procedure

Prothrombin Time (Using CLIA-Waived ProTime Analyzer)

STANDARD PRECAUTIONS:

  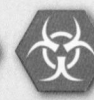

Handwashing   Gloves   Biohazard

PURPOSE:

To properly and safely perform an automated prothrombin time determination to evaluate the clotting time of a drop of blood.

EQUIPMENT/SUPPLIES:

- Gloves
- Biohazard container
- Sharps container
- Capillary puncture equipment
  - 70% isopropyl alcohol
  - Tenderlett lancet
  - 2 × 2 gauze
  - Adhesive bandage
- CLIA-Waived ProTime Analyzer with accessories

(continues)

PROCEDURE STEPS:

1. Assemble and organize equipment and supplies. Check expiration dates. RATIONALE: Being organized helps the process go more smoothly and professionally.

2. Wash hands and put on gloves. RATIONALE: Hand washing and gloving protects the patient and you.

3. Turn on the ProTime analyzer and follow the prompts. Insert the test cuvette into the analyzer. RATIONALE: Turn on the analyzer to warm up the machine; calibrate to maintain quality controls.

4. Introduce yourself by name and credential, identify the patient, and recheck the provider's orders. RATIONALE: Introducing yourself and stating your credentials demonstrates professionalism and helps to reassure the patient. Identifying the patient and rechecking the provider's orders will ensure the proper tests will be performed on the right patient.

5. ***Explain the rationale for performance of the procedure to the patient, showing awareness of the patient's concerns.*** Allay the patient's fears regarding the procedure to help him or her feel safe and comfortable. RATIONALE: Explaining the procedure and allaying the patient's fears will assure the patient that you are concerned about any apprehension he or she may have and that you are open to discussing the patient's concerns.

6. Select the site, prepare the site, and perform the capillary puncture using the Tenderlett lancet. Remember to use gauze to wipe away the first drop. RATIONALE: The Tenderlett lancet contains the reservoir required for use with the ProTime-3.

7. Fill the Tenderlett lancet cup to the fill line and then place it onto the cuvette, which was placed into the machine in step 3. Be sure it is snapped into place. Press the start button. RATIONALE: The Tenderlett cup is calibrated for the analyzer and must be properly placed for the test to run correctly.

8. Apply a gauze compress and ask the patient to hold pressure for 3 to 5 minutes. RATIONALE: A patient having this test performed usually has a delayed clotting time. Assess that the bleeding has stopped and apply bandage. RATIONALE: A patient should never leave your care until the bleeding has stopped.

9. Stay by the analyzer and await a prompt to remove the Tenderlett lancet device. When prompted, immediately remove the device and discard it into a nearby sharps container. RATIONALE: The device must be removed as soon as the clot has formed. This must be done very quickly, within seconds. The Tenderlett device contains a lancet and must be discarded into a sharps container.

10. Read the clotting time in seconds and the INR. Record the results. RATIONALE: Results should be recorded as soon as possible to decrease the chance of error.

11. Notify the provider immediately if the results fall within a critical range. RATIONALE: If the patient has a seriously delayed clotting time, the risk of a serious event occurring (such as a stroke) is greater. The provider must be notified immediately in order to adjust the anticoagulant dosage and/or prescribe other treatment.

12. Disinfect the analyzer according to the manufacturer's instructions, discard all contaminated equipment and supplies into appropriate biohazard waste receptacles, and disinfect the counter space. Remove gloves and wash hands. RATIONALE: Using disinfectants not recommended by the manufacturer could harm the analyzer. Use sharps containers for sharp supplies and red biohazard bags for contaminated gauze and gloves. Washing hands removes residual contamination.

13. Document the procedure in the patient's medical record in the progress notes charting section and complete a lab report. File the lab report in the lab section of the patient's record. RATIONALE: Accurate and timely documentation are important in medical laboratory procedures.

DOCUMENTATION:

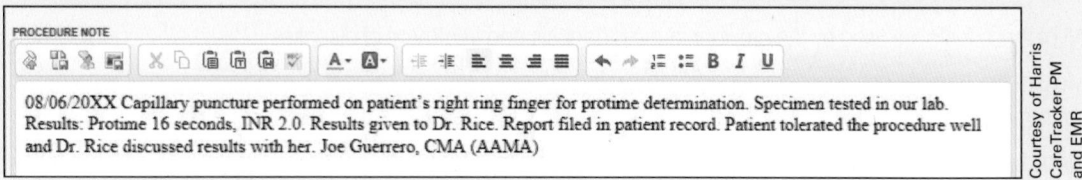

08/06/20XX Capillary puncture performed on patient's right ring finger for protime determination. Specimen tested in our lab. Results: Protime 16 seconds, INR 2.0. Results given to Dr. Rice. Report filed in patient record. Patient tolerated the procedure well and Dr. Rice discussed results with her. Joe Guerrero, CMA (AAMA)

Courtesy of Harris CareTracker PM and EMR

AUTOMATED HEMATOLOGY

Professional

Use of the larger, more sophisticated automated or semiautomated hematology instruments is not categorized as waived testing under CLIA and therefore is not within the medical assistant's scope of practice without further education and training. CLIA has allowed many specific analyzers into the waived category, such as the hemoglobin and protime analyzers. All procedures performed with automated instrumentation are modifications of manual methods. Automated hematology procedures have many advantages over the manual methods. They are faster, less expensive, simple to operate, and accurate. The instruments can be calibrated and lend themselves to control testing. Any laboratory test previously performed manually is now able to be performed using automated devices. Most are equipped with printers that produce hard copy results. Many can store quality-control results and print out quality-control data summary sheets, and they may be able to translate results directly into the patient's EHR.

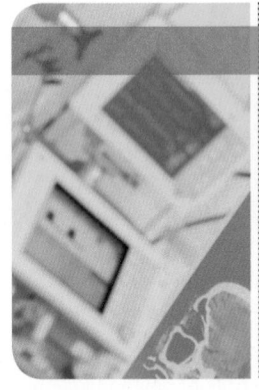

CASE STUDY 40-1

Refer to the scenario at the beginning of the chapter.

CASE STUDY REVIEW

1. What should Gwen do if the clinic buys a new machine for laboratory analysis that she is not familiar with?
2. How can Gwen be sure that she is using the laboratory analyzers properly and that the patient test results are accurate?
3. Who should Gwen consult if she has questions about how to perform a test using an analyzer?

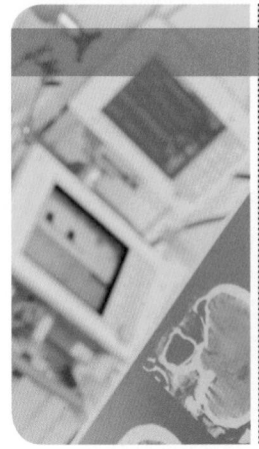

CASE STUDY 40-2

Today is busier than usual at Inner City Health Care. While she is performing an ESR for Jim Marshal, a patient in his late 30s, medical assistant Gwen Carr, CMA (AAMA), is called by Dr. King to help with another patient. She hurriedly places the sedimentation rack on top of an incubator in the sunlight by an open window and leaves to assist Dr. King.

CASE STUDY REVIEW

1. Critique Gwen Carr's technique, including how Gwen can use the attributes of professionalism to improve.
2. Is there another option Gwen has for running the ESR test during a very busy day?
3. How do you think the test results will differ from accurately run ESR tests?

Summary

- Hematology tests are the second most frequently performed tests in the ambulatory care setting.
- Medical assistants must have a knowledge of hematology to accurately and efficiently perform the tests.
- The study of hematology includes hematopoiesis, which is the formation of the blood elements, as well as the hematologic tests and their relation to the pathology of the body.
- This chapter introduced the more common hematologic tests that are performed in the ambulatory care setting, including all the parts of the CBC, the ESR methods, and the erythrocyte indices.
- All of these tests are used by the provider in the diagnosis and treatment of disease.
- Most of the hematology procedures performed in today's ambulatory care setting use some type of automated instrumentation.
- Blood specimens used in the sampling of hematologic procedures are biohazardous material. Be sure to follow Universal and Standard Precautions when you work with these specimens.

CERTIFICATION REVIEW

1. Which of the following is not a cellular component of blood?
   a. Erythrocytes
   b. Leukocytes
   c. Thrombocytes
   d. Erythropoietin
2. The formation of blood cells is defined as which of the following?
   a. Erythropoietin
   b. Hematopoiesis
   c. Mean corpuscular volume
   d. Hemoglobinopathy
   e. Erythrocytosis
3. Sickle cell anemia, a hereditary disease, has which type of hemoglobin?
   a. Hemoglobin S
   b. Hemoglobin A
   c. Hemoglobin E
   d. Hemoglobin C
4. The volume of packed red cells compared with the total volume of the sample is calculated for which test?
   a. Hematocrit
   b. Hemoglobin
   c. MCH
   d. MCV
   e. Sed rate
5. Which of the following is the most common white cell type found in the granulocytic series?
   a. Lymphocyte
   b. Monocyte
   c. Neutrophil
   d. Basophil
6. Erythrocyte indices are used for the diagnosis, classification, and treatment of which conditions?
   a. Infections
   b. Anemias
   c. Inflammatory diseases
   d. Neoplasms
   e. Leukemias

7. Which hematologic test result shows an increase with infections, inflammatory disease, acute stress, and tissue destruction?
   a. Hemoglobin
   b. MCV
   c. Hematocrit
   d. ESR
8. What is the most frequent hemoglobin disease seen in the ambulatory care setting?
   a. Iron deficiency anemia
   b. Sickle cell anemia
   c. Leukemia
   d. Anisocytosis
   e. Hypochromia
9. Which test within a CBC is within the scope of practice of a medical assistant under CLIA's waived test category?
   a. Using a HemoCue to determine a hemoglobin level
   b. Using a hemacytometer to count WBCs manually
   c. Using the Unopette system to count RBCs manually
   d. Using an automated blood analyzer that requires calculations and mixing of reagents
10. The highly sensitive C-reactive protein (hsCRP) test is used for detecting what?
    a. Any type of protein in the blood
    b. Vascular inflammation
    c. Very specific diseases such as lupus
    d. Anemia and leukemia
    e. Heart disease

Urinalysis

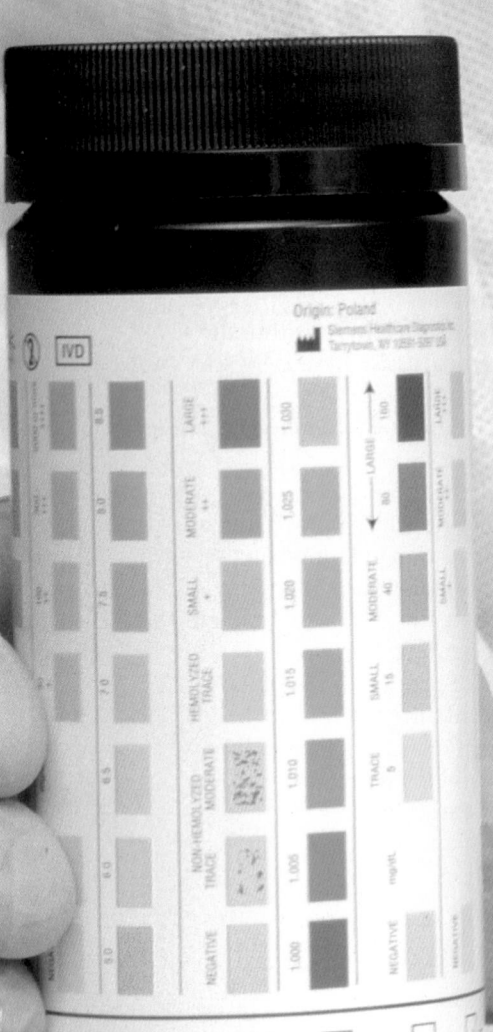

1. Define and spell the key terms as presented in the glossary.
2. Display sensitivity to the patient's rights and feelings in collecting specimens.
3. Explain the rationale for performing a proper clean catch collection to a patient.
4. Explain the process of urine formation.
5. Discuss the importance of safety procedures and quality control when working with urine.
6. Describe the importance of proper collection and preservation of 24-hour urine specimens.
7. Describe the medical assistant's scope of practice regarding performance of a urinalysis.
8. Perform the physical examination of urine.
9. Perform the chemical examination of urine.
10. Identify the proper method of preparing urine sediment for microscopic examination.
11. Identify normal and abnormal structures found during the microscopic examination of urine sediment.

KEY TERMS

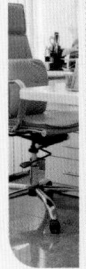

acid–base balance	hematuria	refractometer
amorphous	hemoglobinuria	sediment
bilirubin	ketoacidosis	specific gravity
bilirubinuria	ketones	supernatant
casts	ketonuria	turbid
chain of custody	ketosis	urea
circadian rhythm	midstream	urinary tract infection (UTI)
creatinine	pH	urobilinogen
crystals	quantitative tests	
glucosuria	reagents	

SCENARIO

At Inner City Health Care, clinical medical assistant Gwen Carr, CMA (AAMA), performs many urinalyses. Although urinalysis is a routine procedure, Wanda recognizes its importance as a diagnostic tool, and she performs each test carefully to ensure accurate results. Gwen takes time to instruct patients in the proper collection procedures. She encourages patients to ask questions before collecting the urine sample, and she provides written instructions for easy reference. When she performs the urinalysis, Gwen follows safety and quality control guidelines. By paying attention to the details of the procedure, Gwen does her best to ensure the quality of the urinalysis results.

Chapter Portal

Examination of the urine (urinalysis) has been performed for centuries by medical practitioners as a diagnostic tool for many diseases. Urinalysis refers to the study of urine as an aid in diagnosis or to follow the course of disease. The urine examination is a routine part of most physical examinations.

The routine urinalysis is one of the most frequently performed procedures in the medical office laboratory. Many tests can be performed on one urine sample. This procedure is often ordered

continues

because urine is easily obtained, and much information about the body's metabolism may be gained from the results of this testing. Results can indicate a systemic disease process or renal (kidney) or urinary tract disease.

Practice, experience, and attention to detail are the most important tools in achieving quality results. Following Standard Precautions when working with any body fluid is mandatory.

URINE FORMATION

Before discussing the analysis of urine, it is helpful to understand how urine is formed in the human body. Formation and excretion of urine is the principal way the body excretes water and gets rid of waste. These waste products, if not removed, can rapidly become toxic.

The kidneys are highly specialized organs that eliminates soluble (dissolved in water) waste products of metabolism. There are two kidneys, one on each side of the body. They are about 11 to 12 cm long and 5 to 6 cm wide. The kidneys are shaped like two lima beans with their concave border directed toward the midline of the body. The left kidney is slightly higher than the right (Figure 41-1).

Urine is formed in the kidneys and is excreted from the body by way of the urinary tract system. The kidneys also regulates the fluid outside the cells of the body by eliminating certain fluids and returning other fluids, maintaining a careful balance (homeostasis). In this manner, the body is protected from dramatic changes in fluid volume, acidity and alkalinity (**acid–base balance**), composition, and pressure. The formation of urine is accomplished through three specific processes: filtration, reabsorption, and secretion.

Filtration

The kidneys filters waste products, salts, and excess fluid from the blood. The filtering unit of the kidney is called the glomerulus. The part of the kidney that concentrates the filtered material is called the tubule. Together, the glomerulus and the tubule combine to form the nephron (Figure 41-2).

Most of the work of the kidneys is done by the nephrons. There are approximately one million nephrons in each kidney. Each minute,

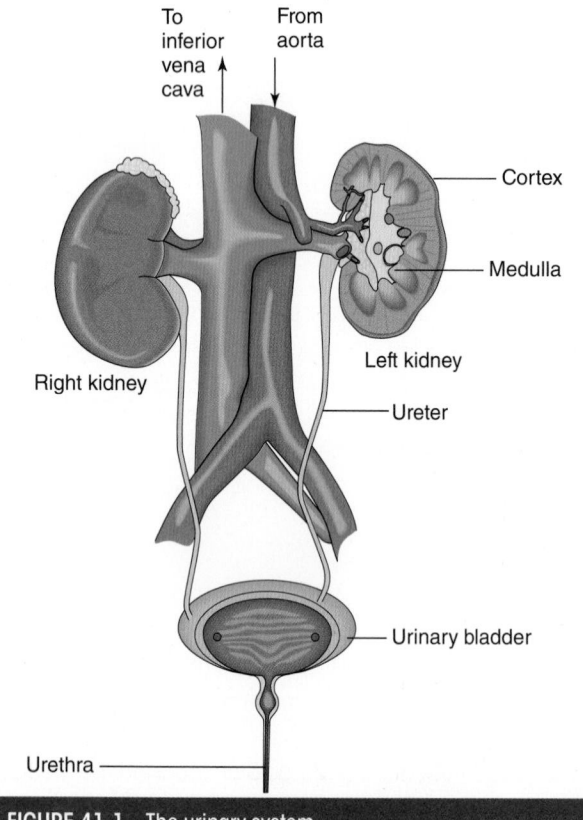

FIGURE 41-1 The urinary system.

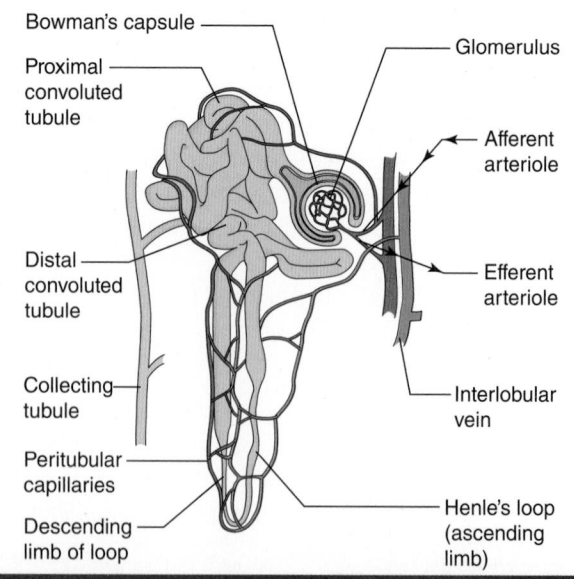

FIGURE 41-2 Parts of the nephron, including the glomerulus.

more than 1,000 mL of blood flows through the kidneys to be cleansed. In the glomerulus, certain substances are filtered out of the blood. The remaining filtrate then passes into the tubule, where various changes occur. Substances filtered out from the body can include water, ammonia, electrolytes, glucose, amino acids, **creatinine**, and **urea**. These wastes leave the body in the eliminated urine.

For example, when people with diabetes have excess glucose in their blood, the body attempts to eliminate the excess glucose through the urine. Routine urinalysis testing will reveal the excess glucose, alerting the provider to the presence of too much glucose. In this manner, diabetes can be investigated; such a result can also be an indication that a patient with diabetes is not taking enough insulin to control the glucose in the blood.

Reabsorption

While passing through the kidneys, some substances may need to be reabsorbed by the blood. Approximately 180 liters of filtrate is produced daily by the body, but only 1 to 2 liters of urine is eliminated from the normally functioning human body. Therefore, much of the filtrate, including water, sodium, chloride, potassium, bicarbonate, glucose, calcium, and amino acids, is reabsorbed into the body.

Under normal conditions, blood cells and most proteins stay in the blood plasma because they are too large to pass through the walls of the capillaries of the glomerulus. If blood cells and excess protein are found in the urine, the provider is alerted that the kidneys are not filtering properly due to an irregular condition affecting the urinary tract.

As long as the concentration of glucose in the blood is less than 180 mg/dL (milligrams per deciliter), the glucose will be completely reabsorbed. If the level increases to more than 180 mg/dL, the glucose is not reabsorbed. Substances such as glucose that are reabsorbed in relation to their concentration in the blood are known as threshold substances. Homeostasis usually requires glucose and protein to be almost completely reabsorbed, whereas other threshold substances such as creatinine, amino acids, potassium, sodium, and chloride are only partially reabsorbed.

Secretion

Near the end of the blood's journey through the kidneys, specifically in the distal convoluted tubule, other substances that have not already been filtered are secreted into the urine. Such substances as hydrogen and ammonium ions may be secreted into the urine in exchange for sodium. Certain drugs in the blood at this point may also be secreted into the urine.

URINE COMPOSITION

After urine progresses through a healthy kidney, it is approximately 96% water and 4% dissolved substances, most of which come from either dietary intake or metabolic waste products. These substances are primarily urea, salt, sulfates, and phosphates. Abnormal constituents of urine include red and white blood cells, fat, glucose, casts, bile, acetone, and hemoglobin (Table 41-1).

When certain disease processes occur in the human body, the following changes in urine production and composition can occur:

- The amount of urine excreted can increase or decrease.
- Urine color can change.
- Urine appearance can vary.
- Urine odor can change.
- Cells can be present in urine.
- Chemical constituents in urine can change.
- Urine concentration (specific gravity) may vary.

TABLE 41-1

NORMAL AND ABNORMAL SUBSTANCES IN URINE

NORMAL	ABNORMAL
Urea	Bile
Uric acid	Blood
Creatinine	Fat
Sodium	Glucose
Potassium	Protein
Ammonium	White blood cells
Sulfate	Urobilinogen
Chloride	Microorganisms (bacteria, parasites)

SAFETY

Safety

The federal government has set up guidelines to ensure the safety of everyone working in the health care field and for the protection of our environment. These guidelines are now referred to as OSHA's Standard Precautions. Other terms used to describe care when handling infectious materials are Transmission-Based Precautions and biohazard precautions. OSHA's Chemical Hygiene Plan covers safety precautions when using chemical in the medical laboratory (see Chapter 37).

Some precautions to use when handling urine specimens include:

- Treat all specimens as if they were infectious, handling them with gloved hands.

- Avoid splashes or creation of aerosols when handling or disposing of urine specimens. Wearing face shields will prevent splashes from getting into the eyes, nose, or mouth.

- Store urine specimens appropriately in a designated refrigerator that contains no food or drink items.
- Dispose of urine appropriately, possibly in a designated sink (run water to wash the specimen into the drain) or toilet.

QUALITY CONTROL

As in every area of the laboratory, every effort must be made by health care professionals to produce test results free from error. Regulatory agencies depend on facilities that perform laboratory tests such as urinalysis to maintain standards that will ensure reliable results. Quality control (QC) programs are an important part of urine testing to ensure accurate and reliable result and they must be incorporated into every urine testing procedure. Because many of the tests are interpreted by visual examination, the QC procedures are dependent on the expertise of the person performing the examination. See the "Quality Control Guidelines" Quick Reference Guide for more information on the general QC procedures that should be followed.

⧉ QUICK REFERENCE GUIDE

Quality Control Guidelines

- ☐ Check expiration date of all **reagents** (test chemicals) used in testing.
- ☐ Follow manufacturer's guidelines for storage of reagents and testing supplies.
- ☐ Test urine as soon as possible, not letting it cool.
- ☐ Take care to not contaminate testing supplies and reagent strips.
- ☐ Use correct amounts of urine when testing.
- ☐ Use correct timing when testing chemical constituents of urine.
- ☐ Test positive and negative control samples exactly as you test patient samples.
- ☐ Maintain equipment and machinery and ensure correct calibration.
- ☐ Keep records of QC measures.

CLINICAL LABORATORY IMPROVEMENT AMENDMENTS (CLIA)

Legal

The regulations under CLIA are discussed in Chapter 37. Several CLIA regulations apply to the medical assistant performing urine testing. They include:

- Appropriate training in the methodology of the test being performed
- Understanding of urine-testing QC procedures
- Proficiency in the use of instrumentation; being able to troubleshoot problems
- Knowledge of the stability and proper storage of reagents (substances involved in urine testing)
- Awareness of factors that influence test results
- Knowledge of how to verify test results

The microscopic examination of urine is designated by CLIA to be a PPMP (provider-performed microscopy procedure) and therefore must be performed by a provider. The medical assistant is trained and able to prepare the slide for viewing and reading by the provider. The medical assistant should always take the opportunity to view the slide and discuss the finding with the provider as part of professional development and continued education.

URINE CONTAINERS

The first step toward achieving proper results during laboratory testing is proper collection of the specimen to be tested. There are a variety of containers (Figure 41-3) used for urine collection, including nonsterile containers for random specimens (urinalysis), sterile containers for cultures (testing specimens for growth of bacteria), and 24-hour collection containers with added preservatives.

Just before handing the urine specimen cup to the patient, label the cup with the patient's name,

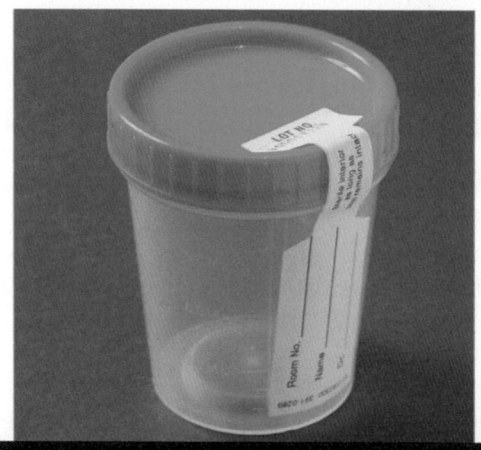

FIGURE 41-3 Urine collection containers should be calibrated and clear, and they should have a secure lid.

the date, and the time. Some facilities require more information, so follow the protocol of your facility. Always use a permanent marker so the information stays clear. Always label the cup, not the lid. This practice ensures that the specimen will not be separated from the label if the lid is removed. If the patient is unable to procure a specimen, discard the cup and then give the patient a new cup if the patient is later able to give a specimen.

When using electronic medical records, computer-generated labels can be printed. One label can be applied to the cup and other labels used for additional tests ordered, if appropriate. An example of an additional lab test is a culture and sensitivity of the urine, as explained later in this chapter.

Occasionally, a patient will bring a sample with him or her in a generic container from home. General recommendations are to provide the patient with a new urine specimen cup and request a fresh sample. The exception to this rule would be if the patient has brought a "first morning void" specimen in an appropriate container as directed by the provider.

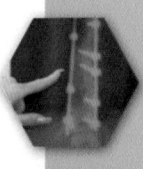

Critical Thinking

1. Why does CLIA differentiate laboratory tests into separate categories?
2. In a urinalysis, why is the microscopic examination not in CLIA's waived category?

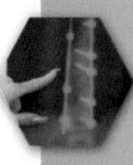

Critical Thinking

1. Which tests can be performed on urine that is not in a sterile container and why?
2. What would you say to a patient who brings in a urine specimen from home in a clean baby food jar?

URINE COLLECTION

Urine Specimen Types

Professional

Patients may have questions about how a specimen should be collected. The medical assistant must be able to give proper instructions using common terms that the patient will be able to understand. Following are common types of urine specimens that providers frequently might order.

Random (Spot) Specimen. Random (spot) urine samples are specimens that can be obtained at any time and are the most common collection performed in the outpatient setting. Random simply means that there is no particular time placed on the collection. Patients are requested to give a specimen whenever they are present for their appointment. If the patient has already voided, not knowing a specimen would be required, the medical assistant may offer the patient several cups of water in an attempt to procure another specimen. Because the kidneys constantly produce urine, the patient should be able to provide another specimen within 15 to 20 minutes of drinking several cups of water.

First Morning Void Specimen. The first morning void is typically the most concentrated specimen and has a higher acid pH (which helps preserve the cellular components). It is preferred, but because it is less convenient, it is seldom ordered unless the patient is an inpatient or is in some other controlled setting.

Fasting/Timed Specimens. A fasting (going without food and drink except water) urine specimen is ordered less often than a random specimen. The provider may want to measure a urinary substance without interference from food intake. Some providers may require an overnight fast. Others may ask the patient to have a meal and then urinate four hours later.

It is up to the medical assistant to give the patient proper instruction as to how to collect a fasting, or timed, specimen. Written directions given to the patient in addition to oral instructions are best. A regular urinalysis container can be used for a fasting specimen. It does not require a sterile container.

Twenty-Four-Hour Specimen. Urine varies in its concentration of certain substances at different times during any 24-hour period of **circadian rhythm** (waking and sleeping) and the intake of food and water. Therefore, a 24-hour specimen is sometimes requested when **quantitative tests** (measuring the amount) for different substances are desired. The results of this type of collection then will be expressed in *units per 24 hours*. Some commonly tested substances include sodium, potassium, calcium, and creatinine.

The container used to collect this amount of urine should be of adequate size. Usually a one-gallon, dark-colored plastic bottle is used (Figure 41-4). The 24-hour container and instructions may be mailed to the patient, or the patient may pick them up at the laboratory.

Urine collected over a 24-hour period may be refrigerated between collections. After the collection is complete, it must be returned to the medical laboratory as soon as possible.

Safety

For measuring urine constituents, preservatives need to be added to the 24-hour urine bottle before the collection begins. Without the preservative, the urine constituents may break down and be impossible to quantify. Some preservatives are strong acids or bases. Examples of preservatives used include thymol, toluene, and certain acids. As with all laboratory chemicals, the medical assistant and the patient should avoid contact between the preservative and the skin. The urine specimen should be collected into a smaller container and then poured carefully into the main container. Vapors must not be inhaled when adding the specimen to the container. The patient's written instructions should contain a warning about avoiding contact with preservatives.

Collection Methods

In addition to ordering the type of urine specimen desired (random, fasting, 24-hour), the

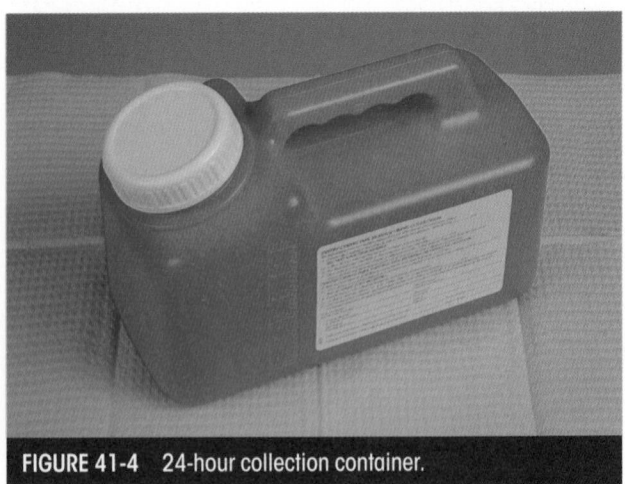

FIGURE 41-4 24-hour collection container.

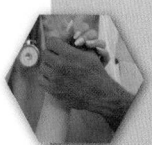

Patient Education

24-Hour Urine Collection

1. When giving a patient any type of instructions, make sure that the patient understands the importance of each step. Always provide written instructions as well as oral. Emphasize that failing to follow the instructions will cause the results to be invalid, requiring another collection.

2. The patient begins a 24-hour collection by emptying the bladder and not keeping the specimen. The container is then labeled with the time of bladder emptying. Patients generally start the collection between 6 and 8 pm, but any 24-hour period is acceptable.

3. Explain that each time the patient urinates within the 24-hour period, the urine is transferred into the collection container.

4. Instruct the patient to refrigerate the container between urinations if required.

5. Explain that at the end of the 24-hour period, the patient should urinate and transfer the urine into the container. The exact time should be written on the label as the "ended" or "completed" time.

6. The most common errors in the 24-hour urine specimen collection are the inclusion of the first voided specimen and the discarding of one or more of the voided specimens during the 24-hour period. Be sure the patient understands these steps.

provider might also order a certain type of collection method to collect the specific sample. These methods include clean-catch midstream and catheterized collection.

Procedure

Clean-Catch Midstream Collection. To avoid as much contamination as possible when collecting a specimen, providers prefer that the patient cleanse the genital area before collection. The clean-catch order means that cleansing towelettes are provided in addition to a urine container. Male patients are directed to cleanse the urethral opening twice with cleansing towelettes, and female patients are directed to cleanse the urethral area with three swipes, using three separate towelettes. (See Procedure 41-1 for complete instructions.) Female patients should also be instructed to notify

---

PROCEDURE 41-1

Procedure

Instructing a Patient in the Collection of a Clean-Catch, Midstream Urine Specimen

PURPOSE:

To instruct a patient on the proper technique of collecting a urine specimen suitable for urinalysis testing.

EQUIPMENT/SUPPLIES:

- Gloves
- Urine cup with a secure lid
- Cleansing towelettes (two for males, three for females)
- Marking pen
- Written instructions posted in restroom

PROCEDURE STEPS:

1. Wash hands and assemble the supplies. RATIONALE: Always wash hands before working with each patient as a means of preventing disease transmission. Being organized ensures that the procedure will be performed in a professional manner.

(continues)

2. ***Introduce yourself by name and credential. Identify the patient,*** and provide for a private area free from distractions. RATIONALE: Identifying the patient ensures that the right patient will have the right procedure. Introducing yourself and stating your credentials provides for a professional rapport with the patient. Providing for a private area ensures that the patient will have the freedom to ask questions and that confidentiality will be maintained. Being in an area that is free from distractions allows you to use a moderate voice volume and still be heard and understood by the patient.

3. Provide the patient with a capped urine cup labeled with his or her name, a pair of gloves, and the cleansing towelettes. RATIONALE: The cup should be labeled (not the cap) prior to giving it to the patient so there is not a chance of a mix-up. Gloves will protect the patient's hands from contamination from the urine and from the genital area. The towelettes will be used for cleansing the area prior to obtaining the sample.

4. Show the patient the written instructions posted in the bathroom. RATIONALE: The patient should always have written instructions in case he or she forgets a step. The instructions should be posted at a level that can be read by the female patient while sitting and by the male patient while standing.

5. ***Speaking to the patient's level of understanding, explain the rationale*** for why the urine sample should be a clean-catch midstream sample and what that means. ***Show awareness of the patient's concerns.*** RATIONALE: When the patient understands the reasons behind the instructions, he or she is much more likely to follow the steps completely.

6. Ask the patient to first wash his or her hands and apply the gloves. RATIONALE: Gloves are worn to protect the patient's hands from contamination.

7. ***Demonstrate professionalism and courtesy to the patient*** while you explain the cleansing process for a clean-catch sample: For the male patient, explain that he is to cleanse the urethral opening twice, using two separate towelettes, before he begins to urinate. For the female patient, explain that she will need to spread her labia and cleanse from front to back first on one side, then the other, and lastly, in the middle. Explain that she is to hold her labia apart until the urine sample is obtained. RATIONALE: Demonstrating professionalism and courtesy will maintain a professional atmosphere and help put the patient at ease, as some patients may become embarrassed with these instructions. Cleansing the urethral opening ensures that the sample will have no or few epithelial cells from the skin. Epithelial cells are quite large and can make the urine difficult to evaluate microscopically because the bacteria and other cells can be hidden behind them.

8. Explain the process of obtaining the midstream specimen: For both the male and the female patient, he or she is to bring the cup into the stream and obtain about half a cup before removing the cup from the stream. RATIONALE: The mid-stream catch is used to further prevent epithelial cells from entering the sample. If the patient were to stop and start the urine flow, the chances of epithelial contamination increase.

9. Explain to the patient that he or she should secure the cap onto the cup. RATIONALE: The secure lid will prevent spillage.

10. The patient may rinse the outside of the capped cup if needed and towel dry it. RATIONALE: Rinsing and drying the outside of the cup will remove any urine that may be present.

11. The patient should be instructed as to where to place the specimen cup. Using a paper towel as a barrier, the cup may be returned to the medical assistant or placed in the lab receptacle as directed. RATIONALE: Some clinics have a pass-through door to the laboratory with a shelf for the patient to place the specimen, and in some clinics, the sample may be handed to the medical assistant. The paper towel creates a barrier between the specimen and the hand.

12. The patient is to then remove the gloves, dispose of them into the red bag waste receptacle, and wash his or her hands. RATIONALE: Contaminated waste should always go into red bag receptacles. Hands should be washed to remove any residual powder from the gloves and/or contamination that may have touched the hands.

13. ***Ask the patient if he or she has any questions and provide appropriate responses.*** RATIONALE: Soliciting questions will encourage the patient to ask if there is something he or she does not understand. Providing appropriate responses will further the patient's understanding and ensure a cleaner specimen.

the medical assistant if they are menstruating during the collection.

After cleansing, the patient should begin to urinate into the toilet. After beginning to urinate, the patient pulls the cup into the urine stream and collects the sample, then removes the cup from the stream and voids the rest of the urine into the toilet. This is called a **midstream** specimen. The midstream urine should be as free of contamination as possible.

Catheterized Collection. Urinary catheterization involves insertion of a sterile flexible tube into the urinary bladder through the urethra. Although urinary catheterization is performed for many reasons, this section discusses only the use of catheterization as a way to obtain a urinary sample (see Chapter 29 for catheterization procedures).

Obtaining a urine specimen by catheterization is required when a completely sterile specimen is needed or when the patient is unable to follow cleansing instructions. The patient may not understand the language, may be mentally unable to comprehend the instructions, or may be physically unable to perform the process. Catheterization is a sterile procedure and is performed only under a provider's order and only by health care professionals who have been adequately trained. Because the urinary bladder is considered a sterile environment, if the catheterization is not performed properly, bacteria may be introduced into the patient's bladder, which can lead to a bladder infection.

CULTURE AND SENSITIVITY OF URINE

Occasionally, the provider will order a culture and sensitivity (C&S) of a urine specimen. The medical assistant is responsible for preparing the sample for transport. A commonly used system is the urine culture and sensitivity transport kit (see Procedure 41-2).

EXAMINATION OF URINE

Urine should be examined in a fresh state, preferably while still warm if possible. However, on rare occasions, the urine sample cannot be tested immediately. If immediate testing is not possible, the urine should be refrigerated at about 4°C (39°F) or stored on ice and tested within 2 hours. Crystals and casts begin to break down after 2 hours. Any time delay allows bacteria to multiply and can lead to inaccurate microbiology results.

PROCEDURE 41-2
Utilizing a Urine Transport System for C&S

Procedure

STANDARD PRECAUTIONS:

 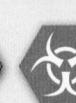  

Handwashing   Gloves   Biohazard   Goggles & Mask   Gown

PURPOSE:

To prepare a urine specimen for transport using a culture and sensitivity transport kit.

EQUIPMENT/SUPPLIES:

- Gloves
- Sterile urine cup and specimen
- Urine culture and sensitivity transport kit
- Laboratory requisition
- Paper towel

(continues)

PROCEDURE STEPS:

1. Wash hands and put on gloves. RATIONALE: Washing hands before any laboratory process prevents contamination of the specimen. Gloving provides personal protection.

2. Assemble equipment and supplies. Place paper towel on the work surface. (Figure 41-5A shows one type of system). RATIONALE: Organizing your work area prevents confusion and error caused by missing supplies.

3. Follow all safety guidelines, being careful not to splash the urine specimen. Wipe up all spills immediately with disinfectant cleaner. RATIONALE: Preventing splashes and spills will prevent exposure to biohazardous substances. Cleaning any spill immediately prevents further contamination and risk for exposure.

4. Examine the specimen for proper labeling, paying attention to detail. RATIONALE: The specimen cup must be properly labeled to ensure QC.

5. Check the urine C&S transport kit expiration date. RATIONALE: If the kit has expired, the contents cannot be guaranteed sterile.

6. Open the urine C&S transport kit package (Figure 41-5B). Remove the cap from the specimen cup, placing the lid upside down on the paper towel. RATIONALE: The cap must be placed upside down to maintain the sterile inner surface.

7. Follow the manufacturer's instructions exactly:

   a. Place the urine tube in the tube adapter (Figure 41-5C) and the specimen straw into the urine within the specimen cup (Figure 41-5D).

   b. Advance urine tube into the adapter, pushing the tube onto the needle while keeping the specimen straw submerged in the urine.

   c. Allow the vacuum in the urine tube to draw up the urine. Fill to the exhaustion of the vacuum within the tube (Figure 41-5E).

   d. Remove the tube and the specimen straw/adapter unit and dispose of it into a biohazard container.

   e. Gently invert the tube 8 to 10 times to mix the preservative within the tube.

8. Label the tube with patient's name, date, time, and other required information. RATIONALE: Labeling with the required information prevents mix-ups of specimens and ensures a quality timeline.

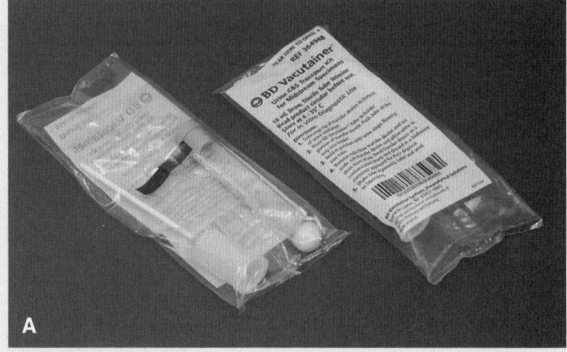

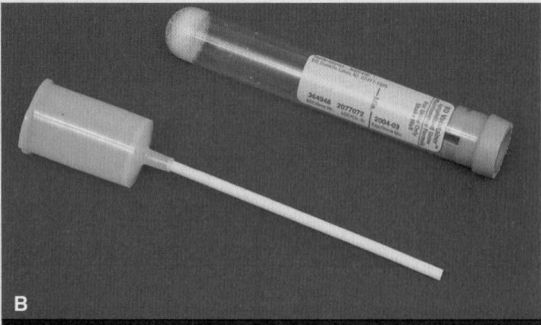

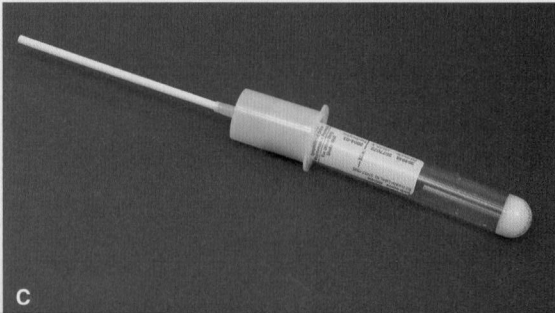

FIGURE 41-5 The urine transport kit for culture and sensitivity. (A) Packaged as a kit. (B) The components of the kit. (C) The tube is connected to the straw and adapter.

(continues)

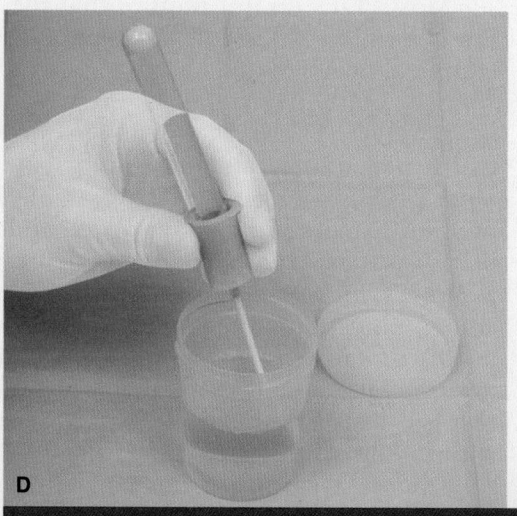 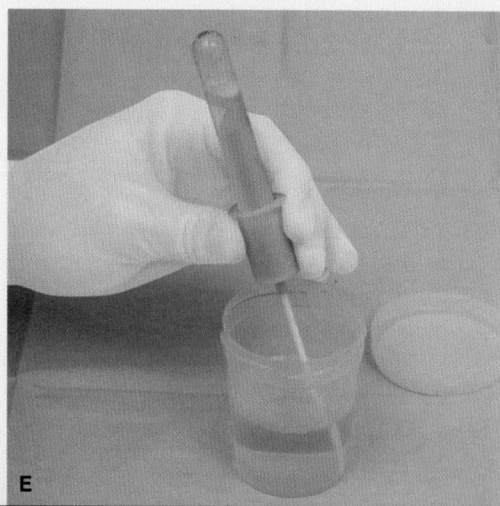

FIGURE 41-5 *(continued)* (D) The end of the straw is placed in the urine (the vacuum tube is not pushed completely onto the adapter until the straw is submerged in the urine). (E) The vacuum in the tube draws up the urine.

9. Dispose of all contaminated supplies, disinfect all surfaces, remove gloves, and wash hands. RATIONALE: Using appropriate disposal techniques and disinfecting all surfaces according to Standard Precautions safely controls biohazard substances.

10. Complete the laboratory requisition and document procedure in the patient's chart or electronic medical record. RATIONALE: Proper documentation ensures the laboratory will have the necessary information and the patient's medical record will be accurate and complete.

DOCUMENTATION:

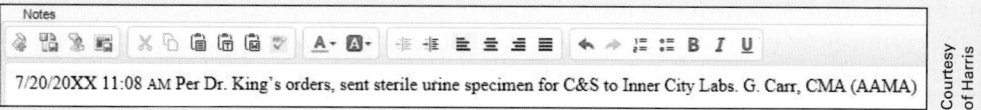

Notes

7/20/20XX 11:08 AM Per Dr. King's orders, sent sterile urine specimen for C&S to Inner City Labs. G. Carr, CMA (AAMA)

Courtesy of Harris CareTracker PM and EMR

The routine urinalysis procedure is composed of three parts:

- *Physical or visual* examination of the urine
- *Chemical* examination of the urine
- *Microscopic* examination of urine sediment

Safety

The medical assistant should wash hands, put on gloves, and follow all safety guidelines when performing any of the following procedures. Some facilities require eye protection when pouring urine or performing any procedure where splashing of urine into the eye could occur. All surface areas in the restroom should be decontaminated immediately after procuring or testing urine specimens.

Physical Examination of Urine

When the medical assistant begins the process of performing a urinalysis, the first step is performing the physical or visual examination. This examination consists of:

- Assessing the volume of the urine specimen, making sure that the amount is sufficient for testing

- Observing and recording the color, appearance, and transparency of the specimen
- Noting any unusual odor
- Measuring the specific gravity of the specimen

Specimen Volume. The first step in performing a urinalysis is to determine if the sample's volume is adequate for testing.

The medical assistant must have enough urine to fill a test tube with at least 10 mL (about 2 teaspoons) of urine with enough leftover in the specimen cup to completely insert and wet a chemical reagent strip and to culture if ordered.

The volume usually requested of the patient is 125 mL or about a half cup, but patients should be assured that samples of much less volume can be tested. If the patient is able to submit only a small volume of urine, the provider will determine the priority of which tests to perform according to the patient's suspected diagnosis. For example, if only a test for protein and glucose is requested, then only enough urine to process the chemical reagent strip portion is needed. However, if a test for microscopic examination of the urine, such as to diagnose a bladder infection, is requested, then a full test tube is needed as well as some extra urine for a culture. These testing criteria are thoroughly discussed later in this chapter.

The provider should be consulted for further direction if the amount of urine submitted is less than needed for the complete urinalysis. The urinalysis report should reflect that the quantity was not sufficient for complete testing. The medical assistant should write "QNS" (quantity not sufficient), where applicable, or follow clinic protocol.

If the patient is able to give less than 10 mL of urine for the test tube, the medical assistant should make a note of the amount of urine used. For example, if the patient provides 5 mL, the medical assistant may go ahead with the microscopic examination of urine but should note on the report that the specimen was only 5 mL. The rationale for this notation becomes clear when you understand that the amount of a substance found in 10 mL of urine will be less in a smaller sample. In other words, if the patient has five white blood cells in 10 mL of urine, he or she might have only two to three white blood cells in 5 mL of urine. Unless the notation is made that

the sample was smaller, the provider may diagnose incorrectly.

Most POLs do not require that the urine volume be noted unless it is less than adequate for a complete urinalysis.

Urine Color. There is a wide range of color in normal urine, usually ranging from a pale yellow to a dark yellow or amber (Figure 41-6). The range of color usually is the result of the concentration of the urine. A darker color generally indicates a more concentrated urine. The color of urine comes from normal metabolic processes, the end products of which are deposited in the urine. After assessing the adequacy of the urine volume, the medical assistant then observes and records the color of the urine.

Diet and certain drugs can add substances to the urine that give it a specific color. The medical assistant should be familiar with common reasons for abnormally colored urine and whether they are pathologic (due to a disease process) or nonpathologic abnormalities. For example, the most common pathologic cause of red urine is the presence of red blood cells, known as **hematuria**. Red blood cells in urine may indicate bleeding in the urinary tract either because of a bladder infection or a kidney stone. A nonpathologic example of abnormally colored urine is the medication phenazopyridine (Pyridium), which can turn the urine bright orange. Table 41-2 lists several urine color variations and possible causes.

Urine Transparency. In order to assess transparency or clarity, the urine should be viewed

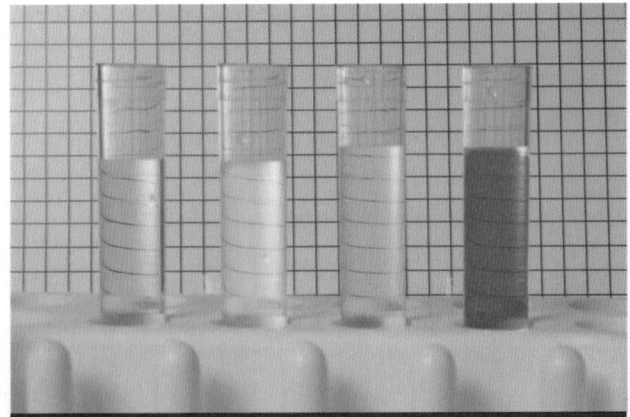

FIGURE 41-6 Normal urine can range in color from straw and yellow, to amber. Abnormal urine (depending on its constituents) can be red, brown, fluorescent orange, and more.

TABLE 41-2

URINE COLORS AND POSSIBLE CAUSES

COLOR	POSSIBLE CAUSE
Straw to yellow	Normal
Orange to amber	Concentrated urine
Colorless	Dilute urine
Deep yellow	Vitamin intake
Bright orange	Drugs, usually phenazopyridine (Pyridium)
Orange-brown	Urochrome/urinbilinogen
Greenish orange	Bilirubin
Smokey	Red blood cells
Wine red/reddish brown	Hemoglobin pigments
Green or blue	Methylene blue

through a clear cup or tube. Urine is considered clear if a line of print can be read through it. Urine transparency normally is not significant by itself. However, it may be helpful when included with the rest of the urinalysis information. Transparency of urine usually is recorded as clear, hazy, cloudy, or **turbid** (opaque) (see Figure 41-7). The descriptive terms used may vary in different facilities.

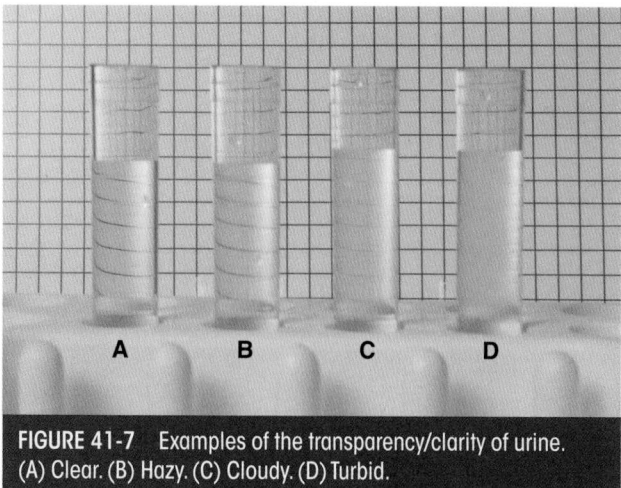

FIGURE 41-7 Examples of the transparency/clarity of urine. (A) Clear. (B) Hazy. (C) Cloudy. (D) Turbid.

There are many causes of cloudy urine, most of which are considered normal. Cloudiness could be attributed to contamination from vaginal discharges, white blood cells, bacteria, or yeast. As urine cools, sometimes crystals form, which may give urine a cloudy appearance.

Urine Odor. With experience, the medical assistant will recognize certain odors in the urine that can indicate specific conditions. Odors, though not recorded on the final laboratory urinalysis report, should not be disregarded. For example, the urine of a patient with diabetes who may have a condition known as **ketoacidosis** may have a sweet odor. Urine full of bacteria will have a foul odor that is easily recognized.

Urine Specific Gravity. **Specific gravity** is defined as the ratio of the weight of a given volume of a substance to the weight of the same volume of distilled water at the same temperature. Distilled water used as the reference point has been given the specific gravity value of 1.000. The specific gravity of urine indicates the concentrations of solids such as phosphates, chlorides, proteins, glucose, and urea that are dissolved in urine.

Variations in urine specific gravity can give the provider diagnostic information. In uncontrolled diabetes, glucose is released into the patient's urine. Glucose molecules are dense and may give the urine a high specific gravity. Another reason for high specific gravity readings is dehydration, because urine becomes more concentrated as the body tries to conserve fluid. In addition, the color of this urine will be darker. In a well-hydrated patient, the specific gravity is low and the color is pale, meaning that the urine is mostly water. The normal range of specific gravity for urine is from 1.005 to 1.030. Specific gravity is highest in the first morning samples because the urine has become concentrated through the night.

Specific gravity is often tested by using either a chemical test strip, a urinometer, or a refractometer. A urinometer is made from a small glass tube weighted to float in a sample of urine (usually 15 mL). The glass tube has been calibrated, and the stem of the tube has been marked accordingly to read 1.000 at the bottom of the meniscus in distilled water at room temperature. The meniscus is the curvature that appears in a liquid's upper surface when the liquid is placed in a container. The medical assistant reads the specific gravity of the urine from the stem at the meniscus. However, the temperature of the urine must be taken into account if it differs from 70°F, which is considered normal room temperature. The buoyancy of a liquid changes with the temperature. If the urine is allowed to come to room temperature, the medical assistant risks the physical and chemical changes that can occur to urine when left for more than 20 minutes. The urinometer is the least accurate and the most difficult to use so it is not recommended as the best option for measuring the weight (specific gravity) of urine.

The most common tool for determining the specific gravity of liquids is the **refractometer** (Figure 41-8). The refractometer measures light as it passes through the urine sample. If the urine sample contains solids and dissolved particles, the refractometer reading is higher. If the urine sample is clearer (such as water), the refractometer reading is lower.

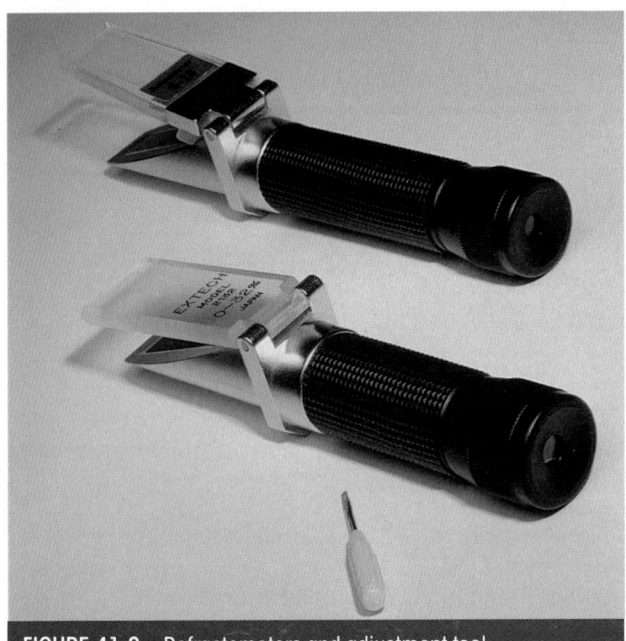

FIGURE 41-8 Refractometers and adjustment tool.

Procedure

The refractometer reading is about 0.002 less than that of the true specific gravity. This slight difference is more than made up for by the ease of using the instrument and the instrument's reliability. This instrument needs only a drop or two of urine, and the result does not have to be adjusted for temperature as long as the temperature is between 60° and 100°F (see Procedure 41-3).

Procedure

PROCEDURE 41-3
Using the Refractometer to Measure Specific Gravity

STANDARD PRECAUTIONS:

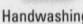    

Handwashing   Gloves   Biohazard   Goggles & Mask   Gown

PURPOSE:

To measure and record the specific gravity of a urine specimen.

NOTE: This procedure is separated from the complete urinalysis for instructional purposes only. The physical examination of urine is always performed along with the chemical analysis and usually includes the microscopic examination as well. For a complete urinalysis, see Procedure 41-4.

EQUIPMENT/SUPPLIES:

- Refractometer and adjustment screw driver
- Urine sample
- Gloves
- Pipettes
- Distilled water

- Lint-free tissues
- Biohazard container
- Disinfectant cleaners
- Urinalysis report form

(continues)

PROCEDURE STEPS:

1. Wash hands and put on gloves. RATIONALE: Washing hands before any laboratory process prevents contamination of the specimen. Gloving provides personal protection.

2. Assemble equipment and supplies. RATIONALE: Organizing your work area prevents confusion and error caused by missing supplies.

3. Follow all safety guidelines, being careful not to splash the urine specimen. Wipe up all spills immediately with disinfectant cleaner. RATIONALE: Preventing splashes and spills will prevent exposure to biohazard substances. Cleaning any spill immediately prevents further contamination and risk for exposure.

4. QC must be performed on the refractometer before every use. This is accomplished by checking the specific gravity of a drop of distilled water:

   a. Clean the surface of the prism and the cover with lint-free tissue and distilled water. Wipe dry.

   b. Depending on the type of refractometer used, you may either apply the drop and then close the cover, or close the cover and apply the drop of distilled water to the notched portion of the cover so it flows over the prism (Figure 41-9A).

   c. With the instrument tilted to allow light to enter, view the scale and read the specific gravity number (Figure 41-9B). Distilled water should be exactly 1.000.

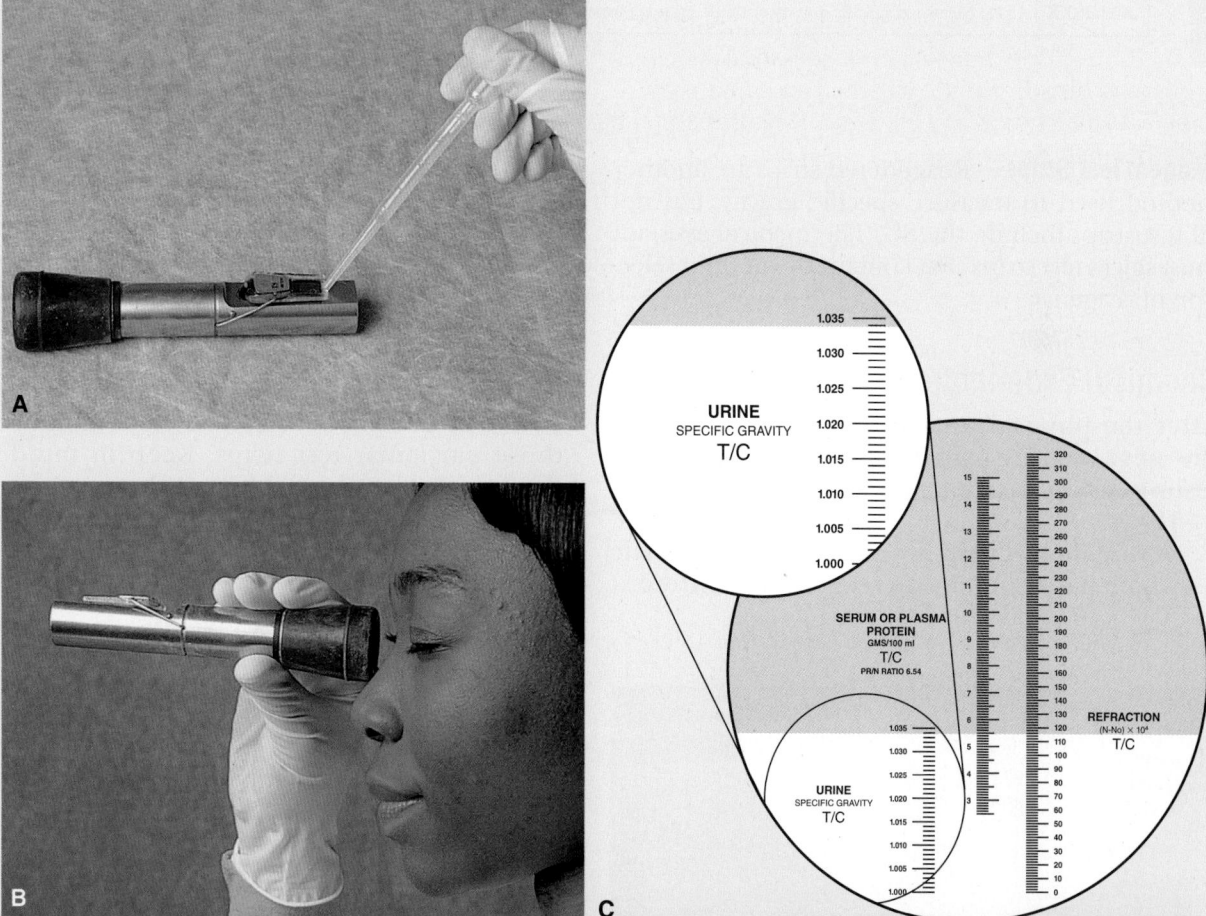

FIGURE 41-9 (A) A pipette or dropper may be used to fill the refractometer with urine. (B) The medical assistant looks through the refractometer. The instrument is held toward a light source. (C) The specific gravity readout.

(continues)

    d. If the QC test shows the refractometer to be calibrated properly, you may record the results on your QC sheet and proceed to test the urine specimen. If the QC test shows the refractometer to be inaccurate, the instrument is not calibrated properly. Use the small adjustment screwdriver to adjust the calibration. Do this adjustment using distilled water until the gauge reads 1.000.

5. Test the urine specimen exactly as the distilled water was tested and record the specific gravity (Figure 41-9C) into the urinalysis report in the patient's health record.

6. Proceed with the rest of the urinalysis (Procedure 41-4).

7. Dispose of the specimen into the toilet or designated sink and all supplies into appropriate biohazard containers. Disinfect all reusable equipment and all surfaces. RATIONALE: Using appropriate disposal techniques and disinfecting all surfaces according to Standard Precautions safely controls all biohazard substances.

8. Remove gloves. Wash hands.

9. Document procedure in patient's chart or electronic medical record.

DOCUMENTATION:

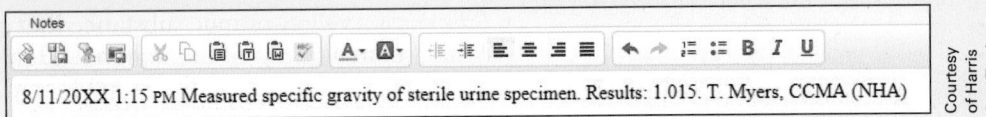

Notes

8/11/20XX 1:15 PM Measured specific gravity of sterile urine specimen. Results: 1.015. T. Myers, CCMA (NHA)

Courtesy of Harris CareTracker PM and EMR

Reagent Test Strips.

Reagent test strips are another method used to measure specific gravity, but not all test strips include the SG. The medical assistant must select test strips that contain the desired selection of reagents.

Chemical Examination of Urine

After the physical testing of a urine specimen, the next step in urinalysis testing is chemical testing using reagent test strips (see Figure 41-10).

A **reagent test strip** is a narrow strip of plastic on which pads containing reagents for different reactions are attached. The reagent test strip is the primary tool used for chemical examination of urine. The pads have reagents to test for many metabolic processes, including kidney and liver functions, urinary tract infection (UTI), and pH balance. The name of the test strips indicates how many tests are included. For example, MultiStix 10 SG and Chemstrip 10 SG indicates there are 10 tests included on those particular test strips. Keep in mind that the more tests available on the reagent test strips, the more expensive the product will be. Table 41-3 lists some tests available on urine reagent strips.

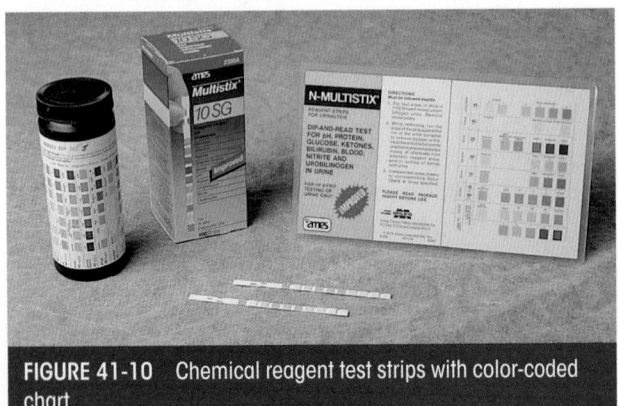

FIGURE 41-10 Chemical reagent test strips with color-coded chart.

TABLE 41-3

CHEMICAL TESTING AVAILABLE ON URINE REAGENT TEST STRIPS

pH	Blood
Protein	Urobilinogen
Glucose	Nitrite
Ketones	Leukocyte esterase
Bilirubin	Specific gravity

Chemicals in Urine

- *Glucose* is the sugar most commonly found in urine. *Glycosuria* and **glucosuria** both are terms that describe the condition of having glucose in urine. Glucose is normally filtered out of urine in the glomerulus of the kidneys and is reabsorbed in the renal tubules. If the body has too much glucose in the blood, the extra will not be reabsorbed and instead will "spill" into the urine. Although diabetes is almost always suspected, further testing is required before a diagnosis of diabetes can be made.

- *pH* is the abbreviation for potential hydrogen ion concentration. The pH test determines if the urine is alkaline or acidic. The scale for pH runs from 0 for the most acidic to 14 for the most alkaline or base. Neutral pH is 7. The pH of urine varies from 4.5 to 8. The kidneys and lungs are responsible for helping the blood stay at its perfect pH level (7.35 to 7.45). The kidneys do this by adjusting the substances they secrete. A person can die if the blood is too acidic (acidosis) or too alkaline (alkalosis). Because there is so little room for deviation in the pH of blood, the kidneys and lungs are constantly adjusting secretions. Many things affect the pH of the urine, from medication and diet to pathological conditions. Diets high in protein, some medications, renal tuberculosis, high fevers, and uncontrolled diabetes can cause acidic urine, whereas alkaline urine can be caused by diets high in vegetables, citrus fruits, dairy products, some medications, and UTIs. Letting a urine specimen sit at room temperature for too long can cause a false high-pH (more alkaline) reading.

- *Protein* (albumin) may be secreted in very small (trace) amounts by the kidneys. The presence of protein in urine (proteinuria) occasionally has a nonpathological basis such as excessive exercise, exposure to extreme heat or cold, or acute emotional stress. Any substantial and/or consistent presence of protein in urine is of concern for renal disease. Proteins are large compounds and can get through the filtering system (glomerulus) of the kidneys only if there has been damage to the glomeruli. Think of a volleyball net that a small golf ball could pass through but not a larger basketball, unless there are holes (damage) to the net. Damage can be caused by many things: diseases, toxins, or systemic conditions such as diabetes and uncontrolled high blood pressure.

- *Ketones* are formed whenever the body uses fat/fatty acids for energy rather than carbohydrates/sugars. This can happen whenever there is a low intake of carbohydrates/sugars such as in dieting and in certain metabolic disorders such as diabetes. In diabetes, the body lacks insulin or is unable to use glucose properly for energy, so it uses fatty acids. Insulin is a chemical that helps the body use glucose for energy, so some people with diabetes replace their insulin. As fats are broken down, ketone bodies form and "spill" into the urine. The presence of ketones in urine is called **ketonuria**. The burning of fats for energy is called **ketosis** or sometimes *lipolysis*. Persons on carbohydrate-careful diets often use chemical reagent test strips to check if their urine contains ketones, thus indicating that their bodies are burning fats. Ketosis should not be confused with ketoacidosis, which is a dangerous condition for people with diabetes and alcoholics.

- *Bilirubin* is a yellow-orange substance that comes from the breakdown of hemoglobin. Hemoglobin is contained within the red blood cells. Because individual RBCs live for only 120 days, they are constantly breaking down and being replaced. When the RBCs "die," the heme part of the hemoglobin circulates in the blood until the liver filters it out. The liver is responsible for changing the heme into a water-soluble substance called bilirubin. Before it gets to the liver, it is called indirect or free bilirubin. After it leaves the liver, it is called direct or conjugated bilirubin. The liver sends the conjugated bilirubin to the gall bladder where it is released with bile into the small intestine. When there is a blockage in the liver or gall bladder ducts or when there is a disorder or disease of the liver, the bilirubin cannot get past the gall bladder to the small intestine, so it continues to circulate in the blood. This excess of bilirubin in the blood can lead to yellow-orange skin called *jaundice*. The body will try to get rid of extra bilirubin through the urine. Hence, any detection of bilirubin in the urine (*bilirubinuria*) can be indicative of a problem in the liver and/or gall bladder. Newborn babies can be jaundiced because their systems are not mature enough to get rid of the bile. Because bilirubin breaks down in sunlight, we treat jaundiced babies with special "bili-lights" to help them break down the bilirubin in their skin. Knowing that bilirubin is so unstable, we need to protect it from light in our urine samples, another good reason to test urine samples immediately. Keep in mind that further testing is required before a diagnosis can be made, because bilirubinuria is a symptom, not a disease.

- *Hematuria* is the presence of blood in the urine. If the blood in the urine is not from a nonpathogenic source, such as contamination from menstruation, it is indicative of a bladder infection (often called a **urinary tract infection** [UTI]), irritation of the urinary tract from a kidney stone, or, rarely, a neoplasm. Many chemical reagent test strips differentiate between hemoglobin and intact red blood cells. Hemoglobin in urine is called **hemoglobinuria** and can indicate pathogenic conditions such as severe infectious diseases, transfusion reactions, and hemolytic anemias. A nonpathogenic cause of hemoglobinuria occurs when the urine is allowed to sit too long, so any RBCs present start breaking down, thus releasing their hemoglobin. Sometimes the chemical reagent test strips indicate the presence of blood in the urine, but no blood cells are seen during the microscopic examination. This is an example of hemoglobin being present rather than intact RBCs. The presence of blood in urine is considered along with the patient's symptoms and other tests to arrive at a definitive diagnosis.
- **Urobilinogen** is a substance formed when bacteria in the digestive tract breaks down bilirubin. A very small percentage is excreted in the urine and is increased in liver disease. Urobilinogen gives color to feces.
- *Nitrite* forms in urine when certain pathogenic bacteria are present. These specific bacteria convert normal nitrate in urine to abnormal nitrite; thus, nitrite in urine is always indicative of the presence of these pathogenic bacteria in sufficient quantities to cause a bladder infection. Whenever nitrite is positive in a urine sample, white blood cells, bacteria, and often red blood cells also will be seen. The provider often orders a urine culture to determine the type of bacteria and the best medication to eradicate it.
- *Leukocytes* are white blood cells, which may be present in infected urine. Chapter 39 discusses leukocytes in detail. The chemical reagent test strips will detect only esterase (a leukocyte enzyme) but not the specific WBC, so a microscopic examination is still important as is a urine culture and sensitivity test. These results along with the patient's symptoms will help the provider diagnose and treat a UTI.
- *Specific gravity* (SG) has been discussed previously in this chapter and is available as a test option on many brands of chemical reagent test strips. The normal SG for urine is between 1.005 (very dilute urine) to 1.030 (concentrated urine).

Reagent Test Strip Quality Control. Reagent test strips are easy to use, but the complexity of the chemical testing should not be overlooked (see Quick Reference Guide).

» QUICK REFERENCE GUIDE

Reagent Test Strip Quality Control

☐	Never use outdated reagent test strips.
☐	Do not expose reagent test strips to direct sunlight, moisture, or excessive heat.
☐	Follow the manufacturer's instruction for storage.
☐	Do not remove strips from original container except at time of use.
☐	Since reagent pads are colored, employees should be tested for color-blindness.
☐	Use only the color chart accompanying the test strips for accuracy.
☐	Test within the time required.

TABLE 41-4

REAGENT STRIP SENSITIVITY

TEST	RANGE	NORMAL VALUE
pH	5 to 9	5 to 8
Protein	Negative to positive*	Negative
Glucose	Negative to >1,000 mg/dL	Negative
Ketone	Negative to >80 mg/dL	Negative
Bilirubin	Negative to large	Negative
Blood	Negative to large	Negative
Leukocyte esterase	Negative to large	Negative
Nitrites	Negative to positive	Negative
Urobilinogen	0.2 to 8.0 mg/dL	2.0 mg/dL
Specific gravity	1.000 to 1.035	Varies greatly

*Note that positive results in a newborn for glucose, ketone, and protein are considered critical values and should be reported to the provider immediately.

When reporting results, it is important to use the proper units and terms as directed by your laboratory. An example of the sensitivity of the reagent strips is shown in Table 41-4.

Automated urine analyzers (Figure 41-11A–H) capable of timing and reading the test strip are available. Automated urine analyzers are easy to operate, CLIA-waived, and more accurate because they reduce human error. Many such devices will also connect electronically to patient management systems, eliminating the need for manual documentation of the test results.

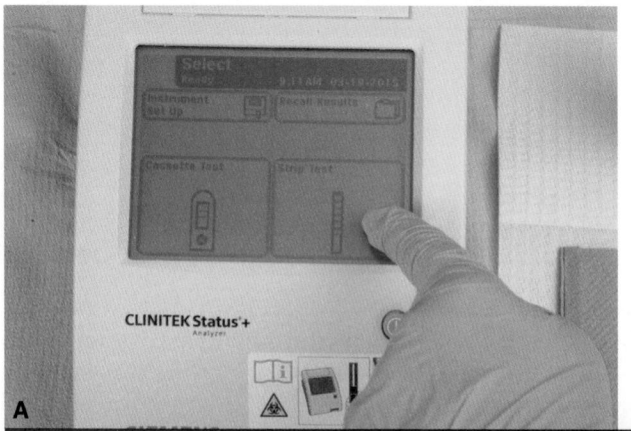
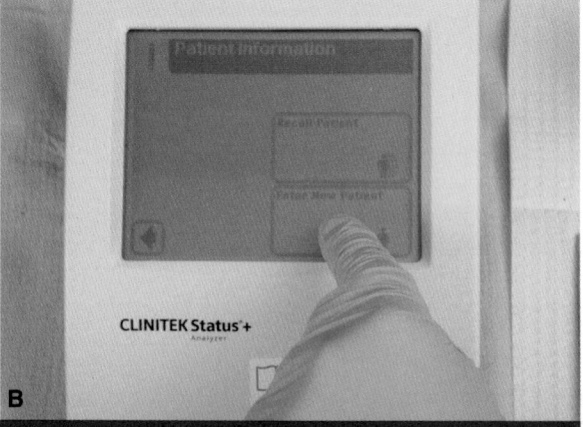

FIGURE 41-11 (A) After mixing urine in the tube, turn the machine on and select Strip Test. (B) Enter the operator and patient information.

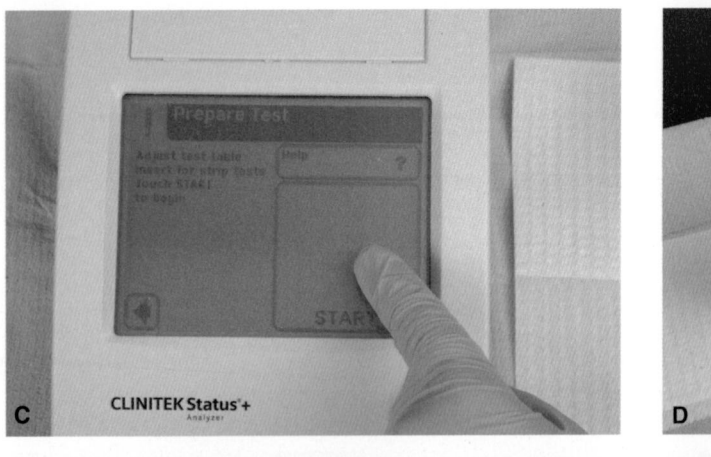

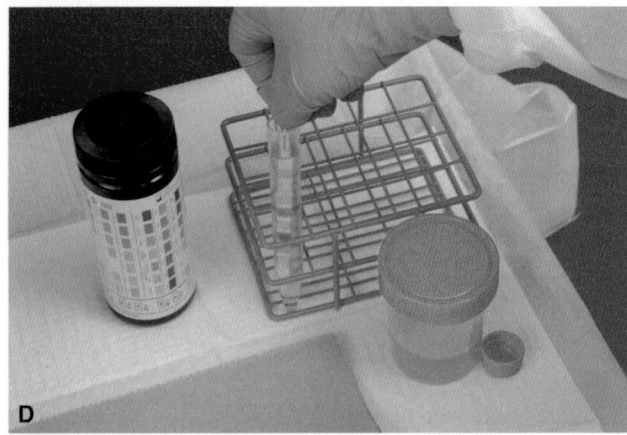

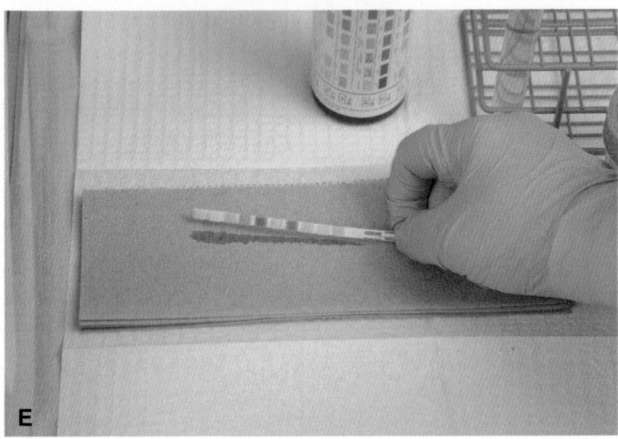

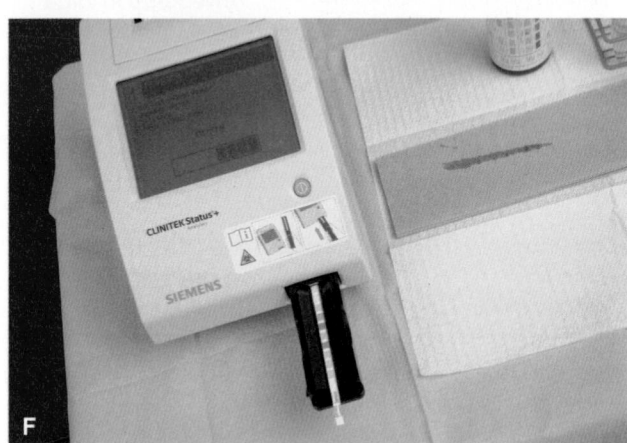

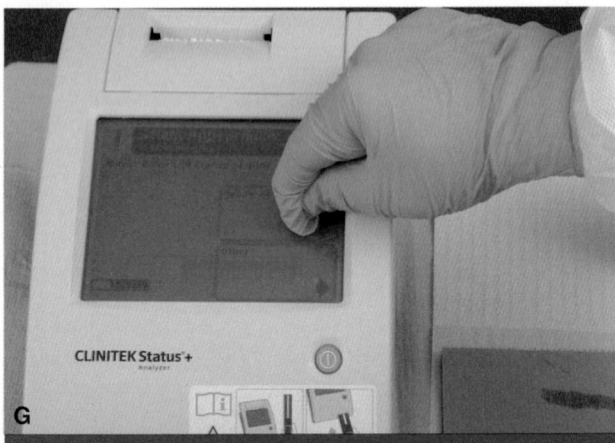

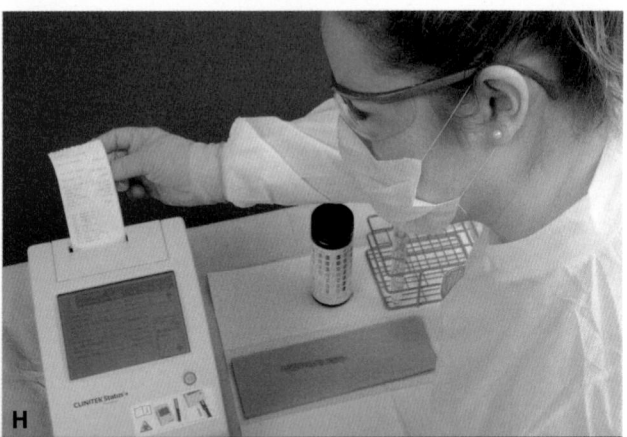

FIGURE 41-11 *(continued)* (C) Select the Start button. (D) Immediately dip the test strip into the urine. (E) Place the strip on its side against a paper towel or blot the pads with gauze. (F) Immediately place the strip on the machine's test strip holder. (G) Enter the color and clarity of urine. (H) The U/A test results will appear in the LCD window and will print out.

Microscopic Examination of Urine Sediment

In addition to the physical and chemical examination of urine, the medical assistant should be familiar with the microscopic examination of urine. CLIA considers the microscopic examination of urine to be a provider-performed microscopy procedure (PPMP) and not within the category of waived tests. Nevertheless, the medical assistant must be able to properly centrifuge the specimen and set up a slide of the urine sediment for the provider to examine. It is recommended that

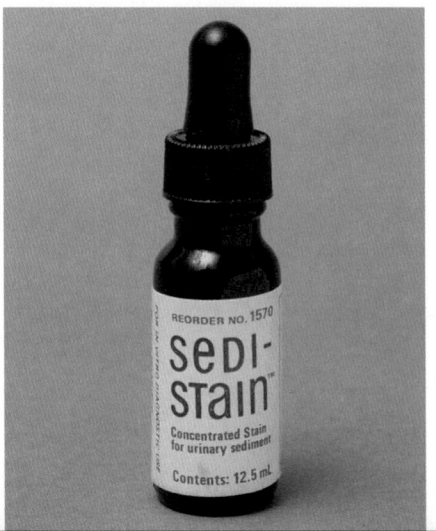

FIGURE 41-12 Sedi-Stain is an example of a stain used in laboratories.

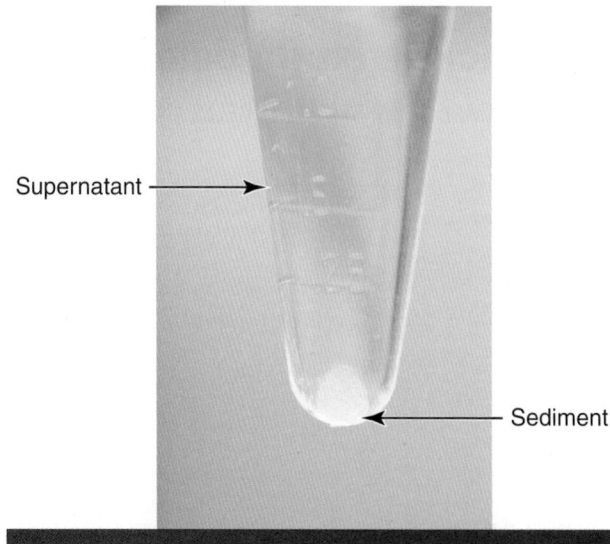

FIGURE 41-13 Example of a tube of urine after centrifugation.

Supernatant

Sediment

the medical assistant have a working knowledge of all urine sediment components, the pathologic significance of the components, and how to report the presence of sediment components. The **sediment** (insoluble material) at the bottom of the centrifuge tube is used for the microscopic examination (see Chapter 38 for proper use of the microscope).

One of the most important items to have on hand when performing a microscopic urine examination is a urine color atlas. It takes years to be able to correctly identify abnormal components of urine. A color atlas should always be available to the medical assistant to help with identification.

Some laboratories make use of urine stains to add color to certain structures in the urine sediment. Sedi-Stain is an example of such a stain (Figure 41-12).

Sediment. Sediment is obtained by centrifuging a sample of urine. The solid substances, such as cells and crystals, are forced to the bottom of the test tube, leaving clear fluid called **supernatant** on the top (Figure 41-13). The supernatant urine is carefully poured off. Most urine test tubes are specifically formed to assist in the process of pouring off all but 1 mL of the supernatant fluid. This is accomplished by quickly inverting the tube completely upside down (do not shake the tube in this position). When returned to the upright position, the 1 mL of fluid will be present in the bottom of the tube, together with the urine sediment. This is the perfect amount of supernatant fluid to resuspend the sediment. Try the inversion process first

with plain water until you are able to perform it easily. After the supernatant has been poured off, the sediment needs to be resuspended or mixed back into the 1 mL of fluid. Resuspend the sediment by gently tapping the tube on the counter or flicking it with your finger until the sediment and cellular components have all been mixed and resuspended in the fluid. A drop of sediment is then placed on a slide and examined microscopically.

Microscopic Examination of Urine. When viewing a normal urine specimen, the medical assistant may see very little under the microscope. Squamous epithelial cells may be seen, especially in women. These cells have no medical significance because they are skin cells continuously sloughed off into the urine. They are generally reported as few, moderate, or many. If the provider sees many epithelial cells in the urine specimen, it is indicative that the specimen is contaminated with skin cells. Better education of the patient of the reasons for and the technique of a clean-catch midstream collection should result in a less contaminated specimen.

Abnormal Urine Sediment Cells and Microorganisms. Microscopic examination of the urine sediment may show one or more of the cells and microorganisms shown in the following Quick Reference Guide.

Some of the more common findings in diseased conditions are red blood cells (hematuria), white blood cells, and bacteria, all of which, depending on the clinical examination, can indicate a urinary tract infection (UTI), kidney stones, or trauma.

QUICK REFERENCE GUIDE

ABNORMAL URINE SEDIMENT CELLS AND MICROORGANISMS

Element	Description
Red blood cells 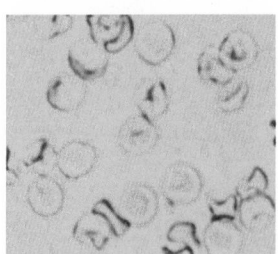	Red blood cells appear as pale, light-refractive disks when seen under high power. Large amounts of red blood cells in urine (hematuria) indicate disease or trauma. These cells are counted in a microscopic field (high-power field [HPF]) and reported as cells counted per HPF (e.g., 10/HPF).
White blood cells 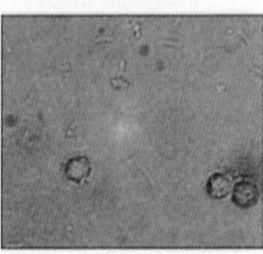	A few white blood cells can appear in normal urine. More than four white blood cells in urine often indicate a UTI. White blood cells are slightly larger than red blood cells, may appear granular, and have a visible nucleus (the red blood cell has no nucleus). White blood cells are reported in the same manner as red blood cells.
Renal tubular epithelial cells 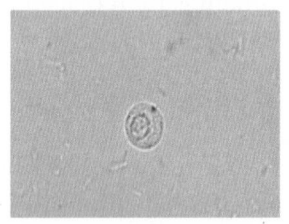 Bayer Healthcare Diagnostic Division, Norwood, MA	Renal tubular epithelial cells can indicate kidney disease if they are present in large numbers. They can be confused with both white blood cells and other epithelial cells. Renal and vaginal epithelial cells are smaller than squamous epithelial cells. Renal epithelia are rounder and vaginal epithelia are more oblong with pointed ends. They are also reported in the same manner as white and red blood cells.
Bacteria 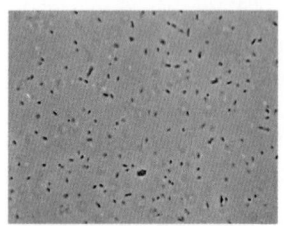 Bayer Healthcare Diagnostic Division, Norwood, MA	Bacteria can appear as tiny round or rod-shaped objects. Rod-shaped bacteria are generally easier to see because round bacteria may appear as amorphous, or shapeless, material. Bacteria often seem to be shaking or vibrating. This is called Brownian movement and is caused by the molecules of water bumping against the bacteria. Bacteria can be very active, actually moving across the microscopic field. If many bacteria are seen and the specimen is not an obviously contaminated specimen, the indication is usually a UTI. Bacteria can be reported as few, moderate, or many. If both rod-shaped and round bacteria are seen in the same specimen, they may be reported as mixed bacteria. Mixed bacteria may indicate a contaminated specimen. The provider will consider the patient's symptoms in addition to the results of the urinalysis to make a diagnosis and will often order a C&S of the urine.

(continues)

Element	Description
Yeast Bayer Healthcare Diagnostic Division, Norwood, MA	Yeast cells may be present in urine, possibly indicating a yeast infection in the urinary tract. Yeast cells are smaller than red blood cells but may appear similar to them. Yeasts are round and can be observed to be budding. To distinguish between yeast and red blood cells, a drop of dilute acetic acid is added to the urine sediment. The acetic acid will cause the red blood cells to hemolyze, making the yeast more easily viewed. The most common yeast found is *Candida albicans.* Yeasts are reported as the amount per HPF.
Parasites Bayer Healthcare Diagnostic Division, Norwood, MA	The most frequently seen parasite in urine is *Trichomonas vaginalis. Trichomonas* is a parasite that can infect the urinary tract and is often recognized by the movement of its tail (flagella). Always check with a provider or someone more familiar with these organisms before reporting the specimen as positive for *Trichomonas.*
Sperm Bayer Healthcare Diagnostic Division, Norwood, MA	Sperm is reported when seen in male and female urine. Normal sperm have oval bodies with one long, thin flagella.
Artifacts **Starch granules** Bayer Healthcare Diagnostic Division, Norwood, MA **Cotton fibers** Bayer Healthcare Diagnostic Division, Norwood, MA	Hair, fibers, powder, and oil are among the substances that may appear in urine sediment as a result of contamination during collection or later. If a structure cannot be identified using a good urine atlas, it probably is an artifact. A urine atlas will show illustrations of artifacts. If in doubt, get an expert opinion.

(continues)

Element	Description
Crystals in Urinary Sediment	
Triple phosphate *Bayer Healthcare Diagnostic Division, Norwood, MA*	This is a normal, colorless crystal. It is found in neutral alkaline urine.
Calcium oxalate *Bayer Healthcare Diagnostic Division, Norwood, MA*	This is a normal crustal made up of colorless squares with an "X" shape in the center. It is seen in renal calculi and foods high in oxalic acid.
Ammonium biurate *Bayer Healthcare Diagnostic Division, Norwood, MA*	This is a normal, yellow-brown crystal. It is seen in old specimens and ammonia produced by bacteria.
Casts in Urinary Sediment	
Hyaline *Bayer Healthcare Diagnostic Division, Norwood, MA*	Rare hyaline casts can be seen in normal urine but increase with any kidney disease. They can also be seen as a result of fever, emotional stress, or strenuous exercise. Hyaline casts are nearly transparent and can be difficult to see under the microscope without some light adjustment.
Granular *Bayer Healthcare Diagnostic Division, Norwood, MA*	Granular casts contain remnants of disintegrated cells that appear as fine or coarse granules.

(continues)

Element	Description
Cellular 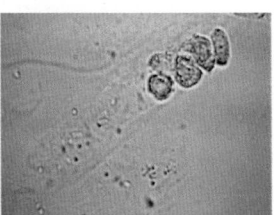 Bayer Healthcare Diagnostic Division, Norwood, MA	Cellular casts may contain epithelial cells, red blood cells, or white blood cells.

Sometimes yeast or *Trichomonas vaginalis* parasites are seen in pathological conditions. Yeast cells look a lot like RBCs but are smaller and can often be seen to be "budding" or separating. *Trichomonas* is often recognized by the movement of its tail (flagella). There may also be oil droplets, hair, cotton fibers, and **amorphous** (shapeless) and other incidental materials that are of no clinical concern. Bacteria in urine will often be very active, shaking or vibrating across the microscopic field. This is called Brownian movement and is caused by the molecules of water bumping against the bacteria. Sperm may be seen, especially in male urine. Sperm have oval bodies with one long, thin flagella.

Urine **crystals**, caused by concentrations of various elements, are interesting and attractive but may either be incidental, due to medication, or indicative of a kidney disease or condition.

Urinary **casts** are formed when protein accumulates and precipitates in the kidney tubules and are then washed into the urine. They are cylindrical with rounded or flat ends and are classified according to the substances inside them.

PROCEDURE 41-4
Performing a Complete Urinalysis

Procedure

STANDARD PRECAUTIONS:

 Handwashing
 Gloves
 Biohazard
 Goggles & Mask
 Gown

PURPOSE:

To perform a complete urinalysis, including the physical, chemical, and microscopic examination within 30 minutes of obtaining the specimen.

EQUIPMENT/SUPPLIES:

- Gloves
- Permanent marker
- Urine specimen
- Refractometer
- Reagent test strips and color chart
- Urine test tubes
- Centrifuge
- Microscope
- Microscope slides
- Coverslips
- Disposable pipettes

(continues)

- Sedi-Stain (optional)
- Urine atlas
- Urine atlas guide
- Urinalysis report form

- Biohazard container
- Sharps container
- Disinfectant cleaner

PROCEDURE STEPS:

1. Wash hands and put on gloves. RATIONALE: Washing hands before any laboratory process prevents contamination of the specimen. Gloving provides personal protection.

2. Assemble equipment and supplies. RATIONALE: Organizing your work area prevents confusion and error caused by missing supplies.

3. Follow all safety guidelines, being careful not to splash the urine specimen. Wipe up all spills immediately with disinfectant cleaner. RATIONALE: Preventing splashes and spills will prevent exposure to biohazard substances. Cleaning any spill immediately prevents further contamination and risk for exposure.

4. Examine the specimen for proper labeling, ***paying attention to detail.*** The specimen should be labeled on the cup, not the lid. RATIONALE: If the specimen is not labeled, the identity of the patient is unknown. The specimen should be labeled on the cup rather than the lid, because the lid can be removed from the specimen and mixed up with other lids.

5. Ensure the lid is securely tightened and mix the urine thoroughly. RATIONALE: Securing the lid will prevent leaking of urine while mixing. Mixing the specimen will suspend all particles and cellular components in the specimen so that the urine that is poured into the centrifuge tube contains a good sampling of the specimen.

Physical Analysis of Urine

6. Measure and note the amount of urine in the specimen if it is less than 10 mL. The amount of the specimen does not have to be noted if it is more than 10 mL. RATIONALE: If the sample is less than 10 mL, it is considered less than the default amount for testing. If a sample is less than the default quantity, the amount should be noted on the report. If the quantity is too small to perform the test ordered, the report should be marked as "QNS" (quantity not sufficient).

7. Visually assess the urine color, preferably against a light background, and note the color. RATIONALE: Urine color names should come only from accepted color descriptors, not from arbitrary names.

8. Assess the clarity of the urine by holding the urine tube against a white background with good lighting and observe it for cloudiness. Determine if it is clear, slightly cloudy, cloudy, or very cloudy/turbid. RATIONALE: The clarity of the urine is useful in predicting the presence of contaminants such as skin cells, mucus, and other debris.

9. Measure and record the specific gravity using the preferred method (Procedure 41-3). RATIONALE: The specific gravity is a way to determine the concentration of dissolved particles within the sample and is part of the physical examination of urine.

Chemical Analysis of Urine

10. Prior to performing the chemical analysis, label a urine centrifuge tube with the patient's name and pour 10 mL into the tube for the microscopic examination. Set aside in the centrifuge. RATIONALE: Setting this aliquot aside ensures that it is not contaminated by the chemicals of the test strips or the process of the chemical examination.

11. Select the appropriate reagent test strips and read and follow the manufacturer's instructions. RATIONALE: Each manufacturer will provide specific instructions related to their product. Even manufacturers whose test strips you are already familiar with could change their instructions. The package insert should be read carefully every time a new package is used.

12. Remove a test strip from the container and replace the cap tightly. RATIONALE: Strips are adversely affected by light and moisture and should always be kept sterile in the original container with the lid securely on.

(continues)

13. Immerse the test strip completely in the well-mixed urine and remove it immediately (Figure 41-14A). While removing the test strip from the cup, tap it gently onto a paper towel to remove excess urine (Figure 41-14B). RATIONALE: Removing the excess urine prevents the specimen from cross-contamination of adjacent chemical pads on the strip, which can cause inaccurate results.

14. Properly time the test for each test pad. RATIONALE: Proper timing is essential for accurate results. The manufacturer's instructions will clearly list the proper time for each test.

15. Holding the test strip close to the container (or chart) but not touching it, compare the color of the pads on the test strip with the color guides on the container (or chart) (Figure 41-14C). RATIONALE: Touching the chart or container with the wet test strip will contaminate the chart/container with urine. If this accidentally happens, be sure to disinfect the surface.

16. Record the results on the urinalysis report form or in the patient's electronic medical record.

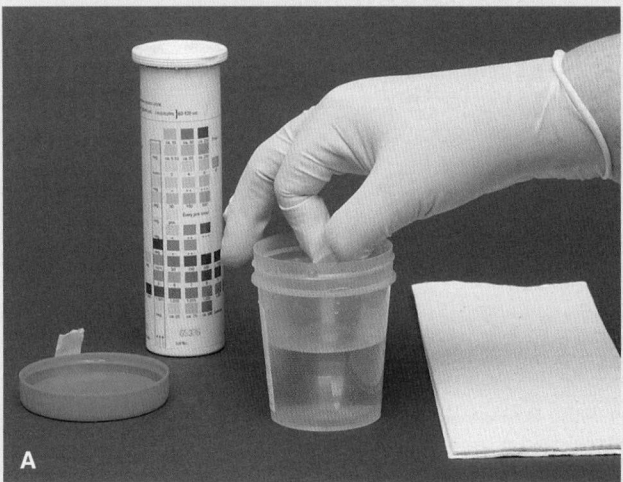

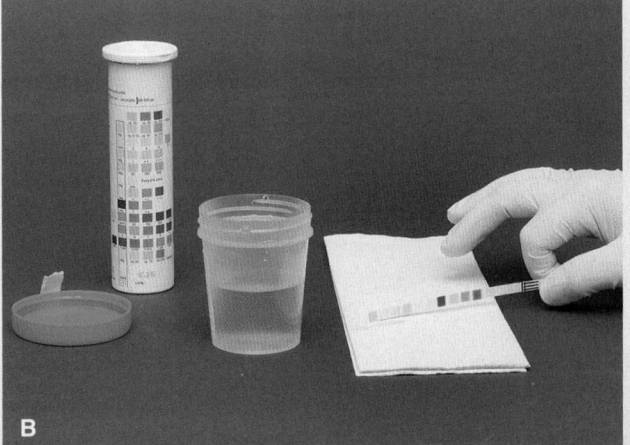
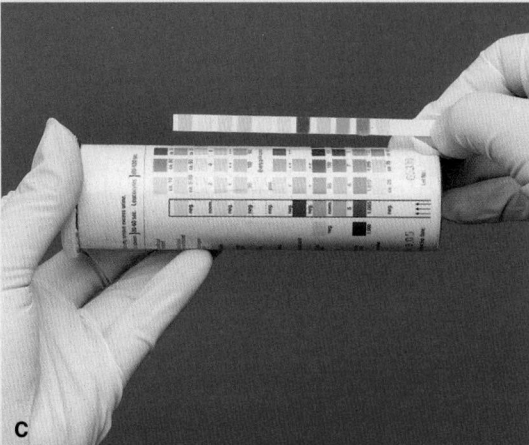

FIGURE 41-14 Performing a chemical examination of urine. (A) Immerse the reagent strip into the urine. (B) Remove the strip and tap it lightly on a paper towel to remove excess urine. (C) Read the strip by matching the color on the strip to the color chart. Take care not to touch the strip onto the color chart.

(continues)

Microscopic Examination of Urine

17. Centrifuge 10 mL of urine at 1,500 g (revolutions per minute) for 5 minutes. Be sure to balance the centrifuge and securely close and lock the lid. RATIONALE: Centrifugation forces the sediment to the bottom of the tube. Balancing and locking the lid ensures safety during centrifugation.

18. After centrifugation, pour off the supernatant, leaving about 1 mL in the bottom of the tube. Add two drops of Sedi-Stain if desired. Remix the sediment by tapping gently on the counter or with your fingernail. RATIONALE: The test will be performed on the sediment only so the excess supernatant is not needed. Sedi-Stain colors the cells and other elements for easier viewing.

19. Place a drop of the well-mixed sediment onto a clean microscope slide. Cover with a coverslip by holding the coverslip at an angle to the drop, bringing the edge close to the drop until the urine spreads along the edge of the coverslip, and then gently lower the coverslip onto the drop. Keep the tube. RATIONALE: Using this technique to place the coverslip onto the specimen will prevent air pockets from forming. Keep the tube in the event that a fresh slide needs to be prepared.

20. Place the slide onto the microscope stage but do not leave the light on. RATIONALE: Do not leave the light on because this will heat the slide and destroy the specimen.

21. Alert the provider that the slide is ready for viewing. RATIONALE: The microscopic examination is considered by CLIA to be in the moderately complex test category of PPMP. *Working within your scope of practice,* you are encouraged to view and discuss the microscopic examination with the provider as part of your professional development and continuing education. If you do view the slide before the provider views it, do not leave the light on. If the slide dries before the provider can view it, prepare a fresh slide.

22. **NOTE:** The following steps are included so the medical assistant can learn to examine urine microscopically even though the provider must perform the actual assessment.

    a. When examining urine sediment, it is important to keep the light subdued by lowering the condenser and to constantly vary the fine focus adjustment to view the structures that are faint. Proper lighting and focus adjustments take a great deal of practice.

    b. Scan the sediment using a 100× (low-power) magnification. A 100× magnification is achieved by using the 10× objective lens (The eyepiece lens [10×] multiplied by the objective lens [10×] equals a 100× magnification).

    c. View 10 to 15 fields and around the edges of the slide for casts. Casts are often forced to the edges. It may be necessary to use the 40× objective (400× magnification) to identify the casts.

    d. Scan the slide using the 40× objective The eyepiece lens (10×) multiplied by the objective lens (40×) equals a magnification of 400× for other cells and formed elements. The count is obtained by averaging the number of each formed element or cell in 10 to 15 visualized fields.

23. After the provider is finished with the specimen and the patient has left the clinic, dispose of the specimen into the toilet or designated sink and all used supplies into appropriate biohazard containers. Disinfect all reusable equipment and all surfaces. Remove gloves and wash hands. RATIONALE: Using appropriate disposal techniques and disinfecting all surfaces according to Standard Precautions safely controls all biohazard substances. Remember that microscopic slides and coverslips are glass and should be placed into an appropriate biohazard sharps container.

24. File the completed laboratory report form into the laboratory section of the patient's chart or electronic medical record and document the procedure.

DOCUMENTATION:

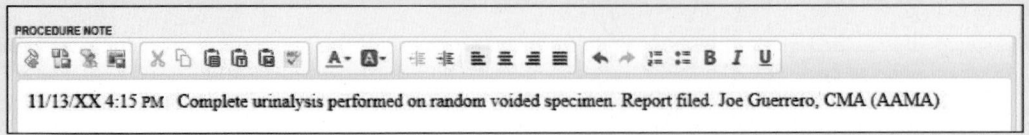

PROCEDURE NOTE

11/13/XX 4:15 PM   Complete urinalysis performed on random voided specimen. Report filed. Joe Guerrero, CMA (AAMA)

Urinalysis Report

When using electronic medical records, test results are entered directly into the patient's medical record on the computer (Figure 41-15). The report will contain the patient's name, the type of urine specimen (voided or catheterized and whether it was a clean-catch midstream specimen), the provider who ordered the urinalysis, the medical assistant performing the physical and chemical portions of the urinalysis, the date and time the specimen was obtained and the date and time it was tested, and the findings.

Patient Name	DOB	Age	Gender	Report Status: **Final**
Morgan, Jane W	**1/22/1955**	**58**	**F**	Reported: **11/11/20XX**
Ordering Provider				Accession:
Winston Lewis				Collected: **7/30/20XX**

Abnormal or Normal	Test	Results	Abnormal Results	Units	Reference Range
Urinalysis dipstick panel in Urine by Automated test strip					
A	**Clarity of Urine**		**Cloudy**		**Clear**
N	Ketones [Mass/volume] in Urine by Automated test strip	Negative			Negative
A	**Nitrite [Presence] in Urine by Automated test strip**		**Positive**		**Negative**
A	**Hemoglobin [Mass/volume] in Urine by Automated test strip**		**Trace**		**None**
N	pH of Urine by Automated test strip	7.5			5.0–9.0
A	**Protein [Mass/volume] in Urine by Automated test strip**		**Trace**		**Negative**
N	Urobilinogen [Mass/volume] in Urine by Automated test strip	Normal			Normal
N	Specific gravity of Urine by Automated test strip	1.030			< 1.030
N	Bilirubin [Mass/volume] in Urine by Automated test strip	Negative			Negative
N	Glucose [Mass/volume] in Urine by Automated test strip	Negative		mg/dL	Negative
N	Color of Urine	Dark Yellow			Yellow

FIGURE 41-15 Urinalysis test results printed from an electronic medical record.

DRUG SCREENING

Testing for drugs is common during job interview processes. Some clinics specialize in occupational health, offering preemployment physicals including drug screening. The actual test might be CLIA-waived, but there are detailed protocols and legal documentations that need to be strictly adhered to. The POL should be certified to perform drug testing, and all clinical personnel should receive special training. A **chain of custody** must take place so that the specimen is guarded against tampering and to guarantee the integrity of the specimen.

Some basic criteria in the chain of custody process are as follows:

- When the patient arrives, he or she must show photo ID, which is copied. The copy is signed.
- The patient signs a consent form for the testing and completes a questionnaire.
- The urine collection cup has a built-in thermometer to ensure the urine is fresh and is at body temperature.
- The patient is asked to leave coats and bags with the clinic personnel, and these items should be secured.
- The bathroom and patient are inspected for chemicals and/or urine samples that do not belong to the patient.
- In the case of a legal court-ordered drug test, the collection of the urine is monitored. Monitoring may occur in all drug testing, depending on clinic policy.
- After the sample is collected, the temperature is recorded and the sample is sealed and secured for transport to a testing facility. The patient signs to verify that the sample is his or hers.
- If a CLIA-waived test kit is used in the POL, a test strip is dipped into the urine, and the reagent will react qualitatively (positive, negative, or sometimes inconclusive) for various substances during a specific amount of time. Inconclusive samples must be tested further.

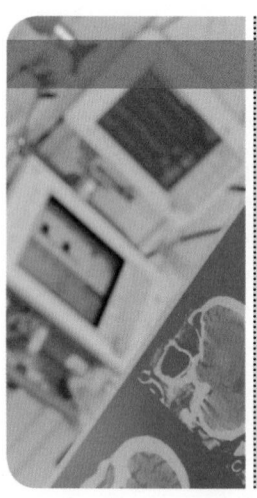

CASE STUDY 41-1

Refer to the scenario at the beginning of the chapter. Gwen is careful to prepare her patient properly so she gets a good sample, she pays attention to the details so that the test is run properly, and she cares about the quality of the results.

CASE STUDY REVIEW

1. What is the worst that can happen if the patient does not give a good clean-catch midstream urine sample?
2. What might happen if the reagents Gwen uses are outdated or have not been stored properly?
3. If Gwen does not care about the quality of the urine tests, how does that reflect on the rest of Gwen's work?

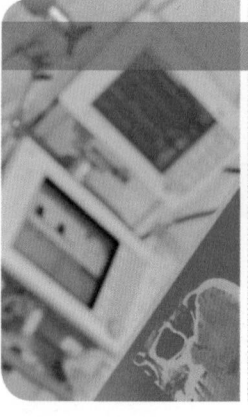

CASE STUDY 41-2

Linda Sterns came to Inner City Health Care today because she is experiencing frequent urination, itching, and burning when urinating. Dr. King ordered a urinalysis, which clinical medical assistant Thomas Myers, CCMA (NHA), is performing. Thomas notes that the urine has a cloudy appearance and the chemical reagent test strip tests positive for nitrites. Thomas confers with Dr. King, who instructs him to prepare a slide for a microscopic examination of the specimen.

CASE STUDY REVIEW

1. Why might Dr. King want to examine this specimen microscopically?
2. How would the findings be reported?

Summary

- Providers order a variety of tests on urine to help them determine or rule out certain abnormalities to make a correct diagnosis and prescribe treatment.

- Urine is formed as blood is filtered through the kidneys. Substances such as by-products of metabolism, mineral excesses, cells, bacteria, parasites, crystals, and casts can be found in the urine during examination.

- Medical assistants need to understand the proper collection techniques for urine specimens in order to instruct patients on the proper collection procedures.

- It is important for the medical assistant to understand and adhere to the quality control and safety guidelines involved with collecting and handling specimens, preservatives, and reagents.

- Medical assistants perform the physical and chemical examination of urine and prepare the urine sample for the provider to perform the microscopic examination.

- Medical assistants are trained in the performance of all phases of the urinalysis.

- Medical assistants must always project a professional image and be able to use appropriate communication and active listening skills when providing care to patients.

Study for Success

To reinforce your knowledge and skills of information presented in this chapter:

- Review the *Key Terms* and *Learning Outcomes*
- Consider the *Critical Thinking* features and *Case Studies* and discuss your conclusions
- Answer the questions in the *Certification Review*

Procedure

- Perform the *Procedures* using the *Competency Assessment Checklists* on the *Student Companion Website*

CERTIFICATION REVIEW

1. What three processes are involved in the formation of urine?
   a. Filtration, suspension, absorption
   b. Secretion, absorption, formation
   c. Filtration, formation, secretion
   d. Filtration, secretion, reabsorption

2. What are the three basic parts of a typical urine examination?
   a. Volumetric, chemical, macroscopic
   b. Pathologic, chemical, confirmatory
   c. Physical, chemical, microscopic
   d. Random, 24-hour, catheterized
   e. Clean-catch, midstream, random

3. What is the specimen of choice for routine urinalysis?
   a. Sterile
   b. Clean-catch
   c. Catheterized
   d. Timed

4. A patient with diabetes will normally have an excess of what substance in the urine?
   a. Hemoglobin
   b. Glucose
   c. Insulin
   d. Sodium
   e. Protein

5. What is the most common way of doing a chemical analysis of urine in a provider's office?
   a. Reagent test strip
   b. Microscopic examination
   c. Culture test
   d. Urinometer

6. Which substance or structure is automatically considered abnormal when found in urine?
   a. Phosphates
   b. Urea
   c. Blood
   d. Salt
   e. Crystals

7. What safety guideline is important to follow during a routine urinalysis?
   a. Use the same pipette for all patients' urine samples
   b. Allow urine to sit at room temperature to ferment the urine properties
   c. Once tested, urine can be disposed of by the janitorial service
   d. Treat all specimens as if they were infectious
8. Which casts are considered fairly normal in urine?
   a. Hyaline
   b. Red blood cell
   c. White blood cell
   d. Bacterial
   e. Tubular
9. Specific gravity of urine can be measured using which of the following?
   a. Urinometer
   b. Refractometer
   c. Chemical reagent strip
   d. All of these
10. If a urine specimen is labeled "QNS," what does it refer to?
    a. Quality not sufficient
    b. Quality not specific
    c. Quantity not sufficient
    d. Quantity not specific
    e. Quantity not specified

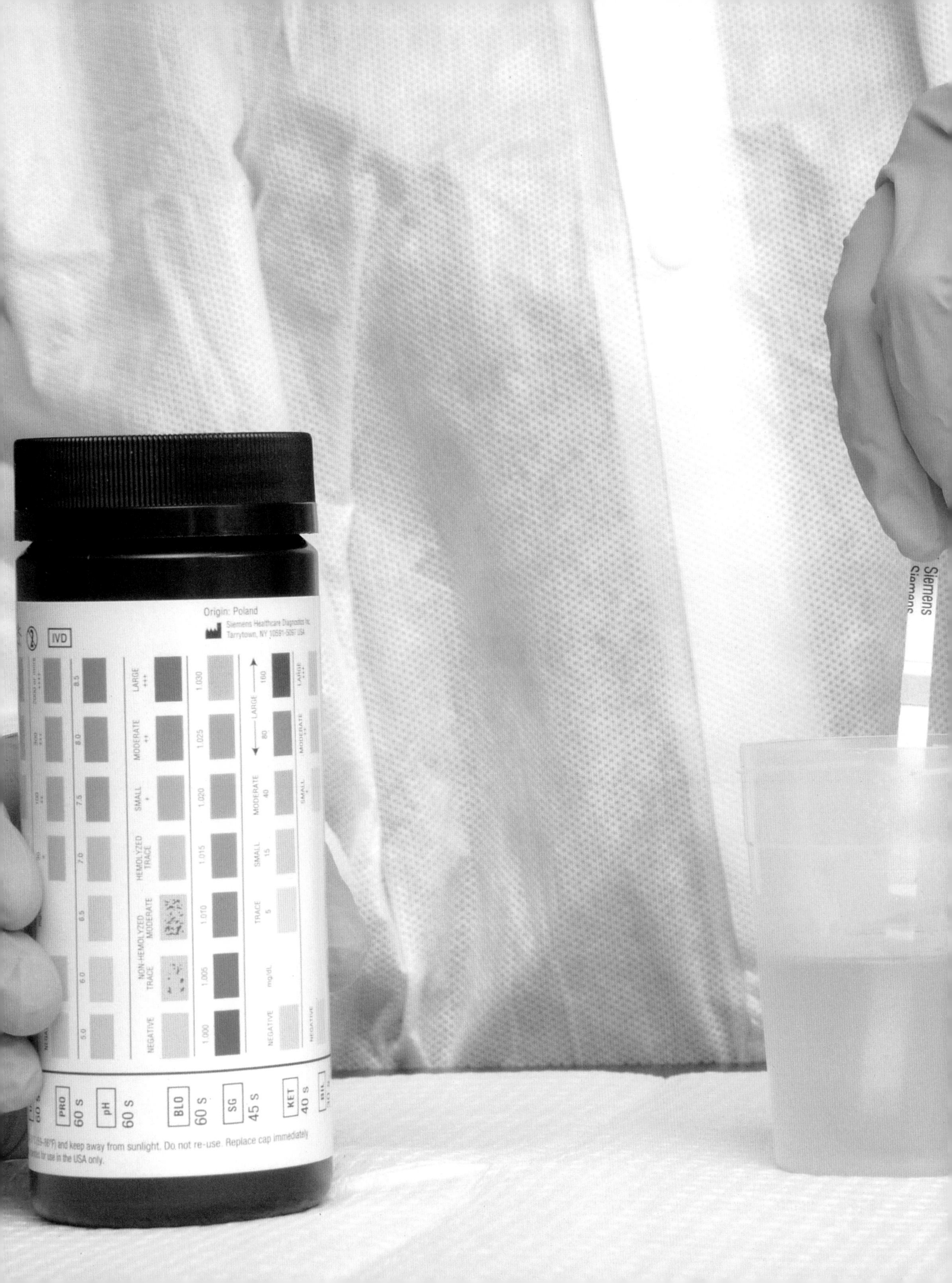
Origin: Poland
Siemens Healthcare Diagnostics Inc.
Tarrytown, NY 10591-5097 USA
IVD
PRO
60 s
pH
60 s
BLO
60 s
SG
45 s
KET
40 s
and keep away from sunlight. Do not re-use. Replace cap immediately
Siemens

CHAPTER 42

Basic Microbiology

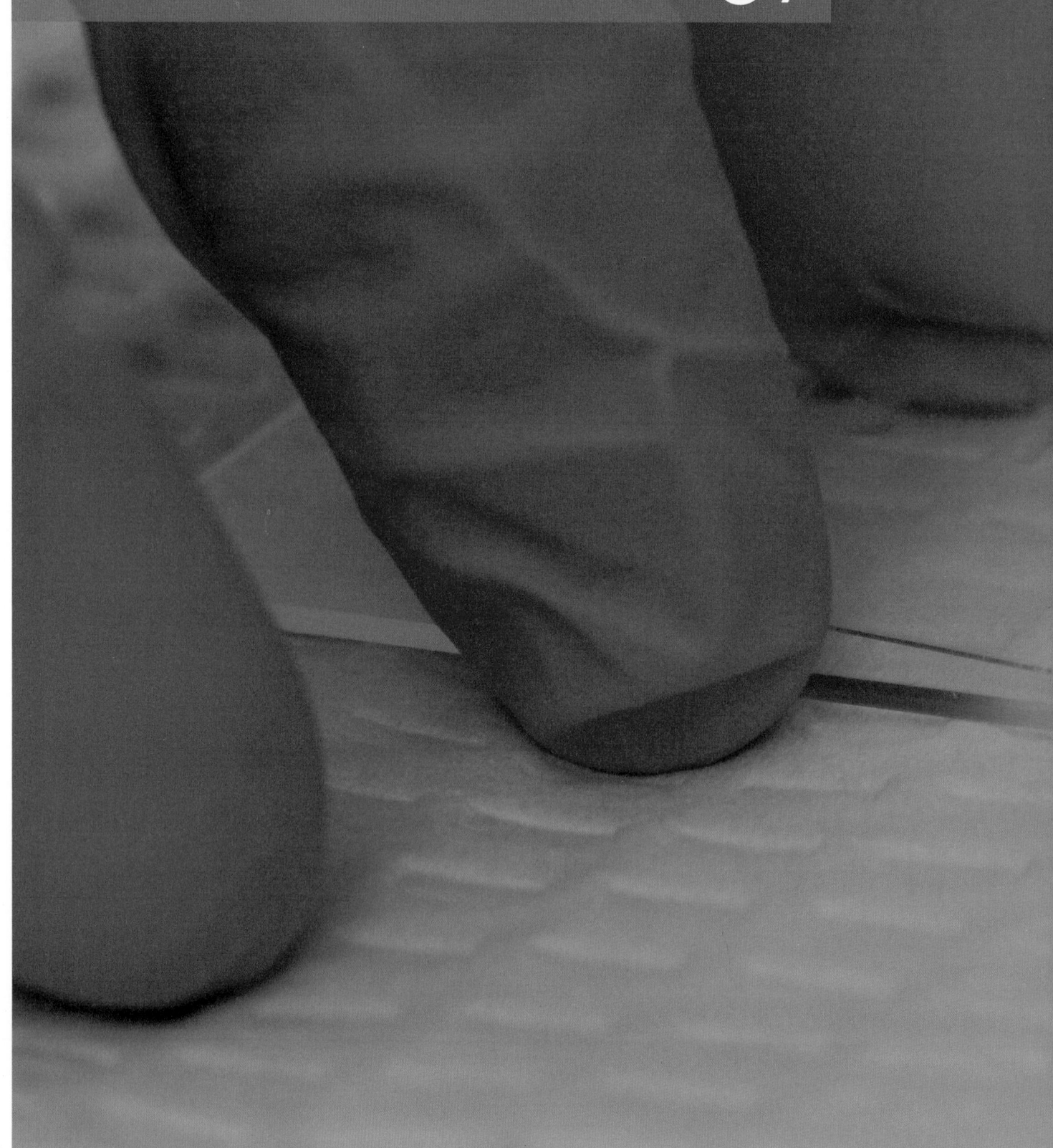

1. Define and spell the key terms as presented in the glossary.
2. Identify the most common microbiology laboratory equipment and state their uses within the microbiology laboratory.
3. Discuss the importance of safety procedures and quality control when working with microbiologic specimens.
4. Display sensitivity to the patient's rights and feelings in collecting specimens.
5. Explain foodborne illnesses, preventative measures, symptoms, and treatments.
6. Compare and contrast bacteria, viruses, fungi, and parasites.
7. Explain the types of microbiology specimens collected in the POL and how they are collected.
8. Describe the medical assistant's scope of practice within microbiology laboratory procedures.
9. Explain the concept of staining slides to microscopically observe microorganisms.
10. Discuss the purpose and advantages of wet mount and KOH slides.
11. Demonstrate inoculating culture specimens to media plates.
12. Describe the significance of sensitivity testing.
13. Identify two parasites and two fungi that can be observed in the POL and the disease conditions that they cause.

KEY TERMS

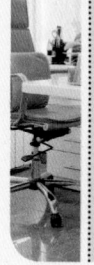

aerobic	incubate	potassium hydroxide (KOH)
aerosols	inoculate	species
agar	morphology	spores
anaerobic	mycology	virology
broth tubes	nomenclature	wet mount
expectorate	normal flora	Wood's lamp
genus	nosocomial	
Gram stain	ova	

SCENARIO

To aid in diagnosing and treating patients, the providers at Inner City Health Care order tests to identify disease-causing bacteria, fungi, viruses, and parasites. Some of these tests, such as the quick tests for group A *Streptococcus,* are performed in the office laboratory, whereas other tests are sent to a reference laboratory. Regardless of where the test will be performed, medical assistant Joe Guerrero, CMA (AAMA), follows all safety precautions when handling specimens. He checks the test manufacturer's or laboratory's procedures and carefully completes each step. By following all safety guidelines and test procedures, Joe ensures his and others' safety. He also obtains a high-quality specimen for testing.

The word *microbiology* comes from the Greek words *micro* ("small") and *bios* ("living"). The field of medical microbiology includes the study of pathogenic organisms such as bacteria, viruses, fungi, and parasites (Figure 42-1). This chapter discusses processes for obtaining specimens, allowing the pathogen to **incubate** (or grow) in culture media for identification, diagnosing disease, and treating disease.

Although most microbiology testing is complicated and usually performed in regional and larger laboratories, many CLIA-waived test kits are being developed to allow for quicker diagnosis and treatments. As more waived tests become available and the role of the medical assistant expands, you must develop even more skill in accurately obtaining specimens and properly processing those specimens by following testing protocol exactly.

Since communicable diseases are caused by pathogenic microorganisms, safety while working with them in the laboratory is crucial. Following Standard Precautions when working with any body fluid is mandatory.

THE MEDICAL ASSISTANT'S ROLE IN THE MICROBIOLOGY LABORATORY

The role of the medical assistant in microbiology within the physicians' office laboratory (POL) is to obtain specimens, test specimens within the Clinical Laboratory Improvement Act (CLIA)–waived category, prepare slides for microscopic examination by the provider, and prepare cultures as required for transport to an outside laboratory.

We, as medical assistants, must be careful to ensure that the specimen for culture was taken with sterile supplies, handled properly, prepared as required, and delivered to the outside testing laboratory within the optimum timeframe.

Many quick and simple to perform CLIA-waived test kits are currently available to test for microbiologic pathogens. The test kits, although designed to be less complicated than most laboratory methods, still require attention to detail for accurate results.

MICROBIOLOGY

All living forms are alike in that their cells contain a nuclear material referred to as DNA (deoxyribonucleic acid), which carries special genetic information. All microorganisms have certain growth requirements and all are able to reproduce themselves except the virus, which needs to invade a living host cell in order to reproduce. **Virology** (the study of viruses), bacteriology, parasitology, and **mycology** (the study of fungi) (see Figure 42-1) are all discussed later in this chapter as well as in Chapter 21.

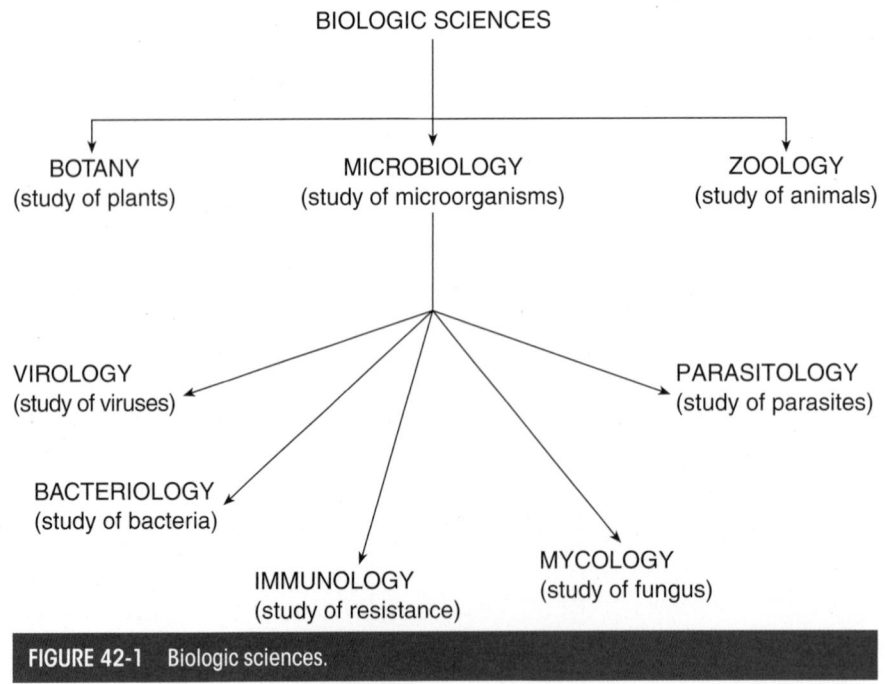

BIOLOGIC SCIENCES

BOTANY
(study of plants)

MICROBIOLOGY
(study of microorganisms)

ZOOLOGY
(study of animals)

VIROLOGY
(study of viruses)

PARASITOLOGY
(study of parasites)

BACTERIOLOGY
(study of bacteria)

IMMUNOLOGY
(study of resistance)

MYCOLOGY
(study of fungus)

FIGURE 42-1 Biologic sciences.

EQUIPMENT

Basic equipment needed in a microbiology department of a clinic or a POL varies depending on the size of the facility and the tests performed. Most POLs have the following equipment.

Autoclave

An autoclave (Figure 42-2) is used in the POL to sterilize instruments that may have been contaminated while processing specimens. It can also be used to sterilize contaminated materials prior to disposal. The setting of 15 PSI (pounds per square inch) and a temperature of 121°C for 15 to 20 minutes is sufficient to kill infectious agents, spores, viruses, and contaminants. Many laboratories use presterilized and disposable instruments but still use autoclaves for killing pathogenic specimens prior to disposal. (See Chapters 21 and 30 for more information on operation of the autoclave and its uses.)

Microscope

An important piece of equipment for the POL or clinic is the microscope. This instrument is used to view organisms that cannot be seen with the naked eye on a prepared slide. Skill in using the microscope is necessary to gain information from studying the slide. The microscope is a delicate instrument and should be cared for properly as stated by the manufacturer (see Chapter 38 for more information on the use and care of the microscope).

Safety Hood

Safety

Aerosols are airborne particles that can be released into the air when culturing. They are potentially dangerous if inhaled. Some laboratories, especially if aerosols are used,

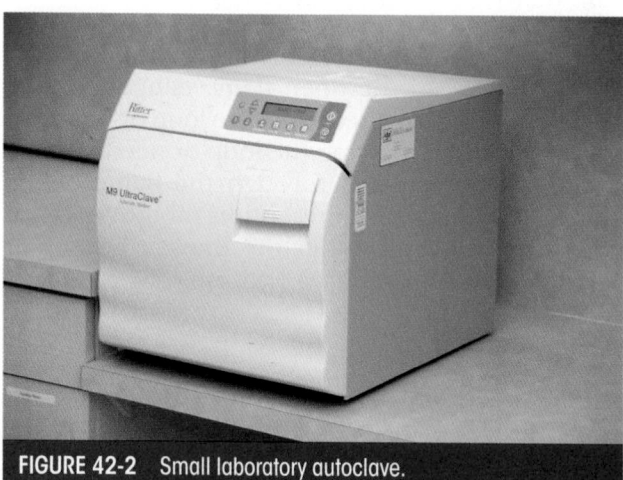

FIGURE 42-2 Small laboratory autoclave.

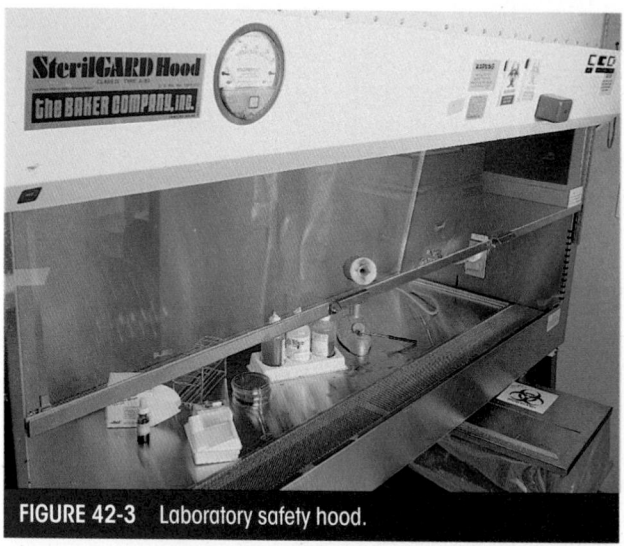

FIGURE 42-3 Laboratory safety hood.

will have a safety hood (Figure 42-3). By using the safety hood, the health care worker is separated from the specimen by a glass in front of the face, with fumes and aerosols suctioned into the hood. The use of a safety hood is mandatory when performing a culture on a specimen with a potential aerosol. Aerosols are particularly dangerous in fungus cultures. It is a good idea to use the safety hood with foul-smelling specimens to minimize odors. Tuberculosis is an example of a disease caused by bacteria that travel by aerosol from person to person.

Incubator

The incubator is an apparatus that can maintain a constant temperature of 35 to 37°C. Most organisms, whether **aerobic** (grows well in oxygen) or **anaerobic** (will not grow well or at all in oxygen), grow at these temperatures. Some bacteria grow best at lower temperatures and some bacteria require a higher temperature for optimum growth. Temperature requirements must be met for adequate growth. (Refer to Chapter 21 for growth requirements of microorganisms.)

Anaerobic Equipment

Certain types of cultures, such as deep-wound cultures, could contain anaerobic (requiring an oxygen-free environment) pathogens. To grow anaerobic bacteria, the absence of oxygen is achieved by using something as simple as a candle jar (Figure 42-4) into which the inoculated petri dish is placed with a lighted candle. When the airtight cover is put on the jar, the burning of the candle will use up the available oxygen and generate carbon dioxide, creating the anaerobic environment. Organisms such as *Neisseria*

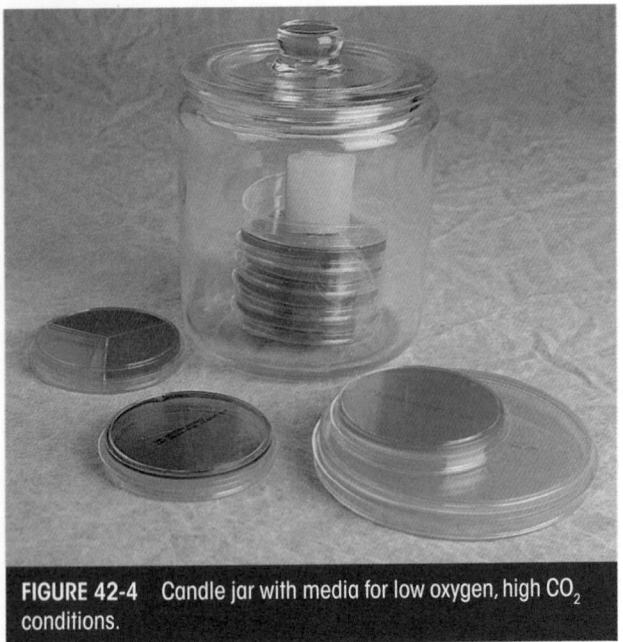

FIGURE 42-4 Candle jar with media for low oxygen, high CO_2 conditions.

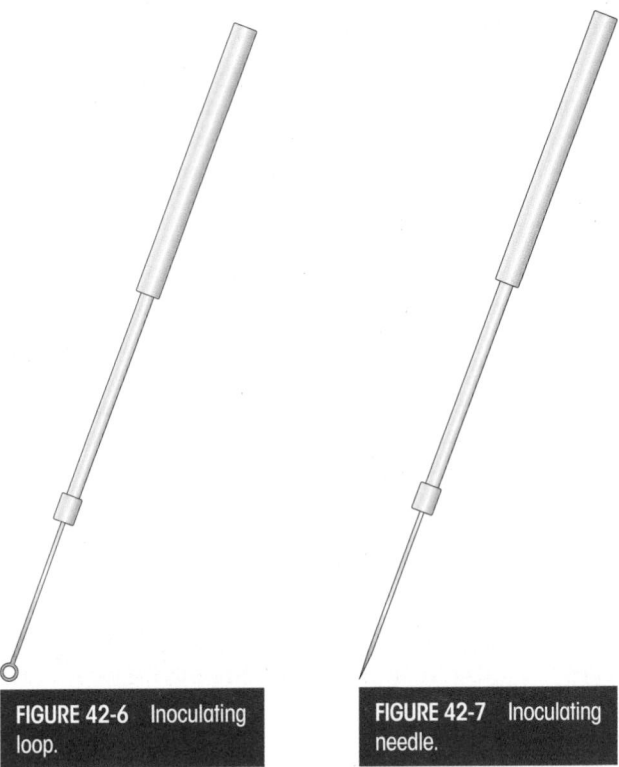

FIGURE 42-6 Inoculating loop.

FIGURE 42-7 Inoculating needle.

gonorrhoeae, which causes gonorrhea, need a high carbon dioxide atmosphere to survive.

Another method of maintaining an anaerobic condition is a specialized jar called a gas pack jar (Figure 42-5). This jar contains a foil pack that, when activated, gives off carbon dioxide, decreasing the oxygen in the jar.

Inoculating Equipment

An *inoculating loop* (Figure 42-6) is a piece of wire with a rounded end and a handle at the other end. An *inoculating needle* (Figure 42-7) is similar to the loop but has a straight end. Both the loop and the needle are used to **inoculate** (introduce) organisms onto a culture medium in a plate or broth. The loop is usually preferred when inoculating liquid onto the surface of a culture media and the needle is used for a deep "stab" inoculation of more solid bacteria colonies. If it is made of wire, the loop or needle can be heated to sterilize it before and after use. As an alternative, sterile plastic disposable loops or needles can be used. These are for one-time use and are disposed of in the biohazard waste container.

Incinerator

Incineration is the quickest method of sterilizing the inoculating loop and needle. This can be accomplished by using an electrical incinerator (Figure 42-8) or a Bunsen burner (less popular today because of the open flame danger). Sterilization before and after using the loop or needle is accomplished by placing the loop or needle in the incinerator or passing through the flame of the Bunsen burner. Extreme caution should be taken when working with either the Bunsen burner or incinerator to avoid burns or fires.

Culture Media

In the microbiology laboratory the term *media* refers to a host of substances used to foster the growth of bacteria (Figure 42-9). Culture media is explained in detail later in this chapter.

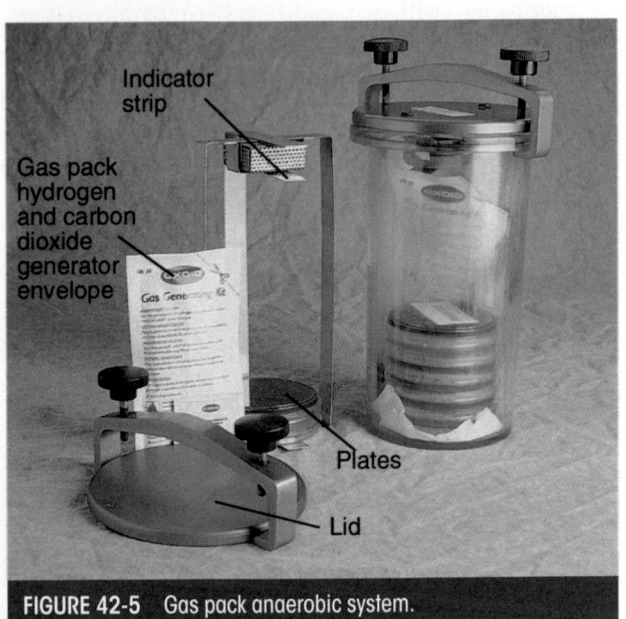

Indicator strip

Gas pack hydrogen and carbon dioxide generator envelope

Plates

Lid

FIGURE 42-5 Gas pack anaerobic system.

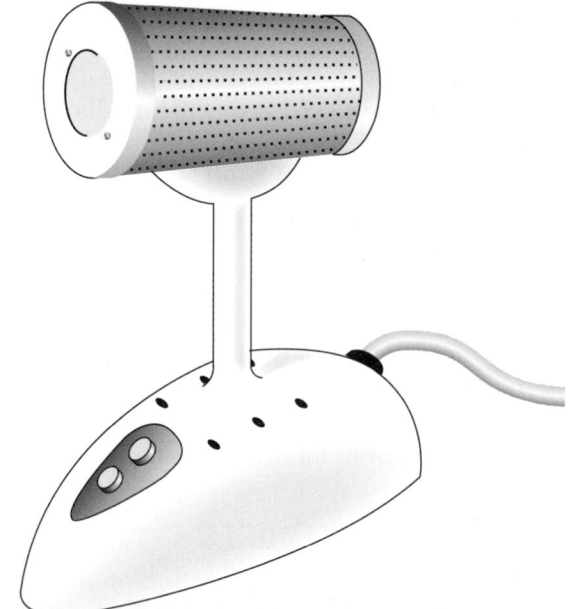

FIGURE 42-8 Electric incinerator.

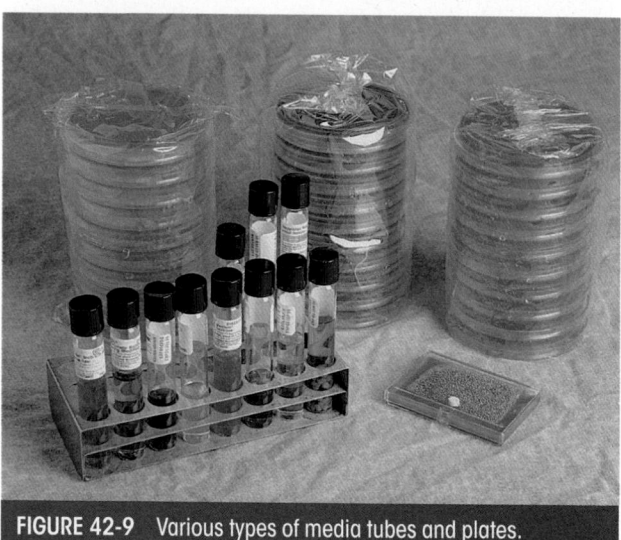

FIGURE 42-9 Various types of media tubes and plates.

Refrigerator

A refrigerator is needed in the POL to store certain materials, such as media and testing kits that need a temperature of 2 to 8°C. Food and drink should never be stored in the refrigerator with any specimens, kits, or media.

SAFETY WHEN HANDLING MICROBIOLOGY SPECIMENS

Safety

Safety should be practiced in every area of the clinical laboratory at all times. Microbiology specimens can be especially dangerous because of potential pathogens, so

following safety rules will reduce danger to all clinical and laboratory personnel. There is never any eating, smoking, drinking, or putting objects into the mouth while working with microbiology specimens or in the laboratory area itself. Eyes, noses, and mouths should not be touched. The practice of washing hands several times a day should become a habit. Some important safety measures are discussed in this section, with more detailed discussions in Chapters 21 and 37.

Personal Protective Equipment

Personal protective equipment (PPE) such as a buttoned laboratory coat or apron, safety goggles, and gloves, should be worn at all times when processing microbiology specimens, and all PPE should be removed when leaving the work area. At times, personnel performing microbiology testing will work behind a shield to avoid splashes and spatters of blood and body fluids, and use a safety fume hood to avoid inhalation of aerosol pathogens.

Standard Precautions must be strictly adhered to while obtaining and processing specimens and everyone handling specimens (including couriers, receptionists, and laboratory assistants) should wear gloves to protect themselves from leakage of the container and contamination with a pathogenic organism.

Work Area

The counters where specimens are processed and set up should be cleaned with a strong germicide before and after daily use and immediately after a spill. Pathogens could be present where microbiology specimens are cultivated. This area should be dust free and clean at all times. Care should be taken to maintain a clean and uncluttered work area.

Specimen Handling

Sometimes patients will bring microbiology specimens to the POL or clinic to be processed, so the medical assistant should look for leaks and contamination on the outside of the transporting containers. It is a good practice always to wear gloves when receiving specimens. Most specimens will arrive in a plastic bag to avoid danger to laboratory personnel. When sending specimens to an outside laboratory to be processed, it is important to use the appropriate container to avoid contamination. All specimens should be handled as if they were contaminated with pathogens. See Chapter 21 for more information on Standard Precautions.

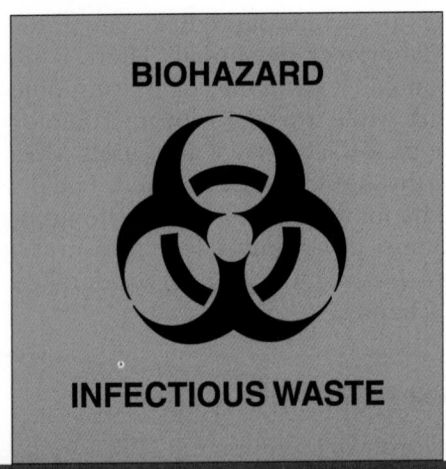

FIGURE 42-10 Biohazard symbol.

Disposal of Waste and Spills

Facilities are required to have a written plan for disposal of dangerous biohazard waste and that plan should be strictly followed. Biohazard waste generally is placed in red bags marked with the universal biohazard symbol (Figure 42-10). Most clinics and POLs employ an outside agency to dispose of waste. It is extremely important that biohazard waste is not placed with regular waste and disposal guidelines are followed according to federal and state guidelines.

If a spill should occur, follow the agency's or employer's rules for cleanup and disposal. Generally, a 5% phenol or a 10% bleach solution can be used effectively.

QUALITY CONTROL

Although quality control is practiced in all areas of the clinical laboratory, the microbiology department has equipment, media, and reagents that need quality-control checks with almost every test. The following list details some measures that are a part of a quality-control program in microbiology:

- All equipment with temperature controls should be monitored daily.
- The microscopes should be cleaned and kept dust free.
- Testing for microorganism identification is often accomplished with the use of a special kit. When using kits for different tests, the positive and negative controls must be run at all times. Before use, the expiration date should be checked.

- Media of all types should not be used past the shelf life and should be stored at the proper temperatures. Your POL should have a list of which bacteria to use on specific media for optimum growth. This list can be found in your laboratory manual.
- The laboratory manual should be updated periodically.
- All chemicals or reagents with Safety Data Sheets (SDSs) should be available to reference when working with a chemical that is not familiar to you.
- All quality control testing should be documented in proper laboratory logs.

COLLECTION PROCEDURES

When a provider needs identification of an organism that is causing an infection, he or she orders a culture from that site. The culture specimen should be collected properly and delivered within a reasonable period. The results of the culture will depend on the quality of the original specimen. All specimens obtained for identification of infectious organisms must be taken from the site of the infection, not the surrounding area.

Once the specimen is collected correctly, it should be placed in the appropriate container and delivered to the laboratory soon after collection. Many organisms will die if not kept moist. Transport media can have a moistening agent to keep the specimen from drying out.

If a specimen comes into the laboratory in an improper container or has not been delivered within a reasonable period soon after collection, it must be rejected and another specimen obtained. The container in which the specimen has been placed should be sterile, and the right type should be used for a specific culture. Sterile containers are used for most collections, with the exception of stool collection containers, which do not have to be sterile. The culturette swab system is a self-contained plastic tube with a sterile swab used to collect the specimen. The swab is then placed back into the tube. The tube contains a medium that keeps the swab moist and preserves the specimen for testing (Figure 42-11).

The laboratory's success in isolating the causative pathogens depends on the following factors:

1. Proper collection from infection site
2. Collection of specimen during infectious period
3. Sufficient amount of specimen
4. Appropriate specimen container

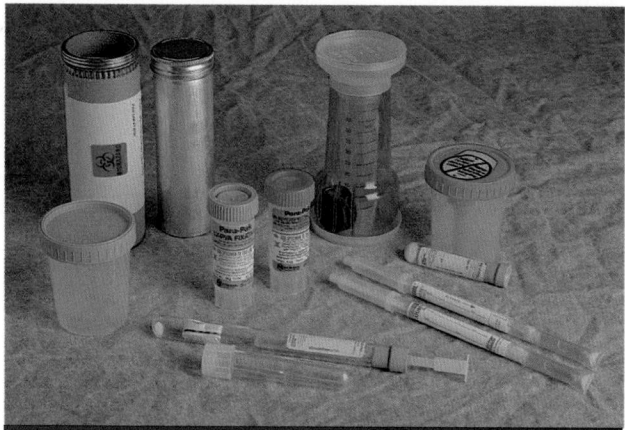

FIGURE 42-11 Various collection and transport containers for bacteriologic specimens.

Urine Cultures

Patients should be instructed to obtain a clean-catch urine specimen in a sterile container. A clean-catch midstream specimen is obtained by first cleaning the genital area and then urinating midstream into a specimen container. Details of this procedure are found in Chapter 41, Procedure 41-1. Patients should be given clear instructions so that a quality specimen for culturing can be obtained.

Sometimes a urinary catheterization is done to collect a sterile urine specimen for culture. Sterile technique is followed and the urine is collected into a sterile container. (See Chapter 29 for more information on urinary catheterization.)

Throat Cultures

Procedure

When taking a throat specimen for culture, explain to the patient that a throat culture is necessary to identify certain organisms. Be sure to tell the patient that there may be some momentary discomfort in obtaining the specimen, especially if his or her throat is sore. Answer all questions about the process of obtaining the specimen. Throat culture specimens are taken using the culturette swab. As mentioned in the previous section, the culturette contains a sterile swab and growth medium for moisture to keep the bacteria viable (see Procedure 42-1).

5. Appropriate transport medium or inoculation onto proper media and placement in correct atmosphere to ensure growth
6. Specimen labeled properly
7. Specimen delivered to the laboratory in a minimal amount of time
8. Specimen collected before the administration of antibiotics

Competency

When collecting specimens, it is important that the medical assistant carefully follow the instructions as designated in the laboratory manual.

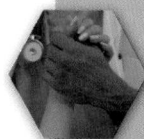

Patient Education

As you obtain throat cultures from patients, you may want to give them some helpful advice concerning their condition. Generally, when a person has a sore throat, it is associated with other respiratory symptoms as well. The following suggestions may provide some relief from discomfort and help patients toward better health.

1. Advise patients to drink plenty of liquids, especially water, and to eat sensibly from the basic food groups.

2. Urge patients to get extra rest and dress comfortably (according to the weather/temperature outside).

3. Suggest use of gargles or throat lozenges (or both) to relieve painful sore throat.

4. Remind patients to avoid tobacco/smoking.

5. Instruct patients to cough/sneeze into tissue and discard into proper waste container wherever they are to prevent the spread of microorganisms. Because sewer waste is treated and disinfected, flushing a contaminated tissue is an effective method of disposal.

6. Remind patients to refrain from sharing drinking glasses and tableware and from intimate contact such as kissing while they are infected and still contagious. All eating utensils should be sanitized in hot water after use to avoid the spread of contagious diseases. Perhaps the most important educational advice is reminding patients to wash their hands frequently.

Procedure

Obtaining a Throat Specimen for Culture

STANDARD PRECAUTIONS:

Handwashing

Gloves

Goggles &
Mask

PURPOSE:

To obtain secretions from the nasopharynx and tonsillar area as a means of identifying a pathogenic microorganism.

EQUIPMENT/SUPPLIES:

- Tongue depressor
- Culturette system with culture swab and collection media tube
- Label and requisition form
- Gloves and face shield
- Good light source
- Biohazard transport bag

PROCEDURE STEPS:

1. Introduce yourself by name and credential and identify the patient. RATIONALE: Identifying yourself helps establish professional trust and rapport with the patient.

2. ***Explain to the patient the rationale for performance of the procedure, showing awareness of the patient's concerns related to the procedure.*** RATIONALE: Explaining the procedure and allaying the patient's concerns will assure the patient that you are concerned about any apprehension he or she may have and that you are open to discussing the concerns.

3. Have an emesis basin and tissues ready. RATIONALE: You will want to be prepared in case the patient spits up or vomits.

4. Have the patient in a sitting position. RATIONALE: The patient in a sitting position will facilitate better visualization of the throat area.

5. Wash hands, gather supplies, and apply gloves and face shield. RATIONALE: Washing hands before any patient contact will eliminate contamination. Gathering equipment before beginning the procedure ensures less chance of errors caused by missing supplies. Gloves and a face shield will offer personal protection in case the patient coughs, spits up, or vomits.

6. Ask the patient to open his or her mouth wide and then adjust the light source. RATIONALE: A widely opened mouth and properly adjusted light source will facilitate better visualization of the throat area.

7. Remove the culture swab from the culturette tube using sterile technique. RATIONALE: Using sterile technique maintains the sterility of the swab, which results in a quality specimen for culture.

8. Ask the patient to say "ah." Gently press the front of the tongue with the tongue depressor and swab the back of the throat and tonsillar area. Concentrate primarily on any red, raw areas, and pustules. Take care to not touch the swab on the inside of the cheeks or on the tongue (Figure 42-12A). RATIONALE: Having the patient say "ah" lowers the back of the tongue. Gently pressing the front of the tongue reminds the patient

(continues)

to keep the mouth opened and assists in keeping the back of the tongue down without causing a gag reflex. Swabbing only the tonsillar area and the back of the throat without touching the inside of the cheeks or the tongue ensures that the specimen will contain mostly the bacterial infectious agent (*Streptococci*), if present, and not normal mouth flora or other contaminants. The red, raw areas and pustules will most likely contain the greatest concentration of *Streptococci*.

9. Place the swab back into the culturette tube using sterile technique and crush the glass capsule containing the culture media (Figure 42-12B). (*NOTE:* Some culturette systems require that the swab puncture a membrane to release the media within the tube. Follow the manufacturer's instructions.) RATIONALE: Using sterile technique avoids contaminating the specimen and having the specimen contaminate any other area. Crushing the glass capsule (or piercing the culture membrane) releases the culture medium, which will maintain the optimum environment for the specimen until it is tested at the regional laboratory.

10. ***Paying attention to detail,*** clearly label the culturette tube according to the POL policy and requirements (Figure 42-12C). RATIONALE: Proper and timely labeling of all specimens ensures that samples will not be mixed up with other patient samples.

11. Ensure patient comfort and answer any questions related to the testing. ***Provide appropriate responses and feedback.*** RATIONALE: Ensuring patient comfort and answering questions will establish professional rapport.

12. Discard contaminated supplies into a biohazard waste container. Disinfect all work surfaces. Remove gloves and face shield and discard appropriately. RATIONALE: Following Standard Precautions when disposing of contaminated supplies and disinfecting work surfaces will eliminate biohazard contaminations.

13. Wash hands. RATIONALE: Gloves protect hands from most but not all infectious microorganisms. Washing hands will remove residual powders and latex.

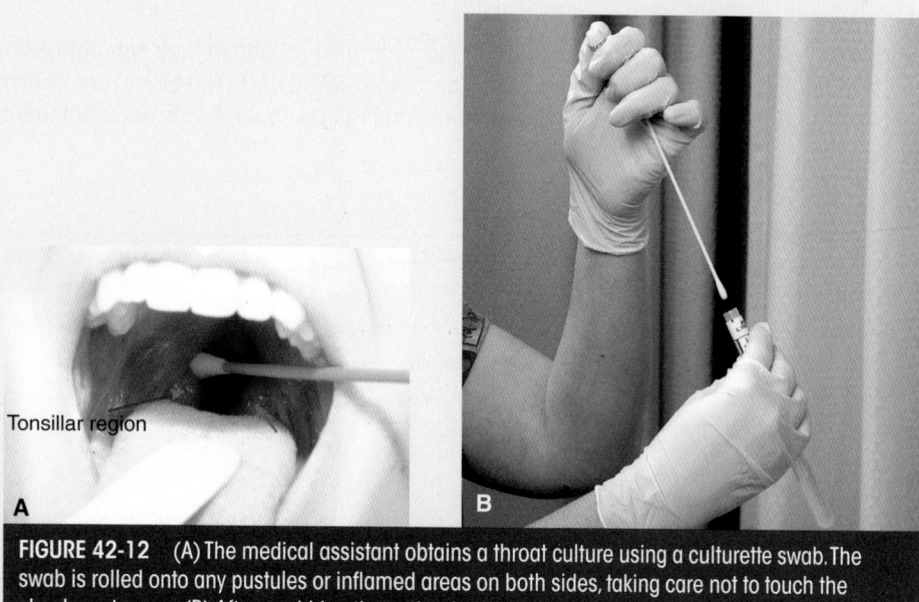

Tonsillar region

A

B

FIGURE 42-12 (A) The medical assistant obtains a throat culture using a culturette swab. The swab is rolled onto any pustules or inflamed areas on both sides, taking care not to touch the cheeks or tongue. (B) After swabbing the patient's throat, the medical assistant returns the swab to the culturette, which contains the moist medium.

(continues)

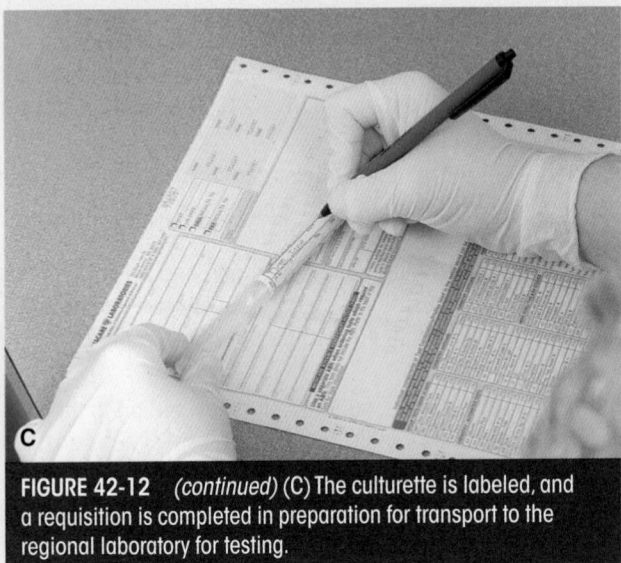

FIGURE 42-12 *(continued)* (C) The culturette is labeled, and a requisition is completed in preparation for transport to the regional laboratory for testing.

14. Complete the laboratory requisition in the presence of the patient and record procedure in patient's chart or electronic medical record. (If performing a rapid strep test, follow the manufacturer's instructions exactly and be sure to also run the controls test.) RATIONALE: Completing the laboratory requisition properly and in the presence of the patient will give the regional laboratory accurate information regarding the patient and the specimen. Any questions about the patient's contact information or insurance can be answered immediately if the patient is present. Completing the requisition in the presence of the patient also ensures the right form accompanies the patient's sample. Charting the procedure will establish a timeline and document the procedure.

15. Place the specimen and the requisition in the biohazard transport bag in their separate compartments and notify the laboratory that the specimen is ready for pick up. RATIONALE: The biohazard transport bag has separate compartments to keep the specimen from coming into contact with, and contaminating, the requisition.

DOCUMENTATION:

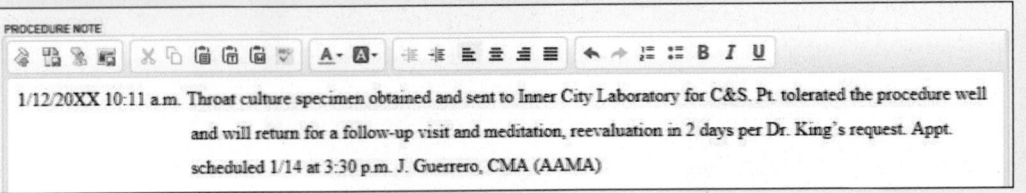

PROCEDURE NOTE

1/12/20XX 10:11 a.m. Throat culture specimen obtained and sent to Inner City Laboratory for C&S. Pt. tolerated the procedure well and will return for a follow-up visit and meditation, reevaluation in 2 days per Dr. King's request. Appt. scheduled 1/14 at 3:30 p.m. J. Guerrero, CMA (AAMA)

Courtesy of Harris CareTracker PM and EMR

Nasopharyngeal Cultures

A nasopharyngeal swab may be requested with a throat culture. This is collected with a swab on a thin wire. A separate swab may be used for each nostril. The patient tilts back the head, and a separate swab is gently inserted into each nostril. The swab is then placed into a sterile tube and kept at room temperature for transport to the laboratory.

Wound Cultures

Procedure

When culturing a wound, a sterile needle might be used to aspirate pus-filled fluid from the wound, or a swab is used. It is important to get the swab deep into the wound without touching the surrounding skin. Specimens for wound cultures often are placed in anaerobic transport medium, especially if the wound is not superficial (see Procedure 42-2).

Perform a Wound Specimen Collection

Procedure

STANDARD PRECAUTIONS:

Handwashing   Gloves   Biohazard

PURPOSE:

To obtain a wound culture from a patient, using sterile technique.

EQUIPMENT/SUPPLIES:

- Sterile culturette
- Gloves
- Other personal protective equipment as required by the collection procedure
- Pen
- Patient chart/EHR

PROCEDURE STEPS:

1. Assemble necessary supplies for collection of the specimen and confirm that the culturette is not expired.
2. Introduce yourself and identify the patient. ***Explain the rationale for performing the procedure, showing awareness of the patient's concerns.*** Answer any questions the patient might have and assist the patient into a comfortable position before you proceed.
3. Verify the provider's order.
4. Wash your hands and apply appropriate PPE.
5. Remove the sterile swab from the sleeve.
6. Collect an adequate specimen without touching any other area except for the exudate and gently rolling the swab in the affected area (Figure 42-13). RATIONALE: Touching the skin or edges of the wound could contaminate the swab and interfere with the results.

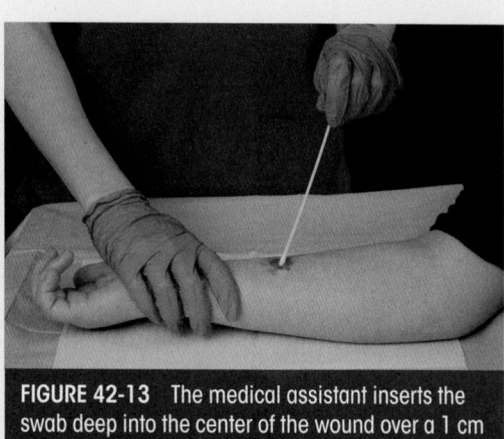

FIGURE 42-13 The medical assistant inserts the swab deep into the center of the wound over a 1 cm area for five seconds.

(continues)

7. Reinsert the sterile swab in the sleeve and break the ampule. RATIONALE: The swab must be protected from drying.

8. Record the patient information on the culturette (not the wrapper); if required, complete a lab requisition form for an outside laboratory.

9. Remove gloves, wash hands, and put on new gloves. Clean and dress the wound according to the provider's orders.

10. Properly dispose of contaminated equipment.

11. Remove PPE and wash your hands.

12. Correctly document the procedure in the patient's medical record.

DOCUMENTATION:

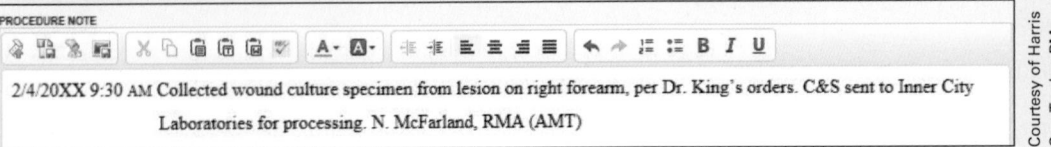

PROCEDURE NOTE

2/4/20XX 9:30 AM Collected wound culture specimen from lesion on right forearm, per Dr. King's orders. C&S sent to Inner City Laboratories for processing. N. McFarland, RMA (AMT)

Courtesy of Harris CareTracker PM and EMR

Sputum Cultures

For sputum specimens to be collected correctly, the patient should cough deeply and **expectorate** into the sterile container (Figure 42-14). The specimen should be a first morning specimen and placed into a sterile container designed to protect all who handle the specimen from contamination. Most sputum collections are performed by respiratory therapists in hospital laboratories.

Stool Cultures

Stool specimens are brought to the laboratory for various tests. If the stool is to be examined for **ova** (eggs) or parasites, the specimen should be as fresh as possible. Special containers (Figure 42-15) are provided to the patient for stool collection to test for ova and parasites. The collection containers for stool cultures do not have to be sterile, but they must be clean and have a tight-fitting lid. Stool specimens must be kept at between room temperature and body temperature. Refrigeration may destroy the parasites within the specimen.

Procedure

For bacterial cultures of stool (as well as for ova and parasites), several different specimens may be sent for testing at different times (see Procedure 42-3).

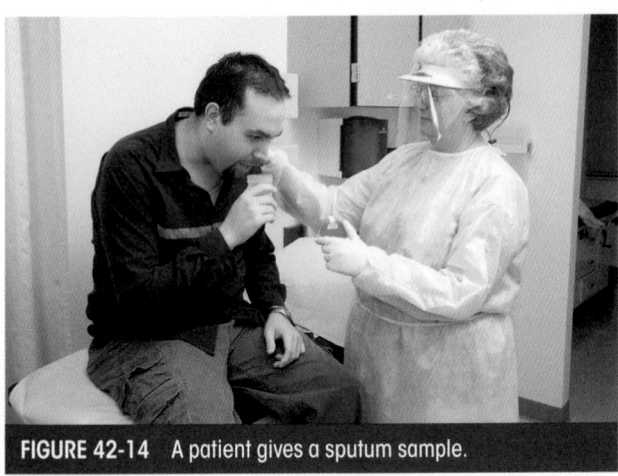

FIGURE 42-14 A patient gives a sputum sample.

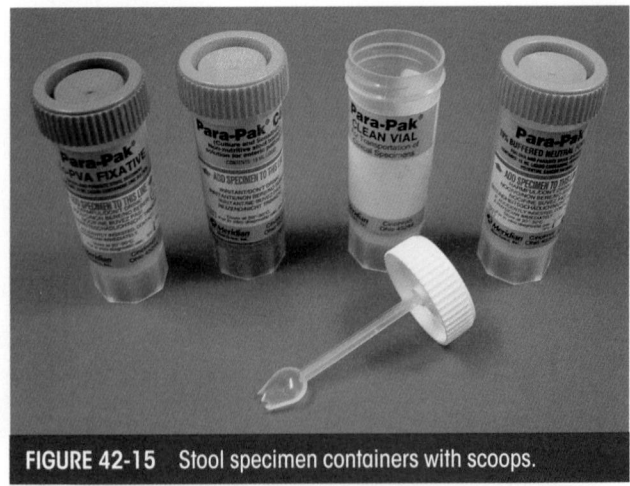

FIGURE 42-15 Stool specimen containers with scoops.

PROCEDURE 42-3

Procedure

Instructing a Patient on Obtaining a Fecal Specimen

STANDARD PRECAUTIONS:

Handwashing

Gloves

Biohazard

PURPOSE:

To instruct a patient in the correct collection of a fecal sample.

EQUIPMENT/SUPPLIES:

- Gloves
- Biohazard transfer bag
- Container and collection scoop
- Special laboratory manual instructions if needed (depending on the test being performed)
- Laboratory requisition form

PROCEDURE STEPS:

1. Assemble and organize equipment and supplies. RATIONALE: Being organized helps the process go more smoothly and professionally.

2. Introduce yourself by name and credential and identify the patient. RATIONALE: Identifying the patient ensures that you have the right patient.

3. Speaking to the patient's level of understanding, ***explain the rationale for performance of the procedure, showing awareness of the patient's concerns.*** Provide written instructions as well. RATIONALE: Explaining the procedure in a manner the patient understands reassures him or her and helps ensure his or her cooperation. Demonstrating professionalism will help maintain a professional atmosphere and may help put the patient at ease, as some patients may become embarrassed with these instructions. The written instructions will assist patients in following the proper procedure.

4. Give the patient the labeled specimen container, instructing him or her to acquire a small amount of stool using the scoop, then tightly secure the lid. RATIONALE: Labeling the container rather than the lid will ensure that the specimen will not be mixed up with another patient's sample in the laboratory. The sturdy lid will prevent leakage of the specimen during transport (see Figure 42-15).

5. Caution the patient to avoid contaminating the stool specimen with urine. RATIONALE: Urine may interfere with the test.

6. Give the patient a biohazard transport bag and instructions on which pocket to put the specimen in and how to secure the bag. The medical assistant can place the laboratory requisition into the other pocket. RATIONALE: Using a biohazard transport bag and properly sealing it will prevent contamination during transport to the laboratory. Keeping the requisition in a separate pocket from the specimen further prevents contamination of the paperwork.

7. The patient should be prepared to transport the specimen to the laboratory as soon as possible while keeping the specimen at or just below body temperature. RATIONALE: If the stool is being tested for parasites and their eggs (ova and parasite, commonly called O&P), the laboratory will want to test the parasites while they are still viable.

(continues)

8. Ask the patient if he or she has any questions and provide appropriate responses. ***Demonstrate professionalism and courtesy while answering questions.*** RATIONALE: Soliciting questions will encourage the patient to ask a question if there is something he or she doesn't understand. Providing appropriate responses will further the patient's understanding and ensure a cleaner specimen.

9. Document that the instructions were given to the patient, both orally and in writing. RATIONALE: Proper documentation serves as a record for future reference.

DOCUMENTATION:

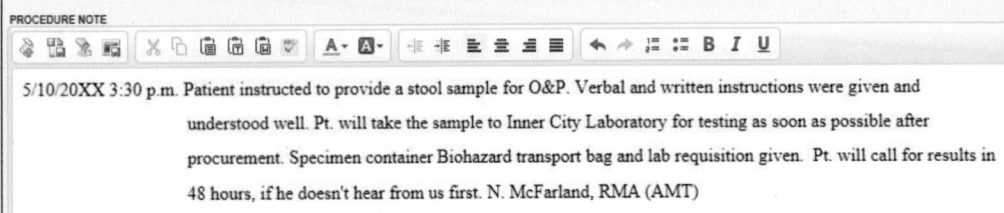

PROCEDURE NOTE

5/10/20XX 3:30 p.m. Patient instructed to provide a stool sample for O&P. Verbal and written instructions were given and understood well. Pt. will take the sample to Inner City Laboratory for testing as soon as possible after procurement. Specimen container Biohazard transport bag and lab requisition given. Pt. will call for results in 48 hours, if he doesn't hear from us first. N. McFarland, RMA (AMT)

Courtesy of Harris CareTracker PM and EMR

Cerebrospinal Fluid (CSF) Cultures

The provider obtains CSF by doing a sterile lumbar puncture (see Procedure 29-1). Before the culture is set up, the tube should be placed in an incubator or left at room temperature. Refrigeration of spinal fluid can kill two common meningitis-causing bacteria, *Haemophilus influenzae* and *Neisseria meningitidis*. CSF culture is a STAT order for processing, and the medical assistant is responsible for calling the laboratory for immediate pickup.

Blood Cultures

Human blood is free from bacteria in a healthy human. If blood does become contaminated with bacteria, septicemia (septic blood infection) can result. Blood cultures are collected by the same means as regular blood collection, with special considerations to avoid any contamination of the blood. A variety of collection devices are available for collecting blood cultures, all requiring careful sterile techniques (see Procedure 39-5).

FOODBORNE ILLNESSES

Foodborne illnesses from bacterial and viral infections and parasites are a huge health care concern in the United States, and they are becoming even more prevalent with the increase of international travel.

The CDC estimates there are about 48 million cases of "food poisoning" each year in the United States. Many people are afflicted without being aware and the infection is self-limiting. Still others are hospitalized, and an estimated 3,000 deaths occur each year as a result of foodborne illnesses.

The most well-known agents that cause foodborne illnesses are *Campylobacter*, *Clostridium botulinum* (botulism), *Cryptosporidium*, *Cyclospora*, *Escherichia coli*, hepatitis A virus, *Listeria*, norovirus, *Salmonella*, *Shigella*, *Staphylococcus aureus*, *Vibrio parahaemolyticus*, and *Vibrio vulnificus*. Some of these foodborne illnesses are contracted from raw or undercooked meats and seafood, some from contaminated food handlers, and some from unwashed produce.

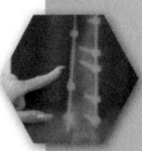

Critical Thinking

A patient presents with diarrhea and vomiting that has lasted for 14 hours. She has vomited 4 times and has had diarrhea every 20 minutes. She is weak, has nausea and a dry mouth, is confused and shaking and has a headache. She has not urinated in several hours although she is sipping water. She has had insulin dependent diabetes for several years, but is otherwise in good health. What laboratory test would be most effective in diagnosing her problem? What are the most important immediate treatments for her?

Symptoms range from mild to severe diarrhea, nausea, vomiting, abdominal pain, fever, and the resulting dehydration, headaches, and flu-like symptoms. Diagnostic evaluations include stool cultures, blood tests, and following the symptoms. Treatments involve antibacterial medications and treating the accompanying symptoms.

VIROLOGY (VIRUSES) IN THE MEDICAL LABORATORY

Viruses are special microorganisms in several ways:

1. Viruses are too small to be seen with a standard microscope. An electron microscope must be used. Comparing the size of a bacteria to a virus would be like comparing a 10-story building to a human being.

2. Viruses are all pathogenic. Bacteria, on the other hand, are mostly harmless.

3. Viruses are not able to reproduce at all by themselves. Viruses must invade other living cells to take over and reproduce, killing the host cell in the process.

4. Viruses are often named for the region, country, or ethnicity where they were first discovered. For example, the Ebola virus first emerged in Sudan and Zaire in 1976, and was named after the Ebola River in Zaire. There is much controversy among nations and cultures because of this practice. No ethnicity, religion, gender, or geographic area wants their name attached to a deadly disease, and so the World Health Organization (WHO) continues to try to settle these naming controversies.

5. Perhaps the most important difference between viruses and other microbes is that there are few treatments available for viruses. Some antiviral medications are being developed, but often viral infections just have to take their course while symptoms are treated.

Identifying and Diagnosing Viral Infections

Many viral infections are tentatively diagnosed by patient symptoms and by the process of eliminating other pathogens. Specific diagnosis of a viral infection can be done in several ways in the medical laboratory. These tests are complicated and not performed in most POLs. Below are some of the ways viral infections can be diagnosed.

1. When a person contracts a pathogen, the immune system creates a specific antibody to fight that particular pathogen. A common way to determine if a person has been exposed to a virus is to run an antibody blood test. Chapter 21 explains immunity in more detail.

2. When a virus infects a cell, viral antigens develop on the cell surface. Tests are performed on tissue samples to detect viral antigens.

3. Culturing is also a way of determining the presence of a virus, but only by viewing how the virus changes the cells in the culture. This process can take weeks.

4. Viral DNA and RNA can also be detected in tissue or body fluid samples.

5. Rapid tests have been developed and are most widely used for diagnosing influenza.

BACTERIOLOGY (BACTERIA) IN THE MEDICAL LABORATORY

Bacterial **nomenclature** (naming) is a two-part system. Two Greek or Latin names are used, the first name being the **genus**, which is capitalized. The second name is the **species**, which is not capitalized. These names may reflect a characteristic of a bacterium or names of places or persons associated with the discovery of the microorganism. For example, *Salmonella typhi* was discovered by an American microbiologist named Salmon. The bacterium causes typhoid fever.

Cell Structures and Behaviors of Bacteria

The bacterial cell is a single-celled organism with a jelly-like cytoplasmic cell membrane, a cell wall, and a nucleus. Figure 42-16 illustrates a basic bacterial cell. Not all bacteria possess flagella for motility, as some are not motile. The cell grows by taking in materials from the environment. After a certain amount of growth, the bacterial cell divides itself into two parts. This reproduction process is called mitosis.

Eighty percent of all bacteria are harmless and necessary for our bodily functions. In healthy individuals, several types of bacteria are found naturally in various parts of the body. These natural bacteria are called **normal flora**. These organisms are always present and help with the body's immune system, digestion, and maintenance of optimum environment balance.

This chapter concentrates on the pathogenic bacteria, those that cause diseases to humans.

Some bacteria can encapsulate themselves in protein, providing protection from antibiotic

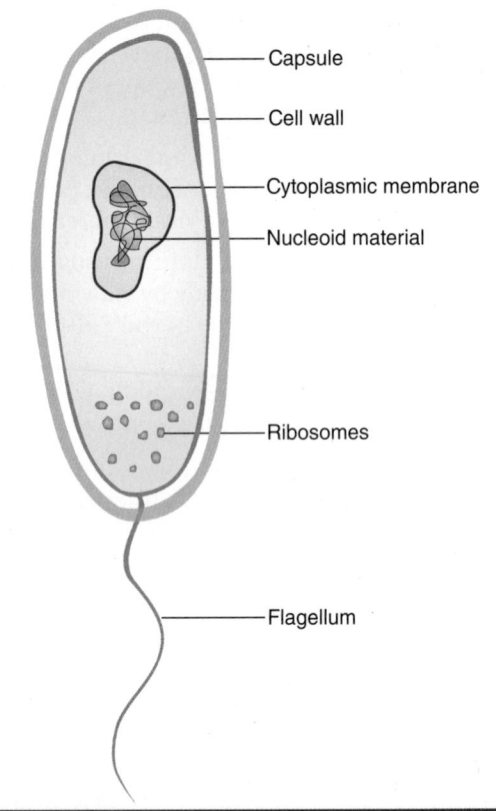

FIGURE 42-16   Basic bacterial cell.

Capsule
Cell wall
Cytoplasmic membrane
Nucleoid material
Ribosomes
Flagellum

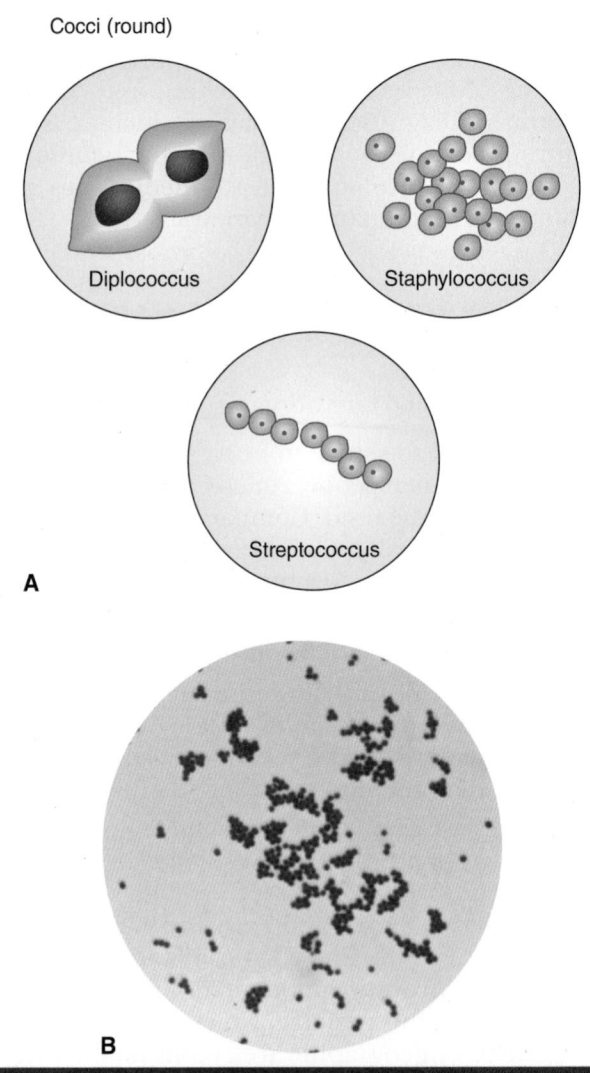

Cocci (round)

Diplococcus

Staphylococcus

Streptococcus

A

B

FIGURE 42-17   (A) Cocci (round). (B) Cocci, as seen through a microscope.

penetration and white blood cell attack. Once encapsulated they are called **spores** and are in an inactive state that can help bacteria resist chemicals, freezing, drying, radiation, and heating. Bacterial spores are so resistant they can live 150,000 years and can survive in dust. Tetanus is an example of a disease caused by bacteria that create spores.

Morphology of Bacteria

Each genus of bacteria has a characteristic **morphology** (shape and appearance), which helps in its identification. Bacteria have three basic morphologies:

1. Cocci (Figure 42-17) are round and occur in clusters, pairs, singles, and tetrads (groups of three). They are nonmotile microorganisms (i.e., they do not move on their own accord).
2. Bacilli are rod shaped and can have rounded, straight, or pointed ends (Figure 42-18). Some bacilli have flagella that give the bacteria motility (movement).
3. Spirilla are spiral-shaped bacteria that have one to many turns (Figure 42-19). Most spirilla are motile.

Identifying Bacteria

There are usually two procedures involved in properly identifying bacteria: the culture and the microscopic examination. The culture method allows us to see how bacteria behave when grown in an appropriate culture medium. We can also apply antibiotics to the petri dish to test the bacteria's resistance or sensitivity patterns. The microscopic examination involves applying bacteria to a slide, applying stains if appropriate, and then viewing stained or unstained bacteria through the microscope.

Gram Stains. Although the medical assistant will not actually perform the staining process, the information is included here to aid in understanding

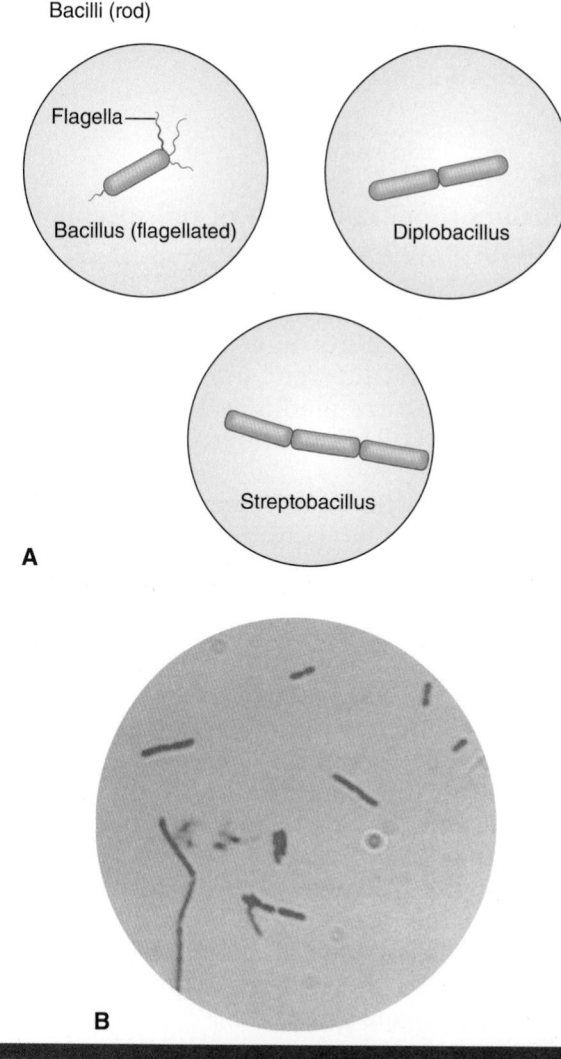

Bacilli (rod)

Flagella

Bacillus (flagellated)

Diplobacillus

Streptobacillus

A

B

FIGURE 42-18 (A) Bacilli (rod-shaped). (B) Bacilli, as seen through a microscope.

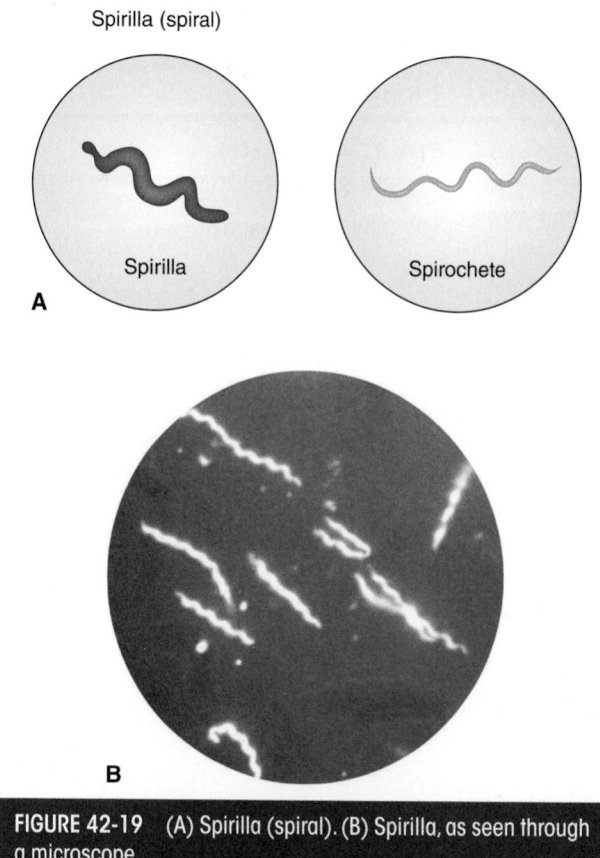

Spirilla (spiral)

Spirilla

Spirochete

A

B

FIGURE 42-19 (A) Spirilla (spiral). (B) Spirilla, as seen through a microscope.

the staining processes. It is important for medical assistants to be familiar with the processes and the terminology related to staining and microscopic identification of bacteria to better serve their patients, providers, and colleagues.

The **Gram stain** was developed in 1884 by Dr. Hans Christian Gram. More than a century later, this famous stain is still in use with little variation. Gram stains are applied to bacteria to differentiate them into two basic groups, either gram positive or gram negative. Gram-positive bacteria have a thicker membrane than gram-negative bacteria, resulting in the gram-positive bacteria taking on a deep purple color. Gram-negative bacteria have a tough outer membrane and stain a lighter pink color. There are some bacteria that resist dyes. These bacteria are called acid-fast bacteria and

heat is applied during staining to help identify them.

Gram-positive bacteria are more susceptible to antibiotics, whereas gram-negative bacteria are resistant to antibiotics; therefore, diseases caused by gram-negative bacteria are more difficult to treat. Both gram-positive and gram-negative bacteria can cause diseases in the same areas of the body such as the lungs, digestive tract, and wounds, but in order to treat the infection effectively, the exact identity of the bacteria needs to be revealed. You may recognize some of the names of the bacteria in Table 42-1.

Wet Mount Slides. Bacteria may also be microscopically examined in a living state, without staining. Characteristics that can be studied by this method include motility, shape, and arrangement of organisms. Since living organisms will not live long in dry conditions, especially near the heat of the microscope light, the bacteria need to be suspended in a liquid. This is called a **wet mount**. (See Chapter 25 and Procedure 25-3 for more information.)

Although microscopy is not a CLIA-waived test, the medical assistant is responsible for setting up

TABLE 42-1

BACTERIAL DISEASES

GRAM-NEGATIVE BACTERIAL DISEASES

Conjunctivitis

Gastroenteritis

Gonorrhea

Meningitis

Nasopharyngitis

Otitis media

Pelvic inflammatory disease

Pneumonia

Rocky Mountain spotted fever

Typhus

Urethritis

GRAM POSITIVE BACTERIAL DISEASES

Endocarditis

Osteomyelitis

Pneumonia

Septic arthritis

Skin infections

Staph food poisoning

Toxic shock syndrome

the slide and can certainly view the slides microscopically and discuss the findings with the provider as a learning exercise.

For vaginal secretions, a swab of the vaginal discharge is placed in a sterile tube containing normal saline and mixed, then a drop is place on the slide for viewing. For stool or other bacterial specimens, a small amount of specimen is mixed with a drop of normal saline then viewed under a microscope.

KOH (Potassium Hydroxide) Preparation. Another type of wet preparation uses a 10% solution of **potassium hydroxide (KOH)** in a wet preparation for the study of fungi and bacterial spores. Since KOH destroys bacteria and epithelial cells, it should only be added after viewing the bacteria. Clearing away the bacteria and epithelial cells allows the fungi and spores to be more easily seen. The slide is prepared by using fragments of human hair, skin, or nails that could have fungus. KOH wet mounts are also useful for examining other body fluids such as vaginal swabs. After adding a drop of 10% KOH and a coverslip, the slide should sit at room temperature for about a half hour to allow the bacteria and epithelial cells to dissolve (see Chapter 25 and Procedure 25-3).

Culture Media

After the proper collection of the specimen, it is kept alive and encouraged to grow by placing the specimen into appropriate culture media. The medium is **agar**, a gelatin-like substance, mixed with nutrients. Since each type of bacteria prefers different nutrients, there are a variety of culture media available, usually in prepared petri dishes provided by the reference laboratory.

Other growth requirements of different organisms must be considered also, such as moisture, temperature, and oxygen and carbon dioxide levels. Organisms that are sensitive to drying must be put into transport medium immediately after collection. Aerobic bacteria grow only in the presence of oxygen. Anaerobic bacteria live and grow in the absence of oxygen. If an anaerobic organism is kept in an aerobic atmosphere while being transported to the reference laboratory, it will probably not survive. Special anaerobic transport systems should be used, and the instructions are provided by the reference laboratory.

Table 42-2 lists some common bacteria, the diseases they cause, their oxygen requirements, and whether they create spores.

Charts listing the proper media to set up for specific types of cultures generally are prominently displayed in the setup area of most microbiology laboratories.

Media Classification. There are several classifications of media, including:

- *Basic*. Basic media are used for general purposes and do not contain added nutrients. They will support the growth of many gram-negative and gram-positive organisms.
- *Differential*. Differential media contain substances that alter the appearance of some types of organisms and not other types.
- *Selective*. Selective media support the growth of one type of organism while inhibiting the growth of another. This is done by the addition of a salt, dye, chemical, or antibiotic. A hektoen enteric (HE) plate for the growth of *Salmonella* and *Shigella* is a selective type of medium.

TABLE 42-2

COMMON BACTERIA, DISEASES, SPORE-FORMING ABILITY, AND OXYGEN REQUIREMENTS

ORGANISM	DISEASE	SPORE FORMING?	OXYGEN REQUIREMENTS
Streptococcus	Strep throat	No	Aerobic
Neisseria gonorrhoeae	Gonorrhea	No	Anaerobic
Salmonella	Food poisoning	Yes	Anaerobic
Staphylococcus	Infections, boils	No	Aerobic
Escherichia coli	Urinary tract infection	No	Aerobic
Clostridium	Botulism	Yes	CO_2

- *Enriched.* This type of medium contains substances that inhibit certain bacteria from growing. These media work well with cultures from sites that possess normal flora, such as the throat. The normal flora is inhibited, and pathogenic bacteria are encouraged to grow. Blood agar and chocolate agar are examples of enriched media.

Inoculating the Media. After selecting the correct medium for the culture and observing the specimen to make sure it is properly collected, the specimen is inoculated onto the medium. If the specimen is on a swab, the swab is rolled directly onto the upper quadrant of the agar plate. If the specimen is a sputum or liquid, it is inoculated onto the plate with a loop.

The inoculum is spread back and forth in a sweeping motion with a flamed (sterilized) loop or needle.

After the agar plate has been inoculated and properly labeled, it should be turned upside down and placed in the proper environment for growth. By turning the agar upside down, any condensation that forms from bacterial growth will be on the inside lid.

Test tubes with liquid nutrient broths may also be used for culturing bacteria. These **broth tubes** have screw-on caps that must not be screwed on too tightly because gas production by some organisms can break the tube.

Inoculating for a colony count is a streaking technique used to plate urine cultures, especially. A special calibrated urine loop is used to make the first streak, followed by a second streak that goes across the entire length of the initial streak. Then another complete streaking is placed over the original streaks after rotating the plate (Figure 42-20). This method distributes the bacteria thinly, isolating bacterial colonies to give the provider a clearer

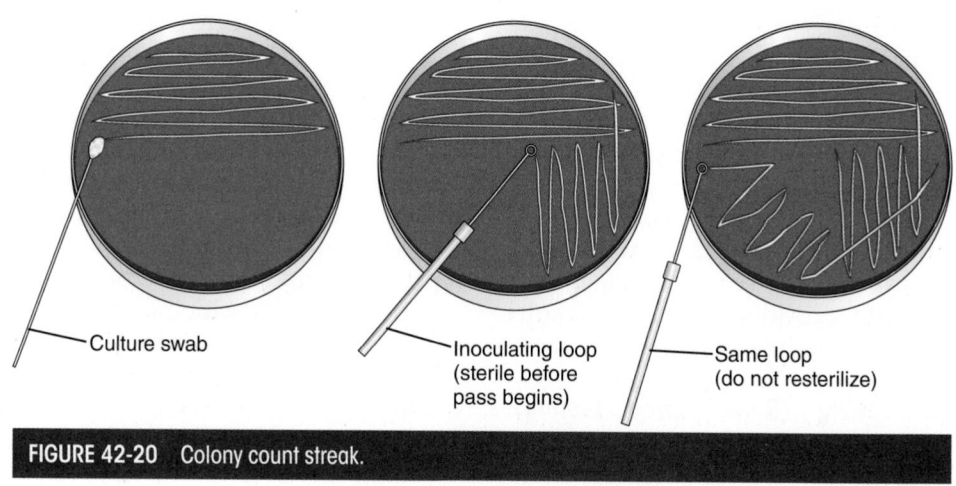

Culture swab

Inoculating loop
(sterile before
pass begins)

Same loop
(do not resterilize)

FIGURE 42-20 Colony count streak.

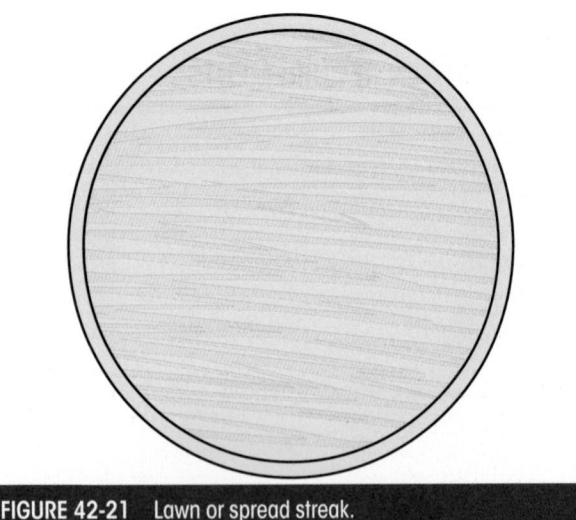

FIGURE 42-21   Lawn or spread streak.

idea of how many colonies of bacteria are present. This is especially useful when working with bacterial cultures, since there can be more than one pathogen growing in the culture. For instance, a wound culture may have both gram-positive and gram-negative organisms growing. It is also necessary at times to separate the pathogenic bacteria from the normal flora, as in throat and sputum cultures.

Other types of streaking include the lawn streak. This streaking technique is used to place an organism over an entire area of an agar plate for sensitivity testing. The bacteria are spread over the entire plate using a swab (Figure 42-21), streaking over the entire area several times from different angles. After the streaking has been completed, the culture of organisms is exposed to various antibiotics to determine sensitivity or resistance. Refer to the Sensitivity Testing section later in this chapter for more information.

Test Kits for Rapid Identification

The age of high technology and computerized equipment has also made inroads into microbiology laboratories, clinics, and POLs. Many traditional methods of identifying bacteria have been replaced by rapid identification test kits.

Rapid test systems, which are usually CLIA-waived, give a quick identification, are economical, and allow the provider to start treatment sooner. Rapid tests allow the provider to receive results while the patient is still in the office.

***Streptococcus* Screening (Rapid Strep Testing).** Throat swabs for the detection of group A *Streptococcus* infection (strep throat) usually are tested in the

POL using a self-contained kit that produces quick results. Performing rapid strep tests is well within the medical assistant's scope under CLIA's waived test category. It is important to identify this gram-positive *Streptococcus* as soon as possible because the bacteria can cause serious damage (i.e., kidney and heart valve damage) if not treated immediately with antibiotics. Viral infections of the throat are usually not treated and will resolve on their own.

The results are based on color development of a spot on the test filter. Test results are available in minutes. Although these tests are quick and convenient, as with any medical procedure, quality controls are critical for accuracy and the following rules should be followed strictly:

- Read and understand the manufacturer's instructions and directions before starting the test.
- Never use outdated materials.
- Observe all safety guidelines and precautions.
- Use the correct swab to take the throat culture. Some cottons and chemicals on the swab will interfere with the test reagents. If possible, use the swabs provided with the kit.
- Always run the positive and negative control together with the patient's actual test.

If a patient has symptoms of an infected throat and the slide test is negative, the provider may additionally order a general throat culture to make sure there is no other infection present. A list of all the CLIA-waived rapid tests is available at the CDC website (http://www.cdc.gov) using the search words "Waived Tests."

Sensitivity Testing

When a patient has had multiple bacterial infections and the provider is trying to determine the best and most effective antibiotic to prescribe or when a bacterial infection is not responding to the currently prescribed antibiotic, the provider will order a culture and sensitivity (C&S) test. The antibiotic that is effective against the culture bacteria is reported as "sensitive to," and the antibiotics that are not effective will be reported as "resistant to," meaning that the bacteria is sensitive to some antibiotics and resistant to others.

To determine which antibiotic will destroy the culture bacteria, the technician uses an apparatus to place small discs on the culture plate. The discs contain various antibiotics. The antibiotic to which the bacteria are sensitive will become surrounded by an area of no growth (Figure 42-22).

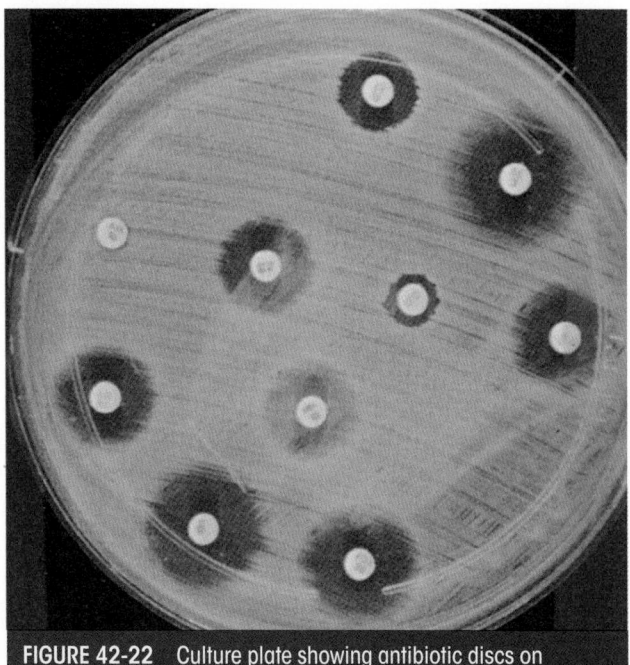

FIGURE 42-22 Culture plate showing antibiotic discs on bacteria. Note the one antibiotic disc in the left area that the bacteria are totally "resistant to." Most of the other antibiotics have carrying degrees of effectiveness and would be labeled "sensitive to." The one just right of the center area is barely effective and would be reported as "intermediate."

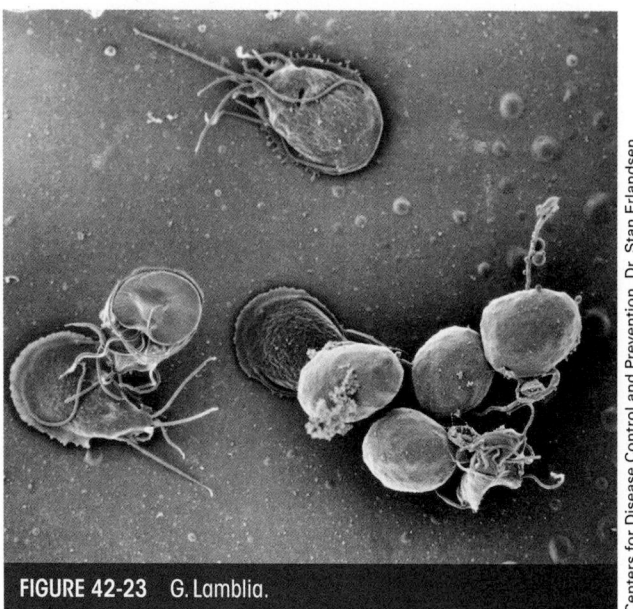

FIGURE 42-23 G. Lamblia.

Centers for Disease Control and Prevention, Dr. Stan Erlandsen

PARASITOLOGY (PARASITES) IN THE MEDICAL LABORATORY

With increased international travel and more public awareness, we are beginning to see and diagnose more parasitic infections. The field of parasitology is a vast one with many different types of parasites. They range from extremely small microscopic ones to those that are large and macroscopic. Parasites have varying life cycles. The degree of severity of illness depends on which parasite enters the human body and infects it. Parasites can be found in the blood, urine, or feces. The more common ones are found in the feces.

Different geographic areas have different types of parasites. As people travel, so do parasites. Resettled immigrant populations may be infected with a parasite previously unseen in a geographic area. World travelers can also bring back rare parasitic infections from their adventures. Many parasites such as giardia (Figure 42-23) enter the human body through contaminated food or drink. Refer to Figure 42-24 for the life cycle of a commonly ingested intestinal parasite, giardia.

Even though parasitology tests are performed by medical technologists rather than medical assistants, the medical assistant must be able to properly obtain the sample, instruct the patient on how to properly obtain the sample (such as a stool sample), and ensure that the patient is prepared properly, understands how and where to transport the specimen, how to maintain the proper temperature of the specimen, and even how quickly the specimen must be returned to the laboratory.

Specimen Collection

Intestinal parasites are the most prevalent type of parasite in the United States. As discussed earlier in this chapter, stool samples are required for examination for the parasite and its eggs (ova and parasite, or O&P). Providers' clinics will have specific instructions and containers when an ova and parasite examination is requested (see Procedure 42-3). When the specimen is sent for testing, it should be labeled correctly with the patient's name, date, and time of the specimen. To help aid in identification, it is important to know if the patient has been traveling, to what area of the world, and what is suspected by the provider. Ideally the patient will transport the specimen directly to the laboratory for testing.

Common Parasites

Some of the more common parasites identified in the POL are *Giardia lamblia* (see Figure 42-23); *Enterobius vermicularis,* the causative organism of

Giardiasis
(Giardia intestinalis)

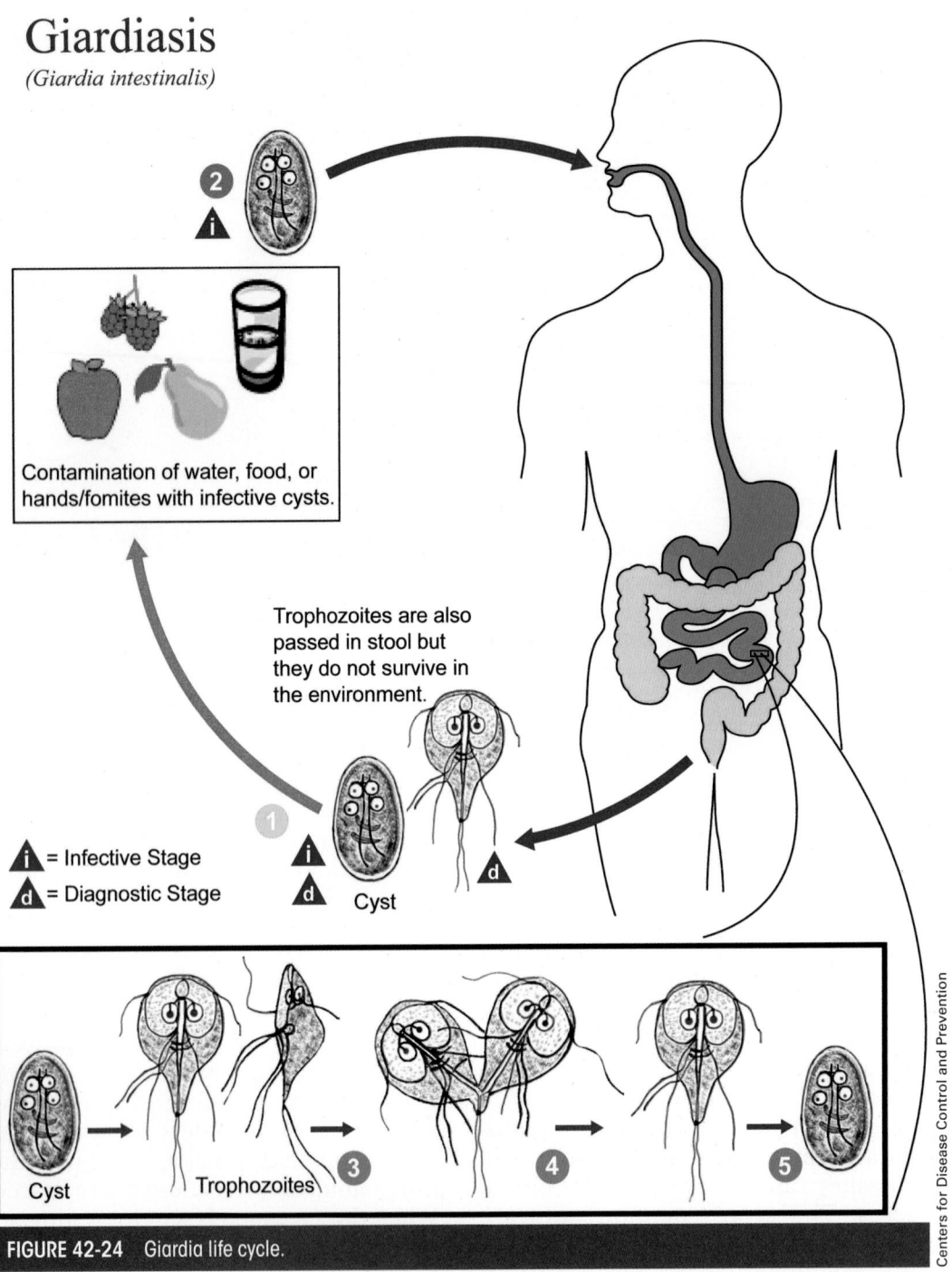

Contamination of water, food, or hands/fomites with infective cysts.

Trophozoites are also passed in stool but they do not survive in the environment.

i = Infective Stage
d = Diagnostic Stage

Cyst

Cyst   Trophozoites

Centers for Disease Control and Prevention

FIGURE 42-24   *Giardia* life cycle.

pinworm infection (Figure 42-25); and *Trichomonas vaginalis* (Figure 42-26), a parasite that infects the urogenital tracts of men and women. Of course the complete list of parasites that infest the human body is much more extensive.

Giardia lamblia is a parasite spread through the fecal–oral route (see Figure 42-24). Giardiasis infection is higher in areas where sanitation and clean water are less available. The organism is resistant to the chlorine levels in tap water and survives well in mountain streams, hence the nicknames of beaver fever and backpacker's diarrhea for the illness it causes. Usual symptoms include diarrhea and multiple gastrointestinal complaints. Stool cultures for ova and parasites (O&P) are the diagnostic tests of choice, and the infection responds well to antibiotics, antiparasitic medications, and antiprotozoal agents.

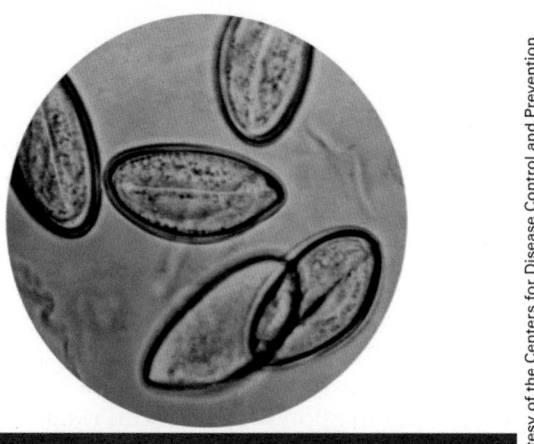

FIGURE 42-25 Pinworm ova, as seen through a microscope.

Courtesy of the Centers for Disease Control and Prevention, Atlanta, GA

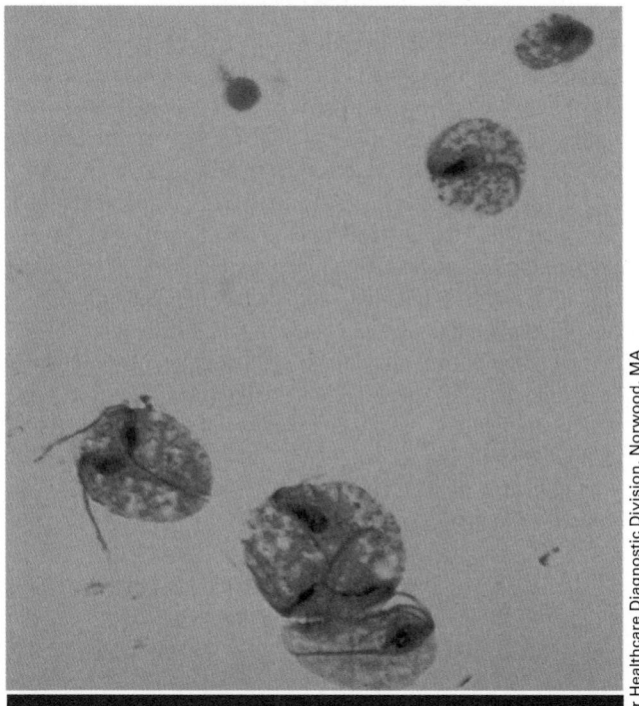

FIGURE 42-26 Trichomonas in stained urine sediment.

Bayer Healthcare Diagnostic Division, Norwood, MA

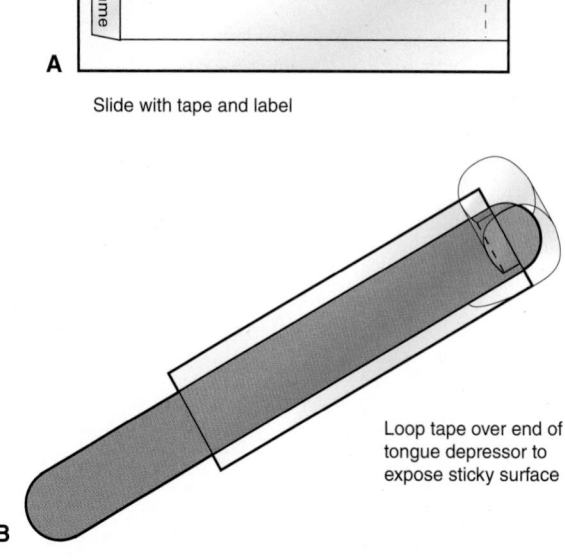

A   Slide with tape and label

B   Loop tape over end of tongue depressor to expose sticky surface

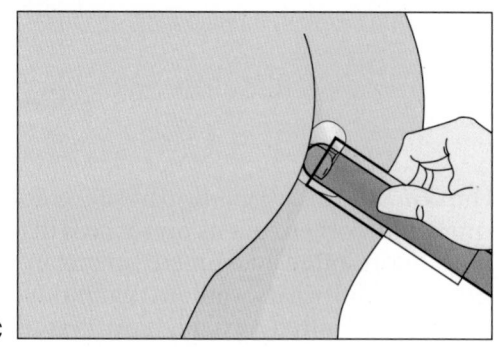

C   Press sticky surfaces against perianal areas

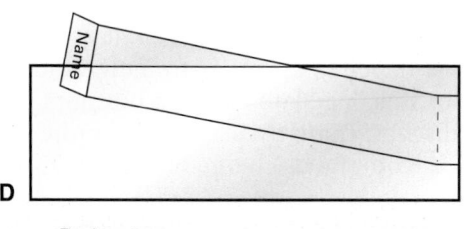

D   Replace tape

FIGURE 42-27 Technique for preparing and using a cellophane tape pinworm paddle.

Enterobius vermicularis, or pinworm, is found worldwide, predominantly in children. The adult worm is shaped like a pin. Pinworm infection can cause severe itching, irritability, and insomnia, depending on the severity of the infection. The adult female worm migrates to the anus at night, depositing ova (eggs) that cause itching during hatching. At times, the adult worm can be found around the anus and in the stool. The adult worm measures approximately 7 to 12 mm long. The egg is the infectious stage of the parasite.

To diagnose the presence of the parasite, either the adult worm or the egg have to be located

in the specimen. A negative diagnosis is confirmed after several negative tests are performed. The specimen is obtained by placing a cellophane tape swab sticky side down to the skin around the anal area. The tape is placed on a slide and brought to the laboratory for examination. The best time for obtaining a sample is during the night or immediately upon awakening when the worms are depositing eggs at the anal area (Figure 42-27).

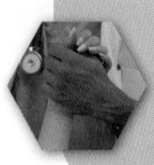
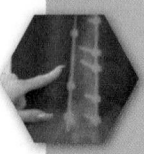
The *Trichomonas vaginalis* parasite is found in both men and women, but its presence is diagnosed five times more often in women (men can harbor the organism for years without symptoms). This parasite is transmitted sexually and because men can harbor it and have no symptoms, it is recommended that both partners be treated. This will prevent the ongoing reinfection of the female patient. The organism belongs to the flagellate class (i.e., it possesses flagella) and is extremely motile. Infection with this flagellate causes a purulent yellowish green discharge and dysuria. The parasite sample is obtained from the discharge or urine.

MYCOLOGY (FUNGI) IN THE MEDICAL LABORATORY

The field of mycology and the fungi that cause infections is extensive. Although most identification and sensitivity testing for fungal organisms takes place in larger laboratories and specific reference laboratories, identification of two common fungal infections can be made quickly in the clinic or POL.

The genus *Candida* has several species that cause yeast infections in the body. *Candida* species are also present in the environment around us. They present a particular problem in the health care setting, where they can cause serious **nosocomial** infections, that is, infections caused by

hospital and medical procedures. Equipment can be easily contaminated with *Candida* organisms.

Yeast infections commonly are found on the moist areas of the body and in the subcutaneous tissue. An infection with yeast can range from mild to serious. *Candida albicans* is the causative agent of vaginal yeast infections. In diagnosing, the swabbed specimen is examined microscopically for the characteristic budding yeast forms. If the specimen is fluid and clear, it is placed on a slide with a drop of saline. If the specimen is thick, it should be mixed with a drop of 10% KOH on the slide to clear away debris. Once the slide is prepared, it is examined microscopically.

Another group of significant fungi that can be generally identified are dermatophytes. These fungi cause infections on the hair, skin, and nails. The microscopic structure of these fungi is detailed. Some of the fungi that cause dermatophytic infections can be diagnosed using a **Wood's lamp**. This is a lamp with an ultraviolet light. Some dermatophytes will fluoresce (glow brightly) under this light.

Mycotic infections can also be identified through culture and kit identification systems. As a safety precaution, fungi can produce heavy aerosols and should be processed and observed under a safety hood. Figure 42-28 shows the fungus that causes psoriasis infections.

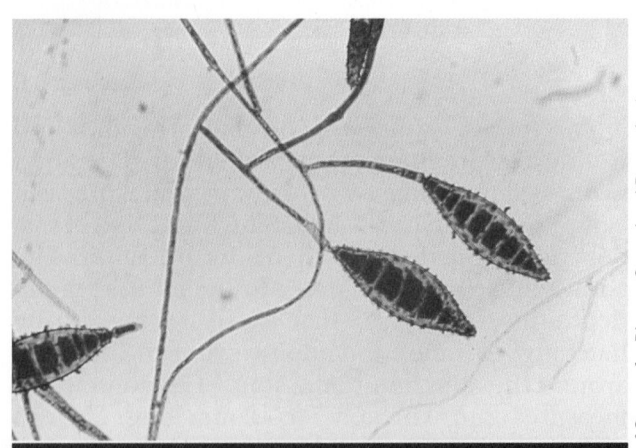

FIGURE 42-28 Microsporum canis is the fungus that causes psoriasis.

Courtesy of Centers for Disease Control and Prevention/ Dr. Lucille K. Georg

CASE STUDY 42-1

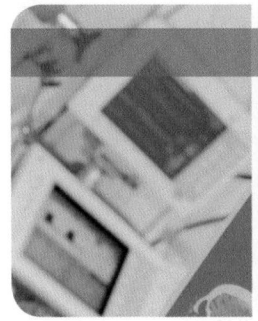

Refer to the scenario at the beginning of the chapter. You can see that Joe is very careful with all safety precautions when handling specimens.

CASE STUDY REVIEW

1. Name a few diseases Joe could contract from the specimens he handles.
2. Discuss the methods of transfer those diseases would take during transmission.

CASE STUDY 42-2

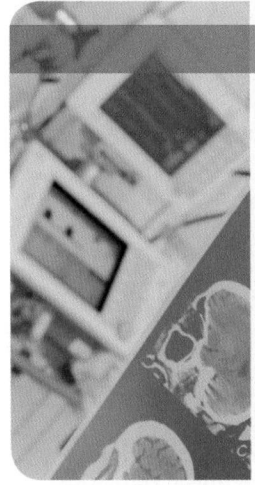

Mary O'Keefe has brought her 3-year-old son Chris to Inner City Health Care with a temperature of 102°F and an extremely sore and red throat. He is irritable and crying. After examining Chris, Dr. King orders a quick test for group A *Streptococcus*. Medical assistant Joe Guerrero, CMA (AAMA), has a difficult time acquiring the throat swab for the test because of Chris's condition. The test is run, and the results are negative. •

CASE STUDY REVIEW

1. How can Joe display his professionalism skills while obtaining the sample?
2. What could be some reasons the test result is negative?
3. What other procedure can be done to diagnose strep throat?
4. How would the test in question 3 be set up?

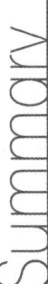

Summary

- The field of microbiology is vast. Many microorganisms are pathogenic and can cause serious infection in patients.
- The proper culturing and identification of such organisms is an important aspect of the successful treatment of patients.
- All specimens that are processed in the POL should be handled carefully and all safety guidelines should be followed.
- For the pathogen to be identified correctly the utmost care must be taken in obtaining the culture without cross-contamination. Sterile equipment should be used.
- When growing a culture specimen, the correct media and incubation process must be used correctly to identify the pathogen.
- Often, a sensitivity test will be requested together with the culture. The information from this test will guide the provider in selecting the appropriate treatment for the patient.
- POLs vary in the type and number of cultures that are performed on the premises and those that are sent out to a reference laboratory.
- In addition to performing bacterial identification, some POLs perform parasitology and mycology tests on a limited basis.
- When performing mycology tests, it is important to work under a safety hood to minimize the risk for exposure to spores from the fungal specimens.
- Of utmost importance is the careful adherence to quality-control guidelines. These procedures ensure the integrity of the test results.

Study for Success

To reinforce your knowledge and skills of information presented in this chapter:

- Review the *Key Terms* and *Learning Outcomes*
- Consider the *Critical Thinking* features and *Case Studies* and discuss your conclusions
- Answer the questions in the *Certification Review*

- Perform the *Procedures* using the *Competency Assessment Checklists* on the *Student Companion Website*

Procedure

CERTIFICATION REVIEW

1. Which of the following structures is *not* part of all bacterial cells?
   a. Nucleus
   b. Ribosome
   c. Spore
   d. Cell wall

2. Which of the following is an example of nonselective media?
   a. Media that contain a substance that alters the appearance of some organisms
   b. Media that will support the growth of all organisms and does not alter their appearance
   c. Media that support the growth of one type of organism and inhibit the growth of other types of organism
   d. Media that separate the bacteria into selective groups
   e. Media that identify the biochemical activity of some organisms

3. When a CSF culture cannot be set up immediately, it should be placed in the incubator or remain at room temperature as opposed to being placed in the refrigerator because some organisms are affected by a low temperature. What is an example of this type of organism?
   a. *Beta streptococci*
   b. *Neisseria meningitidis*
   c. *Streptococcus pneumoniae*
   d. *Staphylococcus aureus*

4. What is the best method of obtaining a specimen of anaerobic organisms?
   a. Swab deep and place into an anaerobic container
   b. Make a lawn-streaked petri dish of the purulent material for later identification
   c. Aspirate purulent fluid and place into a test tube
   d. Swab around the wound and place into an anaerobic container
   e. Take as any other specimen for culture

5. Which of the following statements best describes parasitic infections?
   a. In the United States we have access to clean drinking water and sanitary conditions so parasitic infections are rare.
   b. Parasitic infections are always immediately evident with gastrointestinal symptoms such as diarrhea, nausea, and fatigue.
   c. Parasitic infections do not affect wealthy and/or educated individuals.
   d. Parasitic infections can infect anyone in the United States through water, food, skin, and body openings.

6. What is the best treatment for a parasitic infection?
   a. Total and complete isolation of the infected person
   b. Place the patient into a hyperbolic chamber to kill any anaerobic microorganisms
   c. Hospitalization and IV antibiotics
   d. Antibiotics, antiparasitics, and/or antiprotozoal medications and treating other symptoms as appropriate
   e. Let the infection run its course; the diarrhea and vomiting will rid the body of the parasite

7. When studying the form and structure of an organism, what are you studying?
   a. Bacteriology
   b. Morphology
   c. Microbiology
   d. Parasitology

8. An autoclave must be operated at 121°C and 15 PSI for how long to be effective?
   a. 15 to 20 minutes
   b. 20 to 30 minutes
   c. 30 to 45 minutes
   d. 60 minutes
   e. Only until the temperature reaches 270°F and the air is gone from the chamber

9. Which organism requires a high level of carbon dioxide to survive and grow?
   a. *Escherichia coli*
   b. *Nesseria gonorrhoeae*
   c. *Staphylococcus*
   d. All of these

10. Which parasitic infection is also called pinworm?
   a. *Escherichia coli*
   b. *Pseudomonas aeruginosa*
   c. *Candida albicans*
   d. *Enterobius vermicularis*
   e. *Trichomonas vaginalis*

CHAPTER 43

Specialty Laboratory Tests

1. Define and spell the key terms as presented in the glossary.
2. Demonstrate respect for diversity in approaching patients and families.
3. Discuss quality-control issues related to handling laboratory specimens.
4. Explain the types of waived specialty tests performed in the POL and how specimens are collected.
5. Obtain capillary blood specimens for PKU and glucose testing.
6. Select appropriate PPE for potentially infectious situations.
7. Perform CLIA-waived chemistry tests for infectious mononucleosis and cholesterol.
8. Distinguish between normal and abnormal test results.
9. Explain the concept of the hemoglobin A1c test and contrast it with daily glucometer testing.

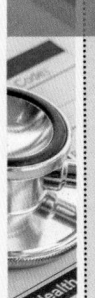

KEY TERMS

ABO blood group	induration
bilirubin	low-density lipoprotein (LDL)
blood urea nitrogen (BUN)	Mantoux test
cholesterol	phenylketonuria (PKU)
Guthrie screening test	purified protein derivative (PPD)
high-density lipoprotein (HDL)	Rh factor
human chorionic gonadotropin (hCG)	triglycerides

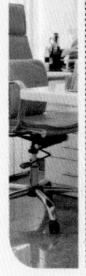

SCENARIO

Nancy McFarland, RMA (AMT), has worked at Inner City Health Care for more than 5 years. In that time, Nancy has become proficient in obtaining specimens from patients for various laboratory tests. Nancy enjoys the work and finds it extremely challenging. She also realizes that communicating with patients to help them understand why their specimens are necessary for testing is just as important as being skillful in collecting and testing the specimens. Nancy has found that when she explains the reason the specimen is needed in terms patients can understand, they are often less fearful, which helps them relax. This can be especially helpful when collecting blood specimens.

Chapter Portal

An increasing number of tests are performed in the ambulatory care setting, many of them by the medical assistant. To meet these new demands, the medical assistant must have a strong background in a variety of areas, including medical terminology, Clinical Laboratory Improvement Amendments (CLIA) regulations, laboratory safety procedures, and specimen collection. Because many procedures require collection of a blood specimen, the medical assistant must also be an excellent phlebotomist. Good record-keeping and communications skills round out the requirements. A quality-control program is necessary to ensure that the results are accurate and reliable. This will require a commitment on the part of the medical assistant to maintain the highest standards throughout the process.

A variety of specialty tests are covered in this chapter, including testing for pregnancy, infectious mononucleosis, tuberculosis (TB), and phenylketonuria (PKU), as well as blood types, hemoglobin A1c, and prothrombin time. This chapter also discusses the chemistry of blood, including chemistry panels, blood glucose, cholesterol, triglycerides, and other specialty laboratory tests such as semen analysis.

URINE PREGNANCY TESTS

Pregnancy tests are used when pregnancy is suspected. Pregnancy tests may also be used to rule out pregnancy before prescribing birth control pills, radiograph studies, and certain antibiotics or other drugs, and for female patients who are to undergo surgery.

Pregnancy testing is based on detection of **human chorionic gonadotropin (hCG)**, a hormone secreted by the placenta that can be detected in the serum of pregnant women as early as 5 days after conception, and in the urine about 11 days after. During pregnancy, hCG levels peak at about 8 to 11 weeks, then decrease to lower but detectable levels for the remainder of the pregnancy.

Commercial/Home Urine Pregnancy Tests

Procedure

A variety of accurate and easy-to-use commercial tests are available for use in the medical office. Manufacturers of pregnancy test kits have designed them to be sensitive, to be easy to perform and interpret, and to give rapid results. Pregnancy tests are one of many tests available for purchase as an over-the-counter product. However, results of tests performed at home should be confirmed by a laboratory test using appropriate quality-control measures and properly trained personnel. CLIA has granted waived status to all urine pregnancy tests that use visual color comparison and to many automated chemistry analyzers for hCG in urine. Medical assistants qualify for the category of waived tests (COW) within the physicians' office laboratory (POL) (see Procedure 43-1).

False-Positive Pregnancy Test Results

A positive reaction to any pregnancy test does not necessarily indicate a normal pregnancy; such a situation is referred to providing a false-positive result. Detection of hCG can also indicate such abnormal conditions as an ectopic pregnancy; a developing hydatidiform mole of the uterus; choriocarcinoma; or cancer of the lung, stomach, uterus, pancreas, colon, or breast.

Quality Control. Kits must be stored and used at the temperature directed by the manufacturer. Most kits contain a built-in control; however, appropriate positive and negative urine controls must always be run with patient specimens. Kits and reagents must not be used after the expiration date. Manufacturer's instructions must be followed precisely for the particular test used.

INFECTIOUS MONONUCLEOSIS

Infectious mononucleosis (IM) is a contagious disease of the herpes family (human herpes virus 4 [HHV-4]) that may have vague clinical symptoms and can mimic other diseases. Blood or serology tests are often the basis for an early diagnosis of the disease and may also be used to follow the course of the disease.

IM is commonly called mono or the kissing disease. The disease is a result of infection, through saliva, of the lymphocytes by the Epstein-Barr virus (EBV). EBV is common in our population. By 5 years of age, approximately 50% of the population is infected, a number that increases to 90% to 95% in adults. After the primary infection, the virus establishes a lifelong latency. The infectious virus may be isolated from saliva for several months, whereas antigens may be detected for life. In addition to causing IM, EBV has been implicated in other diseases such as nasopharyngeal carcinoma (NPC) and chronic fatigue syndrome.

Transmission of EBV

Transmission of EBV IM is primarily by saliva, and it may be spread by the sharing of drinking glasses and less often by blood transfusion. The disease is moderately contagious and is transmitted approximately 10% to 38% of the time in close social groups. In the home or in the hospital, careful hand washing and not sharing drinking or eating utensils will help prevent transmission of the virus.

Symptoms of IM

Mononucleosis is seen most often in children and young adults. Incubation may vary from 4 to 50 days; however, 7 to 14 days is the average. Infection in younger children is usually asymptomatic or manifests minor symptoms such as pharyngitis, otitis media, bronchitis, and other upper respiratory discomforts.

Classic symptoms usually occur when the primary infection is delayed until the second decade of life. IM is most often observed in the 15- to 25-year-old age group. Symptoms usually begin with a fever and swollen glands lasting for 3 to 5 days. Over the next 7 to 20 days, the patient may develop a headache; malaise; chest pain; cough; tonsillitis; rash; soft, swollen lymph nodes; and swollen spleen. While the spleen is enlarged, the patient is advised to curtail activity, especially contact sports and rough activities, to prevent the rare, but serious, rupture of the spleen. Symptoms usually persist for 1 to 2 weeks

Performing Pregnancy Test

Procedure

STANDARD PRECAUTIONS:

Handwashing Gloves Biohazard Goggles & Mask Gown

PURPOSE:

To perform the waived category visual determination test to detect hCG in urine to determine positive or negative pregnancy results.

EQUIPMENT/SUPPLIES:

- Gloves
- Urine specimen
- Stopwatch
- Disinfectant
- Biohazard container
- hCG negative and positive urine controls
- Pregnancy test kit

PROCEDURE STEPS:

1. Wash hands and put on gloves. RATIONALE: While working with body fluids, such as urine, gloves should be worn as personal protection.

2. Assemble all equipment and supplies. RATIONALE: Organizing all equipment and supplies before running the test will eliminate errors caused by missing supplies.

3. ***Paying attention to detail,*** perform the test following the manufacturer's instructions. The following steps are intentionally general so a variety of kits can be used. RATIONALE: The manufacturer's instructions will differ from kit to kit. It is important, as a quality-assurance measure, for the instructions to be read and understood thoroughly. Any questions must be directed to the manufacturer.

   a. Determine materials are at room temperature.

   b. Apply urine to the test unit using dispenser provided (Figure 43-1A).

   c. Wait appropriate time interval (use stopwatch to time test).

   d. Apply first reagent/antibody to test unit using dispenser provided.

   e. Observe color development after appropriate time interval.

   f. Stop reaction.

   g. Consult manufacturer's package insert to interpret test results (Figure 43-1B).

4. Record the results of the test on a laboratory report form following laboratory policy. RATIONALE: Interpretation of results may differ from kit to kit according to the manufacturer's design, and even though laboratory processes are the same, policies and forms will differ from laboratory to laboratory.

5. Repeat steps with both positive and negative urine controls (Figures 43-1C). RATIONALE: Controls are performed to ensure the quality of the reagents and testing supplies. If a positive control test does not show a positive result, then something is wrong with the reagent or the testing supplies. If the control test is not accurate, the patient's test will not be accurate either.

(continues)

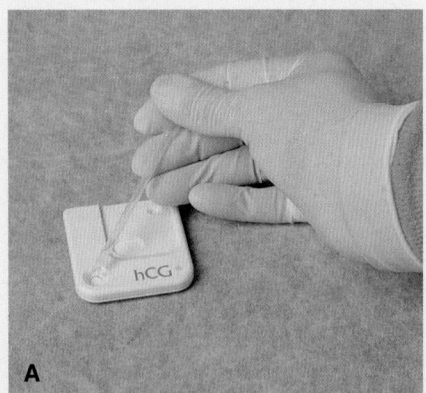
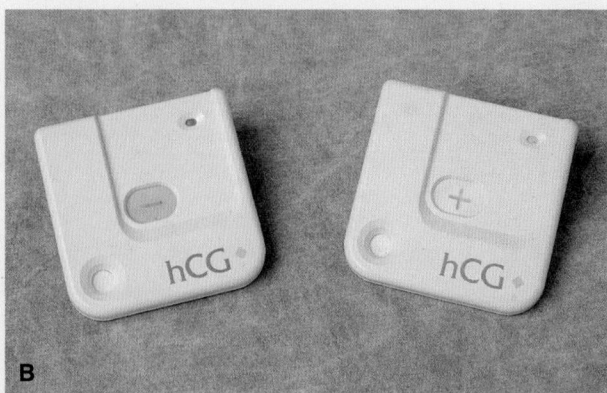
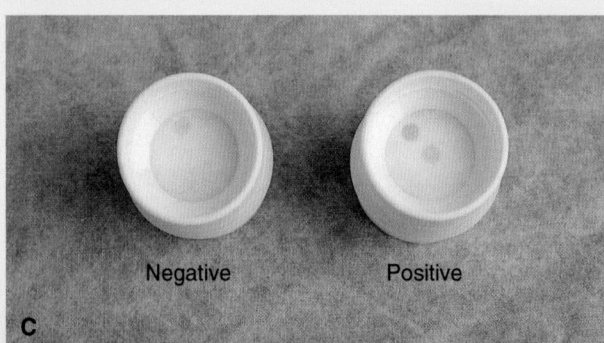

Negative   Positive

FIGURE 43-1 (A) Urine is placed in the test unit according to the manufacturer's instructions. (B) The package instructions specify how the test is to be interpreted. A common indication is with a negative sign (left) and a positive sign (right). (C) Control tests must be performed according to the manufacturer's instructions. The results of the positive and negative controls test are shown.

6. Disinfect reusable equipment. Discard disposable supplies into the biohazard container. Dispose of the specimen per laboratory policy. Clean work area with disinfectant. RATIONALE: Follow Standard Precautions and laboratory policies for disposal of biohazard substances and disinfection of supplies/equipment.

7. Remove gloves and discard into the biohazard container. Wash hands. RATIONALE: Gloves protect hands from most but not all microorganisms. Hands should always be washed after removal of gloves to ensure complete protection and to remove glove powders and latex residue.

8. Document procedure in patient's chart or EHR. Complete a lab report. After the provider has initialed the report, it should be filed in the lab section of the patient's chart. RATIONALE: Documentation should refer the reader to the test result in the laboratory section of patient's health record.

DOCUMENTATION:

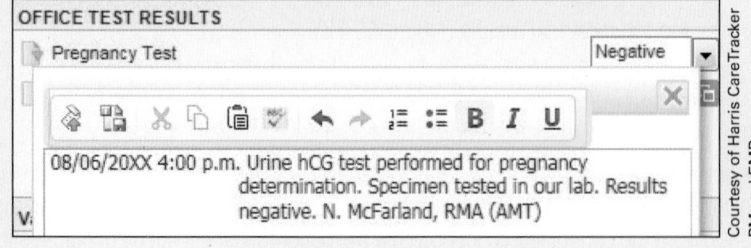

Courtesy of Harris CareTracker PM and EMR

and in more serious cases may last for more than a month.

Treatment of IM

Because there are currently no effective drugs available for EBV, IM treatment is primarily palliative, or supportive. Although a vaccine is not yet available, some important work in that direction is ongoing.

Diagnosis of IM

To properly diagnose IM, the provider must consider blood and serology test results together with the patient's symptoms.

Blood Test for IM. The hematologic tests for IM include white blood cell count and evaluation of the patient's lymphocytes. In IM, lymphocytosis, or increase in lymphocytes, usually occurs, and large numbers of lymphocytes (greater than 20%) have an unusual or atypical appearance.

Serologic Test for IM. Persons with IM produce antibodies by the sixth to tenth day of the illness. Detection of antibodies combined with the blood tests and patient symptoms provide the basis for the diagnosis of IM. The serum test is usually positive after the first week of illness. However, if test results are negative, the test should be repeated a week later if clinical symptoms are still present.

CLIA-Waived IM Tests

Procedure

Several manufacturers have produced CLIA-waived test kits suitable for use by the medical assistant in the POL (see Procedure 43-2).

Kits for IM usually provide all the necessary reagents, materials, and controls. The laboratory must obtain only the specimen to be tested, which is usually a small sample of the patient's plasma or serum or a drop of capillary blood.

PROCEDURE 43-2

Procedure

Performing an Infectious Mononucleosis Test

STANDARD PRECAUTIONS:

   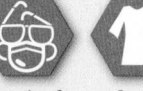 

Handwashing   Gloves   Biohazard   Goggles & Mask   Gown

PURPOSE:

To perform an accurate test of serum or plasma to detect the presence or absence of antibodies of infectious mononucleosis (IM).

EQUIPMENT/SUPPLIES:

- Gloves
- Serum or plasma specimen
- Stopwatch or lab timer
- Surface disinfectant
- CLIA-waived test kit for IM
- Biohazard container

PROCEDURE STEPS:

NOTE: These instructions are intentionally general so a variety of test kits may be considered. The manufacturer's specific instructions will differ from kit to kit. It is important, as a quality-assurance measure, for the instructions to be thoroughly read and understood before performing the test. Any instructions not clearly understood should be clarified with the manufacturer.

(continues)

1. Wash hands and put on gloves. RATIONALE: While working with body fluids, such as urine, gloves should be worn as personal protection.

2. Assemble all equipment and supplies. RATIONALE: Organizing all equipment and supplies before running the test will eliminate errors caused by missing supplies.

3. *Paying attention to detail,* perform the test according to the manufacturer's instructions exactly. RATIONALE: The manufacturer's instructions will vary with each specific kit. Quality results are assured only when instructions are followed precisely.

4. Record the results on a laboratory report form following laboratory policy. RATIONALE: Even though laboratory processes are the same, policies and forms will differ from laboratory to laboratory.

5. Repeat the test procedure using positive and negative controls. RATIONALE: Controls are performed to ensure the quality of the reagents and testing supplies. If a positive control test does not show a positive result, then something is wrong with the reagent or the testing supplies. If the control test is not accurate, the patient's test will not be accurate either.

6. Discard contaminated materials into the biohazard container. Dispose of the specimen appropriately and disinfect reusable materials. Clean the work area with disinfectant. RATIONALE: Follow Standard Precautions and laboratory policies for disposal of biohazard substances and disinfection of supplies/equipment.

7. Remove gloves and discard into the biohazard container. Wash hands. RATIONALE: Gloves protect hands from most but not all microorganisms. Hands should always be washed after removal of gloves to ensure complete protection and to remove glove powders and latex residue.

8. Document results in the patient's chart or EHR. Complete a lab report. After the provider has initialed the report, it should be filed in the lab section of the patient's chart. RATIONALE: Documentation should refer the reader to the test result in the laboratory section of the patient's chart.

DOCUMENTATION:

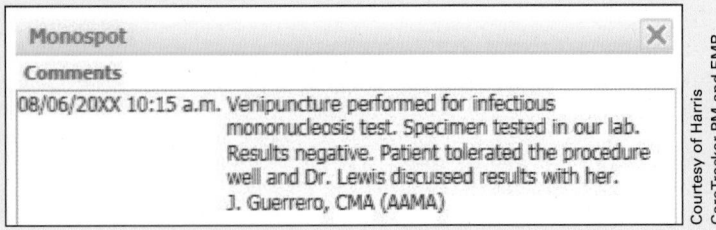

Monospot	✕
Comments	
08/06/20XX 10:15 a.m. Venipuncture performed for infectious mononucleosis test. Specimen tested in our lab. Results negative. Patient tolerated the procedure well and Dr. Lewis discussed results with her. J. Guerrero, CMA (AAMA)	

Courtesy of Harris CareTracker PM and EMR

PROTHROMBIN TIME

Prothrombin time, which is also called protime, PT, and international normalized ratio (INR), is a test of blood's clotting ability. It is used often for people who are taking anticoagulant medications such as Coumadin (warfarin).

Coumadin targets vitamin K molecules and is influenced by dietary intake of vitamin K. This influence makes it an unstable treatment and regular monitoring is needed to make sure it is effective but not overly thinning the blood.

The desired levels of INR are 2.0 to 3.0. Refer to Chapter 40 for more information on coagulation studies and Procedure 40-4 for the process of running a prothrombin time test.

BLOOD TYPING

Blood types are based on the presence or absence of certain antigens on the surface of red blood cells (RBCs). Antibodies are protein molecules that are found in serum; they are also referred to as immunoglobulins (Ig). When RBC antigens and antibodies react, they cause the RBCs to agglutinate (clump). This process, called hemagglutination reactions, are used in the typing of blood. The two major categories of blood typing are for the **ABO blood group** and the **Rh factor**. The ABO blood group consists of type A, type B, type AB, and type O. Within each of these types are the Rh factors, either Rh-positive (factor present) or Rh-negative (no factor).

The ABO and Rh systems place certain restrictions on how blood can be transfused from one individual to another. Depending on their blood type, individuals with a particular RBC antigen may have antibodies against the other types (Table 43-1). An incompatible blood transfusion results when the antigens of the donor RBCs react with the antibodies of the recipient RBCs. This is a potentially life-threatening situation that varies in severity from mild fever to anaphylaxis with severe intravascular hemolysis. Although ABO and Rh typing does not completely rule out the possibility of reaction, it greatly reduces the chances.

ABO Blood Typing

ABO blood typing is determined by the presence or absence of two major antigens, A and B. All people have one of the four blood group categories: A, B, AB, or O. People with group A red blood cells have A antigens, group B red blood cells have B antigens, group AB red blood cells have antigens for both A and B, and group O red blood cells lack both A and B antigens. Naturally occurring antibodies to the other antigen types are found in the serum.

Figure 43-2 illustrates how RBCs are tested for blood type. In the example, type O blood would have no reaction to either anti-A or anti-B, whereas type AB blood would have a reaction to both. By process of elimination, one can determine which type the specimen is. Because type O blood has neither antigens nor Rh factor, it is considered to be the universal donor. Type AB⁺ blood has both

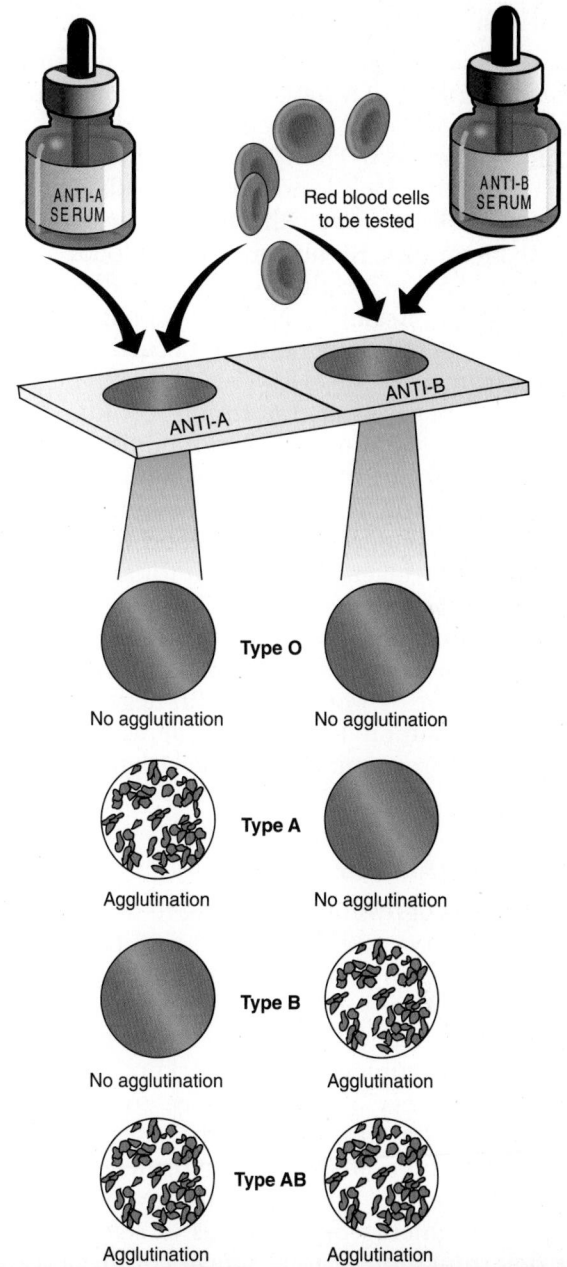

FIGURE 43-2 Blood typing the ABO groups.

antigens and an Rh factor so it is considered to be the universal recipient.

ABO type can be determined by the slide or tube method. The tube method is now most often used for blood typing. Because neither method is considered to be in the waived category by CLIA, they usually are not performed in the POL. Even if the patient carries a card listing his or her blood type, the patient's blood will be retested as a precaution. This is called a blood cross and match test. Nevertheless, it is a good idea to know your individual blood type and Rh factor.

TABLE 43-1

ANTIGENS AND ANTIBODIES IN ABO AND RH BLOOD SYSTEMS

BLOOD GROUP/TYPE	ANTIGEN ON RBC	SERUM ANTIBODIES
O (universal donor)	None	Anti-A and anti-B
A	A	Anti-B
B	B	Anti-A
AB (universal recipient)	A and B	None
Rh⁺	D	No anti-D*
Rh⁻	None	No anti-D*

*There are no naturally occurring antibodies to the Rh system.

Rh Blood Factor

The Rh blood factor test is routinely performed together with ABO typing. The Rh system is named for the rhesus monkey used in experiments that led to its discovery. The Rh factor is found on the surface of RBCs. People possessing the Rh factor are said to have Rh-positive (Rh⁺) blood. Those without the Rh factor have Rh-negative (Rh⁻) blood.

About 85% of North Americans are Rh positive; 15% are Rh negative. Neither Rh-negative nor Rh-positive people have naturally occurring Rh antibodies in their blood. However, if an Rh-negative individual receives a transfusion of Rh-positive blood, he or she will develop antibodies to it and will have a serious transfusion reaction. Nowadays, this medical error is very rare. The antibodies can take 2 weeks to develop. Both blood type and Rh factor must be taken into account for safe and successful transfusions.

Rh blood typing is also performed on pregnant women to determine the mother's Rh blood type and Rh factor. A woman with Rh-negative blood must take caution because problems can occur during the pregnancy. Reference Chapter 25 for more details.

SEMEN ANALYSIS

With the progression of managed health care, more primary care providers are performing semen analysis in their offices to determine sperm cell counts before referring patients to fertility specialists. Examination of semen is also performed as part of a complete fertility workup, to evaluate the effectiveness of a vasectomy, to determine paternity, and to substantiate rape cases.

When semen analysis is performed as part of a fertility workup, the procedure involves macroscopic and microscopic analysis of seminal fluid for determination of total sperm count, percentage of motility, amount of semen, liquefaction time, pH, presence of white blood cells, fructose level, and percentage of normally formed sperm cells (Table 43-2). All male individuals will have variable sperm counts; therefore, a single analysis is insufficient. To achieve a reasonable estimate of these factors, the seminal analysis should be repeated at least three times over a 2-month period. A complete analysis will also include an evaluation of the partner's cervical secretions and sperm survival. This involves determining the ability of sperm to penetrate the mucus and maintain motility.

Postvasectomy semen analysis (PVSA) is done a few weeks after surgery. If sperm cells are present

TABLE 43-2

SAMPLE SEMEN ANALYSIS

TEST	NORMAL RANGE	SAMPLE PATIENT VALUE
Volume	1.5 to 5 mL	2.5 mL
Appearance	White, viscid, opaque	Opaque
Liquification time	30 minutes	30 minutes
pH	7.7 to 8.0	7.12
Total count	50 to 300 million	150 million
% normal sperm	At least 80%	88%
% motility	At least 60%	64%

at that time, then follow-up analysis is required. Waived PVSA kits are now available for home use or use in the POL. The patient is not considered sterile until he has returned *two* samples, at least 1 week apart, that demonstrate no sperm, viable or dead. This typically will take several weeks. Until that time, an alternative method of birth control must be used.

Semen Composition

Semen is a composite solution produced by the testes and the accessory male reproductive organs. It consists primarily of spermatozoa suspended in seminal plasma. Because there is considerable variation in composition between different portions of the fluid as ejaculated, it is important to collect the entire sample. Refer to the Patient Education box for instructions to give to the male patient before semen analysis.

Altering Factors in Semen Analysis

Many factors can alter the results of semen analysis. Several drugs reduce sperm count, as do certain conditions such as orchitis (inflammation of the testes), testicular atrophy, and obstruction of the vas deferens. Cigarette smoking is associated with a decrease in the volume of semen, whereas coffee drinking results in increased sperm density and an increase in the percentage of cells with abnormal morphology. Fever may temporarily suppress the count. Although research suggests

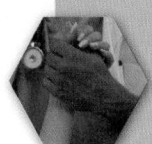

Patient Education

The following instructions should be given to male patients when a semen sample is required for analysis:

1. Advise the patient to avoid consumption of alcohol for several days before the test. He should also avoid ejaculation for 3 days before collection of the semen sample.

2. Provide the patient with instructions and a container. The entire sample should be collected in a clean, dry, glass bottle that has been labeled, including the date and time. The sample is collected by masturbation or interrupted coitus at home, or it may be collected at the medical office of the laboratory. A condom should never be used to collect a semen specimen due to the spermicide content.

3. Specimens for complete fertility analysis collected outside the laboratory must be brought to the laboratory within 30 minutes. Postvasectomy specimens should be brought to the laboratory within 1 hour of collection.

4. The sample must be transported to the laboratory at 37°C (98.6°F). Low temperature during transport will decrease the motility of sperm. Temperature that is too warm could destroy the sperm. Keeping the sample close to the body during transport might be the best advice.

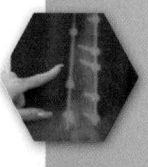

Critical Thinking

Since the sperm sample in a fertility analysis needs to be maintained at internal body temperature until tested, what options would be available for the male patient who lives 40 miles from the laboratory?

that consumption of alcohol may or may not affect sperm function as measured by semen analysis, as a precaution, the patient is instructed to avoid alcohol for several days before testing.

Men with sperm counts lower than 15 million per milliliter of semen are considered infertile. Patients with aspermia (no sperm) or oligospermia (low sperm count, ≤20 million/mL) should be endocrinologically evaluated for pituitary, testicular, adrenal, or thyroid abnormalities.

PHENYLKETONURIA TEST

Communication

Phenylketonuria (PKU) is an inherited condition in which a baby does not have the enzyme that metabolizes the phenylalanine amino acid into tyrosine amino acid properly. Phenylalanine is present in milk and other dairy proteins. If the baby has PKU, phenylalanine can build up in his or her brain and other organs and cause irreversible intellectual disability, loss of muscle coordination, and other

serious disorders. Diagnosis should be made early so that the baby can be put on a diet low in proteins. The baby should be tested at about 2 days old and again at 7 to 14 days old. Although a phenylalanine-restricted diet will prevent intellectual disability, it will not cure the underlying condition. Routine screening of newborns for PKU is mandatory in all states and may be performed in the hospital or the medical office. The medical assistant's role is to properly explain the procedure to the infant's parents and to collect the blood specimen for analysis.

Many other tests can be performed using the blood sample sent on the PKU card, including tests for congenital hypothyroidism (CH), congenital adrenal hyperplasia (CAH), galactosemia, sickle cell disease, and others. The tests that are performed depend on individual state requirements.

Blood Testing for PKU

Excess phenylalanine can be detected in blood or in urine. Normal levels of phenylalanine are less than 2 mg/deciliter (dL); more than 4 mg/dL is considered elevated. The **Guthrie screening test** is used to evaluate blood and is considered more accurate than urine tests. Phenylalanine can be detected in the blood of infants with PKU after 3 to 4 days on a breast milk or formula milk diet. Testing of breast-fed infants is delayed a few days because of the lack of phenylalanine in colostrum, the first breast milk. Colostrum is produced for the first 2 to 3 days after birth and is rich in antibodies, protein, and calories. True breast milk production begins after this time. Positive results from blood testing are confirmed by measuring serum phenylalanine and tyrosine levels. Infants with PKU have increasing phenylalanine levels (>4 mg/dL) and decreasing tyrosine levels (<0.6 mg/dL).

Procedure

The Guthrie test was developed to screen for phenylalanine in the blood, and the first test is usually performed before the infant is discharged from the hospital. However, with managed care and the trend toward very short hospital stays for newborns, many pediatricians' offices are now performing this first test. Even though it may seem that testing for PKU right after birth wouldn't be needed because the newborn hasn't had time to digest phenylalanine, some babies will show positive PKU and other abnormalities. Unfortunately, some babies do not get their 2-week checkup, making this first PKU in the hospital all the more important. Capillary blood is collected from a heelstick onto a filter paper test card and sent to the laboratory for testing (see Procedure 43-3). Patient, provider, and test information, together with the blood samples, are placed directly on the laboratory test card, which is typically provided by most state Departments of Health (Figure 43-3).

Factors That May Influence the Guthrie Test. The following factors may influence the Guthrie test:

- Feeding problems such as vomiting may result in a false-negative result.
- Failure to ingest sufficient phenylalanine—testing before 3 to 4 days of the beginning of a milk diet—will result in a false-negative reaction.
- Premature infants may give false-positive test results because of a delay in the development of certain liver enzymes.
- Drugs such as salicylates, aspirin, or antibiotics taken by the mother (if breast-feeding) or the child may interfere with test results.

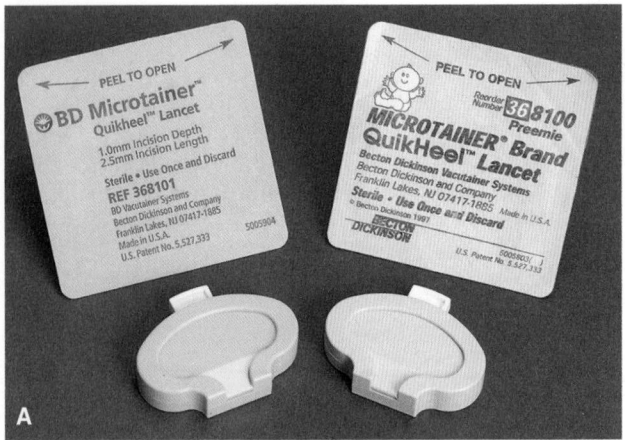

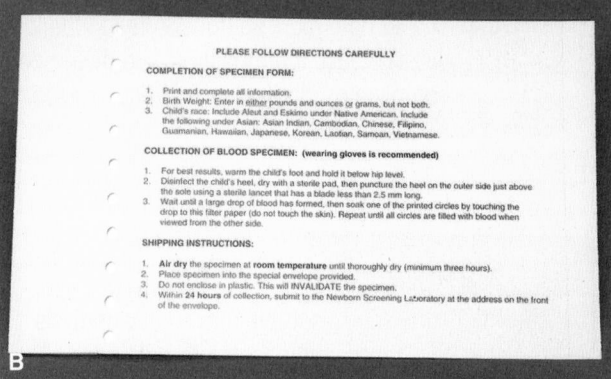

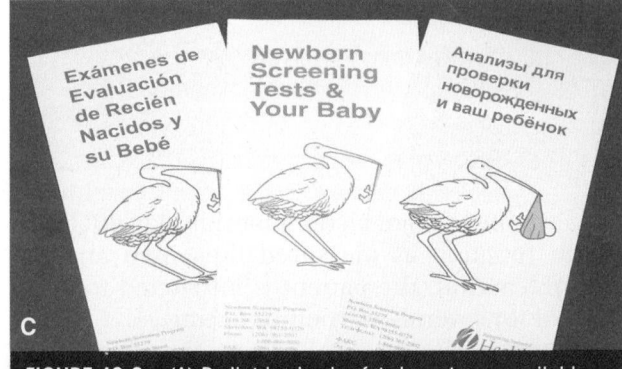

FIGURE 43-3 (A) Pediatric-sized safety lancets are available to vary the depth of the puncture. (B) The back of the PKU test card provides detailed instructions on performing the test and completing the card correctly. (C) Patient information and permission forms are available in a variety of languages.

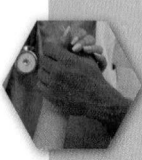

Patient Education

Infants who test positive for PKU require a restricted phenylalanine diet for normal development to occur. Parents will need to have an appointment with a dietician to understand fully what foods the baby can and cannot eat. The diet will include a suitable milk substitute. Blood and urine tests will be necessary periodically to monitor the special diet.

Women who have PKU and become pregnant must be especially careful to avoid phenylalanine during pregnancy.

Procedure

Obtaining Blood Specimen for Phenylketonuria (PKU) Test

STANDARD PRECAUTIONS:

Handwashing   Gloves   Biohazard   Goggles & Mask

PURPOSE:

To obtain a blood specimen using a PKU test card or filter paper to determine phenylalanine levels in newborns who are at least 3 days old.

EQUIPMENT/SUPPLIES:

- Gloves
- PKU filter paper test card and mailing envelope
- Alcohol swabs
- Gauze pads
- Sterile pediatric-sized lancet
- Biohazard waste container
- Official information pamphlet

PROCEDURE STEPS:

1. Wash hands and put on gloves. RATIONALE: While working with body fluids, gloves should be worn as personal protection.

2. Identify the infant. Introduce yourself by name and credential and identify the patient and the parent(s). RATIONALE: Introducing yourself and stating your credentials will demonstrate professionalism and will help ensure the parent's cooperation. Identifying the patient and his or her parent will ensure that you have the right patient.

3. *Speaking to the parent's level of understanding, explain the rationale for performance of the procedure, showing awareness of the parent's concerns.* Provide written information as well. *Demonstrate professionalism and courtesy while you explain.* RATIONALE: Explaining the procedure in a manner the parent understands reassures him or her and helps ensure cooperation. Demonstrating professionalism will help maintain a professional atmosphere and may help put the parent at ease, as some parents may become apprehensive with this procedure. The written information is helpful to the parents and required by law.

4. Select and clean an appropriate puncture site (Figure 43-4A). Allow the alcohol to dry before the puncture. RATIONALE: Cleaning the site before puncture will remove any powders, oils, lotions, and contaminates. Allowing the alcohol to dry prevents the stick from stinging.

5. Grasp the infant's foot, taking care not to touch the cleansed area. Make a puncture approximately 1 to 2 mm deep in the infant's heel, ensuring the infant's lateral, or side, portion of the heel pad is used. A pediatric-sized lancet, which limits the depth of puncture, should be used (Figure 43-4B). If possible, recent puncture sites should always be avoided (see Procedure 39-6, Capillary Puncture).

6. Wipe away the first drop of blood with a gauze pad. RATIONALE: The first drop is diluted with alcohol and should not be collected for the test. Using a gauze pad rather than a cotton ball is preferred because the cotton ball may leave tiny fibers on the puncture site. The fibers may encourage clotting, which will interfere with obtaining sufficient specimen for the test.

7. To collect blood for the test, press the back side of the filter paper test card against the infant's heel while exerting gentle pressure on the heel (Figure 43-4C). The drop of blood should be large enough to completely fill and soak through the circle. *Do not* layer multiple blood drops within a single circle. Completely fill all of the circles on the test card. RATIONALE: Failure to do so will require a retest.

(continues)

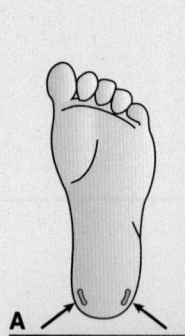
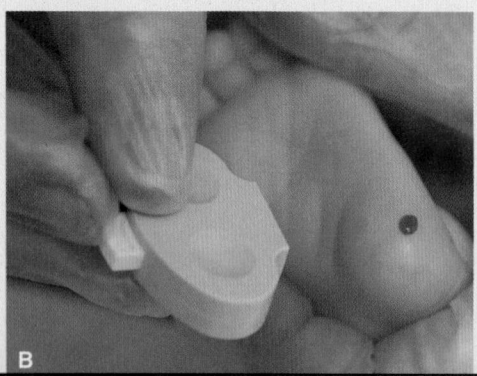
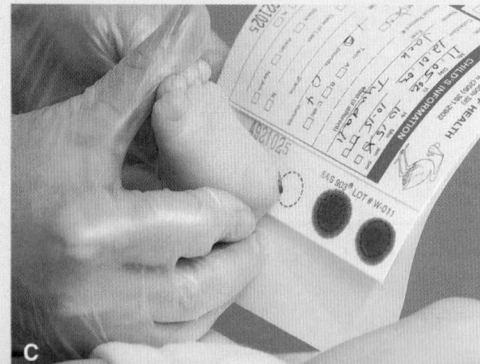

FIGURE 43-4 (A) Capillary blood collections sites on an infant's heel. (B) The infant's foot should be held securely with the nondominant hand while the dominant hand uses the pediatric lancet to perform the capillary heelstick. (C) Drops of blood are transferred from the capillary heelstick puncture site to the PKU filter card, completely filling all the circles.

8. Hold a gauze pad over the puncture and apply gentle pressure until the bleeding stops. Do not apply a bandage. RATIONALE: The bleeding should be stopped before the patient is released from your care. Bandages are discouraged because they can be a choking hazard for infants and toddlers.

9. Properly dispose of all waste in the biohazard container. RATIONALE: Follow Standard Precautions and laboratory policies for disposal of biohazard substances and disinfection of supplies/equipment.

10. Remove the gloves and wash hands. RATIONALE: Gloves protect hands from most but not all microorganisms. Hands should always be washed after removal of gloves to ensure complete protection and to remove glove powders.

11. Ask the parent if he or she has any questions and provide appropriate responses. RATIONALE: Soliciting questions will encourage the parent to ask if there is something he or she doesn't understand. Providing appropriate responses will further the parent's understanding and ensure a more cooperative follow-up.

12. Allow the PKU test card to completely dry on a nonabsorbent surface at room temperature. This will take about 2 hours. If collecting more than one card, *do not* lay one card on another when drying. RATIONALE: This could cause cross-contamination of blood between the cards.

13. After the test card is dry, complete the PKU test card with all patient and provider information. RATIONALE: Allowing the blood to dry thoroughly before further handling lessens the chances of contaminating other parts of the form.

14. Place the test card in the mailer envelope and send it to the laboratory within 2 days. RATIONALE: It is important that the completed card be mailed quickly to eliminate the breakdown of the contents within the specimen and to obtain the results as soon as possible to begin treatment if necessary.

15. Document the procedure in the patient's chart. When test results are returned, they should be initialed by the provider and placed in the lab section of the patient's chart. RATIONALE: Documentation should refer the reader to the test result in the laboratory section of the patient's chart.

DOCUMENTATION:

PROCEDURE NOTE

06/27/20XX 10:54 a.m. Capillary puncture performed on lateral aspect of left heel for PKU testing. Pt. is 12 days old, currently taking no medication, and is not ill. Pt. tolerated the procedure well and adequate specimen was obtained. PKU card completed and mailed. N. McFarland, RMA (AMT)

07/10/20XX 4:16 p.m. PKU test results received and initialed by Dr. King and filed in the laboratory section of the patient's medical record. The patient's parents were notified of the negative results per Dr. King's instructions. N. McFarland, RMA (AMT)

Courtesy of Harris CareTracker PM and EMR

TUBERCULOSIS

Despite efforts to control its spread, 9.6 million people around the world contracted tuberculosis (TB) infections in 2014 (10,000 of those in the United States), and 1.5 million people died from TB infection. The Advisory Council for Elimination of Tuberculosis, an independent group of TB-control experts, recommends screening all patients who fall into high-risk groups, or those who associate with high-risk groups, such as health care workers, including medical assistants. See the "Current Family Practice Recommendations for TB Testing" Patient Education feature in this chapter for a more complete list.

Cause of TB

Infectious TB is caused by the small rod-shaped bacterium *Mycobacterium tuberculosis*. This aerobic bacterium is nonmotile and has a high content of lipid in its cell wall, making it difficult to stain using basic dyes. For this reason, a special method called Ziehl-Neelsen was developed and is used as a tool for identification of mycobacteria. Mycobacteria will retain the red stain in the presence of acid alcohol and are therefore referred to as acid-fast.

Resistance in Mycobacteria

Mycobacteria exhibit an unusual degree of resistance on many fronts. They are able to tolerate drying and the effects of many disinfectants. Mycobacteria also show resistance to most antibiotics, making these infections difficult to treat. To help overcome bacterial resistance to antimicrobial agents, patients take two or three drugs for a period of 6 to 9 months. The most common drug used to fight TB is isoniazid (INH). Other drugs used are rifampin, pyrazinamide, ethambutol, and streptomycin.

Transmission of Infectious TB

Infectious TB is highly contagious, but is not spread by casual contact or even sharing drinks or kissing. Seventy-five percent of new cases occur by inhalation of cough-produced airborne droplets from symptomatic or asymptomatic persons. Crowded conditions contribute to this transmission. TB often is associated with poverty, poor nutrition, and crowded conditions such as those often seen in prisons and psychiatric health hospitals.

Diagnosis of TB

TB diagnosis differentiates between active and inactive TB, and the treatments differ. Active

---

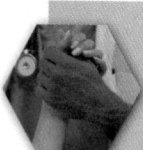

Patient Education

Current Family Practice Recommendations for TB Testing

TB screening is recommended for:

- Close contacts of those with known or suspected TB.

- Persons infected with HIV.

- Intravenous drug users or users of other illicit drugs.

- Chronically ill patients with conditions or diseases that increase the risk for progressing from latent to active TB. Risk factors include diabetes, high-dose steroids, immunosuppressive therapy, chronic renal failure, lymphoma, leukemia, other cancer, weight loss to more than 10% below ideal weight, silicosis, gastrectomy, and jejunoileal bypass.

- Foreign-born persons and those arriving within the last 5 years from countries that have a high incidence of TB.

- Residents and employees of high-risk institutions, such as correctional facilities, nursing homes, psychiatric institutions, and homeless shelters.

- Health care workers, especially those caring for patients at high risk.

- Medically underserved and low-income populations.

- Infants, children, and adolescents exposed to adults at high risk.

TB is a serious and contagious condition that requires isolation of the patient and aggressive treatment with several drugs over several months. TB can live in the body without causing illness, a period when it is referred to as latent or inactive TB. If the person becomes weakened through another illness or injury, the latent TB can become active, taking advantage of the person's weakened state.

Patients exhibiting a positive or questionable **purified protein derivative (PPD)** reaction should have a chest X-ray to detect active TB. A tuberculin skin test (TST), or a sputum sample might also be indicated. Reasons for a positive reaction to PPD are varied. First and most obvious is that the patient has been exposed to TB or has an active case of TB. Persons with an old, inactive case will also give a positive skin test, as will persons who have been vaccinated with BCG. BCG (bacille Calmette-Guerin) is a vaccine used in Europe and South America to help prevent childhood cases of TB. Persons who receive BCG may have a positive skin reaction for a minimum of 4 years and much longer in many cases. Many immigrants will show positive PPD because of a BCG vaccination.

Screening for TB: Skin Testing

Legal

Integrity

Screening for TB may be performed as part of a routine medical examination or as a prerequisite for school or employment. In states where medical assistants can legally perform injections, they may be responsible for administration and interpretation of the skin test. The most accurate method used is the **Mantoux test** (for more information, see the "Mantoux Test" Quick Reference Guide). The tine test, which is a multiple-puncture test, may still be used in some areas but is no longer recommended by the American Academy of Pediatrics. Both the Mantoux and the tine methods use tuberculin, also referred to as PPD, which is a filtrate of tuberculin cultures that are used for skin testing. Persons who have been exposed to TB will develop a hypersensitive response to PPD resulting in the formation of an induration. An induration is a hard, raised area on the skin that is the result of sensitized lymphocytes migrating to the site of the injection. It is important to keep in mind that a positive skin test does not distinguish between active and inactive cases of TB. The medical assistant's role is to measure the size of the induration and report the findings to the provider, who will

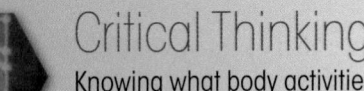
assess the results. Because of the possible severity of the reaction, it is not recommended that the PPD skin test be administered to persons who have had a positive reaction in the past.

THYROID

The thyroid gland is an endocrine gland located in the throat and is responsible for producing thyroid hormones. The thyroid gland takes in iodine to produce its two hormones, thyroxine (T4) and triiodothyronine (T3), and is the only gland in the body that can absorb iodine. There are many critical functions regulated by T3 and T4 (with chemical assistance from other endocrine glands) such as breathing, heart rate, body weight, muscle strength, energy, mood, temperature, cholesterol levels, menstrual cycles, the nervous system, and many more.

Thyroid Functioning Test

We test T3 and T4 levels in the blood if patient symptoms indicate an irregularity. TSH (thyroid stimulating hormone from the pituitary gland) is usually tested with T4. Both T3 and T4/TSH should stay within a therapeutic range as determined by the individual laboratory. If these tests are outside the normal ranges, the provider will order further tests and may prescribe medication. These tests are performed by laboratory technicians, but the medical assistant can draw the sample and educate the patient as delegated by the provider.

BLOOD GLUCOSE

Glucose is the principal and almost exclusive carbohydrate found circulating in blood. It may also be detected in urine, cerebrospinal fluid, and semen. Glucose serves as an energy source for the body. Excess glucose is converted into glycogen for short-term storage in the liver and muscle cells, and as adipose tissue (body fat) for long-term storage. Tests for blood glucose levels are commonly performed in the medical

The Mantoux Test

In the Mantoux test, 0.1 mL of 5 TU (toxin unit) strength PPD is injected intradermally using a 1 mL tuberculin syringe. A short (½ inch), 26- or 27-gauge needle is used. Care must be taken to inject the PPD so that a wheal forms (Figure 43-5). If the injection is too deep, it will be impossible to form the wheal. If the injection is too shallow, the PPD may leak onto the skin. Either of these two errors would invalidate the test results. It is also important to draw exactly 0.1 mL of the PPD, because too much or too little will lead to erroneous test results. Refer to Procedure 35-7 for the complete injection procedure for the Mantoux test.

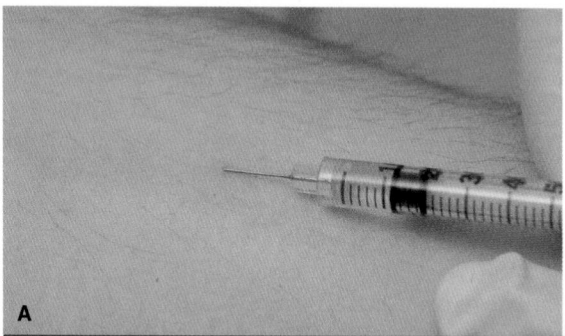 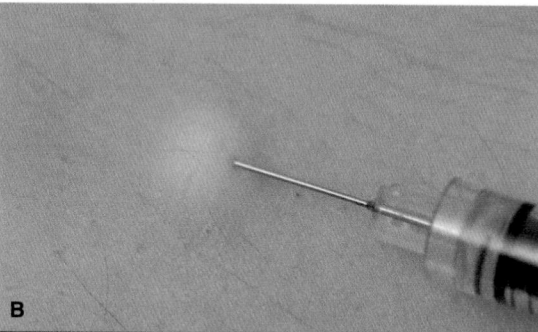

FIGURE 43-5　(A) Gently insert the needle just under the skin surface at about a 5-degree angle with the bevel up. Imbed the entire bevel. Slowly and carefully inject the medication. (B) A wheal should appear as a whitish raised bump.

≫ READING THE RESULTS OF THE MANTOUX TB TEST

The patient will have been instructed to return within 48 to 72 hours for an examination of the Mantoux injection site. If the patient delays the return visit more than 72 hours, the results cannot be properly determined.

Gently feel and measure the **induration** (the hard raised area) (Figure 43-6). Do not include the area of redness or erythema in the measurement. Some patients will show swelling or localized raised hives and complain of itching at the injection site. These responses are not true indurations but rather are localized allergic reactions to the protein derivative and should not be misinterpreted as a positive response to the Mantoux test. Alert the physician to any unusual reactions. Do not repeat the Mantoux test if an allergic reaction has occurred.

The size of the induration is recorded for the provider to assess and determine further testing, as follows:

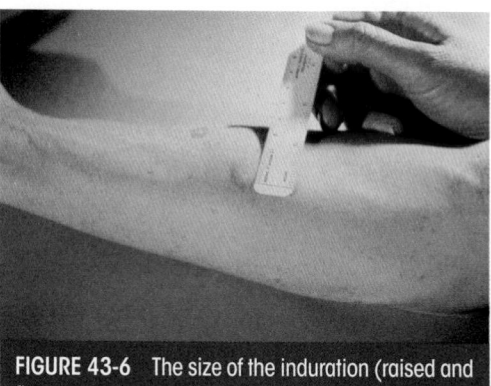

FIGURE 43-6　The size of the induration (raised and firm area, not the redness) is measured as shown.

Courtesy of CDC/Donald Kopanoff

Induration	Description
	Positive reaction for past or present infection: 10 mm or more duration
	Doubtful reaction: 5 to 10 mm duration; considered positive among persons who have had recent contact with active TB, persons who are HIV positive, persons with a chest X-ray consistent with healed TB
	Negative reaction: without induration or less than 5 mm

office. The results are used to screen for carbohydrate disorders such as hypoglycemia (low blood glucose level) and hyperglycemia (high blood glucose level), both of which can occur in diabetes mellitus. A variety of testing methods have been developed to diagnose, evaluate, and monitor abnormalities in carbohydrate metabolism. They include fasting blood glucose (FBG) and the oral glucose tolerance test (OGTT). All tests are discussed here, but the FBG is preferred as the first step in the clinical setting because it is easier and faster to perform, more convenient and acceptable to patients, and less expensive.

Blood glucose concentrations rise after a meal and are regulated by the action of several hormones, including insulin and glucagon. Both insulin and glucagon are produced by the pancreas. Insulin is secreted by pancreatic cells in response to increased glucose levels and aids with the entry of glucose into cells for conversion into energy. Insulin is also required for proper storage of glucose (which is first converted into glycogen) in the liver and in muscle cells. Glucagon is secreted by the pancreas when blood sugar levels decrease and triggers the breakdown of glycogen to help increase and regulate blood sugar levels (see Figure 43-7).

Fasting Blood Glucose

Evaluation of FBG levels is commonly used to screen for diabetes mellitus. Diabetes mellitus is a type of carbohydrate disorder characterized by insulin deficiency (or no insulin) and a state of hyperglycemia.

The normal fasting value of glucose ranges from 70 to 110 mg/100 mL (mg/dL). Table 43-3 lists preferred serum glucose values. A value of 120 mg/dL glucose is the dividing point between healthy and hyperglycemic individuals. Generally, increased glucose levels can indicate diabetes mellitus, and further testing might be indicated.

Hemoglobin A1c

Hemoglobin A1c (HbA1c), or glycosylated hemoglobin, determination is a blood test that measures an average of glucose in the blood over the past few months, giving providers a better picture of how well the diabetic patient has maintained a healthy serum glucose level (Figure 43-8).

Glycosylated hemoglobin is a stable molecule formed when sugar and hemoglobin bind together on the RBC. When the RBC is first formed, it contains no glucose. If glucose is present at increased levels in the blood, the excess enters the RBC and attaches (glycates) to the hemoglobin within the cell. The more glucose present, the more glucose becomes attached. Most RBCs live about 120 days and maintain the glycated state throughout the life of the cell. The HbA1c test measures how much glucose has attached to the RBCs, giving an average of the glucose in the blood over about 3 months. See Table 43-3 for HbA1c preferred values.

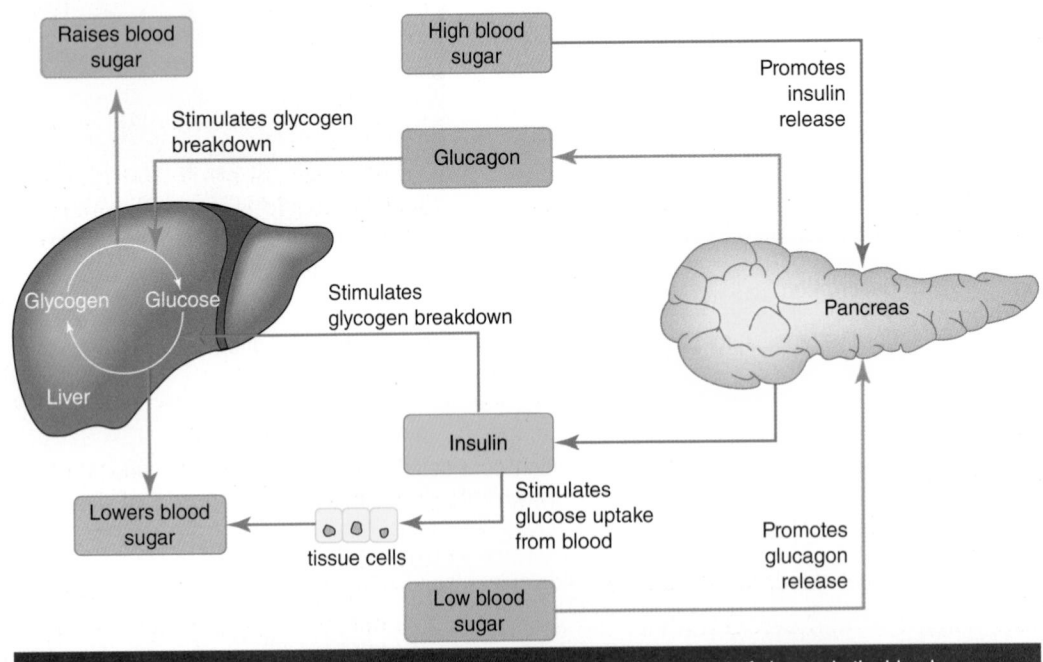

FIGURE 43-7 The pancreas and liver work together to help regulate the amount of glucose in the blood.

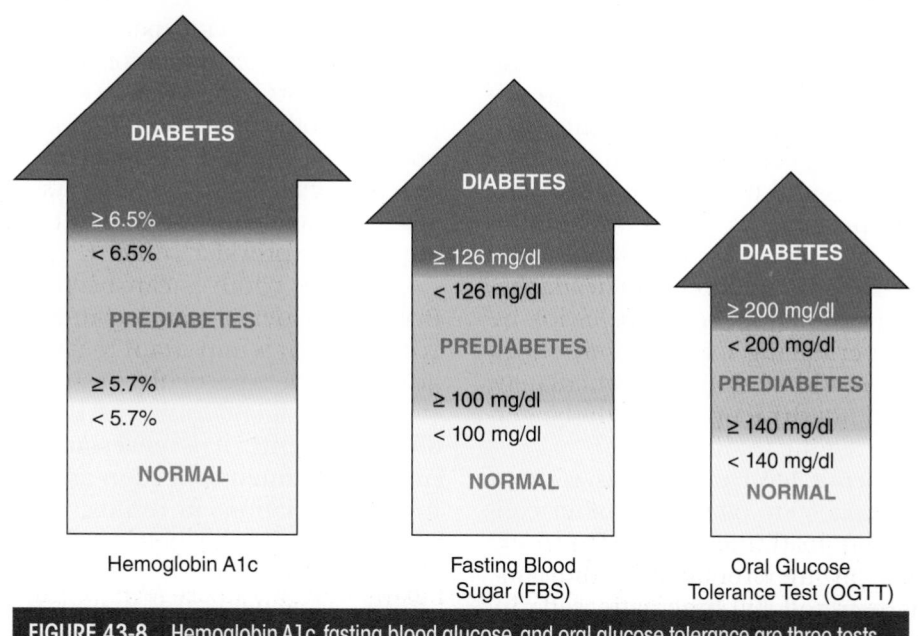

DIABETES
≥ 6.5%
< 6.5%
PREDIABETES
≥ 5.7%
< 5.7%
NORMAL

Hemoglobin A1c

DIABETES
≥ 126 mg/dl
< 126 mg/dl
PREDIABETES
≥ 100 mg/dl
< 100 mg/dl
NORMAL

Fasting Blood
Sugar (FBS)

DIABETES
≥ 200 mg/dl
< 200 mg/dl
PREDIABETES
≥ 140 mg/dl
< 140 mg/dl
NORMAL

Oral Glucose
Tolerance Test (OGTT)

FIGURE 43-8 Hemoglobin A1c, fasting blood glucose, and oral glucose tolerance are three tests that are used to determine blood glucose levels.

What the hemoglobin A1c value does not do is indicate whether the patient has experienced hyperglycemia or hypoglycemia over that time frame because day-to-day readings of glucose levels are not provided; thus, it is not useful in adjusting insulin. Having the patient monitor his or her blood glucose level with a meter and keep a daily diary is a good way to look at his or her day-to-day blood glucose levels. Both tests are useful tools in helping manage diabetes.

Another advantage of hemoglobin A1c is that the patient does not need to fast for this test.

TABLE 43-3

REFERENCE VALUES FOR BLOOD GLUCOSE LEVEL

TEST	PREFERRED GLUCOSE VALUES
Hemoglobin A1c	Less than 5.7% without diabetes Less than 7.0% with diabetes
Fasting serum glucose	70 to 100 mg/dL without diabetes 80 to 130 mg/dL with diabetes
Two-hour postprandial and oral glucose tolerance test	Less than 140 mg/dL without diabetes Less than 180 mg/dL with diabetes

Values vary slightly between laboratories depending on the testing method used.

Two-Hour Postprandial Blood Glucose Test

The 2-hour postprandial (after eating) evaluation of blood glucose level is not often used to diagnose diabetes but is useful in evaluating appropriate insulin dosage. The patient with diabetes takes insulin with a meal, then, exactly two hours after beginning the meal, checks his or her blood glucose level. In a healthy person, the glucose has returned to a normal level, but it may still be elevated in people with diabetes. An elevated 2-hour postprandial test may indicate that the insulin dosage needs to be adjusted.

Oral Glucose Tolerance Test

The oral glucose tolerance test glucose tolerance test (OGTT) provides more detailed information that can be used to assess insulin response to glucose and to diagnose diabetes. This test is often used to diagnose gestational diabetes (diabetes during pregnancy).

After fasting for 8 hours, the patient is given a glucose solution (a process called glucose loading). Blood glucose levels are tested every 30 to 60 minutes for 3 to 6 hours. These measurements help determine the patient's ability to deal with increased glucose. During the test, the patient must not ingest anything (other than the solution) except water. The patient must also abstain from smoking, because smoking acts as a stimulant and increases blood glucose levels. The patient must also refrain from chewing gum, which stimulates the digestive process and also may add sugar to his or her system. Physical activity should be strongly discouraged because activity can activate sugar utilization in the body and affect the test results. Sedentary activity level is suggested.

During the second and third hours of the test, the patient may experience weakness, slight faintness, and perspiration. These are all normal symptoms. If, however, the patient develops a headache, faints, or displays irrational speech or behavior, he or she may be experiencing hypoglycemic shock and the provider should be notified immediately. The patient should not drive or work with dangerous equipment during the testing hours.

The blood glucose level of patients without diabetes usually peaks 30 to 60 minutes after consumption of the test load at 160 to 180 mg/dL and returns to the fasting level after 2 to 3 hours. Patients with diabetes will still have increased glucose levels at the end of the test.

Automated Methods of Glucose Analysis

Several types of glucose analyzers are available that are suitable for POLs or small clinical laboratories. Many of these operate on the principle of reflectance photometry and use adaptations of the enzymatic methods of glucose analysis. One example of an instrument suitable for small laboratories is the DCS 2000 used to test hemoglobin A1c (Figure 43-9).

A variety of inexpensive, handheld glucose meters that are designed for home use are also suitable for use in point-of-care (POC) testing or in the provider's office. See the following Patient Education box for some criteria for patients to consider when purchasing an at-home testing system. Most of these are also suitable for use in point-of-care (POC) testing or in the provider's office (Figure 43-10).

Glucose controls can be purchased to check instrument performance. Since each glucometer is different, it is important to use test materials that are made for a particular instrument, such as test strips and reagents, only with that instrument. With all instruments, it is necessary to use consistent proper specimen collection and testing technique to avoid variations in results; procedure steps are not interchangeable between instruments.

 The medical assistant is sometimes responsible for providing education to patients on how to use glucometers, including maintenance and calibration of the meter. It is

Initiative

important that the medical assistant who works with patients with diabetes become familiar with a variety of meters and their differences and similarities.

Photometry Analyzers. The HemoCue blood glucose system is a professional laboratory-grade compact glucose analyzer based on the principle of photometry (Figure 43-11). The system consists of a compact photometer and disposable microcuvettes. The self-filling microcuvette automatically draws 5 µL of blood from a capillary puncture into its reaction chamber. The microcuvette is then placed into the holder and pushed into the photometer. The glucose concentration in milligrams per deciliter (mg/dL) is displayed in one to four minutes. This system is ideal for POLs and POC testing because of the stability of calibration and the minimal operator training required.

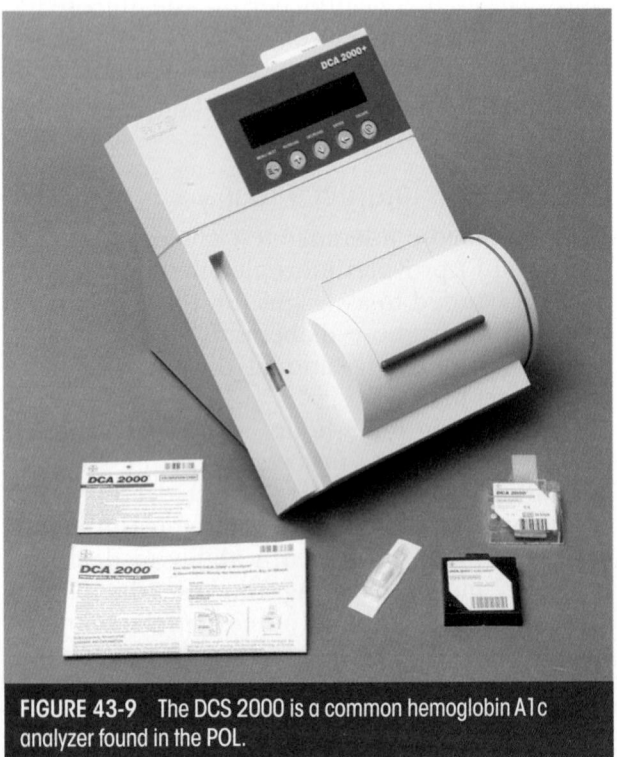

FIGURE 43-9 The DCS 2000 is a common hemoglobin A1c analyzer found in the POL.

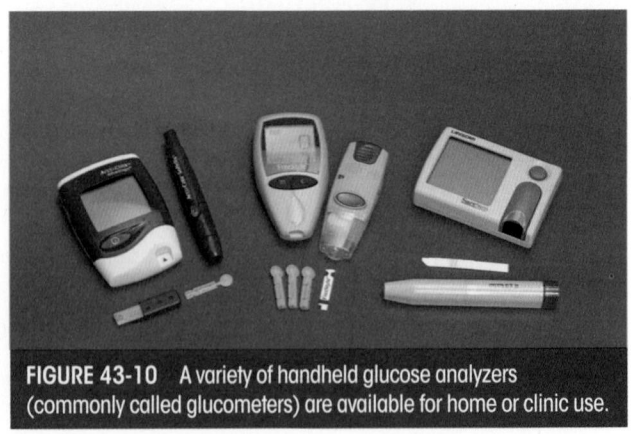

FIGURE 43-10 A variety of handheld glucose analyzers (commonly called glucometers) are available for home or clinic use.

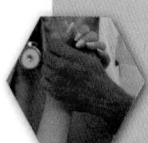

Patient Education

Let your patient know there are many glucose meters available to choose from. All of them use the typical process of a drop of blood applied to a disposable test strip that is then inserted into the meter. The unit measures how much glucose is in the sample. All the meters display the result. Some meters allow a much smaller sample to be used and allow the sample to be taken from sites other than the fingertip (alternate site testing). Some meters record and store a number of test results, and some meters can connect to a personal computer to store results and print them out. Most models have automatic timing, error codes and signals, and barcode readers to help with calibration. Some meters have a large display screen or spoken instructions for people with visual impairments. In choosing a meter, the patient should consider the following:

- Cost per strip
- Amount of blood needed for testing
- Overall size and portability
- Cost of the meter
- Ability to store test results in memory
- Ability to test sites other than fingertip
- Other personal preferences

Many manufacturers offer free meters with the purchase of the test strips. Your clinic may be given free meters to give to patients together with a few sample strips in hopes the patient will continue to use that meter and purchase the strips. Unfortunately, the meters given to patients might not be the best choice for them, but the patients will continue to use them because their doctor provided them. Be sure to let patients know that there are many choices, and that the free meter you are giving them is not necessarily an endorsement of one meter over another.

Reflectance Photometry Analyzers. Several glucose analyzers are available that are based on reflectance photometry. Blood from a fingerstick, serum, or plasma is applied to the reagent area of a test strip. The glucose in the sample reacts with the reagents in the pad(s), causing a color to form. The more glucose present in the sample, the darker or more intense the color. At the appropriate time, the strip is inserted into the test chamber and light is directed onto the test area. The amount of light reflected from the colored test area is measured by the photometer and converted to a digital readout showing the glucose concentration in milligrams per deciliter (mg/dL). Most instruments give results in 1 to 3 minutes. Instructions included with the test strips must be followed carefully for reliable test results (see Procedure 43-4).

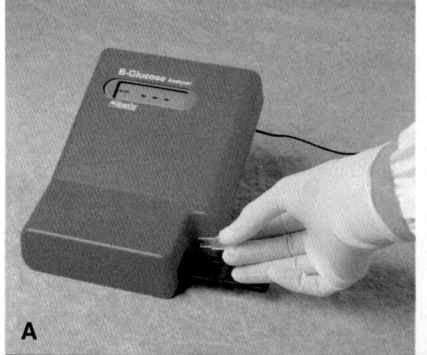 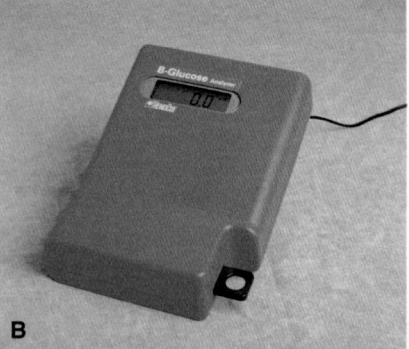 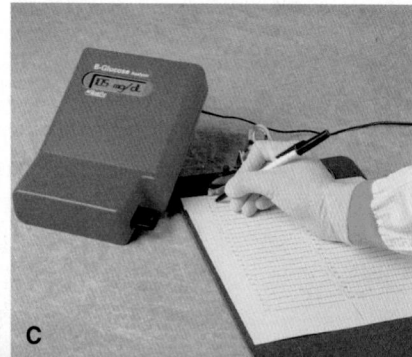

FIGURE 43-11 The HemoCue Blood Glucose System. (A) The patient's blood specimen is placed on the microcuvette. The microcuvette is inserted into its holder and pushed into the photometer. (B) Specimen is allowed to remain in the analyzer until test is completed. (C) When the analyzer has completed the test, the results are displayed and recorded.

PROCEDURE 43-4

Procedure

Measuring Blood Glucose Using an Automated Analyzer

STANDARD PRECAUTIONS:

Handwashing

Gloves

Biohazard

Goggles & Mask

PURPOSE:

To measure blood glucose.

EQUIPMENT/SUPPLIES:

- Gloves
- Safety lancet
- Alcohol swabs
- Glucose analyzer
- Adhesive strip

- 2 × 2 gauze
- Control solutions for glucose analyzer
- Test strips for glucose analyzer
- Laboratory tissue

PROCEDURE STEPS:

1. Review the manufacturer's manual for the specific glucose analyzer being used, ***paying attention to detail***. Turn on the analyzer. RATIONALE: Always read and follow the manufacturer's instructions exactly for your particular analyzer to ensure accurate results.

2. Clean the work area and assemble all materials and supplies. RATIONALE: Organizing all equipment and supplies before running the test will eliminate errors caused by missing supplies.

3. Wash hands. Put on gloves. RATIONALE: Washing your hands ensures that your skin is clean before gloving and decreases contaminants. Applying personal protection equipment when working with body fluids will lessen the chances of exposure to dangerous biohazard substances.

4. Record the control ranges, control lot number, and test strip lot number. RATIONALE: Recording the lot numbers and control ranges is another type of quality-assurance measure and is required by CLIA for many automated tests.

5. Perform the check test and the control test according to the manufacturer's instructions. If both tests are within range, proceed to the glucose test. Repeat both tests if either is out of acceptable range. RATIONALE: Controls are performed to ensure the quality of the reagents and testing supplies. If a positive control test does not show a positive result, then something is wrong with the reagent or the testing supplies. If the control test is not accurate, the patient's test will not be accurate either.

6. Remove a test strip from the bottle and replace the lid. RATIONALE: Replacing the lid securely ensures that the reagents are protected from light and moisture.

7. Insert the test strip into the test chamber. Some analyzers require the sample be applied to the test strip prior to inserting the test strip into the machine. RATIONALE: Follow the manufacturer's instructions for proper use of test kits.

8. Perform a capillary puncture (see Procedure 39-6). Wipe the first drop with gauze. RATIONALE: Wiping the first drop away lessens the amount of tissue fluid in the specimen.

9. Apply a large drop of blood to the test strip. RATIONALE: The test requires a large drop of blood for accurate results. Let a large drop form before applying it to the test device.

10. While the test is running, check the puncture site. If the bleeding has stopped, apply an adhesive strip. RATIONALE: The test will take time to compute, allowing you time to treat the patient.

(continues)

11. After the appropriate time interval has passed, read the glucose concentration. RATIONALE: The test requires an appropriate amount of time for accurate results.

12. Properly dispose of all waste in a biohazard waste container. RATIONALE: Follow Standard Precautions and laboratory policies for disposal of biohazard substances and disinfection of supplies/equipment.

13. Remove gloves and wash hands. RATIONALE: Gloves protect hands from most but not all microorganisms. Hands should always be washed after removal of gloves to ensure complete protection and to remove glove powders.

14. Document the procedure in the progress notes section of the patient's medical record. Document the results of the test, which then go to the provider for his or her initials. RATIONALE: The results should always be initialed by the provider.

DOCUMENTATION:

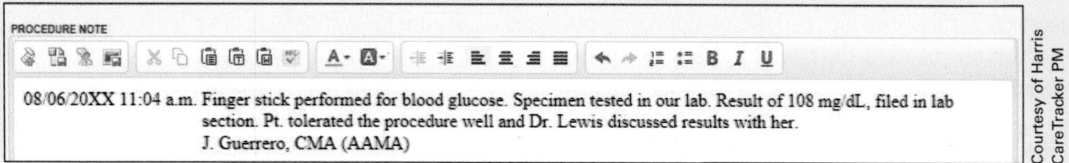

PROCEDURE NOTE

08/06/20XX 11:04 a.m. Finger stick performed for blood glucose. Specimen tested in our lab. Result of 108 mg/dL, filed in lab section. Pt. tolerated the procedure well and Dr. Lewis discussed results with her.
J. Guerrero, CMA (AAMA)

Courtesy of Harris CareTracker PM and EMR

CHOLESTEROL, LIPIDS, AND SYSTEMIC INFLAMMATION

Procedure

Cholesterol is a fatty compound that is essential for many vital life functions and is a normal constituent of blood. Although it is required for life, excess cholesterol is not a necessary part of the diet, except in babies and children. Sufficient quantities are manufactured by the body from carbohydrates and other fats. Excess cholesterol is linked to coronary (heart) artery disease. According to the American Heart Association and the National Institutes of Health, cholesterol should not be restricted in babies and toddlers since fats and cholesterol are important for normal growth and development. Babies and very young children should be on healthy diets, though, containing unsaturated and polyunsaturated oils and fats. From about 4 or 5 years old, they can be transitioned to heart-healthy foods such as nonfat milk. To help reduce the risk for coronary artery disease, nutritionists and agencies such as the American Heart Association and the National Cholesterol Education Program advise that fats make up no more than 30% of the total intake of calories daily, and that the concentration of cholesterol in blood not exceed 200 mg/dL. Cholesterol of 240 mg/dL or greater is considered to present a high risk for heart disease. Cholesterol levels between 200 and 239 mg/dL are considered borderline. Several CLIA-waived cholesterol test kits are available for quick screening purposes (see Procedure 43-5).

The Chemistry of Cholesterol

The cholesterol molecule consists of carbon, hydrogen, and oxygen. Cholesterol is a saturated fatty acid. *Saturated* refers to the number of hydrogen atoms attached to the molecule. The more saturated the fat, the more solid it is at room temperature. Fats of animal origin, for example, butter and animal fat, are saturated and are solid at room temperature. Monounsaturated and polyunsaturated fats are liquid at room temperature. Research into coronary artery disease has shown that saturated fats tend to increase levels of blood cholesterol. Monounsaturated fats (olive and peanut oils) do not change blood cholesterol levels, and polyunsaturated fats (corn, safflower, sunflower, and many fish oils) tend to reduce those levels.

Functions of Cholesterol

The human body is efficient at manufacturing cholesterol. The liver is the main organ that produces cholesterol. Other cells throughout the body use cholesterol to manufacture steroid hormones. In addition, cholesterol is an important component of bile and cellular membranes. Although the

PROCEDURE 43-5

Procedure

Performing Cholesterol Testing

STANDARD PRECAUTIONS:

 Handwashing   Gloves    Biohazard    Goggles & Mask

PURPOSE:

To measure cholesterol and triglycerides for monitoring purposes. *NOTE:* The following steps are intentionally general so a variety of kits can be used. The manufacturer's instructions will differ from kit to kit. It is important, as a quality-assurance measure, for the instructions to be read and understood thoroughly. Any questions must be directed to the manufacturer.

EQUIPMENT/SUPPLIES:

- Gloves
- Blood collecting equipment
- Pipettes with disposable tips
- Chlorine bleach
- CLIA-waived commercial kit for manual determination of cholesterol

- Controls and standards
- Marking pen
- Biohazard container

PROCEDURE STEPS:

1. Assemble all necessary equipment and materials. RATIONALE: Organizing all equipment and supplies before running the test will eliminate errors caused by missing supplies and will show the patient a more professional process.

2. Wash hands; apply gloves. RATIONALE: Washing your hands ensures that your skin is clean before gloving and decreases contaminants. Applying personal protective equipment when working with body fluids will lessen the chances of exposure to dangerous biohazard substances.

3. Obtain a blood sample from the patient, either by fingerstick or venipuncture, depending on the manufacturer's instructions (see Chapter 39). RATIONALE: Always read and follow the manufacturer's instructions to ensure accurate results.

4. *Paying attention to detail,* follow the manufacturer's instructions to perform the cholesterol test. Be sure to run the controls also. RATIONALE: Following all manufacturer's instructions will ensure accurate test results. Controls are performed to ensure the quality of the reagents and testing supplies. If the control test is not accurate, the patient's test will not be accurate either.

5. Properly dispose of all waste in the biohazard container. RATIONALE: Follow Standard Precautions when disposing of sharps and biohazard and contaminated waste.

6. Record the results of the test on a laboratory report form and document the procedure in the patient's chart. After the provider has initialed the report, file it in the patient's chart. RATIONALE: The chart note should refer the reader to the laboratory section of the patient's chart.

DOCUMENTATION:

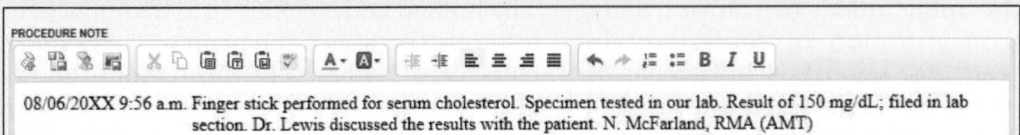

08/06/20XX 9:56 a.m. Finger stick performed for serum cholesterol. Specimen tested in our lab. Result of 150 mg/dL; filed in lab section. Dr. Lewis discussed the results with the patient. N. McFarland, RMA (AMT)

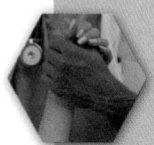

Patient Education

Following your provider's instructions, educate your patients about factors that can influence their blood cholesterol levels:

- *Age and sex.* Cholesterol levels naturally increase as we age, and women experiencing menopause often will experience an increase in their LDL levels.
- *Heredity and family history.* High cholesterol often runs in families. Studies are still in process about the role genetics plays in cholesterol levels.
- *Weight.* Gaining weight increases cholesterol levels in the blood, and losing weight helps to reduce cholesterol levels.
- *Exercise.* Regular physical exercise may reduce LDL levels, as well as increase HDL levels.

body is efficient at making cholesterol, it is not as easily degraded and may accumulate in the body, where it can reach dangerous levels.

In addition to what the body produces, humans take in additional cholesterol through the ingestion of meat, eggs, and dairy products (Figure 43-12). The liver metabolizes cholesterol to its free form, which is then bound to lipoprotein (fat + protein) and transported through the blood. Over time, excess cholesterol in the diet can result in a gradual increase of cholesterol concentration in the blood, which can lead to all sorts of health problems, including cardiovascular conditions. Some of the excess is stored in the liver (a main cause of non-alcoholic fatty liver), whereas some is deposited on the walls of blood vessels, causing atherosclerosis (a narrowing of the arteries due to buildup of plaque) and hardening of the arteries (arterosclerosis).

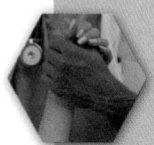

FIGURE 43-12   Cholesterol is created by the liver or obtained through animal sources of food such as meat, eggs, and dairy products.

Since the coronary (heart) arteries are smaller than most other arteries of the body, they are more susceptible to becoming blocked. Blockage of coronary arteries is the most common cause of myocardial infarction (heart attack).

Lipoproteins and Cholesterol Transport

Two kinds of lipoprotein are involved in the transport of cholesterol through the body: **high-density lipoprotein (HDL)** and **low-density lipoprotein (LDL)**. Cholesterol bound to HDL is transported to the liver, where it is excreted in the form of bile. HDL is sometimes referred to as good cholesterol. LDL cholesterol is deposited in the tissues as fat and inside the walls of blood vessels, and it is referred to as bad cholesterol. High levels of LDL are associated with an increased risk for coronary artery disease. Desirable values for HDL and LDL are shown in Table 43-4. Levels of HDL and LDL are influenced by many factors, both genetic and environmental. It is possible to increase HDL levels through a combination of weight loss, a diet low in saturated fats, exercise, and cessation of smoking.

Blood cholesterol may be reported as total cholesterol or as total cholesterol and the HDL and LDL fractions. Cholesterol screening is used to help identify patients who are at a high risk for heart disease.

Cholesterol testing is part of a lipid profile that also evaluates lipoproteins and triglycerides to help identify patients at a high risk for heart disease.

Triglycerides

Triglycerides are a type of lipid found in the blood, and they serve as a source of energy. Fatty acids and glycerol from foods are converted into

TABLE 43-4

VALUES FOR CHOLESTEROL, HDL, LDL, AND TRIGLYCERIDES

MEASUREMENT	VALUES (MG/DL)
Triglycerides	
Desirable	<150
Borderline high	150 to 199
High	200 to 499
Very high	>500
Total cholesterol (with no other risk factors such as hypertension and/or diabetes)	
Desirable	<200
Less desirable	200 to 239
At risk	>240
HDL (good cholesterol)	
Desirable	>60
At risk for women	<50
At risk for men	<40
LDL (bad cholesterol)	
Desirable	<100
Borderline risk	130 to 160
High risk	>190

triglycerides by the liver. When triglyceride levels in the blood are excessive, they are deposited throughout the body as adipose tissue (commonly known as fat). Triglycerides are transported within the bloodstream by LDL and very low-density lipoproteins (VLDLs).

Many factors influence serum triglyceride levels. Serum triglyceride concentration will increase moderately after eating a meal containing fat, peaking 4 to 5 hours later. Increased concentrations of triglycerides are associated with an increased risk for coronary and vascular disease. Desirable values for triglycerides are shown in Table 43-4.

Inflammation

With the escalating rates of heart disease in the United States, and the seemingly ineffective treatments of dietary changes and medications, there has been a shift in focus to systemic inflammation as the predominant cause of heart disease. It has long been determined that inflammation causes cholesterol plaque to accumulate in the arteries. The simple causes of systemic inflammation are said to be due to bacteria, viruses, toxins, and certain types of foods, namely, processed, prepackaged foods and foods high in sugars and omega-6 fatty acids.

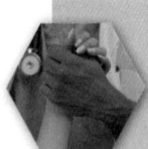

Patient Education

The Simple Scoop on Cholesterol

Cholesterol can be a confusing subject to try to explain to patients. Here is a very basic explanation that may help them:

Our bodies need cholesterol and we get it in two ways. We eat it and our liver manufactures it. Our liver manufactures plenty of cholesterol, so we do not need to eat it (except as babies and young children). There is only one source of cholesterol in our food: animal products (meat, eggs, and dairy). Vegetables, fruits, and grains naturally contain no cholesterol, although they may contain oils.

Our bodies have cholesterol transporters called high-density lipoproteins (HDLs) and low-density lipoproteins (LDLs).

HDLs (sometimes called healthy lipoproteins) carry cholesterol to the liver where they can be released into the stool as bile. We want high levels of HDLs so we can get rid of excess cholesterol.

LDLs (sometimes referred to as lousy lipoproteins) carry cholesterol to our tissues and blood vessels, where they are stored and can cause problems such as blocked arteries, fatty liver, and obesity. We want low levels of LDLs so we can have less risk for heart disease and arterial disease.

Fats and oils can also be confusing. Saturated fats are solid at room temperature and come from animal fats and butter and from manufactured products such as hydrogenated fats. These are the worst fats. Unsaturated fats, which are liquid at room temperature, may be in two forms: monounsaturated fats (*mono* means "single") and polyunsaturated fats (*poly* means "many"). Monounsaturated fats such as olive and peanut oils do not affect blood cholesterol levels, whereas polyunsaturated fats such as corn, safflower, sunflower, and fish oils will actually reduce blood cholesterol levels.

Triglycerides are a type of lipid found in our blood, and they provide energy. If we have too many in our blood, they are also stored in our tissues as fat. The liver converts some of our foods (fatty acids and glycerol) into triglycerides.

Omega-6 oils are used in overly processed foods to sustain shelf life. The consumption of many omega-6 oils causes an imbalance with the healthier omega-3 oils. The ratio should be a 3:1, rather than the more common 15:1 or higher. Overeating overly processed, prepackaged foods loaded with omega-6 oils and sugars often leads to obesity, which can lead to inflammation, high blood pressure, heart disease, diabetes, and even Alzheimer disease. Simply put, we were never meant to consume overly processed, prepackaged food products and should return to eating foods in their natural state.

C-reactive protein (CRP) and the more sensitive hs-CRP are blood tests to determine systemic inflammation and are currently being used in conjunction with traditional cholesterol blood tests and patient assessment to determine cardiac risk. Because CRP is an inflammation indicator, it can also be elevated as a result of acute arthritis and infections.

BLOOD CHEMISTRY TESTS

There are many natural chemicals in blood. The amounts of those chemicals are controlled by the efficiency of the body's organs and organ systems and certainly by environmental factors such as diet, smoking, drugs, and activity, as well as genetic composition.

The provider can order a general chemistry panel (BMP or CMP) or specific panels. As mentioned previously, a panel is a series of tests related to a body system, organ, or function. In interpreting a chemistry panel, the provider can determine pathology or malfunctions within a particular organ.

This chapter discusses each component of blood chemistry tests briefly and explains some of the conditions and diseases that can cause these chemical tests to be abnormal. Keep in mind that all laboratory chemistry tests can vary slightly from laboratory to laboratory. Also remember that no one test, just like no one symptom, will make a diagnosis independent of other clues. The provider is considering laboratory tests together with the clinical picture, patient symptoms, and many other data in finalizing a diagnosis or diagnoses.

Alanine Aminotransferase (ALT)

ALT is an enzyme found in liver tissue. A high level indicates liver damage. A normal ALT level is less than 45 units/L.

Albumin

Most of the protein in plasma is albumin. It is responsible for transporting many small molecules (such as calcium, drugs, and bilirubin). It is synthesized in the liver; thus, low levels of albumin may indicate liver disease. It may also result from kidney disease, because the kidney is allowing too much albumin to spill into the urine. Low albumin may also be caused by malnutrition or a low-protein diet. A normal albumin level is 3.4 to 5.4 mg/dL.

Alkaline Phosphatase (ALP)

ALP is an enzyme. It is present in all our body tissues but mostly in the liver and bone. When levels are high in the blood, liver or bone disease must be suspected. A normal ALP level is 44 to 147 IU/L.

Aspartate Aminotransferase (AST)

AST is found in the muscle cells (heart and skeletal muscles) and in the liver. High levels cannot specifically indicate liver disease, but AST values are considered together with other liver enzymes. AST is also used to monitor patients who have had heart muscle damage (such as heart attacks), but it is not the best or only enzyme tested for that purpose. A normal AST level is 10 to 34 IU/L.

Bilirubin, Total and Direct

Bilirubin is a yellow-orange substance that comes from the breakdown of hemoglobin. Hemoglobin is contained within the RBCs. Because individual RBCs live for only 120 days, they are constantly breaking down and being replaced. When the RBCs die, the heme part of the hemoglobin circulates in the blood until the liver filters it out. The liver is responsible for changing the heme into a water-soluble substance called bilirubin. Before it reaches the liver, it is called indirect or free bilirubin. After it leaves the liver, it is called direct or conjugated bilirubin. The liver sends the conjugated bilirubin to the gallbladder, where it is released with bile into the small intestine. Bilirubin gives feces its characteristic color. When there is a blockage in the liver/gallbladder ducts or a disorder/disease of the liver, the bilirubin cannot get past the gallbladder to the small intestine, so it continues to circulate in the blood. The body will try to get rid of extra bilirubin through the urine. Hence, any detection of bilirubin in the urine (bilirubinuria) can be indicative of a problem in the liver or gallbladder. When the bilirubin level increases, it causes the skin and whites of the eyes to become yellow. This condition is called jaundice. Newborn babies can be jaundiced because their systems are not sophisticated enough to get rid of the bile. Because bilirubin breaks down in sunlight, babies with jaundice are treated with special "bili-lights" that mimic sunshine to help them break down the bilirubin in their skin. The total bilirubin test will indicate problems in the liver and the hepatic system. Notice the total bilirubin test is in the general panel and the direct bilirubin test is part of the hepatic panel. Some types of general blood problems can cause high levels of bilirubin because more blood cells are breaking down than usual. Normal bilirubin ranges are as follows:

Total bilirubin	0.1 to 0.2 mg/dL
Indirect bilirubin	0.1 to 0.7 mg/dL
Direct bilirubin	0.1 to 0.3 mg/dL
Newborn total bilirubin	1 to 12 mg/dL

Blood Urea Nitrogen Test

The **blood urea nitrogen (BUN)** test measures the concentration of urea in blood. The amount of urea in blood reflects the metabolic function of the liver and the excretory function of the kidneys. Most renal diseases result in inadequate excretion of urea from the body; therefore, increased concentrations of urea appear in the blood. BUN is one of several tests, including creatinine, that are used to screen for renal disease and is especially useful for evaluating glomerular function.

Excess protein in the diet is not stored in the body but is metabolized (catalyzed) for energy production. Urea is the nitrogenous end product of protein catabolism and is produced in the liver. It is deposited in the blood and carried to the kidneys for excretion. Surplus urea is measured as BUN. Normal values of urea vary but in adults range between 8 and 25 mg/dL; concentrations greater than 100 mg/dL indicate serious impairment of renal function. A slightly elevated BUN can indicate dehydration.

Calcium

All the cells in the human body need calcium for many functions. It is a critical element for bones, muscles, and the nervous system. Too much calcium can cause the muscles and nerves to become hyperactive, whereas too little calcium can cause the muscles and nerves not to function at all.

Muscle cramps (charlie horses) are often caused by low calcium. Calcium needs to be maintained within certain levels in the blood. If we eat more calcium than we need, the excess is stored in the bones.

If our diets are low in calcium, the needed amount is pulled from the bones. The storage of excess calcium becomes less efficient as women lose estrogen; hence, women are at a greater risk than men to develop osteoporosis. Supplements of calcium may be recommended and the amounts supervised by the health care provider. A normal serum calcium level is 8.5 to 10.2 mg/dL.

Chloride

Chloride is an electrolyte. Its main function is to help with the electrical impulses of the cells. Chloride works closely with sodium. Changes in either sodium or chloride levels usually affect the other. A normal chloride level is 96 to 106 mEq/L.

Carbon Dioxide (CO_2)

Measuring CO_2 actually is measuring bicarbonate. This test is part of an arterial blood gas analysis. The kidneys are the main organs responsible for balancing CO_2. Anything that throws off the body's metabolic balance (e.g., excessive vomiting and diarrhea) can affect the CO_2 levels. The CO_2 levels in the blood are influenced by kidney and lung function. Normal CO_2 is 20 to 29 mEq/L.

Creatinine

Creatinine forms when muscle (creatine) breaks down. Logically, these levels will vary depending on the patient's size and muscularity. This test is used to determine kidney function, and is especially important for patients on diabetic or hypertension medications. A normal creatinine level is 0.8 to 1.4 mg/dL.

Gamma Glutamyltransferase (GGT)

The highest concentrations of GGT are in the liver and kidney. Abnormal levels usually indicate diseases of the liver, kidney, or bone. GGT is used in conjunction with other enzymes, especially ALP, to diagnose diseases. A normal GGT level is 0 to 51 IU/L.

Lactate Dehydrogenase (LDH)

LDH is an enzyme found in many organs, especially the liver, heart, kidneys, brain, skeletal muscles, and lungs. Abnormal levels indicate tissue damage but are not specific by themselves. Like all enzymes, LDH is examined in conjunction with other tests. A normal LDH level is 105 to 133 IU/L.

Phosphorus (Phosphate)

Phosphorus works closely with calcium, another electrolyte. Phosphorus values are used to assist in the proper assessment of calcium levels and to detect endocrine and kidney disorders. Phosphorus levels are related to uncontrolled diabetes and malnourished conditions. A normal phosphorus level is 2.4 to 4.1 mg/dL.

Potassium (K)

Potassium is an electrolyte and is critical to muscle and nerve function and for the transportation of nutrients and cellular wastes across cellular membranes. Abnormal levels of potassium can cause heart muscle irregularities and, if severe, can lead to cardiac arrest. Potassium is controlled by aldosterone, a hormone. Uncontrolled diabetes or excessive vomiting/diarrhea can cause abnormal potassium levels. Patients taking certain diuretics (such as Lasix [furosemide]) should be observed for low potassium. A normal potassium level is 3.7 to 5.2 mEq/L.

Sodium

Sodium is an electrolyte and works closely with chloride. Dietary intake of sodium is usually sufficient, and the kidney can excrete the excess. Sodium is closely related to fluid balance and retention. A normal sodium level is 135 to 145 mEq/L.

Total Protein

Total protein is a measurement of protein in the blood serum and can reflect the nutritional state of the body, the health of the liver and kidneys, and many conditions. If the total protein is abnormal, more specific tests will need to be performed to find out exactly the source of the problem. Of course, if the total protein is abnormal, other tests might show some abnormal levels, too. A normal total protein level is 6.0 to 8.3 mg/dL.

Uric Acid

Uric acid is created when purine is metabolized. It is usually secreted by the kidneys, but too much can build up as crystals in the body and seem to settle in the largest dependent joint, the great toe. This is known as gout. A normal uric acid level is 3.0 to 7.0 mg/dL.

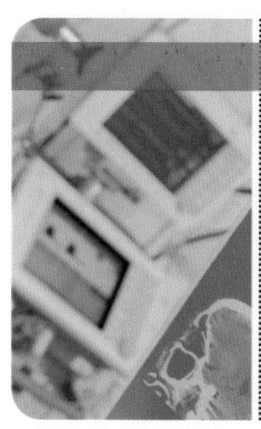

CASE STUDY 43-1

Refer to the scenario at the beginning of the chapter.

Nancy takes pride in paying attention to every detail when performing lab tests. She is also committed to explaining processes to her patients and increasing their comfort level.

CASE STUDY REVIEW

1. What are some key points to adhere to when performing testing using a CLIA-waived test kit to ensure accuracy?

2. What are some specific ways you can utilize your professionalism skills so a patient will have confidence in your abilities?

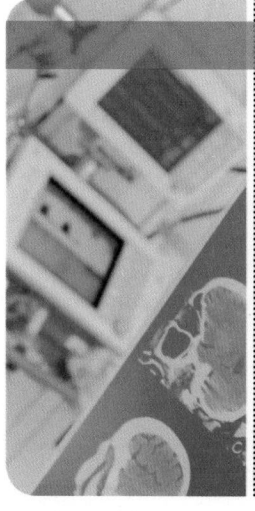

CASE STUDY 43-2

Joe Guerrero, CMA (AAMA), a clinical medical assistant at Inner City Health Care, has performed many venipunctures during his training at college, throughout his practicum, and since his employment at the clinic. He has not, however, performed a heelstick capillary draw since he was in college and even then he practiced on a doll. Until now another medical assistant in the clinic was doing all the heelstick capillary draws for PKU testing, but Joe is ready to start performing them himself. He is concerned and understandably nervous about performing this procedure on an infant.

CASE STUDY REVIEW

1. What course of action should Joe take to prepare himself for performing a procedure that he has not done in several years?

2. Once Joe feels he is technically ready to perform the PKU blood test, what should he do to ensure that the procedure goes well?

Summary

- Knowledge and understanding of terminology are important when dealing with laboratory testing.
- Professional communication skills and respect for patient needs are key to successful laboratory testing.
- Accurate laboratory test results rely on proper specimen collection, handling, and testing protocol.
- Many CLIA-waived test kits and automated methods are available for the POL.
- The medical assistant's knowledge of pathology and testing purposes are crucial to quality patient service.
- The medical assistant must be able to distinguish between normal and abnormal test results.
- Safety procedures and Standard Precautions must be observed at all times and include the proper disposal of infectious materials and reagents. Gloves and goggles are always used when obtaining samples and while performing the actual test.
- Careful documentation by the medical assistant will help the provider in the diagnosis of the patient.

Study for Success

To reinforce your knowledge and skills of information presented in this chapter:

- Review the *Key Terms* and *Learning Outcomes*
- Consider the *Critical Thinking* features and *Case Studies* and discuss your conclusions
- Answer the questions in the *Certification Review*

Procedure

- Perform the *Procedures* using the *Competency Assessment Checklists* on the *Student Companion Website*

CERTIFICATION REVIEW

1. In addition to pregnancy, a positive hCG test can be found in each of the following pathologic conditions except what?
   a. Ectopic pregnancy
   b. Hydatidiform mole of the uterus
   c. Pelvic inflammatory disease
   d. Cancer of the lung
2. If a urine sample for a pregnancy test cannot be tested immediately, it may be stored in what way for 24 hours?
   a. Room temperature, 25°C
   b. Body temperature, 37°C
   c. Fortunately, temperature of the specimen in not an issue
   d. Frozen
   e. Refrigerated at 4°C

3. What disease is sometimes called kissing disease?
   a. Tuberculosis
   b. Infectious mononucleosis
   c. Hemolytic anemia
   d. Hypoglycemia
4. Serum or blood would be the specimen for all but which of the following tests?
   a. ABO typing
   b. EBV
   c. Cholesterol
   d. hCG hormone
   e. All of these
5. Which of the following statements is incorrect regarding blood type?
   a. Type A RBCs have A antigens on the cell.
   b. Type B RBCs have B antigens on the cell.
   c. Type O RBCs have A and B antigens on the cell.
   d. Type AB RBCs have both A and B antigens on the cell.

6. Which of the following is a true statement about Rh factor?
   a. Rh factor is a rare blood type.
   b. Rh factor is present on all RBCs.
   c. Rh factor was discovered by experiments on rhesus monkeys.
   d. People without Rh factor on their RBCs have naturally occurring antibodies called anti-D in their plasma.
   e. Women with Rh factor cannot have more than one child without severe complications.

7. When instructing a patient in the correct collection of a specimen for semen analysis, all of the following should be considered except what?
   a. Avoid the consumption of alcohol several days before the test
   b. Collection of semen into a condom is unacceptable
   c. Specimen should be transported to the laboratory at 37°C within 30 minutes of collection
   d. Avoid the consumption of fats several days before the test

8. Testing for PKU is done on which patients?
   a. Newborns
   b. Children 1 to 3 years of age
   c. Teenagers
   d. Adults older than 40 years
   e. All patients throughout the life cycle

9. What is the best site location for a tuberculin Mantoux test?
   a. Back of the hand
   b. Forearm 3 to 4 inches from bend of arm
   c. ½ inch above the back of the knee
   d. Upper part of the arm in the deltoid muscle

10. A patient with hypoglycemia would have what blood glucose level?
   a. 50 to 70 mg/dL
   b. 70 to 110 mg/dL
   c. 110 to 150 mg/dL
   d. 150 to 200 mg/dL
   e. 200 to 300 mg/dL

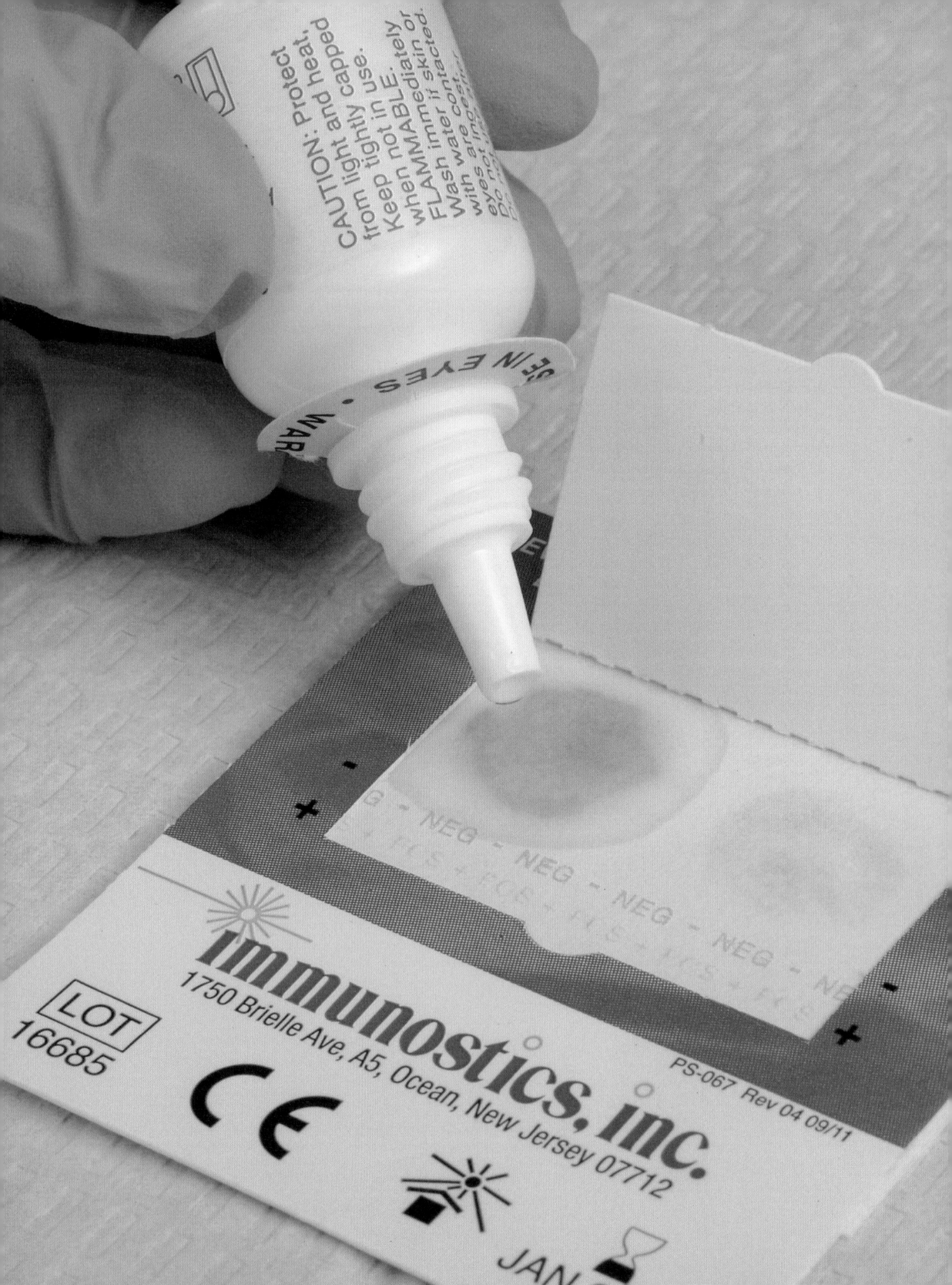

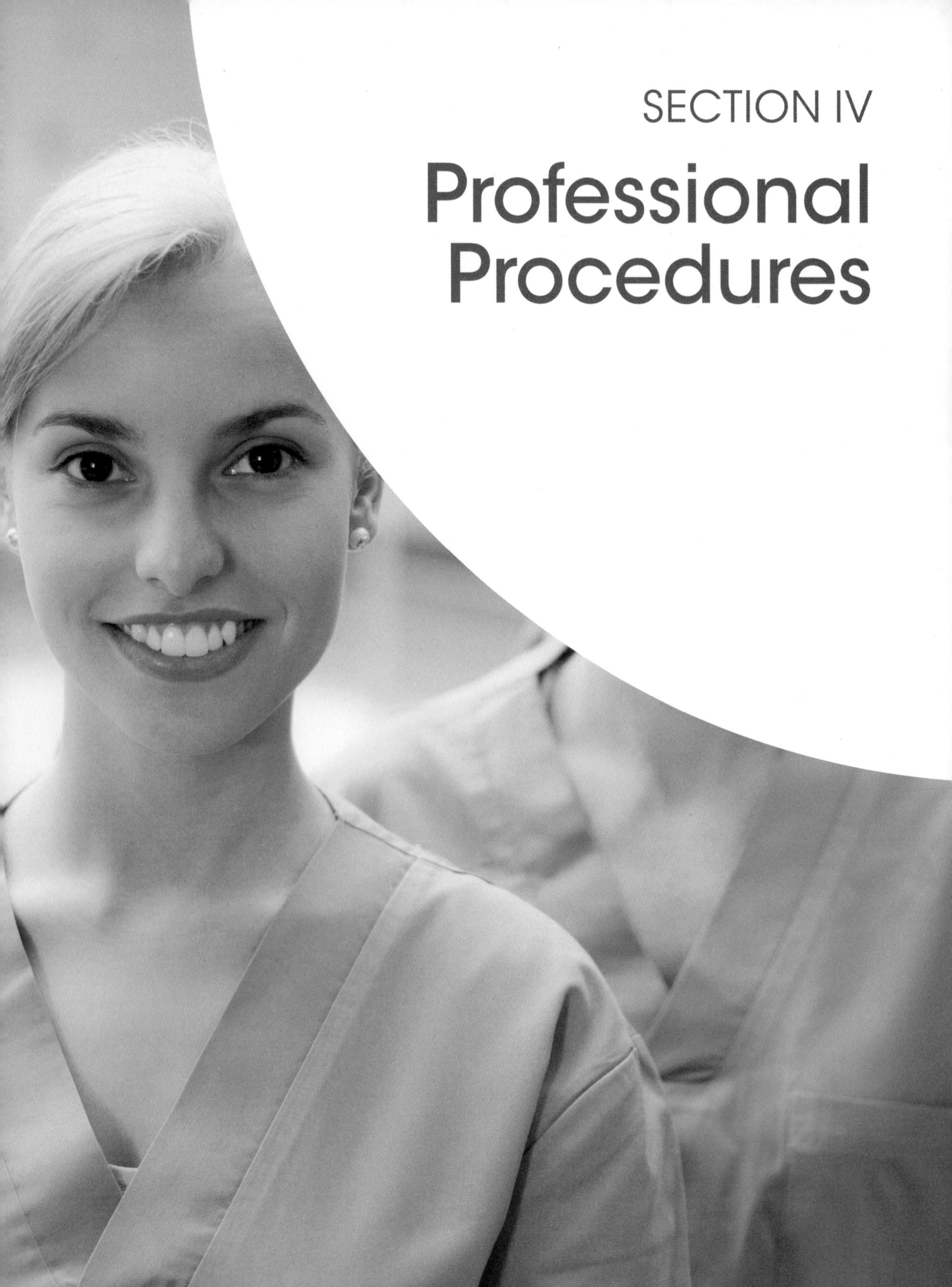

SECTION IV

Professional
Procedures

UNIT X
CLINIC AND HUMAN RESOURCES MANAGEMENT

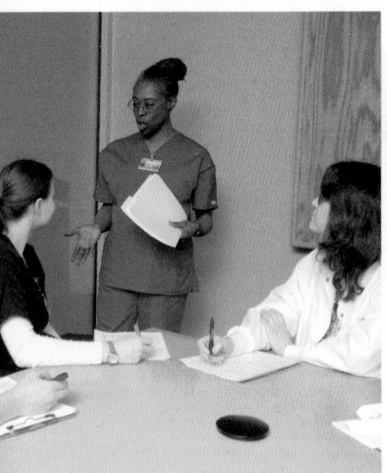
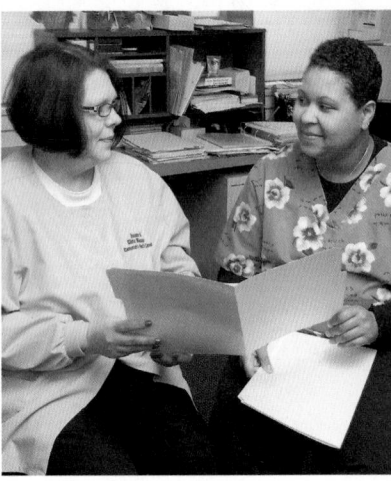
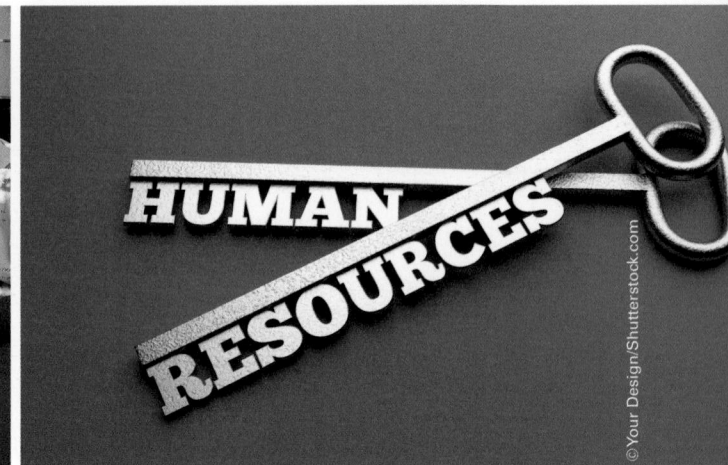

©Your Design/Shutterstock.com

ATTRIBUTES OF PROFESSIONALISM

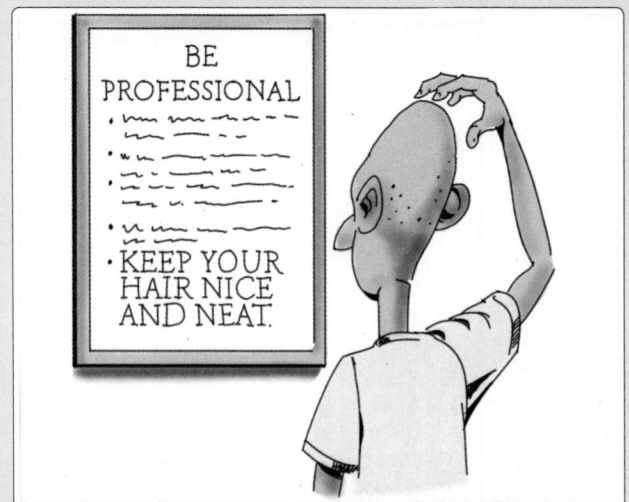

Many experienced and professional medical assistants find themselves in the role of management, often moving into that position through their clinic employment and familiarity with all aspects of the clinic operation. Management responsibilities mean not only carrying the burden of understanding each facet of the operation, even stepping into the role of an employee when necessary, but also shouldering the responsibility of directing, facilitating, and monitoring employee productivity and patient satisfaction. As a professional manager you will support staff members, carry out the wishes of providers, and treat everyone equitably. Personnel will be fully oriented to their positions, evaluated on a regular and predetermined basis, and provided with opportunities for expansion of their role in the clinic.

Listed below are a series of questions for you to ask yourself, to serve as a professionalism checklist.

As you interact with patients and colleagues, these questions will help to guide you in the professional behavior that is expected every day from medical assistants.

Ask Yourself

COMMUNICATION
- [ ] Do I apply active listening skills?
- [ ] Do I display professionalism through written and verbal communication?
- [ ] Do I demonstrate appropriate nonverbal communication?
- [ ] Do I display appropriate body language?
- [ ] Does my knowledge allow me to speak easily with all members of the health care team?

PRESENTATION
- [ ] Am I dressed and groomed appropriately?
- [ ] Do I display a positive attitude?
- [ ] Do I display a calm, professional, and caring manner?

COMPETENCY
- [ ] Do I pay attention to detail?
- [ ] Do I ask questions if I am out of my comfort zone or do not have the experience to carry out tasks?
- [ ] Do I display sound judgment?
- [ ] Am I knowledgeable and accountable?

INITIATIVE
- [ ] Do I show initiative?
- [ ] Have I developed a strategic plan to achieve my goals? Is my plan realistic?
- [ ] Do I seek out opportunities to expand my knowledge base?
- [ ] Am I flexible and dependable?

INTEGRITY
- [ ] Do I demonstrate the principles of self-boundaries?
- [ ] Do I work within my scope of practice?
- [ ] Do I demonstrate respect for individual diversity?
- [ ] Do I recognize the impact personal ethics and morals have on the delivery of health care?
- [ ] Do I protect and maintain confidentiality?
- [ ] Do I maintain moral and ethical standards?
- [ ] Do I do the "right thing" even when no one is observing?

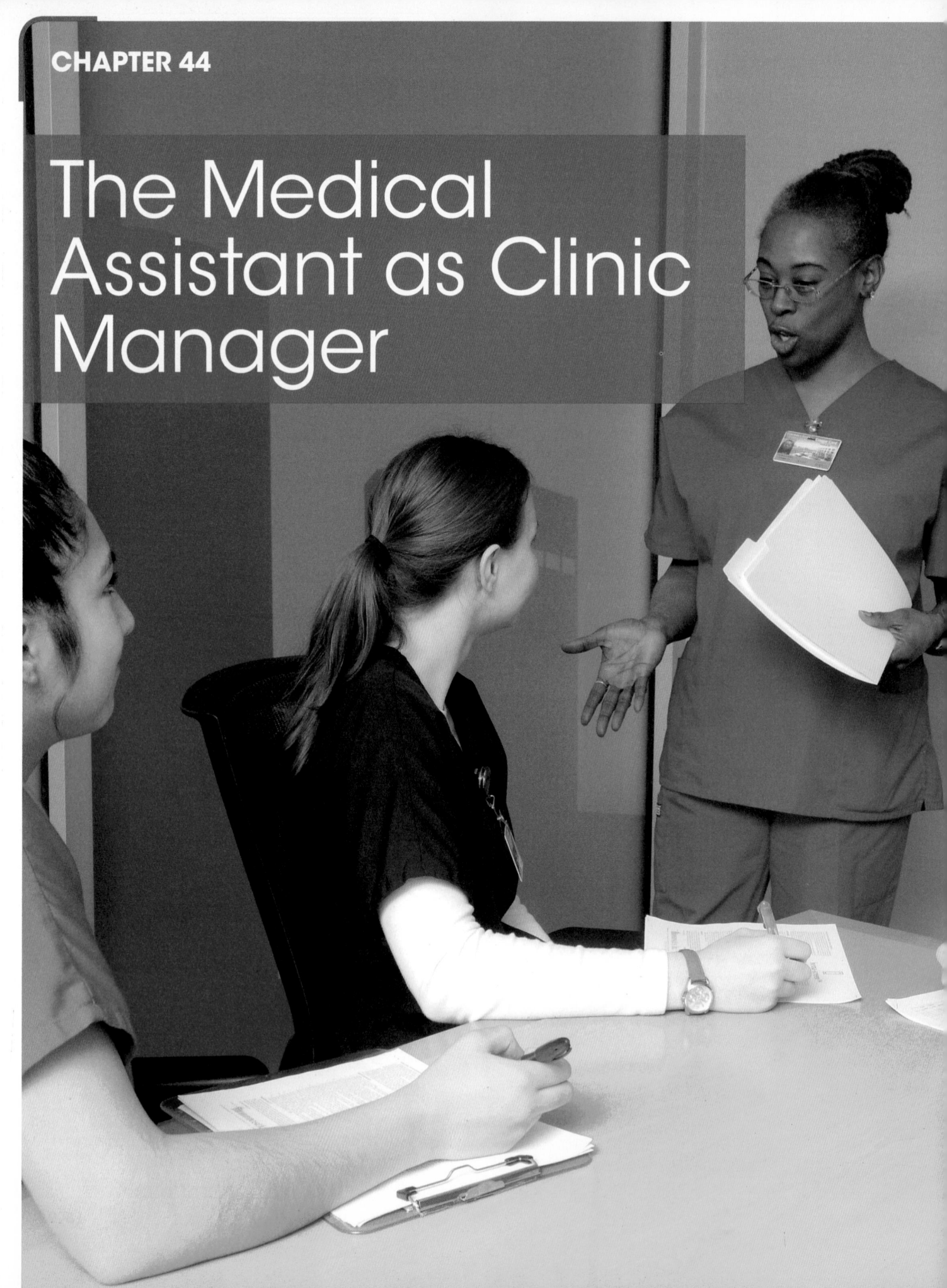

CHAPTER 44

The Medical Assistant as Clinic Manager

1. Define and spell the key terms as presented in the glossary.
2. Describe the qualities of a manager.
3. Discuss characteristics of managers and leaders.
4. Differentiate between authoritarian and participatory management styles.
5. Describe management by walking around and its usefulness in ambulatory care settings.
6. Recall a minimum of four common risks and risk-control measures.
7. List three benefits of a teamwork approach.
8. Discuss the importance of a meeting agenda.
9. Describe appropriate evaluation tools for employees.
10. Recall effective methods of resolving conflict.
11. Identify the steps required to make travel arrangements.
12. Define the term *itinerary* and list important information the itinerary should contain.
13. List three methods of increasing productivity and efficient time management.
14. Describe the purpose of a procedure manual.
15. Discuss the impact of HIPAA's privacy policy in ambulatory care settings.
16. Describe the general concept of marketing and recall at least three marketing tools.
17. Discuss the role of social media in the medical clinic.
18. Describe the purpose and benefit of marketing.
19. Discuss the steps involved in the inventory of administrative and clinical supplies and equipment.
20. Discuss the steps involved in administrative and clinical equipment calibration and maintenance.

KEY TERMS

agenda	itinerary	procedure manual
ancillary services	liability	professional liability insurance
authoritarian style	malpractice	profit sharing
benchmark	management by walking around (MBWA)	risk management
benefit		salary review
blogging	marketing	self-actualization
bond	mentor	shadow
brainstorming	minutes	social media
conflict resolution	negligence	subordinate
embezzle	nonretaliation provision	teamwork
fringe benefits	participatory style	work statement
"going bare"	practicum	

SCENARIO

Marilyn Johnson, CMA (AAMA), has been employed by Inner City Health Care for the past 8 years. Three years ago, she was promoted to the position of clinic manager when the facility added a second clinic for its associates in a nearby suburb. Marilyn has a baccalaureate degree in business administration. Her responsibilities at the clinic include various duties involving personnel, finances, and efficiency.

The drive to improve the productivity of the medical clinic, precipitated by managed care, Medicare, and insurance limits placed on fees, has broadened the scope of employment options and job marketability for medical assistants. This has created an opportunity for medical assistants to advance to the position of clinic manager.

In small clinics, the position of clinic manager may include the duties of the human resources (HR) representative; in larger clinics, these positions will be independent. This book treats them as separate positions (see Chapter 45). In larger facilities, the clinic manager will coordinate with the HR representative to train and manage administrative and clinical staff.

THE MEDICAL ASSISTANT AS CLINIC MANAGER

The manager of a medical clinic or ambulatory care facility can have vast and diverse responsibilities. This chapter covers the following clinic manager duties:

1. Manage and encourage IT services, relationships, and collaboration, ensuring the clinic EHR and relevant staff are kept updated and are involved in system protocols as appropriate

2. Make travel arrangements and prepare an itinerary

3. Arrange and maintain practice insurance and develop risk management strategies

4. Supervise clinic personnel

5. Approve financial transactions and account disposition; generate financial reports as needed

6. Supervise the purchase and storage of clinic supplies

7. Prepare staff meeting agendas, conduct the meetings, and record minutes

8. Supervise the purchase, repair, and maintenance of clinic equipment

9. Assist in improving work flow and time management

10. Create and update the clinic procedure manual, Material Safety Data Sheets (MSDS), and Health Insurance Portability and Accountability Act (HIPAA) manual

11. Prepare patient education materials and arrange patient/community education workshops as needed

QUALITIES OF A MANAGER

Professional

Your technical skills may be what got you noticed, hired, and ultimately promoted, but that will not be enough as a clinic manager. As a manager, you will also need to have talent with "soft" skills that will help you succeed in working with your staff using different approaches.

A clinic manager should not feel the need to be superior to employees but should strive to develop a synergistic organization. The best manager is like an orchestra conductor. He or she constructively blends together the skills and abilities of diverse people to produce a smooth and efficient team. The result is an organization with greater capability than would be achievable by the individuals acting independently.

The clinic manager should have two overarching goals:

- Get the job done
- Make the process enjoyable

Management styles are expected to change significantly in the forthcoming years. By 2017, there will be five generations in the workforce simultaneously. As Generation Z (born in the 1990s) enters the work force, and with the Baby Boomer generation (born between 1946 and 1964) still working and gradually retiring, the challenges of managing varying ethics and working styles of these generations will become very real.

New approaches to making the most of time management, adapting to different employees, finding ways to enable collaboration across generations, and creatively gapping those bridges will become increasingly important. Clinic managers will need to understand that each individual has his or her own set of skills, and with the potential of up to a 50-year age difference in the work environment, being able to co-mingle and use cross-skills to the benefit of all will emerge as useful tools.

Emerging technologies offer an opportunity for the younger generation to teach how to use these products in the work place effectively. In turn, the older generation has much to offer by instilling the value of interpersonal communication, and building sound relationships with co-workers based on experience and longevity.

There is a unique opportunity for the co-mingling of these skilled generations to mutually benefit each other in the workplace.

A good clinic manager needs to be two persons in one body: manager and leader. The two functions are different, and the good manager will use some of each persona in meeting objectives. Table 44-1 lists the characteristics of a manager and a leader.

Good managers are leaders, providing their coworkers with vision, guidance, and a feeling of ownership in the process. They do these things without threats, usually through the power of their personal charisma. It is also important that managers clearly convey their expectations to their employees. Possibly nothing leads to ill feeling between the manager and an employee more than failure to let the employee know what is expected of him or her. Furthermore, a lack of expectations stifles career growth and organizational vitality. Good leaders need to blend many admirable personality traits of leadership to be successful and still control the resources entrusted to them.

Before proceeding with a listing of qualities of a manager/leader, a rule that defines almost all of the ethical qualities needs to be mentioned. This rule is *Treat others as you would like to be treated.* Commonly known as the Golden Rule, it will make the difference between a manager who is successful and one who fails miserably. The rule needs no explanation and will serve any manager well in any circumstance.

Qualities needed by a manager/leader include the following:

- *Effective communication skills.* Communication skills include written and oral methods. The manager must communicate clearly, diplomatically, tactfully, and with respect for the feelings of others.

- *Fair-mindedness.* It is important to always be fair with co-workers. Decisions that impact one fellow employee create a ripple effect. That is, you may have to make the same decision for another employee at another time. Decisions should be based, as much as possible, on the assumption that what is granted to one employee will be granted to others in similar situations. This approach will decrease the risk for being accused of playing favorites or being unfair.

- *Objectivity.* The clinic manager must be able to view challenges without bias or prejudice. For example, when promotions are made, the clinic manager must be able to focus on the job description criteria and individual qualifications without introducing personal preference.

- *Organizational skills.* Being organized includes being able to prioritize tasks, working efficiently and methodically. Know when and be willing to delegate tasks when others have the expertise and time to complete the task within the timelines.

- *People skills.* The clinic manager must like people in general and enjoy working with them. Building confidence and self-esteem in others and being interested in promoting constructive relationships are essential qualities of the clinic manager. The ability to function as an effective team leader provides a role model for other staff members to emulate.

- *Problem-solving skills.* The clinic manager must be a problem solver. This may include being creative and doing away with old paradigms and traditional approaches to solving a problem. When difficult issues arise, focus on the situation, issue, or behavior, not on the person. A discussion about solving the problem without laying blame is much more productive. Positive solutions may be more readily attained when discussing what was observed rather than what was told by someone else.

TABLE 44-1

DIFFERENCES BETWEEN A MANAGER AND A LEADER

MANAGER	LEADER
Organizes and allocates talent and resources	Provides vision and goals, setting reasonable and clear standards
Plans and budgets using available resources	Communicates direction; promotes teamwork and creativity to reach goals
Controls and solves problems, with the ability to adapt to changes seamlessly	Is an inspiring and motivating influence, able to mentor and direct in ways that keep the team moving forward
Establishes structure by organizing, staffing, and implementing policies and procedures	Overcomes resistance to change and resolves barriers
Consistently achieves goals and targets	Is the role model and go-to for the team

- *Technical expertise.* Have a working knowledge of each procedure performed in the clinic, although it is not necessary to be the acknowledged technical expert. In the medical environment, there are many changes, including updates to laws, insurance guidelines, and various business challenges that occur frequently. A good clinic manager is continually learning and encourages **subordinates** to seek opportunities to continue their education and advance their technical skills.

- *Truthfulness.* Lead by example! If an honest mistake is made, be the first to admit to the error and seek the best solution for preventing it from happening again. Respond honestly to requests. For example, two staff members ask for the same day off. The clinic manager will make the decision that only one member may have the day off and will review the policy manual to determine the appropriate criteria for designating whose request will be granted.

Clinic Manager Attitude

Professional

Many managers share a common enemy—themselves. The part of ourselves that is our enemy is our mind and the outlook we have on the world. People who succeed attribute positive results to their own actions. People who underachieve or fail usually attribute negative results to someone else or to chance, over which they have no control. Because underachievers feel helpless to affect results, psychologists conclude that their motivation to succeed is diminished. A low achiever would be unlikely to have a personal risk management system in place. He or she would feel he or she could not affect events. The more positive person could easily take steps to avoid these problems.

The effect of a negative mindset does not stop with failure to accept responsibility for the things that happen to each of us, it continues on. Unless we change our outlook, we lower our expectations and begin accepting the mediocre. Individuals who feel they are helpless to affect events become afraid of success as well as failure, and they subconsciously find a way to fail to avoid the challenges success will bring.

How do you change your mindset? The following are a few suggestions considered helpful:

- Come to terms with what you would have to change if you are to be successful, and be ready for the change.
- Identify what you really want to achieve.

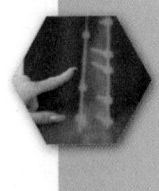
Critical Thinking

How does the clinic manager begin to develop good working relationships with community service organizations to better serve and provide for patients' health care needs? How would this improve the quality of public relations?

- Put your goals in writing using positive terms (say "I will," not "I'll try").
- Begin with small, achievable goals.
- Eliminate poor habits such as procrastination.
- Tune out negative thoughts and focus on positive thoughts.

We are what we think we are. Be careful of your mindset, it can derail you and your job as a manager.

Professionalism

Professional

The medical assistant as clinic manager must exhibit professional behavior at all times. He or she must be courteous and diplomatic and demonstrate a responsible and positive attitude. All verbal and written communications should be accurate and correct and should follow appropriate guidelines. The clinic manager should demonstrate knowledge of federal and state health care legislation and regulations and must perform within legal and ethical boundaries. All documentation must be performed appropriately.

The clinic manager serves as a liaison between the provider, the patient, and other professionals. Therefore, professional demeanor in all respects must be followed. It is not uncommon to be called on to locate community resources and information for patients and employers. A good working relationship with community service organizations fosters the sharing of information vital to your patients' health care needs and promotes quality public relations. Review Procedure 11-5 for specific information on how this is done.

MANAGEMENT STYLES

There are many books written on management styles; however, it is possible to break all of them down into two basic styles, each with an infinite number of variations. Instead of discussing the intricacies of these management styles, for the purpose of this book, we will take a straightforward view and look at only the fundamental styles: authoritarian and participatory. We will also examine a third management technique called, managing by walking around (MBWA), which is, an effective method for keeping abreast of what is going on in an organization and is making a positive comeback in the era of email, texting, and lack of face-to-face interaction due to technology.

Authoritarian Style

A Manager who adopts the **authoritarian style** of management exercises his or her authority over those that report to him or her as a means to achieve goals. Without seeking or considering the input of the staff members, this manager controls the decision making, controls policies, and puts operational plans in place. While this style may seem regimented and inflexible, there are workplace environments where this is beneficial.

For example, in a medical clinic, there is a tendency for there to exist targeted areas of specialty tasks within the support staff. These may be accomplished by just a handful of people, or an extensive group of individuals with focused areas of responsibility. Such is the case in the roles of administrative front desk staff, those working in coding and billing, the clinical staff (including medical assistants, laboratory and diagnostic technicians, physician assistants, and nurse practitioners), in essence, every member that provides a total patient care experience within a clinic. While each member has a specific function, the whole is very much interdependent, and the work flow needs to have a beginning, middle, and end in order for all the parts to be cohesive and accomplish goals for the patient's care, as well as proper reimbursement for the clinic. At the same time, everything must be done within compliance requirements.

Authoritarian management needs to be executed carefully; otherwise, staff may begin to feel resentment and tasks may seem too rote or rigid. This style can foster absenteeism and high turnover, results which can be devastating to the efficient operation of a clinic where every staff member's contribution is of utmost importance. As previously mentioned, each facet of the tasks collectively done by the entire staff are interdependent in the medical environment, creating an opportunity to actually blend management styles to best utilize resources, achieve goals, and maintain a motivated staff.

Participatory Style

A manager who utilizes the **participatory style** of management encourages input and feedback from those that report to him or her. Decision making, policies, and operational plans will at least in part include the suggestions, opinions, and views of those on staff. As an operational whole, each staff member feels that he or she can or has made a contribution, and this increases the sense of value within a team effort. Additionally, the staff can more easily take ownership of the goals, and make adjustments with the assistance of the manager when fine-tuning is necessary. As with any management style, care must be taken with this approach as well. While this style encourages contributions, there will be those that do not contribute, those that are overeager, and in the end, not everyone's ideas can be implemented. Risk of alienating those whose ideas are not used and resentment for others who minimally participate can create unique challenges. However, the opportunity to blend authoritarian and participatory styles can positively influence the needed interdependency in a clinic, where each person's responsibilities have a direct impact on the total care of the patient and smooth operation of the business.

Management by Walking Around

Management by walking around (MBWA) is not really a management style but rather a technique for keeping the manager informed and promoting face-to-face conversations, obtaining feedback, and listening to staff ideas or comments. This style consists of just what the title says—the manager walks around looking at what is going on in the organization and talks with employees. The manager must be careful to make sure his or her motives are not to micromanage and to convey this to the staff.

To this end, some tips are offered here to make the most of using the MBWA technique effectively in the medical clinic.

- *Make this part of a routine, and stay consistent.* When staff see you on a regular basis, and not once a month or only when there is time, the MBWA becomes part of the management

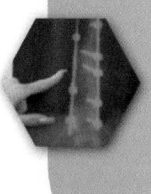

Critical Thinking

How would you make the medical clinic (administrative and clinical space) safe for employees and nonemployees (e.g., patients, venders, visitors)? List as many considerations as possible.

culture in the clinic. This does not mean that a set day and time needs to be adhered to, but rather, simply a consistent habit of stopping by work areas to chat, see how things are going, and gather ideas. You will get more candid and useful information by dropping in unexpectedly, when the staff member was not prepared for your visit.

- *Make it worthwhile.* If you will be stopping by, then make it a point to ask for ideas on improvement, suggestions, and also acknowledge a good idea when presented. When a good idea or suggestion is implemented, give credit where due without showing favoritism. Encourage support from staff that curbs resentment but still allows recognition.

- *Follow up on questions and concerns.* If you are presented with an issue for which you do not have an immediate solution or response, take the time to follow up and get back with an answer in a timely fashion. The staff will appreciate that you have not forgotten or given less than your full attention to a problem they are experiencing.

- *Stick to fact-finding.* Do not utilize MBWA as a means to identify procedures incorrectly done, criticize, or discipline staff if problems are identified by you during the walk around. These should be noted and addressed in a different setting and time, appropriate to the circumstances.

The idea of the MBWA technique is to build rapport and keep on top of the state of the organization through staff feedback. Keep to this objective. Employees are more likely to be engaged and productive when they see the manager and have an opportunity to speak with you frequently than if they do not. We are now in a time where managing people is taking place through email, texting, and formal staff meetings, and the manager can literally be a person always in her office and not easily accessible. Even with an open door policy, most staff are reluctant to initiate a discussion as opposed to having a touch-base visit that takes place frequently in their own work area.

RISK MANAGEMENT

The clinic manager should formulate a **risk management** procedure that assesses risks to which he or she and the organization are exposed and take steps to develop

contingencies that minimize probable risks. Some common risks and risk-control measures are:

- *Loss of a critical employee.* Have cross-training of employees to permit them to assume the duties of an employee who is ill or terminates his or her employment.

- *Failure of a supplier or contractor.* Maintain sufficient inventory to permit contracting with a secondary supplier before critical shortages occur. Monitor the status of orders so that you are aware of any failures in delivery before they have a negative impact and so that supplies can be obtained from a second source. Have a list of secondary sources.

- *Accidental disclosure of confidential information through error or unauthorized entry.* Have protocols in place regarding breach of confidentiality and defining steps to be taken in the event information is compromised. Define protocols to patients alerting them to the unlikely but potential possibility of accidental disclosure. Notify patients immediately if confidential information is compromised and work with them for resolution.

- *Computer failure.* Back up the system regularly. Have a secondary system that permits the clinic to operate until repairs are effected. Have a maintenance contract in place with a reputable firm permitting overnight repair.

- *Injury to a staff member or nonemployee.* Continually review safety procedures and conduct safety surveys. Have adequate liability insurance for the medical clinic.

- *Managerial position change.* Continuously network with friends and associates to permit you to rapidly seek a new position before experiencing a job loss. It's always easier to get a job while you still have a job.

Incident reports are required to notify managers of events involving injuries to patients, visitors, or staff; medical errors or omissions; breach of confidential information; and potentially dangerous conditions associated with facilities or equipment. This report signals the risk manager to implement existing protocols to minimize risk. Medical incident reports are confidential and cannot be released to anyone without a signed release of information agreement. The medical incident report form is an administrative document and is not considered part of the medical record. Procedure 44-1 provides steps for completing a medical incident report.

Procedure

Completing a Medical Incident Report

PURPOSE:

To complete an accurate medical incident report providing all legally required information and to submit it in a timely manner.

EQUIPMENT/SUPPLIES:

- Appropriate medical incident report form
- Computer with Incident Report Software
- Notes taken regarding incident

PROCEDURE STEPS:

1. Report situations that were harmful by discussing the incident with the employee(s) involved and read notes of pertinent information. Ask those who witnessed the incident to describe when, where, and what they saw in their own words. RATIONALE: Provides an understanding of what happened and ensures all the information needed is documented.

2. *Pay attention to detail* when completing the clinic-approved medical incident report form. A single-sheet, multiple-copy form is best. The form should contain basic patient identification data, a checklist of different incidents, and a space for written comments. RATIONALE: Ensures that all information needed is documented.

3. The person completing the incident report form should be the individual who witnessed the incident, first discovered the incident, or is most familiar with the incident. RATIONALE: This ensures the most accurate recording of the incident.

4. Each section of the form must be completed. The incident description should be a brief narrative consisting of an objective description of the facts but should not draw any conclusions. Quotes should be used when appropriate with any unwitnessed incidents (e.g., "Patient states . . ."). The name(s) of any witnesses should be included on the report as well as employees directly involved in the incident. RATIONALE: To provide unbiased information without making judgments.

5. *Implement time management principles.* Incident reports must be submitted in a timely manner to the appropriate administrator or office following protocol identified in the procedure manual for the clinic. RATIONALE: Ensures that appropriate documentation and action is taken for follow-up.

IMPORTANCE OF TEAMWORK

The use of **teamwork** to improve the efficiency of the clinic at first may seem incongruent to your desire to improve clinic efficiency, because it seems that several people are now involved in solving a problem that you as the manager should solve and explain. Teamwork builds morale and actually results in getting more accomplished with the resources you have because the team members develop ownership of the solution to a problem and want to make it work. When it works, it flatters them and builds their esteem.

The efficiency of a team results from collectively working together to plan how to "work smarter" and how to dovetail tasks and support each other so that wasted effort is avoided. To achieve all of these things, a team not only must be given the responsibility and the authority to plan and execute their plan to solve a problem, but they must know your expectations for them. Sometimes this means that you, the clinic manager, must stick your neck out for them. They will reward you handsomely for doing so. For more information on how to build a successful team, see the "Importance of Teamwork" Quick Reference Guide.

Importance of Teamwork

Category 1:

Getting the team started.
Successful teamwork is the result of a clear vision, specific goals, and a well-planned strategy on the part of the team leader.

The team leader must ensure that individual team members understand and support the specifics of the problem they are being asked to solve. To achieve this, the team should create a **"work statement"** to outline the goals and objectives to be achieved, and the sequential order of tasks to be completed in order to achieve the stated goals.

The team leader should allow the wider team to develop the work statement in order to foster team ownership of the stated goals, but the leader must also ensure that the goals remain focused on solving the problem at hand. The team leader must manage differences of opinion to maintain a cohesive team.

Once a work statement has been developed, a timetable should be established for achieving results. Clear standards that must be maintained in order to solve the problem should also be identified. The wider team should be involved in setting the standards and timetable, with the leader's direction.

Category 2:

Problem solving.
This stage is also known as **"brainstorming"** a solution. Brainstorming allows everyone to contribute solutions without consideration for practicality or flaws, then organizing ideas after everyone has had a chance to speak.

The team will next organize and prioritize the solution, creating a list of the solutions in descending order from those having the greatest impact and the lowest cost or implementation difficulty to those of least impact.

Once brainstorming is complete, solutions are evaluated for practicality and correctness. The goal is to arrive at the best workable solution.

The team leader prepares a needs assessment and **"benchmarks"** the clinic to other facilities to see how others accomplish these tasks as a way to generate ideas and view the solutions from another perspective.

Category 3:

Implement the solution.
Putting the solution in place involves the team working out a detailed plan and accompanying schedule to assist in implementation by assigned team members.

Any remaining problems are assigned to subteams that will meet to further solve these issues just as the primary team did. The entire team continues to meet periodically to address problems and find resolutions.

Assignments are made, and resources, funds, and equipment are made available to the team and defined for their use.

Category 4:

Recognition.
In order to develop a team spirit and sense of **"self-actualization"** within the clinic, a successful team should be acknowledged for its efforts. This may include a dinner or luncheon for the team members, or other appropriate recognition from the team leader or other supervisory person as applies.

SUPERVISING PERSONNEL

Creating an atmosphere in which open and honest communication can take place is critical to supervising personnel. This type of communication may be encouraged through the establishment of regular staff meetings, with each staff member sharing ideas for improvement and areas of concern. Eliciting the help of others in problem-solving strategies promotes harmony (Figure 44-1).

Staff and Team Meetings

The clinic manager usually initiates the staff and team meeting idea and should officiate at such meetings. Failure of the clinic manager to be present may convey a message that the meeting is an event not worthy of attention. It is important that the clinic manager be familiar with basic parliamentary procedures. The purchase of books such as *Robert's Rules of Order* or *Parliamentary Procedure at a Glance* is an excellent investment.

Procedure

Successful staff and team meetings are announced well in advance or on established timelines to enable the majority of

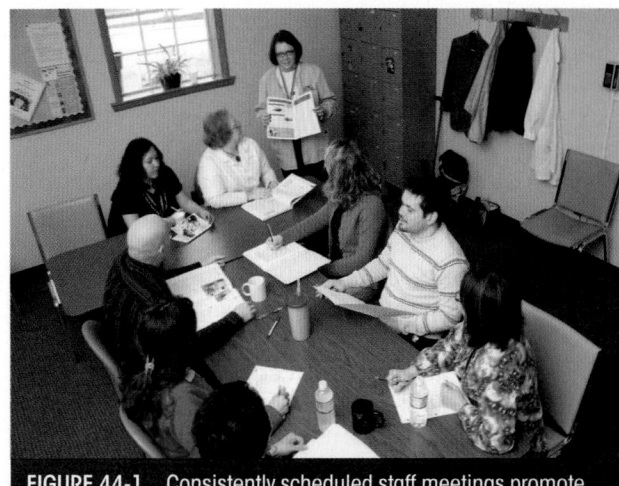

FIGURE 44-1 Consistently scheduled staff meetings promote communication and harmony among the health care team.

clinic personnel to attend. An **agenda** identifying the subjects to be covered during a given meeting should be issued before the meeting so that each attendee arrives prepared with input or questions relevant to the topics. Procedure 44-2 outlines the procedural steps for preparing a meeting agenda.

PROCEDURE 44-2

Procedure

Preparing a Meeting Agenda

PURPOSE:

To prepare a meeting agenda, a list of specific items to be discussed or acted on, to maintain the focus of the group and allow business to be transacted in a timely fashion.

EQUIPMENT/SUPPLIES:

- List of participants
- Order of business
- Names of individuals giving reports
- Names of any guest speakers
- Computer and paper to print agendas

PROCEDURE STEPS:

1. ***Paying attention to detail,*** reserve proposed date, time, and place of meeting. RATIONALE: Ensures that the facilities are available for the meeting.

2. Collect information for meeting agenda by previewing the previous meeting's minutes for old business items, checking with others for report items, and determining any new business items. RATIONALE: Ensures that all old and new business items have been identified.

3. Prepare a hard copy of the agenda and have it approved by the chair of the meeting. RATIONALE: Confirmation by the chair of the agenda content ensures that agenda is correct and complete.

4. ***Implementing time management principles,*** send agenda to meeting participants a few days in advance of the meeting. RATIONALE: Permits participants to prepare for the meeting by completing any tasks required and preparing any necessary documentation.

Figure 44-2 shows a sample agenda. Each meeting should end with opportunity for nonagenda items to be discussed or suggested for inclusion in the next meeting. The meeting should have a fixed time to end.

A written record in the form of **minutes** should be maintained and sent to all team members regardless of whether they attended the meeting. This policy keeps all members informed about policy changes and decisions that impact the clinic operations. The minutes also trigger a reminder for any new procedures or revisions to be made in the procedure manual. See Chapter 14 for additional information related to agendas and minutes.

The minutes for a staff and team meeting should record action plans under each agenda topic. Summarize all action items agreed to in the meeting in one section of the minutes. This facilitates easy access to information at a later date should it be required.

The date, time, and place of the next meeting should be included. The person preparing the minutes should always sign them. A copy of the minutes should always be maintained in a book for easy reference.

Conflict Resolution

Professional

Conflict resolution, or managing conflict in the work place, is a time-consuming and necessary task not only for the clinic manager, but the providers as well. Conflicts can arise between staff members and providers, patient and provider, and even between the health care staff and the patient or patient's family. These conflicts can escalate to litigation or even violent reactions. Conflicts have a direct impact on morale; clinic efficiency; and ultimately, patient care. Without resolution, high turnover and lack of proper work environment will create serious setbacks for the clinic as a whole.

The hostile work environment has been given significant attention in recent years, and action is available for those who feel that they are working in such an environment. Abusive behavior by other employees, managers, supervisors, or even providers may take the form of a condescending attitude, ridicule, inappropriate comments or jokes, sexual harassment, threats, and fear. This type of behavior in the workplace is now less tolerated, if at all, and an organization can be held responsible for allowing the hostile work environment to continue and failing to act.

While volumes of material have been written about successful conflict management, the most helpful preventative measure is to have an office code of conduct in place. By establishing clinic policies for all members of the medical staff, these rules make it easier to correct and administer discipline where necessary. By imposing limits on unacceptable behavior, and delineating the path to discipline through a chain of command, everyone understands the process to resolution, and can often intercept and solve issues at a lower level.

Another useful tip is to recognize how conflict starts in the first place and put preventative measures in place to avoid it. Misunderstandings, lack of communication, favoritism, inequality of any kind, unreasonable expectations, and unfair or inappropriate criticism are just a few of the

---

AGENDA

STAFF MEETING Wednesday, February 16, 20XX
2:00 PM — Conference Room

1. Read and approve minutes of last meeting
2. Reports
   A. Satellite facility — Marilyn Johnson
   B. Patient flow — Joe Guerrero
   C.
3. Discussion of new telephone system
4. Unfinished Business
   A. Review new procedure manual pages
   B.
5. New Business
   A. Appoint committee for design of new marketing brochure
   B.
6. Open discussion and/or topics for next meeting's agenda
7. Set next meeting time
8. Adjourn

FIGURE 44-2 Sample meeting agenda.

workplace triggers to watch for. Taking others for granted, not keeping promises, not accepting responsibility for mistakes, and personal issues interfering with work objectives and time management are also areas that can create conflict.

The following are some guidelines that may be helpful in preventing conflicts:

- Listen to your employees. What do they say? What do they communicate non-verbally?

- Manage by walking around and talking to your employees.

- Do not tolerate negative comments or actions among employees.

- Encourage an open-door policy for concerns and complaints.

- Be a role model for all employees. Practice what you preach.

- Keep confidences and treat each person with respect and understanding.

When conflicts arise, do not avoid taking immediate action to resolve the issue even if it appears to be superficially resolved. It will resurface at the first instance of stress between the individuals.

A good manager/leader will stay level and cool headed when confronted with conflict. Listening carefully, avoiding accusations or taking sides, and even repeating the issue in their your own words to show you they are understanding the problem are sound approaches to assisting with the situation. Should the conflict not be easily resolved, allow it to rest for the day, and come back to it when emotions are better able to be controlled, but do so within a day or two at most. Prolonging the issue can exacerbate the situation, with unfavorable results.

When dealing with conflict, the most difficult emotion to control is anger. It is often a self-fueling mood that will cause one to say things that were not meant or take action without thinking of the consequences. Intervening early is the best course of action, and truly understanding the problem is the first and most necessary step to successfully defusing the situation.

When addressing conflict between a provider or a supervisor and an employee, mediation is the only appropriate approach. In all other instances the best approach is to use a confrontational approach. The two persons having a conflict are brought together and asked to express their conflicting opinions without interruption. The purpose is to communicate what each perceives to be the problem. If an obvious solution that is acceptable to both parties does not appear, the manager must insist that the parties come up with an acceptable solution to the conflict. (This latter step is not appropriate for conflicts between an employee and a superior in the organization.) In doing so both parties have ownership of the resolution.

Harassment in the Workplace

Harassment consists of verbal or physical behavior/conduct that is (a) unwelcome; (b) based on a protected class (e.g., race, sex, age, national origin, veteran status, or sexual orientation); (c) severe or pervasive; and (d) has a negative impact or creates a hostile environment. As mentioned previously, as a manager, you are legally responsible for ensuring nondiscrimination and preventing harassment. You, as a manager, may be innocent of any kind of sexual harassment yourself, but if the workplace you manage is construed as hostile by any one of your employees and you do not take appropriate action, you and your clinic can be held liable in a court of law.

Legal

When an employee contacts you or you become aware of harassment, you should immediately contact your Human Resources Equal Opportunity Office (EOO). If your facility does not have an EOO, you should collect facts and confront the offending individuals or group, clearly notifying them that the offensive behavior must stop immediately. A report of the incident should be placed in the file of the offending individuals, with a written warning that a future incident will result in termination.

The manager must carefully evaluate the facts surrounding an incident. It is not uncommon for innocent events to be perceived as harassment. When there is conflict between people who are in some way different from each other, simple misunderstandings can be perceived as harassment. Blatant harassment is far less common than this kind of muddled interaction. Although some situations do involve malicious intent, many are largely the result of poor communication, and it is the manager's responsibility to differentiate between the two.

Every employer needs a written comprehensive policy that prohibits all types of harassment. The policy needs to include a definition of what could constitute harassment or create a hostile work environment, information on who to report to, and a **nonretaliation provision**. A nonretaliation provision provides protection to an employee or applicant from being retaliated against due to participation in filing a complaint regarding discrimination, or participating in an investigation or lawsuit. This would include being fired, demoted, passed up for promotion, or being harassed. For example, it is illegal to refuse to promote an employee based on discrimination charges filed by the individual, even if later it was determined that no such discrimination took place.

The law forbids retaliation when it comes to any aspect of employment, including hiring, firing, pay, job assignments, promotions, layoff, training, fringe benefits, and any other term or condition of employment. The harassment Policies and Procedures must be made available to all employees.

Assimilating New Personnel

The goal in the assimilation of new personnel into the workplace is to make it happen as seamlessly as possible. The clinic manager and HR representative usually assume this task jointly, with the clinic manager being responsible for orientation in medical protocols and procedures, and the HR representative handling orientation regarding medical practice rules and regulations and any legal implications.

New Personnel Orientation. The new personnel orientation process consists of orienting and training new employees in the medical protocols and procedures unique to the practice. If the procedure manual is detailed and accurate, this manual becomes a guide for new employees.

It is important to introduce new employees to other staff members and to assign a **mentor** who can respond to questions that new employees may raise. Sometimes the individual leaving a position still is present and is asked to assist in the orientation process. This is especially beneficial if there is a good working relationship between the employee who is leaving and the management of the practice. Depending on the responsibilities of the new employee, a supervisor may be asked to monitor all procedures for a period for accuracy, safety, and patient protection.

The orientation should clearly present what is expected of new employees and explain that, at the end of their probationary period, their performance will be evaluated to determine if full-time employment will be offered. The same procedures followed for new employees should be followed for student practicums, with the exception that expectations and the evaluation process may vary.

Probation and Evaluation. It is common for a new employee to be placed on probation for 60 to 90 days. During this period, both the employee and supervisory personnel determine if the position is a suitable match for both employer and employee. Near the end of the probation period, the employee should be officially evaluated to determine how competently he or she is performing the assigned tasks/duties. The employee should also be given an opportunity to express his or her personal thoughts relative to job satisfaction. Figure 44-3 shows a sample probationary

---

PROBATIONARY EMPLOYEE EVALUATION FORM

Name _____

Hire Date _____

Job Title _____

Pay Rate_____ Supervisor _____

Do you recommend the employee continue in employment?

_____ Yes   _____ No

Please state your reasons for whatever action you recommend. Use the guidelines below to make your decision.

1. Has the employee required more training than is normally needed for the job?

2. Has the employee grasped this job with very little training?

3. Is the employee performing at, above, or below (circle one) the standard for this job?

4. If below, when do you expect the employee to reach the standard?

5. Does the employee get along well with all staff members?

6. Has the employee maintained a good attendance record and a good work attitude?

7. Has the employee expressed any dissatisfactions?

_____ _____
Supervisor's Signature   Date

FIGURE 44-3 Sample probationary employee evaluation.

employee evaluation form. The evaluation becomes part of the employee's personnel record at the end of the probation period.

Supervising Student Practicums. The student **practicum** is a transitional stage that provides opportunities for the student to apply theory learned in the classroom to a health care setting through practical, hands-on experience. Some institutions use the term *externship* or *internship*, and still others operate through a cooperative education program. The number of hours for the practicum are predetermined together with criteria for site selection and tasks to be performed by the student.

The clinic manager should schedule an information interview with the student before the practicum begins. During this time, the expectations of the clinic manager and the student may be established. A tour of the facility and introductions to key personnel aid the student in feeling more comfortable the first day of "work."

Because the student will be writing in medical records where correct spelling is mandatory or may be scheduling appointments and must write telephone numbers without transposition, some pretesting may be offered. By giving a spelling test of 10 commonly used medical terms or verbally stating five telephone numbers for the student to write down, an immediate evaluation is attained.

The clinic manager should directly supervise or identify someone else to supervise the student. During the first few days of the practicum, the student may simply **shadow** the supervisor, learning the routine, provider preferences, and protocols for that particular clinic. As the student begins to feel comfortable in the new environment, minimal tasks should be assigned. Based on the student's ability to follow directions and perform tasks, increased skill–level tasks may be added.

The supervisor will direct and evaluate the student's progress; schedule activities that will provide experience in all aspects of medical assisting, including administrative, clinical, and laboratory procedures; maintain accurate records of attendance and hours "worked"; and communicate the student's progress to the medical assisting supervisor from the educational institution.

When working with students, it is important to remember that they still have much to learn and will need lots of reassuring guidance. When you take time to explain each step and to provide the rationale for each, students will learn more quickly. Demonstrating new or different techniques and approaches helps students by providing them with options that they may find more comfortable.

Remember that this type of learning is stressful. The student is not yet accustomed to communication with a "real" patient, let alone working with a provider. Your role as clinic manager is to reduce as much stress as possible for everyone concerned. Introduce the student to the patient and ask the patient's permission to allow the student to perform a procedure. Many patients will be tolerant when they realize the circumstances and will be quite cooperative.

Employees with Chemical Dependencies or Emotional Problems

Employees with chemical dependencies or emotional problems are ill and are to be treated as such. Approach the situation constructively rather than punitively. Make a commitment to the employee, to the rest of the staff, and to the patients that at no time will patient care be put at risk. Help an employee with a problem to find the support and counseling necessary. No staff member should be permitted to remain on the premise with impaired judgment while under the influence of alcohol or controlled substances. If chemical dependency treatment is necessary, make accommodation as seems appropriate or is warranted. Everyone occasionally feels discouraged and distressed. Hopefully, the provider-employer and the manager are able to recognize problems before they become too serious.

It has been said that one in four individuals will experience some form of a mental health problem during the course of a year. Work-related stress is the base cause of a significant degree of mental strain. Plan for and create a work environment that reduces as much stress as possible. Actions to consider may include the following:

1. Properly educate and train all employees for their positions.

2. Encourage teamwork and reward those who help each other.

3. Mandate "break periods" in the day for each employee.

4. Create a pleasant work environment (plants, water, music, and so on).

5. Establish a blowing off steam place for when employees are especially frustrated.

6. Take everyone out for lunch at least once a quarter.

7. Have regular staff meetings to discuss employee concerns and clinic improvements.

8. Celebrate birthdays and special occasions (e.g., length of service).

Keep in mind that a happy employee who feels valued in his or her position will stay much longer than someone who is unhappy and does not feel valued.

Evaluating Employees and Planning Salary Review

It is important that all employees know whether they are performing their job as expected and know how they can improve their performance if necessary.

Performance Evaluation. Not only is evaluation of employees necessary during the probation period, but it is necessary for current employees as well. Evaluations should be performed no less than once a year on the anniversary of the hire date. Some clinic managers may wish to evaluate an employee more often, especially if a problem has surfaced in an evaluation.

The evaluation may take many forms; it can be formal or informal; it may involve more than one person. The results of the evaluation, however, must be a part of the employee's personnel record. For that reason, a formal evaluation is preferred. Many practices use a written evaluation that requires that the employee evaluate himself or herself before meeting with the clinic manager (Figure 44-4). The clinic manager uses the same form for evaluation. During the meeting, notes are compared as the evaluation is conducted.

The climate of the performance evaluation should be comfortable and provide privacy (Figure 44-5). The meeting should be friendly, but the employee must sense the importance of the evaluation. Do not allow any disagreements to escalate into arguments during the evaluation. Without reading the employee's self-evaluation, ask the employee to tell about the self-assessment. Acknowledge the employee's point of view and identify where you agree or differ from the self-assessment. Be prepared to describe specific examples of positive performance and negative performance.

When negative performance is identified, ask the employee for possible solutions. Then a plan can be determined to alter the negative performance. In this way, a trusting atmosphere is established in that both of you are working together for a solution that will benefit the medical practice. Always look for and seek a win–win situation whenever possible. The action plan determined should then be evaluated at the next performance evaluation.

At the close of the evaluation, always express your confidence in the individual to make any changes necessary, offer assistance where needed, and thank the employee for participating. End any evaluation with a positive statement about some portion of the employee's performance.

There are occasions when reviews are performed more frequently than annually. A review would occur 2 to 3 months after a significant promotion to measure how things are progressing. Reviews occur more often when general performance falls well short of past efforts or a serious error in judgment has been made. This type of review may end with a reprimand; a warning to correct the problem by a given date; or possibly, immediate dismissal. Document any steps to be taken to correct a problem and any reason that is cause for dismissal.

Salary Review. Although the practice is common in some areas, it may be better not to tie salary increases or bonuses with the annual performance evaluation. Conduct the **salary review** at the beginning of the new year separate from performance evaluations.

Salary review is important. Unfortunately, in smaller medical clinic and ambulatory care settings, the review of salary may have to be raised by the employee. Provider-employers tend to forget that their employees have been with them for over a year without a raise or a discussion of financial remuneration. If this is the case, it is perfectly acceptable for the employee to raise the issue on a yearly basis. However, the best approach is for the clinic manager to conduct salary reviews at the beginning or end of each calendar year.

Data should be collected before a salary review. The clinic manager should network with other clinic managers in the local area to determine wages and salaries for comparable individuals with comparable skills. Remember, also, that it is far more cost effective to reward good employees with a salary increase than it is to train a new employee who commands a lesser salary than current employees. Reward employees well and provide benefits that encourage them to stay with the practice. Employees who stay with the practice for a long time not only fully understand

PERFORMANCE REVIEW FORM

_____   _____
Employee Name   Title

_____   _____
Supervisor   Department

TYPE OF REVIEW (Check One)

_____ Quarterly

_____ Annual

_____ Probation

_____ Other _____

Review Period Covered _____ to _____

PERFORMANCE DEFINITIONS (To be used for general performance rating and job specific criteria rating)

5 = Outstanding	Performance that is clearly superior, beyond the call of duty, or substantially above standard level. Seldom attained level of performance but achievable.
4 = Above Standard	Very commendable performance; exceeds the norm for the job.
3 = Standard	Competent and consistent performance; expected level of activity and performance for the job. Most often rating received.
2 = Below Standard	Performance needs improvement. This level of performance is unacceptable; needs improvement to meet the standards for the job.
	Employee new to the job: Performance might receive below standard rating due to lack of job knowledge and is expected to improve with experience.
	Experienced employee: Performance is below acceptable level and requires direction and/or counsel.
1 = Unsatisfactory	Performance is unacceptable. Job activity is clearly and substantially lacking in quality, quantity, or timeliness. May also not be meeting cost or budget constraints. Needs much improvement to meet the standards for the job.

(office use only)	FINAL RATING: CHECK ONE (clinic use only)
EVALUATION SUMMARY	_____ Merit Increase Recommended
Total I _____	_____ No Merit Increase—Satisfactory Performance/No Growth
Total II _____	_____ No Merit Increase (Probationary/Special Evaluation)
	_____ No Merit Increase (Performance Probation)
	_____ Re-evaluate in 90 Days for Unsatisfactory or in 180 Days for Needed Improvement

GENERAL PERFORMANCE RATING (PART I)

General Criteria	Rating	Comments Supporting Rating
1. **Patient Relations:** How well does the employee communicate a "we care" image to the patients, visitors, providers, and fellow employees?		
2. **Work Responsibilities:** Evaluate the employee's work relative to quality, quantity, and timeliness.		
3. **Teamwork:** Does the employee have a team spirit? Does the employee interact well with coworkers/supervisor/manager?		(continues)

FIGURE 44-4 Sample performance review form.

General Criteria	Rating	Comments Supporting Rating
4. **Adaptability:** Is the employee open to change and new ideas? Does the employee remain flexible to changes in routine, workload, and assignments?		
5. **Personal Appearance:** How well does the employee maintain appropriate personal appearance, including proper attire, hygiene?		
6. **Communication:** Does the employee communicate well? Is information given and received clearly? Does he/she have good verbal and written skills?		
7. **Dependability:** Can the employee be relied upon for good attendance? Does the employee perform and follow through on work without supervisory intervention or assistance?		

Subtotal I _____ ÷7 General Criteria = _____

JOB-SPECIFIC CRITERIA RATING (PART II) (To be used with Job Description attached)

Responsibility and Standard	Rating	Comments Supporting Rating
Complete a section for each responsibility listed on the employee's job description.		

Subtotal II _____ ÷ _____ = _____
job duties

Contributions made since last review:

_____

_____

Education or training received since last review:

_____

_____

Action to be taken based on performance:

_____

_____

_____

Comments:

_____

_____

_____

_____	_____
Employee Signature	Date
_____	_____
Supervisor Signature	Date
_____	_____
Provider Signature	Date

FIGURE 44-4 Sample performance review form. *(continued)*

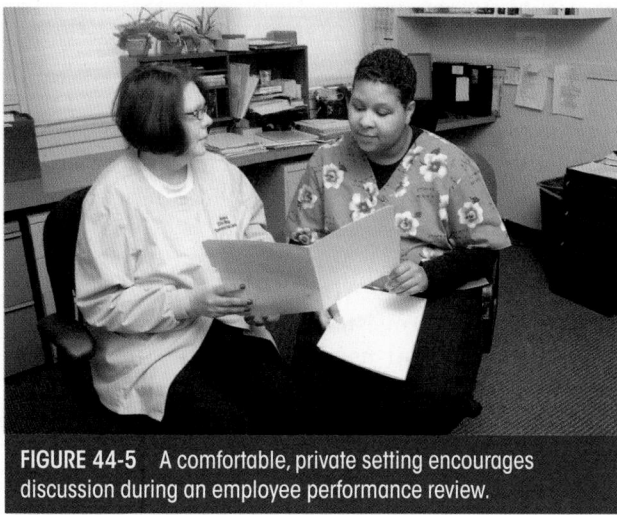
FIGURE 44-5 A comfortable, private setting encourages discussion during an employee performance review.

how best to serve their provider-employers, they have established a relationship with patients that is beneficial.

How much of a raise is to be awarded at the time of salary review is difficult to determine and depends on many factors that might include the profits of the year, the patient load, the workload, and the current cost of living.

The critical shortage of health care employees today is reflected in the shortage of medical assistants across the country. Advertisements for individuals to work in ambulatory care settings tell the story. A consideration worth mentioning is that often the salary does not match the education, experience, and special training required of someone working in the health care field. Educators often hear, "Why would I spend a year or more in education to be paid what I would make working in a fast food restaurant?" Because it is costly in time and resources to replace employees, it is best to invest that cost into a fair and just salary increase for valued employees.

Dismissing Employees

Most clinic/human resource managers do not enjoy rating the performance of other employees, particularly when difficult topics are involved and it may be necessary to dismiss an employee. However, the written performance evaluation actually establishes the format for such a dismissal when necessary and is more likely to remove the emotion from the situation. Involuntary dismissal is still difficult when it is necessary.

Involuntary Dismissal. Involuntary dismissal results from two primary causes: poor performance or serious violation of clinic policies or job descriptions. When it becomes apparent to the clinic manager that the effectiveness of an employee is dropping well below expectations, it will be known in the annual review or a performance review may be called. The review allows the employee to be informed of the shortcomings, to explain any reasons for the present situation, and to determine a plan to alleviate the problem. If the problem is a serious one, probation is usually invoked and any lack of significant improvement in the time provided results in immediate dismissal.

When the problem is a violation of either clinic policy or procedures, both a verbal and a written warning are given to the employee. Involuntary dismissal follows if the situation persists. Dismissal may be immediate if the action is a serious violation of policy. Serious violations depend on the clinic practice, but some causes for immediate dismissal include theft, making fraudulent claims against insurance, placing the patient in jeopardy by not practicing safe techniques, and breach of patient confidentiality.

Some key points to keep in mind when dismissal is necessary are:

1. Make the dismissal in private.
2. Take no longer than 10 minutes for the dismissal.
3. Be direct, firm, and to the point in identifying reasons.
4. Do not engage in an in-depth discussion of performance.
5. Explain terms of dismissal (keys, clearing out area of personal items, final paperwork).
6. Listen to the employee's opinion and emotions; it is not necessary to agree.
7. Accompany the employee to his or her desk to pack his or her belongings.
8. Escort the employee out of the facility; do not allow him or her to finish the work of the day.

Voluntary Dismissal. Other reasons for dismissal may be more pleasant. Changes in personnel occur for many good reasons, and people to voluntarily leave their jobs. They may relocate, seek advancement at another facility, or simply have personal reasons for leaving. These employees will give their manager proper notice and will be able to turn their current projects and duties over to their replacements. They have time to say good-bye to their friends and leave with a good feeling about their employment.

PROCEDURE MANUAL

The **procedure manual** provides detailed information relative to the performance of tasks within the facility in which one is employed. Each procedure manual should be designed for that specific clinic setting and should satisfy its requirements.

The procedure manual serves as a guide to the employee assigned a specific task and may also be useful in evaluating the employee's performance. If a temporary employee is assigned the task, the procedure manual will be invaluable in ensuring that each procedure is completed as outlined.

The provider(s) and the clinic manager should have copies of the procedure manual, and all employees should have access to the procedure manual. Copies of individual sections may be given to the employee responsible for the task; the employee should be instructed to follow these guidelines and told that they may be used as employee evaluation tools. If all employees have access to the clinic computer system, the procedure manual can be made available in electronic format.

Organization of the Procedure Manual

It is best to use a loose-leaf binder with separator pages denoting each procedure. Many clinic managers find it helpful to divide the binder into administrative and clinical sections with subdivisions for each primary task performed (Table 44-2).

Procedure

To facilitate using the procedure manual, a consistent format should be developed and used throughout the manual. Each procedure should be a step-by-step outline or list of steps to be taken to complete a task as desired in that facility. Providing the rationale for a step, when appropriate, enhances the learning process, especially for new staff members. Material Safety Data Sheets (MSDS) are required to be maintained in the clinic and available for personnel to reference at any time. MSDS must be compiled for all chemicals considered hazardous and maintained in an appropriate manual. Some clinics opt to maintain these records in a separate tabbed section of the procedure manual. Others choose to maintain a separate MSDS manual. The information must be reviewed and updated on a regular basis. See Chapter 38 for detailed information regarding MSDS. Procedure 44-3 provides steps for developing and maintaining a procedure manual.

TABLE 44-2

ORGANIZING THE PROCEDURE MANUAL

ADMINISTRATIVE SECTION	CLINICAL SECTION	ADMINISTRATIVE/CLINICAL SECTIONS
Personnel Management	Physical Examinations	HIPAA and ADA compliance
Communication (oral and written)	Infection Control	Creating a Safe Environment
Patient Scheduling	Collecting Specimens	Evacuation Procedures
Records Management	Laboratory Procedures	Emergency Codes
Financial Management	Surgical Asepsis	Fire Safety
Facility and Equipment Management	Emergencies	Fire Extinguisher Safety
	Material Safety Data Sheets (MSDS)	Response to National Disaster or Emergency
	OSHA	Medical Assistant Response to Disaster Preparedness
	CLIA '88	

PROCEDURE 44-3

Procedure

Developing and Maintaining a Procedure Manual

PURPOSE:

To develop and maintain a comprehensive, up-to-date procedure manual covering each clinical, technical, and administrative procedure in the clinic, with step-by-step directions and rationales for performing each task.

EQUIPMENT/SUPPLIES:

- Computer (electronic storage allows changes and revisions to be made easily)
- Binder, such as a three-ring binder
- Paper
- Standard procedure manual format

PROCEDURE STEPS:

1. *Pay attention to detail* by writing step-by-step procedures and rationales for each clinical, technical, and administrative function. Each procedure is written by experienced employees close to the function and then reviewed by a supervisor and clinic manager. Rationales help employees understand **why** something is done. RATIONALE: Establishes consistent guidelines to be followed.

2. Include regular maintenance instructions and flow sheets for cleaning, servicing, and calibrating of all clinic equipment, both in the clinical and in the administrative areas. RATIONALE: Equipment needs to be cleaned and maintained on a regular basis to ensure it is working properly and that it lasts as long as needed. Some manufacturer guarantees and service contracts require regular cleaning and maintenance, especially on new and leased equipment. Instructions are necessary so that the task can be performed properly. The flow sheets provide documentation of dates the equipment was cleaned, serviced, and/or calibrated and the person who performed the task.

3. Include local and out-of-the-area resources for clinical and administrative staff, providers, and patients. Provide a listing in each area with contact information and services provided. RATIONALE: The procedures and instructions listed in the procedure manual should provide supporting documentation needed for accomplishing each task. For example, if the clinic requires that local public transportation resources be given to each patient who needs transportation, the procedure manual has a listing of transportation available in the area with telephone numbers and schedules. This document could either be printed from the computer or photocopied from the manual and provided to the patient.

4. *Recognize the importance of local, state, and federal legislation and regulations* that are related to processes performed in both clinical and administrative areas. RATIONALE: Having a listing of the rules and regulations assists in performing those regulated duties correctly and legally.

5. Include the clinic procedures and flow sheets for taking inventory in each of the areas and instructions on ordering procedures. RATIONALE: When a clinic has processes clearly written for managing inventory and ordering equipment and supplies, the clinic is less likely to run out of needed items and may even be able to take advantage of discounts offered by manufacturers.

6. Collect the procedures into the Clinic Procedure Manual. RATIONALE: Provides a reference guide with step-by-step instructions and examples where appropriate.

7. Store one complete manual in a common library area. Provide a completed copy to the provider-employer and the clinic manager. Distribute appropriate sections to the various departments. RATIONALE: Provides a reference guide with step-by-step instructions and examples where appropriate.

8. Review the procedure manual annually and add any new procedures, delete or modify as necessary, and indicate the revision date (e.g., Rev. 10/12/XX). RATIONALE: Maintains current clinic protocols.

Updating and Reviewing the Procedure Manual

When new procedures are added to the clinic routine, a new procedure page should be developed immediately. The new page is useful as an educational tool or job aid while team members are learning new techniques.

An annual page-by-page review should be done to ascertain if each procedure is still being used and to ensure that each page is correct in each detail and satisfies all criteria established by the staff personnel. This contributes to an efficient clinic and gives all employees a sense of pride and satisfaction that they are performing within the scope of their training and to their greatest potential. The procedure manual should be reviewed by personnel performing the various tasks, and their suggestions should be evaluated and incorporated into the revisions when appropriate. All new procedure pages and revisions should be dated (e.g., Rev. 02/15/XX).

HIPAA IMPLICATIONS

HIPAA regulations require each clinic to develop a separate HIPAA manual that is in either an electronic form or a paper manual. The manual spells out all policies and procedures of the practice and security management measures; identifies the security officer; addresses workforce security issues, information access concerns, security awareness and training, security incidents, and contingency plans; evaluates security effectiveness; and contains copies of all business associate contracts.

The HIPAA manual must be available to all employees and updated on a regular basis. During an audit, the clinic manager will be asked to produce the HIPAA manual for review and to establish compliance with all regulations. All documentation of policies and procedures are to be kept for 6 years even if the wording has changed or a particular policy or procedure has been eliminated. If an incident is under investigation, this allows an investigator to go back to what a policy said 6 years ago.

TRAVEL ARRANGEMENTS

The clinic manager may be asked to make travel arrangements for providers going on vacation or to conventions, symposiums, or out-of-town seminars and continuing medical education (CME) courses. If the providers do a fair amount of travel or if they live in a metropolitan area, they may use the services of a travel agent. Attention to detail is extremely important in preventing travel disruptions.

Read carefully the instructions for completing registration forms, complete them online, or, mail them as quickly as possible to secure reservations to conventions. Next, make hotel and travel arrangements. General information regarding the provider's travel preferences should be maintained in a file and referred to when making travel arrangements. Helpful information to maintain in this file includes:

- Name of travel agents used in the past
- Provider's or clinic credit card numbers (though this information must be properly safeguarded)
- Transportation preferences
- Preferred airline, class of travel, seating choice
- Hotel/motel accommodations (bed size, suite, studio, connecting rooms, price range, amenities)

Next, contact the travel agent and identify the destination, date and time for departure and return, number traveling in party, and seating preference. A travel agent can assist with rental car and hotel accommodations, if needed. Take your time and pay attention to details. When tickets are received, always check to see that all departure and arrival times match what is needed and that a confirmation number has been provided for car rentals and hotel arrangements.

The Internet can be used to search for the lowest-cost air, auto, and lodging reservations. The procedures do not require extensive knowledge of travel and airline reservation protocols. Searching for information on the Internet requires the use of a search engine if you do not already have a list of favorite travel Web sites. Once you refine your search, you may have choices such as Travelocity.com, Expedia.com, or Priceline.com. Select the desired Web sites and follow its instructions.

 Procedure 44-4 outlines the steps for making travel arrangements via the Internet.

PROCEDURE 44-4

Making Travel Arrangements via the Internet

Procedure

PURPOSE:
To use the Internet to make travel arrangements for the provider.

EQUIPMENT/SUPPLIES:

- Travel plan
- Computer
- Provider's or clinic's credit card to pay for reservations.

PROCEDURE STEPS:

1. *Paying attention to detail,* confirm the planned trip: date, time, and place for departure and arrival; preferred mode of transportation (plane, train, bus, car); number of travelers; preferred lodging type and price range; and whether travelers' checks are required. RATIONALE: Confirming pertinent travel details ensures that correct arrangements will be made.

2. Go to the computer and access the Internet.

3. *Show initiative* by selecting a search engine to locate Web sites using the key term "air fares." Web sites may provide links to air fares, auto reservations, and hotel/motel reservations. Follow Web site instructions for making arrangements. Review and copy confirmation of your transaction. RATIONALE: The Internet can be a time saver and a cost effective way of securing travel arrangements.

4. Pick up tickets or arrange for their delivery, if necessary. Tickets purchased on the Internet can be mailed or picked up at an airport, or they can be electronic tickets.

5. Make additional copies of the itinerary or create the itinerary. The itinerary should list date and time of departures and arrivals, including flight numbers and seat assignments. Note the mode of transportation to lodging (shuttle, bus, car, taxi). Include name, address, and telephone number of lodgings and meeting places.

6. Maintain one copy of the itinerary in the clinic file.

7. Give several copies of the itinerary to the provider. RATIONALE: Ensures that a copy is on file with the clinic and that there are sufficient copies for the traveler(s) and families.

Itinerary

If you have used a travel agent in making the travel arrangements, the agency most likely will provide several copies of the **itinerary**. An itinerary is a detailed plan for a proposed trip. The clinic should maintain one copy of the itinerary in case the provider must be reached for emergencies. The provider should have one copy to carry with him or her and a copy to leave with family members. You may need to develop the itinerary if you have made the travel arrangements via computer. Figure 44-6 shows a sample travel itinerary.

Important information to be included on any itinerary includes:

- *Air travel.* Departure and arrival date and time, meals, airline name and telephone number, airport
- *Car rental.* Name, telephone number, confirmation number
- *Hotel/motel.* Name, confirmation number, dates, telephone number
- *Meeting location.* Name, address, room number, telephone number

TRAVEL ITINERARY

James Whitney, MD
Inner City Health Care
400 Inner City Way
Seattle, WA 98400

15 Sept 20XX   INVOICE: 880133795

29 Sept Friday
USAIR   630   Coach Class   Equip-Boeing 757 Jet
LV: Seattle   11:55P   Nonstop   Miles-2125   Confirmed
AR: Pittsburgh   7:23A   Elapsed time-4:28   Arrival Date-30Sept
                                                            Seat-31C

30 Sept-Saturday
Alamo   1 Compact 2/4 DR   Drop-101CT   Confirmed
Pickup-Pittsburgh   Pittsburgh Airport   Chg-USD .00
Rate-   59.98   Base rate   Guaranteed   Extra Hr 10.00-UN
Phone-412-472-5060

                                    Confirmation-1870649

01 Oct Sunday
USAIR   1419   Coach Class   Equip-Boeing 737 Jet
LV: Pittsburgh   3:05P   Nonstop   Miles-2125   Confirmed
AR: Seattle   5:27P   Elapsed time-5:22
Lunch   Seat-20A

Ticket Number/s:
Whitney/James   3570933   BA Card $461.00
        Air Transportation $416.36   Tax   44.64   TOTAL $461.00
                                                    Sub Total $461.00
                                                    Credit Card Payment $461.00-
                                                    Amount Due   0.00

TICKET IS NON REFUNDABLE. TRIP INSURANCE IS AVAILABLE. RECONFIRM ALL FLTS 24 HRS PRIOR TO DEPARTURE

FIGURE 44-6 Sample travel itinerary.

TIME MANAGEMENT

Initiative

Time management is an item of critical importance to the manager. You may have upward of 20 staff members putting demands on your time, and added to this are vendors, your superiors, business associates, and a host of others. A manager has not a moment to lose in the day, so managing time makes the difference between a normal 8- or 10-hour day and a 15-hour or more day. The following suggestions are some proven means of managing your time whether in management or as a salaried employee.

- *Handle items once.* Once the mail is opened, sorted, and prioritized, try to handle it only once more, when action is taken with it. Picking it up, reading it, and setting it down again without taking action is a real waste of time.

- *Develop a to-do list.* At the end of each day prepare a list of things you plan to complete the next day and try to work down this list. Prioritize the list by importance or by practical order.

- *Guard your time.* Schedule meetings with personnel and vendors so that they do not fragment your time, making you have to re-start a task and get up to speed over and over again. Although modern management practice is to have an open-door policy with employees, this does not mean you should allow them to come into your office whenever they think about it. Have them schedule time with you. Make them think about what they want to discuss and do not let them monopolize your time. This is also true of meeting with vendors; require vendors to schedule ahead a time to meet with you.

- *Delegate work.* Assign others or a team to perform some of the functions discussed in this chapter. Having a team prepare weekly work schedules and vacation schedules results in less bickering and feelings of favoritism that you would have to spend time defusing if you made the schedules yourself. This does not mean that you do not have to approve them and, in some instances, make the hard decisions, but it results in your people having ownership in the decisions.

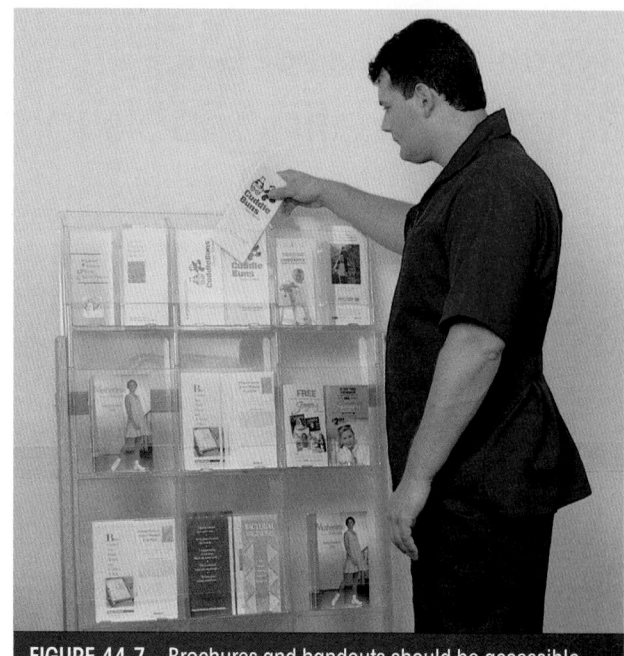

FIGURE 44-7 Brochures and handouts should be accessible and inviting to patients and clinic visitors.

MARKETING FUNCTIONS

Communication

Effective communication skills are essential in the management of the ambulatory care setting. These skills are used by the clinic manager inside the ambulatory care setting to establish friendly, professional relationships with colleagues and patients. Communication is just as critical when relating to external audiences, such as other organizations, potential new patients, and community members. Developing relationships outside the clinic is often called marketing, a concept that clinic managers may use to enhance the image and visibility of an ambulatory care setting while also providing benefits to patients, potential patients, and the neighboring community.

In its broadest sense, **marketing** can be defined as the process by which the provider of services makes the consumer aware of the scope and quality of these services. Although marketing is a tool traditionally used by for-profit organizations to promote and sell products and services, it has become increasingly acceptable among health care organizations, whether they are for- or not-for-profit.

Marketing functions and materials are diverse and can include presence on social media sites, seminars and workshops, patient education brochures (Figure 44-7), brochures that describe the ambulatory care setting and its scope of services, HIPAA policies, newsletters, press releases, and special events such as open houses or participation in community health care events. Depending on the size and resources of the medical clinic, the manager may choose to use all or some of these tools.

Legal   Diversity

When producing written material and organizing events, it is essential that ethical guidelines be respected at all times. Marketing tools should be appropriate, in good taste, and designed to quietly enhance the reputation of the clinic. Cultural issues should always be considered. For example, patient education brochures for a practice with many Spanish-speaking patients should be produced in bilingual editions, with English on one side and Spanish on the other. Legal issues are important as well; when presenting material of a medical nature, it is extremely important that information be accurate and up to date.

Effective marketing is a valuable tool for the clinic manager, especially as managed care calls on all health care professionals to become more competitive to survive. Marketing can increase visibility and credibility. The effective manager enlists the talents and skills of the entire team in developing a marketing plan. (See the "Marketing Tools in the Medical Environment" Quick Reference Guide.)

Marketing Tools in the Medical Environment

Brochures.
Patient education brochures can address a variety of topics. Specialized procedures, surgeries, and common diseases and syndromes that are explained in simple terms can aid in understanding and patient preparation when needed. This information must always be updated. Clinic brochures describe the clinic, HIPAA policies, insurance and payment information, provider profiles, and scope of services for the patient. Cultural issues should be considered by providing material in multiple languages, as applicable to the practice.

Seminars and workshops.
In clinics where patient education, procedure preparation, or obtaining more information before making medical decisions is important, seminars and workshops are effective tools for providing expert advice. These tools meet patient and community needs by providing a forum for health care professionals and patients to interact. Popular topics include hypertension, diabetes, eating disorders and bariatric surgery, joint replacement, and pain management. Audiovisuals, presentations, handouts, brochures, and anatomical models or samples can elaborate on and enhance seminar content, helping patients remember what was said.

Category 1:

Internal marketing tools.
Marketing tools specific to the functions of the clinic and services provided are often presented in the form of brochures, seminars, and workshops.

Newsletters.
Newsletters are more focused on the individual practice and its philosophies. Newsletters can be sent to the clinic's mailing list, or there are online services that offer newsletter creation and then the newsletters can be sent by email. This is an optimal way to offer health-related articles, including clinic updates such as policy changes, staff introductions, and insurance information. Typically released biannually or quarterly, newsletters can be made available in the waiting room.

Web sites and e-zines.
Having access to clinic information and resources, such as registration forms, portal login, and other clinic-related materials any time of day or night is necessary in our technology-driven world. Web sites also provide a place to present medical information in the form of articles, videos, and interactive tools for current and potential patients. E-zines are online magazines that can be released on Web sites or emailed to a patient base on a regular basis, and can also be archived for future reference.

Category 3:

External marketing tools.
Educating the public on various medical topics and procedures often goes hand in hand with the subtle promotion of a clinic when using marketing tools. Whether a clinic specializes in a particular area of medicine, emphasizes preventative measures for better health, or introduces new treatment or surgery options, external marketing provides a platform to accomplish these goals while also giving the community options for local health care professionals providing these services.

Special events.
Medicine is a collaborative effort, and special events such as health fairs, community events, and open houses offer an opportunity to join with other organizations to promote wellness. These events are usually well attended and offer the perfect place to discuss clinic services as well as new medical technology and procedures. They're also a great way provide information directly to the community.

Press releases.
Releasing information through local publications and even some online resources requires a press release. The press release follows a particular format for submission, and is almost exclusively accepted in digital form through email or online forms to editors. They are a way to announce clinic expansions, new equipment, providers joining the practice, or add-on services and affiliations with area facilities.

Social media.
Digital forms of communication have made social media such as Facebook, Twitter, and blogging not only necessary marketing tools, but excellent ways to keep information updated and available to patients and visitors seeking information. Video and photo sharing sites, such as Instagram, can be used to present medical information as a tool in patient education. In the clinic, providers often have an archive of videos handy on tablets, smart phones, and on the exam room PC that visually explain diseases, surgeries, and procedure preparation in addition to traditional anatomical models and drawings.

SOCIAL MEDIA AND THE MEDICAL CLINIC

Social media is an instrument of communication enabling communication in both directions. The telephone was an early means of social communication, but its reach to a mass audience was limited. Reading a newspaper or listening to a report on the radio does not allow the user to interact. This is where, on a very basic level, social media stands apart. It does allow a Web site visitor to interact with the site and with other visitors on the site. Social media can take on many different forms. Definitions of some of these social media forms are:

- *Webinar.* A seminar or lecture delivered over the Internet. It can be one-way (webcast) or with audience interaction.

- *Social networking.* Interact by adding friends, commenting on profiles, and joining groups and having discussions. Facebook and LinkedIn are examples of this form of social media, as are Twitter and Instagram on a micro scale.

- *Blogs.* A Web site on which an individual or group of users record opinions and information in a more conversational and informal manner, called blogging.

- *Social photo and video sharing.* Interact by sharing photos or videos and commenting on user submissions. YouTube and Instagram are examples of this form.

- *Wikis.* Interact by adding articles and editing existing articles. Wikipedia is an example of this form.

- *Social news.* Interact by voting on articles and submitting comments. Examples include Reddit and Digg.

The social media revolution has forever carried over to business. A purposeful and carefully designed social media strategy must become an integral part of any modern, complete, and directed business plan or job-seeking strategy.

Social media gives you a voice and a way to communicate with patients and potential consumers, to find qualified employees, and to verify the background of persons seeking employment with your organization. It personalizes the medical clinic and helps you to spread your message in a relaxed and conversational way. Social media projects your clinic as a personality. You want the clinic to become a respected source of information to the patient. According to a study highlighted by the American Academy of Family Physicians' (AAFP) social media guide, more than 70% of primary care physicians and oncologists use social media at least once a month to explore or contribute health information. Purpose, direction, consistent updating, and posting of relevant content will go a long way in making social media sites places where time is well spent by visitors. The main focus should be on providing an source of information for patients, caregivers, and families. As time has proven, many people seek out information on the Internet by searching their symptoms and concerns, and overwhelm themselves and cause anxiety in an effort to self-educate. Social media provides the perfect platform for the medical community to present facts and reasonable data, and encourage the patient to consult with a medical professional in the clinic in order to properly address health concerns.

You must always remember that in no way should social media be a place for offering medical advice. However, the effort to present accurate, valuable information that gently guides the patient to the correct and safest course of action while providing an enjoyable and more personalized experience can be achieved.

The power of social networking as a marketing tool is illustrated by response buttons on Facebook such as the "Like" button. The "Like" button links your Web site to the visitor's Facebook profile if he or she Likes your site. Your site, through his or her profile, becomes a living testimonial to your product or organization. In addition, you have the ability to publish updates to the user. One contact now becomes hundreds.

Many clinic managers are perplexed over whether social networking should be allowed by employees while at work. Many managers have a perception of employees hanging out on cyberspace wasting time. Experts on the subject do not support this perception. They feel that social networking can contribute to team building and can motivate employees, especially in small companies where the staff may be isolated from each other. The result has been increased productivity in most instances. Prohibition of social networking can result in the loss of valued employees. The answer to the question probably lies between total prohibition and uncontrolled use resulting in abuse. If social networking is allowed on the job, protocols should be in place to prevent HIPAA violations, to define where and when social networking is acceptable, and to prohibit bullying of colleagues. A manager must use caution in monitoring employee actions online to avoid overstepping legal boundaries.

RECORDS AND FINANCIAL MANAGEMENT

Providers entrust a great deal of responsibility to their medical clinic managers. The daily payments received through the mail and clinic visits must be processed and prepared for banking. Clinic expenses must be processed and paid in a timely fashion to capitalize on any discounts available. Employee requirements and records such as Social Security records; Withholding Allowance Certificates (W-4 forms) indicating the number of exemptions claimed (Figure 44-8); and Employment Eligibility Verification Forms (Form I-9) ensuring that all persons employed are either U.S. citizens, lawfully admitted immigrants, or citizens of other countries authorized to work in the United States must be completed and filed with the appropriate federal agencies. Also, state and local tax records must be maintained for each employee.

Electronic Health Records and the Clinic Manager

The practice management (PM) system and electronic medical record (EMR) discussed in Chapter 10 is the nerve center for the clinic manager as he or she orchestrates a smooth-running organization. It provides all of the data needed by the clinic manager at the click of a mouse or a few keystrokes. Table 44-3 lists sample data types and the resulting actions by the manager.

Payroll Processing

In some cases, it is the clinic manager's responsibility to prepare payroll checks for each employee and record all deductions withheld. A W-2 form (Figure 44-9) summarizing all earnings and deductions for the year must be prepared for each employee by January 31 of the following year. The Social Security Administration must receive a summary report of W-2 forms each year.

Legal

To comply with all federal, state, and local governmental regulations, it is important that the clinic manager who processes payroll maintain complete,

TABLE 44-3

CLINIC MANAGER ACTIONS IN RESPONSE TO PM AND EMR DATA

DATA	ACTION BY CLINIC MANAGER
Staffing requirements and appointment schedules	Hire or terminate employees, obtain additional clinic space and equipment, adjust vacation schedules
Equipment and supplies requests, and inventory data	Issue purchase orders, authorize payment of invoices, secure vendors and suppliers, negotiate maintenance contracts
Financial and billing reports	Practice financial status reports, instructions for coding and billing on past due accounts, actions on billing denied due to coding errors
Employee time sheets	Payroll authorization, corrective actions for missed work
Medical records	Review if patient demographics and HIPAA requirements are current
Personnel data	Progress reviews, salary reviews, W-4 forms, corrective actions, licenses, malpractice insurance contracts

up-to-date records on every employee. This information should be gathered from new employees and updated every year, including any changes in employee status. For more specific information regarding printed and electronic filing forms, consult the Internal Revenue Service Web site (http://www.irs.gov) for detailed instructions. It is a good idea to have employees update their W-4 form each year in case they want to adjust their deductions or make any other change. To accomplish this, many payroll managers include a new W-4 form with the first paycheck at the beginning of each year. Every employee file should contain the employee's Social Security number; number of exemptions claimed on the W-4 form; employee's gross salary; and all deductions withheld for all taxes, including Social Security, federal, state, local, and unemployment tax (where applicable), and disability insurance (where applicable).

Form W-4 (2016)

Purpose. Complete Form W-4 so that your employer can withhold the correct federal income tax from your pay. Consider completing a new Form W-4 each year and when your personal or financial situation changes.

Exemption from withholding. If you are exempt, complete **only** lines 1, 2, 3, 4, and 7 and sign the form to validate it. Your exemption for 2016 expires February 15, 2017. See Pub. 505, Tax Withholding and Estimated Tax.

Note: If another person can claim you as a dependent on his or her tax return, you cannot claim exemption from withholding if your income exceeds $1,050 and includes more than $350 of unearned income (for example, interest and dividends).

Exceptions. An employee may be able to claim exemption from withholding even if the employee is a dependent, if the employee:

• Is age 65 or older,

• Is blind, or

• Will claim adjustments to income; tax credits; or itemized deductions, on his or her tax return.

The exceptions do not apply to supplemental wages greater than $1,000,000.

Basic instructions. If you are not exempt, complete the **Personal Allowances Worksheet** below. The worksheets on page 2 further adjust your withholding allowances based on itemized deductions, certain credits, adjustments to income, or two-earners/multiple jobs situations.

Complete all worksheets that apply. However, you may claim fewer (or zero) allowances. For regular wages, withholding must be based on allowances you claimed and may not be a flat amount or percentage of wages.

Head of household. Generally, you can claim head of household filing status on your tax return only if you are unmarried and pay more than 50% of the costs of keeping up a home for yourself and your dependent(s) or other qualifying individuals. See Pub. 501, Exemptions, Standard Deduction, and Filing Information, for information.

Tax credits. You can take projected tax credits into account in figuring your allowable number of withholding allowances. Credits for child or dependent care expenses and the child tax credit may be claimed using the **Personal Allowances Worksheet** below. See Pub. 505 for information on converting your other credits into withholding allowances.

Nonwage income. If you have a large amount of nonwage income, such as interest or dividends, consider making estimated tax payments using Form 1040-ES, Estimated Tax for Individuals. Otherwise, you may owe additional tax. If you have pension or annuity income, see Pub. 505 to find out if you should adjust your withholding on Form W-4 or W-4P.

Two earners or multiple jobs. If you have a working spouse or more than one job, figure the total number of allowances you are entitled to claim on all jobs using worksheets from only one Form W-4. Your withholding usually will be most accurate when all allowances are claimed on the Form W-4 for the highest paying job and zero allowances are claimed on the others. See Pub. 505 for details.

Nonresident alien. If you are a nonresident alien, see Notice 1392, Supplemental Form W-4 Instructions for Nonresident Aliens, before completing this form.

Check your withholding. After your Form W-4 takes effect, use Pub. 505 to see how the amount you are having withheld compares to your projected total tax for 2016. See Pub. 505, especially if your earnings exceed $130,000 (Single) or $180,000 (Married).

Future developments. Information about any future developments affecting Form W-4 (such as legislation enacted after we release it) will be posted at *www.irs.gov/w4*.

Personal Allowances Worksheet (Keep for your records.)

A   Enter "1" for **yourself** if no one else can claim you as a dependent . . . .   **A** _____

B   Enter "1" if: {
• You are single and have only one job; or
• You are married, have only one job, and your spouse does not work; or
• Your wages from a second job or your spouse's wages (or the total of both) are $1,500 or less. } . .   **B** _____

C   Enter "1" for your **spouse.** But, you may choose to enter "-0-" if you are married and have either a working spouse or more than one job. (Entering "-0-" may help you avoid having too little tax withheld.) . . . .   **C** _____

D   Enter number of **dependents** (other than your spouse or yourself) you will claim on your tax return . . . . .   **D** _____

E   Enter "1" if you will file as **head of household** on your tax return (see conditions under **Head of household** above) . .   **E** _____

F   Enter "1" if you have at least $2,000 of **child or dependent care expenses** for which you plan to claim a credit . . .   **F** _____
    (**Note:** Do **not** include child support payments. See Pub. 503, Child and Dependent Care Expenses, for details.)

G   **Child Tax Credit** (including additional child tax credit). See Pub. 972, Child Tax Credit, for more information.
    • If your total income will be less than $70,000 ($100,000 if married), enter "2" for each eligible child; then **less** "1" if you have two to four eligible children or **less** "2" if you have five or more eligible children.
    • If your total income will be between $70,000 and $84,000 ($100,000 and $119,000 if married), enter "1" for each eligible child . .   **G** _____

H   Add lines A through G and enter total here. (**Note:** This may be different from the number of exemptions you claim on your tax return.) ▶ **H** _____

For accuracy, **complete all worksheets that apply.**
• If you plan to **itemize** or **claim adjustments to income** and want to reduce your withholding, see the **Deductions and Adjustments Worksheet** on page 2.
• If you are **single and have more than one job** or are **married and you and your spouse both work** and the combined earnings from all jobs exceed $50,000 ($20,000 if married), see the **Two-Earners/Multiple Jobs Worksheet** on page 2 to avoid having too little tax withheld.
• If **neither** of the above situations applies, **stop here** and enter the number from line H on line 5 of Form W-4 below.

---------------------------- **Separate here and give Form W-4 to your employer. Keep the top part for your records.** ----------------------------

Form **W-4**
Department of the Treasury
Internal Revenue Service

Employee's Withholding Allowance Certificate

▶ Whether you are entitled to claim a certain number of allowances or exemption from withholding is subject to review by the IRS. Your employer may be required to send a copy of this form to the IRS.

OMB No. 1545-0074

2016

1 Your first name and middle initial	Last name	2 **Your social security number**

Home address (number and street or rural route)	3 ☐ Single ☐ Married ☐ Married, but withhold at higher Single rate.
City or town, state, and ZIP code	**Note:** If married, but legally separated, or spouse is a nonresident alien, check the "Single" box.

4   If your last name differs from that shown on your social security card, check here. You must call 1-800-772-1213 for a replacement card. ▶ ☐

5	Total number of allowances you are claiming (from line **H** above **or** from the applicable worksheet on page 2)	5	
6	Additional amount, if any, you want withheld from each paycheck	6	$

7   I claim exemption from withholding for 2016, and I certify that I meet **both** of the following conditions for exemption.
• Last year I had a right to a refund of **all** federal income tax withheld because I had **no** tax liability, **and**
• This year I expect a refund of **all** federal income tax withheld because I expect to have **no** tax liability.
If you meet both conditions, write "Exempt" here . . . . ▶   7 _____

Under penalties of perjury, I declare that I have examined this certificate and, to the best of my knowledge and belief, it is true, correct, and complete.

Employee's signature
(This form is not valid unless you sign it.) ▶

Date ▶

8 Employer's name and address (Employer: Complete lines 8 and 10 only if sending to the IRS.)	9 Office code (optional)	10 Employer identification number (EIN)

For Privacy Act and Paperwork Reduction Act Notice, see page 2.   Cat. No. 10220Q   Form **W-4** (2016)

FIGURE 44-8   Form W-4 indicates the number of exemptions claimed by the employee for income tax purposes.

Deductions and Adjustments Worksheet

Note: Use this worksheet *only* if you plan to itemize deductions or claim certain credits or adjustments to income.

1	Enter an estimate of your 2016 itemized deductions. These include qualifying home mortgage interest, charitable contributions, state and local taxes, medical expenses in excess of 10% (7.5% if either you or your spouse was born before January 2, 1952) of your income, and miscellaneous deductions. For 2016, you may have to reduce your itemized deductions if your income is over $311,300 and you are married filing jointly or are a qualifying widow(er); $285,350 if you are head of household; $259,400 if you are single and not head of household or a qualifying widow(er); or $155,650 if you are married filing separately. See Pub. 505 for details . . .	**1**	$ _____
2	Enter: { $12,600 if married filing jointly or qualifying widow(er) / $9,300 if head of household / $6,300 if single or married filing separately }	**2**	$ _____
3	**Subtract** line 2 from line 1. If zero or less, enter "-0-"	**3**	$ _____
4	Enter an estimate of your 2016 adjustments to income and any additional standard deduction (see Pub. 505)	**4**	$ _____
5	**Add** lines 3 and 4 and enter the total. (Include any amount for credits from the *Converting Credits to Withholding Allowances for 2016 Form W-4* worksheet in Pub. 505.)	**5**	$ _____
6	Enter an estimate of your 2016 nonwage income (such as dividends or interest)	**6**	$ _____
7	**Subtract** line 6 from line 5. If zero or less, enter "-0-"	**7**	$ _____
8	**Divide** the amount on line 7 by $4,050 and enter the result here. Drop any fraction	**8**	_____
9	Enter the number from the **Personal Allowances Worksheet,** line H, page 1	**9**	_____
10	**Add** lines 8 and 9 and enter the total here. If you plan to use the **Two-Earners/Multiple Jobs Worksheet,** also enter this total on line 1 below. Otherwise, **stop here** and enter this total on Form W-4, line 5, page 1	**10**	_____

Two-Earners/Multiple Jobs Worksheet (See *Two earners or multiple jobs* on page 1.)

Note: Use this worksheet *only* if the instructions under line H on page 1 direct you here.

1	Enter the number from line H, page 1 (or from line 10 above if you used the **Deductions and Adjustments Worksheet**)	**1**	_____
2	Find the number in **Table 1** below that applies to the **LOWEST** paying job and enter it here. **However,** if you are married filing jointly and wages from the highest paying job are $65,000 or less, do not enter more than "3"	**2**	_____
3	If line 1 is **more than or equal to** line 2, subtract line 2 from line 1. Enter the result here (if zero, enter "-0-") and on Form W-4, line 5, page 1. **Do not** use the rest of this worksheet	**3**	_____

Note: If line 1 is **less than** line 2, enter "-0-" on Form W-4, line 5, page 1. Complete lines 4 through 9 below to figure the additional withholding amount necessary to avoid a year-end tax bill.

4	Enter the number from line 2 of this worksheet	**4**	_____
5	Enter the number from line 1 of this worksheet	**5**	_____
6	**Subtract** line 5 from line 4	**6**	_____
7	Find the amount in **Table 2** below that applies to the **HIGHEST** paying job and enter it here	**7**	$ _____
8	**Multiply** line 7 by line 6 and enter the result here. This is the additional annual withholding needed .	**8**	$ _____
9	Divide line 8 by the number of pay periods remaining in 2016. For example, divide by 25 if you are paid every two weeks and you complete this form on a date in January when there are 25 pay periods remaining in 2016. Enter the result here and on Form W-4, line 6, page 1. This is the additional amount to be withheld from each paycheck	**9**	$ _____

Table 1

Married Filing Jointly		All Others	
If wages from **LOWEST** paying job are—	Enter on line 2 above	If wages from **LOWEST** paying job are—	Enter on line 2 above
$0 - $6,000	0	$0 - $9,000	0
6,001 - 14,000	1	9,001 - 17,000	1
14,001 - 25,000	2	17,001 - 26,000	2
25,001 - 27,000	3	26,001 - 34,000	3
27,001 - 35,000	4	34,001 - 44,000	4
35,001 - 44,000	5	44,001 - 75,000	5
44,001 - 55,000	6	75,001 - 85,000	6
55,001 - 65,000	7	85,001 - 110,000	7
65,001 - 75,000	8	110,001 - 125,000	8
75,001 - 80,000	9	125,001 - 140,000	9
80,001 - 100,000	10	140,001 and over	10
100,001 - 115,000	11		
115,001 - 130,000	12		
130,001 - 140,000	13		
140,001 - 150,000	14		
150,001 and over	15		

Table 2

Married Filing Jointly		All Others	
If wages from **HIGHEST** paying job are—	Enter on line 7 above	If wages from **HIGHEST** paying job are—	Enter on line 7 above
$0 - $75,000	$610	$0 - $38,000	$610
75,001 - 135,000	1,010	38,001 - 85,000	1,010
135,001 - 205,000	1,130	85,001 - 185,000	1,130
205,001 - 360,000	1,340	185,001 - 400,000	1,340
360,001 - 405,000	1,420	400,001 and over	1,600
405,001 and over	1,600		

FIGURE 44-8 Form W-4 indicates the number of exemptions claimed by the employee for income tax purposes. *(continued)*

22222	Void ☐	**a** Employee's social security number	For Official Use Only ▶ OMB No. 1545-0008	

b Employer identification number (EIN)		**1** Wages, tips, other compensation	**2** Federal income tax withheld
c Employer's name, address, and ZIP code		**3** Social security wages	**4** Social security tax withheld
		5 Medicare wages and tips	**6** Medicare tax withheld
		7 Social security tips	**8** Allocated tips
d Control number		**9**	**10** Dependent care benefits
e Employee's first name and initial / Last name / Suff.		**11** Nonqualified plans	**12a** See instructions for box 12
		13 Statutory employee ☐ Retirement plan ☐ Third-party sick pay ☐	**12b**
		14 Other	**12c**
			12d
f Employee's address and ZIP code			

15 State	Employer's state ID number	**16** State wages, tips, etc.	**17** State income tax	**18** Local wages, tips, etc.	**19** Local income tax	**20** Locality name

Form **W-2** Wage and Tax Statement **2016**

Copy A For Social Security Administration — Send this entire page with
Form W-3 to the Social Security Administration; photocopies are **not** acceptable.

Do Not Cut, Fold, or Staple Forms on This Page

Department of the Treasury—Internal Revenue Service
For Privacy Act and Paperwork Reduction Act Notice, see the separate instructions.

Cat. No. 10134D

© U.S. Internal Revenue Service

FIGURE 44-9 Form W-2 summarizes all earnings and deductions for the year and must be prepared for each employee by January 31 of the following year.

To process payroll, the provider's clinic must have a federal tax reporting number, obtained from the Internal Revenue Service. In some states, a state employer number also is needed.

Preparing Payroll Checks.

When preparing payroll checks, it is important to keep a record of all tax and insurance amounts deducted from an employee's earnings. For those clinics that still operate on a manual bookkeeping system, the write-it-once system is one of the most efficient ways to accurately maintain these records. Payroll records should include:

- Employee name, address, and telephone number
- Social Security number
- Date of employment

Each paycheck stub should contain:

- Number of hours worked, including regular and overtime (if hourly)
- Dates of pay period
- Date of check
- Gross salary

- Itemized deductions for federal income tax, Social Security (FICA) tax, state tax, and city or local tax
- Itemized deductions for health insurance and disability insurance
- Other deductions such as uniforms, loan payments, and so on
- Net salary (gross earnings minus taxes and deductions)

Figuring Employee Taxes.

When figuring federal income taxes and Social Security taxes, use the "Circular E", also known as Publication 15, which contains federal income tax tables provided by the Internal Revenue Service. Federal tax is based on amount earned, marital status, number of exemptions claimed, and length of pay period. State and city or local taxes are typically a percentage of the gross earnings.

Legal

All federal and state taxes withheld must be paid on a quarterly basis to the appropriate government offices. These monies should be accompanied by the required reporting forms. It is important to observe deposit requirements for withheld income tax and Social Security and Medicare taxes. These requirements, which change frequently, are listed in the Federal Employer's Tax Guide, available from the U.S. Government Printing Office, Internal Revenue Service (or online at http://www.irs.gov).

Additionally, there are third-party providers that offer software and support for payroll preparation, tax filing, and even direct deposit. Examples include ADP and Paychex. Implementing the services of a private book-keeper or accountant to tend to these responsibilities is another solution when performing in-house payroll is not feasible.

Managing Benefits and Other Responsibilities. **Benefits**, or additional remuneration to the salary earned by full-time employees, must be managed and records maintained for each employee. Examples of benefits include paid vacation, paid holidays, health/dental insurance, disability insurance, **profit-sharing** options, and complimentary health care. Some ambulatory care settings may refer to all or some of these benefits as **fringe benefits**.

Other responsibilities of the clinic manager include maintaining a personnel file for each employee, providing his or her history with the facility, application for the current position, evaluations, promotions, problems, awards, entitlements, legal forms required by state and federal agencies, and so on. All Occupational Safety and Health Administration (OSHA) data, hazard material training and documentation, HIPAA training documentation, cardiopulmonary resuscitation (CPR) certifications, immunization records, AIDS education, and confidentiality agreements must be recorded and maintained.

FACILITY AND EQUIPMENT MANAGEMENT

Safety

The physical plant or building must be observed and maintained with safety being a key ingredient. It should be the responsibility of each staff member to report to the clinic manager any facility repairs that require attention and suggest replacement or recommend new pieces of equipment as required by the practice to support the health care needs of its population.

The clinic manager usually is responsible for maintenance of the clinic and may hire **ancillary services** to provide janitorial and laundry services, dispose of hazardous materials, and maintain aquariums or plants that may enhance the environment of the facility. The clinic manager must be cognitive of the importance of patient confidentiality when ancillary services are present. Ancillary services must not view confidential material. A signed business associate agreement must be on file for each ancillary service contracted.

Magazine subscriptions and health-related literature for the reception area are the responsibility of the clinic manager. Selections should be made carefully, keeping in mind the interests of the patients and their cultures. These materials should not be kept once they become dog-eared, torn, or outdated. The use of plastic protectors and appropriate storage shelving aid in keeping the area and materials tidy.

The clinic manager, together with the provider, is responsible for facility improvements, including any necessary repairs, decorating and color scheme, and floor plan suggestions. The wise clinic manager does not make these decisions independently but asks for suggestions from staff members. Remember, the team-building approach adds a cohesive element to any clinic environment.

Administrative and Clinical Inventory of Supplies and Equipment

All administrative and clinical supplies and equipment in the facility must be inventoried. Maintaining a sufficient inventory of administrative and medical supplies requires implementation of a system for taking inventory of supplies frequently enough to permit placing and receiving an order before a shortage occurs. Large facilities frequently use the PM system to inventory items that normally would be billed as part of a procedure, but this will not identify routinely used medical and administrative supplies.

Medical clinics operate on a budget, so comparison shopping is prudent. Many companies have online catalogs with full descriptions and prices of their products. The cost of an item is not the only consideration when purchasing inventory. Consider the following:

- Warranties
- Bulk orders
- Maintenance agreements
- Quality and durability
- Personal preferences
- Cost factors

Online ordering via the Internet can save time and money. When placing orders, select those suppliers with secure Web sites; it is generally safe to use credit cards with these vendors. Supplies also can be ordered through hard copy catalogs. Review Chapter 18 for specifics in completing a purchase order. Benchmarking with other medical clinics nets valuable information in determining reputable vendors.

Competency

When an order is received, it must be opened and checked properly. Look first for the packing slip, which lists the items ordered and the items shipped. Verify that no items have been substituted or back-ordered. Each item unpacked must be checked against the packing slip to be sure there are no discrepancies. Write the date the shipment was received, who verified it, and any follow-up information. The new stock should be stored appropriately.

Some items purchased come with a warranty. A warranty usually is activated online at the vendor's Web site or by using a warranty card packaged with the purchased item. Warranty cards are similar to postcards and establish the purchase date and name and address of the purchaser. The returned warranty information provides the vendor with information should it be necessary to notify the buyer of recalls or defective parts. It is also proof of purchase and gives the length of time the warranty is in effect.

Procedure

It is important to create a file or a digital file, such as a spreadsheet, for each piece of equipment in the medical clinic. Information in this file should include:

- Date of purchase and original receipt
- Manufacturer name, address, and telephone number
- Model number and owner's manual
- Technical support information and telephone number
- Warranty information
- Service agreement
- Date last serviced
- Routine maintenance or calibration information

The steps for inventorying supplies and equipment for administrative and clinical needs are given in Procedure 44-5.

PROCEDURE 44-5

Procedure

Performing an Inventory of Equipment and Supplies

PURPOSE:

To develop an inventory of expendable administrative and clinical supplies in a medical clinic.

EQUIPMENT/SUPPLIES:

- Computer
- Printout of most recent inventory spreadsheet, listing items by storage location, name and identification code, number of items, minimum quantity requiring reorder, date and quantity of last reorder, expiration dates of items, if any
- Clipboard, pad of reorder forms, pen or pencil

PROCEDURE STEPS:

1. *Paying attention to detail,* compare number of items on hand corresponding to each name or code identification number with the printout, and write in the new inventory number on the printout. RATIONALE: Determines what is on hand and what needs to be ordered.

2. If the number of any item is less than the minimum quantity, fill out a reorder form listing completely the name, identification number, and quantity required.

3. Repeat the previous step for each storage location on the inventory printout sheet.

4. After completing the inventory, enter the new inventory information, including date of inventory, quantity, and date of reorder request, into the computer database. RATIONALE: Determines what needs to be ordered.

5. Forward the reorder forms to the person responsible for purchasing. RATIONALE: Forwards information to the person responsible for reordering supplies and equipment.

   NOTE: If the clinic uses handheld computers on a wireless network, all information can be entered directly into the computer record while doing the inventory, making unnecessary the reentry and preparation of reorder forms. If the handheld computer is not networked, it will be necessary to download or sync the data after completing the inventory.

Administrative and Clinical Equipment Calibration and Maintenance

Administrative and clinical equipment must be cleaned, calibrated, and maintained on a regular basis. Most clinics use a computer spreadsheet or relational-type database, depending on the size of the facility. The database identifies the equipment by name or type, its assigned facility identification number, location in the facility, warranty expiration date, service period, dates when service and calibration were last performed, and when the next service or calibration will be required. The database also may identify service contracts for equipment not maintained or calibrated by facility personnel and information on equipment service contractors such as contacts, phone numbers, and addresses. The database is backed up by a paper file containing operation manuals, warranty information, and service contracts.

Administrative equipment such as computers should be cleaned and maintained regularly. Review Chapter 10 for suggestions on routine maintenance. Telephones as well as any other pieces of administrative equipment should be cleaned and working order checked.

Procedure

Laboratory and clinical equipment must be maintained and quality-control measures utilized. Calibration checks are required for a number of pieces of equipment: sphygmomanometers and centrifuges, to name two. Microscopes and various types of scopes used during physical examinations and specialty procedures contain light sources that must be checked before each use. A replacement supply of bulbs should be available. See Chapter 38 for more information on quality control and safety in the medical laboratory. Assigning a clinical laboratory manager to oversee the equipment is a good idea. Procedure 44-6 provides steps for routine maintenance and calibration of clinical equipment.

The clinic storage areas should be well maintained, and each item should always be put back in its place with lids replaced properly to prevent any accidents. Medication storage requires special attention. Many medications must be stored at certain temperatures, kept dry, or stored in dark, airtight containers. All medications, including samples, must be kept out of patient access areas. Narcotics should always be stored in a separate locked cabinet. A daily inventory should be maintained.

PROCEDURE 44-6

Procedure

Performing Routine Maintenance and Calibration of Clinical Equipment

PURPOSE:

To ensure the operability and calibration of clinical equipment.

EQUIPMENT/SUPPLIES:

- Equipment list with maintenance or calibration requirements
- Clipboard, pen with black ink, maintenance log and service calendar log forms, deficiency tags
- Access to operation and service manuals of equipment to be serviced
- Access to any necessary maintenance tools and supplies

PROCEDURE STEPS:

1. Locate the number assigned by the clinic manager to identify the equipment being serviced, and verify serial number, manufacturer/maker, technical support phone number, warranty information, and last date of service. RATIONALE: Provides medical assistant with all information needed for maintenance and servicing of equipment.

2. *Paying attention to detail,* visually inspect each piece of equipment associated with the clinical area.

   - *Practicing risk management principles,* check for any frayed electrical cords, loose connections, or safety issues such as tripping hazards associated with electrical cords.

   - Clean each item according to manufacturer specifications, and replace light bulbs and batteries if necessary.

   RATIONALE: Equipment works more efficiently when clean and all parts are working properly.

(continues)

3. Check to ensure the equipment meets operational/calibration standards as defined in the operation and service manual. Recalibrate the equipment following the instructions in the manual if required. RATIONALE: Calibration standards must be maintained for correct results.

4. Follow necessary safety precautions and tag any equipment not meeting operational standards and report the deficiency. RATIONALE: Equipment must be either replaced or repaired to ensure proper results.

5. Fill out and sign the maintenance record sheet if the equipment meets operations standards. RATIONALE: Documents routine maintenance was performed.

6. ***Paying attention to detail,*** complete documentation form by verifying information for each piece of equipment serviced and/or calibrated. Complete the appropriate information for service using the Service Calendar Log form. RATIONALE: Documents what has been done and the date completed.

NOTE: The equipment list, maintenance records, and deficiency reports may be included in the PM system of many practices.

Documentation Example:

Maintenance Log

Name of Equipment	Serial Number	Mfg/ Maker	Technical Support Phone Number	Purchase Date	Service Plan	Last Serviced	Completed By
EKG #8	80462	HP	xxx-xxx-xxxx	1/20/XX	On file	6/12/xx	bql
Centrifuge #3	79031	HP	xxx-xxx-xxxx	7/20/XX	On file	6/12/xx	bql

Service Calendar Log Form

January	February	March	April	May	June	July	August	September	October	November	December

LIABILITY COVERAGE AND BONDING

Legal

Negligence is performing an act that a reasonable and prudent provider would not perform or failure to perform an act that a reasonable and prudent provider would perform. The common term used to describe professional **liability** or legal responsibility today is **malpractice**. It is much easier to prevent malpractice than to defend it in litigation; therefore every effort should be taken to prevent negligence. Events that could result in a malpractice litigation invariably will occur from time to time in even the best of medical clinics. When such an incident occurs, complete honesty with the patient and insurance carrier is the best policy. Protocols should be implemented or existing ones revised to prevent any future occurrences, and all steps necessary to minimize risk to the patient should be taken.

Insurance policies specifically designed to protect the provider's assets in the event a liability claim is filed and awarded in the patient's favor are available. Any provider not carrying such insurance is said to be **"going bare"** and would personally be responsible for any court costs, damages, and attorney fees if a malpractice suit were lost.

Practicing medical assistants should carry **professional liability insurance** for protection. Medical assistants who are members of the American Association of Medical Assistants (AAMA) have the option of purchasing personal and professional insurance through the organization at corporate rates.

Some providers carry their employees on their policies. If this is the case, always ask to see the policy and verify that your name is printed on the policy—no name indicates no coverage. The manager may need to see that professional liability insurance has been purchased, all appropriate names are listed, and the premiums are paid in a timely fashion.

Professional liability insurance is important if the provider-employer is sued. In this event, the provider and the medical assistant could be named in the suit. If the case were lost, both the provider and the medical assistant could be liable.

Individuals who are responsible for handling financial records and money in the medical clinic may be bonded. A **bond** is purchased for a cash value in an employee's name that ensures that the provider will recover the amount of loss in the event that an employee **embezzles** funds. It is the clinic manager or the HR manager's responsibility to ask prospective employees if they are bondable. Individuals who are not bondable may not be the best candidates for the position.

LEGAL ISSUES

Legal

The clinic manager must be aware of and follow all state and federal regulations impacting the practice. Information related to the Clinical Laboratory Improvement Amendments of 1988 (CLIA '88) and the Occupational Safety and Health Administration (OSHA) can be found in Chapter 37. Federal regulations related to provider clinic laboratories (POLs) are discussed in Chapter 37. The Centers for Medicare and Medicaid Services Web site also is helpful (http://www.cms.gov).

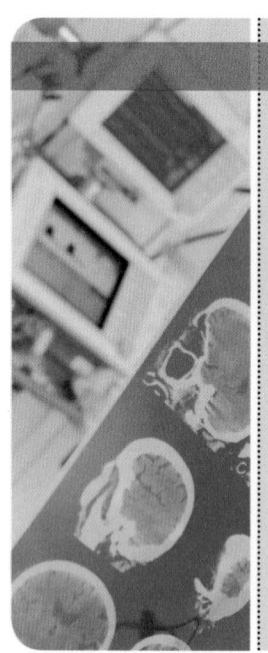

CASE STUDY 44-1

Refer to the scenario at the beginning of the chapter.

Drs. Lewis and King have requested sigmoidoscopy procedures to be scheduled for two different patients. The patients are scheduled. Both patients are put on a strict diet and pretest protocol for several days to prepare for the procedures. The day of the appointments, Marilyn Johnson, CMA (AAMA), and clinic manager, discovers that the two sigmoidoscopy procedures have been scheduled at the same time. The problem is that the clinic has only one sigmoidoscope available.

CASE STUDY REVIEW

1. Form two groups to discuss problem-solving solutions. Assume that rescheduling either of the patients is not an acceptable solution because of the patients' pretest protocol. The patients would be upset if the procedure could not be performed due to a scheduling problem.

2. How could this problem have been avoided?

3. Both patients have been told about the scheduling problem and one is upset and argumentative. What role should the clinic manager assume in this predicament?

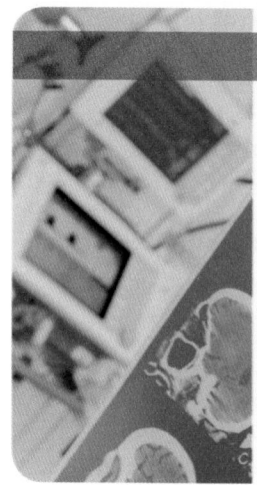

CASE STUDY 44-2

Ellen Armstrong, CMAS (AMT), the clinic administrative medical assistant, speaks privately with Marilyn Johnson, the clinic manager and the person responsible for personnel. Ellen has a suspicious lump in her breast. She has seen both her internist and a surgeon for evaluation. Next week, she will have the lump removed, perhaps even a complete mastectomy. Ellen is concerned about the time she will need to be away from the clinic.

CASE STUDY REVIEW

1. Identify the first and immediate concerns to be addressed.
2. What action might be taken to help both Ellen and the clinic manager address these concerns?
3. Is it helpful to plan for the best results, the worst results, or both?

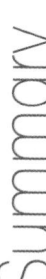

Summary

- The clinic manager oversees the operations and staff of the clinic and keeps it running smoothly. The role of clinic manager varies greatly depending on the size of the medical practice and the provider's trust in the manager's competency level.

- You should know the qualities of a good manager, including management styles and how to utilize them.

- Formulating risk management procedures to assess and minimize common risks is the duty of the clinic manager.

- The clinical manager must effectively utilize teamwork in the clinic for daily operations, including using recognition as a tool to motivate and develop a team, and using a team for problem solving.

- The clinic manager must use effective supervisory techniques to manage orientation of new personnel as well as discipline and evaluate staff, including proper dismissal methods.

- Time management guidelines that make the most of every work day by increasing productivity should be developed by the clinic manger.

- Marketing strategies for the benefit of the clinic and patients include enhancing the visibility, promotion, and image of the clinic; providing services in the form of patient seminars, support groups, and informational sessions that highlight clinic services and educate the patient; and using social media as a communication and marketing tool.

- The clinic manager is responsible for payroll and managing benefits, or monitoring outsourced payroll services; facility and equipment management, including managing inventory and ordering; and staying current on state and federal regulations that impact the clinic and practice.

Study for Success

To reinforce your knowledge and skills of information presented in this chapter:

- Review the *Key Terms* and *Learning Outcomes*

- Consider the *Critical Thinking* features and *Case Studies* and discuss your conclusions

- Answer the questions in the *Certification Review*

- Perform the *Procedures* using the *Competency Assessment Checklists* on the *Student Companion Website*

Procedure

CERTIFICATION REVIEW

1. What must individual team members do in order for teamwork to be successful?
   a. Do as they are told by the clinic manager
   b. Not ask why they are doing something a certain way
   c. Understand and support the task
   d. Think independently and solve the problem on their own

2. What is the purpose of meeting minutes?
   a. They should address each agenda topic and include a brief summary of discussions, actions taken, name of each person making a motion, the exact wording of motions, and motion approval or defeat.
   b. They are a detailed plan for a proposed trip.
   c. They include information regarding mode of transportation and lodging reservations.
   d. They must follow parliamentary procedures.
   e. They are not important and minutes do not need to be recorded.

3. What is it important to consider when working with practicum students?
   a. They should have expert knowledge about their field.
   b. They do not need supervision when working with a patient.
   c. They are experienced with working on real patients.
   d. They have much to learn.

4. Which of the following statements is *not* correct regarding a student practicum?
   a. It is a transitional stage that provides opportunities for students to apply theory learned in the classroom to a health care setting through hands-on experience.
   b. It assumes that the student is an employee who does not need to be introduced to patients.
   c. It may require the student to shadow another medical assistant for a few days.
   d. It involves an evaluation of the student's progress.
   e. Students gain valuable experience.

5. What is a procedure manual?
   a. It is a detailed plan for a proposed trip.
   b. It provides detailed information regarding mode of transportation and lodging reservations.
   c. It provides detailed information relative to the performance of tasks within the health care facility.
   d. It summarizes action details of staff meetings.

6. Developing relationships outside the clinic is often referred to as what?
   a. Marketing
   b. Benchmarking
   c. Advertising
   d. Sales
   e. A way to find a job

7. Which of the following does *not* involve record and financial management?
   a. Payroll processing
   b. Preparing payroll checks
   c. Figuring taxes
   d. Equipment and supplies maintenance

8. How must controlled substances be handled?
   a. They must be kept separate from other drugs.
   b. They must be stored in a separate locked cabinet.
   c. They are recorded in a book that is maintained daily.
   d. All of these
   e. Only a and c

9. What is the purpose of the procedure manual?
   a. To serve as a guide to the employee assigned a specific task.
   b. It may be used in evaluating the employee's performance.
   c. It is invaluable in assuring that each procedure is completed as outlined.
   d. It should be generic so that any clinic could follow the procedures.

10. What is a benefit of social media in the medical clinic?
    a. It provides another way to communicate with patients and potential consumers.
    b. It provides a way to find employees and to verify the background of persons seeking employment.
    c. It projects your clinic's personality.
    d. It can send notices and reminders to patients on various topics.
    e. All of these

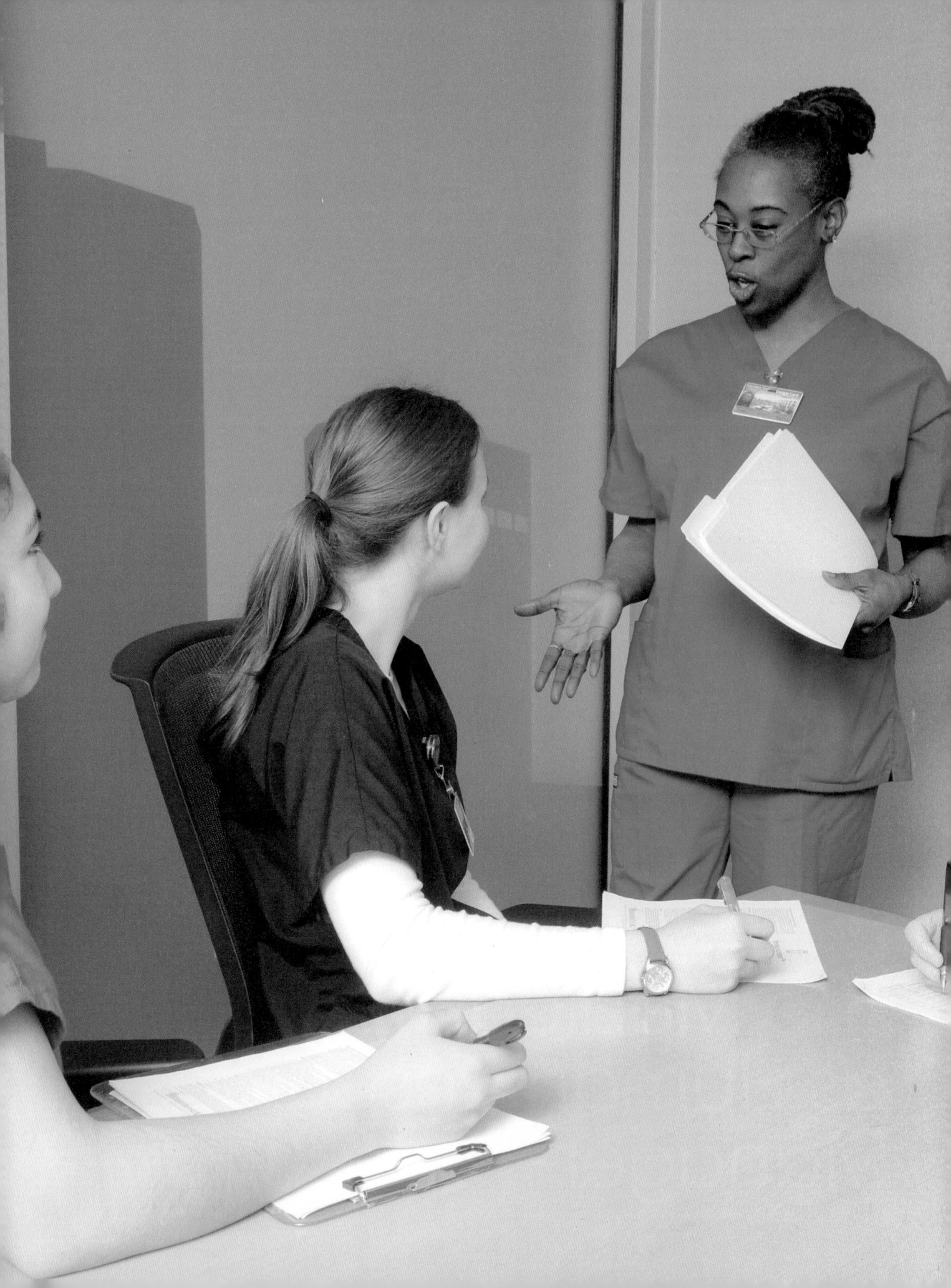

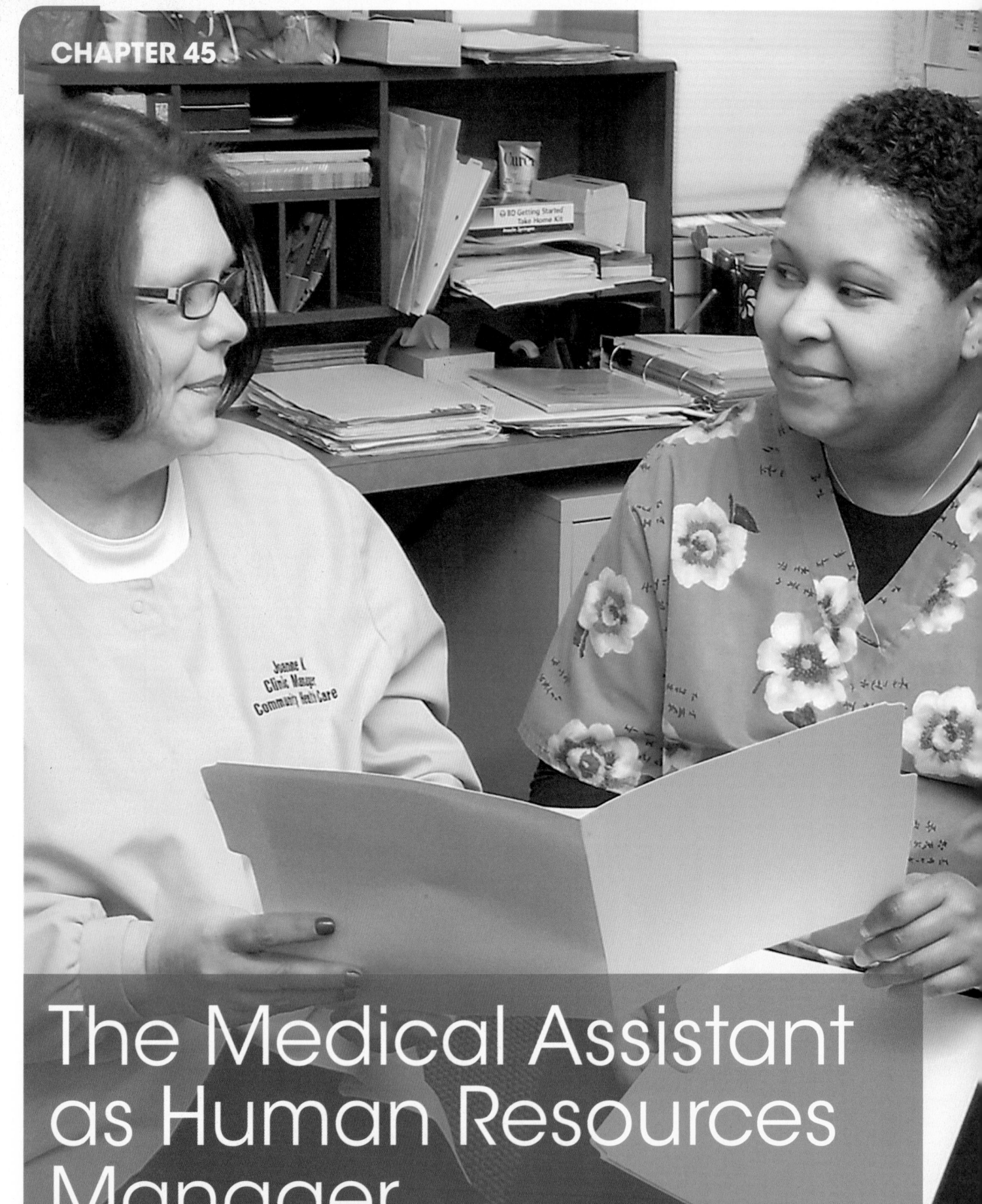

CHAPTER 45

The Medical Assistant as Human Resources Manager

1. Define and spell the key terms as presented in the glossary.
2. Interpret the role of the human resources manager.
3. Explain the function of the clinic policy manual.
4. Analyze methods of recruiting employees for a medical practice.
5. Conduct an employment interview.
6. Categorize items to keep in an employee's personnel record.
7. List and define a minimum of four laws related to personnel management.
8. Discuss possible methods for evaluating employees.
9. Compare and contrast voluntary and involuntary separations.
10. Recall continuing education possibilities for employees.

KEY TERMS

Boomer generation
exit interview
Generation X
Generation Y
Generation Z

involuntary dismissals
letter of resignation
LGBT (lesbian, gay, bisexual, transgender)
overtime
probation

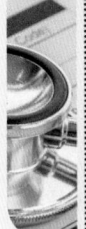

SCENARIO

Inner City Health Care has been open for close to 20 years, and it has seen many changes in the clinic and the neighborhood it serves. A recent and private conference with the clinic manager, the human resources manager, and two of the doctors revealed a conflict. The older of the two doctors has a strong negative opinion about the **LGBT (lesbian, gay, bisexual, transgender)** community. Two men were recently seen in the clinic by this provider. One was quite ill; the other, his partner, was very concerned. While a complete examination was given to the ill patient, the doctor sighed in relief when his blood workup showed suspected probable lymphocytic leukemia and he was able to make a referral to a nearby oncology clinic for the patient's treatment. Because Inner City Health Care practices in a state where there are not laws against discrimination of LGBT patients, it appears that an ethical dilemma must be addressed by the clinic staff.

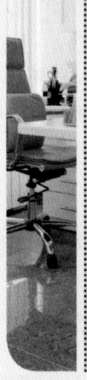

Chapter Portal

A s you near the end of your studies and preparations to enter the field of health care, it is helpful for you to know how human resource managers are likely to function in the hiring process.

The medical assistant's employment responsibilities are many and varied. As you learned in Chapter 44, often they become clinic managers and assume a quite different function in the medical setting once they have been employed in the field and gained sufficient experience. The size of the ambulatory care setting and the number of employees likely determines if a human resources (HR) manager is a part of the practice. Whether the HR manager heads an HR department in a large, corporate medical setting with the title Human Resources Manager, or is a medical assistant/clinic manager who has HR responsibilities, there are some common tasks assigned as specific HR duties.

TASKS PERFORMED BY THE HUMAN RESOURCES MANAGER

A search for employment is likely to involve interactions with individuals with the title of Human Resources Manager. It can be helpful to understand that position and the corresponding responsibilities when applying for a position. Tasks usually assigned to the HR manager include determining job descriptions for, hiring, and orienting employees; maintaining employee personnel records that include credentials and continuing education units (CEUs); and managing employee separations. With today's quest for greater clinic efficiency and the tremendous increase in federal and state regulatory requirements, the skills required of an HR manager have greatly broadened. Former responsibilities have been expanded to include preparing the policy manual, scheduling employee evaluations, preventing and investigating discrimination and harassment claims, and complying with regulatory agencies. The HR manager also assists in providing training and educational opportunities for employees so they are current in all aspects of quality patient care. Today's HR manager must seek to improve employee satisfaction and retention as well as foster accountability. The majority of today's work force will have several positions prior to retirement and are less likely to stay with one practice during their work years than previous workers; therefore, job satisfaction is an important key to retention.

Increasingly, HR managers are expected to be able to support the organization's efforts that focus on productivity, service, and quality. In a climate in which there are too few persons for the positions to be filled and the delivery methods for health care are changing almost daily, productivity, service, and quality are essential to a successful practice. It becomes the responsibility of the HR manager to see that every employee's productivity level is high, that the service is A+, and that quality is at the highest level. Today's customers, the patients, often choose their health care provider, even within their health insurance limitations, on the basis of service and quality.

Competency   Integrity

The position of HR manager now requires a higher level of education and experience to better grasp the legal and regulatory aspects of personnel management. The HR manager also must have excellent people skills, a strong sense of fairness, and the ability to resolve conflicts. None of this is accomplished in a vacuum. It requires working in close cooperation with the clinic manager and the employer(s).

This chapter discusses these responsibilities in the following separate but overlapping functions:

1. Creating and updating the clinic policy manual
2. Recruiting and hiring clinic personnel
3. Orienting new personnel
4. Scheduling salary reviews
5. Conducting exit interviews
6. Maintaining personnel records
7. Complying with all state and federal regulations regarding personnel
8. Planning/providing employee training and education
9. Maintaining records of credentials, licensure, certifications, and CEUs, such as cardiopulmonary resuscitation (CPR)

THE CLINIC POLICY MANUAL

The procedure manual described in Chapter 44 identifies specific methods and steps in performing tasks. The policy manual provides more general guidelines for clinic practices and will be introduced to new employees very quickly following the hiring process. See Table 45-1 for a brief summary of each type of manual. The policy manual identifies clear guidelines and directions required of all employees. It also defines appropriate expectations and boundaries of the employment relationship. Having written policies means not having to determine policy on a case-by-case basis. Policy manuals will vary based on the size of the practice or

TABLE 45-1

POSSIBLE CONTENT OF POLICY AND PROCEDURE MANUALS

POLICY MANUAL	PROCEDURE MANUAL
Mission statement	Details of procedures performed
Employer(s) biographic data	Administrative procedures
Employment issues	Clinical procedures
Wages, salaries, and benefits	Safety issues
Employee conduct	Asepsis
Confidentiality guidelines	Safety Data Sheets
HIPAA compliance	Emergency protocol

problems to be addressed, but some common topics include the mission statement of the practice, biographic data on each provider, employment policies, wage and salary policies, benefits to be awarded, and employee conduct expectations.

Establishing and stating the mission of the practice clearly identifies the goals and objectives to be sought by each employee. Having biographic data of each provider helps employees to respond to queries from patients about a provider's experience, education, and interests.

Legal

Employment policies might include statements on equal employment opportunity, job requirements for particular positions and to whom each person reports, recruitment and selection procedures, orientation of new employees, probation, and dismissal. Wage and salary policies should be in writing. How are employees classified? What are the working hours, how is overtime compensated, and how are salary increases determined? What benefits (medical, retirement, vacation, holidays, sick leave, and profit sharing) does the practice have? The answers to such questions are part of the policy manual. A discussion of employee conduct

is another component of the policy manual. A statement regarding the strict confidentiality of all information received in the practice is essential in this area of the policy manual and often includes a form requiring a signature from the new hire assuring he or she fully understands the consequences of any breach in confidentiality. Guidelines should be established about uniforms, dress codes, appearance, and personal hygiene. Can an employee hold a second job outside the practice? Are staff members responsible for housekeeping duties? Is updated certification required? If so, what accommodations are made for continuing education requirements?

Procedure

A computerized policy manual ensures it is an easy task to make any changes and updates. Any changes made are to be shared with employees so that everyone is up to date on policies. Having a policy manual with clearly written directives helps employees understand the expectations and boundaries of the employment relationship. The policy manual is reviewed with each new employee and updated on a regular basis. Procedure 45-1 provides details on developing and maintaining a policy manual.

PROCEDURE 45-1

Developing and Maintaining a Policy Manual

Procedure

PURPOSE:

To develop and maintain a comprehensive, up-to-date policy manual of all clinic policies relating to employee practices, benefits, clinic conduct, and so on.

EQUIPMENT/SUPPLIES:

- Computer
- Binder, such as a three-ring

- Paper
- Standard policy manual format

PROCEDURE STEPS:

1. Develop precise, written clinic policies detailing all necessary information pertaining to the staff and their positions. The information should include benefits, vacation, sick leave, hours, dress codes, evaluations, rules of conduct, and grounds for dismissal. RATIONALE: Well-defined policies clearly outlined for each employee are necessary for efficient and effective staff operations.

2. Identify procedures for reimbursing overtime, preventing discrimination and harassment, creating a safe working environment, and allowing for jury duty.

3. Include a policy statement related to rules of conduct.

4. Identify steps to follow should an employee become disabled during employment.

5. Determine what employee opportunities for continuing education, if any, will be reimbursed; include requirements for recertification or licensure.

(continues)

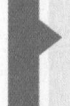

6. Provide a copy of the policy manual for each employee. RATIONALE: Each employee is made aware of facility policies.

7. Review and update the policy manual regularly. Add or delete items as necessary, dating each revised page. RATIONALE: Policy manual will always be current.

RECRUITING AND HIRING CLINIC PERSONNEL

The majority of employees in ambulatory and primary care centers are full-time, part-time, or occasionally independent contractor employees. Full-time employees generally work 30 hours or more per week; part-time employees work less than 30 hours per week. Either may be paid by the hour. Full-time employees may be salaried and exempt from overtime regulations. Most part-time employees are paid by the hour. Benefits are often different between full- and part-time employees. Independent contractors who are employed usually work with the facility to perform specific predetermined tasks at a predetermined rate of pay for the services provided and are not eligible for benefits from the clinic.

Before recruiting and hiring personnel to fill positions within the medical facility, the HR manager and employers must understand exactly what the role and responsibilities of the position are by having a current job description for the position. They must follow a recruiting policy that is effective and fair and that observes all appropriate laws and regulations.

Job Descriptions

Before any position is filled, a job description must be in place. This usually is created cooperatively by the clinic manager and the employer(s). Once the job qualifications are defined, the lead personnel and HR manager can begin efforts to fill the position.

In daily operations, most job descriptions are on file, but if the situation involves a new or greatly expanded clinic, a complete set of job descriptions is needed before recruiting can begin. Even when a written description is on file, it should be reviewed when a new employee is to be hired. The person who is leaving the position is often an excellent resource to assess the accuracy of the current job description and any changes that should be made.

Procedure

The job description must include basic qualifications necessary for the position and have enough information to provide both the supervisor and the employee with a clear outline of what the position entails (Figure 45-1). Necessary work experience, skills, education, and any special certification or licensure that is expected is to be identified in the job description. Procedure 45-2 provides details on preparing job descriptions.

JOB DESCRIPTION

POSITION TITLE:
Administrative Medical Assistant

REPORTS TO:
Clinic Manager and Provider-Employer(s)

RESPONSIBILITIES AND DUTIES:
- Be a therapeutic and helpful receptionist
  1. Answer telephone as quickly as possible, hopefully by the second ring
  2. Greet all patients warmly and with a helpful attitude
- Manage time efficiently with appropriate scheduling for patients and professional staff
  1. Schedule patients according to their needs, scheduling guidelines, staff availability, and equipment readiness
  2. Call to remind patients of their visit the day before appointment
- Respond to patient requests on the telephone and in person
  1. Ascertain reason for request
  2. Satisfy patient request or refer patient to one who can
- Prepare patient charts for professional staff
  1. Print schedules and encounter forms
  2. Pull patient charts late afternoon the day before appointment; print as necessary
  3. Check charts for completeness
  4. Attach encounter form when patient arrives to check in

AUTHORITY BOUNDARIES:
The Clinic Manager will assist in answering questions. Remember that it is better to ask than to make an error. Screening concerns not identified in a policy/procedure manual also can be directed to the clinical medical assisting staff.

POSITION REQUIREMENTS:
Two years' experience and/or graduate of a medical assistant program. CMA (AAMA), RMA, or CMAS preferred.

FIGURE 45-1 Sample job description for administrative medical assistant.

PROCEDURE 45-2

Preparing a Job Description

PURPOSE:

To provide a precise definition of the tasks assigned to a job; to determine the expectations and level of competency required; and to specify the experience, training, and education needed to perform the job for purposes of recruiting and performance evaluation.

EQUIPMENT/SUPPLIES:

- Computer
- Paper
- Standard job description format

PROCEDURE STEPS:

1. Describe each task that creates the job. RATIONALE: A detailed job description identifies clear expectations for each employee.
2. List special medical, technical, or clerical skills required.
3. Determine the level of education, instruction, and experience required for the position.
4. Determine where the job fits in the overall structure of the practice.
5. Specify any unusual working conditions (hours, locations, and so on) that may apply.
6. Describe career path opportunities.

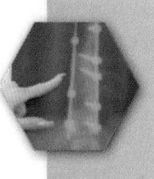

Critical Thinking

Identify proper qualifications for an administrative medical assistant in a fairly large ambulatory care setting. Determine what work experience might qualify versus what work experience is preferred. Identify possible certifications that might be helpful. Explain.

Another important point with respect to the job description is that a review and update of the description should be done every year. Most positions change constantly, whether from a minor shifting of duties or the addition of some new technical procedure or device. Without updating a job description, a person with the wrong qualifications may be recruited to fill a vacancy.

When seeking employment, it is most helpful to understand the job description for the position being sought and to make certain that your qualifications fit that description.

Recruiting

A major challenge facing the HR manager today is recruitment. Medical assisting is among the top 10 occupations where expected employment growth is much faster than average for all occupations. According to the U.S. Department of Labor, Bureau of Labor Statistics, employment for medical assistants is likely to grow 23% from 2014 to 2024. One reason for this demand is the aging of the U.S. population and the demands made upon primary and ambulatory care providers. Medical assistants with formal education, instruction, and appropriate certification will be in high demand. When employers have been unsuccessful in recruiting qualified medical assistants, they have turned to contracting for some work, such as transcription and billing.

Once the hiring need is determined, the HR manager begins the recruitment process. Networking is a highly effective method of finding employees. Networking is a process in which people of similar interests exchange information in social, business, or professional relationships. A survey conducted by Jobvite in 2014 indicated that nearly 75% of companies use social media networks to recruit employees. LinkedIn was the most popular, followed by Facebook. The HR manager may network with members of the American Association of Medical Assistants (AAMA) and express an interest in a new employee for an open position. Current employees are often excellent resources because they may know of a qualified person who is looking for a position. The majority of candidates will come through referrals such as these as well as internal transfers.

The medical assistant departments of nearby colleges are another good resource. Medical assisting students may find employment through their practicum experience near the end of their coursework. Individuals who volunteer to shadow, follow, or work in a facility are often seen as potential employees. Although newspaper advertisements or Craigslist may generate many résumés, they are only marginally effective as search tools. It is often far too time consuming to review the large volume of applications generated by this approach. There are a number of medical employment Internet sites that identify positions for medical assistant personnel, often in specific locales.

Preparing to Interview Applicants

Once several applicants have expressed interest in the position, preparation for the interview begins. The HR manager is likely to have a number of résumés to consider. Some applicants may have already completed a job application if they dropped off a résumé. The résumés and applications can be reviewed together. Some important points to remember in reading these documents follow.

When considering education, look beyond the degree earned. Look for a good performance record at school and the kinds of supplemental education achieved. Does attendance at seminars and short-course training programs relate to your position needs? When reading a person's work history, make note of any unexplained gaps in employment. You may want to ask specific questions in the interview. Has advancement been gained in each new position? Are the responsibilities and duties of the applicant's positions explained, or will questions need to be asked of the prospective employee?

Look for information that indicates if this candidate really enjoys the kind of work setting you have. Is the applicant comfortable serving the infirm? Can you truly identify the level of skill from the descriptions, or are the applicant's skills descriptions vague? The cover letter, if one is included, should address the specifics required

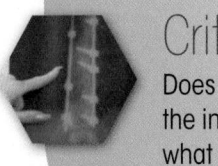

Critical Thinking

Does your job search preparation fit with the information identified above? If not, what might you do now to make a change so that it will fit?

of your position. Does the person display a negative or a positive attitude? Do not excuse any errors or unprofessional appearance in the job application or the résumé. Each should be perfect in all aspects. An individual who is careless in this respect is likely to be careless in the position.

Some applications will be discarded when compared to the preceding guidelines. With the remaining candidates, determine who is to be interviewed and make telephone calls to establish interviews. You may make note of the quality of speaking skills, especially if this person will be using the telephone in the position. Make an interview appointment date with only those who seem truly interested in the position during your telephone conversation.

The Employment Interview

The employment interview is usually conducted by only one person if second interviews are anticipated. The provider-employer, clinic manager, or another employee may be present at either the first or the second interview, however (Figure 45-2). The interviewer(s) will want to review the application and résumé before the interview for particular

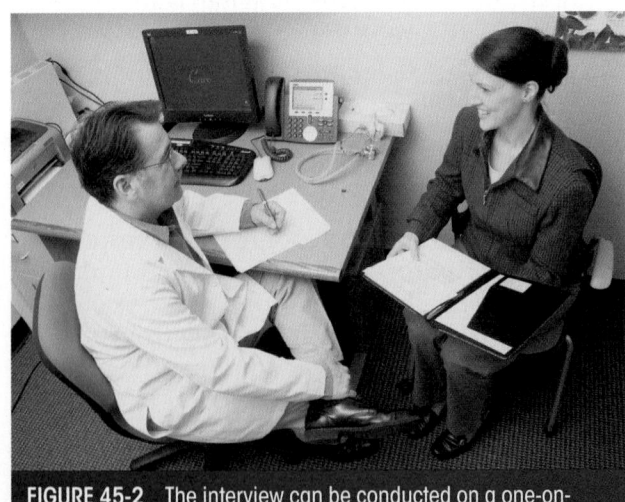

FIGURE 45-2 The interview can be conducted on a one-on-one basis with only the applicant and one staff member or with several staff members meeting with the applicant at once.

points to ask the candidate. Before the interview, those doing the interviewing should establish a set of questions for all of the applicants. These predetermined questions will help avoid one applicant being given advantages over another and will help ensure continuity throughout all the interviews. An interview worksheet is an excellent tool to use to make certain that the interview process is fair and equitable with each candidate. The worksheet should provide enough room for notes taken during the interview.

Suggested items for the interview worksheet are:

- Applicant's name
- Telephone number
- Education and experience
- Work experience
- Special skills
- Professional demeanor
- Voice and mannerisms specific to position
- Questions and responses
- Ability to problem solve when given a scenario
- Any health-related or work-related problems applicant discloses
- Interviewer's personal impressions and recommendations

Conduct interviews in a quiet and private setting. Do not schedule interviews back to back without time to collect your thoughts or to allow you to compare notes with others participating in the interview. Ask job-related questions. For example:

- Describe your last position. What did you like best about it? What did you like least? What is most important to you about a position?
- Describe your administrative and clinical skills.

Refer to Chapter 47 for some more sample questions. Let the applicant do the most of the talking.

Legal Any questions related to age, sex, race, religion, or national origin are inappropriate. Recall from Chapter 6 that currently 22 states prohibit discrimination based on sexual orientation as well. Inquiries about medical history, drug use, or arrest records may not be made. Keep your questions related to performance on the job. If you may want to bond this employee, you may ask candidates if they have been bonded before or are willing to be bonded. It may be best to leave salary discussions for a second interview, but it can also be helpful to determine if applicants' salary expectations are in line with what you can offer. A question such as "What salary are you expecting?" is appropriate. Do not make a job offer until all the candidates selected for interviews have been interviewed, and do not prejudge someone on any factor other than the person's qualifications presented during or after the interview.

At the close of the interview, let the applicant know when a decision will be made or whether a second interview will be conducted and how notification will be made. A tour of the facility and introduction to key staff members may be offered but are not necessary at the time of the first interview. Finally, thank the applicant for participating in the interview and being interested in the position.

Selecting the Finalists

Shortly after the final interview is completed, the HR manager should talk with all the others involved in the interviews to select the top candidates. This is done by comparing notes and impressions from the interviews and by taking into consideration the ability of a candidate to work with patients and colleagues who might have a variety of problems and cultural backgrounds. The next step is to check references from former employers, supervisors, co-workers, and instructors. A large corporate medical practice may even have a consent form each candidate is asked to sign that gives permission to check references and call former employers and instructors. You may need to recognize, however, that even with a signed release from a potential new employee, many organizations and businesses restrict the release of reference information to only name, dates of employment, and title of position served. Telephone checks for references are an excellent strategy because you receive an immediate response. If you stress confidentiality when you make the contact, it will be more likely that the person will respond candidly to your questions. When possible, always check with more than one reference and former employer to get a more accurate assessment of the candidate. All reference information is to be kept confidential. A sample telephone reference check form is shown in Figure 45-3.

A checklist of questions to ask might include:

1. What were the dates of employment of (name of applicant) at your firm?
2. Describe the position held.
3. Reason for leaving the position?

4. Strong points of the employee?

5. Limitations of the employee?

6. Can you comment on attendance and dependability?

7. Would you rehire?

8. Anything else we should know about this candidate?

TELEPHONE REFERENCE

Name of Applicant _____

Person Contacted _____

Position and Name of Business _____

_____

Telephone Number _____

Relationship to Applicant _____

- May I verify the employment history of (applicant's name) who is applying for a position with our medical clinic?

  _____, _____ to _____, _____

- Describe the responsibilities held by this individual.

- Identify the salary _____

- What are this individual's strong points?

- What are this individual's weak points?

- Describe this individual's overall attitude toward the position and toward patients.

- Please comment on dependability and attendance.

- Given the opportunity, would you rehire? Why or why not?

- Why did this individual leave the position?

- Describe personal and professional growth this individual made while in your firm.

- Is there anything else you would like to tell us?

Reference call made by _____

Date _____

FIGURE 45-3 Sample form to use for telephone references.

Offer the position when a first-choice candidate has been determined and indicate when a response is needed. Be prepared with a second-choice candidate should the preferred candidate respond negatively. At the time of the offer, the candidate should understand the salary offered, the starting date, the practice policies, and the benefits. When a candidate has accepted the position, a confirmation letter should be written that clearly spells out details discussed earlier. Give specific instructions on when and where the new employee should report the first day on the job. If practical, the employee should be given the policy and procedure manuals to read. Employers are required by federal law to verify that all employees are authorized to work. This is done by having the candidate complete an Eligibility Verification (I-9) form (see Case Study 45-1).

 For the unsuccessful applicants, send a letter explaining "We have selected another candidate whose qualifications and experience more closely meet our needs at this time. We would like to keep your résumé on file should another suitable position become available." Copies of these letters, as well as the interview checklists, should be kept for a minimum of 6 months should any questions arise regarding your choice of candidate. Procedure 45-3 provides details on interviewing.

ORIENTING NEW PERSONNEL

 Orienting new employees is usually the responsibility of both the clinic manager and lead personnel who are most likely to work the closest with the new employee. It is common for a new employee to be placed on **probation** for 30 to 60 days, during which time both the employee and supervisory personnel may determine if the environment and the position are satisfactory for the employee. Procedure 45-4 outlines how to orient personnel.

Elements important to orientation include introducing the new employee to other staff members, assigning a mentor who can respond to questions, and making the employee aware of the procedures to be performed in this new position. If the procedure manual is detailed and accurate, this manual now becomes the daily guide for the new employee. Sometimes the individual leaving a position may still be present and is asked to assist in the orientation process. This is especially beneficial if there is a good working relationship between the employee who is leaving and the management of the practice. Depending on the responsibilities

PROCEDURE 45-3

Procedure

Conducting Interviews

PURPOSE:

To screen applicants for training, experience, and characteristics to select the best candidate to fill the position vacancy.

PROCEDURE STEPS:

1. Review résumés and applications received.
2. Select candidates who most closely match the education and experience being sought.
3. Develop a strategic plan for conducting the interviews by creating an interview worksheet for each candidate listing points to cover.
4. Select an interview team; this team should always include the HR or clinic manager and the immediate supervisor to whom the candidate will report.
5. Call personally to schedule interviews. RATIONALE: This allows you to judge the applicant's telephone manners and voice.
6. Maintain ethical standards by reminding the interviewers of various legal restrictions concerning questions to be asked.
7. Conduct interviews in a private, quiet setting. RATIONALE: Careful interviewing of potential employees is an important step in hiring the best candidate for the position.
8. Put the applicant at ease by beginning with an overview of the practice and staff, briefly describing the job, and answering preliminary questions.
9. Ask questions about the applicant's work experience and educational background using the résumé and interview worksheet as a guide.
10. Provide the most promising applicants additional information on benefits and a tour of the clinic, if practical.
11. Applicant's general salary requirements may be discussed, but avoid discussion of a specific salary until a formal offer is tendered.
12. Inform the applicants when a decision will be made and thank each for participating in the interview.
13. Do not make a job offer until all the candidates have been interviewed.
14. Check references of all prospective employees.
15. Establish a second interview between the provider-employer(s) and the qualified candidate if necessary.
16. Confirm accepted job offers in writing, specifying details of the offer and acceptance. RATIONALE: A written document provides proof of hiring and employment details.
17. Show respect by notifying all unsuccessful applicants by letter when the position has been filled. RATIONALE: Makes a positive statement to those not hired and keeps the doors open for future employment possibilities.

of the new employee, a supervisor may be asked to monitor for a period all the new employee's procedures for accuracy, safety, and patient protection. During the probation period, the employee should be officially evaluated by the clinic manager.

Generational Expectations

Today's HR managers will employ several different generations in their facility and must strive for a cohesive team among the generations. **Generation X** is defined as those born between 1966 and 1976; **Generation Y** (also known as the Millennial generation) was born between 1977 and 1994; and **Generation Z**, which is just now entering the work force, was born between 1995 and 2012. Search for information on Generation X at http://www.pewresearch.org and a summary of the "Gen Y and Gen Z Global Workplace Expectations Study" at http://millennialbranding.com.

Generation Xers are usually more moderate politically and socially than Generations Y and Z. They are fairly comfortable with technology, but

Orienting Personnel

Procedure

PURPOSE:

To acquaint new employees with clinic policies, staff, what the job encompasses, procedures to be performed, and job performance expectations.

PROCEDURE STEPS:

1. Tour the facilities and introduce the clinic staff.
2. Complete employee-related documents and explain their purpose.
3. Explain the benefits program.
4. Present the clinic policy manual and discuss its key elements.
5. Review federal and state regulatory precautions for medical facilities.
6. Review the job description.
7. Explain and demonstrate procedures to be performed and the use of procedure manuals supporting these procedures.
8. Demonstrate the use of any specialized equipment.
9. Assign a mentor from the staff to help with the orientation. RATIONALE: Without proper orientation and training, even the best new employee can fail.

worry about having enough money in retirement. They have learned, however, to be self-reliant, and often loyal to one employer.

It is interesting to note that both Generations Y and Z expect to have a number of job placements before retirement. Money is also not always the driving force in their job-related decisions; generally, these workers seek job advancement and satisfaction over salary. While both Generations Y and Z are quite comfortable in the world of electronic media and production, they increasingly see the value of face-to-face interaction.

The **Boomer generation**, born between 1955 and 1965, may still struggle with the vast advancement of technology in all aspects of their work. They will marvel at how much simpler the modern EKG machine is than what they first used, and are delighted in the bookkeeping and accounting software that keeps track of financial matters so easily. However, while they may seek members of Generations X, Y, and Z for assistance with technology, they likely will have a better understanding of the basic concepts behind these more modern and electronically enhanced methods than either Generation Y or Z.

EVALUATING EMPLOYEES

There are a number of reasons for regular predetermined performance reviews of employees. The review process is an opportunity to check employee compliance with the job description, motivate an employee to a higher level of performance, suggest possible areas of development for an employee, and—perhaps most important—communicate with an employee about job satisfaction and possible changes to be made.

Often, evaluations include a rating scale from 1 to 5 for these and many other qualities to be evaluated. However, there is increasing evidence to discourage such a scale, mostly because many employers tend to score in the middle and because it leaves so much to individual interpretation. To foster communication, motivate, and encourage improvement of employees at the time of evaluation, consider a different piece to add to the guidelines. Both the employer and the employee might be asked to perform an ABC. *A* stands for "What is Awesome about this job or person?" *B* is "What could be Better?" and *C* is "What would you like to Change?" The more standard evaluation format can simply include a straight yes or no—the employee either satisfactorily meets the criteria or does not. However, the ABC method allows for an expansion to include the information an evaluation really hopes to reveal.

DISMISSING EMPLOYEES

The function of employee dismissal or separation falls mostly to the clinic manager; however, in a large facility with an HR representative, discussing dismissal or separation with that individual can be quite beneficial. Such a discussion ensures that all the information necessary is in place before a separation. There are voluntary and involuntary separations or dismissals.

Voluntary separations usually occur when an employee is relocating, advancing to another position elsewhere, retiring, or leaving for other personal reasons. A letter of resignation is usually submitted to both the clinic manager and the HR representative. These employees will give their manager proper notice and may be able to turn current projects and duties over to their replacements. There is also time to say good-bye to their colleagues and have a good feeling about their employment.

Involuntary dismissals or separations usually occur when an employee's performance is poor or there has been a serious violation of the clinic policies or job description. The clinic manager is aware of poor performance through the probationary reviews. Verbal and written warnings must be given to the employee and are to be well documented. Dismissal can be immediate if there is a serious breach of clinic policy. The HR director can provide necessary detail to the clinic manager and/or provider(s) regarding when and if immediate dismissal is recommended. If a clinic manager expects any serious difficulties with an employee during an immediate dismissal, the HR director or another person appointed to assist should be present when the employee is notified (see Chapter 44 for a more detailed discussion).

Exit Interview

An **exit interview** is an excellent opportunity for the employee who voluntarily leaves a practice and the HR manager to discuss the positive and negative aspects of the job and what changes might be made for a new person coming into the facility. A sample exit interview form is shown in Figure 45-4. It also allows the opportunity for the employee to ask for a letter of reference or to view the personnel file before leaving. In a voluntary separation, a **letter of resignation** for the personnel file is necessary.

Any separation process, voluntary or involuntary, must include a statement in the personnel file. For involuntary separation, be certain that the reasons for the dismissal are well documented in an honest, nonjudgmental statement. State only the facts in the personnel file; do not state opinion. Remember that employees have the right to view their personnel file at any time.

Employers are always to be informed of any dismissal as quickly as possible. As indicated above, some may be involved in the actual dismissal process.

EXIT INTERVIEW FORM

1. What did you like and dislike about the work you have been doing?
   (Including: support on the job; opportunity for personal growth; recognition and rewards)

2. What kind of people have you found the providers, your immediate supervisor, and co-workers to be?
   (Including: attitude; fairness; scheduling and assignment of work; work expectations; technical competence; assistance and guidance available; team spirit)

3. What is your view of our management practices and policies?
   (Including: clarity and fairness of practice policies; communications; management and staff)

4. How have you felt about performance appraisals, your salary and benefits?
   (Including: adequacy of salary; regularity and fairness of appraisals)

5. What are your principal reasons for leaving the practice?
   (Including: primary dissatisfactions; job or personal changes)

6. In what areas do you feel we need to improve?

Interviewer signature: _____ Date _____

Employee signature: _____ Date _____

FIGURE 45-4 Sample exit interview form.

From Ricardo, M. (1992). Personnel management handbook (2nd ed.). New York: The McGraw-Hill Companies, Inc. Copyright 1992. Reprinted with permission.

MAINTAINING PERSONNEL RECORDS

An important aspect of the responsibilities of the HR manager is maintaining personnel records. All documentation and correspondence related to each employee from application to dismissal, ranging from awards to reprimands and including formal reviews, must be kept in the confidential personnel file. Access to this file is limited to certain management personnel and the employee. Not all of these people are allowed to see the entire file. These files are usually kept for a period of 3 to 5 years after employees leave the practice. Some of the personnel files may be maintained electronically on the computer. However, access to those files must be protected so that only those with authorized access are able to open the files or make changes to them.

Such a file also includes the kind of information normally maintained for payroll and business practices. That information includes the name, address, telephone number, and Social Security number of the employee. The position title, date of beginning employment, rate of pay (hourly or otherwise), total overtime pay, deductions or additions to wages, wages paid each pay period, and the date the employee leaves the practice also are included.

COMPLYING WITH PERSONNEL LAWS

Only a brief introduction to the laws related to the ambulatory care setting are given in this section; therefore, this text is not meant to be a legal guide for an HR manager. The practice attorney should always be contacted if there is any question regarding personnel laws, which may vary in some states depending on the size of the practice.

Overtime must be addressed in each practice. Who is reimbursed for overtime and how is that reimbursement determined? Typically, administrative medical assistants, insurance billers, medical transcriptionists, and clinical medical assistants are likely to be eligible to be paid overtime. Overtime pay at a rate of not less than one and one-half times the regular rate of pay after a 40-hour work week is standard. Each week stands alone and one week cannot compensate for another. If the practice does not want to be involved in contentious overtime situations, require that any overtime be preauthorized in advance.

The Equal Pay Act of 1963 prevents wage discrimination for jobs that require equal skill, effort, and responsibility. The Civil Rights Act of 1964 prevents employers from discriminating against individuals on the basis of race, color, religion, sex, age, or national origin, and a number of states also consider discrimination based on sexual orientation illegal (see Chapter 6). Refer to Case Study 45-1 for an example of this dilemma.

Sexual harassment violates Title VII of the Civil Rights Act. Steps must be taken to ensure that all employees are working in an atmosphere that is not hostile, where sexual gestures, the presence of pornographic or offensive materials, or obscene language are not allowed either from patients or others in the clinic (see Chapter 6).

Employees have a right to expect safe working conditions. The Occupational Safety and Health Act (OSH Act) was established to prevent injuries and illnesses resulting from unsafe or unhealthy working conditions (see Chapter 21 for a detailed discussion of the standards and requirements, especially in the section on bloodborne pathogens, that went into effect in 1992). Compliance with this law requires that each employee be aware of possible risks associated with chemical hazards and how to protect themselves. Because there are many of these hazards in a medical practice, compliance and protection for employees are extremely important, and training sessions should be held in this area.

The Immigration Reform Act requires employers to verify the right of employees to work in the United States. Documentation acceptable for verification is a Social Security card or birth certificate. The U.S. Citizenship and Immigration Services will provide instructions and a form for employees and employers to complete, commonly referred to as the I-9 or Employment Eligibility Verification form (see Case Study 45-2)

Employers cannot discriminate against or otherwise condemn any full-time employee for jury duty. Although the employer does not have to continue pay during jury duty, the employee cannot lose seniority, insurance, or other benefits. Many employers continue an employee's full pay during the time of service on a jury because the reimbursement from the government for jury service is minimal. This is a way to benefit employees and encourage good citizenship.

The preceding discussion is by no means comprehensive but does include personnel regulations most likely to affect a medical practice. Any concerns should be directed to the practice's attorney.

SPECIAL POLICY CONSIDERATIONS

Several other managerial issues may arise in a medical setting for which the clinic manager and the HR manager will have to plan. These can include policies for temporary employees, rules of conduct, avoiding discrimination, and having a support system in place for employees who need physical or emotional help.

Temporary Employees

Temporary employees who may be employed for 90 days or less include students who are serving an internship or practicum from a local college and are practicing their skills for when they will be on the job. They should be reviewed on a regular basis in cooperation with their college supervisor. Give them as much actual hands-on experience as possible; they are potential future employees. Accommodating students in the practice is a two-way benefit. Students learn what reality is in the ambulatory care setting and are able to practice newly developed skills. Current staff members in the facility are "sharpened" by the students' presence. Teaching and monitoring someone's actions always results in sharpening and rethinking the skills of the current staff. Many HR directors and managers depend on these programs for future job applicants.

Smoking Policy

Smoking on the premises of a health care facility is generally prohibited. Additionally, some states and cities have laws that restrict smoking. When a policy is established, it should cover everyone—employers, employees, *and* patients. The objective is to have a policy that is workable and enforceable, promotes health, encourages employee morale and productivity, and sets examples for patients.

Discrimination

Legal

The Americans with Disabilities Act (ADA) and the Americans with Disabilities Act Amendments Act (ADAAA) of 2008 prohibit discrimination against people with disabilities by all private employers with 15 or more employees. Some states may further prohibit discrimination in facilities with a much smaller size workforce. *All* public entities are prohibited from discriminating against qualified individuals with disabilities. The ADA establishes guidelines prohibiting discrimination against a "qualified individual with a disability" in regard to employment. The 2008 Amendment made it easier for an individual to establish a disability. Someone with a disability who satisfies the skills necessary for the job; has the experience, education, and any other job requirements; and who, with reasonable accommodation, can perform the job cannot be discriminated against. Employers often find that persons with disabilities are their finest employees.

Persons who are HIV positive or have AIDS are included in the guidelines set forth by the ADA. Persons with HIV/AIDS cannot be discriminated against. It can be assumed that if a safe working environment is provided where all employees follow the rules for Standard Precautions, then reasonable accommodation has been made for the person with HIV or AIDS.

An employer cannot refuse a job to a qualified person based on the belief that in the future the employee may become too ill to work. The hiring decision must be based on the individual's ability to perform the functions of the position at the present time. If a current employee reveals to the manager that he or she is HIV positive or has AIDS, that information must be kept confidential and must be kept apart from the general personnel file. The manager may choose to hold a discussion at that time of what accommodations might be needed in the future.

PROVIDING/PLANNING EMPLOYEE INSTRUCTION AND EDUCATION

Health care changes daily—new procedures are established, better techniques are discovered for performing a particular task, and so on. Major changes regularly occur in medical insurance. Computer systems are updated or new software is added. A more sophisticated telephone system is installed to make certain patients are responded to promptly. New state or federal regulations mandate additional education or compliance in safety. New medications become available that providers may prescribe and employees must understand. All this demands that employees receive continuing and constant updates in their area of employment.

Instruction and education may be accomplished within the practice or outside the practice. When an employee is a member of a professional organization such as the American Association of Medical Assistants, many monthly meetings include continuing education opportunities. Recertification of all medical assistants is to be encouraged and supported financially, if required. Numerous seminars and conferences held throughout the country may be beneficial to employees. Local hospitals often have continuing education opportunities that may be beneficial. Managers will keep abreast of these opportunities and encourage employees to attend. Any continuing education opportunity that may benefit the employee on the job and the medical practice itself should ideally be paid for by the employer(s). Credentialed employees will always need to update skills and earn CEUs to maintain their credentials in active status. An important function of HR is to make CEUs opportunities available to employees.

It is often best to provide employee instruction and education within the facility when the necessary instruction is specific to the medical practice. For instance, instruction on new computer software is apt to be specific to the particular setting. When sophisticated new equipment is purchased, companies often provide in-house instruction for the individuals who will be using the equipment. Take advantage of as many of those opportunities as are available and for as many of your employees as possible. When the instruction is quite expensive or time consuming, make certain at least one person receives the instruction. Then have that individual teach others as appropriate. Whenever possible, provide instruction outside of regular hours when patients are not being seen—before the clinic opens or after the clinic closes or during a lunch period. Always pay employees for any time served over their regular working hours. Offer certificates for any in-services.

Careful attention to continuing education and instruction for employees will pay for itself many times over again. The more confident and secure employees feel in the skills they are expected to perform, the more satisfied the practice's patients will be.

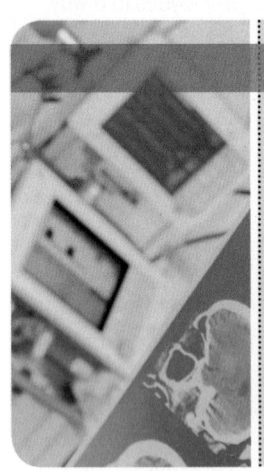

CASE STUDY 45-1

Refer to the scenario at the beginning of this chapter.

CASE STUDY REVIEW

1. Is there a legal issue here, an ethical issue, or both? If so, identify.
2. Should a policy be written to identify how the clinic is to respond to similar patient needs? Explain.
3. Do you agree with the provider's hesitation and relief? Justify your response.
4. If a clinic policy developed is opposite of your beliefs, what will you do? Might the scenario be different if the patient involved was a long-time patient of the clinic whose lifestyle was not known?

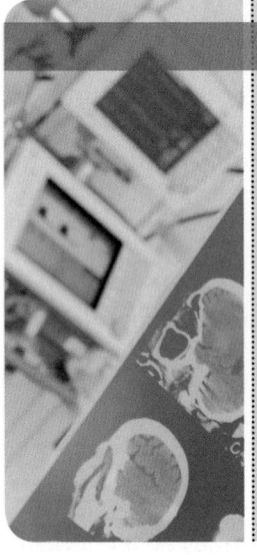

CASE STUDY 45-2

Ellen Armstrong, CMAS (AMT), is an administrative medical assistant at Inner City Health Care. The HR manager has suggested that she might expand her skills and learn some of the procedures related to the hiring process. A new medical assistant who specializes in nutrition is coming on board. Ellen has been asked to make certain his I-9 form is completed appropriately. The HR manager tells Ellen that she will need to download the latest form for the new employee to complete.

CASE STUDY REVIEW

1. Ellen knows that the I-9 is a government form verifying employment eligibility. What keywords might she use in her Internet search to find the form?
2. Once the form has been located, identify the specific rules necessary in completion of the form. What document in List A would a number of prospective employees most likely have?
3. In what area of the clinic might you post the lists of acceptable documents for the I-9 form?
4. With what agency is the form filed on successful completion?

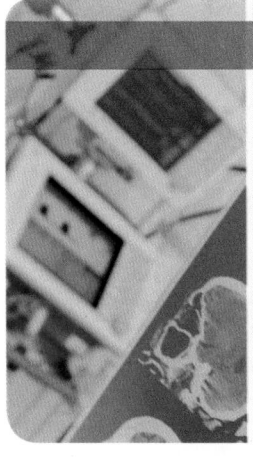

CASE STUDY 45-3

Charles Kensington has just been hired as the HR manager in a large metropolitan clinic. In studying the policy manual, he notes that there is no defined policy for sick leave or bereavement leave. Consider the steps he might take to write such a policy.

CASE STUDY REVIEW

1. To whom should he speak regarding what currently occurs when an employee is ill or when there is a death in the family?
2. What might Charles consider in writing this policy?
3. How should a policy be approved once it is written?
4. What parameters would you suggest for the policy?

Summary

- HR management is a challenge and includes many different tasks.
- Policy manuals assist the management team in recruiting, hiring, and maintaining the employees in the organization.
- The HR manager who is successful will hire the right people for the open positions and monitor employees in a way that enables and encourages them to give the best patient care possible.
- Managing personnel records will include everything from application to dismissal, all reviews, and salary documents.
- HR management must be able to comply with personnel laws, enforce policies, manage temporary employees, prevent discrimination, and provide necessary employee instruction and education.
- The HR manager will always have variety on the job and will have the satisfaction of watching a health care team function smoothly and efficiently.

Study for Success

To reinforce your knowledge and skills of information presented in this chapter:

- Review the *Key Terms* and *Learning Outcomes*
- Consider the *Critical Thinking* features and *Case Studies* and discuss your conclusions
    - Answer the questions in the *Certification Review*
    - 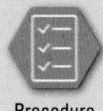 Perform the *Procedures* using the *Competency Assessment Checklists* on the *Student Companion Website*

Procedure

CERTIFICATION REVIEW

1. What is a fitting description of HR managers?
   a. They need no special education for the position; experience is sufficient.
   b. They may work longer hours and are responsible for hiring and orienting personnel.
   c. They need legal education to understand labor laws.
   d. Their most important task is to keep the providers out of trouble with employees and patients.

2. Which of the following questions may be asked in an interview?
   a. How old are you?
   b. Have you ever been arrested?
   c. Can you supply a driver's license or a Social Security card?
   d. Do you plan to start a family soon?
   e. Do you have someone to care for your children should they become ill?

3. When a candidate has been accepted for a position, what will the HR manager need to do?
   a. Call the candidate to determine what salary is preferred
   b. Write a letter defining the position details and intent to hire
   c. Check references provided by the candidate
   d. Notify patients of a staff change
4. What is commonly known about overtime hours in the medical facility?
   a. They are to be expected as part of the position.
   b. They do not require prior authorization.
   c. They are usually paid at no less than one and one-half times the regular pay rate.
   d. They are paid only to managers.
   e. They are a sign that the facility is sadly understaffed.
5. Who will the HR manager work with most closely?
   a. The clinic patients and the provider-employer(s)
   b. The clinic manager and county health department
   c. All employees except management
   d. The provider-employer(s), clinic manager, and employees
   e. Only the provider(s) with whom all HR matters are settled
6. Walter, one of the clinic medical assistants has been called to a two-week jury duty assignment. What discussion will he have with HR?
   a. He will be told he cannot serve; the clinic is far too busy.
   b. He will have to find a part-time replacement while he serves.
   c. HR will quickly make plans for a replacement during the days he must serve, pay his full salary, and encourage his participation.
   d. The HR manager will request a hardship excuse from jury duty for Walter.
   e. HR will need to have other employees pick up Walter's duties.
7. What resources are best for recruiting medical employees?
   a. Students in a business college
   b. Newspaper advertisements
   c. Networking sources
   d. The state's unemployment office
8. How will employees receive the instruction/education necessary to remain current in their positions?
   a. They will need to seek that instruction after hours and not expect reimbursement.
   b. They will already be current and up-to-date in the health care field.
   c. They should be paid for any time required and served over regular working hours.
   d. Training is usually done during lunch hours, and hopefully the providers will arrange for lunch.
   e. They will get sufficient updating from their professional associations.
9. Which of the following statements regarding personnel records is accurate?
   a. They are usually kept for 3 to 5 years after employment ends and may include payroll data.
   b. They are available for anyone to view, but are kept locked away.
   c. They will not include any papers related to anything other than employment.
   d. They are available only to HR and the provider(s).
10. Which of the following statements is true regarding dismissal or separation?
    a. It may be voluntary or involuntary and is always documented.
    b. It is always permanent.
    c. It will not require an exit interview.
    d. It requires a letter of referral.
    e. It upsets everyone and is to be kept private.

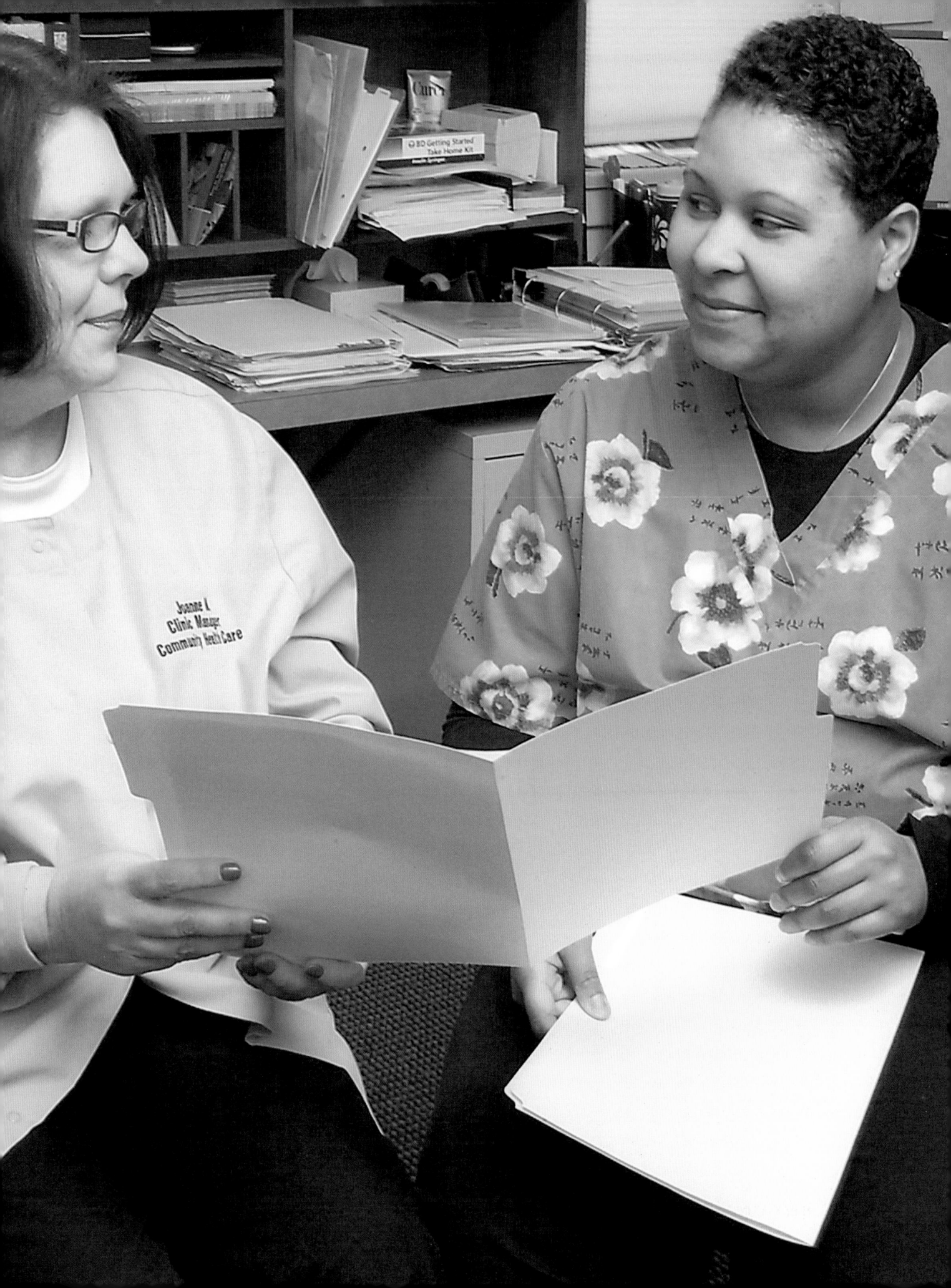

UNIT XI
ENTRY INTO THE PROFESSION

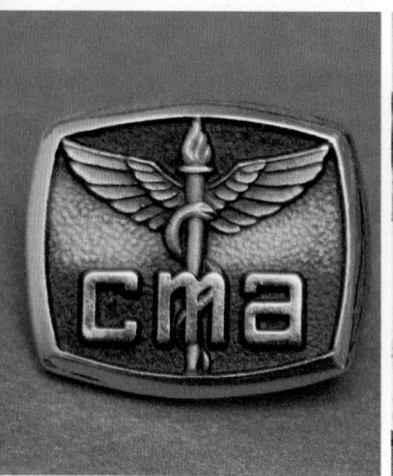
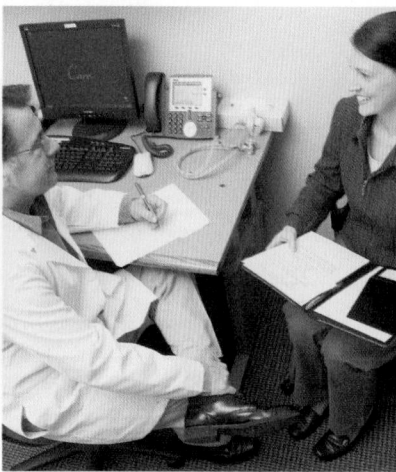
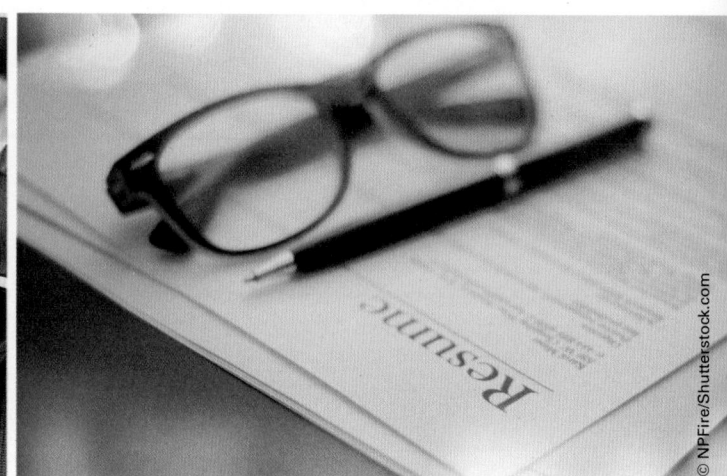

© NPFire/Shutterstock.com

ATTRIBUTES OF PROFESSIONALISM

The medical assisting profession continues to be one of the fastest growing professions in the United States, with increasing numbers of career-oriented candidates entering the profession annually. Therefore, it is important that you develop ways to uniquely present yourself and your skill set to a potential employer. Successfully passing the national certification examination and receiving a medical assisting credential is one way to establish your professionalism. Achieving certification acknowledges that you have standard entry-level knowledge and skills, while continuing to maintain the credential demonstrates a lifelong commitment to professional development.

Securing employment as a certified medical assistant is your first job. Developing a comprehensive job search strategy that includes self-assessment, résumé preparation, interview techniques, and follow-up is a key component to successful employment. Each component of your strategy demonstrates professionalism through communication, presentation, competency, initiative, and integrity.

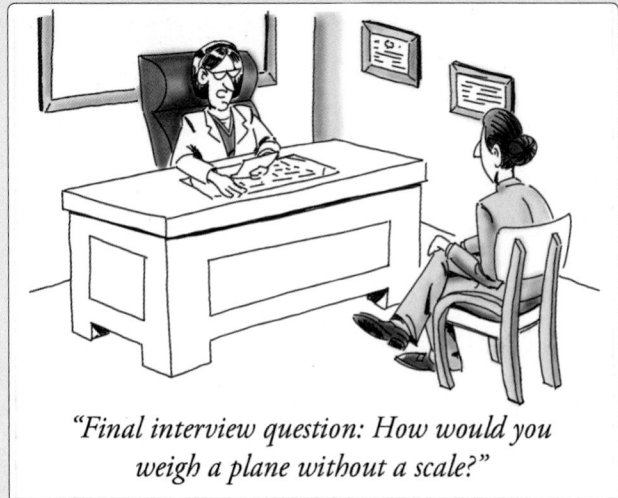

"Final interview question: How would you weigh a plane without a scale?"

Listed below are a series of questions for you to ask yourself, to serve as a professionalism checklist as you prepare for your future career as a medical assistant. As you interact with patients and colleagues, these questions will help to guide you in the characteristics and behaviors that are expected every day from professional medical assistants.

Ask Yourself

COMMUNICATION
- [ ] Do I apply active listening skills?
- [ ] Do I display professionalism through written and verbal communication?
- [ ] Do I demonstrate appropriate nonverbal communication?
- [ ] Do I display appropriate body language?
- [ ] Does my knowledge allow me to speak easily with all members of the health care team?

PRESENTATION
- [ ] Am I dressed and groomed appropriately?
- [ ] Do I display a positive attitude?
- [ ] Do I display a calm, professional, and caring manner?

COMPETENCY
- [ ] Do I pay attention to detail?
- [ ] Do I ask questions if I am out of my comfort zone or do not have the experience to carry out tasks?
- [ ] Do I display sound judgment?
- [ ] Am I knowledgeable and accountable?

INITIATIVE
- [ ] Do I show initiative?
- [ ] Have I developed a strategic plan to achieve my goals? Is my plan realistic?
- [ ] Do I seek out opportunities to expand my knowledge base?
- [ ] Am I flexible and dependable?

INTEGRITY
- [ ] Do I demonstrate the principles of self-boundaries?
- [ ] Do I work within my scope of practice?
- [ ] Do I demonstrate respect for individual diversity?
- [ ] Do I recognize the impact personal ethics and morals have on the delivery of health care?
- [ ] Do I protect and maintain confidentiality?
- [ ] Do I maintain moral and ethical standards?
- [ ] Do I do the "right thing" even when no one is observing?

CHAPTER 46

Preparing for Medical Assisting Credentials

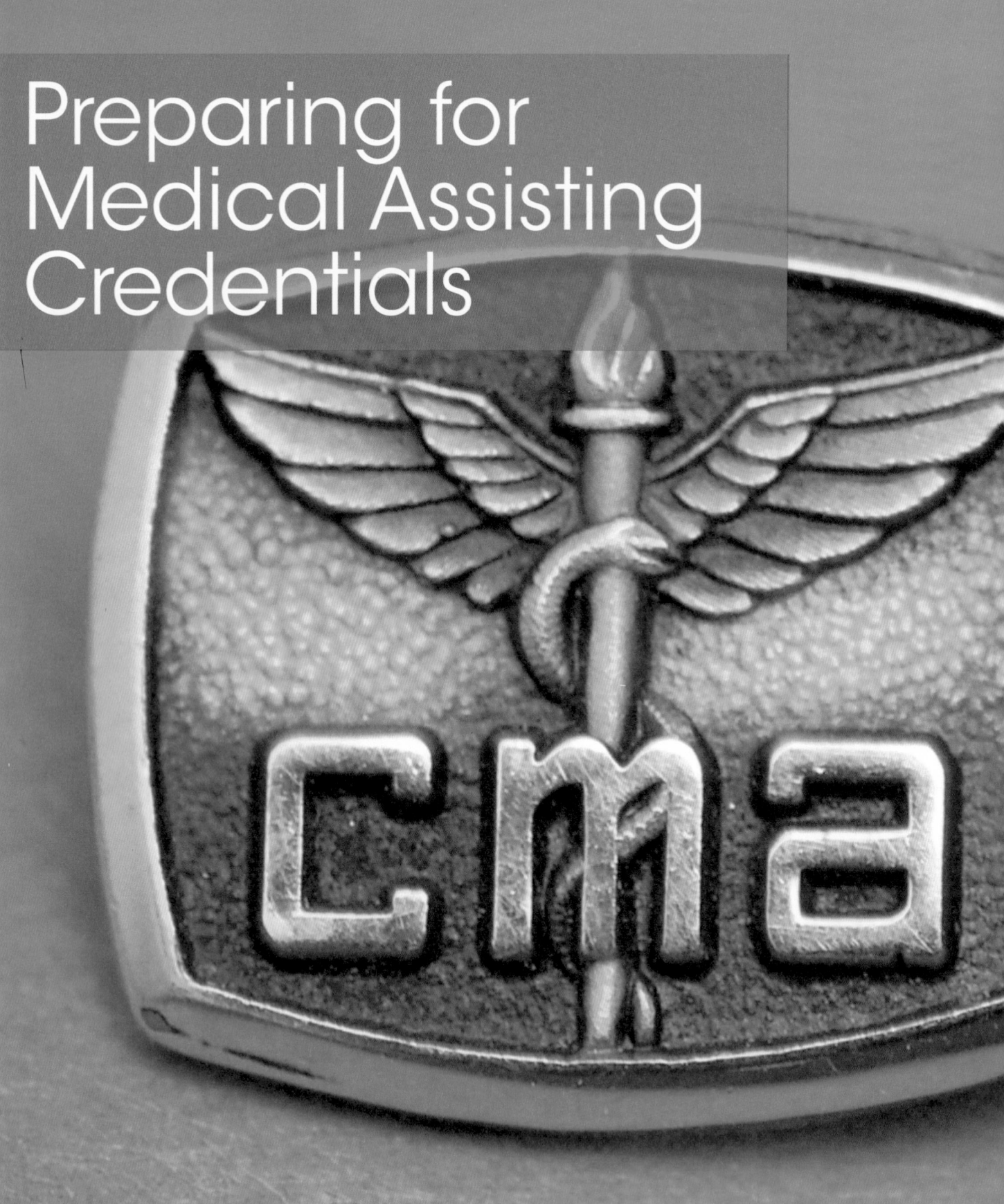

1. Define and spell all of the key terms as presented in this chapter.

2. Discuss the purpose of certification and the importance of recertification.

3. Develop a plan and study schedule to sit for a medical assistant certification examination.

4. Compare the various agencies providing medical assisting certification.

5. Discuss the role of the Commission on Accreditation of Allied Health Education Programs (CAAHEP), the AAMA Endowment, and the Medical Assisting Education Review Board (MAERB).

6. Analyze the differences between a registered medical assistant and a certified medical administrative specialist.

7. Identify and describe the two medical assisting credentials available through the National Healthcareer Association (NHA).

8. Identify the benefits of medical assistant certification and registration.

9. Describe several methods for pursuing continuing education opportunities through each accrediting agency.

10. Examine professional organizations and the value they offer you as a medical assistant.

KEY TERMS

Accrediting Bureau of Health Education Schools (ABHES)

American Association of Medical Assistants (AAMA)

American Medical Technologists (AMT)

certification

certification examination

Certified Clinical Medical Assistant (CCMA [NHA])

Certified Medical Administrative Assistant (CMAA [NHA])

Certified Medical Administrative Specialist (CMAS [AMT])

Certified Medical Assistant (CMA [AAMA])

Commission on Accreditation of Allied Health Education Programs (CAAHEP)

continuing education units (CEUs)

National Healthcareer Association (NHA)

recertification

Registered Medical Assistant (RMA [AMT])

SCENARIO

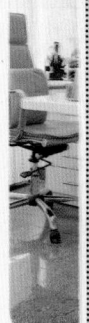

Dr. Ray Reynolds currently is the senior provider at Inner City Health Care, a multiprovider clinic. When he began his practice years ago, however, he had a private practice and employed one full-time and two part-time medical assistants. Dr. Reynolds felt the practice ran smoothly, except when an assistant had to be replaced. Retraining a new person consumed a great deal of valuable time. Even if the new employee came with experience from another medical practice, the procedures still required retraining.

Dr. Reynolds now finds that when he needs to replace a medical assistant, he looks at the applicants' résumés and interviews only those candidates who are credentialed medical assistants. The practice is too busy to spend time training and retraining new employees.

Forty years ago, medical assistants were trained on the job by the practitioner with whom they were employed. With no established criteria for evaluating such training, quality control varied. This chapter will present the purpose of certification, certifying agencies, and preparation for certification examinations.

PURPOSE OF CERTIFICATION

Certification is intended to set a consistent minimum standard for evaluating an individual's professional competence as a medical assistant. The medical assisting profession continues to be one of the fastest growing occupations in the United States. Because of the demand for skilled medical assistants, increasing numbers of career-oriented candidates enter this profession annually. Certification acknowledges the professional has standard entry-level knowledge and skills. The Certifying Board of AAMA recently received accreditation from the International Accreditation Service (IAS). This achievement establishes AAMA as the most respected and credible personnel certification organization for the medical assisting profession.

Successfully passing a certification examination builds personal self-esteem, confidence, and a positive attitude in performing the responsibilities assigned. (See Chapter 1 for more history regarding certification.) Other benefits of certification include help in your career advancement and compensation. Hiring providers view credentialed medical assistants as professionals who have shown proficiency in entry-level skills. Individuals who are competent and interested in continued learning experiences are more apt to be rewarded with promotions and salary increases. Maintaining the credential demonstrates a lifelong commitment to professional development. The graduate medical assistant has a goal and challenge to which to aspire, first by earning the credential and second by maintaining the credential through continuing education and recertification.

Some certifying agencies offer student membership into their organizations. This avenue provides excellent opportunities to network and be mentored by fellow professionals, to enroll in continuing education programs, and to receive many other membership perks. For example, students enrolled as American Association of Medical Assistants (AAMA) members before their graduation date are eligible for reduced student membership rates. Once they are a student member, they may stay at the student rate for 1 year after graduation if they do not choose to be an active or associate member and pay the higher dues amount. The additional year of membership at the reduced rate helps the recent graduate maintain membership while finding a job and becoming established in their career.

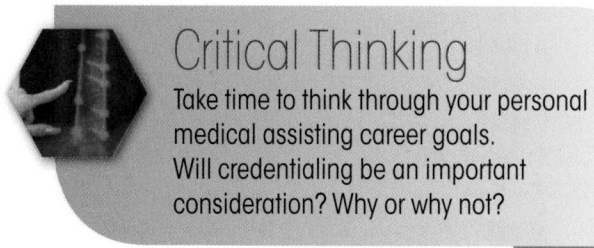

Critical Thinking

Take time to think through your personal medical assisting career goals. Will credentialing be an important consideration? Why or why not?

CERTIFICATION AGENCIES

The **American Association of Medical Assistants (AAMA)** offers examinations to certify the **Certified Medical Assistant (CMA [AAMA])**. The **American Medical Technologists (AMT)** offers examinations to certify the **Registered Medical Assistant (RMA [AMT])** and the **Certified Medical Administrative Specialist (CMAS [AMT])**. The **National Healthcareer Association (NHA)** is another agency offering certification to health care professionals. These professionals include the **Certified Clinical Medical Assistant (CCMA [NHA])** and the **Certified Medical Administrative Assistant (CMAA [NHA])**. See Table 46-1 for a comparison of the various certifying agencies for medical assisting.

When responding to advertisements or during the interview process, "certified medical assistants" are responsible to make clear to prospective employers which credential they have been awarded.

TABLE 46-1

COMPARISON OF AGENCIES PROVIDING MA CERTIFICATION

CERTIFICATION DETAILS			
Certifying agency	American Association of Medical Assistants (AAMA)	American Medical Technologists (AMT)	National Healthcareer Association (NHA)
Credential	CMA (AAMA)	RMA (AMT) or CMAS (AMT)	CCMA (NHA) or CMAA (NHA)
Certification exam	Computer-based national exam; administered through Prometric testing centers (www.prometric.com)	Computer-based national exam offered at Pearson Vue testing centers (www.pearsonvue.com); or paper exam by appointment	National exam; can be taken online or as a paper exam
Exam format	200 multiple-choice questions selected from topics listed on the Content Outline for the CMA (AAMA) Maximum test time is 195 minutes	210 multiple-choice questions covering topics related to clinical, administrative, and general subjects 2.5 hours to complete Immediate pass/fail notification Reschedule within 24 hours if failed Four lifetime attempts allowed	200 multiple-choice questions Separate tests for CCMA and CMAA (exam completion time approximately 90 minutes)
Continuing education	AAMA-approved CEUs: 60 units every five years 10 clinical 10 administrative 10 general 30 discretionary	Certification Continuation Program (CCP): 30 points every three years AMT and AMTIE* offer several CE options for points	Continued Education (CE) Program: 10 NHA-approved continuing education credits every two years

*American Medical Technologists Institute For Excellence (AMTIE)

PREPARING FOR CERTIFICATION EXAMINATIONS

Preparation for the examination requires planning, scheduling, and discipline. It is important to plan well in advance to ensure confidence and a passing score to earn your credential. If you are sitting for the examination immediately upon graduation, your preparation time for the examination may only allow 2 to 3 months. If you have been out of school for some time or your work experience has been very specialized, you may need longer to prepare for the examination.

During the planning stage, determine the date you want to sit for the examination. Check with the appropriate Web site or call the appropriate examination department to obtain the current application form. The application form contains information such as dates, times, and locations of test sites; policies regarding deadlines; incomplete applications; examination verification information; and information regarding study guides.

It is important to consider having a study group or partner. The right study environment can be invaluable to your success for several reasons. First, it is important to select a study partner or group who shares your commitment to a successful outcome and who plans to sit for the examination on or near the same date you have selected. A study partner can also give you some accountability for keeping to the planned schedule.

Once it has been determined when and where you will sit for the examination and who your study partner(s), if any, will be, a meeting should be scheduled to discuss the review/study approach. It may be that your group will decide to review/study each subject provided in the Curriculum Content Outline accompanying the application. Other groups review/study only those areas in which they feel less confident. A plan that meets the needs of each group member and that all can agree to works best.

Meeting once or twice a week helps the group stay focused and on task. Independent study should be done throughout the week. During the independent study time, each group member may be asked to write 10 multiple-choice questions relevant to the week's study topic. Answers to these questions should be on a separate page. Some find it helpful to also provide the rationale or textbook page number that supports their answer. When the group meets, a discussion of the study topic could take place and copies of the questions could be distributed for answering. The questions could then be corrected and discussion of any questionable or missed answers could take place.

Once a schedule has been established and agreed on, discipline is required. It is critical that each group member spend time individually preparing for the next group meeting. Someone should be put in charge of each group meeting to keep the event from turning into a social gathering. To help with this, it is a good idea to set a specific time limit for the study/review session. If individuals want to visit after the session, they are free to do that without disrupting the purpose of the session. All members should be committed to being prepared and attending each scheduled review/study session.

AMERICAN ASSOCIATION OF MEDICAL ASSISTANTS (AAMA)

The AAMA is an organization whose objective is to promote skills and professionalism, protect the medical assistants' right to practice, and encourage consistent health care delivery through professional certification. The AAMA is a sponsoring member of the **Commission on Accreditation of Allied Health Education Programs (CAAHEP)**. CAAHEP establishes the standards for medical assisting programs and is the issuing body of the accreditation for AAMA. (See Chapter 1 for the history of AAMA).

Only graduates of medical assistant programs accredited by CAAHEP and the **Accrediting Bureau of Health Education Schools (ABHES)** may sit for the AAMA Certified Medical Assistant exam. To locate CAAHEP medical assisting information, go to www.aama-ntl.org and follow the drop-down menu for specific information. To locate ABHES registered medical assisting information, go to www.americanmedtech.org and follow the drop-down menu for specific information. The AAMA Endowment is a nonprofit corporation that provides funding for two purposes:

- Awarding of scholarships to students in CAAHEP-accredited medical assisting education programs
- Accrediting medical assisting education programs through CAAHEP

The Medical Assisting Education Review Board (MAERB) operates under the authority of the endowment and evaluates medical assisting programs according to standards adopted by the endowment and CAAHEP. The MAERB recommends programs to CAAHEP for accreditation. The MAERB also reviews standards for medical assisting curricula, conducts accreditation workshops for educators, and provides medical assisting educators with current information about CAAHEP, accreditation laws, policies, and practices.

Certified Medical Assistant (AAMA) Examination Format and Content

The AAMA **certification examination** is a comprehensive test of the knowledge actually used in today's medical clinic. The content is drawn from an in-depth analysis of the numerous tasks practicing medical assistants perform on a daily basis.

Examination questions are formulated by the Certifying Board's Task Force for Test Construction (TFTC). This group is composed of practicing medical assistants, providers, and medical assisting educators from across the United States. The TFTC updates the examination annually to reflect changes in medical assistants' day-to-day responsibilities, as well as the latest developments in medical knowledge and technology.

The three major areas tested include:

1. *General.* Psychology, Communication; Professionalism; Medical Terminology; Medical Law/Regulatory Guidelines; Medical Ethics; and Risk Management, Quality Assurance, and Safety
2. *Administrative.* Medical Reception, Patient Navigator/Advocate, Medical Business Practices, Establish Patient Medical Record, Scheduling Appointments, and Practice Finances
3. *Clinical.* Anatomy and Physiology, Infection Control, Patient Intake and Documentation of Care, Patient Preparation and Assisting the Provider, Nutrition, and Collecting and Processing Specimens

Certified Medical Assistant (AAMA) Application Process

Candidates should read all instructions carefully before completing the application form. Incomplete or incorrect applications will not be processed and will be returned to the candidate. Postmark deadlines for applications, cancellations, and examination location changes are strictly enforced.

Applications are available from the AAMA Certification Department, 7999 Eagle Way, Chicago, IL 60678-1079, or may be downloaded from the AAMA Web site (www.aama-ntl.org) or completed online.

When completing a printed application, it is recommended that the application be sent by certified mail, return receipt requested to verify delivery. The application must be typewritten or printed using black ink only. Be sure the application is signed and dated properly and the eligibility category section is completed appropriately. Applications take up to 45 days after the postmark date to process.

Tear off the application page from the instruction pamphlet. Do not mail the instructions back with the application. Keep this information for future reference together with a copy of everything submitted, including a copy of your completed application and payment check or money order. If you are paying by Visa or MasterCard, provide the requested information at the top of the application.

Certified Medical Assistant (AAMA) Examination Scheduling and Administration

The CMA (AAMA) certification examination is offered via computer-based testing (CBT). Candidates whose applications are accepted will receive a Scheduling Permit containing instructions for making a testing appointment, and will be able to select locations and flexible testing times at Prometric test centers throughout the United States. To schedule examination appointments, candidates go to www.prometric.com and select a test center and appointment test time. Centers are open 9:00 AM to 5:00 PM Monday through Saturday. An email confirming your appointment will be sent to you.

Photo identification is required for admission to the examination. Candidates are not permitted to bring any items except identification into the examination area. All exam candidates will receive

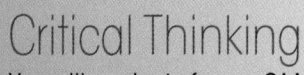

Critical Thinking

You will graduate from a CAAHEP-accredited program in June and want to sit for the CMA examination the last Saturday of June (the same month in which you graduate). Go to the AAMA Web site and determine when your application must be postmarked for acceptance for this test date. What is the date the online application must be completed?

an unofficial pass/fail result immediately upon completion of the exam. An official report of your scores will be mailed within 6 to 10 weeks after the exam date.

Certified Medical Assistant (AAMA) Recertification

All newly certified and recertifying CMAs (AAMA) will be current through the end of the calendar month of initial certification or most recent recertification for 60 months.

Recertification can be achieved either by reexamination or by **continuing education units (CEUs)**. Recertification units are evaluated on supportive documentation and relevancy to medical assisting as defined by the AAMA *Medical Assistant Role Delineation Study* or the *Content Outline for the Certification/Recertification Examination*.

A total of 60 units is necessary to recertify the CMA (AAMA) credential. A minimum of 10 units is required in each category: general, administrative, and clinical. The remaining 30 units can be accumulated in any of the three content areas or from any combination of the three categories. At least 30 of the required 60 recertification units must be accumulated from AAMA-approved CEUs. If desired, all 60 units may be AAMA CEUs.

Applicants who accumulate all 60 units through AAMA CEUs, and in the correct content areas, can order a recertification over the telephone. Application fees still apply; however, an application form is not required. All CMAs employed or seeking employment must have current certified status to use the CMA (AAMA) credential.

Continuing education courses are offered by local, state, and national AAMA groups. Guided study programs are also available through AAMA's Quest for Excellence program. *CMA Today*, the official bimonthly publication of AAMA, provides articles designated for CEUs.

A CMA (AAMA) need not be a member of the AAMA nor currently employed to recertify. The entire recertification by continuing education instructions and application can be downloaded from AAMA's Web site (www.aama-ntl.org). Review of recertification applications can take up to 90 days. If all criteria are met, recertification is granted. The date that the application was postmarked to the AAMA Executive Office will be the date of recertification.

CEU Documentation. On successfully passing the certification examination and earning the CMA (AAMA) credential, one should begin to document all CEUs earned. It is important to have the following information for CEU documentation:

- Complete date of the activity
- Sponsor (group or organization issuing the credit for the continuing education activity)
- Program title
- Amount and type of credit earned (e.g., CEU, CME, contact hour or college credit)
- Recertification units (AAMA CEUs or other credit)
- Units per content area (general, administrative, clinical)

A copy of the handbook *Recertify your CMA (AAMA) Credential* may be downloaded from www.aama-ntl.org. A sample continuing education verification form as well as a blank form is included for your convenience. Recertification is made much easier when this form is documented completely and kept up to date.

AMERICAN MEDICAL TECHNOLOGISTS (AMT)

The American Medical Technologists (AMT) awards the registered medical assistant RMA (AMT) credential to individuals graduating from ABHES-accredited medical assisting programs who successfully pass their examination. ABHES is recognized by the U.S. Department of Education for accreditation of postsecondary schools offering traditional instruction as well as instruction by distance delivery.

The AMT also offers certification for the certified medical administrative specialist (CMAS). The CMAS (AMT) is employed primarily in the administrative area of provider clinics or hospitals.

They must understand and use medical terminology properly and be skilled in all administrative tasks performed in health care settings. Each individual state decides the scope of practice for the CMAS (AMT), with most states not requiring licensure.

Additional information regarding CMAS (AMT) education requirements, duties performed, working conditions, employment outlook, and estimated earnings can be found online at www.americanmedtech.org.

Registered Medical Assistant (AMT) Examination Format and Content

AMT certification examinations are intended to evaluate the competence of entry-level practitioners. The Education, Qualifications, and Standards Committee of American Medical Technologists develops registered medical assistant RMA (AMT) examinations. The medical assistant committee writes test questions and reviews questions submitted from other sources (e.g., instructors, experts, practitioners, and other individuals associated with the medical assistant profession). The medical assistant committee also determines certification requirements and addresses standard-setting issues related to the credential. Once test construction has been completed, the examination is reviewed and approved by the AMT Board of Directors.

Examinees are required to select the single best answer; multiple answers for a single item are scored as incorrect. Test questions may require examinees to recall facts, interpret graphic illustrations and information presented in case studies, analyze situations, or solve problems. The approximate percentage of questions in each content area is as follows:

1. General Medical Assisting Knowledge—41.0%
   - Anatomy and Physiology
   - Medical Terminology
   - Medical Law
   - Medical Ethics
   - Human Relations
   - Patient Education

2. Administrative Medical Assisting—24.0%
   - Insurance
   - Financial bookkeeping
   - Medical secretarial-administrative medical assistant

3. Clinical Medical Assisting—35.0%

- Asepsis
- Sterilization
- Instruments
- Vital signs
- Physical examinations
- Clinical pharmacology
- Minor surgery
- Therapeutic modalities
- Laboratory procedures
- Electrocardiography
- First aid

Registered Medical Assistant (AMT) Application Process

The following criteria have been established for applicants sitting for the RMA (AMT) examination:

1. Applicant shall be of good moral character and at least 18 years of age.
2. Applicant shall be a graduate of an accredited high school or acceptable equivalent.
3. Applicant must meet one of the following requirements:

   a. Applicant shall be a graduate of a:

   - Medical assisting program that holds programmatic accreditation by (or is in a postsecondary school or college that holds institutional accreditation by) the ABHES or the CAAHEP.
   - Medical assisting program in a postsecondary school or college that has institutional accreditation by a Regional Accrediting Commission or by a national accrediting organization approved by the U.S. Department of Education. That program must include a minimum of 720 clock hours (or equivalent) of training in medical assisting skills (including a clinical practicum of no less than 160 hours).
   - Formal medical services training program of the U.S. Armed Forces.

   b. Applicant shall have been employed in the profession of medical assisting for a minimum of 5 years, no more than 2 years of which may have been as an instructor in a postsecondary medical assisting program.

4. Applicants applying under criteria 3 a or b *must* take and pass the AMT certification examination for RMA.

The AMT Board of Directors has further determined that applicants who have passed a generalist medical assistant certification examination offered by another medical assisting certification body (provided that examination has been approved for this purpose by the AMT Board of Directors), who have been working in the medical assisting field for 3 of the past 5 years, and who meet all other AMT training and experience requirements may be considered for RMA (AMT) certification without further examination. Applications and a useful handbook for the AMT candidate can be downloaded from AMT's Web site at (www.american-medtech.com).

Registered Medical Assistant (AMT) Examination Scheduling and Administration

All applications must be completed online or printed clearly except for the signatures required. All ancillary documentation must also be submitted (e.g., application fee; proof of high school graduation or equivalent; and official final transcripts stating graduation from medical assistant school, college, or training program [with school seal affixed or notarized]).

When the AMT registrar has received the application and all required information, an authorization letter containing a toll-free number is mailed to you. You can then contact Pearson Vue locations at www.pearsonvue.com/amt to schedule a date and time to take the examination. Two forms of valid identification are required, both bearing your signature and at least one bearing your photo. Photo identification is limited to a driver's license, state-issued identification card, military identification, or passport.

All AMT registration examination tests are available in paper-and-pencil format or in computerized formats at over 200 locations in the United States, its territories, and Canada. Tests can be scheduled daily except Sundays and holidays. Both formats are identical in length; however, experience has shown the computerized test takes less time to complete. Your computerized test score is displayed moments after you complete your test. A paper copy of your result is provided to you before you leave the testing center.

Registered Medical Assistant (AMT) Recertification

The AMT has established the Certification Continuation Program (CCP) for continuing education points. Certification will be suspended following a 30-day grace period if proper documentation is not submitted. Each RMA (AMT) is required to accumulate 30 points, which must be turned in every 3 years for recertification. You can use the AMTrax mobile app to record and track your activities for submission. You may view and print your record at any time using date ranges. Retaking the RMA examination is not an option for reinstatement or recertification.

NATIONAL HEALTHCAREER ASSOCIATION (NHA)

The National Healthcareer Association (NHA) also offers national certification examinations for health care professionals. Certified programs are accredited by the National Commission for Certifying Agencies (NCCA), a division of the Institute for Credentialing Excellence (ICE). NHA works with educational institutions throughout the country on curriculum development, competency testing, and preparation and administration of their examination and offers a continuing education (CE) program.

Certified Clinical Medical Assistant and Certified Medical Administrative Assistant Examination Format and Content

The NHA certifies the Certified Clinical Medical Assistant (CCMA [NHA]) and the Certified Medical Administrative Assistant (CMAA [NHA]) among other health career professions. Criteria for taking NHA certification examinations include one of the following: The applicant must have a high school diploma and have recently successfully completed an NHA-approved training program or the applicant must have either a high school diploma or equivalency and have recently worked in the field of certification for a minimum of 1 year as a full-time employee. Work experience must be documented in writing and signed by the director or employer.

The NHA offers several methods to help prepare candidates for their national certification examination. All students applying for NHA certification examination receive NHA study guides. The examination is offered in traditional pencil-and-paper formats or can be taken online at any of the approved locations.

Certified Clinical Medical Assistant and Certified Medical Administrative Assistant Application Process

There are four ways to apply for the NHA national certification examination:

- Online using www.nhanow.com. Go directly to the secured registration page and submit the registration form using Visa, MasterCard, Discover, American Express, or school voucher.
- The registration form can be downloaded and printed. Once it is filled out completely, it can be mailed along with payment. Address and mail to:

  National Healthcareer Association
  7 Ridgedale Avenue, Suite 203
  Cedar Knolls, NJ 07927

- The completed registration form can be faxed to the NHA with credit card information or school voucher. The fax number is 1-973-644-4797.
- Telephone the Customer Service Department at 1-800-449-9092. You can then complete the registration over the phone. You will need your credit card number and expiration date or school voucher accessible for payment information.

Certified Clinical Medical Assistant and Certified Medical Administrative Assistant Examination Scheduling and Administration

The NHA examination can be scheduled at any of the approved locations:

- *Training schools/colleges.* Check with your school for details.
- *Testing sites.* There are more than 550 PSI/LaserGrade testing sites nationwide.
- Experienced individuals can take examinations at their place of employment.

NOTE: All examinations are required to have an exam proctor present.

Certified Clinical Medical Assistant and Certified Medical Administrative Assistant Recertification

NHA offers a Continuing Education (CE) Program to make the process of continuing education more convenient for the health care professional. Courses in this program can be taken at your convenience at home. New industry standards require that each NHA-certified health care professional complete 10 CE credits every 2 years.

In the event that certification expires, reinstatement is permitted within a year of the expiration date. If reinstatement is initiated within a year of the expiration date, the individual must submit evidence of 15 completed CE credits and pay a renewal and reinstatement fee. After a year from the expiration date, reinstatement is not permitted and the individual must apply and take the certification examination again to become recertified.

Applicants who pass the examination will be nationally certified as recognized by the NHA. They will receive a certification certificate suitable for framing and a wallet-size ID certification card containing their national certification number. CE credits will be reviewed by NHA, and a sticker to apply to the certification ID card will be mailed if the credits are accepted.

PROFESSIONAL ORGANIZATIONS

Professional

Professional organizations have evolved to establish standards by which medical assistants and medical assisting programs are evaluated. Programs accredited by agencies must meet certain criteria, and students must pass national examinations to become certified. Medical assistants are not licensed and need not be certified to meet employment requirements; however, those certified are viewed as professionals with entry-level skills and a commitment to continuing education.

American Association of Medical Assistants (AAMA)

The AAMA was instrumental in defining the scope of training required for the profession and developed standards and guidelines by which programs could become accredited and the medical assistant credentialed. Membership in the AAMA offers many benefits, including the following:

- Medical assisting news and health care information through the bimonthly magazine *CMA Today*
- CEUs for AAMA activities entered in the Continuing Education Registry and access to your transcript online
- Educational events provided by local chapters, state societies, and national meetings
- Answers to legal questions regarding job-related issues
- If eligible, application for the prestigious CMA examination at a reduced fee

- Discounts on car rentals, conventions, workshop and seminar fees, and self-study courses
- Opportunity to network with other practicing medical assistants

American Medical Technologists (AMT)

The AMT is another nonprofit certification agency and professional membership association representing allied health care individuals. It certifies medical assistants by awarding the RMA (AMT) national credential to those candidates successfully satisfying requirements. AMT has many local chapters, state societies, and a Uniform Services Committee. Each of these societies meets regularly and annually for a national convention.

AMT benefits and services include:

- Continuing education through the *Journal of Continuing Education Topics & Issues*, which is published three times a year
- AMT's Institute for Excellence (AMTIE), which monitors continuing education credits and sends a "report card" each year
- Four scholarships available to members who want to return to school and five scholarships for current students enrolled in allied health care programs
- State societies that offer opportunities for continuing education, activities, and networking
- Peer recognition through AMT's prestigious RMA (AMT) credential
- Personal discount programs

National Healthcareer Association (NHA)

The NHA serves as a reliable resource for up-to-date information on health career opportunities, training programs, education opportunities, and industry forecasts. The NHA newsletter *The NHA Today* is well respected and provides current trends, articles, and information regarding the health care field.

NHA benefits and services include:

- National certification
- Continuing education opportunities
- Collaboration with educational institutions in curriculum development and competency testing
- Annual Continuing Education Program
- Elite Membership Program that puts you in touch with a team of placement specialists to expand job opportunities

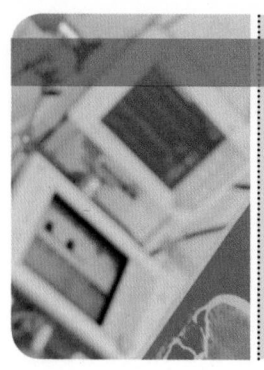

CASE STUDY 46-1

Refer to the scenario at the beginning of the chapter.

CASE STUDY REVIEW

1. Discuss the advantages of certification to the medical assistant.
2. Discuss the advantages of certification to the provider.
3. How does certification set a consistent minimum standard for evaluating professional competence as a medical assistant?

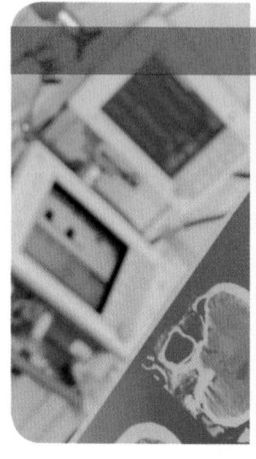

CASE STUDY 46-2

It is May, and Nancy McFarland, who graduated from an ABHES-accredited program 4.5 years ago, is beginning to research the procedures and requirements for taking the RMA (AMT) examination. Nancy completed her internship at Inner City Health Care and was hired to work there full time (35 hours per week) when she graduated.

CASE STUDY REVIEW

1. If Nancy wants to take the examination in January, what is the procedure for applying?
2. Nancy is setting up a study schedule. She plans to review course textbooks and tests, purchase a study guide, and set up a study group. Develop a simple study schedule.
3. What criteria should Nancy consider when asking people to join her study group?

Summary

- The purpose of certification is to establish a minimum standard for evaluating an individual's professional competence and acknowledges standard entry-level knowledge and skills as a medical assistant.

- Strategies for preparing for the certification examination include determining the date to sit for the examination, completing the application process, selecting study partner(s), establishing a meeting schedule and itinerary, and appointing a meeting facilitator.

- The objective of AAMA is to promote skills and professionalism, protect medical assistants' right to practice, and encourage consistent health care delivery through certification. CAAHEP establishes the standards for medical assisting programs, and is the issuing body of accreditation for AAMA. The Endowment is a nonprofit corporation that provides funds for scholarships and accreditation of medical assisting education programs through CAAHEP. MAERB operates under the authority of the Endowment and evaluates medical assisting programs and recommends programs for CAAHEP accreditation. It also reviews standards for medical assisting curricula; conducts accreditation workshops for educators; and provides educators with current information regarding accreditation laws, policies, and practices.

- Candidates sitting for CMA (AAMA) credentialing must pass a computer-based national test administered through Prometric testing centers. Sixty CEUs in specific categories are required every 5 years to maintain accreditation.

- Candidates sitting for the RMA (AMT) and the CMAS (AMT) credentials must pass a computer-based national test administered through Pearson Vue testing centers. Thirty points every 3 years are required to maintain certification.

- Candidates sitting for the CCMA (NHA) and the CMAA (NHA) credentials must pass an online test. Ten NHA-approved credits every 2 years are required to maintain certification.

- Professional organizations offer current news and health information; continuing education options; local, state and nation chapters; discount programs; and networking and employment opportunities.

CERTIFICATION REVIEW

1. What should the goal and challenge of each graduating medical assistant be?
   a. Find employment
   b. Have a good benefit package
   c. Possess entry-level skills
   d. Earn the CMA/RMA credential and maintain it

2. Which statement is true of the certification examination?
   a. It is a comprehensive test based on tasks medical assistants perform daily.
   b. It contains all true/false questions.
   c. It is developed by the AMTIE.
   d. It is developed by the NBME.
   e. It is developed by CAAHEP.

3. Which of the following is *not* a benefit of membership in a professional organization such as AAMA or AMT?
   a. Answers to legal questions regarding job-related issues
   b. Legal advice regarding divorce
   c. Nationwide networking opportunities
   d. Professional journal publications

4. Which of the following is valid for recertification of the CMA (AAMA) credential?
   a. Submitting work experience
   b. Reexamination or CEU method
   c. Submitting on-the-job training
   d. Submitting military training
   e. Submitting practicum experience

5. To keep the RMA (AMT) credential current, an individual must complete which of the following?
   a. 10 credits every 2 years
   b. 30 points every 3 years
   c. 30 points every 5 years
   d. 60 points every 5 years

6. The RMA was established by which of the following organizations?
   a. ABHES
   b. CAAHEP
   c. AMT
   d. AAMA
   e. NHA

7. The NHA offers medical assisting certification for which of the following?
   a. CMA
   b. RMA
   c. CCMA and CMAA
   d. CMAS

8. Which answer is true of the RMA examinations?
   a. They are offered at Pearson Vue locations.
   b. They are offered twice a year.
   c. They are offered three times a year.
   d. They are offered six times a year.
   e. They are offered at Prometric locations.

9. Which credential may *only* graduates of CAAHEP- and ABHES-accredited medical assisting programs earn?
   a. CCMA (NHA)
   b. CMAS (AMT)
   c. CMA (AAMA)
   d. CMAA (NHA)

10. To retain certification, industry standards require that each NHA-certified health care professional complete which of the following?
    a. 10 credits every 2 years
    b. 30 points every 3 years
    c. 30 points every 5 years
    d. 10 credits every 5 years
    e. 10 credits every 3 years

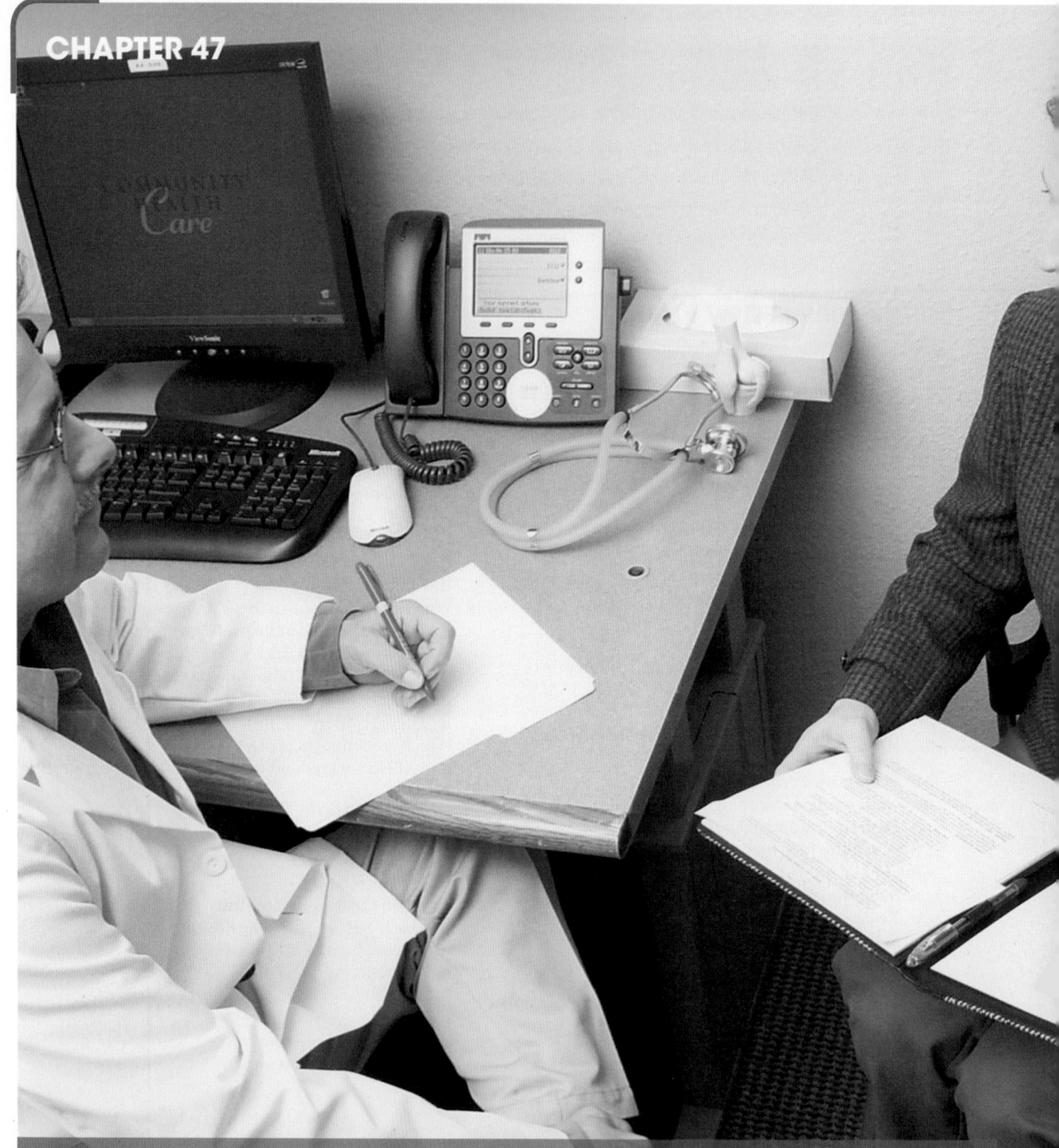

CHAPTER 47

Employment Strategies

1. Define and spell the key terms as presented in the glossary.
2. List the steps involved in job analysis and research.
3. Describe a contact tracker and its usefulness.
4. Formulate three examples of accomplishment statements.
5. Differentiate chronologic, functional, targeted, online profile, and e-résumé.
6. Identify the purpose and content of a cover letter.
7. Demonstrate effective ways to anticipate and respond to an interviewer's questions.
8. Describe appropriate overall appearance and dress for an interview.
9. Identify the benefits of writing a follow-up letter.

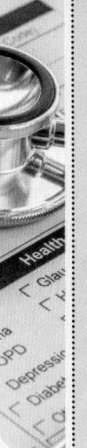

KEY TERMS

accomplishment statements	Internet blogs
application/cover letter	interview
application form	keywords
career objective	networking
chronologic résumé	profile
contact tracker	references
direct skills	résumé
e-résumé	social media
functional résumé	targeted résumé
headline	transferable skills

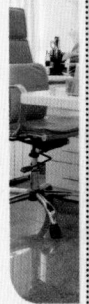

SCENARIO

Eun Mee Soo, RMA (AMT), is a graduate of an accredited medical assisting program and recently passed the national certification examination. While attending school, Eun Mee was employed part-time as a sales representative in one of the city's prestigious clothing stores. She has no medical work experience except her practicum at Inner City Health Care. She is now preparing her résumé and beginning her job search. Eun Mee plans to move out of state (she always dreamed of moving north), so she will also be looking for a new apartment. All of these changes are a bit unsettling for Eun Mee. She is beginning to wonder if she should defer relocating at this time and stay close to home until she feels more secure.

Chapter Portal

The work-a-day world is very different from what you have experienced in school. In the work world, your success or failure will not be determined by passing tests at the completion of an instructional course. Success will be based upon your attitude and performance on a day-to-day basis, sometimes under difficult and stressful conditions. This chapter will focus on helping you plan a job search strategy and prepare a résumé that presents you as a qualified candidate for the job, and it will walk you through the steps to a successful interview.

DEVELOPING A STRATEGY

It is best to begin developing your job search strategy early in your training as a medical assistant. If you have not started this phase, determine to begin today by developing a strategy that is realistic, recognizing that you and a hundred other medical assistants may be applying for the same job. How are *you* different from every other person applying for this job? The following sections will help make *you* stand out, be different, and hopefully be successful in your job search.

Attitude and Mindset

Professional

One important quality an employer looks for in employees is their attitude. Your attitude is not something you turn on and off or learn in school. It is the result of your innate personality combined with the events that mold you during your life. Your instructors and acquaintances have a significant impact over who you are. Your attitude is reflected by how you react to:

1. Taking direction
2. Seeking excellence or doing just enough to get by
3. Meeting your employer's needs, not just looking forward to payday
4. Assuming responsibility for your actions versus considering your problems to be someone else's fault

An employer will zero in on a negative attitude and eliminate you as a candidate almost immediately. While formal training is important and you can be retrained to do things the way a new employer desires, your attitude takes time to change and requires a willingness to make the change. Develop a strategy to cultivate a positive attitude while you are still in school. This is a time when you will have professional guidance and resources, as well as excellent role models to emulate.

Self-Assessment

Before starting to explore employment opportunities that are right for you, focus on yourself and build a picture of your strengths and weaknesses, what motivates you, how you relate to other people in the workplace, and how you cope with stress. The assessment should not be totally based on your own conclusions, but will require obtaining the opinions of your peers, instructors, and friends as well.

What are your strengths and weaknesses? Review your work or prior employment experience, academic studies, and outside interests as well as those things you have found difficult or challenging. Ask yourself—would I be willing to do that all day every working day? Could I obtain additional training to make myself more competent in a given task where I am weak?

What do I enjoy? Starting with the items you noted as strengths, rank them in order of how much you like doing them. Do a similar ranking of the items that are weaknesses. Make a separate list of the recreational activities you enjoy. From your list of strengths and weaknesses, build a job description for your ideal job. From your list of recreational activities, evaluate where you would like to live to continue those activities. Repeat this procedure to create a list of several jobs and locations you would enjoy.

Evaluate your working style. As part of the self-assessment, you should evaluate what direct and transferable skills you have that will make you a contributing member of the medical team. **Direct skills** are the medical skills and procedures you have acquired in school and developed proficiency in during the practicum experience. **Transferable skills** are those skills that would be useful in a wide variety of professions and may have been perfected during the education process or learned in employment settings. Leadership, communication, writing, computer literacy, keyboarding, linguistics, and spelling are some examples of transferable skills.

Think about what work environment you find most suited to your personality. Do you enjoy working with people or working alone? Are you a self-starter or do you require supervision? Do you perform well in a stressful environment? Identify what motivates you. What type of manger do you want to work for: authoritarian or participatory? When you interview, you need to interview your potential employer to determine the style of management you will encounter.

What is your salary requirement? The salary of a medical assistant varies with location, proficiency in skills, credentials, and experience. As of 2016, the national median salary is $30,135 per year, ranging from $20,021 to $41,900. As part of your preparation for seeking a position, assess your salary needs and the salary schedule in your location. You may be asked as part of the interview what salary you expect. You also need to consider the benefits offered by the employer. If your employer does not provide medical coverage, for example, this will be an expense you will need to take into consideration. Likewise, while retirement may be a long way off, an IRA plan is part of the salary compensation requiring consideration.

Research clinic profile. Is this a specialty clinic and would you enjoy working in this specialty? Evaluate what the clinic does and compare that with your moral and ethical standards. For example, if the clinic performed abortions or certain types of birth control procedures, would you be comfortable assisting?

Is there opportunity for advancement in the future? Consider where you want to be in your career in 5 or 10 years. Evaluate the opportunity for advancement at a particular clinic, or what the current and future job market looks like in a specific geographic location.

Initiative

Your employment strategy does not end with landing a position. Once hired, continue to prepare for the next step in your career. Be active in technical organizations and professional groups that help you develop future contacts. Most job opportunities are developed through **networking** or personal referrals. Prepare yourself for a more responsible position by broadening your skills. Interview for positions that advance your career even when you are currently satisfied. The key is to gain as much exposure as possible, as you may need it in the future.

THE JOB SEARCH

Many of your instructors may have contacts with prospective employers through practicum sites, and your school may have an employment office that posts employment opportunities. Take advantage of every opportunity to let people know you are looking for a job. Consider speaking with your primary care provider, your dentist, and other professionals such as your hair and nail specialists. You never know where a good lead will come from. Personal networking and **social media** will be critical to your job search.

Person-to-person networking is the linking together of individuals who, through trust and relationship-building that is genuine and authentic, advertise for one another. It should be a major part of your job search and should begin during your practicum experience. Let your practicum supervisor know your employment availability and ask if there are current or future job openings for which you might qualify. During the practicum experience, take full advantage of every opportunity to demonstrate your skills, to learn new skills, and to be a team member.

Networking also develops through student memberships and participation in AAMA, AMT, or other professional organizations. Student membership discounts are offered by these organizations and opportunities to participate in leadership roles, continuing education sessions, and observing professional behaviors are just a few of the benefits of membership. Professional organizations provide exposure through local, state, and national functions. (See Chapter 46 for additional information about professional organizations.)

Social media is currently used by more than 95% of employers seeking to fill positions with qualified applicants. Employers use social media to post positions and check the background and attitude of applicants. In today's technological setting, the first thing recruiters and employers will do is investigate you online. Be aware of any and all postings online, as they are there for the entire world to view.

LinkedIn is probably the number one site for professional networking and job search, used by over 94% of recruiters. Facebook, used by 65% of recruiters, is the largest social network and can be used to network with city, school, or workplace associates to make your position availability public knowledge. Twitter, used by 55% of recruiters, is another networking option. Participation in professional **Internet blogs** such as LinkedIn discussion groups is yet another social media avenue to explore during your job search. By establishing your own Web site, you can post your résumé, portfolio, and letters of recommendation. This platform can also be used to highlight specific skills such as critical thinking, communication, and professionalism. You will want to be sure that all information is accurate and well supported.

In order to effectively use social media, you will need to establish a professional profile and participate intelligently in group activities to establish a business-like online presence for yourself. Your online **profile** should demonstrate professional experience, tenure, and accomplished skills. It should include a summary that highlights the qualities and personal attributes that make you a good fit for the companies and organizations you are targeting. The summary can include real situations from your classroom experiences or related jobs and should include keyword-rich content. See the "Keyword Descriptors" Quick Reference Guide for a list of effective keywords that can be used in your professional profile.

Awards and Affiliations

Accrediting Bureau of Health Education Schools (ABHES)

American Association of Medical Assistants (AAMA)

American Medical Technologists (AMT)

Associate in Applied Science degree (AAS)

Cardiopulmonary resuscitation (CPR)

Certification examination

Certified Clinical Medical Assistant CCMA ((NHA)

Certified Medical Administrative Assistant CMAA (NHA)

Certified Medical Administrative Specialist CMAS (AMT)

Certified Medical Assistant CMA (AAMA)

Commission on Accreditation of Allied Health Education Programs (CAAHEP)

Continuing education units (CEUs)

National Healthcareer Association (NHA)

Registered Medical Assistant RMA (AMT)

Sample: After earning an associate in applied science (AAS) degree, sat for the certification examination and was awarded the Certified Clinical Medical Assistant (CCMA) credential from the National Healthcareer Association.

Direct Skills

Bilingual	First aid	Patient navigator/advocate	Safety issues
Charting	Infection control		Scheduling
Coding	Injections	Patient preparation	Surgical asepsis
Communication	Insurance	Pharmacology	Telephone techniques
Data entry	Interpersonal skills	Processing specimens	Valued
Diagnostic testing	Laboratory	Quality assurance	Venipuncture
Documentation of care	Medical asepsis	Reception	Vital signs
EKGs	Medical terminology	Regulatory guidelines	X-rays
Emergency management	Patient intake	Risk management	

Sample: Utilized bilingual skills to aid diverse populations to feel valued and understood during medical encounters.

Power Verbs

Assembled	Communicated	Expedited	Increased
Assessed	Compiled	Evaluated	Integrated
Assigned	Computed	Exhibited	Interpreted
Attended	Contributed	Facilitated	Justified
Budgeted	Created	Formalized	Logged
Catalogued	Delegated	Generated	Maintained
Classified	Developed	Greeted	Measured
Charted	Documented	Headed	Modified
Coded	Established	Identified	Negotiated
Collected	Evaluated	Implemented	Observed

(continues)

Operated	Recommended	Scheduled	Taught
Organized	Reconciled	Selected	Telephoned
Participated	Regulated	Served as	Trained
Perfected	Requested	Solicited	Transferred
Prepared	Responsible for	Streamlined	Verified
Procured	Retrieved	Summarized	
Proofread	Revised	Supervised	

Sample: Streamlined procedure-scheduling through the use of computer technology, decreasing patient wait time from 6 to 2 days.

Transferrable Skills

Analyzed	Enumerated	Inventoried	Specified
Accommodated	Established	Maximized	Solicited
Bilingual skills	Evaluated	Mobilized	Summarized
Brainstormed	Facilitated	People skills	Time management skills
Communication skills	Implemented	Processed	Validated
Conducted	Improvised	Quantified	Verified
Demonstrated	Incorporated	Realized	Welcomed
Displayed	Instituted	Rejuvenated	

Sample: Implemented time management skills learned while working as a server in my last position.

As part of a serious job search, you should contact many individuals and will need some means of recording the contacts, their responses, and your actions. Figure 47-1 shows a helpful sample **contact tracker**. It should be used to prevent confusion and to keep track of valuable information and action

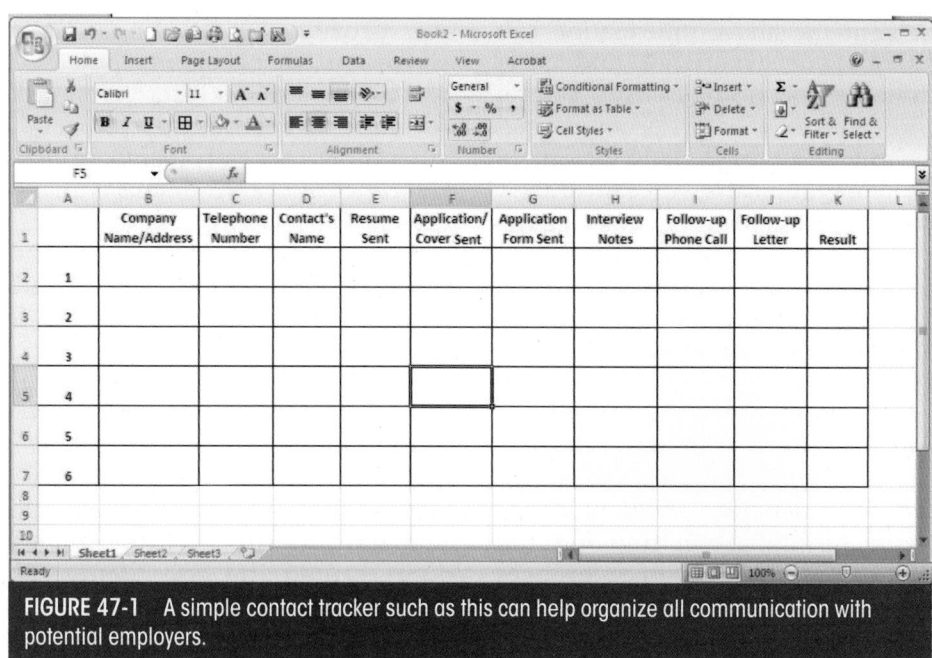

FIGURE 47-1 A simple contact tracker such as this can help organize all communication with potential employers.

items. Copy or design your own contact tracker form and document all pertinent information regarding your job search contacts.

RÉSUMÉ PREPARATION OR ONLINE PROFILE

A **résumé** is a brief presentation of your qualifications and experience in your chosen career. You need to capture in words the most important qualities and characteristics to communicate a clear vision both online and offline of who you are. Your message should be tailored to your target audience. Try to answer the following questions:

- What is your vision for the job that you are seeking?
- What are your guiding principles? (Being all you can be, decisive, driven, enjoy challenges, team-worker, etc.)
- What are your short and long-range goals?
- What are your job-specific attributes? (Use keyword-rich content.)
- What are your core technical strengths and accomplishments?
- Who is your target audience and what they are looking for in a candidate?
- What will differentiate you from your competition?
- Did you emphasize your value to the organization and position yourself as a good fit to meet the employers' needs?

How you present the above information can vary depending on your experience and background. The following section discusses several résumé styles. Regardless of style, accuracy and truthfulness are the most important factors to remember. One typographical error can destroy all you are trying to accomplish. Gross exaggerations or outright lies about your academic and employment experience are usually discovered through social media, references, or your answer to interview questions. Lies could cost you the job (see Table 47-1).

At some point, you may be asked for a list of **references** to aid the future employer in assessing the accuracy of résumé content. References should be listed on a separate sheet of paper that matches your résumé paper and has the same letterhead. Select a variety of references

TABLE 47-1

TOP 10 LIES ON RÉSUMÉS

TOP 10 SERIOUS LIES ON RÉSUMÉS	TOP 10 WHITE LIES ON RÉSUMÉS
School awarding degree	Communication skills
Foreign language fluency	Job duties in former positions
Degree received	Presentation skills
College major	Research skills
GPA	References
Work history	Computer skills
Recognition	Salary
Portfolio of projects	Graduation year
Position held (job title)	Professional memberships
College minor	Career growth

Source: http://fortune.com/2014/09/10/resume-lies-are-on-the-rise/

to be included with your résumé. An individual who knows you well or has worked with you long enough to make an honest assessment and recommendation regarding your employment history and qualifications is an excellent reference. Professional references such as a former instructor, provider, practicum supervisor, or fellow coworker are excellent choices. Use only non-related persons as references, unless you have a formal work relationship with a relative.

Always ask permission to use someone as a reference *before* the name is printed on the reference list. Verify the correct spelling of the reference's name, as well as his or her correct title, place of employment and position, and email address and telephone number for prospective employers.

Help your references aid you in obtaining an interview and employment. A personal visit or telephone call to discuss your career objectives and how you plan to conduct your job search will be helpful. Ask for any suggestions they may have to offer. Provide them with a copy of your résumé and cover letter. This helps your references visualize the position for which you are applying and picture how you may benefit that employer.

Keep in touch with references. Check back to see what prospective employers have called and types of questions asked. Add information or notes to your contact tracker. Knowing what questions employers ask of your references may produce some valuable pointers for your next letter, résumé, or interview. Finally, thank your references. They will appreciate knowing how you are doing and that you value their assistance.

Résumé Styles

Procedure

Various résumé styles have been developed, each having specific advantages and disadvantages. Choose the style or combination of styles that best describes your strengths and ability to do the job. It may be advantageous to check with the human resource department of the facility to which you are applying to determine if they have a résumé style preference. Many facilities accept only online résumés and have specific guidelines to be followed. The objective of an online résumé or online profile is different from a paper résumé. The online résumé is not tailored to a specific job, but is designed to tell who you are and to sell your personality and general qualifications. The paper résumé is designed to sell what you can do for a potential employer. If you obtain an interview from an online résumé or profile, you should also have a job-specific paper résumé and reference list available to leave with the interviewer if requested. See Procedure 47-1 for steps to prepare a résumé.

Chronologic Résumé. Your **chronologic résumé** should be organized so that the most important information you want to share is the first thing the reader sees. If your job experience is your greatest asset and may set you apart from other applicants, put your work history and job skills first. If your education and training is your best professional feature, put your education and training first. Some medical managers and human resources directors take only 10 seconds to scan a résumé. You want them to see clearly and quickly what you have to offer.

The chronologic résumé is advantageous when:

- The position is in a highly traditional field, such as teaching, law, or health care, where specific employers are of paramount interest

- You are staying in the same field as prior jobs
- Job history shows real growth and development
- Prior titles are impressive

The chronologic résumé is *not* advantageous when:

- Your work history is spotty
- You are changing career goals
- You have been in the same job for many years
- You are looking for your first job

Figure 47-2 illustrates a chronologic résumé.

Functional Résumé. The **functional résumé** highlights specialty areas of accomplishment and strengths. It allows you to organize them in an order that supports your work objective.

The functional résumé is advantageous when:

- Your experience can be sorted into areas of function, for example, administrative, clinical, supervisory
- You are changing careers
- You are reentering the job market after an absence
- Your career path or growth is not clear from a chronologic listing
- You have had a variety of different, apparently unconnected, work experiences
- Much of your work has been volunteer, freelance, or temporary
- You want to eliminate repetition of descriptions of job duties
- You have extensive specialized experience

The functional résumé is *not* advantageous when:

- You want to emphasize a management growth pattern
- Your most recent employers are highly prestigious and the specific employers are of paramount interest

A sample of a functional résumé for a person reentering the job market is shown in Figure 47-3.

Targeted Résumé. The **targeted résumé** is best for focusing on a clear, specific job target. It should contain a **career objective** and list your skills, capabilities, and any supporting accomplishments related

ASHLEY JACKSON, CMA (AAMA)
2031 Craig Street ~ Renton, Washington 98055

Work: 206-878-1545 Cell: 206-835-9879
Home: 253-838-6690 email: asjack@pinetree.com

WORK EXPERIENCE

September, 20XX–Present GROUP HEALTH COOPERATIVE
Directed support for a dermatology/surgery practice.
Patient preparation.
Medical and surgical asepsis.
Assist with sterile procedures.
Patient follow-up.

June, 20XX–August, 20XX VALLEY INTERNAL MEDICINE
Clinical responsibilities.
Assisted with surgeries in ambulatory care setting.
Patient preparation.
Medical and surgical asepsis.
Assisted with sterile procedures.

March, 20XX–June, 20XX VALLEY INTERNAL MEDICINE
Medical Assistant Practicum
Administrative duties and clinical responsibilities utilizing all medical assisting skills, including patient induction, chief complaint, vital signs, patient preparation, EKGs, medical and surgical asepsis, and sterile procedures.

EDUCATION/CERTIFICATION

Associate in Applied Science degree, June, 20XX, Highline Community College, Des Moines, Washington 98198-9800.

Certified Medical Assistant (AAMA), June, 20XX.

FIGURE 47-2 Sample chronologic résumé.

to that objective. **Accomplishment statements** begin with power verbs and give a brief description of what you did and the demonstrable results that were produced. The targeted résumé style enables graduating students to list classes related to their career objective, grade point average, student awards, and achievements. This information adds substance to a résumé when work experience is minimal and should be at the beginning of the résumé because it is your most significant asset.

The targeted résumé is advantageous when:

- You are very clear about your job target
- You have had a variety of experiences that appear unrelated to each other but that include skills that you can use in a skills list related to your job target
- You can go in several directions and want a different résumé for each
- You are just starting your career and have little experience but know what you want, and are clear about your capabilities

The targeted résumé is *not* advantageous when:

- You want to use one résumé for several different applications
- You are not clear about your abilities and accomplishments

JOAN BISHOP, RMA (AMT)
4320 Sprig Street
Renton, Washington 98055

Work: 206-878-1545   Cell: 206-835-9879
Home: 253-838-6690   email: jbishop@abc.net

TEACHING:

Instructed community groups on issues related to child abuse.

Taught volunteers how to set up community program for victims of domestic violence.

Conducted workshops for parents of abused children.

Instructed public school teachers on signs and symptoms of potential and actual child abuse.

COUNSELING:

Consulted with parents for probable child abuse and suggested courses of action.

Worked with social workers on individual cases, in both urban and suburban settings.

Counseled single parents on appropriate coping behaviors.

Handled pre-take interviewing of many individual abused children.

ORGANIZATION/COORDINATION:

Coordinated transition of children between original home and foster home.

Served as liaison between community health agencies and schools.

Wrote proposal to state for county funds to educate single parents and teachers.

WORK HISTORY:

20XX–20XX   Community Mental Health Center, Tacoma, Washington
                         Volunteer Coordinator—Child Abuse Program

20XX–20XX   C.A.R.E.—Child-Abuse Rescue-Education, Trenton, New Jersey
                         County Representative

EDUCATION:

20XX   B.S. Sociology, Douglass College, New Brunswick, New Jersey

FIGURE 47-3 Sample functional résumé. This style is useful for a person reentering the job market.

Figures 47-4A and 47-4B show samples of targeted résumés.

Online Profile. An online profile may have to follow specified rules. For example, a LinkedIn profile should employ the following tips to appear more professional:

- Establish a custom LinkedIn URL.
- Use a clear, friendly, and appropriate professional action photo of yourself. Written permission will be required if a patient is included in your action photo such as the photo used in the example.

- Make your **headline** promote your skills like a news headline. As an example, "Medical Assistant" is common and does not separate you from the other job seekers. A more exciting and enticing headline might be "Patient Friendly and Proactive Paraprofessional."

ASHLEY JACKSON, CMA (AAMA)
2031 Craig Street ~ Renton, Washington 98055

Work: 206-878-1545   Cell: 206-835-9879
Home: 253-838-6690   email: asjack@pinetree.com

CAREER OBJECTIVES: To obtain a position as a medical assistant in an ambulatory care/surgery facility that allows use and development of clinical skills.

ACHIEVEMENTS:
Certified Medical Assistant.
Graduate of an accredited medical assistant program accredited by the Commission on Accreditation of Allied Health Education Programs (CAAHEP).
Experienced in providing assistance with surgeries in an ambulatory care setting.
Excellent communication and interpersonal skills.

SKILLS AND CAPABILITIES:
Post-surgery patient follow-up.
Patient induction.
Vital signs.
Patient preparation.
EKGs.
Medical and surgical asepsis.
Sterile procedures.

WORK HISTORY:
September, 20XX to present   Group Health Cooperative, Seattle, WA
                             Surgical Medical Assistant.
June, 20XX–August, 20XX   Valley Internal Medicine, Renton, WA
                             Clinical Medical Assistant.
March 20XX–June, 20XX   Valley Internal Medicine, Renton, WA
                             Practicum Student/Trainee.

EDUCATION/CERTIFICATION:
Associate in Applied Science Degree, Highline Community College.
Certified Medical Assistant (AAMA).

AFFILIATIONS:
American Association of Medical Assistants.

FIGURE 47-4A Sample targeted résumé. This style is useful when focusing on a specific job target.

- Use action words in your target job description to show your passion for the job you are seeking.
- Your work summary should be around three to five short paragraphs, preferably with a bulleted section in the middle. It should walk the reader through your work passions, key skills, and unique qualifications. It should also list the various facilities you have had exposure to over the years. Highlight past results in your summary.
- Avoid buzzword such as *experienced* (say in what), *team player* (more specific language would be *led a team to develop office protocols*), *references available on request* (it is obvious they are). Be specific and personable.
- Highlight your achievements

Ashley Jackson, CMA (AAMA)
1321 Craig Street
Renton, Washington 98055
(253) 838-6690
Cell (206) 835-9879
Asjackson@pinetree.com

Professional Profile

Eager to utilize my medical assisting knowledge and skills in an
ambulatory/surgery facility that allows further development of clinical skills.
- Dedicated to meeting the needs of individual patients at their level of need.
- Committed team member approach to care delivered to patients.

What People Say:

"Ashley's positive attitude is a strong asset as it helps guide her actions, thoughts, and words. Ashley uses her strong knowledge base to make critical thinking choices."
    Stephanie Young, CMA (AAMA)
    Group Health Cooperative

"Ashley builds strong relationships with her co-workers, supervisors, providers, and patients. She shows interest in their lives and models respect, kindness, and empathy. She truly cares about people."
    Martha Marshall, RN
    Valley Internal Medicine

"Ashley's clinical critical thinking skills are excellent. She is competent and works well with others to see that quality care is provided to each patient in an efficient and timely manner."
    Donald Blackburn, PA
    Valley Internal Medicine

Education, Honors, and Certification

Associate in Applied Science
Highline Community College, Des Moines, Washington
Overall GPA: 3.9
Dean's List
Current Red Cross First Aid and CPR cards
Certified Medical Assistant (AAMA)
President SeaTac Chapter of AAMA

Work Experience

Group Health Cooperative Seattle, Washington
September, 20XX to present
- Post-surgery patient follow-up
- Patient induction
- Vital signs
- Patient preparation
- EKGs
- Medical and surgical asepsis
- Sterile procedures

Valley Internal Medical, Renton, Washington
June, 20XX to August, 2011
- EKGs
- Patient preparation
- Medical and surgical asepsis
- Surgical procedures

FIGURE 47-4B Sample of a more creative targeted résumé.

- Do not leave the current job entry blank. Put something like *Full-Time Student/Medical Assistant* in the current job block, and in the company block use something like *In Transition* or *Seeking Opportunity*. Many search engines will skip you if you leave a blank.

- Use the additional profiles section to showcase outside activities that are appropriate.
- Request LinkedIn recommendations from people who have complimented you on your work. As appropriate, have them highlight your skills. (See Figure 47-5.)

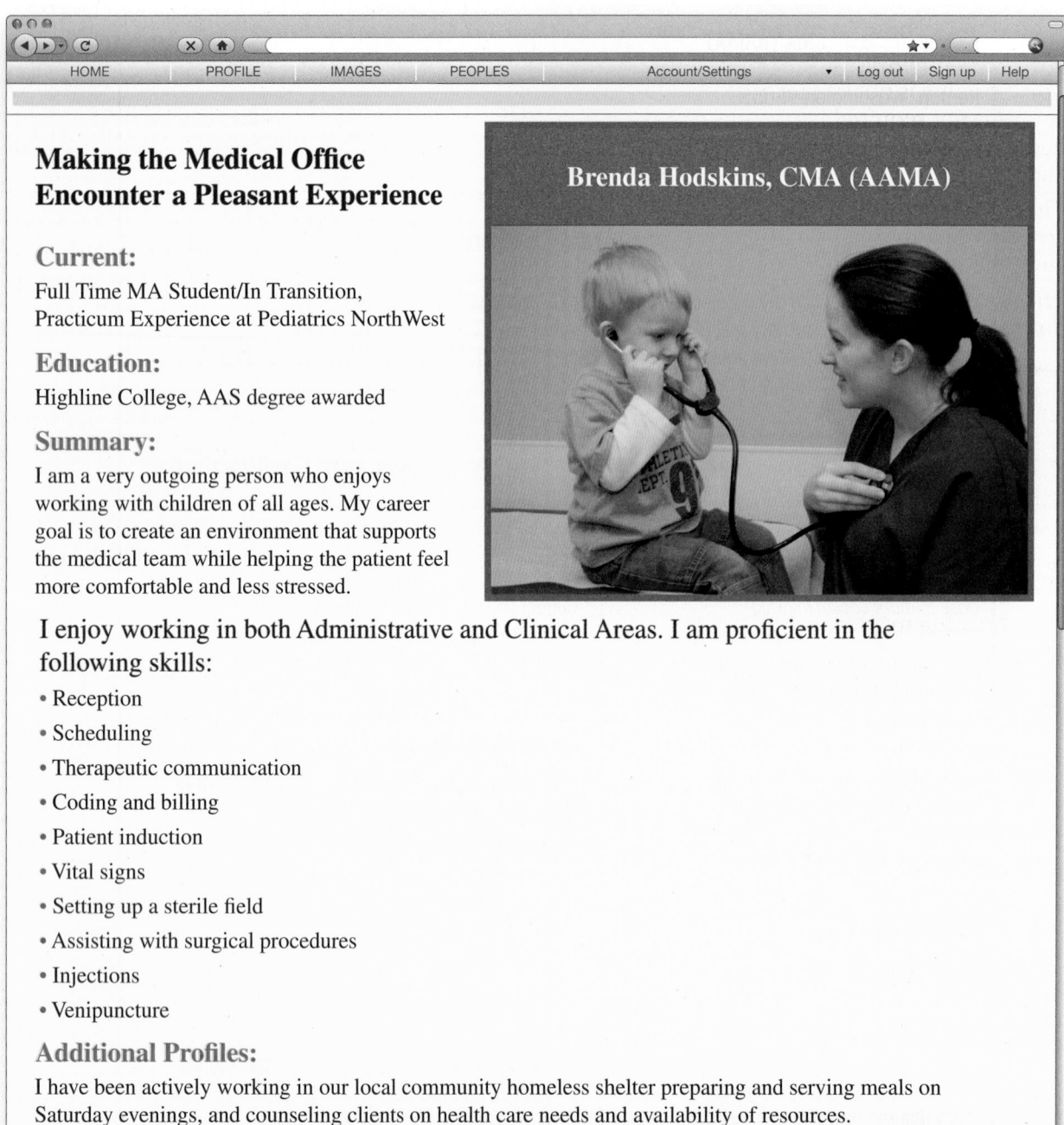

Making the Medical Office Encounter a Pleasant Experience

Brenda Hodskins, CMA (AAMA)

Current:

Full Time MA Student/In Transition,
Practicum Experience at Pediatrics NorthWest

Education:

Highline College, AAS degree awarded

Summary:

I am a very outgoing person who enjoys working with children of all ages. My career goal is to create an environment that supports the medical team while helping the patient feel more comfortable and less stressed.

I enjoy working in both Administrative and Clinical Areas. I am proficient in the following skills:

- Reception
- Scheduling
- Therapeutic communication
- Coding and billing
- Patient induction
- Vital signs
- Setting up a sterile field
- Assisting with surgical procedures
- Injections
- Venipuncture

Additional Profiles:

I have been actively working in our local community homeless shelter preparing and serving meals on Saturday evenings, and counseling clients on health care needs and availability of resources.

FIGURE 47-5 Sample online profile.

E-Résumé. An electronic résumé, also known as an **e-résumé**, is electronically delivered via email, submitted to Internet job boards, or placed on Web pages. When employers post jobs on their own Web sites, they generally expect job seekers to respond electronically.

Special care must be taken when preparing the e-résumé, as many employers place résumés directly into searchable databases. The following points should be considered:

- Formatting must be removed before the résumé can be placed in a database. Submitting a formatted résumé may cause it to be eliminated.

- Submit a text résumé, also known as a text-based résumé, plain-text résumé, or ASCII text résumé. These variations are preferred when submitting résumés electronically.

- The e-résumé is not visually appealing. Eye appeal is not required because its main purpose is to be placed into a keyword-searchable database.

- The text résumé is not vulnerable to viruses and is compatible across computer programs and platforms.

- The text résumé is versatile and can be used for:

  - Posting on job boards
  - Pasting piece-by-piece into the profile forms of job boards, such as Monster.com
  - Pasting into the body of an email to be sent to prospective employers
  - Converting to a Web-based HTML résumé
  - Sending as an attachment to prospective employers
  - Converting to a scannable résumé

Employers are often inundated with résumés from job seekers each time they advertise a position opening. Therefore, in an effort to save time and to determine the best-qualified candidates for the position, employers digitize the résumés to create an electronic résumé. Using software to search for specific **keywords** that relate to the position, the number of candidates can quickly be narrowed. If you apply for a job with a company that searches databases for keywords and your résumé does not conform, you may not be considered for the position.

How do you determine keywords? Begin scrutinizing employment ads and list keywords repeatedly mentioned in association with jobs that interest you. Nouns that relate to the skills and experience the employer is looking for will quickly surface. Keywords may include job-specific skills/profession-specific words, technologic terms and descriptions of technical expertise, job titles, certifications, types of degrees, awards received, and professional organization memberships.

Keywords should be used throughout the résumé, but they should be front loaded. Front loaded means to use as many keyword descriptors as possible in the first 100 words of the résumé. A good goal is to aim for 25 to 35 keyword descriptors. This may be achieved by using synonyms, various forms of the keyword, and both the spelled-out and acronym versions of common terms. If a person reviews the résumé, he or she will see enough keywords to process it through the software search. (Refer back to the "Keyword Descriptors" Quick Reference Guide for suggested keywords.)

PROCEDURE 47-1

Preparing a Résumé

Procedure

PURPOSE:

To prepare a résumé that presents you as a uniquely qualified candidate for a specific employment opportunity. The résumé should document your education, experience, and skills for the position to which you are applying.

EQUIPMENT /SUPPLIES:

- Computer and printer
- High-quality paper and matching envelope
- Dictionary and thesaurus
- Names, titles, addresses, telephone numbers, and email addresses of educational institutions and past employers

PROCEDURAL STEPS:

1. Check with the human resource department of a prospective employer to see if they have a résumé style preference. Many accept only online resumes.

(continues)

2. Select the résumé style, or combination of styles, that best showcases your experience and skills to a prospective employer. RATIONALE: Demonstrates your professionalism and competence level.

3. Create a letterhead that includes your legal name, address, telephone number, cell number, work telephone number, email address, and social media contact information (e.g., LinkedIn). RATIONALE: Provides all of the pertinent information a prospective employer needs to contact you.

4. Itemize your educational experience beginning with the most recent or present date, following the format for the résumé style selected.

5. List all significant employment experience beginning with the most recent or present date following the format for the résumé style selected.

6. Include other relevant information such as certifications; first aid, CPR, AIDS, or AED training; achievements; GPA and awards; memberships in professional organizations such as AAMA, AMT, NHA; community service; and volunteer programs. RATIONALE: Steps 4 through 6 provide an overall picture of the competence, skills, and professionalism you have to offer to your future employer. Be sure to front load your résumé with as many keyword descriptors as possible. Mention all direct and transferrable skills and use accomplishment statements in your narrative. This provides a clear picture of what you have to offer an employer and demonstrates your professionalism and communication skills.

7. Proofread carefully for any errors or omissions. Be sure the information is accurate and truthful. RATIONALE: Check to be sure that the grammar, spelling, punctuation, and capitalization are correct. Review the résumé carefully to ensure you have been honest and not misled an employer. Proofread several times and ask a trustworthy person that knows you well to read your résumé for accuracy and correctness in all respects.

8. Print résumé on good quality paper, at least 20- to 24-pound stock with a watermark. Choose a shade of white, cream, or gray bond paper. RATIONALE: To distinguish yourself from other candidates and to present a professional image.

9. Convert your résumé into PDF format to ensure formatting remains consistent with the printed version of your résumé.

10. Update your contact tracker. RATIONALE: To maintain current status on any and all employment opportunities.

APPLICATION/COVER LETTERS

The **application/cover letter** is a means of introducing yourself and submitting your résumé to a potential employer in response to an unsolicited application or job posting, with the goal of obtaining an interview. A well-written cover letter highlights your qualifications and experience for employment and enhances the information contained within your résumé. It should reflect how your skills satisfy the employer's needs. The letter should follow a standard business style and should not be more than one page in length. (Review Chapter 14.) It should be printed on the same type of paper as the résumé.

Because this may be your first contact with a potential employer, the letter should sell you and describe your intentions regarding employment, display your personality, and create interest in reading your enclosed résumé.

Some guidelines to follow in writing the application/cover letter include:

1. Address your letter to a specific individual whenever possible. You may need to make a telephone call to obtain the name, title, and correct spelling.

2. Keep the letter concise, use correct grammar and spelling, and follow standard business letter format (formality is key).

3. The first paragraph should state your reason for writing and focus the reader's attention. It should not give as a reason "in response to a help wanted ad" or "referral from a network contact."

4. The second paragraph should identify how your education, experience, and qualifications relate to the job and refer to the enclosed résumé.

5. The last paragraph should close with a request for an interview.

6. Have someone with management experience review your cover letter. This could be your practicum supervisor, an instructor, a friend, or an acquaintance who is in a supervisory position.

7. Do not reproduce cover letters. An original letter should be sent to each individual.

8. The cover letter should be placed on top of the résumé and mailed in a business-size envelope that matches its contents or in an 8½-by-11 manila envelope containing your return address.

9. Do not staple the cover letter to the résumé.

A sample of an application/cover letter is shown in Figure 47-6A.

An alternate example of an application/cover letter using Information Mapping® to highlight and draw attention to specific information in your letter is shown in Figure 47-6B. This format is considered easier to read because the focus is on specific blocks of information. In addition, its uniqueness draws attention to your letter and may result in your being selected when competition is keen.

2031 Craig Street
Renton, Washington 98055
August 22, 20XX

Sarah Molles, Manager
Seattle Group Health Cooperative
304 Fourth Avenue
Seattle, Washington 98124-1716

Dear Ms. Molles:

I am interested in the medical assistant position to assist in a dermatology surgery practice. I meet the qualifications and would like to be considered for the position.

I am currently a certified clinical medical assistant certified through the National Healthcareer Association (NHA). I have experience as a clinical assistant in an internal medicine clinic and have excellent communication and interpersonal skills.

I will be available for an interview Tuesday and Thursday afternoons from 1:00 p.m. to 4:00 p.m. I will call you next Thursday to set up an appointment for an interview.

Yours truly,

Porscha Dolan, CCMA (NHA)

Enclosure, Résumé

FIGURE 47-6A   Sample application/cover letter.

2031 Craig Street
Renton, Washington 98055
August 22, 20XX

Sarah Molles, Manager
Seattle Group Health Cooperative
304 Fourth Avenue
Seattle, Washington 98124-1716

SUBJECT: SURGICAL MEDICAL ASSISTANT POSITION

Background	I am interested in the medical assistant position to assist in a dermatology surgery practice. I meet the qualifications and would like to be considered for the position.
Qualifications	I am currently a certified medical assistant graduated from a 2-year program accredited by the Commission on Accreditation of Allied Health Education Programs (CAAHEP). I have experience as a clinical assistant in an internal medicine clinic and have excellent communication and interpersonal skills.
Requested Action	I will be available for an interview Tuesday and Thursday afternoons from 1:00 p.m. to 4:00 p.m. I will call you next Thursday to set up an appointment for an interview.

Yours truly,

Ashley Jackson, CMA (AAMA)

Enclosure, Résumé

FIGURE 47-6B Sample information mapped application/cover letter.

COMPLETING THE APPLICATION FORM

Sooner or later during the job search you will be asked to complete an **application form**. In most cases this will be an online activity. How well you complete this task may be a key factor in obtaining an interview and that first job.

Reading through the application form questions, you may be tempted to write "See résumé" rather than repeat pertinent information already contained within your résumé. Do not fall into this pitfall. Answer every item completely. The application is organized in the manner that suits the clinic, whereas individual résumés are organized in a variety of ways. Finding specific information on a résumé is more time consuming for the clinic, whereas finding the same information on the job application is easy and quick because they know where to look for it. Read all the directions carefully. Look for seemingly insignificant directions placed at the top or bottom of the page that state "Print Carefully," "Complete in Your Own Hand-writing," or "Please Type." Employers may use this to assess your ability to read and follow directions and pay attention to detail.

If the application is to be handwritten, use black ink to complete the form. Black ink is considered legal, often is an indelible (permanent) ink, and is more legible if the form must be duplicated. Concentrate when completing the form and be sure to print clearly and make no errors. When possible, copy the application before beginning in case an error is made.

The current trend is toward online application forms. These forms are prepared by keying information into the appropriate spaces or blocks by using a computer. The completed forms are printed and mailed to the prospective employer or sent electronically. Sending electronically is increasingly the preferred method. All of the concerns relative to care in following instructions, providing complete and accurate information, and proofreading the application for any errors before sending are applicable.

If you are asked to list experience but the application does not specify "paid experience," be sure to list any volunteer or practicum experience that relates to the position you are seeking. Volunteer work can be important as an indicator of your willingness to work, your ability to serve the public, and your organizational skills.

You may be asked to complete the application form "on the spot." Plan ahead for this event and carry a completed copy of your résumé, reference list, and application/cover letter with you. These documents should provide all the information needed to complete the application form and may be submitted with the application form. This demonstrates to the potential employer your seriousness and preparedness for finding a job. Also carry with you information not included in your résumé, such as which years you attended high school and your salary history. A pocket spelling wordbook or dictionary may be a useful tool to carry for those who find spelling challenging.

THE INTERVIEW PROCESS

Professional

If your application/cover letter, résumé, and application form have made a favorable impression with the organization, you may be invited for an interview. An **interview** is a meeting in which you and the interviewer discuss the employment opportunities within that particular organization. It is the interviewer's responsibility to determine if you are the right fit to be a part of the team. The interviewer uses the interview process to assess appearance, attitude, and dependability. The interviewer also tries to verify that you have been honest in the skills you claim to have mastered. You, on the other hand, are selling your qualifications and assessing if this is an organization in which you want to be employed.

Being well prepared for the interview will increase your self-confidence and ability to focus during the actual interview. Knowing that your application/cover letter, résumé, and references all support your career goal and objectives allows you time to concentrate on interview preparation and presentation.

The Look of Success

The look of success begins with the outward appearance. First impressions are lasting, so strive for a favorable, professional look from head to toe. Appropriate conservative attire is important. Remember, your goal is to sell your professional abilities.

Hair should be clean and healthy looking, and worn in an appropriate style for the ambulatory care setting. Long hair should be worn off the collar in perhaps a French braid or twist. Strive for a neat, professional style.

The skin should have a healthy glow. Consultation with a cosmetician may prove helpful in solving skin problems or may provide an opportunity for trying new products. A basic understanding of your personal skin type and selection of cosmetics that complement your skin tone aid in the presentation of a professional appearance. The natural look is most appropriate for the medical clinic.

A daily shower and use of personal hygiene products is advised. Remember to use caution where perfumes and scents are concerned because many magnify when the body is under stress and the scent may be offensive or cause allergic reactions in others. Smokers should be aware that smoke odor carries in their hair, skin, and clothing. This odor may not be acceptable in health care settings.

Fingernails should be short and oval shaped or have rounded corners. Only clear nail polish should be worn in the ambulatory care setting if you are not working in the clinical area. Nail polish that is chipped or cracked must be removed or replaced immediately because it creates crevices in which pathogens may hide, multiply, and spread.

First impressions are lasting, so make yours professional in all respects. Smart casual attire is appropriate for both men and women. This consists of a skirt and blouse or a tailored pantsuit for women and slacks and dress shirt with or without a tie for men. Pay attention to details such as your accessories and shoe selection. Accessories should be small and tasteful. Shoes should be clean, polished, and in good repair. They should fit properly and be comfortable and easy to walk in (Figure 47-7). Women may carry a small purse if necessary. Be sure that your cell phone is turned off before entering the clinic.

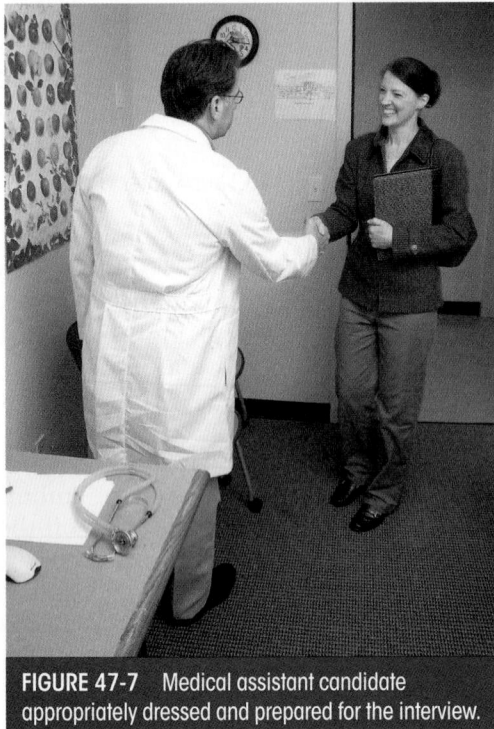

FIGURE 47-7 Medical assistant candidate appropriately dressed and prepared for the interview.

When you feel well and know that you look good, you project a confident and professional appearance. In other words, you are professionally poised. *Webster's Dictionary* defines *poise* as balance and stability; ease and dignity of manner. Personal poise combines all of the previously mentioned body appearances plus smoothness of movement and physical flexibility.

Preparing for the Interview

Before the interview takes place, carefully research the organization offering the position. Study the organization's mission statement, financial reports, future projections, and any other information available. Be prepared to relate your skills and interests to the needs of this organization. In other words, what can you contribute and why should they hire you? The interview is your opportunity to sell yourself and identify ways in which you can benefit the employer.

A portfolio is recommended in which to keep an extra copy of your résumé, reference list, application, and cover letter. An interviewer may ask for these documents especially if you have applied online. You should also have copies of letters of recommendation, a copy of your transcript from the schools you attended, and copies of any certificates such as AIDS training, first aid,

CPR, and AED training. These items should not be presented unless dictated by events that take place during the interview. You might also have with you the name of the interviewer and a copy of any questions you plan to ask the interviewer. A last-minute review will refocus your thoughts before you go into the interview. Keep your list available for quick reference in the event your mind goes blank when you are asked if you have questions.

To arrive 5 to 10 minutes early, check a map for directions or make a trip the day before your interview. Try to travel about the same time as you would for the interview so you have an idea of the time it takes, traffic flow, construction areas encountered, and parking availability. Plan for inclement weather (raincoat, umbrella, shoes). It is a good idea to make a quick trip to the restroom on arrival to change shoes or recheck your appearance.

Introduce yourself confidently to the administrative medical assistant and identify by name the person you wish to see and the time of your appointment. Always arrive alone. The employer wants to see you and sense your self-reliance and responsibility. While you wait, try to relax and observe the clinic setting, other employees, what they are wearing, and their manner of conducting business. This may be helpful to you during the interview and in making a decision to work there.

The following Quick Reference Guide lists reasons employers do not hire applicants.

The Actual Interview

When you enter an interviewer's office, think of yourself as a guest and take your cues from him or her. Most interviewers will introduce themselves and extend a hand. A firm handshake, responding by introducing yourself, and smiling confidently convey a positive professional image. Remain standing until you are invited to be seated. Keep

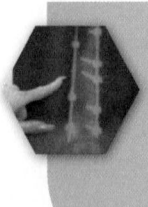

Critical Thinking

If you are a smoker, how can you minimize the smoke odor carried on your person before you go on a job interview? Make a list and prioritize each suggestion into a plan of action.

Reasons for Employers Not Hiring

Employers in business were asked to list reasons for not hiring a job seeker. Given in rank order (from most unwanted to least unwanted), the 15 biggest gripes are as follows:

1. Poor appearance (not dressed properly, poorly groomed)
2. Acting like a know-it-all
3. Cannot express self clearly; poor voice, diction, grammar
4. Lack of planning for work—no purpose or goals
5. Lack of confidence or poise
6. No interest in or enthusiasm for the job
7. Not active in school extracurricular programs
8. Interested only in the best dollar offer
9. Poor school record (academic, attendance)
10. Unwilling to start at the bottom
11. Making excuses, hedges on unfavorable record
12. No tact
13. Not mature
14. No curiosity about the job
15. Critical of past employers

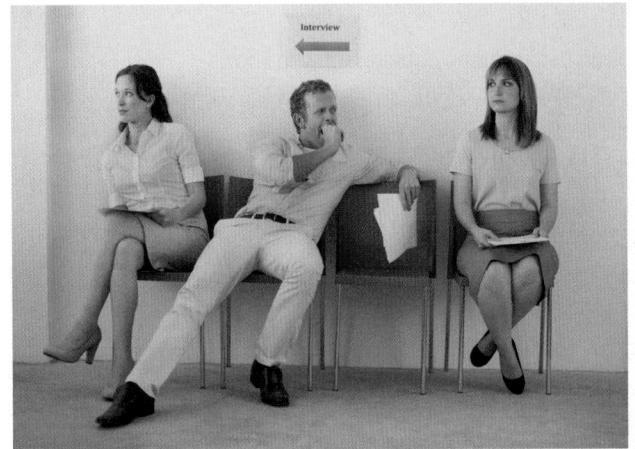

© PeopleImages.com/gettyimages.com

your personal items on your lap or place them on the floor near your chair. Do not invade the interviewer's territory by placing your things on the desk.

Sit erect in the chair with your feet flat on the floor or cross only your ankles. Avoid nervous mannerisms while you speak and maintain good eye contact, but do not stare the interviewer down. Be natural and positive about the position, organization, and yourself. Present a professional image by using medical terminology when responding to questions or providing information. Observe the interviewer carefully for cues. Respond to questions completely, trying not to repeat yourself or give more information than was requested.

Be prepared for the kinds of questions that may be asked during the interview process. Ask yourself, "If I were the employer, what would I want to know about the applicant?" Examples of standard questions asked by most employers are provided in the following Quick Reference Guide. Consider how you would respond to each question.

Remember that the interviewer is asking questions to determine if you are qualified for the position and if you are the kind of person who will fit into the organization. *Think* before answering questions; try to provide the information requested in a positive and professional manner. Do not respond with slang terms. *Listen* carefully so that you understand what information the question is requesting. *Ask* for clarification if you are uncertain. This demonstrates your ability to be open enough to ask questions when in doubt.

Typical Questions Asked During An Interview

- I see from your résumé you graduated from ___ college. What did that college have to offer that others didn't?
- What subjects did you enjoy the most and why?
- What do you see yourself doing 5 years from now?
- What salary do you expect and what do you think it will be in 5 or 10 years?
- What do you consider to be your greatest strengths and weaknesses?
- How do you think a friend or professor who knows you well would describe you?
- What qualifications do you have that make you think you would be successful in this position?
- In what ways do you think you can make a contribution to our organization?
- What two or three accomplishments have given you the most satisfaction?
- What didn't you like about your last employer?
- How well do you work under pressure?
- Will you be able to work overtime occasionally?
- How do you respond to criticism?
- How would you respond if a patient or coworker made advances toward you?
- How would you handle following procedures with which you do not agree?
- Describe a specific medical procedure.
- Do you have any questions you would like to ask?
- How would you establish credibility quickly with our team?
- What attracted you to this clinic?
- What is the last book you read?
- Why should we hire you?
- What is your personal mission statement?

INTERVIEW
☑ Experience
☑ Communication
☑ Education
☑ Skills

© iQoncept/shutterstock.com

Interviewing the Employer

The worst thing that can happen to an entry-level employee is to be hired and then have to quit or be fired because of a conflict with the employer. The interview process is a two-way street. You, the interviewee, should also interview the potential employer. The following are danger signs of an employer who could make your work life very difficult:

- Disrespectful behavior during the interview toward other staff members or you
- Signs of insecurity by the manager
- Lack of enthusiasm toward the organization
- Signs of being highly stressed
- Negative attitude in statements
- Arrogance or answers own questions
- Uses the pronoun *I* excessively

You have to "read" the interviewer because some of the signs listed could be attributed to a "bad day." If too many signals are showing or, after prudent questioning on your part, you still have concerns, perhaps you should look for employment elsewhere to avoid the possibility of damaging your future career.

Following are a few questions you might ask the interviewer to resolve some of these concerns raised by observations:

- How would you describe the clinic culture?
- How do you handle differing opinions on how best to accomplish tasks?
- How are employee accomplishments recognized?
- What is the leadership style at the clinic?
- What is the attitude toward professional growth and educational opportunities?

Answers to these questions will help you determine if the clinic culture is one you can embrace.

Closing the Interview

By observing the interviewer and listening carefully, you will be able to determine when the interviewer feels he or she has enough information about you to make a decision. Usually during the closing the interviewer asks if you have any additional questions. This is your opportunity to collect information helpful in making a decision to accept or decline an offer. Your questions provide another opportunity to sell yourself, show that you have done your homework about the organization, and have listened carefully during the interview. Select three or four questions that will help you the most.

Questions about the organization are excellent choices. Examples are:

- What are the opportunities for advancement with this organization?
- I read that your organization has educational benefits. Could you explain briefly how that program works?
- You mentioned in-house training programs for employees. Could you give one or two examples?

You may also have some questions about the job itself. Examples of these types of questions are:

- Is this a newly created position? If so, what results are you hoping to see?
- Was the last person in this position promoted? What contributed to his or her advancement?

- What do you consider the most difficult task on this job?
- What are the lines of authority for this position?

Do not use this question time to ask about salary, sick leave, vacations, or retirement benefits. At this point, your focus should be on the value and skills you can contribute to the organization. These questions may be asked during a second interview or when a position is offered.

Before you leave, thank the interviewer for taking time to discuss the position with you. If you definitely are interested in the position, ask to be considered as a candidate for the position. If follow-up procedures have not been explained, now is the time to ask when the final selection will be made and how you will be notified. A firm handshake as you leave, a pleasant smile, and confidence as you exit will leave a professional picture in the interviewer's mind.

INTERVIEW FOLLOW-UP

Following up after the interview is essential. Remember to update your contact tracker with the date and method of your follow-up. If a question caught you off-guard, formulate a response for future interviews. It is now time to telephone your references to let them know the name of the organization and the person's name with whom you interviewed, something about the position, and your qualifications. Share any information that will help your references support you in obtaining the position.

Follow-Up Letter

Procedure

Take time to write a follow-up letter or handwritten note to the interviewer a day or two after your interview to thank him or her for the time spent interviewing you. The handwritten note should be a simple professional-looking thank you blank note card used to express your appreciation for the interview. Handwriting should neat and aligned evenly. A request to be considered for the position may be reiterated if you truly are interested in the position. The follow-up letter should be written in standard business format and printed on the same paper as your application/cover letter, references, and résumé. Be sure that all spelling and grammar are correct (see Procedure 47-2).

The follow-up letter provides another opportunity to express your interest in the organization and the position. You can briefly emphasize the experience and skills you have to offer and again request to be considered a candidate for the position.

Record the mailing date on your contact tracker and keep a copy of the letter in a file with other

PROCEDURE 47-2

Prepare an Interview Follow-Up Letter

Procedure

PURPOSE:

To write an error-free follow-up letter or handwritten thank you note in appreciation for a job interview and to express continued interest in the position posted.

EQUIPMENT/SUPPLIES:

- Computer and printer
- High-quality paper and envelope
- Addressee's name, title, and address
- Dictionary and thesaurus

PROCEDURAL STEPS:

1. Collect the needed equipment and information required to write the letter.

2. Follow standard business format for writing the letter. If handwriting a note, be sure to use good penmanship. RATIONALE: Following up after an interview provides yet another opportunity to express your interest in the position, to briefly emphasize the experience and skills you can contribute, and to request being considered for the position.

3. Proofread carefully to be sure that the grammar, spelling, punctuation, and capitalization are correct. RATIONALE: To present a professional image and an error-free résumé.

4. Print the letter on good quality paper, at least 20- to 24-pound stock with a watermark. Choose a shade of white, cream, or gray bond paper. RATIONALE: To distinguish yourself from other candidates and to present a professional image.

5. Sign the letter and place the original in the addressed envelope to be mailed.

6. Update your contact tracker and maintain a copy of the letter in your file. RATIONALE: To maintain current status on any and all employment opportunities.

---

information about the organization. Figure 47-8 shows a sample follow-up letter.

Follow Up by Telephone

Allow a few days for your follow-up letter to reach the interviewer. If you do not hear from the interviewer within a week or by the designated time established during the interview, you may call to ask if you are still being considered for the position or if a decision has been made.

Speak directly into the mouthpiece of the telephone using good diction and voice volume. Identify yourself and provide some information to aid the interviewer in recalling who you are. Perhaps mentioning the date you interviewed will suffice. Be polite and professional, and remember to thank the individual for speaking with you. At the end of the conversation say good-bye and wait until the other person hangs up before you break the connection. Log the telephone call and its response on your contact tracker for future reference.

AFTER YOU ARE EMPLOYED

You are now a newly employed medical assistant. What do you do now to advance your career? Following are some suggestions:

- Make sure your workstation is set up and you have what you need to do the job.
- Practice good time management skills.
- Try to allow time for emergencies, which will occur.
- Do not be a know-it-all; ask other employees how they do things around here.
- Get to know colleagues and be part of the team.
- Seek feedback on how you are doing your job.
- Create a professional image.

Dealing with Difficult People

Sooner or later you will encounter co-workers who could be described as just plain "jerks." Jerks may

2031 Craig Street
Renton, Washington 98055
August 28, 20XX

Sarah Molles, Manager
Seattle Group Health Cooperative
304 Fourth Avenue
Seattle, Washington 98124-1716

Dear Ms. Molles,

Thank you for scheduling a personal interview with me last Wednesday, August 26, at 9:45AM. I enjoyed discussing the medical assistant position open in one of your dermatology surgery practices. I would like to be considered for the position.

After talking with you, I feel my qualifications match closely with those you requested. My communication and interpersonal skills are excellent and a necessary ingredient for any medical assistant.

I look forward to hearing from you September 5 as you mentioned during the interview. If there are any questions I may answer, please telephone me.

Sincerely,

Ashley Jackson, CMA (AAMA)
(206) 255-1365

FIGURE 47-8 Sample follow-up letter.

be defined as persons who use power to belittle and ridicule people who work under them. These people may be foul-mouthed, power hungry, bullies, uncouth, or unethical. There are several ways to free yourself from jerks:

- Check out emotionally (attempt to ignore the comments); indifference is an underrated virtue.
- Try to move to a different position within the organization.
- If all else fails, change jobs.

Getting a Raise

One of the main reasons people do not get a raise is because they do not ask. This is particularly true of professional women. It has been reported that less than half ask for a raise or promotion within the first 12-month working period. Of those that ask, almost three quarters received a raise or promotion. After taking into consideration the wages of persons with similar job descriptions and experience, if your salary appears to be lagging, you should not feel uncomfortable asking for a raise at your next favorable performance review.

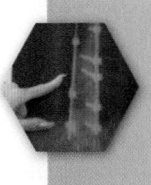

Critical Thinking

As you begin to prepare for a job interview, how can you prepare yourself to reflect a professional image, attitude, and demeanor, and verbal and nonverbal communication skills, as well as articulately describe your skills and abilities to fit the position to which you are applying? Develop a complete written checklist and review it before each interview.

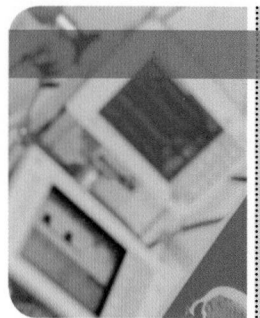

CASE STUDY 47-1

Refer to the scenario at the beginning of the chapter.

CASE STUDY REVIEW

1. Which résumé style represents Eun Mee best and why?
2. List transferable skills that Eun Mee may want to include in her résumé.
3. What is the purpose of an accomplishment statement? Provide examples Eun Mee might use.

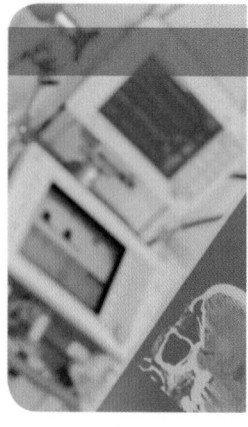

CASE STUDY 47-2

Drs. Lewis and King are part of a multi-provider family practitioner clinic. They are in need of a new medical assistant to take the place of one who will be leaving at the end of the month. They have scheduled interviews with five applicants. Eun Mee Soo is the first candidate to be interviewed.

CASE STUDY REVIEW

1. Eun Mee wants to bring some papers to the interview. What is the best way to do this? What paperwork would be appropriate to bring with her?
2. Why should Eun Mee arrive 5 to 10 minutes early for the interview?
3. How should Eun Mee enter the room?

Summary

- Begin the job search while still in school and look for ways to distinguish yourself from other applicants.
- Remember that attitude and mindset are important qualities employers look for.
- Self-analysis aids in the overall picture of who you are and what you are looking for in an employment package. In addition, it helps with résumé and interview techniques.
- Choose the résumé style that best reflects what you have to offer a future employer. Use keyword descriptors to describe the skills and attributes you possess.
- Your employment package should include a well-written, accurate résumé, reference sheet, and application/cover letter. Complete the application form if requested to do so. Include copies of any pertinent awards, certifications, and letters of recommendation in your employment package.
- Dress for success for the interview and be prepared by preplanning answers to questions that may be asked or that you may want to ask.
- Interview follow-up may include a thank you letter and/or a telephone call.

Study for Success

To reinforce your knowledge and skills of information presented in this chapter:

- Review the *Key Terms* and *Learning Outcomes*
- Consider the *Critical Thinking* features and *Case Studies* and discuss your conclusions
- Answer the questions in the *Certification Review*

Procedure

- Perform the *Procedures* using the *Competency Assessment Checklists* on the *Student Companion Website*

CERTIFICATION REVIEW

1. Which response best describes a résumé?
   a. It is a summary or brief account of your qualifications and progress in your career.
   b. It is also known as a contact tracker.
   c. It always includes references.
   d. It is known as an e-résumé.

2. Which of the following statements is true of references?
   a. References must always be listed on the résumé.
   b. A reference should be a relative.
   c. A reference should be someone who likes you and your work but may not be a good communicator.
   d. A reference should be someone who knows you or has worked with you long enough to make an honest assessment of your capabilities and integrity.
   e. References must only be persons with whom you have worked.

3. When is it advantageous to use the targeted résumé style?
   a. When prior titles are impressive
   b. When reentering the job market after an absence
   c. When you are just starting your career and have little experience
   d. When you have extensive specialized experience

4. Which of the following is true of the application/cover letter?
   a. It is a detailed data sheet describing your vital information, education, and experience.
   b. It introduces you to a prospective employer and captures their interest in you as a candidate for the position.
   c. It lists individuals who can vouch for you.
   d. It should be lengthy and detailed.
   e. It thanks the employer for reviewing your résumé.

5. Which of the following is true of the interview?
   a. It does not require much thought or preparation.
   b. It requires you to think before answering questions, listen carefully, and ask for clarification if uncertain of the question.
   c. It provides time to ask questions about salary, vacation, and benefits.
   d. It does not require any follow-up.

6. Which task is *not* involved in self-assessment?
   a. Compiling a list of potential employers
   b. Identifying your strengths and weaknesses
   c. Listing things you enjoy
   d. Researching the clinic profile
   e. Evaluating your work style

7. What is the purpose of a résumé?
   a. To sell yourself
   b. To provide references
   c. To assist in maintaining your contact tracker
   d. To provide an opportunity to use social media

8. Which social media avenue is the number one networking site for the job search?
   a. The Internet
   b. Internet blogs
   c. Facebook
   d. LinkedIn
   e. Twitter

9. Which of the following best describes the term *accomplishment statement*?
   a. It is comprised of keywords descriptors that give a brief description of what you did and the results produced.
   b. It is a list of contacts and their responses and your actions.
   c. It is a list of who you know or have worked with.
   d. It is a brief account of your qualifications and progress in your career.

10. Which of the following responses is not included in follow-up after the interview?
    a. Telephoning references to update them
    b. Sending a follow-up letter to the interviewer
    c. Asking references to call the interviewer and put in a good word for you
    d. Following up with the interviewer by telephone
    e. Updating contact tracker information

APPENDIX A
Common Health Care Abbreviations and Symbols

AAMA	American Association of Medical Assistants
AAP	American Academy of Pediatrics
AAPC	American Academy of Professional Coders
ab	abortion
abd	abdomen
ABE	acute bacterial endocarditis
ABG	arterial blood gases
ABHES	Accrediting Bureau of Health Education Schools
ABO	blood grouping system
ac	acute
	before meals (ante cibum)
AC	alternating current
ACA	Affordable Care Act
ACAP	Alliance of Claims Assistance Professionals
ACIP	Advisory Committee on Immunization Practices
ACO	Accountable Care Organization
ACOG	American Congress of Obstetricians and Gynecologists
ACS	American Cancer Society
ACTH	adrenocorticotropic hormone
ADA	Americans with Disabilities Act
ADAAA	Americans with Disabilities Act Amendments Act of 2008
ADAD	autosomal dominant Alzheimer's disease
ADHD	attention deficit hyperactivity disorder
ADL	activities of daily living
ad lib	as desired
adm	admission
ADR	alternative dispute resolution
AED	automated external defibrillator
AES	Advanced Encryption Standard
Afib	atrial fibrillation
AFP	alpha-fetoprotein
AHA	American Heart Association
AHD	arteriosclerotic heart disease
	atherosclerotic heart disease
AHDI	Association for Healthcare Documentation Integrity
AHIMA	American Health Information Management Association
AIDS	acquired immunodeficiency syndrome
AIIR	airborne infection isolation room

Alb	albumin
ALP	alkaline phosphatase
ALT	alanine aminotransferase
	argon laser trabeculoplasty
AM	before noon (ante meridiem)
AMA	against medical advice
	American Medical Association
AMBA	American Medical Billing Association
AMI	acute myocardial infarction
amt	amount
AMT	American Medical Technologists
AMTIE	American Medical Technologists Institute for Excellence
ant	anterior
ante	before
AP	anterior/posterios
A&P	anatomy and physiology
	anterior and posterior
	auscultation and palpation
	auscultation and percussion
APC	ambulatory payment classifications
APGAR	appearance, pulse, grimace, activity, and respiration
Apps	applications
Aq	water (aqua)
A/R	accounts receivable
ARDS	acute (or adult) respiratory distress syndrome
ARRA	American Recovery and Reinvestment Act
ARU	automated routing unit
ASA	acetylsalicylic acid
ASAP	as soon as possible
ASC	atypical squamous cell
ASCAD	arteriosclerotic coronary artery disease
	athrosclerotic coronary artery disease
ASC US	atypical squamous cell of uncertain significance
ASCVD	arteriosclerotic cardiovascular disease
	atherosclerotic cardiovascular disease
ASD	autism spectrum disorder
ASRT	American Society of Radiologic Technologists
AST	aspartate aminotransferase
AV	atrioventricular
A&W	alive and well
Ax	axillary

Ba	barium
BaE	barium enema
BBB	bundle branch block
BC	birth control
BC/BS	Blue Cross/Blue Shield
BCP	birth control pills
BE	bacterial endocarditis
BHRT	bioidentical hormone replacement therapy
bid	twice a day
bil	bilateral
BM	basal metabolism
	bowel movement
BMI	body mass index
BMR	basal metabolism rate
BNA	budget neutrality adjuster
BNP	B-type natriuretic peptide
BP	blood pressure
B/P	blood pressure
BPH	benign prostatic hypertrophy
BRCA1	breast cancer susceptibility protein mutations 1
BRCA2	breast cancer susceptibility protein mutations 2
BS	blood sugar
	bowel sounds
	breath sounds
BSA	body surface area
BSE	bovine spongiform encephalopathy
	breast self-exam
BSL	blood sugar level
BSN	bowel sounds normal
BSO	bilateral salpingo-oophorectomy
BSR	blood sedimentation rate
BUN	blood urea nitrogen
BW	birth weight
	blood work
	body weight
Bx	biopsy
C	Celsius
	Centigrade
	cup
C1	first cervical vertebra
Ca	calcium
CA	cancer
	carcinoma
CAAHEP	Commission on Accreditation of Allied Health Education Programs
CAD	computer-aided detection
	coronary artery disease
CAHD	coronary arteriosclerotic heart disease
	coronary athersclerotic heart disease
CAM	complementary and alternative medicine
caps	capsules
CARE	Consistency, Accuracy, Responsibility, and Excellence in Medical Imaging and Radiation Therapy Act of 2013
CAT	computerized axial tomography
cath	catheterization
CBC	complete blood count
CBT	computer-based testing

CC	chief complaint
CCA	Certified Coding Associate
CCHIT	Certification Commission for Health Information Technology
CCMA (AMT)	Certified Clinical Medical Assistant through American Medical Technologists
CCP	Certification Continuation Program
CCR	continuity of care record
CCS	Certified Coding Specialist
CCS-P	Certified Coding Specialist–Physician-Based
CCT	cardiac computerized tomography
CCU	coronary care unit
C&D	cystoscopy and dilation
CDC	U.S. Centers for Disease Control and Prevention
CE	continuing education
CEA	carcinoembryonic antigen
cerv	cervical
	cervix
CEU	continuing education unit
CF	conversion factor
CHAMPVA	Civilian Health and Medical Program of the Department of Veterans Administration
CHD	childhood disease
	congenital heart disease
	congestive heart disease
	coronary heart disease
CHEDDAR	chief complaint, history, examination, details of problems, drugs and dosages, assessment, return visit if applicable
CHF	congestive heart failure
CHO	carbohydrate
CHP	Chemical Hygiene Plan
CIN	cervical intraepithelial neoplasia
CJD	Creutzfeldt-Jakob disease
ck	check
Cl	chlorine
cldy	cloudy
CLIA	Clinical Laboratory Improvement Amendments
cm	centimeter
CMA (AAMA)	Certified Medical Assistant through the American Association of Medical Assistants
CMAA (NHA)	Certified Medical Administrative Assistant through the National Healthcareer Association
CMAS (AMT)	Certified Medical Administrative Specialist through American Medical Technologists
CME	continuing medical education
CMR	cardiac magnetic resonance
CMS	Centers for Medicare and Medicaid Services
CMT	Certified Medical Transcriptionist
CNS	central nervous system
C/O	complains of
CO_2	carbon dioxide
COB	coordination of benefits
COPD	chronic obstructive pulmonary disease
COW	Certificate of Waiver
CPAP	continuous positive airway pressure
CPC	Certified Professional Coder
CPC-A	Certified Professional Coder–Apprentice

CPC-H	Certified Professional Coder–Hospital	DPM	doctor of podiatric medicine
CPC-HA	Certified Professional Coder–Hospital Apprentice	DPT	diphtheria, pertussis, and tetanus
CPE	complete physical exam	Dr	doctor
CPR	cardiopulmonary resuscitation	DR	delivery room
CPT	Current Procedural Terminology	DRGs	diagnosis-related groups
CPU	central processing unit	DS	discharge summary
CR	computed radiography	DSD	dry sterile dressing
CRB	Curriculum Review Board	dsg	dressing
crit	hematocrit	DT	delirium tremens
CRP	C-reactive protein	DTaP	diphtheria and tetanus toxoids and acellular pertussis vaccine, pediatric formulation
CS	cerebrospinal		
	cesarean section	DTR	deep tendon reflex
C&S	culture and sensitivity	D&V	diarrhea and vomiting
CSF	cerebrospinal fluid	DW	distilled water
CT	computerized tomography	D/W	dextrose in water
CVA	cerebrovascular accident	dx	diagnosis
CVE	capsule video endoscopy	DXA	dual-energy X-ray absorptiometry
CVP	central venous pressure		
CVS	chorionic villus sampling	ea	each
cx	cervix	EAP	extensible authentication protocol
CXR	chest X-ray	EBV	Epstein–Barr virus
cysto	cystoscopic examination	ECC	emergency cardiac care
	cystoscopy	ECG	electrocardiogram
		echo	echocardiogram
			echoencephalogram
DACUM	developing a curriculum	E. coli	Escherichia coli
DARP	data, assessment, response, plan	ECT	electroconvulsive therapy
d/c	discharge		electronic claims transmission
	discontinue	ED	erectile dysfunction
DC	doctor of chiropractic		emergency department
	discontinue	EDB	expected date of birth
	discharge	EDC	estimated date of confinement
D&C	dilation and curettage		expected date of confinement
DDS	doctor of dentistry	EDD	estimated date of delivery
DEA	U.S. Drug Enforcement Agency		expected date of delivery
DEERS	Defense Enrollment Eligibility Reporting System	EEG	electroencephalogram
		EENT	eyes, ears, nose, and throat
del	delivery	e.g.	for example
DES	diethylstilbestrol	EGD	esophagogastric duodenoscopy
DHHS	U.S. Department of Health and Human Services	EHR	electronic health record
		EKG	electrocardiogram
diab	diabetic	elix	elixir
	diabetes	email	electronic mail
diag	diagnosis	EMG	electromyography
diff	differential white blood cell count	EMR	electronic medical record
dil	dilute	EMS	emergency medical service
Disp	dispense	ENT	ear, nose, and throat
dL	deciliter	EO	ethylene oxide
DM	diabetes mellitus	EOB	explanation of benefits
DNA	deoxyribonucleic acid	eos	eosinophil
	does not apply	EPA	Environmental Protection Agency
DNR	do not resuscitate	EPCA-2	early prostate cancer antigen-2
DO	doctor of osteopathy	EPO	Exclusive Provider Organization
DOA	dead on arrival	eq	equivalent
DOB	date of birth	ER	emergency room
DOD	date of death	ERCP	endoscopic retrograde cholangiopancreatography
DOE	dyspnea on exertion		
dos	dosage	ERT	estrogen replacement therapy
DPI	dry powder inhaler	ERV	expiratory reserve volume

ESR	erythrocyte sedimentation rate
ESRD	end-stage renal disease
EST	electroshock therapy
exam	examination
ext	extract
F	Fahrenheit
FAM	fertility awareness methods
FAS	fetal alcohol syndrome
FAST	face drooping, arm weakness, speech, time to call 911
fax	facsimile
FBS	fasting blood sugar
FDA	U.S. Food and Drug Administration
Fe	iron
FECA	Federal Employees Compensation Act Program
FEF	forced expiratory flow
FEV	forced expiratory volume
FGM	female genital mutilation
FH	family history
FHR	fetal heart rate
FHS	fetal heart sound
fl	fluid
fl oz	fluid ounce
FLMA	Family and Medical Leave Act
FMP	first menstrual period
FP	family practice
freq	Frequent
FSH	follicle-stimulating hormone
ft	foot
FTA	fluorescent treponemal antibody
FTP	file transfer protocol
FTT	failure to thrive
FVC	forced vital capacity
fx	fracture
g	gram
G	Gravida
	gauge
gal	gallon
GB	gallbladder
GC	gonococcus
	gonorrhea
GERD	gastroesophageal reflux disease
GGT	gamma glutamyltransferase
GI	gastrointestinal
GIFT	gamete intrafallopian transfer
Gm	gram
GP	general practice
GPCI	Geographic Practice Cost Index
gr	grain
grav	pregnancy
GTH	gonadotropic hormone
GTT	glucose tolerance test
gtt(s)	drop (drops)
GU	genitourinary
GYN	gynecology

h	hour
HAART	highly active antiretroviral therapy
HAI	health care–associated infection
HAV	hepatitis A
HBIG	hepatitis B immune globulin
HBP	high blood pressure
HBV	hepatitis B
HCFA	U.S. Health Care Financing Administration
hCG	human chorionic gonadotropin
HCl	hydrochloric acid
HCP	health care provider
HCPCS	Healthcare Common Procedure Coding System
Hct	hematocrit
HCV	hepatitis C
HCVD	hypertensive cardiovascular disease
HDL	high-density lipoprotein
HDV	hepatitis D
HEENT	head, eyes, ears, nose, and throat
HEPA	high-efficiency particulate air
HEV	hepatitis E
Hgb	hemoglobin
HGP	Human Genome Project
H&H	hemoglobin and hematocrit
Hib	*haemophilus influenza* type b
HIC number	the identification number of a Medicare beneficiary issued by CMS or the RRB
HIDA scan	hepatobiliary iminodiacetic acid scan
HIPAA	Health Insurance Portability and Accountability Act
HIV	human immunodeficiency virus
HITECH	Health Information Technology for Economic and Clinical Health Act
HMO	health maintenance organization
H/O	history of
H₂O	water
H&P	history and physical
HPI	history of present illness
HPV	human papillomavirus
HR	human resources
HRS	Healthcare Reimbursement Specialist
HRT	hormone replacement therapy
HSV1	herpes simplex virus 1
HSV2	herpes simplex virus 2
ht	height
HT	hormone therapy
hx	history
Hz	Hertz
IBS	irritable bowel syndrome
ICCU	intensive coronary care unit
ICD	implantable cardioverter-defibrillator
ICD-9-CM	International Classification of Diseases, 9th revision, Clinical Modification
ICD-10-CM	International Classification of Diseases, 10th revision, Clinical Modification
ICU	intensive care unit

ID	intradermal	LE	lupus erythematosus
I&D	incision and drainage	LEEP	loop electrosurgical excision procedure
IDDM	insulin-dependent diabetes mellitus	LGBT	lesbian, gay, bisexual, transgender
IDS	integrated delivery system	LHRH	luteinizing hormone-releasing hormone
IIS	immunization information system	Liq	liquid
IM	internal medicine	LL	left leg
	intramuscular	LLQ	lower left quadrant
	infectious mononucleosis	LMP	last menstrual period
imp	impression	LP	lumbar puncture
IN	intranasal	LRQ	lower right quadrant
inf	infusion	LUQ	left upper quadrant
Inj	injection	L&W	living and well
INR	international normalization ratio	lymphs	lymphocytes
I&O	intake and output		
IOM	Institute of Medicine	M	male
IP	inpatient	m	meter
IPA	independent provider association	MA	medical allowable
IPV	inactive poliovirus	Mac	Macintosh (Apple computer)
	intimate partner violence	MBCD	management by coaching and development
IPPB	intermittent positive pressure breathing	MBCE	management by competitive edge
IPPS	inpatient prospective payment systems	MBDM	management by decision models
ISMP	Institute of Safe Medicine Practices	MBP	management by performance
ISP	Internet service provider	MBS	management by styles
IT	information technology	MBWA	management by wandering around
IUD	intrauterine device	MBWS	management by work simplification
IV	intravenous	mcg	microgram
IVF	in vitro fertilization	MCHC	mean corpuscular hemoglobin and red cell indices
IVP	intravenous pyelogram	MCO	managed care organization
		MCV	mean corpuscular volume and red cell indices
JAAMT	*Journal of the American Association for Medical Transcription*	MD	doctor of medicine
			muscular dystrophy
JAMA	*Journal of the American Medical Association*	MEF	mean expiratory flow
JCAHO	Joint Commission on Accreditation of Healthcare Organizations	MDI	metered dose inhaler
		MDR	minimum daily requirement
		med	medicine
K	potassium	mEq	milliequivalents
kg	kilogram	MFS	Medicare fee schedule
KOH	potassium hydroxide	mg	milligram
KUB	kidney, ureter, and bladder	MH	marital history
kV	Kilovolt		medical history
KVO	keep vein open		menstrual history
		MHT	menopausal hormonal therapy
l	length	MHx	medical history
L	liter	MI	maturation index
LA	left atrium		myocardial infarction
	lactic acid	MICE	motion, ice, compression and elevation
	left arm	mL	milliliter
L&A	light and accommodation	mm	millimeter
lab	laboratory	mm³	cubic millimeter
lac	laceration	MMA	Medicare Prescription Drug Improvement and Modernization Act
LAC	long arm cast		
LAN	local area network	mm Hg	millimeters of mercury
lap	laparotomy	MMR	measles, mumps, and rubella
LASIK	laser-assisted in-situ keratomileusis	MOM	milk of magnesia
lat	lateral	mono	mononucleosis
lb	pound	MP	menstrual period
LBBB	left bundle branch block	MRC	Medical Reserve Corps
LDH	lactate dehydrogenase		
LDL	low-density lipoprotein		

MRI	magnetic resonance imaging
MRIA	magnetic resonance imaging angiography
MRSA	methicillin-resistant *Staphylococcus aureus*
MS	mitral stenosis
	multiple sclerosis
MSAFP	mother's serum alpha-fetoprotein
MSHA	Mine Safety and Health Administration
MT	medical technologist
	medical transcriptionist
multip	multipara
MVP	mitral valve prolapse
MVV	maximum voluntary ventilation
NA	not applicable
NaCl	sodium chloride
NACP	National Association of Claims Assistance Professionals
NAPPSI	National Alliance for the Primary Prevention of Sharps Injuries
narc	narcotic
NB	newborn
NBSTSA	National Board of Surgical Technology and Surgical Assisting
N/C	no complaints
NCAI	National Coalition for Adult Immunization
ND	doctor of naturopathy
NDC	National Drug Code
NEBA	National Electronic Billers Alliance
NEC	not elsewhere classified
neg	negative
NG	nasogastric
NGU	nongonococcal urethritis
NHA	National Healthcareer Association
NIDA	National Institute on Drug Abuse
NIDDM	noninsulin-dependent diabetes mellitus
NIH	National Institutes of Health
NL	normal limits
NLNA	National League for Nursing Accrediting
NMP	normal menstrual period
noct	at night
Non-PAR	nonparticipating provider
NOS	not otherwise specified
NPI	national provider identification
NPO	nothing by mouth
NR	no refill
	nonreactive
	normal range
	nonspecific
NS	normal saline
	not significant
	not sufficient
NSAID	nonsteroidal anti-inflammatory drug
N&T	nose and throat
N&V	nausea and vomiting
NVD	nausea, vomiting, and diarrhea
O	oral
O_2	oxygen

OB	obstetrics
OB-GYN	obstetrics-gynecology
OC	office call
	on call
	oral contraceptive
occ	occasionally
OCR	Office of Civil Rights
	optical character reader
OGTT	oral glucose tolerance test
OM	office manager
OOB	out of bed
OP	outpatient
O&P	ova and parasites
OPD	outpatient department
OPIM	other potentially infectious material
OPPS	a system that classifies all hospital outpatient services into Ambulatory Payment Classifications for reimbursement
	outpatient prospective payment systems
OPV	oral polio vaccine
OR	operating room
	operative report
ortho	orthopedics
os	mouth
OSHA	U.S. Occupational Safety and Health Administration
OT	occupational therapist
	occupational therapy
OTC	over the counter
OURQ	outer upper right quadrant
OV	office visit
OWCP	Office Workers' Compensation Programs
oz	ounce
P	phosphorus
	pulse
PA	physician's assistant
	posteroanterior
P&A	percussion and auscultation
PAC	phenacetin, aspirin, and codeine
	premature atrial contraction
PACS	picture archiving and communications systems
Pap	Papanicolaou (smear, test)
PAR	participating provider
para	number of pregnancies
para I	primipara
PAT	paroxysmal atrial tachycardia
path	pathology
PBI	protein-bound iodine
pc	after meals
PC	personal computer
PCA	patient-controlled analgesic
PCC	Poison Control Center
PCMH	patient-centered medical home
PCN	penicillin
PCP	primary care provider
PCR	polymerase chain reaction
PCV	packed cell volume

PDA	personal digital assistant	PSDA	Patient Self-Determination Act
PDR	*Physician's Desk Reference*	PSRO	Professional Standards Review Organization
PE	physical examination	pt	patient
peds	pediatrics		pint
PEG	percutaneous endoscopic gastrostomy	PT	physical therapy
	pneumoencephalography		prothrombin time
Peg-IFN	pegylated interferon	PTA	prior to admission
per	by or with	PTCA	percutaneous transluminal coronary angioplasty
PERF	peak expiratory flow rate		
PERRLA	pupils equal, round, regular, react to light, and accommodation	PTT	partial thromboplastin time
		PUBS	percutaneous umbilical blood sampling
PET	positron emission transmission or tomography	pulv	powder
		PVC	premature ventricular contraction
PFT	pulmonary function testing	PVP	photoselective vaporization of the prostate
pH	hydrogen in concentration	px	physical examination
PH	past history		prognosis
	personal history		
	public health	QA	quality assurance
PHI	protected health information	q AM	every morning
PHO	physician-hospital organization	qh	every hour
PI	present illness	q (2, 3, 4)h	every 2, 3, or 4 hours
	pulmonary infarction	qid	four times a day
PID	pelvic inflammatory disease	QISMC	Quality Improvement System for Managed Care
PKU	phenylketonuria		
PM	after noon (post meridiem)	qns	quantity not sufficient
	post mortem (after death)	qt	quart
PMN	polymorphonuclear neutrophils		
PMP	past menstrual period	R	right
PMS	premenstrual syndrome		respirations
PNC	penicillin		rectal
PRNT	plague reduction neutralization test	RA	right arm
PO	postoperative	RAM	random access memory
po	by mouth (per os)	RBC	red blood cell
POB	place of birth	RBC/hpf	red blood cells per high power field
POCT	point of care testing	RBCM	red blood cell mass
POL	physician office laboratory	RBCV	red blood cell volume
POLST	Physician Orders for Life-Sustaining Treatment	RBRVS	Resource-Based Relative Value Scale
		REM	rapid eye movement
POMR	problem-oriented medical record	resp	respiration
pos	positive	Rh	rhesus (factor)
POS	point-of-service	Rh−	rhesus negative
postop	postoperative	Rh+	rhesus positive
PP	present problem	RHD	rheumatic heart disease
	postprandial	RICE	rest, ice, compression, and elevation
PPB	positive pressure breathing	RL	right leg
PPBS	postprandial blood sugar	RLQ	right lower quadrant
PPD	purified protein derivative	RMA (AMT)	Registered Medical Assistant through American Medical Technologists
PPE	personal protective equipment		
PPO	preferred provider organization	RNA	ribonucleic acid
preop	preoperative	R/O	rule out
primip	woman bearing first child	ROA	received on account
prn	as the occasion arises, as necessary	ROM	range of motion
procto	proctoscopy		read-only memory
prog	prognosis	ROS	review of systems
PROM	premature rupture of membranes	ROTA	rotavirus
pro-time	prothrombin time	RPR	rapid plasma reagin test
PRSP	penicillin-resistant *Streptococcus* pneumonia	RSV	respiratory syncytial virus
		RT	radiation therapy
PSA	prostate-specific antigen		

RUQ	right upper quadrant
RV	residual volume
RVUs	relative value units
Rx	prescription
S	subjective data (POMR)
SA	sinoatrial
S&A	sugar and acetone (urine)
SAC	short arm cast
SARS	severe acute respiratory syndrome
SBE	shortness of breath on exertion
	subacute bacterial endocarditis
SDS	safety data sheet
SE	standard error
sed rate	sedimentation rate
segs	segmented neutrophils
seq	sequela
SF	scarlet fever
	spinal fluid
SG	specific gravity
SH	social history
SIDS	sudden infant death syndrome
sig	instructions, directions
sigmoid	sigmoidoscopy
SIL	squamous interepithelial lesion
SMA 12/60	Sequential Multiple Analyzer (12-test serum profile)
SOAP	subjective data, objective data, assessment, and plan
SOAPER	subjective, objective, assessment, plan, education, response
SOAPIER	subjective, objective, assessment, plan, implementation, evaluation, response
SOB	shortness of breath
SOF	signature on file
sol	solution
solv	solvent
SOMR	source-oriented medical record
SOP	standard operating procedure
SOS	if necessary
spec	specimen
sp gr	specific gravity
spont ab	spontaneous abortion
SQ	subcutaneous
SR	sedimentation rate
SS	signs and symptoms
SSI	Supplemental Security Income
SSL	service sockets layer
Staph	*Staphylococcus*
stat	immediately
STD	sexually transmitted disease
Strep	*Streptococcus*
subq	subcutaneous
supp	suppository
surg	surgery
sx	signs
	symptoms
sym	symptoms
syr	syrup

T	temperature
T3	tri-iodothyronine
T4	thyroxine
TA	temporal artery
T&A	tonsillectomy and adenoidectomy
tab	tablet
TB	tuberculin
	tuberculosis
Tbs	tablespoon
TC	throat culture
	tissue culture
	total capacity
	total cholesterol
Td	tetanus and diphtheria immunization
TDD	telecommunication device for the deaf
TDM	therapeutic drug monitoring
temp	temperature
TENS	transcutaneous electrical nerve stimulator
TESE	testicular sperm extraction
TFTC	Task Force for Test Construction
ther	therapy
therap	therapeutic
TIA	transient ischemic attack
tid	three times a day
TIG	tetanus immune globulin
tinct	tincture
TKO	to keep open
TLC	tender loving care
	total lung capacity
TLS	transport layer security
TMJ	temporomandibular joint
top	topically
TOPV	trivalent oral poliovirus vaccine
TP	total protein
tPA	tissue plasminogen activator
TPI	treponema pallidum immobilization test
TPMS	Total Practice Management System
TPN	total parenteral nutrition
TPR	temperature, pulse, and respiration
tr	tincture
trig	triglycerides
TSH	thyroid-stimulating hormone
tsp	teaspoon
TSS	toxic shock syndrome
TTY	teletype communications
TUNA	transurethral needle ablation
TURBT	transurethral resection of bladder tumor
TURP	transurethral resection of prostate
tus	cough
Tx or tx	treatment
T&X	type and cross match
Tym	tympanic
UA	urinalysis
UB04	Uniform Bill 04
UCG	urinary chorionic gonadotropin
UCHD	usual childhood diseases
UCR	usual, customary, reasonable
ULQ	upper left quadrant

ung	ointment
UNICEF	United Nations International Children's Emergency Fund
UR	utilization review
urg	urgent
URI	upper respiratory infection
URL	Uniform Resource Locator
urol	urology
URQ	upper right quadrant
URT	upper respiratory tract
URTI	upper respiratory tract infection
USB	universal system bus port
USDA	United States Department of Agriculture
USDE	United States Department of Education
USMLE	United States Medical Licensing Examination
USP	United States Pharmacopoeia
UT	urinary tract
UTI	urinary tract infection
UV	ultraviolet
Vac	vaccine
VAERS	Vaccine Adverse Event Reporting System
vag	vagina
	vaginal
VD	venereal disease
VDRL	Venereal Disease Research Laboratory
VIS	vaccine information statement
vit	vitamin
vit cap	vital capacity
VoIP	voice over Internet protocol
vol	volume
VRE	vancomycin-resistant enterococcus
VRS	voice recognition software
VS	vital signs
VSED	voluntarily stop eating and drinking
VT	tidal volume
V tach	ventricular tachycardia
WAN	wide area network
WBC	white blood cell
WCE	wireless capsule endoscopy
WDWN	well developed, well nourished
WHI	Women's Health Initiative
WHO	World Health Organization
WN	well nourished
WNF	well-nourished female
WNL	within normal limits
WNM	well-nourished male

WO	written order
w/o	without
wt	weight
WVE	wireless video endoscopy
x	multiply by
XDR TB	extensively drug-resistant tuberculosis
XR	X-ray
XRA	X-ray angiography
X-ray	radiograph or radiogram
YOB	year of birth
yr	year
ZIG	zoster immunoglobulin

Symbols

*	birth
†	death
♂	male
♀	female
+	positive
−	negative
±	positive or negative, indefinite
÷	divide by
=	equal to
>	greater than
<	less than
×	multiply by
#	number, pound
'	foot, minute
"	inch, second
ā	before
c̄	with
Δ	change
°	degree
Ⓛ	left
p̄	after
q̄	each; every
®	registration
s̄	without
s̄s̄	one-half
x̄	except
	without

GLOSSARY OF TERMS

Note: The equivalent Spanish word follows in parentheses in blue.

abduction (abducción) motion away from the midline of the body (Ch. 32).

ABO blood group (grupo sanguíneo ABO) genetically determined system of antigens found on the surface of erythrocytes. The population can be divided into four ABO blood groups: A, B, AB, and O (Ch. 43).

abortion (aborto) expulsion of the products of conception before viability (Ch. 25).

abrasion (abrasión) a superficial scraping of the epidermis (Ch. 8).

absorption (absorción) the process whereby the drug passes into the body fluids and tissues (Ch. 34).

abuse (abuso) misuse; excessive or improper use, especially of narcotics or psychoactive drugs (Ch. 16, 34).

accession record (numeric system) (registro de entrada [sistema de ordenación por número]) logbook used to assign numbers to correspondence or patients (Ch. 13).

accomplishment statements (declaraciones de logros) statements that begin with a power verb and give a brief description of what you did, and the demonstrable results that were produced (Ch. 47).

accountable care organization (ACO) a group of health care providers (doctors, other primary care providers, clinics, and hospitals) that voluntarily organize in order to provide coordinated and high-quality care to their Medicare patients (Ch. 2).

accounting (contabilidad) system of monitoring the financial status of a facility and the financial results of its activities, providing information for decision making (Ch. 20).

accounts payable (cuentas por pagar) sum owed by a business for services or goods received (Ch. 18); also unwritten promise to pay a supplier for property or merchandise purchased on credit or for a service rendered (Ch. 20).

accounts receivable (cuentas por cobrar) amount owed to a business for services or goods supplied (Ch. 18).

accounts receivable (A/R) ratio assets (relación de cuentas por cobrar a activos) outstanding accounts receivable divided by the average monthly gross income for the past 12 months (Ch. 19, 20).

accreditation (acreditación) process whereby recognition is granted to an educational program for maintaining standards that qualify its graduates for professional practice; to provide with credentials (Ch. 1).

Accrediting Bureau of Health Education Schools (ABHES) (Junta de Acreditación de Escuelas de Educación en Salud [ABHES]) entity accrediting private, postsecondary institutions in the United States which offer allied health education programs as well as programmatic accreditation of medical assistant, medical laboratory technician, and surgical technology programs (Ch. 46).

accrual basis accounting (contabilidad según el principio del devengo) reports income at the time charges are generated (Ch. 20).

acid–base balance (equilibrio ácido-básico) condition that occurs when the net rate at which the body produces acids or bases is equal to the net rate at which acids or bases are excreted (Ch. 41).

acquired immunodeficiency syndrome (AIDS) (síndrome de inmunodeficiencia adquirida [SIDA]) disorder of the immune system caused by a human immunodeficiency virus (HIV), a retrovirus that destroys the body's ability to fight infection. As the disease progresses, the individual becomes overcome by disorders, including cancers and opportunistic infections. There is no known cure for AIDS (Ch. 21).

active listening (escucha activa) received message is paraphrased back to the sender to verify the correct message was decoded (Ch. 4).

activities of daily living (ADL) (actividades de la vida diaria [AVD]) activities usually performed during a typical day that involve caring for oneself, such as eating and brushing teeth (Ch. 32).

acupuncture (acupuntura) treatment to relieve pain and disease by puncturing the skin with thin needles at specific points (Ch. 2).

acute or adult respiratory distress syndrome (ARDS) (Síndrome de dificultad respiratoria aguda o de adulto [ARDS]) a life-threatening condition that occurs when there is severe fluid buildup and hemorrhage in the lungs (Ch. 29).

acute stress (estrés agudo) the most common form of stress; occurs with rapid onset. It comes from demands and pressures of the recent past and anticipated demands and pressures in the future. It is thrilling and exciting in small doses, but too much is exhausting (Ch. 3).

additive (aditivo) any material placed in a tube that maintains or facilitates the integrity and function of the specimen (Ch. 39).

adduction (aducción) motion toward the midline of the body (Ch. 32).

adjustments (ajustes) increases or decreases to patient accounts not due to charges incurred or payments received (Ch. 16, 18).

administer (administrar) to give a medication (Ch. 6, 34, 35).

administrative law (derecho administrativo) establishes agencies that are given the power to make laws and enact regulations (Ch. 6).

aegis (auspicio) sponsorship or protection (Ch. 37).

aerobic (aerobio) organism that requires oxygen for survival and growth (Ch. 21, 42).

aerosolized (aerosolizado) dispensed by means of a mist (Ch. 26).

aerosols (aerosoles) particles from potentially infectious materials that may be released in the air (Ch. 42).

afebrile (afebril) without fever (Ch. 23).

Affordable Care Act (ACA) act signed into law in March 2010 by President Barack Obama with the goal of placing individuals, families, and small businesses in control of their health care (Ch. 1).

agar (agar) a gelatin-like substance extracted from red algae that contains nutrients and moisture for bacteria growth (Ch. 42).

ageism (discriminación por edad) a form of stereotyping that discriminates against individuals on the basis of their age (Ch. 28).

agenda (orden del día) printed list of topics to be discussed during a meeting, sometimes giving time allocation (Ch. 14, 44).

agent (agente) person representing another (Ch. 6).

airborne transmission (transmisión por aire) spread of disease-causing microorganisms through the air (Ch. 21).

aliquot (alícuota) part of the whole specimen that has been taken off for use or storage (Ch. 39).

allergies (alergias) acquired hypersensitivity to a substance (allergen) that does not normally cause a reaction (Ch. 22).

alternative dispute resolution (ADR) (resolución alternativa de conflictos [RAC]) an alternative to trial that encourages the parties to settle their differences out of court (Ch. 6).

amblyopia (ambliopía) a condition in which one eye has stronger vision than the other one. It is a disorder caused by the eye and the brain not working together. Also known as lazy eye (Ch. 29).

ambulation (ambulación) the activity of walking around. To walk, the act of walking (Ch. 32).

ambulatory care setting (entorno de atención ambulatoria) health care environment where services are provided on an outpatient basis. *Ambulatory* is from Latin and means "capable of walking." Examples include the solo provider's office, the group practice, the urgent care center, and the health maintenance organization (Ch. 1, 2).

American Association of Medical Assistants (AAMA) (Asociación Estadounidense de Asistentes Médicos [AAMA])   professional organization dedicated to serving the interests of Certified Medical Assistants (Ch. 46).

American Medical Technologists (AMT) (Tecnólogos Médicos Estadounidenses [AMT])   national organization which credentials health care professionals, including Registered Medical Assistants (RMA) and Certified Medical Administrative Specialists (CMAS) (Ch. 46).

amino acid (aminoácido)   basic structural unit of protein (Ch. 33).

amniocentesis (amniocentesis)   surgical puncture of the amniotic sac to remove fluid for laboratory analysis (Ch. 25).

amniotomy (amniotomía)   artificial rupture of the amniotic sac (Ch. 25).

amoebic dysentery (disentería amébica)   infectious intestinal disease caused by amoebas and characterized by inflammation of the mucous membrane of the colon (Ch. 21).

amorphous (amorfo)   shapeless; possessing no definite form (Ch. 41).

amplified (amplificado)   made larger or enlarged. The amplifier of the electrocardiograph enlarges the electrical impulse activity and the recording can be read more easily (Ch. 36).

amplitude (amplitud)   amount, extent, size, abundance, or fullness (Ch. 36).

anaerobic (anaerobio)   refers to an organism that needs little or no oxygen for survival or growth (Ch. 21, 42).

anaphylaxis (anafilaxia)   hypersensitive state of the body to a foreign protein or drug (Ch. 8, 29, 34).

ancillary services (servicios auxiliares)   professional companies hired to complete a specific job (Ch. 44).

andropause (andropausia)   midlife changes in a male (Ch. 28).

anesthesia (anestesia)   loss of feeling or sensation; an anesthetic is any mechanism that causes anesthesia (Ch. 30).

angina   a symptom of inadequate blood flow to the heart that is evidenced by pain in the chest, arm, neck or a combination of these (Ch. 28).

angina pectoris   see angina (Ch. 36).

angiogram (angiograma)   series of X-rays of a blood vessel(s) after injection of a radiopaque substance (Ch. 36).

anisocytosis (anisocitosis)   marked variation in the size of cells (Ch. 40).

anorexia [nervosa] (anorexia)   loss of appetite (Ch. 29).

answering services (servicios de respuesta)   services employed to answer the calls of an ambulatory care setting after hours; unlike an answering machine, a live operator answers the call and forwards it appropriately (Ch. 11).

antibodies (anticuerpos)   specific chemicals produced by B cells of the immune system in response to an antigen (Ch. 21).

anticoagulant (anticoagulante)   chemical in a blood tube that prevents the clotting of the blood by removing the calcium from the blood or by stopping the formation of 39).

antigen (antígeno)   substance such as bacteria or other agents that the body recognizes as foreign, the stimulus for antibody production (Ch. 40)

antioxidant (antioxidante)   something that prevents oxidation (Ch. 33).

aphasia (afasia)   the inability to speak (Ch. 29).

apical (apical)   pertaining to the apex of the heart. A site for measuring heart rate with a stethoscope (Ch. 23).

apnea (apnea)   cessation or absence of normal spontaneous breathing (Ch. 23, 35).

appendicular skeleton (esqueleto apendicular)   skeleton that consists of the pectoral and pelvic girdles and the upper and lower extremities. The pelvic girdle attaches the upper extremities to the trunk (Ch. 29).

application/cover letter (solicitud/carta de presentación)   letter used to introduce yourself and your résumé to a prospective employer with the goal of obtaining an interview (Ch. 47).

application form (formulario de solicitud)   form devised by a prospective employer to collect information relative to qualifications, education, and experience in employment (Ch. 47).

application software (software de aplicación)   software that performs a specific data-processing function (Ch. 10).

approximate (aproximar)   to bring together the edges of a wound (Ch. 30).

arbitration (arbitraje)   a form of dispute resolution that allows a neutral party to settle the dispute (Ch. 6).

arrhythmia(s) (arritmia)   deviations from the normal pattern or rhythm of the heartbeat (Ch. 23, 36).

arteriosclerosis (arteriosclerosis)   hardening of the arteries caused by buildup of plaque, a deposit of fatty substances on the artery lining (Ch. 28).

articulating (elocuente)   expressing oneself clearly and distinctly (Ch. 11).

artifact (artefacto)   the signal distortion which interferes with or obscures the interpretation of a study (Ch. 36).

ascorbic acid (ácido ascórbico)   vitamin C (Ch. 33).

aseptic (aséptico)   freedom from any infectious material; absence of microorganisms (Ch. 21).

assay (ensayo)   analysis of a substance to determine constituents and relative proportion of each (Ch. 38).

assets (activos)   properties of value that are owned by a business entity (Ch. 20).

assignment of benefits (asignación de beneficios)   signing over of benefits by the beneficiary to another party (Ch. 16).

assistive device   a walking aid, such as a walker, crutch, or cane (Ch. 32).

associate's degree (Título de técnico)   a degree granted by a junior college at the end of a two-year course (Ch. 1).

Association for Healthcare Documentation Integrity (AHDI) (Asociación para la Integridad de la Documentación del Cuidado de la Salud [AHDI])   professional organization in the field of medical transcription/editing (Ch. 15).

assumptive coding (suposición de codificación)   assuming a positive lab value can be coded as a disease or condition (Ch. 17).

ataxia (ataxia)   defective muscular coordination, primarily seen when attempting voluntary muscular movements (Ch. 24).

atherosclerosis (aterosclerosis)   a form of arteriosclerosis marked by calcium deposits in the arterial linings (Ch. 23).

attributes (atributos)   inherent characteristics (Ch. 1).

auditor (auditor)   a person responsible for determining the final content of a document and the document's correctness in every aspect (Ch. 15).

augment (aumentar)   to add or increase (Ch. 36).

auricle (aurícula)   the external ear; also called pinna (Ch. 29).

auscultation (auscultación)   the diagnostic listening to the sounds of the inner workings of the body using a stethoscope (Ch. 24).

authoritarian style   operates on the premise that most workers cannot make a contribution without being directed (Ch. 44).

autoclave (autoclave)   used to achieve sterilization. The autoclave uses steam under pressure to obtain higher temperatures than can be achieved with boiling (Ch. 30).

automated external defibrillator (AED) (desfibrilador externo automatizado [DEA])   portable, self-contained, automatic device with voice instructions on how to use for individuals in cardiac arrest. It is used externally to electronically "shock" the myocardium into contracting again. Same as cardioversion (Ch. 8).

automated routing unit (ARU) (enrutador automático [ARU])   telephone system that answers a call and uses a recorded voice to identify departments or services (Ch. 11).

autopsy report (informe de autopsia)   also called an autopsy protocol, a necropsy report, or a medical examiner report. Autopsies are performed to determine the cause of death or to ascertain and confirm disease presence (Ch. 15).

avascularized (avascularized)   lacking blood or lymphatic vessels (Ch. 30).

avulsion (avulsión) an open wound in which the skin is torn off and bleeding is profuse (Ch. 8).

axial skeleton (esqueleto axial) consists of bones that lie around the center of the body (Ch. 29).

axilla the space below the shoulder joint where nerves and blood vessels enter the upper arm (Ch. 32).

bachelor's degree (licenciatura) four-year academic degree conferred by colleges and universities (Ch. 1).

bacilli (bacilo) one of the three classifications of bacteria; rod shaped (Ch. 21).

bacterial vaginosis (vaginosis bacteriana) an overgrowth of normal vaginal bacteria that results in an abnormal discharge (Ch. 25).

balance (balancear) amount owed (N); to verify posting accuracy (V); records difference between debit and credit columns (Ch. 18).

balance sheet (balance general) itemized statement of assets, liabilities, and equity; a statement of financial condition (Ch. 20).

balanitis (balanitis) the swelling and/or inflammation of the glans penis (Ch. 27).

bandages (venda) nonsterile gauze or other material applied over a sterile dressing to protect and immobilize (Ch. 8).

bariatrics (bariátrica) the branch of medicine that deals with prevention, control, and treatment of obesity (Ch. 29).

barriers (barreras) obstacles that exist to protect an individual from contact with blood or other potentially infected materials. Called personal protective equipment (PPE), barriers include gloves, masks, face shields, laboratory coats, protective eyewear, and gowns (Ch. 21).

Bartholin gland (glándula de Bartolino) one of two small mucous glands located at the vaginal opening at the base of the labia majora (Ch. 25).

basal metabolic rate (BMR) (índice metabólico basal) level of energy required when the body is at rest (Ch. 33).

baseline (valor de referencia) known or initial measurement against which future measurements are compared (Ch. 23); also, flat, horizontal line that separates the various waves of the ECG cycle (Ch. 36).

baseline values see baseline (Ch. 38).

basophils (basófilo) granulocytic white blood cells that mediate inflammation, mediate the allergic–antigen response, and release histamine to increase inflammation. They are the least common of the white blood cells (Ch. 40).

Bell's palsy temporary paralysis of the 7th cranial nerve due to damage or trauma (Ch. 29).

benchmark (comparador de rendimiento) making a comparison among different organizations relative to how they accomplish tasks, such as office computerization, file system organization, and employee remuneration (Ch. 44).

beneficiary (beneficiario) person under a policy eligible to receive benefits (Ch. 16).

benefit (beneficio) remuneration that is in addition to salary (Ch. 44).

benefit period (período de beneficios) the specified time during which benefits will be paid under certain types of health insurance coverages (Ch. 16).

benign prostatic hyperplasia (BPH) enlarged prostate gland that is not cancerous in origin (Ch. 27).

beriberi (beriberi) disease caused by a deficiency in vitamin B (thiamin); characterized by headaches, depression, anorexia, constipation, tachycardia, edema, and heart failure (Ch. 33).

Betadine (Betadine) brand of povidone-iodine solution used as a skin antiseptic. Betadine is also available in a scrub (soap) solution (Ch. 30).

bias (sesgo) slant toward a particular belief (Ch. 4).

bilirubin (bilirrubina) orange-yellow pigment that forms from the breakdown of hemoglobin in aged or damaged red blood cells. Bilirubin usually travels in the bloodstream to the liver, where it is converted to a water-soluble form and is excreted into the bile (Ch. 41, 43).

bilirubinuria (bilirrubinuria) the presence of bilirubin in urine (Ch. 41).

bimanual examination (examen bimanual) an examination performed by the provider using two hands to examine the internal pelvic organs. Two fingers of one hand are inserted into the vagina and the other hand presses on the outside of the abdominal wall. Shape, consistency, and position of the pelvic organs can be determined (Ch. 25).

bioequivalent (bioequivalentes) as it relates to pharmacokinetics, two compounds of the same active ingredients that are equally bioavailable and produce the same desired effect on the body (Ch. 34).

bioethics (bioética) branch of medical ethics concerned with moral issues resulting from high technology and sophisticated medical research. Social issues such as genetic engineering, abortion, and fetal tissue research raise important bioethical questions (Ch. 7).

biopharmaceuticals (productos biofarmacéuticos) a pharmaceutical agent that is extracted from, manufactured in, or semisynthesized from a biologic product using biotechnology (Ch. 34).

biopsy (biopsia) removal of a small piece of living tissue from an organ or other part of the body for microscopic examination to confirm or establish a diagnosis (Ch. 29, 38).

biotransformation (biotransformación) the chemical alteration that a drug undergoes in the body, usually in the liver (Ch. 34).

bipolar (bipolar) having two poles or processes (Ch. 36).

birthday rule (regla del cumpleaños) method to determine which of two or more health insurance policies covering a dependent child will be primary; that parent with the birthday falling first in the calendar year has the primary policy (Ch. 16).

blind copy (copia oculta) protects the privacy of email. Other recipients cannot identify who else may have received the transmitted message (Ch. 14).

blogging (blogging) using a digital platform for expressing thoughts, ideas, experiences, or observations (Ch. 44).

bloodborne pathogen (patógeno transmitido por la sangre) microorganism capable of causing disease and is found in blood or components of blood (Ch. 21).

blood urea nitrogen (BUN) (nitrógeno ureico en sangre [BUN]) nitrogen in the blood in the form of urea. The level of nitrogen in the blood is an indicator of kidney function (Ch. 43).

body fluid (líquido corporal) any secretion or excretion from the human body such as vaginal, cerebrospinal, synovial, pleural, pericardial, peritoneal, amniotic, sputum, and saliva (Ch. 37).

body language (lenguaje corporal) nonverbal communication that includes wordless clues and unconscious body movements, gestures, and facial expressions that accompany verbal messages (Ch. 4).

body mechanics (mecánica corporal) practice of using certain key muscle groups together with correct body alignment to avoid injury when lifting or moving heavy or awkward objects (Ch. 32).

body surface area (BSA) (área de superficie corporal [ASC]) a highly accurate method for calculating medication dosages for infants and children up to 12 years of age (Ch. 35).

bond (fianza) binding agreement with an employee ensuring recovery of financial loss should funds be stolen or embezzled (Ch. 44).

bond paper (papel bond) durable, strong paper usually used for correspondence (Ch. 14).

bone densitometry (la densitometría ósea) a radiographic procedure to measure the mineral concentration and structure of bone. Used primarily to diagnose osteoporosis (Ch. 31).

Boomer generation (generación de Boomer) individuals born from 1955–1965 (Ch 45).

bradycardia (sinus) (bradicardia [sinusal]) slow (less than 60 beats per minute), but regular heartbeat (Ch. 23, 36).

bradypnea (bradipnea) abnormally slowed respiratory rate (Ch. 23).

brainstorming (tormenta de ideas) process of developing ideas through a synergistic interaction among participants in an environment free of criticism (Ch. 44).

Braxton-Hicks (Braxton-Hicks) irregular, intermittent, and painless uterine contractions; also known as false labor (Ch. 25).

breast self-examination (BSE) a screening examination to detect early changes or signs of malignancy that can be performed at home by the woman, not the provider (Ch. 25).

bronchodilator (broncodilatador)   a drug that expands the bronchial tubes (Ch. 29).

broth tubes (tubos de caldo)   tubes filled with a broth substance that will support the growth of certain microorganisms (Ch. 42).

bruits (ruidos)   sound of venous or arterial origin heard on auscultation (Ch. 24).

buffer words (palabras de relleno)   expendable words used while answering the telephone (Ch. 11).

buffy coat (capa leucocitaria)   layer of white blood cells and platelets that forms at the interface between the plasma and red blood cells in a centrifuged microhematocrit tube of blood containing an anticoagulant (Ch. 40).

bulbourethral glands (glándulas bulbouretrales)   located internally at the base of the penis and are part of the male reproductive system. These glands are responsible for the manufacture and discharge of a clear viscous secretion known as preejaculate. This fluid lubricates the urethra in preparation for ejaculation (Ch. 27). In females these mucous producing glands are located on each side, slightly to the posterior of the vaginal opening (Ch. 31).

bulimia (bulimia)   a syndrome in which an individual binges on food and then purges by inducing vomiting (Ch. 29, 33).

bundled codes (códigos agrupados)   a grouping of several services that are directly related to a specific procedure and are paid as one (Ch. 17).

burnout (agotamiento profesional)   a state of fatigue or frustration brought about by a devotion to a cause, a way of life, or a relationship that failed to produce the expected reward (Ch. 3).

cachectic (caquéctico)   describes a state of ill health, malnutrition, and wasting (Ch. 33).

calibration (calibración)   determination of the accuracy of an instrument by comparing the information provided with an accepted standard known to be accurate (Ch. 36, 37).

calorie(s) (caloría)   unit of heat. The large calorie is used in discussion of human nutrition. The large calorie is also expressed as the kilogram calorie (kcal), equal to 1,000 small calories (Ch. 33).

candidiasis (candidiasis)   infection of the skin or mucous membrane with any species of the fungi *Candida* (Ch. 25, 42).

capitation (capitación)   use of the number of members enrolled in a plan to determine salary of the provider; the provider is paid a fixed fee for each member no matter how many times that member is seen by the provider (Ch. 16).

caption (leyenda)   method of designation used on file guides (Ch. 13).

carbuncle (ántrax)   necrotizing infection of skin and tissue composed of a cluster of boils (Ch. 29).

carcinoma in situ (carcinoma in situ)   cancer that does not extend beyond the basement membrane (Ch. 25).

cardiac catheterization (cateterismo cardíaco)   passage of a catheter into the heart through an arm or leg vein and blood vessels leading into the heart. The purpose is to obtain cardiac blood samples, detect abnormalities, and determine intracardiac pressure. Contrast medium can be injected and a coronary artery angiogram can be performed (Ch. 36).

cardiac cycle (ciclo cardíaco)   period from the beginning of one heartbeat to the beginning of the next succeeding beat, including systole and diastole. One complete heartbeat (Ch. 36).

cardiogenic (cardiogénico)   a type of shock in which the cardiac muscle is unable to contract and adequately provide blood to the body (Ch. 8).

cardiopulmonary resuscitation (CPR) (reanimación cardiopulmonar [RCP])   combination of rescue breathing and chest compressions performed by a trained individual on a patient experiencing cardiac arrest (Ch. 8).

cardioversion (cardioversión)   conversion of a pathological cardiac rhythm (arrhythmia), such as ventricular fibrillation, to normal sinus rhythm (Ch. 8, 36).

career objective (objetivo profesional)   expresses your career goal and the position for which you are applying (Ch. 47).

carotene (caroteno)   vitamin A (Ch. 33).

carrier (portador)   person who harbors a pathogenic organism and who is capable of transmitting the organism to others (Ch. 21).

cash basis accounting (contabilidad de caja)   reports income at the time money is collected (Ch. 20).

cashier's check (cheque de caja)   bank's own check drawn against the bank's account (Ch. 18).

casts (cilindros)   tiny structures usually formed by deposits of protein or other substances on the walls of renal tubules; in urine, they can indicate kidney disease (Ch. 41).

catalyst (catalizador)   substance that allows a chemical reaction to proceed at a much quicker rate and without as much energy input (Ch. 33).

cataracts (catarata)   opacity of the eye lens that usually occurs from aging, trauma, or disease (Ch. 28).

catheterization (cateterismo)   insertion of a catheter tube into the body for evacuating fluids or injecting fluids into body cavities. In urinary catheterization, the tube is inserted through the urethra into the bladder for withdrawal of urine (Ch. 24).

cathode (cátodo)   a negative electrode from which electrons are emitted (Ch. 31).

caustic (cáustico)   corrosive and burning; destructive to living tissue (Ch. 21, 30).

cautery (cauterio)   destruction of tissue by burning (Ch. 30).

cell-mediated immunity (inmunidad mediada por células)   the regulatory activities of T cells during the specific immune response (Ch. 21).

cellulose (celulosa)   type of indigestible fiber made of carbohydrates found in plants (Ch. 33).

Centers for Medicare and Medicaid Services (CMS) (Centros de Servicios de Medicare y Medicaid [CMS])   formerly known as HCFA. CMS is a federal agency within the U.S. Department of Health and Human Services (DHHS). The agency administers Medicare, Medicaid, and the State Children's Health Insurance Program (SCHIP). CMS also administers the Health Insurance Portability and Accountability Act of 1996 (HIPAA) and Clinical Laboratory Improvement Act of 1988 (CLIA '88) (Ch. 16).

central processing unit (CPU) (unidad de procesamiento central [CPU])   brain of the computer that performs instructions defined by software (Ch. 10).

centrifuge (centrifugador)   a laboratory device that spins tubes using centrifugal force to separate the fluid portion of blood or urine from the formed elements (Ch. 39, 41).

cerebral vascular accident (CVA) (accidente cerebrovascular [ACV])   loss of blood supply to the brain (anoxia); also referred to as a stroke (Ch. 29).

certificate of waiver (COW)   certificate issued to a laboratory to perform only CLIA-waived tests (Ch. 37).

certification (certificación)   guarantees something or someone as being true or as represented by or as meeting a standard (Ch. 1, 46).

certification examination (examen de certificación)   standardized means of evaluating medical assistant competency (Ch. 46).

certified check (cheque certificado)   depositor's own check that the bank has indicated with a date and signature to be good for the amount written (Ch. 18).

Certified Clinical Medical Assistant (CCMA [NHA]) (Asistente Clínico Médico Certificado [CCMA])   an NHA certification for a clinical medical assistant (Ch. 1, 47).

Certified Medical Administrative Assistant (CMAA [NHA]) (Asistente Administrativo Médico Certificado [CMAA])   an NHA certification for a medical administrative assistant (Ch. 1, 46).

Certified Medical Administrative Specialist (CMAS [AMT]) (Especialista Administrativo Médico Certificado [CMAS])   an AMT certification for a medical administrative specialist (Ch. 46).

Certified Medical Assistant (CMA [AAMA]) (Asistente Médico Certificado [CMA (AAMA)])   a medical assistant who has successfully completed the AAMA's national certification examination (Ch. 1, 46).

Certified Medical Transcriptionist (CMT) (Transcriptor Médico Certificado [CMT])   one who has completed a two-part certification examination administered by the Association for Healthcare Documentation Integrity (AHDI) (Ch. 15).

cerumen (cerumen) a substance secreted by glands at the outer third of the ear canal (Ch. 29).

cervical punch biopsy (biopsia cervical en sacabocados) a biopsy of the uterine cervix using an instrument, the end of which is a punch (Ch. 25).

cesarean section (operación cesárea) delivery of fetus through surgical incision into the uterus (Ch. 25).

chain of custody (cadena de custodia) procedures in which the patient and sample are monitored and controlled so that the sample can be directly linked to the patient at all times and verified by the clinical personnel (Ch. 41).

chalazion (pinza de Chalazion) a benign, painless bump or nodule inside the upper or lower eyelid. May result from healed internal styes and form around an oil gland in the tissue of the eyelid resulting in inflammation (Ch. 29).

chart notes (notas clínicas) (also called progress notes) provider's formal or informal notes about presenting problem, physical findings, and plan for treatment for a patient examined in the office, clinic, acute care center, or emergency department (Ch. 15).

check register (registro de cheques) record of checks written; categorized into separate and identified columns (Ch. 20).

CHEDDAR a form of medical documentation that includes:

  C Chief complaint, presenting problems, subjective information

  H History, social and physical, of presenting problem; contributing data

  E Examination; body systems reviewed

  D Details of problem(s) and complaint(s)

  D Drugs and dosages; list of current medications, dosages, frequency

  A Assessment; diagnostic evaluation, further testing, medications

  R Return visit, if applicable (Ch. 22).

cheilosis (queilosis) caused by a deficiency of vitamin B_2 (riboflavin) and characterized by sores on the lips and cracks in the corners of the mouth (Ch. 33).

Cheyne-Stokes (Cheyne-Stoke) regular pattern of irregular breathing rate often seen in children and that may be seen in brain dysfunction (Ch. 23).

chief complaint (CC) (queja principal [QP]) specific symptom or problem for which the patient is seeing the provider today (Ch. 15, 22).

chlamydia (clamidia) a bacterium that causes one of the most prevalent sexually transmitted diseases (Ch. 25).

chlamydiae obligate intracellular parasites that are totally dependent on the host cell for energy (Ch. 21).

cholecalciferol (colecalciferol) vitamin D (Ch. 33).

cholesterol (colesterol) sterol lipid that is widely distributed in animal tissues and ingested in foods containing animal products such as meat, dairy products and eggs. Cholesterol is produced in the liver, is a component of bile, and is needed in limited amounts for body functions (Ch. 43).

chronic stress the response to emotional pressure for a prolonged period over which an individual perceives he or she has no control. Chronic stress can have a serious impact on physical and psychological health (Ch. 3).

chronologic résumé (curriculum vitae cronológico) résumé format used when you have employment experience (Ch. 47).

circadian rhythm (ritmo circadiano) pattern based on a 24-hour cycle emphasizing the repetition of certain physiologic phenomena such as eating and sleeping (Ch. 41).

circumcision (circuncisión) the surgical removal of the foreskin (prepuce) of the penis (Ch. 26).

circumduction (circunducción) circular motion of a body part (Ch. 32).

civil law (derecho civil) law related to actions between individuals (Ch. 6).

claim register (registro de reclamaciones) diary or register of claims submitted to each insurance carrier. When payment is received, the date and amount of payment is entered in the register (Ch. 17).

claustrophobia (claustrofobia) fear of being confined in any space (Ch. 31).

clinical chemistry (química clínica) analysis and study of blood, body fluids, excreta, and tissues in the diagnosis and treatment of disease (Ch. 38).

clinical diagnosis (diagnóstico clínico) identification of a disease by history, laboratory studies, and symptoms (Ch. 22, 38).

closed questions (preguntas cerradas) questions answered with a yes or no (Ch. 4).

cloud computing (computación en la nube) storing program software on servers at a hosting company so that software download is available on demand (Ch. 10).

cluster scheduling (programación de cluster) a method of appointment scheduling which involves grouping or categorizing similar types of visits or procedures on particular days or blocks of time. Also known as specialty scheduling or practice-based scheduling (Ch. 12).

clustering (agrupación) a grouping together of nonverbal messages into statements or conclusions (Ch. 4). Can also be used to describe a scheduling system where patients with similar complaints/conditions are scheduled consecutively (example is scheduling all the allergy injections for 3:00 PM to 4:00 PM every Tuesday and Thursday) (Ch. 12).

CMS 1500 (02/12) (CMS 1500 [02/12]) formerly known as the HCFA 1500 form; the office health insurance claim form for Medicare and Medicaid (Ch. 17).

coach (entrenador de) one responsible for helping patients gain the knowledge, skills, tools, and confidence to become an active participant in the management of their health care. Health coaches may act as advocates or intermediaries in the patient–provider relationship (Ch. 4).

cobalamin (cobalamina) vitamin B_{12} (Ch. 33).

cocci (cocos) bacteria that are round, spherical, oval, or ovoid in shape (Ch 21, 42).

cochlear implantation (implante coclear) an electrical device that receives sounds and transmits the resulting signal to electrodes implanted in the cochlea. The signal stimulates the cochlea and the individual is able to perceive sound (Ch. 26).

coenzyme (coenzima) substance that enhances a catalyst (Ch. 33).

cognitive functioning (funcionamiento cognitivo) awareness with perception, reasoning, judgment, intuition, and memory (Ch. 28).

coinsurance (coseguro) that percentage paid by either the insured party, or the insured's employer (Ch. 16).

collection ratio (relación de cobranza) gross income divided by the amount that could have been collected less disallowances (Ch. 19, 20).

colonoscopy (colonoscopia) visual examination of the colon with a lighted scope (Ch. 29).

colposcopy (colposcopia) visual examination of vaginal and cervical tissues using a colposcope following an abnormal Pap smear. A magnifying lens and powerful lights are used (Ch. 25).

comedones (comedón) blackheads; usually the result of blocked sebaceous glands caused by acne (Ch. 29).

Commission on Accreditation of Allied Health Education Programs (CAAHEP) (Comisión de Acreditación de Programas Educativos Asociados a la Salud [CAAHEP]) entity accrediting over 2,000 educational programs in 20 health sciences professions (Ch. 46).

common law (derecho consuetudinario) refers to laws developed in England and France and brought to the United States by the early settlers; sometimes referred to as judge-made law (Ch. 6).

communicable (transmisible) contagious. Capable of being transmitted from one person to another either directly or indirectly (Ch. 21, 37).

compensation (compensación) overemphasizing of characteristics to make up for a real or imagined failure or handicap (Ch. 4).

competency (competencia) demonstrating mastery of a task, the skill or ability to perform a task (Ch. 1).

complementary and alternative medicine complementary medicine complements or is used with traditional or mainstream medicine. Alternative medicine is used in place of traditional or mainstream medicine. When health care providers cooperate in offering both types of care, the term *integrative medicine* is used (Ch. 2).

complete blood count (CBC) (recuento sanguíneo completo [RSC])   set of hematologic tests consisting of hemoglobin, hematocrit, total white blood cell count including differential, total red blood cell count including indices, and platelets (Ch. 40).

compliance (cumplimiento)   conformity in fulfilling official requirements (Ch. 1).

compounding (composición)   combining two or more substances in definite proportions (Ch. 35).

condylomata (condiloma)   a wart-like lesion of viral origin found on external genitalia or perianal region (Ch. 25).

confidentiality agreement (acuerdo de confidencialidad)   when signed, the agreement signifies that the medical transcriptionist is committed to keeping all patient information confidential (Ch. 15).

conflict resolution (resolución de conflictos)   solving problems between co-workers or any two parties (Ch. 44).

congenital anomalies (anomalías congénitas)   conditions present at the time of birth that deviate from what is considered normal (Ch. 25).

congruency (congruencia)   occurs when the verbal message and the nonverbal message agree (Ch. 4).

conjunctivitis   inflammation or infection of the outer membrane of the eyeball and the inner eyelid (Ch. 26, 29).

constitutional law (derecho constitucional)   consists of laws that are made by the constitution of the United States or individual states (Ch. 6).

consultation report (informe de consulta)   document that reports the findings and advice of another provider requested to see a patient by the attending provider (Ch. 15).

contact tracker (seguidor de contactos)   form used to keep track of employment contact information such as name of employer, name of contact person, address and telephone number, date of first contact, résumé sent, interview date, follow-up information (Ch. 47).

contact transmission (transmisión por contacto)   spread of disease-causing microorganisms by directly or indirectly touching the source of the infection or by touching an object or environmental surface (Ch. 21).

contamination (contaminar)   occurs when something is made unclean; often used to describe a sterile area being made unsterile or exposing a clean area to a pathogenic substance (Ch. 30).

continuing education units (CEU) (unidades de educación continua [UEC])   method for earning points toward recertification (Ch. 46).

contraception (anticoncepción)   voluntary prevention of pregnancy (Ch. 25).

contracting (contraer)   acquiring an infection from pathogens (Ch. 21).

contract law (derecho contractual)   law that refers to agreements between individuals and entities that are binding (Ch. 6).

contracture(s) (contractura)   occurs when the body is in a nonmoving state. The usually flexible connective tissues become stiffened and are replaced with fiber-like tissues (Ch. 32).

contraindication (contraindicación)   any symptom or circumstance indicating that the use of a particular drug is inappropriate when it would otherwise be advisable. For example, the use of alcoholic beverages is a contraindication when the drug Flagyl is prescribed (Ch. 34).

control test (prueba de control)   test of a sample with known results used to compare with the results of a patient's sample (Ch. 38).

controlled substances (sustancias controladas)   drugs that are approved for medical use in the United States and are determined by the government to have a high abuse potential and a high likelihood of dependency (Ch. 34).

coordination of benefits (COB) (coordinación de beneficios [COB])   the provision of an insurance contract that limits benefits to 100% of the cost (Ch. 16).

co-payment (copago)   payment required when a patient is seen by the provider (Ch. 16).

coryza (coriza)   inflammation of the mucous membranes of the nose due to an allergic reaction such as hay fever or a cold (Ch. 21).

cost accounting (contabilidad de costos)   helps to determine what it costs the ambulatory care setting to perform particular services and is an integral part of managerial accounting (Ch. 20).

cost analysis (análisis de costos)   procedure that determines the costs of each service (Ch. 20).

cost ratio (relación de costos)   formula that shows the cost of a procedure or service and helps determine the financial value of maintaining certain services (Ch. 20).

countershock (contrachoque)   application of an electric current to the heart directly or indirectly to alter a disturbance in cardiac rhythm (Ch. 36).

coupling agent (agente de acoplamiento)   an agent used when ultrasonography is used; enhances penetration of sound waves through tissue (Ch. 25).

crash cart or tray (bandeja o carro de parada)   tray or portable cart that contains medications and supplies needed for emergency and first aid procedures (Ch. 8).

C-reactive protein (CRP) (proteína C reactiva [CRP])   screening blood test for inflammation (Ch. 40).

creatinine (creatinina)   chemical waste product formed by muscle metabolism and excreted by the kidneys; when urine filtration is impaired, creatinine is increased in blood, which indicates abnormal kidney function (Ch. 41).

credentialed (acreditado)   a document or certificate proving a person's qualifications (Ch. 1).

credit (crédito)   decreases balance due; column used for entering payments (Ch. 18).

crepitation (crepitación)   grating sound heard on movement of ends of a broken bone (Ch. 8).

criminal law (derecho penal)   law related to wrongs committed against the welfare and safety of society as a whole (Ch. 6).

crossover claim (reclamación de crossover)   A claim that is billed to the supplemental insurer by the regional Medicare fiscal intermediary for providers PAR with Medicare, after Medicare pays its portion (Ch. 16).

cross-reference (referencia cruzada)   notation in a file to direct the reader to a specific record that may be filed under more than one name/subject (e.g., married name/maiden name or foreign names) where the surname is not easily recognizable (Ch. 13).

cryopreservation (crioconservación)   storage of biologic materials (sperm, embryo, tissue, plasma) at extremely cold temperature for use at a later time (Ch. 7).

cryosurgery (criocirugía)   the destruction of tissue by application of extreme cold, silver nitrate, and carbon dioxide (Ch. 25).

cryotherapy (crioterapia)   the use of low temperatures for medical therapy (Ch. 32).

cryptorchidism (criptorquidia)   undescended testicle (Ch. 27).

crystals (crystals)   may be found in normal urine sediment. Though they have no particular significance, they should be noted because they may indicate disease states (Ch. 41).

culture (cultura)   the attitudes and behavior that are characteristic of a particular social group or organization (Ch. 4). Growing bacteria or fungi in media within a laboratory setting for identification of disease (Ch. 42).

culture and sensitivity (cultivo y sensibilidad)   often referred to as C&S. The sample is cultured for bacteria and then is exposed to various antibiotics to determine what the bacteria is sensitive (and resistant) to (Ch. 38, 42).

Current Procedural Terminology (CPT) (Terminología Actual sobre Procedimientos [TAP])   standard codes for procedures and services. Used by most ambulatory care settings in encoding the claim form and recognized by most insurance carriers (Ch. 17).

current reports (informes actuales)   reports such as history and physical examinations that should be complete within 24 hours (Ch. 15).

cyanosis (cianosis) discoloration of the skin due to abnormal amounts of reduced hemoglobin in the blood caused by decreased oxygen and increased carbon dioxide in the blood (Ch. 24).

cystitis (cistitis) inflammation of the bladder (Ch. 28).

cytology (citología) science that deals with the formation, structure, and function of cells (Ch. 38).

DARP (DARP) a problem-oriented medical record charting method that is based on data, assessment, response, and plan (Ch. 22).

data backup (backup de datos) storage of all files, programs, and the operating system necessary to restore the computer in the event of a major failure (Ch. 10).

day sheet (hoja diaria) form used with pegboard system to record daily patient transactions (Ch. 18).

debit (debe) used for entering charges and description of services; column is on the left (Ch. 18).

debris (detritos) remains of broken down or damaged cells or tissues (Ch. 21).

declination form (formulario de rechazo) written formal refusal (Ch. 21).

decode (decodificar) to translate into language that is easily understood; to interpret (Ch. 4).

deductible (deducible) that amount of incurred medical expenses that must be met before the insurance policy will begin to pay (Ch. 16).

deep tendon reflexes (DTRs) (reflejos tendinosos profundos) the rapid contraction of a tendon in response to a rapid tap that demonstrates an intact spinal cord and nerve arc (Ch. 29).

defendant (demandado) person who defends action brought in litigation (Ch. 6).

Defense Enrollment Eligible Reporting System (DEERS) (Sistema de Informes de Elegibilidad para la Inscripción en Defensa [DEERS]) a system operated by the Department of Defense and used by TRICARE contractors to determine and confirm the eligibility of beneficiaries (Ch. 16).

defense mechanisms (mecanismo de defensa) behaviors that protect the psyche from guilt, anxiety, or shame (Ch. 4).

defibrillation (desfibrilación) stopping fibrillation of the heart by use of drugs or by physical means (Ch. 36).

defibrillator (desfibrilador) a machine that delivers an electric current to alter a disturbance in cardiac rhythm (Ch. 36).

defragmentation (desfragmentación) reorganization of information on a hard disk to store files as continuous units rather than as small packets. A computer with little fragmentation of files will operate at a higher speed (Ch. 10).

dementia (demencia) impairment of intellectual function that is progressive and interferes with normal activities (Ch. 28).

demyelination (desmielinización) destruction of the myelin sheath; often a factor in multiple sclerosis (Ch. 29).

denial (rechazo) rejection of or refusal to acknowledge (Ch. 4).

deoxygenated (desoxigenada) blood that is high in carbon dioxide, low in oxygen, and pumped through the heart to the lungs where the carbon dioxide is exchanged for oxygen (Ch. 36).

depolarization (despolarizar) process of reducing to a nonpolarized condition. Generation of an electrical current is enhanced. Electrical activity generated when the atria or ventricles contract (Ch. 36).

deposition (declaración) oral testimony given by an individual with a court reporter and attorneys for both sides present; often used as part of the discovery process (Ch. 6).

dermatophysosis (dermatophysosis) fungal skin infection commonly known as ringworm (Ch. 29).

dexterity (destreza) skill and ease in using the hands (Ch. 1).

diagnosis (diagnóstico) determination of disease or condition (Ch. 17).

diagnosis-related groups (DRGs) (grupos relacionados de diagnóstico) these designations ensure that all given diagnoses are as specific as possible and also justify the length of a patient's stay in the hospital (Ch. 16).

diastole (diástole) one component of blood pressure measurement representing the lowest amount of pressure exerted during the cardiac cycle; the force exerted on the arterial walls during cardiac relaxation (Ch. 23, 36).

diathermies (diathermies) the application of high-frequency electromagnetic currents or ultrasonography to produce heat in body tissue for a therapeutic purpose (Ch. 32).

diethylstilbestrol (DES) (dietilestilbestrol [DES]) a synthetic hormone used therapeutically in menopausal disturbances. It should not be given during pregnancy. It has been related to cervicovaginal malignances in daughters of mothers who had it prescribed for them to treat a threatened abortion. DES has been related to reproductive disorders in males whose mothers took it during pregnancy (Ch. 25).

differential diagnosis (diagnóstico diferencial) diagnosis based on comparison of symptoms of similar diseases (Ch. 38).

digestion (digestión) breaking down of food into smaller particles. It can be either physical or chemical (Ch. 33).

dilation (dilatación) expansion of an orifice or organ (Ch. 25).

diploma (diploma) a document bearing record of graduation from or of a degree conferred by an educational institution (Ch. 1).

diplopia (diplopia) the subjective complaint of seeing two images instead of one; also known as double-vision (Ch 8).

direct skills (habilidades directas) skills that are job specific. Skill in taking a blood pressure reading would be specific to the medical field (Ch. 47).

discharge summary (DS) (resumen de alta médica [DS]) medical reports that document the hospitalization history of a patient (Ch. 15).

discovery (exhibición de pruebas) the time in which both parties are allowed access to all information and evidence related to a legal case; follows the subpoena process (Ch. 6).

dislocation (luxación) displacement of a bone or joint from its normal position (Ch. 8, 29).

dispense (dosificar) prepare and give out a medication to be taken at a later time (Ch. 6, 34, 35).

displacement (desplazamiento) displacing negative feelings onto something or someone else with no significance to the situation (Ch. 4).

disposition (temperamento) temperament, character, personality (Ch. 1).

distribution (distribución) the process whereby the drug is transported from the blood to the intended site of action, site of biotransformation, site of storage, and site of elimination (Ch. 34).

diuretic(s) (diurético) substance that causes less water to be reabsorbed by the kidney and therefore causes water to be excreted from the body (Ch. 33).

DNA (ADN) deoxyribonucleic acid; important nuclear material that carries genetic codes (Ch. 38).

documentation (documentación) written material that accompanies purchased software containing the information necessary for using the software appropriately; sometimes known as the manual (Ch. 10)

donut hole (período sin cobertura) within the Medicare Part D prescription drug program, the donut hole is the phase of coverage in which all costs are covered by the enrollee rather than CMS (Ch. 16).

Doppler (Doppler) a noninvasive technique used with ultrasonography to evaluate blood flow through major arteries and veins of the arms, legs, and neck. It can reveal blood clots or blockages (Ch. 31).

dorsal recumbent (decúbito dorsal) in this position, the patient lays on his or her back (dorsal) face up, legs separated, knees flexed, with feet flat on the table (Ch. 24).

dorsiflexion (dorsiflexión) movement of the foot upward at the ankle joint (Ch. 32).

dosimeter (dosímetro) a device for measuring X-ray output (Ch. 31).

double-booking (doble-reserva) a method of appointment scheduling where two or more patients are given a particular appointment time (Ch. 12).

down-code (baja de codificación) insurance carriers down-code if documentation or codes are ambiguous and reimburse for the lowest possible fee (Ch. 17).

Down syndrome (síndrome de Down) a genetic defect present at birth that is the result of an abnormality of chromosome 21 (Ch. 25).

dressing (apósito) sterile gauze or other material applied directly to a wound to absorb secretions and to protect (Ch. 8).

droplet transmission (transmisión por gotitas) method of spreading disease from respiratory secretions through the air. Spread is usually confined to within 3 feet of the infected patient (Ch. 21).

DTap (diphtheria, tetanus, pertussis) (DTap) a vaccine that protects humans from diphtheria, tetanus, and pertussis (Ch. 26).

durable power of attorney for health care (poder legal duradero para atención médica) legal form that allows a designated person to act on another's behalf in regard to health care choices (Ch. 5, 6).

dysmenorrhea (dismenorrea) painful menses (Ch. 25).

dyspareunia (dispareunia) painful intercourse (Ch. 25).

dysplasia (displasia) abnormal development of tissue (Ch. 25).

dyspnea (disnea) shortness of breath or labored/difficult breathing (Ch. 23, 28).

dysuria (disuria) painful or difficult urination (Ch. 29).

echocardiogram (ecocardiograma) noninvasive diagnostic method that uses ultrasound to visualize internal cardiac structure, including valves (Ch. 31).

eclampsia (eclampsia) complication of pregnancy that includes general edema, hypertension, proteinuria, and convulsions (Ch. 25).

ectopic pregnancy (embarazo ectópico) implementation of the fertilized ovum outside of the uterine cavity (Ch. 25).

edematous (edematoso) abnormal accumulation of fluid in the tissues resulting in swelling (Ch. 39).

editor (corrector) see auditor (Ch. 15).

effacement (borramiento) thinning and shortening of the cervical canal during labor to permit passage of fetus (Ch. 25).

effleurage (effleurage) deep or gentle stroking massage (Ch. 32).

EHR (RSE) see electronic health record (Ch. 10).

ejaculation (la eyaculación) ejection of seminal fluid and sperm during male orgasm (Ch. 27).

electrocardiogram (electrocardiograma) record of the electrical activity of the heart; showing P, QRS, and T waves (Ch. 36).

electrocardiograph (electrocardiografio) instrument for recording the electrical activity of the heart (Ch. 36).

electrocardiography (electrocardiografía) process of recording the electrical activity originating of the heart (Ch. 36).

electrocautery (electrocauterización) control of bleeding using an instrument that is electrically heated (Ch. 8).

electrochemical gradient (gradiente electroquímico) the formation of electrical signals that allow information to flow through the nervous system (Ch. 32).

electrode (electrodo) also known as a sensor. Used to conduct electricity from the body to the electrocardiograph (Ch. 36).

electrolyte (electrolito) substance that conducts electricity whose components are important in maintaining fluid and acid–base balance (Ch. 33, 36, 38).

electromyography (EMG) (electromiografía) recording of the electrical activity of muscle tissue, using electrodes attached to the skin or inserted into the muscle (Ch. 32).

electronic check (cheque electrónico) electronic version of a paper check, used to make payments online (Ch. 18).

electronic health record (EHR) (registro de salud electrónico [RSE]) a patient's electronic medical records from multiple sources combined into one master database (Ch. 10).

electronic mail (email) (correo electrónico) the process of sending, receiving, storing, and forwarding messages in digital form over computer networks (Ch. 11).

electronic medical record (EMR) (registro médico electrónico [RME]) patient medical record from a single medical practice, hospital, or pharmacy (Ch. 10, 15).

electrosurgery (electrocirugía) uses an electric current in a concentrated area to either cut or destroy tissue whenever pathologic examination is not required (Ch. 30).

elimination (eliminación) the process whereby a drug is excreted from the body. Elimination occurs via the gastrointestinal tract, respiratory tract, skin, mucous membranes, and mammary glands (Ch. 34).

emancipated minors (menor emancipado) persons under age 18 years who are financially responsible for themselves and free of parental care (Ch. 6).

embezzle (malversar) appropriate fraudulently to one's own use (Ch. 44).

emergency medical services (EMS) (servicios médicos de emergencia [SME]) a local network of police, fire, and medical personnel trained to respond to emergency situations. In many communities, the system is activated by calling 911 (Ch. 8).

empathy (empatía) ability to be objectively aware of and have insight into another's feelings, emotions, and behaviors, and to be aware of the significance and meaning of these to the other person (Ch. 1).

EMR (RME) see electronic medical record (Ch. 10).

encephalitis (encephalitis) inflammation of the brain tissue. It is usually a viral infection but may be caused in some cases by bacterial, fungal, parasitic, or rickettsial infections (Ch. 29).

encode (encoding) (codificar [codificación]) creating a message to be sent (Ch. 4).

encounter form (formulario de visita) formerly known as a charge slip or superbill. A copy of the encounter form is given to the patient after seeing the provider. It identifies the procedures performed, diagnoses, charges, and when to return (Ch. 17, 18).

encryption (cifrado) the process of coding email to render the transmission essentially secure (Ch. 11).

encryption technology (tecnología de cifrado) converts information into code; used to protect privacy and confidentiality of individuals in computer software (Ch. 12).

endometriosis (endometriosis) occurs when tissue that resembles the endometrium invades various locations in the pelvic cavity and elsewhere (Ch. 25).

endoscope (endoscopia) an instrument or device that is used to observe the inside of a hollow organ or cavity (Ch. 30).

enunciation (dicción) speaking clearly; articulating (Ch. 11).

eosinophils (eosinófilos) granulocytic white blood cells with red eosin-stained granules in the cytoplasm. They are elevated in cases of allergies (Ch. 40).

epidemic (epidemia) an infectious disease that attacks many persons at the same time in the same location (Ch. 21).

epidemiology (epidemiología) field of science that studies the history, cause, and patterns of infectious diseases (Ch. 21).

epididymitis (epididimitis) inflammation of the tubes on the testis (Ch. 27).

epinephrine (epinefrina) used to treat allergic reactions (Ch. 9); also known as adrenaline. Epinephrine is manufactured as a chemical (pharmaceutical preparation) and is often mixed with local anesthetics for use as a vasoconstrictor in minor surgery (Ch. 30).

episodic stress (tensión episódica) occurs when individuals take on too many tasks, becoming overwhelmed by all of the demands, and are unable to satisfy all of the demands (Ch. 3).

epispadias (epispadias) a condition at birth in which the opening of the urethra is not at the tip of the penis, but on the upper penile surface (Ch. 27).

epistaxis (epistaxis) acute hemorrhage from the nostril, nasal cavity, or nasopharynx. Also known as a nose bleed (Ch. 29).

erectile dysfunction (ED) (disfunción eréctil [DE]) impotence; occurs when a man is unable to achieve or to sustain an erection of the penis during sexual intercourse (Ch. 27).

erection (la erección) penile rigidity as a result of sexual or other types of stimulation (Ch. 27).

e-résumé (curriculum vitae electrónico) electronic résumés may be delivered electronically via email, submitted to Internet job boards, or placed on Web pages (Ch. 47).

ergonomics (ergonomía) scientific study of work and space, including factors that influence worker productivity and that affect workers' health (Ch. 10).

erosion (erosión) destruction of the superficial layer of tissue by trauma, ulceration, or inflammation (Ch. 25).

erythema (eritema) redness or inflammation of the skin or mucous membranes that is the result of dilatation and congestion of superficial capillaries (Ch. 29).

erythrocyte indices (índices de eritrocitos) three equations that provide information about the sizes and hemoglobin content of red blood cells. These include the mean corpuscular (cell) volume, mean corpuscular hemoglobin, and mean corpuscular hemoglobin concentration (Ch. 40).

erythrocyte sedimentation rate (velocidad de eritrosedimentación) measurement of how far the red cells settle in a vertical sample of blood in one hour. Also called sed rate and ESR (Ch. 40).

erythrocytes (eritrocito) red blood cells, one of the formed elements of the blood (Ch. 39, 40).

erythropoietin (eritropoyetina) hormone that causes production of new red blood cells (Ch. 40).

esophagitis (esofagitis) inflammation that may damage tissues of the esophagus (Ch. 28).

Ethernet (Ethernet) references the networking of computers using metallic conductors or hard wires (Ch. 10).

ethics (ética) defined in terms of what is morally right and wrong; ethics will differ from person to person; often defined by a code or creed as in the Code of Ethics from the American Association of Medical Assistants (AAMA) (Ch. 7).

eupnea (eupnea) normal breathing (Ch. 23).

euthanasia (la eutanasia) causing death of someone who is suffering from an incurable and painful disease or who is in an irreversible coma (Ch. 7).

eversion (eversión) moving a body part outward (Ch. 32).

exclusion (exclusión) specific disease or condition listed in an insurance policy for which the policy will not pay (Ch. 16).

exclusive provider organization (EPO) (organización de proveedor exclusivo [EPO]) a closed-panel preferred organization (PPO) plan where enrollees receive no benefits if they opt to receive care from a provider who is not in the EPO (Ch. 16).

excoriated (excoriación) scratches or superficial abrasions of the skin (Ch. 21).

excretions (excreción) waste matter. The elimination of waste products from the body (Ch. 21, 37).

exit interview (entrevista de salida) opportunity for departing employees to provide their positive and negative opinions of the position and facility (Ch. 45).

expectorate (expectorar) act of coughing up material from airways that lead to the lungs (Ch. 21, 42).

expert witness (testigo experto) individual with highly specialized knowledge and skills in a particular area who testifies to a standard of care (Ch. 6).

explanation of benefits (EOB) (explicación de beneficios [EDB]) insurance report that is sent with claim payments explaining the reimbursement of the insurance carrier (Ch. 16, 17).

explicit (explícito) fully revealed or expressed without ambiguity or vagueness, leaving no question as to intent (Ch. 8).

expressed consent (consentimiento expreso) permission given either verbally or in writing (Ch 6).

expressed contract (contrato explícito) written or verbal contract that specifically describes what each party in the contract will do (Ch. 6).

extension (extensión) straightening of a body part (Ch. 32).

external respiration (respiración externa) ventilation of the lungs when the exchange of oxygen and carbon dioxide takes place (Ch. 29).

externship (práctica laboral) transition stage between the classroom and actual employment; may also be referred to as internship or practicum (Ch. 1).

extracellular (extracelular) pertaining to the environment outside of a body cell (Ch. 33).

exudate(s) (exudados) accumulated fluid in a cavity; an oozing of pus; matter that penetrates through vessel walls into adjoining tissue (Ch. 26, 30).

facilitate (facilitar) to make an action or process easier (Ch. 1).

Fair Debt Collection Practice Act (FDCPA) (Ley sobre Prácticas Justas para el Cobro de Deudas) 1977 federal law that outlines collection practices (Ch. 19).

fat-soluble vitamins (soluble en lípidos) pertaining to substances that are hydrophobic and therefore dissolve better in fat (Ch. 33).

fax (facsimile) (fax [facsímilx]) machine that sends documents from one location to another by way of telephone lines (Ch. 11).

febrile (febril) having a fever (Ch. 23).

felony (delito mayor) a serious crime such as murder, larceny (thefts of large sums of money), assault, and rape (Ch. 6).

female genital mutilation (FGM) (mutilación genital femenina) Partial or complete removal of the clitoris; partial or total removal of the labia minora and/or labia majora; narrowing the vaginal opening by creating a covering seal; and the pricking, piercing, or cauterizing of genitals (Ch. 7).

fenestrated (fenestrado) having openings. A sterile, fenestrated drape is used in surgery. It has an opening in it to expose only the operative site. The remainder of the drape covers the patient and is a sterile area (Ch. 30).

fenestrated drape (paño fenestrado) a type of drape with an opening, usually round, that can be placed with the opening over a particular body area; used in surgery and for proctologic examinations (Ch. 24).

fibromyalgia discomfort of muscles, tendons, ligaments, and soft tissues brought on by trauma, strain, and emotional stress (Ch. 29).

financial accounting (contabilidad financiera) provides information primarily for entities external to the organization such as the government (Ch. 20).

firewall (cortafuegos) hardware device or software program designed to prevent unauthorized access to a computer system (Ch. 10).

first aid (primeros auxilios) immediate (or first) care provided to persons who are suddenly ill or injured; first aid is typically followed by more comprehensive care and treatment (Ch. 8).

fiscal intermediary (intermediario fiscal) local administrator for Medicare (Ch. 16).

fixed cost (costo fijo) cost that does not vary in total as the number of patients vary (Ch. 20).

flag (indicador de mensaje) method of identifying a blank space or a question regarding dictator's meaning by attaching a note or marker to indicate the question (Ch. 15).

flexion (flexión) bending of a body part (Ch. 32).

fluoroscope (fluoroscope) a device consisting of a screen; mounts separately or with an X-ray tube that shows the images of objects interposed between the table and the screen (Ch. 31).

folic acid (ácido fólico) one of the B-complex vitamins (Ch. 33).

fomite (fómite) substance that absorbs and transmits infectious material; for example, contaminated items such as equipment (Ch. 21).

fontanels (fontanelas) soft spots lying between the cranial bones of the skull of a fetus, newborn, and infant (Ch. 26).

formalin (formalina) an aqueous solution of 37% formaldehyde (Ch. 25).

form letter (carta tipo) letter containing the same content in the body but sent to different individuals (Ch. 14).

Fowler's (Fowler) patient sits in a position with the back of the examination table raised to either 45 degrees (semi-Fowler's) or 90 degrees (high Fowler's). Legs rest flat on the table. A pillow may be placed under the knees. This position is used for patients having cardiovascular or respiratory problems to facilitate their breathing, and for examination of the upper body and head (Ch. 24).

fracture (fractura) break in a bone. There are several types of fractures, but all are classified as either open or closed fractures (Ch. 8).

fraud (fraude) deliberate misrepresentation of facts (Ch. 16).

frenulum (frenillo) of the tongue, a fold of mucous membrane located under the tongue attaching the tongue to the floor of the mouth (Ch. 23).

frequency (frecuencia) urinating frequently (Ch. 29).

friable (friable) easily broken (Ch. 30).

fringe benefits (beneficio complementario) benefits above and beyond salary to which an employee may be entitled. Examples include health and life insurance, paid vacation, sick days, personal days, and tuition reimbursement for courses related to employment (Ch. 44).

fulgurated (fulgurado) destroyed by electric current (Ch. 25).

full block letter (carta de bloque completo) major letter style in which all lines begin flush with the left margin. This style is suggested for offices desiring a contemporary-looking, efficient letter (Ch. 14).

fume hood (campana de humo) type of hood or barrier used in the laboratory to capture chemical vapors and fumes and move them away from health care workers and into a building's exhaust fan system (Ch. 37).

functional résumé (curriculum vitae funcional) résumé format used to highlight specialty areas of accomplishment and strengths (Ch. 47).

furuncle (forúnculo) localized, suppurative staphylococcal skin infection originating in a gland or hair follicle (Ch. 29).

gait (marcha) manner or style of walking including rhythm and speed (Ch. 32).

gait belt (cinturón de marcha) safety belt worn by the patient around the waist that provides a firm handhold for the caregiver when transferring the patient or when assisting in ambulation (Ch. 32).

galvanometer (galvanómetro) mechanism in the electrocardiograph that changes the voltage into a mechanical motion for recording purposes (Ch. 36).

gamma globulin (gamma globulina) antibody that is produced by the body in response to foreign substances such as bacteria, viruses, and cancerous cells. Also known as immunoglobins (Ch. 29).

Generation X (Generación X) individuals born from 1966 to 1976 (Ch. 45).

Generation Y (Generación Y) Individuals born from 1977 to 1994; also known as the Millennial generation (Ch. 45).

Generation Z (Generación Z) Individuals born from 1995 to 2012 (Ch. 45).

genetic engineering (ingeniería genética) alteration, manipulation, replacement, or repair of genetic material (Ch. 7).

genitalia (genitales) the reproductive organs, internal and external (Ch. 25).

genotype (genotipo) the genetic constitution of an organism (DNA sequence) (Ch. 21).

genus (género) first Greek or Latin name given to a microorganism; always capitalized (Ch. 42).

geriatrician (geriatra) a medical doctor who is specially trained to meet the unique health care needs of older adults (Ch. 28).

geriatrics (geriatría) the branch of medicine concerned with the problems of aging (Ch. 28).

gerontology (gerontología) the scientific study of the problems associated with aging (Ch. 28).

gestation (gestación) period of development from fertilization to birth (Ch. 25).

gestational diabetes (diabetes gestacional) diabetes that first manifests clinically during pregnancy. It usually subsides after delivery (Ch. 25).

gingivitis (la gingivitis) inflammation of the gums (Ch. 32).

glaucoma (glaucoma) condition caused by increased intraocular pressure due to a buildup of aqueous humor. This results in mild visual disturbances with little or no pain but can lead to severe visual impairment if untreated (Ch. 28, 29).

Global Harmonized System (GHS) defines and classifies chemical hazards and communicates around the world for health and safety. Pictograms is an important part of the system to lessen language barriers

glossitis inflammation of the tongue (Ch. 32).

glucosuria (glucosuria) the presence of glucose in urine (also correct is glycosuria) (Ch. 41).

glycogen (glicógeno) carbohydrate form used for storage of sugar in the body (Ch. 33).

goal (meta) result or achievement toward which effort is directed (Ch. 3).

"going bare" ("estar desprotegido") said of a provider who does not carry professional liability insurance (Ch. 44).

goniometer (goniómetro) instrument used to measure the angle of a joint's range of motion (Ch. 32).

goniometry (goniometría) measurement of joint motion (Ch. 32).

Good Samaritan laws (leyes del Buen Samaritano) laws designed to protect individuals from legal action when rendering emergency medical aid, without compensation, within the areas of their training and expertise (Ch. 8, 11).

gout (la gota) form of arthritis caused by metabolic disturbances in purine metabolism resulting in uric acid crystal deposits in the joints. Causes periodic attacks of arthritis pain and joint inflammation (Ch. 29).

Gram stain (tinción de Gram) named for its inventor, Hans Christian Gram, and is, most common stain used in microbiology to observe gross morphologic features of bacteria; a differential stain, allowing differentiation between Gram-negative and Gram-positive organisms (Ch. 42).

gravidity (gravidez) total number of pregnancies a woman has had regardless of duration, including a present one (Ch. 25).

gross contamination (contaminación importante) highly infectious material present (Ch. 21).

gross examination (examen macroscópico) viewing specimens with the naked eye (Ch. 15).

guarantor (garante) the person identified as responsible for payment of the bill (Ch. 18).

Guthrie screening test (prueba de detección de Guthrie) also known as newborn screening test; diagnostic test for the detection of phenylketonuria (PKU) (Ch. 43).

hardware (hardware) physical equipment used by the computer system to process data (Ch. 10).

headline (titular) The words or phrases used in a profile that promote qualifications and skills that distinguish an application from others (Ch. 47).

Healthcare Common Procedure Coding System (HCPCS) (Sistema de Códigos de Procedimientos Comunes de la Atención Médica [HCPCS]) a coding system consisting of the CPT, national codes (level II), and local codes (level III); previously known as HCFA Common Procedure Coding System (Ch. 17).

health care directive (directiva salud) A document that allows a patient to appoint an agent to make health care decisions in the event the patient is unable to do so (Ch. 5).

Health Insurance Portability and Accountability Act (HIPAA) (Ley de Portabilidad y Responsabilidad de Seguros de Salud [HIPAA]) government rules, regulations, and procedures resulting from legislation designed to protect the confidentiality of patient information (Ch. 6, 15).

health maintenance organization (HMO) (organización de mantenimiento de la salud [HMO]) type of managed care operation that is typically set up as a for-profit corporation with salaried employees. HMOs "with walls" offer a range of medical services under one roof; HMOs "without walls" typically contract with providers in the community to provide patient services for an agreed-upon fee (Ch. 2, 16).

helminths (helmintos) a general term meaning "worms" (Ch. 21).

hematochezia (hematochezia) bright red blood present in feces (Ch. 29).

hematocrit (hematocrito) percentage of red blood cells within a specimen of anticoagulated whole blood (Ch. 40).

hematology (hematología) study of blood and the blood-forming tissues (Ch. 38, 39, 40).

hematoma (hematoma) a bruise, accumulation of blood in tissues. Sometimes around the venipuncture site during or after venipuncture caused by the leakage of blood from where the needle punctured the vein (Ch. 39).

hematopoiesis (hematopoyesis) formation of blood cells (Ch. 40).

hematuria (hematuria) abnormal presence of blood in urine, symptomatic of many disorders of the genitourinary system and renal diseases (Ch. 29, 41).

hemiplegia (hemiplejía) paralysis of one side of the body (Ch. 32).

hemoconcentration (hemoconcentración) decrease of fluid with an increase of blood cells caused by leaving the tourniquet on the arm longer than one minute, resulting in inaccurate blood samples (Ch. 39).

hemoglobin (hemoglobina) protein molecule within the red blood cell that transports oxygen. Also helps maintain pH of blood (Ch. 40).

hemoglobinopathies (hemoglobinopatía) inherited diseases resulting from the formation of one abnormal hemoglobin molecule within the normal chain of four (Ch. 40).

hemoglobinuria (hemoglobinuria) hemoglobin in urine, which indicates an unusual breakdown of RBCs within the bloodstream (Ch. 41).

hemolysis (hemólisis) rupturing and destruction of the red blood cells during the process of blood collection. The serum or plasma becomes contaminated and has a reddish color (Ch. 33, 39).

hemolyzed (hemolizada) rupture of red blood cells (Ch. 39).

hemoptysis (hemoptisis) spitting up of blood arising from the mouth, larynx, trachea, bronchi, or lungs characterized by a sudden attack of coughing with production of bloody sputum (Ch. 29).

hemostasis (hemostasia) the process that stops bleeding; either a natural balancing process of the body or by mechanical means (such as using a hemostat instrument to clamp a blood vessel) (Ch. 40).

Hibiclens (Hibiclens) brand of antiseptic soap solution (Ch. 30).

HIC number (número HIC) The identification number of a Medicare beneficiary issued by CMS or the RRB (Ch. 16).

Hierarchy of Needs (jerarquía de necesidades) needs that are arranged in a specific order or rank; sequential arrangement. Associated with Abraham Maslow (Ch. 4).

high-context communication (comunicación de alto contexto) communication style that involves great reliance on body language, reference to objects in the environment, and culturally relevant phraseology to convey an idea. Relies on the listener knowing related events through close association with the speaker or culture (Ch. 4).

high-density lipoprotein (HDL) (lipoproteína de alta densidad [HDL]) lipoprotein in the blood composed primarily of protein; removes cholesterol from peripheral tissues and transports them to the liver for excretion (Ch. 43).

histology (histología) study of a tissue biopsy sample for the determination of disease (Ch. 38).

history and physical examination report (H&P) (informe de historia clínicay examen físico [H&P]) report of patient's history and physical examination to document reason for visit (Ch. 15).

history of the present illness (HPI) (antecedentes de enfermedad actual [AEA]) the chronologic description of the development of the patient's illness (Ch. 15).

Holter monitor (monitor Holter) a portable continuous recording of cardiac activity for a 24-hour period (Ch. 36).

homeopathy (homeopatía) a healing modality that uses diluted doses of certain substances to create an "energy imprint" in the body to bring about a cure (Ch. 2).

homeostasis (homeostasia) state of equilibrium of internal environment (Ch. 33).

hordeolum (hordéolo) inflamed sebaceous gland of the eyelid caused by bacterial infection; stye (Ch. 29).

hospital outpatient prospective payment system (OPPS) (sistema de pago prospectivo de hospital para pacientes ambulatorios) A system that classifies all hospital outpatient services into Ambulatory Payment Classifications for reimbursement (Ch. 16).

human chorionic gonadotropin (hCG) (gonadotropina coriónica humana [hCG]) hormone secreted by the trophoblast after fertilization of the ovum. It may be detected in the blood and urine of pregnant women (Ch. 25, 43).

humoral immunity (inmunidad humoral) immunity mediated by antibodies in body fluids such as plasma and lymph (Ch. 21).

human immunodeficiency virus (HIV) (virus de la inmunodeficiencia humana [VIH]) virus causing AIDS; it is a retrovirus that ultimately destroys immune system cells (Ch. 21).

hyaline (hialino) transparent, clear; hyaline casts consist of mucuprotein, they are transparent and often difficult to see in unstained urine (Ch. 41).

hydrocele (hidrocele) swelling of the scrotum due to painless buildup of watery fluid around one or both testes (Ch. 27).

hydrocollator pack (paquete de hidrocolator) pack filled with gel that is warmed in a water bath (Ch. 32).

hydrogenated (hidrogenado) an unsaturated fat that is combined with hydrogen (Ch. 33).

hypercalcemia (hipercalcemia) elevated level of calcium in the blood (Ch. 33).

hyperemesis gravidarum (hiperemesis gravídica) severe nausea and vomiting during pregnancy with inability to eat; may lead to severe dehydration (Ch. 25).

hyperextension (hiperextensión) position of maximum extension, or extending a body part beyond its normal limits (Ch. 32).

hyperglycemia (hiperglucemia) increased levels of blood glucose. Hyperglycemia does not necessarily mean that the patient is diabetic but may be an indication of prediabetes (Ch. 8).

hyperkalemia (hipercaliemia) elevated level of potassium in the blood (Ch. 33).

hypermagnesemia (hipermagnesemia) elevated magnesium in the blood (Ch. 33).

hypernatremia (hipernatremia) elevated sodium in the blood (Ch. 33).

hyperopia (hipermetropía) farsightedness. Caused when the eyeball is irregularly shaped (shortened); the image is focused behind the retina, causing distance vision to be unclear (Ch. 29).

hyperphosphatemia elevated level of phosphorus in the blood (Ch. 33).

hyperpnea (hiperpnea) increased respiratory rate and depth as seen in exercise, pain, fever, and hysteria (Ch. 23).

hypertension (hipertensión) blood pressure that is consistently greater than 140/90 mm Hg (Ch. 23).

hyperthermia (hipertermia) body temperature above normal range; an unusually high fever (Ch. 28).

hyperthyroidism (hipertiroidismo) an overactive thyroid gland which causes an increase in thyroid hormone being released.

hyperventilation (hiperventilación) ventilation rate that is greater than metabolically necessary, potentially leading to alkalosis (Ch. 23).

hypocalcemia (hipocalcemia) decreased level of calcium in the blood (Ch. 33).

hypochromic (hipocrómico) less color than normal (Ch. 40).

hypoglycemia (hipoglucemia) state of having a lower than normal blood glucose level (Ch. 8).

hypogonadism (hipogonadismo) when the testes produce little or no testosterone (Ch. 27).

hypokalemia (hipokalemia) decreased level of potassium in the blood (Ch. 33).

hypomagnesemia (hipomagnesemia) decreased level of magnesium in the blood (Ch. 33).

hyponatremia (hiponatremia) decreased level of sodium in the blood (Ch. 33).

hypophosphatemia (hipofosfatemia) decreased level of phosphorus in the blood (Ch. 33).

hypospadias (hypospadias) a condition at birth in which the opening of the urethra is not at the tip of the penis, but on the underside (Ch. 27).

hypotension (hipotensión)   abnormally low blood pressure resulting in inadequate tissue profusion and oxygenation (Ch. 23).

hypothermia (hipotermia)   extremely dangerous cold-related condition that can result in death if the individual does not receive care and if the progression of hypothermia is not reversed. Symptoms include shivering, cold skin, and confusion (Ch. 8, 28).

hypothyroidism (hipotiroidismo)   an underactive thyroid gland which causes a decrease in thyroid hormone being released.

hypoventilation (hipoventilación)   decrease in respiration rate with shallow depth of respiration (Ch. 23).

hypovolemic (hipovolémico)   a type of shock in which the body has lost blood or fluid volume to such an extent that there is not enough circulating volume to fill the ventricles. The heart attempts to compensate by increasing the heart rate (Ch. 8).

hypoxemia (hipoxemia)   lack of oxygen in the blood (Ch. 35).

hypoxia (hypoxia)   oxygen deficiency (Ch. 8, 25).

hysterosalpingogram (histerosalpingograma)   X-ray of uterus and fallopian tubes using a contrast medium (Ch. 25).

idiopathic (idiopático)   any illness or condition with an unknown cause that arises spontaneously (Ch. 23).

immune system (sistema inmunitario)   body's strong line of defense against invading microorganisms. The body recognizes foreign substances such as microorganisms and produces substances to fight them off. Antibodies, white blood cells, digestive enzymes, and resistance of the skin are some examples (Ch. 21).

immunoglobulins (inmunoglobulinas)   family of proteins capable of acting as antibodies, thereby protecting individuals from pathogenic microorganisms; also, antibodies produced by the cells of the immune response system (Ch. 21).

immunohematology (inmunohematología)   study of blood group antigens and antibodies; blood banking (Ch. 38).

immunology (inmunología)   the study of the components of the immune system and their function (Ch. 38).

immunomodulator (inmunomodulador)   a substance that has the ability to change immune responses (Ch. 21).

immunosuppressed (inmunosuprimido)   refers to a patient whose immune system is unhealthy because of disease, medication, and/ or genetics; these patients can be particularly susceptible to attack by microorganisms (Ch. 21).

implantable cardioverter/defibrillator (ICD) (cardioversor/ desfibrilador)   an implantable device used for life-threatening arrhythmias. Its purpose is to shock the heart out of the arrhythmia and into a more normal sinus rhythm (Ch. 31, 36).

implicit (implícito)   capable of being understood from something else though unexpressed; implied (Ch. 8).

implied consent (consentimiento implícito)   consent assumed by the health care provider, typically in an emergency that threatens the patient's life. Implied consent also occurs in more subtle ways in the health care environment; for example, when a patient willingly rolls up the sleeve to receive an injection (Ch. 6).

implied contract (contrato implícito)   contract indicated by actions rather than words (Ch. 6).

improvise (improvisar)   to make, invent, or arrange in an unplanned or spontaneous manner (Ch. 1).

incision (incisión)   a surgical cut made into the skin or tissue (Ch. 8).

income statement (estado de resultados)   financial statement showing net profit or loss (Ch. 20).

incompetence (incompetencia)   a legal term indicating a person who is not able to manage his/her affairs due to a low I.Q., mental deterioration, illness or psychosis, or it may sometimes indicate physical disability (Ch. 6).

incontinence (incontinencia)   uncontrollable loss of urine or feces (Ch. 28).

increments (increment)   increases or additions in number, size, or extent (Ch. 24).

incubate (incubar)   allowing a pathogen to grow in culture media (Ch. 42).

independent provider association (IPA) (Asociación Independiente de Médicos [IPA])   independent network of physicians in private practice who contract with the association to treat patients for an agreed-upon fee (Ch. 2, 16).

indexing (indexar)   selecting the name, subject, or number under which to file a record and determining the order in which the units should be considered (Ch. 13).

indirect statements (declaraciones indirectas)   means of eliciting a response from a patient by turning a question into a statement of interest (Ch. 4).

infection (infección)   invasion of pathogens into living tissue (Ch. 30).

infection control (control de infecciones)   methods to eliminate or reduce the transmission of infectious microorganisms (Ch. 21).

infectious agents (agentes infeccioso)   pathogens responsible for a specific infectious disease (Ch. 21).

inflammation (inflamación)   the normal nonspecific immune response by the body to any type of injury (trauma, bacterial, viral, and temperature extremes) (Ch. 30).

inflammatory response (respuesta inflamatoria)   body's defense against the threat of infection or trauma. Characterized by redness, pain, heat, and swelling (Ch. 21).

informed consent (consentimiento informado)   consent given by the patient who is made aware of any procedure to be performed, its risks, expected outcomes, and alternatives (Ch. 6, 30).

inhalers (inhaladors)   devices that are used to deliver medication into the lungs and are most often used to treat asthma (Ch. 29).

inner-directed people (personas con autodeterminación)   people who decide for themselves what they want to do with their lives (Ch. 3).

inoculate (inocular)   to place colonies of microorganisms onto nutrient media for culture testing (Ch. 42).

input device (dispositivo de entrada)   a device used to input data into a computer (Ch. 10).

integrated delivery system (IDS) (sistema de prestación de servicios médicos integrado [IDS])   a health care organization of affiliated provider sites combined under a single ownership that offers the full spectrum of managed health care (Ch. 16).

integrative medicine (medicina integradora)   brings together two or more treatment modalities so they function as a harmonious whole, as seen in alternative forms of health care (Ch. 2).

internal respiration (respiración interna)   passage of oxygen from the blood into the cells (Ch. 29).

International Classification of Diseases, 9th Revision, Clinical Modification **(ICD-9-CM) (Clasificación Internacional de Enfermedades, 9.ª Revisión, Modificación Clínica [CIE-9-MC])**   standard diagnosis codes used to identify a patient's medical problem. Used by most ambulatory care settings in encoding the claim form and recognized by most insurance carriers (Ch. 17).

International Classification of Diseases, 10th Revision, Clinical Modification **(ICD-10-CM) (Clasificación Internacional de Enfermedades, 10.ª Revisión, Modificación Clínica [CIE-10-MC])**   a classification system developed by the National Center for Health Statistics (NCHS) as a clinical modification to the ICD-10 system developed by the World Health Organization (WHO), primarily as a unique system for use in the United States for morbidity and mortality reporting (Ch. 17).

International Classification of Diseases, 10th Revision, Procedure Coding System **(ICD-10-PCS) (Clasificación Internacional de Enfermedades, 10.ª Revisión, sistema de codificación de procedimiento)**   developed by the United States as mandated by the Health Insurance Portability and Accountability Act for reporting inpatient procedures (Ch. 17).

Internet (Internet)   a worldwide publicly accessible network of networks and computers (Ch. 10).

Internet blog (blogs de Internet)   A Web site or web page updated regularly by one person or a small group. It is often written in conversational style and discusses one or more specific topics. The blog is usually interactive, allowing visitors to leave comments (Ch. 47).

internship (pasantía)   transition stage between classroom and employment (Ch. 1).

interrogatory (interrogatorio)   a written set of questions that must be answered, under oath, within a specific time period; part of the discovery process (Ch. 6).

interview (entrevista) meeting in which you and the interviewer discuss employment opportunities and strengths you can contribute to the organization (Ch. 47).

intimate partner violence (IPV) (violencia de pareja [IPV]) refers to violence or abuse between a spouse or former spouse; boyfriend, girlfriend or former boyfriend/girlfriend; and same-sex or heterosexual intimate partner or former same-sex or heterosexual intimate partner (Ch. 6, 7).

intracellular (intracelulares) "inside the cell"; located or occurring inside a cell (Ch. 21).

intraepithelial (intraepitelial) within the epithelium (Ch. 25).

intravenous pyelogram (IVP) (pielograma intravenoso) radiographic study of the kidneys, ureters, and bladder using a contrast medium (Ch. 29).

inversion (inversión) moving a body part inward (Ch. 32).

in vitro fertilization (IVF) (fertilización in vitro [IVF]) the ovum is fertilized in a culture dish, allowed to grow, and then implanted into the uterus (Ch. 7).

involuntary dismissals (despido involuntario) termination of employment based on poor job performance or violation of office policies (Ch. 45).

involutes (involuciona) when the uterus returns to normal size and shape after childbirth (Ch. 25).

ionizing radiation (radiación ionizante) X-ray beams (Ch. 31).

ischemia (isquemia) local and temporary lack of blood to an organ or part caused by obstruction of circulation (Ch. 36).

isoelectric (isoeléctrico) having equal electrical potentials. It is represented on the ECG as the flat horizontal line, the baseline (Ch. 36).

isolation (aislamiento) separating a patient with certain infections or communicable diseases from other individuals (Ch. 21).

isolation categories (categorías de aislamiento) system of seven categories developed by the Centers for Disease Control and Prevention (CDC) that isolates patients according to known infections. These categories have been condensed into three Transmission-Based Precautions based on air, contact, and droplet routes of transmission (Ch. 21).

isopropyl alcohol (alcohol isopropílico) commonly called rubbing alcohol; 70% alcohol solution commonly used as a cleaner (Ch. 30).

isotope (isótopo) a chemical element (Ch. 31).

itinerary (itinerario) detailed written plan of a proposed trip (Ch. 44).

jargon (jerga) words, phrases, or terminology specific to a profession (Ch. 11).

jaundice (ictericia) yellow discolorization of the skin and sclera caused by excess bilirubin in the blood (Ch. 24).

ketoacidosis (cetoacidosis) accumulation of ketones in the body, occurring primarily as a complication of diabetes mellitus; if left untreated, it could cause a coma (Ch. 8, 41).

ketones (cetonas) chemical compound produced during an increased metabolism of fat; also, test on a reagent strip (Ch. 41).

ketonuria (cetonuria) having ketones in urine (Ch. 41).

ketosis (cetosis) a condition of the body burning fatty acids for energy in the absence of appropriate glucose/carbohydrates; may be referred to as lipolysis (Ch. 41).

key (keyed) (mecanografiar) to input data by keystrokes on a computer keyboard (Ch. 14).

key unit (unidad clave) first indexing unit of the filing segment (Ch. 13).

keywords (palabras clave) words that relate to a job-specific position. Keywords may be job-specific skills or profession-specific words (Ch. 47).

kinesics (cinésica) study of body language (Ch. 4).

labile (lábil) a specimen that is easily broken down (Ch. 37).

labyrinthitis (laberintitis) inflammation of inner ear or labyrinth (Ch. 24).

laceration (laceración) tears or splits in the skin or tissues caused by trauma (Ch. 8).

Lamaze (Lamaze) a method of childbirth which teaches the mother about the physiology of childbirth and techniques of relaxation, concentration, and breathing (Ch. 25).

laparoscopy (laparoscopía) a procedure in which a lighted instrument is used to view the inside of the pelvic cavity (Ch. 25).

lead wire (alambre guía) a conductor attached to an electrocardiograph. Consists of limb leads and chest leads (Ch. 36).

ledger (libro mayor) record of charges, payments, and adjustments for individual patient or family (Ch. 18).

lesion (lesión) injury or wound. A circumscribed area of tissue that has been altered pathologically (Ch. 29).

letter of resignation (carta de renuncia) letter informing the current employer of the employee's decision to resign from a current position (Ch. 45).

leukocyte esterase (esterasa leucocitaria) an enzyme produced by leukocytes; test on a reagent strip that indicates the presence of white blood cells in the urinary tract (Ch. 41).

leukocytes (leucocito) white blood cells; one of the formed elements of blood (Ch. 39, 40).

LGBT (LGBT) common abbreviation to refer to individuals who are lesbian, gay, bisexual, or transgender (Ch. 45).

liability (pasivo) debts and financial obligations for which one is responsible (Ch. 20); legal responsibility (Ch. 44).

libel (calumnia) false and malicious writing about another constituting a defamation of character (Ch. 6).

libido (libido) sexual drive (Ch. 27).

license (licencia) permission by competent authority (the state) to engage in a profession; permission to act (Ch. 1); permission statement authorizing the use of copyrighted computer software (Ch. 10).

licensure (matrícula) granting of licenses to practice a profession (Ch. 1).

ligature (ligadura) length of suture thread without a needle, used for tying off vessels during surgery (Ch. 30).

limiting charge (limitación de carga) The dollar amount up to 115% of the Medicare allowed amount that can be charged to the patient by a Medicare non-PAR provider (Ch. 16).

lithotomy (litotomía) patient lays on the back similar to the dorsal recumbent position except the buttocks should be as close to the bottom edge of the table as possible, and feet are placed in stirrups attached to the foot of the table (Ch. 24).

litigation (litigio) court action (Ch. 6).

lochia (loquios) discharge from the uterus of blood, mucus, and tissue during the period after childbirth (Ch. 25).

long-range goals (metas a largo plazo) achievements that may take three to five years to accomplish (Ch. 3).

low-context communication (comunicación de bajo contexto) communication style that uses few environmental or cultural idioms to convey an idea or concept. Ideas are spelled out explicitly (Ch. 4).

low-density lipoprotein (LDL) (lipoproteína de baja densidad [LDL]) lipoprotein in the blood composed primarily of cholesterol. The cholesterol carried by LDL may be deposited in peripheral tissues and is associated with an increased risk for heart disease (Ch. 43).

lumen (luz) the space within an artery, vein, intestine, needles, and catheter or tube (Ch. 23).

lymphadenopathy (linfadenopatía) chronic enlargement or swelling of lymph nodes due to a disease process (Ch. 21).

lymphocyte (linfocito) white blood cell with a dense nonsegmented nucleus and lacking granules in the cytoplasm; functions to combat viruses and coordinate the immune response, making antibodies (Ch. 40).

lyophilized (liofilizado) the process of rapidly freezing a substance at extremely low temperatures and then dehydrating the substance in a high vacuum (freeze drying) (Ch. 26).

macroallocation (macroasignación) of scarce medical resources; decisions are made by Congress, health systems agencies, and insurance companies (Ch. 7).

macrocytic (macrocítico)   term that describes a larger than normal cell (Ch. 40).

macular degeneration (degeneración macular)   degeneration of the macula area of the retina caused by aging; a leading cause of visual impairment in people older than 50 years, making it difficult to do fine work (Ch. 28).

magnetic resonance imaging (la proyección de imagen de resonancia magnética)   a method of medical imaging that measures the response of tissues to a magnetic field and radio waves resulting in images of tissues and organs of the body (Ch. 31).

major medical (médicos mayores)   Insurance that covers catastrophic expenses resulting from illness or injury (Ch. 16).

major mineral (mineral principal)   mineral that is required in large amounts by the body (Ch. 33).

malabsorption (malabsorción)   inadequate absorption of nutrients from the intestinal tract (Ch. 29).

malaise (malestar)   discomfort, uneasiness, or indisposition, often indicative of infection (Ch. 21, 29).

malaria (paludismo)   acute infectious disease caused by the presence of protozoan parasites within the red blood cells; usually comes from the bite of a female mosquito (Ch. 21).

male infertility (infertilidad masculine)   low sperm production, abnormal sperm function (Ch. 27).

malfeasance (fechoría)   conduct that is illegal or contrary to an official's obligations (Ch. 6).

malpractice (mala praxis)   professional negligence (Ch. 6, 44).

mammogram (mamografía)   A radiographic technique that allows imaging of the breast tissue to evaluate for abnormalities (Ch. 31).

managed care operation (establecimiento de atención administrada)   any health care setting or delivery system that is designed to reduce the cost of care while still providing access to care (Ch. 2).

managed care organization (MCO) (organización de atención administrada [MCO])   a health insurance organization that adheres to the principles of strong dependence on selective contracting with providers, the use of primary care physicians, prospective and retrospective utilization management, use of treatment guidelines for high cost chronic disorders, and an emphasis on preventive care, education, and patient compliance with treatment plans (Ch. 16).

management by walking around (MBWA) (gestión itinerante [MBWA])   a technique for keeping managers informed about the health of their organization (Ch. 44).

managerial accounting (contabilidad administrativa)   generates financial information that can enable more efficient internal management (Ch. 20).

manometer (manómetro)   device for measuring a liquid or gaseous pressure. The measurement is expressed in millimeters of mercury or water (Ch. 23).

Mantoux test (prueba de Mantoux)   test for tuberculosis involving the intracutaneous injection of purified protein derivative (see PPD) (Ch. 43).

marketing (comercialización)   process by which the provider of services makes the consumer aware of the scope and quality of those services. Marketing tools might include public relations, brochures, patient education seminars, and newsletters (Ch. 44).

masking (ocultamiento)   attempt to conceal or repress true feelings or the message (Ch. 4).

matrix (matriz)   to establish an appointment matrix, a provider's unavailable time slots are marked with an X. Patients are not scheduled during those times (Ch. 12).

mature minor (menor maduro)   a person, usually younger than 18 years, who is able to understand and appreciate the consequences of treatment despite his or her young age (Ch. 6).

Mayo stand(s)/instrument tray(s) (mesa de Mayo)   portable metal tray table used for setting up small sterile fields for minor surgery and procedures (Ch. 30).

meaningful use (uso significativo)   a Centers for Medicare and Medicaid (CMS) program that awards incentives for using certified electronic health records (EHR) to improve patient care (Ch. 13).

meconium (meconio)   first feces of a newborn (Ch. 25).

mediation (mediación)   dispute resolution that allows a facilitator to help the two parties settle their differences and come to an acceptable solution (Ch. 6).

medical asepsis (asepsia médica)   clean and free from infection (Ch. 21, 37).

medical necessity (necesidad médica)   the likelihood that a proposed health care service will have a reasonable beneficial effect on the patient's physical condition and quality of life at a specific point in his or her illness or lifetime. The concept that procedures are eligible for reimbursement only as a covered benefit when they are performed for a specific diagnosis or specified frequency (Ch. 17).

medical transcriptionist (transcriptor médico)   A specialist that listens to voice recordings dictated by health care providers and create medical records in the proper format for the type of document (Ch. 15).

medically indigent (médicamente indigente)   refers to those individuals unable to pay for their own medical coverage (Ch. 6).

Medicare Part A (Medicare Parte A)   benefits covering inpatient hospital and skilled nursing facilities, hospice care, and blood transfusion (Ch. 16).

Medicare Part B (Medicare Parte B)   benefits covering outpatient hospital and health care provider services (Ch. 16).

Medicare Part C (Medicare Parte C)   commonly referred to as Medicare advantage plans. These plans are approved by Medicare and are run by private companies (Ch. 16).

Medicare Part D (Medicare Parte D)   prescription drug coverage by Medicare (Ch. 16).

Medigap policy (póliza de Medigap)   an individual plan covering the patient's Medicare deductible and co-pay obligations that fulfills the federal government standards for Medicare supplemental insurance (Ch. 16).

megaloblastic anemia (anemia megaloblástica)   a type of anemia characterized by many large immature and dysfunctional red blood cells (Ch. 33).

memorandum (memorándum)   interoffice correspondence, usually referred to as a memo (Ch. 14).

memory (memoria)   refers to storage of computer data. Memory can be volatile (lost when computer is turned off) or nonvolatile (permanently written to storage device) (Ch. 10).

meningitis (meningitis)   inflammation of the delicate tissues that cover the brain and spinal cord. It may be caused by bacterial, viral, or fungal infection (Ch. 29).

meniscus (menisco)   curvature appearing in a liquid's upper surface when a liquid is placed in a container (Ch. 23, 35).

menopausal hormone therapy (MHT) (terapia hormonal para la menopausia)   when natural hormones are symptomatically absent and hormones from outside the body are ingested to elevate levels (Ch. 25).

menopause (menopausia)   the cessation of menstruation usually occurring between 45 and 55 years of age (Ch. 28).

mensuration (medición)   a method of examination using the process of measuring. The measurements of height and weight, the length of a limb, and the amount of flexion and extension of an extremity are all forms of mensuration (Ch. 24).

mentor (mentor)   person assigned or requested to assist in training, guiding, or coaching another (Ch. 44).

metabolism (metabolismo)   total of all changes, chemical and physical, that take place in the body (Ch. 33).

metered dose inhaler (inhalador de dosis medida)   a device used to deliver a prescribed amount of medication to the respiratory tract, especially the lungs (Ch. 29).

metrorrhagia (metrorragia)   uterine bleeding at irregular intervals (Ch. 25).

mHealth (mHealth)   a term that stands for mobile health, which refers to the practice of medicine supported by mobile devices (Ch. 11).

microallocation (microasignación)   of scarce medical resources; decisions are made by providers and individual members of the health care team (Ch. 7).

microbiology (microbiología) branch of biology dealing with the study of microscopic forms of life (Ch. 38).

microcytic (microcítico) term describing a smaller than normal cell (Ch. 40).

microorganisms (microorganismo) microscopic living creatures capable of transmission and reproduction in specific circumstances (Ch. 21).

microscopic examination (examen microscópico) viewing a specimen with the aid of a microscope (Ch. 15, 38).

midstream (mitad de micción) urine sample collected in the middle of a flow of urine (Ch. 41).

minor (menor) person who has not reached the age of majority, usually 18 years (Ch. 6).

minutes (actas) written record of topics discussed and actions taken during meeting sessions (Ch. 14, 44).

misdemeanor (contravención) a lesser crime; misdemeanors vary from state to state in their definition. Punishment is usually probation or a time of public service and a fine (Ch. 6).

misfeasance (irregularidad) a civil law term referring to a lawful act that is improperly or unlawfully executed (Ch. 6).

modalities (modalidades) physical agents such as heat, cold, light, water, and electricity used to treat muscular or joint malfunction (Ch. 32).

modified block letter, indented (carta estilo bloque modificado, con sangría) modified letter style with indented paragraphs. Paragraphs in this style of letter may be indented five spaces (Ch. 14).

modified block letter, standard (carta estilo bloque modificado, estándar) major letter style where all lines begin at the left margin with the exception of the date line, complimentary closure, and keyed signature. The exceptions usually begin at the center position or a few spaces to the right of center (Ch. 14).

modified wave scheduling (planificación en olas modificada) system where multiple patients are scheduled at the beginning of each hour, followed by single appointments every 10 to 20 minutes the rest of the hour (Ch. 12).

modifiers (modificador) additional codes that may be added to a five-digit CPT code to further explain the service provided (Ch. 17).

modulated (modulado) speech that varies in pitch and intensity (Ch. 11).

money market savings accounts (cuentas de ahorro del mercado monetario) bank accounts that pay a higher interest rate (money market rate) than standard savings accounts and permit writing a limited number of checks (Ch. 18).

monocytes (monocito) white blood cells without cytoplasmic granules that have a large convoluted nonsegmented nucleus; responsible for phagocytosis of pathogens and assisting in antibody formation (Ch. 40).

morbidity (morbilidad) number of cases of disease in a specific population (Ch. 17, 21).

morbid obesity (obesidad mórbida) obesity so severe that it can result in serious diseases (Ch. 29).

morphology (morfología) form and structure of an organism (Ch. 42).

mortality (mortalidad) the ratio of the number of deaths to a given population (Ch. 17, 21).

motherboard (tarjeta madre) printed circuit containing the inner connections of a digital computer including the CPU, RAM and ROM memory, and other support systems. It provides connectivity to input and output systems (Ch. 10).

mounting (montaje) process of applying in sequence a portion of each of the 12 leads of the ECG recording onto a commercially prepared mounting form or plain sheet of paper as part of the patient's permanent record (Ch. 36).

multigravida (multigrávida) a woman who has been pregnant more than once (Ch. 25).

mycology (micología) study of fungi (Ch. 38, 42).

myocardial infarction (infarto de miocardio) a heart attack; usually caused by a blockage of one or more of the coronary arteries (Ch. 8, 36).

myopia (miopía) nearsightedness; caused by an elongated (shaped) eyeball and the image is focused in the front of the retina resulting in the inability to focus on objects at a distance (Ch. 29).

myringotomy (miringotomía) incision into the tympanic membrane; part of the treatment for otitis media (Ch. 26).

Nägele's rule (regla de Nägele) usual method for calculating expected date of birth (Ch. 25).

narrative charting (trazado de la narrative) a chronologic account in paragraphs describing client status, procedures, interventions and treatments, and client's response (Ch. 22).

National Healthcareer Association (NHA) (Asociación Nacional de Profesiones de Salud [NHA]) an association that offers national certification examinations for health care professionals. NHA works with educational institutions on curriculum development, competency testing, and preparation and administration of their examination for certification (Ch. 46).

navigator (navigator) works in conjunction with the medical home health care team (Ch. 4).

nebulizer (nebulizador) an apparatus that changes the medication for asthma from a liquid form into a mist for ease of inhaling the medication into the lungs (Ch. 29).

negligence (negligencia) failure to exercise a certain standard of care (Ch. 6, 44).

neonatal (neonatal) pertaining to a newborn (Ch. 25).

neonate (neonato) a newborn (Ch. 26).

networking (conexión en red) connecting two or more computers together to share files and hardware. The system is called a network (Ch. 10); process in which people of similar interests exchange information in social, business, or professional relationships (Ch. 47).

neurogenic (neurogénico) a type of shock in which there is injury or trauma to the nervous system causing the loss of tone in the vessels resulting in massive dilation of arterioles and venuoles. This results in a dramatic drop in blood pressure (Ch. 8).

neutrophils (neutrófilo) the most common type of granulocytic white blood cell (Ch. 40).

nevi (nevos) plural of the medical term *nevus*, meaning mole (Ch. 30).

nevus (nevo) a mole (Ch. 28).

niacin (niacina) one of the B-complex vitamins (Ch. 33).

nocturia (nocturia) excessive urination during the night (Ch. 27, 29).

nomenclature (nomenclatura) naming (Ch. 42).

nomenclature systems (sistemas de nomenclatura) provide terms that follow preestablished naming conventions; a disease nomenclature is a listing of the proper name for each disease entity with its specific code number (Ch. 17).

nomogram (nomograma) graph that shows the relation among numeric values. Body surface area (BSA) of a patient can be estimated by its use (Ch. 35).

noncompliant (inobservancia) describes one who fails to follow a required command or instruction (Ch. 6).

nonfeasance (omisión) a civil law term referring to the failure to perform an act, official duty, or legal requirement (Ch. 6).

noninvasive procedure (procedimiento no invasivo) a procedure that does require penetrating the skin or a body opening (Ch. 31, 36).

nonretaliation provision (disposición de no represalias) provides protection to an employee or applicant from being retaliated against due to participation in filing a complaint regarding discrimination, or participating in an investigation or lawsuit (Ch. 44).

normal flora (flora normal) microorganisms that are normally present in a specific site (Ch. 21, 42).

normal saline (solución salina normal) a solution of sodium chloride (salt) and distilled water. It has the same osmotic pressure as blood serum. It is also known as isotonic or physiologic saline (Ch. 8).

normal sinus rhythm (ritmo sinusal normal) term used to describe the heart's rhythm when it is within the normal range (Ch. 36).

normochromic (normocrómico) of normal color, in this case, when referring to red blood cells (Ch. 40).

normocytic (normocítico) term that describes a normal-sized cell (Ch. 40).

nosocomial (intrahospitalaria) infection acquired in a health care setting (hospital, clinic, nursing home) (Ch. 21, 42).

notary (notary public) (escribano público) someone with the legal capacity to witness and certify documents; can take depositions (Ch. 18).

nullipara (nulípara) a woman who has not carried a pregnancy to the stage of viability (Ch. 25).

nutrient (nutriente) ingested substance that helps the body stay in its homeostatic state (Ch. 33).

nutrition (nutrición) a complex process by which a plant or animal takes in, breaks into usable segments, and utilizes nutrients to sustain life (Ch. 33).

nystagmus (nistagmo) continuous involuntary movement of the eyes (Ch. 29).

objective (objetivo) a patient sign that is visible, palpable, or measurable by an observer (Ch. 22).

occlusion (oclusión) closure of a passage (Ch. 8).

old reports (informes anteriores) reports such as a discharge summary that should be completed within 71 hours (Ch. 15).

oliguria (oliguria) decrease in urine output (Ch. 29).

one-handed technique (técnica con una sola mano) a scooping technique for covering a dirty needle with its cover using only one hand, therefore decreasing the risk of needle stick in the absence of a biohazard container (Ch. 21).

open-ended questions (preguntas abiertas) questions that encourage verbalization and response; questions that seek a response beyond a simple yes or no (Ch. 4).

operating system (OS) (sistema operativo [SO]) software used to control the computer and its peripheral equipment. Also referred to as system software (Ch. 10).

operative report (OR) (informe quirúrgico [OR]) medical report that chronicles the details of a surgical procedure (Ch. 15).

opportunistic infection (infección oportunista) an infection that results from a defective immune system that cannot defend itself from pathogens normally found in the environment (Ch. 21).

optical character recognition (OCR) (reconocimiento óptico de caracteres) U.S. Postal Service's computerized scanner that reads addresses printed on letter mail. If the information is properly formatted, then the OCR will find a match in its address files and print a bar code on the lower right edge of the envelope (Ch. 14).

orchiectomy (orquidectomía) surgical excision of a testicle (Ch. 27).

organomercurial (compuestos organomercuriales) any mercury-containing organic compound (Ch. 26).

orthopnea (ortopnea) difficulty breathing in any position other than an upright position (Ch. 23).

oscilloscope (osciloscopio) an electronic device used for recording electrical activity of the heart, brain, and muscular tissues (Ch. 31, 36).

osteoporosis (osteoporosis) a thinning of the long bones, pelvic bones, and vertebrae (Ch. 28, 31).

otitis media (otitis media) acute infection of the middle ear usually caused by bacteria. Symptoms are pain, fever, discharge, and decreased hearing acuity (Ch. 29).

otoscope (otoscopio) instrument used to examine the external ear canal and tympanic membrane (Ch. 29).

outer-directed people (personas influenciables) people who let events, other people, or environmental factors dictate their behavior (Ch. 3).

out guide or sheet (señalador o marcador) card, folder, or slip of paper inserted temporarily in the files to replace a record that has been retrieved from the files (Ch. 13).

output device (dispositivo de salida) a device used to output data from a computer. Includes printers, faxes, data storage drivers, screens, and plotters (Ch. 10).

outsourcing (subcontratación) the practice of contracting with a service outside of the clinic or hospital to a company where the task can be accomplished at a lower cost and with a faster turnaround time (Ch. 15).

ova (óvulos) eggs; in laboratory setting, usually refers to eggs of a parasite (Ch. 42).

overtime (horas extra) money paid at a rate of not less than one and one-half times the regular rate of pay after a 40-hour work week is completed (Ch. 45).

owner's equity (patrimonio neto) amount by which business assets exceed business liabilities. Also called net worth, proprietorship, and capital (Ch. 20).

oxidation (oxidación) process of a substance combining with oxygen (Ch. 33).

oximetry (oximetría) a method of measuring oxygen saturation in a noninvasive manner (Ch. 29).

oxytocin (oxitocina) a pituitary hormone that stimulates the muscles of the uterus to contract, thus inducing labor (Ch. 25).

palliative (paliativa) refers to measures taken to relieve symptoms of disease (Ch. 5, 21, 31).

pallor (palidez) lack of color, paleness (Ch. 24).

palpate (palpar) to feel with fingertips, to search for a vein through touch (Ch. 39).

palpation (palpación) an examination of the body using touch; often used to help verify observations (Ch. 24).

panel (panel) a series of tests related to a particular organ or organ system of body function. For example, a liver panel would check many different functions of the liver. Previously called a profile (Ch. 38).

Pap (Papanicolaou) test (prueba de Papanicolaou) screening exam to detect the presence of abnormal cervical cells (Ch. 25).

paracentesis (paracentesis) puncture of a cavity for removal of fluid (Ch. 21).

parasitology (parasitología) study of organisms (parasites and their eggs) that live within or on another organism and at the expense of that organism (Ch. 38).

parasympathetic nervous system (sistema nervioso parasimpático) part of the autonomic nervous system that returns the body to its normal state after stress has subsided (Ch. 3).

parenteral (parenteral) injection of a liquid substance into the body via a route other than the alimentary canal (Ch. 21, 35).

parity (paridad) carrying a pregnancy to the point of viability regardless of the outcome (Ch. 25).

participatory style operates on the premise that the worker is capable and wants to do a good job (Ch. 44).

parturition (parir) the process of giving birth (Ch. 25).

patch (parche) modification to software to fix deficiencies in the software. Frequently downloaded from the software supplier's Web site or from floppy disks provided by the supplier (Ch. 10).

patency (la permeabilidad) open, not blocked (Ch. 25).

pathogens (patógeno) disease causing microorganisms (Ch. 21, 42).

pathology report (informe de patología) medical reports generated to describe the gross and microscopic examinations performed during a surgical procedure (Ch. 15).

patient-centered medical home (PCMH) (hogar médico centrado en el paciente) a model of care that responds to each patient's unique needs through: (1) making a personal and coordinating physician available for care; (2) providing comprehensive care at all stages of life; (3) practicing culturally sensitive, integrated and coordinate care while focusing on quality and safety; and (4) enhancing patients' access to care. As of 2016, PCMH recognition and accreditation is not available in all states (Ch. 2).

patient portal system (sistema de portal del paciente) secure Web sites or applications combined with other software, such as an EMR, that allow patients to have convenient 24-hour access to interact and communicate with their health care providers (Ch. 11).

Patient Self-Determination Act (PSDA) (Ley de Autodeterminación del Paciente [PSDA]) the Act that includes the advance directive giving patients the right to be involved in their health care decisions (Ch. 6).

patient service centers (centros de servicio al paciente) satellite laboratory facilities located in convenient areas for patients where specimens can be collected or dropped off (Ch. 38).

payee (beneficiario) person named on a check who is to receive the amount indicated (Ch. 18).

peak (pico) the opposite of *trough*, this is the point at which a drug is at its highest level in the body, usually about 30 minutes after administration. In lab tests, the peak would tell the provider the strongest influence the drug would have on the body at that particular dose (Ch. 38).

pegboard system (sistema de tablero de clavijas) most commonly used manual medical accounts receivable system (Ch. 18).

pellagra (pelagra) disease caused by a deficiency in vitamin B$_3$ (nicotinic acid) characterized by sores on the skin, diarrhea, anxiety, confusion, and death if not treated (Ch. 33).

pelvic inflammatory disease (enfermedad inflamatoria pélvica) infection of uterus, fallopian tubes, and adjacent pelvic structures; most common causes are gonorrhea and chlamydia, spread as sexually transmitted diseases (Ch. 25).

percussion (percusión) the process of eliciting sounds from the body by tapping with either a percussion hammer or fingers. The vibrations and sounds from underlying organs and cavities can be felt and heard (Ch. 24).

percutaneous transluminal coronary angioplasty (PTCA) (angioplastía transluminal coronaria percutánea [PTCA]) a procedure that widens a narrowed or blocked coronary artery (Ch. 36).

peripheral (periférico) away from the center of the body (Ch. 23).

pernicious anemia (anemia perniciosa) chronic anemia caused by lack of hydrochloric acid in the stomach; weakness, fatigue, tingling of extremities, and even heart failure can result; vitamin B$_{12}$ injections are the treatment for this condition (Ch. 28, 33).

petrissage (petrissage) a kneading movement in massage (Ch. 32).

petty cash (caja chica) small sum kept on hand for minor or unexpected expenses (Ch. 18).

Peyronie disease (enfermedad de Peyronie) curvature of the penis during erection (Ch. 27).

pH (pH) scale that indicates the relative alkalinity or acidity of a solution; measurement of hydrogen ion concentration (Ch. 41).

pharmacogenomics (farmacogenómica) the study of the response of the body to various chemical compounds based on an individual's genetic inheritance (Ch. 34).

pharmacokinetics (farmacocinética) refers to the way a drug is handled by the body (Ch. 35).

pharmacology (farmacología) study of drugs; the science concerned with the history, origin, sources, physical and chemical properties, and uses of drugs and their effects on living organisms (Ch. 34).

pharmazooticals (fármacos derivados de animales) drugs obtained from tissues such as the adrenal glands of animals (Ch. 34).

phenylketonuria (PKU) (fenilcetonuria [FCU]) a hereditary disease caused by the body's inability to oxidize the amino acid phenylalanine. If not discovered and treated early, brain damage can occur, causing severe intellectual disability and other serious permanent disabilities (Ch. 26, 43).

phimosis (fimosis) tightening of the foreskin that does not allow retraction (Ch. 27).

phishing (suplantación de identidad) a practice where the recipient of email is directed to go to a Web site to provide information to his or her bank, the IRS, or other official organization. The Web site is actually a fake made to resemble the real thing, and when information is given, it goes to the consumer fraud criminal (Ch. 10).

phlebotomy (flebotomía) process of collecting blood (Ch. 39).

photophobia (fotofobia) extreme sensitivity to light (Ch. 33).

physiatry (fisiatría) a medical specialty that treats a wide variety of medical conditions affecting the brain, spinal cord, nerves, bones, joints, ligaments, muscles, and tendons (Ch. 32).

physician's office laboratory (POL) (laboratorio del consultorio del medico [POL]) laboratory within a physician's office where common office laboratory tests are performed (Ch. 38).

phytomedicines (fitomedicinas) herbs used as medicinal plants. They contain plant material as their active ingredient (Ch. 35).

placenta abruptio (desprendimiento de la placenta) sudden and abrupt separation of the placenta from uterine wall (Ch. 25).

placenta previa (placenta previa) occurs when the placenta lies low in the uterus and can partially or completely cover the cervical os (Ch. 25).

plaintiff (demandante) person bringing charges in litigation (Ch. 6).

plantar flexion (flexión plantar) occurs when the foot moves downward at the ankle (Ch. 32).

plasma (plasma) fluid portion of blood from a tube containing anticoagulant. This fluid contains fibrinogen (Ch. 39).

point-of-care testing (POCT) also known as near-patient testing or bedside testing, as it brings the portable laboratory services directly to where the patient is located, wherever that may be (Ch. 38).

point-of-service (POS) device (dispositivo de punto de servicio [POS]) device allowing direct communication between a medical office and the health care plan's computer (Ch. 17).

point-of-service (POS) plan (plan de punto de servicio [POS]) a plan that allows direct communication between a medical office and the health insurance company (Ch. 16).

polycystic (poliquístico) many cysts; as in polycystic ovarian syndrome in which the ovary is enlarged and has many fluid-filled sacs (Ch. 25).

polyps (pólipo) tumors with a stem found in the nose, uterus, bladder, colon, or rectum (Ch. 29).

port (puerto) shortened term for *portal*—an entry way. When related to intravenous therapy, it is a type of adapter that can serve as an additional means for infusing fluids or medications. The port can be attached to the primary tubing. The port has a needleless entry site (Ch. 35).

portfolio (cartera) notebook or file containing examples of materials commonly used (Ch. 14).

positron emission tomography (PET) (tomografía por emisión de positrones [PET]) a radiographic procedure that uses a computer and a radioactive substance. The radioactive substance is injected into the patient's body and gives off charged particles. They combine with particles in the patient's body to produce color images that reveal the amount of metabolic activity in an organ or structure (Ch. 31).

postcoital (poscoital) period of time following (after) sexual intercourse (Ch. 25).

posting (asiento) recording financial transactions into a bookkeeping or accounting system (Ch. 18).

potassium hydroxide (KOH) (hidróxido de potasio [KOH]) 10% solution placed on vaginal smears, as well as skin scrapings, hair, and other dry substances, to dissolve excess debris. This clears the vision field for better viewing of fungi and spores (Ch. 42).

practice-based scheduling (programación basada en la práctica) see cluster scheduling (Ch. 12).

practice management (prácticas de gestión) type of health care software, often intertwined with EMR and used in the day-to-day financial and administrative operations of a medical clinic (Ch. 10).

practicum (práctica) transitional stage providing opportunity to apply theory learned in the classroom to a health care setting through practical, hands-on experience (Ch. 1, 44).

preauthorization (autorización previa) obtaining an insurance carrier's consent to proceed with patient care and treatment. Unless authorization is obtained, insurance carriers may not pay benefits for specific problems (Ch. 16).

precedents (precedentes) refers to rulings made at an earlier time and include decisions made in a court, interpretations of a constitution, and statutory law decisions (Ch. 6).

precipitate (precipitado) substance in the form of fine particles that separates from a solution if allowed to stand for a time (Ch. 35).

precordial (precordial) pertaining to the area on the anterior surface of the body overlying the heart (Ch. 36).

preeclampsia (preeclampsia) a complication of pregnancy characterized by generalized edema, hypertension, and proteinuria (Ch. 25).

preference cards (tarjetas de preferencia)   a method of noting a provider's preferred method of conducting a procedure that includes positioning, medication(s), instrumentation, room setup, and so on (Ch. 30).

preferred provider organization (PPO) (organización de proveedor preferido [PPO])   organization of providers who network together to offer discounts to purchasers of health care insurance (Ch. 2, 16).

prejudice (prejuicio)   opinion or judgment that is formed before all the facts are known (Ch. 4).

prenatal (prenatal)   time period between fertilization and birth (Ch. 25).

prepuce (prepucio)   a free fold of skin that covers the head of the penis or clitoris (Ch. 27).

presbycusis (presbiacusia)   progressive loss of hearing caused by the normal aging process (Ch. 28).

presbyopia (presbicia)   farsightedness caused by loss of elasticity of the lens of the eye, occurring typically in middle and old age (Ch. 28, 29).

prescribe (recetar)   to order or recommend the use of a drug, diet, or other form of therapy (Ch. 6, 34).

present problem (PP) (problema presente [PP])   see chief complaint (CC) (Ch. 15).

preservative (conservante)   chemical added to food to keep it fresh longer or added to urine to preserve it for testing (Ch. 33).

priapism (priapismo)   an erection lasting more than four hours; can occur with or without sexual stimulation (Ch. 27).

primary care provider (PCP) (médico de atención primaria [PCP])   primary care provider for a patient; all care is coordinated through the PCP (Ch. 16).

primigravidas (primigrávidas)   women who are pregnant for the first time (Ch. 25).

privileged (privilegiada)   confidential information that may only be communicated with the patient's permission or by court order (Ch. 15).

probate court (tribunal sucesorio)   court that administers estates and validates wills (Ch. 19).

probation (período de prueba)   period during which the employee and supervisory personnel may determine if both the environment and the position are satisfactory for the employee (Ch. 45).

problem-oriented medical record (POMR) (historia clínica orientada al problema [POMR])   a type of patient chart recordkeeping that uses a sheet at a prominent location in the chart to list vital identification data. Patient medical problems are identified by a number that corresponds to the charting; for example, bronchitis is #1, a broken wrist is #2, and so forth (Ch. 13, 22).

procedure manual (manual de procedimientos)   manual providing detailed information relative to the performance of tasks within the job description (Ch. 44).

processed food (alimentos procesados)   food that is no longer in a whole, natural state; cooked or packaged with parts removed or ingredients added (Ch. 33).

proctologic (proctologic)   the branch of medicine dealing with diseases of the rectum and the anus (Ch. 24).

professionalism (profesionalismo)   the qualities that characterize or distinguish a professional person who conforms to the technical and ethical standards of the profession (Ch. 1).

professional liability insurance (seguro de responsabilidad profesional)   insurance policy designed to protect assets in the event a claim for damages resulting from negligence is filed and awarded (Ch. 44).

proficiency testing (prueba de aptitud)   sample tests performed in a clinical laboratory to determine with what degree of accuracy tests are being performed. Testing samples are checked in the same manner as patient specimens (Ch. 37).

profile (perfil)   a brief written description providing information describing your personality, qualifications, and skills for an employment position (Ch. 47).

profit sharing (participación en las ganancias)   sharing in the financial profits, gains, and benefits of an organization (Ch. 44).

progress notes (notas de evolución)   also called chart notes. Provider's formal or informal notes about presenting problem, physical findings, and plan for treatment for a patient examined in the office, clinic, acute care center, or emergency department (Ch. 15).

projection (proyección)   act of placing one's own feelings on another (Ch. 4).

pronation (pronación)   occurs when the arm moves so the palm is down (Ch. 32).

prone (prono)   in this position, the patient is instructed to lay face down on the table with head turned to side; arms may be placed above the head or along the side of the body. The drape must cover from the mid-chest area to the legs (Ch. 24).

proofread (revisar)   to read a document to verify the accuracy of content and that correct grammar, spelling, punctuation, and capitalization were used (Ch. 14).

proprietary (empresa de propiedad privada)   privately owned and managed facility, a profit-making organization (Ch. 1).

prostaglandins (prostaglandinas)   modulators of biochemical activity in tissues (Ch. 25).

prostatectomy (prostatectomía)   surgical removal of all or a portion of the prostate (Ch. 27).

prostate-specific antigen (PSA) (antígeno prostático específico)   protein produced by prostatic cells that when elevated may indicate prostatic cancer (Ch. 27).

prostatitis (prostatitis)   an inflammation of the prostate gland (Ch. 27).

proteinuria (proteinuria)   protein in the urine (Ch. 29).

protime (tiempo de protrombina)   method of monitoring coagulation time (Ch. 40).

protozoa (protozoos)   one-celled animals divided into four groups: amoebae, flagellates, ciliates, and coccidia (Ch. 21).

provider-performed microscopy procedures (PPMP) (procedimiento de microscopia realizada por el proveedor [PPM])   a CLIA term for those microscopic examinations that require the expertise of a physician or mid-level provider qualified in microscopic examinations. The PPMP is part of the CLIA's moderately complex category of tests (Ch. 37).

pruritus (prurito)   itchiness (Ch. 21, 29, 34).

puerperium (puerperio)   the period from the end of the third stage of labor until involution of uterus is complete, usually 3 to 6 weeks (Ch. 25).

pulse oximeter (oxímetro de pulso)   a device (similar to a clip) that can be attached to a finger or bridge of the nose. It measures oxygen concentration in the blood (Ch. 23).

puncture (punción)   a wound caused by an object piercing the skin and underlying soft tissues that creates a small hole (Ch. 8).

purging (purga)   method of maintaining order in files by separating active from inactive and closed files (Ch. 13).

purified protein derivative (PPD) (derivado proteico purificado [DPP])   filtrate obtained from *Mycobacterium* cultures used for intradermal testing for tuberculosis (Ch. 43).

pyorrhea (piorrea)   discharge of pus from the gums, around the teeth (Ch. 24).

pyrexia (pirexia)   fever (Ch. 23).

pyridoxine (piridoxina)   vitamin B_6 (Ch. 33).

pyuria (piuria)   pus in the urine (Ch. 29).

qualitative tests (prueba cualitativa)   analyses to identify quality or characteristics of components, such as size, shape, and maturity of cells (Ch. 38).

quality assurance (QA) (aseguramiento de calidad [QA])   process to provide accurate, complete, consistent health care documentation in a timely manner while making every reasonable effort to resolve inconsistencies, inaccuracies, risk management issues, and other problems (Ch. 15, 37).

quality control (control de calidad)   measures used to monitor the processing of laboratory specimens. Include proper use, storage, handling, stability, expiration dates, and indications for measuring precision and accuracy of analytic processes (Ch. 37).

quantitative tests (prueba cuantitativa) analyses that can identify quantity or actual number counts such as counting the number of blood cells (Ch. 38, 41).

RACE (RACE) an acronym that stands for Remove patients from area, activate Alarm, Contain the fire and smoke, and Extinguish if safe to do so (Ch. 9).

radioactive (radioactivo) emits rays or particles from nucleus (Ch. 31).

radiograph (radiografía) the film on which an image is produced through exposure to X-rays (Ch. 31).

radiology and imaging reports (informes de radiología y de diagnóstico por imágenes) medical reports that describe the findings and interpretations of the radiologist (Ch. 15).

radiolucent (radiolúcido) allowing X-rays to pass through. A dark area appears on the radiograph (Ch. 31).

radionuclides (radionúclidos) atoms that disintegrate by emitting electromagnetic radiation (Ch. 31).

radiopaque (radiopaco) impenetrable to X-rays. A light area appears on the radiograph (Ch. 31).

radiopharmaceuticals (sustancias radiofarmacéuticas) radioactive chemicals used in testing the location, size, outline, or function of tissue, organs, vessels, or body fluids (Ch. 31).

rales (estertores) abnormal bubbling or crackling sound heard by auscultation during the inspiratory phase of respiration (Ch. 23).

range of motion (ROM) (amplitud de movimiento [ROM]) amount of movement that is present in a joint (Ch. 32).

ratchets (trinquetes) locking mechanisms on the handles of many surgical instruments (Ch. 30).

rationalization (racionalización) act of justification, usually illogically, that one uses to keep from facing the truth of the situation (Ch. 4).

reagent (reactivo) chemical substance that detects or synthesizes other substances in a chemical reaction; used in laboratory analyses because it is known to react in a specific way (Ch. 38).

reagent test strip (tira de prueba reactiva) narrow strip of plastic on which pads containing reagents are attached; used in the urinalysis chemical examination to detect glucose, bilirubin, ketones, specific gravity, blood, pH, urobilinogen, nitrites, and leukocyte esterase and other substances (Ch. 41).

reception (recepción) the area of a medical clinic where patients are received and greeted. It should never be referred to as a "waiting area" (Ch. 9).

recertification (nueva certificación) documentation submitted to support continued education for maintaining a professional credential (Ch. 46).

reference laboratories (laboratorios de referencia) independent, regionally located laboratories used by hospitals for complex, expensive, or specialized tests (Ch. 38).

reference ranges (rangos de referencia) also referred to as normal value, normal range, or reference value; range of values that includes 95% of test results for a normal healthy population (Ch. 38).

references (referencias) during the job application process, individuals who have known or worked with a person long enough to make an honest assessment and recommendation regarding the person's employment history (Ch. 47).

referral (remisión) term used by managed care facilities for authorization for someone other than the patient's primary care provider to treat the patient (Ch. 16).

refractometer (refractómetro) instrument that measures the refractive index of a substance or solution; used in the urinalysis physical examination to measure the urine specimen's specific gravity (Ch. 41).

Registered Medical Assistant (RMA [AMT]) (Asistente Médico Matriculado [RMA]) credential awarded for successfully passing the AMT examination (Ch. 1, 46).

Registered Medical Transcriptionist (RMT) (transcriptor médico registrado [RMT]) credential awarded following completion of a two-part certification examination administered by the Association for Healthcare Documentation Integrity (AHDI) (Ch. 15).

regression (regresión) moving back to a former stage to escape conflict or fear (Ch. 4).

regulated waste (residuos regulados) any waste that contains infectious material that would pose a threat due to possible transmission of pathogenic microorganisms (Ch. 21).

rehabilitative medicine (medicina de rehabilitación) field of medical disciplines that seeks to use physical and mechanical agents to restore an individual or body part to normal or near-normal function after an illness or injury (Ch. 32).

reimbursement (reembolso) payment (Ch. 37).

remittance advice (aviso de pago) summarizes all of the benefits paid to a provider within a particular period of time; includes all of the patients covered by a specific insurance company for the time period (Ch. 16).

repolarization (repolarización) reestablishment of a polarized state in a muscle after contraction (Ch. 36).

repression (represión) occurs when one copes with an overwhelming situation by temporarily forgetting it; temporary amnesia (Ch. 4).

requisitions (solicitud) request form sent with a specimen specifying tests to be performed on the specimen; most common tests are separated into logical categories with additional space for writing special requests (Ch. 37, 38).

rescue breathing (respiración de rescate) performed on individuals in respiratory arrest, rescue breathing is a mouth-to-mouth (using appropriate protective equipment) or mouth-to-nose procedure that provides oxygen to the patient until emergency personnel arrive (Ch. 8).

residual urine (orina residual) amount of urine remaining in bladder immediately after voiding; seen with hyperplasia of prostate (Ch. 28).

resistance (resistencia) ability of the immune system to resist or withstand an infectious disease (Ch. 21).

resource-based relative value scale (RBRVS) (escala de valores relativos basada en recursos [RBRVS]) basis for the Medicare fee schedule (Ch. 16).

respiratory syncytial virus (RSV) (virus sincitial respiratorio) a very common virus that leads to mild, cold-like symptoms in adults and older healthy children. It can be more serious in young babies, especially those in certain high-risk groups (Ch. 26).

résumé (curriculum vitae) written summary data sheet or brief account of qualifications and progress in your chosen career (Ch. 47).

retention (retención) urine held in the bladder; inability to empty the bladder (Ch. 27).

reticulocyte (reticulocito) an erythrocyte that is released from the bone marrow before it is mature; retains some of its nucleus material (Ch. 40).

retrolental fibroplasia (fibroplasia retrolenticular) disease of blood vessels of retina in newborns (Ch. 35).

review of systems (ROS) (revisión de sistemas [ROS]) inquires about the system directly related to the problems identified in the history of the present illness (Ch. 15).

Rh factor (factor Rh) blood factor indicating the presence or absence of the Rh antigen on the surface of human erythrocytes (Ch. 43).

rhizotomy (rizotomía) a procedure in which nerve fibers are damaged to block pain (Ch. 29).

rhonchi (roncus) breath sounds that are low-pitched wheezes resembling snoring when auscultated using a stethoscope. They are present continuously during inspiration and expiration (Ch. 23).

rhythm strip (tira de ritmo) ECG recording of a single lead, usually lead II, that is used to determine the rhythm of the heartbeat. An arrhythmia can more easily seen in a rhythm strip verses a twelve-lead ecg tracing because it is run longer per provider's request (Ch. 36).

riboflavin (riboflavina) vitamin B_2 (Ch. 33).

rickettsiae (rickettsiae) intracellular parasitic small nonmotive bacteria (Ch. 21).

risk management (gestión de riesgos) techniques adhered to in the ambulatory care setting that keep the practice, its environment, and its procedures as safe for the patient as possible. Proper risk management also reduces the possibility of negligence that leads to torts and malpractice suits (Ch. 6, 8, 15, 44).

roadblock (obstáculo) Any barrier that blocks therapeutic communication (Ch. 4).

rosacea (rosácea) a chronic skin condition characterized by pustules, papules, erythema, and hyperplasia. Its cause is unknown (Ch. 29).

rotation (rotación) occurs when a body part is turned around its axis (Ch. 32).

rouleaux (rouleaux) RBCs form aggregates that look like rolls or stacks of coins. This phenomenon is evident in inflammatory conditions (Ch. 40).

safety data sheet (SDS) (hoja de datos de seguridad) document listing chemical safety information, product name, hazardous ingredients, fire and explosive tendencies, health hazards, emergency and first aid procedures, spill or leak procedures, protection and control measures, and special precautions (Ch 37).

salary review (revisión de salario) process by which the employee is informed of his or her revised base pay rate (Ch. 44).

salicylates (salicilatos) aspirin-type drugs that can cause ulcers because of their irritation to the gastrointestinal tract (Ch. 29).

saturated fats (grasa saturada) fats that are typically solid at room temperature, most commonly found in animal products such as butter, milk, cream, and eggs as well as coconut and palm oils (Ch. 33).

scleroderma (esclerodermia) slowly progressing disease characterized by deposition of fibrous connective tissue in the skin and in internal organs (Ch. 24).

scope of practice (ámbito de práctica) the range of clinical procedures and activities that are allowed by law for a profession (Ch. 1).

screening (prueba de detección) evaluating patient symptoms to determine emergent needs. Sometimes used to determine the next best course of action when assisting a provider in giving appropriate patient care (Ch. 11, 12).

secretion (secreción) substance produced by the cells of glandular organs from materials in the blood (Ch. 21, 37).

scrotum (escroto) a soft tissue structure that holds the testes (Ch. 27).

scurvy (escorbuto) a deficiency in vitamin C characterized by the abnormal formation of bones and teeth. Signs of hemorrhage can appear, such as bruising (Ch. 33).

Secure Sockets Layer (SSL) (capa de sockets seguros) a protocol designed to allow secure Web-based transfer of data using encryption (Ch. 10).

sediment (sedimento) insoluble material that settles to the bottom of a liquid; material examined in the urinalysis microscopic examination (Ch. 41).

self-actualization (autorealización) being all that you can be; developing your full potential and experiencing fulfillment (Ch. 3, 44).

self-insurance (autoseguro) insurance carried by large companies, nonprofit organizations, and government to reduce costs and gain more control of their finances. Each plan differs in coverage and claim filing requirements (Ch. 16).

sensor (sensor) term used to describe a metallic-coated paper tab that is applied to the patient's body in preparation for an ECG (also known as electrode). Sensors are placed on specific locations on the skin, then attached to the ECG with wires. The sensors conduct electricity from the patient to the ECG machine (Ch. 36).

sensorineural (neurosensorial) related to permanent hearing loss that results from damage or malformation of the middle ear and auditory nerve (Ch. 26).

septic (sepsis) Overwhelming infection that occurs most often in critically ill patients. Chemicals are released into the bloodstream that cause vasodilatation and other organic products that are harmful to the organs and tissues. The vasodilation and decreased ability of the cells and tissues to utilize oxygen is the basis for this type of shock (Ch. 8).

serum (suero) liquid portion of blood obtained after blood has been allowed to clot (Ch. 38, 39).

server (servidor) computer with massive hard drive capacity that is used to link other computers together so that data can be shared by multiple users. A computer system in an ambulatory care facility is likely to be linked or networked with a central server (Ch. 10).

severe acute respiratory syndrome (SARS) (síndrome respiratorio agudo y grave [SARS]) a viral outbreak of a respiratory illness first reported in Asia in 2003; spread by close person-to-person contact and characterized by fever and respiratory symptoms (Ch. 21).

shadow (aprendizaje por observación) follow a supervisor or delegated subordinate to learn facility protocol (Ch. 44).

sharps (objetos filosos) needles, scalpels, or other sharp instruments that are capable of causing a penetrating or puncture wound of the skin (Ch. 21).

shock (shock) potentially serious condition in which the circulatory system is not providing enough blood to all parts of the body, causing the body's organs to fail to function properly (Ch. 8).

short-range goals (metas a corto plazo) created when long-range goals are dissected and reassembled into smaller, more manageable time segments (Ch. 3).

sickle cell anemia (anemia drepanocítica) an inherited blood disorder that may shorten life span (Ch. 25).

sigmoidoscopy (sigmoidoscopía) a diagnostic examination of the interior of the sigmoid colon (Ch. 29).

simplified letter (carta simplificada) major letter style recommended by the Administrative Management Society that omits the salutation and complimentary closure. All lines are keyed flush with the left margin. In medical offices, this style is most often used when sending a form letter (Ch. 14).

Sims' (sims) in this position, the patient is instructed to lay on the left side; the left arm and shoulder may be drawn back behind the body. The left knee is slightly flexed to support the body, and the right knee is flexed sharply (Ch. 24).

sitz bath (baño de asiento) a warm water bath, in which only the hips and buttocks are immersed (Ch. 30).

slander (calumnia) false and malicious words about another constituting a defamation of character (Ch. 6).

smartphone (teléfono inteligente) a mobile device that is used as a phone and has many functionalities of a computer (Ch. 11).

Snellen chart (gráfica de Snellen) consists of the alphabet letters in various combinations starting at the top with a large E, and letters of descending size by line toward the bottom. Each line is labeled with the visual acuity measurement (Ch. 29).

SOAP/SOAPI/SOAPER/SOAPIER a form of medical documentation that includes all or a portion of the following:

- **S** Subjective data; patient's complaint in his or her own words
- **O** Objective, observable, measurable findings
- **A** Assessment, probable diagnosis based on subjective and objective factors
- **P** Plan for treatment, medications, instructions, return visit information
- **I** Implementation, or how the actions were carried out
- **E** Education for the patient
- **R** Response of patient to education and care given or Revision of the plan (Ch. 13, 22).

social media (medios sociales) forms of electronic communication such as Web sites or blogs that enable users to share content or to participate in social networking, sharing ideas, and personal messages (Ch. 44, 47).

solvent (solvente) producing a solution, dissolving (Ch. 21).

sonographer (ecografista) professionally trained individual capable of performing the ultrasound examination (Ch. 36).

source-oriented medical record (SOMR) (historia clínica orientada a la fuente [SOMR]) a type of patient chart record-keeping that includes separate sections for different sources of patient information, such as laboratory reports, pathology reports, and progress notes (Ch. 13, 22).

species (especie) second Greek or Latin name given to microorganisms; the species name is not capitalized (Ch. 42).

specific gravity (densidad específica) ratio of weight of a given volume of a substance to the weight of the same volume of distilled water at the same temperature; test often performed during the urinalysis physical examination; can also be tested by reagent strip (Ch. 41).

spermatic cord (cordón espermático) bundle of fibers, nerves, the vas deferens, testicular artery, and a network of veins forming a cord (Ch. 27).

spermatogenesis (espermatogénesis) the formation of mature sperm (Ch. 27).

spermatozoa (espermatozoides) mature, mobile male sex cells (Ch. 27).

spill kit (kit para derrames) commercially packaged materials consisting of supplies and equipment needed to clean up a spill of a biohazardous substance (Ch. 21).

spirometry (espirometría) test to measure the air capacity of the lungs (Ch. 29).

splint (férula) any device used to immobilize a body part. Often used by EMS personnel (Ch. 8).

spores (esporas) an inactive state of some bacteria in which they are encapsulated in protein. The encapsulation protects them from heat, chemicals, freezing, desiccation, and radiation and antibiotics. Spores can live for thousands of years with no nutrients. When spores are exposed to fertile human tissue they can become activated and grow. Tetanus is one type of bacteria that creates spores (Ch. 42).

sprain (esguince) injury to a joint, often an ankle, knee, or wrist, that involves a tearing of the ligaments. Most sprains are minor and heal quickly; others are more severe, include swelling, and may not heal properly if the patient continues to put stress on the affected joint (Ch. 8).

sputum (esputo) substance from the respiratory tract expelled by coughing (Ch. 21).

Standard Precautions guidelines recommended by the CDC to prevent the spread of microorganisms through direct or indirect contact. Contact precautions include the donning of gown, gloves, and mask if there is to be contact with the patient or prolonged contact with their environment. This is in addition to Standard Precautions (Ch. 21).

Standard Precautions (Precauciones Estándar) precautions developed in 1996 by the Centers for Disease Control and Prevention (CDC) that augment Universal Precautions and body substance isolation practices. They provide a wider range of protection and are used any time there is contact with blood, moist body fluid (except perspiration), mucous membranes, or nonintact skin. They are designed to protect all health care providers, patients, and visitors (Ch. 8, 21).

stat report (informe de tendencia) a medical report requested of medical transcription that should be returned within 2-4 hours (Ch. 15).

status asthmaticus (estado asmático) severe episode of asthma that does not respond to ordinary treatment (Ch. 35).

status epilepticus (estado epiléptico) a continuous seizure that is prolonged, or two or more seizures without a recovery period between them. Status epilepticus is associated with significant morbidity and mortality (Ch. 8).

statute of limitations (ley de prescripción) statute that defines the period in which legal action can take place (Ch. 19).

statutory law (derecho estatutario) refers to the body of laws established by states (Ch. 6).

steam sterilization (esterilización por vapor) the most widely used method of sterilization used in the medical office. An autoclave, basically a pressure cooker, is used to achieve sterilization (Ch. 30).

sterile field (campo estéril) an area that is considered sterile, usually designated by a sterile drape. The area contains sterile supplies and instruments needed for a particular sterile procedure or surgery (Ch. 30).

stertorous (estertoroso) snoring sound heard with labored breathing (Ch. 23).

stomatitis (estomatitis) inflammation of the mouth associated with chemotherapy. Can include swelling, redness, halitosis, and ulcerations (Ch. 31).

strabismus (estrabismo) disorder of the eye in which optic axes cannot be directed to the same object (cross-eye) (Ch. 29).

strain (distensión) injury to the soft tissue between joints that involves the tearing of muscles or tendons. Strains often occur in the neck, back, and thigh muscles (Ch. 8).

stream scheduling (programación ininterrumpida) system where patients are seen on a continuous basis throughout the day (e.g., at 15-, 30-, or 60-minute intervals), with each patient having a distinct appointment time (Ch. 12).

stress (estrés) body's response to change; can be manifested in a variety of ways, including changes in blood pressure, changes in heart rate, and onset of headache (Ch. 3).

stressors (factores estresantes) demands to change that cause stress (Ch. 3).

strictures (estenosis) narrowing of a tube-like structure such as the esophagus or urethra (Ch. 30).

stridor (estridor) crowing sound heard on inspiration, the result of an upper airway obstruction (Ch. 23).

stylus (estilete) heated slender wire of the electrocardiograph that melts the wax off of the ECG paper during the recording (Ch. 36).

subjective (subjetivo) symptom that is felt by the patient but not observable by others (Ch. 22).

sublimation (sublimación) occurs when a socially unacceptable impulse is redirected into one that is socially acceptable (Ch. 4).

subordinates (subordinado) in an organization, people under the direction of (reporting to) a person of greater authority (Ch. 44).

subpoena (citación) written command designating a person to appear in court under penalty for failure to appear (Ch. 6).

subscriber (suscriptor) A term used by some insurance plans to describe the policyholder or insured (Ch. 16).

sudoriferous (sudorípara) a gland located in the epidermis that secrets sweat (Ch. 29).

superbill (superbill) see encounter form (Ch. 17).

supernatant (sobrenadante) urine that appears above the sediment when centrifuged; poured off before sediment is examined in the urinalysis microscopic examination (Ch. 41).

supination (supinación) occurs when the arm is moved so the palm is up (Ch. 32).

supine (supina) this position is assumed when patient is laying flat facing up. It is used for examination of the anterior surface of the body from head to toe (Ch. 24).

supine hypotension (hipotensión supina) a condition that may occur when a pregnant woman is lying in supine position; the heavy, large uterus presses on the inferior vena cava and aorta, reducing blood flow back to the heart (Ch. 25).

suppression (supresión) occurs when one deliberately refuses to acknowledge something that causes mental pain or suffering (Ch. 4).

suppurant (supurante) an agent causing pus formation (Ch. 30).

suppurative (supurativo) producing or associated with the generation of pus (Ch. 26).

surge protection (protección contra sobretensiones) protection of the fragile electronics from spikes in electrical voltage that occur on electric distribution lines (Ch. 10).

surgical asepsis (asepsia quirúrgica) procedures that render objects sterile; techniques to maintain sterile conditions during invasive procedures (Ch. 30).

surrogate (sustituto) substitute; someone who substitutes for another (Ch. 7).

suture (sutura) surgical material or thread; may describe the act of sewing with the surgical thread and needle (Ch. 30).

swaged (estampada) a surgical needle that has been attached, during manufacturing, to a length of suture material (Ch. 30).

symbols (símbolos) instructional guides assisting with the coding process (Ch. 17).

symmetry (simetría) correspondence in shape, size, and position of body parts on opposite sides of the body (Ch. 24).

sympathetic nervous system (sistema nervioso simpático) large part of the autonomic nervous system that prepares the body for fight or flight (Ch. 3).

syncope (síncope) fainting (Ch. 8, 26, 36).

system software (software de sistema) see operating system (Ch. 10).

systole (sístole) one component of blood pressure measurement representing the highest amount of pressure exerted during the cardiac cycle; the force exerted on the arterial walls during cardiac contraction (Ch. 23, 36).

tachycardia, sinus (taquicardia sinusal) abnormally rapid heartbeat greater than 100 beats/minute. A type of cardiac arrhythmia (Ch. 23, 36).

tachypnea (taquipnea) abnormal increased rate of breathing (Ch. 23).

targeted résumé (curriculum vitae dirigido al objetivo) résumé format utilized when focusing on a clear, specific job target (Ch. 47).

Tay-Sachs (Tay-Sachs) an inherited disease that is usually fatal (Ch. 25).

teamwork (trabajo en equipo) persons synergistically working together (Ch. 44).

telemedicine (telemedicina) the remote delivery of health care by means of telecommunication (Ch. 11).

test cable (cable de prueba) accessory device that attaches between the Holter monitor and the electrocardiograph to check for correct waveform and lack of artifact (Ch. 36).

testes (testículos) the plural form of testis; the oval-shaped male reproductive organs, resting in the scrotum, that produce and store sperm and are the major source of the male hormone, testosterone (Ch. 27).

testicular torsion (torsión testicular) a twisting of the spermatic cord (Ch. 27).

thalassemia (talasemia) a hereditary anemia that may be fatal (Ch. 25).

thallium stress test (prueba de esfuerzo con talio) chemical element given intravenously and used in cardiac stress tests. The radioisotope localizes in the myocardium, and a scanning device picks up the distribution of the thallium and can identify blockages in the coronary arteries. An accurate test for coronary artery disease (Ch. 36).

therapeutic communication (comunicación terapéutica) use of specific and well-defined professional communication skills to create a feeling of comfort for patients even when difficult or unpleasant information must be exchanged (Ch. 4).

therapeutic drug monitoring (TDM) (monitoreo de fármacos terapéuticos [TDM]) periodic blood tests to determine the effectiveness of a particular drug. Drugs will have a therapeutic level that must be attained in order for the drug to be therapeutic or effective. If the blood level of the drug is below the range of therapeutic effectiveness, the provider will probably increase the dosage. Likewise, if the drug is above the therapeutic range, the provider will probably lower the dosage (Ch. 38).

thermotherapy (termoterapia) use of heat to treat a physical condition (Ch. 32).

thiamin (tiamina) vitamin B_1 (Ch. 33).

thixotropic gel (gel tixotrópico) gel material capable of forming an interface between the cells and fluid portion of the blood as a result of centrifugation (Ch. 39).

thrombocytes (platelets) (trombocito) cellular fragments of megataryocyte; plays an important role in blood coagulation, hemostasis, and clot formation (Ch. 39, 40).

thrombocytopenia (trombocitopenia) a deficiency of platelets in blood, which causes bleeding and slow blood clotting (Ch. 40).

thrombocytosis (trombocitosis) a condition of too many platelets, which can result in blood clots (Ch. 40).

tic douloureux (tic douloureaux) inflammation of the trigeminal nerve, cranial nerve number five (Ch. 29).

tickler file (archivo de recordatorios) system to remind of action to be taken on a certain date (Ch. 13).

time focus (enfoque en el tiempo) defines the period of time that is important and to which an individual's actions are directed or oriented (Ch. 4).

tinea pedis (tiña pedis) medical term for athlete's foot that is caused by a fungus (Ch. 29).

tinnitus (tinnitus) ringing or buzzing sound in the ear (Ch. 24, 33).

titer (título) measurement of amount of antibody present against a particular antigen (Ch. 25).

tocopherol (tocoferol) vitamin E (Ch. 33).

tonic-clonic phase (fase tónico clónica) muscular stiffening followed by the rapid and rhythmic jerking of the extremities during a seizure (Ch. 8).

tort (agravio) wrongful act that results in injury to one person by another (Ch. 6).

tort law (derecho de responsabilidad civil) law that stems from torts, or wrongful acts that cause harm to one person, by another (Ch. 6).

tourniquet (torniquete) device used to facilitate vein prominence (Ch. 8, 39).

toxicology (toxicología) tests for toxic substances in blood and monitors drug usage, therapeutic levels of medication, or toxicity of drugs being used (Ch. 38).

trabeculoplasty (trabeculoplastia) a very focused beam of light to treat the drainage angle of the eye, easing the flow of ocular fluid and decreasing the pressure in the eye (Ch. 29).

trace mineral (oligomineral) mineral required by the body in small amounts (Ch. 33).

tracing (trazado) graphic record, usually of an event that changes with time, as with the electrical activity of the heart (Ch. 36).

traditional indemnity insurance (seguro de responsabilidad civil tradicional) A type of insurance that provides coverage on a fee-for-service basis (FFS). There is usually a deductible and a co-payment or co-insurance (Ch. 16).

transdermal (transdérmico) system of medication delivery that consists of a small adhesive patch that may be applied to intact skin near the treatment site (Ch. 34).

transducer (transductor) device that converts one form of energy to another. During an ultrasound procedure, the transducer picks up echoes and converts them to electrical energy. The energy is transformed into digitalized images that can be viewed and printed. Photographs of the image can be taken (Ch. 31, 36).

transferable skills (habilidades transferibles) skills that would be used in a host of different and unrelated occupations. Keyboarding skill is an example of a transferable skill. It could be used by a secretary, data entry clerk, medical assistant, or clothing manufacturer (Ch. 47).

transient ischemic attack (ataque isquémico transitorio) temporary interference with blood flow to brain; may last only a few moments or several hours; neurologic symptoms occur (Ch. 28).

Transmission-Based Precautions (Precauciones Basadas en la Transmisión) second tier of Centers for Disease Control and Prevention (CDC) guidelines that applies to specific categories of patients and that includes air, contact, and droplet precautions. Transmission-Based Precautions are always used in addition to Standard Precautions (Ch. 21).

transurethral resection of the prostate (TURP) (resección transuretral de la próstata) removal of prostate tissue using a device inserted through the urethra (Ch. 27).

Trendelenburg (Trendelenburg) a supine position in which the patient's head is angled 15 to 30 degrees below the level of the feet (Ch. 24).

triage (triage) screening to determine which patient is treated first when two or more patients present with emergencies simultaneously (Ch. 8).

trial balance (saldo de comprobación) created by totaling debit balances and credit balances to confirm that total debits equal total credits (Ch. 20).

TRICARE (TRICARE) formerly the Civilian Health and Medical Program for Uniformed Services (CHAMPUS). TRICARE offers HMO, PPO, and fee-for-service medical insurance for dependents of active duty and retired military personnel and dependents of personnel who died while on active duty (Ch. 16).

trichomoniasis (tricomoniasis) infestation with a *Trichomonas* parasite, which may be transmitted through sexual intercourse (Ch. 21, 25).

triglycerides (triglicéridos) form of fat in the bloodstream that functions to store energy; an overabundance can cause of cardiovascular disease (Ch. 43).

trimester (trimestre) three months; one third of the gestational period of pregnancy (Ch. 25).

triple option plan (plan de opción triple) a managed care model allowing enrollees the option of traditional, HMO, or PPO health plans (Ch. 16).

trough (valle) the opposite of *peak*, this is the point at which the drug is at its lowest level in the body. Usually this occurs just before the next dose is administered. In lab tests, the trough will tell the physician the weakest influence the drug would have on the body at that particular dose (Ch. 38).

Truth-in-Lending Act (Ley de Veracidad en los Préstamos) also known as the Consumer Credit Protection Act of 1968; an act requiring providers of installment credit to state the charges in writing and to express the interest as an annual rate (Ch. 19).

tubal ligation (ligadura de trompas) female surgical sterilization procedure that severs and seals the female fallopian tubes (Ch 7).

turbid (turbio) opaque, not clear. Used to describe urine that is cloudy (Ch. 41).

turnaround time (TAT) (plazo de entrega) specific time limit established for completion of medical reports (Ch. 15).

tympanostomy (timpanostomía) placement of a tube through the tympanic membrane to allow ventilation of the middle ear; part of the treatment for otitis media (Ch. 26, 29).

ulcer (úlceras) gradual disturbance of the skin and underlying tissues due to an underlying process; for example, prolonged pressure that interrupts tissue oxygenation or the pressure that occurs from increased venous pressure in vascular disease (Ch. 8).

ultrasonic cleaner (limpiador ultrasónico) machine that uses the energy of high-frequency sound waves that agitate to sanitize instruments before sterilization (Ch. 21).

ultrasonography (ecografía) process of placing a handheld transducer against a body area to be tested. The transducer sends sound waves through the skin and the various internal organs. When echoes are formed and sent back, the transducer converts them into electrical energy. This energy is transformed into a picture on a monitor or printed on paper. Photographs of the images can be taken and become part of the patient's permanent record (Ch. 25, 36).

ultrasound (ultrasonido) uses high-frequency sound waves for therapeutic reasons to generate heat in deep tissue (Ch. 32).

unbundling (desagregación) refers to separating the components of a procedure and reporting them as billable codes with charges to increase reimbursement rates (Ch. 17).

undoing (reparación) partaking in actions designed to make amends to cancel out inappropriate behavior (Ch. 4).

Uniform Bill 04 (UB04) (Factura Uniforme 04 [UB04]) unique billing form used extensively by acute care facilities for processing inpatient and outpatient claims (Ch. 17).

URL (uniform resource locater) (localizador uniforme de recursos [URL]) the address that defines the route to a file on the Web or any other Internet facility (Ch. 11).

unipolar (unipolar) having or pertaining to a one-pole process (Ch. 36).

unit (unidad) each part of a name (business or person), words, or numbers that will be indexed and coded for filing (Ch. 13).

unit dose (dosis unitaria) premeasured amount of medication, individually packaged on a per-dose basis (Ch. 35).

universal emergency medical identification symbol (símbolo universal de identificación médica para emergencias) identification sometimes carried by individuals to identify health problems they have (Ch. 8).

Universal Precautions (Precauciones Universales) guidelines established by the Centers for Disease Control and Prevention (CDC) to protect health care workers from infectious diseases (Ch. 21).

up-coding (sobrecodificación) also known as code creep, overcoding, and overbilling. Up-coding occurs when the insurance carrier deliberately bills a higher rate service than what was performed to obtain greater reimbursements (Ch. 17).

urea (urea) principal end product of protein metabolism (Ch. 41).

urgency (urgencia) the need to urinate immediately (Ch. 29).

urinary tract infection (UTI) (infección del tracto urinario [ITU]) also referred to as a bladder infection (Ch. 41).

urobilinogen (urobilinógeno) colorless compound produced in the intestine after the breakdown by bacteria of bilirubin (Ch. 41).

urticaria (urticaria) hives (Ch. 29, 34).

usual, customary, and reasonable (UCR) (usual, acostumbrado y razonable [UCR]) fee schedule often used by Medicare and some insurance carriers. *Usual* refers to the fee typically charged by a provider for certain procedures; *customary* is based on the average charge for a specific procedure by all providers practicing the same specialty in a defined geographic region; and *reasonable* refers to the mid-range of fees charged for this procedure (Ch. 16).

utilization review (UR) (revisión de utilización [RU]) review of medical services to determine they are necessary before they can be performed (Ch. 20).

vaccines (vacuna) pharmacologic agents capable of producing artificial active immunity (Ch. 21).

variable cost (costo variable) cost that varies in direct proportion to volume (Ch. 20).

varicocele (variocele) dilatation of veins found in the male spermatic cord (Ch. 27).

vas deferens (conducto deferente) a muscular tube that connects the testes with the urethra (Ch. 27).

vasectomy (vasectomía) male surgical sterilization procedure that severs and cuts each vas deferens (Ch. 7, 27).

vasoconstriction (vasoconstricción) narrowing or constricting of blood vessels (Ch. 32, 33).

vasodilation (vasodilatación) relaxation of blood vessels, with decreased blood pressure (Ch. 33).

vector (vector) a carrier of disease, usually an insect, that is the causative organism of disease from infected to noninfected individuals (Ch. 21).

venipuncture (venopunción) puncturing into a vein with a needle to obtain a blood sample (Ch. 39).

vertigo (vértigo) the sensation of moving around in space; dizziness, lightheadedness (Ch. 24).

vesicles (vesículas) blisters or other elevations on the skin (Ch. 25).

viability (viable) ability to live, grow, and develop after birth; usually 24 weeks or greater than 1 pound (Ch. 25).

virology (virología) study of viruses (Ch. 38, 42).

virulence (virulencia) an organism's relative power and degree of pathogenicity (Ch. 21).

viscosity (viscosidad) degree of thickness of a liquid (Ch. 39).

vitiligo (vitíligo) skin disorder characterized by smooth white spots on various areas of the body (Ch. 24).

Voice over Internet Protocol (VoIP) (protocolo de voz por Internet [VoIP]) the real-time transmission of voice signals over the Internet or Internet Protocol (IP) network (Ch. 11).

voice recognition software (VRS) (software de reconocimiento de voz) software that translates voice commands and is used in place of a mouse and keyboard (Ch. 15).

volatile (volátil) easily evaporated (Ch. 30).

voucher check (cheque con comprobante) check with detachable form used to detail reason check is drawn; commonly used for payroll checks (Ch. 18).

waived (prueba de baja complejidad) term used to describe a category of clinical laboratory tests that are simple, unvarying, and require a minimum of judgment and interpretation (Ch. 37).

watermark (sello de agua) design incorporated in paper during the papermaking process that is visible when the paper is held up to the light (Ch. 14).

water-soluble vitamins (soluble en agua) Vitamins that can be dissolved in water and are carried to the body's tissues but are not stored in the body. Examples include vitamin C and the b vitamins (Ch. 33).

wave scheduling (planificación en olas) system where patients are scheduled for the first half hour of every hour and then are seen throughout the hour (Ch. 12).

Wernicke-Korsakoff syndrome (síndrome de Wernicke-Korsakoff) a syndrome whose symptoms include a clinical triad of confusion, ataxia, and nystagmus caused by a deficiency of vitamin B_1 (thiamine) (Ch. 33).

wet mount (preparación en fresco) a method of adding liquid, usually saline or potassium hydrochloride, to a specimen on a slide for examination and preservation. The specimen is placed on a slide and one drop of saline (for diagnosis of trichomonas vaginalis) or potassium hydroxide (for diagnosis of vaginal yeast infections) is applied and mixes with the specimen. It is then covered with a coverslip and examined microscopically (Ch. 25, 42).

wheezes (sibilancia) high-pitched musical sound heard on expiration, often the result of an obstruction or narrowing of respiratory passages (Ch. 24).

Wood's lamp (lámpara de Wood) special light used to detect organisms that fluoresce such as certain fungi, bacteria, and parasites. Scabies and ringworm are two examples. Scratches in the eye may be detected using a Wood's lamp after the eye has been stained with a fluorescent dye. Also used in determining margin dissection of melanoma (Ch. 42).

Wood's lamp examination diagnostic test in which the skin or hair is examined while exposed to the black light emitted by a Wood's lamp (Ch. 29).

Workers' Compensation insurance (seguro de indemnización por accidentes de trabajo) medical and paycheck insurance for workers who sustain injuries associated with their employment (Ch. 16).

work statement (declaración de trabajo) concise description of the work you plan to accomplish (Ch. 44).

wound (herida) a break in the continuity of soft parts of body structures caused by violence or trauma to tissues. In an open wound, skin is broken, as in a laceration, abrasion, avulsion, or incision. In a closed wound, skin is not broken, as in contusion, ecchymosis, or hematoma (Ch. 8).

xerophthalmia (xeroftalmía) dry, lusterless mucous membranes of the eyes (Ch. 33).

ZIP+4 (ZIP+4) standard zip code plus four additional digits that identify a postal delivery area. Mail will be processed more efficiently and effectively with the use of the ZIP+4 code in the address (Ch. 14).

REFERENCES/BIBLIOGRAPHY

GENERAL REFERENCES

Acello, B., & Hegner, B. R. (2016). *Nursing assistant: A nursing process approach* (11th ed.). Clifton Park, NY: Cengage Learning.

Altman, G. B. (2004). *Delmar's fundamentals and advanced nursing skills* (2nd ed.). Clifton Park, NY: Cengage Learning.

Blesi, M. (2017). *Medical assisting: Administrative and clinical competencies* (8th ed.). Clifton Park, NY: Cengage Learning.

Delaune, S. C., & Ladner, P. K (2011). *Fundamentals of nursing standards and practice* (4th ed.). Clifton Park, NY: Cengage Learning.

French, L. L. (2018). *Administrative medical assisting* (8th ed.). Clifton Park, NY: Cengage Learning.

Green, M. A. (2016). *3-2-1 Code It!* (5th ed.) Clifton Park, NY: Cengage Learning.

Ingenix. (2003). *HIPAA tool kit.* Salt Lake City, UT: St. Anthony's Publishing/Medicode.

Josephson, D. L. (2004). *Intravenous infusion therapy for nurses: Principles and practices* (2nd ed.). Clifton Park, NY: Cengage Learning.

Krager, D., & Krager, C. (2005). *HIPAA for medical clinic personnel.* Clifton Park, NY: Cengage Learning.

Lewis, M. A., Tamparo, C. D., & Tatro, B. (2012). *Medical law, ethics, and bioethics for health professions* (7th ed.). Philadelphia: F. A. Davis.

Moisio, M. A. (2014). *A guide to health insurance billing* (4th ed.). Clifton Park, NY: Cengage Learning.

Rice, J. (2017). *Principles of pharmacology for medical assisting* (6th ed.). Clifton Park, NY: Cengage Learning.

Simmers, L. (2014). *DHO health science* (8th ed.). Clifton Park, NY: Cengage Learning.

Spratto, G. R., & Woods, A. L. (2016). *PDR nurse's drug handbook.* Clifton Park, NY: Delmar Cengage Learning.

Tamparo, C. D. (2016). *Diseases of the human body* (6th ed.). Philadelphia: F. A. Davis.

Tamparo, C. D., & Lindh, W. Q. (2017). *Therapeutic communications for health care professionals.* (4th ed.) Clifton Park, NY: Cengage Learning.

Venes, D. (2013). *Taber's cyclopedic medical dictionary* (22nd ed.). Philadelphia: F. A. Davis.

Walters, N. J., Estridge, B. H., & Reynold, A. P. (2012). *Basic Clinical Laboratory Techniques* (6th ed.) Clifton Park, NY: Cengage Learning.

SECTION I: GENERAL PROCEDURES

UNIT I: INTRODUCTION TO MEDICAL ASSISTING AND HEALTH PROFESSIONS

Chapter 1: The Medical Assisting Profession

American Association of Medical Assistants. http://www.aama-ntl.org

American Medical Technologists. http://www.americanmedtech.org

Balasa, D. (2000, January/February). Securing the future for medical assistants to practice. Professional Medical Assistant, 6–7.

Balasa, D. (2003). Vigilance is key to protecting practice rights. CMA Today, 36(4). Retrieved May 4, 2016 from http://www.aama-ntl.org/cmatoday/archives

Balasa, D. (2005). CARE bill gains momentum in Congress. CMA Today, 38(4). http://www.aama-ntl.org/cmatoday/archives

Balasa, D. (2012). Frequent questions about medical assistant's scope of practice. CMA Today, 45(2). http://www.aama-ntl.org/CMAToday/archives/publicaffairs/details.aspx?ArticleID=886

Bureau of Labor Statistics, Occupational Employment Statistics. Medical assistants. Retrieved May 10, 2016 from http://www.bls.gov/oes/current/oes319092.htm

Carli, L. L., LaFleur, S. J., Loeber, C. C., Connell, F., & Geiser, R. (1995). Nonverbal behavior, gender, and influence. Journal of Personality and Social Psychology, 68(6), 1030–1041.

Congress.gov. H.R.1146: Consistency, Accuracy, Responsibility, and Excellence in Medical Imaging and Radiation Therapy Act of 2013. Retrieved May 12, 2016 from https://www.congress.gov/bill/113th-congress/house-bill/1146/all-actions?overview=closed

McCarty, M. (2003, March). The lawful scope of a medical assistant's practice. AMT Events. http://hws.hrsa.gov/default.aspx?category=Auxiliary+Health&occu=Medical+Assistants http://www.bls.gov/oco/ocos164.htm

National Healthcareer Association. http://www.nhanow.com

Chapter 2: Health Care Settings and the Health Care Team

American Board of Medical Specialties & Subspecialties. (2016). Approved ABMS specialty & subspecialty certificates. http://www.abms.org/

Commonwealth Fund. (2015, August). Primary care providers' views of recent trends in health care delivery and payment. http://www.commonwealthfund.org/publications/issue-briefs/2015/aug/primary-care-providers-views-delivery-payment

National Center for Complementary and Integrative Health. (2010). Credentialing: Understanding the education, training, regulation, and licensing of complementary health practitioners. http://nccam.nih.gov/health/decisions/credentialing.htm

Creswell, J. (2014). Race is on to profit from rise of urgent care. New York Times Business Day. http://www.nytimes.com/2014/07/10/business/race-is-on-to-profit-from-rise-of-urgent-care.html?_r=0

American Medical Association. (2013). Health care careers directory, 20129–20130. Chicago: Author.

Miles, C. J. (2014, June). Concierge medicine: An alternative to insurance. Association of Mature American Citizens. http://amac.us/concierge-medicine-alternative-insurance/

National Committee for Quality Assurance (NCQA). The future of patient-centered medical homes: Foundation for a better health care system. http://www.ncqa.org/Portals/0/Public%20Policy/2014%20Comment%20Letters/The_Future_of_PCMH.pdf

Urgent Care Association of America. (2015). Industry FAQs. http://www.ucaoa.org/?page=IndustryFAQs

UNIT II: THE THERAPEUTIC APPROACH

Chapter 3: Coping Skills for the Medical Assistant

About.com. (n.d.). What you need to know about stress management. http://stress.about.com

American Institute of Stress. Stress effects. Retrieved April 4, 2016 from http://www.stress.org/stress-effects/

HelpGuide.org. (2016, June). Preventing burnout. http://www.helpguide.org/articles/stress/preventing-burnout.htm

HelpGuide.org. (n.d.). Understanding stress. Retrieved April 4, 2016 http://www.helpguide.org/mental/stress.htm

Mayo Clinic. (n.d.). Job burnout: How to spot it and take action. Retrieved April 4, 2016 http://www.mayoclinic.org/healthy-lifestyle/adult-health/in-depth/burnout/art-20046642

Milliken, M. E., & Honeycutt, A. (2012). *Understanding human behavior: A guide for health care providers* (8th ed.). Clifton Park, NY: Cengage Learning.

Chapter 4: Therapeutic Communication Skills

EuroMed Info. (n.d.). Doing a cultural assessment. http://www.euromedinfo.eu/doing-a-cultural-assessment.html

EuroMed Info. (n.d.). How culture influences health beliefs. http://www.euromedinfo.eu/how-culture-influences-health-beliefs.html/

Humes, K. R., Jones, N. A., & Ramirez, R. R. (2011, March). Overview of race and Hispanic origins: 2010. 2010 Census Briefs. Washington, DC: U.S. Census Bureau. http://www.census.gov/prod/cen2010/briefs/c2010br-02.pdf

Luckmann, J. (2000). *Transcultural communication in health care.* Clifton Park, NY: Cengage Learning.

Novickas, R. (2014, January/February). Helping hands: Reach out to deaf and hearing-impaired patients. CMA Today.

Pew Research Center. (2013). 45% say Muslim Americans face "a lot" of discrimination: After Boston, little change in views of Islam and violence. http://www.people-press.org/files/legacy-pdf/5-7-13%201Islam%20Release.pdf

Purnell, L. D. (2014) *Culturally competent health care.* Philadelphia: F.A. Davis.

Chapter 5: The Therapeutic Approach to the Patient with a Life-Threatening Illness

Back, A., Arnold, R., & Tulsky, J. (2010). *Mastering communication with seriously ill patients.* New York: Cambridge University Press.

Callinan, K. (2016). End-of-life care. Are we ready for real reform? Compassion & Choices. https://www.compassionandchoices.org/2016/01/28/end-of-life-care-are-we-ready-for-real-reform/

Kübler-Ross, E., & Kessler, D. (2005). *On grief and grieving.* New York: Scribner.

Purnell, L., & Paulanka, B. (2008). *Transcultural health care: A culturally competent approach.* Philadelphia: F. A. Davis.

WebMD. (2016, February). HIV & AIDS: How they're different. http://www.webmd.com/hiv-aids/difference_between_hiv_aids

UNIT III: RESPONSIBLE MEDICAL PRACTICE

Chapter 6: Legal Considerations

Centers for Disease Control and Prevention. (2016). 2016 Nationally notifiable conditions. http://wwwn.cdc.gov/nndss/conditions/notifiable/2016/

Centers for Medicare and Medicaid Services. (n.d.). Patient's bill of rights. https://www.cms.gov/CCIIO/Programs-and-Initiatives/Health-Insurance-Market-Reforms/Patients-Bill-of-Rights.html

Compassion & Choices. (2016, February 2). Durable power of attorney for health care: How to make the selection. https://www.compassionandchoices.org/durable-power-of-attorney-for-healthcare-how-to-make-the-selection/

Drug Policy Alliance. (2013, May). Removing marijuana from the Controlled Substances Act. http://www.drugpolicy.org/sites/default/files/DPA_Fact%20sheet_Marijuana%20Reclassification_May%202013.pdf

MedlinePlus. (2015, May 1). Reportable diseases. https://www.nlm.nih.gov/medlineplus/ency/article/001929.htm

National Healthcare Decisions Day (NHDD). (n.d.). Advance care planning resources. http://www.nhdd.org/public-resources/#where-can-i-get-an-advance-directive

Physician Orders for Life-Sustaining Treatment Paradigm. (n.d.). What is POLST? http://www.polst.org/about-the-national-polst-paradigm/what-is-polst/

U.S. Department of Health and Human Services. (2015, August 28). About the law, health care. http://www.hhs.gov/healthcare/about-the-law/read-the-law/index.html

U.S. Department of Labor. (n.d.). Family and Medical Leave Act. http://www.dol.gov/whd/fmla/spouse/

Washington State Medical Association (WSMA). (2007). Durable power of attorney for health care, health care directive, and POLST. http://www.wsma.org

World Health Organization. (n.d.). Understanding and addressing violence against women. http://www.who.int/reproductivehealth/topics/violence/vaw_series/en/

Chapter 7: Ethical Considerations

Aliesch, S. (ed.). (2016, Spring). Document and discuss. Compassion and Choices Magazine, 4–5.

American Medical Association. (2016, April 10). Code of medical ethics: Current opinions of the council on ethical and judicial affairs. http://www.ama-assn.org; http://www.ama.assn.org/ama/pub/physician-resources/medikcal-ethics/code-medical-ethics.page

Blanchard, K., & Peale, N. V. (1988). *The power of ethical management.* New York: William Morrow and Company, Inc.

Collins, S., Gunja, M., & Beutel, S. (2015, September). New U.S. Census data show the number of uninsured americans dropped by 8.8 million. Commonwealth Fund Blog, Commonwealth Fund. U.S. Census Bureau, 2013 and 2014 Current Population Survey Reports.

Covey, S. R. (2015). The 7 habits of managers. Audio CD. Franklin Covey on Brilliance Audio.

Covey, S. R. (1991). *Principle-centered leadership.* New York: Simon & Schuster.

Gold, J. (2014, January 29). In cities, the average doctor wait-time is 18.5 days. Wonkblog, Washington Post.

Patient Bill of Rights and Responsibilities. (2012, October). John Hopkins Medicine, John Hopkins Hospital, Baltimore, MD. http://www.hopkinsmedicine.org/the_johns_hopkins_hospital/

Planned Parenthood. (2016, April). The U.S. Supreme Court: Your boss can now decide if you can have access to birth control coverage. https://www.plannedparenthoodaction-org/blog/supreme-court-bosses-can-deny-birth-control-coverage-employees

Smith, S. (2014, April). Happening now. CNN. http://www.cnn.com/2014/04/10/health/tissue-engineering-success/

Stewart, K. (2015, October 8). At Catholic hospitals, a "right to life" but not a right to death. Retrieved April 18, 2016 from http://www.thenation.com/.../at-catholic-hospitals-a-right-to-life-but...

World Health Organization. (2011). An update on WHO's work on female genital mutilation (FGM) progress report. Retrieved from WHO_11.18_eng.pdf, April 14, 2016.

Chapter 8: Emergency Procedures and First Aid

American Heart Association. (2016). Hands only CPR. http://cpr.heart.org/AHAECC/CPRAndECC/Programs/HandsOnlyCPR/UCM_473196_Hands-Only-CPR.jsp

American Heart Association. (2015). Adult Basic Life Support. https://ebooks.heart.org//epubreader/bls-provider-manual-ebook#

American Heart Association. (n.d.). Advanced Cardio-vascular Life Support. http://www.heart.org/HEARTORG/CPRAndECC/HealthcareTraining/AdvancedCardiovascularLifeSupportACLS/Advanced-Cardiovascular-Life-Support-ACLS_UCM_001280_SubHomePage.jsp

American National Red Cross. (2001). *Staywell.* St. Louis, MO: Mosby.

American Red Cross. (2005). CPR and emergency cardiac care: New CPR guidelines for professionals and nonprofessionals. http://www.redcross.org/cpr.html

Emergency Nurses Association. (n.d.). Use of tourniquets for control of extremity bleeding. Retrieved May 16, 2016 from https://www.ena.org/practice-research/Practice/Documents/TIPSTourniquets.pdf.

Epilepsy Foundation. (2013, July). What is a tonic-clonic seizure? http://www.epilepsy.com/learn/types-seizures/myoclonic-seizures

Medical Reserve Corps. (2008). Emergency medical care. http://www.medicalreservecorps.gov

MedlinePlus. (2015, January 11). Gastrointestinal bleeding. http://www.nlm.nih.gov/medlineplus/ency/article/003133.htm

National Institutes of Health. (2008). New CPR guidelines. http://www.health.nih.gov

SECTION II: ADMINISTRATIVE PROCEDURES

UNIT IV: INTEGRATED ADMINISTRATIVE PROCEDURES

Chapter 9: Creating the Facility Environment

Azoulay, R. (2009). *Music, the breath and health: Advances in integrative music therapy.* New York: Satchnote Press.

Barker, J., Pocock, E., Huber, C., & Black Associates. The future of ambulatory care. American Institute of Architects. http://www.aia.org/practicing/groups/kc/AIAB086508

Cama, R. (2009). *Evidence-based healthcare design.* New York: John Wiley & Sons.

Centers for Disease Control and Prevention. (n.d.). Emergency preparedness and response. http://emergency.cdc.gov/preparedness/kit/disasters/

Healthcare Designed. (n.d.). Interior design + architecture for healthcare. https://healthcaredesigned.wordpress.com/category/healthcare-design-architecture/

Purnell, L. D. (2014) *Guide to culturally competent health care.* Philadelphia: F. A. Davis Publishers.

TGBA Architects. (n.d.). Medical office building and clinic design. www.tgbarchitects.com/medical-clinic-architects.php

U.S. Department of Labor, Occupational Safety and Health Administration. (n.d.). Fire extinguisher basics. https://www.osha.gov/SLTC/etools/evacuation/portable.html

U.S. Department of Labor, Occupational Safety and Health Administration. (n.d.). How to plan for workplace emergencies and evacuations. http://www.osha.gov/Publications/osha3088.html

Chapter 10: Computers in the Medical Clinic

American Medical Association. (2015). E-5.07 confidentiality: Computers. http://www.ama-assn.org

Centers for Disease Control and Prevention. (2012, September 1). Self-study modules on tuberculosis measures to protect patient confidentiality. http://www.cdc.gov/tb/education/ssmodules/module7/ss7reading4.htm

GFI Blog. (2015, February 18). Most vulnerable operating systems and applications in 2014. http://www.gfi.com/blog/most-vulnerable-operating-systems-and-applications-in-2014/

Heller, M. (2017). *Clinical medical assisting: A professional, field smart approach to the workplace* (2nd ed.). Clifton Park, NY: Cengage Learning.

Storage Craft. (n.d.). Data storage lifespans: How long will media really last? https://www.storagecraft.com/blog/data-storage-lifespan/

U.S. Department of Health and Human Services. (2014, August 7). More physicians and hospitals are using EHRs than before. http://www.hhs.gov/about/news/2014/08/07/more-physicians-and-hospitals-are-using-ehrs-than-before.html

Chapter 11: Telecommunications

Administrative Arts. (n.d.). How to be a great assistant. http://administrativearts.com/welcome-to-administrative-arts/

HiMSS. (n.d.). Using patient portals to achieve meaningful use. http://www.himss.org/using-patient-portals-achieve-meaningful-use-ep-edition?ItemNumber=35966

HIPAA Journal. (n.d.). FCC confirms rules regarding HIPAA and patient telephone calls. http://www.hipaajournal.com/fcc-confirms-rules-regarding-hipaa-and-patient-telephone-calls-8048/

Chapter 12: Patient Scheduling

See General References

Chapter 13: Medical Records Management

Burt, C. W., Hing, E., & Woodwell, D. (2005). *Electronic medical record use by office-based physicians: United States, 2005.* Hyattsville, MD: U.S. Department of Health and Human Services, Centers for Disease Control and Prevention.

Centers for Medicare and Medicaid Services. (2016, June). Ensuring proper use of electronic health record features and capabilities. https://www.cms.gov/Medicare-Medicaid-Coordination/Fraud-Prevention/Medicaid-Integrity-Education/Downloads/ehr-decision-table.pdf

Hansen, D. (2008). Congress considers mandate for Medicare e-prescribing. http://www.ama-assn.org/amednews/2008/01/07/gvsb0107.htm

Healthcare IT News. (2015, January 15). 12 tips for better EHR usability. http://www.healthcareitnews.com/news/12-tips-better-ehr-usability

HealthIT.gov. (2014, August 29). Benefits of EHRs. https://www.healthit.gov/providers-professionals/why-adopt-ehrs

Medical Economics. (2015, December 10). Last word: Medical records. Creation vs. control. http://medicaleconomics.modernmedicine.com/medical-economics/news/last-word-medical-records-creation-vs-control

Chapter 14: Written Communications

Humphrey, D. D. (2004). *Contemporary medical office procedures* (3rd ed.). Clifton Park, NY: Cengage Learning.

Reed Tinsley. (n.d.). Forms & checklists. http://www.rtacpa.com/forms-checklists

Robert, H. M., III, Evans, W. J., Honemann, D. H., & Balch, T. J. (2000). *Robert's rules of order newly revised* (10th ed.). Cambridge, MA: Perseus.

Terryberry, K. (2005). *Writing for the health profession.* Clifton Park, NY: Cengage Learning.

Villemarie, D., & Villemarie, L. (2005). *Grammar and writing skills for the health professional.* Clifton Park, NY: Cengage Learning.

Chapter 15: Medical Documents

American Association for Medical Transcription. (1990). *AAMT model job description: Medical transcriptionist.* Modesto, CA: American Association for Medical Transcription.

Burns, L., & Maloney, F. (2003). *Medical transcription and terminology: An integrated approach* (2nd ed.). Clifton Park, NY: Cengage Learning.

Conerly-Stewart, D. L., & Ireland, P.A. (2015). *Forrest general medical center: Advanced medical transcription course* (4th ed.). Clifton Park, NY: Cengage Learning.

Ireland, P. A., & Stein, C. (2018). *Hillcrest medical center: Healthcare documentation and medical transcription* (8th ed.). Clifton Park, NY: Cengage Learning.

Tossey, K. L. (1998). The integration of digital photographs into medical transcription. Journal of the American Association for Medical Transcription, 17(6), 19–21.

UNIT V: MANAGING FACILITY FINANCES

Chapter 16: Medical Insurance

Green, M. A., & Rowell, J. C. (2017). *Understanding health insurance: A guide to billing and reimbursement* (13th ed.). Clifton Park, NY: Cengage Learning.

Chapter 17: Medical Coding

American Medical Association. (2016). *Current procedural terminology.* Chicago: American Medical Association.

American Medical Association. (2011). *International classification of diseases, clinical modifications (ICD-9)* (2nd ed., 9th rev.). Chicago: American Medical Association.

Bowie, M. J. (2017). *Understanding ICD-10-CM and ICD-10-PCS: A worktext* (3rd ed.). Clifton Park, NY: Cengage Learning.

Ingenix. (2011). *HCPCS level II.* Salt Lake City, UT: St. Anthony Publishing/Medicode.

Office of Inspector General, U.S. Department of Health and Human Services. (2000). Compliance program guide for individual and small group physician practices. http://oig.hhs.gov/authorities/docs/physcian.pdf

Optum360. (2016). *ICD-10-CM professional for physicians, 2016* (2016 ed.). Providence, RI: Optum360.

Papazian-Boyce, L. M. (2016). *Comprehensive medical coding.* Boston: Pearson.

Sayles, N. B. (2017). *Health information management technology: An applied approach.* Chicago: American Health Information Management Association.

Chapter 18: Daily Financial Practices

Beehive. (n.d.). How to write a personal check. http://www.thebeehive.org

Centers for Medicare and Medicaid Services. (2007). CMS clarifies guidelines for national provider identifier (NPI) deadline implementation. http://www.cms.hhs.gov

Electronic prescriptions. (n.d.). http://www.medisoft.com

Chapter 19: Billing and Collections

Dana Neal's Best Credit. (n.d.). Summary of the Fair Debt Collection Practices Act. http://www.bestcredit.com/summary-of-the-fair-debt-collection-practices-act/

Free Advice Legal. (n.d.). How are estate creditors handled? http://law.freeadvice.com/estate_planning/probate/estate_creditors.htm

IC System. (n.d.). Medical collections services. http://www.icsystem.com/medical-collections-services/

Johnson, J. (1994). *Basic filing procedures for health information management.* Clifton Park, NY: Cengage Learning.

NOLO. (n.d.). What is the difference between Chapter 7 and Chapter 13 bankruptcy? http://www.nolo.com/legal-encyclopedia/what-is-the-difference-between-chapter-7-chapter-13-bankrutpcy.html

Shatzman, B. (n.d.). Medical billing resources: Use better collection techniques to increase patient payments. http://www.mbrbilling.com/blog/bid/138985/Use-Better-Collection-Techniques-To-Increase-Patient-Payments

Chapter 20: Accounting Practices

Droms, W. G. (2003). *Finance and accounting for nonfinancial managers* (2nd ed.). Cambridge, MA: Perseus.

SECTION III: CLINICAL PROCEDURES

UNIT VI: INTEGRATED CLINICAL PROCEDURES

Chapter 21: Infection Control and Medical Asepsis

American Academy of Pediatrics. (2009). Prologue. In L. K. Pickering (ed.), *Red book: Report of the Committee on Infectious Diseases* (28th ed.; pp. 1–2). Elk Grove Village, IL: American Academy of Pediatrics.

American Liver Foundation. (2016). HepC123: Medication regimens according to HCV genotype. http://hepc.liverfoundation.org/treatment/the-basics-about-hepatitis-c-treatment/medication-regimens-according-to-genotype/

Banerlee, R., Schecter, G. F., Flood, J., & Porco, T. C. (2008, October 6). Extensively drug-resistant tuberculosis: New strains, new challenges. U.S. National Library of Medicine. 10.1586/14787210.6.5.713.

Barbee S. L., Weber D. J., Sobsey, M. D., & Rutala, W. A. (1999, May). Inactivation of *Cryptosporidium parvum* oocyst infectivity by disinfection and sterilization processes. Gastrointestinal Endoscopy, 49(5), 605–611.

Blaney, D. D., Daly, E. R., Kirkland, K. B., Tongren, J. E., Kelso, P. T., & Talbot, E. A. (2011, May). Use of alcohol-based hand sanitizers as a risk factor for norovirus outbreaks in long-term care facilities in northern New England, December 2006 to March 2007. American Journal of Infection Control, 39(4), 296–301.

Goldmann, D. A., Weinstein, R. A., Wenzel, R. P., Tablan, O. C., Duma, R. J., Gaynes, R. P., Schlosser, J., & Martone, W. J. (1996). Strategies to prevent and control the emergence and spread of antimicrobial-resistant microorganisms in hospitals: A challenge to hospital leadership. Journal of the American Medical Association, 275(3), 234–240.

Infectious Disease Epidemiology, Prevention and Control Division, STD and HIV Section, Minnesota Department of Health. (2007). Hepatitis B and HIV/AIDS. http://www.health.state.mn.us

Kampf, G., Marschall, S., Eggerstedt, S., & Ostermeyer, C. (2010, March 26). Efficacy of ethanol-based hand foams using clinically relevant amounts: A cross-over controlled study among healthy volunteers. BMC Infectious Diseases, 10, 78.

Merck. (2009). Host defense mechanisms against infection. The Merck Manual for Health Care Professionals. http://www.merckmanuals.com/professional/infectious_diseases/biology_of_infectious_disease/host_defense_mechanisms_against_infection.html

Mount Sinai Hospital, Department of Microbiology. (2007). FAQ: Methods of disease transmission. http://microbiology.mtsinai.on.ca/faq/transmission.shtml

Occupational Safety and Health Administration. (2012, April 12). Bloodborne pathogens: 1910.1030 (Regulations [Standards–29CFR]). Retrieved May 30, 2016 from https://www.osha.gov/pls/oshaweb/owadisp.show_document?p_table=STANDARDS&p_id=10051

Pommerville, J. C. (2004). *Alcamo's fundamentals of microbiology* (7th ed.). Sudbury, MA: Jones and Bartlett.

Saiman, L., et al., Banning artificial nails from health care settings. American Journal of Infection Control, 30(4), 252–254. http://www.ajicjournal.org/article/S0196-6553(02)59151-3/abstract

Siegel, J. D., Rhinehart, E., Jackson, M., Chiarello, L., & the Healthcare Infection Control Practices Advisory Committee. (2007). 2007 Guidelines for isolation precautions: Preventing transmission of infectious agents in healthcare settings. http://www.cdc.gov/hicpac/pdf/isolation/Isolation2007.pdf

Sigma-Aldrich. (2015). Microbiology introduction. http://www.sigmaaldrich.com/technical-documents/articles/microbiology/microbiology-introduction.html

U.S. Department of Health and Human Services, Centers for Disease Control and Prevention. (2015). Healthcare-associated infections (HAIs). http://cdc.gov/hai

U.S. Department of Health and Human Services, Centers for Disease Control and Prevention. (2015). Precautions to prevent spread of MRSA. http://www.cdc.gov/mrsa/healthcare/clinicians/precautions.html

U.S. Department of Health and Human Services, Centers for Disease Control and Prevention. (2014, August 22). Update on recommendations for use of herpes zoster vaccine. Morbidity and Mortality Weekly Report (MMWR), 63(33), 729–731. http://www.cdc.gov/mmwr/preview/mmwrhtml/mm6333a3.htm

U.S. Department of Health and Human Services, Centers for Disease Control and Prevention. (2013). Prevention strategies for seasonal influenza in healthcare settings. http://www.cdc.gov/flu/professionals/infectioncontrol/healthcaresettings.htm

U.S. Department of Health and Human Services, Centers for Disease Control and Prevention (2011). Basic infection control and prevention plan for outpatient oncology settings. Retrieved on May 16, 2016 from http://www.cdc.gov/hai/pdfs/guidelines/basic-infection-control-prevention-plan-2011.pdf

U.S. Department of Health and Human Services, Centers for Disease Control and Prevention (2009). Healthcare Infection Control Practices Advisory Committee (HICPAC). http://www.cdc.gov/hicpac/2007IP/2007ip_part1

U.S. Department of Health and Human Services, Centers for Disease Control and Prevention. (2009). Respiratory hygiene/cough etiquette in healthcare settings. http://www.cdc.gov/flu/professionals/mfectioncontxol/resphygiene.htm

U.S. Department of Health and Human Services, Centers for Disease Control and Prevention. (2004). Facts about pneumonic plague. Retrieved May 22, 2016, from http://www.emergency.cdc.gov/agent/plague/factsheet.asp

U.S. Department of Health and Human Services, Centers for Disease Control and Prevention. (2003). Model plans and programs for the OSHA Bloodborne Pathogens and Hazard Communications standards. https://www.osha.gov/Publications/osha3186.pdf

U.S. Department of Health and Human Services, Centers for Disease Control and Prevention, Garner, J. S., and the Hospital Infection Control Practices Advisory Committee. (1996). Guidelines for isolation precautions in hospitals. Hospital Infection Control Advisory Committee. http://wonder.cdc.gov/wonder/prevguid/p0000419/p0000419.asp#head002002000000000

U.S. Department of Health and Human Services, National Vaccine Program Office (November 9, 2015), U.S. national vaccine plan. http://www.hhs.gov/nvpo/national-vaccine-plan/index.html

U.S. Department of Labor, Occupational Safety and Health Administration. (2011). Hepatitis B vaccination protection. https://www.osha.gov/OshDoc/data_BloodborneFacts/bbfact05.html

Weissman, C., Enari, M., Klohn, D., & Flechsig, E. (2002). Transmission of prions. Proceedings of the National Academy of Sciences, 99(4), 16378–16383. http://www.pnas.org/content/99/suppl.4/16378.full.pdf

World Health Organization. (2015). Global Health Observatory (GHO) data. http://www.who.int/gho/hiv/en/

World Health Organization. (2012). Hepatitis B. http://www.who.int/mediacentre/factsheets/fs204/en/

Chapter 22: The Patient History and Documentation

Brent, N. J. (2001). *Other torts and civil rights. In Nurses and the law: A guide to principles and applications* (2nd ed.; pp. 114–115, 127–128). Philadelphia: W. B. Saunders Company.

California State University–Chico. (n.d.). JCAHO Do Not Use list. http://www.csuchico.edu

Catalano, L. A. (2014). What you need to know about electronic documentation. American Nurse Today, 9(11), 24–46.

Smalls, H. (2009). Of counsel: Documentation do's and don'ts. Neonatal Network, 28(2), 133–135.

The Joint Commission. (2015). Facts about the official "Do Not Use" list of abbreviations. https://www.jointcommission.org/facts_about_do_not_use_list/

U.S. Department of Health and Human Services, Centers for Disease Control and Prevention.

(2006, October 12). Recommended adult immunization schedule by age group and medical conditions: United States, 2006–2007. Summary published by the Advisory Committee on Immunization Practices. http://www.cdc.gov

Chapter 23: Vital Signs and Measurements

A.D.A.M. Medical Encyclopedia. (2011). Narcolepsy: Daytime sleep disorder; cataplexy. http://www.ncbi.nlm.nih.gov/pubmedhealth/PMH0001805/

American Heart Association. (2016, March 23). Understanding blood pressure readings. http://www.heart.org/HEARTORG/Conditions/HighBloodPressure/AboutHighBloodPressure/Understanding-Blood-Pressure-Readings_UCM_301764_Article.jsp#.V274hvkrLIU

American Heart Association. (n.d.). All about heart rate (pulse). http://www.heart.org/HEARTORG/Conditions/More/MyHeartand-StrokeNews/All-About-Heart-Rate-Pulse_UCM_438850_Article.jsp

Dieckmann, R., Brownstein, D., & Gausche-Hill, M. (eds). (2000). *Pediatric education for prehospital professionals* (pp. 43–45). Sudbury, MA: Jones & Bartlett, American Academy of Pediatrics.

Emedicine Health. (2016). Pediatric vital signs. http://www.emedicinehealth.com/pediatric_vital_signs/article_em.htm

Environmental Protection Agency. (2016, March 23). Use of mercury and mercury compounds in products and processes. EPA ICR No. 2532.01, OMB Control No. 2070-NEW. https://www.federalregister.gov/articles/2016/03/30/2016-07174/agency-information-collection-activities-proposed-new-collection-epa-icr-no-253201-comment-request#h-9

Mayo Clinic. (2015, September 12). Diseases and conditions: Fever. http://www.mayoclinic.org/diseases-conditions/fever/in-depth/thermometers/art-20046737

Millikan, G. A. (1942). The oximeter: An instrument for measuring continuously oxygen-saturation of arterial blood in man. Review of Scientific Instruments, 13, 434–444.

O'Rourke, M., & Frolich, D. (1999). Pulse pressure: Is this a clinically useful risk factor? Hypertension, 34, 372–374.

Shimbo, D., Muntner, P., Mann, D., Barr, R. G., Tang, W., Post, W., & Shea, S. (2011, April 15). Association of left ventricular hypertrophy with incident hypertension: The multi-ethnic study of atherosclerosis. American Journal of Epidemiology, 173(8), 898–905.

Welch Allyn. (2006). Normal body temperatures. https://intl.welchallyn.com/documents/Thermometry/SM2556_Rev_B_Temp_Chart_Card_OLC.pdf

Wilkins, R. L., Dexter, J. R., & Smith, J. R. (1984). Survey of adventitious lung sound terminology in case reports. Chest, 85(4), 523–525. doi:10.1378/chest.85.4.523. PMID 6705583. http://chestjournal.org/cgi/content/abstract/85/4/523

World Health Organization. (2013). WHO calls for the phase out of mercury fever thermometers and blood pressure measuring devices by 2020. http://www.who.int/mediacentre/news/notes/2013/mercury-medical-devices-20131011/en/

Chapter 24: The Physical Examination

See General References

UNIT VII: ASSISTING AND SPECIALTY EXAMINATIONS AND PROCEDURES

Chapter 25: Obstetrics and Gynecology

Agency for Healthcare Research and Quality. (n.d). Advancing excellence in health care: Breast cancer screening. http://www.guideline.gov/content.aspx?id=34275#Section420

American Cancer Society. (2016). Guidelines for the early detection of cancer. http://www.cancer.org/healthy/findcancerearly/cancerscreeningguidelines/american-cancer-society-guidelines-for-the-early-detection-of-cancer

American Cancer Society. (2011). *Breast cancer: Early detection*. Atlanta, GA: American Cancer Society. http://www.cancer.org/cancer/breastcancer/index

American College of Obstetricians and Gynecologists, Committee on Gynecologic Practice and the American Society for Reproductive Medicine Practice Committee. (2012, August). Committee opinion: Compounded bioidentical menopausal hormone therapy. Number 532, August 2012 (Reaffirmed 2014, Replaces No. 387, November 2007 and No. 322, November 2005). Retrieved on June 4, 2015 from http://www.acog.org/Resources-And-Publications/Committee-Opinions/Committee-on-Gynecologic-Practice/Compounded-Bioidentical-Menopausal-Hormone-Therapy

Centers for Disease Control and Prevention. (n.d.). Genital HPV infection: CDC fact sheet. http://www.cdc.gov/std/HPV/STDFact-HPV.htm

Centers for Disease Control and Prevention. (n.d.). Human papillomavirus (HPV). http://www.cdc.gov/hpv/vaccine.html

Centers for Disease Control and Prevention, Division of Nutrition, Physical Activity and Obesity. (2015, June 4). Healthy pregnant or postpartum women. Retrieved on May 30, 2016 from http://www.cdc.gov/physicalactivity/basics/pregnancy/

Emory Healthcare. (n.d.). Prenatal visit schedule. http://www.emoryhealthcare.org/maternity-center/patient-information/prenatal-visit-schedule.html

Ghidini, A. (n.d.). Fetal blood sampling: Technique and complications. http://www.uptodate.com/home/index.html

Jørgensen, K. J., & Gotzche, P. C. (2016). Breast cancer screening: Benefit or harm? Journal of the American Medical Association, 315(13), 1402. doi:10.1001/jama.2015.19126

Littleton, L. Y., & Engebretson, J. C. (2002). *Maternal, neonatal, and women's health nursing.* Clifton Park, NY: Cengage Learning.

Mayo Clinic. (n.d.). Hormone therapy: Is it right for you? http://www.mayoclinic.com/health/hormone-therapy/WO00046/

Morrison, R. W., & Lett, S. M. (2007). *Human papillomavirus (HPV) vaccine for VFC-eligible girls now available (memorandum).* Jamaica Plain, MA: Commonwealth of Massachusetts, Executive Office of Health and Human Services, Department of Public Health, State Laboratory Institute. http://www.cdc.gov/hpv/vaccine.html

National Cancer Institute. (2011, December 5). Menopausal hormone therapy and cancer. http://www.cancer.gov/about-cancer/causes-prevention/risk/hormones/mht-fact-sheet

National Cancer Institute. (2007). Tamoxifen: Questions and answers. Retrieved August 29, 2007, from http://www.cancer.gov/cancertopics/factsheet/therapy/tamoxifen

National Cancer Institute. (2008, February 14). Fact Sheet 4.21: Human papillomavirus (HPV) vaccines. Questions and answers. www.cancer.gov/cancertopics/factsheet/prevention/HPV-vaccine

Queensland Health. (n.d.). Cultural dimensions of pregnancy, birth and post-natal care. https://www.health.qld.gov.au/multicultural/support_tools/14MCSR-pregnancy.pdf

Roberts, J. M., & Cooper, D. B. (2001). Series, preeclampsia trio: Pathogenesis and genetics of preeclampsia. Lancet, 357, 53–56.

U.S. Department of Health and Human Services, U.S. Food and Drug Administration. (2014, December 4). FDA approves Gardasil 9 for prevention of certain cancers caused by five additional types of HPV. Retrieved on June 4, 2016 from http://www.fda.gov/NewsEvents/Newsroom/PressAnnouncements/ucm426485.htm

Walsh, T., Casadei, S., Coats, K. H., Swisher, E., Stray, S. M., Higgins, J., & King, M-C. (2006). Spectrum of mutations in BRCA1, BRCA2, CHEK2, and TP53 in families at high risk of breast cancer. Journal of the American Medical Association, 295(12), 1379–1388.

Chapter 26: Pediatrics

Ambroz, K. G., & Eilber, W. (2003). An enhanced method of pediatric urine collection. Internet Journal of Emergency Medicine, 1(1).

Centers for Disease Control and Prevention. (2016, March 22). ACIP vaccine recommendations. http://www.cdc.gov/vaccines/hcp/acip-recs/index.html

Centers for Disease Control and Prevention. (2016, July 28). U.S. selected practice recommendations for contraceptive use. Morbidity and Mortality Weekly Report. http://www.cdc.gov/mmwr/cme/conted.html

Centers for Disease Control and Prevention. (n.d.). Childhood development. http://www.cdc.gov/ncbddd/childdevelopment/positiveparenting/toddlers.html

Centers for Disease Control and Prevention. (n.d.). General recommendations on immunization: Recommendations of the Advisory Committee on Immunization Practices (ACIP). http://www.cdc.gov/mmwr/pdf/rr/rr6002.pdf

Centers for Disease Control and Prevention. (n.d.). Parent's guide to childhood immunizations. http://www.cdc.gov/vaccines/pubs/parents-guide/downloads/parents-guide-508.pdf

Centers for Disease Control and Prevention. (2007, January). National health and nutrition examination survey (NHANES): Anthropometry procedures manual. http://www.cdc.gov/nchs/data/nhanes/nhanes_09_10/BodyMeasures_09.pdf

Clifton, J. C. (2007). Mercury exposure and public health. In *Pediatric clinics of North America* (pp. 237–269). National Library of Medicine and the National Institutes of Health. http://www.pubmed.gov

Mandleco, B. L. (2004). *Growth and development handbook: Newborn through adolescent.* Clifton Park, NY: Cengage Learning.

Pediatrics for Medical Students. (2016, April 21). Pediatric vital signs reference chart. http://www.pedscases.com/sites/default/files/Vital%20Signs%20Reference%20Chart%201.2_1.pdf

Potts, N. L., & Mandleco, B. L. (2012). *Pediatric nursing: Caring for children and their families* (3rd ed.). Clifton Park, NY: Cengage Learning.

Price, C. S., Thompson, W. W., Goodson, B., et al. (2010, October). Prenatal and infant exposure to thimerosal from vaccines and immunoglobins and risk of autism. Pediatrics, 126(4), 656–664.

Sirotnak, A. P., & Pataki, C. (n.d.). Failure to thrive clinical presentation. http://emedicine.medscape.com/article/915575-clinical#b4

Chapter 27: Male Reproductive System

American Cancer Society. (2016). Key statistics for prostate cancer. http://www.cancer.org/cancer/prostatecancer/detailedguide/prostate-cancer-key-statistics

Crooks, R., & Baur, K. (2016). *Our sexuality* (13th ed.). Belmont, CA: Wadsworth.

Centers for Disease Control and Prevention. (2015, February). Facts about hypospadias. Retrieved December 19, 2015, from http://www.cdc.gov/ncbddd/birthdefects/hypospadias.html

Faiman, C. (2012). Male hypogonadism. http://www.clevelandclinicmeded.com/medicalpubs/diseasemanagement/endocrinology/male-hypogonadism/

Ferro, F., Lais, A., Matarazzo, E., Capozza, N., & Caione, P. (1996). Retractile testis and gliding testis: Two distinct clinical entities. http://www.ncbi.nlm.nih.gov/pubmed/8966651

Harvard Health Publications. (2011, April 26). Harvard experts discuss surgical options for benign prostatic hyperplasia. http://www.harvardprostateknowledge.org/harvard-experts-discuss-surgical-options-for-benign-prostatic-hyperplasia

Litwin, M., Nied, R., & Dihanani, N. (1998). Health-related quality of life in men with erectile dysfunction. http://www.ncbi.nlm.nih.gov/pmc/articles/PMC1496922/

University of California–San Francisco. (n.d.). Phimosis. https://urology.ucsf.edu/patient-care/children/phimosis

Warner, J. (ed.). (2007). Erectile dysfunction. http://www.webmd.com/sexual-conditions/guide/mens-sexual-problems

WebMD. (n.d.). Common male sexual problems: Erectile dysfunction. http://www.webmd.com/sexual-conditions/guide/mens-sexual-problems

Williams, M., & Schellhammer, P. F. Testicular seminoma. http://emedicine.medscape.com/article/437966-overview

Chapter 28: Gerontology

Administration on Aging. (n.d.). Aging statistics. http://www.aoa.acl.gov/aging_statistics/index.aspx

Cox, H. (2001). *Later life: The realities of aging* (5th ed.). Upper Saddle River, NJ: Prentice Hall.

Hogstel, M. O. (2001). *Gerontology: Nursing care of the older adult.* Clifton Park, NY: Cengage Learning.

Lodge, H. S. (2007, March 6). You can stop "normal" aging. Parade Magazine.

Markson, E., & Hollis-Sawyer, G. (2000). *Readings in social gerontology.* Los Angeles: Roxbury.

Perls, T. (2007). Simple steps may slow aging. Consumer Reports on Health, 19, 1–4.

World Health Organization. (2015, September). Ten facts on ageing and health. http://www.who.int/features/factfiles/ageing/en/

Chapter 29: Examinations and Procedures of Body Systems

ALS Association. (2016). Symptoms and diagnosis. http://www.alsa.org/about-als/symptoms.html

Alzheimer's Association. (2016). Medications for memory loss. http://www.alz.org/alzheimers_disease_standard_prescriptions.asp

American Cancer Society. (2014, February). FDA clears camera-in-a-pill for people who could not complete colonoscopy. http://www.cancer.org/cancer/news/fda-clears-camera-in-a-pill-for-people-who-could-not-complete-colonoscopy

American Cancer Society. (2011). Stomach cancer. http://www.cancer.org/Cancer/StomachCancer/DetailedGuide/stomach-cancer-diagnosis

American Family Physician. (n.d.). Metered dose inhalers and how to use them correctly. http://www.aafp.org/afp/20010815/603.html

Borowitz, D., Robinson, K. A., Rosenfeld, M., et al. (2009). Cystic Fibrosis Foundation evidence-based guidelines for management of infants with cystic fibrosis. Journal of Pediatrics, 155(6 Suppl), S73–S93.

Cambridge Color Test Handbook. (2011, January). https://sites.oxy.edu/clint/physio/article/CAMBRIDGECOLOURTESTHandbook.pdf

Cancer Research Institute. (2009). Conquering melanoma: Prevent it, spot it, treat it. http://www.cancerresearch.org/resources/conquering-melanoma/p2.html

Centers for Disease Control and Prevention. (2011). General information about TB blood tests. http://www.cdc.gov/tb/topic/testing/bloodtest.htm

Centers for Disease Control and Prevention. (2011). Rabies: Diagnosis in humans. http://www.cdc.gov/rabies/diagnosis/animals-humans.html

Chernecky, C. C., & Berger, B. J. (2008). *Laboratory tests and diagnostic procedures* (5th ed.). Philadelphia: Saunders Elsevier.

COPD Foundation. (n.d.). Chronic obstructive pulmonary disease overview and treatment overview. http://www.copdfoundation.org

Donohoe Dennison, R. (2000). *Pass CCRN!* (2nd ed.). St. Louis, MO: Mosby.

Farley, A., & McLafferty, E. (2008). Lumbar puncture. Nursing Standards, 22(22), 46–48.

Feldman, E. L. (2007). Amyotrophic lateral sclerosis and other motor neuron diseases. In L. Goldman & D. Ausiello (eds.), *Cecil textbook of medicine* (23rd ed.; Chapter 435). Philadelphia: Saunders Elsevier.

Gallager, C. (2009). Parkinson's disease. In D. Rakel (ed.), *Integrative medicine* (2nd ed.). Philadelphia: Saunders Elsevier.

Goldberg, S. (2004). *The four-minute neurologic exam.* Miami, FL: MedMaster Publishing Co.

Green, P. H., & Cellier, C. (2007). Celiac disease. New England Journal of Medicine, 357, 1731–1743.

Kline, J. A., & Runyon, M. S. (2007, June). Pulmonary embolism and deep venous thrombosis. In J. A. Marx, R. S. Hockenberger, & R. M. Walls (eds.), *Rosen's emergency medicine concepts and clinical practice* (6th ed.; Vol. 2; pp. 1368–1382).

Middleton, F. A., & Tillery, S. I. H. (2003). Cerebellum. In L. Nadel (ed.), *The encyclopedia of cognitive science* (pp. 467–475). London: Macmillan.

National Eye Institute. (2015, September). Facts about age-related macular degeneration. https://nei.nih.gov/health/maculardegen/armd_facts

National Eye Institute. (2015, February). Facts about color blindness. https://nei.nih.gov/health/color_blindness/facts_about

National Heart, Lung, and Blood Institute. (2011). What is cardiomyopathy? http://www.nhlbi.nih.gov/health/health-topics/topics/cm/

National Heart, Lung, and Blood Institute. (2007). Section 4: Managing asthma long term overview (pp. 277–280). http://www.nhlbi.nih.gov/

National Multiple Sclerosis Society. (2016). Diagnosing MS. http://www.nationalmssociety.org/Symptoms-Diagnosis/Diagnosing-MS

Neighbors, M., & Tannehill-Jones, R. (2015). *Human diseases* (4th ed.). Clifton Park, NY: Cengage Learning.

Robinson, P. D., Cooper, P., & Ranganathan, S. C. (2009, September). Evidence-based management of paediatric primary spontaneous pneumothorax. Paediatric Respiratory Reviews, 10(3), 110–117.

Roe, S. (2003). *Delmar's clinical nursing skills and concepts.* Clifton Park, NY: Cengage Learning.

U.S. Department of Health and Human Services, National Institutes of Health. (2010). Alzheimer's disease medication fact sheets. www.nia.nih.gov/alzheimers/publication/alzheimers-disease-medications-fact-sheet

U.S. National Library of Medicine, PubMed Health. (2011). Myasthenia gravis. www.ncbi.nlm.nih.gov/pubmedhealth/PMH0001731/

WebMD. (n.d.). Asthma guide, overview and facts, treatment and self-care. http://www.webmd.com/asthma/guide/asthma-overview-facts

WebMD. (n.d.). Examinations and tests for COPD. http://www.webmd.com

Wilt, T. J., Niewoehner, D., Kim, C., Kane, R. L., Linabery, A., Tacklind, J., Macdonald, R., & Rutks, I. Agency for Healthcare Research and Quality. (2008) Use of spirometry for case finding, diagnosis, and management of chronic obstructive pulmonary disease (COPD): Summary. Retrieved September 23, 2016 from http://www.ncbi.nlm.nih.gov/books/NBK11854

UNIT VIII: ADVANCED TECHNIQUES AND PROCEDURES

Chapter 30: Assisting with Minor Surgery

Alguire, P., & Mathes, B. (1998). Skin biopsy techniques for the internist. Journal of General Internal Medicine, 13(1), 46–54. http://www.ncbi.nlm.nih.gov/pmc/articles/PMC1496896/

Association of Surgical Technologists, Inc. (2012). *Surgical technology for the surgical technologist* (5th ed.). Clifton Park, NY: Cengage Learning.

McCarty, M. N. (2012, June). The lawful scope of practice of medical assistants: 2012 update. AMT Events, pp. 110–119. http://isgweb.aorn.org/ISGWeb/downloads/CEA10011-4003.pdf

Phillips, N. (2004). *Barry and Kohn's operating room technique* (10th ed.). St. Louis, MO: Mosby.

U.S. Department of Health and Human Services, Centers for Disease Control and Prevention (2011, latest update). Guideline for prevention of surgical site infection, 1999. http://www.cdc.gov/ncidod/dhqp/pdf/guidelines/SSI.pdf

U.S. Food and Drug Administration. (2011). Liquid chemical sterilization. http://www.fda.gov/MedicalDevices/ProductsandMedical-Procedures/GeneralHospitalDevicesandSupplies/ucm208018.htm

Chapter 31: Diagnostic Imaging

Carlton, R. R., & Adler, A. M. (2001). *Principles of radiographic imaging: An art and a science* (5th ed.). Clifton Park, NY: Cengage Learning.

Cornuelle, A., & Gronefeld, D. (1998). *Radiographic anatomy and positioning: An integrated approach.* Stanford, CT: Appleton and Lange.

Cowling, C. (1998). *Radiographic positioning procedures, Vol. 2: Advanced imaging procedures.* Clifton Park, NY: Delmar Cengage Learning.

Gingold, E. (2014). Modern fluoroscopy imaging systems. http://www.imagewisely.org/imaging-modalities/fluoroscopy/articles/gingold-modern-systems

Library of Congress. (2013). H.R.1146: Consistency, Accuracy, Responsibility, and Excellence in Medical Imaging and Radiation Therapy Act of 2013. https://www.congress.gov/bill/113th-congress/house-bill/1146/text

Mettler, F. A., Jr., & Guiberteau, M. J. (2012). *Essentials of nuclear medicine imaging* (6th ed.). Philadelphia: W. B. Saunders.

Orenstein, B. W. (2006). Hot issues: MRI and implantable devices. Radiology Today, 7(4), 8.

RadiologyInfo.org. (2016). Bone densitometry. http://www.radiologyinfo.org/en/info.cfm?pg=dexa

U.S. Food and Drug Administration. (2016, March 25). Radiation-emitting products. http://www.fda.gov/Radiation-EmittingProducts/RadiationSafety/RadiationDoseReduction/ucm299354.htm

White, C. D., Zieve, D., & Ogilvie, I. (n.d.). Bone mineral density test. MedlinePlus Medical Encyclopedia. http://www.nlm.nih.gov/medlineplus/ency/article/007197.htm

Chapter 32: Rehabilitation and Therapeutic Modalities

Beck, F. (2006). *Theory and practice of therapeutic massage* (4th ed.). Clifton Park, NY: Delmar Cengage Learning.

Hausswirth, C., Louis, J., Bieuzen, F., Pournot, H., Fournier, J., Filliard, J-R., & Brisswalter, J. (2011). Effects of whole-body cryotherapy vs. far-infrared vs. passive modalities on recovery from exercise-induced muscle damage in highly-trained runners. PLOS ONE, 6(12), e27749. doi:10.1371/journal.pone.0027749. ISSN 1932-6203. PMC 3233540. PMID 22163272.

Mayo Clinic. (2016). Slide show: Tips for choosing and using canes. http://www.mayoclinic.org/healthy-lifestyle/healthy-aging/multimedia/canes/sls-20077060

O'Sullivan, S. B., & Schmitz, T. (2006). *Physical rehabilitation: Assessment and treatment* (5th ed.). Philadelphia: F. A. Davis.

Weiss, R. C. (2009). *Physical therapy aide: A work text* (3rd ed.). Clifton Park, NY: Cengage Learning.

Chapter 33: Nutrition in Health and Disease

American College of Allergy, Asthma, and Immunology. (2014). Types of food allergy. http://acaai.org/allergies/types/food-allergies

American Heart Association. (2015). Trans fats. http://www.heart.org/HEARTORG/HealthyLiving/HealthyEating/Nutrition/Trans-Fats_UCM_301120_Article.jsp#.V50wiaIorv8

American Heart Association. (2014). Know your fats. http://www.heart.org/HEARTORG/Conditions/Cholesterol/PreventionTreatmentofHighCholesterol/Know-Your-Fats_UCM_305628_Article.jsp#.V54ojqIorv8

Centers for Disease Control and Prevention, (2013). Obesity: United States, 1999–2010. http://www.cdc.gov/mmwr/preview/mmwrhtml/su6203a20.htm

Centers for Disease Control and Prevention. (n.d.). Childhood obesity facts. http://www.cdc.gov/healthyyouth/obesity/facts.htm

Chang, L., & Nierenburg, C. (n.d.). Healthy kitchens: How much protein do you need? http://www.webmd.com/diet/healthy-kitchen-11/how-much-protein

Cleveland Clinic. (2015, May 11). Diseases and conditions: Lactose intolerance. http://my.clevelandclinic.org/health/diseases_conditions/hic_Lactose_Intolerance

Consumer Reports. (2015). Is Ephedra legal? Consumer Reports investigates. http://www.consumer-reports.org

DeBruyne, L. K., Pinna, K., & Whitney, E. N. (2016). *Nutrition and diet therapy* (9th ed.). Clifton Park, NY: Delmar Cengage Learning.

The FPIES Foundation. (2016, March 1). About food protein–induced enterocolitis syndrome. http://fpiesfoundation.org/about-fpies-3/

Jacobson, M. T. (2014). Protein: Are you getting enough? http://www.webmd.com/food-recipes/protein

Lawson, H. (2014). American Academy of Nutrition and Dietetics: Children need carbohydrates. http://www.eatright.org/resource/food/nutrition/dietary-guidelines-and-myplate/children-need-carbohydrates

Mayo Clinic. (2016, September 2). Diseases and conditions: Lactose intolerance. http://www.mayoclinic.org/diseases-conditions/lactose-intolerance/basics/definition/con-20027906

Mayo Clinic Staff. (2014). Nutrition and healthy eating. http://www.mayoclinic.org/healthy-lifestyle/nutrition-and-healthy-eating/in-depth/carbohydrates/art-20045705?pg=2

Medical News Today. (2015, July 7). Is a gluten-free diet good for our health? http://www.medicalnewstoday.com/articles/288406.php

Nutrients Review. (n.d.) Carbohydrates. http://www.nutrientsreview.com/carbs

Nutrients Review. (n.d.). Monosaccharides. http://www.nutrientsreview.com/carbs/monosaccharides-simple-sugars.html

Richardson, M. (2004). Calcium absorption in post-menopausal women. Harvard Women's Health Watch, 5, 1–3.

University of Maryland Medical Center. (2016). Vitamin B1 (thiamine). http://umm.edu/health/medical/altmed/supplement/vitamin-b1-thiamine

University of Maryland Medical Center. (2016). Vitamin B2 (riboflavin). http://umm.edu/health/medical/altmed/supplement/vitamin-b2-riboflavin

University of Maryland Medical Center. (2016). Vitamin B5 (pantothenic acid). http://umm.edu/health/medical/altmed/supplement/vitamin-b5-pantothenic-acid

University of Maryland Medical Center. (2016). Vitamin H (biotin). http://umm.edu/health/medical/altmed/supplement/vitamin-h-biotin

University of Oregon, Linus Pauling Institute. (2016). Calcium. http://lpi.oregonstate.edu/mic/minerals/calcium#deficiency

University of Oregon, Linus Pauling Institute. (2016). Iron. http://lpi.oregonstate.edu/mic/minerals/iron#function

University of Oregon, Linus Pauling Institute. (2016). Magnesium. http://lpi.oregonstate.edu/mic/minerals/magnesium

University of Oregon, Linus Pauling Institute. (2016). Micronutrient Information Center. http://lpi.oregonstate.edu/mic/vitamins/vitamin-K

University of Oregon, Linus Pauling Institute. (2016). Phosphorus. http://lpi.oregonstate.edu/mic/minerals/phosphorus

University of Oregon, Linus Pauling Institute. (2016). Sodium (chloride). http://lpi.oregonstate.edu/mic/minerals/sodium

U.S. Department of Human Services, National Institutes of Health. (2016). Thiamin fact sheet for health professionals. https://ods.od.nih.gov/factsheets/Thiamin-HealthProfessional/

U.S. Department of Human Services, National Institutes of Health. (2016). Vitamin B6: Dietary supplement fact sheet. https://ods.od.nih.gov/factsheets/VitaminB6-HealthProfessional/#h3

Vitamin D Council. (n.d.). What is vitamin D? https://www.vitamindcouncil.org/about-vitamin-d/what-is-vitamin-d/

World Health Organization. (2016). Micronutrient deficiencies. http://www.who.int/nutrition/topics/vad/en/

Zeratsky, K. (2016), Nutrition and healthy eating. http://www.mayoclinic.org/healthy-lifestyle/nutrition-and-healthy-eating/expert-answers/fat-grams/faq-20058496

Chapter 34: Basic Pharmacology

Broderick, M. (2003, September). Spotting drug abuse. RN Magazine, 66(9), 48–53.

Centers for Disease Control and Prevention. (2007). Public emergency preparedness and response. http://www.bt.cdc.gov

Consumer Healthcare Products Association. (n.d.). FAQs about the OTC Review. http://www.chpa.org/FAQsOTCReview.aspx

Drug Topics. (2007). Facts & figures. http://drugtopics.modernmedicine.com

FDAReview.org, a project of the Independent Institute. (2016). The drug development and approval process. http://www.fdareview.org/03_drug_development.php

Green, E. D., & Guyer, M. S. (2011, February 10). Charting a course for genomic medicine from base pairs to bedside. Nature, 204–214. https://www.genome.gov/pages/about/planning/2011nhgris-trategicplan.pdf

Human Genome Project Information. (2011). Pharmacogenomics. http://www.ornl.gov/sci/techresources/Human_Genome/medicine/pharma.shtml

Medical Board of California, Department of Consumer Affairs. (2010). Medical assistants: Frequently asked questions. http://www.mbc.ca.gov/allied/medical_assistants_questions.html

MedicineNet.com. (2005). Wonder drugs using pharmazooticals. http://www.medicinenet.com/script/main/art.asp?articlekey=52324

Pharmaceutical Research and Manufacturers of America. (2015). Biopharmaceutical research & development: The process behind new medicine. http://www.phrma.org/sites/default/files/pdf/rd_brochure_022307.pdf

UC Davis Health System, Center for Professional Practice of Nursing. (n.d.). Crash carts and their typical contents and indications. http://ucdmc.ucdavis.edu/cne/resources/clinical_skills_refresher/crash_cart/index.html

U.S. Department of Justice, Drug Enforcement Administration, Office of Diversion Control. (2014). Title 21 Code of Federal Regulations. Part 1304. Records and reports of registrants, §1304.11 Inventory requirements. http://www.deadiversion.usdoj.gov/21cfr/cfr/1304/1304_11.htm

U.S. Drug Enforcement Agency (DEA). (2007). Drugs of abuse publication chart. http://www.justice.gov/dea/docs/drugs_of_abuse_2011.pdf

U.S. Food and Drug Administration, Department of Health and Human Services. (2004, February 6). FDA issues regulations prohibiting sale of dietary supplements containing ephedrine alkaloids and reiterates: It advises that consumers stop using these products. Retrieved on September 23, 2016 from http://www.fda.gov/NewsEvents/Newsroom/PressAnnouncements/2004/ucm108242.htm

U.S. Food and Drug Administration, Department of Health and Human Services. (2014, July 18). Frequently asked questions on patents and exclusivity. http://www.fda.gov/Drugs/DevelopmentApprovalProcess/ucm079031.htm#How%20many%20years%20is%20a%20patent%20granted%20for

U.S. Food and Drug Administration, Department of Health and Human Services. (2015, June 4). How to dispose of unused medicines. http://www.fda.gov/forconsumers/consumerupdates/ucm101653.htm

Vicinanzo, A. (2015, April 23). Biological terrorist attack on US an "urgent and serious threat." Homeland Security Today. http://www.hstoday.us/briefings/daily-news-analysis/single-article/biological-terrorist-attack-on-us-an-urgent-and-serious-threat/0ce6ebf3524d83c537b1f4f0cc578547.html

Weisman, R. (2014, November 18). Cost of bringing drug to market tops $2.5b, research finds. Boston Globe. https://www.bostonglobe.com/business/2014/11/18/cost-bringing-prescription-drug-market-tops-billion-tufts-research-center-estimates/6mPph8maRxzcvftWjr7HUN/story.html

Wooten, J. M. (2003, April). Medicine cabinet staples are not without risks. RN Magazine, 66(4), 96.

World Health Organization. (n.d.). Health aspects of biological and chemical weapons. http://www.who.int

Chapter 35: Calculation of Medication Dosage and Medication Administration

Balasa, D. A. (2008). New roles for the certified medical assistant to enhance quality and effectiveness of care. Journal of Medical Practice Management. http://www.aama-ntl.org/resources/library/JMPM_New_Roles_CMAs.pdf

Centers for Disease Control and Prevention. (2006). Health care workers and regulations regarding safety needles. http://www.cdc.gov/medicationsafety/

Centers for Disease Control and Prevention, Division of Health Care Quality Promotion. (2004, February). Workbook for designing, implementing, and evaluating a sharps injury prevention program. http://cdc.gov/sharpsafety/wk_info.html

Centers for Medicare and Medicaid Services. (2010). Eligible professionals meaningful use core measures. http://www.cms.gov/Regulations-and-Guidance/Legislation/EHRIncentivePrograms/downloads/4_e-prescribing.pdf

eNotes. (2014, March 3). Why would someone use an intramuscular injection over another kind? http://www.enotes.com/intramuscular-injection-reference/intramuscular-injection

Joslin Diabetes Center. (n.d.). Insulin A to Z: A guide on different types of insulin. http://www.joslin.org/info/insulin_a_to_z_a_guide_on_different_types_of_insulin.html

Newton M., Newtown, D. W., & Fudin, J. (1992). Reviewing the big three injection routes. Nursing, 22, 34–42

Nursing Times. (2008, December 16). Are techniques used for intramuscular injection based on research evidence? https://www.nursingtimes.net/clinical-archive/cardiology/are-techniques-used-for-intramuscular-injection-based-on-research-evidence/1952004.article

Open Clinical Knowledge Management for Medical Care. (2006). CPOE: Computer physician order entry systems. www.openclinical.org/cpoe.html

UNC Health Care and UNC School of Medicine Newsroom. (2016, March 14). Scientists create painless patch of insulin-producing beta cells to control diabetes. http://news.unchealthcare.org/news/2016/march/scientists-create-painless-patch-of-insulin-producing-beta-cells-to-control-diabetes

U.S. Department of Health and Human Services, National Institute of Diabetes and Digestive and Kidney Diseases. (2014, February). Types of diabetes. https://www.niddk.nih.gov/health-information/diabetes/types

Whitley, H. W. (2008). Sex-based differences in drug activity. American Family Physician, 80(11), 1254–1258.

Chapter 36: Cardiac Procedures

American Heart Association. (n.d.). Heartsaver AED. http://www.americanheart.org

Fozzard, H. A., Haber, E., Jennings, R. B., et al. (eds.). (1991). The heart and cardiovascular system (p. 2193). New York: Raven Press.

Passanisi, C. (2001). Electrocardiology essentials. Clifton Park, NY: Cengage Learning.

Pearlman, J. D., & Linn, E. C. (2011). Imaging in coronary artery disease. MedScape Reference: Drugs, Diseases & Procedures. http://emedicine.medscape.com/article/349040-overview

Van Belle, E., Bauters, C., Asahara, T., & Isne, J. M. (1998). Endothelial regrowth after arterial injury: From vascular repair to therapeutics. Cardiovascular Research, 38(1), 54–68, http://cardiovascres.oxfordjournals.org/content/38/1/54.full

UNIT IX: LABORATORY PROCEDURES

Chapter 37: Regulatory Guidelines for Safety and Quality in the Medical Laboratory

Centers for Medicare and Medicaid Services. (2016, May 24). Clinical Laboratory Improvement Amendments. https://www.cms.gov/Regulations-and-Guidance/Legislation/CLIA/index.html?redirect=/clia/

Centers for Medicare and Medicaid Services. (2016, March 28). Infection prevention & control guidelines & recommendations. http://www.cdc.gov/oralhealth/infectioncontrol/guidelines/index.htm

Centers for Medicare and Medicaid Services. (n.d.). CMS form 116. http://www.cms.hhs.gov

National Fire Protection Association. (n.d.). Codes and standards. http://www.nfpa.org/codes-and-standards/all-codes-and-standards/list-of-codes-and-standards?mode=code&code=170

U.S. Department of Labor, Occupational Safety and Health Administration. (n.d.). Foundation of workplace chemical safety programs. https://www.osha.gov/dsg/hazcom/global.html

U.S. Department of Labor, Occupational Safety and Health Administration. (n.d.). Hazard communication standard: Safety data sheets. https://www.osha.gov/Publications/OSHA3514.html

U.S. Department of Labor, Occupational Safety and Health Administration. (n.d.). OSHA law & regulations. https://www.osha.gov/law-regs.html

Chapter 38: Introduction to the Medical Laboratory

American Association for Clinical Chemistry. (2013, November 1). Harmonization of clinical laboratory test results. https://www.aacc.org/health-and-science-policy/advocacy/position-statements/2013/harmonization-of-clinical-laboratory-test-results

Lab Tests Online. (n.d.). Understanding laboratory tests as a patient and as a health care professional. https://labtestsonline.org

Chapter 39: Phlebotomy: Venipuncture and Capillary Puncture

See General References

Chapter 40: Hematology

See General References

Chapter 41: Urinalysis

See General References

Chapter 42: Basic Microbiology

U.S. Department of Health and Human Services, Centers for Disease Control and Prevention. (n.d.). Intestinal parasites. http://www.cdc.gov/foodsafety/foodborne-germs.html

U.S. Food and Drug Administration. (n.d.). Databases. http://www.fda.gov/search/databases.html

Chapter 43: Specialty Laboratory Tests

U.S. Food and Drug Administration. (n.d.). Databases. http://www.fda.gov/search/databases.html

SECTION IV: PROFESSIONAL PROCEDURES

UNIT X: CLINIC AND HUMAN RESOURCES MANAGEMENT

Chapter 44: The Medical Assistant as Clinic Manager

Colbert, B. J. (2006). *Workplace readiness for health occupations* (2nd ed.). Clifton Park, NY: Cengage Learning.

Facebook. (n.d.). "Like" button. http://developers.facebook.com/docs/opengraph/

Nations, D. (n.d.). What is social media? What are social media sites? http://webtrends.about.com/od/web20/a/social-media.htm

Sobell, S. (2011, June). Social networking @ work: The costro connection.

Chapter 45: The Medical Assistant as Human Resources Manager

Schawbel, D. (2014). Comparing Gen Y and Gen Z workplace expectations: Millennial Branding and Randstad US release first worldwide study. http://millennialbranding.com/2014/geny-genz-global-workplace-expectations-study/

Smith, B. E., & Ricci, C. Healthcare trends 2015: White paper. https://www.besmith.com/thought-leadership/white-papers/healthcare-trends-2015

UNIT XI: ENTRY INTO THE PROFESSION

Chapter 46: Preparing for Medical Assisting Credentials

American Association of Medical Assistants. (2015). Recertify your CMA (AAMA) credential. http://www.aama-ntl.org

American Association of Medical Assistants. (n.d.). FAQs on CMA (AAMA) certification. http://www.aama-ntl.org

American Medical Technologists. (n.d.). AMT certification: A guide to allied health certification. http://www.americanmedtech.org

National Healthcareer Association. (n.d.). NHA national certification examination. http://www.nhanow.com

Chapter 47: Employment Strategies

CBS News. (2011, September 1). The best career strategy ever. http://www.cbsnews.com/news/the-best-career-strategy-ever/

Daily Muse. (n.d.). The 31 best LinkedIn profile tips for job seekers. https://www.themuse.com/advice/the-31-best-linkedin-profile-tips-for-job-seekers

Fletcher, L. (n.d.). How to write a LinkedIn profile. http://www.blueskyresumes.com/free-resume-help/article/how-to-write-a-linkedin-profile/

Imperial College London Business School. (n.d.). Career strategy. http://www3.imperial.ac.uk/pls/portallive/docs/1/50325698.PDF

Job-Hunt. (n.d.). Guide to Facebook for job search. http://www.job-hunt.org/social-networking/facebook-job-search/facebook-job-search.shtml

Job-Hunt. (n.d.). Guide to using LinkedIn for job search. http://www.job-hunt.org/social-networking/LinkedIn-job-search/LinkedIn-job-search.shtml

Job-Hunt. (n.d.). Personal branding makes your LinkedIn summary dazzle. http://www.job-hunt.org/personal-branding/branded-linkedin-summary.shtml

Job-Hunt. (n.d.). 10-step personal branding worksheet. http://www.job-hunt.org/personal-branding/personal-branding-worksheet.shtml

PayScale. (n.d.). Medical assistant salary (United States). http://www.payscale.com/research/US/Job=Medical_Assistant/Hourly_Rate

Schawbel, D. (2016, April). 7 secrets to getting your next job using social media. http://mashable.com/2009/01/05/job-search-secrets/

Social Media Defined. (2016, April). LinkedIn defined. http://www.socialmediadefined.com/2009/01/30/linkedin-defined/

INDEX

Note: Page references in **bold type** refer to boxes, procedures, figures, and tables.

A

AAMA. *See* American Association of Medical Assistants (AAMA)
Abbreviations
    common medical, 1496–1504
    for patient charts, 561, **563**
    for prescriptions, 1098–1100, **1099**, **1100**
    of states, **327**
    of street suffixes, **327**
Abdominal aortic aneurysm, **840**
Abdominal examination, **622**, 625
ABO blood typing, 1372–1373, **1373**
Abortion, 131, 647
Abscess, **779**, **781**
Abuse
    child, 111, 126, **127**, 722–723
    elder, 112, 126, **127**, 766
    ethical issues related to, 126
    intimate partner, 112–113, 126, **127**
Accountability, 13
Accounting practices
    accounts payable, 460–461
    accounts receivable trial balance, 460, **461**
    cost analysis and, 462
    day-end summary, 459–460
    disbursement records, 460–461
    double-entry system, 458
    financial records and, 462
    function of, 460–461
    income earned reporting, 463–465, **463**, **464**
    legal and ethical guidelines for, 465–466
    pegboard system and, 413, **414**, 415, 416, 458
    PMS, 458–459
    single-entry system, 458
    use of computer service bureau for, 459
Accounts payable, 460
Accounts receivable ratio, 446, 465
Accounts receivable trial balance, 460, **461**
Accreditation
    ABHES, 8
    CAAHEP, 8, 175
Accrediting Bureau of Health Education Schools (ABHES), 8, 34, 1462
Accrual basis, 463
Acme stage, of infectious disease, 490
Acne, **779**, **781**
Activated charcoal, **1082**
Active files, 298
Active listening, 58, 71
Acupressure, **31**
Acupuncture, 29
Acute respiratory distress syndrome (ARDS), **826**, **829**
Acute stage, of infectious disease, 490
Acute stress, 43
Acute viral hepatitis diseases, 497, **499**
Additives, 1243, **1243**, **1244**, 1244, **1245**
Adenocarcinomas, 670
Administrative law, 97
    examples of, 97–102
Administrative Simplification Compliance Act (ASCA) (2005), 402
Adolescents
    growth and development in, **703**
    nutrition for, 1044–1045
Adrenaline, **1082**

Adson, 923
Adults, ethical issues related to, 128
Advanced Beneficiary Notification (ABN), 411, 936
Advance directives
    explanation of, 113–114
Advanced Registered Nurse Practitioners (ARNPs), 35
Adverse reactions, 697
Aerosols, 722
Afebrile, 571
Affordable Care Act (ACA), 97–98
Agar, 1356
Age
    communication and, 62, **63–64**
    cultural diversity in calculation of, 548
Aged reports, 343
Agenda. *See* Meeting agenda
Aging. *See also* Gerontology; Older adults
    facts about, 753, **753**
    health in, 769–770
    memory impairment and, 765–766
AIDS, 84, 497. *See also* HIV/AIDS
Airborne precautions, **505**
Airborne transmission, 484, 503
Alanine aminotransferase (ALT), 1391
Albumin, 1391
Albuterol, **1082**
Alcohol-based hand rubs (ABHR), **527**
Alcohol use
    effects of, **1089**
    during pregnancy, 650
Aliquot, 1248
Alkaline phosphatase (ALP), 1391
Allergenic extracts, 1151–1152
Allergies, food, 1050–1051
Allergy skin testing, 778
Allied Bureau of Health Education Schools (ABHES), 1462
Allied health professionals
    health unit coordinators as, 33
    job descriptions for various, **32–33**
    medical assistants as, 31–33
    medical laboratory technologists as, 33, **33**
    nurses as, 34–35
    pharmacists as, 34
    pharmacy technicians as, 34, **34**
    phlebotomists as, 34
    physical therapists as, **32–33**, 34
    physical therapy assistants as, 34
    physicians assistants as, 35
    registered dietitians as, 34
Alphabetic filing system, 290, **291**
Alpha-fetoprotein test, 645
Alpha-Z filing system, 289, **289–290**
Alternative dispute resolution (ADR), 109
Alternative medicine, 31, **31**
Alzheimer's disease, **784**
Amblyopia, **796**
Ambulation, 999, **1000–1002**
Ambulatory care settings. *See also* Computerized medical clinics
    boutique or concierge practices as, 24–25
    design and environment in, 183, 187–189, **188–189**
    educational materials in, 187
    emergencies in, 138–139
    explanation of, 21–22
    group practices as, 23
    legal compliance in, 189–190
    managed care operations as, 24
    medical assistants in, 7

Ambulatory care settings (*Continued*)
   overview of, 183
   predictions for future, 196–197
   procedure to close, 196
   procedure to open, 195
   reception area in, **185–187**, 185–187
   safety issues for, 190–195, **192–194**
   urgent care centers as, 24
   welcoming environment in, 184
American Association of Medical Assistants (AAMA)
   background of, **14**, 14–15, 1467
   certification offered by, 14, 17, 1460, 1462–1464
   code of ethics of, 120, **120**, 123–124
   continuing education and, 14–15
   educational and certification standards of, 19
   liability insurance offered by, 108
   medical assistant definition of, 6, 7
American Chiropractic Association, code of ethics, 124
American Heart Association, 173, **174**
American Medical Association (AMA)
   code of ethics, 120, **120**, 124
   confidentiality policy of, 217
American Medical Technologists (AMT)
   certification offered by, 15, **15**, 1460, 1464–1466
   function of, 15, 1467
   on scope of practice, 17
American Recovery and Reinvestment Act (2009) (ARRA), 213, 279
Americans with Disabilities Act (1990) (ADA)
   explanation of, 99
   facility design and, 184, 189–190
   telephone communications and, 241
Amniocentesis, 645–647
Amniotic fluid, 507
Amoebic dysentery, 481
Amorphous, **1326**
Amphetamine, **1086**
Amplified DNA probe test, 681
Ampules, **1124–1126**
Amyl nitrite, **1088**
Amyotropic lateral sclerosis (ALS), **784**, **787**
Anabolic steroids, **1088**
Anaerobic equipment, 1341–1342, **1342**
Analgesic, **1073**
Anaphylaxis, 1079
Ancillary services, 1430
Andropause, 764
Anemia, 761, **845**, **847**, 1285
Aneroid manometers, 593
Aneroid sphygmomanometer, 593
Anesthesia, 381, 932
Anesthesiologist assistants (AAs), **32**
Anesthetics, 932–934, **934**, **1073**
Angina pectoris, **840**, **844**, **1176**
Angiography, 793, **975**, **976**
Anorexia nervosa, 49, **858**, **866**, 1044–1045
Answering machines, 242
Answering services, 242
Antacids, **1073**
Anthrax, **532**, 1083
Antianxiety medications, **1073**
Antiarrythmic medication, **1073**
Antibacterial creams, 932
Antibiotic-resistant bacteria, **485**, 486
Antibiotics, **1074**
Antibodies, 487, 488
Anticholesterol medication, **1074**
Anticholinergic medication, **1074**
Anticoagulants, **1074**, 1238, 1243, 1244
Anticonvulsants, **1074**
Antidepressants, **1075**
Antidiarrheals, **1075**
Antidote, **1075**
Antiemetics, **1075**
Antihistamines, **1075**
Antihyperlipidemic medication, **1075**
Antihypertensives, **1075**

Antiinflammatories, **1076**
Antineoplastic medication, **1076**
Antioxidants, 1030, 1035–1036
Antipsychotics, **1075**
Antipyretic medication, **1076**
Antitussive medication, **1076**
Antiulcer medication, **1077**
Antiviral medication, **1077**
Antivirus protection programs (computer), 209–210
APGAR Score, **649**, 688
Aphasia, 781
Apical pulse, 585, **587–588**, **714–715**
Apnea, 590, 591
Appearance. *See* Personal appearance
Appendicitis, **858**, **866**
Appendicular skeleton, 847
Application/cover letters, 1484–1485, **1485**, **1486**
Application forms, 1486–1487
Appointment matrix, 261–262, **262–263**
Appointments. *See* Patient scheduling
Apps, 211, 308
Aquamatic K-Pad, 1014
Arbitration, 109
Archival storage, medical record, 301
Arms, examination of, **622**
Arm splints, 160
Arrhythmias, 585, 1188
Arteriosclerosis, **840**, 1047
Articulation, 223
Artifacts
   AC interference, 1174, **1175**
   in urine, **1327**
Artificial insemination, 130
Ascorbic acid, 1030, **1035**
Asepsis, 45
   medical, 45, 524–525, **525–527**, 528, **529**, 530–531, **903**, 903–904
   surgical, 900, **903**, 903–904
Aspartate aminotransferase (AST), 1391
Aspiration, of joint fluid, **963–964**
Assisted reproductive technology (ART), 130, 649–650
Assisted suicide, 82, 132
Assistive devices
   canes as, 1008–1009
   crutches as, 1007–1008
   explanation of, 1004
   types of, **1004–1006**
   walkers as, 1007
   wheelchairs as, 1009, **1009**
Associate's degree, 8
Association for Healthcare Documentation Integrity (AHDI), 335, 336
Asthma, 721, **826**, **829**
Astigmatism, **796**, **801**
Atherosclerosis, 592, 1047
Athlete's foot, **779**, **781**
Athletic trainers (ATs), **32**
Atrial fibrillation, **1179**
Atropine, **1082**
Attitude, 12, 1472
Atypical squamous cells (ASCs), 670
Audiometry, **818–819**
Augmented leads, 1168–1169
Aural temperature, **575–576**, 580, 712
Auscultation, 613
Auscultatory gap, 595
Authoritarian managers, 1405
Authorization for Release of Health Care Information Form, **542**
Autoclave, 907–912, **909–916**, 1341, **1341**
Automated external defibrillator (AED), 173, **174**, 1181
Automated hematology, 1302
Automated routing units (ARUs), 242
Automated urine analyzers, 1322–1323, **1323–1324**
Automatic electrocardiograph machines, 1165
Autopsy reports, 342, **343**
Avascular necrosis, **848**
Avian influenza, 474

Avulsion, **937**
Axial skeleton, 847
Axillary crutches, 1007
Axillary temperature, 580, **582–583**, 712

B

Bachelor's degree, 8
Bacilli, 1354, **1355**
Back pain, **851**, **852**
Bacteria
    cell structure for, 1353–1354, **1354**
    drug-resistant, **485**, 486
    explanation of, 478, 481
    identifying, 1354–1356
    media to identify, 1356–1357, **1357**
    microscopic examination of, 1353–1358, **1355**
    morphology, 1354
    in urine, 1317, **1326**
Bacterial diseases, common, **481**
Balance sheets, 462
Balanitis, 733
Bandages, 149, 151, **151**, 932, **933**, **934**
Banking procedures
    for checking accounts, 423–424, **425–429**
    for online banking, 421
    for savings accounts, 423
Bankruptcy, patient, 452
Bank statements, 427, **429**, 430, **430**
Bariatrics, 880–881
Bariatric surgery, 880
Barium enema, **878**, **977**
Barium swallow test, **863**, **878**, **976**, **977**
Bartholin glands, 666, **677**
Basophils, **1293**
Battery, 106
Bell's palsy, **784**, **787**
Benadryl, **1082**
Benign prostatic hyperplasia, 733, 735–736
Benign prostatic hypertrophy, 733, 735–736
Benzodiazepines, **1085**
Betadine, 932
Bethesda system, 666
Bias, communication and, 62, 64
Bilirubin, 1321, 1391–1392
Bilirubinuria, 1321
Billing. *See also* Collections; Daily financial practices
    cycle system of, 445, **445**
    for insurance carriers, 447–448
    monthly, 445, **445**
    for past-due accounts, 445
    patient statements and, 443–445, **444**
    payment at time of service policy and, 440–442
    policies for, 440
    Truth-in-Lending Act and, 442, **442**
Bill of Rights, 96, 97–98
Bimanual pelvic examination, **668**, **669**
Bioethics, 127–128, 131
Biohazard labels, 523, **523**
Biohazardous waste, 1343, **1343**
Bioidentical hormone replacement therapy (BHRT), 673
Biopsies
    explanation of, **1218**
    of kidney, 885
    of skin, 778
Bioterrorism, 532–533, **532–533**, 1083
Biotin, **1034**
Bipolar leads, 1168
Birth control, 129–131
Birth control pills, 651, **655**, **656**
Blanchard, Kenneth, 122
Bleeding
    control of, **152–153**
    external, 167
    internal, 168
Blogs, 1425, 1473

Blood
    from capillary puncture, 1270–1271
    cellular components of, 1236–1237, **1238**
    hazard communication for, 523, **523**
    infection control and, 507
    in urine, 1322
Blood and lymph system
    diagnostic procedures for, 839, 844
    disorders of, **845–846**, **847**
    function of, 839, 844
Bloodborne pathogens, 475, 515–516, 518
Bloodborne Pathogen Standard (Occupational Safety and Health
    Administration), 515–516, **520–523**, 1246
Blood chemistry tests, 1391–1393
Blood clotting, **1243**
Blood collection, 1238–1239, **1239**, **1240**. *See also* Phlebotomy
Blood culture, 1265, **1265**, **1266–1268**, 1352
Blood glucose, 1380, 1382–1385
Blood glucose tests, 1380, 1382–1385, **1382–1384**, **1386–1387**
Blood incompatibility, 650
Blood pressure
    abnormalities in, 598–599, **598**
    in children, 717
    equipment to measure, 592–594, **592–594**
    explanation of, 591–592
    normal, 598
    procedure to measure, 594–595, **596–597**, **589–590**
    recording, 595
Blood typing tests, 1372–1374, **1373**
Blood urea nitrogen (BUN), 884, 1392
Blue Cross/Blue Shield (BC/BS), 360
Bluetooth, 208
Body fluids, 507
Body language, 59. *See also* Nonverbal communication
Body mass index (BMI), **881**
Body mechanics, 994, **995**
Body movements, 619
Body surface area (BSA), 1101, 1113, **1114**
Body temperature. *See also* Thermometers
    aural, 580
    in children, 712
    explanation of, 570–571
    measurement of, **579–583**
    method to record, 583–584
    oral, 576, 578, **579–580**, 580
    rectal and axillary, 580, **581–583**
    terms used to describe, 571, **572**
Bonding, 466
Bonds, 1434
Bone cancer, **848**
Bone densitometry, 981
Bookkeeping, 413–414, **414**, 458–459. *See also* Accounting practices
Boomer generation, 1448
Botulism, **532**, 1083
Boutique medical practices, 24–25
Bradycardia, 585
Bradypnea, 590
Braille, 190, **190**
Brainstorming, **1408**
Brand-name drugs, 1061
Braxton-Hicks contractions, 650
Breast cancer, **677**
Breast examinations, **622**, 625, **663**, 663–666, **664–665**
Breast-feeding, 1043
Breast milk, 507
Breast self-examination (BSE), **663**, 663, **664–665**, 665–666
Breathing emergencies, 172–173, 175
Breath odors, 619–620
Breath sounds, 591
Brochures, 1423, **1423**
Bronchitis, **826**, **829**
Bronchodilators, **1077**
Broth tubes, 1357
Bruits, 613
Bubonic plague, 1083
Buffy coat, 1238
Building. *See* Facility environment

Bulbourethral glands, **734**, **735**
Bulimia, 49, **858**, **866**, 1044
Bundled codes, 389
Burnout, 48–49. *See also* Stress
Burns
  classification of, 151, **154**
  explanation of, 151, 153
  first-aid for, 153, **155–156**
  types of, 154, 156
Bursitis, **851**, **852**
Bush, George W., 131, 279
Business letters. *See also* Written communication
  for collection purposes, 448–449, **449**, **450**
  components of, 308–313, **311**, **312**
  misused words in, 306, **307**
  proofreading of, 307–308, **308**
  spelling in, 306, **307**
  styles for, 313–314, **315**, **316**
  supplies for, 314–321
  writing tips for, 306
Butryl nitrite, **1088**
Butterfly needle collection system, **1261**, 1261, **1262–1265**

C

Calcium, **1037**, 1039, 1392
Callus, **779**, **781**
Calories, 1026
Cancer
  of blood, **845–846**, **847**
  bone, **848**
  breast, **677**
  cervical, **677**
  colon, **859**, **866**, 874, 1048
  endometrial, **677**
  lung, **828**, **829**
  ovarian, 674
  pancreatic, **864**, **867**
  penile, 738
  prostate, **734**, 739
  rectal, **865**, **867**
  skin, **779–782**
  stomach, **865**, **867**
  testicular, **733**, 739–740
  therapeutic diets for, 1048
  therapeutic response to patients with, 83–84
  urinary bladder, **882**, **884**
Candida, 1362
Candida albicans, 1362
Candidiasis, **677**
Canes, 1008–1009
Cannibis, **1088**
Cannon, Walter, 42
Capillary puncture, 1270–1272, **1271–1276**
Capillary specimen, **1275–1276**
Capitation, 374
Capsule video endoscopy (CVE), 868, **871**
Carbohydrates, 1023–1024, **1024**, 1026, **1029**, **1042**
Carbon dioxide (CO_2), 1392
Cardiac ablation, 1188
Cardiac arrhythmias, 1176–1177
Cardiac cycle, 1162–1163, **1163**
Cardiac electricity, **1168**
Cardiomyopathy, **841**
Cardiopulmonary resuscitation (CPR), 113, 172, 173, **174**, 175
Cardiovascular disease, 1047–1048
Cardiovascular system, in older adults, 761
Cardioversion, 1181
CARE (March 30, 2013), 17, 972
Caregiving, cultural diversity and, **68**, 69
Carpal tunnel syndrome, 215, **784**, **848**, **852**
Cash
  on hand, 424–425
  petty, 432
Cash basis, 463
Cashier's checks, 423

Casts, 853, **853**, **854–856**, **1328–1329**
Catalyst, 1030
Cataract, **796**, **801**
Catheterization. *See* Urinary catheterization
Catheterized urine collection, 1313
Cautery, 916–917
Celiac disease, **858**, **866**
Cell-mediated immunity, 487
Cell structure, 1353–1354, **1354**
Cellulose, 1040
Centers for Disease Control and Prevention (CDC)
  immunization guidelines of, 689
  infection control and, 513–514, 528, 531, 1196
Centers for Medicare and Medicaid Services (CMS), 362, 462, 1103, 1199
Central European diet, **1052**
Central processing unit (CPU), 204, 214
Centrifuge, 1212
Cerebral vascular accident (CVA), **172**, **785**, **787**
Cerebrospinal fluid aspiration, **788–790**
Cerebrospinal fluid (CSF), 507, 1352
Certificate of Training, **1206**
Certificate of Waver (COW) laboratories, **1183**
Certification
  AAMA, 14, 17, 1460, 1462–1464
  agencies granting, 1460, **1461**
  AMT, 15, **15**, 1464–1466
  CCMA, 16, 1466–1467
  CMA, **7**, 14, **14**
  CMAA, 16
  CMAs, **7**, 15
  examinations for, 1460–1462
  function of, 14, 16, **16**
  NCCT, 16, **16**
  NCMA, 16
  NHA, 15–16, 1466–1467
  purpose of, 1460
  RMA, **8**, 15
Certification Commission for Health Information Technology
  (CCHIT), 213
Certified clinical medical assistant (CCMA), 1460, 1466–1467
Certified medical administrative assistant (CMAA), 1460,
  1466–1467
Certified medical administrative specialist (CMAS), 15
Certified medical assistants (CMAs), 7, 14, **14**, 1460, 1462–1464
Cerumen, 814
Cervical cancer, **677**
Cervical cap, 651, **653**, **655**
Cervical cone biopsy, 678
Cervical intraepithelial neoplasia (CIN), 666
Cervical punch biopsy, 674, 678
Chalazion, **796**
Charts. *See* Patient charts
Checking accounts, 423–424
Checkout system, file, 297
Check register, 461
Checks
  acceptance of, 425–426
  lost or stolen, 426
  method to deposit, 424, **425**, **426**
  nonsufficient funds, **427**
  types of, 423–424
  writing and recording, 427, **428–430**
CHEDDAR charting approach, 548–549
Chemical burns, 154
Chemical "cold" sterilization, 930, **905–907**
Chemical Hygiene Plan (CHP), 1201–1203, **1203–1205**, 1206
Chemical Inventory Form, **1203**
Chemicals, avoiding exposure to, 1206–1207
Chemical sterilization, 905, 930
Chemical tissue destruction, 917
Chemical urinalysis, **1319**, **1320**, 1320–1323, **1323–1329**, **1329–1332**
Chemotherapy, 47
Chest, examination of, **622**, 625
Chest circumference, 606, 709, **711**
Cheyne-Stokes, 590
Chicken pox, **496**
Chief complaint (CC), 338

principles of, 524
standard precautions and, 142, 483, **502–503**
Infection cycle
  explanation of, 476, **477**
  infectious agents and, 476–478, 481–483
  mode of transmission and, 483–484
  portal of entry and, 484
  portal of exit and, 483
  reservoir and, 483
  susceptible host and, 484–486
Infections
  incision and drainage of, **961–962**
  nosocomial, 1362
Infectious diseases, **1196**. *See also specific diseases*
  agents of, 476–478, 481–483
  body's defense mechanisms to fight, 486–489
  causes of, 475–476
  common bacterial, **481, 482**
  common viral, **478**
  examples of, **491–496**
  fungal, **483**
  immunizations for, 476, **479–480**
  impact of, 475
  overview of, 474
  reporting requirements for, 500, **500**
  stages of, 489–490
  standard precautions for, 501, **502–506**, 503, 507–508, **508–514**, 513–514
    (*See also* Infection control)
  transmission of, **477**, 483–484, 490, **491–496**, 503
Infectious mononucleosis tests, **845**, 1368, 1371
Infectious waste, disposal of, 513, **514**
Infertility, 649–650, 670–671, 737–738
Inflammation, 487, 937, **938**, 1293, 1390–1391
Inflammatory response, 487
Influenza, **491, 829**
Informed consent
  explanation of, 106–107, 936
  implied, 107
  legal incompetence and, 107
Inhalants, **1088–1089**
Inhalation medications, 1080, 1152–1155, **1153, 1154**
Inhalers, 837, 839, 1152
Initiative, **9**, 12–13
Injectable anesthetics, 932–933
Injections. *See also* Immunizations
  basic guidelines for, **1122–1123**, 1142
  intradermal, **1122–1123**, 1135, 1136
  intramuscular, 696, **696**, **1122–1123**, 1136
  subcutaneous, **696, 1122–1123**, 1135, **1136**
Inner-directed people, 47
Inoculating equipment, 1342, **1342**
Inoculating needle, 1342, **1342**
Insect stings, 162, 165–166
Inside address, 310
Inspection, 612–613
Instruments. *See also* Equipment/supplies
  care of, 927–930
  categories of, 920–927, **921–930**
  checking quality of, 1219
  explanation of, 920
  sterilization of, **912–916**
Insulin, **1082**, 1108, **1109**, 1382
Insurance. *See* Medical insurance
Insurance coding. *See* Medical insurance coding
Insurance fraud/abuse, 375
Integrated delivery systems (IDSs), 360
Integrative medicine, 29–30
Integrity, **9**, 13
Integumentary system. *See also* Skin
  allergy skin testing and, 778
  disorders of, **779–781**
  explanation of, 777–778, **777**
  in older adults, 759
  skin tests for, 778, **781**
Intentional torts, 105
Interactive videoconferencing, 248–249
Internal bleeding, 168

International Classification of Diseases 9th Revision, Clinical Modification (ICD-9-CM), 384,
  10th Revision, Clinical Modification (ICD-10-CM), 384–386, **387–388**
International direct distance dialing (IDDD), 239
International normalized ratio (INR), 1372
Internal Revenue Service, 97
Internet
  explanation of, 207
  secure sites on, 210, **210**
  security issues related to, 208–210
  travel arrangements using, 1420
  virus protection and, 209–210
Interpretive electrocardiograph, 1166
Interrogatory, 109
Interviews
  cultural awareness during, 539, 544
  employment, 1442–1446, **1446, 1447**, 1487–1491, **1488, 1489, 1490**
  patient, 539, **543**, 543–545
  techniques for, 72–73
Intestinal protozoa, **483**, 1359
Intimate partner violence (IPV), 112–113, 126
Intradermal injections
  administration of, **1122–1123**
  of purified protein derivative, **1142–1144**
Intradermal test, 778
Intramuscular injections
  administration of, **1122–1123, 1147–1149**
  explanation of, 696, **696**
  marking correct site for, 1136, **1137–1141**
  site selection for, 1135–1136
  Z-track method for, 1149, **1149–1151**
Intrauterine device (IUD)
  explanation of, **656, 657**
  insertion of, **654, 656, 657**
Intravenous pyelogram (IVP), 735, 884, **885**
Intravenous therapy, 1133–1135, **1134**
Invasion of privacy, 106
Invasive, 1213
In vitro fertilization (IVF), 130, 649
Involuntary dismissal, 1417, 1449
Iron, 1039
Iron deficiency anemia, 1285
Irritable bowel syndrome (IBS), **864, 867**
Ischemia, **1176**
Islamic diet, **1054**
Isoelectric line, 1162
Isolation categories (Centers for Disease Control), 514
Isopropyl alcohol, 932
Isuprel, **1082**
Italian diet, **1052**
Itinerary, 1421

J

Japanese diet, **1053**
Jaundice, 620, 1391
Jenner, Edward, 475
Jewish diet, **1053**
Job application/cover letters, 1484–1486, **1485, 1486**
Job application forms, 1486–1487
Job descriptions, **1442**, 1442–1443, **1443**
Job hunting. *See* Employment strategies
Job instability, 46
Job interviews, 1442–1446, **1446, 1447**, 1487–1491, **1488, 1489, 1490**
Job résumés, 1476–1483, **1478–1484**
Job search, 1473, 1476
Joint fluid aspiration, **963–964**
Joint movement, **1010, 1011**, 1011
Judicial branch of government, 96

K

Ketoacidosis, 1317
Ketones, 1321
Ketonuria, 1321
Ketosis, 1321

Pneumonic plague, 1083
Pneumothorax, **828**, **829**
Point-of-care testing (POCT), 1214
Point-of-service (POS) device, 403, **404**
Point-of-service (POS) plans, 361
Poison Control Center, 162
Poisoning, 162
Policy manuals, 1440–1441, **1441–1442**
Polycystic kidneys, **882**, **884**
Polysaccharides, 1023
Poor, care of, 126
Position, 60–61, **60**
Positioning, 614, 617
Positron emission tomography (PET), 793, 981–982, **982**
Post-lumbar puncture, **791**
Postoperative instructions, 936
Postpartum period, 651
Postscript, 313
Posture, 60, 216–217, 223, 619, 994, **995**
Postvasectomy semen analysis (PVSA), 1374
Potassium, **1037–1038**, 1039
Potassium hydroxide (KOH), 679, 1356
Power medication, reconstituting, **1127–1129**
The Power of Ethical Management (Blanchard/Peale), 122
Power verbs, 1478
Practice-based scheduling, 255
Practice management (PM), 212–213, **212**
    for telephone calls, 231
Practicums, student, 8, 1413
Preauthorization, 370–371
Precertification, 370–371
Precipitate, 1115
Precordial leads, 1169–1170
Preeclampsia, 637
Preexisting conditions, 356
Preferred provider organizations (PPOs), 21, 361
Pregnancy
    alcohol intake during, 650
    cultural considerations during, 640, **641**
    cultural difference in views of, 636–637
    initial prenatal visits during, 637, **639**, 640, **640**, **644–645**
    normal uterine, **637**
    nutrition and, 1043
    patient education on, 638, **640**
    return prenatal visits during, 642, **642**, **644–645**, 645–647, **646**
    x-rays and, 972–973
Pregnancy complications
    abortion/interruption of pregnancy as, 647
    blood incompatibility as, 650
    eclampsia as, 647
    ectopic pregnancy as, **640**, 647
    gestational diabetes as, 637, 647–648
    hyperemesis gravidarum as, 648
    placenta previa as, 648, **648**
    preeclampsia as, 637
Pregnancy tests, 1368, **1369–1370**
Prejudice, 62, 64
Premature atrial contraction (PAC), **1178**
Premature ventricular contraction (PVC), **1180**
Premenstrual syndrome (PMS), **677**
Prenatal history, 642, 645–647
Prenatal tests, 638, **639**
Prenatal visits
    initial, 637–638, **639**, 640, **640**, **644–645**
    return, 642, **642**, **644–645**, 645–647, **646**
Presbyopia, **801**, 802
Preschoolers, **701**. *See also* Children
Prescriptions. *See also* Medications
    abbreviations and symbols used on, 1098–1100, **1099**, **1100**
    for controlled substances, 1098, **1098**
    electronic, 1066
    explanation of, 1097–1100, **1097**, **1098**
Presentation, **9**, 10–12
Present problem (PP), 338
Press releases, 1423, **1424**
Pretrial conference, 109
Preventive maintenance, 1220

Priapism, 738–739
Primary survey, for emergency assessment, **139**, 140, **141**
Principle-centered leadership, 121–122
Principle-Centered Leadership (Covey), 121
Prions, 482
Privacy. *See also* Confidentiality
    computer security and, 208–210
    invasion of, 106, 189
Probation, 1412, **1412**, 1413, 1446
Problem-oriented medical records (POMRs), 282–283, 559–560
Procedure manual, 1418, **1418**, **1419**, 1420
Procedures. *See* Examinations
Proctologic table, **616**
Proctosigmoidoscopy, **871**, **872**
Prodromal stage, of infectious disease, 490
Professional fees, 125
Professionalism
    collections and, 452–453
    explanation of, 6, **9–11**
    in medical transcription, 345
    in telecommunications, 249
Professional liability insurance, 108, 1434
Professional organizations, 1467
Proficiency tests, 1220
Prefilling syringes, 694
Progestin, 672
Program software, 207
Progress notes, 337, **337**
Prone position, **616**
Proofreader's marks, **308**
Proofreading, 307–308, **308**
Proportion, 1103–1104
Proportional method, to calculate medication dosage, 1107, 1111
Proprietary schools, 7
Prostaglandins, 650
Prostate
    disorders of, 733, 735–736, 739
    explanation of, 733
Prostate cancer, **735**, 739
Prostatitis, **735**, 739
Protected health information (PHI), 99, 244, 540
Protein, 1025–1026, **1029**, 1321, 1393
Prothrombin time, **1300–1301**, 1372
Provider-performed microscopy procedures (PPMPs), 1197, 1198, **1198**
Pruritus, 778, 1079
Psoriasis, **779**, **780**
Public duties, 111–113
Puerperium, 637. *See also* Postpartum period
Puerto Rican diet, **1052**
Pulmonary embolism (PE), **828**, **829**
Pulse oximeters, 594, **594**, 836–837, **836**, **837**
Pulse pressure, 595
Pulse/pulse rate
    abnormalities in, 585
    in children, 712
    explanation of, 584
    in infants, **714–715**
    measurement and evaluation of, 585, **586–588**
    method to record, 585
Pulse sites, **584**, 584–585
Puncture, **937**
Purging, record, 298
Purified protein derivative (PPD), 1380
P wave, 1163
Pyelonephritis, **883**, **884**
Pyridoxine, **1034**, 1035

Q

Qualitative tests, **1216**
Quality assurance (QA), 333, 1197
Quality control, in microbiology laboratory, 1344
Quantitative tests, **1216**
Quinlan, Karen Ann, 132

Therapeutic diets. *See also* Nutrition
  for cancer, 1048
  for diabetics, 1046–1047
  explanation of, 1045
  for individuals with cardiovascular disease, 1047–1048
  for weight control, 1045–1046
Therapeutic drug monitoring (TDM), 1213
Therapeutic exercises
  electromyography as, 1012
  electrostimulation of muscle as, 1012
  muscle testing, 1011
  range of motion, 1010–1011, **1010**
  types of, 1011–1012
Therapeutic modalities
  explanation of, 1012
  heat and cold as, 1012–1013
  massage therapy as, 1015–1017, **1016**
  moist and dry cold as, 1014–1015
  moist and dry heat as, 1013–1014
  ultrasound as, 1015
Thermometers. *See also* Body temperature
  cleaning and storing, 584
  disposable, 573
  electronic and digital, 573–574, **573**, **579–580**, **713–714**
  phaseout of mercury, 571, 573, **577**
  temporal artery, 574, 576, **577–578**
  tympanic, 574
Thermotherapy, 1012
Thiamin, **1032–1034**
ThinPrep Pap Test, **668**
Third-degree burns, **154**, **156**
Third-party guidelines, 391–392, **393**
Third-party payers, 445
Thixotropic separator gel, 1244, **1245**
Throat, examination of, **622**, 624–625
Throat cultures, 1345, **1346–1348**
Thrombocytes, 1237, 1282. *See also* Platelets
Thrombocytopenia, 1295
Thrombocytosis, 1295
Thrombophlebitis, **843**, **844**
Thyroid functioning test, 1380
Thyroxine (T4) test, 1380
Tic douloureux, **786**, **787**
Tickler files, 296–297, **297**
Time focus, 69
Time management, 1422–1423
Tine test, 1380
Title VII of Civil Rights Act (1964), 98
Toddlers. *See also* Children
  growth and development in, **701**
Tonsillitis, 720, **828**, **829**
Topical spray anesthetics, 934
Torts
  common, 105–106
  explanation of, 104, 105
  negligence and, 105
  standard of care and scope of practice and, 104–105
Practice management system (PMS)
  for accounting, 458–459
Total protein, 1393
Touch, 61, 185
Tourniquets, 149, 1245–1246, **1246**, 1248–1249, **1249**
Towel clamps, 924, **926**
Toxicology department, **1216**, **1218**
Toxicology tests, **1218**
Toxic shock syndrome (TSS), **495**
TPMS. *See* Total practice management system (TPMS)
Trace minerals, 1040
Traditional indemnity insurance, 358, 360
Transcription. *See* Medical transcription
Transcutaneous electric nerve stimulation (TENS), 1012
Transdermal system of medication delivery, 1080, **1081**
Transducer, 1187
Transferable skills, 1472
Transmission-Based Precautions, **1196**
Trans unsaturated fatty acids, **836**, 1024, **1026**

Transurethral resection of the prostate (TURP), **734**, **736**, 736
Transverse fracture, **853**
Travel arrangements, 1420, 1421, **1421**, **1422**
Traveler's checks, 423
Treadmill stress test, **1186**, 1186–1187
Trendelenburg position, 616
Trial, 109–110
TRICARE, 366
Trichomonas, **678**, 679
Trichomonas vaginalis, 1360, **1361**, 1362
Trichomoniasis, 481, **677**
Triglycerides, 1024, **1024**, 1389–1390
Triiodothyronine (T3) test, 1380
Trimester, 645
Triple option plans, 361
Trough, 1213
Trust, 71
Truth-in-Lending Act (1968), 442, **442**
Tubal ligation, 130, **654**
Tuberculosis (TB), 45, 47, **495**, **828–829**, 1375–1376
Tuberculosis tests, **1379**, 1379–1380
Tularemia, 1083
Turnaround time (TAT), 343
T wave, 1163
Two-hour postprandial blood glucose test, 1383
24-hour urine collection, 1310, **1311**
Tympanic thermometers, 574, **575–576**
Tympanometry, 815
Tympanostomy, 815

U

Ultrasonic cleaning, 528, **529**, 929–930
Ultrasonography, 1187
Ultrasound
  for diagnostic imaging, 645–647, **984**, 984–985
  as therapeutic modality, 1015
Unbundling, 389
Uniform Anatomical Gift Act (1968), 101
Uniform Bill 04 form, 401–402, **401**
Unipolar leads, 1168
United States Pharmacopeia/National Formulary, 1071
Universal Blood and Body Fluid Precautions, **1196**
Universal Precautions (Centers for Disease Control), 514
Universal Serial Bus (USB) port, 204, 206
Urea, 1307
Urgent care centers, 24
Uric acid, 1393
Urinalysis
  chemical, **1320**, 1320–1323, **1323–1332**
  collection methods for, 1310–1311, **1311–1312**, 1313
  culture and sensitivity transport kit for, **1313–1315**
  drug screening and, 1334
  explanation of, 881, 1214, 1305
  federal regulations and, 1309
  patient instructions for, **1311–1312**
  procedure for complete, **1239–1332**
  quality control for, 1308, **1308**
  reporting results of, 1333, **1333**
  safety precautions for, 1308
  specific gravity, **1318–1320**
  urine examination and, 1313, 1315–1318
Urinalysis department, 1216
Urinalysis tests, **1217**
Urinary bladder cancer, **882**, **884**
Urinary catheterization
  explanation of, 614, 885–887, **886**, **887**
  of females, **891–892**
  of males, **888–890**
Urinary system
  conditions and disorders of, 881, **882–884**
  description of, 881, 1305, **1306**
  diagnostic tests for, 881, 884–885
  diseases and disorders of, **883**, 884–885, 1321, **1326**
  in older adults, 763

World Health Organization (WHO), 528
Wound culture, 1348
Wound specimen collection, 1349–1350
Wounds
    application of sterile adhesive skin closure strips to, **957–958**
    care of, 936–938, **937**, **938**
    closed, **149**, **938**
    healing of, 148–151, **149–151**
    irrigation of, **950–952**
    open, 148, **937**
Written communication. *See also* Business letters
    components of, 308–313, **311**, **312**
    guidelines for, 306–308
    legal and ethical issues related to, 327
    as medical document, 340, 341, **344**
    in medical records, 299–300
    meeting agendas as, 323, **324**
    meeting minutes as, 323–324, **325**
    memoranda as, 321, 323, **323**
    preparing and composing, **309–310**
    processing incoming, 324–327
    processing outgoing, **318–323**, 324–327, **326**, **327**
    styles for, 313–314, **315–317**
    supplies for, 314–321
    types of, 323, **323**, **324**, **325**

X

X-rays. *See also* Diagnostic imaging
    contrast media and, 975, **976**
    equipment for, 973–975, **974**
    flat plate, 984
    function of, 972
    patient preparation for, 975
    safety procedures for, 972–973

Y

Yeast cells, **1327**
Yeast infections, 1362

Z

Zen macrobiotic diet, **1054**
Zinc, 1040
ZIP+4, 326
Z-track intramuscular injection technique, 1149, **1149–1151**